Varney's Midwifery

Fifth Edition

Edited by

Tekoa L. King, CNM, MPH, FACNM
Deputy Editor, *Journal of Midwifery &*
   Women's Health
Health Sciences Clinical Professor
Department of Family Health Care Nursing
School of Nursing
University of California, San Francisco
San Francisco, California

Mary C. Brucker, CNM, PhD, FACNM
Editor, *Nursing for Women's Health*
Assistant Professor, Adjunct Track
School of Nursing & Health Studies
Georgetown University
Washington, DC

Jan M. Kriebs, CNM, MSN, FACNM
Assistant Professor and Director,
   Midwifery
Department of Obstetrics, Gynecology,
   and Reproductive Sciences
University of Maryland School
   of Medicine
Baltimore, Maryland

Jenifer O. Fahey, CNM, MSN, MPH
Assistant Professor
Department of Obstetrics, Gynecology,
   and Reproductive Sciences
University of Maryland School
   of Medicine
Baltimore, Maryland

Carolyn L. Gegor, CNM, MS, FACNM
Assistant Professor
Nurse-Midwifery & Women's Health
   Nurse Practitioner Program
School of Nursing & Health Sciences
Georgetown University
Washington, DC

Helen Varney, CNM, DHL (Hon.), MSN, FACNM
Professor Emerita
Yale University School of Nursing
New Haven, Connecticut

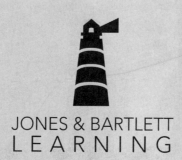

JONES & BARTLETT
LEARNING

World Headquarters
Jones & Bartlett Learning
5 Wall Street
Burlington, MA 01803
978-443-5000
info@jblearning.com
www.jblearning.com

Jones & Bartlett Learning books and products are available through most bookstores and online booksellers. To contact Jones & Bartlett Learning directly, call 800-832-0034, fax 978-443-8000, or visit our website, www.jblearning.com.

Production Credits

Chief Executive Officer: Ty Field
President: James Homer
Chief Product Officer: Eduardo Moura
Executive Publisher: William Brottmiller
Senior Editor: Amanda Harvey
Associate Acquisitions Editor: Teresa Reilly
Associate Managing Editor: Sara Bempkins
Editorial Assistant: Rebecca Myrick
Production Manager: Carolyn Rogers Pershouse

Marketing Communications Manager: Katie Hennessy
Art Development Editor: Joanna Lundeen
Photo Research and Permissions Coordinator: Joseph Veiga
VP, Manufacturing and Inventory Control: Therese Connell
Composition: Arlene Apone
Cover Design: Karen LeDuc and Kristin E. Parker
Cover Image: © style_TTT/ShutterStock, Inc.
Printing and Binding: Edwards Brothers Malloy
Cover Printing: Edwards Brothers Malloy

Library of Congress Cataloging-in-Publication Data
Varney's midwifery / edited by Tekoa L. King, Mary C. Brucker, Jenifer O. Fahey, Jan M. Kriebs, Carolyn L. Gegor, Helen Varney Burst.
-- Fifth edition.
      p. ; cm.
Midwifery
Preceded by Varney's midwifery / Helen Varney, Jan M. Kriebs, Carolyn L. Gegor. 4th ed. c2004.
Includes bibliographical references and index.
ISBN 978-1-284-02541-5 (hbk.)
I. Varney, Helen, editor of compilation. II. King, Tekoa L., editor of compilation. III. Brucker, Mary C., editor of compilation. IV. Fahey, Jenifer, editor of compilation. V. Kriebs, Jan M., editor of compilation. VI. Varney, Helen. Varney's midwifery. Preceded by (work): VII. Title: Midwifery.
[DNLM: 1. Nurse Midwives. 2. Midwifery. 3. Obstetrical Nursing. 4. Women's Health. WY 157]
RG950
618.2--dc23
                    2013032431

6048

Printed in the United States of America
17 16 15 14 13   10 9 8 7 6 5 4 3 2 1

Dedication

*This book is dedicated to Helen Varney Burst,
CNM, MSN, DHL (Hon), FACNM.*

Helen Varney Burst authored the first edition of this text, which was published in 1989 and originally titled *Nurse-Midwifery*. This book was the first text written for modern midwives in the Western Hemisphere. One of the hallmarks of a profession is a codified body of knowledge, yet prior to the publication of this book, midwives cobbled together British midwifery texts, United States medical textbooks, and various shared modules and articles in order to learn about the healthcare services we offer to women. In the preface for the first edition Helen Varney Burst wrote, "This book was written because it needed to be written."

Over the course of several previous editions, this text has translated and applied the universal principles of midwifery and it has become the quintessential midwifery textbook in the United States. Now appropriately titled *Varney's Midwifery*, the book is considered the cornerstone for midwifery education. Furthermore, it has been translated into several other languages and is used in the education and training of midwives globally.

Varney's Midwifery is just one aspect of the midwifery career that Helen Varney Burst has pursued. Many midwives today know Helen Varney Burst only through her eponymous text. Yet it was her background of many years in midwifery practice, as an active member of the midwifery community (including being president of the American College of Nurse-Midwives), and as a midwifery author that enabled her to write with such clarity and vision.

Helen Varney Burst is one of the most generous individuals we have met. She is the epitome of a midwife of intelligence, articulation, and altruism. She will quickly mention many midwives and others who helped her with the production of the previous editions of *Varney's Midwifery*, but it is her voice that permeates the chapters and her dedication that saw it to fruition. Every page bore her fingerprint. After the fourth edition, she personally chose to pass the torch on for future editions, yet her standard had been set. This heartfelt dedication is only one of a list of well-deserved honors and is given with sincere gratitude. Her legacy will continue and be felt for generations and editions to come of *Varney's Midwifery*. It is through *Varney's Midwifery* that all midwives can truly say they are "Helen's students."

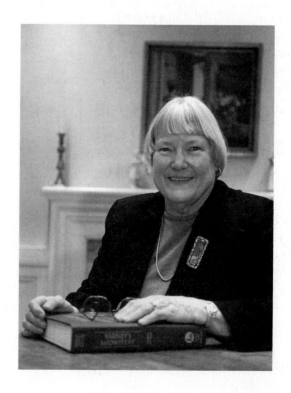

Brief Contents

Contents

Part IV   Antepartum 597

Promotion of Health During Pregnancy

Joyce E. Roberts

Part VII   Newborn   1183

Welcoming the Newborn
Lily Hsia

Preface

Today, midwives practice in all areas of women's health and in all settings involved with women's healthcare services. This text is intended to provide the basis for full scope midwifery practice especially the scientific underpinning and therapeutic interventions that have changed since the last edition was published.

Like its predecessors, the text is divided into sections that address the profession of midwifery, primary care, antepartum, intrapartum, postpartum, and newborn. In addition, each section has new chapters that reflect current midwifery practice. For example, there has been an explosion in genetics, and prenatal care now includes choices that women must make about a variety of tests.

In this edition, chapters on anatomy and physiology precede each section in order to reduce redundancies while providing the needed science proximate to the management chapters. The previously titled "Skills" chapters have been placed as appendices to the chapter to which they pertain for ease of use.

It can be noted that this edition has many contributors. The authors were chosen for their expertise and also to reflect variations in geography and practice settings. Each section also contains an introduction by a nationally known midwife. Finally, we are delighted that this, the fifth edition, will be the first one available digitally. Every effort has been made to offer current information without errors, but should any be found, they are ours. Any

and all corrections, comments, and suggestions are encouraged.

As we highlight the new, it is also important to acknowledge the old because the basic structure or "bones" of this book are the essential characteristics that make it the quintessential text for midwifery in the United States. The midwifery management process can be found in the boxes that outline management of specific conditions. There has been a deliberate intention to maintain midwifery language and approach to care throughout. In the United States and globally midwives practice in settings that range from low-resource to high-resource. The text and appendices have been written to describe techniques that can be used in any setting.

The fifth edition of *Varney's Midwifery* could not have been "born" without the tremendous outpouring of help and support from everyone involved. Busy expert midwife authors responded positively to unreasonable deadlines and multiple revisions. And their practice partners covered call, taught extra classes, and did whatever else they could to help. We also thank all the midwifery students, who helped authors by contributing class time discussing how a particular topic should be framed, providing proofreading, and helping find necessary research and other sources.

In summary, this edition of *Varney's Midwifery* truly reflects the practice, profession, and professionals that make midwifery today.

Acknowledgments

To Bill, Kya, Tim, Todd, Deepa, and Simon Thomas who was born just as this book was being born. The support each of you offered while I was working on this book was more than I can thank you for. Kya, being with you as you gave birth to Simon and watching you become a mother made reading these chapters richer than I could have imagined. And to Mary who is the best partner one could ever hope to have. In the end, it comes back to you, Bill, with all my love.

Tekoa L. King

To all those who made this possible: the woman we serve, the students who learn, and the midwives who care. And to my friends and family, especially Nancy, Linda, Cathy, and Ted who tolerated my absences physically or mentally while the book was being written. And of course to Tekoa, who is the best.

Mary C. Brucker

With thanks and gratitude to my midwifery partners, who have shared their wisdom and caring over many years; to my family: Robert, Juniper, William and Michael; and as always, to David, whose support makes all things possible.

Jan M. Kriebs

I have truly stood on the shoulders of giants during this project. Helen, you have been my mentor and inspiration since my first day as a student-midwife. Thank you. Jan, Carolyn, Tekoa, and Mary, I am so grateful for your support (both the gentle guidance and the tough love) as I find my way as an author and editor. A debt of gratitude to my practice partners who have given to this book behind the scenes in ways for which I will never be able to adequately thank them. Thank you to my husband, Sean, and my mother, Judy, who always give me support, wise counsel, and help me find the energy and extra hours in which to work, study, and write. Finally, to Ana and Ellie, my amazing daughters, who are always so generous of their time with mommy, thank you, and I love you.

Jenifer O. Fahey

For Helen Varney Burst, who invited and mentored me to carry on this book, my appreciation is endless. To the students of the Georgetown Nurse-Midwifery Program, I offer gratitude that you challenged me to expand my knowledge and to broaden my approach to learning. I am in awe of your brilliance, sensitivity to women and families, and commitment to midwifery. Watching your progression from idealistic new students to passionate, critically thinking CNMs has been an unparalleled experience for me. You have taught me what this book should truly be, and shown me the wisdom and knowledge it has already imparted. To my husband Andy, and daughters, Stacey and Brittany, without you, I would be unable to realize my dream of devoting my time and talents to midwifery. You have my love forever.

Carolyn L. Gegor

Contributors

Cindy M. Anderson, WHNP-BC, PhD, FAAN
Associate Professor
University of North Dakota
Grand Forks, North Dakota

Melissa D. Avery, CNM, PhD, FACNM, FAAN
Professor, School of Nursing
University of Minnesota
Minneapolis, Minnesota

Alice J. Bailes, CNM, MSN, FACNM
Co-Founder, BirthCare & Women's Health, Ltd
Alexandria, Virginia

Mary K. Barger, CNM, PhD, MPH, FACNM
Associate Professor
University of San Diego
San Diego, California

Mary C. Brucker, CNM, PhD, FACNM
Editor, *Nursing for Women's Health*
Assistant Professor Adjunct Track
Georgetown University School of Nursing
    & Health Studies
Washington, DC

Anne Z. Cockerham, CNM, WHNM-BC, PhD
Course Coordinator
Frontier Nursing University
Hyden, Kentucky

Susanna Rose Cohen, CNM, MSN
Assistant Professor
University of Utah
Salt Lake City, Utah

Michelle R. Collins, CNM, PhD
Associate Professor
Vanderbilt University
Nashville, Tennessee

Ann F. Cowlin, MA, CSM, CCE
Yale University Athletic Department
New Haven, Connecticut

Michelle R. Davidson, CNM, CFN, PhD
Associate Professor
George Mason University
Fairfax, Virginia

Jennifer M. Demma, CNM, MSN
Clinical Faculty Director
Georgetown University School of Nursing
    & Health Studies
Washington, District of Columbia

Dawn C. Durain, CNM, MPH, FACNM
Senior Lecturer, Associate Program Director
University of Pennsylvania
Philadelphia, Pennsylvania

Ladan Eshkevari, CRNA, LAc, PhD
Associate Professor and Assistant Program
    Director, Nurse Anesthesia Program
Georgetown University School of Nursing
    & Health Studies
Washington, District of Columbia

Jenifer O. Fahey, CNM, MSN, MPH
Assistant Professor
University of Maryland School of Medicine
Baltimore, Maryland

Mary Ann Faucher, CNM, PhD, FACNM
Associate Professor
Baylor University-Louise Herrington
    School of Nursing
Dallas, Texas

Carolyn L. Gegor, CNM, MS, FACNM
Assistant Professor
Georgetown University, School of Nursing
    & Health Studies
Washington, District of Columbia

Karen Trister Grace, CNM, MSN
Interim Program Director
Georgetown University School of Nursing
    & Health Studies
Washington, District of Columbia

Barbara W. Graves, CNM, MN, MPH, FACNM
Director
Baystate Midwifery Education Program
Springfield, Massachusetts

Sharon L. Holley, CNM, DNP
Assistant Professor
Vanderbilt University
Nashville, Tennessee

Lily Hsia, CNM, CPNP, MS, FACNM
Former Chairperson and Associate Professor
SUNY Downstate Medical Center
Brooklyn, New York

Linda A. Hunter, CNM, EdD, FACNM
Clinical Assistant Professor
Warren Alpert Medical School
Brown University
Women & Infants Hospital
Providence, Rhode Island

Marsha E. Jackson, CNM, MSN, FACNM
Director and Co-Founder
BirthCare & Women's Health, Ltd
Alexandria, Virginia

Cynthia Jensen, RN, MS, CNS
Neonatal Outreach Educator
University of California, San Francisco
Benioff Children's Hospital
San Francisco, California

Ruth Johnson, CNM, MSN, MPA
Advanced Practice Psychiatric Nurse,
    Certified Nurse-Midwife
Massachusetts General Hospital
Wellesley, Massachusetts

Ira Kantrowitz-Gordon, CNM, PhD
Senior Lecturer, Director Nurse-Midwifery
    Education Program
University of Washington
Seattle, Washington

Deborah Brandt Karsnitz, CNM, DNP, FACNM
Course Coordinator
Frontier Nursing University
Hyden, Kentucky

Holly Powell Kennedy, CNM, PhD, FACNM, FAAN
Helen Varney Professor of Midwifery
Yale University
New Haven, Connecticut

Joyce L, King, CNM, FNP, PhD, FACNM
Associate Professor
Emory University
Atlanta, Georgia

Tekoa L. King, CNM, MPH, FACNM
Deputy Editor, *Journal of Midwifery
    & Women's Health*
Health Sciences Clinical Professor
University of California, San Francisco
San Francisco, California

Jan M. Kriebs, CNM, MSN, FACNM
Assistant Professor, Director, Midwifery Division
University of Maryland School of Medicine
Baltimore, Maryland

Gwen A. Latendresse, CNM, PhD
Assistant Professor
University of Utah
Salt Lake City, Utah

Janet L. Lewis, CNM, MSN, MA
Senior Lecturer
University of Pennsylvania
Philadelphia, Pennsylvania

Frances E. Likis, CNM, NP, DrPH, FACNM, FAAN
Editor-in-Chief, *Journal of Midwifery
    & Women's Health*
Senior Investigator, Vanderbilt University
    Evidence-Based Practice Center
Nashville, Tennessee

Lisa Kane Low, CNM, PhD, FACNM
Associate Professor
University of Michigan
Ann Arbor, Michigan

Nancy K. Lowe, CNM, PhD, FACNM, FAAN
Professor and Chair
College of Nursing University of Colorado
Aurora, Colorado

**Margaret (Peg) Marshall, CNM, MPH,
    EdD, FACNM**
Senior Technical Advisor
USAID
Washington, DC

William F. McCool, CNM, PhD, FACNM
Associate Clinical Professor, Director of
    Midwifery Graduate Program
University of Pennsylvania
Philadelphia, Pennsylvania

Mary Kathleen McHugh, CNM, MSN, FACNM
Assistant Professor
Georgetown University School of Nursing and
    Health Studies
Washington, District of Columbia

Tonia L. Moore-Davis, CNM, MSN
Instructor of Clinical Nursing
Vanderbilt University School of Nursing
Nashville, Tennessee

Patricia Aikins Murphy, CNM, DrPH, FACNM
Deputy Editor, *Journal of Midwifery*
    & Women's Health
Professor
University of Utah
Salt Lake City, Utah

Deborah L. Narrigan, CNM, MSN
Project Coordinator, Better Birth Outcomes
Vanderbilt University School of Nursing
Nashville, Tennessee

Jeremy L. Neal, CNM, PhD
Assistant Professor
The Ohio State University College of Nursing
Columbus, Ohio

Kathryn M. Osborne, CNM, PhD, FACNM
Course Coordinator
Frontier Nursing University
Hyden, Kentucky

Lisa L. Paine, CNM, DrPH, FACNM
Principal & Senior Consultant
The Hutchinson Dyer Group
Cambridge, Massachusetts

Julia C. Phillippi, CNM, PhD, FACNM
Assistant Professor
Vanderbilt University School of Nursing
Nashville, Tennessee

Nancy Jo Reedy, CNM, MPH, FACNM
Adjunct Instructor, Clinical Faculty Advisor
Georgetown University School of Nursing and
    Health Studies
Washington, District of Columbia

Joyce E. Roberts, CNM, PhD, FACNM, FAAN
Professor (Retired)
University of Michigan
Ann Arbor, Michigan

Judith P. Rooks, CNM, MPH, MS, FACNM
Past President, American College of Nurse-Midwives
Portland, Oregon

Sharon L. Ryan, CNM, DNP
Clinical Assistant Professor, Director Nurse-
    Midwifery and Women's Health Specialty Tracks
The Ohio State University College of Nursing
Columbus, Ohio

Mavis N. Schorn, CNM, PHD, FACNM
Associate Professor, Assistant Dean for Academics
Vanderbilt University
Nashville, Tennessee

Celeste R. Thomas, CNM, MS
Instructor (Clinical)
University of Utah
Salt Lake City, Utah

Joyce E. Thompson, CNM, DrPH, FACNM, FAAN
International Midwifery Consultant
Professor Emerita
University of Pennsylvania
Philadelphia, Pennsylvania

Kimberly K. Trout, CNM, PhD
Program Director, Associate Professor
Georgetown University School of Nursing
    & Health Studies
Washington, District of Columbia

Helen Varney, CNM, MSN, DHL (Hon.), FACNM
Professor Emerita
Yale University School of Nursing
New Haven, Connecticut

**Saraswathi M. Vedam, RN, CNM, MSN, FACNM,
    Sci D (hc)**
Associate Professor
University of British Columbia
Vancouver, British Columbia

Deanne R. Williams, CNM, MS, FACNM
Advanced Practice Clinical Coordinator
Intermountain Healthcare, Inc.
Salt Lake City, Utah

Erin M. Wright, CNM, MS
Instructor
University of Maryland School of Medicine
Baltimore, Maryland

Midwifery

Midwifery Revealed: Introducing the Profession

When Helen Varney Burst received an honorary doctorate from Georgetown University in 1987, midwifery was characterized as an ancient profession reborn in contemporary society. The three introductory chapters in this fifth edition of *Varney's Midwifery* carefully render midwifery past and present and set the stage for the future. In doing so, they expose the science, value, complexities, and politics of midwifery. Has the practice of midwifery always been so hard? I expect the answer is "yes and no." By itself, the very nature of midwifery work is hard. However, it is the context in which midwifery is situated that adds to both the challenges and the joys of being a midwife. The authors of these introductory chapters capture this extraordinarily well, leaving the reader with a sense of awe at the tenacity, resilience, and grit of midwives and the profession of midwifery. My advice to any individual who does not embrace these three prerequisites after reading the first three chapters is to find another profession. For those who sign on, my message is "Welcome to our world—you will not be disappointed!"

Helen Varney Burst begins the fifth edition by portraying the history and profession of midwifery in the United States. I was a student when the second edition of her book was current, and

I remain amazed at the growth of our profession over those 30 years, so artfully presented in this chapter. Midwifery has an intricate and confusing professional history in the United States that reflects our vast, immigrant nation, the domination of medicine, religious beliefs, economics, and the low status of women, among other factors. Burst carefully traces these influences to help us understand midwifery today. She unravels a puzzle to expose our vulnerabilities and our strengths. Reputations are earned, and the status of midwifery partially reflects our history and our investment in excellence. Over time, and within a changing landscape, midwifery has adopted a professional stature not accessible to our early predecessors. This has required organization, setting and maintaining standards for education and practice, astute record-keeping, and state and federal regulation. It has also required negotiation and collaboration with colleagues who might think differently, within and outside of the profession, thus creating a very different—and, I believe, positive—future for midwifery than our foremothers faced in this country.

Deanne Williams, Susanna Cohen, and Celeste Thomas ground us firmly in present-day midwifery in the second chapter. Building on midwives' remarkable history, they help the reader understand the fundamentals that guide our profession, including accreditation of education, certification of knowledge, regulatory requirements, and scope of practice. They detail the evolution of theory to describe the work of midwifery and the multiple roles a midwife might assume, as entrepreneur, educator, clinician, and scientist. Today's professional midwife requires an astute knowledge base in order to practice using best evidence; skills to provide effective, safe, ethical, and comforting care; political savvy; emotional intelligence; and an eagle eye to track changing trends in health care. The midwife cannot and should not practice in isolation, and the authors use the wise words of Louden to note the relationship between the high standards of midwifery and low maternal mortality, especially when cordial relationships with physicians are maintained. Their review of the evidence is clear: Midwifery has exceptional outcomes is representative of the best care possible.

Peg Marshall and Joyce Thompson take us on a global spin to understand the world in which women live, birth, and die, as well as the role of midwifery in caring for them and their children throughout the world. Women who do not have access to family planning or qualified healthcare providers tend to have poor health outcomes and are more likely to die in childbirth. Their chances diminish when they live in societies where women are not valued. Even in the United States, there is stark difference along racial lines in maternal mortality rates, and the rate of maternal mortality grew disturbingly high from 1987 to 2007. When a mother dies, her children are more likely to die—women are the roots of a healthy society. The authors of this chapter describe the vast international work done to support safe motherhood. Midwifery is often at the heart of these efforts. Their exquisite depiction of international midwifery situates U.S. midwives within a global community. It forces us to see beyond our borders, comparing ourselves to international standards, and to consider midwifery's role in caring for women across the global community.

These introductory chapters made me proud to be part of our midwifery heritage, and humbled to walk among the great midwives that make up our profession. As midwives we hold the trust of each woman who comes to us for care, and it is our responsibility to assure her that our care is stellar. Burst quotes a biblical midwife—"Fear not"—who seeks to reassure a woman during her labor. I would echo those words to all midwives, and especially our students: Midwifery is strong and is working day by day with women to strengthen their health and, through them, the health of the world.

Holly Powell Kennedy

CHAPTER

1

The History and Profession of Midwifery in the United States

HELEN VARNEY BURST

And it came to pass, when she was in hard labour, that the midwife said unto her, Fear not....[1]

The voice of this midwife echoes down to us through history from antiquity. Midwifery is as old as the history of *Homo sapiens*. Fulfilling its meaning of "with woman," midwifery has survived through the centuries as birth—the renewal of life—continues through the ages. Midwives are referred to in many ancient texts, including Chinese, Greek, Roman, Egyptian, and Hebrew texts as well as ancient writings from India, South America, and Africa. It is meaningful that the first known words spoken by a midwife are "fear not."

Definitions and Practice

Today midwifery is an internationally recognized profession with practitioners throughout the world. The following international definition of a midwife and scope of practice was adopted by the International Confederation of Midwives (ICM) during a Council meeting in 2011 and supersedes previous versions:

> A midwife is a person who has successfully completed a midwifery education programme that is duly recognized in the country where it is located and that is based on the ICM *Essential Competencies for Basic Midwifery Practice* and the framework of the ICM *Global Standards for Midwifery Education*; who has acquired the requisite qualifications to be registered and/or legally

licensed to practice midwifery and use the title "midwife"; and who demonstrates competency in the practice of midwifery.

Scope of Practice

The midwife is recognised as a responsible and accountable professional who works in partnership with women to give the necessary support, care and advice during pregnancy, labour and the postpartum period, to conduct births on the midwife's own responsibility and to provide care for the newborn and the infant. This care includes preventative measures, the promotion of normal birth, the detection of complications in mother and child, the accessing of medical care or other appropriate assistance and the carrying out of emergency measures.

The midwife has an important task in health counselling and education, not only for the woman, but also within the family and the community. This work should involve antenatal education and preparation for parenthood and may extend to women's health, sexual or reproductive health and child care. A midwife may practise in any setting including the home, community, hospitals, clinics or health units.[2]

In the United States, midwifery education that meets the standards of the American College of Nurse-Midwives (ACNM) goes beyond the scope of practice defined by ICM to include the primary health care of newborns and of women from puberty through senescence.[3,4] The ACNM defines midwifery and the scope of practice of certified nurse-midwives (CNMs) and certified midwives (CMs) as follows:

> Midwifery as practiced by certified nurse-midwives (CNMs®) and certified midwives (CMs®) encompasses a full range of primary health care services for women from adolescence beyond menopause. These services include the independent provision of primary care, gynecologic and family planning services, preconception care, care during pregnancy, childbirth and the postpartum period, care of the normal newborn during the first 28 days of life, and treatment of male partners for sexually transmitted infections. Midwives provide initial and ongoing comprehensive assessment, diagnosis and treatment. They conduct physical examinations; prescribe medications including controlled substances and contraceptive methods; admit, manage and discharge patients; order and interpret laboratory and diagnostic tests and order the use of medical devices. Midwifery care also includes health promotion, disease prevention, and individualized wellness education and counseling. These services are provided in partnership with women and families in diverse settings such as ambulatory care clinics, private offices, community and public health systems, homes, hospitals and birth centers.[5]

The American College of Nurse-Midwives defines CNMs and CMs as follows:

> CNMs are educated in two disciplines: midwifery and nursing. They earn graduate degrees, complete a midwifery education program accredited by the Accreditation Commission for Midwifery Education (ACME), and pass a national certification examination administered by the American Midwifery Certification Board (AMCB) to receive the professional designation of CNM.[5]

> CMs are educated in the discipline of midwifery. They earn graduate degrees, meet health and science education requirements, complete a midwifery education program accredited by ACME, and pass the same national certification examination as CNMs to receive the professional designation of CM.[5]

Certification gives official recognition to an individual who has met professional standards for safe practice and protects the public. Certification is conferred upon an individual who has met eligibility requirements for and successfully passed the national certification examination of the ACNM-designated certifying agent, currently the American Midwifery Certification Board (AMCB; formerly the ACNM Certification Council). As of January 1, 2011, all CNMs/CMs have time-limited certificates and must renew their certification every 5 years by meeting specific continuing education requirements. Those CNMs/CMs who are permanently retired from practice are in a different category of certification that identifies this nonpractice status. AMCB certification differentiates certified nurse-midwives and certified midwives, and their broad scope of practice, from other types of midwives.[6]

Beliefs Characterizing Midwifery

A number of beliefs are central to midwifery practice and characterize the health care given by midwives. Collectively, these beliefs and their implementation constitute the midwifery model of care. These beliefs include facilitation of natural processes and nonintervention in normal processes; continuity of care; promotion and implementation of family-centered maternity care; advocacy for the woman and her rights and responsibilities; and education of women to facilitate their knowledgeable participation and decision making in their health care and for understanding their bodily processes. Midwives also support preventive health care, the reduction of maternal and infant mortality and morbidity, the role of the midwife within the community, and the contribution of midwifery within the healthcare system. These beliefs are expressed in the Hallmarks of Midwifery in the ACNM Core Competencies for Basic Midwifery Practice.[4]

The philosophy of the American College of Nurse-Midwives states beliefs that support and provide a base for the characteristics of health care given by nurse-midwives:

> We, the midwives of the American College of Nurse-Midwives, affirm the power and strength of women and the importance of their health in the well-being of families, communities and nations. We believe in the basic human rights of all persons, recognizing

that women often incur an undue burden of risk when these rights are violated.

We believe every person has a right to:
- Equitable, ethical, accessible quality health care that promotes healing and health
- Health care that respects human dignity, individuality and diversity among groups
- Complete and accurate information to make informed health care decisions
- Self-determination and active participation in health care decisions
- Involvement of a woman's designated family members, to the extent desired, in all health care experiences

We believe the best model of health care for a woman and her family:
- Promotes a continuous and compassionate partnership
- Acknowledges a person's life experiences and knowledge
- Includes individualized methods of care and healing guided by the best evidence available
- Involves therapeutic use of human presence and skillful communication

We honor the normalcy of women's lifecycle events. We believe in:
- Watchful waiting and non-intervention in normal processes
- Appropriate use of interventions and technology for current or potential health problems
- Consultation, collaboration and referral with other members of the health care team as needed to provide optimal health care

We affirm that midwifery care incorporates these qualities and that women's health care needs are well-served through midwifery care.

Finally, we value formal education, life-long individual learning, and the development and application of research to guide ethical and competent midwifery practice. These beliefs and values provide the foundation for commitment to individual and collective leadership at the community, state, national and international level to improve the health of women and their families worldwide.[7]

Individual CNMs and CMs also articulate these beliefs when writing about their practice or service philosophy or presenting to the public or teaching students. Nancy Fleming, CNM, PhD, captured the spirit and substance of a discussion in 1993 by the ACNM Board of Directors of the elements that distinguish midwifery when she wrote *The Heart of Midwifery*:

> The heart of midwifery care for women and newborns lies more in the nature of that care than in its specific components. Midwifery practice has a firm foundation in the critical thought process and is focused on the prevention of disease and the promotion of health, taking the best from the disciplines of midwifery, nursing, public health, and medicine to provide safe, holistic care.
>
> Midwives are partners with women in the provision of health care, engaging in a dynamic reevaluation of each woman's unique health needs.
>
> Midwives would rather nurture a woman's progress with hands-on care than diagnose her problems from afar,
>
> …rather listen than lecture,
>
> …rather teach a health principle than treat an illness,
>
> …rather empower a woman to join in decision making than decide for her,
>
> …rather urge her to speak for herself than to be her advocate,
>
> …rather instill a woman with trust in her body than demonstrate the midwife's technical proficiency
>
> although midwives will do all these things when necessary.
>
> Midwifery is a profession born of a woman's vision, nurtured in an understanding of women's developmental phases, and committed to assuring women in all populations that it is their birthright to be part of this unique care.[8]

These beliefs have had practical application throughout the history of nurse-midwifery in the United States. Through the Maternity Center Association in New York City, nurse-midwives were active in the

1930s in the provision of prenatal care and parent education; they were in the forefront of the early movements in the 1940s related to family-centered maternity care, natural childbirth, and preparation for childbirth and parenthood. In the 1950s and 1960s, nurse-midwives led the efforts to promote breastfeeding, rooming-in, and the inclusion of fathers or significant others in hospital labor and delivery rooms. They also provided leadership in the development of birth centers in the late 1970s and the birth center movement in the 1980s.

More recently, nurse-midwives have been involved in key veins of research. The development of the Optimality Index—United States (adapted from an Optimality Index used in the Netherlands) was undertaken by Patricia Aikens Murphy, CNM, DrPH, and Judith Fullerton, CNM, PhD; it "measures the process of care and associated outcomes in a single index."[9] Moreover, the qualitative research done by Holly Kennedy, CNM, PhD, has identified the practice characteristics and processes of exemplary midwives. From her research, Dr. Kennedy developed a model of exemplary midwifery care that, in her words, "provides structure for future research on the unique aspects of midwifery care to support its correlation with excellent outcomes and value in health care economics."[10]

Early History of Midwifery in the United States

For the purposes of this text, the history of midwifery in the United States begins with the arrival of colonists in the New World. Midwives were among the first women to settle the colonies. Although there were midwives among the Native Americans, their history has not been extensively researched.

Midwives were considered vital to colonial community life and were treated with dignity. Special courtesies were extended to midwives, and arrangements were made to provide them with housing, land, food, and salary as payment for their services. This information is noted in town records and charters of the mid-seventeenth century. Birth-related services, however, were just one of many healthcare contributions colonial midwives made to the community. They also often functioned as herbalists, veterinarians, and nurses who tended the sick and the dying and prepared the body after death.[11]

During antebellum slavery from 1800 until the Civil War, the African American midwife provided midwifery and healthcare herbalist services for both black and white women on plantations. Midwives were valued slaves. A slave midwife contributed financially to her owner both as a cost saving for the plantation she was on and through payments for her services on other plantations made to her owner.[12]

During the nineteenth century, pioneer women crossed the plains in covered wagons, followed the Oregon and Santa Fe trails, settled the "Wild West," and bore children with the assistance of other women in the wagon trains, forts, or settlements who functioned as midwives in the situation.[13] Mormon history documents the honorable role and heroic work of midwives during that group's trek from Illinois to Utah in 1846 and 1847.[14]

Despite the initial honor accorded midwives in the colonies and their importance to other segments of the population through the years, a series of factors reduced midwifery from a respected profession to one in disrepute by the early twentieth century. These factors included religious attitudes, economic demands, replacement by physicians, lack of access to education, lack of organization or legal recognition, an influx of immigrants, and the low status of women.

Factors Leading to the Decline of Midwifery: Seventeenth to Late Nineteenth Centuries

Religious restrictions plagued midwives from the beginning. Most of the early midwives came from England, where in the seventeenth century the licensing of midwives took place under the auspices of the Church of England. Criteria were moralistically judgmental; they emphasized good character and granted the ability to denounce sins and to baptize. The midwives' oath included a vow to pressure the mother into naming the true father. The results of such actions were not always appreciated. Conversely, in the Puritan communities, midwives were often suspected of witchcraft, especially if a malformed baby was born.

By the early eighteenth century, there was no organization or authority to establish guidelines for fees. Compensation was not always adequate, so practicing midwifery was no longer economically feasible for many women. This was especially true in the rapidly growing towns and cities.

In European society in the late eighteenth century, it was fashionable to have male midwives (physicians) for lying-in. This trend soon crossed the ocean, where physicians capitalized on it. Historian

Claire Fox offers this analysis of the historical roots of antipathy toward the midwife:

> As the practice of medicine became highly competitive, physicians and medical students were advised that their presence at a delivery would insure the entire family as grateful patients thereafter. For example, the outspoken and highly influential Dr. Walter Channing, of Harvard, objected strongly to the practice of midwifery by women in his "Remarks on the Employment of Females as Practitioners in Midwifery," (1820) and pointed out that "Women seldom forget a practitioner who has conducted them tenderly and safely through parturition—they feel a familiarity with him, a confidence and reliance upon him which is of the most essential mutual advantage....It is principally on this account that the practice of midwifery becomes desirable to physicians. It is this which ensures to them the permanency and security of all their other business.[15]

Male physicians thus replaced female midwives.

The eighteenth and nineteenth centuries marked a time of rapid development in medical and nursing science and of discoveries and teaching pertinent to obstetric practice. These developments included the end of the Chamberlen family secret of forceps and subsequent refinement of these instruments, technical advances that decreased the risks involved in cesarean section, pioneering efforts in obstetric anesthesia, conquest of puerperal fever, emergence of modern nursing in the 1860s, and inclusion of obstetrics in medical practice. Physician promises of relief from pain during childbirth, the use of chloroform by Queen Victoria during childbirth in 1850, the corresponding evolution of understanding of the nervous system with the development of spinal methods of analgesia and anesthesia,[16] the need for women receiving obstetric analgesia and anesthesia to be in the hospital, and the lack of access to hospitals by midwives all contributed to decreased use of midwives.

The observations and teachings of William Smellie (1697–1763), who developed teaching manikins and kept meticulous records of his patients, identified the mechanisms of labor and refuted any number of myths and misconceptions. The anatomical studies of William Hunter (1718–1783) included discoveries pertaining to the lymphatic system, placental circulation, and pregnant uterus. William Shippen, Jr. (1736–1808), the first lecturer on obstetrics, and Samuel Bard (1742–1821), author of the first American textbook on obstetrics, are credited with promoting obstetrical teaching in the United States. All made measurable contributions to the science and art of obstetrics.[17,18]

These developments, new knowledge, and teachings were not accessible to the midwife because of the relative isolation of midwives from one another and the lack of schools, national organizations, journals, legal recognition, or other means of communication among midwives. Any one of these structures would have provided a channel for learning. Without them, the knowledge and practice of the midwife became sadly out-of-date even as advanced medicine and modern nursing came to the fore.

Further, women were not considered to have the mental capacity for higher learning and were deliberately excluded from admission to organizations devoted to higher learning. Historian Judy Litoff writes:

> The development of formal medical education in America...provided potential male midwives with a decided advantage over their female counterparts. By the end of the eighteenth century, four medical schools, all restricted to male students, had been established on American soil. This meant that women were being systematically excluded from attaining a medical education at the precise time when knowledge of the scientific advances in obstetrics would have enabled them to become more competent midwives. Once this process had begun, it became increasingly difficult for midwives to keep up with the medical discoveries of the nineteenth century which eventually brought about the development of modern obstetrics.[19]

The Early Twentieth Century

The Industrial Revolution at the end of the nineteenth century brought an influx of immigrants from a number of European countries who formed pockets of cultural communities within cities. Each such community had its own midwives who came from the "old country." The vast majority were well-prepared midwives in their own country[20] but had the combined problems of not speaking English and not having access to the existing healthcare system. Their African American counterparts in the rural South also could not gain access to the formal healthcare system and were poorly educated because of racism and Jim Crow segregation laws. These "granny" midwives frequently passed the practice of midwifery from mother to daughter, learned through experience, and relied heavily on patience, home remedies, and prayer, as these were the only resources available to them and the women they served.

There were also Caucasian "granny" midwives such as those in Appalachia[21] and in the Ozarks of Southern Missouri.[22] In California and the Southwest, women of Spanish descent—*Californiana* midwives and Mexican *parteras* (midwives)—served their communities in multiple capacities.[23] In Hawaii and the Pacific Northwest were immigrant educated *Sanba* midwives from Japan.[24] Lack of licensure, organization, formal education programs, and a means by which to communicate with one another, as well as the scientific developments and social factors, combined to prevent midwives in all parts of the United States from having access to the official healthcare system during this era.

The low status of women in general at the beginning of the twentieth century also affected the education and work of midwives. Norma Swenson, in her analysis of social factors affecting the history of midwifery in the United States, makes the following comments:

> But the final and I think more significant point was that the status of women at the turn of the century was at a particularly low ebb. At that point in time women were regarded as economically exploitable but at the same time socially and politically incompetent, in the sense that they were perceived as being unfit to exercise good judgment concerning their own affairs or the affairs of others, and in fact were legally prevented from doing so. Paternal domination of home and society was at an all-time high.
>
> It was then in this kind of atmosphere that midwives were outlawed and women were, therefore, in effect blamed for the appalling conditions under which mothers and babies died at that time, when in fact women were powerless to control social conditions, and coped as midwives as well as they could with circumstances which were largely the product of a man-made industrial and social revolution.[25]

The "Midwife Problem"

In 1906, a study was done on midwifery practice in New York City. The study specifically looked at ethnicity, length of time in the United States, age,

level of education, ability to speak English, midwifery training, indication of economic status, personal and environmental cleanliness, length of time in practice, scope of practice (i.e., inclusion of complications in childbearing, criminal abortion), and contents and cleanliness of the midwifery bag. The study was conducted by a nurse under the auspices of the Public Health Committee of the Association of Neighborhood Workers (an organization of social workers). However, the discussion overstated the findings and the report ended with a diatribe that concluded that 42% (more than 43,000 mothers) of the total number of births reported for 1905 in greater New York were attended by "incompetent, ignorant, unclean midwives."[26] Although the midwives were no more responsible than the physicians for the high maternal and infant mortality rates at that time, they bore the brunt of the blame.[27] This report generated a debate over what became known as the "midwife problem."

All too soon, the various factors that contributed to the decline and disrepute of midwifery converged. Between 1912 and 1914, the licensing and practice of midwives became a topic of heated debate. During this time, medical schools began to include obstetrics in their curricula, and by 1930, obstetrics had become an established medical specialty. Obstetric care began to move out of the home and into the hospital, and laws were passed to regulate the practice of the indigenous midwives.

On one side of the debate were a majority who believed that all midwifery should be abolished; on the other side were those who believed midwives could perform a valuable function. The former feared the status midwives would gain if they achieved legal recognition and promoted the idea that improving the practice of midwives was an impossible task. Those in favor of continuing midwives' practice suggested that midwifery was a feasible option if these providers were given proper training, licensing, and supervision.

One significant event that influenced the outcome of the debate over the "midwife problem" took place while the debate raged. This event grew out of reality. Some states had already passed laws granting legal recognition to midwives that included requirements and specifications aimed at control of their practice. These laws were passed in an effort to reduce high mortality rates, as it was evident that the medical profession could not assume the entire task of obstetric care. In the South, licensure, education, and supervision of African American midwives was facilitated by the Sheppard-Towner Act from 1921 to 1929.[28] This legislation assigned money, administered through the

Children's Bureau, for providing better maternal–infant care. Included in the Act was the specification that public health nurses should be employed for the instruction of untrained midwives.

As a result of laws to regulate midwifery practice, a number of midwifery schools were established. The best known of these institutions were the Bellevue School of Midwifery in New York City and the Preston Retreat Hospital in Philadelphia. The Bellevue School of Midwifery, designed to instruct immigrant midwives in meeting requirements for practice, operated from 1911 until 1935, when it was closed by order of the New York City Commissioner of Hospitals, a physician. In his opinion, changing social and medical standards rendered the school superfluous and an unnecessary expense to the city. To support his action, he cited a decrease in the number of midwives as deliveries in hospitals had increased to 81% of all births in New York City.[29] The Preston Retreat was a maternity hospital founded in 1836. In 1916, a practical nurse education program was started there, and in 1923 a course in midwifery was introduced that eventually had both practical nurses and registered nurses for students. Enrollment dwindled, but the midwifery course continued until 1960. It is not known when registered nurses (RNs) were first admitted to the course.[30]

Although midwives were first placed under physician control in Illinois in 1896, the word "supervision" in relation to their practice does not appear until the 1907 report of the 1906 study of midwifery in New York City and subsequently in New York City statutes the following year. Thereafter, "supervision" appeared with increasing frequency in both the literature and regulations, and the concept was well established by the time nurse-midwives came into existence in the United States during the 1920s and 1930s.[31]

The debate over the "midwife problem" culminated in the legal registration, regulation, and restriction of midwives and the practice of midwifery; the introduction of nurse-midwives from Europe; and the development of nurse-midwifery in the United States. However, the price for the introduction of nurse-midwifery in the United States was the loss of autonomy that midwives originally had in exchange for credibility and access to the healthcare system.[32]

When nurse-midwifery began in the United States in the 1920s, it faced rancorous opposition. The profession was allowed to exist *only* if it was attached to nursing and *under* the auspices of medical supervision and control. It is necessary to be knowledgeable about this context within which nurse-midwifery developed to understand that the compromises made at that time were necessary for midwifery to survive in the United States. Those compromises made nearly a century ago still influence current-day philosophical, interprofessional, and practice issues.[32]

The Start of Nurse-Midwifery

The early supporters and proponents of midwifery clearly saw that midwifery, on its own, would not be able to survive as a profession in the United States. The concept of nurse-midwifery was first promoted around 1911–1914. The combination of nursing and midwifery represented a natural marriage of women's professions. Nursing was an established profession with access to the healthcare system; it was also a means by which women could obtain an education. The idea was to teach nurses to perform midwifery services in normal cases. Nursing was interested in midwifery from a public health viewpoint because maternity care was abysmal at that time. Even opponents of midwifery were supportive of nurse-midwifery as a lesser evil.[32]

The first two decades of the twentieth century are notable for the recognition of the woeful inadequacy of maternity care and subsequent actions taken to improve this care. The establishment of the Children's Bureau in Washington, D.C., in 1912 and the Maternity Center Association in New York City in 1918 had an immense influence on improvements in maternal–infant health care and the introduction of nurse-midwifery.

The Children's Bureau

In 1903, Lillian Wald, a nurse and founder of the Henry Street Settlement and the Visiting Nurse Association in New York City, suggested the formation of a federal children's bureau. President Theodore Roosevelt recommended a bill to establish such a bureau in 1909, but it was not until 1912 that the U.S. Congress passed a bill, which President Taft signed, establishing the Children's Bureau.

The stated purpose of the Children's Bureau was to investigate and report "upon all matters pertaining to the welfare of children and child life among all classes of our people."[33] The first act of the Children's Bureau was to conduct a study of infant deaths, which, according to available statistics, documented an infant mortality rate of approximately 124 deaths per 1000 live births.[27] It is to the Children's Bureau's credit that in analyzing the data from its first study, the organization identified the inescapable link between infant health and maternal health during the maternity cycle. The Children's Bureau then conducted studies of maternal mortality and conclusively established the importance of early and continuous prenatal care in reducing both maternal and infant mortality.[34] Thanks to the publication of this information, the idea of prenatal care gained respectability and the concept of health care throughout the intraconceptional period began to grow.

The Maternity Center Association

In 1915, the New York City Health Commissioner made another study of maternal and infant mortality. The findings of this study, which again demonstrated the connection between mortality and lack of prenatal care, led to the formation of a plan whereby the city was zoned and a maternity center was established in each zone. The first such maternity center opened in 1917. The need for central organization quickly became evident, and the Maternity Center Association (MCA) was established in 1918. By 1920, MCA had 30 maternity centers in New York City. From this network grew MCA's first endeavors in developing teaching materials and educational exhibits for use by individuals and agencies. In 1921, the association decided to concentrate its efforts on a demonstration of providing complete maternity care in one district and to cease the scattered efforts being carried out in its many centers, although some of the other clinics were maintained for a while longer. This decision was based on the belief that most nursing agencies and hospitals caring for families were now giving sufficient emphasis to prenatal care in their healthcare services.[35]

In the meantime, MCA and the Henry Street Visiting Nurse Association collaborated on a study that illustrated the value of specialized maternity care within a generalized public health nursing program. Subsequently, MCA embarked on an intensive educational program in maternity care for both the public and professional health personnel, especially physicians and public health nurses. When requests for assistance on this front from all over the country became too numerous to accommodate them all in New York City, MCA developed Maternity Institutes, taught by a traveling MCA nurse equipped with a duplicate of the teaching materials used at MCA. By 1935, half of all employed public health nurses in the country had attended a Maternity Institute either in their own community or in New York City.[35,36]

MCA also expanded its efforts beyond New York City to supply information about the need for maternity care to expectant parents throughout the United States. Mother's Day was dedicated to this endeavor for several years, with an emphasis on saving mothers' lives. The mayors of cities made Mother's Day proclamations regarding saving mothers' lives, and ministers preached their Mother's Day sermons on the subject, using packets of educational materials sent by MCA.[36]

On the basis of its demonstration of the benefits of providing complete maternity care, its collaboration with the Henry Street Visiting Nurse Association, the study of maternity care in other countries, and the enthusiasm of public health nurses who had attended the Maternity Institutes, MCA concluded that there was a need to prepare nurses to handle normal obstetric care and discussed opening a school of nurse-midwifery. This idea was temporarily thwarted in the early 1920s by bitter opposition from both medicine and nursing and by a lack of cooperation from the New York City Commissioner of Welfare.[36]

In the meantime, Mary Breckinridge was preparing to introduce nurse-midwives from Europe. Nurse-midwives had proved their effectiveness in European countries, where they were an established part of the healthcare system.

The Frontier Nursing Service

The first nurse-midwives to practice in the United States were British-trained nurse-midwives brought to this country in 1925 by Mary Breckinridge as part of her plan to provide health care for families in the remote rural areas of the Kentucky mountains. This endeavor was organized as the Kentucky Committee for Mothers and Babies in May 1925; through a change in its articles of incorporation, it became the Frontier Nursing Service (FNS) in 1928.[37] Thus FNS traces its history back to, and dates itself from, 1925.

Mary Breckinridge was admirably suited for the task she undertook. Her qualifications included a family background and upbringing that gave her a wealth of influential contacts. Her professional preparation as a registered nurse at St. Luke's Hospital in New York City; study of public health at Teacher's College, Columbia University; and work as a traveling lecturer for the Children's Bureau[38] had brought her into contact with advocates for public health nurses becoming midwives and related developments in New York City. She also trained as a state-certified midwife in England. Mrs. Breckenridge conducted a carefully self-designed program of observation and study of the Highlands and Islands Medical and Nursing Service in Scotland, concentrating on the Outer Hebrides, with further study in England. From this background and her experiences abroad, she developed a plan involving outpost nursing centers staffed by nurse-midwives and backed by a medical director located at a small, local, rural hospital. Her program was to be administered by a director, overseen by an executive committee and board of trustees, and supported by local committees throughout the United States. Before the work began, a survey of births and deaths in the region where the nurse-midwives planned to work was conducted to provide baseline data for subsequent statistics and research. In her book *Wide Neighborhoods*,[37] Mary Breckinridge wrote in fascinating detail of the myriad activities, people, concerns, and problems involved in bringing her plan to fruition.

The work and record of the Frontier Nursing Service (**Figure 1-1**) are legendary. The records kept during the earlier years were in accord with a statistical system set up by the Carnegie Corporation and tabulated by statisticians from the Metropolitan Life Insurance Company. In 1951, the FNS statistics showed that 8596 registered nurse-midwifery clients had been delivered since 1925, 6533 of whom were delivered in mostly primitive homes, with a gross maternal death rate of 1.2 per 1000 (or 12 per 10,000 live births) for the 25 years studied.[37(p311)] This mortality rate was in contrast to national maternal mortality rates of 66.1 per 10,000 live births in 1931, 37.6 per 10,000 live births in 1940, and 8.3 per 10,000 live births in 1950.[39] The total number of FNS maternal deaths was 11, which included 2 deaths that were actually due to cardiac conditions but occurred within the puerperal period. Subtracting those 2 deaths gives FNS a puerperal death rate of 9.1 per 10,000 live births—far less than the national puerperal death rate of 34 deaths per 10,000 live births among white women for the same period (1925–1954), during which there were 10,000 FNS confinements.[40]

In addition to providing maternity care, the FNS brought a comprehensive scope of healthcare services to its target rural population. These services included general dental, pediatric, medical, and surgical services; general eye, tonsil, and worm treatment services; special tuberculosis and trachoma services; and social services supported by Alpha Omicron Pi, the national sorority of social workers, as its national philanthropic project.[37]

World War II had a large impact on the Frontier Nursing Service, both in staffing levels and in the direction the war mandated for nurse-midwifery education at FNS. Great Britain had been both the source of British nurse-midwives working in the Frontier Nursing Service and the provider of midwifery education for U.S. registered nurses, who were sent to Great Britain for their education and returned to work at FNS. With the advent of war, the British nurse-midwives wanted to return to their homeland to be of service to their country. It became evident that a long-deferred plan for an educational program in nurse-midwifery in the United States had to be instituted immediately.

The Frontier Graduate School of Midwifery started with a class of two students in November

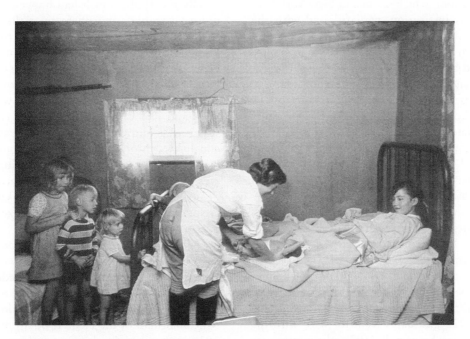

Figure 1-1 A nurse-midwife of the Frontier Nursing Service in a home in Kentucky, circa 1950.
Source: Reproduced by permission from Frontier Nursing Service, Hyden, Kentucky.

1939.[37(p324)] In 1970, the school changed its name to the Frontier School of Midwifery and Family Nursing (FSMFN) when a Family Nurse Practitioner Program was begun. This program closed in 1991 and then was resurrected in 1999 as the Community-Based Family Nursing Education Program (CFNP), and in 2011 the institution was renamed Frontier Nursing University. In the meantime, midwifery education at FNS continued without pause, and in 1989 became the Community-Based Nurse-Midwifery Education Program (CNEP). In 2004, FSMFN was accredited as an independent graduate school by the Southern Association of Colleges and Schools. This was followed in 2005 by institutional accreditation for the school and continuing programmatic accreditation for the nurse-midwifery program by the American College of Nurse-Midwives and programmatic accreditation by the National League for Nursing for the nurse practitioner programs.

Although FNS started the first nurse-midwifery service in the United States, it did not have the first nurse-midwifery education program in the United States.

The Early Nurse-Midwifery Education Programs

The Manhattan Midwifery School

The first school established specifically to educate graduate nurses to be midwives was the Manhattan Midwifery School, which opened in New York City in 1925. This institution was affiliated with the Manhattan Maternity and Dispensary, a hospital specializing in maternity care. The midwifery course was initiated by Emily A. Porter who was a registered nurse and superintendent of the hospital. The program was placed under the jurisdiction of the hospital's School of Nursing. Plans for this program were formulated during 1924, and there were three graduates from the 4-month course in 1925. The 1927 Annual Report of the Manhattan Maternity and Dispensary states that "this is the only school in the country offering such a course at present."

In 1928, Mary M. Richardson, RN, BS, a public health nurse who was a graduate of St. Luke's Hospital in New York City and of Columbia University Teachers' College, and who had studied midwifery at the Hospital for Mothers and Babies in London, became the Directress of the School of Nursing and the course in midwifery. Two of the program's 1928 graduates went to work with the Frontier Nursing Service. By 1929, the course was

6 months in length. The 1931 annual report, however, noted that Mary Richardson had left as Directress of Nursing to return to public health work and that the course had ended:

> The Midwifery Course for graduate nurses started in 1925 has been discontinued during the last year as it was becoming more and more difficult to get enough District cases to take care of the needs of Medical Students.... It was the first and only Midwifery School for graduate nurses in the country. We are glad to hear that a similar one has recently been opened in New York City—The Lobenstine Midwifery Clinic to which we may refer our many applicants.[41]

There were at least 18 graduates of the Manhattan Midwifery School.[41]

The Lobenstine Midwifery School

The School of the Association for the Promotion and Standardization of Midwifery was more commonly known as the Lobenstine Midwifery School, named for one of the charter members, Dr. Ralph Waldo Lobenstine. The Association for the Promotion and Standardization of Midwifery was the creation of Maternity Center Association, which was convinced of the need for nurse-midwives whose preparation would combine U.S. education in obstetric nursing with the education received by the professional European midwife.[42]

By the 1930s, much had happened to create a more favorable atmosphere since the abortive attempt by MCA in the early 1920s to establish a nurse-midwifery education program. There was growing recognition of how obstetric conditions in the United States compared poorly with those in other countries, which had much lower mortality rates and well-organized systems of educated and supervised midwives. Publicity spread about the conclusive proof gathered by the Frontier Nursing Service of the value of a system utilizing nurse-midwives, the work of MCA in parent education, and its demonstration with the Henry Street Visiting Nurse Association of the value of specialized maternity nursing care.

The Association for the Promotion and Standardization of Midwifery was incorporated in early 1931 by three members of the medical board of the Maternity Center Association and its general director, Hazel Corbin, RN. Ralph Waldo Lobenstine, MD, chairman of the medical board of MCA since 1918, was one of the charter members, as was Mary

Breckinridge, director of the Frontier Nursing Service. Lobenstine worked tirelessly until his death in 1931 to bring about the establishment of nurse-midwifery services and education. The determination of the members of the Association for the Promotion and Standardization of Midwifery and the financial support of a group of 60 former patients and friends of Lobenstine led to the establishment of the Lobenstine Midwifery Clinic, Inc., in November 1931.[42]

The nurse-midwifery services provided through the clinic consisted of prenatal care and patient education at the clinic, intrapartum and postpartum care in the woman's home except when hospitalization was required for medical reasons, and postpartum checkups at 14 days and 6 weeks in the clinic. Four attending obstetricians provided their services at medical clinics and round-the-clock consultation and, if necessary, were present in the woman's home for delivery. During the 26 years the Lobenstine Clinic provided clinical services (1932–1958), a total of 7099 births were attended, of which 6116 took place in women's homes. The maternal mortality rate of the clinic was 0.9 per 1000 live births, as contrasted to a maternal death rate of 10.4 per 1000 live births for the same geographic district as a whole and 1.2 per 1000 live births for a leading hospital in New York City at that time.[42]

Organizational and administrative details of the clinic were worked out and a curriculum was designed for the school. The latter was guided by British curricula but modified to meet the needs, cultural patterns, and healthcare systems in the United States. Hattie Hemschemeyer, RN, BS, MA, a public health nurse educator, was named director of the Lobenstine Midwifery Clinic and School. Rose McNaught, RN, CM, a public health nurse who had obtained her midwifery preparation in London and then returned to work at the Frontier Nursing Service, was loaned to Lobenstine by FNS to help develop the program. She joined the Lobenstine staff as a clinician and faculty member. The school opened in September 1932 and had six graduates in 1933, including Hattie Hemschemeyer.

By 1934, the memorial funds that had been pledged to establish and maintain the school and clinic for 3 years were exhausted. Therefore, in 1934, MCA and the Lobenstine Midwifery Clinic consolidated under the name and auspices of Maternity Center Association, which also assumed administrative and financial responsibility for the School of the Association for the Promotion and Standardization of Midwifery.[42] Thus MCA traces the history of its school of nurse-midwifery back to 1932.

The Maternity Center Association School of Nurse-Midwifery (**Figure 1-2**) graduated 320 students between 1933 and 1959, utilizing the services provided by the Lobenstine Clinic for educational purposes. In 1958, it moved inside a major medical and educational institution, and was established in the Downstate Medical Center, State University of New York in Brooklyn, New York; students used Kings County Hospital for clinical experience. This move was facilitated by Hazel Corbin, RN, executive director of MCA; Marion Strachan, CNM, BS, MA, director of the nurse-midwifery program; and Louis Hellman, MD, chairman and professor of obstetrics and gynecology at Downstate Medical Center and Kings County Hospital.

Subsequent Early Education Programs

Today, almost all of the nurse-midwifery and midwifery education programs that are accredited by the Accreditation Commission of Midwifery Education of the American College of Nurse-Midwives can trace their beginnings to the Maternity Center Association's School of Nurse-Midwifery because they were started by either graduates or students of graduates of the MCA program. The exception is the FNS Frontier Graduate School of Midwifery and a handful of programs started by Frontier Nursing Service graduates.[43]

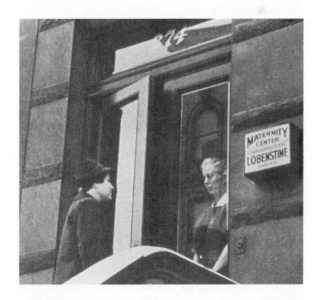

Figure 1-2 A new nurse-midwifery student (Margaret Thomas) in the 1930s being greeted by faculty member Rose McNaught at the Maternity Center Association Lobenstine Clinic and School.
Source: Reproduced by permission from Maternity Center Association, New York, New York.

By the end of the 1950s, seven nurse-midwifery education programs were in operation in the United States. They are listed here with their starting dates, names, and locations as of 1960:

> 1932: School of the Association for the Promotion and Standardization of Midwifery (became the Maternity Center Association School of Nurse-Midwifery in 1934; affiliated with Downstate Medical Center, State University of New York, and Kings County Hospital, Brooklyn, New York, in 1958; also includes an early affiliation of MCA and Kings County Hospital with Johns Hopkins University during 1958–1960)
>
> 1939: Frontier Graduate School of Midwifery of the Frontier Nursing Service, Hyden, Kentucky
>
> 1945: Catholic Maternity Institute School of Nurse-Midwifery, Santa Fe, New Mexico
>
> 1947: Catholic University of America, Washington, DC (affiliated with Catholic Maternity Institute)
>
> 1955: Columbia University Graduate Program in Maternity Nursing, New York City, New York
>
> 1956: The Johns Hopkins University Nurse-Midwifery Program, Baltimore, Maryland
>
> 1956: Yale University Graduate Maternal and Newborn Health Nursing Program, New Haven, Connecticut

Three of these programs subsequently closed: Catholic Maternity Institute (1968); Catholic University of America (1968), which has the distinction of being the first nurse-midwifery education program to be part of a master's degree program; and the Johns Hopkins University Nurse-Midwifery Program (1981). In addition to the closure of the Manhattan Midwifery School in 1931 and the Preston Retreat School of Midwifery in 1960, two other schools opened and closed during the 1940s:

> 1941–1946: The Tuskegee School of Nurse-Midwifery in Tuskegee, Alabama; a joint project of the Macon County Health Department, the Children's Bureau, the Julius Rosenwald Fund, Tuskegee University (although not officially part of Tuskegee University), and the Alabama State Department of Health. Graduated 31 students.[44]
>
> 1942–1943: The Flint-Goodridge School of Nurse-Midwifery in New Orleans, Louisiana; in connection with Flint-Goodridge Hospital and Dillard University.

The Flint-Goodridge School of Nurse Midwifery graduated two students[45] and has the distinction of being the first nurse-midwifery program to be affiliated with a university.

The 1940s and 1950s

The early graduates from MCA went into a variety of positions, with their only common denominator being their goal of improving maternity care. The majority of graduates either practiced or taught clinical nurse-midwifery in MCA or FNS programs or became involved with various aspects of public health. A number of nurse-midwives in public health went to work in state health departments in positions designed for the supervision and teaching of indigenous midwives. These positions were in keeping with one of the original purposes of the Sheppard Towner Act—that public health nurses be employed for the instruction of untrained midwives. As many of the early MCA graduates were also public health nurses, they were ideally prepared for working in rural maternity care, where the majority of indigenous midwives practiced.

Other graduates held positions as maternal–child health consultants for state boards of health or within the federal bureaucracy. Still other graduates became involved in the nurse-midwifery education programs at Tuskegee Institute in Alabama and the Flint-Goodridge School in Louisiana.

In 1944, members of the Medical Mission Sisters (a Roman Catholic order) who were graduates of the MCA program started the Catholic Maternity Institute (CMI) in Santa Fe, New Mexico. Births took place in the home or in La Casita, the first nurse-midwifery birth center. In 1947 Catholic University of America affiliated with CMI in order for nurses to study nurse-midwifery as a specialty in their master's degree program, thus becoming the first university-based nurse-midwifery program.

In the middle and late 1940s, graduates of MCA at Yale University were central figures in developing the concept and practice of rooming-in and in studying the effects of natural (prepared) childbirth and family-centered supportive care on a woman's prenatal, intrapartum, and postpartum experience.

The 1950s saw the development of three more educational programs by MCA graduates, at Columbia University, Johns Hopkins University, and Yale University. Maternity Center Association was directly involved in initiating two of these programs (Columbia and Johns Hopkins) by sending nurse-midwives to start them. The 1950s also saw the founding of the American College of Nurse-Midwifery. The history of this professional organization is detailed later in this chapter.

In the 1940s and 1950s, there was considerable demand for nurse-midwives to serve as nursing educators in maternity nursing; to fill nursing service staff, supervisory, and consultant positions in hospital obstetrics departments; and to act as consultants in federal and international health organizations. These employment possibilities, combined with a lack of opportunities for clinical nurse-midwifery practice, created the situation in which a large percentage of the early graduate nurse-midwives did not actually practice clinical nurse-midwifery. In a 1954 survey, 147 nurse-midwives identified 426 job positions they had held since graduation. Of these 426 job positions, 27% involved being a staff nurse-midwife.[46]

The 1960s

Opportunities to practice clinical nurse-midwifery were severely limited for a nurse-midwife graduating in the early 1960s. Only two states and one city legally recognized the practice of nurse-midwifery at that time: New Mexico, Kentucky, and New York City. Another state, Maryland, had nurse-midwives practicing under an old granny midwife law.

In brief, a graduate could join the faculty of one of the existing nurse-midwifery education programs; practice at Catholic Maternity Institute in Santa Fe, Frontier Nursing Service in Kentucky, Baltimore City Hospital and Johns Hopkins University in Baltimore, or Kings County Hospital or Cumberland Hospital in New York City; or go to an overseas mission field. A few other isolated service positions or projects existed but generally were not well known or, as in the case of the Madera County project in California, offered only short-term employment by virtue of being demonstration projects. Therefore, the majority of graduates of that era went into teaching, supervisory, administrative, or consultative positions in related fields. This situation led to the need for refresher programs for nurse-midwives wanting to return to the practice of clinical nurse-midwifery when, less than a decade later, service sites in which to practice expanded rapidly.

In the late 1950s and the 1960s, nurse-midwives made a deliberate and concerted effort to get into hospitals, as that was where the majority of births (approximately 70% at that time) now took place. The movement of nurse-midwives into hospitals brought concepts of family-centered maternity care

and a consumer advocate to childbearing women who gave birth in hospitals. During this era, nurse-midwives began working in both in-hospital and out-of-hospital settings.

By 1967, approximately 23% of 468 employed nurse-midwives who responded to a questionnaire[47] were actually practicing clinical nurse-midwifery. This number represented a substantial increase from the 11% practicing in 1963. Of the 468 employed nurse-midwives who responded to the 1967 survey, 103 (22%) worked in foreign countries, mostly through church missions or international health organizations. Fifty-six percent of the employed nurse-midwives were in service areas related to maternity care but were not working clinically as nurse-midwives; 75% held positions above the staff level. Of the 23% who actually practiced nurse-midwifery, 35% were also on the faculties of schools of nurse-midwifery; 53% provided nurse-midwifery services throughout the maternity cycle; and the remaining 12% functioned as nurse-midwives in one or more—but not all—phases of the maternity cycle.

Development of opportunities to practice clinical nurse-midwifery remained slow into the late 1960s. It was not until 1968, when nurse-midwives were employed in the Maternal–Infant Care (MIC) nurse-midwifery program in New York City to practice in community clinics linked with hospitals, that previously unheard-of employment opportunities for nurse-midwives to practice midwifery began to become available.[48] The first nurse-midwife to practice within the Indian Health Service started her job in 1969.[49]

Five nurse-midwifery education programs opened in the 1960s, four of which subsequently closed (the second date is the closing date):

1960–1981: University of Puerto Rico/Caparra Heights District Hospital, San Juan, Puerto Rico

1963–1972: New York Medical College Graduate School of Nursing Nurse-Midwifery Program, New York City

1965: University of Utah Graduate Maternal-Infant Nursing Program, Salt Lake City, Utah

1966–1975: Ponce District Hospital, Ponce, Puerto Rico

1969–1985: University of Mississippi Medical Center Nurse-Midwifery Program, Jackson, Mississippi

A number of obstacles contributed to this slow development in practice and education. Paramount among these were misconceptions and stereotypes regarding nurse-midwives. These misconceptions led to outright hostility by some, even as some other professionals supported nurse-midwifery. Both hostility and support emanated from the professional groups with whom nurse-midwives most closely work: physicians and nurses.

Following are some of the stereotypes and misconceptions often heard during that period of time that hindered the development of nurse-midwifery in the 1960s, as well as the factual rebuttals given at that time:

- *Stereotype:* Midwives are untrained and unskilled. Frequently, when only the "midwife" part of the term "nurse-midwife" is used, a negative image of the good-hearted, loving, but untrained midwife of past history is engendered. It leads to the irrational conclusion that nurse-midwives are an uneducated menace representing a backward step into illiteracy in the provision of maternal–infant health care.

- *Fact:* The term "nurse-midwife" actually specifies exactly who and what a nurse-midwife is. Either part of the name alone does not fully describe the unique profession of the nurse-midwife in the United States. The nurse part recognizes the prerequisite education in nursing, differentiates the nurse-midwife from the historical or contemporary lay midwife, and assures a continuing emphasis on patient education, support, and counseling. All certified nurse-midwives are registered nurses. Half of the nurse-midwifery education programs are offered in schools granting a master's degree. The midwife part of the name recognizes the additional specialized preparation and functioning of the nurse-midwife, tempers the medical focus in normal obstetrics, and identifies the nurse-midwife with professional midwife counterparts the world over.

- *Misconception:* Nurse-midwives are trying to be "little doctors." In general, physicians think that nurse-midwives do not know "their place," while nurses think that nurse-midwives have "sold out" to physicians and are, therefore, "traitors to nursing."

- *Fact:* Nurse-midwifery is a clearly defined profession that includes a scope of practice, which overlaps with both nursing and medicine. Nurse-midwives believe fervently in who they are, what they have to offer, and what they can do. Nurse-midwives are experts in the normal childbearing cycle. They wish to be precisely who they are and to do precisely what they do—that is, to encourage and facilitate natural, normal childbearing processes with a minimum of intervention; to educate, support, and instigate personal and family growth; to foster self-confidence and independence; to dispel fear; and to provide a calm atmosphere of acceptance and caring. Nurse-midwives are neither sell-outs nor traitors to either nursing or medicine. Instead, they realistically recognize the need for having the support of both the nursing and the medical professions for real growth in nurse-midwifery to take place. For the benefit of mothers and babies, nurse-midwives continue to seek accord with both.

The 1970s

In the late 1960s and early 1970s, everything changed. Suddenly nurse-midwifery was not only acceptable but inundated with requests for practitioners and berated for the lack of nurse-midwives to meet the demand. Thus the late 1960s and early 1970s were a time of rapid development in nurse-midwifery, with widespread proliferation of nurse-midwifery services and educational programs that continued through the decade.

By the end of the 1970s, there were 22 basic nurse-midwifery education programs in the United States; in 10 years, the number of programs was double the number developed during the preceding 37 years. Fifteen new programs opened during this period of time, of which seven subsequently closed (the second date is the closing date):

1972: University of Illinois at Chicago Nurse-Midwifery Program

1971–1975: Loma Linda University Nurse-Midwifery Program, California

1973: University of Minnesota Nurse-Midwifery Program, Minneapolis

1973: Medical University of South Carolina Nurse-Midwifery Program, Charleston

1973: Georgetown University Nurse-Midwifery Program, Washington, DC

1973–1984: St. Louis University Graduate Program in Nurse-Midwifery, Missouri

1973–1985: Meharry Medical College Nurse-Midwifery Program, Nashville, Tennessee

1974–1998: University of Kentucky Nurse-Midwifery Program, Lexington

1975: University of Medicine and Dentistry of New Jersey Nurse-Midwifery Program, Newark

1975–1995: University of California, San Diego Nurse-Midwifery Program

1974–1997: U.S. Air Force Nurse-Midwifery Program, Andrews Air Force Base, Maryland

1976: Emory University Nurse-Midwifery Program, Atlanta, Georgia

1977–1985: University of Arizona Nurse-Midwifery Program, Tucson

1978: University of Miami Nurse-Midwifery Program, Florida

1978: San Francisco General Hospital/University of California San Francisco Interdepartmental Nurse-Midwifery Education Program

The proliferation of educational programs overextended the existing resources for clinical experience for students. A workshop of nurse-midwifery education and service directors focusing on their interdependence was held in 1973. The group divided into task forces to make recommendations for solutions to the serious lack of clinical experience available to students. These recommendations were forwarded from the workshop to the ACNM Board of Directors.[50] Nurse-midwives cooperated with one another in the provision of clinical facilities and clinical faculty for educational purposes. This effort meant sacrifice for the preservation of the profession on the part of those midwives for whom their own direct care of women, babies, and families is their greatest satisfaction.

A number of factors contributed to this unprecedented growth in nurse-midwifery education and practice sites:

- Official recognition by organized obstetrics. A joint statement in 1971 by the American College of Obstetricians and Gynecologists, the Nurses Association of the American College of Obstetricians and Gynecologists, and the American College of Nurse-Midwives recognized and supported the development and utilization of nurse-midwives. Recognition was for the practice of nurse-midwifery within "teams of physicians, nurse-midwives, obstetric registered nurses and other health personnel...directed by a qualified obstetrician-gynecologist...for the complete care and management of *uncomplicated maternity* patients."[51]

- Increased visibility and involvement of the women's movement and feminism. Women's increased feelings of self-worth and self-confidence led to a natural alliance between women, who wanted to participate in and be responsible for their childbearing experience, and nurse-midwives, who facilitate the natural and normal processes, provide family-centered care, and promote parental self-determination.

- Recognition by the consumer. An increasing number of articles about the "new midwife" were published in major magazines such as *Redbook*, *Newsweek*, *Life*, and *McCall's*; in Sunday news magazines; and in newspapers such as the *New York Times* and the *Wall Street Journal*. Greater consumer awareness and the satisfaction of those experiencing nurse-midwifery care and writing about it led to consumer demand for nurse-midwifery services.

- Use of nurse-midwives in federally funded projects such as Maternal–Infant Care (MIC), Family Planning monies (314E), the Agency for International Development (AID), and demonstration projects geared toward improving maternal–infant health care and providing family planning services. Through these projects, other healthcare professionals became familiar with nurse-midwifery. This familiarity dispelled misconceptions, and many physicians and nurses subsequently became ardent supporters of nurse-midwifery.

- Childbearing by the children of the post–World War II baby boomers during the mid-1960s and 1970s. There was not a sufficient supply of obstetricians to care for all of the childbearing women in the country during this second baby boom. This shortage, combined with the small number of general practitioners doing obstetrics, led to policy analyses on how best to use the optimal capabilities of each healthcare worker and promoted the obstetric interdisciplinary team concept as articulated in the 1971 joint statement mentioned earlier.

- Demonstration of the efficacy of the obstetric interdisciplinary team concept. The effectiveness of nurse-midwives had been statistically proven many times since the first studies of the Frontier Nursing Service,[37, 39, 40] by the Madera County Demonstration Program in California in the 1960s,[52] and in every service where nurse-midwives had worked. The team concept was demonstrated in Mississippi, where infant mortality was cut in half in Holmes County in the early 1970s.[53]

- The involvement of nurse-midwives in inter-conception health care (i.e., family planning, human sexuality, and gynecologic screening) and in neonatal care including promotion of parenting. The ability of nurse-midwives to provide care throughout the childbearing cycle facilitates the provision of continuity of care to new families.

The two different credentialing mechanisms for national certification as a certified nurse-midwife (credentialing of the individual) and for the accreditation of nurse-midwifery education programs (credentialing of the education program) were well established by the early 1970s. A decade later, ACNM certification was recognized by the National Commission of Health Certifying Agencies. The ACNM Division of Accreditation (DOA) was first recognized by the U.S. Department of Education (USDOE) as a national accrediting body in 1982. Recognition has been renewed as proscribed by the USDOE ever since.

The first private practice with nurse-midwives began in the early 1970s.[54] With the consumer "discovery" of the nurse-midwife came a burgeoning of private practice nurse-midwives, and another inhibiting misconception was laid to rest:

- *Misconception:* Nurse-midwives are less expensive than physicians and their care is not as good as the care offered by physicians. This is why nurse-midwives are hired to care for the indigent and those persons who cannot pay for healthcare services.

- *Fact:* This misconception arose from the fact that in prior decades, nurse-midwifery practices were mainly situated in large medical centers and city hospitals serving the medically indigent or in remote rural areas with few physicians. This initial concentration of nurse-midwives in settings serving women from lower socioeconomic groups occurred because the nurse-midwife's professional services were welcomed first in areas where help was most desperately needed. By the mid-1970s, nurse-midwives were in practice with physicians all over the country, taking care of families from all socioeconomic brackets. According to a 1976–1977 survey by the American College of Nurse-Midwives,[55] approximately 26% of all nurse-midwives practicing nurse-midwifery worked in some form of private practice arrangement.

Nurse-midwives were well accepted by women, who often preferred to have a nurse-midwife in attendance at their birth as long as their condition did not require the physician member of the team. This preference is largely a result of the time the nurse-midwife spends explaining and teaching during the office visits, the commitment of the nurse-midwife to the woman throughout labor, and the practical application of the beliefs of the nurse-midwife in promoting a family-centered, normal childbearing experience.

During the 1970s, nurse-midwifery had become not only acceptable but also desirable and demanded. After years of struggling for existence, nurse-midwives now faced the problem of a severe shortage of supply to meet the demand both from within the established healthcare system and from a small but growing number of consumers who were dissatisfied with the health care provided by the "official" system. These consumers desired care outside of the system, and looked to nurse-midwives for support and services. Inability by the small total number of nurse-midwives to respond to both demands and provide a sufficient number of childbirth alternatives (e.g., hospital birthing rooms, childbirth centers, or carefully selected home births) led to further dissatisfaction on the part of the consumer with professional health care and fostered the development of often untrained lay midwives or birth attendants, along with a do-it-yourself movement.

Lay midwifery developed in the 1970s in response to disenchanted childbirth consumers who wanted to give birth to their babies outside of the hospital. The term *lay midwifery* in the 1970s and 1980s referred to all non-nurse-midwives, whose preparation in midwifery was highly variable. Lay midwifery struggled with its early identity as these providers disagreed sharply among themselves regarding the desirability of formal education, standards, credentialing, and regulation.

A number of groups and organizations supportive of lay midwifery and home birth sprang up during the 1970s: the National Association of Parents and Professionals for Safe Alternatives in Childbirth (NAPSAC), Home Oriented Maternity Experience (HOME), Association of Childbirth at Home International (ACHI), and the National Midwives Association (NMA). Existing organizations such as the International Childbirth Education Association (ICEA) and La Leche League added their support. The first national meeting of lay midwives took place in 1977 in El Paso, Texas.

The 1980s

By the 1980s, nurse-midwives were practicing in the full range of possible arenas—from clinics and federally funded programs to health maintenance organizations (HMOs) and hospitals, from being employed by physicians to employing the physicians—and providing a full range of services, from in-hospital birth services to out-of-hospital birth services or a mix of both, to provide continuity of care between settings. By this time, nurse-midwives were perceived to be competitors of physicians for the obstetric healthcare dollar. Supportive physicians continued to enable nurse-midwifery practice by providing necessary physician consultation, collaboration, and referral systems. Opposing physicians tried to restrict the growth of nurse-midwifery through state legislative battles over statutory recognition of nurse-midwives, mandated third-party reimbursement, and prescriptive authority; denial of hospital practice privileges; and pressure on supportive physicians vis-à-vis their malpractice insurance. The entire situation was exacerbated by an overabundance of physicians—a trend that would continue for the foreseeable future. In the view of many physicians, nurse-midwives were no longer needed.

An investigative congressional hearing into the problems faced by nurse-midwives was held in 1980,[56] and the Federal Trade Commission became actively concerned about possible and real restraint-of-trade issues.[57] At the same time, healthcare costs had become unacceptably high and some nurse-midwifery services were demonstrating that they were cost-effective.[58]

A survey of nurse-midwives in 1971 showed that 37% of the respondents were in the direct practice of nurse-midwifery, compared with 23% in 1967 and 18% of those nurse-midwives practicing in the United States in 1963. By 1976–1977, 51% of 1218 respondents living in the United States and replying to a questionnaire[55] were practicing clinical nurse-midwifery. In the 15 years from 1963 to 1978, active nurse-midwifery services increased from six services in 3 states and New York City to multiple services in 35 states, with more in planning stages. By 1982, 67% of 1584 survey participants living in the United States stated they were practicing clinical nurse-midwifery.[59] In 1984, nurse-midwives were practicing in all 50 states; by 1988, nearly 80% of the respondents to an ACNM survey were in nurse-midwifery practice and education.[60] The legal recognition of nurse-midwifery had spread from 3 states and New York City in 1963 with its legal status in the other states largely unknown, to a very clear legal status in all 50 states and 4 jurisdictions (District of Columbia, Guam, Puerto Rico, and the Virgin Islands) as a result of extensive and intensive work by the legislation committee of the American College of Nurse-Midwives.

The late 1970s and early 1980s also saw the rapid development of out-of-hospital childbirth centers, with Maternity Center Association spearheading this movement. Twelve nurse-midwifery education programs opened during the 1980s, 7 of which subsequently closed (the second date is the closing date):

1980: University of Colorado, Denver

1980: University of Pennsylvania, Philadelphia

1981: Oregon Health Sciences Center, Portland

1981–2003: University of Southern California, Los Angeles

1982–1988: Rush University/St. Luke's Medical Center, Chicago, Illinois

1982–1987: Stanford University, Stanford, California

1982: University of Florida, Gainesville

1983: Case Western Reserve University, Frances Payne Bolton School of Nursing, Cleveland, Ohio

1983–1999: University of California, San Francisco/University of California, San Diego Intercampus Nurse-Midwifery Program

1984–2003: Baylor College of Medicine, Houston, Texas

1987–1998: Education Program Associates, San Jose, California

1989–2006: Parkland Hospital/Texas Women's University, Dallas, Texas

In 1982, Midwives Alliance of North America (MANA) was organized for representation of lay midwives including those in Canada and Mexico as well as the United States. The midwifery membership in MANA is diverse; it includes anyone who chooses to call herself, or rarely himself, a midwife and reflects a complete range of educational preparation and experience. MANA established an Interim Registry Board (IRB) in 1986 to create an examination and maintain a registry of midwives who passed the examination. Taking the examination was voluntary.

The 1990s

The 1990s witnessed another growth spurt in nurse-midwifery education programs, with an unprecedented 26 programs opening. This growth spurt was in part a result of states' recognizing the quality and cost-effectiveness of nurse-midwifery care and funding local programs. During the 1980s and 1990s, the number of programs again doubled, so that by the end of the twentieth century 45 ACNM-accredited basic nurse-midwifery education programs existed, one of which was also an accredited basic midwifery education program. A listing of all the current education programs accredited by the ACNM Division of Accreditation can be obtained from the ACNM website (www.midwife.org).[61] Ten of the 26 programs that opened during the 1990s subsequently closed.

The ACNM set the goal of having 10,000 certified nurse-midwives by 2001. In 1995, slightly more than 5000 had been certified. With the increased number of new programs, the growing number of students in existing programs, and the advent of community-based distance-learning programs, the trajectory to reach the 2001 goal was on target; in mid-2001, the total number of persons ever certified as nurse-midwives was 9327. Distance learning came into its own in the late 1980s and 1990s. The idea was first envisioned for nurse-midwifery education in the 1970s but took a quantum leap forward when combined with web-based technologies in the late 1980s.[62,63]

The healthcare system started to move in the direction of managed care in the early 1990s. As this movement gathered steam, nurse-midwives once again found themselves struggling to be recognized and "at the table" both nationally and locally for far-reaching decisions affecting the healthcare system and nurse-midwifery practice. Practical preparation for establishing nurse-midwifery practices and services increasingly focused on business aspects of a practice, including marketing, budgets, financial concerns and policy issues, methods of determining productivity, billing and coding, and effective business practices. Responding to the needs for practical guidance, the Nurse-Midwifery Service Directors Network published *An Administrative Manual for Nurse-Midwifery Services*. For its part, in addition to offering its long-existing *Guidelines for Establishing a Nurse-Midwifery Practice*, the ACNM put together a marketing packet for CNMs and handbooks on managed care and managed care contracting. In 1996, the Midwifery Business Institute was started by nurse-midwives at the University of Michigan School of Nursing and the University of Michigan Health System; both institutions co-sponsor this periodic conference.

In 1989, the ACNM board of directors stated that "The ACNM will actively explore, through the DOA [Division of Accreditation], the testing of non-nurse professional midwifery educational routes." In 1990, the DOA determined that to address the charge from the board of directors, it was necessary to first identify those nurse competencies that were assumed to be brought by a registered nurse to a nurse-midwifery education program. The DOA completed this task in 1994. These competencies were then combined with specified prerequisite courses into an ACNM DOA document entitled *Skills, Knowledge, Competencies, and Health Sciences Prerequisite to Midwifery Practice*.[64]

In 1994, the ACNM, in response to requests from state regulatory agencies, took a leadership role in setting the standards for the credentialing of non-nurse professional midwives. The immediate impetus for this effort was the growing use of licensed healthcare professionals—most often physician assistants—to practice midwifery without educational preparation or credentialing for this role. Using, at a minimum, the same criteria specified for nurse-midwifery education programs, the ACNM DOA developed criteria for basic midwifery education programs for non-nurse midwives, and the ACNM Certification Council committed itself to the testing and certification of graduates from ACNM DOA-accredited midwifery programs who would receive the credential of Certified Midwife (CM).[64] These midwives meet the same endpoint academic and clinical objectives as nurse-midwives. The first education program for non-nurse (direct-entry) midwives preaccredited by the ACNM DOA was established in 1996. The program launched its first graduates in 1997, and in 1999 it was fully accredited. Three other direct-entry midwifery programs have since been preaccredited by the ACNM DOA.

In 1991, the National Coalition of Midwifery Educators, an organization separate from MANA and the MANA Education Committee, formed the Midwifery Education and Accreditation Council (MEAC). MEAC organized and defined itself in terms of accrediting education of direct-entry midwives in the maternity cycle and out-of-hospital—especially home birth—practice. It developed standards and criteria that reflect the core competencies and guiding principles set by the Midwives Alliance of North America.

The examination of the Interim Registry Board (IRB) of MANA was first administered in 1991. In 1992, the IRB separated from MANA and incorporated as the North American Registry of Midwives (NARM). Midwives credentialed by NARM are Certified Professional Midwives (CPM).

Credentialed midwifery at the beginning of the millennium now encompassed both nurse-midwives and two types of non-nurse (direct-entry) mid-wives, leading to three sets of initials: certified nurse-midwives and certified midwives, who were credentialed by ACNM, and certified professional midwives, who are credentialed by NARM. The two types of direct-entry midwives (CMs and CPMs) have different educational processes and two very different scopes of practice. Both are well defined and distinguishable from the noncredentialed lay midwife.

The 2000s

By 2011, the number of CNMs and CMs ever certified had more than doubled during the previous 15 years, to reach 11,546 CNMs and CMs.[65] The proliferation of education programs slowed, however, as 12 programs closed during the 2000s (9 of which were part of the 26 that had opened during the 1990s); another 5 new programs opened, however, bringing the total number of ACNM-accredited programs to 39 in 2011.

The National Center for Health Statistics first began collecting data on midwifery-attended births in 1975; in 1989, it revised the birth certificate data collection form to distinguish CNM-attended births from births attended by other midwives. CMs are now included with CNMs in birth certificate data.[66] The number of CNM-attended births has risen from 132,286 births in 1989 to 313,516 births in 2009, representing 7.6% of all births.[65–67] The proportion of vaginal births attended by CNMs/CMs, however, is 11.8%.[66] This discrepancy in proportions is thought to be due, at least in part, to the rapid growth in cesarean deliveries[68] and means that now CNMs/CMs attend 1 in 9 vaginal births.[66] In 2009, 96.1% of CNM/CM-attended births occurred in the hospital, 2% in freestanding birth centers, and 1.8% in the home.[65]

Legislative issues continued to be of highest priority for nurse-midwives in the 2000s. By mid-year 2008, nurse-midwives had prescription writing authority in all 50 states.[68] Other state-level legislation focused on removal of supervisory verbiage in licensure laws, reimbursement, liability insurance, and removal of barriers to practice and access. The Committee for the Advancement of Midwifery Practice (CAMP) was created in New York state in 2000 to expand licensure of CMs with full-scope practice, equivalent to CNMs, to all 50 states. Top federal legislative issues throughout the decade included obtaining an equitable Medicare reimbursement rate to improve access by CNMs/CMs to vulnerable populations, federal funding of ACNM-accredited education programs, and support of improving quality and reducing disparities in access to women's healthcare services.

By 2002, the *Joint Statement of Practice Relations Between Obstetrician-Gynecologists and Certified Nurse-Midwives/Certified Midwives* had evolved through the 1980s and 1990s to now emphasize mutual respect, equivalency, and a collaborative relationship.[69,70] The most recent *Joint Statement* in 2011 builds on the 2002 *Joint Statement* to highlight the promotion of evidence-based practice, acknowledge that CNMs/CMs are licensed independent providers, and states that obstetrician/gynecologists and CNMs/CMs should receive equivalent third-party reimbursement.[71,72]

Throughout the decades, the work of nurse-midwives has been documented and facilitated by what was first the ACNM Research and Statistics Committee and eventually became the Division of Research in 1988.[73,74] This work and the studies done form a body of knowledge, provide evidence for midwifery care, guide policy, inform legislative efforts and legislators, and facilitate national and international networking.

The 2000s was another time of media coverage not only in newspapers and magazines, but also documentaries promoting midwifery.[75] In addition, a number of nurse-midwives authored books, including both novels and memoirs.[76] The ACNM published *Every Baby Magazine;* established Midwives PAC and publishes a monthly on-line newsletter, *The Advocate,* on federal and state advocacy; and joined with other organizations in an advocacy such as the Coalition for Patient's Rights. Childbirth Connection (formerly known as Maternity Center Association) continues to provide leadership in improving the quality of maternity care through research, education, advocacy, and work with other organizations in producing influential reports, such as *Evidence-Based Maternity Care: What It Is and What It Can Achieve* in 2008.[77] Childbirth Connection was also the catalyst for the creation of the Transforming Maternity Care Project, which convened a Vision Team in 2008 to produce a document titled *2020 Vision for a High-Quality, High-Value Maternity Care System.* This document formed the basis for the development of a blueprint of strategies during a 2009 symposium. Opportunities for action to bring about transformation in maternity care have been identified, and there is ongoing monitoring of progress. Access to the project and details can be found at the following website: www.transform.childbirthconnection.org.

In May 2001, the U.S. Department of Education renewed its recognition of the ACNM Division of Accreditation for preaccreditation and accreditation of nurse-midwifery education programs, and also recognized the expansion of the scope of its activities to include preaccreditation and accreditation of direct-entry midwifery education for the non-nurse. In addition, the DOA was recognized as an institutional accreditor in 2006.[78] In 2008, the name of the DOA changed to the Accreditation Commission for Midwifery Education (ACME).

The Midwifery Education and Accreditation Council (MEAC) also applied for and received recognition from the U.S. Department of Education as an accrediting body in January 2001. MEAC-accredited programs prepare graduates for the examination of the North American Registry of Midwives (NARM) and recognition as a CPM. In 2005, MEAC initiated the Outreach to Educators Project, which evolved into the Association of Midwifery Educators (AME) in 2006.

In 2001, the National Association of Certified Professional Midwives was formed with the purpose of establishing a professional organization and setting national practice standards for CPMs.

The American College of Nurse-Midwives

The American College of Nurse-Midwives is the national professional organization for CNMs and CMs. Its mission is "to establish midwifery as the standard of care for women. We lead the profession through education, clinical practice, research, and advocacy."[79] Incorporated in 1955, the ACNM was founded as the outgrowth of a series of circumstances that rendered its creation necessary.

Early efforts to organize nurse-midwives met with difficulties. An organizational meeting in 1940, chaired by Hattie Hemschemeyer, Director of the Maternity Center Association School of Nurse-Midwifery, resulted in the formation of the National Association of Certified Nurse Midwives (NACNM). Bylaws were written, but the organization never evolved. A 1944 meeting of nurse-midwives, again called by Hattie Hemschemeyer to discuss formation of a national organization, led the group to reject the option of establishing a new organization as financially and time/effort prohibitive. The group also rejected the option of working to make the FNS-related American Association of Nurse-Midwives (AANM) become the national organization they envisioned because the AANM "did not admit colored nurse-midwives."[80] Instead, the group accepted an offer from the integrated National Organization of Public Health Nurses (NOPHN) to establish a section within NOPHN for nurse-midwives.[80]

As a section of NOPHN, nurse-midwives could define themselves, share information and knowledge, and start the process of setting education and practice standards for the profession. In 1949, the nurse-midwifery section published the first national descriptive data gathered about nurse-midwives.[81] NOPHN was dissolved in 1952 following a general reorganization of U.S. national nursing organizations. While NOPHN was absorbed into the American Nurses Association (ANA) and the National League for Nursing (NLN), these organizations did not make any provision for a recognizable entity of nurse-midwives. Instead, the nurse-midwives were assigned to the ANA's Maternal and Child Health Council and the NLN's Interdivisional Council, which encompassed the areas of obstetrics, pediatrics, orthopedics, crippled children, and school nursing. The membership and concerns of the NLN council were simply too broad to serve as a forum or voice for nurse-midwifery. Moreover, being part of the ANA's Council would have meant that nurses who were not midwives would be making decisions about nurse-midwifery practice and education. Ironically, even though nurse-midwives were in positions of leadership in maternal–child nursing in educational, professional, and federal organizations pertaining to health care, they were rarely recognized as specifically being nurse-midwives.

The Committee on Organization

As the identity of nurse-midwives could not be maintained in either the ANA or the NLN, the nurse-midwives present at an ANA convention in the spring of 1954 agreed to establish the Committee on Organization. Sister M. Theophane Shoemaker, the director of the Catholic Maternity Center in Santa Fe, New Mexico, was chair of the committee.

The Committee on Organization, though claiming its progress was slow and tedious, had within 2 months identified reasons for organizing; discussed ways in which organization could be accomplished; written a definition of a nurse-midwife; identified the functions of a new organization if one was to be established; set educational standards for nurse-midwifery schools, including a statement of purpose and basic admission requirements; designed and mailed a questionnaire to locate nurse-midwives and ascertain their desire to organize; written and mailed two of the eventual six *Organization Bulletins of The*

Committee on Organization;[82] and organized a meeting of nurse-midwives for December 1954. Forty-six nurse-midwives attended that meeting, during which they reviewed the work done thus far, discussed the results of the questionnaire (to which 147 nurse-midwives had replied), and approved the definition of a nurse-midwife and a statement of purpose of a nurse-midwifery organization. The major issue, however, was how organization could be accomplished. Four possible options had been identified:

1. Organization within the American Nurses Association as a conference group
2. Organization within the National League for Nursing as a council
3. Reorganization of the American Association of Nurse-Midwives into a national organization
4. Formation of an entirely new organization of nurse-midwives to be known as the American College of Nurse-Midwifery

The American Association of Nurse-Midwives had been started in 1929 as the Kentucky State Association of Midwives, incorporated by nurse-midwives working with the Frontier Nursing Service. Mary Breckinridge, then director of the FNS, was the continuing president of AANM during her lifetime. At that time, the organization's function was akin to that of an alumnae association, although membership was not limited to alumnae. Efforts to reach out to the AANM to persuade its members to reorganize were made by Sr. Theophane Shoemaker and Hattie Hemschemeyer. Mary Breckinridge, however, stood firm in her belief that nurse-midwives should be part of the nursing organizations and that the structure of the AANM would not change.[80] The AANM, therefore, was eliminated as a possible option based on its members' analysis and statement of preference not to be considered.

The remaining options were either to organize within one of the national nursing organizations or to create a new organization. This decision was deferred until letters requesting a conference group and a council, respectively, were submitted to, and replies were received from, the ANA and NLN. The letters were approved during the meeting.

The NLN expressed interest and concern but pointed out that its bylaws for organization of a council would not meet the needs of the nurse-midwives. The reply from the ANA was not encouraging. This organization was interested in a plan to establish an interdisciplinary committee of the ANA and the NLN, with additional representatives from the public, to study the improvement of the care of mothers and children. The nurse-midwives could be a part of this committee. Sister Theophane Shoemaker identified the basic issue of being part of a larger nursing organization in a letter to Hattie Hemschemeyer: "We still would not have autonomy in setting up standards of education and practice. And the definition of ourselves would depend upon ANA's decision."[83]

This information was published in the fourth *Organization Bulletin*, along with the plans for the next meeting of the Committee on Organization and a request for comments regarding what was emerging as the obvious direction for organization. At its meeting in May 1955, the Committee on Organization voted unanimously to proceed with the formation of the American College of Nurse-Midwifery. Those present based their action on the facts that all the other options had essentially been ruled out, that 133 of the 147 nurse-midwives answering the questionnaire had responded positively to the idea of belonging to a new organization of nurse-midwives, that formation of a separate organization obviously seemed to be the only way that nurse-midwives could work together and accomplish the goals that had been delineated in the statement of purposes, and that only one response had been received to the request for comments regarding this direction. The Committee on Organization had done such a splendid job of keeping all the nurse-midwives informed and involved that there was nothing further to be said.

The Committee on Organization then began working to incorporate and establish the new organization. The incorporation of the American College of Nurse-Midwifery took place on November 7, 1955, in the state of New Mexico. New Mexico was chosen because it was one of the few states in which nurse-midwives were practicing and incorporation there involved the least amount of red tape, time, and expense.

The ACNM as an Organization

The first annual meeting of the American College of Nurse-Midwifery was held November 12 and 13, 1955, in Kansas City, Missouri. Hattie Hemschemeyer, Director of the Maternity Center Association School of Nurse-Midwifery, was elected the first president of the ACNM. In her first message to members in the *Bulletin of the American College of Nurse-Midwifery,* she wrote about the driving force and movement of nurse-midwifery in terms that remain equally valid today:

The College must select carefully the work it undertakes and then do well the work it has undertaken. We need to work with dedication and conviction....

We have a pioneer job to do, and if we work as well and as constructively in a group as we have in the past as individuals, we can help to improve professional competence, provide better service and educational programs, and make fuller use of resources. The future looks bright.[84]

On the ACNM's 10th anniversary, Hemschemeyer stated, "Our identity as a College gives us fundamental rights and grave responsibilities."[85]

In 1956, both the American College of Nurse-Midwifery and the American Association of Nurse-Midwives were accepted into the International Confederation of Midwives (ICM) upon the recommendation of England and Scotland and the unanimous vote of the executive council of the ICM. In 1969, the American Association of Nurse-Midwives merged with the American College of Nurse-Midwifery to form the American College of Nurse-Midwives. In October 1972, the American College of Nurse-Midwives hosted the triennial congress of the ICM in Washington, DC, when Lucille Woodville, then nursing consultant to the Bureau of Indian Health Affairs and past president of the ACNM (1969–1971), was president of the ICM (1969–1972).

The objectives of the American College of Nurse-Midwives, first expressed in the Articles of Incorporation in 1955, and approved as "specific purposes" in the Articles of Incorporation and Bylaws in the May 2008 revision of the Bylaws, reflect both nurse-midwifery's concern for quality health care for women and infants and the assumption of the "grave responsibilities" alluded to by Hattie Hemschemeyer:

Article II. Purposes and Limitations. Section C. Specific Purposes:

Consistent with the ACNM Articles of Incorporation and these Bylaws, ACNM is empowered to:

1. foster and promote excellence in the practice of midwifery and the education of midwives;
2. facilitate the advancement and awareness of excellence in midwifery practice and education, including care of women through the life span and practices which foster public safety;
3. support midwives, other women's health professionals, and students through educational activities, professional conferences, written publications, and other means;
4. engage in and support research activities relating to the profession of midwifery and women's health;
5. develop and disseminate standards for midwifery practice as provided by CNMs and CMs;
6. disseminate a comprehensive body of knowledge concerning women's health and the practice of midwifery, through continuing education activities, professional conferences, written publications, and other means;
7. foster the development and support of midwives, midwifery practice and education, and midwifery professional organizations internationally, and to promote improved access to quality maternal and newborn care in all countries;
8. support quality services to members concerning business and clinical issues, and provide guidance on credentialing, legislative and regulatory issues;
9. establish and support accreditation of CNM/CM educational programs, and facilitate the continuing education of midwives;
10. provide a recognized forum for the free exchange of ideas and information related to the midwifery profession and women's health issues;
11. serve as a source of information to the public and to government agencies concerning excellence in midwifery and women's health care practices and services;
12. support the development and recognition of qualified individuals involved in midwifery practice, education, scholarship, and policy;
13. support and foster cooperation among midwives and other women's health care clinicians, educators, students, and organizations, including research organizations, government bodies, educational institutions, and other organizations in the United States and internationally;
14. foster consensus for professional policies and practices related to midwifery practice and education;

15. support and foster appropriate professional licensure regulations and legislation related to midwifery and women's health issues;
16. speak for the profession of midwifery in relation to issues affecting the professional affairs of CNMs and CMs; and
17. engage in all other corporate activities permitted by law.[86]

The seal of the ACNM (**Figure 1-3**) reflects basic philosophical beliefs of nurse-midwifery. Rita Kroska, CNM, PhD, who designed the seal in 1955, interprets its symbols as follows:

The large shield is comprised of four symbols: a small shield of stars and stripes exemplify the United States of America; three intertwined circles exemplify the family with the lower circle containing crosshatching to illustrate the crib containing the child; a tripod with flames rising exemplifies continuance and warmth in dedication to the American family; and, lastly, the large shield contains an undulating band above the tripod but beneath the smaller shield and circles. The undulation portrays movement, persistence, steadiness, and steadfastness to the word written within. That word is VIVANT, an expletive in French, which means Let Them Live! It is there to fill out the sentence of the symbols, to give emphasis short of exclamatory oath, that of unremitting dedication to safeguarding and promoting the health and wellbeing of family life, particularly the mother and infant.

The large shield is encircled by a ribboned band containing the inscription, "AMERICAN COLLEGE OF NURSE-MIDWIVES, NEW MEXICO, Nov. 7, 1955."

Originally, between 1955 and 1969, the word "nurse-midwives" was "nurse-midwifery," and without the year 1929 included within the inscription. The two changes took place in 1969 when the American Association of Nurse-Midwives with headquarters at the Frontier Nursing Service in Wendover, Kentucky, and the American College of Nurse-Midwifery joined and became the American College of Nurse-Midwives. The year 1929 was the founding of the American Association of Nurse-Midwives.[87]

The A.C.N.M. Foundation

The A.C.N.M. Foundation was established in 1967 as a nonprofit, tax-exempt organization that collaborates closely with and complements the goals of the ACNM.

Its mission is to promote excellence in health care for women, infants, and families worldwide through the support of midwifery.[88] The A.C.N.M. Foundation supported critical early developments within the ACNM, such as the first national certifying examination; the first portable exhibit about nurse-midwives; workshops on nurse-midwifery education, clinical practice, and the approval process; and means for publicizing nurse-midwifery and the ACNM. The Foundation has sponsored, published, and disseminated significant reports, studies, surveys, educational materials, and research. It distributes numerous midwifery scholarships and awards.[89] The ACNM would not have been able to accomplish all that it has without the support of the A.C.N.M. Foundation and the dedication of its board of trustees.

Activities of the ACNM

The membership of the American College of Nurse-Midwives has been characterized from the beginning by dedication, commitment, hard work, articulateness, personal sacrifice, vision, and pioneering spirit. The annals of the ACNM's brief history are peopled with creative giants who were also willing to do the necessary detail work while dipping into their own pocketbooks to finance it. Starting with a charter membership of 124, the ACNM had grown to a membership of 860 by its twentieth anniversary in 1975. By 1980 the membership, including students, had increased to more than 1500, by 1984 to 2534, by 1995 to more than 5000, and by the end of 2002

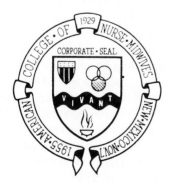

Figure 1-3 The seal of the American College of Nurse-Midwives.
Source: Reproduced by permission of the American College of Nurse-Midwives.

there were more than 7000 CNM, CM, and student members. Seventeen nurse-midwives attended the first annual meeting in Kansas City in 1955; 291 members attended the twentieth annual meeting in Jackson, Mississippi, in 1975. Convention attendance first passed the 1000 mark with 863 members and 138 guests at the 1984 Philadelphia meeting, and more than 2000 people attended the Washington, D.C., meeting in 2000.

The rapid expansion of nurse-midwifery and proliferation of nurse-midwives placed stress on the professional organization. The total number of nurse-midwives and the membership of the ACNM experienced a sevenfold increase during the first 20 years of the organization's existence, tripled during the next 10 years, and tripled again during the next 20 years by the time of the 50th anniversary of the ACNM in 2005.

The organization faced the challenge of having to change from a small, intimate group of hardworking, dedicated nurse-midwives with a relatively simple organizational structure to a large group with an organizational structure and management style that could cope with a rapid increase in membership without losing its dedication and ideals. This was achieved with a major restructuring and revision of the ACNM bylaws in 1974. The organization went from determination of policy by a simple majority vote by the members attending the annual meeting to decision making being placed in the hands of a representative-style board of directors of volunteer nurse-midwives made up of nationally elected officers and six regionally elected representatives. The board of directors was, and continues to be, kept informed by the work of the ACNM membership committees and divisions and the expressed will of those in attendance at the annual meeting.

The second restructuring and revision of the ACNM bylaws occurred in 2008. The membership had again increased (sixfold), and the organization needed a structure that could respond nimbly in the modern era of instant communication, shifting healthcare policy, and changing membership needs while continuing to retain its values. This bylaws revision followed several years of thought about restructuring, identification of strategic priorities, and a values proposition survey. Major changes included the redefinition of associate members as individuals other than a CNM/CM interested in supporting the mission and purposes of ACNM and all CNMs/CMs as active members; the creation of state affiliates, replacing the previous local chapter system, and CNM/CM partner organizations; and the creation of a president-elect and a student representative on the board of directors.

The ACNM continues to be a volunteer membership organization, as CNMs/CMs believe strongly in their right to involvement and participation in the direction, values, and policies of their profession. The membership and the ACNM as a whole are supported by a professional staff. The ACNM has undergirded every aspect of nurse-midwifery and midwifery for CNMs and CMs: education, practice, recognition, legislation, credentialing, insurance, communication, research, and interprofessional and interorganizational relationships.

Recent examples of interprofessional and interorganizational endeavors reflect the organization's vigor. Since 2009, the ACNM has participated in the planning and implementation of a Home Birth Consensus Summit that was held in October 2011 with representatives from other professional stakeholder organizations, including Midwives Alliance of North America, American Congress of Obstetricians and Gynecologists, American Academy of Pediatrics, National Association of Certified Professional Midwives, Association of Women's Health, Obstetric, and Neonatal Nurses, and Childbirth Connection. A follow-up summit was held in April 2013.[90] In addition, in June 2012, the midwifery membership organizations in the United States released a document, *Supporting Healthy and Normal Physiologic Childbirth: A Consensus Statement by ACNM, MANA, and NACPM.* This document summarizes the evidence for the benefits of normal physiologic childbirth, and identifies factors that facilitate or disrupt physiologic childbirth.

The productivity of the membership of the American College of Nurse-Midwives since its founding in 1955 is inspirational, and the group's history is peopled with visionaries, committed hard-working implementers, and talented contributors. In 1994, the ACNM established the Fellows of the American College of Nurse-Midwives (FACNM). Membership in this group is an honor bestowed upon those midwives whose demonstrated leadership, clinical excellence, outstanding scholarship, and professional achievement have merited special recognition both within and outside of the midwifery profession. The mission of FACNM is to serve the ACNM in a consultative and advisory capacity.

The ACNM has also supported international efforts through its Department of Global Outreach (DGO). Established in 1981, the DGO has implemented projects and provided technical assistance in more than 30 developing countries. A major project of the DGO has been the writing of the *Life-Saving Skills Manual for Midwives.*[91] Now in its fourth edition (originally published in 2008), it forms the basis for life-saving skills training programs and projects in Ghana, Indonesia, Nigeria, Uganda, and Vietnam. The work of technical editors—an extensive number of external reviewers representing more than 10 countries—and field-testing have made this training effort of healthcare providers truly life-saving. A corollary has been the development of the family-focused, community-based *Home Based Life Saving Skills Guidelines and Manual*[92] to further reduce maternal and neonatal mortality. Field-tested in India, Ethiopia, Vietnam, Gaza, and the West Bank, it forms the foundation for competency-based training of women and men within a community within the context of their culture and the social context of childbirth within that society.

The founding of the ACNM was described as follows: "To support individual efforts the nurse-midwives have banded together....This provides them with an official mouthpiece for education, a base for common planning and discussion."[93] Almost a century ago, the lack of any national organizations, journals, system of education, legal recognition, or access to the healthcare system led to the "midwife problem and debate." Today the ACNM provides or works for all of these mechanisms of survival and speaks for the profession of nurse-midwifery and midwifery as practiced by CNMs and CMs.

● ● ● References

1. *The Holy Bible.* Genesis 35:17.

2. *International Definition of the Midwife.* Adopted by the International Confederation of Midwives Council meeting, June 15, 2011. Supersedes the ICM "Definition of the Midwife" 1972 and its amendments of 1990 and 2005.

3. ACNM position statements: *Certified Nurse-Midwives and Certified Midwives as Primary Care Providers/ Case Managers,* 1992, revised 1994 and 1997; and *Midwives Are Primary Care Providers and Leaders of Maternity Care Homes,* June 2012.

4. *Core Competencies for Basic Midwifery Practice.* Approved by the ACNM Board of Directors, June 1, 2007; updated January 15, 2008, and June 2012.

5. *Definition of Midwifery and Scope of Practice of Certified Nurse-Midwives and Certified Midwives.* Approved by the ACNM Board of Directors, February 6, 2012. Supersedes all previous definitions.

6. See AMCB website (www.amcbmidwife.org) for further information and history.

7. *Philosophy of the American College of Nurse-Midwives.* Revised September 2004.

8. Nancy Fleming was Secretary of the ACNM board of directors at the time. The discussion was part of a visionary planning summit conceptualized and convened by Joyce Thompson, CNM, DrPH, then president of ACNM.

9. Murphy PA, Fullerton JT. Measuring outcomes of midwifery care: development of an instrument to assess optimality. *J Midwifery Women's Health.* 2001;46(5):274-284.

10. Kennedy HP. A model of exemplary midwifery practice: results of a Delphi study. *J Midwifery Women's Health.* 2000;45(1):4-19.

11. See, for example, Ulrich LT. *A Midwife's Tale: The Life of Martha Ballard Based on Her Diary, 1785-1812.* New York: Alfred A. Knopf; 1990.

12. Webber T. The African American midwife during antebellum slavery. In: Diers D, ed. *Celebrating the Contributions of Academic Midwifery.* New Haven, CT: Yale University School of Nursing; 2005:84-91.

13. Raffloer K. *The Experience of Childbirth on the Oregon Trail: A Search for the Presence of Midwives* [Master's thesis]. New Haven, CT: Yale University School of Nursing; 1999.

14. See, for example, Smart DT, ed. *Mormon Midwife: The 1846-1888 Diaries of Patty Bartlett Sessions.* Logan, UT: Utah State University Press; 1997.

15. Fox CG. Toward a sound historical basis for nurse-midwifery. *Bull Am Coll Nurse-Midwifery.* 1969;14(3):76-82.

16. Pomerantz M. *Factors Contributing to the Widespread Use of Epidurals for Pain Relief in Childbirth* [Master's thesis]. New Haven, CT: Yale University School of Nursing; 1999.

17. Thoms H. *Our Obstetrical Heritage: The Story of Safe Childbirth.* Hamden, CT: Shoe String Press; 1960.

18. Speert H. *Obstetric and Gynecology: A History and Iconography, Revised Second Edition of Iconographia Gyniatrica.* San Francisco: Norman Publishing; 1994.

19. Litoff JB. *American Midwives: 1860 to the Present.* Westport, CT: Greenwood Press; 1978:9.

20. Dawley K. The campaign to eliminate the midwife. *Am J Nurs.* 2000;100(10):53.

21. Litoff JB. Forgotten women: American midwives at the turn of the twentieth century. *Historian.* 1978;40(2):235-251.

22. Perry DS. The early midwives of Missouri. *J Nurse-Midwifery.* 1983;28(6):15-22.

23. Manocchio RT. Tending communities, crossing cultures: midwives in 19th century California. *J Midwifery Women's Health.* 2008;53(1):75-81.

24. Smith SL. *Japanese American Midwives: Culture, Community, and Health Politics, 1880-1950*. Chicago: University of Illinois Press; 2005.

25. Swenson N. The role of the nurse-midwife on the health team as viewed by the family. *Bull Am Coll Nurse-Midwifery*. 1968;13(4):125-133.

26. Crowell FE. The midwives of New York. *Charities and the Commons*. January 1907;17:667-677. In Litoff JB. *The American Midwife Debate: A Sourcebook on Its Modern Origins*. Westport, CT: Greenwood Press; 1986:36-49.

27. Litoff JB. *The American Midwife Debate: A Sourcebook on Its Modern Origins*. Westport, CT: Greenwood Press; 1986:5-10.

28. Pressley BD. *Granny Midwives in South Carolina: The State's Regulation and Education of a Vocational Cadre of Traditional Midwives 1910-1940* [Master's thesis]. New Haven, CT: Yale University School of Nursing; 2001.

29. New York State Department of Health. Bellevue School for Midwives to close. *Health News*. May 6, 1935. This article quotes an article in the *New York Herald-Tribune* giving the reason for closure.

30. Dawley K. E-mail communication to Jill Cassells; November 6, 1999.

31. Grady SD. *Midwifery and Professional Autonomy in the Early Twentieth Century* [Master's thesis]. New Haven, CT: Yale University School of Nursing; 1994.

32. Varney Burst H. From numerous speeches given on the history of nurse-midwifery, 1991 to present.

33. Lindenmeyer K. *"A Right to childhood": The U.S. Children's Bureau and Child Welfare, 1912-46*. Urbana: University of Illinois Press; 1997.

34. Corbin H. Historical development of nurse-midwifery in this country and present trends. *Bull Am Coll Nurse-Midwifery*. 1959;4(1):13-26.

35. Maternity Center Association. *Maternity Center Association Log: 1915-1980*. New York: Maternity Center Association; 1980.

36. Maternity Center Association. *Maternity Center Association: 1918-1943*. New York: Maternity Center Association; 1943.

37. Breckinridge M. *Wide Neighborhoods: A Story of the Frontier Nursing Service*. New York: Harper; 1952.

38. Cockerham AZ, Keeling AW. *Rooted in the Mountains, Reaching to the World: Stories of Nursing and Midwifery at Kentucky's Frontier School, 1939-1989*. Louisville, KY: Butler Books; 2012.

39. National Office of Vital Statistics; Public Health Service; Department of Health, Education, and Welfare. *Vital Statistics of the United States, Vol. I, 1950*. Washington, DC: National Office of Vital Statistics; 1954.

40. Metropolitan Life Insurance Company. Summary of the tenth thousand confinement records of the Frontier Nursing Service. *Frontier Nursing Service Quart Bull* Spring 1958;33(4). Reprinted in *Bull Am Coll Nurse-Midwives*. 1960;5:1-9.

41. Cassells J. *The Manhattan Midwifery School* [Master's thesis]. New Haven, CT: Yale University School of Nursing; 2000.

42. Maternity Center Association. *Twenty Years of Nurse-Midwifery: 1933-1953*. New York: Maternity Center Association; 1955.

43. Varney Burst H, Thompson J. Genealogic origins of nurse-midwifery education programs in the United States. *J Midwifery Women's Health*. 2003;48(6):464-472.

44. Canty L. *The Graduates of the Tuskegee School of Nurse-Midwifery* [Master's thesis]. New Haven, CT: Yale University School of Nursing; 1994.

45. Horch J. *The Flint-Goodridge School of Nurse-Midwifery* [Master's thesis]. New Haven, CT: Yale University School of Nursing; 2002.

46. The Committee on Organization. *Bulletin of the Committee on Organization*. November 1954;1(3).

47. American College of Nurse-Midwifery. *Descriptive Data, Nurse-Midwives—U.S.A.,1968*. Washington, DC: American College of Nurse-Midwifery; 1968.

48. Lang D. Providing maternity care through a nurse-midwifery service program. *Nurs Clin North Am*. 1969;4:509.

49. Landwehr GA. *Nurse-Midwifery Within the Indian Health Service: 1965-1980* [Master's thesis]. New Haven, CT: Yale University School of Nursing; 2002.

50. American College of Nurse-Midwives. *Responding to the Demands for Nurse-Midwives in the United States: A Workshop Report*. Washington, DC: American College of Nurse-Midwives; March 8-10, 1973.

51. *Joint Statement on Maternity Care, 1971*. Approved by the American College of Nurse-Midwives, American College of Obstetricians and Gynecologists, and Nurses Association of the American College of Obstetricians and Gynecologists; 1971.

52. Levy BS, Wilkinson FS, Marine WM. Reducing neonatal mortality rate with nurse-midwives. *Am J Obstet Gynecol*. 1971;109:50-58.

53. Meglen MC. Nurse-midwife program in the Southeast cuts mortality rates. *Contemp OB/GYN*. 1976;8:79.

54. Burnett JE Jr. A physician-sponsored community nurse-midwife program. *Obstet Gynecol*. 1979;40(5):719-723.

55. American College of Nurse-Midwives. *Nurse-Midwifery in the United States: 1976-1977*. Washington, DC: American College of Nurse-Midwives; 1978.

56. Transcript of the testimony given to the Subcommittee on Oversight and Investigation, Interstate and Foreign Commerce Committee, U.S. House of Representatives. Washington, DC; December 18, 1980.

57. Bailey PP. Nurse-midwifery and the Federal Trade Commission. *J Nurse-Midwifery.* 1984;29(5):311-315.

58. Cherry J, Foster JC. Comparison of hospital charges generated by certified nurse-midwives' and physicians' clients. *J Nurse-Midwifery.* 1982;27(1):7-11.

59. American College of Nurse-Midwives. *Nurse-Midwifery in the United States: 1982.* Washington, DC: American College of Nurse-Midwives; 1984.

60. Lehrman EJ, Paine LL. Trends in nurse-midwifery: results of the 1988 ACNM Division of Research mini-survey. *J Nurse-Midwifery.* 1990;35(4):192203.

61. American College of Nurse-Midwifery Midwifery education programs. Available at: http://www.midwife.org/rp/edumap.cfm. Accessed October 10, 2012.

62. Varney Burst H. The history of nurse-midwifery education. *J Midwifery Women's Health.* 2005;50(2):129-137.

63. Osborne K, Stone S, Ernst E. The development of the community-based nurse-midwifery education program: an innovation in distance learning. *J Midwifery Women's Health.* 2005;50(2):138-145.

64. Burst HV. An update on the credentialing of midwives by the ACNM. *J. Nurse-Midwifery.* 1995;40(3):290-296.

65. American College of Nurse-Midwives. *Essential Facts about Midwives.* Silver Springs, MD: American College of Nurse-Midwives; updated December 2011. Available at: http://www.midwife.org/Essential-Facts-about-Midwives. Accessed October 4, 2012.

66. DeClercq EJ. Trends in midwife-attended births in the United States, 1989-2009. *J Midwifery Women's Health.* 2012;57:321-326.

67. American College of Nurse-Midwives. *Fact Sheet: Essential Facts About Midwives.* Silver Springs, MD: American College of Nurse-Midwives; June 2008.

68. Declercq E. Trends in CNM-attended births, 1990-2004. *J Midwifery Women's Health.* 2007;52(1):87-88.

69. American College of Obstetricians and Gynecologists and American College of Nurse-Midwives. *Joint Statement of Practice Relations Between Obstetrician-Gynecologists and Certified Nurse-Midwives/Certified Midwives.* October 1, 2002.

70. Shah MA. The president's pen: make way for a new ACNM/ACOG joint statement. *Quickening.* September/October 2002.

71. American College of Obstetricians and Gynecologists and American College of Nurse-Midwives. *Joint Statement of Practice Relations Between Obstetrician-Gynecologists and Certified Nurse-Midwives/Certified Midwives.* February 2011.

72. Kennedy HP. Cross-discipline and collaborative dialogue. *Quickening.* Spring 2011;42(2):3.

73. Kennedy HP. Reflections on the past and future of midwifery research. *J Midwifery Women's Health.* 2005;50(2):110-112.

74. Raisler J, Kennedy H. Midwifery care of poor and vulnerable women, 1925-2003. *J Midwifery Women's Health.* 2005;50(2):113-121.

75. For example, the documentary *The Business of Being Born.* Ricki Lake, executive producer, and Abby Epstein, director. 2008.

76. For example, Letts E. *Quality of Care.* New York: Penguin New American Library Accent Novels; 2005. Harman P. *The Blue Cotton Gown: A Midwife's Memoir.* Boston: Beacon Press; 2008. Muhlhahn C. *Labor of Love: A Midwife's Memoir.* New York: Kaplan; 2009.

77. Sakala C, Corry M. *Evidence-Based Maternity Care: What It Is and What It Can Achieve.* New York: Milbank Memorial Fund; 2008.

78. Carrington B, Varney Burst H. The American College of Nurse-Midwives' dream becomes reality: the Division of Accreditation. *J Midwifery Women's Health.* 2005;50(2):146-153.

79. American College of Nurse-Midwives. ACNM vision, mission, and core values. Updated April 2012. Available at: http://www.midwife.org/ACNM/files/ACNMLibraryData/UPLOADFILENAME/000000000269/ACNM%20Vision%20Mission%20Core%20Values%20April%202012.pdf. Accessed October 4, 2012.

80. Dawley KL. *Leaving the Nest: Nurse-Midwifery in the United States 1940-1980* [Doctoral dissertation]. Philadelphia, PA: University of Pennsylvania; 2001:94.

81. Nurse-midwifery today. *Public Health Nurs.* May 1949.

82. Committee on Organization. *Bulletin of the Committee on Organization.* Vol. 1, No. 1-3, May-November 1954; Vol. 2, No. 1-3, April-October 1955.

83. Sister Theophane Shoemaker to Hattie Hemschemeyer. Letter dated February 23, 1955.

84. Hemschemeyer H. Sends message to members. *Bull Am Coll Nurse-Midwifery.* 1956;1(2):5-6.

85. Hemschemeyer H. Report of the first president of the American College of Nurse-Midwifery. *Bull Am Coll Nurse-Midwifery.* 1965;10(1):4-10.

86. American College of Nurse-Midwives. *Articles of Incorporation and Bylaws.* Approved May 2008. Available at: http://www.midwife.org/documents/ACNMBylaws2008reformattedfinal21110.pdf. Accessed October 4, 2012.

87. Kroska R. The emblem of the American College of Nurse-Midwives. *J Nurse-Midwifery*. 1973;18(3): 23-24.

88. See American College of Nurse-Midwives website (www.acnm.org) for further information.

89. *The A.C.N.M. Foundation: 1967-1992 Happy 25th Birthday!* [Brochure]. 1992.

90. For additional information, see www.homebirth summit.org.

91. Marshall MA, Buffington ST, Beck DR, Clark PA. *Life-Saving Skills Manual for Midwives*, 4th ed. Silver Spring, MD: American College of Nurse-Midwives; 2008.

92. Buffington S, Sibley L, Beck D, Armbruster D. *Home Based Life Saving Skills*. Silver Spring, MD: American College of Nurse-Midwives; 2003.

93. Editorial. *Bull Am Coll Nurse-Midwifery*. 1959;4(2): 37-38.

● ● ● Bibliography

American College of Nurse-Midwifery. *Descriptive Data, Nurse-Midwives—U.S.A., 1963*. New York: American College of Nurse-Midwifery; 1963.

American College of Nurse-Midwifery. *Descriptive Data, Nurse-Midwives—U.S.A., 1968*. New York: American College of Nurse-Midwifery; 1968.

American College of Nurse-Midwives. *Descriptive Data, Nurse-Midwives—U.S.A., 1971*. New York: American College of Nurse-Midwives; 1971.

American College of Nurse-Midwives. *Nurse-Midwifery in the United States: 1976-1977*. Washington, DC: American College of Nurse-Midwives; 1978.

American College of Nurse-Midwives. *Nurse-Midwifery in the United States: 1982*. Washington, DC: American College of Nurse-Midwives; 1984.

American College of Nurse-Midwives. *Responding to the Demands for Nurse-Midwives in the United States: A Workshop Report*. Washington, DC: American College of Nurse-Midwives; March 8-10, 1973.

American College of Nurse-Midwives. *What Is a Nurse-Midwife?* Washington, DC: American College of Nurse-Midwives; 1978.

Arney W. *Power and the Profession of Obstetrics*. Chicago: University of Chicago Press; 1982.

Bailey PP. Nurse-midwifery and the Federal Trade Commission. *J Nurse-Midwifery*. 1984;29(5):311-315.

Borst C. *Catching Babies: The Professionalization of Childbirth, 1870-1920*. Cambridge, MA: Harvard University Press; 1996.

Breckinridge M. *Wide Neighborhoods: A Story of the Frontier Nursing Service*. New York: Harper; 1952.

Browne HE, Isaacs G. The Frontier Nursing Service. *Am J Obstet Gynecol*. 1976;124:16.

Buffington S, Sibley L, Beck D, Armbruster D. *Home Based Life Saving Skills*. Silver Spring, MD: American College of Nurse-Midwives; 2003.

Burnett JE Jr. A physician-sponsored community nurse-midwife program. *Obstet Gynecol*. 1972;40:719.

Burst HV. The American College of Nurse-Midwives: a professional organization. *J Nurse-Midwifery*. 1980;25(1): 4-6.

Burst HV. Harmonious unity. *J Nurse-Midwifery*. 1977; 22:10.

Burst HV. The influence of consumers on the birthing movement. In Strawn J, ed. *Topics in Clinical Nursing: Rehumanizing the Acute Care Setting*. 1983;5(3):42-54.

Burst HV. Our three-ring circus. *J Nurse-Midwifery*. 1978;23:11.

Burst HV. An update on the credentialing of midwives by the ACNM. *J Nurse-Midwifery*. 1995;40(3):290-296.

Cameron J. *The History and Development of Midwifery in the United States: Can Maternity Nursing Meet Today's Challenge?* Columbus, OH: Ross Laboratories; 1967.

Canty L. *The Graduates of the Tuskegee School of Nurse-Midwifery* [Master's thesis]. New Haven, CT: Yale University School of Nursing; 1994.

Carrington B, Varney Burst H. The American College of Nurse-Midwives' dream becomes reality: the Division of Accreditation. *J Midwifery Women's Health*. 2005; 50(2):146-153.

Cassells J. *The Manhattan Midwifery School* [Master's thesis]. New Haven, CT: Yale University School of Nursing; 2000.

Cavero C. Modern midwifery: complicated rebirth of an ancient art. *Fam Community Health*. 1979;2(3):29-39.

Chaney JA. Birthing in early America. *J Nurse-Midwifery*. 1980;25(2):5-13.

Cherry J, Foster JC. Comparison of hospital charges generated by certified nurse-midwives' and physicians' clients. *J Nurse-Midwifery*. 1982;27(1):7-11.

Cockerham AZ, Keeling AW. *Rooted in the Mountains, Reaching to the World: Stories of Nursing and Midwifery at Kentucky's Frontier School, 1939-1989*. Louisville, KY: Butler Books; 2012.

Cohn S, Cuddihy N, Kraus N, Tom S. Legislation and nurse-midwifery practice in the USA [Special legislative issue]. *J Nurse-Midwifery*. 1984;29(2).

Committee on Organization. *Organization Bulletin*. Vol. 1, No. 1-3, May-November 1954; Vol. 2, No. 1-3, April-October 1955.

Corbin H. *Forty-Fifth Annual Report*. New York: Maternity Center Association; 1963.

Corbin H. Historical development of nurse-midwifery in this country and present trends. *Bull Am Coll Nurse-Midwifery.* 1959;4(1):13-26.

Crowe-Carraco C. Mary Breckinridge and the Frontier Nursing Service. *Register of the Kentucky Historical Society.* July 1978.

Crowell FE. The midwives of New York. *Charities and the Commons.* January 1907;17:667-677. In: Litoff JB. *The American Midwife Debate: A Sourcebook on Its Modern Origins.* Westport, CT: Greenwood Press; 1986:36-49.

Dawley K. The campaign to eliminate the midwife. *Am J Nurs.* 2000;100(10):53.

Dawley KL. *Leaving the Nest: Nurse-Midwifery in the United States 1940-1980* [Doctoral dissertation]. Philadelphia, PA: University of Pennsylvania; 2001:94.

Dawley K, Varney Burst H. The American College of Nurse-Midwives and its antecedents: a historic time line. *J Midwifery Women's Health.* 2005;50(1):16-22.

Declercq E. Trends in CNM-attended births, 1990-2004. *J Midwifery Women's Health.* 2007;52(1):87-88.

Diers D, Burst HV. Effectiveness of policy related research: nurse-midwifery as case study. *Image.* 1983;15(3):68-74.

Ernst EK. Tomorrow's child. *J Nurse-Midwifery.* 1979; 24(5):7-12.

Ernst EKM, Gordon KA. Fifty-three years of home birth experience at the Frontier Nursing Service, Kentucky: 1925-1978. In: Stewart L, Stewart D. *Compulsory Hospitalization: Freedom of Choice in Childbirth? Vol. 2.* Marble Hill, MO: NAPSAC Publications; 1979.

Forman AM, Cooper EM. Legislation and nurse-midwifery practice in the USA: report on a survey conducted by the legislation committee of the American College of Nurse-Midwives. *J Nurse-Midwifery.* 1976;21(2):1-57.

Fox CG. Toward a sound historical basis for nurse-midwifery. *Bull Am Coll Nurse-Midwifery.* 1969;14(3): 76-82.

Gatewood TS, Stewart RB. Obstetricians and nurse-midwives: the team approach in private practice. *Am J Obstet Gynecol.* 1975;123:35.

Grady SD. *Midwifery and Professional Autonomy in the Early Twentieth Century* [Master's thesis]. New Haven, CT: Yale University School of Nursing; 1994.

Harris D. The development of nurse-midwifery in New York City. *Bull Am Coll Nurse-Midwifery.* 1969;14(1):4-12.

Hellman, L. M., and O'Brien, F. B. Nurse-midwifery: an experiment in maternity care. *Obstet. Gynecol.* 24:343-349, 1964.

Hellman LM. Nurse-midwifery in the United States. *Obstet Gynecol.* 1967;30:883.

Hemschemeyer H. Report of the first president of the American College of Nurse-Midwifery. *Bull Am Coll Nurse-Midwifery.* 1965;10(1):4-10.

Hemschemeyer H. Sends message to members. *Bull Am Coll Nurse-Midwifery.* 1956;1(2):5-6.

Hogan A. A tribute to the pioneers. *J Nurse-Midwifery.* 1975;20(2):6-11.

Horch J. *The Flint-Goodridge School of Nurse-Midwifery* [Master's thesis]. New Haven, CT: Yale University School of Nursing; 2002.

Hosford E. Alternative patterns of nurse-midwifery care: III. The home birth movement. *J Nurse-Midwifery.* 1976;21(3):27-30.

Kennedy HP. A model of exemplary midwifery practice: results of a Delphi study. *J Midwifery Women's Health.* 2000;45(1):4-19.

Kennedy H. Reflections on the past and future of midwifery research. *J Midwifery Women's Health.* 2005;50(2): 110-112.

Kroska R. The emblem of the American College of Nurse-Midwives. *J Nurse-Midwifery.* 1973;18(3):23-24.

Landwehr GA. *Nurse-Midwifery Within the Indian Health Service: 1965-1980* [Master's thesis]. New Haven, CT: Yale University School of Nursing; 2002.

Lang D. The American College of Nurse-Midwives: what is the future for certified nurse-midwives? in hospitals? childbearing centers? homebirths? In: Stewart L, Stewart D. *21st Century Obstetrics Now!* Marble Hill, MO: NAPSAC; 1977:89-104.

Lang D. Modern midwifery. In: Dickason EJ, Schult MO. *Maternal and Infant Care,* 2nd ed. New York: McGraw-Hill; 1979:145-147.

Lang D. Providing maternity care through a nurse-midwifery service program. *Nurs Clin North Am.* 1969;4:509.

Lazarus W, Levine ES, Lewin LS. *Competition Among Health Practitioners: The Influence of the Medical Profession on the Health Manpower Market. Vol. 1: Executive Summary and Final Report; Vol. 2: The Childbearing Center Case Study.* Washington, DC: Federal Trade Commission; February 1981.

Leavitt JW. *Brought to Bed: Childbearing in America, 1750-1950.* New York: Oxford University Press; 1986.

Lehrman EJ, Paine LL. Trends in nurse-midwifery: results of the 1988 ACNM Division of Research mini-survey. *J Nurse-Midwifery.* 1990;35(4):192-203.

Levy BS, Wilkinson FS, Marine WM. Reducing neonatal mortality rate with nurse-midwives. *Am J Obstet Gynecol.* 1971;109:50.

Litoff JB. *The American Midwife Debate: A Sourcebook on Its Modern Origins.* Westport, CT: Greenwood Press; 1986.

Litoff JB. *American Midwives: 1860 to the Present.* Westport, CT: Greenwood Press; 1978.

Litoff JB. Forgotten women: American midwives at the turn of the twentieth century. *Historian.* 1978;40(2): 235-251.

Litoff JB. The midwife throughout history. *J Nurse-Midwifery*. 1982;27(6):3-11.

Lubic RW. Evaluation of an out-of-hospital maternity center for low risk patients. In: Aiken LH. *Hospital Policy and Nursing Practice*. New York: McGraw-Hill; 1980.

Lubic RW. The nurse-midwife joins the obstetrical team. *Bull Am Coll Nurse-Midwives*. 1972;27(3):73-77.

Lubic RW, Ernst EKM. The childbearing center: an alternative to conventional care. *Nurs Outlook*. 1978;26:754.

Manocchio RT. Tending communities, crossing cultures: midwives in 19th century California. *J Midwifery Women's Health*. 2008;53(1):75-81.

Marshall MA, Buffington ST, Beck DR, Clark PA. *Life-Saving Skills Manual for Midwives*, 4th ed. Silver Spring, MD: American College of Nurse-Midwives; 2008.

Maternity Center Association. *Maternity Center Association, 1918-1943*. New York: Maternity Center Association; 1943.

Maternity Center Association. *Maternity Center Association Log: 1915-1980*. New York: Maternity Center Association; 1980.

Maternity Center Association. *Twenty Years of Nurse-Midwifery, 1933-1953*. New York: Maternity Center Association; 1955.

Meglen, M. C. Nurse-midwife program in the Southeast cuts mortality rates. *Contemporary OB/GYN* 1976;8:79.

Meglen MC, Burst HV. Nurse-midwives make a difference. *Nurs Outlook*. 1974;22:382.

Metropolitan Life Insurance Company. Summary of the tenth thousand confinement records of the Frontier Nursing Service. *Frontier Nursing Service Quart Bull*. Spring 1958;33(4). Reprinted in *Bull Am Coll Nurse-Midwives*. 1960;5:1-9.

Murphy PA, Fullerton JT. Measuring outcomes of midwifery care: development of an instrument to assess optimality. *J Midwifery Women's Health*. 2001;46(5):274-284.

Nurse-midwifery today. *Public Health Nurs*. May 1949.

Osborne K, Stone S, Ernst E. The development of the community-based nurse-midwifery education program: an innovation in distance learning. *J Midwifery Women's Health*. 2005;50(2):138-145.

Perry DS. The early midwives of Missouri. *J Nurse-Midwifery*. 1983;28(6):15-22.

Pomerantz M. *Factors Contributing to the Widespread Use of Epidurals for Pain Relief in Childbirth* [Master's thesis]. New Haven, CT: Yale University School of Nursing; 1999.

Pressley Byrd D. *Granny Midwives in South Carolina: The State's Regulation and Education of a Vocational Cadre of Traditional Midwives 1910-1940* [Master's thesis]. New Haven, CT: Yale University School of Nursing; 2001.

Raffloer K. *The Experience of Childbirth on the Oregon Trail: A Search for the Presence of Midwives* [Master's thesis]. New Haven, CT: Yale University School of Nursing; 1999.

Raisler J, Kennedy H. Midwifery care of poor and vulnerable women, 1925-2003. *J Midwifery Women's Health*. 2005;50(2):113-121.

Robinson S. A historical development of midwifery in the black community: 1600-1940. *J Nurse-Midwifery*. 1984;29(4):247-250.

Rooks JB. American nurse-midwifery: are we making an impact? *J Nurse-Midwifery*. 1978;23:15-19.

Rooks JP. *Midwifery and Childbirth in America*. Philadelphia: Temple University Press; 1997.

Rooks J. Nurse-midwifery: the window is wide open. *Am J Nurs* 1990:90(12):30-36.

Rooks J, Fischman S. American nurse-midwifery practice in 1976-1977: reflections of 50 years of growth and development. *Am J Public Health*. 1980;70:990-996.

Roush RE. The development of midwifery: male and female, yesterday and today. *J Nurse-Midwifery*. 1979;24(3):27-37.

Sakala C, Corry M. *Evidence-Based Maternity Care: What It Is and What It Can Achieve*. New York: Milbank Memorial Fund; 2008.

Schlinger H. *Circle of Midwives: Organized Midwifery in North America*. New York: Hilary Schlinger; 1992.

Shah MA. The president's pen: make way for a new ACNM/ACOG joint statement. *Quickening*. September/October 2002.

Sharp ES. Nurse-midwifery education: its successes, failures, and future. *J Nurse-Midwifery*. 1983;28(2):17-23.

Shoemaker M. (Agnes Reinders). *History of Nurse-Midwifery in the United States*. Washington, DC: Catholic University of America Press; 1947.

Smart DT, ed. *Mormon Midwife: The 1846-1888 Diaries of Patty Bartlett Sessions*. Logan, UT: Utah State University Press; 1997.

Smith MC, Holmes LJ. *Listen to Me Good: The Life Story of an Alabama Midwife*. Columbus, OH: Ohio State University Press; 1996.

Smith SL. *Japanese American Midwives: Culture, Community, and Health Politics, 1880-1950*. Chicago: University of Illinois Press; 2005.

Speert H. *Obstetric and Gynecology: A History and Iconography, Revised Second Edition of Iconographia Gyniatrica*. San Francisco: Norman Publishing; 1994.

Swenson N. The role of the nurse-midwife on the health team as viewed by the family. *Bull Am Coll Nurse-Midwifery*. 1968;13(4):125.

Thiede HA. Interdisciplinary MCH teams can function within the system with proper planning. *Am J Dis Child*. 1974;127:633.

Thiede HA. A presumptuous experiment in rural maternal-child health care. *Am J Obstet Gynecol*. 1971;111: 736.

Thomas MW. *The Practice of Nurse-Midwifery in the United States*. Washington, DC: Children's Bureau, U.S. Department of Health, Education, and Welfare; 1965.

Thoms H. *Our Obstetrical Heritage: The Story of Safe Childbirth*. Hamden, CT: Shoe String Press; 1960.

Tom SA. The evolution of nurse-midwifery: 1900-1960. *J Nurse-Midwifery*. 1982;27(4):4-13.

Transcript of the testimony given to the Subcommittee on Oversight and Investigation, Interstate and Foreign Commerce Committee, U.S. House of Representatives. Washington, DC; December 18, 1980.

Ulrich LT. *A Midwife's Tale: The Life of Martha Ballard, Based on Her Diary, 1785-1812*. New York: Knopf; 1990.

Varney H. *Nurse-Midwifery*. Boston: Blackwell Scientific Publishing; 1980.

Varney Burst H. The history of nurse-midwifery education. *J Midwifery Women's Health*. 2005;50(2):129-137.

Varney Burst H, Thompson J. Genealogic origins of nurse-midwifery education programs in the United States. *J Midwifery Women's Health*. 2003;48(6):464-472.

Webber T. The African American midwife during antebellum slavery. In: Diers D, ed. *Celebrating the Contributions of Academic Midwifery*. New Haven, CT: Yale University School of Nursing; 2005:84-91.

Wertz RW, Wertz DC. *Lying-in: A History of Childbirth in America*. New York: Free Press; 1977.

Wiedenbach E. Nurse-midwifery: purpose, practice, and opportunity. *Nurs Outlook*. 1960;8:256.

Williams HV. *Nursing, Nurse-Midwifery, and the History of Nurse-Midwifery in the United States* [Unpublished paper]. 1969.

Williams SR. *Divine Rebel: The Life of Anne Marbury Hutchinson*. New York: Holt, Rinehart, and Winston; 1981.

Wilson KT. *Physicians Instrumental in the Development of Nurse-Midwifery in the United States, 1915-1939* [Master's thesis]. New Haven, CT: Yale University School of Nursing; 1995.

CHAPTER

2

Professional Midwifery Today

DEANNE R. WILLIAMS

SUSANNA R. COHEN

CELESTE R. THOMAS

Introduction

Midwifery in the twenty-first century is a profession that is deeply rooted in service to both women who are vulnerable to poor pregnancy outcomes and the preservation of a childbirth experience that honors the normal process of birth as well as the transformational power of the childbearing experience. While midwives maintain their commitment to provide individualized care responsive to the needs of the woman, they are also increasingly recognized as key players in a global community of healthcare professionals who improve the lives of mothers and babies. This expanded allegiance—from the individual, to the profession, to women wherever they need care—is reflected throughout this text and is the primary focus of this chapter.

Midwifery in the United States, as represented by certified nurse-midwives, certified midwives, and certified professional midwives, is a dynamic profession. The scope of midwifery practice has expanded, as has the core knowledge needed to provide safe care and to participate as members of an interdisciplinary team. Likewise, civil society has expanded its expectations for healthcare professionals, and midwives have responded by adopting new standards for their profession.

The essential characteristics of a profession are measurable, interconnected, and commonly recognized. A profession has the following properties: (1) specialized knowledge typically obtained at the college level (graduation from a nationally accredited education program and earning a degree); (2) legal recognition (federal and state laws); (3) self-organized

with a commitment to serve (professional membership organizations); (4) standards of competency (e.g., certification by a nationally recognized certification agency); (5) established standards of practice; and (6) adheres to ethical standards.

Although this chapter will not contribute directly to the clinical competence that students and midwives seek early in their careers, it does put midwifery practice into a societal context via a review of these essential characteristics that make midwifery a profession. This is the environment that graduates enter as they come to understand that being a safe, legal, independent, and successful midwife requires more than clinical competence.

The Professional Paradigm: Midwifery in the Twenty-First Century

Along with the more detailed information about the history of midwifery that was presented in the introductory chapter, **Box 2-1** provides a list of some of the seminal events in the development of modern midwifery in the United States and acknowledges a few of the key individuals, groups, and events that have helped develop midwifery into a profession today.[1,2]

Types of Professional Midwives

Most midwives have been asked the following questions about their profession: What is the difference among a certified nurse-midwife (CNM), a certified midwife (CM), and a certified professional midwife (CPM)? What is a lay midwife?

BOX 2-1 Evolution of the Profession of Midwifery in the United States

1925:   Mary Breckinridge opens the Frontier Nursing Service (FNS) in Hyden, Kentucky—the first nurse-midwifery service.

1929:   FNS nurse-midwives organize the American Association of Nurse-Midwives.

1931:   Lobenstine Midwifery School opens—the first nurse-midwifery education program.

1955:   ACNM incorporated.

1956:   Yale University School of Nursing opens a nurse-midwifery program.

1965:   ACNM accredits education programs.

1960s– Counterculture, feminism, and grassroots rejection of over-medicalization of birth and increased
1970s: conversation about home birth; childbearing women share their very personal experiences comparing traditional medical care with midwifery care.

1970:   First edition of *Our Bodies, Ourselves* published. The ninth edition was published in 2011. This book has been a strong supporter of midwifery since its beginnings and includes many midwives as contributing authors.

1971:   First CNM credential issued based on national examination.

1975:   Publication of *Spiritual Midwifery* by Ina May Gaskin. This book introduced a generation of women to natural childbirth while giving voice to childbirth's spiritual components.

1977:   The Maternity Center of El Paso opens—the first direct-entry education program for lay midwives.

1977:   The first gathering of lay midwives in El Paso, Texas.

1978:   ACNM's *Core Competencies for Basic Nurse-Midwifery Practice* published.

1982:   Founding of MANA.

1989:   MANA establishes the Interim Registry Board to explore a national registry exam; this later becomes NARM.

1990:   ACNM's first *Code of Ethics* published.

1993:   ICM's first *Code of Ethics* published.

1994:   MANA's *Core Competencies for Basic Midwifery Practice* published.

1994:   First CPM credential issued.

1994:   ACNM endorses development of the CM credential.

1998:   First CM credential issued.

1999:   Baccalaureate degree required for CNM.

2000:   NACPM founded.

2010:   Graduate degree required for CNM/CM.

Over time these efforts have been supported by the following parties:

- Community activists who set out to improve the quality of care for special populations, especially those composed of those individuals who because of age, race, ethnicity, or socioeconomic status are considered vulnerable
- Military leaders who identified nurse-midwives as qualified providers who could help make up for difficulty in recruiting physicians
- Birth collectives that wanted to train their own midwives
- Epidemiologists who looked beyond care provided by physicians, discovered midwifery, and published research on midwifery outcomes
- Elected public officials who pushed motivated midwives to get their policies in order, codified those policies, and then resisted attempts by organized medicine to make midwifery illegal

ACNM = American College of Nurse-Midwives; CM = certified midwife; CNM = certified nurse-midwife; CPM = certified professional midwife; ICM = International Confederation of Midwives; MANA = Midwives Alliance of North America; NACPM = National Association of Certified Professional Midwives; NARM = North American Registry of Midwives.

A direct-entry midwife? A licensed midwife? An indigenous midwife? While the answers to these questions are evolving, and they can be both confusing and controversial, an exploration of the similarities and differences between midwives is important to the profession (**Table 2-1**).

Terms such as "lay midwife" and "direct-entry midwife" do not have a common definition. For some, the term "lay midwife" describes an individual who has no formal education as a midwife, while others use this term to refer to a midwife who is not recognized by a government entity. The term "direct-entry midwife" typically refers to a midwife who has entered the profession without first becoming a nurse. In some states, direct-entry and licensed midwife are categories of licensure that are separate from the licensure of CNMs. The terms "traditional midwife," "community midwife," and "indigenous midwife" acknowledge the women or men who follow traditional customs as they attend births in their community. These midwives work in areas that have limited access to the formal education and well-staffed hospitals found in larger cities. Traditional midwives often are elders who are influential and trusted because they practice in concert with local belief systems. Examples include

Table 2-1	Types of Midwives in the United States		
	Certified Nurse-Midwife	**Certified Midwife** (CM does not have to be an RN)	**Certified Professional Midwife**
Education	Nationally accredited education programs Graduate degree Increase in number of programs that require doctoral degree	Nationally accredited education programs Graduate degree	Nationally accredited education programs
Certification	Nationally recognized certification exam Must graduate from accredited program Graduate degree required	Nationally recognized certification exam Must graduate from accredited program Graduate degree required	Nationally recognized certification exam Minimum requirement: high school diploma or equivalent CNMs and CMs may qualify to take the certification exam
Scope of practice	Obstetrics (hospital and out-of-hospital births), well-woman gynecology, newborn, prescriptive authority	Obstetrics (hospital and out-of-hospital births), well-woman gynecology, newborn, prescriptive authority	Primary maternity care of healthy women experiencing normal pregnancies Specialize in home and out-of-hospital births
Licensure	50 states and 3 territories	3 states	Recognized by licensure in 16 states and by permit or certification in 3 additional states
Challenges	Licensure and scope of practice vary from state to state Some states do not recognize independent practice	Licensure and scope of practice vary from state to state Some states do not recognize independent practice Not recognized in Medicare rules	Illegal in 12 states Licensure and scope of practice vary from state to state Not recognized in Medicare rules
Standard-setting professional organizations	ACNM AMCB ACME	ACNM ACMB ACME	NACPM NARM MEAC MANA

ACNM = American College of Nurse-Midwives; AMCB = American Midwifery Certification Board; ACME = Accreditation Commission on Midwifery Education; NACPM = National Association of Certified Professional Midwives; NARM = North American Registry of Midwives; MEAC = Midwifery Education Accreditation Council;MANA = Midwives Alliance of North America ; RN = registered nurse.

aboriginal midwives in Canada and *comodronas* in Guatemala.

In the United States, the midwifery community was divided for many years between nurse-midwives and lay midwives. Prior to the 1990s, many midwives who were not CNMs resisted becoming nurses to be eligible for midwifery education programs and were opposed to adopting national standards for education and certification. This resistance partially stemmed from concern that the next steps would be a formal education requirement that did not recognize apprenticeship education and state licensure. Concern also arose that national standards would permit non-midwives to define the midwife's scope of practice. Being a "lay midwife" and attending home births was seen by some as the ultimate in independent practice and a source of pride.

The CPM credential, first issued in 1994, was originally developed to provide competency-based certification for midwives who were primarily apprentice trained in out-of-hospital birth. The natural consequences of creating the CPM certification examination were the obligation to ensure that those who take the exam meet common standards for education and practice and the creation of a structure within which to discipline those who do not perform in a manner consistent with the standards. CPMs now have national standards for education, certification, and practice; are seeking licensure in all states; and are pursuing reimbursement from both government and nongovernment insurance companies.

When all nurse-midwives were required to be experienced nurses prior to entering midwifery education, it was difficult for CNMs to consider other routes to midwifery as equivalent to their own. In 1991, the board of directors of the American College of Nurse-Midwives (ACNM) endorsed the development of an alternative educational path to midwifery that did not require a nursing degree, leading to the CM credential. Over the next 7 years, the requirements to accredit education programs and certify graduates who were not registered nurses were designed and tested to ensure that after graduation and certification, one could not distinguish between the knowledge and skills of a CNM and a CM. The first CM credential, which required passing the same certification examination that is offered to nurse-midwives, was issued in 1998.

Although significant variations between CPMs, CNMs, and CMs still exist (as summarized in Table 2-1), the interaction between the three professional membership organizations for midwives—the ACNM, the Midwives Alliance of North America (MANA), and the National Association of Certified Professional Midwives (NACPM)—now focuses more on common values and goals than on differences. It is increasingly clear that in the United States, where the consumer is unlikely to understand the difference between midwives with different credentials, each individual who uses the title "midwife" assumes responsibility for the image of the entire profession.

Evolution of the Profession of Midwifery

> I found…that wherever a city, a country, a region, or a nation had developed a system of maternal care which was firmly based on a body of trained, licensed, regulated and respected midwives (especially when the midwives worked in close and cordial co-operation with doctors), the standard of maternal care was at its highest and maternal mortality was at its lowest. I cannot think of an exception to that rule…[3]

The Early Years: The Trailblazers

The scope of practice of CNMs and CMs as defined by the ACNM and recognized in federal and state laws has changed over the years. The early nurse-midwifery "trailblazers" (1930s to 1950s)[2] who predated the 1955 incorporation of the American College of Nurse-Midwifery (changed to Midwives in 1969) would probably be surprised to learn that today's CNMs and CMs provide more than just maternity care to women and are working in very specialized women's healthcare clinics. The small number of home births attended by CNMs/CMs might also surprise the trailblazers. They might also wonder why today's CNMs/CMs sometimes have to fight to be recognized as primary care providers, given that primary care was an essential component of the public health nursing practiced by those who added midwifery training to become nurse-midwives.

Building the Profession: The Fence Builders

Lessons learned from the successes and failures of the CNM trailblazers served as guideposts for the "fence builders."[4] The fence builders wrote ACNM standards for the education, certification, and practice of midwives, launched a peer-reviewed journal (*Journal of Nurse-Midwifery*, whose name was changed to *Journal of Midwifery & Women's Health* in 1999), created a network of midwives supporting midwifery-owned businesses and offered their services to help save women's lives and educate midwives in low-resource countries. More recent accomplishments that depended upon the work of the early fence builders include legislation that (1) protects the right of women to choose midwifery care (1997); (2) ensures Medicare payment for maternity care provided by nurse-midwives (1988); (3) expands this coverage to full-scope nurse-midwifery care (1993); and (4) now provides for Medicare payments to CNMs that are equal to payments made to physicians (2011).

CPMs have also evolved over time. There are now three standard-setting professional organizations that work to move the CPM profession forward: MANA, founded in 1982; the North American Registry of Midwives (NARM), founded in 1994; and NACPM, founded in 2000. One unique aspect of these organizations is that they represent midwives from very diverse clinical and educational experiences and, therefore, it is not easy to summarize their evolution over time. Judith P. Rooks, in her landmark book, *Midwifery and Childbirth in America,* stated that these midwives "developed as part of the social and cultural ferment of the late 1960s" and "invented themselves in rural communes, religious communities, and the nooks and crannies of urban counterculture enclaves."[2]

After the late 1960s, these midwives faced a number of challenges: (1) their lack of credentials and illegal status in some states; (2) different educational processes, which range from pure apprenticeship to private 3-year schools; (3) negative publicity accompanying bad outcomes at home births that may have been attended by midwives with insufficient training who have not undergone recognized educational processes for direct-entry midwives; and (4) the negative stereotype that midwives in general are less competent than physicians.[1]

Members of MANA realized that the only way to convince the public and the government of their professionalism and avoid legal persecution was to create a standardized national certification process. In response, the NARM certification exam and CPM credential were created. The CPM credential is "open to midwives educated through all possible routes, including apprenticeship, self-study, formal vocational programs, university training, and all combinations thereof."[1]

Midwifery Now: The Tower Builders

Midwives in the twenty-first century must fill the role of "tower builders"[4] by continuing to help the profession, in all of its diversity, meet the growing demand for midwifery care in a digital world. These midwives will carry the profession, and its low-technology, high-touch roots into a high-technology world characterized by more integrated healthcare delivery systems. Like the midwifery trailblazers and fence builders, today's midwives must also be "protectors." They must continue to distinguish the midwifery profession from the professions of nursing and medicine and expand the evidence base that defines the best practices in midwifery.

Few of these labor-intensive accomplishments would have ever moved from internal ideals to cultural norms without consumer support. From the Maternity Center Association (now Childbirth Connection) to Citizens for Midwifery, consumers have provided inspiration, influence, and financial resources to promote and protect access to midwifery care.[5,6] The list of individuals who created a public demand and stood beside midwifery during some very difficult times is long.

Characteristics of the Midwifery Profession

To protect the profession from those who resist increasing access to midwifery care by suggesting that midwives are undereducated, outdated, or unprofessional, it is important for midwives to be able to answer a critical question: What makes one a professional? According to Ament, "in the United States, the overall objective of protecting the public welfare…is accomplished through three interdependent mechanisms: 1) a prescribed, accredited course of study; 2) national certification; and 3) governmental, usually state or other jurisdiction, licensure."[7] Thus a professional must show evidence of attending an accredited education program, attaining national certification, and becoming licensed by all the appropriate legal jurisdictions. Midwifery leaders and healthcare researchers have also described additional "characteristics of professionalism" that are less easily measured, but considered to be integral to the specific profession of midwifery.

Core Competencies

Core competencies delineate the fundamental knowledge, skills, and behaviors expected of members of the profession. They serve as the reference point for standardization of the curricula for otherwise diverse education programs, the criteria for accrediting education programs that are not all within colleges of nursing, and the development of the certification examination. These competencies inform regulatory agencies, consumers, and employers of what, at a minimum, can be expected from those who meet the criteria to use the professional credential.

The first ACNM Core Competencies for Basic Midwifery Practice were published in 1978, although some concepts could be found in earlier midwifery documents.[8] The core competencies have been updated regularly to reflect changes in the profession, including the decision to educate and certify midwives who do not have a nursing education, previously mentioned as the CM.

First published in 1994, the MANA Core Competencies for Basic Midwifery Practice are referenced for the CPM certification exam and the Midwifery Education Accreditation Council (MEAC) accreditation process.[9]

Using core competencies as a measurement of a student's success enables education programs to recognize that many individuals enter midwifery programs with preexisting skills and enables the students to focus their studies on new areas, rather than repeating already learned information. In addition, clear, meaningful competencies reassure the public as well as the midwifery community that all accredited programs graduate well-prepared individuals.

Accreditation

Earning a college degree is a significant measure of success in the United States. It represents knowledge obtained in an institution that adheres to national standards that are established to ensure preparation of students who are well educated, by qualified faculty in their chosen field. Students, employers, and consumers want to know that a degree reflects mastery of a prescribed set of knowledge and skills.

To increase the value of formal education and to protect students from fraud, the federal government and professional organizations have established standards for institutions of higher education that address the learning environment, content of the curriculum, and qualifications of faculty. In the case of midwifery, the Accreditation Commission for Midwifery Education (ACME) has been recognized by the U.S. Department of Education as a programmatic accrediting agency since 1982 for nurse-midwifery education programs and since 1994 for direct-entry midwifery programs. Maintaining midwifery accreditation standards that are separate from those required for nursing education has allowed the CNM/CM profession to self-regulate, maintain a strong public voice for improving access to midwifery care, and influence public policy that affects the health of women and families.

The U.S. Secretary of Education recognizes the MEAC, established in 1991, as a national accrediting agency for direct-entry midwifery education programs. MEAC-accredited programs, which may or may not be affiliated with an institution of higher education, prepare students to take the CPM examination.

Certification

For CNMs and CMs, certification—passing an examination that measures mastery of fundamental knowledge needed for safe practice that is obtained through a recognized program of study—is required to obtain a state license to practice, to obtain hospital staff privileges, and to qualify for reimbursement from government and private health insurance plans. The criteria for taking the exam, the content of the exam, and the requirements for maintaining certification are developed under the auspices of organizations that do not serve as advocates for the profession. While members of the profession can serve as expert advisors, certification organizations work to protect the recipients of care and follow the standards established by the National Commission for Certifying Agencies. CNMs have been certified by examination since 1971, CPMs since 1994, and CMs since 1998.

State Regulation

The assumption of responsibility for the life and health of another individual—or individuals, in the case of the maternal–fetal dyad—comprises a legal and social contract with multiple contingency clauses. State legislators have responsibility for protecting citizens from unsafe healthcare practitioners and do so by establishing, via state laws, the rules that govern practice. State agencies are charged with adopting regulations that further clarify the rules. A typical state midwifery practice act will establish (1) qualifications for initial and renewed licensure, (2) scope of practice, (3) relationship with physicians, (4) prescriptive authority with special requirements related to prescribing controlled substances, and (5) definitions of unlawful or unprofessional conduct. Because the laws governing licensure must be handled through the legislative process, they are subject to the influence of multiple stakeholders; moreover, the process of getting a bill passed can be unpredictable. As a result, there is variation in midwifery scopes of practice and requirements for licensure or authorization to practice from state to state. Some state practice acts are not entirely consistent with the standards of practice endorsed by professional midwifery organizations and taught in accredited midwifery education programs. Despite this discrepancy, the licensed midwife is expected to follow the rules and regulations for whatever method of authorization he or she is granted by the state. The practice of midwifery can also be subject to state and federal laws governing Medicare and Medicaid payment, prescriptive authority, controlled substances, and licensing of freestanding birth centers.

Midwifery Scope of Practice

An individual's scope of practice is determined by several factors, including legal jurisdictions, institutional policy, and individual education and training. Most laws governing midwifery practice define the clinical or professional relationship between midwives and consulting physicians. At their best, the laws support midwifery independent practice and collaborative management; at their worst, they require direct physician supervision of midwives. The rules and regulations governing midwifery practice usually are available on state-sponsored websites. Professional organizations such as ACNM and MANA provide online summaries of all the state midwifery laws. A recent review by Osborne summarized current state regulations regarding prescriptive authority for midwives.[10]

Midwives who attend births in a hospital and some birth centers are required to be credentialed and privileged by the healthcare facility prior to caring for women in that setting. Bylaws, as established by the healthcare facility, define the requirements for obtaining privileges, the responsibilities of those who are granted privileges, specific procedures that may be performed by the individual providers, protections offered to those who are privileged, and grounds for removal of privileges. These bylaws may also specify the role and responsibilities of the midwife in relation to consulting physician(s) and the responsibilities of the physician in relationship to collaborating midwives. All privileged providers are expected to adhere to institution bylaws, even when they are more restrictive than the state law.

The Professional: The Exemplary Midwife

Professions also assume responsibility for setting their own standards of performance. As is often noted, there is a difference between being a member of a profession and being a "professional." As Kennedy has stated, the "midwife's professionalism is a key factor in empowering women during the childbearing process."[11] Thus, to be a professional, one must know how professionalism is defined and measured.

Kennedy identified three dimensions of midwifery professionalism:

1. The *dimension of therapeutics*, which illustrates how and why the midwife chooses and uses specific therapies when providing care

2. The *dimension of caring*, which reflects how the midwife demonstrates that she cares for, and about, the woman

3. The *dimension of the profession*, which examines how midwifery might be enhanced and accepted by "exemplary" practice[11]

Kennedy divided the dimension of therapeutics into two qualities that must be held in balance: supporting the normalcy of birth, while simultaneously maintaining vigilance and attention to detail, intervening only when necessary. "This process of supporting normalcy could aptly be described as the art of doing 'nothing' well."[11]

The dimension of caring is demonstrated by "1) respecting the uniqueness of the woman and family; and 2) creation of a setting that is respectful and reflects the woman's needs."[11] Midwives explore and honor each individual woman's personal history and cultural context. They work in partnership with women with the goal of providing emotional support and strengthening self-confidence.

Some qualities identified by Kennedy as linked to the dimension of caring include "an unwavering integrity and honesty, compassion and understanding, the ability to communicate effectively, and flexibility."[11] Midwives are emotion-workers. They support the emotional journey of women through health care. For example, midwives support the birthing woman while also identifying and managing their own emotions in order to best meet the needs of the woman, including situations in which the woman may be fearful. The professional midwife then works to minimize her fear. In addition to creating an emotional setting that meets the woman's needs, exemplary midwives are experts at creating safe emotional settings. Midwives who care for women in labor are experts in protecting the sacred physical birth space. Using skills that make midwifery a unique profession, they help to create a peaceful environment that is the most conducive to the birth process, maternal satisfaction, and mother–child bonding in the immediate postpartum period.

The dimension of the profession focuses on "the delineation, promotion, and sustenance of midwifery as a professional role."[11] Midwives demonstrate this dimension through evidence-based practice, quality and peer review, continuing education, commitment to and passion for the profession, and nurturing and caring for themselves. The exemplary midwife's focus is not just on the individual woman or birth; in addition, the midwife is driven to foster the profession and advocate for improving women's health care locally and globally.

Midwifery Within the U.S. Healthcare System

The quintessential midwifery role is provider of direct care to women. The other chapters in this text detail how that role is fulfilled. Additional roles inherent in midwifery include researcher, educator, policymaker, and business manager, among others. Thus the practice of midwifery is not solely devoted to direct patient care, but rather encompasses a variety of other activities.

Improving the health of women is a personal, communal, and political responsibility, and midwives work wherever women need them. While many midwives attend births and provide women's health services, they may also work as entrepreneurs, educators, and researchers. In all of these settings, midwives collaborate with a variety of team members.

In clinical practice, midwives may work for large hospitals or healthcare systems in metropolitan areas,

in small private practices in rural communities, and anywhere in between. Midwives may attend births in homes, freestanding birth centers, or hospitals. They may be self-employed in a private business, or they may be employees of physicians or healthcare organizations. They may provide care to women from vulnerable populations or to women with extensive social and financial resources. Midwives can limit their practice to women with needs that are age or disease specific, such as family planning, infertility, obstetric triage, menopause, incontinence, or pelvic pain, or they can provide a general range of services.

Since the 1960s, the majority of CNMs, and now CMs, who attend births have done so in hospitals and freestanding birth centers, whereas the vast majority of CPMs attend births in homes or freestanding birth centers. Although these trends may continue for a while, the future may present more workplace opportunities for all midwives.

In 1989, the Centers for Disease Control and Prevention (CDC) began collecting data on nurse-midwife–attended births. Since then, there has been a steady increase in the number of women having vaginal births attended by CNMs and CMs, and in 39 states an overall increase in the proportion of births attended by midwives (**Figure 2-1**).[12,13]

Historically, the percentage of out-of-hospital births (including birth center and home births) declined from 44% in 1940 to 1% in 1969, and

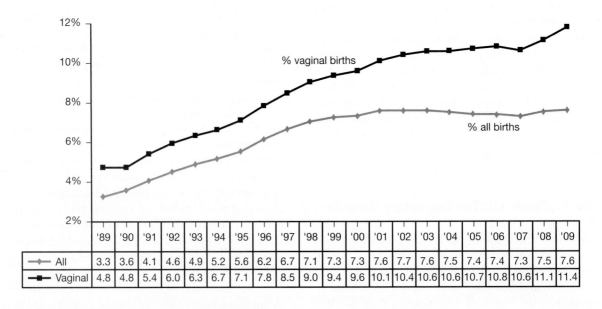

	'89	'90	'91	'92	'93	'94	'95	'96	'97	'98	'99	'00	'01	'02	'03	'04	'05	'06	'07	'08	'09
All	3.3	3.6	4.1	4.6	4.9	5.2	5.6	6.2	6.7	7.1	7.3	7.3	7.6	7.7	7.6	7.5	7.4	7.4	7.3	7.5	7.6
Vaginal	4.8	4.8	5.4	6.0	6.3	6.7	7.1	7.8	8.5	9.0	9.4	9.6	10.1	10.4	10.6	10.6	10.7	10.8	10.6	11.1	11.4

Figure 2-1 Percentage of live births attended by certified nurse-midwives, 1989-2009.
Source: Martin JA, Hamilton BE, Ventura SJ, et al. Births: Final Data for 2010. *National Vital Statistics Reports,* Vol. 61, No. 1. Hyattsville, MD: National Center for Health Statistics; 2012.

remained stable until recently. The majority of out-of-hospital births occur at home. According to the National Center for Health Statistics (NCHS), from 2004 to 2009, U.S. home births increased from 0.56% to 0.72%—a 29% increase.[14]

The Employee

With so many opportunities, the typical midwife seeking a job searches for a position that is a good match to his or her experience, personality, skill set, and lifestyle. When evaluating the positives and negatives of any job, it is important to review several other aspects of the business that may contribute to success or frustration. These aspects may include availability of and relationship with collaborative physicians, ancillary support (e.g., billing, patient flow), retirement benefits, reimbursement for professional expenses (e.g., licenses, certification, continuing education), and payment for malpractice premiums. It is important to determine whether the malpractice coverage is an occurrence policy or a claims-made policy. An occurrence policy covers claims that *occur* during the life of the policy, whereas a claims-made policy covers only claims that are *made* during the life of the policy. A claims-made policy requires the insured to purchase extended coverage, termed a tail or prior acts policy, if employment changes. Who pays the cost of the extension—which may be 1.5 times the annual premium—is an important consideration, especially when the midwife is an employee. Ament provides a post-job-interview rating tool that facilitates an objective measure of the match between the midwife's expectations and the practice characteristics (**Table 2-2**).[7]

Whether or not a prospective employer offers a formal contract, asking for confirmation in writing of offered remuneration and job specifics is a wise request. If asked to sign a contract, it may be important for the professional to consult with an attorney. Even if a contract is considered non-negotiable, the midwife should thoroughly understand the content prior to signing. **Box 2-2** provides a list of topics that should be discussed prior to accepting a position.

The Entrepreneur

Most midwives consider midwifery to be a vocation. Thus it can be challenging to think of midwifery as "a business"—yet all midwives need to understand the basic principles of running a successful business. There is a growing need for midwives to become accomplished administrators and business managers. Even job hunting is a business skill.

Many midwives have, either independently or in groups, become business owners. The opportunity to

Table 2-2	Postinterview Evaluation for a Midwife		
Rate your responses to the following questions:			
1 = acceptable 2 = unsure 3 = unacceptable			
Practice philosophy	1	2	3
Patient volume	1	2	3
Patient demographics	1	2	3
Patient outcomes	1	2	3
Productivity requirements	1	2	3
Clinical hours	1	2	3
Practice partners	1	2	3
Support staff	1	2	3
Practice facilities	1	2	3
Birth facilities	1	2	3
Nonclinical responsibilities	1	2	3
Availability of resources	1	2	3
Orientation	1	2	3

Source: Ament L. *Professional Issues in Midwifery*. Sudbury, MA: Jones and Bartlett; 2007.

avoid the limitations imposed by the business model or clinical guidelines developed by others, such as physicians, hospitals, and community clinics, can be very tempting, and in some cases, it may be a necessity. While many midwifery-owned businesses have succeeded in spite of inadequate planning or limited resources, the advice offered by successful entrepreneurs is consistent—namely, consult experts, invest in marketing, develop competence in billing, and collect data. Each of these aspects of running an independent midwifery practice is an important factor that can facilitate long-term success.

Business Advice from Experts

It is unwise to open a business without seeking the expertise of, at a minimum, an attorney and an accountant. The legal structure of a midwifery business (e.g., sole proprietorship, partnership, or limited liability company) will have short- and long-term personal and financial consequences. Midwife business owners should be experts on the laws and regulations that govern midwifery practice, but must also know how the laws governing medical practice, the corporate practice of medicine, and pharmacy regulations impact their plans. Midwives providing care during out-of-hospital births must comply with health department regulations, birth center requirements, building codes, and a variety of business regulations.

BOX 2-2 Contract Negotiations

1. *Type of Position: salary, hourly?*
2. *Benefits*
   a. Salary
   b. Health, dental, optical insurance
   c. Paid vacation (#)
   d. Paid sick leave (#)
   e. Paid holidays (#)
   f. Life insurance, retirement annuity
3. *Other Professional Benefits*
   a. Tuition reimbursement
   b. Expense account/continuing education costs and paid time off
   c. Professional membership dues
   d. Professional journal subscriptions
   e. Professional licenses
   f. Pager/cell phone
   g. Mileage
   h. Bonuses
      i. Productivity by volume or
      ii. Productivity by effectiveness
   i. Malpractice insurance
      i. Amount of coverage
      ii. Personal policy or rider
      iii. Tail
4. *Other*
   a. Work hours: office, call, administrative time, committee or other responsibilities
   b. Paid for overtime?
   c. Scheduling of appointments: how many per day, time per visit
   d. Productivity data
   e. Length of orientation
   f. Employee handbook

Contract

1. Position description
2. Work hours/expectations
3. How evaluated? When? By whom?
4. Salary (and benefits)
5. Duration of contract
6. Amendment and modification agreement
7. Restrictive clause?
8. Termination of contract conditions
   a. Of the person
   b. Of the position
   c. Length of notice
   d. Compensation

Source: Ament L. *Professional Issues in Midwifery*. Sudbury, MA: Jones and Bartlett; 2007.

Midwives who employ others must determine how they will compensate those employees and follow the relevant employment tax codes and antidiscrimination policies. Beyond malpractice coverage, new business owners are often surprised to learn how many insurance policies need to be purchased and how many business contracts need to be finalized. In all of these areas, good advice can save money, protect investments, and enable midwives to provide care for women.

Preparing a business plan and seeking guidance from an accountant on the costs of doing business provide clarity for all involved and are requirements when seeking loans to help establish a business. Elements in a business plan are listed in **Box 2-3**. The time spent attending to details and establishing a reporting system that provides regular feedback on revenues versus expenses provides a way to measure success for the entire team and relieves pressure when the unexpected happens.

In a country that places a high value on independent business ownership, many types of support exist

BOX 2-3 Business Planning

Benefits of a Business Plan

- Makes you think about many aspects you might not have considered
- Helps to solidify ideas into an organized format
- Clarifies the role of others: collaborating physicians, other health professionals
- Serves as a benchmark for actual performance

Business Plans Help You To

- Quantify resources
- Evaluate finances
- Prioritize objectives

Elements of a Business Plan

- Cover page
- Executive summary
- Practice organization
- Market analysis
- Market plan
- Regulatory issues
- Facility and space requirements
- Equipment requirements
- Accounting, taxes
- Financial data
- Time lines

Source: Ament L. *Professional Issues in Midwifery*. Sudbury, MA: Jones and Bartlett; 2007.

for small business owners, including information on how to formulate business plans and where to apply for small business loans. Midwives who are business owners often agree to mentor the next entrepreneur. The Midwifery Business Network is an organization of midwives who are committed to sharing information, providing support to midwives interested in the business aspects of midwifery practice, and increasing the number of midwife-owned services.[15] The Midwifery Business Network sponsors an annual fall conference and has published an *Administrative Manual for Midwifery Practices*.[16] Other business guides also exist in areas outside of midwifery, which may provide additional useful information.[17]

Midwifery services that are not independent businesses still have business or administrative aspects of importance. Even a two-person service has to reach an agreement on scheduling, compensation, records management, monitoring of financial statements, negotiation of collaborative agreements with physicians, peer review, and strategies to handle personal and professional adversity. Services that reside in large corporations may inherit many of these decisions and struggle to have a voice in changes that directly influence their practices. While responsibilities for the success of the service are shared, there must be a designated leader or service director who serves as the primary contact with the corporation, assumes responsibility for participating on department- or corporate-level committees, is able to describe the success of the service in corporate terms, and knows how to move an agenda within the organization. Midwives place a high value on building relationships with women and on positive feedback from the individuals for whom they provide care. Those skills can be extrapolated into the business arena and will serve the midwives well.

Marketing

Many advisors encourage early attention to a marketing plan. Without a coherent, consumer-friendly message about the services offered and an identified medium for reaching the target population, the business may not be able to sustain itself. Not every service can cover the cost of a logo and four-color brochures, but all midwives can develop marketing skills. For example, the organized, scientific, lecture approach may intimidate some women, while others may look for messages that midwifery practice is evidence based and provides adequate safeguards in the event of major complications.

Professional organizations may be a ready source of marketing advice and materials. Indeed, many are involved in national marketing campaigns that can be adapted to local settings. Both ACNM and MANA, for example, have marketing campaigns that can be adapted for local audiences.

Billing for Services

No matter what size the business, every employee should be able to describe the source of revenue that covers employee salaries and know how to support that revenue stream. When the services provided by a midwife are billable, then the midwife must clearly document the services provided and complete a form to initiate the billing process. The midwife also is responsible for fulfilling the requirements for documentation that support the billing codes. For example, the amount paid for an exam will vary based on the intensity of the exam as measured by the number of systems included in the physical assessment, the types of problems identified, and the amount of time spent providing and coordinating care. If this content is not thoroughly documented in the healthcare record, payment may be reduced or even denied.

However the billing gets done, service directors are usually responsible for establishing a system of checks and balances that monitors the accuracy and timeliness of the billing process and limits the opportunity for embezzlement or insurance fraud. The time and money spent establishing a viable medical record and billing system are necessary outlays to ensure the ongoing success of the business.

Data Collection

Lessons learned from Mary Breckenridge, who gathered local data prior to opening the Frontier Nursing Service, continue to serve the midwifery profession well. These lessons include the power of local data, including baseline descriptive data before opening a service, descriptive and outcome data from the first day of operation, assistance from researchers, and dissemination of the findings. A number of readily accessible mechanisms for collecting and collating practice-specific and national data exist that describe the care provided by midwives. Members of ACNM can join in the ACNM Benchmarking Project,[18] which allows participants to examine their practices and compare them to other like practices across the United States. The MANA Division of Research, with its MANAStats system, and the American Association of Birth Centers, with its Uniform Data Set, both have developed web-based data collection tools that can be used by individuals and contribute to a national database on the outcomes of midwifery care.[19,20]

The Educator

All midwives are educators. Policymakers, potential employers, and consumers all need to learn what is unique and valuable about the midwifery approach to care. Women need to learn how to care for their own bodies and how to safely prepare for puberty, pregnancy, menopause, and all the points in between. Consumer-oriented materials often are used for this purpose, and may be written by midwives. For example, the *Journal of Midwifery & Women's Health* regularly publishes a patient education handout titled *Share with Women*. This series of copyright-free handouts targeted to women reviews important clinical topics using appropriate language and illustrations for lower health literacy.

Some midwives educate others to be midwives. All midwives in practice are encouraged to clinically teach and precept students. There are approximately 40 midwifery education programs accredited by ACME with numerous midwives on faculty. Directors of these programs meet twice a year through their association, known as Directors of Midwifery Education (DOME). It is by "midwifing" individuals to develop skills in the cognitive, affective, and psychomotor domains that the midwifery profession continues to flourish. The legacy of midwifery also depends on socialization of midwifery students into the role and responsibilities of the midwife.

The Researcher and User of Research

Sackett et al. concisely defined evidence-based practice (EBP) in 2000 as the "integration of the best research evidence with clinical expertise and patient values."[21] Not all midwives need to actively conduct research, but all need to understand relevant research and implement evidence-based care. The systematic use of evidence in the field of obstetrics usually is dated to the 1989 publication of the two-volume book, *Effective Care in Pregnancy and Childbirth* (1989).[22] In this ground-breaking treatise, the authors combed through existing obstetric research articles and identified those clinical practices supported by research as well as those practices that the evidence did not support.

Several databases that summarize the most recent evidence on a multitude of clinical topics are available to women's healthcare providers. One important evidence-based database is the Cochrane Library (named for Archie Cochrane a physician and pioneer in the area of evidence-based medicine). The Cochrane Library contains several databases, including the Cochrane Database of Systematic Reviews.[23] Other sources of research that midwives often use include PubMed, the Up-to-Date Database, and DynaMed. Anderson and Stone, in their textbook, outlined the steps for locating the evidence for a particular clinical scenario (**Box 2-4**).[24] It is of note that these steps are similar to the midwifery management process as discussed in the *Introduction to the Care of Women* chapter.

When gathering information, it is important to remember that "not all evidence is created equal." Once all the research data have been gathered, the findings need to be compared and contrasted. Evidence then is evaluated as to its strength. The clinically applicability of the recommendations are ultimately based on the strength of the evidence (**Figure 2-2**).[25]

The Collaborator: Member of an Interprofessional Healthcare Team

All healthcare providers work within a healthcare system that includes professionals who have different scopes of practice, different professional cultures, and different professional roles. The factors that make interprofessional relationships work well become especially pertinent for midwives when a woman develops complications or conditions that lie beyond the scope of midwifery practice. Although it has long been recognized that interprofessional teams provide better care than single-disciplinary groups for patients with complex medical needs,[26] interprofessional collaboration and communication have only recently been the focus of education, research, and clinical initiatives.[27,28]

BOX 2-4 Methodology for Finding the Evidence

1. Identify the clinical problem.
2. Formulate a focused, answerable question following the PICO format (problem, intervention, comparison, outcomes).
3. Locate relevant and appropriate resources.
4. Critically appraise the information.
5. Implement and integrate the evidence into clinical practice.
6. Communicate the information (to the woman, her family, and to other providers).

Source: Adapted from Anderson BA, Stone SE. *Best Practices in Midwifery.* New York: Springer; 2013.

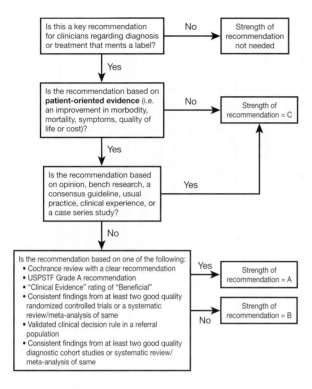

Figure 2-2 Algorithm for evaluation of strength of evidence and determination of recommendation.

Source: Reprinted with permission from Ebell MH, Siwek J, Weiss BD, et al. Strength of recommendation taxonomy (SORT): a patient-centered approach to grading evidence in the medical literature. *J Am Board Fam Pract.* 2004;17(1):59-67.

The patient safety movement has shined a light on the most recent focus on interprofessional collaboration and the need to improve communication between healthcare providers. In the 1999 groundbreaking Institute of Medicine (IOM) report *To Err Is Human*, it was estimated that 45,000 to 98,000 patients die each year in U.S. hospitals due to medical errors.[29] Subsequent medical error and patient safety reports have highlighted poor communication and inadequate team coordination as the source of many of these medical errors. For example, a Joint Commission sentinel event analysis on preventing infant death and injury during birth identified communication problems as the root cause of the healthcare delivery error in 72% of the cases analyzed.[30] Fifty-five percent of the organizations studied cited organizational culture, including "hierarchy and intimidation, failure to function as a team, and failure to follow the chain-of-communication," as commonly encountered barriers to effective communication and teamwork.[30]

In the years following these publications, much work has been done on identifying ways to foster and support teamwork in healthcare delivery. Successful

interprofessional collaboration in obstetrics, for example, has been associated with improved patient outcomes, a high degree of patient satisfaction, fewer cesarean sections, and lower costs.[31]

The Definitions of Collaborative Care

According to the International Confederation of Midwives (ICM) Essential Competencies for Basic Midwifery Practice, "The midwife…works collaboratively (teamwork) with other health workers to improve the delivery of services to women and families."[32] Moreover, "[t]he midwife has the skill and/or ability to…identify deviations from normal during the course of pregnancy and initiate the referral process for conditions that require higher levels of intervention."[32]

ACNM recognizes that midwives are independent practitioners who function within a complex medical system, which includes collaboration with multiple healthcare professionals, to ensure the health and safety of women and their newborns.[33] The levels of collaborative management as defined by ACNM include consultation, collaboration, and referral, and the definitions for each of these levels often serve as guidelines for similar language within state laws and hospital bylaws (**Table 2-3**).[34]

The 2011 ACNM and American College of Obstetricians and Gynecologists (ACOG) Joint Statement of Practice Relations Between Obstetrician-Gynecologists and Certified Nurse-Midwives/Certified Midwives declares that "health care is most effective when it occurs in a system that facilitates communication across care settings an among providers."[35] MANA, NARM, and NACPM have all published documents that address the relationship between CPMs and physicians.[36] In these documents, midwifery practice is described as autonomous and CPMs are expected to collaborate, refer, and transfer care in critical situations.

Essential Components of Collaboration

Interprofessional collaboration can be a challenging endeavor. In 2011, a group of experts from several professional associations published a white paper that itemized recommended core competencies for interprofessional collaboration within four competency domains: (1) roles and responsibilities for collaborative practice, (2) values and ethics for interprofessional practice, (3) interprofessional communication, and (4) interprofessional teamwork and team-based care.[27, 28,37] In addition, several authors have identified essential components of successful collaboration, which are summarized in **Box 2-5**.[27,28,37–40]

Table 2-3   The Continuum of Collaborative Management in Midwifery Care

Level of Collaborative Management	Definition	Primary Responsibility for Patient	Midwife's Role	Collaborator's Role	Comments
Consultation (With a provider of any specialty)	"The process whereby a CNM or CM seeks the advice or opinion of a physician or another member of the health care team."	Midwife	Primary provider	Advisor/consultant	Prepare for the consultation Know the woman's medical history Review the basics of management of the diagnosis or problem Understand the social and psychosocial factors underlying her health Understand your practice setting and scope of practice Remember the Midwifery Management Process
Collaboration	"The process whereby a CNM or CM and physician jointly manage the care of a woman or newborn who has become medically, gynecologically or obstetrically complicated."	Co-management (depending on the severity of the complication, the midwife may remain the primary care provider)	Normal processes, coordination of care, continuity with patient	Care for the obstetric, gynecologic, or neonatal complications	Use interprofessional communication techniques such as SBAR and closed-loop communication Clearly delineate roles to ensure all aspects of the plan of care (POC) are considered Communicate with the woman and her family about the relationship
Referral[a]	"The process by which the CNM or CM directs the client to a physician or another health care professional for management of a particular problem or aspect of the client's care."	Physician or other referral provider	Coordination of care, ensure timely and full transfer of care, continuity of services	Assumes the primary responsibility for care of the patient	Ensure that referral/transfer is the best POC for the patient Ensure that the woman understands that she has been transferred to another provider's care and that she has access to appointment and contact information Consider potential problem of patient abandonment and/or "punting" of difficult-to-care-for women Use interprofessional communication techniques like the handoff

SBAR = situation, background, assessment, recommendation.

[a] Referral in this continuum refers to transfer of care. Referral in the context of insurance is providing a patient with a reference to a specialty provider.

Source: Definitions adapted from American College of Nurse-Midwives. *Collaborative Management in Midwifery Practice for Medical, Gynecological and Obstetrical Conditions.* Silver Spring, MD: American College of Nurse-Midwives; 1997.

BOX 2-5 Essential Components of Successful Collaboration and Teamwork[a]

1. Professional competence in each member of the team (common body of knowledge, shared language, similarities in treatment modalities)
2. Common orientation to the patient as the primary unit of attention
3. Shared mental model: every member of the team can anticipate and predict the needs of the others
4. Recognition and acknowledgment of interdependence among all members of the team
5. Interprofessional respect and mutual trust
6. Formal system of communication between providers
7. Effective communication based on the goal of reaching consensus (an interest in solutions that maximize the contributions of all parties)
8. Mutual performance monitoring (identification of mistakes and provision of feedback within team to facilitate self-correction)
9. Identified team leader for each situation
10. Situation monitoring and adaptability as the situation changes
11. Ability to shift work responsibilities as needed to under-utilized team members

[a]This list is compiled from different analyses of essential characteristics for teams in general and teams in specific urgent or emergency situations. It is not designed to be complete or placed in rank order, but rather to give the reader a description of some characteristics that are essential for successful interprofessional team function. Midwives are always members of interprofessional teams.

Sources: Adapted from Interprofessional Education Collaborative Expert Panel. *Core Competencies for Interprofessional Collaborative Practice: Report of an Expert Panel.* Washington, DC: Interprofessional Education Collaborative; 2011; Ivey S. A model for teaching about interdisciplinary practice. *J Allied Health.* 1988;17:189-195; King TL, Laros RK, Parer JT. Interprofessional collaborative practice in obstetrics and midwifery. *Obstet Gynecol N Amer.* 2012;39:411-422.

Teamwork

Teamwork and communication are skills that can be learned.[41–43] Although patient outcomes following simulation training have not yet fully been determined, it appears that simulation training improves teamwork, team coordination, and interprofessional communication.[41,43]

The U.S. Agency for Healthcare Research and Quality (AHRQ) has developed a series of materials and training curricula, collectively titled TeamSTEPPS, which can be used in healthcare settings to help foster successful teamwork.[39,44,45] The TeamSTEPPs curricula emphasize the development of four core competencies: communication, mutual support, situation monitoring, and leadership.

Communication Techniques for Successful Collaboration

Direct and deliberate communication techniques include the *SBAR, closed-loop communication,* and *the handoff.*

The SBAR—an acronym for Situation, Background, Assessment, and Recommendation—is structured communication tool that has been shown to significantly improve the quality of communication between healthcare providers and to reduce medical errors.[46] The SBAR approach omits the nonessential elements of a woman's history, distills the most pertinent information, and clarifies what is needed. The midwife can use the SBAR approach to obtain a consultation from a specialist (**Box 2-6**) or to communicate during an emergency (**Box 2-7**).

In closed-loop communication, the midwife directs the message to a particular team member, the team member repeats the order or request aloud, and the midwife confirms that the team member heard correctly. This communication allows the whole team to hear the orders and correct any errors before the orders are executed. Closed-loop communication tools such as the *call-out* and the *check-back* can be used to communicate critical information to all members of the team, thereby allowing them to anticipate what will be needed next, but use of such tools also requires that team members communicate what they intend to do with the information.

When transferring care from one provider to another, an official handoff includes the transfer of information along with primary care responsibility; this step provides an opportunity to clarify information, confirm understanding, and discuss the management plan. The handoff can occur between two midwives or between the midwife and the referral physician when a transfer of care is indicated. The goal of the handoff is to give the new primary provider all of the information needed to safely care for the woman and her family. **Figure 2-3** provides an example of a handoff form.

Communication skills such as the SBAR, closed-loop communication, and the handoff are like any clinical skill—they must be practiced and adapted to individual settings.

BOX 2-6 SBAR Used for a Consultation

The midwife at a clinic is caring for a woman at 33 weeks' gestation who was previously diagnosed with gestational diabetes type 1A. When reading the woman's blood glucose log, the midwife observes that more than 20% of her values are high. She calls the consulting maternal–fetal medicine physician and gives this consult SBAR.

S: I want to consult with you about a woman with uncontrolled gestational diabetes.

B: Maria Gonzalez is a 24-year-old G1P0 at 33 weeks by LMP consistent by 19-week ultrasound. Her 1-hour GTT was 150 and her 3-hour GLT had 2 elevated values. She was sent to the diabetes education center and received diet and glucose monitoring education. Over the last 2 weeks, 20% of her values are out of range, with five fasting levels between 100 and 110 and five 2-hour postprandial levels higher than 150, the highest being 180. She had a reactive NST today, the fetus is size equal to dates, and her urinalysis was negative for glucose.

A: Diabetes diet is inadequate to control glucose levels and I believe she needs medication.

R: I would like your recommendation for medication therapy and schedule her to see you for a consultation in the next few days.

BOX 2-7 SBAR Used in an Emergency Situation

The midwife at a small community hospital is caring for a woman who is bleeding heavily immediately after giving birth. She has called for physician assistance from a provider in the next room. When the physician arrives, the midwife says:

S: This woman is having a postpartum hemorrhage.

B: Marta gave birth to her fifth child 15 minutes ago over an intact perineum. Her total EBL is 800 mL. She has received 40 IU of oxytocin (Pitocin), 0.2 mg of ergonovine (Methergine), and 800 mcg of misoprostol per rectum (Cytotec). The placenta appeared intact, and there are no clots in the lower uterine segment.

A: She has severe uterine atony, and I think I feel some placental tissue in the anterior portion of the fundus.

R: Can you please put on some gloves and assist me?

The Policymaker

The building blocks of the midwifery profession (standards for education, certification, and practice) open many doors for midwives to contribute to the development of public and private policy. For the profession as a whole to thrive, each midwife must walk through these doors. Federal, state, and institutional policies determine which healthcare services and birth settings are available to women as well as who will be reimbursed and at what rate. Which education programs receive government funding to support faculty and students is also a matter of policy. Hospitals, clinics, and employers all write policies that influence access to midwifery care.

Members of the midwifery profession, primarily serving in a volunteer capacity, wrote the vast majority of the original policies that define the profession of midwifery. Even today, professional organizations remain dependent upon a high level of volunteer effort to keep these policies relevant. Meeting the policy needs of the profession primarily represents a labor of love and a dogged determination to turn a vision into reality.

Many of the successful midwifery policymakers will confess to initially not seeing the need for this work, doubting their own abilities, or hoping someone else would do it.[47] It was discovered that becoming a policymaker is a learned behavior; thus the midwifery profession is now filled with successful midwife role models, and guidance on how to make this transition is readily available (**Box 2-8**).

In spite of many past successes, much policy work remains to be done. Some physician associations are opposed to laws that recognize advanced practice clinicians as independent providers, instead advocating for required physician supervision. Many state laws governing the practice of nurse-midwifery need to be changed to permit independent practice.

As of 2012, CPMs could not be licensed to practice in more than 30 states, and CMs could not be licensed in 47 states. Major decisions are also looming: should CNMs seek more midwifery practice acts that are separate from nursing and include their CM colleagues or stay under the advanced practice registered nurse (APRN) umbrella; can CNMs/CMs and CPMs be licensed under the same practice act; should CPMs be required to earn a college degree; should CNMs/CMs be required to earn a doctoral degree; and will the U.S. Congress pass healthcare legislation that moves the profession forward or backward—either outcome is always a possibility.

Professional Ethics in Midwifery

Midwives must be well versed in the ethics involved in all healthcare interactions.[48,49] The subject of professional ethics in health care is complex, and the introduction presented here is not a comprehensive review of this important topic. Additional resources that address health literacy, health numeracy, values clarification, options counseling, the interface between legal and ethical issues, and ways to communicate risk are listed at the end of this chapter.

An ethical framework for practice, beginning with the concept of accountability, is critical to the continuation of midwifery as an independent and respected profession.[7,50] Ethical guidelines encourage self-regulation, foster professional identity, protect midwives and clients, and serve as a measure of professional maturity.[51]

Ethics is defined as a guiding set of principles that inform actions.[51] The ACNM Code of Ethics was first published in 1990, and the ICM ethical code was introduced in 1993. These documents, as well as the MANA Statement of Values, provide guidance for the ethical behavior of midwives in various roles, including caring for women and their families, education, research, public policy, business management, and financial organization of health services.[52,53] A number of other organizations have published statements on "the rights" of individuals who receive health care—a concept that is inherent in most statements on ethical principles. In 2004, the Childbirth Connection (formerly the Maternity Association) revised *The Rights of Childbearing Women*; this document applies widely accepted principles of human rights to maternity care.[54]

Bioethical Principles

Four broad ethical principles define modern bioethics—the ethics of working with or caring for human beings. They include respect for autonomy, nonmaleficence (do no harm), beneficence (do good), and justice (**Table 2-4**).[55, 56]

Respecting an individual's privacy, ensuring confidentiality, encouraging shared decision making, and providing for informed decision making are all extensions of these bioethical principles. Research has shown that when healthcare providers do not respect these rights, their behavior may be seen as a form of abuse and could lead to psychological trauma for the woman.[57] Healthcare professionals can also experience ethical dilemmas when the application of one ethical principle appears to contradict a second principle.

Table 2-4	Bioethical Principles	
Bioethical Principle	**Definition**	**Midwifery Application**
Autonomy	Self-determination	The midwife respects the right of the woman to make decisions regarding her care.
Beneficence	Do good	The midwife acts in a way that promotes the woman's best interests and well-being.
Nonmaleficence	Do no harm	The midwife avoids any actions that cause harm to the woman or her infant.
Justice	Fairness	The midwife accords the woman her due rights and treats all women equally.

Source: Adapted from Mighty HE, Fahey J. Clinical ethics in obstetrics and gynecology. In *Obstetrics and Gynecology: The Essentials of Clinical Care.* Stuttgart, Germany: Thieme Publishers; 2010:517-526.

Privacy and Confidentiality

Protection of a woman's privacy is not simply ethical; in most cases it is mandated by the Health Insurance Portability and Accountability Act of 1996 (HIPAA). When working in collaboration with other healthcare providers, only those parts of the health information that are immediately pertinent to the individual's care should be disclosed, and the woman should be personally notified if the midwife desires to contact a consultant about the woman's health.

Family members, partners, or friends are often present during office visits or in a birthing site. It is important to confirm that the woman has given permission before information is shared when others are present. A midwife must also be careful to not discuss client information in places where third parties might overhear. Emails, faxes, digital records, the Internet, and social media can all be sources that lead to inadvertent but serious breaches in confidentiality. Family members should not automatically be used as translators when a woman does not speak the same language as the midwife.

Informed Consent and Informed Decision Making

The concept of informed decision making or informed consent (as it is often referred to legally) evolved through a number of court decisions and government regulations. In the 1950s and 1960s, U.S. courts began to mandate that consent be obtained before surgery. The 1970s saw an explosion of court rulings provided legal guidance regarding informed decision making.[58]

The ethical concept underlying informed consent includes client understanding of the recommended treatment and her free consent to that treatment.[59] The minimum required components of informed consent are sixfold: (1) diagnosis or assessment, (2) purpose of the proposed treatment or procedure, (3) possible risks of the treatment, (4) possible benefits of the treatment, (5) alternative treatments and the risks and benefits of those alternatives, and (6) possible benefits and risks of not receiving the treatment or procedure. The assumption underlying informed consent is that the individual is capable of understanding the content of the discussion so that self-determination may be protected and supported.

The legal interpretation of informed consent centers on disclosure and liability—did the individual receive enough information to consent to a procedure to protect the provider from being sued? This legal interpretation has been the cited as one reason for the creation of consent forms.

Some midwives and others prefer to use the term "informed decision making" for this process, as it encompasses both informed consent and informed refusal. Foster identified three essential components of informed decision making: (1) *knowing* or understanding, (2) *competency*, and (3) *voluntary* permission.[51] The ethical/moral interpretation of informed decision making centers on autonomous choice—was the woman able to exercise her right to decide what happens to her body? The ethical obligation is often a higher standard than what is mandated by the law.

Facilitating informed or shared decision making is a process that may take place over several visits and conversations. Women need time to process information and ask questions. Healthcare consumers may not always be familiar with complicated language and may need concrete explanations to understand the information well enough to make a decision. A woman's cognitive ability or the presence of physical, medical, intellectual, or developmental disabilities must be taken into consideration as well. If a woman is deemed incapable or incompetent, then a responsible individual must decide for her.

Women may also experience personal circumstances that curtail their ability to make a decision voluntarily. The ACNM Code of Ethics identifies some of these circumstances: pressure from family members, the midwife, or other care providers; aspects of the environment such as lack of privacy; lack of funding; restriction of healthcare access; or an abusive relationship.[57] The midwife must assess these factors and also take into account the cultural context when determining whether the woman is able to make a decision on her own volition at any given time.[58,60] **Box 2-9** identifies some practical considerations for addressing a potential ethical issue.

Ethical Dilemmas

The ACNM Code of Ethics states:

> The conflict of two or more moral obligations in a particular situation necessitates deliberate ethical analysis and decision making, including weighing and balancing principles and preferably involving and achieving consensus among all affected parties.[52]

For example, one healthcare provider's attempt to "do good," such as performing a cesarean section birth for a diagnosis of failure to progress, might be interpreted by the recipient of care as "doing harm"—in this case, performing surgery without adequate time waiting for a vaginal birth. Equally challenging is the fact that obstetrics is a field in which the professional attending birth has two patients, the mother and the fetus, whose interests may not be in equipoise.[56] However, a woman's right to autonomy does not change because she is pregnant. The consensus of modern medical ethics is that the duty owed to the fetus may be different from that owed to the mother, and the duty to both change depending on the gestational age and maternal condition(s).[61] A few example ethical scenarios are presented in **Box 2-10**.

BOX 2-9 Ethics: A Midwife's Quick Checklist

- Are the woman's wishes clear?
- Does the woman have the capacity to consent to, or refuse, treatment?
- Are there disagreements involving family members or partners?
- Is the woman's current plan of care appropriate?
- Is her health information being protected?
- Can you identify resource or fairness issues?

Source: Adapted from Sokol DK. Ethics man: rethinking ward rounds. *BMJ.* 2009;338:571.

BOX 2-10 Ethical Scenarios

Ethical Scenario 1

A woman with a low-risk pregnancy is "miserable" and requests an induction at 37 weeks' gestation. She and is adamant that she will go elsewhere for her care if the midwife will not induce her. The midwife validates the woman's feelings and explains the risks of elective induction but supports the position that induction at 37 weeks is not recommended.

The midwife knows that the benefits to the woman and fetus are maximized (**beneficence**) and harm is minimized (**nonmaleficence**) when labor begins on its own. This professional must weigh this information with the principle of **autonomy**, the woman's right to make an informed decision about her body and fetus.

Ethical Scenario 2

A woman presents for her first visit of the pregnancy and tells the midwife that she is uninsured and does not have many financial resources. Normally the midwife counsels women extensively about their genetic options in pregnancy at the first visit. It becomes clear to the midwife in the course of their conversation that the woman would never be able to afford any of the costly genetic testing and wonders if counseling should be performed. The midwife decides to counsel this woman in the same manner as any other woman.

The midwife's decision to counsel this woman regardless of her ability to afford genetic testing illustrates the principle of **justice**.

Evidence for Midwifery Care

Recent systematic reviews have demonstrated that not only is midwifery-led care (care in which the primary provider is the midwife) equivalent to the care provided by physicians, but on many outcome measures it has proved to be superior. A 2008 Cochrane meta-analysis reviewed 11 trials including 12,276 women, and found several statistically significant differences in outcomes for those women who received midwife-led care (**Table 2-5**).[62] All of the studies included in this systematic review were randomized, controlled trials; in addition, the studies were not limited to one country. The findings noted that midwife-led care included less prenatal hospitalization, less regional analgesia, fewer episiotomies, and fewer instrument deliveries. In addition, women who were cared for in a system of midwife-led care were more likely to experience no intrapartum analgesia/anaesthesia, a spontaneous vaginal birth, feeling in control during childbirth, attendance at birth by a known midwife, and initiation of breastfeeding. Finally, the newborns of women who had midwife-led care were more likely to have a shorter length of hospital stay. The authors concluded that "most women should be offered midwife-led models of care

Table 2-5	Systematic Review of Midwife-Led Care, 2008		
Outcome or Subgroup Title	**Number of Studies**	**Number of Participants**	**Statistical Measure with 95% Confidence Interval**
Significant Risk Reductions Found			
Duration of postnatal hospital stay (days)	2	1944	Mean difference = −0.14 [−0.33, 0.04]
Mean labor length (hours)	2	1614	Mean difference = −0.27 [−0.18, 0.72]
Mean length of neonatal hospital stay (days)	2	259	Mean difference = −2.00 [−2.15, −1.85]
Antenatal hospitalization	5	4337	RR = 0.90 [0.81, 0.99]
Fetal loss/neonatal death before 24 weeks	8	9890	RR = 0.79 [0.65, 0.97]
Overall fetal loss and neonatal death	10	11806	RR = 0.83 [0.70, 1.00]
Instrumental vaginal birth (forceps/vacuum)	10	11724	RR = 0.86 [0.78, 0.96]
Episiotomy	11	11872	RR = 0.82 [0.77, 0.88]
Admission to special care nursery/neonatal intensive care unit	10	11782	RR = 0.92 [0.81, 1.05]
Neonatal convulsions (as defined by trial authors)	1	1216	RR = 0.33 [0.01, 8.03]
Regional analgesia (epidural/spinal)	11	11892	RR = 0.81 [0.73, 0.91]
Opiate analgesia	9	10197	RR = 0.88 [0.78, 1.00]
Significant Increases Found			
Attendance at birth by known midwife	6	5225	RR = 7.84 [4.15, 14.81]
High perceptions of control during labor and childbirth	1	471	RR = 1.74 [1.32, 2.30]
No intrapartum analgesia/anaesthesia	5	7039	RR = 1.16 [1.05, 1.29]
Breastfeeding initiation	1	405	RR = 1.35 [1.03, 1.76]

RR = relative risk.

Source: Adapted from Hatem M, Sandall J, Devane D, et al. Midwife-led versus other models of care for childbearing women. *Cochrane Database Syst Rev.* 2008;4(CD004667). doi: 10.1002/14651858.CD004667.pub2.

and women should be encouraged to ask for this option although caution should be exercised in applying this advice to women with substantial medical or obstetric complications."[62]

Similar results were highlighted in a 2011 systematic review that examined outcomes for APRNs in the United States. For the purposes of this study, the authors defined certified nurse-midwives as APRNs, and their birth outcomes from 1990 to 2008 were examined separately from those of other groups of providers.[63] This review summarized the results from all levels of studies, including observational studies, and studies were limited to the United States. A high level of evidence was found that certified nurse-midwives, when compared to physicians, had lower rates of cesarean section birth, episiotomy, operative delivery, labor analgesia, and perineal lacerations, and equivalent rates of labor augmentation, low Apgar scores, and low-birth-weight infants. The systematic review also demonstrated a moderate level of evidence that nurse-midwives have lower rates of epidural use and induction of labor, comparable or higher rates of vaginal births, comparable or lower rates of newborn intensive care unit admissions, and higher rates of breastfeeding among women who received care from these professionals (**Table 2-6**).[63]

In addition to these two large reviews, numerous other published research studies have focused on specific practices of midwives that may account for these differing maternal and neonatal outcomes. In 2012, ACNM updated a PowerPoint slide set titled "The Pearls of Midwifery," which translates the latest evidence in a manner that can be easily communicated to other providers, or to women and their families (**Box 2-11**).[64]

Traditional Practices and New Evidence

Many of the practices promoted by midwives have a "tradition of use" but no modern research evidence to determine either their risks or their benefits. International meetings of midwives often reveal indigenous or population-specific common birth practices that have not been systematically evaluated. These situations, where the evidence for best practice is not available, provide the midwife with the opportunity to describe, without endorsing, local practices and the customs that surround them; identify potential risks and benefits, particularly if adopted in different locations; promote critical thinking about the wisdom of adopting the new approach; and develop a research project to study the practice.

Midwifery has a long tradition that includes learning by watchful waiting; sharing empirical knowledge via oral traditions; defining and protecting the normal, nonmedicalized birth process; and actively challenging "the evidence." These characteristics have served women well, especially when research is conducted to evaluate the midwifery approach. Examples where midwives have had a strong influence in the evolution of best practices include elimination of routine episiotomies,[65] redefinition of the Friedman labor curve,[66] promotion of early and prolonged breastfeeding for neonatal and maternal health,[67] delayed cord clamping,[68] immediate skin-to-skin contact between mother and newborn,[69] water immersion during labor,[70] and nonpharmacologic methods of pain control.[71]

Midwife scholars and researchers can be the link between women and the evidence. Many care practices have already been studied and either validated or refuted, while many others need motivated, informed midwives to conduct systematic reviews.

Conclusion

This chapter describes the midwifery profession now. Midwifery is an evolving profession with a strong, inspirational foundation; a mature infrastructure to promote policies that improve access to high-quality midwifery care; highly educated individuals who are defining best practice; and plenty of unfulfilled potential. Midwives have demonstrated their capacity to do the hard work of profession building, critically evaluate traditional models of care, challenge policies based on flawed research, and pursue a more just healthcare delivery system. How the profession changes and grows will reflect who the new midwives are, what brings them to the profession, who educates them, and how much they are willing to give to individual women, to the profession of midwifery, and to the process of creating a world where all women receive the best care possible.

> I think of midwifery as a seed full of potential—a seed that will grow into a lush blossoming tree with green branches and plenty of ripe fruit for nurturing women, babies and families. (Marina Alzugaray, MS, LM, CNM)

Table 2-6	A Systematic Review of Outcomes Provided by Certified Nurse-Midwives, 1990–2008, United States			
Outcome	**Number of Studies**	**Comments**	**Grade of Evidence**	**Summary**
Breastfeeding	3 studies (0 RCT)	All favored CNMs	Moderate	Higher breastfeeding rates among women cared for by CNMs compared to other providers
Cesarean section births	15 studies (1 RCT)	Only the RCT did not have significant difference, but it was a 1992 study with rates less than 10%; 13 of 15 other studies favored CNMs and the others showed equivalency	High	Lower rates of cesarean section births for women cared for by CNMs than physician providers
Epidural anesthesia	10 studies (0 RCT)	Nine of 10 observational studies noted CNMs used less epidural anesthesia than physicians	Moderate	Less epidural use by women cared for by CNMs than other providers
Episiotomy	8 studies (1 RCT)	Consistency among studies	High	Episiotomy rates lower for women cared for by CNMs than other providers in all studies
Labor analgesia	6 studies (1 RCT)	All women had access, but less analgesia was used by women under CNM care	High	Less analgesia use by women cared by CNMs than other providers
Labor augmentation	9 studies (1 RCT)	Only one observational study did not favor CNMs; it was from single institution Otherwise, findings were consistent, especially with the RCT	High	Lower or comparable use of labor augmentation for women cared for by CNMs and other providers
Labor induction	9 studies (0 RCT)	No RCT; 7 of 9 studies favored CNMs (similar to labor augmentation)	Moderate	Comparable or lower rates of labor induction for women cared for by CNMs compared to other providers
Low Apgar births	11 studies (1 RCT)	Most studies define a low Apgar score as < 7 Studies included some focusing only on low-risk births; others included high-risk births and inconsistent use of statistical control	High	Comparable Apgar scores among newborns of women cared for by CNMs than physician providers
Low birth weight (< 2500 g)	8 studies (1 RCT)	Six studies reported no difference; the other two favored CNMs	High	Comparable rates of low-birth-weight neonates of women care for by CNMs and other providers
NICU admission	5 studies (0 RCT)	Lack of RCT and inconsistent statistics; no study found a higher rate of admission and two reported lower rates for CNMs	Moderate	Comparable or lower rates of NICU admission for newborns of women cared for by CNMs compared to other providers
Perineal lacerations	6 studies (1 RCT)	All studies favored CNMs	High	Rates of third- and fourth-degree perineal lacerations lower for women cared for by CNMs than other providers
Vaginal birth after cesarean birth (VBAC)	5 studies (0 RCT)	Four of 5 studies favored CNMs; the other showed no difference	Moderate	Comparable or higher rates of VBAC for women cared for by CNMs compared to other providers
Vaginal operative births (forceps, vacuum, or both)	8 studies (1 RCT)	RCT similar for forceps; lower for CNMs with vacuum Five of 6 studies favored CNMs	High	Lower or comparable rates of vaginal operative births for women cared for by CNMs and other providers

CNM = certified nurse-midwife; NICU = neonatal intensive care unit; RCT = randomized controlled trial; VBAC = vaginal birth afte cesarean.

Source: Adapted from Newhouse RP, Stanik-Hutt J, White KM, et al. Advanced practice nurse outcomes 1990-2008: a systematic review. *Nurs Econ.* 2011;29(5):230-250.

BOX 2-11 Midwifery Pearls

- Oral nutrition in labor is safe and optimizes outcomes
- Ambulation and freedom of movement in labor are safe, are more satisfying for women, and facilitate the process of labor
- Hydrotherapy is safe and effective in decreasing pain during active labor
- Continuous labor support should be the standard of care for all laboring women
- Intermittent auscultation should be the standard of care for low-risk women
- Do not routinely artificially rupture the membranes
- Second stage management should be individualized and support an initial period of passive descent and self-directed open-glottis pushing
- There is no evidence to support routine episiotomy or aggressive perineal massage at birth
- Delayed cord clamping improves neonatal outcomes
- Immediate skin-to-skin contact after birth promotes thermoregulation, improves initial breastfeeding, and facilitates early maternal-infant bonding
- Out-of-hospital birth is safe for low-risk women

Source: Adapted from American College of Nurse-Midwives. Evidence-based practice: pearls of midwifery: a presentation by the American College of Nurse-Midwives, Washington, DC, 2010. Available at: http://www.midwife.org/Pearls. Accessed December 11, 2012.

References

1. Davis-Floyd R, Johnson CB. *Mainstreaming Midwives: The Politics of Change.* Oxford, UK: Routledge; 2006.

2. Rooks JP. *Midwifery and Childbirth in America.* Philadelphia, PA: Temple University Press; 1997.

3. Louden I. *Death in Childbirth: An International Study of Maternal Care and Maternal Mortality 1800-1950.* Oxford, UK: Clarendon Press; 1992.

4. Sharp E. Nurse-midwifery education: its successes, failures and future. *J Midwifery Women's Health.* 1983;28(2):17-23.

5. Childbirth Connection. Available at: http://www.childbirthconnection.org. Accessed November 6, 2012.

6. Citizens for Midwifery. Available at: http://cfmidwifery.org/index.aspx. Accessed November 6, 2012.

7. Ament LA. *Professional Issues in Midwifery.* Sudbury, MA: Jones and Bartlett; 2007.

8. American College of Nurse-Midwives. *Core Competencies for Basic Midwifery Practice.* Silver Spring, MD: American College of Nurse-Midwives; 2012. Available at: http://www.midwife.org/ACNM/files/ACNMLibraryData/UPLOADFILENAME/000000000050/Core%20Comptencies%20Dec%20 2012.pdf. Accessed June 16, 2013.

9. Midwives Alliance of North America. Core competencies for basic midwifery practice. 2011. Available at: http://mana.org/manacore.html. Accessed November 6, 2012.

10. Osborne K. Regulation of prescriptive authority for certified nurse-midwives and certified midwives. *J Midwifery Women's Health.* 2011;56:543-556.

11. Kennedy HP. A model of exemplary midwifery practice: results of a Delphi study. *J Midwifery Women's Health.* 2000;45(1):4-19.

12. Declerq E. Trends in midwife-attended births in the United States, 1989-2009. *J Midwifery Women's Health.* 2012;57(4):321-326.

13. Martin JA, Hamilton BE, Ventura SJ, et al. Births: *Final Data for 2010. National Vital Statistics Reports,* Vol. 61, No. 1. Hyattsville, MD: National Center for Health Statistics; 2012.

14. Centers for Disease Control and Prevention. NCHS data brief: home births in the United States, 1990-2009. Available at: http://www.cdc.gov/nchs/data/databriefs/db84.htm. Accessed November 6, 2012.

15. Midwifery Business Network. Available at: http://www.midwiferybusinessnetwork.com. Accessed November 6, 2012.

16. Midwifery Business Network. Administrative manual for midwifery practices. Available at: https://member.midwife.org/members_online/members/viewitem.asp?item=MBN1&catalog=PUB&pn=1&af=ACNM. Accessed November 6, 2012.

17. Buppert C. *Nurse Practitioner's Business Practice and Legal Guide.* 4th ed. Burlington, MA: Jones & Bartlett Learning; 2012.

18. American College of Nurse-Midwives. ACNM benchmarking project. Available at: http://www.midwife.org/Benchmarking. Accessed November 6, 2012.

19. Midwives Alliance of North American. MANAStats. Available at: https://www.manastats.org/help_public_about. Accessed November 6, 2012.

20. American Association of Birth Centers. Uniform data set (UDS). Available at: http://www.birthcenters.org/data-collection. Accessed November 6, 2012.

21. Sackett DL, Straus SE, Richardson WS, Rosenberg WM, Haynes RB. *Evidence-Based Medicine: How to Practice and Teach EBM.* 2nd ed. Edinburgh, Scotland: Churchill Livingstone; 2000.

22. Chalmer I, Enkin M, Marc JM, Keirse C. *Effective Care in Pregnancy and Childbirth*. Oxford, UK: Oxford University Press;1989.

23. Cochrane Database of Systematic Reviews. Available at: http://www.cochrane.org. Accessed November 6, 2012.

24. Anderson BA, Stone SE. *Best Practices in Midwifery*. New York: Springer; 2013.

25. Ebell MH, Siwek J, Weiss BD, et al. Strength of recommendation taxonomy (SORT): a patient-centered approach to grading evidence in the medical literature. *J Am Board Fam Pract*. 2004;17(1):59-67.

26. Baldwin DC Jr. Some historical notes on interdisciplinary and interprofessional education and practice in health care in the USA. *J Interprof Care*. 1996;21(suppl 1):23-37.

27. Avery M, Montgomery O, Sbrandl-Salutz E. Essential components of successful collaborative maternity care models. *Obstet Gynecol North Am*. 2012;39:423-434.

28. King TL, Laros RK, Parer JT. Interprofessional collaborative practice in obstetrics and midwifery. *Obstet Gynecol North Am*. 2012;39:411-422.

29. Kohn LT, Corrigan JM, Donaldson MS. *To Err Is Human: Building a Safer Health System*. Washington, DC: National Academy Press; 2000.

30. The Joint Commission. *Sentinel Event Alert: Preventing Infant Death and Injury During Delivery* (Issue no. 30). Oakbrook Terrace, IL: The Joint Commission; 2004. Available at: http://www.jointcommission.org/assets/1/18/SEA_30.PDF. Accessed February 19, 2012.

31. Jackson DJ, Lang JM, Swartz WH, et al. Outcomes, safety, and resource utilization in a collaborative care birth center program compared with traditional physician-based perinatal care. *Am J Public Health*. 2003;93:999-1006.

32. International Confederation of Midwives. Global standards for midwifery regulation 2010. 2011. Available at: http://www.internationalmidwives.org/Portals/5/2011/Global%20Standards/GLOBAL%20STANDARDS%20FOR%20MIDWIFERY%20REGULATION%20ENG.pdf. Accessed November 6, 2012.

33. American College of Nurse-Midwives. Independent midwifery practice. 2012. Available at: http://www.midwife.org/index.asp?bid=59&cat=3&button=Search. Accessed November 6, 2012.

34. American College of Nurse-Midwives. *Collaborative Management in Midwifery Practice for Medical, Gynecological and Obstetrical Conditions*. Silver Spring, MD: American College of Nurse-Midwives; 1997.

35. American College of Nurse-Midwives. *Joint Statement of Practice Relations Between Obstetrician-Gynecologists and Certified Nurse-Midwives/Certified Midwives*. Silver Spring, MD: American College of Nurse-Midwives; 2011.

36. Midwives Alliance of North America. *Midwives Model of Care. Midwifery Task Force 1996-2001*. Raleigh, NC: Midwives Alliance of North America; 2001. Available at: http://mana.org/definitions.html. Accessed February 19, 2012.

37. Interprofessional Education Collaborative Expert Panel. *Core Competencies for Interprofessional Collaborative Practice: Report of an Expert Panel*. Washington, DC: Interprofessional Education Collaborative; 2011.

38. Ivey S. A model for teaching about interdisciplinary practice. *J Allied Health*. 1988;17:189-195.

39. King TL, Laros RK, Parer JT. Interprofessional collaborative practice in obstetrics and midwifery. *Obstet Gynecol N Amer*. 2012;39:411-422.

40. King H, Battles J, Baker DP, et al. TeamSTEPPS: team strategies and tools to enhance performance and patient safety. Agency for Healthcare Research and Quality. Available at: http://www.ahrq.gov/downloads/pub/advances2/vol3/Advances-King_1.pdf. Accessed November 6, 2012.

41. Merien AER, van der Ven J, Mol BW, Houterman S, Oei SG. Multidisciplinary team training in a simulation setting for acute obstetric emergencies: a systematic review. *Obstet Gynecol*. 2010;115(5):1021-1031.

42. Crofts JF, Ellis D, Draycott TJ, Winter C, Hunt LP, Akande VA. Change in knowledge of midwives and obstetricians following obstetric emergency training: a randomized controlled trail of local hospital, simulation center and teamwork training. *BJOG*. 2007;114:1534-1541.

43. Robertson B, Schumacher L, Gosman G, Kanfer R, Kelley M, DeVita M. Simulation-based crisis team training for multidisciplinary obstetric providers. *Simulation in Healthcare*. 2009;4(2):77-83.

44. Baker DP, Gustafson S, Beaubien J, Salas E, Barach P. *Medical Teamwork and Patient Safety: The Evidence-Based Relation Literature Review*. Rockville, MD: Agency for Healthcare Research and Quality; 2005. Available at: http://www.ahrq.gov/qual/medteam. Accessed February 19, 2012.

45. Miller LA. Patient safety and teamwork in perinatal care: resources for clinicians. *J Perinat Neonat Nurs*. 2005;19(1):46-51.

46. Vardaman JM, Cornell P, Gondo MB, et al. Beyond communication: the role of standardized protocols in a changing health care environment. *Health Care Manage Rev*. 2012;37(1):88-97.

47. Williams DR. We need to say in unison: We are midwives and we do policy! Editorial. *J Midwifery Women's Health*. 2008;53(2):101-102.

48. Thompson JB. A human rights framework for midwifery care. *J Midwifery Women's Health*. 2004;49(3):175-176.

49. Thompson JB, King TL. A code of ethics for midwives. *J Midwifery Women's Health.* 2004;49(3):263-265.

50. Thompson HO, Thompson JE. Toward a professional ethic. *J Nurse-Midwifery.* 1987;32(1):105-110.

51. Foster IR, Lasser J. *Professional Ethics in Midwifery Practice.* Sudbury, MA: Jones and Bartlett; 2011.

52. American College of Nurse-Midwives. *Code of Ethics with Explanatory Statements.* Silver Spring, MD: American College of Nurse-Midwives; 2008.

53. Midwives Alliance of North America. *Statement of Values and Ethics.* Washington, DC: Midwives Alliance of North America; 2010.

54. Childbirth Connection. The rights of childbearing women. 2004. Available at: http://www.childbirth connection.org/article.asp?ck=10084&ClickedLink= 0&area=27. Accessed October 1, 2012.

55. Beauchamp TL, Childress, JF. *Principles of Biomedical Ethics.* 5th ed. New York: Oxford University Press; 2001.

56. Mighty HE, Fahey J. Clinical ethics in obstetrics and gynecology. In *Obstetrics and Gynecology: The Essentials of Clinical Care.* Stuttgart, Germany: Thieme Publishers; 2010:517-526.

57. Hodges S. Abuse in hospital-based birth settings. *J Perinatal Educ.* 2009;18(4):8-11.

58. Beauchamp TL. Informed consent: its history, meaning, and present challenges. *Cambridge Q Healthcare Ethics.* 2011;20:515-523.

59. Ethical decision making in obstetrics and gynecology. ACOG Committee Opinion no. 390. American College of Obstetricians and Gynecologists. *Obstet Gynecol.* 2007;110:1479-1487.

60. Sokol DK. Ethics man: rethinking ward rounds. *BMJ.* 2009;338:571.

61. Yeo GSH, Lim ML. Maternal and fetal best interests in day-to-day obstetrics. *Ann Acad Med Singapore.* 2011;40:43-49.

62. Hatem M, Sandall J, Devane D, et al. Midwife-led versus other models of care for childbearing women. *Cochrane Database Syst Rev.* 2008;4(CD004667). doi: 10.1002/14651858.CD004667.pub2.

63. Newhouse RP, Stanik-Hutt J, White KM, et al. Advanced practice nurse outcomes 1990-2008: a systematic review. *Nurs Econ.* 2011;29(5):230-250.

64. American College of Nurse-Midwives. Evidence-based practice: pearls of midwifery: a presentation by the American College of Nurse-Midwives, Washington, DC, 2010. Available at: http://www.midwife.org /Pearls. Accessed December 11, 2012.

65. Carroli G, Mignini L. Episiotomy for vaginal birth. *Cochrane Database Syst Rev.* 2009;1:CD000081. doi: 10.1002/14651858.CD000081.pub2.

66. Albers LL, Schiff M, Gorwoda JG. The length of active labor in normal pregnancies. *Obstet Gynecol.* 1996;87:355-359.

67. Horta BL, Bahl R, Martines JC, Victoria CG. *Evidence on the Long-Term Effects of Breastfeeding: Systemic Review and Meta-analyses.* Geneva, Switzerland: World Health Organization; 2007. Available at: http://whqlibdoc.who.int/publications /2007/9789241595230_eng.pdf. Accessed November 6, 2012.

68. Mercer JS, Vohr BR, McGrath MM, et al. Delayed cord clamping in very preterm infants reduces the incidence of intraventricular hemorrhage and late-onset sepsis: a randomized, controlled trial. *Pediatrics.* 2006;117(4):1235-1242.

69. Moore ER, Anderson GC, Bergman N, Dowswell T. Early skin-to-skin contact for mothers and their healthy newborn infants. *Cochrane Database Syst Rev.* 2012;5:CD003519. doi: 10.1002/14651858. CD003519.pub3.

70. Cluett ER, Burns E. Immersion in water in labour and birth. *Cochrane Database Syst Rev.* 2009;2:CD000111. doi: 10.1002/14651858.CD000111.pub3.

71. Simkin PP, O'Hara M. Nonpharmacologic relief of pain during labor: systematic reviews of five methods. *Am J Obstet Gynecol.* 2002;186(suppl 5):S131-S159.

• • • Additional Resources

Professional Midwifery Organizations and Policy Statements

Accreditation Commission for Midwifery Education. Available at: http://www.midwife.org/Accreditation. Accessed December 14, 2012.

American Association of Birth Centers. Available at: http ://www.birthcenters.org. Accessed December 12, 2012.

American College of Nurse-Midwives. *Definition of Midwifery and Scope of Practice of Certified Nurse-Midwives and Certified Midwives.* Silver Springs, MD: American College of Nurse-Midwives; 2011.

American College of Nurse-Midwives, NACPM, MANA joint statement on physiologic childbirth. Available at: http://www.nacpm.org/documents/Normal-Physiologic -Birth-Statement.pdf. Accessed August 24, 2012.

American Midwifery Certification Board. Available at: http://www.amcbmidwife.org/index.php. Accessed December 12, 2012.

International Confederation of Midwives. Essential competencies for basic midwifery practice 2010. 2011. Available at: http://www.internationalmidwives.org/Portals/5/2011 /DB%202011/Essential%20Competencies%20ENG.pdf. Accessed November 6, 2012.

International Confederation of Midwives. Global standards for midwifery education 2010. 2011. Available at: http://www.internationalmidwives.org/Portals/5/2011 /DB%202011/MIDWIFERY%20EDUCATION%20 PREFACE%20&%20STANDARDS%20ENG.pdf. Accessed November 6, 2012.

International Confederation of Midwives. Global standards for midwifery regulation 2010. 2011. Available at: http://www.internationalmidwives.org/Portals/5/2011/Global%20Standards/GLOBAL%20STANDARDS%20FOR%20MIDWIFERY%20REGULATION%20ENG.pdf. Accessed November 6, 2012.

Midwives Alliance of North America. Core competencies for basic midwifery practice 2011. Available at: http://mana.org/manacore.html. Accessed December 12, 2012.

Midwives Alliance of North America. Direct-entry midwifery state-by-state legal status. May 11, 2011. Available at: http://mana.org/statechart.html. Accessed August 24, 2012.

National Association of Professional Midwives. Standards for practice. Available at: http://www.nacpm.org/index.html. Accessed December 12, 2012.

North American Registry of Midwives. History of CPM exam and date of first CPM certificate. Available at: http://narm.org/certification/history-of-the-development-of-the-cpm/. Accessed September 26, 2012.

Business of Midwifery

Fennel KS. Medicare billing for certified nurse-midwifery services. *OB-Gyn Coding Alert*. September 24, 2012. Available at: http://www.supercoder.com/coding-newsletters/my-ob-gyn-coding-alert/medicare-billing-for-certified-nurse-midwifery-services-article. Accessed December 13, 2012.

Slager J, ed. *An Administrative Manual for Midwifery Practices*. 3rd ed. Hebron, KY: Midwifery Business Network; 2006.

Improving Maternal Health

Day-Stirk F, Fauveau V. The state of the world's midwifery: making the invisible visible. *Int J Gynecol Obstet*. 2012;119:S39-S41.

Interprofessional Collaborative Practice

American College of Nurse-Midwives. *Collaborative Management in Midwifery Practice for Medical, Gynecological and Obstetrical Conditions*. Silver Springs, MD: American College of Nurse-Midwives; 1997.

American College of Nurse-Midwives. *Definition of Midwifery and Scope of Practice of Certified Nurse-Midwives and Certified Midwives*. Silver Springs, MD: American College of Nurse-Midwives; 2011.

Beckett DC, Kipnis G. Collaborative communication: integrating SBAR to improve quality/patient safety outcomes. *J Healthcare Qual*. 2009;31:19-28.

Dunsford J. Improving patient safety with SBAR. *Nurs Women's Health*. 2009;13(5):385-390.

Interprofessional Education Collaborative Expert Panel. *Core Competencies for Interprofessional Collaborative Practice: Report of an Expert Panel*. Washington, DC: Interprofessional Education Collaborative; 2011.

Kohn LT, Corrigan JM, Donaldson MS. *To Err Is Human: Building a Safer Health System*. Washington, DC: National Academy Press; 2000.

Veltman L, Larison K. PURE conversations: enhancing communication and teamwork. *J Healthcare Risk Manage*. 2007;27(2):41-45.

In addition, see the following themed journal issues:

Clinical Parameters of Midwifery Practice. *J Midwifery Women's Health*. 2000;49(6).

Collaborative Practice in Obstetrics and Gynecology. *Obstet Clin North Am*. 2012;39. This issue includes 12 articles that address interprofessional collaborative practice between midwives and other healthcare providers. Guest editors were Holly P. Kennedy, CNM, PhD, and Richard Waldman, MD.

Ethics in Midwifery

American College of Obstetricians and Gynecologists. *Informed Consent*. Committee Opinion no. 439. August 2009.

Chervenak FA, McCullough LB. The fetus as a patient: an essential ethical concept for maternal–fetal medicine. *J Matern Fetal Med*. 1996;5:115-119.

Kukla R, Kuppermann M, Little M, Lyerly AD. Finding autonomy in birth. *Bioethics*. 2009;23(1):1-8.

Sharp ES. Ethics in reproductive health care: a midwifery perspective. *J Nurse Midwifery*. 1998;43(3):235-245.

Thompson FE. Moving from codes of ethics to ethical relationships for midwifery practice. *Nurs Ethics*. 2002;9(5):522-536.

Vardaman JM, Cornell P, Gondo MB, et al. Beyond communication: the role of standardized protocols in a changing health care environment. *Health Care Manage Rev*. 2012;37(1):88-97.

In addition, see the following themed journal issues:

Ethics in Midwifery and Women's Health. *J Midwifery Women's Health*. 2004;49(3):173-280.

Evidence-Based Practice

Ip S, Chung M, Raman G, Chew P, et al. *Breastfeeding and Maternal and Infant Health Outcomes in Developed Countries*. Rockville, MD: Agency for Healthcare Research and Quality; 2007. Available at: http://www.ncbi.nlm.nih.gov/books/NBK38337. Accessed November 6, 2012.

Johnson KC, Davis BA. Outcomes of planned home births with certified professional midwives: large prospective study in North America. *BMJ*. 2005;330:1416.

McDonald SJ, Middleton P. Effect of timing of umbilical cord clamping of term infants on maternal and neonatal outcomes. *Cochrane Database Syst Rev*. 2008;2:CD004074. doi: 10.1002/14651858.CD004074.pub2.

CHAPTER

3

International Midwifery and Safe Motherhood

MARGARET A. MARSHALL

JOYCE E. THOMPSON

Introduction

Midwifery—"an ancient profession reborn in contemporary society"[1]—is by its very nature global. Midwives have been with women since the beginning of civilization and have been integral members of immigrant groups during migration to new lands. The professional midwifery workforce is responding to the needs of women today. The most compelling reason for understanding the international nature of midwifery is the ever-increasing demand for promoting basic human rights, especially for girls and women—including the right to a safe and secure reproductive life.[2,3]

Although midwifery practice in many parts of the world includes care of women through the entire lifespan, this chapter primarily focuses on midwifery during the maternity period because these skills are recognized as inherent components of midwifery practice. An overview of the reproductive health needs of women and girls in low-resource settings and the role of midwifery care in meeting women's needs globally is presented. A Safe Motherhood approach is described as an illustration of an international collaborative strategy that focuses on the global problem of maternal mortality. Midwives are the key health professionals in efforts to make pregnancy, birth, and the newborn period safe and to promote the health and well-being of girls and women worldwide.

The Health of Women and Children: The Foundation for a Nation's Health

Search for a Common Language

The health of a nation is directly related to maternal and child health. To describe and compare health statistics, a common language must be used. **Table 3-1** lists the terms and definitions of key health indices that are used by all countries to report measures of reproductive health.[4-7]

Controversy exists regarding collection and interpretation of data within countries. For example, in countries with weak surveillance and vital records systems, rates are calculated through mathematical modeling with wide confidence intervals. As surveillance systems continue to improve through personnel training and improved web-based and e-mobile data collection systems, the quality of data should improve markedly. Unfortunately, many women never enter the healthcare system during pregnancy, even when gravely ill and, therefore, deaths and disabilities are not well captured in vital statistics, surveillance data, or other records. When making comparisons over time or from one country to another, it is important to know not only the standard definition of a measure, but also how the statistics are collected and reported within the country.[7]

Maternal Mortality Rate and Maternal Mortality Ratio

In 1997, the World Health Organization(WHO) International Classification of Diseases revised the

Table 3-1	Maternal/Child Health Indices
Term	**Definition and Explanations**
Maternal mortality	Death of a woman while pregnant or within 42 days of termination of pregnancy, irrespective of the duration and the site of pregnancy, from any cause related to or aggravated by the pregnancy itself or its management, but not from accidental or incidental causes.[5]
Accidental or incidental causes of maternal mortality	Those causes that result in death irrespective of pregnancy, such as traffic accidents, gunshot wounds, and poisonings.
Late maternal death	"Death of a woman from direct or indirect obstetric causes, more than 42 days but less than one year after termination of pregnancy." This designation is used more frequently in developed countries where the technology permits keeping the woman alive more than 42 days, even though her death is related to childbirth.[5]
Direct obstetrical death/ direct maternal deaths	"Deaths resulting from obstetrical complications of the pregnancy state (pregnancy, labor, and puerperium), from interventions, omissions, incorrect treatment, or from a chain of events resulting from any of the above." In the 2012 modification to the WHO International Classification of Diseases (ICD10), deaths from suicide, puerperal psychosis, and postpartum depression were moved to the category of direct maternal deaths, although this definition has not yet been universally adopted.
Indirect obstetric deaths	Deaths resulting from previous existing disease or disease that developed during pregnancy and that were not due to direct causes, but were aggravated by physiologic effects of pregnancy.
Maternal mortality rate	The number of women who die while pregnant or within the first 42 days after pregnancy, from any cause related to or aggravated by pregnancy, per 100,000 women of reproductive age in a given year. This rate is difficult to obtain and often not used in low-resource areas such as developing countries.[5]
Maternal mortality ratio	"Number of women who die while pregnant or up to and including 42 days after giving birth, from any cause related to or aggravated by pregnancy, per 100,000 live births in a given year." The ratio is the method most commonly used to express trends within a country and to make cross-country comparisons.
Lifetime risk of maternal death	"Risk of an individual woman dying from pregnancy or childbirth during her life and calculated by multiplying the maternal mortality rate by 30, or the number of years of exposure to pregnancy between ages 15 and 44." Calculations are based on maternal mortality and fertility rates in the country.[7,8] This method recognizes that women of high fertility or women lacking in universal access to effective family planning have an extremely high risk of dying as a result of pregnancy or childbirth as they are repeatedly exposed to the risk of pregnancy.
Incidence	Measure of the number of individuals in a population who have developed a new condition within a particular period in time—for example, the number of births in the United States in 2012. The measure can be expressed as absolute number, percentage, or ratio.
Prevalence	Measure of the number of individuals in a population found to have a specific condition. Prevalence is calculated by comparing the number of people found to have the condition to the total number of people studied—for example, the percentage of pregnant women who are currently HIV positive in a country. Prevalence is usually expressed as a percentage or the number of cases per 10,000 or 100,000 individuals.
Unmet need for family planning	A calculation derived from identifying the number of women, either married or in a union, who are not using contraception, are fertile, and desire to stop childbearing/postpone next birth for at least 2 years, plus the number of currently pregnant or postpartum women who are carrying an unwanted or mistimed pregnancy, plus women in postpartum amenorrhea who are not using contraception and, at the time they became pregnant, had wanted to delay or prevent the pregnancy, divided by total number of women of reproductive age (15–49 years) who are married or in a union, with total multiplied by 100.
Neonatal morality rate	Number of deaths of a newborn in the first 28 days of life per 1000 live births.

Table 3-1	Maternal/Child Health Indices *(continued)*
Term	**Definition and Explanations**
Infant mortality rate	Number of infants dying before reaching 1 year of life per 1000 live births in a given year.
Perinatal mortality rate[a]	The sum of fetal deaths (more than 20 weeks' gestation) plus neonatal deaths (within the first 28 days after birth) during a year divided by the sum of live births plus fetal deaths during that year. Expressed per 1000 live births plus fetal deaths.
Under-5 mortality rate	Probability that an infant will die before reaching the age of 5 if subject to current age-specific mortality rates, per 1000 live births.

[a]There are three definitions of perinatal death rate in use today. One uses neonatal deaths within 7 days, one uses neonatal death within 28 days, and one uses fetal death as a gestation more than 28 weeks.

Sources: Adapted from World Health Organization. *International Classification of Diseases.* Geneva, Switzerland: WHO; 1987:9; Pattinson R, Say L, Souza JP, Van den Broek N, Rooney C, on behalf of the WHO Working Group on Maternal Mortality and Morbidity Classifications. WHO maternal death and near-miss classifications. *Bull WHO.* 2009;877:734; Barfield WD and the Committee on Fetus and Newborn. Standard terminology for fetal, infant, and perinatal deaths. *Pediatrics.* 2011;128:177-181; Herz B, Measham AR. *The Safe Motherhood Initiative: Proposals for Action.* World Bank Discussion Paper No. 9. Washington, DC: World Bank; 1987.

definition of maternal mortality *rate* to include deaths within 1 full year, instead of 42 days, after the termination of pregnancy. Due to the difficulty in obtaining this information, most countries do not use the 1-year rate; instead, 42 days is utilized. The advantage of using the maternal mortality rate (rather than the ratio) is that it compares maternal deaths with all women in a given population who are at risk of dying related to pregnancy. In a society with a reliable system of gathering data, the maternal mortality rate accurately reflects deaths that are related to a pregnancy.

In most developing countries, however, the census data are too old or inaccurate for use in maternal mortality rates or one of the terms used in the calculation may be defined differently. The term "reproductive age" is used in the denominator to calculate the maternal mortality rate. Countries use a variety of age ranges—for example, 10–54 years, 15–54 years, or 15–49 years—to define reproductive age, thereby limiting comparability of data.

Because the maternal mortality rate is difficult to obtain, the maternal mortality *ratio* (MMR) is used more frequently. The MMR is the number of maternal deaths per 100,000 live births in a given period of time. Births are comparatively easy to count compared to the number of women who are of reproductive age. Therefore, the MMR is the method most commonly used to express trends within a country and to make cross-country comparisons, especially in developing countries and/or low-resource sites. Betrán et al. conducted a systematic review of maternal mortality in 141 countries.[8] Using standard regression models, they found that (1) the proportion of births assisted by a skilled attendant, (2) the infant mortality rate, and (3) national per capita expenditures on health were three factors strongly related to maternal mortality

worldwide.[9] **Figure 3-1** provides a map illustrating the global maternal mortality ratios in 2010.[10]

The WHO International Classification of Diseases (ICD10) was modified again in 2012. Deaths resulting from suicide, puerperal psychosis, and postpartum depression were moved to the category of direct maternal deaths. Many countries have not adopted this new recommendation, especially given that it inflates the numerator used to calculate mortality ratios. Therefore, two ratios may be reported for some countries.[6]

Another way in which multicountry analysis of maternal mortality can be expressed is lifetime risk. The lifetime risk of maternal death is simply the risk of an individual woman dying from pregnancy or childbirth during her life. The MMR is multiplied by 30, the number of years of exposure to pregnancy between ages 15 and 44. A lifetime risk of 1 in 3000 represents a low risk of dying from pregnancy and childbirth, while 1 in 100 is a high risk.[7,8] **Table 3-2** presents regional data on the lifetime risk of a woman dying during her childbearing years.[10]

As difficult as it is to obtain accurate maternal mortality data, morbidity data collection is even more elusive. Mortality data measure a single event or incidence. Morbidity data, by comparison, is much less likely to be recorded, suffers from a lack of standard case definitions, and frequently involves several comorbidities (e.g., one woman with multiple conditions such as severe anemia, vesico-vaginal fistula, repeated urinary tract infections, and clinical depression).

Lack of clear definitions can adversely affect a woman's health. Definitions are crucial because they dictate which treatment protocol will be used. Some terms do not have a standard definition that is shared

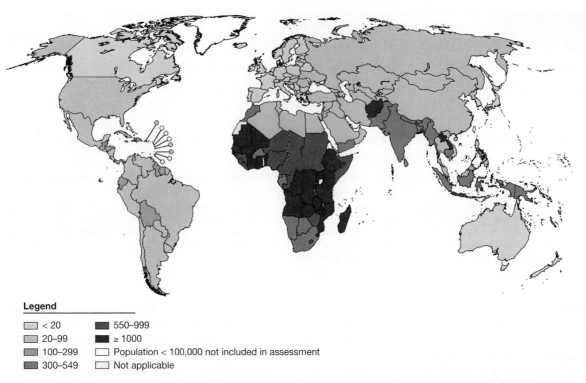

Legend

☐ < 20	■ 550–999
☐ 20–99	■ ≥ 1000
■ 100–299	☐ Population < 100,000 not included in assessment
■ 300–549	☐ Not applicable

The boundaries and names shown and the designations used on this map do not imply the expression of any opinion whatsoever on the part of the WHO concerning the legal status of any country, territory, city or area or of its authorities, or concerning the delimitation of its frontiers or boundaries.
Dotted lines and dashed lines on maps represent approximate border lines for which there may not yet be full agreement.

Figure 3-1 Maternal mortality ratio (per 100,000 live births), 2010.
Source: Data from: *Trends in Maternal Mortality: 1990-2010.* www.who.int/reproductivehealth/publications/monitoring/9789241503631/en/index .html. Figure 1, page 33. Used by permission. Map image © iStockphoto/Thinkstock

by other countries. Other terms, such as "postpartum hemorrhage," have a standard definition (i.e., more than 500 mL blood loss), but the definition is inadequate to designate morbidity or cause of mortality. A woman entering labor with a hemoglobin level of 12 g/dL may tolerate blood loss of 500 mL with few symptoms, yet another woman entering labor with a hemoglobin of 46 g may die after a 300 mL blood loss.

Data regarding women of reproductive age who are not pregnant also can be difficult to obtain. Estimates of unmet family planning needs are directly associated with poor reproductive outcomes in a country.[10] Despite considerable advances in the provision of both modern and traditional family planning services over the past 50 years, millions of women in the developing world who desire to delay or avoid pregnancy are not using any family planning method, largely because they do not have access, they fear side effects, or their families object. These women are not accessing care and, therefore, numbers that reflect the magnitude of the problem are difficult to obtain.

Health indices are important reflections of a country's neonatal/infant/child health as well. Children represent the future of a country, and their health is an important predictor for the health of a nation. Common measurements include newborn or infant mortality rates based on age. As with maternal measurements, neonatal morbidity often is difficult to identify. Some of the more common diseases that result in death of a child in developing countries are rarely major problems in developed countries. Malaria, malnutrition, and neonatal tetanus, for example, can be fatal simply depending upon where a child is born.

Maternal Mortality: The Global Situation

Since 1982, WHO has systematically reviewed indexed medical literature, non-indexed publications, and reports from national and local authorities regarding maternal mortality and maternity care

Table 3-2	Estimates of Women's Lifetime Risk of Death from Pregnancy and Childbirth by United Nations Millennium Development Goal Region, 2010
Region	**Lifetime Risk of Maternal Death**
World	1 in 180
Developed regions	1 in 3800
Developing regions	1 in 150
Sub-Saharan Africa	1 in 39
Latin America and Caribbean	1 in 520
Eastern Asia[a]	1 in 1700
Southern Asia[b]	1 in 160
Southeastern Asia[c]	1 in 290
Western Asia[d]	1 in 430

[a]China, Democratic People's Republic of Korea, Mongolia, Republic of Korea.

[b]Afghanistan, Bangladesh, Bhutan, India, Iran (Islamic Republic of), Maldives, Nepal, Pakistan, Sri Lanka.

[c]Cambodia, Indonesia, Lao People's Democratic Republic, Malaysia, Myanmar, Philippines, Singapore, Thailand, Timor-Leste, Vietnam.

[d]Bahrain, Iraq, Jordan, Kuwait, Lebanon, Oman, Qatar, Saudi Arabia, Syrian Arab Republic, Turkey, United Arab Emirates, West Bank and Gaza Strip (territory), Yemen.

Source: Adapted from World Health Organization, UNICEF, United Nations Fund for Population Activities. Trends in maternal morbidity and mortality 1990–2010. Available at: http://www.who.int /reproductivehealth/publications/monitoring/9789241503631 /en/index.html. Accessed December 25, 2012.

BOX 3-1 Brief Facts Regarding Maternal Death

- Ninety-nine percent of all maternal deaths occur in developing countries.
- Maternal mortality is higher in women living in rural areas and among poorer communities.
- Young adolescents face a higher risk of complications and death as a result of pregnancy compared to older women.
- Every day, approximately 800 women die from preventable causes related to pregnancy and childbirth.
- More than half of all maternal deaths occur in sub-Saharan Africa, and almost one-third occur in South Asia.
- The maternal mortality ratio in developing countries is 240 per 100,000 live births versus 16 per 100,000 in developed countries.
- A woman's lifetime risk of maternal death is 1 in 150 in developing countries versus 1 in 3800 in developed countries.
- Skilled care before, during, and after childbirth can save the lives of women and newborns.
- Only 46% of women in low-income countries benefit from skilled care during childbirth. This means that millions of births are not attended by a midwife, a physician, or a trained nurse.
- Maternal health and newborn health are closely linked. More than 3 million newborns die every year, and an additional 26 million fetuses are stillborn.

Source: Adapted from World Health Organization. Maternal mortality fact sheet. Fact sheet No. 348. May 2012. Available at: http://www.who.int/mediacentre/factsheets/fs348/en /index.html. Accessed September 12, 2012.

coverage worldwide. In 1996, WHO reported that almost 600,000 women died of pregnancy-related causes per year, most of which were preventable.[11,12] Since then, maternal mortality has dropped by almost 50%, yet approximately 800 women die every day from preventable causes related to pregnancy and childbirth, with 99% of these women dying in developing countries.[13] Today, more than 50% of maternal deaths occur in just six countries: India, Nigeria, Pakistan, Afghanistan, Ethiopia, and Democratic Republic of the Congo.[14] Box 3-1 presents brief facts regarding maternal and newborn health on a global scale.

Causes of Maternal Mortality

In developing countries, the five major direct causes of maternal death are (1) hemorrhage, (2) sepsis, (3) pregnancy-induced hypertension, (4) unsafe abortion, and (5) obstructed labor.[15] However, when considering maternal mortality, a far wider scope of health problems, including maternal trauma, chronic disease, and reduced energy output, have profound ramifications for the woman, her family, and the economy, and these influences cannot be ignored. Worldwide, women die during pregnancy from diseases for which prevention and treatment strategies exist. For example, in Nigeria, 11% of maternal deaths are caused by malaria.[16] Other common causes of death in women include tetanus, tuberculosis, and HIV/AIDS. In 2011, approximately 34.2 million individuals worldwide were HIV positive, of whom only 8 million were receiving antiretroviral therapy.

Of the estimated 1.5 million pregnant women living with HIV, 57% received effective antiretroviral drugs to avoid mother-to-child transmission. Without antiretroviral therapy, the mother-to-child transmission rate ranges from 15% to 45%—a consequence that could be prevented or significantly decreased.[17]

A Destiny of Reproductive Risk

For many women, their destiny of reproductive risk begins at birth. Health risks for women are potentiated or increased by culture, education, geography, and low social status.[18] Lack of education prevents girls and women from reaching their full potential, and healthcare access and treatments can be limited for females. When the education, class, religion, race, or dominant language of the healthcare provider and the woman differ, misunderstandings, disrespect, and abuse become relatively common.[19]

Cultural factors that limit access to care tend to be poorly documented. Use of faith healers, local herbs, over-the-counter treatments, and unqualified practitioners who claim unearned health credentials can complicate access to appropriate care in a timely fashion. When individuals believe disease is caused by black magic or lack of faith, orthodox medical services based on belief in the germ theory are not seen as a solution. Cultural factors also include the existing norms that denigrate the status of women, with the consequence of interfering with a woman's decisions regarding health care.

The Road to Maternal Death: Unmet Family Planning Needs

Women who are unable to access the family planning and control the child spacing they desire can have many unintended pregnancies. An estimated 47,000 women die as a result of unsafe abortions every year. Unsafe abortions account for approximately 13% of total maternal mortality every year, and the annual unsafe abortion rate (14 per 1000 women age 15–49) remained unchanged from 1990 to 2008. It is estimated that approximately one-third of maternal deaths could be prevented by universal access to effective family planning.[20]

Not only does unintended pregnancy expose women to all the usual risks of pregnancy complications and ultimately death, but evidence indicates that as abortion laws become increasingly restrictive (e.g., in Central America and Peru) deaths from suicide—particularly among adolescents—rise. Ongoing studies are seeking to evaluate the strength of this association.[21] In 2012, women in sub-Saharan Africa accounted for 59% of all women with unmet needs for family planning services and 91% of unintended pregnancies.[22] Addressing the unmet need for modern family planning would result in 26 million fewer induced abortions every year in the developing world.[23]

The Three Delays

Once an obstetric emergency occurs, its cause can be analyzed within the framework of the "three delays," which collectively prevent timely, high-quality care from reaching those most in need:

1. Delay in recognition that there is a problem and making the decision to seek care
2. Delay in reaching the appropriate level of care once the problem or complication has been recognized
3. Delay in receiving the appropriate care after arrival at the service site[24]

Box 3-2 illustrates the reality of delays that midwives in resource-poor settings encounter on a daily basis.

Factors related to inadequate supplies, transport to a referral center, surgical capability, blood banks, and money with which to access available healthcare services contribute to poor outcomes for women in developing countries. These factors have been categorized as the "enabling environment or system of care," as distinct from the person who provides needed care.[25] When a supportive environment is available, skilled providers may render safe, high-quality care in any site: home, maternity home, birth center, health post, district hospital, or referral hospital. The supportive environment at each level of care plays an important role in rendering emergency obstetric services when required; in its absence, no site is as safe as it might be. In summary, maternal mortality represents only the tip of the mountain of health problems for women, even as it provides an important surrogate for the health of the nation.

Unintended Consequences of Maternal Mortality: Child Mortality

Child mortality is intimately related to maternal mortality and morbidity, especially for neonates. In 2011, 6.9 million children under 5 years of age worldwide died, which translates into approximately 19,000 children each day or almost 800 every hour. Progress on this front has been made in recent decades, but, similar to the problem of maternal mortality, progress in reducing child mortality is unequally distributed across regions and countries and within countries. Ten countries have been recognized as being responsible for two-thirds of stillbirths, neonatal,

---

BOX 3-2 Voice of a West African Midwife

The patient was a 36-year-old gravida 4 para 3 with one live baby. She had been attended since 12 weeks of pregnancy. (She was my friend and came from this very village.) The patient came in with labor pains at 6 p.m. onset. 1 p.m. P.V. [vaginal examination] done. Os was 2 cm dilated. Membranes intact. Labor progressed well. Patient delivered spontaneously a live female infant at 1:15 a.m. The placenta appeared to be complete but the membranes were ragged. Patient started bleeding. IV 500 cc set up with Pitocin. External bimanual compression done without effect. Manual removal [uterine exploration] done. Only blood clots expelled. Internal bimanual compression done without effect. Another IV 1000 mL set up and the patient was transferred. There were transportation difficulties and the road is very bad. It took us 4 hours 10 minutes to travel a 35 km journey. The patient received 2500 mL of IV fluids but very unfortunately the IV got infiltrated on the way; but due to the bad road I could not get the vein. All attempts to start the IV again failed. The patient expired at the hospital before the doctor arrived. EBL 2500 cc. I collapsed at the hospital. They gave me Valium 20 mg and put me in a bed. I was not aware for some time. I cried and felt very bad. They talked to me and explained that they sometimes have such women die at their hospital with everything. I did not feel confident and competent. Sometimes when I think about it now I cry.

This rural midwife trained in Life-Saving Skills had organized the traditional birth attendants in the seven villages around her to come to her maternity home for continuing education and to refer their patients with problems. Note that once the bad road was graded, travel time was decreased from 4 hours 10 minutes to less than an hour and a half.

Source: Marshall MA. Ghana Registered Midwives Association continuing education project—Carnegie Corporation grant B SOU, final evaluation report. Unpublished evaluation of Life-Saving Skills Training Project, 1992. [Permission given by midwife for publication of her story.]

---

and maternal deaths (**Table 3-3**), and intensive philanthropic attention has been focused on this subset of high-priority countries.[26]

Maternal Death in the United States Today

Most pregnant women in the United States can anticipate a safe birth and healthy newborn. However, in 2007 (the latest year for which data are available), there were 548 maternal deaths in the United States. Although markedly lower than the ratio seen in developing countries, this number represents a maternal mortality ratio of 12.7, almost double the ratio of 6.6 identified in 1987. The etiology of this increase in maternal deaths (**Figure 3-2**) is not totally understood.[27] Changes in coding and classification of maternal deaths over the years are likely to account for part of the increase, but other factors may include differences in pregnancy-related conditions, and access to and use of high-quality services.[28] Major racial disparities in maternal mortality have existed since the 1940s.[29,30] Non-Hispanic black women die at almost three times the rate of non-Hispanic white women.

The major direct causes of maternal death in the United States are hypertension (preeclampsia, eclampsia), hemorrhage of pregnancy, placenta previa, and abortions. The indirect causes of death usually are preexisting medical conditions that complicate pregnancy.[31] For example, the increasing rates of obesity and type 2 diabetes in the United States have ramifications for women who become pregnant.

Compared to other countries, the United States ranks 39th globally in maternal mortality ratio, in contrast to Australia (4), Japan (9), and Canada (11). The increases in MMR in the United States are matched by rising mortality ratios in Afghanistan, Zimbabwe, and eight low-income countries, as well as the developed nations of Canada and Norway.[15]

Strategies Designed to Reduce Maternal Mortality

Countries and groups worldwide have developed strategies designed to decrease the numbers of women dying from preventable causes. Foremost among these are the Millennium Development Goals (MDG) and Safe Motherhood Initiatives. Other strategies have been more focused on specific aspects of the problem, such as increasing numbers of midwives or other skilled providers.

Table 3-3	Top Ten Countries for Absolute Number of Stillbirths, Maternal Deaths, and Neonatal Deaths, 2008		
	Rank for Number of Stillbirths	Rank for Number of Maternal Deaths	Rank for Number of Neonatal Deaths
India	1	1	1
Nigeria	2	2	2
Pakistan	3	7	3
China	4	12	4
Bangladesh	5	8	7
Democratic Republic of the Congo	6	3	5
Ethiopia	7	5	6
Indonesia	8	9	8
Tanzania	9	6	10
Afghanistan	10	4	9
Total	1.8 million stillbirths— 66% of worldwide total	221,000 maternal deaths— 62% of worldwide total	2.4 million neonatal deaths— 67% of worldwide total

Source: Reprinted with permission from Lawn JE, Blencowe D, Pattinson R, et al. for *The Lancet*'s Stillbirths Series steering committee. Stillbirths: Where? When? Why? How to make the data count? *Lancet.* 2011;377:1448-1463.

Millennium Development Goals

In 2000, the leaders of 189 members states of the United Nations' (UN) General Assembly issued a Millennium Declaration that addressed the principles of human dignity, equality and equity, peace and security and disarmament, poverty eradication, gender equality and empowerment of women, human rights, democracy and good governance, protecting the common environment and protecting the vulnerable, such as women and children.[32] Eight goals[33] with concrete benchmarks (targets) for tackling the effects of extreme poverty were approved; these eight MDGs are listed in **Box 3-3**. Goals 4, 5, and 6 are generally considered the "health" goals. However, goals 1, 2, and 3 also are integral for the improvement of the overall health of women and their newborns/children.[34–36]

The targets for each MDG can be found on the United Nations website, along with the progress made to date, including predictions regarding which countries will meet each target by 2015.[37] Sub-Saharan Africa and South Asia are falling short of the targets, especially in maternal health.[38,39] The MDG targets for goals 4 and 5 listed in **Box 3-4** include the reduction of maternal mortality by 75% between 1990 and 2015.

The development and use of the MDGs represents a critical step toward organizing, implementing, and evaluating different strategies to decrease maternal and child mortality and morbidity. These goals provide the focus for specific interventions and collaborations among interested parties and enhance political will. Nevertheless, it has become clear that reducing the number of maternal and child deaths will not be a simple undertaking, nor is there a magic bullet to solve the problem.

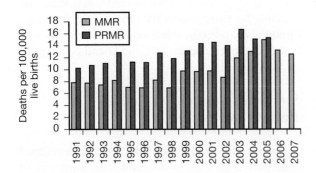

Figure 3-2 Maternal mortality ratios (MMRs), 1991–2007, and pregnancy-related mortality rates (PRMRs), 1991–2005, United States.
Source: Reprinted with permission from Callaghan WM. Overview of maternal mortality in the United States. *Semin Perinatol.* 2012;36(1): 2-6.

BOX 3-3 Millennium Development Goals

1. Eradicate extreme poverty and hunger
2. Achieve universal primary education
3. Promote gender equality and empower women
4. Reduce child mortality
5. Improve maternal health
6. Combat HIV/AIDS, malaria, and other diseases
7. Ensure environmental sustainability
8. Develop global partnership for development

Source: Adapted from *The Millennium Development Goals Report 2013*. Available at: http://www.un.org/millennium goals/pdf/report-2013/mdg-report-2013-english.pdf. Accessed July 6, 2013.

BOX 3-4 Targets of Millennium Development Goals 4 and 5

Goal 4: Reduce Child Mortality

Target 4.A: Reduce by two-thirds, between 1990 and 2015, the under-5 mortality rate.

Goal 5: Improve Maternal Health

Target 5.A: Reduce by three quarters, between 1990 and 2015, the maternal mortality ratio.

Target 5.B: Achieve, by 2015, universal access to reproductive health.

Source: Adapted from Millennium Development Goals indicators. Available at: http://mdgs.un.org/unsd/mdg/host .aspx?Content=indicators/officiallist.htm. Accessed December 25, 2012.

Safe Motherhood Initiatives

"Safe Motherhood" is a term commonly used in the global community. However, there is no full definition of the concept. The following is the authors' contemporary definition that combines several found in the literature over the years and their own international work:

> Safe Motherhood begins with the basic human right of having it be safe to be a girl and a woman in any society. This means that no woman should die or be harmed by pregnancy or birth. Therefore, Safe Motherhood requires availability, acceptability, and easy access to a competent healthcare provider for a woman's prenatal, birth, postpartum, family planning, and other reproductive health needs. It also requires an enabling environment of care for childbearing with a functional health system, adequate supplies and equipment, transport to referral facilities when needed, timely evidence-based action taken to address any threat to the life of the woman or her newborn, and the political will to make the health of childbearing women and newborns a priority.

Table 3-4 lists the key organizations that promote and work toward Safe Motherhood internationally. Some consortia have been formed to address Safe Motherhood directly; other organizations have expanded into the area of reduction of maternal deaths in their quests to promote health, social justice, and other related projects.

Specific Strategies for Reducing Global Maternal and Neonatal Mortality

A Skilled Provider at Birth

The inverse correlation between presence of a skilled birth attendants and maternal mortality is well established.[40] One of the process indicators used to measure progress in attaining the MDG goals 4 and 5 is the proportion of births attended by skilled personnel.[41,42] However, it is not expected that the MDG goals will be met given that the current decline in MMR is approximately 3.1% annually.[43] This fact has resulted in mobilized resources and policies designed to increase the number of fully qualified midwives.

Currently only 54% of women globally have access to skilled care during childbirth.[45] In some countries today, only 1 in 5 women have a skilled attendant present at their birth.[44,46] Persons who are skilled providers are those who have midwifery skills (physicians, midwives, or nurses), whether or not they are educated as midwives.[46] An important distinction differentiates between a *trained* provider and a *skilled* provider. A trained provider may have as little formal education as a 5-day training program for a traditional birth attendant (TBA) and may not consistently recognize emergencies or have the skills to manage an obstetric emergency.

Historically, much time and effort have been invested in the training of TBAs, based on the theory that TBAs are an available resource and that this investment would lower the incidence of maternal deaths. More than 30 years of study has shown that such training has not contributed significantly to a

Table 3-4	Organizations Promoting Safe Motherhood	
Organization	**Purpose/Mission/Goal**	**Comments**
World Health Organization (WHO) 1948–present	Attainment by all people of the highest possible level of health.	Founding member of Safe Motherhood Initiative. Board member of PMNCH. Tracks indicators of maternal/newborn/child health. Provides practice guidelines for sexual and reproductive health.
International Confederation of Midwives (ICM) 1919–present	To advance worldwide the goals and aspirations of midwives in the attainment of improved outcomes for women, their newborns, and families during the childbearing cycle, using the ICM midwifery philosophy and model of care.	Sets standards for international midwifery: Core Documents (e.g., *Definition of a Midwife*) and other resources. Involved in global Safe Motherhood initiatives since 1987. Board member of PMNCH. Joint statement on skilled birth attendants.
International Federation of Gynecology and Obstetrics (FIGO) 1954–present	To promote the well-being of women and to raise the standard of practice in obstetrics and gynecology.	FIGO Save the Mothers Fund Project and the FIGO-LOGIC Gates project. Board member of PMNCH. Publishes *State of World's Women* annually.
American College of Nurse-Midwives (ACNM) 1955–present *Department of Global Outreach* 1981–present *Safe Motherhood Initiative-USA* 1997–early 2000s	Midwives working to strengthen midwifery globally as a means to promote the health and well-being of women and infants worldwide. Safe Motherhood begins with having it be safe to be a girl and a woman in our society.	International resources: • *Life-Saving Skills Manual for Midwives* • *Home-Based Life Saving Skills* Strengthen midwifery associations globally and other technical assistance. Partnership to advocate for reduction of needless maternal deaths in the United States.
Safe Motherhood Interagency Group (IAG) 1987–2003 Partnership for Maternal and Newborn Health (PMNH) 2003–2004 Child Survival Partnership (CS) 2004–2005	To mobilize and inform governments and others on the continuing problem of maternal and newborn mortality and disability in many areas of the world. To offer strategic directions, expert technical advice, and informational resources to promote maternal–newborn health. To promote child health throughout the world.	Evolving partnerships of key stakeholders concerned with maternal and newborn health, then child health, globally. Provide expert technical advice, advocacy, and support primarily for resource-poor nations. Family Care International (FCI) created a website to serve as repository of resources on Safe Motherhood, along with fact sheets and briefing cards. Currently FCI is the lead partner responsible for PMNCH's advocacy activities.
Partnership for Maternal, Newborn, and Child Health (PMNCH) 2005–present	To mobilize and monitor political will, global resources, and effective interventions in support of health systems and communities to improve survival and well-being of women, newborns, and children.	Partners: More than 350 worldwide. 14-member board: UN agencies, bilateral donors, Ministries of Health, foundations, NGOs, academics, and international maternal–child health associations. Emphasis is on country-led, country-driven initiatives with increased commitment to primary health care and human rights. Two-dimensional continuum of care: (1) Time: adolescence through motherhood and (2) Place: households to communities to health facilities.

Table 3-4	Organizations Promoting Safe Motherhood *(continued)*	
Organization	**Purpose/Mission/Goal**	**Comments**
United Nations (UN) 1948–present	In 2000, 189 member states agreed to the Millennium Declaration.	Adopted eight MDGs with specific targets for measurement of progress and benchmarks for achievement by 2015.
		MDGs 4 (child health) and 5 (maternal health) directly address health of women and children.
		MDGs 1–3 indirectly address the health of women and children.
White Ribbon Alliance (WRA) for Safe Motherhood 1999–present	To raise awareness of the need to make pregnancy and childbirth safe for all women in both developed and developing countries.	International coalition of more than 150 countries and 15 national alliances.
		The white ribbon symbol is dedicated to the memory of all girls and women who have died needlessly in pregnancy and childbirth.
Women Deliver conferences 2007–present	Global advocacy organization bringing together voices from around the world to call for action to improve the health and well-being of girls and women.	Theme: "Invest in women—It pays!"
		Conferences (2007, 2010, 2013) bring education, health, development, equity, human rights, poverty reduction, and micro-finance sectors together to mobilize increased funding allocations for maternal health.

MDG = Millennium Development Goal; NGO = nongovernmental organization.

reduction in maternal mortality for births that take place in the home.[45,46] However, there is limited evidence that indicates the number of stillbirths and newborn deaths is reduced when TBAs refer women to higher levels of care prenatally and for birth.[47] It is important to understand that these findings are not an indictment of TBAs. It is unreasonable to expect that community women, no matter how skilled and loving, can effect great change when working within a system riddled with poor transportation, lack of emergency funds, inadequate blood safety, and poor referral institutions. The improvement of maternity care is a systemic problem requiring multiple levels of preparedness and active community awareness and participation.

Many nations have promoted moving childbirth into institutions as an answer to maternal mortality. But experience has shown that the site of birth is not the critical factor. The linchpin of improved maternal outcomes is introducing skilled providers at every level of care. However, even the presence of a skilled provider, although essential, is not sufficient to save women's lives without an enabling environment of care.

Preventing Neonatal Morbidity/Mortality

Each year approximately 4 million neonatal deaths occur globally, accounting for 40% of all deaths of children younger than 5 years of age. Approximately 85% of newborn deaths are due to infections, birth trauma, and prematurity. The remaining deaths result from a variety of causes, including 7% due to neonatal tetanus. Thus 450 newborns die every hour from conditions that are largely preventable with well-known low-technology interventions.[27] There is a core of evidence-based interventions that impacts newborn mortality. If applied with 99% coverage, these care interventions could reduce newborn mortality by 72%. Such interventions include kangaroo care (skin-to-skin contact) for premature infants, use of corticosteroids for women in premature labor, exclusive breastfeeding, clean birth practices, and community case management for close newborn follow-up.[47]

Approximately 50% of neonatal deaths occur in the first 24 hours of life, and 75% of deaths occur in the first week of life (**Figure 3-3**).[48] **Table 3-5** summarizes strategies to improve newborn health.[49,50]

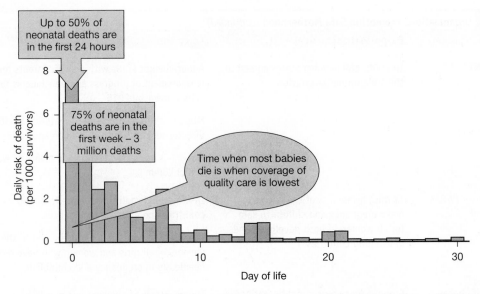

Deaths in first 24 hours are recorded as occurring on day 0 or possibly day 1, depending on the interpretation of the question and coding of the response. Preference for reporting certain days (7, 14, 21, and 30) is apparent.

Figure 3-3 Neonatal deaths by day for first month of life.
Source: Adapted from Lawn JE, Cousens S, Zupan J; Lancet Neonatal Survival Steering Team. 4 million neonatal deaths: When? Where? Why? *Lancet.* 2005;365(9462):891-900.

Global Partners Involved in Safe Motherhood Initiatives

Safe Motherhood Interagency Group

The worldwide Safe Motherhood Inter-Agency Group (IAG) was launched in 1987 in Nairobi, Kenya. The goal of this groundbreaking meeting was to raise awareness, alert the international community to the silent tragedy of maternal mortality, and mobilize efforts and resources on behalf of women. At the 1990 World Summit for Children, 166 nations signed on to the action plan goals, one of which was to reduce maternal mortality by 50% by the year 2000.[51]

The founding members of IAG included WHO, UNICEF, the United Nations Fund for Population Activities (UNFPA), the World Bank, the Population Council, and the International Planned Parenthood Federation. In 1999, a decision was made to add the two major health professional groups, the International Confederation of Midwives (ICM) and the International Federation of Gynecology and Obstetrics (FIGO), as well as two regional Safe Motherhood groups. The Secretariat for the IAG was located at Family Care International in New York City and has been housed at WHO in Geneva, Switzerland, since the group was expanded into the current Partnership for Maternal, Newborn and Child Health in 2005.

The primary objectives of the various Safe Motherhood partnerships are to mobilize and inform governments and others about the continuing problem of maternal and newborn mortality and disability in many areas of the world; to offer strategic directions for intervention to promote maternal, newborn, and child health based on expert technical advice; and to provide a variety of informational tools and resources, such as fact sheets and briefing cards, which can be used to promote Safe Motherhood and newborn health throughout the world.

In 1998, a meeting in Colombo, Sri Lanka, was held to celebrate the 10th anniversary of the global Safe Motherhood Initiative. The focus of this meeting was to identify those interventions that had been successful in reducing maternal death and disability, to define needs and priorities including cost-effective strategies, and to determine future action needed to promote safer pregnancy and birth in the world (**Box 3-5**). These strategies remain relevant today.[52]

The 10 action messages have been used to focus subsequent Safe Motherhood IAG activities, beginning with an emphasis on skilled attendance at birth and later adding an emphasis on the prevention of unsafe abortion. Since 2007, these advocacy Safe

Table 3-5	Strategies to Improve Newborn Health
Time in Childbearing Cycle	**Special Attention**
Care of Future Pregnancies	
Improve the health and status of women	Promote safer sexual practices
Improve the nutrition of girls	Provide opportunities for female education
Discourage early marriage and early childbearing	
Care During Pregnancy	
Improve the nutrition of pregnant women	Monitor and treat pregnancy complications such as anemia, preeclampsia, and bleeding
Immunize against tetanus	
Screen and treat infections, especially syphilis and malaria	Promote voluntary counseling and testing for HIV
Improve communication and counseling: birth preparedness, awareness of danger signs, and immediate and exclusive breastfeeding	Reduce the risk of mother-to-child transmission (MTCT) of HIV
Care at Time of Birth	
Ensure skilled care at delivery	Recognize danger signs in both mother and baby and avoid delay in seeking care and referral
Provide for clean delivery, clean hands, clean delivery surface, clean cord cutting, tying and stump care, and clean clothes	Recognize and resuscitate asphyxiated babies immediately
Keep the newborn warm; dry and wrap baby immediately, including head cover, or put skin-to-skin with mother and cover	Pay special attention to warmth, feeding, and hygiene practices with preterm and low-birth-weight babies.
Initiate immediate, exclusive breastfeeding, at least within 1 hour	
Provide prophylactic eye care, as appropriate	
Care After Birth	
Ensure early postnatal contact with skin-to-skin contact	Recognize danger signs in both mother and newborn, particularly of infections, and avoid delay in seeking care and referral
Promote continued exclusive breastfeeding	
Maintain hygiene to prevent infection; ensure clean cord care and counsel mother on general hygiene practices, such as hand washing	Support HIV-positive mothers to make appropriate, sustainable choices about feeding
Provide immunizations such as Bacillus Calmette-Guérin (BCG) vaccine, oral polio vaccine (OPV), and hepatitis B vaccine, as appropriate	Continue to pay special attention to warmth, feeding, and hygienic practices for low-birth-weight babies

Source: Adapted from Costello A. *State of the world's newborns: a report from saving newborn lives.* Washington, DC: Save the Children; 2001:9

Motherhood projects have expanded into *Women Deliver* conferences to bring together governments, civil society, and the private sector to share advances in improving maternal health, and the lives of girls and women generally, focused on achieving the targets of MDG 5. The theme, "Invest in women—It pays!" evokes the concept that when a society spends money to improve the lives of women, children, and families, the benefits result in sustainable development for that society.[53]

Family Care International (FCI) continues to serve as an information clearinghouse related to Safe Motherhood information, including the production of an annotated bibliography of Safe Motherhood, and also has activities and publications related to the Skilled Care Initiative, maternal health, and advocacy for women and their health. FCI launched the Safe Motherhood Partners Listserv in 2000 to improve coordination and collaboration among a range of organizations that share the commitment to make

---

BOX 3-5 Ten Action Messages from the Sri Lanka Meeting on Safe Motherhood Initiatives

1. Advance safe motherhood through human rights.

2. Empower women; ensure choices.

3. Safe motherhood is a vital economic and social investment.

4. Delay marriage and first birth.

5. Every pregnancy faces risks.

6. Ensure skilled attendance at delivery.

7. Improve access to quality reproductive health services.

8. Prevent unwanted pregnancy and address unsafe abortion.

9. Measure progress.

10. The power of partnership.

Source: Adapted from Family Care International. Safe Motherhood: a review. Available at: http://www.familycareintl.org /UserFiles/File/SM%20A%20Review_%20Full_Report _FINAL.pdf. Accessed December 27, 2012.

---

pregnancy and birth safe for all women and newborns. This listserv is now part of the Partnership for Maternal, Newborn, and Child Health.

Partnership for Safe Motherhood and Newborn Health

In 2001, the Safe Motherhood IAG moved toward becoming a more inclusive organization and mobilized significant financial resources directed toward improving the health and well-being of childbearing women, their newborns, and young children. The Partnership for Safe Motherhood and Newborn Health (PSMNH) was officially launched in 2003 and included all former Safe Motherhood IAG members, in addition to representatives from the U.S. Agency for International Development (USAID), Department for International Development of the United Kingdom, Save the Children, Initiative for Maternal Mortality Programme Assessment (IMMPACT), White Ribbon Alliance, UN Foundation, Asian Development Bank, Norwegian Ministry of Foreign Affairs, and the Maternal Newborn Health (MNH) project of Johns Hopkins University. The future of Safe Motherhood became stronger with this combination of major

donors, bilateral agencies, and universities, as well as international provider groups.

In 2004, a separate Child Survival partnership was formed, and it became apparent that there was an urgent need for coordination of global efforts in maternal, newborn, and child health toward achieving MDGs 4 and 5 to avoid overlap of efforts and make efficient use of new and existing resources. Thus, in 2005, the Partnership for Maternal, Newborn and Child Health (PMNCH) was formed. The global PMNCH joins maternal, newborn, and child health advocates into an alliance with more than 350 members led by a 14-member Steering Committee (Board) and supported by a Secretariat housed at WHO. The Conceptual and Institutional Framework of the PMNCH focuses on a two-dimensional continuum of care in time (from prepregnancy through pregnancy, childbirth, and the crucial early days and years of life) and place (between homes and health systems, including linkages between various levels of health facilities).[54] One of the hallmarks of the PMNCH is its emphasis on country-led, country-driven initiatives with an increased commitment to primary health care. The power of partnership has resulted in increased resources available to address MDGs 4 and 5.

Safe Motherhood Initiative—USA

In 1996, the voting members at the American College of Nurse-Midwives (ACNM) annual business meeting unanimously endorsed the establishment of a Task Force on Safe Motherhood to focus on maternal death and disability in the United States, noting that this was an important problem in the United States as well as throughout many areas of the world. From this early endeavor, the Safe Motherhood Initiative—USA (SMI-USA) was born in 1997. The founding partners included ACNM, the Midwives Alliance of North America, the American College of Obstetricians and Gynecologists, the March of Dimes, the National Black Women's Health Project, and the National Coalition of Hispanic Health and Human Services Organization. Technical support and expertise were contributed by the Centers for Disease Control and Prevention (CDC) and the Maternal–Child Health Bureau of the U.S. Department of Health and Human Services. The vision of SMI-USA agreed to by the founding and subsequent partners stated that:

> All pregnancies are intended.
>
> All women will complete childbirth strengthened.
>
> No woman will die or be harmed as a result of being pregnant.

SMI-USA no longer exists as an official group due to changing priorities within the various participating organizations, but its brief history is an example of what midwives can do by working collaboratively with other organizations in the United States to promote safe motherhood.

White Ribbon Alliance for Safe Motherhood

The goal of the White Ribbon Alliance is to raise awareness of the need to make pregnancy and childbirth safe for all women in both developed and developing countries. Since its global launch in 1999 during the International Confederation of Midwives (ICM) Congress in the Philippines, the White Ribbon Alliance for Safe Motherhood has become a rapidly growing global movement with members in more than 150 countries and 15 national alliances as of 2012. This organization is now a leader among the agencies holding governments and institutions accountable for the tragedy of maternal mortality.[55] The White Ribbon Alliance for Safe Motherhood is a grassroots movement that builds alliances, strengthens capacity, influences policies, harnesses resources, and inspires action to save the lives of women and newborns around the world. Its effectiveness comes from the fact that the White Ribbon Alliance is a broad-based, collaborative effort among international nongovernmental organizations (INGOs), government agencies, local nongovernmental organizations (NGOs), and community-based organizations in resource-limited countries to decrease maternal mortality through shared resources and experiences.

The organization members attempt to assist in the development of coalitions, usually called Safe Motherhood Initiatives or White Ribbon Alliances, in all countries of the world. Activities undertaken to date include provision of advice and technical assistance to groups in developing countries wishing to start their own White Ribbon Alliance, an electronic newsletter to share experiences and lessons learned, development of a social mobilization field guide on how to start a Safe Motherhood coalition, and awarding annual prizes in conjunction with the Global Health Council, a U.S.-based NGO working on international health issues, to those groups making a substantial contribution to the health of childbearing women through their own national alliances. The white ribbon icon is a symbol of remembrance for all those women who have died during pregnancy, birth, or the postpartum period.

A recent emphasis by the White Ribbon Alliance is on disrespect and abuse suffered by childbearing women. Studies show that midwives, other providers, and family are at times responsible for cruel and harmful treatment when women are at their most vulnerable. The White Ribbon Alliance is championing a movement with human rights advocates and other partners to highlight and address these abuses.[20]

World Health Organization

The World Health Organization is a major player in the global health arena. The WHO constitution states that "Health is a state of complete physical, mental and social well-being and not merely the absence of disease or infirmity."[56]

WHO works diligently to achieve its primary objective—the attainment by all people of the highest possible level of health—by acting as the directing and coordinating authority on international health work. Its core functions[57] are listed in **Box 3-6**.

WHO works with specialized agencies, such as the CDC in the United States, for the eradication of epidemic, endemic, and other diseases. It also established and revises as needed the international nomenclatures of diseases, causes of death, and public health practices. WHO advocates and promotes maternal and child health and welfare, mental health, health services, health personnel preparation, and deployment strategies, and it conducts research in the field of health in cooperation with member states and designated centers of excellence, such as the WHO Collaborating Centers in Nursing and Midwifery.

BOX 3-6 Core Functions of the World Health Organization

1. Providing leadership on matters critical to health and engaging in partnerships where joint action is needed
2. Shaping the research agenda and stimulating the generation, translation, and dissemination of valuable knowledge
3. Setting norms and standards, and promoting and monitoring their implementation
4. Articulating ethical and evidence-based policy options
5. Providing technical support, catalyzing change, and building sustainable institutional capacity
6. Monitoring the health situation and assessing health trends

Source: Adapted from World Health Organization. *11th general programme of work: 2006–2015.* Geneva, Switzerland: WHO; 2006.

WHO's global headquarters is located in Geneva, Switzerland, with regional and country offices throughout the world. WHO has six distinct regions, each of which has a regional office. Every WHO regional office has a post for a nursing/midwifery advisor, although nurses without midwifery credentials often fill these posts. WHO consists of "member states"—generally countries with membership in the United Nations that agree to the conditions set forth in the WHO constitution, including the payment of assessed financial quotas.

WHO's overall organization-wide priorities since 1987 have included an emphasis on maternal health, beginning with the launch of the global Safe Motherhood Initiative in 1987. Resources such as videos (e.g., *Why Did Mrs. X Die?* and *Opening the Gates to Life*), manuals (e.g., *Mother–Baby Package*[58]), and educational standards (e.g., the *Midwifery Education Modules*[59]) have all come from the Division of Reproductive Health, the technical arm of WHO. In 1998, World Health Day was dedicated to Safe Motherhood, and maternal health received global attention in a new way. WHO publishes annual reports on the world's health, and several of these reports have focused on women and children. The 2005 World Health Report, *Making Every Mother and Child Count*, focused on the midwife as the prototype skilled attendant,[60] and the 2006 World Health Report, *Working Together for Health*, emphasized the need for an additional 330,000 new midwives to meet the demand for coverage in maternal health.[61]

In 1999, WHO, UNFPA, UNICEF, and the World Bank issued a joint statement for reducing maternal mortality. The new emphasis in this document was acknowledgment that Safe Motherhood can be achieved through the promotion and support of basic human rights, including empowering women to make choices in their reproductive lives with the support of their families and communities, and ensuring access to quality maternal health services, with birth attended by skilled personnel with midwifery skills, along with timely access to emergency obstetric care should severe complications arise.[62]

The need for greater collaboration in the global effort to ensure healthy outcomes for all childbearing women and their newborns is the current theme of WHO, ICM, FIGO, PMNCH, and the White Ribbon Alliance. WHO has long recognized the value of a well-educated midwife in reducing maternal death and disability.[63] From 1948 to the present time, the World Health Assembly (WHA) has adopted a series of resolutions aimed at strengthening nursing and midwifery with the goal of achieving health for all.[64] Midwives have held key positions within WHO Geneva as technical experts in the Safe Motherhood and Making Pregnancy Safer programs of work, and they have worked with ICM, ICN, and FIGO on the development of training materials for midwives and physicians. These modules were updated and a 2011 publication, *Strengthening Midwifery Toolkit*,[65] is available on the WHO website; the latter includes chapters on midwifery education, regulation, supervision, and evaluation. Individual midwives have held technical advisory positions within WHO over the years. WHO was one of the partners that participated in the development of the *State of the World's Midwifery* report in 2011.[66]

A 2011 resolution ensured that nursing and midwifery are included in national health plans and policymaking and any efforts to expand the human resources for health. This action and other WHO activities recognize the valuable role that professional midwives play in any effort to improve the health of women, especially childbearing women.

The WHO Global Advisory Group on Nursing and Midwifery (GAGNM) was established several years ago to advise the Director General on key policies and programs for nursing and midwifery that pertain to health systems and the social determinants of health.[67] During the past decade, its emphasis has been on developing the human resources needed for health and the Millennium Development Goals. GAGNM members also participated with WHO and its partners in developing *Strategic Directions for Strengthening Nursing and Midwifery Services (2011–2015)*, a document that provides a framework for collaborative action to "improve health outcomes for individuals, families and communities through the provision of competent, culturally sensitive, evidence based nursing and midwifery services."[68]

International Federation of Gynecology and Obstetrics

FIGO is the only worldwide organization that allows obstetricians and gynecologists from national societies to be grouped together in an international membership organization. FIGO was founded in 1954; as of 2012, there were 124 national societies in membership representing obstetrician-gynecologists around the world.[69] The mission of FIGO is to promote the well-being of women and to raise the standard of practice in obstetrics and gynecology.

Among the major FIGO activities related to Safe Motherhood were the organization of the FIGO Save the Mothers Fund Project, along with the

Leadership in Obstetrics and Gynecology for Impact and Change (LOGIC) project.[70] Designed to reduce maternal mortality in developing countries, these projects work primarily through the "twinning" of obstetrics and gynecology societies in developed and developing countries. Of interest to midwives is FIGO's *World Report on Women's Health*, which is published every three years. This supplement to the *International Journal of Gynecology and Obstetrics* represents a comprehensive overview of issues in women's health.

International Midwifery

International Confederation of Midwives

The ICM is a global federation of midwifery associations. The ICM is the only international midwifery association that has won formal recognition by the United Nations as an NGO, receiving its first UN accreditation in January 1957.[71] From modest European beginnings in the early 1900s, the ICM has expanded to include 108 midwifery associations in membership from 98 countries, representing an estimated 250,000 midwives worldwide by 2012.[72] The ACNM was accepted into membership of the ICM in 1956.

The aim of the ICM is "to advance worldwide the goals and aspirations of midwives in the attainment of improved outcomes for women, their newborns and families during the childbearing cycle, using the ICM midwifery philosophy and model of care."[73] The first ICM *Vision* statement, adopted in 1993, focused on the importance of empowering healthy women and midwives who would work together to create healthy societies.

All members of the ICM are either independent associations of midwives or autonomously governed midwives' groups within other organizations, such as nursing or obstetric societies. Associations can be considered for membership when their midwife-members meet the criteria contained within the most current *ICM Definition of the Midwife*.[74] Since the mid-1950s, ICM member associations have been grouped together in four geographic regions: Africa, Americas, Asia-Pacific, and Europe.

The current ICM *Vision* states, "ICM envisions a world where every childbearing woman has access to a midwife's care for herself and her newborn."[73] The *Mission* of the ICM, as revised in 2008, is "To strengthen member associations and to advance the profession of midwifery globally by promoting midwives as the specialists in the care of childbearing women and in keeping birth normal in order to enhance the health of women, their newborns and their families."[73]

Since the early 1990s, ICM's strategic actions to achieve the *Vision* have focused on three primary goals with strategic objectives: (1) address women's health globally, (2) promote and strengthen the midwifery profession, and (3) promote the aims of the ICM internationally.[75] During the 2008 ICM Council, the strategic objectives under each goal were prioritized, giving the greatest emphasis to strengthening of midwifery education, including the role of the midwife as educator, and strengthening of and support for midwives' professional autonomy by developing mechanisms that enable midwifery education, regulation, and practice to be designed and governed primarily by midwives.[76] The renewed emphasis on midwifery education and autonomy resulted in the "three pillars" of ICM: education, regulation, and association strengthening.[77]

Core Documents of ICM

The ICM sets standards for international midwifery through the work of its committees, task forces, and consultants, based on the mandates from the ICM Council of Delegates that represents each member association and is responsible for all policy decisions. The most recent core documents include the updated ICM *Definition of the Midwife* (2011), the ICM *Vision* (2008) and *Mission* (2008), the *ICM International Code of Ethics for Midwives* (2008), the ICM *Philosophy and Model of Care* (2008), the updated ICM *Essential Competencies for Basic Midwifery Practice* (2013), and the new ICM *Global Standards for Midwifery Education and Guidelines* (2010), and ICM *Global Standards for Midwifery Regulation* (2011). All of these core documents can be found on the ICM website.[78] Collectively, these documents form a framework for strengthening midwifery globally so that the health of women and newborns can be improved. Midwives interested in working or currently working internationally need to understand and use these documents as appropriate in their work.

The ICM's definition of a midwife helps to clarify who is a fully qualified midwife, given that many individuals use the title "midwife" in various countries but not all midwives are prepared in accord with the ICM definition and core documents. It is estimated that approximately one-half of the world's professional midwives are also nurses, constituting dual professional qualification. The *International Definition of the Midwife*, first developed in 1972 in conjunction with WHO and FIGO, has been one of the most important documents that the ICM has ever issued. This definition was updated in 1991 and again in 2002 and 2005, primarily to modernize its language and to reflect more clearly the self-governance and autonomy of midwifery. In 2011, another milestone was reached with an update that reflects adherence to the core ICM documents and results in a fully qualified midwife.[74] The 2011 revised ICM *International Definition of the Midwife*[79] is presented in *The History and Profession of Midwifery in the United State*s chapter. The scope of midwifery practice was separated from the actual definition of a midwife for clarity and can also be found in *The History and Profession of Midwifery in the United States* chapter.

ICM initiated a formal process in January 1996 through which a global statement of essential (i.e., "basic" or "core") competencies for midwifery practice was developed and reviewed for relevance to the political, educational, and practice environments of ICM-member countries; this statement was later field-tested in 22 different countries (**Box 3-7**).[80] A total of 214 individual knowledge, skills, and professional behaviors within six domains (e.g., antepartum, intrapartum) were presented for consideration and comment by midwifery educators, senior midwifery students, practicing midwives, and regulators of midwifery practice.

It was during this field-testing that both the type of midwifery education and the scope of midwifery practice were addressed. Within this sample, slightly more than 40% of education programs were exclusively midwifery education without requiring nursing, 30% were based on nursing first, and 20% integrated nursing and midwifery content. The scope of practice ranged from care during pregnancy and childbirth only to care for women from adolescence to senescence, with births attended in all settings. Some noticeable differences were found based on regions of the world, with midwives in southern tier low-resource nations—such as in sub-Saharan Africa, where the midwife is often the only health professional in the area—having a wider scope of practice than midwives in many developed countries.[80]

During 2009–2010, the competencies were reviewed and a seventh competency was added that addressed "abortion-related services," resulting in the adoption of the ICM *Essential Competencies for Basic Midwifery Practice* in 2010. The majority of the evidence-based competencies with 268 knowledge, skills and professional behaviors are considered to be *basic or core*—that is, those that should

---

BOX 3-7 International Confederation of Midwives Essential Competencies for Basic Midwifery Practice 2010, Revised 2013

1. Midwives have the requisite knowledge and skills from obstetrics, neonatology, the social sciences, public health and ethics that form the basis of high quality, culturally relevant, appropriate care for women, newborns, and childbearing families.
2. Midwives provide high quality, culturally sensitive health education and services to all in the community in order to promote healthy family life, planned pregnancies and positive parenting.
3. Midwives provide high quality antenatal care to maximize health during pregnancy and that includes early detection and treatment or referral of selected complications.
4. Midwives provide high quality, culturally sensitive care during labour, conduct a clean and safe birth and handle selected emergency situations to maximize the health of women and their newborns.
5. Midwives provide comprehensive, high quality, culturally sensitive postpartum care for women.
6. Midwives provide high quality, comprehensive care for the essentially healthy infant from birth to two months of age.
7. Midwives provide a range of individualised, culturally sensitive abortion-related care services for women requiring or experiencing pregnancy termination or loss that are congruent with applicable laws and regulations and in accord with national protocols.

Source: Adapted from The International Confederation of Midwives. *Essential Competencies for Basic Midwifery Practice.* Available at: http://internationalmidwives .org/assets/uploads/documents/CoreDocuments/ICM %20Essential%20Competencies%20for%20Basic%20 Midwifery%20Practice%202010,%20revised%202013.pdf. Accessed July 6, 2013.

---

be an expected outcome of midwifery preservice education. Other items are designated as *additional*, meaning those that could be performed by midwives who elect a broader scope of practice, allowing for variation in the preparation and practice of midwifery throughout the world based on the needs of the local community and/or nation.[79] A 2010 survey of 58 low-resource countries found that more than 25% of the programs surveyed did not meet the 2010 ICM *Global Standards for Midwifery Education.*[66]

The first set of global standards for preservice midwifery education using a modified Delphi survey to obtain consensus from midwives and other experts on the minimum expectations for a midwifery education program was developed in 2009–2010. Major decisions included determining a minimum of 3 years to be required for an exclusively midwifery program and 18 months post registration (e.g., nursing, clinical officer) following secondary education. A set of *Companion Guidelines* was also developed to help countries implement and evaluate education standards.

A consensus process was used to develop ideal standards for the regulation of midwifery as an autonomous profession, taking advantage of regional meetings.[82] Each of these documents was adopted by the ICM Council in 2011.

ICM Congresses and Conferences

The ICM Triennial Congresses are meetings in which midwives from all over the world gather to share knowledge, ideas, and experience. The congresses have been the primary activity and financial strength of ICM since 1919, with the exception of the World War II years. The series of triennial meetings has been uninterrupted since 1954. In the mid-1990s, the ICM designated May 5 each year as the International Day of the Midwife. The ICM Council sets the theme for activities during each triennium within the context of Safe Motherhood and women's health, focusing on the role of midwives. Member associations are active during this annual event and often raise funds to support attendance by midwives from resource-poor nations at ICM conferences and congresses.

The partnership between ICM and UNFPA resulted in the recent publication, *The State of the World's Midwifery 2011: Delivering Health, Saving Lives*. This publication, which is supported by 28 other agencies, is the first report since the 1970s to document the status of the midwifery workforce. It addresses 58 countries with high rates of maternal, fetal, and newborn mortality. The intent of this report is that policymakers and governments will recognize the value of midwifery care in reducing maternal and newborn deaths while also working with midwives to increase access, coverage, and quality of maternity services.[66] Another major publication of the ICM is a peer-reviewed journal, *International Journal of Childbirth*, which was inaugurated in 2011 in both electronic and paper formats; subscriptions are available from the ICM website.

ICM holds a permanent seat on the PMNCH board. One of ICM's key influences in the expanded global partnership was the conceptual framework emphasizing the key role that healthy women play in the development of any nation, and the belief that to be healthy, women need to be accorded full human rights and should not fear death when giving birth.[55]

American College of Nurse-Midwives International Activities

The ACNM has had a strong international orientation since its inception. The group's founders came from primarily European midwifery traditions, and early midwifery graduates often served as missionaries worldwide. A significant percentage of ACNM members have overseas work experience. ACNM has also had a long history of active involvement in ICM, sharing core documents, providing consultants and leaders of task forces, and frequently providing leadership by filling the roles of Regional Representatives or Board of Management officers.

In 1981, ACNM developed a home within the organization for the conduct of international projects. In the early 1990s, the Special Projects Section began to incorporate a number of Safe Motherhood projects. The *Life-Saving Skills Manual for Midwives* by Marshall and Buffington (1998) was developed, piloted in Ghana, and then taught in more than 20 countries. The manual has been translated into multiple languages, and currently is in its fourth edition.[83] The Home Based Life Saving Skills (HBLSS) program was developed to address community-based needs. Both Life-Saving Skills (LSS) and HBLSS are competency-based curricula. LSS trains skilled providers to manage obstetric emergencies and decrease both morbidity and mortality. HBLSS seeks to reduce maternal and neonatal mortality by increasing awareness and access to emergency life-saving measures within the community and home.[84] HBLSS trains women and their families to identify obstetric emergencies. The LSS and HBLSS curricula are based on the Community Partnership Model, which describes a continuum of life-saving care that is required to ensure survival once an emergency occurs[85] (**Figure 3-4**). Take Action cards (**Figure 3-5**)[86] are used as references for recognizing an emergency and actions that can help prevent morbidity and death once a particular type of emergency occurs.

In 2000, the Special Project Section became the ACNM Department of Global Outreach. The work

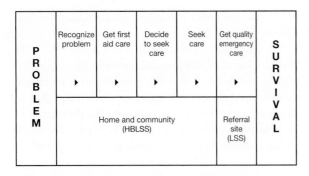

Figure 3-4 Home Based Life Saving Skills and Life Saving Skills: The pathway to survival.

Source: Reprinted with permission from Sibley LM, Buffington ST. Building community partnerships for safer motherhood: home based life saving skills. At a Glance. January 2003. NGO Networks for Health. Available at: http://pdf.usaid.gov/pdf_docs/PNACS822.pdf. Accessed December 20, 2012.

of the Department of Global Outreach includes international projects such as those focusing on training in LSS, HBLSS, postpartum and postabortion care, midwifery association strengthening, family planning, maternal-to-child HIV transmission, family-centered maternity care, and domestic violence. In its first 20 years of work, ACNM efforts have involved more than 30 countries.

A new ACNM Division of Global Health was established in 2010. This division provides ACNM members with the opportunity to share their international expertise and work on projects that complement and support staff efforts in the Department of Global Outreach. The Division of Global Health serves as the coordinating body within the organization for global research, education, networking, and communication across the membership.

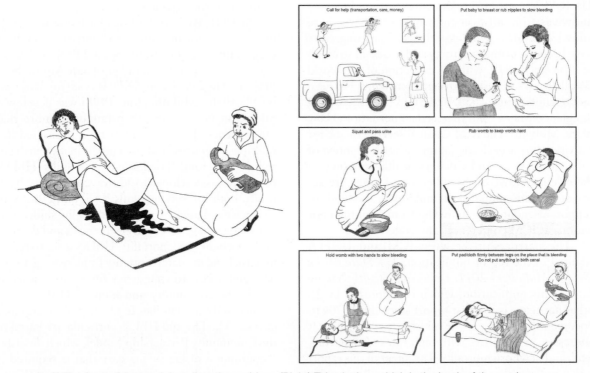

(Left) The front of the card describes the problem. (Right) Take Action, which is the back of the card, shows the steps taken to mitigate the problem.

Figure 3-5 Home Based Life Saving Skills: Take action card on bleeding too much after baby is born.
Source: Reprinted with permission from American College of Nurse-Midwives. *HBLSS Take Action Card Booklet.* 2nd ed. Silver Spring, MD: American College of Nurse-Midwives; 2010.

Beyond Borders: Midwives Working Internationally

Midwifery students and practitioners who are interested in international midwifery and Safe Motherhood/women's health often wonder what they need to do to follow through on these interests. First and foremost, they need to successfully complete their midwifery basic education and practice to gain confidence in their ability to work in a variety of situations with women from a variety of cultures. Individuals can contact the ACNM Department of Global Outreach or join the ACNM Division of Global Health to discover what other midwives are doing throughout the world.

Among the most important criteria for international work in midwifery is excellence in both practice and teaching. Expertise takes time to develop and is built upon ongoing midwifery experience. Effective international work also requires expert communication skills, cultural sensitivity, and awareness of the impact of personal values and value biases about others who are "different." Individuals inevitably view the world through a personal "value lens"—and must understand that though there are some universal values, such as respect for human dignity, many other values are not shared from one culture to another, from one country to another, or from one person to another in the same country. The person with unexamined values can be a menace to others, for lack of insight into oneself often means the unconscious imposition of one's personal values on others—too often inappropriately.

Future Trends and Challenges in International Midwifery

The evolution of midwifery practice internationally has undergone a series of major changes. A profession that began primarily by attending women during their labors and births and providing several days' postpartum care has added on a full range of services, including prenatal care, newborn care, family planning, health-oriented gynecologic care, preconception care, care of the menopausal woman, primary care, and care of some common medical conditions. These services have always been delivered in a variety of worksites—home, clinic, and hospital. The challenges for the midwife in addressing international care, especially Safe Motherhood, involve several areas: policy, clinical practice, and community-based approaches to social mobilization.

Policy Development/Volunteerism

Midwifery associations in various countries have made major gains over the past 30 years by becoming involved in policy development. It is critical that midwives do not slide into the expectation that others will recognize the value of the profession. Volunteerism is difficult with modern busy lives and competing priorities. Nevertheless, volunteerism is an integral part to the midwifery commitment to the needs of mothers and newborns around the world.

Clinical Practice

Midwifery clinical practice always evolves. As painful as it may be for those who are comfortable with the current scope of practice, flexibility is the key to embracing changing conditions and priorities. Expanded emergency skills as well as dealing with all areas of AIDS prevention and care, epidemics, displaced populations, post-trauma war survivors, environmental hazards, terrorism, and war all challenge the creativity and resilience of midwives.

Community-Based Approaches

One of the ongoing challenges for midwives concerned with health of women is how to better address community factors. Midwives need skills in advocacy, social mobilization, participatory learning methodologies, utilization of positive deviance approaches, and other strategies. Advocacy can affect policy, which in turn directly affects the lives of women. Social mobilization that brings community awareness to the barriers to safer pregnancy and development of community solutions to community problems can have lasting positive effects. Individuals and groups both inside and outside countries are investing heavily in new technologies to make high-quality care more accessible. Innovations are being embraced by funders but must be adopted by the community in question. Midwives can facilitate adoption of new innovations when appropriate. Examples of current technologies under development or newly in use are found in **Box 3-8**.[87]

Participatory learning activities are techniques developed by agricultural workers to involve community members in examining all sides of a problem and seeing how multiple inputs can help bring about a solution. The goal is to encourage various levels and groupings of stakeholders to contribute in practical

---

BOX 3-8 Suggested New Technologies for International Use

- Vaccines against malaria, tuberculosis, and AIDS
- An antishock Neoprene pressure garment to prevent/treat shock from acute blood loss
- A marking pen impregnated with chemicals to detect protein in the urine when drops are placed on a piece of paper
- A disposable single-dose "blister" attached to a needle for one-time administration of oxytocin, pediatric antibiotics, and other medications, permitting administration of emergency drugs in a community setting by community members with accurate dosage
- Baby blankets with embedded heated paraffin to maintain temperature regulation for fragile, premature, or ill infants during transport to appropriate level of care
- A colorimeter attached to each box of vaccines or other medications, which turns color when safe temperature limits in the cold chain have been exceeded, impacting vaccine quality
- Insecticide-treated bednets and curtains for the prevention of malaria
- Global positioning systems (GPS) technology utilized for locating the ill for transport and mapping of disease prevalence
- Mobile phone technology for summoning emergency assistance, reporting surveillance data (e.g., maternal or newborn deaths, incidence of reportable diseases such as avian influenza, and Ebola), and collecting vital records data
- Phones to send messages to pregnant women according to their stage of pregnancy
- Games with family planning and human sexuality information targeted to adolescents

---

ways. In contrast, positive deviance is a strategy that analyzes how positive behavior has survived in the face of cultural and family pressures. For example, if a few families in a village have refused the community standard to have their daughters circumcised, studying how they have succeeded in a pressured environment can yield helpful information in developing a strategy to eliminate female genital mutilation. Applying strategies such as participatory learning activities and positive deviance facilitates implementation of profound changes at the community level.

Conclusion

Many epigrams exist that illustrate the importance of women and mothers, such as "Women hold up half the sky." Yet all too many women suffer from the inability to attain their potential in the world, both in developed and developing countries. One example of a major activity to promote health for individual women, societies, and nations is to address maternal mortality through collaborative efforts such as Safe Motherhood projects. Another example is recognition of midwives and midwifery skills as essential for promoting the health of women. Midwives have the power to make a profound impact on the survival of women, mothers, and infants globally. Beginning with the best educational preparation, maintaining competence, and listening and responding to, while never becoming complacent about, maternal mortality and morbidity are guidelines for midwives today. Women, families, and the world depend on midwives.

● ● ● References

1. Mercer JM. Honorary doctorate citation for Helen Varney Burst. Georgetown University, May 23, 1987.
2. Fathalla MF. Health and being a mother in the twenty-first century. *Intl J Obstet Gynecol.* 2007;98(3):195-199.
3. Thompson J, Thompson H. Ethical aspects of care. In: Walsh L V. *Midwifery: Community-Based Care During the Childbearing Year.* Philadelphia, PA: Saunders; 2001:489-490.
4. World Health Organization. *International Classification of Diseases.* Geneva, Switzerland: WHO; 2010. Available at: http://www.who.int/classifications/icd/en. Accessed July 6, 2013.
5. Pattinson R, Say L, Souza JP, Van den Broek N, Rooney C, on behalf of the WHO Working Group on Maternal Mortality and Morbidity Classifications. WHO maternal death and near-miss classifications. *Bull WHO.* 2009;877:734.
6. Barfield WD and the Committee on Fetus and Newborn. Standard terminology for fetal, infant, and perinatal deaths. *Pediatrics.* 2011;128:177-181.
7. Herz B, Measham AR. *The Safe Motherhood Initiative: Proposals for Action.* World Bank Discussion Paper No. 9. Washington, DC: World Bank; 1987.
8. Betrán AP, Wojdyla D, Posner SF, Gülmezoglu AM. National estimates for maternal mortality: an analysis based on the WHO systematic review of maternal mortality and morbidity. *Biomed Central Pub Health.* 2005;5:131.

9. World Health Organization, UNICEF, United Nations Fund for Population Activities. Trends in maternal morbidity and mortality 1990-2010. Available at: http://www.who.int/reproductivehealth/publications /monitoring/9789241503631/en/index.html. Accessed December 25, 2012.

10. World Health Organization. Unmet family planning needs. Available at: www.who.int/reproductivehealth /topics/family_planning/unmet_need_fp/en/index .html. Accessed September 12, 2012.

11. World Health Organization, United Nations Fund for Population Activities, UNICEF, World Bank. *Reduction of Maternal Mortality: A Joint WHO/UNFPA/UNICEF/ World Bank Statement*. Geneva: WHO; 1999:25.

12. World Health Organization. *Revised 1990 Estimates of Maternal Mortality: A New Approach by WHO and UNICEF*. Geneva, Switzerland: WHO; April 1996.

13. World Health Organization. Maternal mortality fact sheet. Fact sheet No. 348. May 2012. Available at: http://www.who.int/mediacentre/factsheets/fs348/en /index.html. Accessed September 12, 2012.

14. Hogan MC, Foreman KJ, Naghavi M, et al. Maternal mortality for 181 countries, 1980-2008: a systematic analysis of progress towards Millennium Development Goal 5. *Lancet*. 2010;375:1609-1623.

15. Nour NM. An introduction to maternal mortality. *Rev Obstet Gynecol*. 2008;1(2):77-81.

16. UNICEF Nigeria: at a glance. Available at: http://www .unicef.org/infobycountry/nigeria_statistics.html. Accessed December 25, 2012.

17. WHO HIV/AIDS fact sheet No. 360. July 2012. Available at: http://www.who.int/mediacentre/fact sheets/fs360/en/index.html. Accessed September 17, 2012.

18. Evans EC. A review of cultural influences on maternal mortality in the developing world *Midwifery*. November 10, 2012. Epub ahead of print.

19. Bowser D, Hill K. *Exploring Evidence for Disrespect and Abuse in Facility-Based Childbirth: Report of a Landscape Analysis*. USAID-TRAction Project. Harvard School of Public Health and University Research Co., LLC. September 17, 2010.

20. Campbell O, Graham W. Strategies for reducing maternal mortality: getting on with what works. *Lancet*. 2006:368:1284-1299.

21. Personal communication, Dr. Virginia Camacho, United Nations Fund for Population Activities, Senior Regional Reproductive Health Advisor, May 7, 2012.

22. Singh S, Darroch JE, Ashford JE, Vassloff M. *Adding It Up: The Costs and Benefits of Investing in Family Planning and Maternal and Newborn Health*. New York: Guttmacher Institute and United Nations Population Fund; 2009.

23. United Nations Fund for Population Activities. Fact sheet: contraception saves lives. July 5, 2012. Available at: http://www.unfpa.org/webdav/site/global/shared /documents/Reproductive%20Health/Fact%20Sheets /Contraceptives_UNFPA%20Fact%20Sheet_July%20 5%202012.pdf. Accessed September 17, 2012.

24. Thaddeus S, Maine D. Too far to walk: maternal mortality in context. *Soc Sci Med*. 1994;38:1091-1110.

25. Family Care International. *Saving Lives: Skilled Attendance at Childbirth*. Background paper. New York: FCI, in collaboration with Safe Motherhood Inter-Agency Group; 2001.

26. Lawn JE, Blencowe D, Pattinson R, et al. for *The Lancet*'s Stillbirths Series steering committee. Stillbirths: Where? When? Why? How to make the data count? *Lancet*. 2011;377:1448-1463.

27. Callaghan WM. Overview of maternal mortality in the United States. *Semin Perinatol*. 2012;36(1):2-6.

28. Berg C, Callaghan WM, Syverson C, Henderson Z. Pregnancy-related mortality in the United States, 1998 to 2005. *Obstet Gynecol*. 2010;116(6):1302-1309.

29. Centers for Disease Control and Prevention (CDC). Differences in maternal mortality among black and white women—United States, 1990. *MMWR*. 1995;44(1):6-7, 13-14.

30. King JC. Maternal mortality in the United States: why is it important and what are we doing about it? *Semin Perinatol*. 2012;36(1):14-18. doi: 10.1053 /j.semperi.2011.09.004.

31. Xu J, Kochanek K, Murphy S, Tejada-Vera B. Deaths: final data for 2007. *Natl Vital Stat Rep*. May 2010;58(19). Hyattsville, MD: National Center for Health Statistics.

32. United Nations. *Millennium Declaration*. New York: UN; 2000. Available at: http://www.un.org/millennium /declaration/ares552e.htm. Accessed December 25, 2012.

33. *The Millennium Development Goals Report 2013*. Available at: http://www.un.org/millenniumgoals/pdf /report-2013/mdg-report-2013-english.pdf. Accessed July 6, 2013.

34. Thompson JB. Poverty, development, and women: Why should we care? *JOGNN*. 2007;36(6):523-530.

35. Tyer-Viola L, Cesario SK. Addressing poverty, education and gender equality to improve the health of women worldwide. *JOGNN*. 2010;39:580-589.

36. Diaz-Granados N, Pitzul J, Dorado LM, et al. Monitoring gender equity in health using gender sensitive indicators: a cross national study. *Women's Health*. 2011;20:140-153.

37. Lozano R, Wang H, Foreman KJ, et al. Progress towards Millennium Development Goals 4 and 5 on maternal and child mortality: an updated systematic analysis. *Lancet*. 2011;378(9797):1139-1165.

38. Ekechi C, Wolman Y, de Bernis L. Maternal and newborn health road maps: a review of progress in 33 sub-Saharan African countries, 2008-2009. *Reprod Health Matt.* 2012;20(39):164-168.

39. Maclean GD. An historical overview of the first two decades of striving towards Safe Motherhood. *Sex Reprod Healthcare.* 2010;1:7-14.

40. Rosskam E, Pariyo G, Hounton S, Alga H. Increasing skilled birth attendance through midwifery workforce management. *Int J Health Plann Manage.* October 14, 2012. Epub ahead of print.

41. World Health Organization. Achieving Millennium Development Goal 5: target 5A and 5B on reducing maternal mortality and achieving universal access to reproductive health. Available at: http://whqlibdoc .who.int/hq/2009/WHO_RHR_09.06_eng.pdf. Accessed September 8, 2012.

42. Hardee K, Gay J, Blanc AK. Maternal mortality: neglected dimensions of Safe Motherhood in the developing world. *Global Pub Health.* 2012:1-15.

43. Mbizvo MT, Say L. Global progress and potentially effective policy responses to reduce maternal mortality. *Int J Gynaecol Obstet.* 2012;119(suppl 1):S9-S12.

44. United Nations. Millennium Development Goals indicators: percent skilled health personnel. Available at: http://mdgs.un.org/unsd/mdg/SeriesDetail.aspx ?srid=570. Accessed December 25, 2012.

45. World Health Organization. Making pregnancy safer: the critical role of the skilled attendant. A joint statement by WHO, ICM, and FIGO. WHO; 2004. Available at: http://whqlibdoc.who.int/publications /2004/9241591692.pdf. Accessed January 22, 2013.

46. Sibley LM, Sipe TA, Barry D. Traditional birth attendant training for improving health behaviours and pregnancy outcomes. *Cochrane Database System Rev.* 2012;8:CD005460. doi: 10.1002/14651858. CD005460.pub3.

47. Adam T, Lim SS, Mehta S, et al. Cost effectiveness analysis of strategies for maternal and neonatal health in developing countries. *BMJ.* 2005;331:1107. Available at: http://bmj.com/cgi/content/full/331/7525/1107. Accessed October 5, 2012.

48. March of Dimes, PMNCH, Save the Children, WHO. *Born Too Soon: The Global Action Report on Preterm Birth.* Eds. CP Howson, MV Kinney, JE Lawn. Geneva, Switzerland: WHO; 2012.

49. Lawn JE, Cousens S, Zupan J; Lancet Neonatal Survival Steering Team. 4 million neonatal deaths: When? Where? Why? *Lancet.* 2005;365(9462): 891-900.

50. Costello A. *State of the World's Newborns: A Report from Saving Newborn Lives.* Washington, DC: Save the Children; 2001:9.

51. Ross SR. *Promoting Quality Maternal and Newborn Care: A Reference Manual for Program Managers.* Washington, DC: Cooperative for Assistance and Relief Everywhere (CARE); 1998.

52. Family Care International. Safe Motherhood: a review. Available at: http://www.familycareintl.org/UserFiles /File/SM%20A%20Review_%20Full_Report _FINAL.pdf. Accessed December 27, 2012.

53. Women Deliver. Available at: http://www.women deliver.org/about. Accessed December 25, 2012.

54. Partnership for Maternal, Newborn, and Child Health. Conceptual and institutional framework. Available at: http://www.who.int/pmnch/activities/cif /conceptualandinstframework.pdf. Accessed December 25, 2012.

55. White Ribbon Alliance. Available at: http://www.white ribbonalliance.org. Accessed December 25, 2012.

56. United Nations. *Charter, Article 57: World Health Organization.* New York: UN; 1948.

57. World Health Organization. *11th General Programme of Work: 2006-2015.* Geneva, Switzerland: WHO; 2006.

58. World Health Organization. *The Mother–Baby Package.* Geneva, Switzerland: WHO; 1994.

59. World Health Organization. *Midwifery Education Modules* (2nd ed.). Geneva, Switzerland: WHO; 2006. Available at: http://www.who.int/maternal_child_ adolescent/documents/9241546662/en/index.html. Accessed December 25, 2012.

60. World Health Organization. *World Health Report 2005: Make Every Mother and Child Count.* Geneva, Switzerland: WHO; 2005.

61. World Health Organization. *World Health Report 2006: Working Together for Health.* Geneva, Switzerland: WHO; 2006. Available at: http://www.who.int/whr /2006/en/index.html. Accessed December 25, 2012.

62. World Health Organization, United Nations Fund for Population Activities, UNICEF, World Bank. *Reduction of Maternal Mortality: A Joint WHO/ UNFPA/UNICEF/World Bank Statement.* Geneva, Switzerland: WHO; 1999.

63. World Health Organization. Midwives to the world. *World Health: The Magazine of the World Health Organization 50th year.* March-April 1997;2. See also World Health Organization. Nursing and midwifery programme at WHO. Available at: http://www.who .int/hrh/nursing_midwifery/en. Accessed December 25, 2012.

64. Vonderheid SC, Al-Gasser N. World Health Organization and global health policy. *J Nurs Scholarship.* 2002;34(2):109-110.

65. World Health Organization. *Strengthening Midwifery Toolkit.* Geneva: WHO; 2011. Available at: http ://www.who.int/maternal_child_adolescent/documents /strenthening_midwifery_toolkit/en/index.html. Accessed December 25, 2012.

66. United Nations Fund for Population Activities. State of the world's midwifery. 2011. Available at: http://www.unfpa.org/sowmy/report/home.html. Accessed December 25, 2012.

67. Thompson JE. The WHO Global Advisory Group on Nursing and Midwifery (GAGNM). *J Nurs Scholarship*. 2002;34(2):111-113.

68. World Health Organization. Strategic directions for strengthening nursing and midwifery services 2011-2015. Available at: http://www.who.int/hrh/resources/nmsd/en/index.html. Accessed December 25, 2012.

69. Federation of International Gynecology and Obstetrics. Available at: http://www.figo.org. Accessed December 25, 2012.

70. Federation of International Gynecology and Obstetrics. LOGIC initiative. Available at: http://www.figo.org/projects/LOGIC_initiative. Accessed December 25, 2012.

71. Candau MO. Letter to Executive Secretary, International Confederation of Midwives. January 10, 1957. [Letter referring to the decision of the WHO Executive Board to admit ICM into official relations with WHO as a nongovernmental organization. Copy available upon request from author.]

72. International Confederation of Midwives. Available at: http://www.internationalmidwives.org. Accessed December 25, 2012.

73. International Confederation of Midwives. Mission and vision. Available at: http://www.internationalmidwives.org/Whoweare/AboutICM/tabid/225/Default.aspx. Accessed September 3, 2012.

74. International Confederation of Midwives. International definition of a midwife. 2011. Available at: http://www.internationalmidwives.org/Portals/5/2011/Definition%20of%20the%20Midwife%20-%202011.pdf. Accessed September 3, 2012.

75. International Confederation of Midwives. Articles of association. 2010. Available at: http://www.internationalmidwives.org/Portals/5/2011/DB%202011/ICM%20Constitution%20--%20June%202010.pdf. Accessed September 3, 2012.

76. International Confederation of Midwives. ICM Council minutes 2008. [Copy available upon request from author.]

77. Lynch B. ICM president's address to ICM Council. June 14, 2011. [Copy available upon request from author.]

78. International Confederation of Midwives. Core documents. Available at: http://www.internationalmidwives.org/Whatwedo/Policyandpractice/CoreDocuments/tabid/322/Default.aspx. Accessed December 25, 2012.

79. International Confederation of Midwives. Essential competencies for basic midwifery. Available at: http://www.unfpa.org/sowmy/resources/docs/standards/en/R430_ICM_2011_Essential_Competencies_2010_ENG.pdf. Accessed December 25, 2012.

80. Fullerton JT, Brogan K. *Essential Competencies for Midwifery Practice: A Project Report and Survey Analysis*. The Hague: ICM; 2002.

81. Fullerton JT, Severino R, Brogan K, Thompson JE. Essential competencies of midwifery practice. Phase II: Affirmation of the competency statements. *Midwifery*. September 2003;19.

82. Fullerton JT, Thompson JE, Pairman S, Moyo N. The International Confederation of Midwives: a global framework for midwifery education, regulation and professional practice. *Int J Childbirth*. 2011;1(3):145-158.

83. Buffington ST, Beck DR, Clark PA. *Life-Saving Skills Manual*. 4th ed. Silver Spring, MD: American College of Nurse-Midwives; 2008.

84. Sibley L, Buffington SD, Beck D, Armbruster D. Home-based life saving skills: promoting safe motherhood through innovative community-based interventions. *J Midwifery Women's Health*. 2001;46:258-266.

85. Sibley LM, Buffington ST. Building community partnerships for safer motherhood: home based life saving skills. *At a Glance*. January 2003. NGO Networks for Health. Available at: http://pdf.usaid.gov/pdf_docs/PNACS822.pdf. Accessed December 20, 2012.

86. American College of Nurse-Midwives. *HBLSS Take Action Card Booklet*. 2nd ed. Silver Spring, MD: American College of Nurse-Midwives; 2010.

87. Tureski KE. Big choices on a small screen: can mobile games really spark change? *Frontlines*. September/October 2012;30-33.

● ● ● **Additional Resources**

Alan Guttmacher Institute:
http://www.guttmacher.org

American College of Nurse-Midwives (ACNM):
http://www.midwife.org

Centers for Disease Control and Prevention (CDC):
http://www.cdc.gov

Every Woman Every Child Global Strategy 2010:
http://www.everywomaneverychild.org

Family Care International (FCI):
http://www.familycareintl.org/en/home

International Confederation of Midwives (ICM):
http://www.internationalmidwives.org

International Council of Nurses (ICN):
http://www.icn.ch

International Federation of Gynecology and Obstetrics (FIGO):
http://www.figo.org

International Pediatric Association (IPA):
http://www.ipa-world.org

International Planned Parenthood Federation:
http://www.ippf.org

Joint United Nations Programme on HIV/AIDS
(UNAIDS):
http://www.unaids.org

Midwives Alliance of North America (MANA):
http://www.mana.org

Partnership for Maternal, Newborn and Child Health:
http://www.pmnch.org

Population Council:
http://www.popcouncil.org

Reproline:
http://www.reproline.jhu.edu

Save the Children; Saving Newborn Lives:
http://www.savethechildren.org

United Nations Fund for Population Activities
(UNFPA):
http://www.unfpa.org

United Nations Children's Fund (UNICEF):
http://www.unicef.org

White Ribbon Alliance:
http://www.whiteribbonalliance.org

Women Deliver:
 http://www.womendeliver.org

World Bank:
http://www.worldbank.org

World Health Organization (WHO):
http://www.who.int

II

Primary Care

Midwives as Primary Care Providers

Midwives today have an unprecedented opportunity to improve the health and well-being of women and families through primary care. Now more than ever, the midwife's role in primary care must be embraced by midwives themselves, the populations they serve, the health settings within which they practice, and the policymakers responsible for ensuring the health of this nation's people. The chapters in this section review primary care topics that are critical for clinical practice.

The evolution of the primary care provider role for midwives in the United States might seem like recent history, but its roots harken back decades, if not centuries. By the early 1970s, content had been added to the formal midwifery curricula regarding family planning, which ushered in a role that expanded beyond the maternity cycle to include well-woman care before and after pregnancy.[1] By the 1990s, competencies in primary care were added to midwifery education and practice standards.[2]

In 1992, the American College of Nurse-Midwives (ACNM) issued its first formal statement declaring that certified nurse-midwives (CNMs) provide primary care for women and newborns.[3] This statement coincided with publication of the results of a landmark prospective study than showed 7 of 10 visits made to CNMs were by women or infants vulnerable to poor access or poor outcomes by virtue of their race, ethnicity, age, education, income, immigration status, or place of residence.[4] By the end of the twentieth century, it had become clear that midwives can make primary care services more available when they are integral members of the primary care workforce.

Most recently, the midwife's primary care role has been solidified with passage of the Patient Protection and Affordable Care Act in 2010. This legislation includes comprehensive insurance reforms and a federal commitment to increase the availability of primary care services. Federal recognition of the midwife's primary care role is further evidenced by primary care workforce expansion efforts that include midwives, Medicaid/Medicare program payment for midwifery services, federal funding for education programs that prepare midwives as primary care providers, and federal employee insurance coverage for midwifery services.

Current core competencies for basic midwifery practice specify the primary care content for which midwives are responsible.[2] In 2012, ACNM issued a policy statement that reaffirmed the role of midwives in primary care. This statement also affirmed midwives' roles within the patient-centered medical home, a relatively new model that incorporates improved quality of care strategies, promotes communication, and enhances efficient delivery of care in a multidisciplinary model—with the patient at the center of the partnership.[5]

Midwifery care is focused on normalcy, and the *Nutrition, Health Promotion and Health Maintenance*, and *Common Conditions in Primary Care* chapters in this text present the knowledge needed to help all women of all ages maintain and facilitate health. Yet women who receive primary care from midwives experience a range of health inequities that influence their health and well-being and can lead to health disparities. This reality compels the midwife to have an understanding of the social and economic determinants of health.

Attention to race and ethnic diversity is a priority because of changing U.S. demographics and the glaring disparities in health outcomes experienced by women and children of color. Yet other aspects of diversity within populations cared for by midwives are equally expansive and include populations for which inequality in access and health disparities are well documented: young or old age, low education and low literacy, low income, religious affiliation, disability status, sexual minority status, and place of residence (especially remote, rural, or urban areas).

To bring about health equity in access, outcomes, and quality, midwives must become culturally proficient primary care providers and, when possible, emerge as leaders in this area. To do so, midwives must embark on a personal and professional journey. Cultural humility is an essential first step in the development of the cultural competence skills needed for the practice of effective primary care.[6] Midwives must commit to the practice of cultural humility—a lifelong process of self-critique, self-awareness, and reflection. By examining their own worldview, rather than focusing solely on the client's belief system and culturally specific traits, the midwife will appreciate those intrinsic qualities that enable individuals to attain health, happiness, and wholeness. With this understanding, the midwife can adapt primary care practice to be more patient centered and, as such, more effective. Likewise, the midwife can advance on the cultural competence continuum toward the ultimate goal of cultural proficiency.

Regardless of the practice setting, midwives are certain to encounter women who experience health inequality in any number of ways, including poor access to primary care and mental health care. Nearly half of women nationwide live in a primary care provider shortage area.[7] By joining ranks with their foremothers who practiced primary care midwifery for disenfranchised women and families with poor or no access to even the most basic health care, midwives today who embrace the primary care role and commit to advancing cultural proficiency can and will make lasting improvements in the health of the entire nation.

Lisa L. Paine

● ● ● References

1. Rooks JP. *Midwifery and Childbirth in America.* Philadelphia, PA: Temple University Press; 1997.

2. American College of Nurse-Midwives. *Core Competencies for Basic Midwifery Practice.* Silver Spring, MD: ACNM; December 2012.

3. American College of Nurse-Midwives. *Position Statement: Certified Nurse-Midwives and Certified Midwifes as Primary Care Providers/Case Managers.* Washington, DC: ACNM; 1992; revised 1994, 1997.

4. Paine LL, Lang JM, Strobino DM, et al. Characteristics of nurse-midwife patients and visits, 1991. *Am J Pub Health.* 1999;89(6):906-909.

5. American College of Nurse-Midwives. *Position Statement: Midwives Are Primary Care Providers and Leaders of Maternity Care Homes: Certified Nurse-Midwives and Certified Midwives as Primary Care Providers/Case Managers.* Silver Spring, MD: ACNM; June 2012.

6. Tervalon M, Murray-Garcia J. Cultural humility versus cultural competence: a critical distinction in defining physician training outcomes in multicultural education. *J Heath Care Poor Underserved.* 1998;9(2):117-125

7. James CV, Salginicoff A, Thomas M, Ranji U, Lillie-Blanton, Wyn R. *Putting Women's Health Care Disparities on the Map: Examining Racial and Ethnic Disparities at the State Level.* Menlo Park, CA: Kaiser Family Foundation; 2009:1-104.

An Introduction to the Care of Women

JAN M. KRIEBS

Midwife Means "With Woman"

Midwifery is both art and science—and above all midwifery is care for women and their families. As discussed in the first chapter of this text, midwifery in the United States has grown from local efforts to care for women with few resources, into a well-respected profession that offers women primary care and gynecologic services, as well as maternity and birth care, including newborn care. These services are provided in interdisciplinary settings because midwives rely on the skills of gynecologists and obstetricians, nurses, social workers, and other health professionals, just as they rely on other midwives for their respective expertise. One key to understanding midwifery care is to recognize the interweaving of skills and knowledge from many sources, and the willingness to work with others to achieve the best possible health outcomes for a woman.

The evidence-based studies and expert opinions that underpin the science of midwifery are the same as those from which medicine and nursing draw their understanding of health care. In brief, most clinicians practice similarly, often based on the preferences and experience of those who have taught them. Unfortunately, relatively few of the expert recommendations on which clinicians rely are drawn from high-quality research.

The flawed perception that guidelines are consistently based on solid evidence and lack bias has been acknowledged.[1] For example, the American College of Obstetricians and Gynecologists has documented that fewer than one-third of its Practice Bulletins are based on "good and consistent" evidence.[2] Further, much of pregnancy care cannot be evaluated safely and ethically using the types of research recognized as being most rigorous. Midwifery research continues to account for only a small percentage of the work being done in women's health, although an increasing number of scholars are contributing knowledge in this area. Examples range from the development of Centering Pregnancy as a model of care to the research done on delayed cord-clamping after birth.[3,4] Deciphering the evidence, acknowledging the quality of information from which recommendations are made, and recognizing biases—both from midwives and others—are all key components of midwifery care.

Midwifery is distinguished by characteristics that define a partnership with women. A willingness to listen; sensitivity to cultural, sexual, and generational issues; informed/shared decision making; the patience to be "with women"—all combine with professional behaviors to describe midwifery practice. This chapter addresses both clinical tasks and professional behaviors. In these pages, the goal is to identify those core skills needed to be a midwife.

Essential skills begin with an understanding of the midwifery management process. Developed by midwifery education programs in Mississippi and New Jersey in the mid-1970s,[5,6] its seven steps serve as a guide to the process of care at an individual level and offer an opportunity to evaluate the effectiveness of care (**Box 4-1**). The midwifery management process emphasizes the midwife's responsibility as an independent care provider and is based on the scientific process. The overlap with the common flow of an individual healthcare visit is obvious; this process

BOX 4-1 The Midwifery Management Process

1. Investigate by obtaining all necessary data for complete evaluation of the woman or newborn.

2. Make an accurate identification of problems or diagnoses and healthcare needs based on correct interpretation of the data.

3. Anticipate other potential problems or diagnoses that might be expected because of the identified problems or diagnoses.

4. Evaluate the need for immediate midwife or physician intervention and/or for consultation or collaborative management with other healthcare team members, as dictated by the condition of the woman or newborn.

5. Develop a comprehensive plan of care that is supported by explanations of valid rationale underlying the decisions made and is based on the preceding steps.

6. Assume responsibility for the efficient and safe implementation of the plan of care.

7. Evaluate the effectiveness of the care given, recycling appropriately through the management process for any aspect of care that has been ineffective.

also recognizes that most care is provided not in discrete sessions but rather over time, and that continuity over time is essential to improve quality of care.

Communication

Use of Language

Learning to listen to one's own words and see one's physical position relative to others is a skill like any other. Both speech and body language affect the relationship between midwife and the woman receiving care. Among other things, this means that word choice needs to be appropriate for the woman's educational and cultural background. The midwife has to move to where the woman is in terms of understanding; by beginning there, both can move together to identify and discuss a problem. The language that any healthcare provider spends years mastering is not the common tongue.

Start where the woman is—you'll get further.

Active listening is an essential skill. It requires the patience to allow a woman to tell her own story with minimal interruptions or directive language. Asking open-ended questions gives a woman a chance to put into her own words what is concerning her. When one listens actively, one focuses on what is being said, reflects back what one hears, and verifies that both participants in the conversation share understanding. Waiting silently to encourage additional information; paraphrasing an unclear statement by asking, "I think you mean _____. Is that correct?"; reflecting back, such as by saying, "I hear you saying _____."; and providing reassurance that the woman's information is important are all critical tools. Validating understanding of a problem described by a woman is essential—it is all too easy to misunderstand her real concern. Further, the woman needs to believe that what she says will be held in confidence, and that she may say anything she needs to safely. Active listening also incorporates a nonverbal component, including eye contact, leaning toward a person rather than away from her, having an open body position that suggests acceptance, avoiding closed positioning (e.g., not crossing the arms), and maintaining a professional facial expression.

Another tool for listening to oneself in professional conversations is to address the four gates of speech that are part of the mystical Sufi tradition. Among several phrasings, the following are appropriate when considering how communication in a professional setting affects the woman's ability to hear what is being said. The midwife's words should answer the following four questions:

1. *Is it truthful?* If not, there is no need to say it.

2. *Is it kind?* Many of the topics that need to be discussed require kindness to make it possible for the listener to accept unpalatable advice. Kindness is not ignoring a problem, nor is it patronizing the woman. For example, there are many ways to tell someone she weighs too much and needs to lose weight. Compare "You're obese and you need to eat less" with "I'm concerned that your weight is harming your health." Which of these statements will be more likely to lead to accepting a referral to a nutritionist?

3. *Is it necessary?* Preventing damage from diabetes or hypertension may hinge on the woman accepting the referral and actively participating in improving her health.

4. *Is it appropriate?* In one sense, discussing weight management is always appropriate, but what if the woman has come to be treated

for a sexually transmitted infection (STI)? Perhaps weight loss is not the concern she needs to focus on today.

Addressing Sensitive Concerns

Midwives deal with some of the most intimate and personal aspects of a woman's life. Her choice of partner, her decisions about childbearing, and her sexual experiences constitute one theme. Her risk for being exposed to violence, whether physically, sexually, or emotionally, is another theme. The acceptability of her lifestyle or habits, her exposure to infections, her literacy level, and whether she even has a home are all topics that can and will come up during midwifery care.

Women experience stigma for many reasons. When a person has been exposed to negative reactions in the community enough times, the individual tends to withdraw from creating opportunities to be stigmatized. It is the midwife's job to create a safe environment, where questions can be asked and answered, and where help can be sought and offered. When greeting a woman or family in the office, when providing care, and when discussing choices, watch for physical or verbal cues that suggest that another topic needs to be addressed.

Approaching the Woman

The first steps in any clinical encounter usually occur before the midwife and a woman meet. Somehow, the woman has found the practice, made an appointment, been checked in for her visit, and possibly been seen by a nurse or medical assistant. She has observed whether the setting is professional and the furnishings are in good repair. Although it is not the purpose of this chapter to discuss practice management, all of these events have shaped the woman's first impressions of her midwife and of midwifery. Seemingly simple choices about work flow, such as whether the woman is seen first in an office or undressed on an exam table, say something about mutual respect. Just as when making a home visit, the midwife looks for clues about the woman's lifestyle and health of her family; likewise, the woman seeks clues about the midwife's practice and professionalism.

The first professional question during a visit is always a variant of "Why do you come in to see us today?" Before asking this question, however, mutual introductions should take place. Think of the relationship forged during this encounter as a framework for the care that the woman will receive. The woman should be seated comfortably and with adequate personal space. The midwife's position should promote direct eye contact. Asking, "How are you today?" or "How are you feeling?" establishes concern for her as an individual. Listening to her answer assists her in establishing trust in midwifery care.

From a compliance or payment perspective, the order of the visit's elements encapsulates the essential components of care. While compliance refers to legal requirements (such as Medicare regulations) and payment refers to what must be done to receive compensation from insurers, both have standards that must be met. Some visits will be tightly problem focused; some will be comprehensive examinations. Both types of visits follow the same sequence. All begin with the same question: "Why do you come in to see us today?" The answer establishes the chief concern of the woman—that is, the reason for the visit. Sometimes other, more pressing problems will become apparent during the conversation or examination, but this question is the starting point.

The structural components of the visit include the following: chart review of previous records and test results, history, and review of systems; the examination and any office-based tests; the assessment and diagnosis; and the decision making about future visits, tests, and treatment plus the discussion, teaching, and guidance offered to the woman. **Appendix 4A** reviews standard precautions that are an essential component of any healthcare visit.

Collecting the Medical History

When collecting a medical history, the midwife first considers the purpose of the visit. If the woman has come for a comprehensive or general reason, the history obtained will be broader than if the visit were problem focused. Consider a new obstetric visit, which will include a complete personal, social, and family history, as well as genetic risks, and contrast it with a triage visit for nausea and vomiting of pregnancy that will focus on the current concern, asking about exposure to spoiled food and infectious contacts, allergies, gastrointestinal disorders, and problems with nausea in prior pregnancies.

The general principle is to work from the least invasive questions to those that require more personal exposure. When one question at a time is asked, and there is a pause to wait for each response, information is less likely to be confused or omitted. Establishing and maintaining an easy flow of dialogue and a nonjudgmental manner promotes open exchange of information. A woman should be advised that some questions are very personal, and that she is not required to answer ones that she does not wish to discuss. It may be necessary to ask particularly sensitive questions on more than one occasion before the woman is able to give a full answer. An example of a situation that may require such treatment is that of prior abuse, as discussed later in this chapter. **Appendix 4B** provides a review of the complete health history.

> Always ask yourself, What is the next question I should ask? What haven't I considered?

Review of Systems

The review of systems (ROS) bridges the divide between prior medical history and today's examination. It includes recent signs and symptoms the woman has noticed, such as burning on urination or a rash. The ROS combines with the history to open up more extensive lines of questioning. In many practices, the ROS is a checklist given to a woman to complete while waiting. During a focused visit, the ROS may be part of the conversation during the examination. When questions are asked well, this part of the encounter can identify further areas of concern or topics for education.

The Physical Examination

Most examinations in women's health are screening examinations, unless the midwife is serving as the primary care provider (PCP) and the history or ROS has identified additional potential health problems that need to be explored in depth. Screening physical examinations abbreviate the detail that can be elicited when every organ system is fully evaluated. **Appendix 4C** outlines a comprehensive physical examination.

By tradition, a woman's initial health assessment, whether she is pregnant or not, is comprehensive, meaning that it includes all the major organ systems. Women who see their midwife regularly and have another provider designated as a PCP can receive a "single system" examination that targets and more completely evaluates the genitourinary and reproductive systems. In that case, the thyroid, breasts, abdomen, and pelvis are examined fully, but other systems are not addressed. Because the breast and pelvic examinations are key to any women's health assessment, these components of the physical examination are reviewed in **Appendices 4D and 4E**.

In-Office Laboratory Testing

A final part of the office examination is the completion of any in-office tests to be performed. Among those tests commonly performed in midwifery offices are urine dipstick, wet mount, potassium hydroxide to test for the presence of yeast, pregnancy tests, and fern tests (**Appendix 4F**). The Clinical Laboratory Improvement Amendments of 1988 (CLIA) regulate tests performed in an office (42 CFR part 493).[7] The CLIA regulations are federal regulatory standards for all clinical laboratory tests done on humans in all settings except research protocols. CLIA identifies three categories of laboratory tests based on the complexity of test methodology: (1) waived tests, (2) tests of moderate complexity, and (3) tests of high complexity. Waived tests are those that are accurate (i.e., the likelihood of erroneous results is negligible), pose little risk of harm if performed incorrectly, and have been cleared by the Food and Drug Administration (FDA) to be performed at home. Examples of waived tests and tests of moderate complexity are listed in **Table 4-1**. When both home and professional versions of a waived test (e.g., pregnancy tests) are available, the FDA must approve the professional version for waiver separately.[8]

If *only* waived tests will be performed in an office, then a Certificate of Waiver can be obtained to license the office laboratory. The Centers for Medicare and Medicaid Services provides explanations of the waiver process and requirements on its website.[9] CLIA tests that are of moderate and high complexity require further registration and documentation. Provider-performed microscopy, for example, is considered a subcategory of moderate-complexity testing. Information on obtaining a license for an office laboratory can be found in the current CLIA regulations.[10]

Establishing a Differential Diagnosis: Making an Assessment

When all the information available during the visit has been gathered, the midwife makes an assessment based on a differential diagnosis. The "differential"

Table 4-1	CLIA Testing Categories: Waived and Moderately Complex
CLIA Waived Tests	**CLIA Tests of Moderate Complexity**
Dipstick or tablet reagent urinalysis (nonautomated) for bilirubin, glucose, hemoglobin, ketones, leucocytes, nitrates, pH, protein, specific gravity, and urobilinogen	Provider-performed microscopy: all direct wet-mount preparations for the presence or absence of bacteria, fungi, parasites, and human cellular elements
Fecal occult blood	All potassium hydroxide (KOH) preparations
Ovulation tests: visual color comparison tests for luteinizing hormone	Postcoital direct, qualitative examinations of vaginal or cervical mucus
Urine pregnancy tests: visual color comparison tests	Qualitative semen analysis (limited to the presence or absence of sperm and detection of motility)
Blood glucose by glucose monitoring devices cleared by the FDA specifically for home use	Fern tests
	Pinworm examinations
	Urine sediment examinations
	Nasal smears for granulocytes
	Fecal leukocyte examinations

summarizes the various conditions, disorders, and health problems that might be the cause of each identified concern. It is sometimes very straightforward—for example, assuming a woman has come for an annual examination, she is in good health, and her only questions were about choosing a birth control method, the assessment addresses her normal examination and the contraceptive counseling or initiation of a method that is appropriate. At other times, the differential diagnosis can be quite complex. Right lower quadrant abdominal pain in a woman in early pregnancy might be appendicitis, an ectopic pregnancy, a corpus luteum cyst, or any of many other possible disorders. Those conditions that are most dangerous are the first differentials considered followed by those that are most common. The symptoms, history, and examination findings are considered to determine the most likely cause.

Sometimes the initial differential diagnosis will be descriptive rather than diagnostic. In the second example in the preceding paragraph, ectopic pregnancy will always be the first condition considered, as it can cause irremediable harm to the woman. The differential diagnosis suggests avenues for further testing or evaluation and helps to direct the plan. Again following the example of the woman with right lower quadrant (RLQ) pain in early pregnancy, the initial diagnosis is descriptive: RLQ pain in pregnancy. The first tests ordered should be a pelvic ultrasound and a quantitative level of serum human chorionic gonadotropin (hCG).

Creating a Plan

The plan should always include any lab work or procedures ordered, any medications prescribed, and the date of the next visit. For midwives, however, the plan never includes just these three items. Among the "hallmarks of midwifery" are health education, counseling, and guidance.[11] Every plan for every woman includes documentation ensuring that these aspects of care were addressed. The reputation of midwifery rests in part on midwives' ability to be available for support, knowledge, and clarity of information. The education and counseling is sometimes just-in-time teaching, such as what a group B *Streptococcus* (GBS) screening culture is and why it is being done at the 36-week prenatal visit; at other times, it consists of information that addresses long-term plans—for example, the new Pap smear guidelines and why the intervals are changing. The plan also includes information that will lead to informed decision making.

Informed Consent and Shared Decision Making

Informed consent and *informed refusal* are the traditional terms for documenting a woman's agreement or disagreement with a procedure or plan of care. Ethically and legally, obtaining informed consent is the responsibility of all healthcare providers.[12] Educational and financial status have been shown to affect clients' preferences for shared or directed decision making; as the disparity between care provider and client widens, the information provided and path to a decision change.[13] For the most effective results, the process should be thought of in terms of informed decision making, as the process allows for the woman to question and/or decline treatment in whole or part. **Box 4-2** summarizes the essential components of informed consent.

Health Literacy and Health Numeracy

The midwifery approach to informed decision making must address the woman in language she can understand, with explanations that are clear and do not omit factual information that is important. Health literacy is defined by the U.S. Department of Health and Human Services as "the degree to which individuals have the capacity to obtain, process, and understand basic health information and services needed to make appropriate health decisions."[14] Approximately half of the U.S. adult population has low health literacy.[15] Low health literacy is consistently associated with more hospitalizations and lower use of preventative

services such as mammography and vaccinations. Although educational attainment frequently is used as a proxy for health literacy, many individuals actually read and, more importantly, comprehend at levels below their formal educational level.

Health numeracy, which is the degree to which individuals understand quantitative and probabilistic health information, is an important component of health literacy.[16] Ways to increase the likelihood that a woman will understand the probability of an event include using absolute numbers in place of percentages, relative risks, or risk ratios;[17] avoiding the words "rare," "unlikely," "uncommon," and "unusual," as these are imprecise concepts subject to individual interpretation; and using small denominators and whole numbers.[18] For example, "1 in 4" is more easily understood than "25 out of 100" or "25%."

Shared Decision Making

The midwife is responsible for providing good information; the woman is responsible for considering the alternatives, asking questions, and making the decision. There are only rare occasions where professional judgment can override a woman's consent; most of these involve potentially fatal emergencies requiring rapid action. Even then, there are limitations on action—some decisions require consent of a family member or even court approval.

Shared decision making is different from presenting risks and benefits. This type of woman-centered decision making can occur only when clear communication of risk, benefits, and the range of available options is presented. Then the woman is able to make her decision within the context of her personal values and beliefs and preferences. Midwives have the responsibility to verify that women are pleased with the amount and type of information received, and feel that their needs have been addressed during a visit.

Ethical behavior requires that no harm be done (nonmaleficence), that the midwife acts for the good of the family or community involved (beneficence), that all persons are treated equally (justice), and that the woman be able to make a choice (autonomy). It is sometimes difficult to accept that the choice a woman makes is not the one a midwife is comfortable with, or even an option under consideration.

When a midwife cannot or does not provide a requested service, the obligation is to advise the

---

BOX 4-2 Essential Elements of Informed Consent or Informed Refusal

- The known or possible diagnosis
- The nature and purpose of the proposed treatment or procedure
- The benefits and risks associated with the recommended plan
- Complications and side effects (include both common and severe)
- Likelihood of success for this individual
- Reasonable alternatives available
- Benefits and risks associated with the alternatives
- Possible consequences of not following the proposed plan of care
- Assessment of the person's understanding and agreement

woman about resources in an unbiased manner. No midwife should act in a way that violates her or his understanding of safety for the woman and evidence-based care. Likewise, no midwife should withhold information or care based on her or his personal beliefs. The woman's ability to choose is impaired where the line between personal beliefs and professional actions is drawn.

Cultural Competence

"Culture is an integrated pattern of human behavior that includes the thoughts, communications, actions, customs, beliefs, values, and institutions associated wholly or partially with racial, ethnic, or linguistic groups as well as religious, spiritual, biological, geographical or sociological characteristics. Culture is dynamic in nature and individuals may identify with multiple cultures over the course of their lifetimes."[19]

Importantly, culture is more than racial and ethnic groups. An individual's culture has multiple diverse components including factors such as religion, gender identification, and occupation, just to name a few. To provide health care, midwives must understand the importance of each woman's cultural frame of reference. Culturally competent practice is particularly important for midwives because midwives often serve women who are from disadvantaged cultures in one way or another.

It is also important to remember that health care is a cultural construct as well—emerging from beliefs about the characteristics of disease and the impact on the human body—thus, culture is a primary factor in the provision of health services that influences both the provider and the receiver of care.

There are many different definitions of cultural competence and several related terms such as *cultural humility, cultural sensitivity,* and *cultural awareness.*[20] Each of these definitions and terms describe part of a broader concept. The definition used by the United States Department of Health and Human Resources Office of Minority Health states that cultural competence is "a set of congruent behaviors, attitudes, and policies that come together in a system, agency, or among professionals that enables effective work in cross-cultural situations."[19] Cultural competence refers to a healthcare provider's ability to honor and respect beliefs, interpersonal styles, attitudes, and behaviors of the women served. Cultural competence in health care must be incorporated at all levels—from policy and administration to clinical practice. To begin to understand the concept of culture and the plethora of world views that each person brings to a situation, it is important to keep the following three points in mind:

1. Culture is not static; it is dynamic and ever changing; the cultural practices that individuals remember and practice from their country or place of origin are often different from the practices that are occurring in that same place today.

2. Culture, language, ethnicity, and race are not the only determinants of a person's values, beliefs, and behaviors. Occupation, socioeconomic status, cultural upbringing, and educational level have an influence on how individuals define and view themselves.

3. In describing any culture or cultural practice, within-group differences are as great as across group differences. In other words, no culture and no ethnic, linguistic, or racial group is monolithic. There are wide variations in attitudes, beliefs, and behaviors. To assume that people who share a common culture and language are alike is to make a dangerous mistake.[21]

The "cultural competence continuum" can help midwives meet the health care needs of a culturally diverse population. The "cultural competence continuum" (**Figure 4-1**) describes six distinct levels of competence, ranging from destructiveness to proficiency. The cultural competence continuum is especially helpful in the identification of cultural deficits and the targeting of areas in need of development and improvement. The cultural competence continuum also provides a framework for the recognition of practitioner and service intervention biases.[22] Becoming a culturally competent provider requires a series of steps. The first is recognizing where one is on the continuum and moving forward. The second is a life-long commitment to the process. The characteristics of culturally competent healthcare practitioners are listed in **Box 4-3**. Additional resources for cultural competence are listed at the end of this chapter.

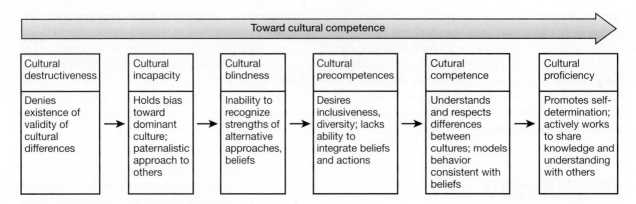

Figure 4-1 Cultural competence continuum.
Source: Adapted from Cross TL, Bazron BJ, Dennis KW, et al. *The Cultural Competence Continuum: Toward a Culturally Competent System of Care: A Monograph on Effective Services for Minority Children Who Are Severely Mentally Disturbed.* Washington, DC: Georgetown University Child Development Center; 1989:13; Doyle EI, Faucher MA. Pharmaceutical therapy in midwifery practice: a culturally competent approach. *J Midwifery Women's Health.* 2002;47:122-129.

BOX 4-3 Characteristics of Culturally Competent Practitioners

- Move from cultural unawareness to an awareness and sensitivity of their own cultural heritage.

- Recognize their own values and biases and are aware of how they may affect clients from other cultures.

- Demonstrate comfort with cultural differences that exist between themselves and clients.

- Know specifics about the particular cultural groups they are working with.

- Understand the historical events that may have caused harm to a particular cultural group.

- Respect and are aware of the unique needs of clients from diverse communities.

- Understand the importance of diversity within as well as between cultures.

- Endeavor to learn more about cultural communities through client interactions, participation in cultural diversity dynamics, and consultations with community experts.

- Make a continuous effort to understand a client's point of view.

- Demonstrate flexibility and tolerance of ambiguity, and are nonjudgmental.

- Maintain a sense of humor and an open mind.

- Demonstrate a willingness to relinquish control in clinical encounters, to risk failure, and to look within for the source of frustration, anger, and resistance.

- Acknowledge that the process is as important as the product.

Source: Randall-David, E. *Culturally Competent HIV Counseling and Education.* Rockville, MD: DHHS Maternal and Child Health Bureau, 1994.

Conclusion

The expert midwife has mastered the skills of history taking, examination, diagnosis, and treatment. She or he has become comfortable teaching, guiding, and caring for women throughout their lives. Using solid evidence as a base for decisions and focusing on safety for women will have become second nature. Equally important, the expert midwife has moved beyond simple performance of the necessary elements of care to a level where each woman is viewed as an individual and as a member of her community, to respect different cultures, become culturally competent in delivering healthcare services, and to truly believe that all women deserve midwifery care.

• • • References

1. Sniderman AD, Furberg CD. Why guideline-making requires reform. *JAMA*. 2009;301(4):429-431.

2. Wright JD, Pawar N, Gonzalez J, et al. Scientific evidence underlying the American College of Obstetricians and Gynecologists' Practice Bulletins. *Obstet Gynecol*. 2011;118(3):505-512.

3. Novick G, Sadler LS, Kennedy HP, et al. Women's experience of group prenatal care. *Qual Health Res*. 2011;21(1):97-116.

4. Mercer JS, Vohr BR, Erickson-Owens DA, et al. Seven-month developmental outcomes of very low birth weight infants enrolled in a randomized controlled trial of delayed versus immediate cord clamping. *J Perinatol*. 2010;30(1):11-16.

5. University of Mississippi Medical Center, Nurse-Midwifery Education Program. *Management Process*. Jackson, MS: Author; 1972-1973.

6. College of Medicine and Dentistry of New Jersey, New Jersey Medical School, Nurse-Midwifery Education Program. *Management Process*. Newark, NJ: 1975.

7. Centers for Disease Control and Prevention. Clinical laboratory Improvement Amendments: CLIA regulations. Updated April 5, 2012. Available at: http://wwwn.cdc.gov/clia/regs/toc.aspx. Accessed October 8, 2012.

8. United States Food and Drug Administration. Medical devices: CLIA waivers. Updated June 6, 2009. Available at: http://www.fda.gov/medicaldevices/device regulationandguidance/ivdregulatoryassistance /ucm124202.htm. Accessed October 8, 2012.

9. Centers for Medicare and Medicaid Services. Clinical Laboratory Improvement Amendments (CLIA): how to obtain a CLIA Certificate of Waiver. Available at: http://www.cms.gov/Regulations-and-Guidance/Legislation/CLIA/downloads/HowObtainCertificateofWaiver.pdf. Accessed October 8, 2012.

10. Centers for Disease Control and Prevention. CLIA provider performed microscopy. Updated July 7, 2004. Available at: http://wwwn.cdc.gov/clia/ppm.aspx. Accessed October 8, 2012.

11. American College of Nurse-Midwives. Core competencies for basic midwifery practice. Available at: http://www.midwife.org/ACNM/files/ACNMLibraryData/UPLOADFILENAME/000000000050/Core%20Competencies%20June%202012.pdf. Accessed October 8, 2012.

12. Paterick TJ, Carson GV, Allen MC, Paterick TE. Medical informed consent: general considerations for physicians. *Mayo Clin Proc*. 2008;83(3):313-319.

13. Verlinde EE, De Laender N, De Maesschalck S, et al. The social gradient in doctor–patient communication. *Int J Equity Health*. 2012;11:12.

14. U.S. Department of Health and Human Services. *Healthy People 2010: Understanding and Improving Health*, 2nd ed. Washington, DC: U.S. Government Printing Office; November 2000.

15. Nelson W, Reyna VF, Fagerlin A, et al. Clinical implications of numeracy: theory and practice. *Ann Behav Med*. 2008;35(3):261-274.

16. Golbeck AL, Ahlers-Schmidt CR, Paschal AM, et al. A definition and operational framework for health numeracy. *Am J Prev Med*. 2005;29(4):375-376.

17. Galesic M, Gigerenzer G, Straubinger N. Natural frequencies help older adults and people with low numeracy to evaluate medical screening tests. *Med Decis Making*. 2009;29(3):368-371.

18. Edwards A, Elwyn G, Mulley A. Explaining risks: turning numerical data into meaningful pictures. *BMJ*. 2002;324(7341):827-830.

19. U.S. Department of Health and Human Services. Office of Minority Health. What Is Cultural Competency? Available at: http://minorityhealth.hhs.gov/templates/browse.aspx?lvl=2&lvlID=11. Accessed July 7, 2013.

20. Jesse DE, Kirkpatrick MK. Catching the spirit of cultural care: A midwifery exemplar. *J Midwifery Women's Health*. 2013;58:49-56.

21. Lynch E, Hanson M,J eds. *Developing Cross Cultural Competence: A Guide for Working with Children and Their Families*. 3rd ed. Baltimore, MD: Paul H Brooks Publishing; 2004.

22. Cross TL, Bazron BJ, Dennis KW, et al. *The Cultural Competence Continuum: Toward a Culturally Competent System of Care: A Monograph on Effective Services for Minority Children Who Are Severely Mentally Disturbed*. Washington, DC: Georgetown University Child Development Center; 1989:13.

23. Randall-David, E. Culturally *Competent HIV Counseling and Education*. Rockville, MD: DHHS Maternal and Child Health Bureau; 1994.

• • • **Additional Resources**

Berkowitz B. Cultural aspects in the care of the orthodox Jewish woman. *J Midwifery Women's Health*. 2008;53: 62-67.

Brach C, Fraser, Director for the Agency for Health Care Research and Quality. Can cultural competency reduce racial and ethnic health disparities: A review and conceptual model. *Medical Care Res Rev*. 2000;57(suppl. 1): 181-217.

Callister, LC. Culturally competent care of women and newborns: Knowledge, attitude, and skills. *J Obstet Gynecol Neonatal Nurs*. 2001;30(2):209-215.

Cioffi J, Dip G. Caring for women from culturally diverse backgrounds: Midwives experiences. *J Midwifery Women's Health*. 2004;49:437-442.

DeWalt DA, Callahan LF, Hawk VH, et al. Health Literacy Universal Precautions Toolkit. (Prepared by North Carolina Network Consortium, The Cecil G. Sheps Center for Health Services Research, The University of North Carolina at Chapel Hill, under Contract No. HHSA290200710014.) AHRQ Publication No. 10-0046-EF) Rockville, MD: Agency for Healthcare Research and Quality; April 2010.

Doyle E, Faucher MA. Pharmaceutical therapy in midwifery practice: A culturally competent approach. *J Midwifery Women's Health*. 2002;47:122-120

Dutton L, Koenig K, Fennie K. Gynecologic care of the female-to-male transgender man. *J Midwifery Women's Health*. 2008;53:331-337.

Fadiman, A. *The Spirit Catches You and You Fall Down*. New York: Farrar, Straus, and Giroux; 1997.

Hindin PK. Intimate partner violence screening practices of certified nurse-midwives. *J Midwifery Women's Health*. 2006;51:216-221.

Rorie, JL, Paine, LL, Barger, MK. Primary care for women: Cultural competence in primary care services. *J Nurse-Midwifery*. 1996;41(2):92-100.

U.S. Department of Health and Human Services, Offices of Minority Health. *National Culturally and Linguistically Appropriate Services (CLAS) Standards in Health Care, Executive Summary*. 2010. Available at: https://www .thinkculturalhealth.hhs.gov/Content/clas.asp. Accessed July 7, 2013.

U.S. Department of Health and Human Services. *Culture, Language, and Health Literacy*. Available at: http://www .hrsa.gov/culturalcompetence/index.html. Accessed July 7, 2013.

4A

Standard Precautions

Healthcare-associated infections (HAIs) are any infections that individuals acquire while receiving direct services. Although activities designed to prevent HAIs were originally targeted toward protection for consumers, healthcare workers are also at risk for HAIs. Therefore, knowledge and institution of standard precautions that protect both the women and families for whom midwives provide care, as well as the midwives themselves, are a core standard of practice.

Standard precautions are the essential activities that should be employed by all healthcare workers in all healthcare settings for the purpose of preventing HAIs without regard to specific infection risks. Standard precautions are the most basic level of infection control and have four components: (1) hand hygiene, (2) use of personal protective devices, (3) safe injection practices, and (4) respiratory hygiene/cough etiquette.

Standard precautions[1] are sometimes viewed as interfering with the close relationship valued both by midwives and women. However, they are also the most effective method of preventing *both* parties from accidentally being exposed to infection. On some occasions it is the midwife who is more at risk when caring for a woman with an infection than the woman herself. Standard precautions are not limited to the hospital environment, although some accommodations to precautions are observed in ambulatory settings.[2] For example, complete contact precautions are not always possible when someone presents with an open lesion that was not disclosed previously.

Standard Precautions

1. Hand hygiene is to be performed before and after every encounter with an individual, regardless of the healthcare environment—hospital, home, birth center, or office. Alcohol-based cleaners are effective against a wider spectrum of pathogens than soap and water and are preferred unless the hands are visibly soiled. Soap and water are always used when any dirt, blood, or body fluids are visible.[3]

2. Gloves are worn for vaginal examinations; collection of cultures; birth; phlebotomy; finger and heel sticks; handling the newborn before the baby is washed and dried; and handling of any sanitary or bed pads, clothing, linens, or other items soiled with body fluids. Hand hygiene is always performed after glove removal.

3. Personal protective equipment (PPE) is used to prevent exposure of skin and mucous membranes (eyes, nose, mouth) to blood, amniotic fluid, vaginal secretions, semen, repeated contact with breast milk, and body fluids or secretions containing visible blood. PPE can include gloves, cover gowns or aprons, masks, protective eyewear, foot covers, and mouthpieces or other barriers for use during resuscitation.

4. Safety needles have mechanisms built in to protect providers from accidental needle

punctures. Blunt tipped needles are advised for drawing up fluids from a vial to minimize needle sticks associated with sharp needles. Both safety syringes/needles and blunt needles should be used whenever available. Needles are *not* to be recapped, removed from disposable syringes, bent, broken, or otherwise manipulated by hand after use. All sharp needles and disposable instruments are placed in puncture-resistant disposal containers located in the immediate area, but outside the reach of visiting children.

5. Respiratory hygiene is observed to protect against respiratory and other droplet infections. This includes provision of tissues, masks, and hand cleaner in all healthcare settings; a reminder to women and their family members who are ill to cover coughs or sneezes and utilize the provided supplies; and seeing that all healthcare staff also observe these precautions.

• • • References

1. Siegel JD, Rhinehart E, Jackson M, et al. 2007 guideline for isolation precautions: preventing transmission of infectious agents in healthcare settings. Available at: http://wwhttp://www.cdc.gov/hicpac/pdf/isolation/Isolation2007.pdfw.cdc.gov/ncidod/dhqp/pdf/isolation2007.pdf. Accessed October 7, 2012.

2. Centers for Disease Control and Prevention, National Center for Emerging and Zoonotic Infectious Diseases. Guide to infection prevention for outpatient settings: minimum expectations for safe care 2011. Available at: http://www.cdc.gov/HAI/pdfs/guidelines/standatds-of-ambulatory-care-7-2011.pdf. Accessed September 29, 2012.

3. Centers for Disease Control and Prevention. Guideline for hand hygiene in health-care settings: recommendations of the Healthcare Infection Control Practices Advisory Committee and the HICPAC/SHEA/APIC/IDSA Hand Hygiene Task Force. *MMWR*. 2002; 51(No. RR-16):1-56. Available at: http://www.cdc.gov/mmwr/PDF/rr/rr5116.pdf. Accessed October 7, 2012.

4B

Collecting a Medical History

In women's health, the chief concerns are frequently focused on reproductive or gynecologic concerns. This does not mean that the medical, surgical, or family history can be omitted. A woman's overall health influences healthcare decision making, as prior illnesses and surgeries may affect which type of examination is needed and which medications can be prescribed. Family history may open up a discussion about future health risks. For midwives with an active primary care practice, many general health concerns, elicited in the history and review of systems, may also be addressed during routine examinations.

History of the Present Illness

After determining the chief concern for a visit, the next step is to inquire about the history of the present illness (HPI). This is often a misnomer—for example, a chief concern of "I need my Pap test and birth control pills" leads to an HPI that addresses how the woman is managing her contraception and her satisfaction with her current method (and possibly to a discussion of screening recommendations). A chief concern that begins with abnormal uterine bleeding leads to the more traditional assessment of the history of the woman's current symptoms. A common mnemonic for the questions asked about a medical problem is OLD CARTS (Onset, Location/radiation, Duration, Character, Aggravating factors, Relieving factors, Timing, and Severity). These questions can be followed by "What has changed now that made you come in?" or "How did you decide it was time to come in?"

The Medical and Surgical History

A medical and surgical history includes review of all the organ systems, mental health, common infections, blood transfusions, injuries and traumas, and surgeries (**Table 4B-1**). The list in Table 4B-1 is not comprehensive, but does include questions that are frequently or specifically germane in a woman's health examination. Clearly, any other problems that are identified should also be investigated.

Some commonly asked questions include the following:

1. Have you ever had a major illness—for example, any breathing problems, stomach or liver problems, or any bladder infections?

2. Are there any others you can think of?

3. Have you ever had to have any special tests or procedures?

4. Have you ever been admitted to the hospital because you were sick? When was that? Why were you in the hospital?

5. Who has been taking care of you for (problem)? Have they suggested you see anyone else?

For the woman who is seen on a regular basis, asking whether there has been any change in her health, and possibly reminding her of what she previously reported, can assist with time management during the visit.

Table 4B-1	Past Medical and Surgical History		
1. Neurologic Migraine headaches Other types of headaches Epilepsy or seizure disorders Multiple sclerosis	**2. Skin** Chronic skin conditions	**3. Respiratory** Asthma Tuberculosis	**4. Cardiovascular** Hypertension Hyperlipidemia CVA Myocardial infarction
5. Breast Does she check her breasts regularly? Biopsy, cyst or adenoma removal Breast enlargement, reduction or reconstruction Other breast problems	**6. Gastrointestinal** GERD Chronic diarrhea or constipation Cholecystectomy Appendectomy Bariatric surgery	**7. Genitourinary** Frequent UTIs Genital tract infections STIs Hysterectomy, myomectomy, oophorectomy Postchildbirth repair Cervical LEEP, cone biopsy Maternal DES exposure	**8. Musculoskeletal** Arthritis, Any limitations of motion
9. Hematologic Sickle cell, hemoglobinopathies Anemia Bleeding disorders	**10. Endocrine** Thyroid disorders Diabetes	**11. Infections** Childhood infections Vaccinations, especially TDaP and influenza Chronic illnesses—HIV, hepatitis B or C, herpes PID Endometritis	**12. Psychological** Depression Postpartum depression Other mental disorders
13. Allergies Drug Environmental Food	**14. Medications** Prescription Vitamins Over the counter Herbal, homeopathic, nutritional or other supplements	**15. Other** Surgeries Physical trauma Injuries	**16. Risk of violence:** **physical, sexual, or emotional** Violence: current/past Abusive behavior: current/past

Abbreviations: CVA= cerebral vascular accident; DES = diethylstilbesterol; GERD = Gastroesophageal reflux disease; LEEP = loop electrosurgical excision procedure; PID = pelvic inflammatory disease; STI = sexually transmitted infection; UTI = urinary tract infection.

Social History

The social history, like the sexual history, brings up topics that may be embarrassing or even threatening to some women (**Table 4B-2**). Ask these questions in a quiet, professional tone, and respect the woman's need to avoid certain answers. Relationship questions should be asked in a pattern that allows women to reveal relationships that are more complicated than "single" or "married with children."

Gynecologic and Obstetric History

This area is a natural progression after the general history is taken, and some of the items mentioned previously need not be reasked if the answer is already recorded. Listen for answers to questions not yet asked and try to remember them (**Table 4B-3**).

Sexual History

The core questions have been asked as part of the gynecologic history—age at first coitus, number and gender of partners, current status—but a number of other questions should be asked when appropriate to the visit. Do not expect women to volunteer these answers unless the questions are asked (**Table 4B-4**).

Table 4B-2	Social History		
1. Relationship status With a partner Married—keep in mind that this is no longer a "heterosexual only" question in some states Single Widowed, separated, or divorced	**2. Diet** Eating habits, history of eating disorders Diet recall Any food restrictions—vegetarian or vegan, religious, cultural limitations	**3. Substance use** Caffeine Tobacco Alcohol Illicit drugs Use of others' prescriptions	
4. Employment/student status	**5. Hazardous exposures at work or home**	**6. Regular physical activity**	
7. Seat belt use	**8. Guns or weapons in home**		

Table 4B-3	Gynecologic and Obstetric History		
1. Last menstrual period and last regular menstrual period	**2. Age at menarche, timing of menstrual cycles** Any irregularity of timing Amount and duration Premenstrual symptoms Dysmenorrhea Endometriosis	**3. Perimenopausal symptoms** Age at menopause—surgical or natural Use of hormone therapy	**4. Pap smear history** Abnormal Pap test Colposcopy Cervical treatment or surgery
5. Contraceptive history* Types used Duration of use Any problems	**6. Age at onset of sexual activity** See Sexual History in Table 4B-4.	**7. Pregnancy** G/P-TPAL Gravida (number of pregnancies) Para (number of births); T: term; P: preterm; A: spontaneous or elective abortions; L: number of living children Ectopic and multiple pregnancies Problems with pregnancies, births, or recovery Genetic testing Postpartum depression	**8. Other** Infertility Childbearing plans

*If a woman has had only women partners, she may have had no need for contraception, but may have still chosen to use hormonal contraception for other benefits.

Family History

Family histories assist in identifying risk factors and genetic concerns. Some concerns may be medical; other factors may relate to psychological or social concerns. First- and second-degree relatives are most important. Minimum components include the elements listed in **Table 4B-5** for parents, siblings, grandparents.

The final question in the history should be some variant of "Is there anything else I should have asked you today?" or alternatively "Is there anything else I should know or that you want to share with me?"

Review of Systems

The review of systems (ROS) acts as a bridge from the past to the present. It is a structured inquiry about current symptoms or concerns related to each body system. This part of the exam serves as a check for symptoms that the woman may be experiencing but has not yet mentioned. **Table 4B-6** is an example of a self-administered ROS form that women can complete while waiting for the visit. In some practices, a standard screening tool for depression such as the PHQ-9 is also provided for clients to fill out privately before the visit. Alternatively, you may complete an ROS as you do the physical examination, asking the woman about symptoms as the examination progresses.

Table 4B-4	Sexual History	
1. Sexually active (yes/no) If no, have you ever been sexually active?	**2. If yes:** Are your sex partners men, women, or both? In recent months, how many sex partners have you had?	**3. Monogamous with current partner (yes/no)**
4. Comfortable with frequency and types of sexual activity (yes/no)	**5. Patterns of sexual behavior** Frequency Type of sexual practices	**6. Specific problems:** Decreased libido Vaginal dryness, lack of lubrication Pain on penetration or with certain positions Insufficient foreplay Partner disregard of her sexual preferences
7. Problems of partner Impotence Delayed or premature ejaculation Sexually related violence	**8. Do you or your partner use any protection against sexually transmitted diseases? (yes/no)** If yes: What kind of protection and how often do you use it? If no: Could you tell me the reason?	**9. Have you ever been diagnosed with a sexually transmitted disease? (yes/no)** If yes: When? How were you treated? Have you had any recurring symptoms?
10. Has your partner ever been diagnosed with a sexually transmitted disease? (yes/no) If yes: When? How was he or she treated? Were you tested for the same sexually transmitted disease? **13. Do you have any other questions about sexual health or sexual practices that you want to discuss today?**	**11. Have you ever been tested for HIV or other sexually transmitted diseases? Would you like to be tested?**	**12. Are you using contraception or practicing any kind of birth control?**

Table 4B-5	Family History	
1. Parents and siblings Living or dead Age at death Cause of death	**2. Chronic disorders** Heart disease—especially coronary artery disease Diabetes Cancer—especially breast, reproductive, or colon	**3. Genetic problems** Birth defects Mental retardation

Table 4B-6	Review of Systems

Please mark any of the following that are bothering you now or within the last 2 weeks.

1. Constitutional:
❑ weight loss ❑ weight gain
❑ fatigue ❑ fever
❑ change in appetite

2. Neurologic:
❑ dizziness ❑ seizures
❑ numbness ❑ trouble walking
❑ memory problems
❑ headaches ❑ fainting

3. Skin:
❑ rash ❑ sore ❑ dry skin
❑ moles
❑ acne ❑ eczema

4. Eyes:
❑ double vision
❑ vision changes
❑ spots before eyes
❑ glasses/contacts

5. Ears, nose, throat:
❑ sinus problems
❑ hearing problems
❑ earaches
❑ ringing in ears
❑ sore throat ❑ mouth sores
❑ dental problems

6. Respiratory:
❑ painful breathing ❑ wheezing
❑ short of breath
❑ chronic cough ❑ spitting up blood

7. Cardiovascular:
❑ chest pain or pressure
❑ leg swelling
❑ difficulty breathing when active
❑ rapid or irregular heartbeat

8. Breasts:
❑ pain in breast ❑ breast lump
❑ nipple discharge

9. Gastrointestinal:
❑ frequent diarrhea
❑ bloody stools
❑ nausea/vomiting ❑ constipation
❑ passing gas or stool involuntarily

10. Genitourinary:
❑ blood in urine ❑ pain with urination
❑ frequent urination
❑ incomplete emptying of bladder
❑ unintended urine leaking
❑ leaking urine with cough or lifting
❑ abnormal vaginal bleeding
❑ painful periods ❑ pain with sex
❑ premenstrual symptoms (PMS)
❑ abnormal vaginal discharge
❑ hot flashes

11. Muscle and skeletal:
❑ muscle weakness ❑ spasms
❑ muscle or joint pain
❑ frequent falls

12. Hematologic and lymphatic:
❑ frequent bruising
❑ enlarged lymph nodes
❑ cuts that do not stop bleeding

13. Endocrine:
❑ hair loss
❑ heat/cold intolerance
❑ abnormal thirst ❑ hot flashes

14. Psychiatric:
❑ mood swings ❑ frequent crying
❑ anxiety ❑ trouble sleeping
❑ thoughts of hurting yourself or
   someone else

15. Allergies:
❑ hay fever ❑ hives
❑ seasonal allergies
❑ latex allergy
❑ food allergies

4C

The Physical Examination

As with the medical history, this description of the physical examination focuses on those aspects most significant for women's health. Be alert for any inconsistency between the woman's history and the physical examination.

Review of General Principles

1. As with every healthcare visit, hand washing is essential immediately prior to beginning the examination. Alcohol-based gels and/or foams are appropriate.

2. Ask the woman whether she has any area in particular she wants to have examined.

3. Drape the woman in such a way that only the area being examined is exposed. Let your approach and touch show respect for her body as well as respect for her right to modesty and privacy.

4. The examination should progress from head to toe, and minimize the times the woman has to change position (**Table 4C-1**).

5. Talk as you go, both to let her know what is happening next and to share reassuring findings. Let her know if any part of the examination will be uncomfortable.

6. Use a touch that is as firm as needed to elicit accurate information.

7. Share your findings with the woman. If she is anxious about something that you find to be normal, describe why the examination is normal.

8. Discuss physical changes that may be abnormal with the woman briefly during the examination and in more detail after she is dressed at the end of the visit.

Table 4C-1	**Physical Examination**

1. Constitutional Findings

Measured height and weight, body mass index (BMI)

Vital signs: blood pressure, pulse, respiratory rate, temperature

General appearance, grooming, cleanliness

2. Neurologic:

Orientation to time, place, person

Cranial nerves (visible alterations)

Mood and affect

Depression score (if formal assessment done)

3. Skin

Normal tone and turgor

Rashes, boils, or lesions

4. Head and Neck:

Eyes with pupils equal and responsive to light and accomodation (PERLA)

Dental care needed

Thyroid

Enlargement of lymph nodes

5. Respiratory:

Lung sounds

Respiratory effort

6. Cardiovascular:

Heart rate and rhythm

Audible murmurs or extra heart sounds

Pulses

Varicosities

7. Neurologic:

Orientation to time, place, person

Cranial nerves (visible alterations)

Mood and affect

Depression score (if formal assessment done)

8. Gastrointestinal:

Abdominal tone, guarding, rigidity

Bowel sounds

Size of liver and spleen, masses

Hernias, inguinal lymph nodes

Rectum (hemorrhoids, fissure)

9. Genitourinary (see Appendix 4E)

Costovertebral angle tenderness (CVAT) (see figure in the *Common Conditions in Primary Care* chapter)

Suprapubic tenderness

10. Musculoskeletal:

Spinal deformity

Range of motion

Deep tendon reflex (DTR); see **Box 4C-1**

Clonus (see box in the *Complications During Labor and Birth* chapter)

BOX 4C-1 Deep Tendon Reflexes

Deep tendon reflexes (DTRs) are also known as stretch reflexes because they are elicited by briefly stretching a muscle by tapping its tendon briskly. The brisk tap stimulates a sensory nerve impulse that travels through the reflex arc and ends with stimulation of the muscle in a brief contraction. This brief contraction causes a corresponding brief movement, or jerk, of the anatomical body part affected by the contraction of muscle. Therefore it is necessary, for each reflex tested, to know the name and location of the tendon to tap, the muscle in which to feel the contraction, and the anatomical body part in which to observe the jerk.

Significance and Charting

Hyperactive deep tendon reflexes are indicative of disease of the upper motor neutron or pyramidal tract. Hypoactive or absent deep tendon reflexes are indicative of a number of diseases. If you observe either condition, you should consult with a physician.

Reflexes are evaluated on a scale of 0 to 4+ as follows:

0 = absent; no response

1+ = decreased; diminished; sluggish

2+ = normal; average

3+ = brisk

4+ = very brisk; hyperactive
        (usually associated with clonus)

Reflexes designated 1+ are low-normal reflexes; 3+ reflexes are more brisk than the average reflex response and indicate the possible but not absolute presence of disease; 0 and 4+ reflexes are definitely abnormal and indicate disease requiring physician consultation. Reflexes should be symmetrical for homologous muscles and symmetry should be noted in the charting.

If only one or two of the reflexes is evaluated bilaterally, then the charting would reflect which one. For example: Quadriceps and biceps deep tendon reflexes (DTR)—2+ and symmetrical or Quadriceps DTR—3+, no clonus, symmetrical

Procedure

1. General:
   a. Symmetry is determined by comparing the reflex response on one side with the same reflex response on the other side.
   b. In testing reflexes, you should if possible palpate the muscle of the reflex being tested while tapping its tendon.
   c. The limb to be tested should be in a flexed or semiflexed position.
   d. The woman should be as relaxed as possible. If necessary, in the event the woman's reflexes appear absent or symmetrically diminished, use the technique of the reinforcement, which involves isometric contraction of muscles other than those being tested. For example, while testing leg reflexes, ask the woman to interlock her fingers and pull in opposite directions with her eyes closed; or when testing arm reflexes, have the woman clench her teeth or squeeze her thigh with the opposite hand, again with her eyes closed. The woman must be sufficiently relaxed for a deep tendon reflex to be elicited. Reinforcement works in two ways: (1) it distracts the woman and thereby causes relaxation; (2) the deliberate contraction of different muscles from those being tested may increase reflex activity. A reflex is not considered absent unless it cannot be elicited while using the technique of reinforcement.
   e. Tap the tendon briskly. A reflex hammer is most useful for this purpose. If a reflex hammer is not available the edge of your stethoscope or, for the quadriceps reflex, even the tips of your fingers suddenly striking the tendon may suffice. A brisk tap produces a sudden additional stretch of the tendon. The reflex hammer, when held loosely and swung in an arc using wrist action, provides just the right force and briskness.
   f. Position the woman so her limbs are symmetrical.
2. Eliciting the biceps reflex:
   a. Feel for the tendon of the biceps brachii muscle in the bend of the elbow. This can be identified by bending the woman's arm up and down at the elbow.
   b. Place the thumb of one of your hands firmly on the tendon.
   c. Position the woman's arm so it is partially flexed at the elbow and either resting in her lap or supported on your arm (the same arm as the thump you are using).
   d. Tap the tendon indirectly by striking your thumb with the pointed end of the reflex hammer.
5. Eliciting the quadriceps (knee-jerk) reflex:
   a. Position the woman so that her knees are somewhat flexed. If the woman is lying down, support her knees in the flexed position with your hand under her knees so her lower leg is relaxed. It is not necessary for the woman's foot to be off the bed. If the woman is sitting, be sure that her legs dangle over the edge of the examining table or bed, that her weight is on her buttocks and thighs, and that her feet are not resting on any object or the floor.

4D

Breast Examination

Clinical examination of the breasts takes place while taking into consideration any concerns expressed by the woman, any relevant personal or family history, and review of any prior records or reports. Routine formal breast self-examination is no longer recommended, but rather has been replaced by "breast awareness" as a way to recognize abnormal changes between clinical evaluations. There is no consensus about the frequency and effectiveness of clinical breast examinations[1–3]; for more information on breast evaluation and diagnosis, see the *Breast Conditions* chapter.

Procedure for Breast Examination

1. Wash hands prior to beginning the examination.

2. The woman should be seated on the examining table so that she is facing the examiner. Her chest area should be entirely exposed. Throughout the examination, use the drape or gown to cover any parts of the woman's body not being examined.

3. Have the woman sit erect, facing the examiner. Look at the breasts with her arms loose at her sides, raised overhead, and then with her hands on her hips so that her elbows are extended 90 degrees from the plane of her abdomen. Ask her to lean forward to check that the breasts hang freely.

   - With her arms raised, the pectoral fascia is elevated. If there is a carcinoma that has attached to the fascia, the breast may show an indentation in the contour or skin retraction. When her hands are pressed against her hips, the pectoral muscles contract and if there is a carcinoma that is fixed to the underlying fascia, the breast may elevate more than expected or skin dimpling or nipple deviation may occur. Similarly, when leaning over, the breasts will normally fall freely away from the chest but may exhibit asymmetry or retraction if the fibrosis of a breast lesion is present.

   - Note any visible scars.

4. Palpate the lymph nodes above and below the clavicle on both sides.

5. Ask the woman to lie supine on the table, and have her raise one arm and fold it behind her head or across her forehead.

   - If she has expressed concern about a possible mass or lesion, the opposite breast should be examined first.

6. Gently palpate the axillary lymph nodes. Move your palpating hand within the axilla to press anteriorly for the pectoral nodes, posteriorly for the subscapular nodes, along the upper arm for the lateral brachial nodes, and deep in the middle for the central axillary nodes (**Figure 4D-1**).

   - Small isolated lymph nodes that are palpable may reflect irritation from shaving or a localized infection. They should be reevaluated within 1 month.

SUPERFICIAL (SURFACE) LYMPHATICS

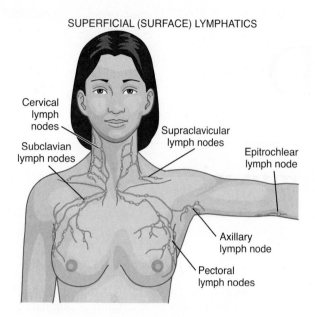

Cervical lymph nodes

Subclavian lymph nodes

Supraclavicular lymph nodes

Epitrochlear lymph node

Axillary lymph node

Pectoral lymph nodes

Figure 4D-1 Lymph nodes in the superficial region of the chest and the axillary region.

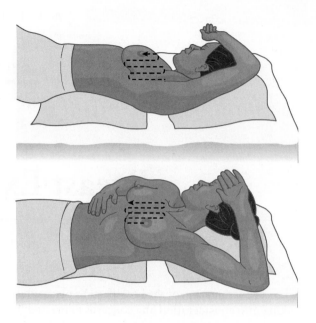

Figure 4D-2 Direction of palpation for the clinical breast examination.

7. Inspect the appearance of the nipples and areolae.
   - Nipples may be erect, flat, or inverted. The appearance changes with reproductive maturity, pregnancy, breastfeeding, and aging.
   - Spontaneous discharge, cracking, lesions, and bleeding are abnormal.
   - Do not squeeze the nipple in an attempt to elicit discharge.

8. Inspect the appearance of the breasts.
   - Skin texture and appearance change over time.
   - Edema, redness, retracted or collapsed areas, visible sores, and masses are all abnormal observations.

9. The most effective pattern for clinical breast examination works up and down the breast, beginning under the axilla and working toward the sternum, and from the clavicle to below the inframammary ridge (**Figure 4D-2**).

10. Palpate each breast for texture and masses. Using the flat surface of the fingers, gently palpate each area being assessed with a circular motion (**Figure 4D-3**) .

11. The full depth of the breast to the underlying rib cage is examined (**Figure 4D-4**).
   - Breast tissue has texture. Some young women will have very smooth tissue, while an older woman who has breastfed may

have an all-over nodular texture. The texture of the breast should be consistent.
   - Prior to the menses, coarse nodularity or firmness may be more noticeable.
   - Palpable masses of any kind need to be evaluated further (**Figure 4D-5**).

12. While performing the breast evaluation, the examiner describes what is being felt and explains how a woman can recognize breast changes. If the woman wishes to learn self-examination, this is the appropriate time to illustrate the procedure.

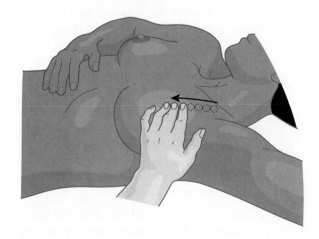

Figure 4D-3 Palpation technique for clinical breast examination.

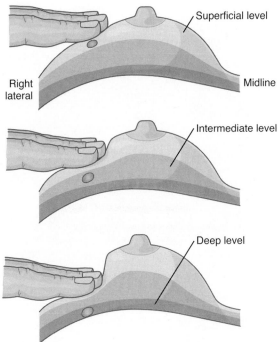

Apply pressure in a circular motion with the pads of your fingers to increasing levels, making three circles: superficial, intermediate, and deep pressure.

Figure 4D-4 Palpating breast tissue to three different levels of pressure.

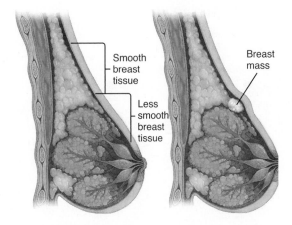

Figure 4D-5 "Lumpy" breast texture versus a mass.

• • • References

1. American College of Obstetricians and Gynecologists Practice Bulletin No. 122. Breast cancer screening. *Obstet Gynecol.* 2011;118(2P1):372-382.

2. U.S. Preventive Services Task Force. Screening for breast cancer: U.S. Preventive Services Task Force recommendation statement. *Ann Intern Med.* 2009; 151(10):716-726, W-236.

3. Barton MD, Harris R, Fletcher SW. Does this patient have breast cancer? The screening clinical breast examination: should it be done? how? *JAMA.* 1999; 282:1270-1280.

4E

Pelvic Examination

The pelvic examination is performed based on a woman's reported concerns, personal history, and family history. Prior to beginning the pelvic examination, the midwife should determine whether or not the woman previously has had a pelvic examination, and if she has any concerns, questions, or history of problems during a pelvic exam. Prior to any procedure, discussing what is involved is essential. Although this appendix will describe both a pelvic and speculum examination, the midwife should remember that not all women will need a speculum examination with a pelvic examination.

During and after a pelvic examination, the choice of words and personal facial expressions should be used with intention. Helping the woman to remain calm and presenting a professional demeanor throughout are important behaviors. A woman's face usually will convey her level of comfort and sometimes if she has questions. Therefore, visualization of both faces, midwife and woman, should be unobstructed throughout the procedure. It is always preferable to have a chaperone when performing a pelvic examination; this person assures the woman that no untoward or unprofessional activity is likely. Pragmatically the chaperone also can hand equipment and receive specimens to facilitate the procedure.

1. Before beginning an examination, the woman should be offered the opportunity to empty her bladder.

2. It is assumed that, similar to prior to any physical examination, the midwife performs hand hygiene, preferably in front of the woman in order to reassure her. To minimize the risk

for contamination of the room with vaginal secretions, assemble all necessary equipment prior to beginning the examination. This includes taking lids off containers and opening any packages needed.

3. When the woman is gowned for the examination, she should move to the end of the examining table and rest her feet in the stirrups or on the lowered section of the table. Her buttocks should extend just beyond the end of the table, so that her perineum is at the edge of the table to facilitate easier insertion of the speculum (**Figure 4E-1**). Her arms should be relaxed at her sides or across her abdomen. Some women will be more comfortable in a semi-reclining position. The drape sheet should be adjusted as needed for modesty and some midwives advocate draping so that the woman's knees are covered and only the pelvic area uncovered.

a. Before proceeding further with the examination, as well as at any point during the procedure when the woman demonstrates potential discomfort, the midwife should verify that the woman does not feel physically uncomfortable.

4. Adjustment of the light is usually done before gloving and speculum selection. The speculum should be the correct size and mechanically functional.

   - Place the speculum and any needed supplies for the examination on a clean surface. In some practices, the speculums are placed on

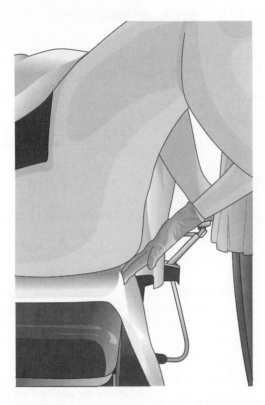

Figure 4E-1 Positioning a woman for a pelvic examination.

clean areas with heating pads beneath them to warm, but not heat, the instruments.

o How to glove for this examination is controversial:

a. Some midwives double glove both hands, and remove the outermost glove if it touches the woman or any secretions.

b. Others double glove only the hand that will be used for the internal examination. The first glove is then removed after internal contact.

c. In the past, it was common to use one glove only, which was placed on the hand that performed the internal examination. However, with the advent of universal precautions, most midwives also glove the hand that performs the external/abdominal portion of the examination. The important factor is that the midwife continuously is

aware of hand cleanliness. Cross-contamination can occur easily, especially by touching equipment, the light, or the clean area on the table after touching the woman's perineum. It is also helpful to be cautious with language and not call the gloved hand for the internal exam "dirty."

5. Correct choice of a speculum can both facilitate visualization and decrease the woman's discomfort. Specula come in many sizes and designs. Pederson specula are straight sided; Graves models have a "duck-billed" shape that increases visualization of the vaginal vault and fornices when lax musculature or submucosal fat impedes visualization of the upper vagina. Narrow (virginal) specula and shorter pediatric specula are also available for use whenever conditions require a smaller device. **Figure 4E-2** shows the variety of specula available. Disposable plastic specula are similar in shape to the Pederson metal specula.

External Inspection of the Genitalia

1. Ask the woman to allow her knees fall apart, and to relax her hip and thigh muscles.

• When the legs and buttocks are relaxed, there is less likelihood that the vaginal muscles will be tightened against the speculum.

• The woman is reminded that she should speak immediately if she is having pain or needs the exam to stop.

• Gently touch the inside of the woman's thigh with the back of the gloved hand before proceeding with the examination and let her know before the introitus or vagina are touched.

2. Inspection of the external genitalia (**Figure 4E-3**). Separate the labia majora and inspect the labia minora. Then separate the labia minora and inspect the clitoris, the inside of the labia minora, vestibule, urethral orifice, and vaginal introitus. **Table 4E-1** lists observations to be noted.

• Inspect the Skene's glands and urethra for normal appearance, irritation, swelling, lesions, redness, or discharge. Separate the

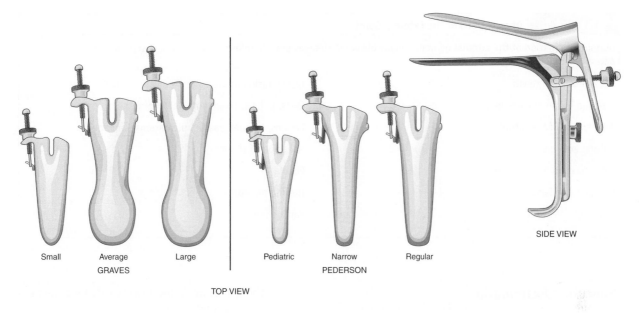

Figure 4E-2 Common vaginal speculum types.

labia; insert one finger into the vagina, palm up; and sweep down the Skene's glands at each side of the urethra toward the introitus. Pressing directly upward onto the urethra, again sweep from the apex of the vagina toward the introitus to elicit discharge from the urethra if present.

- Inspect the Bartholin's glands for masses, fluctuation, redness, heat, or pain, with one finger in the vagina and the other fingers and thumb outside the vagina. Palpate the entire area, usually by gently palpating the tissue between the thumb and the index finger, both sides of the vaginal opening in turn. Pay particular attention to the posterolateral portion of the labia majora.

- Inspecting the glands before performing the speculum examination increases the likelihood that any discharge will be noted.

- This sequence also allows for smooth transition to the speculum examination.

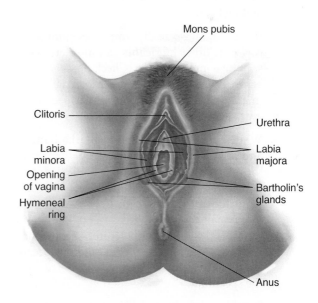

Figure 4E-3 Normal external genitalia.

Table 4E-1	Observations of the External Genitalia

During examination of the external genitalia, many observed changes provide information of clinical significance. Assess the following:

Pattern of hair growth	Discoloration or bruising
Size and shape of each area	Cysts, polyps, condyloma, or other growths
Appearance of the introitus	Lesions, fissures, rashes, ulcerations, crusting
Clitoral enlargement	Adhesion of tissues
Inflammation or irritation	Fistula
Swelling or edema	Uterine prolapse
Scarring	Varicosities

Speculum Examination

1. Start with use of the hand to be designated for use with equipment. Verify that the speculum previously chosen is appropriate in size and that it is warm (skin temperature). If not, discard the glove on the hand that has palpated the external genitalia, rectify the situation, and reglove.

2. If needed, lubricate the warm speculum with water, as other lubricants can interfere with specimen interpretation. Check the speculum before using it to make sure the locking knobs (metal speculum) or latch (plastic speculum) work correctly.

3. While holding the speculum by the handle and securing the two blades together with the index finger across the top blade to avoid inadvertent opening and increasing the size/diameter of the device, have the two fingers that remained in the vagina after palpation of the labia positioned in the posterior introitus. If needed, the fingers may be slightly spread apart to create a visible space for insertion of the speculum.

4. Provide gentle downward pressure with the two fingers and guide the speculum blades between the two fingers into the vagina. The speculum should enter and be removed from the vagina at a 45-degree angle so the speculum avoids touching the sensitive anterior structures (e.g., urethra, clitoris). As the speculum enters the vagina, at a 45-degree angle, slowly begin to remove the fingers as the speculum slides downward along the posterior vaginal wall.

5. Rotate the speculum to a horizontal position as it moves toward the posterior portion of the vagina. Do not open the bills until the speculum is fully inserted.

6. Maintaining downward pressure, withdraw the speculum slightly and open it only as much as is needed to visualize the cervix using the thumb piece.

   - The most common cervical position is tilted slightly posterior, so placing the speculum behind the cervix and gently opening it is the technique most likely to identify the cervix with minimal discomfort for the woman.

7. When the cervix is visible, insert the speculum slightly deeper to stabilize and improve visibility, and then use the screws or latch (on a plastic speculum) to fix the open position of the speculum. The anterior blade of a metal speculum can be adjusted if a larger area needs to be created.

   - Note any discharge, cysts, polyps, lesions or masses, vascularity, erosion, or eversion.

8. It is at this point that specimens are collected if needed.

After collecting specimens, rotate the speculum to visualize the anterior and posterior walls of the vagina. Many midwives will perform this inspection as they slowly remove the speculum. Note that the speculum blades can be allowed to fall together after clearing the cervix. The speculum should be rotated back at a 45-degree angle as it nears the vaginal introitus and then gently removed.

A

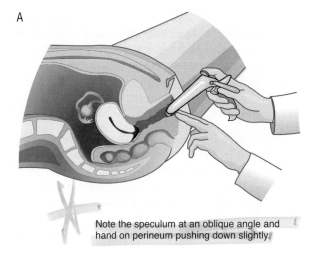

Note the speculum at an oblique angle and hand on perineum pushing down slightly.

B

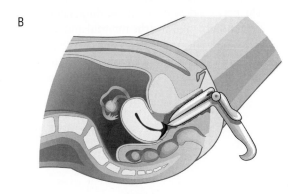

C

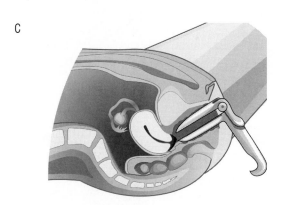

Figure 4E-4 Speculum examination: (A) Position of the hands and speculum at insertion (speculum at oblique angle); (B) speculum inserted along the posterior wall of the vagina; (C) speculum open to visualize cervix.

Source: Parts B and C from Schuiling KD, Likis FE (eds.). *Women's Gynecologic Health.* 2nd ed. Burlington, MA: Jones & Bartlett Learning; 2013.

Bimanual Examination

1. If necessary, discard gloves and don a new one/pair. Apply water-based gel to the fingers of the gloved hand that will be inserted into the vagina.

2. This portion of the examination is performed with two fingers in the vagina, unless the introitus is too tight or the woman too uncomfortable to tolerate more than one finger.

   ◆ Keep the thumb of the examining hand tucked to one side or folded into the palm to avoid unintentional pressure on the clitoris and to allow the fingers to reach further into the vagina.

3. Pressing gently downward, insert two fingers and place them along the posterior wall of the vagina.

4. Press downward firmly to open the vagina and ask the woman to bear down, observing for the bulge of a cystocele or urethrocele. Observe for uterine descent associated with prolapse.

5. Spreading the examining fingers apart, the woman should be asked to bear down a second time, and posterior bulging associated with a rectocele or enterocele is observed if present.

6. Ask the woman to tighten her vaginal muscles around the vaginal fingers.

   ◆ Kegel's exercises can be taught at this point.

7. Sweep the vaginal fingers around the walls to assess for masses or lesions such as cysts, polyps, or condyloma.

8. When the fingers reach the cervix, they should be moved circumferentially around the cervix.

   ◆ Assess for size, consistency, smoothness, shape, mobility, and dilation.

9. Move the cervix gently side to side between two fingers to assess for cervical motion tenderness.

10. Place the external hand above the symphysis and press downward and forward toward the vaginal hand with the palmar surface of the fingers. With the vaginal hand, lift upward directly against the cervix to bring the uterine fundus in contact with the hand on the abdomen. Press both hands together gently

to outline an anteverted or anteflexed uterus. The uterus should move smoothly between the hands. If necessary, reposition the abdominal hand farther up the abdomen to locate the fundus.

11. Note the position of the uterus (anteverted, retroverted, anteflexed, retroflexed, military). Also note shape, size, consistency, mobility, tenderness, or presence of any masses.

12. If the uterus is not identified, repeat the maneuver with the vaginal fingers on either side of the cervix (**Figure 4E-5** illustrates uterine positions).

13. If the uterine position is still not palpated, it may be in a military or posterior position. With fingers in the vagina above and below the uterus, press inward with the external hand and assess as much of the lower portion of the uterus as is possible.

14. To assess the adnexa, place the external hand in the area between the iliac crest of the innominate bone and the abdominal midline midway between the level of the umbilicus and the symphysis pubis. Use the flats of the palmar surface of fingers on the abdomen to press deeply downward and obliquely toward the symphysis pubis and toward the fingers in the vagina.

15. With the vaginal hand, the palm should face upward. Both of the examining fingers in the vagina are placed in the lateral vaginal fornix corresponding to the side (right or left) that the abdominal hand is positioned to examine. Press the fingers deeply inward and upward toward the abdominal hand as far as possible.

16. Palpate the entire area between the uterus and the pelvic sidewalls with a sliding, gentle, but firm touch, pressing the internal and abdominal hands toward each other as they synchronously move together from the abdominal area above the pelvic brim downward toward the symphysis.

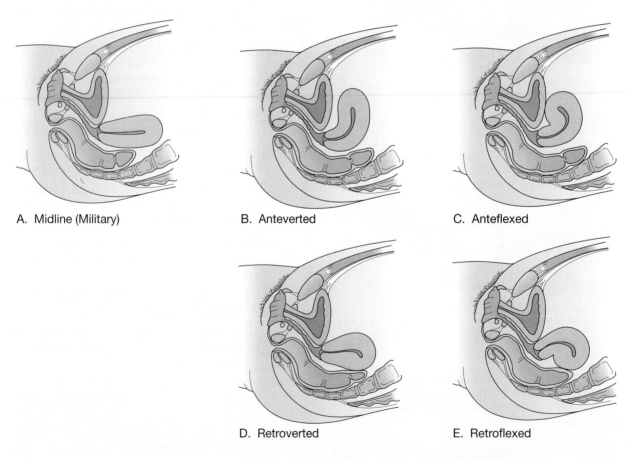

A. Midline (Military)   B. Anteverted   C. Anteflexed

D. Retroverted   E. Retroflexed

Figure 4E-5 Uterine positions: (A) midline, (B) anteverted, (C) anteflexed, (D) retroverted, (E) retroflexed.

Source: Kriebs JM, Gegor CL. *Varney's Pocket Midwife.* 2nd ed. Sudbury, MA: Jones and Bartlett; 2005.

Rectovaginal Examination

1. Before attempting a rectovaginal examination, the midwife should explain why the examination is indicated—to further evaluate the uterus and adnexa or to check for fistula. Offer reassurance that if the woman can relax, the examination should not be painful.

2. Change current gloves and lubricate the examining fingers.

3. Insert a gloved index finger into the woman's vagina. Ask the woman to bear down, and gently insert the middle finger into the rectum.

4. Palpate the area of the anorectal junction and just above it. Ask the woman to tighten and relax her rectal sphincter.

   ◆ This position allows for assessment of sphincter tone and for internal hemorrhoids.

5. As both vaginal and rectal examining fingers slide as far as they will reach, palpate half of the rectal wall, sweeping the examining finger back and forth as the distance is covered methodically. Asking the woman to bear down extends the area that can be reached and makes the procedure more comfortable for her.

6. When a uterus is retroverted or retroflexed, the posterior side of the uterus may be palpated. Palpate as much of the posterior side of the uterus as possible with the rectal examining finger.

7. As the vaginal and rectal fingers are withdrawn, the other half of the rectal wall is examined as in step 5.

8. Remove gloves and discard them. Perform hand hygiene.

9. Assist the woman to a sitting position and offer her cleansing wipes and tissues with which to clean herself.

4F

Collecting Urinary, Vaginal, Cervical, and Rectal Specimens for Testing and Interpretation of Saline and KOH Slides

Specimens collected during obstetric and gynecologic examinations are used to test for infections, risk of preterm labor, rupture of the membranes, and cervical cancer. In all cases, standard precautions are used to prevent provider exposure to blood and body fluids. The order of specimen collection is determined by the purpose and type of specimen collected.

General Principles for Specimen Collection

1. Care is always taken during examination to avoid cross-contamination—either of the equipment and supplies or of the woman and clinical specimens—by the appropriate use of gloves and clean or sterile technique, and by attention to surroundings.

2. Avoiding the use of gel when collecting specimens improves detection. The gel can interfere with testing by obscuring the collection site, altering the pH of a specimen, and making microscopy less accurate. Only warm water should be used to moisten a speculum.

3. The usual order of specimen collection is as follows:

    A. Voided urine

    B. Vaginal swab for culture/nucleic acid amplification tests (NAAT)

    C. Vaginal swab for pH, saline, or KOH

    D. Endocervical swab for NAAT or culture

    E. Papanicolaou testing

Procedure for Collecting Urine Specimens

Urine specimens can be used for urinalysis, urine culture, and nucleic acid amplification technology (NAAT) for *Neisseria gonorrhoeae* and *Chlamydia trachomatis*.

1. Determine whether a catheterized specimen is necessary before collecting the specimen. Examples of times when this might be necessary are after rupture of the membranes, during the early postpartum period, when it will be difficult for the woman to adequately clean the area, or whenever a definitive measurement of urinary protein, leukocytes, or erythrocytes is necessary.

2. If performing a bladder catheter collection:

    A. Open the sterile catheter and leave it in the sterile wrap.

    B. Don sterile gloves.

    C. Place the end of the catheter where the urine will come out into a sterile collection device.

    D. Holding the labia away from the urethra, cleanse the periurethral and vaginal area with soap (not disinfectant, which may interfere with culture). Wipe from front to back, and repeat twice, using a clean pad each time.

    E. Using aseptic technique, insert the catheter tipped with water-based lubricant into the urethra until urine is returned (usually 4–5 cm).

F. Remove the catheter from the urethra when you have enough urine for the specimen or when urine no longer drains, depending on the purpose of the procedure.

G. Cap the sterile collection device without contaminating the inside by touching it.

H. Remove gloves.

I. Label the sterile collection device.

Procedure for Collecting and Interpreting Wet Mount and Potassium Hydroxide Specimens for Vaginal Infections[1,2]

In the United States, microscopy for the diagnosis of infection or rupture of the amniotic membranes falls under the Clinical Laboratory Improvement Amendments of 1988 (CLIA). These federal regulations, which mandate improved quality controls, include requirements for competence in provider-performed microscopy. The Centers for Medicare and Medicaid Services is responsible for these regulations; more information is available at http://wwwn.cdc.gov/clia/regs/toc.aspx.[3] As with any procedure that has the potential for exposure to blood or other body fluids, standard precautions are always observed. The first step is knowing how to use the microscope (**Box 4F-1**)

Saline specimens are used for the direct visualization of vaginal yeasts, trichomonads, and clue cells typical of bacterial vaginosis. Assessment of the presence or absence of lactobacilli and white blood cells can also aid diagnosis. A sample placed in potassium hydroxide (KOH) is used to visualize yeasts. The KOH destroys the cell walls of bacteria and epithelial cells, but not the cell walls of fungi. KOH can also be collected for use in the "whiff" test, to identify release of amines when a bacterial vaginosis specimen is exposed to an alkaline solution.

1. Prepare a test tube with 0.5–1 mL of normal saline; if a separate tube will be collected for KOH testing, place the same amount of KOH in the second tube. Saline is preferred over distilled water to help preserve the living specimen long enough for examination.

2. Insert a moistened speculum into the vagina and visualize the cervix.

3. As the speculum is inserted and positioned, note the appearance of the perineum, vaginal mucosa, cervical epithelium, and any discharge. The discharge is categorized by quantity, color, consistency, and odor.

4. Using a sterile cotton swab, collect a sample of fluid from the posterior fornix and/or from the vaginal wall. If necessary, a second swab may be used to obtain an adequate sample.

5. Place the swab into the tube containing saline and rotate it vigorously.

6. Repeat to collect a sample for KOH preparation as needed.

7. Specimens are evaluated as soon as possible, preferably within 15 minutes.

8. Wearing gloves, use the swab to place a drop of fluid containing each specimen on a clean slide. Avoid touching the surface of the slide as much as possible. It is preferable to use a second slide when collecting for KOH, to prevent contamination of the saline specimen.

9. Place a cover slip over each specimen. Hold the cover slip by the edges. The cover slip should be placed at a 45-degree angle and lowered slowly, to minimize air bubbles (**Figure 4F-1**).

    ◆ Fingerprints, lint, and dust can be misidentified as part of the specimen. Keeping the slide as clean as possible and carefully focusing on the edge of the cover slide will assist in finding the correct viewing plane.

10. If the cover slip is floating because the specimen is too thick, a small piece of lint-free paper can be used to absorb some of the excess.

BOX 4F-1 Use of the Optical Microscope

An optical microscope can be used to facilitate diagnosis in the clinical setting. Proper microscope maintenance—minimizing exposure to dust by covering the microscope when not in use, cleaning the eyepiece and objective lenses with compressed air and a lint-free paper wipe, and wiping down mechanical components with a microfiber or other lint-free cloth—will preserve the quality of images. Prior to using a microscope for the first time, familiarity with the light source, adjustment of the fine and coarse focus knobs, technique for moving the slide on the mount, and the powers available for viewing a specimen is necessary. Most modern microscopes will have a 10× eyepiece lens and 4×, 10×, and 40× objective lenses. The oil immersion lens is not used for these procedures.

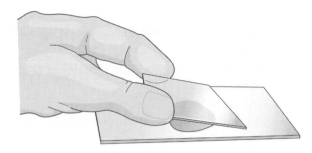

Figure 4F-1 Cover slide placement.

11. The saline slide is inspected first, followed by the KOH slide if needed.

12. Focus on the edge of the cover slip using the low-power lens (10×). At this point, the fine adjustment should be all that is necessary to bring specimens into focus.

13. Examine the specimen by moving the slide back and forth, using the knob or handle provided for that purpose.

    ◆ Enough of the slide must be inspected to provide a correct diagnosis. The entire specimen may need to be viewed because the specimen will not be distributed equally across the slide.

14. Specimens of vaginal secretions are inspected under 40× power. The samples are read as positive or negative, with details of the specific findings as needed.

    ◆ While the 10× lens gives an overview of cells and fungal material present, the 40× lens enables the examiner to identify blood cells, clue cells, bacteria, trichomonads, and yeast hyphae or spores accurately (**Figure 4F-2**). See the *Reproductive Tract and Sexually Transmitted Infections* chapter for discussion of diagnosis of vaginal infections and STIs.

15. Turning off the microscope light, cleaning up spilled material, and properly discarding the sample complete the procedure.

Procedure for Collecting Vaginal or Cervical Specimens for *N. gonorrhoeae* and *C. trachomatis*

Most laboratories now use NAAT or similar DNA-based testing for evaluation of mucopurulent cervicitis and for screening for *N. gonorrhoeae* and

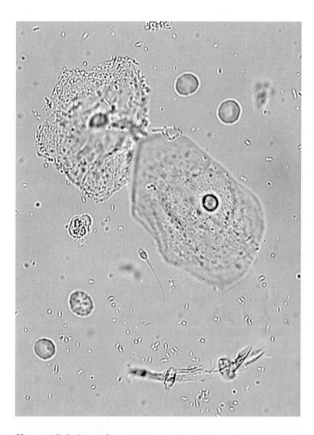

Figure 4F-2 Normal wet mount.

Source: Used with permission from Seattle STD/HIV Prevention Training Center and Cindy Fennell, MS, MT, ASCP

C. trachomatis.[4,5] These tests are the most sensitive available, and their specificity is similar to that of culture. If the product being used is approved for vaginal testing, these specimens are as accurate as cervical ones, and more accurate than urine specimens in women. A provider can collect vaginal swabs, or such samples may be self-collected by the woman. Culture for *N. gonorrhoeae* is utilized as an alternative when these tests are not available or when resistance testing is needed. *Chlamydia* cultures have poor sensitivity and specificity.

1. Insert a moistened speculum into the vagina and visualize the cervix.

2. Note the presence of any discharge or cervical irritation.

3. For a vaginal specimen, swab the upper vaginal wall and posterior fornix for 10–30 seconds with a Dacron swab.

4. For cervical specimens, first use a large swab to remove any mucus discharge obscuring the cervical opening.

5. Insert a sterile Dacron swab into the cervix approximately 2 cm and rotate for 5 seconds. The specimen collected for liquid cytology Papanicolaou tests is adequate for this purpose.

6. Do not allow a cervical swab to touch the vaginal walls while it is being removed.

7. Place the specimen in the transport medium.

Procedure for Performing a Papanicolaou Test

Liquid-based specimen collection, in which the specimen is collected at the cervix, has become the standard where available, due to improved ability to interpret abnormalities. This material can also be used for human papillomavirus (HPV) testing.[6] In a conventional Pap smear, a slide is made directly from the specimen collected at the cervix. An extended-tip spatula plus endocervical brush technique or broom plus endocervical brush has been shown to provide the most accurate results, and should be used whenever available.[7,8] See the discussion of routine cervical cancer testing in the *Health Promotion and Health Maintenance* chapter for more information.

1. Insert a moistened speculum into the vagina and visualize the cervix.

2. If only a Pap test is being performed, a small amount of water-based gel can be used to lubricate the speculum.

3. Using a spatula or broom, sweep the cervix, rotating the spatula or broom 360 degrees to cover the entire ectocervix. An extended-tip spatula is the preferred device. If the squamocolumnar junction is visible, it should be included.

4. Remove the device without touching the vaginal sidewalls; rotate it gently in liquid medium to dislodge the cells, or roll across a clean slide, depending on whether a liquid or dry collection method is used.

5. For dry specimens only: Place one flat side on the top half of the slide and stroke once to the end of the slide. Then turn the spatula or brush over and place the other flat side on the bottom half of the slide and stroke once to the end of the slide. If the specimen is too thick, take the edge of the device and, with a single light stroke down the slide, remove the excess.

6. Insert a cervical brush into the endocervix approximately 2 cm and rotate through 90–180 degrees.

7. Repeat the procedure for processing as in steps 4 and 5.

8. If a dry technique is used, the specimen should immediately be fixed before transport to preserve cellular integrity.

● ● ● **References**

1. American College of Physicians. Wet mount examinations. Available at: http://www.acponline.org/running _practice/mle/wm_exams.htm. Accessed January 4, 2012.

2. Lowe S, Saxe JM. *Microscopic Procedures for Primary Care Providers.* Philadelphia: Lippincott, Williams & Wilkins; 1999.

3. Centers for Disease Control and Prevention. Current CLIA regulations. Available at: http://wwwn.cdc.gov /clia/regs/toc.aspx. Accessed September 29, 2012.

4. Centers for Disease Control and Prevention. Sexually transmitted disease treatment guidelines, 2010. Available at: http://www.cdc.gov/std/treatment/2010 /default.htm. Accessed January 4, 2012.

5. Association of Public Health Laboratories. Laboratory diagnostic testing for *Chlamydia trachomatis* and *Neisseria gonorrhoea.* Available at: http://www .aphl.org/aphlprograms/infectious/std/Documents /CTGCLabGuidelinesMeetingReport.pdf. Accessed January 4, 2012.

6. Hoda RS, Loukeris K, Abdul-Karim FW. Gynecologic cytology on conventional and liquid-based preparations: a comprehensive review of similarities and differences. *Diagn Cytopathol.* April 17, 2012. doi: 10.1002/dc.22842. [Epub ahead of print].

7. Martin-Hirsch PL, Jarvis GG, Kitchener HC, Lilford R. Collection devices for obtaining cervical cytology samples. *Cochrane Database System Rev.* 2011;4.

8. Davis-Devine S, Day SJ, Anderson A, et al. Collection of the BD SurePath Pap Test with a broom device plus endocervical brush improves disease detection when compared to the broom device alone or the spatula plus endocervical brush combination. *CytoJournal.* 2009;6:4. Available at: http://www.cytojournal.com /text.asp?2009/6/1/4/45495. Accessed September 29, 2012.

● ● ● **Additional Resources**

Marchand L, Mundt M, Klein G, Agarwal SC. Optimal collection technique and devices for a quality Pap smear. *Wisc Med J.* 2005;104(6):51-55.

C H A P T E R

5

Pharmacotherapeutics

MARY C. BRUCKER

TEKOA L. KING

Introduction

Throughout history, pregnancy and midwifery have been surrounded in myths. One of the modern myths is that midwives eschew the use of drugs and only use, at most, herbal remedies. In reality, knowledge of pharmacology is necessary for the practice of midwifery in the twenty-first century so that midwives use pharmacotherapeutic agents appropriately. All 50 states grant some type of prescriptive authority to certified nurse-midwives.[1] Prescriptive authority remains less common for certified midwives, as their credential is newer and their numbers fewer. Prescriptive authority is controlled on the state level and ranges from very limited to relatively broad. Many states limit prescriptive authority according to the schedule of controlled substances described later in this chapter. Some prescriptive authority laws are based on specific wording in state licensing laws or practice sites.

As an increasing number of midwives attain prescriptive privileges, knowledge of pharmacology becomes even more important.[1] Although midwives may use a wide repertoire of nonpharmaceutical techniques, there are conditions and situations in which no effective substitutes exist for pharmacologic treatments. One of the greatest challenges to the midwife in clinical practice is maintaining current information about drug indications, doses, side effects, and contraindications.

Throughout this text, specific therapeutic agents are discussed as treatments for various conditions. However, the field of pharmacology is both expansive and ever-changing; thus this chapter presents a wide overview that includes discussion of specific situations such as common drugs used for treating woman who are pregnant or breastfeeding. Although many examples are included in the chapter as illustrations, it should not be assumed that they are exhaustive. Additionally, certain terms—including "drugs," "agents," "medications," and "pharmaceuticals"—are used interchangeably throughout the chapter. The word "drug" does not connote an illicit substance or a licit substance being abused; rather, drugs with abuse potential are specifically designated as such. Drugs are listed by generic name followed by the most common brand name in parentheses.

This chapter has four sections. The first reviews fundamental concepts for midwives with prescriptive authority, including the drug development process, legal requirements for prescriptive authority, and essential information about drug–drug interactions and adverse effects of drugs. The second section reviews essential drug categories most commonly used in midwifery practice. The third and fourth sections describe pharmacologic essentials specific to prescribing drugs for women who are pregnant and women who are lactating.

The Lexicon of Pharmacology

As knowledge in pharmacology has expanded, so has the accompanying lexicon. A prerequisite to understanding drug actions and their effects is the midwife's ability to define the various terms used in pharmacology. Some of these terms are old and established. *Pharmacology* itself means the study of all aspects of drugs. In addition, several more specific terms are employed in the field. *Pharmacokinetics* describes the absorption, distribution, metabolism (biotransformation), and excretion (clearance) of drugs. These factors then determine the amount of the agent available at the target sites for action. *Pharmacodynamics* refers to the action of drugs on the body. The pharmacodynamic action of a drug results from the drug's binding relationship at the receptor site as either an agonist or an antagonist. *Pharmacotherapeutics* is the field focusing on treatment effects of drugs. Additional terms can be found in the pharmacology glossary presented in **Box 5-1**.

Drugs in Modern Society

More than 4 billion prescriptions are written each year in the United States. Each prescription filled can result in a 20% profit to the manufacturer, making the pharmaceutical industry highly profitable.

Most adults in the United States take at least one medication, and many take multiple pharmaceuticals daily.[2] The extensive use of drugs is related to several factors: the increase in their availability; the public belief that drugs are safe, especially over-the-counter products; and the plethora of healthcare providers, pharmacies, and Internet sites that supply drugs. These multiple options mean that an individual may receive drug prescriptions and recommendations from a variety of providers who may be unaware of the other prescribers' actions. Direct-to-customer advertising exposes many more individuals to prescription drugs and proposed therapeutic options of which they might have been previously unaware.[3] In addition to public acceptance of drugs to treat illnesses, there is a growing appreciation of how agents may be used for prophylaxis against various diseases or for general health maintenance. Drugs used for prophylaxis tend to be used for long periods of time. They include blockbuster drugs, such as atorvastatin (Lipitor).

Even individuals who avoid taking specific drugs or agents may constantly be exposed to pharmaceuticals through the food chain or in their daily environment.[4] The results of such exposure, including direct toxic reactions and reproductive toxicology, are beyond the scope of this chapter, although this area is likely to grow in importance.

Drug Development and Regulation

Drugs are labeled in various ways. Specific drugs can be described by the physiochemical property of the drug (e.g., an acid) or by pharmacotherapeutic indication (e.g., sedative). The same drug could be identified by its chemical name [e.g., 2-(2-methyl-5-nitro 1*H*-imidazol1-l-yl)ethanol], its generic name (metronidazole), and its most common brand name (Flagyl).

Drugs formulated as medications are regulated in the United States by the Food and Drug Administration (FDA), one of 12 agencies within the U.S. Department of Health and Human Services. The pharmaceuticals for which the FDA has authority may be obtained by prescription or over the counter.

The FDA also regulates medical devices such as intrauterine contraceptive systems (e.g., ParaGard, Mirena) and biologic agents such as vaccines. The FDA does not regulate dietary supplements, such as St. John's wort, although the agency does track adverse reactions that occur following use of dietary supplements. Similarly, the FDA may require labeling to designate that safety has not been established for cosmetics, although recall of cosmetics is voluntary by the manufacturer.[5]

Drugs that are approved for specific use by the FDA must demonstrate both safety and efficacy for that indication in a series of preapproval studies that are submitted to the FDA for review. The regulation of drugs is administered by the Center for Drug Evaluation and Research (CDER), a subgroup within the FDA that oversees the research, development, manufacture, and marketing of both prescription and over-the-counter (OTC) drugs. After FDA approval, if unexpected risks are detected, CDER takes action to inform the public, change a drug's label, or, when necessary, remove the product from the market. The FDA itself does not develop, manufacture, or test drugs.

Drug manufacturers submit full reports of studies conducted on specific drugs, called clinical trials, so that CDER can evaluate the data and determine if the drug should be approved for a specific indication. This approval commonly is termed FDA labeling. The clinical trials are intended to be appropriately large enough to determine safety and effectiveness. However, sometimes the FDA approves a drug, only to remove it from the marketplace later due to adverse effects that emerge once the drug is in use by a large diverse population or when used in conjunction with other agents. **Box 5-2** identifies the sequencing of studies and subsequent clinical trials that are conducted prior to FDA approval, and **Figure 5-1** illustrates the process.[6]

Historically, women have not been participants in most drug development studies.[7,8] Although there are many reasons for this exclusion, one factor is the changing environment in a woman's body over

BOX 5-1 A Brief Glossary of Pharmacology

Adverse drug reaction Response to a drug that is noxious and unintended, and that occurs at doses normally used for prophylaxis, diagnosis, or therapy of disease or for the modification of physiologic function.

Agonist A drug that binds to a receptor and activates it, producing a pharmacological response.

Antagonist A drug that attenuates the effects of an agonist. Antagonism can be competitive and reversible (i.e., the drug binds reversibly to a region of the receptor in common with the agonist) or competitive and irreversible (i.e., the antagonist binds covalently to the agonist binding site, and no amount of agonist can overcome the inhibition).

Bioavailability Percentage of an administered drug that is available to target tissues.

Bioequivalent Pharmacologically equivalent.

Black box warning A method that the FDA uses to identify unusual harm associated with an agent. Often this warning is added to package inserts after postmarketing studies identify unexpected risks linked to a drug.

Brand name A trademarked name assigned to a drug by its manufacturer. Some brand names are similar to the generic name (e.g., pseudoephedrine/Sudafed); others suggest their indications for use (e.g., Tamiflu).

Chemical name Although rarely used by prescribers and consumers, a name of a drug that describes its chemical composition.

Compounding Mixing or combining ingredients to produce a pharmaceutical agent. Pharmacists may perform compounding to change the form from solid pill to liquid, or it may be done to create a unique dose and combination of products for a specific individual.

Controlled substance Pharmaceuticals as listed in schedules found in U.S. Law 21 U.S.C. §802(32)(A). These agents include opiates as well as nonopiates but generally have a high risk of addiction, often without valid medicinal use. Examples include heroin.

Cosmeceutical A cosmetic product that has medicinal or druglike benefits.

Direct-to-consumer advertising Advertising of selected drugs placed in popular media and directed to the general public as opposed to providers in peer-reviewed journals.

Dispense (furnish) The process of giving a drug to a consumer.

Ecopharmacology Derivation of drugs from plants, especially those found in the rainforest, as well as exploration of pharmacologic implications of pollutants in water that exert pharmaceutical-like effects, most often estrogenic in nature. The latter substances also have been called ecoestrogens or xenoestrogens.

Formulary List of approved or available drugs. It is often used by insurers to identify agents that will be reimbursed or paid for by the insurer.

Generic name A formulation that contains the same active ingredients found in the original brand formulation and is bioequivalent to that formulation.

Half-life The period of time required for the concentration or amount of drug in the body to be reduced to exactly one-half of a given concentration or amount.

Hypersensitivity reaction A state of altered reactivity wherein the body reacts to a foreign substance with an exaggerated immune response; classified as Type I, II, III, or IV depending on the specific pathologic response.

Immunotherapy Treatment of disease by inducing, enhancing, or suppressing an immune response.

Loading dose A larger than normal dose administered as the first in a series of doses, with the other does being equal to each other but smaller than the first. A loading dose is administered to achieve a therapeutic amount in the body more rapidly.

Nutraceutical (functional food) A food or supplement (e.g., folic acid) that has specific health benefits.

Off-label use Prescription or use of a drug for conditions other than those approved by the FDA.

Over-the-counter (OTC) Pharmaceuticals sold without prescriptions.

Pharmacodynamics How drugs produce their effects, such as interactions at a receptor site.

Pharmacogenetics The study of how drugs interact with the genetic makeup of an individual or the genetic response to a drug; this may be one of the first clinical applications derived from the Human Genome Project.

Pharmacogenomics Studies that illustrate similarities and differences in pharmacodynamic and pharmacokinetic mechanisms among various individuals and people of different ethnic backgrounds.

Pharmacokinetics The movement of drugs in the body, specifically encompassing the study of factors that determine the amount of chemical agents at their sites of biologic effect at various times after the agent is administered. Pharmacokinetics is composed of four specific factors: absorption, distribution, metabolism (biotransformation), and excretion (clearance).

Pharmacotherapeutics The field concentrating on the treatment effects of drugs. There are several subsections within pharmacotherapeutics.

Polypharmacy The practice of treating individuals using multidrug regimens. This term generally is accepted to mean administration of five or more drugs.

(continues)

BOX 5-1 A Brief Glossary of Pharmacology *(continued)*

Prescriptive authority Legal ability to prescribe drugs, medical devices, or other regulated healthcare interventions.

Side effect A physiologic response unrelated to the desired drug effects that occurs with therapeutic doses of the medication. Side effects may be beneficial or negative.

Therapeutic window A point at which the plasma drug concentration is between the minimum effective concentration (MEC) in the plasma for obtaining the desired drug action and the mean toxic concentration (MTC).

Toxicology The branch of pharmacology that deals with the nature, effects, and treatments of poisons.

---

the course of the menstrual cycle, which could affect the pharmacokinetics and pharmacodynamics of a drug. Even when women have participated in clinical trials, it has been rare that an analysis of gender differences has been published. Moreover, clinical trials for contraceptives generally do not include many adolescents, as women younger than the age of 18 are considered pediatric patients. Pediatrics itself is a difficult area in which to conduct clinical trials because of the inherent problems obtaining informed consent.

Although the FDA approves drugs for specific indications, once it is marketed the same drug may be prescribed for another use—a phenomenon is called "off-label use." Examples abound regarding off-label use.[9] For instance, the most commonly used tocolytic in the United States is magnesium sulfate, yet it is not FDA approved for that indication. Methotrexate (Rheumatrex)—a folic acid antagonist used as a chemotherapeutic agent—has a marked predilection for destruction of trophoblastic tissue and is used off label for medical treatment of an unruptured ectopic pregnancy. Midwives should recognize that off-label use, though it remains common, should not be undertaken capriciously. A legal liability potentially exists, especially if the drug is not yet widely accepted in practice for the off-label indication.

Controlled Substances

The U.S. Drug Enforcement Administration (DEA) was established in 1973 within the Department of Justice. This agency has a special role in the regulation of prescription drugs that have the potential for abuse, under the 1970 Controlled Substance Act (CSA). The CSA has classified pharmaceuticals that can be abused into one of five schedules based on the substance's medicinal value, harmfulness, and potential for abuse or addiction. Schedule I is reserved for the most dangerous drugs that have no recognized medical use, such as LSD and heroin. Schedule V is the classification used for the least dangerous drugs, such as brand-name antitussives containing small amounts of codeine. Meperidine (Demerol) is a Schedule II agent. Knowledge of these schedules is important for midwives with prescriptive authority because this authority is often limited to specific schedules. **Box 5-3** lists the five schedules for controlled substances.

A registration number issued by the DEA is needed to prescribe a controlled substance. In 1993, the DEA published a regulation that established a new category under which healthcare providers other than physicians, dentists, veterinarians, or podiatrists could receive individual DEA registration numbers

---

BOX 5-2 Phases of the Food and Drug Administration Drug Approval Process

FDA	Phase Description
1	Designed to determine drug dynamics and identify drug metabolites. This phase is usually small and may be omitted if extensive international study has been conducted.
2	Controlled clinical trials to verify effectiveness and basic safety.
3	Randomized clinical trials, usually placebo controlled.
4	Postmarketing clinical trials, usually to gather information about adverse reactions, morbidity, and mortality that can be obtained only in larger groups.

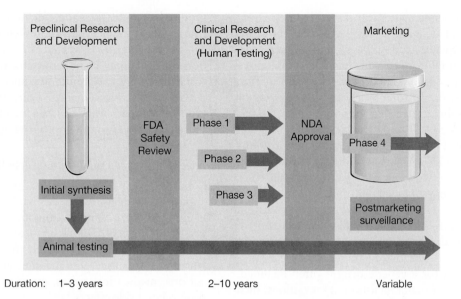

Figure 5-1 Steps required by the FDA for reviewing a new drug.
Source: Hanson GR, Venturelli PJ, Fleckenstein AE. *Drugs and Society.* 11th ed. Sudbury, MA: Jones & Bartlett; 2012.

granting controlled substance prescribing privileges consistent with the authority granted them under state law.[10] Under this regulation, providers such as certified nurse-midwives were given authority to prescribe controlled substances if approved to do so by the state or jurisdiction in which they practice.

The Prescription

Midwives with prescriptive authority have the legal ability to write prescriptions. Although many prescriptions are phoned into a pharmacy or, increasingly, transmitted by electronic means, a midwife needs to know the required components of a prescription.

BOX 5-3 FDA Classification of Controlled Substances

Schedule	Interpretation	Schedule	Interpretation
I	High potential for abuse and no current accepted medical use. Examples are heroin and LSD.	III (cont.)	are barbiturates and preparations containing small quantities of codeine. Prescriptions may be oral or written. Up to five renewals are permitted within 6 months.
II	High potential for abuse. Use may lead to severe physical or psychological dependence. Examples are opioids, amphetamines, short-acting barbiturates, and preparations containing codeine. Prescriptions must be written in ink or typewritten and signed by the practitioner. Verbal prescriptions must be confirmed in writing within 72 hours and may be given only in a genuine emergency. No renewals are permitted.	IV	Low potential for abuse. Examples include chloral hydrate, phenobarbital, and benzodiazepines. Use may lead to limited physical or psychological dependence. Prescriptions may be oral or written. Up to five renewals are permitted within 6 months.
III	Some potential for abuse. Use may lead to low-to-moderate physical dependence or high psychological dependence. Examples	V	Subject to state and local regulations. Abuse potential is low; a prescription may not be required. Examples are antitussive and antidiarrheal medications containing limited quantities of opioids.

All handwritten prescriptions must be legibly written in indelible ink. Every prescription must include the midwife's name, address, and contact information. It is optimal to have the midwife's prescriptive authority number or other identifying information appear either on the top of the prescription order or adjacent to the midwife's signature. In some states, the midwife's collaborating physician's numbers will also be placed on the prescription. All prescriptions are dated, and information about the prescription is placed in the woman's record so that if she loses the prescription, changes pharmacies, or moves, it can be easily retrieved. Only one drug can be written on each prescription blank. Refills, if any, are noted, especially as certain health plans limit coverage of monthly drugs. Permission to substitute a brand-name product for a generic drug is often included. Some authorities maintain lists of abbreviations, such as "TID" for "three times a day," although use of any abbreviations is increasingly discouraged.

The section of the prescription specific to the medication consists of four parts: (1) superscription, (2) inscription, (3) subscription, and (4) signature. The superscription includes the symbol "Rx," although according to World Health Organization guidelines, it is more proper to use the Latin "℞". In any case, the symbol is derived from the Latin word for "recipe" or "take." The inscription specifies the ingredients and their quantities (e.g., nitrofurantoin 100 milligram capsules). The subscription informs the pharmacist how to compound or dispense the medication (e.g., dispense 10 capsules). It is important to avoid decimals and, where necessary, write words in full to avoid misunderstanding. For example, write "levothyroxine 50 micrograms," not "0.050 milligram" or "50 mg." The signature, or "sig," is not that of the prescriber, but represents the Latin "signa" or "mark" that provides the instructions that enable the woman to understand dosages and when to take a drug. The sig should include route, frequency, duration, and any other specific information—for example, "Take 1 capsule by mouth at bedtime for 10 days."

Generally it is recommended that the generic or nonproprietary name be used when a prescription is written. Use of generic names enables the pharmacist to maintain a more limited stock of drugs and/or dispense the least expensive drug. However, if there is a particular reason to prescribe a brand-name drug, the trade name can be added. Some authorities allow generic substitution by the pharmacist and require the addition "Do not substitute," "Dispense as written," or "Brand medically necessary" if that brand, and no other, is to be dispensed. When a specific brand is required, the midwife should document that instruction in the woman's chart along with the rationale. The documentation is created not only for completeness, but also may be necessary for the prescription to be covered by a public insurance program such as Medicaid, various managed care groups, or other types of health insurance. **Figure 5-2** illustrates a sample prescription written appropriately by a midwife.

Adverse Drug Reactions and Adverse Drug Events

Adverse drug reactions (ADRs) are unintended responses to a drug that occur when normal dosing is used. ADRs are quite common.[11,12] The term *adverse drug events* (ADEs) is a more inclusive category connoting any injury that results from the administration of a drug. ADEs includes adverse drug reactions, medication errors, overdoses, and known dose-related side effects.

After a drug has been determined to be safe and effective in preapproval clinical trials, it is prescribed for individuals in a broader population—that is, for a more diverse group than the relatively select group who participated in the clinical trials. Thus adverse effects of drugs are primarily identified during the postmarketing period. The Adverse Event Reporting Program of the FDA collects reports of ADRs via the FDA MedWatch program. Details of how to report an adverse drug reaction are listed in **Box 5-4**.

Adverse drug reactions are classified as either immune or non-immune reactions. Non-immune reactions are predictable. They include drug–drug interactions, drug overdose, and drug toxicity, and commonly occur secondary to known pharmacologic effects or in a dose-related manner. Conversely, immune reactions, which are also called allergic reactions, are unpredictable. The four types of hypersensitivity reactions that cause a drug allergy are listed in **Table 5-1**.

Drug–Drug Reactions

Although most drugs are therapeutic when used alone, adverse reactions may occur when certain drugs are used concomitantly. In some instances, reactions may occur when drugs are taken simultaneously with certain botanical/herbal therapies or even specific foods. It is important to consider such potential reactions when considering drugs for an individual woman.

Most drugs are metabolized via a group of liver enzymes called the cytochrome P-450 family. When a drug undergoes biotransformation via one of the cytochrome P-450 enzymes, it may be altered from a prodrug into an active drug, made inactive, or altered

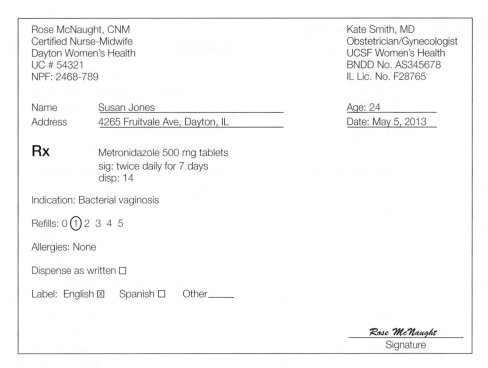

Rose McNaught, CNM
Certified Nurse-Midwife
Dayton Women's Health
UC # 54321
NPF: 2468-789

Kate Smith, MD
Obstetrician/Gynecologist
UCSF Women's Health
BNDD No. AS345678
IL Lic. No. F28765

Name   Susan Jones   Age: 24
Address   4265 Fruitvale Ave, Dayton, IL   Date: May 5, 2013

Rx   Metronidazole 500 mg tablets
              sig: twice daily for 7 days
              disp: 14

Indication: Bacterial vaginosis

Refills: 0 ①2 3 4 5

Allergies: None

Dispense as written ☐

Label: English ☒   Spanish ☐   Other_____

                                        Rose McNaught
                                          Signature

Figure 5-2 A sample prescription.

into a formulation that is more active. For example, codeine is metabolized by CYP2D6 into morphine (the active metabolite of codeine).

Assume drug A and drug B are both metabolized via the same cytochrome P-450 enzyme. When these drugs are taken at the same time, drug A either inhibits or enhances the activity of the cytochrome P-450 enzyme. In turn, metabolism of drug B is either inhibited, which results in higher plasma levels and perhaps overdose, or enhanced (i.e., it is metabolized more rapidly than usual), which results in a reduction of the plasma concentration of the drug, making it less effective. For example, the antifungal drug fluconazole (Diflucan) is an inhibitor of CYP2CP; when it is given to a person who is also taking tolbutamide (Micronase), the plasma concentration of tolbutamide increases and the individual becomes more likely to experience hypoglycemia.[13] In another example, cardiac arrhythmias may occur when one of the macrolides erythromycin (E-base), azithromycin (Zithromax), or clarithromycin (Biaxin) is taken simultaneously with the antifungal ketoconazole (Nizoral).

Some individuals have genetic mutations called polymorphisms that encode for the cytochrome P-450 enzymes. A common polymorphism of CYP2D6 inhibits function of this enzyme. Persons with this polymorphism are poor metabolizers and as such, they can have an exaggerated or toxic response to drugs

BOX 5-4 How to Report an Adverse Drug Reaction

In 1993, the FDA founded *MedWatch,* a reporting system for adverse events or sentinel events. This system includes a computerized information database designed to support postmarketing safety surveillance program for all FDA-approved drug and therapeutic biologic products. Any suspected adverse events or reactions to medications, drug products, or medical devices (other than vaccines or investigational drugs) should be reported using FDA Form 3500 (available online at https://www.accessdata.fda.gov/scripts/medwatch/medwatch-online.htm). Information re-garding the reporting of vaccine-related adverse event reports (VAERS) can be found at https://vaers.hhs.gov/professionals/index.

For individuals who prefer, the MedWatch program can be contacted by phone, fax, or mail, as well as online.

Phone: 1-800-332-1088

Fax: 1-800-FDA-0178

Mail: MedWatch
5600 Fishers Lane
Rockville, MD 20857

Table 5-1	Four Types of Hypersensitivity Reactions	
Type	**Timing of Reaction**	**Examples**
Type 1 (immediate)	Minutes to hours after drug exposure	• Anaphylaxis from exposure to penicillin • Hives following exposure to sulfa drugs • Angioedema from ACE inhibitors
Type 2 (cytotoxic)	Variable	• Transfusion reaction • Hemolytic anemia from penicillin
Type III (immune complex formed)	1–3 weeks after drug exposure	• Drug-induced lupus caused by minocycline (Minocin) • Serum sickness caused by cefaclor (Ceclor)
Type IV (delayed or cell mediated)	2–7 days after drug exposure	• Ampicillin rash • Contact dermatitis caused by topical antihistamine

that are metabolized by CYP2D6. For example, persons with this polymorphism have a fivefold increased risk of adverse reactions when taking metoprolol (Lopressor) compared to persons who do not have this polymorphism.[14] Approximately 5% to 14% of Caucasians, 0% to 5% of Africans, and 0% to 1% of Asians have the polymorphism that results in a lack of CYP2D6 activity.[15] Gene testing for this cytochrome P-450 mutation is available but not yet implemented commonly in practice. This is only one reason why it is important to know all of the medications, including herbs, that a woman is taking before prescribing or recommending other substances.

Drug Resistance

Shortly after drug manufacturers began mass production of penicillin in the 1940s, infections secondary to resistant *Staphylococcus aureus* began to appear. The spread of resistance was rapid.[16] Between 1979 and 1987, only 0.02% of strains of pneumococcus were reported by the Centers for Disease Control and Prevention (CDC) as resistant; by 1994, 6.6% were reported to be resistant. Several factors account for the development and rapid rise of drug-resistant strains of bacteria. One factor is the human complacency that developed in the 1980s when many scientists and clinicians began to view bacterial infection as an easily curable condition. Antimicrobial agents were used liberally, even for conditions for which they were not indicated, such as the common cold.

When susceptible bacteria were eradicated, the few survivors were those that were resistant to the antimicrobial agent. Through natural selection, these microbes then became the predominant microorganism.

Resistant microbes have several mechanisms of action. For example, penicillin resistance is the result of gene action. Because penicillin inhibits enzymes involved in cell wall synthesis, some of the organisms can alter their cell walls so that the antibiotic cannot bind to it. These organisms are called beta-lactamase inhibitors because they produce an enzyme called beta-lactamase that breaks open the beta-lactam ring of the penicillin molecule.[17,18] In contrast, resistance to quinolones involves altering the ability of the drug to penetrate its target.[19]

Bacteria can acquire genes that provide resistance to antimicrobial drugs in one of three ways: (1) spontaneous DNA mutation (e.g., drug-resistant tuberculosis); (2) transformation in which one bacterium assumes DNA from another bacterium (e.g., penicillin-resistant gonorrhea); and (3) resistance acquired from a small circle of DNA called a plasmid that can move from one type of bacterium to another (e.g., shigella). The third type is the most troublesome, because with plasmid acquisition, the bacteria may simultaneously become resistant to several types of drugs.

The rise in drug resistance directly correlates with the trend toward increased use of antimicrobials. Clinicians are advised to use antimicrobials only when these agents are clearly indicated, and to use narrow-spectrum agents when the microorganism is known. Clinicians should also educate women about the appropriate use of antimicrobials, including avoidance of antibacterial soaps and cleansers that may contribute to the problem. The antibacterial agents added to a variety of substances, such as soaps, lotions, and cleaning supplies, can act like antibiotics in the selection of resistant strains of microbes; these products are no more effective than similar agents without the antibacterial additives, and controversy has arisen regarding whether they may contribute to drug resistance.[20]

Regulation of Herbal Therapies

More than 2000 years ago, Hippocrates documented the use of more than 200 herbal remedies. Today, many herbs and botanicals are sold as dietary supplements, even though their actions and safety largely remain unknown. Under the Dietary Supplement Health and Education Act of 1994 (DSHEA), a manufacturer must ensure that its dietary supplement is safe before the product is marketed in the United States.[21] The FDA is responsible for taking action against any unsafe dietary supplement product after it reaches the market. Generally, manufacturers do not register with the FDA, nor do they seek FDA approval before producing or selling dietary supplements. The FDA's postmarketing responsibilities include monitoring safety concerns, such as through voluntary dietary supplement adverse event reporting. The FDA also monitors product information, such as labeling, claims, package inserts, and accompanying literature. The Federal Trade Commission regulates dietary supplement advertising.

Many individuals consume nutritional supplements and herbs, often as a complementary therapy to pharmaceutical treatments. The use of herbs is challenging for midwives, as much of the information available on the Internet or in journals remains anecdotal or reflects expert opinion. Some evidence-based information can be obtained, however. In 1978, a regulatory agency was established in Germany to evaluate the effectiveness of herbal remedies. Called the German Commission E, the group of 24 scientists evaluated studies (clinical, case, field), and prepared scientific monographs. By 2004, only herbs that the German Commission E found to be effective and to carry a low risk of adverse effects were expected to be available in Germany. Although the work generally has been lauded, many common North American herbs are not included in the German registry.[22] The American Botanical Council, based in Texas, has published an English translation of the German monographs.[23]

Currently, the National Center for Complementary and Alternative Medicine (NCCAM) has approximately two dozen studies in process that are comparing herbal remedies to conventional pharmaceutical treatments for specific conditions, such as endometriosis. Publication of the results of these U.S. studies should expand knowledge in the area. Until such solid evidence becomes available, midwives must remain cautious regarding claims involving therapeutic uses of herbs. Many sources simply list possible indications for supplements without any accompanying scientific data.

Pharmacotherapeutics in Primary Care

The drug categories most commonly used in primary care are analgesics, antihistamines, antimicrobials, hormonal formulations used for contraception, and immunizations. It is not possible to review these topics in depth here. Instead, this section simply introduces the reader to analgesics, antimicrobials, and antihistamines—key drug categories that incorporate the pharmacologic principles and clinical implications that are inherent in all drug categories and that are not covered in other chapters of this text. References that have more in-depth information are provided where relevant.

Analgesics

Analgesic medications are categorized as non-opioid analgesics and opioid analgesics. Non-opioid analgesics include aspirin, acetaminophen (Tylenol), and nonsteroidal anti-inflammatory drugs (NSAIDs).[24] Opioid analgesics are a family of drugs with an action similar to morphine.

In the outpatient setting, most of the prescriptions written for analgesia are for formulations that contain a mixture of non-opioid and opioid drugs. It is essential that the prescriber know the mechanism of action, predictable side effects/adverse effects, individual dose variations, maximum daily dose, important drug–drug interactions, and expected response for each medication that is prescribed.

Several different formulations combine an opiate with a non-opiate. For example, the combination of acetaminophen and codeine comes in different strengths of acetaminophen (e.g., Tylenol #1, #2, or #3). In this case, although the drug is usually prescribed on the basis of the 30 mg of codeine in each tablet, the maximum dose is actually limited by the maximum dose of acetaminophen that is safe to take in a 24-hour period. When choosing a specific formulation, the midwife will assess the analgesic capability of a particular formulation and match that to the pain control needs of the woman.[18,25]

Analgesics have pharmacologic effects that are broad and affect many physiologic functions. Consequently, this category of drugs requires that the prescriber be especially aware of side effects and adverse effects. NSAIDs mitigate pain via their ability to inhibit cyclooxygenase (COX), the enzyme responsible for synthesizing prostaglandins.[26,27] Prostaglandins protect gastric mucosa, inhibit platelet aggregation, and stimulate uterine contractions, in addition to mediating the inflammatory response and sensitizing pain receptors. Thus these drugs can have multiple predictable side effects that can also be adverse effects.[28,29]

In the inpatient setting, midwives frequently manage pain as part of their care of women during labor. The analgesic options for this clinical setting are unique because the physiologic characteristics and function of both the parturient and the fetus must be taken into consideration. Until recently, meperidine (Demerol) was the drug most commonly administered to mitigate labor pain. This agent is very lipophilic, however, so it transfers across the placenta readily. Meperidine also has an active metabolite that can cause significant respiratory depression in the neonate several hours after the drug was administered to the laboring woman.[29] Today, short-acting opioids such as fentanyl (Sublimaze) and morphine, which has predictable pharmacokinetics, are used, but only for specific indications.[30] Most women who desire significant pain control during labor rely on epidural analgesia.

Both gender differences and individual differences are noted in the pain response and in the response to many analgesics.[31,32] The various hormonal and genetic reasons underlying these differences have yet to be fully elucidated, and the clinical implications of this knowledge have not yet been fleshed out. In any event, when prescribing analgesic medications, it is important to assess response and be available to change the recommended therapy as needed.

Antimicrobials

Antimicrobial drugs include agents directed against bacteria, fungi, viruses, and parasites. Each type of microorganism targeted by these drugs has a different biochemical structure, and consequently each type of antimicrobial has a different chemical structure and biochemical action. In general, antifungal and antiviral drugs attack protein structures that are not present in human cells, so these drugs are less likely to have adverse side effects. At the other end of the spectrum are parasites, which are multicellular organisms that share many similarities with human cells. Safe and effective antiparasitic drugs are particularly difficult to create.

Antimicrobials and analgesics are the most common prescriptions written in primary care practice. It is important to note that the increasingly problematic rise in drug resistance is directly related to the overuse of antibiotics for conditions that do not actually require an antimicrobial agent.[20,33] Thus the first step when using these agents is to make sure they are required. Eight principles describe the critical clinical considerations prior to prescribing an antimicrobial drug:

1. Confirmation of the presence of an infection through history and physical exam
2. Identification of the pathogen when possible
3. Confirmation of need for antimicrobial as opposed to palliative therapies and infection control measures
4. Understanding of host factors that may influence pharmacodynamics as well as the individual's concerns and resources
5. Selection of an appropriate antimicrobial agent using the dual principles of narrowest spectrum and shortest effective duration possible
6. Knowledge of the pharmacokinetics and pharmacodynamics of selected medications
7. Education of individual and family regarding appropriate use of antimicrobial
8. Appropriate monitoring of the therapeutic response[34]

Antibacterial drugs are either bacteriostatic (i.e., they inhibit bacterial growth) or bacteriocidal (i.e., they kill bacteria) in nature. More generally, these agents are classified by their mechanism of action: (1) they attack the cell wall (penicillins, cephalosporins, and vancomycin); (2) they inhibit or alter protein synthesis (macrolides, tetracycline, and aminoglycosides); or (3) they interfere with bacterial DNA (fluoroquinolones, antiprotozoan drugs, and isoniazid [INH]).

Inappropriate prescribing of antibiotics for viral infections and use of third- and fourth-generation broad-spectrum agents when a narrow-spectrum agent is available are by far the most important problems facing midwives who may be prescribing these agents. There are two critical components to the solution to these problems. First, clinical guidelines are available from most professional associations as well as individual institutions; these guidelines can help the prescriber chose the correct therapy. Second, thorough health education that is both culturally competent and provided at the correct health literacy level is essential. As a corollary to this general rule, when an antimicrobial agent is prescribed, detailed information on dose, timing, specific rules about taking with food or drink, and possible side effects or adverse effects is also part of the required health education.

Antihistamines

Four different types of histamine receptors (H_1, H_2, H_3, H_4) are found in multiple tissue sites within the body. Thus antihistamine drugs have a wide range of actions and uses. These agents are commonly used over-the-counter medications.

H_1 receptors are found in the muscles that line blood vessels (vascular smooth muscle) and in nervous tissue. These receptors are involved in the inflammatory response and allergic reactions. H_2 receptors are located in gastric mucosa. Stimulation of these receptors causes secretion of gastric acid. H_3 and H_4 receptors are found in the brain, heart, eye, breast tissue, and immune cells. These receptors appear to be involved in circadian rhythms, allergic reactions, and perhaps carcinomas, although their exact functions are not yet well elucidated.

Antihistamines that are antagonists at H_1 receptors are used to treat allergic reactions, nausea and vomiting, and motion sickness. First-generation H_1 antihistamines have a duration of action of approximately 4–6 hours. Also, because they cross the blood–brain barrier, they cause sedation—the most common side effect. When sedation is the desired effect, it is important to note that tolerance to sedation develops within a few days. Thus drugs such as diphenhydramine hydrochloride (Benadryl) and doxylamine succinate (Unisom Sleep Tabs) should be taken for a few days only. The other side effect of antihistamines that is of clinical concern relates to their anticholinergic effects. This action causes a drying of mucous membranes, which is helpful in treating allergies, but can also cause urinary retention and blurred vision. The primary contraindications to antihistamines are those wherein sedation or anticholinergic effects would cause adverse outcomes. For example, persons with glaucoma or hyperthyroidism should not use antihistamines.

The second-generation H_1 antihistamines have a longer duration of action, which can be as long as 24 hours. In addition, they are more selective for peripheral H_1 receptors and, therefore, do not cause sedation. The second-generation H_1 antihistamines, however, have more drug–drug interactions than do the first-generation drugs in this category.[35]

The H_2 antihistamines are used to treat gastric disorders wherein hyperacidity is a problem. These antihistamines have very few side effects. Cimetidine (Tagamet) has many drug–drug interactions and, for this reason, is not considered the first H_2 antihistamine of choice. Famotidine (Pepcid AC) is more potent than cimetidine (Tagamet) or ranitidine (Zantac). The most common side effect of these drugs is headache, which occurs in 3% to 5% of persons who take these medications.

Use of Drugs During Pregnancy

Pharmacokinetics in Pregnancy

Pharmacokinetics encompasses the absorption, distribution, metabolism, and excretion of drugs. The myriad physiologic changes that occur during pregnancy affect the pharmacokinetics of any drugs and herbs that the pregnant woman uses.[36] Pregnancy-related changes in pharmacokinetics are summarized in **Table 5-2**.

Transport of Drugs Across the Placenta

Drug distribution is complex during pregnancy, as four separate compartments exist: (1) the fetus, (2) the amniotic fluid, (3) the placenta, and (4) the mother. Each of the compartments affects movement of drugs, and occasionally certain drugs can have a higher concentration in a specific compartment.[37] Placental transfer of drugs can be accomplished by any of the traditional drug transfer methods, whether passive or active.

Passive transfer includes simple diffusion and facilitated diffusion. Neither of these two methods requires energy or allows an agent to be transferred across the membrane to an area of higher drug concentration. Most drugs move across the placenta by simple diffusion, although some take advantage of carrier-mediated mechanisms or use facilitated diffusion. Glucocorticoids and cephalexin (Keflex), for example, are transported via facilitated diffusion. One can assume that this mechanism is intended for endogenous compounds such as hormones and, therefore, is also used to transport drugs that are structurally similar to naturally occurring hormones.[38]

Active transport requires energy; the most common method is pinocytosis, a process during which a portion of the plasma membrane engulfs the drug molecule, creating a type of intracellular vesicle. Because of the energy and time required for pinocytosis, the small number of drugs that cross the placenta using active transport are also similar in structure to endogenous compounds that cross the placenta this way. Digoxin (Lanoxin) and valproic acid (Depakene), for example, cross the placenta via active transport.

Table 5-2	Pregnancy-Related Changes in Pharmacokinetics	
Pharmacokinetic Phase	**Pregnancy Changes**	**Clinical Implications**
Absorption	Increased progesterone production causes decreased intestinal motility and 30%–50% increase in gastric emptying time	Gestational nausea and vomiting may impair absorption
		Slower gastric emptying time may delay onset of drug response
	Gastric pH increases at midgestation	Increased exposure to bacteria in intestine may decrease bioavailability of some drugs
		Calcium and iron bind when ingested concurrently, thereby decreasing absorption of both minerals
Lung absorption	Respiratory minute volume increases approximately 50%	Dose requirements for inhaled drugs are decreased
Transdermal, subcutaneous absorption	Skin perfusion and skin hydration are both increased	Both lipophilic drugs and hydrophilic drugs are more rapidly absorbed transcutaneously
	Enhanced perfusion to muscles	Intramuscular absorption of drugs is more rapid and complete compared to absorption in nonpregnant individuals
Distribution	Plasma volume is expanded by approximately 50%	Hydrophilic drugs have reduced plasma concentration and need to be given in higher doses
	Body fat stores increase by 3–4 kg	Lipophilic drugs that concentrate in body fat may accumulate and prolonged effects could be seen following long-term use
Protein binding	Plasma albumin concentrations are reduced secondary to increased plasma volume	Increased free drug is available for pharmacologic effects
		Drugs that are highly protein bound will have more pharmacologic activity in a pregnant woman
Fetal–maternal distribution	Fetal compartment available for distribution of drugs	Highly lipophilic drugs of low molecular weight and that have low protein binding can accumulate in the fetal compartment
	Fetal circulation is more acidic than the maternal circulation	Basic drugs such as meperidine (Demerol) can have higher concentrations in the fetal compartment than in the maternal circulation secondary to "ion trapping"
	Fetal albumin concentration in plasma increases throughout pregnancy and is 20% higher than maternal concentrations at term	Drugs that are highly bound to albumin can concentrate in the fetus at term
		Most drugs in the fetal compartment tend to be 50%–100% of the concentration in the maternal compartment
Metabolism	Changes in estrogen and progesterone affect cytochrome P-450 enzyme activity	Metabolism of caffeine and theophylline (Theo-Dur) is inhibited or slower
	CYP1A2 is inhibited	Metabolism of sertraline (Zoloft) and metoprolol (Lopressor) is enhanced or faster
	CYP3A4 and CYP2C9 are increased	
Elimination	Glomerular filtration rate increases by 50% throughout pregnancy	More rapid clearance of most all drugs that are eliminated renally

Drug transfer is facilitated by various characteristics of the drug, including its size (molecular weight), lipid solubility, plasma protein binding, and acid versus basic properties. Most drugs have a small molecular weight, usually less than 500 daltons (Da), so they are easily transferred easily across the placenta. Drugs with a molecular weight greater than 500 Da transfer incompletely; those like heparin and insulin, which have a molecular weight greater than 1000 Da, transfer very poorly.[38] Drugs that are more lipophilic cross the placenta more readily than those that are hydrophilic, as the placenta is lipoid in character. A non-ionized state facilitates transfer. When ionized basic drugs such as meperidine (Demerol) cross the placenta, they can accumulate in the fetal liver and adrenal glands and become ion-trapped in the fetus because the fetal circulation is more acidic than the maternal circulation.

Once a drug enters the fetal circulation, it is free to bind with proteins in the fetal plasma. Albumin concentrations in the fetal compartment are higher than in the maternal compartment. Thus some highly protein-bound drugs such as diazepam (Valium) may have an increased fetal effect when compared with their maternal effects.

Drug Dose Alterations in Pregnancy

Some medications may need dosage adjustments over the course of pregnancy. For example, aminoglycosides such as gentamicin (Garamycin), as well as other agents such as ampicillin (Omnipen, Polycillin, Principen) and cefazolin (Rocephin), have lower serum concentrations during pregnancy and therefore, to be effective, the doses of these medications may need to be increased for pregnant women. Ampicillin, in particular, has serum concentrations in pregnant women that are 50% of the serum concentrations seen in nonpregnant women. The clinician may also need to decrease theophylline (Theolair) doses for the asthmatic woman, as serum concentrations of this agent rise in pregnancy.

Teratogenic and Fetotoxic Effects of Drugs

Although most women are aware that they should not take drugs during pregnancy, 50% of all pregnancies are unintended and awareness of pregnancy typically occurs only after embryogenesis has begun.[38] Approximately 20% of pregnant women use a medication at least once that is known to have a risk for causing fetal harm.[29] One of the major concerns specific to pregnancy is whether the drugs used are teratogenic.

Teratology is essentially the study of congenital anomalies and teratogens or any agent that irreversibly alters growth, structure, or function in a developing embryo or fetus. Teratogens include viruses such as rubella, chemicals such as mercury, and drugs such as diethylstilbestrol (DES).[36,39] The term *fetotoxic* is used to describe agents, such as tobacco, that have toxic effects on the fetus and adversely affect growth or development.[36,40] The fetus is mostly likely to be exposed to teratogenic agents in the first trimester and to fetotoxic agents in the second and third trimesters.

Overall, birth defects occur in approximately 1% to 3% of all births. This percentage is often called the "background risk" upon which additional risks are calculated based on family history, past history, and environmental exposure. Only 10% of birth defects can be associated with environmental factors, and the majority of environmental factors are not pharmaceuticals. Drugs and chemical agents such as mercury and pesticides account for approximately 45% of the environmental teratogens involved in congenital anomalies. Drugs alone account for only 2% to 3% of all birth defects.[40,41]

The unique fact about teratogenic medications is that avoiding the teratogen can prevent the associated congenital anomaly. Thus knowledge of teratogenic drugs is essential for the practicing midwife. Fortunately, the number of these agents is relatively small, and even fewer are in common use.

The preimplantation period is considered the "all or nothing" period. If a small number of cells are damaged during this time period, the fetus usually compensates without any damage. Conversely, if a large number of cells are damaged, the embryo will be lost and a spontaneous abortion will occur. The period of organogenesis—between 2 and 8 weeks post fertilization, or 4 to 10 gestational weeks—is the most critical period wherein teratogenic exposures can cause fetal malformations[40] (**Figure 5-3**). A list of drugs that are known to have teratogenic or fetotoxic effects is presented in **Table 5-3**.

FDA Drug Categories

In 1979, the FDA published a list of pregnancy risk categories for prescription and nonprescription drugs, including those with known teratogenic effects. These categories are listed in **Table 5-4**.[42] Although the FDA created the drug categories, the drug manufacturer usually determines which category a particular drug will be assigned.[6]

Unfortunately, these FDA pregnancy categories oversimplify the complexity of what is known and what is not known about drug effects on human fetuses, in several different ways.[43] First, the FDA pregnancy categories suggest that the level of risk increases from Category A to Category X. This is only true somewhat true for Categories A, B, and C. Categories D and X are based on the risk weighed against the evidence of benefit. Thus drugs in Categories D, X, and to some extent C may be associated with a similar risk but are categorized differently based on their different risk–benefit calculations.

Second, the pregnancy categories imply that drugs within one category have a similar risk for reproductive harm to the fetus. This is particularly problematic for Category C, which includes drugs that have demonstrated risks in animal studies and

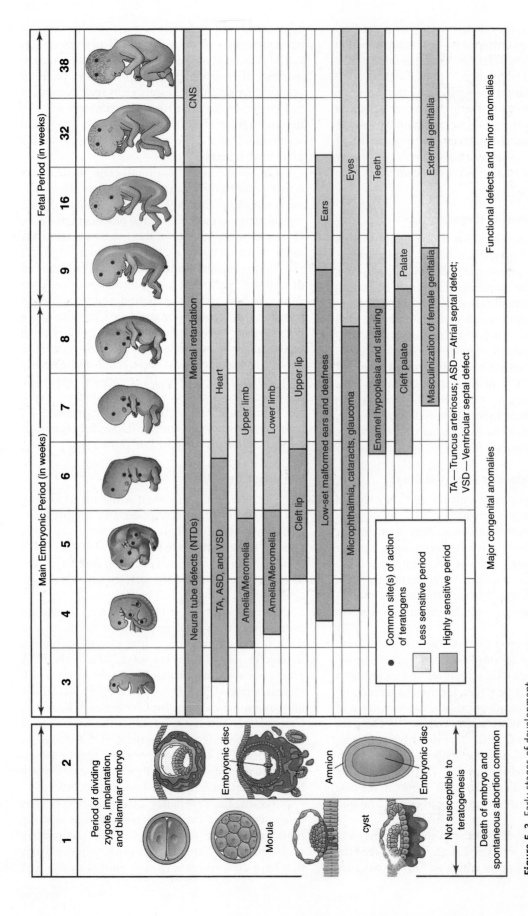

Figure 5-3 Early stages of development.
Source: Reproduced by permission from Moore KL, Persaud TVN. *The Developing Human: Clinically Oriented Embryology.* 6th ed. Philadelphia, PA: W.B. Saunders; 1998.

Table 5-3	Drugs That Have a Teratogenic or Fetotoxic Effect	
Drug Category Name (Brand Name)	**Teratogenic or Fetotoxic Effects**	**Comments**
Androgens and testosterone derivatives: Danocrine (Danazol)	Virilization of females Advanced genital development of males	Dose dependent and based on critical period. Brief exposure rarely is significant. Before 9 weeks' gestation, labioscrotal fusion is common. Incidental, brief exposure usually has minimal risk.
Antibiotics: **Tetracyclines:** Tetracycline (Terramycin) Doxycycline (Adoxa	Abnormalities of teeth discoloration	Critical period is after first trimester. Discoloration of permanent teeth is possible if exposure occurs after 24 weeks' gestation. No well-controlled studies of doxycycline have been performed, but case-controlled studies suggest it is not associated with teratogenic risk. Recommend that doxycycline be used only if it is the only effective agent.
Sulfonamides: Sulfamethoxazole (Bactrim, Septra)	Hyperbilirubinemia in neonate	Contraindicated in third trimester.
Chloramphenicol	Grey syndrome in neonate 2–9 days after therapy administered	Oral chloramphenicol is contraindicated in pregnancy.
Aminoglycosides: Gentamycin (Garamycin) Streptomycin	Neonatal ototoxicity	Streptomycin in high doses used to treat tuberculosis has a clear risk of fetal ototoxicity. The risk associated with gentamycin may be smaller, but this agent is not recommended for use in pregnancy.
Anticonvulsants: Carbamazepine (Tegretol) Phenytoin (Dilantin) Trimethadione (Tridione) Valproic acid (Depakene) Valproate (Depacon)	1% risk of neural tube defect, cardiovascular defects, developmental delays, intrauterine growth restriction Reduced intelligence associated with use of valproic acid or valproate Phenytoin is specifically associated with cardiac defects and cleft palate	Critical period is all trimesters. Risk of neural tube defect is increased, especially when used with other antiepileptic drugs. Risk of neural tube defects is decreased with increased folic acid supplementation. Polytherapy with more than one anticonvulsant increases risk. Newer anticonvulsants such as gabapentin (Neurontin) do not appear to engender a risk of congenital anomaly.
Angiotensin-converting enzyme (ACE) inhibitors: Captopril (Capoten) Enalapril (Vasotec) Lisinopril (Prinivil)	Intrauterine growth restriction Oligohydramnios Renal failure Decreased skull ossification Renal tubular dysgenesis	Risk of growth restriction is approximately 25%, with fetal morbidity of approximately 30%. Risk of adverse effects increases in second and third trimesters (probably due to decreased uteroplacental flow). Beta blockers such as labetalol (Trandate) are safe in pregnancy.
Antidepressants: Fluoxetine (Prozac) Paroxetine (Paxil) Sertraline (Zoloft)	Paroxetine increases risk of cardiac defects 1.5- to 2-fold; the other SSRI-type antidepressants do not appear to have teratogenic effects Exposure in third trimester associated with neonatal withdrawal Persistent pulmonary hypertension noted in case reports	Overall, risks of teratogenic and fetotoxic effects are low. Antidepressants should not be discontinued during pregnancy. If starting antidepressant therapy during pregnancy, avoid paroxetine.

(continues)

Table 5-3	Drugs That Have a Teratogenic or Fetotoxic Effect (continued)	
Drug Category Name (Brand Name)	**Teratogenic or Fetotoxic Effects**	**Comments**
Antineoplastic drugs: Cyclophosphamide (Cytoxan) Methotrexate (Rheumatrex)	Multiple birth defects and spontaneous abortion if used in first trimester	If a woman needs one of these drugs, refer her for consultation with perinatologists and oncologists. Methotrexate is used to treat ectopic pregnancy.
Angiotensin II receptor blockers: Losartan (Cozaar)	Prolonged renal failure and hypotension in the newborn, decreased skull ossification, renal tubular agenesis	Critical period is all trimesters.
Antithyroid drugs: Propylthiouracil (PTU) Methimazole	Fetal and neonatal goiter, fetal hypothyroidism, and aplasia cutis are associated with methimazole but not propylthiouracil	Critical period is all trimesters. Women who need to take antithyroid drugs will generally be counseled to take propylthiouracil. The risk of fetal goiter is approximately 1%–5%.
Aspirin	More than 150 mg/day is associated with prolonged gestation, prolonged labor, bleeding complications in the neonate, premature closure of the ductus arteriosus, and intrauterine growth restriction	Critical period is all trimesters. Although low-dose aspirin may be of benefit for women with antiphospholipid syndrome or lupus, normal adult doses should be avoided.
Benzodiazepines: Alprazolam (Xanax) Chlordiazepoxide (Librium) Diazepam (Valium)	Increased risk of neonatal withdrawal Some studies show increased risk of oral clefts with first-trimester exposure to diazepam	Early data on oral cleft association are controversial. Benzodiazepines are highly lipophilic and have a long half-life in the neonate.
Corticosteroids: Methyl prednisone (Medrol)	Possibly increased risk of oral and cleft defects	Critical period is first trimester. Because the risk is low, oral corticosteroids are used in the first trimester to treat hyperemesis gravidarum and other medical conditions. No risk associated with topical use.
Coumarin (Warfarin)	Bone defects Growth restriction Central nervous system (CNS) defects Developmental delays	15%–25% risk when anticoagulants that impair vitamin K are used, especially between 6 and 9 weeks of gestation. Later use in pregnancy is associated with abruption, CNS defects, stillbirth, and hemorrhage of the fetus/newborn.
Ergot alkaloids: Ergotamine (Cafergot)	Spontaneous abortion Mobius syndrome Intestinal atresia Cerebral developmental abnormalities Low birth weight and preterm birth	Critical period is all trimesters. Sumatriptan (Imitrex): alternative to ergotamine for acute migraine treatment.
Folic acid antagonists: Methotrexate (Rheumatrex) Carbamazepine (Tegretol) Phenytoin (Dilantin) Phenobarbital (Solfoton) Primidone (Mysoline) Trimethoprim (Trimpex)	Spontaneous abortion Neural tube defects Cardiovascular defects Urinary tract defects	Drugs in many different drug categories are folic acid antagonists. Some suggest that risk can be decreased with folic acid supplementation. Trimethoprim is a component of trimethoprim-sulfamethoxazole (Septra), which is commonly used to treat urinary tract infections. This drug should not be given in the first and third trimesters.

Table 5-3	Drugs That Have a Teratogenic or Fetotoxic Effect *(continued)*	
Drug Category Name (Brand Name)	**Teratogenic or Fetotoxic Effects**	**Comments**
Lithium (Lithobid)	Cardiac defects Epstein's anomaly	Absolute risk is small, but alternative drugs should be recommended if possible.
Mifepristone (RU-486)	Antiprogestogen; used as an abortifacient Human data are limited	Primarily used for abortion in combination with misoprostol. Less effective when used alone.
Misoprostol (Cytotec)	Abortion Moebius sequence (brain stem ischemia, vascular disruption) for misoprostol	Potent uterostimulant capable of initiating uterine contractions at all gestational ages.
Nonsteroidal anti-inflammatory drugs: Ibuprofen (Advil) Naproxen (Aleve)	Theorized premature closure of the ductus arteriosus Necrotizing enterocolitis	Contraindicated in general but especially in third trimester.
Retinoids: Isotretinoin (Accutane)	Multiple birth defects, including CNS, cardiac, and endocrine damage	Oral isotretinoin is contraindicated in pregnancy. Topical preparations are unlikely to have serious teratogenic effects but are still contraindicated because other agents can be used.
Statins: Atorvastatin (Lipitor) Lovastatin (Mevacor)	Interfere with cholesterol production Primarily theoretical adverse effects on the fetus	Contraindicated in pregnancy.
Streptomycin and kanamycin	Hearing loss Eighth nerve damage	No ototoxicity has been found with gentamicin or vancomycin.
Thalidomide	Limb deficiencies Cardiac and GI abnormalities	20%–30% risk during critical period (very potent). Used for years before teratogenic effects became obvious. Has caused the belief that all drugs have the potential to be a "new thalidomide." Back on market for oral lesions in HIV, Hansen's disease, TB, and multiple myeloma. STEPS (System for Thalidomide Education and Prescribing Safety) is available online from the manufacturer, Celgene.

drugs for which no animal studies have been conducted.[40,43–45] In fact, each of the categories is heterogeneous with regard to clinical interpretation. For example, only 0.7% of drugs are classified into Category A.[40] Randomized controlled trials (RCTs) of pregnant women to assess risks associated with drugs are ethically questionable and, therefore, are rarely performed. In addition, Category A may suffer from the problem of publication bias, as studies with negative findings are not published as often as studies with positive outcomes. Thus Category A may be used less often than it should secondary to research constraints. Category B has another problem. Classification of a drug into this category can be based on animal studies that document no harm and failure of human studies to document harm or no human studies that show harm.[42] The rigor of safety information based on some human studies or no human studies is not equal, however, so the drugs in this category may have significantly different safety profiles. Categories D and X both include teratogens but differ according to the supposed risks and benefits of their member drugs. For example, some Category D drugs are antiepileptic drugs (AEDs) with known

Table 5-4	FDA Pregnancy Risk Categories for Prescription and Nonprescription Drugs
Category	**Description**
A	Controlled studies in women fail to demonstrate a risk to the fetus in the first trimester (and there is no evidence of a risk in later trimesters), and the possibility of fetal harm appears remote.
B	Either animal reproduction studies have not demonstrated a fetal risk but there are no controlled studies in pregnant women or animal reproduction studies have shown an adverse effect (other than a decrease in fertility) that was not confirmed in controlled studies in women in the first trimester (and there is no evidence of a risk in later trimesters).
C	Either studies in animals have revealed adverse effects on the fetus (teratogenic, embryocidal, or other) or controlled studies in women and animals are not available. Drugs should be given only if the potential benefit justifies the potential risk to the fetus.
D	There is positive evidence of human fetal risk, but the benefits from use in pregnant women may be acceptable despite the risk (e.g., if the drug is needed in a life-threatening situation or for a serious disease for which safer drugs cannot be used or are ineffective).
X	Studies in animals or human beings have demonstrated fetal abnormalities or there is evidence of fetal risk based on human experience, or both, and the risk of the use of the drug in pregnant women clearly outweighs any possible benefit. The drug is contraindicated in women who are or may become pregnant.

Source: Pregnancy labeling. *FDA Drug Bull.* 1979;9:23-24.

teratogenic effects. Even so, these AEDs may be prescribed during pregnancy if they are the only agents effective in controlling seizure activity. Category X is reserved for drugs that are known teratogens and are used to treat disorders for which safe and effective alternative nonteratogenic therapies are available.

In 2008, the FDA proposed a pregnancy and lactation section of drug labeling that omits the letter categories and replaces them with text that is divided into sections addressing clinical considerations, detailed data about risks, and lactation information.[46] It is believed that this system will be adopted in the near future and will replace the current pregnancy categories A, B, C, D, and X.

Despite the fact that the current FDA pregnancy categories lack sufficient specificity, multiple evidence-based sources of reliable information about specific drugs are available on several different websites including the FDA, the Teratogen Information System (TERIS), and the Organization of Teratology Information Specialists (OTIS).

Pharmaceuticals Commonly Used During Pregnancy

At least 50% of all pregnant women are prescribed one or more drugs during pregnancy.[47] Although the majority of these medications are classified into FDA Category A, B, or C, approximately 5% are members of Category D or X.[47] The drug classifications most commonly used during pregnancy include vitamins, antimicrobials, analgesics, and blood

glucose regulators. The sections that follow present a brief review of these categories of pharmaceuticals from which midwives often prescribe or recommend treatments, in order of most frequently to least frequently used.

Vitamins

Prenatal vitamins are multivitamin supplements formulated to provide the vitamins and minerals needed most by pregnant women. In fact, prenatal vitamins are one of the universal symbols of prenatal care, considered essential by both women and their healthcare providers. However, the actual value of vitamin and micronutrient supplements for pregnant women is more nuanced and complex. Although a balanced diet generally provides all the nutrients needed for health during pregnancy, a majority of the women in the United States do not consume a diet that provides all the vitamins and micronutrients needed during pregnancy.[48] This fact is the overall reason why prenatal vitamins are recommended. In addition, evidence indicates that prenatal multivitamins containing additional folic acid have a positive effect in lowering the incidence of several congenital anomalies in addition to neural tube defects.[49]

Multivitamins do have some problems. Calcium interferes with iron absorption, so placing both of these minerals in one vitamin may obviate the overall goal. Many women report significant nausea or gastric upset secondary to the iron in prenatal vitamins—a problem that can be resolved by discontinuing the multivitamin for a period of time, switching to a multivitamin without iron, or sometimes using a different formulation of iron.[50]

The specific vitamins and micronutrients that have documented adverse effects on fetal development if present in insufficient amounts in the diet are folic acid, iron, and iodine.[51] Women who follow vegetarian or vegan diets also need supplemental vitamin B_{12}. There is some evidence that vitamin D supplements may be necessary for women who do not get enough exposure to sunlight[52] and that additional omega-3 fatty acids may improve fetal growth as well as neonatal cognition and visual function although the evidence is not robust enough to recommend either for all women at the time of this writing.[53]

It has been definitively proven that *folic acid* supplementation taken during the 3 months prior to conception and for the first 2 months after conception can reduce the incidence of neural tube defects by approximately 50%.[49,54] Although many dietary sources of folic acid exist, this is the one nutrient that women absorb from supplements better than from dietary sources.[55] Routine supplementation with folic acid is recommended for all women of childbearing years.[56]

Iron is the single most difficult nutrient to obtain via the diet during pregnancy, and iron needs are approximately doubled during pregnancy.[57–59] However, unlike folic acid, routine iron supplementation is controversial. The CDC recommends routine iron supplementation, but other organizations recommend that supplementation be started only for women who do not have normal hemoglobin values.[57–59] Iron supplementation will increase plasma hemoglobin levels but does not have any effect on overall maternal and neonatal outcomes unless iron is used specifically to treat anemia during pregnancy. Iron supplements frequently cause gastrointestinal distress.

Iodine deficiency can cause significant intellectual impairment but is rare in the United States given that table salt and many common foods are routinely fortified with iodine. Nevertheless, many multivitamins contain amounts of iodine that are less than the amount recommended by the American Thyroid Association.[60,61]

Vitamins are not always positive supplements. For example, vitamin A in large doses can be a teratogen. Initially the threshold for adverse effects was thought to be more than 25,000 IU of vitamin A daily, but studies have since shown that cranial neural crest anomalies occur with as little as 10,000 IU daily.[62] Routine supplementation of vitamin A is unnecessary, and, if supplementation is used, it should not exceed 5000 IU daily. Typical prenatal multivitamins contain at least 800 IU of vitamin A. Women should be cautioned not to double or triple their intake of multivitamins in an attempt to get additional folic acid or calcium. Increasing intake of a multiple vitamin increases intake of all of that product's constituents, including vitamin A.

Antimicrobials

Penicillins and *cephalosporins* are among the most commonly prescribed antimicrobials for treatment of various female reproductive infections. Few studies of cephalosporins have been conducted in the first trimester of pregnancy, but no adverse effects have been reported and cephalosporins, like penicillin, belong to the beta-lactam classification of antimicrobial agents. However, because the penicillins and erythromycin have been studied extensively and not found to be associated with teratogenic effects, many experts advocate using them as first-line therapies whenever possible.

Metronidazole (Flagyl) is a well-established antiprotozoal agent and the treatment of choice for *Trichomonas vaginalis* infection and bacterial vaginosis. No teratogenic effect has been found with metronidazole, even though its mechanism of action involves bacterial mutation.[63] The drug is assigned to FDA Category B, yet many providers are hesitant to administer it during the first trimester. Although evidence does not support withholding the drug, the conditions for which it is used generally are not life threatening. Because metronidazole is the most effective drug for the treatment of trichomoniasis, it should be prescribed when indicated.[64]

Quinolones are FDA Category C drugs, but are rarely used in pregnancy because animal studies have demonstrated drug accumulation in the joints with subsequent damage.[65]

Sulfonamides are not teratogenic but require attention to timing. These agents are highly protein bound and can displace bilirubin from binding sites. The most commonly used agents in this category are a combination of sulfamethoxazole and trimethoprim (Bactrim, Septa). Administration of sulfonamides becomes problematic when they are administered near the time of birth because the free bilirubin that is displaced will be in the newborn's circulation. The immature liver is unable to compensate and kernicterus may result from these high plasma levels. Thus sulfonamides should be avoided in the third trimester. One sulfonamide, sulfasalazine (Azulfidine), appears to be an exception. This drug is used primarily for the treatment of ulcerative colitis and Crohn's disease and has a weak effect (if any) on bilirubin.

Tetracyclines are contraindicated in pregnancy because they concentrate in teeth. Children exposed in utero to tetracyclines may have yellowed teeth with poor enamel and vulnerability to caries as well as potential problems with bone growth.

Aminoglycosides include streptomycin, gentamycin (Garamycin), and kanamycin (Kantrex). All are ototoxic drugs that can cause permanent eighth cranial nerve damage. These agents are reserved for grave situations in which their benefits outweigh their risks.

Analgesics

The category of *nonsteroidal anti-inflammatory drugs* technically includes acetaminophen, ibuprofen, and aspirin. In general use, the term NSAIDs refers specifically to the family of drugs similar to ibuprofen (Advil); this is how the term is used in this chapter. Aspirin and NSAIDs have been implicated in disruption of the prostaglandin cascade involved in initiation of labor and, therefore, are linked to post-term pregnancy. NSAIDs can cause premature closure of the ductus arteriosus; indeed, they are employed neonatally for that specific therapeutic effect. Aspirin has been associated with fetal vascular disruptions as well as competition with bilirubin for albumin binding sites. NSAIDs and aspirin should be avoided in pregnancy, especially in the first and third trimesters. An alternative agent without anti-inflammatory action is acetaminophen (Tylenol).[64] Acetaminophen is the analgesic of choice for minor pain during pregnancy.

Opiate analgesics have not been implicated as having teratogenic effects. Caution with their use in pregnancy is based upon fear of addiction, not teratogenicity.

Drugs Used for the Treatment of Medical Conditions During Pregnancy

Although midwives care independently for women without medical or obstetrical complications, they often consult and collaborate in the care of women with medical or obstetrical complications. Thus knowledge of drugs that have teratogenic or fetotoxic effects and that are used in the care of pregnant women who have medical complications is necessary.

Antiepileptic agents pose a distinct challenge to the healthcare provider.[65] Seizure disorders themselves may contribute to teratogenic outcomes. Several older antiepileptic drugs (AEDs) are teratogenic, although the absolute risk of congenital malformations following prenatal exposure is low.[66] Phenytoin (Dilantin) is associated with midline cardiac defects,

hypospadias, neonatal coagulopathy, and neurobehavioral impairment. Carbamazepine (Tegretol), valproate (Depacon), and valproic acid (Depakene) can cause a dysmorphic pattern of minor anomalies, including neural tube defects and midline cardiac defects. Valproate and valproic acid are associated with intellectual impairment, and the congenital anomalies related to this drug appear to be dose dependent.[67] Phenobarbital (Solfoton) has been associated with neurobehavioral impairment and newborn withdrawal syndrome. Newborns exposed in utero to phenytoin (Dilantin), carbamazepine (Tegretol), or phenobarbital (Luminal) are at risk of coagulation problems secondary to drug-induced vitamin K deficiency, and need prompt supplemental vitamin K. Newer-generation antiepileptic drugs such as gabapentin (Neurontin) and lamotrigine (Lamictal) do not appear to have teratogenic effects.[68]

Many mechanisms have been proposed to explain the teratogenicity of anticonvulsant agents. Several of the drugs appear to have antifolate characteristics, and some authorities recommend that women on AEDs should be treated with 4 mg of folic acid both prior to conception and in early pregnancy.[69] The midwife should work closely with maternal–fetal specialists when caring for a woman with a seizure disorder, as treatment requires the choice of the least risky drug, at the lowest dose that controls seizures.

Antidepressants represent another drug category used by many women during pregnancy. The most widely used class of medications to treat depression, bipolar disorder, and anxiety disorders are the selective serotonin reuptake inhibitors (SSRIs) such as fluoxetine (Prozac), paroxetine (Paxil), and sertraline (Zoloft).[70] Untreated depression is associated with several adverse pregnancy outcomes, including preterm birth, postpartum depression, and poor behavioral and mental health outcomes in children.[71] Thus treatment of depression during pregnancy is recommended.[72] Although knowledge about the teratogenic and fetotoxic effects of SSRIs and serotonin norepinephrine reuptake inhibitors (SNRIs) is still being elucidated, there are some associations that women need to be apprised of prior to initiating or continuing therapy during pregnancy.[72,73] Midwives who choose to add these drugs to their individual formulary or manage women who are taking these drugs must know the required screening and diagnostic criteria for depression and other related mental disorders, understand the side effects and adverse effects associated with these agents, appreciate the FDA's "black box" warnings for these drugs, and practice within a setting that provides access to psychiatric services.

Thyroid agents are commonly used during pregnancy. The most common cause of hyperthyroidism is Graves' disease, which occurs secondary to the development of autoantibodies. These autoantibodies bind to the thyroid-stimulating hormone (TSH) receptor on the thyroid gland, which results in excessive production of thyroid hormone. Untreated hyperthyroidism has been linked to spontaneous abortion. The most popular treatment for hyperthyroidism is radioiodine (RAI), which is radioactive iodine that concentrates in the thyroid and destroys thyroid tissue. Radioiodine is contraindicated in pregnancy because it can cross the placenta and destroy the fetal thyroid. Traditionally, propylthiouracil (PTU) has been the drug of choice for hyperthyroidism in pregnancy, as methimazole (Tapazole) has been linked to aplasia cutis in the newborn. More recently this neonatal association has been called into question.[73] Moreover, PTU may result in fetal hypothyroidism when the drug is used in high doses, so close monitoring is required. Women who are taking PTU should be seen by an obstetrician to establish a plan for ultrasound monitoring to assess the fetal thyroid.

The most common etiology of hypothyroidism is Hashimoto's disease, also known as autoimmune thyroiditis. Untreated hypothyroidism can cause fetal mental retardation, preeclampsia, stillbirth, and other adverse obstetric outcomes.[74] Hypothyroidism is treated with levothyroxine (Synthroid), which is synthetic thyroid hormone. Levothyroxine has no adverse effects on the fetus, but the maternal dose may need to be increased by as much as 45% during pregnancy; thus thyroid stimulating hormone (TSH) and free thyroxine (T4) levels are typically assessed once each trimester. The goal is to maintain a euthyroid state during pregnancy.

Antihypertensives are prescribed for women with chronic hypertension. Chronic hypertension is defined as a systolic blood pressure of at least 140 mm Hg or a diastolic blood pressure of 90 mm Hg before pregnancy or in pregnant women prior to 20 weeks' gestation.[75] Angiotensin-converting enzyme (ACE) inhibitors and angiotensin-receptor blockers (ARBs) are contraindicated in pregnancy secondary to an increased risk for teratogenic effects. Use of these drugs in the second and third trimesters is associated with low birth weight, oligohydramnios, and hypoplastic fetal lung development.[75] Atenolol (Tenormin) has been associated with intrauterine growth restriction (IUGR) secondary to reduced placental function. This problem has not been noted following use of the other beta blockers; thus, with the exception of atenolol, beta blockers are the first-line drugs used to treat chronic hypertension in pregnancy. Labetalol (Trandate) is the most commonly used antihypertensive prescribed in the United States today.[75] The other category of antihypertensive drugs that appear safe in pregnancy is the calcium-channel blockers, which include agents such as nifedipine (Procardia XL). Nifedipine is also used as a tocolytic because it inhibits uterine contractions.

Anticoagulants, if needed during pregnancy, should consist of heparin, either regular or low molecular weight, as the drug of choice.[76] Coumarins, including warfarin (Coumadin), easily cross the placenta; when pregnant women take these drugs, approximately one-fourth of their embryos are born with fetal warfarin syndrome (i.e., nasal hypoplasia, optic atrophy, and mental retardation). When the fetus is exposed to coumarins, the results may include cataracts, microcephaly, and microphthalmia, as well as fetal and maternal hemorrhage.

Hypoglycemic agents are another drug category of interest given that women with type 2 diabetes typically use oral hypoglycemic agents when not pregnant. Untreated diabetes is associated with multiple adverse outcomes for both the pregnant woman and her fetus, most of which occur secondary to hyperglycemia. Therefore close glucose control is essential during pregnancy.[77,78] Traditionally women with type 2 diabetes who are pregnant are treated as though they have gestational diabetes and managed with diet, exercise, and injectable insulin. In contrast to oral hypoglycemic agents, insulin is a large molecule and has difficulty crossing the placenta. Therefore, it has been the drug of choice for management of diabetes mellitus during pregnancy.[79] Glyburide (Micronase, Diabeta) and metformin (Glucophage) have recently been the subject of research for treatment of diabetes during pregnancy.[79,80] Glyburide is extensively protein bound and does not cross the placenta in sufficient amounts to affect the fetus. Both glyburide and metformin appear to be safe and effective when used to treat diabetes in pregnancy, but neither is fully endorsed or established in clinical practice as yet.[81]

Pharmaceuticals and Breastfeeding

There is no doubt that breastfeeding is the best method of feeding newborns and young infants. For many lactating women, the need to take a medication during this time presents a concern about infant exposure through their breast milk. Knowledge of how drugs transfer into breast milk and access to reliable resources specific to breastfeeding and drug compatibility will help midwives who care for women during the postpartum period.[82,83] For the majority of drugs, less than 1% of the maternal plasma level of the drug crosses into the breast milk. In addition, binding to the milk proteins or onto the surface of the milk fat globule deters neonatal exposure further, as bound drugs do not passively diffuse out of the newborn's stomach.[84] Other factors that affect the likelihood of drug transfer into breast milk include lipid solubility, low molecular weight, long half-life, and the capacity to remain unbound and non-ionized in the maternal plasma.

The excretion of drugs into breast milk primarily involves passive diffusion through the alveolar/lactocyte cells that line the alveoli, which make up the glandular/secretory tissue within the breast. Most drugs move through these alveolar cells via passive diffusion. Active transport is used by a small number of drugs (e.g., ranitidine [Zantac], nitrofurantoin [Macrobid], acyclovir [Zovirax]). During the first few weeks postpartum, large gaps exist between alveolar cells, facilitating easy transfer of various agents including immunoglobulins. As milk production is established and the alveolar cells expand, the intracellular gaps to close, making drug transfer more difficult.[83] Also, because the majority of milk is produced at the time of feeding and blood flow to the breast is maximized at this time, women should be educated about the timing of peak plasma levels for specific drugs used and counseled to avoid breastfeeding during these times.

One of the most popular approaches used in clinical practice to evaluate drug concentration in breast milk is the milk plasma ratio (M/P). This ratio varies over time as both drug amount and type of milk vary over time, so most drug kinetics is based on a time-averaged ratio or range.[82] The M/P has been calculated for many agents. The majority of drugs have an M/P of 1 or less, indicating that the level of drug in the breast milk is the same as or less than the level in maternal plasma. For example, an M/P of 0.10 indicates that the breast milk contains 10% of the amount of the drug in maternal plasma. Although the M/P can be helpful, this ratio is not clinically relevant unless other factors are considered. For example, a high M/P may not create a problem if the drug poses no harm to the infant. Conversely, a low M/P may be problematic if drug clearance is slow in the neonate or the half-life of the drug is unusually long, exposing the baby to the pharmaceutical over a longer period of time.

In 2001, the American Academy of Pediatrics Committee on Drugs published an evidence-based listing of drug information for breastfeeding that included approximately 400 primary research references.[85] This group currently uses a list of seven categories to rate the threat posed by licit and illicit drugs. Six of the categories include those drugs that (1) are contraindicated, (2) require temporary cessation, (3) are of possible concern, (4) to be used with caution, or (5) compatible with breastfeeding. The additional category includes food and environmental agents.

Fortunately, most drugs commonly used by lactating women are compatible with breastfeeding. Although more research is needed regarding many agents, drug transfer is rarely a reason to discontinue breastfeeding, and the midwife should be encouraged to seek out the most current and reliable information when counseling a woman about the safety of this practice. **Box 5-5** summarizes guidelines for breastfeeding and the use of medications.

Drugs That Stimulate Breast Milk Production: Galactagogues

Breast milk production is controlled by the interplay of two key hormones, oxytocin and prolactin. Nipple stimulation stimulates release of prolactin from the anterior pituitary and release of oxytocin from the posterior pituitary. However, many factors can interfere with successful breastfeeding and

---

BOX 5-5 Guidelines for Breastfeeding and Medication Use

1. Use pharmaceuticals only when necessary.
2. Use the smallest therapeutic dose for the shortest time that is effective.
3. Whenever possible, choose an agent with a short half-life, an agent with a milk plasma ratio of 1 or less, and an agent that is not delivered by sustained release.
4. Arrange the timing of drug dosing so that it is given immediately after nursing or before the infant has a long sleep period.
5. If the drug is contraindicated for infant exposure, pumping and discarding the breast milk may be necessary.
6. Remember, it is rare that a medication is a reason to discontinue breastfeeding.

nipple stimulation. When lactogenesis is not well established, drugs that can stimulate breast milk production are considered. These agents are called galactagogues.

For example, metoclopramide (Reglan) is a dopamine antagonist used for gastrointestinal indications. A side effect of the drug is galactorrhea; thus it is used on an off-label basis to help women increase their milk supply. Metoclopramide tends to have a number of side effects, including fatigue, mental exhaustion, and extrapyramidal effects that produce dystonia, so it is typically used for only a limited duration.[86]

Herbal galactagogues are common. For example, fenugreek (*Trigonella foenum-graecum L.*) has been used for years and is well accepted in many countries, yet data demonstrating its efficacy remain elusive. Studies are ongoing in several areas of the world regarding efficacy of various galactagogues and other herbal remedies. More information about galactagogues can be found in the *Breastfeeding and the Mother–Newborn Dyad* chapter.

Conclusion

Pharmaceutical agents are part of modern life. Pharmacology is an essential area in women's health care, and it is one that continues to grow and challenge providers and women alike. Like any other intervention in a midwife's repertoire, drugs and herbs should be used appropriately and monitored for therapeutic as well as adverse effects. Various publications, both in print and electronic media, have emerged to help with maintaining pharmacologic information. Prominent among these innovations are applications for smart phones that can download information about all FDA-approved medications, including doses, contraindications, cautions, interactions, adverse reactions, cost, and pregnancy categorization. Of course, such resources are only useful when they are updated and consulted regularly.

A single agent is rarely a magic cure for a woman independent of the larger context of her health, social, educational, economic, and other factors. No professional should simply prescribe or recommend any pharmaceutical product without taking such considerations into account. Viewing the woman and her needs holistically is one of the skills of a great midwife. As an ancient Chinese saying states, "It is easy to get a thousand prescriptions, but hard to get one single remedy."

References

1. Osborne K. Regulation of prescriptive authority for certified nurse-midwives and certified midwives: a national overview. *J Midwifery Women's Health.* 2011;56(6):543-557.

2. Institute of Health Care Informatics. The use of medicines in the United States: review of 2010. Available at: http://www.imshealth.com/imshealth/Global/Content/IMS%20Institute/Documents/IHII_UseOfMed_report%20.pdf. Accessed September 8, 2012.

3. Dieringer NJ, Kukkamma L, Somes GW, Shorr RI. Self-reported responsiveness to direct-to-consumer advertising and medication use: results of a national survey. *BMC Health Serv Res.* 2001;11(1):232.

4. Quackenbush R, Hackley B, Dixon J. Screening for pesticide exposure: a case study. *J Midwifery Women's Health.* 2006;51(1):3-11.

5. Title 21 Food and Drug Regulations enforcement policy. Available at: http://www.accessdata.fda.gov/scripts/cdrh/cfdocs/cfcfr/CFRSearch.cfm?fr=7.3. Accessed September 8, 2012.

6. Brucker MC. Modern pharmacology. In: King TL, Brucker MC, eds. *Pharmacology for Women's Health.* Sudbury, MA: Jones and Bartlett; 2011:3-23.

7. Parekh A, Fadiran EO, Uhl K, Throckmorton DC. Adverse effects in women: implications for drug development and regulatory policies. *Expert Rev Clin Pharmacol.* 2011;4(4):453-466.

8. Frederickson M. The drug development process and the pregnant woman. *J Midwifery Women's Health.* 2002;47(6):422-425.

9. Chong YY, Arulkumaran K. Misoprostol: a quarter century of use, abuse and creative misuse. *Obstet Gynecol Surv.* 2004;59(2):128-140.

10. U.S. Department of Justice, Drug and Enforcement Administration, Office of Diversion Control. Mid-level practitioners authorization by state. Available at: http://www.deadiversion.usdoj.gov/drugreg/practioners/index.html. Accessed January 10, 2012.

11. Tharpe N. Adverse drug reactions in women's health care. *J Midwifery Women's Health.* 2011;56(3):205-214.

12. Tache SV, Sonnichsen A, Ashcrofft DM. Prevalence of adverse drug events in ambulatory care: a systematic review. *Ann Pharmacother.* 2011;45(7-8):977-989.

13. Bruggemann RJM, Alffenaar JW, Blijlevens NMA, et al. Clinical relevance of the pharmacokinetic interactions with azol antifungal drugs and other coadministered agents. *Rev Anti-infect Agents.* 2009;48:1441-1446.

14. Zhou SF. Polymorphism of human cytochrome P450 2D6 and its clinical significance. *Clin Pharmacokinetics.* 2009;48(11):689-723.

15. Zhou SF, Liu JP, Chowbay B. Polymorphism of human cytochrome P450 enzymes and its clinical import. *Drug Metabol Rev.* 2009;41(2):89-295.

16. Enright MC, Robinson DA, Randle G, et al. The evolutionary history of methicillin resistant *Staphylococcus aureus* (MRSA). *Proc Natl Acad Sci USA.* 2002;99(11):7687-7692.

17. Drawz SM, Bonomo RA. Three decades of beta-lactamase inhibitors. *Clin Microbiol Rev.* 2010;23(1):160-201.

18. King TL, Mitchell AM, Lannen BJ, Daly M. Anti-infectives. In: King TL, Brucker MC. *Pharmacology for Women's Health.* Sudbury, MA: Jones and Bartlett; 2011:284-286.

19. Hooper D. Emerging mechanisms of fluoroquinolone resistance. *Emerging Infect Dis.* 2001;7(2):337-341.

20. Roe V. Antibiotic resistance: a guide for effective prescribing in women's health. *J Midwifery Women's Health.* 2008;53:216-226.

21. Hoffman FA. Regulation of dietary supplements in the United States: understanding the Dietary Supplement Health and Education Act. *Clin Obstet Gynecol.* 2001;44(4):780-788.

22. Marty AT. The complete German Commission E Monographs. *JAMA.* 1999;281(19):1952.

23. Blumenthal M, Busse W, Goldberg A, et al., eds.; Klein S, Rister R, trans. *Complete German Commission E Monographs: Therapeutic Guide to Herbal Medicines.* Newton, MA: Integrative Medicine Communications; 1998.

24. Munir M, Enany N, Zhang JM. Nonopioid analgesics. *Med Clin North Am.* 2007;91:97-111.

25. Khan MI, Walsh D, Brito-Dellan N. Opioid and adjuvant analgesics: compared and contrasted. *Am J Hosp Palliat Care.* 2011;28(5):378-383.

26. Lowe N, King TL. Labor. In: King TL, Brucker MC, eds. *Pharmacology for Women's Health.* Sudbury, MA: Jones and Bartlett; 2011:1109.

27. van der Bijl P, van der Bijl P Jr. Efficacy, safety and potential clinical roles of the COX-2-specific inhibitors. *Int J Immunopathol Pharmacol.* 2003;16(2 suppl):17-22.

28. Wolfe MM, Lichtenstein DR, Singh G. Gastrointestinal toxicity of nonsteroidal antiinflammatory drugs. *N Engl J Med.* 1999;340:1888-1900.

29. Manns-James L. Pregnancy. In: King TL, Brucker MC, eds. *Pharmacology for Women's Health.* Sudbury, MA: Jones and Bartlett; 2011:1050.

30. Anderson D. A review of systemic opioids commonly used for labor pain relief. *J Midwifery Women's Health.* 2011;56(3):222-239.

31. Craft RM. Sex differences in opioid analgesia: "from mouse to man." *Clin J Pain.* 2003;19:175-186.

32. Sandner-Kiesling A, Eisenach JC. Estrogen reduces efficacy of mu but not kappa-opioid agonist inhibition in response to uterine cervical distention. *Anesthesiology.* 2000;96:375-380.

33. Arnold SR, Straus SE. Interventions to improve antibiotic prescribing practices in ambulatory care. *Cochrane Database System Rev.* 2005;4:CD003539. doi: 10.1002/14651858.CD003539.pub2.

34. Waller DG. Rational prescribing: the principles of drug selection and assessment of efficacy. *Clin Med.* 2005;1(5):26-28.

35. Simons FE, Simons KJ. Histamine and H(1)-antihistamines: celebrating a century of progress. *J Allergy Clin Immunol.* 2011;128(6):1139-1150.

36. Briggs GG. Drug effects on the fetus and breast-fed infant. *Clin Obstet Gynecol.* 2002;45(1):6-21.

37. Syme MR, Paxton JW, Keelan JA. Drug transfer and metabolism by the human placenta. *Clin Pharmacokin.* 2004;43(8):487-514.

38. Wen SW, Yang T, Krewski D, et al. Patterns of pregnancy exposure to prescription FDA C, D and X drugs in a Canadian population. *J Perinatol.* 2008;28:324-329.

39. Hansen WF, Yankowitz J. Pharmacologic therapy for medical disorders during pregnancy. *Clin Obstet Gynecol.* 2002;45(1):13-52.

40. Buhimschi CS, Weiner CP. Medications in pregnancy and lactation: part 1. Teratology. *Obstet Gynecol.* 2009;113(1):166-188. Review. Erratum in: *Obstet Gynecol.* 2009;113(6):1377.

41. Koren G. Fetal risks of maternal pharmacotherapy: identifying signals. *Handb Exp Pharmacol.* 2011;205:285-294.

42. Pregnancy labeling. *FDA Drug Bull.* 1979;9:23-24.

43. Law R. FDA pregnancy risk categories and the CPS: mother risk update. *Can Fam Phys.* 2010;56:239-241.

45. Hansen W, Peacock A, Yankowitz J. Treatment of illnesses in pregnancy and lactation. *J Midwifery Women's Health.* 2002;47(6):409-421.

46. Content and format of labeling for human prescription drug and biological products: requirements for pregnancy and lactation labeling. *Federal Register.* 2008;73(104):30831-30832.

47. Lee E, Maneno MK, Smith L, et al. National patterns of medication use during pregnancy. *Pharmacoepidemiol Drug Safety.* 2006;15:537-545.

48. Skerret PJ, Willett WC. Essentials of health eating: a guide. *J Midwifery Women's Health.* 2010;55(6):492-501.

49. Czeizel AE, Banhidy F. Vitamin supply in pregnancy for prevention of congenital birth defects. *Curr Opin Clin Nutrition Metabolic Care.* 2011;14:291-296.

50. Gill SK, Maltepe C, Koren G. The effectiveness of discontinuing iron-containing prenatal multivitamins on reducing the severity of nausea and vomiting of pregnancy. *J Obstet Gynaecol*. 2009;29(1):13-16.

51. Barger MA. Maternal nutrition and perinatal outcomes. *J Midwifery Women's Health*. 2010;55(6):502-511.

52. Kaludjerovic J, Veith R. Relationship between vitamin D during perinatal development and health. *J Midwifery Women's Health*. 2010;55(6):550-560

53. Jordan RG. Prenatal omega-3 fatty acids: review and recommendations. *J Midwifery Women's Health*. 2010;55(6):520-528.

54. Haider BA, Bhutta ZA. Multiple-micronutrient supplementation for women during pregnancy. *Cochrane Database System Rev*. 2006;4:CD004905. doi: 10.1002/14651858.CD004905.pub2.

55. *Standing Committee on the Scientific Evaluation of Dietary Reference Intakes, Food and Nutrition Board, Institute of Medicine. Dietary Reference Intakes: Folate, Other B Vitamins, and Choline. Washington, DC: National Academy Press; April 17, 1998*. Available at: http://www.nap.edu/openbook.php?record_id=6015&page=196. Accessed January 1, 2010.

56. Wolff T, Witkop CT, Miller T, Syed SB. *Folic Acid Supplementation for the Prevention of Neural Tube Defects: An Update of the Evidence for the U.S. Preventive Services Task Force*. Evidence Synthesis No. 70. AHRQ Publication No. 09-051132-EF-1. Rockville, MD: Agency for Healthcare Research and Quality; May 2009.

57. Centers for Disease Control and Prevention. Recommendations to prevent and control iron deficiency in the United States. *MMWR*. 1998;47:1-29.

58. Pena-Rosas JP, Viteri FE. Effects of routine oral iron supplementation with or without folic acid for women during pregnancy. *Cochrane Database System Rev*. 2006;3:CD004736. doi: 10.1002/14651858.CD004736.pub2.

59. Graves BW, Barger MK. A "conservative" approach to iron supplementation during pregnancy. *J Midwifery Women's Health*. 2001;46:159-166.

60. Public Health Committee of the American Thyroid Association; Becker DV, Braverman LE, Delange F, et al. Iodine supplementation for pregnancy and lactation-United States and Canada: recommendations of the American Thyroid Association. *Thyroid*. 2006;16(10):949-951.

61. Leung AM, Pearce EN, Braverman LE. Iodine nutrition in pregnancy and lactation. *Endocrin Metabol Clin*. 2011;40(4):765-777.

62. Rothman K, More L, Singer J, et al. Teratogenicity of high vitamin A intake. *N Engl J Med*. 1995;333(21):1369-1373.

63. Piper JM, Mitchel EF, Ray WA. Prenatal use of metronidazole and birth defects: no association. *Obstet Gynecol*.1993;82(3):348-352.

64. Buhimschi CS, Weiner CP. Medications in pregnancy and lactation: part 2. Drugs with minimal or unknown human teratogenic effect. *Obstet Gynecol*. 2009;113(2 Pt 1):417-432.

65. Ozyuncu O, Beksac MH, Nemutlu E, et al. Maternal blood and amniotic fluid levels of moxifloxacin, levofloxacin, and cefixime. *J Obstet Gynecol Res*. 2010;36(3):484-487.

66. Lowe SA. Anticonvulsants and drugs for neurological disease. *Best Pract Res Clin Obstet Gynecol*. 2001;15(6):863-876.

67. Banach R, Boskovic R, Einarson T, Koren G. Long-term developmental outcome of children of women with epilepsy, unexposed or exposed prenatally to antiepileptic drugs: a meta-analysis of cohort studies. *Drug Safety*. 2010;33(1):73-79.

68. Molgaard-Nielsen D, Hviid A. Newer-generation antiepileptic drugs and the risk of major birth defects. *JAMA*. 2011;305(19):1996-2002.

69. Hernandez-Diaz S, Werler M, Walker A, Mitchell A. Folic acid antagonists during pregnancy and risk of birth defects. *N Engl J Med*. 2000;343(22):1608-1614.

70. Hackley B, Sharma C, Kedzior A, Sreenivasan S. Managing mental health conditions in primary care. *J Midwifery Women's Health*. 2010;55(1):9-19.

71. Hackley B. Antidepressant medication use in pregnancy. *J Midwifery Women's Health*. 2010;55:90-100.

72. Yonkers KA, Wisner KL, Stewart DE, et al. The management of depression during pregnancy: a report from the American Psychiatric Association and the American College of Obstetricians and Gynecologists. *J Obstet Gynecol*. 2009;114(3):703-713.

73. American College of Obstetricians and Gynecologists. Thyroid disease in pregnancy. ACOG Practice Bulletin. No. 37. *Obstet Gynecol*. 2002;100:387-396.

74. Negro R, Mestman JH. Thyroid disease in pregnancy. *Best Pract Res Clin Endocrinol Metabol*. 2011;25(6):927-943.

75. Seely EW, Ecker J. Chronic hypertension in pregnancy. *N Engl J Med*. 2011;365:439-446.

76. American College of Obstetricians and Gynecologists. Inherited thrombophilias in pregnancy. Practice Bulletin No. 124. *Obstet Gynecol*. 2011;118:730-740.

77. Reedy NJ. Addressing the epidemic: pharmacotherapeutic management of diabetes in women. *J Midwifery Women's Health*. 2002;47(6):471-486.

78. Langer O. Management of gestational diabetes: pharmacologic treatment options and glycemic control. *Encrin Metabol Clin North Am*. 2006;35:53-78.

79. Refuerzo JS. Oral hypoglycemic agents in pregnancy. *Obstet Clin North Am.* 2011;38:227-234.

80. Langer O, Conway D, Berkus M, et al. A comparison of glyburide and insulin in women with gestation diabetes mellitus. *N Engl J Med.* 2000;343(16): 1134-1138.

81. American College of Obstetricians and Gynecologists. Pregestational diabetes mellitus. ACOG Practice Bulletin No. 60. *Obstet Gynecol.* 2005;105:675-685.

82. Ito S. Drug therapy for breast-feeding women. *N Engl J Med.* 2000;343(2):118-121.

83. Hale TW. Breastfeeding mothers. In: King TL, Brucker MC, eds. *Pharmacology for Women's Health.* Sudbury, MA: Jones and Bartlett; 2011:1146.

84. Berlin CM, Briggs GG. Drugs and chemicals in human milk. *Semin Fetal Neonatal Med.* 2005;10:149-159.

85. American Academy of Pediatrics Committee on Drugs. The transfer of drugs and other chemicals into human milk: policy statement. *Pediatrics.* 2001;108(3): 776-789.

86. Gabay MP. Galactogogues: medications that induce lactation. *J Hum Lact.* 2002;18:274-210.

CHAPTER

6

Nutrition

MARY K. BARGER

Nutrition and Health

Health and nutrition are intimately interrelated. Proper nutrition is essential to human growth, development, and well-being. Given that the average woman can expect to live until at least 80 years of age, women should be aware of the increasing evidence that a healthy diet can prevent diseases such as cardiovascular disease (CVD),[1] cancer, adult-onset diabetes, osteoporosis, and age-related vision loss. Measures to reduce this disease burden are relatively simple and well researched: maintaining a healthy weight; eating a well-balanced, nutritious diet; not smoking; and exercising regularly. Unfortunately, instead of adopting healthier diets and lifestyle choices, more than 36% of American women today are obese,[2] and women have decreased their fruit and vegetable intake and increased their moderate alcohol intake.[3]

For midwives to promote changes to counter these negative trends, good nutrition counseling should be incorporated into regular practice so that women can distinguish among the myriad sources of dietary advice. In addition, women need to understand some basic principles of nutrition, appreciate the physiologic response of the body to ingested food, and be familiar with current evidence-based dietary guidelines. This chapter notes that good nutrition is essential at all phases of life, including pregnancy, and that key principles remain the same for women whether they want to lose weight, to gain weight, or to maintain their weight. The basics of nutrition and how what is consumed affects normal physiology are discussed in this chapter. Although understanding individual components of the diet is important for health professionals, counseling women about diet should be positively focused on types of preferable foods to eat and the need to eat a variety of foods, rather than on individual macronutrients and micronutrients.

Principles of Nutrition and Nutrient Recommendations

Nutrients are the chemical components of food. Humans need more than 40 different nutrients for good health. These nutrients are classified as either macronutrients (fats, carbohydrates, and protein) or micronutrients (vitamins and minerals). Water is also a necessary nutrient, but it does not fit into either category. Macronutrients contain calories and are the energy-providing nutrients for the human body. Water, vitamins, and minerals provide no calories but are necessary, although not totally sufficient, for the body to be able to utilize the energy provided by fat, carbohydrates, and protein.

Vitamin and mineral pills have become increasingly popular today, and some women incorrectly think these agents can supply all needed nutrients. Ideally, humans should obtain both macronutrients and micronutrients from a diet composed of a variety of foods rather than from nutritional supplements. This diet must be balanced in a way that prevents nutritional deficiencies and excesses. Variety is essential both to guarantee proper intake of all necessary nutrients and to benefit from the protective effects of certain dietary components against diseases such as cancer and heart disease. Today's research suggests that decreased health risks associated with a good diet are due to combinations of substances in foods and food groups rather than to the effect of any single substance or nutrient.

Nomenclature for Nutritional Standards

Dietary guidelines in 2010 took the important step of recognizing that it is more important to emphasize the types of foods people should eat, rather than concentrating on the individual nutrient levels they should consume. However, labeling on packaged foods regarding the overall nutritive value of a product still can be useful. Therefore, it is important to be familiar with the nomenclature used by various U.S. governmental organizations for nutritional standard setting.

U.S. nutritional standards have two origins: the Institute of Medicine (IOM) Food and Nutrition Board[4] and the Food and Drug Administration (FDA).[5] The Food and Nutrition Board standards were originally developed during World War II as part of an effort to ensure adequate nutrition for members of the armed services. Since then, they have been used to set government policy related to food programs such as the School Lunch Program and food relief efforts globally. The FDA guidelines are more recent and are intended to assist consumers in obtaining recommended nutrients in their diets.

Box 6-1 compares the terms used by the IOM's Food and Nutrition Board and by the FDA.[4,5] An important characteristic of the Daily Reference Intakes (DRIs) is that they not only aim to determine minimum nutrient intake levels necessary to prevent nutritional deficiencies, but also strive to set standards to decrease the incidence of chronic diseases such as osteoporosis and cancer.

Most food labels are based on a "typical" daily 2000-calorie diet. However, the number of calories needed in a day depends on the individual's daily expenditure of calories. Several formulas are available to calculate how many calories an individual needs daily,[6] but clinicians may not have the time to make those calculations. Another option is to use an Internet-based website that calculates the number of calories needed to maintain or lose weight given specific gender, age, height, weight, and daily activity levels (see the list of additional resources at the end of this chapter). According to guidelines issued by the American Heart Association, nonobese women ages 19 to 30 years who are of average stature will need approximately 2000 calories per day to maintain their current weight if they do not engage in physical activity beyond activities of daily living such as work and walking to the bus (sedentary physical activity level). Women who are obese or very active will need more calories to maintain their current weight. Women who are older, or who are trying to lose weight, will require fewer calories.

However, all food is not the same, and calories, therefore, are simply one consideration within a diet. The sections that follow review macronutrients, micronutrients, and the physiologic response to ingested food.

Macronutrients

Fats

Fats are an important a source of energy, providing more calories per gram than either protein or carbohydrates. Fat provides energy at a rate of 9 kcal/g, compared to 4 kcal/g for protein and carbohydrates. Fats are composed of fatty acids and have various roles in the human body, including transport and digestion of the fat-soluble vitamins and components of cell structure. Stored body fat facilitates temperature regulation by serving as insulation and helps to protect vital organs by providing a cushioning effect. In addition, dietary fat intake increases the pleasure of eating and helps signal satiety during a meal.

Since the 1950s, the American Heart Association has urged Americans to eat less fat in their diets, particularly by eliminating cholesterol from red meat and eggs. This campaign has been successful in decreasing fat intake from 45% of total calories to 33%.[7] However, the percentage of calories consumed from fats is *not* linked to chronic diseases; instead, what matters is the *type* of fats consumed. The "fat is bad" campaign that caused people to replace fat calories with generally high glycemic (refined) carbohydrates has been shown to worsen serum lipoprotein levels and is one of the underlying causes of the current obesity and type 2 diabetes epidemic.[8]

Body Fats

Body fats should be distinguished from dietary fat. For example, the cholesterol (a fatlike substance present in all animal tissue) consumed in diet is different than the cholesterol in blood that is measured as part of a lipid panel. Dietary cholesterol is found in foods of animal origin such as meat and eggs, while blood cholesterol is a waxy, fatlike substance manufactured by the body and stored in the liver. Although there is a positive, albeit fairly weak, association between cholesterol dietary intake and actual serum cholesterol levels,[9] the relationship between the two is more complex. For example, eggs—a common source of cholesterol—also are rich in other nutrients that may counterbalance the cholesterol's detrimental effects on the cardiovascular system.

BOX 6-1 U.S. Nutritional Standards

FOOD AND NUTRITION BOARD, INSTITUTE OF MEDICINE

Dietary Reference Intakes (DRIs)

- DRIs not only aim to determine minimum nutrient intake levels necessary to prevent nutritional deficiencies, but also strive to set standards to decrease chronic diseases such as osteoporosis and cancer. This term has more or less supplanted RDAs.
- DRIs are a combination of RDAs and AIs.
- DRIs also specify tolerable upper intake level, recommended dietary allowances, estimated average requirement, and adequate intakes:

Tolerable Upper Intake Level (UL)

- The maximum level of daily nutrient intake that is unlikely to pose risks of adverse health effects to almost all of the individuals in the group for whom it is designed.

Recommended Dietary Allowances (RDAs)

- Developed and updated periodically.
- Set the recommended average intake over a 3- to 7-day period for each nutrient specified.
- Fewer than half of the more than 40 necessary nutrients have an established RDA.
- RDAs are set quite high in order to meet the needs of almost all (97% to 98%) of individuals in a group, so they may be too high for individual needs.

Estimated Average Requirement (EAR)

- The intake value that is estimated to meet the requirement defined by a specified indicator of adequacy in 50% of an age- and gender-specific group. At this level of intake, the remaining 50% of the specified group would not have their needs met.

Adequate Intakes (AIs)

- Used to develop a recommended intake when a scientific basis for establishing the EAR is lacking.

FOOD AND DRUG ADMINISTRATION

Daily Values (DVs) appear on FDA-regulated products.

- DVs are not meant to set levels of nutrients to be consumed every day, but rather to help determine how particular foods fit into an overall healthy diet.
- DVs are calculated based on a diet of 2000 calories (unless otherwise stated).
- DVs are calculated from two sources: daily reference values and reference daily intake.

Daily Reference Values (DRVs)

- Recommended proportions of protein, carbohydrate, and fat in the diet
- Recommended grams per 1000 calories of dietary fiber intake
- Recommended daily maximums for sodium and potassium

Reference Daily Intake (RDI)

- To ensure that the nutritional needs of all age groups are met, the RDI is calculated from the highest DRI for each nutrient.

Sources: Adapted from Food and Nutrition Board. *Dietary Reference Intakes (DRIs): Recommended Intakes for Individuals.* Washington, DC: National Academy of Sciences; 2004, updated 2011; Office of Nutrition, Labeling and Dietary Supplements. *Food Labeling Guide.* College Park, MD: Food and Drug Administration; 2009.

In addition, if someone substitutes an egg for breakfast with a high-glycemic food, such as a large muffin, then more harmful physiologic effects may occur (discussed later in this chapter).

The body uses blood cholesterol to make steroid hormones such as estrogen and progesterone, as described in the *Anatomy and Physiology of the Female Reproductive System* chapter. Blood cholesterol is also required for production of vitamin D and bile, as well as being an important component of cell membranes.

Several subtypes of cholesterol are found in the body, although the two primary ones are low-density lipoprotein (LDL) and high-density lipoprotein (HDL). LDL transports cholesterol out of the liver to other parts of the body. Cells attach to these particles and extract LDL or cholesterol. Excess amounts of LDL promote the production of fatty plaques on arterial walls, causing them to lose elasticity and narrow, resulting in arteriosclerosis. If a plaque breaks free, it may cause a cardiac event such as a heart attack or stroke. LDL often is characterized as "bad" or "lousy" cholesterol. Conversely, HDL carries excess cholesterol away from the arteries and back to the liver; thus it is known as "good" or "healthy" cholesterol. A high level of HDL appears to have a protective effect against coronary heart disease and heart attacks. Exercise is strongly associated with higher levels of HDL in the body and, therefore, with lower risk of cardiovascular disease. In women, unlike in men, the total cholesterol to HDL ratio may be more predictive of the risk for cardiovascular disease than the total cholesterol level.[10]

The latest dietary guidelines recommend keeping daily dietary intake of cholesterol to less than 300 mg per day, and state that serum HDL level should be higher than 35 mg/dL, with a level of 60 mg/dL being optimal. The goal for the total cholesterol to HDL ratio is 5:1, with 3.5:1 being the ideal.

Another way in which fats are transported through the blood to cells is in the form of triglycerides. Serum triglycerides are derived either from consumed fat, especially trans fats, or synthesized de novo by body fat or the liver. The amount of triglycerides synthesized de novo is positively correlated with the consumption of refined carbohydrates. Triglycerides store excess calories as fat and break down stored fat when a source of energy is needed, especially by the brain. Whether a high triglyceride level is an independent cause of heart disease remains controversial, because many individuals with high triglyceride levels also have high LDL and low HDL cholesterol levels, which are known risk factors for heart disease.[11] It does appear, however, that high triglyceride levels are more predictive of cardiovascular disease risk in women than in men and are a risk factor for developing type 2 diabetes, metabolic syndrome, and ischemic stroke in women.[11, 12]

It is recommended that the serum triglycerides remain below 150 mg/dL, although routine screening of triglyceride levels in women who are not at risk for cardiovascular disease is not recommended.[13]

The most recent data from the National Nutrition and Health Examination Survey (NHANES) reveal that serum levels of total cholesterol, LDL, and triglycerides declined and HDL levels increased between 1988 and 2010 in all population subgroups of women, even among those not taking lipid-lowering medications.[14]

Dietary Fats

Dietary fats are characterized by the chemical structure of their fatty acids. They are classified into four types: trans fats, saturated fats, polyunsaturated fats, and monounsaturated fats.

Trans fats Trans fats are produced when vegetable oils are heated in the presence of hydrogen gas and a catalyst, resulting in a partially hydrogenated oil. The advantages of such oils are that they become a solid when cool (easier for transport), they are more stable and unlikely to spoil (prolonged shelf-life), and they can be reheated without breaking down (ideal for making fried foods). Although trans fats are found in small amounts in beef and dairy fat, they are largely consumed from commercially made products. Trans fats are harmful because they elevate LDL cholesterol and lower HDL cholesterol; they also stimulate productions of prostaglandins and other eicosanoids that increase inflammation, platelet aggregation, and vasoconstriction. The combination of these effects results in an increased risk for cardiovascular disease, diabetes, gallstones, weight gain, and ovulatory infertility.[15] The Nurses' Health Study reported that for each 2% increase in calories from trans fats, the risk of coronary heart disease increases 23%.[16] Fortunately, recent publicity about the adverse health effects of trans fats and product labeling requirements have resulted in reformulation of many products to eliminate partially hydrogenated oils. Between 2003 and 2009, average trans fat intake decreased in the United States from 4.6 g/day to 1.3 g/day.[17]

Saturated Fats Saturated fats are derived from both animal and plant sources. These fats often are solid at room temperature and are found in highest amounts in meat fat, butter, whole-milk products, coconut oil, palm oil, and palm kernel oil. Consumption of these fats worsens serum lipoprotein profiles.

Unsaturated Fats As opposed to saturated fats, unsaturated fats have several beneficial roles in the body, including improving serum cholesterol levels, easing inflammation, and stabilizing heart rhythms. These fats are found primarily in vegetable oils, nuts, and seeds, and are liquid at room temperature.

Unsaturated fats are of two types: monounsaturated and polyunsaturated. Monounsaturated fats are found in high concentrations in olives, peanuts, oils such as canola oils, avocados, nuts such as almonds and pecans, and seeds such as pumpkin and sunflower seeds. Polyunsaturated fats are grouped into two types, distinguished by their chemical bonds: omega-6 (n-6) and omega-3 (n-3) fatty acids. Both n-6 and n-3 are considered "essential fatty acids" due to the body's limited ability to produce them and, thus, the need to obtain them from dietary sources. Omega-6 fatty (linoleic) acids are found in safflower, sunflower, corn, soybean, and flaxseed oils, as well as canola oils. Omega-3 fatty acids are found in oily fish such as salmon, mackerel, anchovies, and sardines; algae; and plant sources such as chia and flax seeds, walnuts, and oils such as soybean and canola.

The amount of n-3 fats in the American diet has decreased significantly since the 1950s. This is in part due to changes in the food chain. Today most meat comes from grain-fed animals; relatively speaking, grain-fed animals have less n-3 fats in their meat than grass-fed ones. The consumption of oily fish has also decreased over the same period of time, perhaps due to warnings about heavy metals in fish. Observational studies have shown that the incidence of heart disease mortality, stroke, and mood disorders appears to be correlated with differences in n-3 fat intake.[18] Results from supplementation trials with n-3 fats to prevent heart disease have been somewhat mixed, with some evidence suggesting that such supplements provide secondary prevention among those persons with heart disease, but have a limited effect for prevention of arrhythmias.[19]

In summary, the total amount of calories from fat is unimportant for cardiovascular and general health. What *is* important are the types of fats consumed. Trans fats should be eliminated from the diet as much as possible. Replacing saturated fats with monounsaturated and polyunsaturated fats will provide modest improvements in protection against heart disease. Consumers should be cautious about the foods they choose to substitute for trans fats and saturated fats, as some seemingly healthy alternatives are not necessarily healthier substitutes. Nevertheless, a good recommendation is to reduce consumption of red meat and whole-milk dairy products, increase intake of fish to at least two 6-ounce servings per week, and increase consumption of soy products, nonhydrogenated vegetable oils, and nuts. **Table 6-1** provides the distribution of daily-recommended values of macronutrients for women age 19–30 years, and **Table 6-2** shows the recommended DRIs for women.[4]

Carbohydrates

Carbohydrates, which can be found in grains, vegetables, fruits, and sugars, are the major dietary source of glucose, the body's essential energy for cellular metabolism. All carbohydrates except insoluble fibers are broken down by the body into the basic sugars and absorbed in the bloodstream. Glucose, galactose, and fructose can be used immediately by the body or can be stored in the liver or muscle tissue in the form of glycogen, which is then converted to glucose whenever there is a need for reserve energy.

In the past, carbohydrates have been described as simple or complex, with people being encouraged to eat more complex carbohydrates. However, there is no distinction in this recommendation between the different physiologic consequences that occur after eating different types of complex carbohydrates. Because the amount of insulin that is stimulated in

Table 6-1	Daily Values for Macronutrients for Women 19–30 Years Old	
	Percent Daily Calories [Actual Daily Amount]	
	FDA	**Institute of Medicine**
Fat	30%	20–35%
Saturated fat	< 10%	[ALAP]
Cholesterol	[< 300 mg]	[ALAP]
Trans fat	0	0
Carbohydrates	60%	45–65%
Dietary fiber	[25 g]	[28 g]
Protein	10%	10–35%

ALAP: as little as possible.

Sources: Data from Food and Nutrition Board. *Dietary Reference Intakes (DRIs): Recommended Intakes for Individuals.* Washington, DC: National Academy of Sciences; 2004, updated 2011; Office of Nutrition, Labeling and Dietary Supplements. *Food Labeling Guide.* College Park, MD: Food and Drug Administration; 2009.

Table 6-2	Daily Reference Intakes of Macronutrients for Women				
	Nonpregnant		Pregnancy		
	14–18 Years Old	Adults	Singleton	Multiple	Lactation
Carbohydrate, g	130	130	175	330	210
Fiber, g	26	21–25	28	28	29
Fat, g	ND	ND	ND	156	ND
Protein, g	46	46	71	175	71
Water, L	2.3	2.7	3.0	3.0	3.0

ND: not determined.

Sources: Data from Food and Nutrition Board. *Dietary Reference Intakes (DRIs): Recommended Intakes for Individuals.* Washington, DC: National Academy of Sciences; 2004, updated 2011; Goodnight W, Newman R. Optimal nutrition for improved twin pregnancy outcome. *Obstet Gynecol.* 2009;114(5):1121-1134.

response to carbohydrate intake is a key factor in the body's physiologic response, researchers have developed two measures to assess this response: the glycemic index and the glycemic load.[20]

Glycemic Index The glycemic index (GI) is a measure of the blood glucose response 2 hours after ingesting 50 grams of a food. This index is influenced by the amount of fiber and fat in the consumed food, both of which slow the absorption of the carbohydrate. Therefore, highly processed grains such as white bread, white rice, and semolina-flour pasta have a high index. For example, white rice's glycemic index is 89, compared to 48 for brown rice. Vegetables have a low index due to their fiber content and low natural sugar content; indeed, in some cases, it is hard to even measure their GI. For example, obtaining 50 grams of carbohydrate from broccoli requires ingesting 16 cups. Fruits, although naturally sweet, if consumed as the whole fruit, have a low GI due to the fruit's fiber; for example, an apple has an index of about 10. In general, low-glycemic foods have an index less than 55, whereas those with an index higher than 70 are considered high-glycemic foods.

Glycemic Load When compared to the glycemic index, a better measure of the amount of insulin stimulated by consumption of specific foods is the glycemic load (GL). The GL is calculated as the GI of the food multiplied by the amount consumed, expressed per 100 grams. A low GL is less than 10 and a high GL is higher than 20, with values in between being intermediate. For example, the GI for one cup of brown rice is 45 versus a GL of 18. The same amount of white rice would have a GI of 83 and a GL of 43. This is a typical example, in which

unprocessed grain products stimulate the production of less insulin than do processed foods such as white rice. The same is true for whole fruits as compared to consuming only the juice of the fruit. A person would need to consume 3 to 4 oranges to register the GL of just 8 ounces of orange juice. The GI for a variety of foods has been published[21] and may be obtained online from the University of Sydney in Australia. As discussed previously, ingestion of high-glycemic foods results in worsened lipoprotein profiles, more thrombotic activity, abnormal glucose metabolism, increased inflammation, and more cellular proliferation.

Fiber

Fiber is a type of complex carbohydrate composed of non-starch polysaccharides that cannot be digested by the enzymes in the small intestine. Fiber is characterized as either soluble or insoluble based on its solubility in water. Soluble fiber types include pectin found in fruits, beta-glucans found in oats and barley, and gums found in beans and cereals. Insoluble fiber types include cellulose found in leaves, root vegetables (e.g., beets and carrots), bran, and whole wheat; hemicellulose found in bran and whole grains; and lignin found in plant stems and leaves. The typical American diet is characterized by being low in dietary fiber. Fiber intake among adults in the United States averages approximately 16 grams, or only 60% of recommended amounts.[22] Research has revealed that dietary fiber is associated with a decreased risk of heart disease, most likely through lowering total cholesterol and LDL cholesterol levels, and with decreased risk of type 2 diabetes, diverticulitis, and constipation.[23]

The IOM and U.S. Department of Agriculture (USDA) recommend that carbohydrates compose 45% to 65% of daily caloric intake. Individuals should attempt to maximize their intake of low-glycemic foods rich in fiber, such as whole grains, vegetables, and fruits, and to minimize their intake of high-glycemic foods such as sweetened and energy drinks; refined grains such as white bread, white rice, and russet potatoes; and high-sugar snacks. A desirable intake of fiber for women is 20 to 28 grams per day.

Protein

Protein is the basic component of cells and is needed for cellular growth, replacement, and repair. Enzymes—the substances responsible for controlling the processes that keep the human body functioning smoothly—are composed of protein. Hormones, hemoglobin, and antibodies also are composed partially or entirely of protein. Protein, in turn, is composed of organic compounds known as amino acids. The different arrangements of amino acids into proteins determine the particular properties of each protein.

Approximately 20 amino acids exist that are necessary for human growth and metabolism. The body is able to produce the majority of these necessary amino acids. There are, however, approximately nine amino acids that must be provided by foods—the so-called essential amino acids. Foods of animal origin, such as meat, poultry, fish, eggs, and dairy products, provide all of these essential amino acids and are known as complete proteins. Proteins derived from plants, such as legumes, nuts, and grains, lack certain essential amino acids and, therefore, are termed incomplete proteins. However, a vegetarian diet can supply all of the essential amino acids as long as a variety of plant-based proteins are eaten throughout the day.[24]

Proteins cannot be stored in the body, so they must be consumed daily to avoid the body breaking down nonessential tissue, such as muscle, to supply proteins vital for survival. Recommended protein intake is 0.8 to 1.0 g/kg or 10% to 35% of calories. While protein intake deficiencies are common in the developing world, most persons in the United States consume adequate amounts of protein. The average intakes of women in the United States age 14 to 70 years range from 88 to 109 g/day.[25] No age group in the United States has been found to eat less than 10% of calories as protein, but the highest percentage of calories as protein was 21% among women older than age 70 years. The percentages of adolescents and women older than age 70 years with intakes less than the estimated average requirement were 7.7% and 8.2%, respectively.

The body does not distinguish between animal and plant sources of amino acids. However, protein food sources usually contain other nutrients, such as saturated fat. Evidence from the Nurses' Health Study suggests that substituting plant-based protein for high-glycemic carbohydrates can decrease a woman's risk for heart disease.[26] **Table 6-3** contains a list of foods rich in complete and incomplete proteins.[27]

Table 6-3	Examples of Sample Food Sources of Protein	
Food	**Quantity**	**Amount of Protein (grams)**
Complete Proteins		
Beef, chuck roasted	3 oz	26
Chicken, roasted	3 oz	27
Tuna, fresh	3 oz	25
Pork, center loin	3 oz	23
Beef, lean ground	3 oz	22
Tuna, canned	3 oz	20
Ham	3 oz	19
Chicken breast, deli-type slices	3 oz	17
Salmon	3 oz	17
Scallops	3 oz	17
Cottage cheese	½ cup	14
Eggs	2 large	13
Shrimp	3 oz	12
Yogurt	1 cup	8–12
Milk, any type	1 cup	8
Cheddar cheese	1 oz	7
Incomplete Proteins		
Lentils	1 cup, cooked	18
Beans, cooked (different types)	1 cup	12–15
Tofu, firm	½ c	10
Green peas	1 cup	9
Quinoa, cooked	1 cup	8
Peanut butter	2 Tbsp	8
Peanuts	1 oz	7
Egg noodles, cooked	1 cup	7
Brown rice, cooked	1 cup	5
White rice, cooked	1 cup	4
Bread, whole wheat	1 slice	4
Sunflower seeds	1 oz	4

Source: U.S. Department of Agriculture. USDA National Nutrient Database for Standard Reference, Release 25 online. 2012.

Body's Physiologic Response to Food Intake

Food is a hormonal stimulant more powerful than most drugs. Understanding this reality may be the impetus providers need to spend time with women assessing their diets and helping them to choose better foods. The body's response to food intake depends on the composition of both the macronutrients and the micronutrients ingested. With regard to prevention of inflammation and other processes that promote disease, especially chronic disease, the most important physiologic response to food intake is how much insulin is stimulated. Stimulation of insulin is a direct response to the amount and rate of glucose response from a meal. This glucose response can be measured by estimating the glycemic index of a meal.

Distinguishing high-glycemic meals from low-glycemic meals is important in understanding the body's physiologic response.[20] A high-glycemic meal creates a rapidly rising and high blood glucose response, which results in a similar insulin response. Subsequently, the blood glucose level falls more rapidly than the insulin level decreases, which results in high insulin levels and low glucose and suppression of glucagon. When this occurs, the body responds as if there is adequate glucose, so it suppresses free fatty acids, blocking the body's access to stored fat for energy. Low glucose levels also cause poor brain function, which stimulates the appetite, especially for a high-glycemic meal. After several more hours, to maintain a euglycemic state, skeletal muscles become insulin resistant, decreasing glucose uptake. In turn, free fatty acids and cortisol are secreted to allow access to stored glucose from the liver. In addition, other inflammatory hormones are released, causing oxidative stress and potentially damage from the production of excessive free radicals. Over time, this cycle of increased levels of glucose, insulin, and free fatty acids damages pancreatic beta cells, potentially resulting in type 2 diabetes, as well as affecting other processes associated with a variety of conditions including cardiovascular disease, cancer, neural tube defects, and gallbladder disease.[28]

Eating a diet rich in carbohydrates from whole grains, beans, fruits, and vegetables results in a much more modulated glucose response, in which insulin levels follow but never exceed glucose levels. Therefore, the result is appropriate glucagon stimulation. Over time, as glucose levels decline, stored fat then is available as an alternative energy source until the next meal.

The metabolism of fatty acids results in another important set of physiologic responses. This metabolism leads to the formation of different types of eicosanoids. Eicosanoids are short-acting, powerful, locally acting hormones that aid intracellular communication and regulate cyclic adenosine monophosphate (cAMP), which is needed for peptide hormones to exert their effects in cells. The first identified eicosanoid was prostaglandin, but midwives will recognize other eicosanoids such as prostaglandin E_2, prostaglandin F_2-alpha, and thromboxane, which exist endogenously. These specific agents can dampen cAMP activity as well as exert a pro-inflammatory effect, increase platelet aggregation and cellular proliferation, and cause vasoconstriction. Conversely, the hormones that increase cAMP (e.g., prostacyclin, PGE_1) have the opposite effects. The body needs all of these substances for self-regulation and appropriate functioning. With regard to nutrition, the type of eicosanoid produced, either pro-inflammatory or anti-inflammatory, is influenced by such factors as the presence of insulin, glucagon, omega-3 fatty acids, and trans fats. In brief, the quality of human nutrition encompasses not only the type of food that is consumed, but also the physiologic and chemical responses to it, as well as the presence of viruses and stress.

Micronutrients

Metabolism and use of macronutrients by the body require a host of enzymatic and hormonal processes that are also influenced by the necessary presence of micronutrients—specifically, vitamins and minerals, which for the most part cannot be synthesized by the body.

Vitamins and Minerals

Vitamins are organic substances used by the body as catalysts for intracellular metabolic reactions, whereas minerals are inorganic substances. Vitamins are either fat soluble or water soluble. Both vitamins and minerals are important for healthy bodily functioning. A few of these micronutrients will be highlighted here because they play a special role in women's health or because women in the United States are likely to be deficient in them. Issues related to vitamins and minerals in pregnancy are discussed in the "Nutrition in Pregnancy" section. **Table 6-4** lists the recommended intakes for selected vitamins and minerals in women age 14 to 70 years, the requirements in pregnancy and lactation, and common food sources of these nutrients.

Table 6-4	Recommended Daily Reference Intakes of Vitamins and Micronutrients in Women					
	Nonpregnant Women					
Vitamin/Mineral	**14–18 Years**	**19–50 Years**	**51–70 Years**	**Pregnancy**	**Lactation**	**Dietary Source**
Vitamin A, mcg	700	700	700	770	1200	Yellow/orange vegetables and fruits
Vitamin C, mg	65	75	75	85	120	Citrus fruits
Vitamin D, IU	600	600	600	600–4000*	600–4000*	Fortified dairy
Vitamin E, mg	15	15	15	15	19	Nuts, vegetable oils
Thiamin, mg	1.1	1.1	1.1	1.4	1.4	Pork, enriched grain
Riboflavin, mg	1.1	1.1	1.1	1.4	1.4	Meat, enriched grain
Niacin, mg	14	14	14	18	17	Meat, nuts, legumes
Vitamin B_6, mg	1.2	1.3	1.5	1.9	2.0	Chicken, fish, enriched grains
Folate, mcg	400	400	400	600	500	Leafy vegetables, liver, fortified cereal
Vitamin B_{12}, mcg	2.4	2.4	2.4	2.6	2.8	Animal-based food
Calcium, mg	1300	1000	1200	1300	1300	Dairy
Magnesium, mg	360	320	320	350–360	310–320	Seafood, legumes, grains
Phosphorus, mg	1250	700	700	700	700	Meat
Potassium, g	4.4	4.7	4.7	4.7	5.1	Apricots, figs, nuts, soy, wheat germ
Iodine, mcg	150	150	150	220	290	Iodized salt, seafood
Iron, mg	15	18	8	27	9	Meat, eggs
Choline, mg	400	425	425	450	550	Eggs
Zinc, mg	9	8	8	11	12	Egg yolk, liver, oysters

*Lower values: Institute of Medicine; higher values: Hollis, Wagner.

Sources: Food and Nutrition Board, Institute of Medicine. *Dietary reference intakes (DRIs): Recommended Intakes for Individuals.* Washington, DC: National Academy of Sciences; 2004, updated 2011; Hollis BW, Wagner CL. Vitamin D and pregnancy: skeletal effects, nonskeletal effects, and birth outcomes. *Calcif Tissue Int.* 2013;92(2):128-139.

Vitamins

Fat-Soluble Vitamins

Water-soluble vitamins are excreted from the body and are not stored, whereas fat-soluble vitamins are stored in body fat and, therefore, large doses of these vitamins can have potentially dangerous effects. For example, accumulation of vitamin A, which occurs when this nutrient is ingested as retinol, can result in liver toxicity, visual problems, and increased risk for hip fractures.

Vitamin A is important for vision (especially night vision), a healthy immune system, and cell growth. It is not typically deficient in the U.S. population, but it may be an important nutrient to attend to if working in low-resource countries.

Vitamin D promotes absorption of calcium and phosphate and helps deposit these minerals in teeth and bones, but also plays a role in health beyond bone formation and is involved with regulation of blood pressure, glucose regulation, and modulation of the immune system due to the fact that most body tissues have vitamin D receptors. Vitamin D is a not a true vitamin, as humans synthesize D_3 when the skin is exposed to ultraviolet sunlight. Vitamin D_3

synthesis from sunlight is affected by intensity of sunlight, especially related to latitude and season; the presence of air pollution; and factors that limit the skin's absorptive ability, such as amount of pigmentation, presence of sunscreens, and increasing age. Oily fish and fish liver oils are other sources of vitamin D_3, although absorption is decreased in individuals with intestinal malabsorptive conditions. Vitamin D_2—another form of vitamin D—is derived from plant sterols such as those found in mushrooms. Vitamin D is also consumed through fortified dairy products. Both D_3 and D_2 are inactive forms that require metabolism in the liver to convert the vitamin D to 25(OH)D, the form most commonly used to assess a person's vitamin D levels, followed by metabolism in the kidney to convert it to $1,25(OH)_2D$, the physiologic active form.

Vitamin D deficiency has historically been defined as a serum 25(OH)D concentration less than 10 ng/mL (25 nmol/L), which is the level at which rickets or myopathy develops. In adults, however, low vitamin D can lead to secondary hyperparathyroidism, bone loss, and osteoporosis; thus deficient levels for all populations have been defined at higher levels. Recently the IOM's Food and Nutrition Board conducted a review of vitamin D and its role in health and disease and concluded that the existing evidence was only strong enough to set standards based on bone health outcomes, as there were no randomized studies on other outcomes. Therefore, this organization redefined vitamin D deficiency as concentrations ranging from 30 ng/mL to 20 ng/mL (50 nmol), on the grounds that levels higher than 20 ng/mL are adequate for bone health; at the same time, the IOM increased recommended intakes to 600–800 IU and doubled the upper tolerable level to 4000 IU.[29] Adults who are obese or who take anticonvulsants, glucocorticoids, some antifungals, or AIDS drugs, or who have inflammatory bowel disease or gastric bypass surgery, may require two to three times this dose to achieve healthy levels.[30]

Three facts are important to note in relation to these guidelines. First, modest sun exposure results in a dose of 10,000 to 20,000 IU of vitamin D. Second, the original study that implied toxicity from vitamin D at these lower doses is now considered to be invalid.[31] Lastly, the IOM's assertion that vitamin D deficiency is not prevalent in the U.S. population is not consistent with national data. The Endocrine Society has disagreed with the IOM definition of deficiency and argues that healthy vitamin D levels should remain at or above 30 ng/mL and the upper tolerable level should be 10,000 IU.[30] The Endocrine Society has acknowledged that adults may need to consume 1500–2000 IU daily, double the IOM recommendation, to achieve these levels.[30]

Despite the current controversy about precisely which serum values represent vitamin D deficiency—vitamin D 25(OH)D levels of less than 20 ng/mL (50 nmol) versus less than 30 ng/mL (80 nmol)—there is no question that vitamin D deficiency is prevalent in all ethnic groups of American women. Non-Hispanic black women and Mexican women have particularly low average levels—11 ng/mL and 18.8 ng/mL, respectively.[32]

Water-Soluble Vitamins

Among the water-soluble B vitamins, folic acid (vitamin B_9) has a great import for childbearing women due its role in preventing neural tube defects, which will be discussed in the pregnancy section of this chapter. Folate is essential for RNA and DNA synthesis. Observational studies have found high folate levels to be associated with lower rates of cancer (especially intestinal cancer), cardiovascular disease, and dementia. Supplementation with folate and other B vitamins has proved effective in lowering homocysteine levels, which are associated with cardiovascular disease. However, randomized trials of fairly large populations have not found that vitamin B supplements have decreased the incidence of any of these conditions. Nevertheless, folate deficiency is clearly associated with megaloblastic anemia. Women at risk for megaloblastic anemia include those with poor diets, alcoholics, and those who have malabsorptive disorders or take medications that act as folic acid antagonists (e.g., anticonvulsants, sulfasalazine [Azulfidine]).

Folate is found in liver and leafy greens such as spinach, but the primary dietary source of this micronutrient in the United States is fortified cereal and multivitamin supplements. Folate status can be assessed by either serum folate or RBC folate tests, although the latter is a better indicator of tissue levels or long-term status.

Low and high cut-offs for adequate levels in women are defined as 3 ng/mL (10 nmol/L) and 220 ng/mL (340 nmol/L), respectively. In general, the U.S. population is not folate deficient. Since food fortification began in the mid-1990s, the percentage of the population that is folate deficient in all age and ethnic groups is 1% or less.[33] Although there is little risk of toxicity from high folic acid intake, concern has arisen that consumption of excess amounts could exacerbate the anemia and cognitive symptoms associated with vitamin B_{12} deficiency. Therefore, folic acid supplements of 1 mg or more require a provider prescription.

In summary, most women in the United States have adequate intakes of vitamins, with the exception of vitamin D and, in some subpopulations, folate or vitamin B$_{12}$ (e.g., in the elderly). Nutrition scientists have been learning more about the roles that vitamins play in health beyond the basic understanding achieved in the twentieth century. Randomized trials on the use of vitamin supplements as means to prevent chronic disease have yielded disappointing results, but it may be that, without addressing the content of the entire diet, vitamin supplementation is not powerful enough to overcome the physiologic effects of types and amounts of macronutrients in the diet.

Minerals

Calcium

Calcium is essential not only for healthy bone and teeth formation, but also for nerve conduction, muscle contraction, and blood clotting. Because more than 30% of women in the United States older than the age of 50 years are at risk for bone fracture due to osteoporosis,[34] maximizing peak bone mass through adolescence and early adulthood is essential. Unfortunately, adolescent girls have the lowest total intakes of calcium, 918 mg ± 30 mg, with only 13% to 15% meeting the daily requirement of 1300 mg from both diet and supplements.[35] In addition to calcium's role in building bone mass during adolescence and early adulthood, it is important that women obtain adequate amounts of calcium throughout the lifecycle in order to maintain bone mass. Many older women meet their calcium needs by taking a daily supplement or calcium carbonate antacids. **Table 6-5** lists common food sources of calcium.

Iodine

Iodine is essential for normal thyroid function, and deficiency of this mineral can lead to an enlargement of the thyroid gland known as goiter. Dietary iodine is obtained primarily from iodized salt, fish, and seaweed. From the late 1970s to 2000, iodine levels in the U.S. population declined by 50%, probably due to a combination of decreased salt and fish intake, though levels have since stabilized.[36] It should be noted that the currently popular exotic salts, such as Fleur de Sel and pink salt, are not iodized. The recommended daily intake of iodine is 150 mcg, which would result in a urinary iodine level of 100 mcg/L. The most recent data show that, in general, the U.S. population obtains sufficient iodine, but 34% of childbearing-age women have urinary iodine levels below this threshold, with the highest proportion of such deficiency occurring among non-Hispanic blacks.[36]

Iron

The most common deficiency globally, especially in women, is iron deficiency. Iron is essential to the production of hemoglobin and, therefore, for the transport of oxygen. Eighty percent of the body's iron is found in red blood cells, where it can be measured as hemoglobin. Iron not in red blood cells is stored as ferritin; transferrin is a protein needed for this stored iron to be transported. Nonpregnant women are at risk of anemia because of iron loss during menstruation, coupled with inadequate iron intake or decreased iron stores associated with close spacing of pregnancies. Special populations of women at higher risk for iron-deficiency anemia include those with malabsorption, such as women with inflammatory bowel disease and women who have undergone bariatric surgery. Slightly less than 1 mg of iron is lost daily from the intestine; iron loss is more than 1 mg among women with *Helicobacter pylori* infection, malaria, or with intestinal parasites.

Two forms of iron are found in food: heme and non-heme. Heme iron found in animal products is absorbed more efficiently than non-heme iron. For example, 20% to 30% of heme iron is absorbed, compared to 2% to 10% of non-heme iron. **Table 6-6** lists some common dietary sources of iron. Iron uptake also varies according to the need of a woman's body. If a woman has adequate iron stores, only approximately 10% of ingested iron is absorbed. In the presence of iron deficiency, however, up to 40% of ingested iron can be absorbed.[37]

Some foods or supplements can enhance or inhibit iron absorption, and these items should be discussed when counseling women. Iron uptake enhancers include animal muscle from meat, chicken, or seafood; foods containing vitamin C and, in populations deficient in vitamin A, vitamin A; and fermented vegetables and sauces (e.g., sauerkraut, kimchee, and soy sauce). Iron uptake inhibitors include foods containing phytates (e.g., whole grains, oats, bran, nuts, spinach), phenols (e.g., tea, especially green tea; coffee; cocoa; and red wine), calcium, and soy proteins. Iron absorption also is decreased in the presence of antacids. The presence of pica (persistent and compulsive eating of non-nutritive substances), including excessive consumption of ice, can be either a symptom of anemia or a contributing cause. Frequently, the correction of the anemia will eliminate the pica.

The development of anemia and loss of iron stores follows a progressive course. Adequacy of iron can be measured in several ways. The most commonly

Table 6-5 Examples of Sources of Calcium

	Serving Size	Calcium (mg)		Serving Size	Calcium (mg)
Dairy			**Fruits and Vegetables**		
Yogurt, fruit variety, nonfat	8 oz	345	Orange juice, calcium fortified	6 oz	200
Milk, calcium fortified	8 oz	400	Orange, navel	1	52
Milk, 1%	8 oz.	300	Raisins, seedless	2 oz	28
Lactaid milk	8 oz	300	Broccoli, steamed	½ cup	31
Cheese, American	1 oz	174	Collards, fresh cooked	1 cup	268
Cheese, cheddar	1 oz	204	Collards, frozen, boiled	½ cup	179
Cheese, mozzarella	1 oz	222	Spinach, fresh	1 cup	245
Cottage cheese, nonfat	8 oz	125	Spinach, chopped frozen	½ cup	145
Ice cream	8 oz	176	Kale, fresh, cooked	1 cup	94
Milk, nonfat dry powder	2 Tbsp	104	Mustard greens, fresh	1 cup	165
			Rhubarb, fresh diced	1 cup	105
Seafood			Blackstrap molasses	2 tsp	118
Clams, canned	3 oz	78			
Salmon, pink, canned	3 oz	240	**Nuts, Seeds, and Beans**		
Sardines, canned in oil	2 oz	216	Almonds	1 oz	76
Ocean perch	3 oz	29	Tahini (sesame paste)	1 Tbsp	64
Halibut, baked	3 oz	51	Beans, white, canned	1 cup	191
Shrimp (shelled)	3 oz	60	Beans, navy, canned	1 cup	123
Soy Products			**Cereal**		
Tofu, firm prepared with calcium sulfate	4 oz	253	Oatmeal, instant	1 packet	105
			All Bran (Kellogg)	½ cup	121
Tofu, soft	4 oz	150	Cheerios (General Mills)	1 cup	112
Soy milk	8 oz	300	Total (General Mills)	¾ cup	1000
			Tortilla, corn, 6 in.	1	45
Antacids			Bread, whole wheat	1 slice	30
Tums, regular	1	200			
Tums, extra strength	1	300			

Source: U.S. Department of Agriculture. USDA National Nutrient Database for Standard Reference, Release 25 online. 2012.

available measure is to assess characteristics of the red blood cells (RBCs) such as hemoglobin and to perform a peripheral smear to characterize the RBCs. Biochemical tests that measure earlier stages of iron depletion prior to actual deficiency are serum ferritin and transferrin saturation. The primary laboratory

and clinical findings with differing states of anemia are discussed in the *Prenatal Care* chapter. Although iron-deficiency anemia typically is represented by pale (hypochromic) and small (microcytic) RBCs, changes in RBC morphology occur relatively late in the process.[38]

Table 6-6	Examples of Dietary Sources of Iron	
	Serving Size	Iron (mg)
Breakfast cereals: varies by brand	1 cup	5–18
Prune juice	1 cup	10
Chicken liver	3 oz	8
Beef liver	3 oz	7
Cream of wheat	½ cup	7
Oysters	6	6
Sunflower seed kernels	2 oz	4
Prunes	10	4
Beans: lentils, kidney, garbanzo	2.3 cup	2–3
Beef	3 oz	3
Pork	3 oz	2
Sesame seeds	2 oz	2
Leafy green vegetables, cooked	1 cup	2
Molasses, blackstrap	1 Tbsp	2
Tortilla, wheat/corn, 6 in.	1	1.8/0.7
Chicken	3 oz	1
Plantains, cooked	1 cup	1
Peanut butter	2 Tbsp	0.6

Source: U.S. Department of Agriculture. USDA National Nutrient Database for Standard Reference, Release 25 online. 2012.

According to NHANES data, the overall prevalence of iron-deficiency anemia in U.S. women is 9% among nonpregnant women and twice that among pregnant women. However, this estimate is based on measures of iron stores, such as serum ferritin or transferrin saturation. If hemoglobin, the most widely available measurement method, is used to assess for iron-deficiency anemia, the incidence is lower, approximately 6%.[39] Differences in the use of vitamin supplements by race/ethnicity appear to account for the increased prevalence of anemia among blacks and Hispanics. Approximately 9% to 11% of premenopausal women have been found to be iron deficient.[40]

Women diagnosed with iron-deficiency anemia who increase their dietary consumption of iron-rich foods and avoid taking antacids 2 hours before or 4 hours after meals may be able to correct the problem nutritionally. The other option is iron supplementation. After the addition of 30 to 100 mg of elemental iron on a daily basis, an increase in the reticulocyte count should be noted within 2 weeks and an increase in the hemoglobin within 3 to 4 weeks. Ferrous salts are the first-line choice for oral iron supplementation for the treatment of iron deficiency anemia. Other types of iron supplements are not more effective, do not appear to have a lower side-effect profile, and their cost is approximately four times that of ferrous salts. Because a maximum amount of absorption is possible at one time, divided doses are preferable. Also, separating administration of iron from ingestion of a multivitamin can maximize absorption.

Side effects of iron therapy such as nausea, bloating, abdominal cramping, and constipation are proportional to the dose. Frequently women will discontinue therapy due to these side effects. Women should be counseled about the potential side effects and measures they can take to lessen them. An alternative to daily iron supplementation is taking 120 mg of elemental iron once or twice weekly. It is not recommended that women double their multivitamin supplement in an effort to obtain added iron, as this approach could result in excessive levels of fat-soluble vitamins.

Table 6-7 identifies types of iron supplements and the amounts of elemental iron in each dose. Enteric-coated and slow-release iron formulations are not recommended because iron is absorbed in the small intestine and these products provide iron that is excreted unabsorbed. A key safety issue is that iron supplements—particularly those prescribed prenatally—are the leading cause of childhood poisoning.[41] All women should be cautioned to keep their medications out of the reach of children.

Ideally, these micronutrients should be obtained through intake of a variety of fruits and vegetables each day—at a minimum, five servings per day—and exposure to adequate sunlight. Use of supplements is not a substitute for a healthy diet. While noting that there is little harm in taking a daily multivitamin supplement, the U.S. Preventive Services Task Force (USPSTF) does not currently recommend routine multivitamin/mineral supplementation for the general population for the prevention of chronic diseases such as cardiovascular disease.[42] However, this recommendation does not apply to populations at risk for deficiencies, including women who have undergone gastric bypass and those who have malabsorptive conditions or take medications that can result in lower absorption. Large doses of iron and of vitamins, particularly fat-soluble vitamins, can potentially be hazardous.

Table 6-7	Iron Supplements	
Iron (Fe) Group	**Generic Name (Brand)**	**Dose (Elemental Iron)**
Iron Salts		**(mg)**
Tablets	Iron sulfate (Feosol)	325 (60)
	Iron fumarate (Feostat, Hemocyte)	200 (66)
	Iron gluconate (Fergon)	300 (35)
Liquid	Iron sulfate elixir (Feosol Elixir)	220 (44) per 5 mL
		300 (60) per 5 mL
	Iron gluconate + herbs (Floridex or Floravit— gluten free)	(10) per 10 mL— higher absorption rate
Polysaccharide Iron/Carbonyl Iron		
Tablets	Carbonyl iron (Feosol caplets)	50 (45)
	Polysaccharide iron (Ferrex-150)	150 (150)
Liquid	Carbonyl iron elixir (Prexan)	60 (60) per 5 mL
	Polysaccharide iron elixir (Niferex Elixir)	100 (100) per 5 mL

Dietary Patterns

When discussing nutrition, a healthcare provider will probably be of most value to a woman by emphasizing healthier dietary patterns, which are relevant at any weight and are applicable throughout her life course. The word "diet" is often interpreted by many laypersons too narrowly—that is, to mean "a weight-loss diet"—it may be helpful, therefore, to use a less-familiar term such as "dietary pattern" with a woman when counseling women on nutrition

The Healthy Eating Pyramid developed by faculty in the Department of Nutrition at Harvard School of Public Health, which is based on current nutrition research, is a useful counseling and teaching tool. (**Figure 6-1**).[43] A woman can use the key principles embodied in this pyramid and outlined in **Box 6-2** to create a healthier dietary pattern.[8]

The dietary pattern promoted in the Healthy Eating Pyramid is similar to two other dietary patterns that have been associated with decreases in chronic diseases, especially cardiovascular disease: the Mediterranean diet and the DASH diet.[8] The Mediterranean diet emphasizes eating primarily

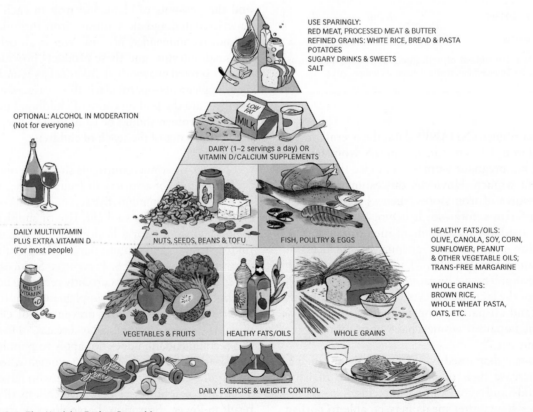

Figure 6-1 The Healthy Eating Pyramid.
Source: Copyright © 2008 Harvard University. For more information about The Healthy Eating Pyramid, please see The Nutrition Source, Department of Nutrition, Harvard School of Public Health, http://www.thenutrtionsource.org and *Eat, Drink, and Be Healthy*, by Walter C. Willett, M.D. and Patrick J. Skerrett (2005), Free Press/Simon & Schuster Inc.

> ### BOX 6-2 Key Principles in the Healthy Eating Pyramid
>
> 1. Choose healthy fats instead of unhealthy fats.
>   - Avoid trans fats; choose monounsaturated and polyunsaturated fats.
> 2. Choose slowly digested carbohydrates over highly refined ones.
>   - Emphasize whole fruits, vegetables, beans, and nuts.
>   - Choose whole grains such as brown rice, bulgur, barley, quinoa, and wheat berries.
> 3. Choose proteins that are plant based at least half of the time, and choose fish, eggs, and poultry the rest of the time, eating little red meat.
> 4. Eat large amounts of fruits and vegetables—a minimum of 5 servings per day.
> 5. Choose low-calorie hydration—water is best.
>   - Drink coffee and tea in moderation.
>   - If milk is part of the diet, choose low-fat types.
>   - Limit juice to one small glass per day.
>   - Avoid high-sugar drinks.
>   - Limit alcohol intake to one glass per day.
> 6. Meet daily recommendations for vitamins and minerals.
> 7. Get daily exercise—30 minutes of brisk walking daily.
>   - Calories expended are important to maintain a healthy weight.
>
> *Source:* Adapted from Skerrett PJ, Willett WC. Essentials of healthy eating: a guide. *J Midwifery Women's Health.* 2010;55(6):492-501.

vegetables, grains, beans, nuts, and seeds, with a serving of fish, poultry, or egg, and small amounts of cheese or yogurt, and obtaining 40% of calories from fats, primarily olive oil. Similarly, the DASH diet emphasizes 8 to 10 servings of fruits and vegetables per day and choosing low-fat/nonfat protein sources; it also limits salt consumption and limits fats to 27% of calories. The DASH diet places less emphasis on the type of fat, except to limit saturated fat to less than 7% of calories. A variant of the DASH diet is the OmniHeart (Optimal Macronutrient Intake Trial to Prevent Heart Disease) diet, which somewhat reduces carbohydrate intake relative to the DASH diet, compensating for the caloric loss either by substituting protein or by substituting unsaturated fat. The investigators who studied the OmniHeart diet documented further lowering of blood pressure, further

improved lipid levels, and further reduced cardiovascular risk compared to the already-healthier standard DASH diet.[44] Finally, the "portfolio" dietary pattern created by researchers at the University of Toronto is primarily a vegetarian diet that appears to reduce LDL levels, but without lowering HDL.[45]

The Healthy Eating Plate graphic[46] (**Figure 6-2**) is an easy method that a midwife can use with women during counseling when discussing their diet patterns and providing direction. Essentially, women can see that half their plate should be occupied by vegetables and fruits (minimum of 5 servings per day), one-quarter with whole grains, and one-quarter with protein, with the addition of a healthy unsaturated fat. It is also important not to ignore fluid intake, especially if it is a high-glycemic, high-calorie intake such as the empty calories found in carbonated beverages.

Weight Management Counseling and Dietary Patterns

Numerous morbidities are associated with obesity: metabolic disorders such as diabetes and polycystic ovarian syndrome, cardiovascular disease, osteoarthritis, and malignancies. Thus it would seem clear that midwives should assist women with obesity and other weight management issues. However, consistent weight management is a very challenging task for many individuals, and, over the years, it remains uncertain whether consistent client weight loss and weight maintenance can be achieved through the kind of low to moderate intensity counseling that a busy clinician can provide.[42] Put differently, while weight loss or maintaining a healthier weight may indeed be an important therapeutic goal, it is only possible when a clinician can provide a brief assessment, targeted conversation, and follow-up with written materials.

When a midwife has limited time, direct referral to a dietician or a specific weight management program may be most helpful. The midwife should seek interventions that are short, precisely targeted, easily administered, understandable to clients, and validated.

Assessment

Assessment customarily begins with a calculation of the woman's body mass index (BMI). Web-based BMI calculators can readily be found on the Internet, but the calculation involves only simple arithmetic and can be done by hand using the formula $BMI = [(\text{weight in pounds}) \div (\text{height in inches})^2] \times 703$ or $BMI = (\text{weight in kilograms}) \div (\text{height in meters})^2$.

For most individuals, including adolescents, a BMI in the "normal" range for their sex is associated

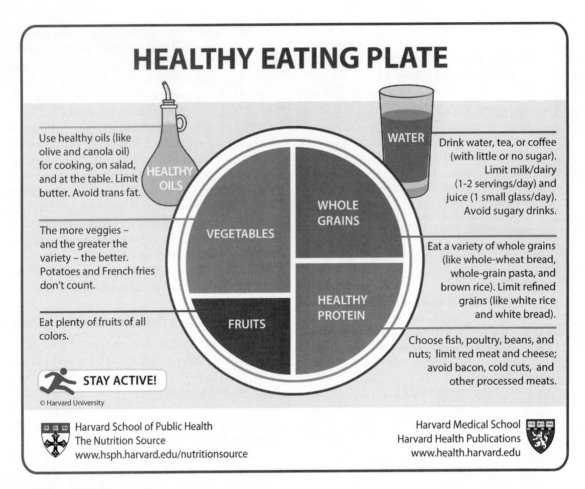

Figure 6-2 The Healthy Eating Plate.
Source: Copyright © 2011 Harvard University. For more information about The Healthy Eating Plate, please see The Nutrition Source, Department of Nutrition, Harvard School of Public Health, http://www.thenutrtionsource.org and Harvard Health Publications, health.harvard.edu.

with a reduced risk of obesity-related morbidities. However, BMI is not as accurate for postmenopausal women, who have typically lost some muscle mass and, therefore, might have a "normal" BMI but be at higher than normal risk. This assessment technique is also clearly inaccurate for body builders or elite athletes, who have much less body fat than average and, therefore, might have a "high" BMI but actually be at normal or even reduced risk. Waist circumference in women more than 35 inches (88 cm) has found to be an additional indicator of increased disease risk. Data reveal that an even better measure to identify persons at risk for cardiovascular disease and diabetes is a waist circumference-to-height ratio of more than 0.5.[47] For example, a waist measure of 37 inches and a height measurement of 65 inches would translate into a ratio of 0.57. The waist-to-height ratio identifies abdominal adiposity in the many different populations in which it has been tested, and the cut-off ratio of 0.5 is applicable in both men and women and in both young and old.

The ease, usefulness, and relative accuracy of the waist-to-height ratio argues strongly for making waist circumference measures a routine part of every health assessment exam.[47]

The 1988 weight management and treatment algorithm from the National Institutes of Health (NIH) and the National Heart, Lung, and Blood Institute (NHLBI), uses BMI as the decision indicator and is available on the Internet.[48] To summarize this algorithm, weight management counseling is not advised if a woman is only overweight but lacks any risk factors for diabetes or cardiovascular disease. However, if she has two risks factors for these and has a BMI higher than 25 or waist circumference larger than 35 inches, or if she has a BMI higher than 30, then she should be asked about her desire to lose weight. If she is ready to make a behavior change, then counseling should be undertaken by the provider. If diet and exercise do not result in weight loss, the clinician should assess the possible reasons for failure and reinforce positive behaviors.

If weight management may be helpful to the woman, the next step should be a brief assessment of her readiness to change. It may be helpful to conceive of the process of weight management as providing cues rather than providing cures. If and when a woman is receptive, she will receive and welcome a supportive and factual weight management conversation, and be able to consider strategies proposed by the midwife as cues to her own behavior and incorporate them into her life. If a woman is not ready to change, attempts to intervene from a healthcare professional will seem irrelevant, irritating, or even threatening to her as an advertisement for a product or behavior in which she has no interest.

Accordingly, a clinician seeing a woman who meets the NIH criteria for weight loss management might use few brief questions to obtain a general concept of where the woman is in her journey using the "stages of change" model. A sample question sequence that is supportive, brief, and factual for the stages of change model is found in **Box 6-3**.

Although it would be ideal to have women complete a 24-hour or 3-day food diary prior to their healthcare visit, and then have the time for the woman and midwife to analyze these data together for macronutrient and micronutrient content, the reality is that busy midwives do not have the time to do this. Another option is to routinely complete a "Starting the Conversation on Healthy Eating" questionnaire, which incorporates questions to assess readiness to change, along with seven questions to assess dietary patterns in all women being seen for an initial or annual visit. This questionnaire is found in **Figure 6-3**.[49] Three response categories exist for each question, and they are scored 0, 1, or 2, starting from left to right, culminating in a range of scores from 0 to 14. Higher scores indicate a poorer dietary pattern. The form includes practical suggestions for each question on how this aspect of eating can be improved. It also includes a section for making goals for changing if a woman is at that stage of change.

A more comprehensive and validated instrument is the easy-to-use "Rapid Eating Assessment for Patients" (REAP), which contains 31 questions. The accompanying "REAP Physician Key for Diet Assessment and Counseling" provides clear directions for further assessment, treatment, and counseling based on responses to each of the questions.[50,51]

All behavioral changes must be made by the woman herself, in a manner that she can freely accept and commit to. Weight is a delicate subject for many women, and repeatedly offering warm support rather than remedies builds trust. When specific plans and strategies seem relevant to discuss, offering

---

BOX 6-3 Sample Question Sequence for the "Stages of Change" Model

"There's no right or wrong answer to this question, but for me to better understand where you are right now, have you been thinking about losing weight?"

[In response to either yes or no] "That's fine." (That is, briefly give support).

[If yes] "Have you been thinking about a plan?"

[If yes] "Is this something you intend to do soon, like within the month, or is this more of a long-term goal?"

"Would you like me to be involved in this process with you, and be a support for you, no matter what happens?"

---

a woman cues to become more active in her weight management rather than imposing cures should be the goal. Cures are imposed; cues are freely accepted or freely put on hold. Finally, if the woman will be seeing the same healthcare provider again, this provider can offer continuing support. It is important for the midwife to take into account and be supportive of weight management failures as well as successes, as both may occur. Repeated, honest, and realistic offers of support "no matter what happens" can help build the needed trust.

While a weight-loss intervention can be part of the nutritional choices made by a woman for herself (in consultation with her healthcare provider), the more fundamental issue remains adopting one of the healthier dietary patterns discussed previously in this chapter. The healthiest and safest weight-loss "diets" usually involve following the same healthier dietary patterns that would be recommended for anyone, with the modification of eating smaller portions, in order to create a slight daily calorie deficit. This calorie deficit should vary with BMI. For women with a BMI in the range of 27–35 who are choosing a healthy weight-loss dietary pattern, it is recommended that they begin by decreasing their caloric intake by 300 to 500 kcal/day in conjunction with adopting or maintaining a healthy dietary pattern. For women with a BMI higher than 35, the recommended decrease in caloric intake is of 500 to 1000 kcal/day. Any weight-loss dietary pattern should not continue for greater than a 6-month period, after which a follow-up assessment with a midwife or

ARE YOU READY TO WORK ON **HEALTHY EATING** DURING YOUR PREGNANCY?
____ I'm ready to make some changes and I would like help
____ I'm not sure if I'm ready to change the way I eat but I would like to start the conversation
____ I'm not ready to change the way I eat at this time

HOW WELL DO YOU EAT?	TIPS TO HELP YOU EAT WELL
How many times a week do you eat food that is fried or high in fat? ☐ Less than 1 ☐ 1–3 ☐ 4 or more	**Eat less fast food.** • If you eat fast food, order grilled chicken, a salad or plain burger.
How many servings of fruit and vegetables do you eat each day? ☐ 5 or more ☐ 3–4 ☐ 2 or less	**Aim for 5 or more servings of fruits and vegetables a day.** • Add a fruit and a vegetable to each meal. • Raw fruits and vegetables are easy snacks.
How many regular sodas, juice or glasses of sweetened beverages do you drink each day? ☐ Less than 1 ☐ 1–2 ☐ 3 or more	**Beverage calories add up.** • Drink water throughout the day. • If you drink milk, switch from whole or 2% to 1% or skim. • Limit soda and other sweet drinks to one or less per day.
How many times a week do you eat beans (like pinto or black beans), chicken or fish? ☐ 3 or more ☐ 1–2 ☐ Less than 1	**Eat more beans, chicken and fish.** • Beans are a great substitute for meat. • Eat up to 12 oz. of low-mercury fish weekly like canned light tuna, salmon or pollock. • Eat baked, broiled, or grilled chicken and fish. • Avoid high mercury fish like shark, swordfish, king mackerel and tilefish.
How many times a week do you eat regular (not low-fat) snack chips or crackers? ☐ 1 or less ☐ 2–3 ☐ 4 or more	**Hold the chips.** • Try popcorn, but limit oil, butter or salt. • Try nuts such as almonds or walnuts, but limit your serving to 2 Tablespoons.
How many times a week do you eat desserts and other sweets? ☐ 1 or less ☐ 2–3 ☐ 4 or more	**Be smart with your sweet tooth.** • Eat smaller amounts of dessert. • Try desserts with less fat and calories like fruit, sherbet or angel food cake.
How many butter, lard and animal fat (visible fat in red meat, chicken skin) do you eat? ☐ Very little ☐ Some ☐ A lot	**Cut back on animal fats.** • Use a small amount of plant-based oils and transfat free margarines. • Season foods with spices and fresh herbs.

0 × (_____) +   1 × (_____) +   2 × (_____) = Total Score _____

IF YOU FEEL THIS WAY	TRY THESE THINGS
Healthy food costs too much.	**Eat well can save you money.** • Eat less meat and more beans. • Eat canned or frozen fruits and vegetables. • Eat at home instead of going out.
Healthy food doesn't taste as good as junk food.	**Don't give up your favorite foods – just eat smaller amounts.** • Try new foods and recipes.
I eat when I'm bored, tired, angry or depressed.	**Find something else to distract you.** • Work on a hobby, call a friend, go for a walk. • Keep only healthy snacks around.
It's hard to be healthy when I eat out.	**Avoid all-you-can-eat places and restaurants that don't offer healthy options.** • Order grilled or low-fat sandwiches and salads instead of fried foods. • Ask for low-fat dressing on the side. • Ask for half portions, share with a friend, or bring leftovers home.
I eat too much at social events.	**You can still eat healthy at social events.** • Eat a healthy snack before you go. • Choose a few things to eat. • Bring healthy dishes to potlucks.
I eat too much when I'm cooking or cleaning.	**Don't just eat because it is there.** • Chew gum or a toothpick. • Ask someone else to put away leftovers while you wash dishes.
I tend to skip regular meals, but snack in front of the TV and throughout the day.	**Make time for regular meals.** • Sit down at the table and eat healthy meals with friends, family and/or co-workers. • Pack lunch and snacks to take to work or for travel.

Figure 6-3 Starting the conversation about healthy eating.

Source: Reprinted from *Journal of Midwifery & Women's Health*, Volume 55, Issue 6, November–December 2010, Elizabeth Widen, RD and Anna Maria Siega-Riz, PhD, RD, Prenatal Nutrition: A Practical Guide for Assessment and Counseling, pp. 540–549, Copyright © 2010 American College of Nurse-Midwives, with permission from Elsevier.

Making a plan
What goal(s) can you set for yourself now? **Before my next visit, I am going to:** ___ Eat fried foods less often ___ Aim to eat 5 or more fruits and vegetables per day ___ Eat smaller portions ___ Instead of regular sodas, juice and sugar sweetened beverages, drink water or skim milk ___ Keep healthy snacks around ___ Other _____

Figure 6-3 Starting the conversation about healthy eating. *(continued)*
Source: Reprinted from *Journal of Midwifery & Women's Health*, Volume 55, Issue 6, November–December 2010, Elizabeth Widen, RD and Anna Maria Siega-Riz, PhD, RD, Prenatal Nutrition: A Practical Guide for Assessment and Counseling, pp. 540–549, Copyright © 2010 American College of Nurse-Midwives, with permission from Elsevier.

other clinician should occur.[48] At the 6-month visit, the clinician can evaluate weight loss, review behaviors the woman has attempted to change, and reinforce these efforts. It is important to initiate plans with the woman to maintain her weight loss, given that weight loss usually plateaus at this time. To reiterate, a midwife can remind a woman that learning and adopting a healthier dietary pattern will be valuable to her throughout her life, whatever her weight, and whatever her health and life goals.

Women who are unable to meet a healthy weight goal with diet and exercise may be candidates for pharmacologic therapy or referral for possible bariatric surgery. Weight-loss drugs work by either suppressing appetite (phentermine [Adipex-P], diethylpropion [Tenuate]) or limiting fat absorption (orlistat [Xenical, Alli]). Three other drugs—two antidepressants (buproprion [Wellbutrin], fluoxetine [Prozac]) and an antiepileptic (topiramate [Topamax])—also achieve weight loss similar to approved weight-loss drugs. Weight loss achieved with these medications after approximately 12 months of use is 3 to 4.5 kg on average.[52]

Currently, there are only three FDA-approved drugs for long-term weight loss: orlistat (Xenical or Alli, over the counter at a lower dose), which has been available for over 10 years, and two newly approved drugs—a phentermine and topiramate combination (Qsymia), which is FDA pregnancy category X, and lorcaserin (Belviq), which is proposed to be a Schedule IV drug due its potential hallucinogenic properties. NHLBI guidelines suggest that candidates for weight-loss drug therapy include women with BMIs higher than 35 and those with BMIs between 30 and 35 who have other comorbidities.

Women with BMIs higher than 40, and women with BMIs between 35 and 40 with a comorbidity such as hypertension, hyperlipidemia, diabetes, or obstructive sleep apnea, and who are unable to lose weight after working with a nutritionist, may benefit from referral to a weight-loss specialist. Bariatric surgery has been shown to be the most successful strategy for weight loss for this population of women.[53]

Eating Disorders as a Type of Eating Pattern Disorder

An estimated 5% to 6% of all women in the United States may have, or have had, some form of eating disorder, although less than half seek treatment for this condition.[54] Primary care providers may not automatically recognize eating disorders. Due to the difficulties of detection and the extremely complex etiology of eating disorders, successful detection, diagnosis, and treatment require a multidisciplinary effort by a team of health professionals, preferably with special education in the field. Although the midwife in a busy practice may lack education for in-depth counseling and treatment of eating disorder, this professional should be able to rule out at least some instances of eating disorders through use of a brief screening and provide follow-up referrals when necessary.

The SCOFF is a brief five-question instrument with a high negative predictive value in the general population. That is, when used among a normal clinical population, the SCOFF questionnaire is not reliable in detecting eating disorder, but it is reliable in ruling it out.[55] "SCOFF" is a mnemonic for the five questions found in the questionnaire. The questions assess whether individuals are making themselves vomit to relieve a feeling of fullness (S); whether they are concerned that they have lost control over what or how much they eat (C); whether they have recently lost a significant amount of weight (15 pounds or more) (O); whether they feel that they are "fat" even when others comment that they are thin (F); and whether they feel that thoughts and feelings about food are dominating their life (F). An answer of "yes" to two or more questions is indicative of an eating disorder. The SCOFF has been validated as an effective screening tool for eating disorders.[55] Persons with some symptoms of disordered eating should be assessed by professionals in more detail.

Nutrition in Pregnancy

Normal pregnancy is a not an inherently fragile event for either the woman or her fetus. This is evidenced by the incidence of relatively robust birth outcomes within rather broad nutritional boundaries. With few exceptions there is little evidence to support an assertion that the addition of a particular nutritional supplement, or combination of them, dramatically improves pregnancy outcomes. Therefore, for reasonably well-nourished populations, perhaps the most important nutritional advice to offer pregnant women is that the types of healthy dietary patterns outlined in this chapter will also generally be the best dietary patterns for pregnancy. A healthcare provider might even take the occasion of a pregnancy to emphasize to a woman that in general, eating healthily for the baby is also eating healthily for herself, and that adopting a healthier dietary pattern during pregnancy can continue after pregnancy as well.

History of Nutritional Guidelines in Pregnancy

Dietary advice during pregnancy has been recorded for centuries. Over time, as our understanding of pregnancy and placental physiology and nutrition science has increased, this nutritional advice has changed. For example, although historical texts occasionally mentioned prohibition from alcohol for pregnant women, fetal alcohol syndrome was not clearly identified until the early 1970s. The knowledge that adequate folic acid one month prior to conception and through the first trimester can prevent neural tube defects has been heralded as the most important nutrition discovery in the last 40 years.

In the 1950s through the 1960s, the basic nutrition advice from physicians to pregnant women was aimed at preventing symptoms of preeclampsia through limiting weight gains to 12 pounds, restricting salt intake, and using diuretics when women developed edema, all without evidence to support these recommendations. We now know that these approaches jeopardized both maternal and fetal health and did nothing to prevent preeclampsia or modulate the severity of the disease.

During the same time, Agnes Higgins developed and implemented a model of nutritional counseling, the *Higgins Intervention Method for Nutritional Rehabilitation During Pregnancy*. Her method assessed the nutrition needs of each pregnant woman based on age, nutritional status, and obstetric factors, and provided the woman with an individualized protein and calorie requirement prescription.[56] This method, which was used for 30 years at the Montreal Diet Dispensary (a Canadian nonprofit agency similar to March of Dimes), demonstrated an ability to decrease low birth weight by 50% and improve outcomes for adolescent and twin pregnancies.[56,57] These outcomes encouraged the March of Dimes to emphasize the role of diet in the prevention of low birth weight and prematurity. Responding to this organization's and others' advocacy, in 1990 the IOM issued nutrition and weight gain guidelines based on an extensive review of the literature and aimed at primarily preventing low birth weight.[58] Thanks to the work of Agnes Higgins, the role of nutrition in successful pregnancies became an important focus for healthcare providers.

Although current general population-based guidelines developed by national organizations make individualized prescriptions unnecessary, they do not replace the importance of taking the time needed to provide individualized nutrition counseling to help women meet these guidelines. The following is a review of specific nutrition requirements and recommendations for pregnant women.

Macronutrients in Pregnancy

Protein

Protein requirements for women during pregnancy and lactation increase from 46 g/day (the recommendation for nonpregnant/nonlactating women) to 71 g/day. In general, this added requirement should not be a problem for women to attain. However, some women have low protein intakes prior to pregnancy and may need special counseling on ways to incorporate more protein into their diet. Women in low-resource settings may have very low protein intakes; in these scenarios, increasing protein, which is frequently the most costly dietary component, can be challenging.

Omega-3 Fatty Acids

Pregnancy and lactation is a time when it may be even more important to encourage increased consumption of omega-3 fatty acids (n-3s), which predominantly come from intake of oily fish. Docosahexaenoic acid (DHA) is the predominant fatty acid found in the brain, retina, and nervous system, and it is also found in large amounts in the placenta. The fetal brain acquires DHA at a rapid rate after the first half of the pregnancy. Studies have documented that children exposed to higher levels of n-3s in utero have better visual acuity, higher intelligence scores, fewer behavioral problems, and less childhood asthma.[59–61] Because the brain continues to develop during infancy and early childhood, the need for adequate n-3 intake continues after birth; thus, for breast milk to have adequate levels to meet this need, the maternal diet must be rich in n-3s. Observational studies support that higher omega-3 intake in pregnancy is associated with less preeclampsia and preterm birth, although the results of supplementation trials have been mixed.[62] There is an emerging body of literature on the role of n-3s in preventing perinatal depression.[63]

The current recommendation is that pregnant women eat two servings (12 ounces) of fish per week. However, this amount may not be sufficient to obtain fetal and neonatal benefits and higher intake of n-3 rich foods may be desirable.[61] Unfortunately, due to concerns regarding ingesting mercury in fish, many pregnant women have significantly decreased their fish consumption in pregnancy.[60] In general, the larger fish species contain more heavy metals. The FDA advises women who plan on becoming pregnant or are pregnant, as well as lactating women, to avoid tilefish, shark, swordfish, and king mackerel, with a further recommendation to limit consumption of albacore tuna to once per week.[64] If a woman cannot eat fish, a supplement that provides 500 mg of eicosapentaenoic acid (EPA) and 300 mg of DHA daily would meet the recommendation of several global health organizations.[65]

Vitamins and Minerals in Pregnancy

There are a few specific pregnancy issues related to vitamin and mineral requirements and supplement use in pregnancy. Prenatal vitamins are prescribed in the United States almost universally. Although the data to support this practice have been weak, it is an expectation of pregnant women that good prenatal care includes prescribing prenatal vitamins. The studies cited in the following sections document that the nutritional intake of specific vitamins is low in at least some populations of U.S. women, thereby increasing the evidence in support of general prenatal vitamin supplementation.

Vitamin A

In pregnancy, excess ingestion of preformed vitamin A (i.e., retinol) of 10,000 IU or more is teratogenic, resulting in cardiac or central nervous system malformations or miscarriage.[66] It is important to check the type of vitamin A and amount provided in a prenatal multivitamin supplement to ensure women will not exceed these limits. Retinol is found in food sources such a chicken and beef liver and cod liver oil. Pregnant women are encouraged to limit retinol ingestion to 5000 IU/day. However, vitamin A as beta-carotene (found in deep yellow and orange vegetables) can be freely ingested. Most manufacturers have replaced retinol with beta-carotene in their prenatal vitamin formulations. Women who are taking a multivitamin that is not a prenatal formulation should be counseled to check the source of vitamin A on the label to ensure that they are not exceeding the safe levels of retinol intake.

Vitamin D

The placenta is rich in vitamin D receptors, and vitamin D regulates gene expression that controls trophoblastic invasion and angiogenesis. In pregnancy, the circulating levels of active vitamin D metabolites are three times higher, but the exact mechanism for this change is unclear.[31] Observational studies have shown that pregnant women with low or deficient vitamin D levels have more bacterial vaginosis, respiratory infections, and preeclampsia prior to 34 weeks, and their infants are at increased risk for multiple sclerosis later in life.[31] The question is whether supplementation in pregnancy can improve serum vitamin D levels and, in turn, improve perinatal outcomes.

Recently, a randomized trial of vitamin D supplementation in pregnancy was undertaken by giving a mixed population of white, black, and Hispanic women doses of 400 IU (the current recommended dose), 2000 IU, and 4000 IU.[31,67,68] The study was powered to examine the safety and effectiveness of larger doses of vitamin D and examined clinical outcomes only as secondary outcomes. The researchers found that women needed 4000 IU as supplements to optimize their vitamin D levels to the study definition of 40 ng/mL (100 nmol/L). There was no evidence of any harm from the higher vitamin D doses, and women who achieved supraphysiologic serum vitamin D levels during the study had no evidence of abnormally high urinary or serum calcium—the major concern regarding vitamin D toxicity. Two significant clinical differences found between the lowest and highest supplemented groups were less gestational hypertension/preeclampsia (8.1% low; 2.6% high) and fewer primary cesarean sections (25.3% low; 14.3% high). The latter finding may reflect the importance of vitamin D on muscle function and supports a previously reported observational study.[69]

The optimal levels of 25(OH)D levels in pregnancy are unclear, although pregnant women in Africa average levels around 150 nmol/L, three times the IOM recommendation.[31] A recent study of vitamin D levels in pregnant women in the upper Midwest showed that 72% of this sample of women had deficient levels, defined as less than 30 ng/mL, with ranges from 41% for white Caucasians to 92% for Middle Easterners.[70]

Folic Acid

Adequate folic acid levels one month prior to conception through the first trimester of pregnancy decreases the risk of neural tube defects (NTDs) by 30% to 50%.[71] Since 1998, when the FDA required fortification of wheat products with folic acid, approximately 1000 fewer infants have been born with NTDs.[71] However, among low-risk women, another one-fourth to one-half of the infants born with NTDs annually could be born without such conditions if their mothers ingested folic acid in the amount of 0.4 mg (400 mcg) per day. Unfortunately, only one in four nonpregnant childbearing-age women in the United States consumes the recommended amount.[72] However, their serum levels may be adequate given fortification of wheat products. Overall, approximately 60% of women are aware of the need for folic acid during pregnancy, but only 17% know that supplements need to be consumed at least one month prior to conception.[73] Relevant knowledge and supplement use are lower among younger women and Hispanic women.

A landmark British study among women with a prior infant with a NTD showed supplementation with 4 mg (1000 times the normal recommended amount) was needed to prevent reoccurrence.[74] This dose should also be prescribed to other high-risk women—a group that includes women with a seizure disorder, those with irritable bowel disease, and possibly those with a BMI higher than 35.[75] Women with malabsorptive syndromes also are classified as high risk, including those women who have undergone bariatric surgery. Women with a multiple gestation need to receive a 1 mg supplement of folic acid as soon as this pregnancy state is recognized.[76]

Iodine

Iodine deficiency in pregnancy is the leading cause of preventable cognitive deficits in the world. Two meta-analyses have shown that prenatal iodine deficiency lowers IQ by 12 to 13 points.[77] The fetal brain is totally dependent on maternal thyroxine for normal development. During pregnancy, iodine requirements increase 50% to meet the need for increased thyroid hormone production. The recommended pregnancy intake for iodine is 220 mcg and 290 mcg during lactation. This intake should result in urinary iodine levels between 150 and 249 mcg/L, which is the World Health Organization's recommendation for pregnancy. Data from 2005–2008 national nutrition examinations showed that an alarming 57% of pregnant women had urinary iodine levels below 150 mcg/L.[36]

Both the American Thyroid Association and the Teratology Society recommend that all pregnant women receive 150 mcg of iodine supplementation daily.[78] A survey of prenatal vitamins found that only slightly more than half contained iodine.[79] Those vitamins with iodine used either potassium iodide or kelp, but the measured amount of iodine is more accurate for those products that use potassium iodide. More than one-third of the kelp type had dose variations of more than 50%, with the majority of such variation due to lower-than-labeled doses.

Iron

Optimal hemoglobin levels in pregnancy are between 9.5 and 12.5 mg/dL. Both low (< 9.0 mg/dL) and high (> 13.0 mg/dL) levels are associated with low birth weight.[80] Although the USPSTF found insufficient evidence to recommend for or against universal iron supplementation in pregnancy,[42] a large meta-analysis demonstrated that routine iron supplementation decreases the incidence of low birth weight and maternal anemia.[80] Conversely, too much iron can harm both the woman and her fetus. The provision of extra iron beyond the 30 mg found in a prenatal vitamin to women without deficiency produces oxidative stress and significantly increases the number of small-for-gestation infants and women with hypertensive disorders.[81] Therefore, the goal of iron supplementation during pregnancy beyond prenatal vitamin supplementation should not be to achieve a high hemoglobin level, but rather to correct a current anemia.

Two special considerations arise regarding iron absorption and screening in pregnancy. The first is the risk of significant anemia. Pregnant women have an increased demand for iron, which increases from 2 mg to 3.5 mg per day.[82] Women of higher parity and with closely spaced pregnancies are at higher risk for anemia, as they may not have had an opportunity to replace their iron stores between pregnancies. The second consideration is that iron absorption increases dramatically during pregnancy, from 7% in the first trimester to 66% in the third trimester.[82]

Also, the normal drop in hemoglobin and hematocrit levels in the second trimester of pregnancy is physiologic, not pathologic.

Current cut-off values for diagnosing anemia in pregnancy are found in **Table 6-8**.[58] Normal values should be adjusted for altitude, smoking, and African American race.

Calcium

The fetus will obtain whatever calcium is needed from the mother. However, women need adequate calcium to maintain healthy bones and teeth. The recommended daily allowance (RDA) for women 19 years or older during pregnancy and lactation is 1000 mg. For adolescents, this requirement is 1300 mg. Evidence demonstrates that calcium supplementation of 1500 to 2000 mg decreases the risk of developing preeclampsia by 30% to 50%, although this effect

Table 6-8	Diagnostic Values for Anemia in Pregnancy	
	Hemoglobin (g/dL)	Hematocrit (%)
Trimester		
First	11	33
Second	10.5	32
Third	11	33
Adjustment for Smoking		
0.5–0.9 pack/day	+ 0.3	+ 1.0
1.0–1.9 pack/day	+ 0.5	+ 1.5
2.0 or more pack/day	+ 0.7	+ 2.0
Adjustment for Altitude		
3000–3999 feet	+ 0.2	+ 0.5
4000–4999 feet	+ 0.3	+ 1.0
5000–5999 feet	+ 0.5	+ 1.5
6000–6999 feet	+ 0.7	+ 2.0
7000–7999 feet	+ 1.0	+ 3.0
8000–8999 feet	+ 1.3	+ 4.0
African American	– 0.8	– 2.5

Source: Committee on Nutritional Status During Pregnancy, Food and Nutrition Board, Institute of Medicine. *Nutrition During Pregnancy and Lactation: An Implementation Guide.* Washington, DC: National Academy Press; 1992.

is strongest in women with inadequate intake of calcium at the onset of pregnancy.[83]

Pregnant Women's Nutrition
Weight Gain

Specific, accurate nutrition counseling during pregnancy remains important because food and patterns of eating can affect maternal and infant outcomes. In particular, a healthcare provider should not assume that a pregnant woman, from any culture, automatically possesses the most helpful nutrition knowledge, or will automatically choose a healthy dietary pattern. In one example, a study including diverse practice settings and providers, including nurse-midwives, found that one-third of the women reported that they had not been told how much weight to gain during their pregnancy.[84] Study findings that women who gained less than the recommended weight—a risk factor for low birth weight—were more likely to have had providers who recommended a weight gain that was too low, or who gave them no target weight, underscore the importance of accurate weight gain recommendations during pregnancy.

In 1990 the IOM issued pregnancy weight gain guidelines aimed at ensuring adequate weight gain to prevent low birth weight. At the time, the weight gain recommended by IOM was higher than the prevailing recommendation of a 12-pound weight gain. Since then, obesity and excessive weight gain in pregnancy has become a public health concern. In 2009, IOM revisited its recommendations in light of accumulated evidence since the early 1990s, with a particular focus on the role of retention of gestational weight gain in the development of long-term obesity in women, and reissued new gestational weight gain guidelines.[85] These weight gain targets were designed to optimize birth outcomes while at the same time limiting problems with postpartum weight retention, a major contributor to obesity in women.[86] Midwives should be familiar with the current recommended pregnancy weight gains by BMI category, as found in the *Prenatal Care* chapter.[85] Women should be provided with information regarding target weight gain for pregnancy and both interval and total weight gain in pregnancy should be tracked. It is preferable to chart weights serially on a graph so that both the provider and the woman have a pictorial representation of weight changes during the pregnancy.

Women who are underweight and do not gain sufficient weight have an increased risk for preterm birth. Conversely, those who gain excessive weight are at risk for gestational diabetes, cesarean birth, and postpartum weight retention.[85] Sharing this information with women may help alter cultural ideas that a larger weight gain is indicative of a healthier pregnancy; these ideas may be particularly prominent in some populations, such as among some African American women.[87]

It is important that women understand that the adage, "eating for two," is not true. Pregnancy requires only an extra 350 to 450 calories per day during the second and third trimesters—far from "eating for two." A midwife should communicate that this additional caloric requirement during pregnancy, which is normally all the additional calories required, is equivalent merely to one extra healthy snack per day, such as the following:

- 2 ounces of cheddar cheese + medium apple
- 1 cup of black beans + 1 corn tortilla
- 8 ounces of skim milk + 1½ tablespoons of peanut butter + banana

Underweight women should be evaluated for eating disorders and may require expert counseling during pregnancy.[88] All women should be provided with an accurate healthy weight gain target for pregnancy based on their BMI, as well as healthy eating information and tracking. Encouraging the pregnant woman to complete forms such as the previously mentioned "Starting the Conversation" or REAP questionnaires, and assessing their results, can be a rapid method to gain valuable information about her current dietary patterns.

Content of a Healthy Diet in Pregnancy

As noted earlier, nutrition can affect physiologic function at the cellular and organ levels. Therefore, it makes theoretical sense that diet can play a powerful role in maintaining a healthy pregnancy. A few randomized trials have demonstrated that women who changed their dietary pattern to eat as recommended by the Healthy Eating Pyramid had fewer preterm births or gestational diabetes.[89, 90]

Also, there is increasing evidence to support the "Barker hypothesis"; in simple terms, it states that a mother's diet while carrying the in utero fetus, at least in some cases, has effects on that individual's entire life, including genetic predispositions for some chronic diseases.[91] The effects of maternal diet may even extend to a child's preferences for foods that the mother ate during pregnancy. Evidence shows that the fetus experiences odors from the amniotic fluid that are flavored by maternal intake, which in turn influences flavor preferences for four of the five basic tastes—sweet, bitter, sour, and umami (savory)—as

well as volatile odors such as those from carrots and garlic.[92] Therefore, a healthy dietary pattern, identical or similar to that outlined in this chapter, would be beneficial or at least innocuous during pregnancy. Because women are more likely to make behavioral changes during pregnancy than at other times, prenatal care is an ideal time to start the conversation about a healthy dietary pattern.

During pregnancy it is not only the food choices, but the frequency of meals that play a key role. The IOM's *Nutrition During Pregnancy and Lactation* recommends that pregnant women eat three meals a day and at least two snacks, and there is substantial research support for this recommendation.[58] Skipping meals, prolonged periods without eating, or fasting can have measurable deleterious effects on the woman, the fetus, and the likelihood of preterm birth.[93,96] Again, not every woman will know this information automatically.

Some pregnant women will want to observe their religion's periods of fasting, even though Catholicism, Judaism, and Islam all customarily exempt a pregnant woman from any obligation to fast. As part of prenatal care, the healthcare provider must elicit this information and provide teaching as required. Some religious women simply assume, without ever consulting their religious authorities, that they must still observe religious fasts while pregnant. Others do not realize that although fasting in other circumstances would be completely innocuous and readily bearable, it can convey physiologic and chemical messages during pregnancy. For instance, the 24-hour Yom Kippur fast is associated with an increase in spontaneous term births.[94]

The other important consideration for pregnant women is avoidance of foodborne illnesses that can adversely affect the woman and/or the fetus. The primary infections of concern are toxoplasmosis, *Listeria monocytogenes*, and brucellosis, due to their devastating fetal effects. All of these infections come from consuming contaminated and raw or undercooked foods. As part of preventing these infections, pregnant women should avoid raw milk products, soft cheeses, smoked seafood that has not been cooked, raw meat or processed delicatessen meat, meat spreads, pates, and hot dogs that have not been reheated. Fruits and vegetables may be contaminated with *Salmonella* or *Escherichia coli* and, therefore, should be thoroughly washed. Raw vegetable sprouts should be avoided, because it appears impossible to thoroughly clean contaminated sprouts. A similar concern is associated with raw or undercooked eggs. Raw seafood and raw shellfish can cause maternal illnesses, which are usually limited to the gastrointestinal tract and, as such are less likely to affect the fetus. Some, although not all, local departments of public health list sushi as a possible source of *L. monocytogenes*. However research evidence currently does not point to a link between sushi and *Listeria*.

Box 6-4 summarizes dietary recommendations during pregnancy.[97] These recommendations can also be found in the *Prenatal Care* chapter.

Mood disorders can affect nutrition and weight gain in pregnancy. Women who are anxious or depressed are more likely to have lower-quality diets that are especially low in micronutrients; consume more calorie-dense, low-nutritious foods; and skip meals.[98] These habits may partially explain the association between depression and low birth weight. This is another reason that pregnant women should be routinely screened for depression.

Special Populations

Vegetarians

The term *vegetarian* can encompass a number of sub-populations: women whose diets include dairy (lacto-vegetarians); those who eat eggs (ova-vegetarians);

and those who eat both dairy and eggs (lacto-ovarians). Individuals who strictly eat only plants can be called vegans. Women who eat any of the vegetarian diets can meet all their nutritional needs in pregnancy and have healthy birth outcomes,[24] although some modifications may be needed. Eating a variety of fruits, vegetables, and grains, as discussed earlier, is key to a nutritiously sound diet.

Studies conducted in four different industrial countries found that pregnant vegetarians did not meet the recommended standard for vitamin B_{12}, iron, folate, and zinc. Lack of folate was surprising, as the recommended amount should be easily obtained with a variety-rich vegetarian diet. Vitamin B_{12} intake can be adequate among those women who consume eggs, dairy products, and fortified foods; without a regular source of B_{12}, however, vegan diets tend to have low levels of this vitamin.[24] Women consuming a vegan diet need to be certain that they are receiving this vitamin from either fortified soy and rice beverages, fortified foods, or nutritional yeast supplements. Fermented soy products are not a source of vitamin B_{12}.

Iron from plant sources is non-heme iron; thus it is less easily absorbed and more foods can inhibit

---

BOX 6-4 Summary of Dietary Recommendations in Pregnancy

- Take folic acid in a multivitamin at least one month prior to conception to prevent neural tube defects.
- Gain the recommended weight for BMI by eating the following:
  - Three meals a day and two snacks to avoid prolonged periods of fasting
  - A diet rich in fruits and vegetables (at least five servings per day) and fiber-rich carbohydrates
  - Limit carbohydrates with a high glycemic index (e.g., fruit juices and sodas)
  - Use monounsaturated fats and avoid trans fats
  - Adequate amounts of protein, especially from plant-based sources
  - At least two servings of omega-3–rich fish (low in mercury) weekly or use an omega-3 supplement
- Ensure adequate intake of these micronutrients:
  - Vitamin A as beta-carotene and limit food sources with retinol such as liver (< 4 oz/week) or cod liver oil
  - Vitamin D from sunshine exposure (amount will vary by geography, BMI, and skin

  pigmentation); if not feasible, supplement with vitamin D_3 (1000-4000 IU depending on intake of vitamin D–fortified dairy products and vitamin D serum levels)
  - Women adhering to strict vegan diets will need B_{12} supplements
  - Iodine through diet or a multivitamin (preferably as potassium iodide)
  - Iron through diet, multivitamin, or additional low-dose supplement if anemic
  - Calcium through diet, with higher levels suggested for women at risk for preeclampsia
- Drink plenty of water as primary source of liquid; avoid alcohol
- Avoid foodborne illnesses that can cause maternal or fetal disease by eating the following:
  - Well-cooked meat, poultry (including eggs), and fish
  - Only pasteurized dairy and fruit juices
  - Avoid soft cheeses, processed fruits, and raw sprouts

Source: Adapted from Barger MK. Maternal nutrition and perinatal outcomes. *J Midwifery Women's Health.* 2010;55(6):502-511.

its absorption than heme iron. Nevertheless, iron can be obtained in a vegetarian diet.

Nonanimal sources of zinc include nuts and beans although, similar to iron, phytates can bind it, thereby preventing absorption of this micronutrient. Another source of zinc is fortified cereals.

If no dairy products are consumed, pregnant women may not have adequate vitamin D levels and, in the absence of sufficient sunlight exposure, may need vitamin D supplements. Iodine, which comes from fish or sea vegetables, will be low if these foods or iodized salt are not part of the diet.

Studies have shown that the fetal cord blood and breast milk from mothers on vegetarian diets is lower in DHA than their counterparts from women who consume a carnivorous diet.[99,100] Women who eat eggs can increase their DHA by consuming DHA-fortified eggs from hens fed microalgae; otherwise, women can consume microalgae-derived DHA supplements.

Women with Limited Resources

Women with limited incomes, mobility, or language barriers may not have access to a variety of healthy foods or the best foods may too expensive. Pregnant adolescents are members of a unique population where understanding their barriers to healthy eating is challenging because they may not be in charge of buying and preparing food in their households. In any setting, but particularly when working with women who have immigrated to the United States, midwives need to become familiar with culturally specific diet patterns so that they can make food suggestions that may be more readily accepted for incorporation into a woman's diet.

Low-income women are at increased risk for dietary deficiencies.[101] The Special Supplemental Nutrition Program for Women, Infants, and Children (WIC)—a food supplement program run by the USDA—is able to provide food resources and excellent cultural-based nutrition education for pregnant women, breastfeeding women, infants, and children younger than the age of 5. Recent changes in WIC policy and the covered food package have resulted in improved access to fresh fruits and vegetables and improved dietary intakes of its participants.[102,103] The WIC program is also able to connect women with other important community resources to help improve their pregnancy outcomes. WIC is not an entitlement program, but rather a grant program that requires reallocation of funding annually. Therefore, changes may occur at any time in the future for the program. As of 2012, more than half of the infants born in the United States received some food through WIC.[104]

Multiple Pregnancies

Twin and higher-order pregnancies result in more perinatal morbidity largely due to the higher rates of prematurity and low birth weight. Therefore, it is essential that fetal growth in utero be maximized, and good maternal nutrition is the best way to accomplish this goal. Because more than one fetus is present in such pregnancies, the physiologic changes in the woman are even greater, requiring increased requirements for both macronutrients and micronutrients.

Weight guidelines for multiple pregnancies are listed in the *Prenatal Care* chapter. Although studies have not provided sufficient evidence related to underweight women, it seems clear that they need to gain at least as much as normal-weight women. What is even more crucial is the pattern of weight gain. A previous study demonstrated that maternal weight gain prior to 28 weeks' gestation accounted for 80% of birth weight in twins.[105] Therefore, early gestational weight gain is crucial to building nutritional stores that the fetuses can use later in pregnancy, whereas "catch-up" weight gain later in pregnancy has less of an impact on fetal growth.

There are no national guidelines for the increases in other nutritional requirements in multiple pregnancies, but extrapolations have been made from singleton to twin pregnancies. Although requirements will vary by prepregnancy BMI, daily requirements for women with a normal BMI include 3000 to 3500 calories, 175 g protein, 330 g carbohydrate, and 156 g fat.[76] The DHA/EPA requirement is suggested to be the same as in singleton pregnancies, although infants from twin pregnancies have lower cord omega-3 fatty acid levels than singletons, which may argue for higher maternal intake of these nutrients. Maternal micronutrient intake should be increased for folic acid (1 mg), vitamin C (1000 mg), vitamin D (1000 IU), magnesium (800 mg), and zinc (30 mg).[76] It is generally recommended that women with multiple fetuses take two prenatal vitamin supplements beginning in the second trimester to obtain needed micronutrients. This recommendation is safe as long as the vitamin A in the supplements is not retinol; if it is retinol, then the dose needs to remain below 10,000 IU.

Lactation and Postpartum Nutrition

Breast milk is the species-specific food for human infants and, therefore, exclusive breastfeeding for the first 6 months of life should be strongly supported by all healthcare providers. Lactation is a time when good nutrition improves the quality of breast milk, thereby enhancing infant nutrition. Lactation requires an added expenditure of energy on the mother's part, ranging from 500 to 700 calories. These calories can come from maternal fat stores and may be an important method of reducing the risk of postpartum weight retention.[106] Two important nutrients mentioned earlier in this chapter are vitamin D and omega-3 fatty acids. Breastfeeding women may need even higher levels of vitamin D to have sufficient vitamin D levels in their breast milk for the infant.[107] DHA is essential to the developing brain and must come from the maternal diet.

Infants at high risk for allergies and atopic eczema have a decreased incidence of these conditions if they are breastfed exclusively for 4 to 6 months.[108] There is no evidence that maternal avoidance of certain foods during pregnancy or lactation decreases the risk of allergies in infants.[108] However, a randomized trial of prenatal fish oil supplementation showed that by the age of 16 years, children whose mothers received the fish oil had a 63% reduced risk for asthma.[109]

Postpartum weight retention is an important health problem for women. Primiparous women and those with high BMIs prior to pregnancy are at greatest risk for excessive weight gain during pregnancy and, subsequently, more gestational weight retention, which is typically defined as more than 5 kg at one year or more postpartum.[110] The average gestational weight retention at one year is 0.5 to 1.5 kg (2–3 lb), although a large variation is noted, with 13% to 20% of women retaining more than 5 kg (11 lb) at the one-year postpartum mark.[110] Studies have shown that among women with normal BMIs at the start of pregnancy, at one year postpartum 6% will have increased to at least an overweight BMI, with more black women moving into a higher category (8–9%).[110]

The evidence on the role of breastfeeding in postpartum weight loss is mixed, probably reflecting studies' poor control for the intensity and duration of lactation. However, a summary review of breastfeeding among women in developed countries showed that exclusively breastfeeding mothers reached their prepregnant weight about 6 months earlier than bottle-feeding mothers, and that a slowing of weight loss is observed when lactation is stopped.[111] Breastfeeding appears to account for 1 kg weight loss at one year postpartum.

Women should be counseled about ways to lose their pregnancy weight after the birth. Even lactating women can safely exercise (45 minutes per day, 4 days per week) and decrease their daily calories by 500 to achieve a safe weight loss of 1 pound per week with no ill effects on their infant's health.[112]

Nutrition, the Menstrual Cycle, and Fertility

Nutrition affects and is affected by the menstrual cycle. Studies suggest that caloric intake varies during the menstrual cycle, peaking once in the luteal phase and once in the follicular phase, and reaching a nadir during menses.[113,114] These changes are thought to coincide with cyclical fluxes in a woman's basal metabolic rate that are affected by hormones. Women also appear to increase their intake of carbohydrates and fat during the luteal phase, and their intake of protein and fat in the follicular phase, when compared to the menstrual phase.[114] Women with premenstrual syndrome have similar intakes as women without this condition, but increase their intakes of non-milk sugars and alcohol in the luteal phase.[115] Women with very low body fat become anovulatory.

According to the Centers for Disease Control and Prevention, 1.5 million married women in the United States are infertile, with four times that number having a reduced fecundity.[116] Women at the extremes in body weight have been shown to have reduced fertility. Therefore, aiming for a healthy body weight is important for improving fertility. Data from the Nurses' Health Study indicate that for women with high BMIs, losing 5% to 10% of body weight may improve ovulation, especially if regular exercise is incorporated into the regimen.[117] Lean women who exercise strenuously should reduce this activity to a moderate level to improve their fertility. Other specific dietary patterns associated with improved ovulatory fertility from the Nurses' Health Study, beyond those emphasized in this chapter such as eliminating trans fats and eating low-glycemic carbohydrates, include choosing more plant-based proteins, and temporarily trading nonfat or low-fat dairy products for the full-fat versions.[117]

Nutrition and Selected Conditions

Cancer

Numerous studies of every type have been undertaken to identify the role of diet in the development of cancer. Most of the intervention trials using supplements with selected vitamins or minerals have been disappointing in terms of their ability to prevent cancer. This fact underlies the USFSTF findings that there is no evidence to support routine vitamin/mineral supplementation to prevent cancer.[42] One reason for these disappointing results has already been argued in this chapter—namely, that the totality of what we eat, including both macronutrients and micronutrients, exerts a powerful physiologic effect, probably more powerful than just providing a supplement without changing a dietary pattern.

That said, there is "conclusive" or "probable" evidence linking some specific nutrition and especially overall body or abdominal fat to certain cancers per continually updated evidenced reviews from the World Cancer Fund and American Institute for Cancer Research.[118] They note strong evidence that the consumption of non-starchy vegetables and fruits is protective against mouth, esophageal, stomach, and lung cancer. Colorectal cancer is the cancer for which the strongest evidence shows that what we eat or do not eat matters. Along with exercise, dietary fiber, garlic, milk, and calcium consumption have preventive effects related to colorectal cancer, whereas consumption of red meat, processed meat, and alcohol along with greater body and abdominal fat increase this risk. Unfortunately, for breast and reproductive cancers, there is not strong evidence for the role of diet, beyond the indication that greater body or abdominal fat increases the risk of postmenopausal breast cancer and endometrial cancer. For premenopausal breast cancer, breastfeeding is protective and alcohol increases risk.

Age-Related Eye Disease

Macular degeneration and cataracts are two conditions that women may develop as they age. Strong evidence shows that consumption of vegetables and fruits rich in lutein and zexanthines, which accumulate in the eye, may protect against free-radical damage to the eye caused by smoking, pollution, sunlight, and metabolism from an unhealthy diet pattern such as consumption of a high-glycemic diet.[119] Spinach, kale, and brightly colored fruits and vegetables are rich in these nutrients.

Special Populations

Adolescents

Adolescence is a period of rapid physical growth and, therefore, high nutritional need. During this time, adolescents gain 40% of their skeletal mass and 50% of their body weight. Inadequate nutrition, especially calcium intake, can compromise their peak bone mass. Unfortunately, the diet pattern of adolescents tends to be poor due to the consumption of calorie-dense, nutrient-poor foods; it is also a time when teenage girls typically stop drinking milk. Of perhaps greatest concern is the four times increased rate of obesity among U.S. children and adolescents.[120] Today, on average 18% of teens are obese, but the rate is nearly one-third of non-Hispanic black girls.

This increase in body fat has both health and social implications.

The age of onset of puberty has dropped in recent decades. The reasons for this may include increased exposure to environmental pollutants and chemicals, stress, and increased body fat in childhood. For every one-point increase in BMI, menstruation occurs 1 month earlier.[121] Stage 2 or greater breast development is now not uncommon at ages 7 and 8, with its rate ranging from 18% to 43%; black girls have a higher rate of this condition than white girls.[121] Beyond body fat, type of food consumed also plays a role in the development of puberty. Onset of puberty was delayed 7 months in children consuming large amounts of plant protein, whereas those with a high intake of animal protein entered puberty 7 months earlier.[122] Greater isoflavone intake (found in soy products, chickpeas, and lentils) delayed breast development by 7 months.[122] Earlier onset of puberty can pose significant self-image and social problems for young children, who may be seen as more socially and emotionally mature than they actually are.

By developing a young girl's trust and conducting the same kind of sensitive assessment as previously outlined to determine whether she is ready to make at least small alterations in her diet or exercise patterns, a midwife can play a role in helping her establish healthier diet patterns for her life. Problem-solving barriers to change for an adolescent must include consideration about where and when food is consumed, especially if in the presence of peers, and her ability to control the kinds of food purchased and prepared at home. The two nutrients essential at this phase of development are calcium and iron, as both of their intakes tend to be low in teens.

Mature Women

As women age, they may find that their abdominal fat and weight increase. Although this change in perimenopausal women is due to a combination of genetics, age, and physical activity, there is evidence that loss of estrogen contributes to the redistribution of fat to the abdominal area in middle age and later.[123] Increased abdominal fat increases women's risk for cardiovascular disease and type 2 diabetes. Mature women also become increasingly at risk for osteoporosis, which makes adequacy of vitamin D and calcium levels important. Therefore, a healthy eating pattern is important to this population of women to maintain their quality of life.

Many studies have focused on the use of individual nutrients, particularly isoflavones, to help manage hot flashes. Unfortunately, most systematic reviews have not found these therapies to be effective when tested against placebo, although many of studies may be of too short duration to adequately test the comparisons.[124]

Conclusion

Research increasingly confirms that good nutrition is essential during all phases of life, and the basic principles of good nutrition remain remarkably consistent throughout the lifecourse. Albeit with some caveats, good nutrition is good nutrition—for women who are pregnant, or who want to lose weight, gain weight, or maintain their weight. The midwife should understand the basics of nutrition and how dietary patterns affect normal physiology. Nutrition counseling should be gently incorporated into a midwife's regular practice so that each woman can understand some basic principles of nutrition, the physiologic response of the body to ingested food, and current evidence-based dietary guidelines. Although understanding individual components of the diet is important for health professionals, counseling a woman about diet should remain positively focused on the types of preferable foods to eat and the need to eat a variety of foods, rather than emphasizing individual macronutrients and micronutrients. Of course, a midwife should also be prepared with nutrition information specific to pregnancy, be alert to the possibility of eating disorders and refer women appropriately in such case, and be ready with encouragement, factual information, and possible referral if a woman indicates a desire to achieve a healthier weight.

• • • References

1. Belin RJ, Greenland P, Allison M, et al. Diet quality and the risk of cardiovascular disease: the Women's Health Initiative (WHI). *Am J Clin Nutr.* 2011;94(1):49-57.

2. Flegal KM, Carroll MD, Ogden CL, Curtin LR. Prevalence and trends in obesity among US adults, 1999-2008. *JAMA.* 2010;303(3):235-241.

3. King DE, Mainous AG 3rd, Carnemolla M, Everett CJ. Adherence to healthy lifestyle habits in US adults, 1988-2006. *Am J Med.* 2009;122(6):528-534.

4. Food and Nutrition Board. *Dietary Reference Intakes (DRIs): Recommended Intakes for Individuals.* Washington, DC: National Academy of Sciences; 2004, updated 2011.

5. Office of Nutrition Labeling, and Dietary Supplements. *Food Labeling Guide.* College Park, MD: Food and Drug Administration; 2009.

6. Widen E, Siega-Riz AM. Prenatal nutrition: a practical guide for assessment and counseling. *J Midwifery Women's Health.* 2010;55(6):540-549.

7. Wright JD, Wang C-Y. Trends in intake of energy and macronutrients in adults from 1999-2000 through 2007-2008. NCHS data brief, no 49. Hyattsville, MD: National Center for Health Statistics; 2010.

8. Skerrett PJ, Willett WC. Essentials of healthy eating: a guide. *J Midwifery Women's Health.* 2010;55(6):492-501.

9. Kratz M. Dietary cholesterol, atherosclerosis and coronary heart disease. *Handb Exp Pharmacol.* 2005(170):195-213.

10. Bass KM, Newschaffer CJ, Klag MJ, Bush TL. Plasma lipoprotein levels as predictors of cardiovascular death in women. *Arch Intern Med.* 1993;153(19):2209-2216.

11. Miller M, Stone NJ, Ballantyne C, et al. Triglycerides and cardiovascular disease: a scientific statement from the American Heart Association. *Circulation.* 2011;123(20):2292-2333.

12. Berger JS, McGinn AP, Howard BV, et al. Lipid and lipoprotein biomarkers and the risk of ischemic stroke in postmenopausal women. *Stroke.* 2012;43(4):958-966.

13. Helfand M, Carson S. Screening for lipid disorders in adults: selective update of 2001 US Preventive Services Task Force. Rockville, MD: Agency for Health Care Quality; August 20, 2008.

14. Carroll MD, Kit BK, Lacher DA, Shero ST, Mussolino ME. Trends in lipids and lipoproteins in US adults, 1988-2010. *JAMA.* 2012;308(15):1545-1554.

15. Chavarro JE, Rich-Edwards JW, Rosner BA, Willett WC. Dietary fatty acid intakes and the risk of ovulatory infertility. *Am J Clin Nutr.* 2007;85(1):231-237.

16. Mozaffarian D, Pischon T, Hankinson SE, et al. Dietary intake of trans fatty acids and systemic inflammation in women. *Am J Clin Nutr.* 2004;79(4):606-612.

17. Doell D, Folmer D, Lee H, Honigfort M, Carberry S. Updated estimate of trans fat intake by the US population. *Food Addit Contam Part A Chem Anal Control Expo Risk Assess.* 2012;29(6):861-874.

18. Hibbeln JR, Nieminen LR, Blasbalg TL, Riggs JA, Lands WE. Healthy intakes of n-3 and n-6 fatty acids: estimations considering worldwide diversity. *Am J Clin Nutr.* 2006;83(6 suppl):1483S-1493S.

19. Khawaja O, Gaziano JM, Djousse L. A meta-analysis of omega-3 fatty acids and incidence of atrial fibrillation. *J Am Coll Nutr.* 2012;31(1):4-13.

20. Ludwig DS. The glycemic index: physiological mechanisms relating to obesity, diabetes, and cardiovascular disease. *JAMA.* 2002;287(18):2414-2423.

21. Brand-Miller JC, Stockmann K, Atkinson F, Petocz P, Denyer G. Glycemic index, postprandial glycemia, and the shape of the curve in healthy subjects: analysis of a database of more than 1,000 foods. *Am J Clin Nutr.* 2009;89(1):97-105.

22. King DE, Mainous AG 3rd, Lambourne CA. Trends in dietary fiber intake in the United States, 1999-2008. *J Acad Nutr Diet.* 2012;112(5):642-648.

23. de Munter JS, Hu FB, Spiegelman D, Franz M, van Dam RM. Whole grain, bran, and germ intake and risk of type 2 diabetes: a prospective cohort study and systematic review. *PLoS Med.* 2007;4(8):e261.

24. Craig WJ, Mangels AR. Position of the American Dietetic Association: vegetarian diets. *J Am Diet Assoc.* 2009;109(7):1266-1282.

25. Fulgoni VL 3rd. Current protein intake in America: analysis of the National Health and Nutrition Examination Survey, 2003-2004. *Am J Clin Nutr.* 2008;87(5):1554S-1557S.

26. Willett WC. Dietary fats and coronary heart disease. *J Intern Med.* 2012;272(1):13-24.

27. U.S. Department of Agriculture. USDA National Nutrient Database for Standard Reference, Release 25 online. 2012.

28. Ludwig DS. Clinical update: the low-glycaemic-index diet. *Lancet.* 2007;369(9565):890-892.

29. Institute of Medicine Food and Nutrition Board. *Dietary Reference Intakes for Calcium and Vitamin D.* Washington, DC: National Academy Press; 2010.

30. Holick MF, Binkley NC, Bischoff-Ferrari HA, et al. Evaluation, treatment, and prevention of vitamin D deficiency: an Endocrine Society clinical practice guideline. *J Clin Endocrinol Metab.* 2011;97(7):1911-1930.

31. Hollis BW, Wagner CL. Vitamin D and pregnancy: skeletal effects, nonskeletal effects, and birth outcomes. *Calcif Tissue Int.* 2013;92(2):128-139.

32. Moshfegh A, Goldman J, Ahuja J, Rhodes D, Lacomb R. *What We Eat in America, NHANES 2005-2006: Usual Nutrient Intakes from Food and Water Compared to 1997 Dietary Reference Intakes for Vitamin D, Calcium, Phosphorus, and Magnesium.* Beltsville, MD: Agriculture Research Service, U.S. Department of Agriculture; 2009.

33. Pfeiffer CM, Hughes JP, Lacher DA, et al. Estimation of trends in serum and RBC folate in the U.S. population from pre- to postfortification using assay-adjusted data from the NHANES 1988-2010. *J Nutr.* 2012; 142(5):886-893.

34. Dawson-Hughes B, Looker AC, Tosteson AN, et al. The potential impact of the National Osteoporosis Foundation guidance on treatment eligibility in the USA: an update in NHANES 2005-2008. *Osteoporos Int.* 2012;23(3):811-820.

35. Bailey RL, Dodd KW, Goldman JA, et al. Estimation of total usual calcium and vitamin D intakes in the United States. *J Nutr.* 2010;140(4):817-822.

36. Caldwell KL, Miller GA, Wang RY, Jain RB, Jones RL. Iodine status of the U.S. population, National Health and Nutrition Examination Survey 2003-2004. *Thyroid.* 2008;18(11):1207-1214.

37. Hallberg L, Bjorn-Rasmussen E. Determination of iron absorption from whole diet: a new two-pool model using two radioiron isotopes given as haem and non-haem iron. *Scand J Haematol.* 1972;9(3):193-197.

38. Schrier SL. Approach to the adult patient with anemia. *UpToDate.* 2012. Available at: www.uptodate.com.

39. Mei Z, Cogswell ME, Looker AC, et al. Assessment of iron status in US pregnant women from the National Health and Nutrition Examination Survey (NHANES), 1999-2006. *Am J Clin Nutr.* 2011;93(6):1312-1320.

40. Looker AC, Dallman PR, Carroll MD, Gunter EW, Johnson CL. Prevalence of iron deficiency in the United States. *JAMA.* 1997;277(12):973-976.

41. Centers for Disease Control. Toddler deaths resulting from ingestion of iron supplements—Los Angeles, 1992-1993. *MMWR.* 1993;42(6):111-113.

42. U.S. Preventive Services Task Force. *Guide to Clinical Preventive Services.* Rockville, MD: Agency for Healthcare Research and Quality; 2012.

43. Willett WC, Skerrett PJ. *Eat, Drink, and Be Healthy: The Harvard Medical School Guide to Healthy Eating.* New York, NY: Free Press/Simon & Schuster; 2005.

44. Appel LJ, Sacks FM, Carey VJ, et al. Effects of protein, monounsaturated fat, and carbohydrate intake on blood pressure and serum lipids: results of the OmniHeart randomized trial. *JAMA.* 2005;294(19): 2455-2464.

45. Jenkins DJ, Jones PJ, Lamarche B, et al. Effect of a dietary portfolio of cholesterol-lowering foods given at 2 levels of intensity of dietary advice on serum lipids in hyperlipidemia: a randomized controlled trial. *JAMA.* 2011;306(8):831-839.

46. The Nutrition Source. Healthy eating plate. Department of Nutrition, Harvard School of Public Health. Available at: www.hsph.harvard.edu/nutritionsource /healthy-eating-plate.

47. Browning LM, Hsieh SD, Ashwell M. A systematic review of waist-to-height ratio as a screening tool for the prediction of cardiovascular disease and diabetes: 0.5 could be a suitable global boundary value. *Nutr Res Rev.* 2010;23(2):247-269.

48. National Heart, Lung and Blood Institute Obesity Educational Initiative Expert Panel. *Clinical Guidelines on the Identification, Evaluation, and Treatment of Overweight and Obese Adults.* NIH Pub No 98-9083. Bethesda, MD: National Institute of Medicine, National Heart, Lung, and Blood Institute; 1998.

49. Paxton AE, Strycker LA, Toobert DJ, Ammerman AS, Glasgow RE. Starting the conversation performance of a brief dietary assessment and intervention tool for health professionals. *Am J Prev Med.* 2011;40(1): 67-71.

50. Gans KM, Risica PM, Wylie-Rosett J, et al. Development and evaluation of the nutrition component of the Rapid Eating and Activity Assessment for

Patients (REAP): a new tool for primary care providers. *J Nutr Educ Behav.* 2006;38(5):286-292.

51. Gans KM, Ross E, Barner CW, Wylie-Rosett J, McMurray J, Eaton C. REAP and WAVE: new tools to rapidly assess/discuss nutrition with patients. *J Nutr.* 2003;133(2):556S-562S.

52. Graves BW. The obesity epidemic: scope of the problem and management strategies. *J Midwifery Women's Health.* 2010;55(6):568-578.

53. Ben-David K, Rossidis G. Bariatric surgery: indications, safety and efficacy. *Curr Pharm Des.* 2011; 17(12):1209-1217.

54. Hudson JI, Hiripi E, Pope HG Jr, Kessler RC. The prevalence and correlates of eating disorders in the National Comorbidity Survey Replication. *Biol Psychiatry.* 2007;61(3):348-358.

55. Luck AJ, Morgan JF, Reid F, et al. The SCOFF questionnaire and clinical interview for eating disorders in general practice: comparative study. *BMJ.* 2002;325(7367):755-756.

56. Higgins AC, Moxley JE, Pencharz PB, Mikolainis D, Dubois S. Impact of the Higgins Nutrition Intervention Program on birth weight: a within-mother analysis. *J Am Diet Assoc.* 1989;89(8):1097-1103.

57. Dubois S, Dougherty C, Duquette MP, Hanley JA, Moutquin JM. Twin pregnancy: the impact of the Higgins Nutrition Intervention Program on maternal and neonatal outcomes. *Am J Clin Nutr.* 1991; 53(6):1397-1403.

58. Committee on Nutritional Status During Pregnancy, Food and Nutrition Board, Institute of Medicine. *Nutrition During Pregnancy and Lactation: An Implementation Guide.* Washington, DC: National Academy Press; 1992.

59. Malcolm CA, McCulloch DL, Montgomery C, Shepherd A, Weaver LT. Maternal docosahexaenoic acid supplementation during pregnancy and visual evoked potential development in term infants: a double blind, prospective, randomised trial. *Arch Dis Child Fetal Neonatal Ed.* 2003;88(5):F383-F390.

60. Oken E, Wright RO, Kleinman KP, et al. Maternal fish consumption, hair mercury, and infant cognition in a U.S. cohort. *Environ Health Perspect.* 2005; 113(10):1376-1380.

61. Hibbeln JR, Davis JM, Steer C, et al. Maternal seafood consumption in pregnancy and neurodevelopmental outcomes in childhood (ALSPAC study): an observational cohort study. *Lancet.* 2007;369(9561):578-585.

62. Jordan RG. Prenatal omega-3 fatty acids: review and recommendations. *J Midwifery Women's Health.* 2010;55(6):520-528.

63. Wojcicki JM, Heyman MB. Maternal omega-3 fatty acid supplementation and risk for perinatal maternal depression. *J Matern Fetal Neonatal Med.* 2011; 24(5):680-686.

64. U.S. Department of Health and Human Services, U.S. Food and Drug Administration. What you need to know about mercury in fish and shellfish: 2004 EPA and FDA advice for women who want to become pregnant, women who are are pregnant, nursing mothers, and young children. 2004. Available at: http://www.fda.gov/food/resourcesforyou/consumers /ucm110591.htm. Accessed May 13, 2013.

65. Simopoulos AP, Leaf A, Salem N Jr. Workshop statement on the essentiality of and recommended dietary intakes for omega-6 and omega-3 fatty acids. *Prostaglandins Leukot Essent Fatty Acids.* 2000;63(3):119-121.

66. Rothman KJ, Moore LL, Singer MR, Nguyen US, Mannino S, Milunsky A. Teratogenicity of high vitamin A intake. *N Engl J Med.* 1995;333(21):1369-1373.

67. Hollis BW, Johnson D, Hulsey TC, Ebeling M, Wagner CL. Vitamin D supplementation during pregnancy: double-blind, randomized clinical trial of safety and effectiveness. *J Bone Miner Res.* 2011;26(10): 2341-2357.

68. Wagner CL, McNeil R, Hamilton SA, et al. A randomized trial of vitamin D supplementation in 2 community health center networks in South Carolina. *Am J Obstet Gynecol.* 2013;208(2):137.e1-137.e13.

69. Merewood A, Mehta SD, Chen TC, Bauchner H, Holick MF. Association between Vitamin D deficiency and primary cesarean section. *J Clin Endocrinol Metab.* 2009;94:940-945.

70. Collins-Fulea C, Klima K, Wegienka GR. Prevalence of low vitamin D levels in an urban midwestern obstetric practice. *J Midwifery Women's Health.* 2012; 57(5):439-444.

71. Centers for Disease Control and Prevention. Spina bifida and anencephaly before and after folic acid mandate—United States, 1995-1996 and 1999-2000. *MMWR.* 2004;53(17):362-365.

72. Tinker SC, Cogswell ME, Devine O, Berry RJ. Folic acid intake among U.S. women aged 15-44 years, National Health and Nutrition Examination Survey, 2003-2006. *Am J Prev Med.* 2010;38(5):534-542.

73. Centers for Disease Control and Prevention. Use of supplements containing folic acid among women of childbearing age—United States, 2007. *MMWR.* 2008;57(1):5-8.

74. MRC Vitamin Study Group. Prevention of neural tube defects: results of the Medical Research Council Vitamin Study. *Lancet.* 1991;338(8760):131-137.

75. Wilson RD, Johnson JA, Wyatt P, et al. Preconceptional vitamin/folic acid supplementation 2007: the use of folic acid in combination with a multivitamin supplement for the prevention of neural tube defects and other congenital anomalies. *J Obstet Gynaecol Can.* 2007;29(12):1003-1026.

76. Goodnight W, Newman R. Optimal nutrition for improved twin pregnancy outcome. *Obstet Gynecol.* 2009;114(5):1121-1134.

77. Zimmermann MB. The effects of iodine deficiency in pregnancy and infancy. *Paediatr Perinat Epidemiol.* 2012;26(suppl 1):108-117.

78. Obican SG, Jahnke GD, Soldin OP, Scialli AR. Teratology Public Affairs Committee position paper: iodine deficiency in pregnancy. *Birth Defects Res A Clin Mol Teratol.* 2012;94(9):677-682.

79. Leung AM, Pearce EN, Braverman LE. Iodine content of prenatal multivitamins in the United States. *N Engl J Med.* 2009;360(9):939-940.

80. Pena-Rosas JP, De-Regil LM, Dowswell T, Viteri FE. Daily oral iron supplementation during pregnancy. *Cochrane Database Syst Rev.* 2012;12:CD004736.

81. Ziaei S, Norrozi M, Faghihzadeh S, Jafarbegloo E. A randomised placebo-controlled trial to determine the effect of iron supplementation on pregnancy outcome in pregnant women with haemoglobin > or = 13.2 g/dl. *BJOG.* 2007;114(6):684-688.

82. Graves BW, Barger MK. A "conservative" approach to iron supplementation during pregnancy. *J Midwifery Women's Health.* 2001;46(3):159-166.

83. Hofmeyr GJ, Atallah AN, Duley L. Calcium supplementation during pregnancy for preventing hypertensive disorders and related problems. *Cochrane Database Syst Rev.* 2009;3:CD001059.

84. Stotland NE, Haas JS, Brawarsky P, Jackson RA, Fuentes-Afflick E, Escobar GJ. Body mass index, provider advice, and target gestational weight gain. *Obstet Gynecol.* 2005;105(3):633-638.

85. National Research Council. *Weight Gain During Pregnancy: Reexamining the Guidelines.* Washington, DC: National Academies Press; 2009.

86. Oken E, Kleinman KP, Belfort MB, Hammitt JK, Gillman MW. Associations of gestational weight gain with short- and longer-term maternal and child health outcomes. *Am J Epidemiol.* 2009;170(2):173-180.

87. Groth SW, Morrison-Beedy D, Meng Y. How pregnant African American women view pregnancy weight gain. *J Obstet Gynecol Neonatal Nurs.* 2012;41(6):798-808.

88. Harris AA. Practical advice for caring for women with eating disorders during the perinatal period. *J Midwifery Women's Health.* 2010;55(6):579-586.

89. Khoury J, Henriksen T, Christophersen B, Tonstad S. Effect of a cholesterol-lowering diet on maternal, cord, and neonatal lipids, and pregnancy outcome: a randomized clinical trial. *Am J Obstetr Gynecol.* 2005;193:1292-1301.

90. Louie JC, Brand-Miller JC, Markovic TP, Ross GP, Moses RG. Glycemic index and pregnancy: a systematic literature review. *J Nutr Metab.* 2010;2010: 282-464.

91. DeBoo HA, Harding JE. The developmental origins of adult disease (Barker) hypothesis. *Austrail N Zealand J Obstet Gynecol.* 2006;46:4-14.

92. Beauchamp GK, Mennella JA. Flavor perception in human infants: development and functional significance. *Digestion.* 2011;83(suppl 1):1-6.

93. Herrmann TS, Siega-Riz AM, Hobel CJ, Aurora C, Dunkel-Schetter C. Prolonged periods without food intake during pregnancy increase risk for elevated maternal corticotropin-releasing hormone concentrations. *Am J Obst Gynecol.* 2001;185:403-412.

94. Kaplan M, Eidelman AI, Aboulafia Y. Fasting and the precipitation of labor. *JAMA.* 1983;250:1317-1318.

95. Mirghani HM, Hamud OA. The effect of maternal diet restriction on pregnancy outcome. *Am J Perinatol.* 2006;23(1):21-24.

96. Siega-Riz AM, Herrmann TS, Savitz DA, Thorp JM. Frequency of eating during pregnancy and its effect on preterm delivery. *Am J Epidemiol.* 2001;153: 647-652.

97. Barger MK. Maternal nutrition and perinatal outcomes. *J Midwifery Women's Health.* 2010;55(6): 502-511.

98. Fowles ER, Stang J, Bryant M, Kim S. Stress, depression, social support, and eating habits reduce diet quality in the first trimester in low-income women: a pilot study. *J Acad Nutr Diet.* 2012;112(10):1619-1625.

99. Lakin V, Haggarty P, Abramovich DR, et al. Dietary intake and tissue concentration of fatty acids in omnivore, vegetarian and diabetic pregnancy. *Prostaglandins Leukot Essent Fatty Acids.* 1998;59(3):209-220.

100. Sanders TA, Reddy S. The influence of a vegetarian diet on the fatty acid composition of human milk and the essential fatty acid status of the infant. *J Pediatr.* 1992;120(4 Pt 2):S71-S77.

101. Kirkpatrick SI, Dodd KW, Reedy J, Krebs-Smith SM. Income and race/ethnicity are associated with adherence to food-based dietary guidance among US adults and children. *J Acad Nutr Diet.* 2012;112(5): 624-635.

102. Havens EK, Martin KS, Yan J, Dauser-Forrest D, Ferris AM. Federal nutrition program changes and healthy food availability. *Am J Prev Med.* 2012;43(4): 419-422.

103. Whaley SE, Ritchie LD, Spector P, Gomez J. Revised WIC food package improves diets of WIC families. *J Nutr Educ Behav.* 2012;44(3):204-209.

104. Food and Nutrition Service, U.S. Department of Agriculture. *About WIC.* 2012. Available at: http ://www.fns.usda.gov/wic/aboutwic. Accessed May 13, 2013.

105. Luke B, Minogue J, Witter FR, Keith LG, Johnson TR. The ideal twin pregnancy: patterns of weight gain, discordancy, and length of gestation. *Am J Obstet Gynecol.* 1993;169(3):588-597.

106. Ostbye T, Krause KM, Swamy GK, Lovelady CA. Effect of breastfeeding on weight retention from one pregnancy to the next: results from the North Carolina WIC program. *Prev Med.* 2010;51(5):368-372.

107. Hollis BW, Wagner CL. The vitamin D requirement during human lactation: the facts and IOM's "utter" failure. *Public Health Nutr.* 2011;14(4):748-749.

108. Sicherer SH, Burks AW. Maternal and infant diets for prevention of allergic diseases: understanding menu changes in 2008. *J Allergy Clin Immunol.* 2008;122(1):29-33.

109. Olsen SF, Osterdal ML, Salvig JD, et al. Fish oil intake compared with olive oil intake in late pregnancy and asthma in the offspring: 16 y of registry-based follow-up from a randomized controlled trial. *Am J Clinl Nutr.* 2008;88(1):165-175.

110. Gunderson EP. Childbearing and obesity in women: weight before, during, and after pregnancy. *Obstet Gynecol Clin North Am.* 2009;36(2):317-332, ix.

111. Ip S, Chung M, Raman G, et al. Breastfeeding and maternal and infant health outcomes in developed countries. *Evid Rep Technol Assess (Full Rep).* 2007(153):1-186.

112. Lovelady CA, Garner KE, Moreno KL, Williams JP. The effect of weight loss in overweight, lactating women on the growth of their infants. *N Engl J Med.* 2000;342(7):449-453.

113. Davidsen L, Vistisen B, Astrup A. Impact of the menstrual cycle on determinants of energy balance: a putative role in weight loss attempts. *Int J Obes.* 2007;31(12):1777-1785.

114. Tucci SA, Murphy LE, Boyland EJ, Dye L, Halford JC. Oral contraceptive effects on food choice during the follicular and luteal phases of the menstrual cycle: a laboratory based study. *Appetite.* 2010;55(3):388-392.

115. Bryant M, Truesdale KP, Dye L. Modest changes in dietary intake across the menstrual cycle: implications for food intake research. *Br J Nutr.* 2006;96(5):888-894.

116. Centers for Disease Control and Prevention. Infertility fastfacts. 2011. Available at: http://wwwcdc gov/nchs/fastats/fertile.htm.

117. Chavarro JE, Willett WC, Skerrett PJ. *The Fertility Diet.* New York: McGraw-Hill; 2008.

118. World Cancer Fund, American Institute for Cancer Research. *Food, Nutrition, Physical Activity and the Prevention of Cancer: A Global Perspective* (2nd ed.). Washington, DC: AICR; 2009.

119. Christen WG, Liu S, Glynn RJ, Gaziano JM, Buring JE. Dietary carotenoids, vitamins C and E, and risk of cataract in women: a prospective study. *Arch Ophthalmol.* 2008;126(1):102-109.

120. Ogden CL, Carrol M. Prevalence of obesity among children and adolescents in the U.S.: trends 1963-1965 through 2007-2008. National Center for Health Statistics; 2010. Available at: http://www.cdc.gov/nchs/data/hestat/obesity_child_07_08/obesity_child_07_08.htm.

121. Biro FM, Greenspan LC, Galvez MP. Puberty in girls of the 21st century. *J Pediatr Adolesc Gynecol.* 2012;25(5):289-294.

122. Cheng G, Buyken AE, Shi L, et al. Beyond overweight: nutrition as an important lifestyle factor influencing timing of puberty. *Nutr Rev.* 2012;70(3):133-152.

123. Toth MJ, Tchernof A, Sites CK, Poehlman ET. Menopause-related changes in body fat distribution. *Ann N Y Acad Sci.* 2000;904:502-506.

124. Lethaby AE, Brown J, Marjoribanks J, Kronenberg F, Roberts H, Eden J. Phytoestrogens for vasomotor menopausal symptoms. *Cochrane Database Syst Rev.* 2007;4:CD001395.

● ● ● **Additional Resources**

Body Mass Calculator (English and Spanish)

- National Institutes of Health: http://www.nhlbi.nih.gov/guidelines/obesity/BMI/bmicalc.htm

BMI Calculator and Calories for Weight Goal

- WebMD: http://www.webmd.com/diet/calc-bmi-plus

Glycemic Index for Foods

- University of Sydney: http://www.glycemicindex.com

Evidenced-Based Nutrition Resources

- CDC Nutrition Topics: http://www.cdc.gov/nutrition/index.html

- Brown University Nutrition Academic Award Center: http://med.brown.edu/nutrition
  - Rapid Eating Assessment for Patients (REAP) tool
  - WAVE Assessment: Tool to assess weight, activity, and variety of foods eaten on one page

- The Nutrition Source, Harvard University School of Public Health: http://www.hsph.harvard.edu/nutritionsource

Patient Handouts About Nutrition

- Share with Women series—*Journal of Midwifery and Women's Health* and ACNM: http://www.midwife.org/Share-With-Women
- Sample of relevant titles:
  - *Vitamin D*
  - *Folic Acid: What's It All About?*
  - *Eating Safely During Pregnancy* (available in Spanish)
  - *Omega-3 Fatty Acids in Pregnancy*
  - *Weight Gain During Pregnancy* (includes graph to chart weight gain against IOM recommendations; available in Spanish)
  - *Women of Size in Pregnancy*

Other Governmental Resources

- USDA My Pyramid: http://www.mypyramid.gov (has interactive tools including for those who are pregnant and breastfeeding)
- USDA Nutrient Database: http://ndb.nal.usda.gov (interactive database to look up nutrient content of fresh and prepared foods)

CHAPTER

7

Health Promotion and Health Maintenance

KATHRYN OSBORNE

ANN F. COWLIN

Introduction

The *International Definition of the Midwife* from the International Confederation of Midwives articulates the key role midwives play in health education and counseling for women, their families, and the community, and clarifies that this role extends beyond pregnancy, into counseling and education on matters pertaining to women's health throughout the world.[1] Similarly, the American College of Nurse-Midwives (ACNM) has identified that wellness counseling, health promotion, and disease prevention are part of the scope of practice of certified nurse-midwives (CNMs) and certified midwives (CMs).[2] Both ACNM and the International Confederation of Midwives (ICM) address elements of health promotion and disease prevention in the essential/core competencies for entry-level midwifery practice,[3,4] and ACNM recognizes health promotion, disease prevention, and health education as hallmarks of the art and science of midwifery.[3] Therefore, it is essential for midwives to include health promotion as a component of the care they provide. This chapter provides information about health promotion and disease prevention services that aid in promoting and maintaining health for women across the lifespan.

The Midwife's Role in Health Promotion

One of the roles of the midwife is to facilitate women in becoming empowered to be active participants in maintaining their own health and partners in health-care decision making.[3,4] Providing women with the tools necessary to maintain optimal health is the essence of health promotion, and is done primarily through counseling and education. Maintaining optimal health also requires the conduct of specific screening at various intervals in a woman's life to ensure early detection of the onset of disease states. Furthermore, to aid women in becoming empowered to maintain their health and the health of their families, within the context of the communities in which women live, requires that midwives remain aware of the health status of the communities in which they live and practice and advocate for policies that promote healthy communities.

Definition of Terms

Participating in health promotion and health maintenance first requires an understanding of a few key concepts and terms. Each of the following concepts/terms is addressed in this chapter.

Health is defined in a number of ways, based largely on the context in which it is used. The World Health Organization (WHO) defines *health* as "a state of complete physical, mental, and social well-being and not merely the absence of disease or infirmity."[5] Alternatively, the Centers for Disease Control and Prevention (CDC) defines *health* as "a human condition with physical, social, and psychological dimensions, each characterized on a continuum with positive and negative poles. Positive health is associated with a capacity to enjoy life and withstand challenges; it is not merely the absence of disease. Negative health is associated with illness, and in the extreme, with premature death."[6] If health is conceptualized as occurring along a continuum, the goal of the midwife in health promotion is to identify each individual woman's health status and provide the preventive services necessary to keep that status moving in a positive direction.

Disease, for the purpose of this chapter, is defined as any disruption in the physical, emotional, or social functioning of a human being that interferes with the individual's capacity to maintain optimal physical, emotional, or social health.

Primary prevention involves the delivery of healthcare services that focus on preventing disease from occurring in a given population and in individuals.[7] Examples of primary preventive services provided for individual women include immunizations, counseling, and education. At the population/community level, primary preventive services include the implementation of policies that promote clean air, clean water, and workplace safety.

Secondary prevention involves the delivery of healthcare services aimed at early detection of disease states as well as early interventions that limit severity and resulting morbidity.[7] Identification of risk factors through a thorough health history and the conduct of routine screening at appropriate intervals in a woman's life are perhaps the most powerful secondary preventive services provided by midwives.

Tertiary prevention involves the delivery of healthcare services that restore optimal function, improve health status, and limit long-term disability following the identification of disease.[7] Although midwives are involved in the delivery of tertiary preventive services (the treatment of disease states), this chapter focuses on the midwife's role in the provision of primary and secondary preventive services for individual women. Delivery of tertiary preventive services is addressed in other chapters throughout this text.

Health Promotion

The United States spends more money on health care than any country in the world.[8] In 2010, the United States spent an average of $8,402 per person on health care, representing approximately 18% of the gross domestic product (GDP).[9] Based on spending trends, it is estimated that by 2017, annual per capita spending on health care will grow to slightly more than $13,000 per person.[8] Despite the fact that health care spending in the United States far exceeds spending in other countries, the United States has poorer health outcomes on most measures than any other developed nation.[8] Reasons for the rapid growth in U.S. healthcare spending are multifaceted, although research suggests that the cost associated with the treatment of chronic diseases, which are often preventable, is a key contributor.[8–10]

The causes of poor health outcomes in the United States are equally complex. Public health leaders, however, point to the lack of attention paid to health promotion as a primary contributor, estimating that 75% of healthcare spending in the United States goes toward the treatment of preventable disease, while only 3% is devoted to preventive services.[10] A substantial body of evidence demonstrates that increasing the delivery of preventive health services to improve population health will lead to reduced healthcare spending,[8,9] increased productivity, and improvements in quality of life.[8–10]

Rising rates of chronic disease include those conditions that are largely consequences of unhealthy behaviors such as obesity.[11] Associated conditions such as type 2 diabetes, cancer, hypertension, and heart disease not only place a financial burden on healthcare delivery systems, but also lead to a higher risk of decreased quality of life and premature death for the individual with the condition.[8,10] Stopping the onset of chronic disease through primary preventive strategies is the leading goal of health promotion. As part of this mission, key components of health promotion include health education and counseling. This chapter addresses counseling and education for women across the lifespan; education and counseling provided specifically to pregnant women are addressed in detail in later in this text.

Education and Counseling

The leading causes of death in women, which include heart disease, cancer, stroke, chronic respiratory disease, and diabetes,[12] are strongly associated with lifestyle-related behaviors. Therefore, modifying behaviors such as inactivity, poor dietary habits, and tobacco use can reduce a woman's risk for disease-related morbidity and early death. To achieve this goal, midwives and other healthcare providers should be aware that counseling and education aimed at improving personal health practices are likely the most effective tools used in health promotion.[13] In turn, it is important to implement this intervention in such a way that the counseling and education are meaningful to each individual woman. Just as midwives individualize their care for women in labor and birth,[14] so, too, must they customize the care provided for health promotion. An individualized education and counseling plan is based primarily on the findings of a thorough health history and physical exam during which the midwife identifies the health risks that need to be addressed.

Learning Theory

The principles of adult learning provide a framework within which health education can be customized to meet each woman's needs. The primary goal of adult learners is to acquire skills and resources that can be applied in their daily lives, rather than simply to acquire information. Adolescents who have begun to take responsibility for making their own lifestyle decisions will also benefit from the self-directed learning that is facilitated using the principles of adult learning, as summarized in **Box 7-1**.[15] For adults, learning is a process for which the "teacher" becomes a facilitator.

Recognizing the external motivators for adult learners is an important first step in establishing a health promotion plan. To best encourage women and girls to make lifestyle changes, a midwife must know what motivates them and must determine their level of commitment or self-efficacy. By investigating why the woman wants to change behavior—that is, what she deems to be the benefit of behavior change—the midwife gains valuable insight into which types of interventions will be most effective in helping a woman achieve her goals. The woman's talents and skills, combined with her existing beliefs, can be incorporated into the approach used to achieve behavior change. For example, when establishing a plan to increase physical activity, it is important to understand that adolescents may be interested in skill

acquisition, helping others, making friends, or physical appearance. Women of all ages may view physical activity as an outlet for stress; as a way to lose weight, prevent weight gain, and tone muscles; as a way to maintain or increase physical strength; as a means by which to meet new friends; or as the best prevention for diseases such as diabetes or hypertension. Within the parameters of these motivations, the midwife can work with each woman to identify types of exercise or activity that the woman feels comfortable incorporating into her life.

Most women are unlikely to benefit from provider-driven teaching, in which the midwife decides what the woman needs to know and when she needs to know it. Instead, women are more likely to understand and implement the information provided during a teaching/counseling session when the learning is woman centered—in other words, when the woman has identified a need to know and readiness to learn, and when the learning builds on the woman's prior experience.

An important component of any teaching and counseling plan is the provision of anticipatory guidance. The advent of the Internet and multiple sources of health information has led to a well-informed population of healthcare consumers. Nevertheless, not all women are fully informed about the wide range of recommended preventive services, and some may not think to investigate a topic that the midwife expects will be of importance. It is, therefore, incumbent upon the midwife to anticipate the healthcare needs of each woman (based on risk factors) and provide individualized counseling about appropriate health services across the lifespan.

What to Address

After determining how to present the information, the next important step is to identify which content to address during a given clinical encounter. Again, using the principles of adult learning, this step is completed with the woman and the midwife acting in a partnership. Women often present to a clinical encounter with specific questions for their healthcare providers. In those instances, it is easy to design a teaching plan based on the explicitly expressed needs of the woman. Whether the woman presents for a lengthy appointment for an annual physical exam or for a brief appointment with a specific concern, it is important for the midwife to honor (and respond to) the learning needs that are identified by the woman, especially when the time spent with the woman is limited. For example, when a visibly overweight woman presents to the clinic with concerns that her partner

---

BOX 7-1 Assumptions Inherent in Adult Learning Theory

- Adults need to know why they need to learn something before learning it.
- The self-concept of adults is heavily dependent upon a move toward self-direction.
- Prior experiences of the learner provide a rich resource for learning.
- Adults typically become ready to learn when they experience a need to cope with a life situation or perform a task.
- Adults' orientation to learning is life centered; education is a process of developing increased competency levels to achieve their full potential.
- The motivation for adult learners is internal rather than external.

Source: Adapted from Knowles MS, Holton EF, Swanson RA. *The Adult Learner* (7th ed.). Burlington, MA: Elsevier; 2011.

has "been with other women" and consequently fears that she has acquired a sexually transmitted infection (STI), the best approach is for the midwife to provide counseling interventions based on the woman's concerns. Such a visit is not the time to discuss a weight management plan, despite the fact that the midwife has recognized weight management as an area of health promotion that needs to be addressed. Following the lead of the woman allows the midwife to capitalize on a teachable moment, immediately address the woman's health concern, and plan for future visits wherein additional learning will more effectively take place.

When designing a teaching/counseling plan, the midwife should include only topics and content for which evidence of effectiveness exists. Time is a precious commodity in a busy practice setting. Moreover, in 2003, the Institute of Medicine issued a report recommending that all health professionals be educated to deliver patient-centered (in this case, woman-centered) care with an emphasis on evidence-based practice.[16] Therefore, the remainder of this section focuses on evidence-based teaching and counseling for women across the lifespan.

Evidence-Based Counseling Interventions

For the past two decades, healthcare providers have been strongly encouraged to participate in what has come to be known as evidence-based practice (EBP) or the delivery of evidence-based care. One of the earliest definitions of evidence-based practice was "the conscientious, explicit, and judicious use of current best evidence in making decisions about the care of individual patients. The practice of evidence-based medicine means integrating individual clinical expertise with the best available clinical evidence from systematic research."[17] Nursing leaders expanded this definition to include the values and preferences of individuals when making decisions about health care.[18] Using this broader definition of EBP, it is important that midwives consider scientific evidence, their own professional experience, and the values and preferences of individual women when establishing a health promotion management plan. These values and preferences include anything that makes an individual woman unique, such as religious and cultural beliefs, literacy levels, and the woman's prior experience and knowledge.

Professional organizations (such as the American Congress of Obstetricians and Gynecologists) and specialty groups (such as the American Cancer Society) have been advancing recommendations regarding preventive services for several decades.

However, it was not until the 1989 publication of *Guide to Clinical Preventive Services* by the U.S. Preventive Services Task Force (USPSTF) that healthcare professionals were provided with recommendations that were based on an unbiased review of scientific evidence. The USPSTF was originally convened in 1984 by the U.S. Public Health Service and is now sponsored by the Agency for Healthcare Research and Quality (AHRQ). Its mission is "to evaluate the benefits of individual services based on age, gender, and risk factors for disease; make recommendations about which preventive services should be incorporated routinely into primary medical care and for which populations; and identify a research agenda for clinical preventive care."[19] The recommendations of the USPSTF now are considered the "gold standard" for clinical preventive services.[19]

Adopting evidence-based practices is not always easy. One of the fundamental ethical principles upon which healthcare delivery is based is the principle of nonmaleficence, which means to do no intentional harm. Healthcare practitioners want and need to know that the care they provide is safe and not harmful for their clients. Consequently, accepting new evidence that suggests an accepted clinical practice may be harmful can be challenging. A classic example can be seen in changes that have occurred in maternity care regarding the routine use of episiotomy. For many decades, physicians, and some midwives, routinely cut episiotomies because they believed that doing so was better for both the woman and neonate. Implementing the current evidence that cutting episiotomies is more likely to cause harm than is a spontaneous perineal tear has required maternity care providers to accept the need to change practice.

Similarly, in 2009, the USPSTF published new recommendations for breast cancer screening, which included a recommendation *against* teaching women to do breast self-examination (BSE)—the scientific evidence revealed moderate certainty that the harms associated with teaching BSE outweigh the benefits.[20] Accepting the idea that teaching BSE may be harmful, and accepting the need to change current practice with regard to breast cancer screening, has not been easy. Most midwives have been teaching BSE since they began clinical practice and often can cite examples of women who were adamant that their lives were saved because they found a mass during self-examination. However, implementing evidence-based preventive services requires that midwives establish individualized plans for health promotion that are based on best evidence rather than what they "believe" is best practice.

To aid clinicians in selecting evidence-based approaches, the USPSTF provides recommendations for clinical preventive services, including counseling interventions. Recommendations reflect the strength of the available evidence and the magnitude of net benefit from the intervention (benefit minus harms). Professionals may find minor differences in the grading of evidence by the USPSTF based on the year in which the recommendations were made. Recommendations from 2007 to today are based on categories that have been modified from the pre-2007 scale (Table 7-1). Grade A remains an intervention that should be offered to women. Table 7-2 illustrates the current accompanying level of certainty regarding net benefits.

Although the USPSTF has provided many recommendations, there remain some services for which there is insufficient evidence to make a recommendation. In those instances, clinicians decide whether to use a given service based on their own clinical judgment and women's preferences, and women should be informed about the lack of available evidence (or conflicting evidence) to recommend use of the service. Furthermore, the updating of recommendations is an ongoing process for the USPSTF; as new evidence regarding preventive health services emerges, recommendations are modified to reflect the current body of evidence. Presented here are the major counseling interventions recommended by the USPSTF, as of the time of this text's publication, for women across the lifespan. Readers are advised to regularly review the website of the USPSTF for updates of these recommendations, as well as for the addition of new recommendations for preventive services.

Behavioral Counseling

As previously mentioned, leading causes of death in women are related to lifestyle behaviors such as inactivity, tobacco use, and poor dietary habits. Therefore, most of the counseling interventions that are recommended for women involve the implementation of some type of lifestyle change or avoidance of risky behaviors. *Behavioral counseling interventions* include education, counseling, and other interventions provided in primary care settings that are focused on assisting women to adopt new behaviors, change existing behaviors that lead to poor health

Table 7-1	U.S. Preventive Services Task Force Grade Definitions After May 2007	
Grade	**Definition**	**Suggestions for Practice**
A	The USPSTF recommends the service. There is high certainty that the net benefit is substantial.	Offer or provide this service.
B	The USPSTF recommends the service. There is high certainty that the net benefit is moderate or there is moderate certainty that the net benefit is moderate to substantial.	Offer or provide this service.
C	*Note: The following statement is undergoing revision.* Clinicians may provide this service to selected patients depending on individual circumstances. However, for most individuals without signs or symptoms, there is likely to be only a small benefit from this service.	Offer or provide this service only if other considerations support the offering or providing the service in an individual patient.
D	The USPSTF recommends against the service. There is moderate or high certainty that the service has no net benefit or that the harms outweigh the benefits.	Discourage the use of this service.
I Statement	The USPSTF concludes that the current evidence is insufficient to assess the balance of benefits and harms of the service. Evidence is lacking, of poor quality, or conflicting, and the balance of benefits and harms cannot be determined.	Read the clinical considerations section of USPSTF Recommendation Statement. If the service is offered, patients should understand the uncertainty about the balance of benefits and harms.

Source: U.S. Preventive Services Task Force. Introduction. 2010. Available at: http://www.uspreventiveservicestaskforce.org/intro.htm. Accessed September 15, 2012.

Table 7-2	Levels of Certainty Regarding Evidence of Net Benefit for Health Outcomes
Level of Certainty[*]	**Description**
High	The available evidence usually includes consistent results from well-designed, well-conducted studies in representative primary care populations. These studies assess the effects of the preventive service on health outcomes. This conclusion is therefore unlikely to be strongly affected by the results of future studies.
Moderate	The available evidence is sufficient to determine the effects of the preventive service on health outcomes, but confidence in the estimate is constrained by factors such as the following: <ul><li>The number, size, or quality of individual studies</li><li>Inconsistency of findings across individual studies</li><li>Limited generalizability of findings to routine primary care practice</li><li>Lack of coherence in the chain of evidence</li></ul> As more information becomes available, the magnitude or direction of the observed effect could change, and this change may be large enough to alter the conclusion.
Low	The available evidence is insufficient to assess effects on health outcomes. Evidence is insufficient because of the following factors: <ul><li>The limited number or size of studies</li><li>Important flaws in study design or methods</li><li>Inconsistency of findings across individual studies</li><li>Gaps in the chain of evidence</li><li>Findings not generalizable to routine primary care practice</li><li>Lack of information on important health outcomes</li></ul> More information may allow estimation of effects on health outcomes.

[*]The USPSTF defines certainty as "likelihood that the USPSTF assessment of the net benefit of a preventive service is correct." The net benefit is defined as benefit minus harm of the preventive service as implemented in a general, primary care population. The USPSTF assigns a certainty level based on the nature of the overall evidence available to assess the net benefit of a preventive service.

Source: U.S. Preventive Services Task Force. Introduction. 2010. Available at: http://www.uspreventiveservicestaskforce.org/intro.htm. Accessed September 15, 2012.

outcomes, and maintain behaviors that improve health status.[21]

Alcohol Misuse

According to the CDC, 51.5% of nonpregnant women and 7.6% of pregnant women use alcohol. However, an occasional drink is not the issue. Instead, excessive alcohol intake, either chronically or episodically, can have negative health implications. For example, 15% of nonpregnant women and 1.4% of pregnant women report participating in episodic (binge) drinking, which for women is the consumption of more than three alcoholic beverages on one occasion.[22] The risks associated with excessive alcohol use in women include liver disease, heart disease, brain damage, some forms of cancer, sexual assault, unintended pregnancy and STIs, accidental injury, and premature death.[23] For pregnant women, any consumption of alcohol may lead to fetal alcohol syndrome and other disorders along the fetal alcohol

spectrum.[22,23] Diseases caused by alcohol misuse, including fetal alcohol syndrome, are preventable.

The USPSTF recommends that healthcare providers in primary care settings screen all adults, including pregnant women, for alcohol misuse and provide counseling interventions to reduce misuse. The Task Force found insufficient evidence to recommend for or against screening and counseling interventions for adolescents.[23]

This point of discussion illustrates the difference between screening and assessment: The purpose of *screening* is to identify women who may have a problem with alcohol misuse, while the purpose of *assessment* is to identify the extent of the alcohol problem for women with a positive screen.[24] As primary care providers, the recommendation for midwives is to periodically screen all women and provide a brief intervention to reduce alcohol misuse; women who continue to misuse alcohol may be alcohol dependent and should be referred for further assessment and treatment.[24]

Ideally, screening for alcohol misuse should take place in settings that allow for assessment and follow-up of women with a positive screen. Midwives who work in settings without resources for follow-up care will need to identify healthcare providers in the community (or surrounding area) to whom women with a positive screen can be referred.

Many reliable tools to screen women for alcohol misuse have been developed, though perhaps the most easily and widely used tools recommended for use in primary care settings are the CAGE and T-ACE.[23,25] After assuring the woman that the information she shares will remain confidential, the midwife can administer either of these instruments during the collection of a complete health history or separately for a brief assessment of alcohol misuse.

As is true for the entire health history, it is important to remain nonjudgmental when asking questions about sensitive topics such as alcohol use. Screening for alcohol misuse begins by asking the woman how much alcohol she drinks. If the woman indicates that she never consumes any alcohol, the screen is complete. Documentation in the medical record should include the finding of a negative screen for alcohol misuse and a plan to rescreen in one year. If the woman indicates that she consumes any alcohol, the screen continues using a reliable screening instrument such as the CAGE or T-ACE. The CAGE

instrument has just four questions and is designed to assess lifetime alcohol use (**Box 7-2**). The TACE instrument (**Box 7-3**), also has four questions and is particularly sensitive for identification of prenatal alcohol use.[23,25]

Behavioral counseling interventions are implemented after the woman has been screened for alcohol misuse and vary depending on the findings of the initial screen. All pregnant women and women who are planning a pregnancy should be counseled about the harmful effects of alcohol on the fetus. As no level of alcohol use is considered safe in pregnancy, such counseling should include a recommendation to abstain from any alcohol use during pregnancy.[23]

Women with a positive screen for alcohol misuse should be counseled about the harmful effects of alcohol and referred for further assessment and possible treatment for alcohol abuse. Informing a woman about the finding of a positive screen and the need for referral must be done with sensitivity. The best approach is to tell the woman that her responses to the screening questions raise a concern that her alcohol use may be harmful and that she would benefit from meeting with a provider who specializes in alcohol

---

BOX 7-2 CAGE Questions

C: Have you ever felt you should **cut down** on your drinking?

A: Have people **annoyed** you by criticizing your drinking?

G: Have you ever felt bad or **guilty** about your drinking?

E: Eye opener: Have you ever had a drink first thing in the morning to steady your nerves or to get rid of a hangover?

Two or more positive responses indicate a positive screen.

Source: National Institute on Alcohol Abuse and Alcoholism. Screening tests. n.d. Available at: http://pubs.niaaa.nih .gov/publications/arh28-2/78-79.htm. Accessed October 2, 2012.

BOX 7-3 TACE Instrument

T: Tolerance: How many drinks does it take to make you feel high? (more than two drinks = 2 points)

A: Have people **annoyed** you by criticizing your drinking? (1 point)

C: Have you ever felt you ought to **cut down** on your drinking? (1 point)

E: Eye opener: Have you ever had a drink first thing in the morning to steady your nerves or get rid of a hangover? (1 point)

A score of two or more points indicates a positive screen.

Sources: U.S. Preventive Services Task Force. Screening and behavioral counseling interventions in primary care to reduce alcohol misuse: recommendation statement. 2004. Available at: http://www.uspreventiveservicestaskforce. org/3rduspstf/alcohol/alcomisrs.htm#clinical. Accessed October 2, 2012; National Institute on Alcohol Abuse and Alcoholism. Screening tests. n.d. Available at: http://pubs .niaaa.nih.gov/publications/arh28-2/78-79.htm. Accessed October 2, 2012.

counseling. For example, the midwife might address the referral in the following way:

> One of the things we know about alcohol is that it can cause serious health problems for women who drink more than what is considered safe. For women, having more than seven drinks per week or more than three drinks on one occasion is considered "risky or hazardous" drinking.[23,24] Based on your response to the questions I asked about alcohol use, your use of alcohol may fall into that category of risky or hazardous. It may be that this is not the case, but just to be sure, I would like you to see one of my colleagues who is very skilled at assessing alcohol use and at helping women make changes in their alcohol use before it has a negative effect on their health.

The most effective and efficient behavioral counseling intervention for women in whom risky drinking behaviors have been identified is based on the *Five As* construct (assess, advise, agree, assist, arrange), as outlined in **Box 7-4**.[21] The same approach may also be of value when identifying use of other substances of abuse in addition to alcohol.

Documentation in the woman's record should include the finding of a positive screen for alcohol misuse, a description of the behavioral counseling intervention that was provided and referrals that were made, and the plan for return visits for ongoing support.

Most women who use alcohol do so within the limits that are considered safe. For these women, the goal of behavioral counseling is to prevent the onset of risky or hazardous drinking. Counseling should include reminders about safe use limits and recommendations for abstinence when necessary (such as when pregnant or planning a pregnancy, or when medication use or other health conditions warrant abstinence).[26] Documentation in the health record should include the finding of a negative screen for alcohol misuse and plans to rescreen in one year.

Breastfeeding

The benefits of breastfeeding for mothers and infants are well documented. One of the goals of *Healthy People 2020*—the federal government's national goals for health improvement throughout the United States—is to increase the proportion of infants who are breastfed. Breastfeeding was initiated by 76.9% of the women who gave birth in 2009. During that same year, 47.2% of infants were breastfeeding at

---

BOX 7-4 Five As for Alcohol Misuse

- **Assess** or ask the woman about alcohol use and her desire to change behavior.
- **Advise** the woman to change risky behavior using a personalized approach that includes information about the harmful effects of alcohol use and benefits of changing behavior.
- **Agree upon** treatment goals and approaches to changing behavior.
- **Assist** the woman in achieving agreed upon goals by providing education, support and encouragement, and formal counseling when necessary. This may include helping the woman identify sources of social support for change.
- **Arrange** follow-up visits for ongoing assistance with behavioral change and referral to treatment when necessary.

Although these questions have been developed to conduct a brief intervention for alcohol misuse, the questions can be modified for use with brief interventions to aid women with other behavioral changes such as tobacco use or weight loss.

Source: Whitlock EP, Orleans CT, Pender N, Allan J. Evaluating primary care behavioral counseling interventions: an evidence-based approach. *Am J Prev Med.* 2002;22(4): 267-284.

---

6 months and 25.5% were breastfeeding at 1 year.[27] These figures reflect significant increases over the past several years, largely credited to changes in maternity care practices.[27] The *Healthy People 2020* goals for infant feeding are to increase the proportion of infants who are ever breastfed to 81.9%; the number of infants breastfed at 6 months to 60.6%; and the number of infants breastfed at 1 year to 34.1%.[28]

The USPSTF has recognized that interventions in primary care settings to promote breastfeeding lead to increased rates of breastfeeding initiation as well as increased duration of breastfeeding. Therefore, it recommends interventions during pregnancy and the postpartum period to promote breastfeeding and ongoing support for women who choose to breastfeed.[29] The most effective interventions use combined approaches to breastfeeding support, such as formal education for women and families, direct support and observation of mothers, health professional training in breastfeeding support, and peer support and counseling.[29]

Dental Health

Dental health is often not considered by primary care providers, yet dental disease can have profound adverse implications, such as increasing the risk of cardiovascular disease among all individuals and the risk of preterm birth for women who are pregnant. The last recommendations for counseling interventions to prevent dental disease were established in 1996. Those recommendations were to counsel individuals to floss and brush their teeth daily with a fluoride-containing toothpaste and to regularly see a dental provider.[30] Since that time, there has been no new evidence regarding the primary provider's role in promoting oral health, so the USPSTF has elected to maintain the 1996 recommendation and not modify it.[31]

Dietary Counseling

The benefits of healthy eating and the risks associated with an unhealthy diet are well documented. Of the 10 leading causes of death in women, four are related to diet—namely, heart disease, certain forms of cancer, stroke, and diabetes.[12] Assessing the dietary counseling needs of individual women first requires the collection of a 24- to 48-hour recall diet history to evaluate nutritional and caloric intake, the collection of height and weight data for calculation of body mass index (BMI), and collection of the health history for identification of health risk factors that may be related to diet. The recall diet history is collected by asking the woman to record everything she eats in a 24- to 48-hour period, and then this information is analyzed for caloric intake and nutritional adequacy by the midwife. See the *Nutrition* chapter for a complete discussion of BMI calculation.

A BMI of less than 18.5 is considered "underweight"; a BMI in the range 18.5–24.9 is considered "normal"; a BMI in the range 25–29.9 is considered "overweight"; and a BMI of 30 or higher is considered "obese."[32] Women whose weight is categorized as underweight, overweight, or obese are at increased risk for weight-related morbidity and mortality. Poor dietary intake is a modifiable risk factor for several diseases, including certain forms of cancer and coronary artery disease. As such, improving dietary intake can result in improvements in overall health status, especially for women with additional risk factors (such as hypertension, hyperlipidemia, and family history) for diet-related diseases.[33] The USPSTF recommends intensive behavioral dietary counseling for adults with hyperlipidemia and other risk factors for cardiovascular and diet-related chronic disease.[33] It also recommends

offering women with a BMI of 30 or higher intensive, multicomponent behavioral interventions.[34] The decision to offer diet counseling to women without risk factors for coronary artery disease should be made on an individual basis based on the healthcare needs of the woman.[35]

The *Nutrition* chapter contains a detailed description of dietary recommendations and healthy eating. Similar to the brief intervention for alcohol misuse, the most effective and efficient behavioral counseling interventions for women who are overweight or obese, or who are at increased risk for diet-related disease, are based on the *Five As* construct.[33] The *Five As for Alcohol Misuse* can be modified for use with women who are overweight or obese. Documentation in the health record should include findings of the dietary assessment, health risk assessment, and BMI as well as a description of the counseling that was provided.

Injury Prevention

Unintentional injury is the sixth leading cause of death in women in the United States.[12] Although such injuries are usually related to accidents and, therefore, are difficult to control, the USPSTF recognizes several interventions that can effectively limit the risk for unintentional injury. The USPSTF found insufficient evidence to assess the balance of benefits and harms of counseling individuals about proper use of seat belts and child safety seats, however. One reason for this equivocation is that legislative action and community-based intervention, combined with counseling in the primary care setting, have led to substantial increases in the number of persons in the United States who properly use motor vehicle restraints.[36] Approximately 80% of adults use seat belts, and the rate of proper use of child safety seats is estimated at 90%.[36] Whether routine counseling women in primary care settings would increase proper use rates even further is largely unknown.

Nevertheless, the USPSTF recognizes that in the United States, injuries related to motor vehicle occupancy are the leading cause of death for children, adolescents, and young adults up to age 33 years, and the leading cause of death from accidental injury for individuals of all ages. It estimates the harms from counseling about proper motor vehicle safety restraints to be minimal, if any, and notes that the proper use of safety restraints limits the fatality risk by 45% to 70%.[36] Therefore, in addition to supporting policies and community-based interventions that encourage proper use of motor vehicle restraints, counseling women to use motor vehicle restraints properly is likely to cause no harm and may lead to further reductions in motor vehicle–related injury and death. The most effective behavioral counseling interventions are those that include education, demonstration, and distribution/placement of safety restraints, rather than education alone.[37]

Proper use of adult restraints includes wearing the seat belt at all times and making sure that the lap and shoulder belts are properly positioned across the pelvis and ribcage. The shoulder belt should be placed across the middle of the chest and away from the neck; the lap belt should be secured below the stomach and across the hips.[38] Women who are pregnant should be advised to wear a seat belt at all times, with the shoulder strap laying across the chest (between the breasts) and away from the neck. The lap belt should be secured below the abdomen so that it fits snugly across the hips and pelvic bone, as illustrated in **Figure 7-1**. Pregnant women should be further advised to adjust the seat as far back as possible, such that the foot pedals can be comfortably operated and at least 10 inches is maintained between the chest and the steering wheel.[38] Parents should be counseled about proper use of child restraints; the basic principles are outlined in **Box 7-5**.

The findings of the USPSTF with regard to counseling to reduce the incidence of driving under the influence of alcohol and/or other drugs are similar to the findings relative to counseling individuals about the use of motor vehicle safety restraints. The most effective approach to reduce the number of alcohol-related motor vehicle accidents is to include information about "drinking and driving" in behavioral counseling interventions for those individuals who screen positive for alcohol misuse.[36] The USPSTF estimates the harms associated with counseling intended to prevent alcohol-related motor vehicle accidents in adolescents and adults to be minimal, if any, and notes that alcohol is involved in approximately 40% of all U.S. traffic fatalities.[36] Therefore, counseling women about the danger associated with drinking and driving is likely not harmful and may result in fewer alcohol-related motor vehicle accidents. For adolescents, this counseling should include establishing a plan for alternative transportation when in the company of an impaired driver.

Distracted driving is a relatively newly identified phenomenon, and interventions to prevent morbidity and mortality related to this practice have not been evaluated by the USPSTF. Distracted driving refers to driving while doing other things—most specifically, talking on a cell phone and sending/reading text messages. In 2010, more than 3000 persons were killed in the United States in motor vehicle accidents

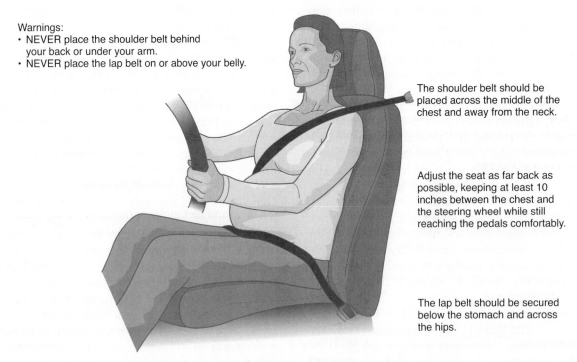

"HOW SHOULD I WEAR A SEAT BELT SAFELY WHILE I'M PREGNANT?"

Warnings:
• NEVER place the shoulder belt behind your back or under your arm.
• NEVER place the lap belt on or above your belly.

The shoulder belt should be placed across the middle of the chest and away from the neck.

Adjust the seat as far back as possible, keeping at least 10 inches between the chest and the steering wheel while still reaching the pedals comfortably.

The lap belt should be secured below the stomach and across the hips.

Figure 7-1 Proper placement of seat belt for women during pregnancy.

caused by distracted driving.[38] As is true for counseling about the dangers associated with drinking and driving, counseling adolescents and adults about the dangers associated with distracted driving, with strong recommendations to refrain from talking on hand-held cell phones and sending/reading text messages, may result in fewer distracted driving–related automobile accidents.

For women age 65 years and older, falls are the leading cause of injury-related death and the most common cause of nonfatal injuries and trauma-related hospitalization.[39] The USPSTF recommends regular exercise or physical therapy for falls prevention in women age 65 years and older.[40] Recommendations for exercise include participation in weight-bearing exercises, leg-strengthening exercises, and exercises that improve balance (such as Tai Chi).[39] Additional recommendations to reduce falls in women age 65 years and older include the identification of, and warnings regarding, medications that cause dizziness or drowsiness; reducing tripping hazards in the home, along with the addition of grab bars and improved lighting; and yearly eye examination with update of corrective lenses as needed.[39]

Physical Activity

Physical fitness is a cornerstone of health and an effective strategy for the reduction of disease.[41] Public health experts recognize that adequate, appropriate physical activity is a factor in the prevention of premature death, heart disease, type 2 diabetes, obesity, infertility, some cancers, osteoporosis, osteoarthritis, falls, and anxiety and depression for both women and men.[42] A total of 150 minutes per week of moderate-intensity exercise is the current minimum recommendation for adults to maintain health and fitness (30 minutes per day at least 5 times per week, or vigorous-intensity physical activity 75 minutes per week).[43] The CDC additionally recommends muscle-strengthening activities on 2 or more days per week that work all major muscle groups.

Support from a healthcare provider can be a significant factor in helping women recognize available resources and make a successful lifestyle change. In addition to the recommendations for counseling about exercise for the prevention of cardiovascular disease, obesity, and falls in older women, counseling about physical activity may be effective in improving overall physical health.[44] This section describes how to assess exercise level, screen for motivation and relevant health factors at various ages, and explore physical activity resources for an individual woman, based on motivation and stage of self-efficacy.

Vital to assessing and counseling women about their exercise regimens is a general understanding of the components of exercise, their effects on health, and which activities provide specific exercise components. **Table 7-3** reviews key points related to this topic.

Exercise intensity is an important consideration when providing counseling. The level of exertion must be safe, yet adequate to accomplish the desired goal. The threshold for effectively improving cardiovascular and metabolic parameters—a key factor in the health benefit of exercise—is activity that is above 3 metabolic equivalents (METs). One MET equals 3.5 mL O_2/kg/min. The more METs the person can tolerate, the greater will be her functional capacity, meaning her ability to metabolize oxygen and recover rapidly following exertion. Functional capacity improves with regular, sustained aerobic exercise. Activities in the MET range of 4–9 are adequate for enhancing functional capacity and are considered moderate at the lower end to vigorous at the higher

Table 7-3	Components of Exercise		
Exercise Component	**Description**	**Effects**	**Examples**
Cardiovascular endurance	Movements that increase pulse, respiration, and metabolic rate	**Chronic:** protection from some disorders and diseases. *Low intensity:* reduction in CVD and events. *Moderate intensity:* greater reduction in CVD and events; some protection from metabolic disorders and cancers; reduction of fat mass, waist/hip ratio, and BMI. *High intensity:* greatest protection from disease and all-cause mortality. **Acute:** feelings of vigor and well-being.	Walking, tai chi, jogging, running, cycling, swimming, aerobics, aerobic dance, step aerobics, dance, rowing
Muscular endurance	High number of repetitions of low-resistance weight training	**Chronic:** improves endurance of target muscle groups; useful for long-endurance, low-intensity repetitious events (e.g., labor/birth). **Acute:** can cause soreness.	Transverse abdominal exercises, squats, pelvic floor exercises
Strength	Overcoming resistance or weight by leverage using muscles as power	Improves health by increasing metabolism and lowering fat mass; increases muscle mass and power; higher intensity allowing fewer repetitions builds more power.	Weight lifting, calisthenics, isometrics (e.g., yoga or ballet), Pilates
Flexibility	Increasing range of motion through dynamic or passive stretching	Can cause injury when done at start of exercise without some aerobic warm-up. When controlled properly, increases range of motion and improves balance and coordination.	Isometrics, passive or held stretches, yoga, dance
Mind/body	Skills that promote mindfulness during active exercise or stress management exercises	Improves balance and coordination for specific events; can produce trophotropic or relaxation response, helping body recover from stress; produces feelings of well-being and ease of mind while still or moving.	Neutral posture and deep breathing, meditation, mindful moving, imagery, relaxation
Combination activities	Activities or classes that include several components	For amateur and competitive athletes and dancers, appropriate amounts provide a wide range of physical and mental health protections.	Most sports, dance, general exercise class, or constructed activity session

CVD = cardiovascular disease.

Source: Reprinted with permission from Cowlin AF. *Basic Pre/Postnatal Fitness Teacher Training Workbook.* Branford, CT: DPT, Inc.; 2010.

end. Activities at or below 3 METs are appropriate for sedentary women who are starting to exercise. Examples of activities and their MET levels are reviewed in **Table 7-4.**[45]

Strength training at or above the threshold level of 8 to 12 repetitions of exercises challenging each of the major muscle groups, two times per week, has been shown to improve metabolic function. Mind/ body or *mindfulness* activities that elicit the *trophotropic effect*, or relaxation response, have been found to provide acute relief of physiologic stress.[46] Activities in these categories include progressive relaxation, meditation, autogenic training, hypnosis, and yoga when a meditative approach is included.

An important first step toward establishing or encouraging an exercise program for women and girls is the collection of a complete history, including a 24- to 48-hour food diary. Specific questions about activity interests and motivation, along with health screening, open up avenues for discussion regarding the types of activities a girl or woman regularly participates in. With the information obtained during a health history, the midwife is able to compile a comprehensive picture of the nutrition status, fitness level, and lifestyle choices of the woman and to assess/categorize her activity levels, as shown in **Box 7-6.**

Prior to initiation of any exercise program, a woman should be screened for medication use,

existence of acute or chronic health conditions, past or current injuries, and lifestyle factors that could affect a girl's or woman's health and ability to exercise. Answers to specific questions about the types of current activities of women and girls allow the midwife to calculate current exertion levels (METs) and the need to alter activity levels. Medical or trauma conditions should be taken into consideration for any adjustments made to an exercise regimen. For the woman who is pregnant, exercise assessment must include identification of conditions that are contraindications to exercise.

While some exercise is beneficial, it is clear that up to a point, the more fit an individual, the greater her protection from all-cause mortality.[47,48] Keeping factors such as BMI, body fat, and waist/hip ratio within a healthy range requires adequate levels of calorie output each week. For a woman with an established exercise habit, the midwife's goal is to support and encourage her participation in a beneficial exercise regimen. For women with little or no current exercise, the midwife's challenge is to help them make small, incremental steps toward an active life

Table 7-4	Examples of Activities and Associated Metabolic Equivalents Levels
METs	**Examples**
Light 2–3 METs	Bowling Gardening Golf Shuffleboard Walking 2 MPH Yoga
Moderate 4–5 METs	Calisthenics (light) Cycling 8–10 MPH Gymnastics Skating 8–9 MPH Volleyball Walking 3–4 MPH
Moderate 6–7 METs	Cycling 11–12 MPH Cross Country Skiing Dancing (moderate) Downhill Skiing Tennis (singles) Walking 4–5 MPH
Heavy 7–9 METs	Aerobic dance Basketball Cycling 12–13 MPH Jogging 5–6 MPH Mountain Climbing Swimming
Heavy 10+ METs	Aerobics (vigorous) Cycling 14+ MPH Handball (fast) Running 6+ MPH Snowshoeing (fast) Swimming (fast)

MET = metabolic equivalents.
Source: Adapted from Ainsworth BE, Haskell WL, Whitt MC, et al. Compendium of physical activities: an update of activity codes and MET intensities. *Med Sci Sports Exerc.* 2000;32:S498-S504

BOX 7-6 Activity Categories for Girls and Women

- **Inactive or sedentary:** no exercise and little or no physical activity such as walking or low-intensity activities of daily living.
- **Low activity level:** low-intensity activities such as fine arts, singing, working at a service or retail store; low-intensity daily activities, such as making a bed, small housework tasks such as loading a dishwasher; one or two 30-minute low-intensity exercise sessions per week, such as yoga or stretching.
- **Moderate activity level:** regular moderate intensity sports, such as cheerleading, drill team, or badminton; moderate-intensity activities of daily living, such as vacuuming or yard work; three or more 30-minute moderate-intensity activities per week, such as vigorous play with young siblings or children, step aerobics, jogging, swimming or dance class.
- **Athlete or dancer:** regular, near daily moderate- to high-intensity physical activity; playing on a school, community or professional sports team, dancing with a dance company, or participating in 4 or more hours of vigorous aerobics per week.

based on motivation and health. If an individual is sedentary or at a low activity level, the next part of the exercise assessment is to determine whether the woman is interested in and committed to becoming more active and to identify any factors that may influence further participation.

Participation in physical activity during adolescence has short-, medium-, and long-term beneficial effects on health. In the short term, exercise aids with identity issues,[49] stress management,[50] and energy balance.[51] In the medium and long term, a number of health factors are affected by physical fitness in adolescence, including the promotion of bone health.[52,53] Current activity threshold guidelines for children and adolescents call for 60 minutes of accumulated moderate to vigorous activity daily.[54]

The habits that young women develop influence their overall health as they age and improve health outcomes for their offspring, especially if continued through the childbearing years. Current activity threshold guidelines for adults include 30 minutes of accumulated moderate activity daily.[54]

Contrary to old myths, regular, moderate to vigorous exercise in pregnancy is safe and generally beneficial for both mother and fetus.[55] Even previously sedentary women can benefit from aerobic conditioning, showing increases in maximal aerobic power and submaximal duration, as well as preservation of anaerobic working capacity in late gestation[56]—all of which are valuable assets during the prolonged endurance test of the first stage of labor, followed by the strength test of the second stage. Women who participate in vigorous activities during pregnancy are more likely to be physically fit in midlife.[57] Recent findings indicate, however, that most pregnant women do not meet the minimum threshold for activity as recommended by the American College of Obstetricians and Gynecologists (ACOG)—that is, 30 minutes of moderate exercise most days of the week.[55] Further, levels of activity tend to decrease during the course of pregnancy, and the daily activities of motherhood pose the greatest obstacle to regular exercise for women.[58] Thus prenatal healthcare providers are encouraged to recommend and support exercise for the women for whom they provide care.[59]

During the 6-week puerperium period, physical activity centers on the immediate recovery from birth, prevention of deconditioning, and coping with adjustments such as breastfeeding and sleep changes. During the extended postpartum period, the focus shifts to further recovery, including structural realignment and weight loss, the psychophysiologic benefits of exercise, and finding social support. All of the new mother's physiologic systems need to recover from the pregnancy and birth. If she had a surgical birth, she may have after-effects from anesthesia and discomfort from major abdominal surgery. If she is breastfeeding, she and her infant have motor skills to acquire as they work out their system. The postpartum woman experiences changes in identity, sleep patterns, and relationships and often may feel that her body is out of balance. Physical activity can have a positive impact on all of these factors[60] and is part of the immediate and continuing recovery care for most other major procedures or surgeries. As a new mother returns to regular, sustained activity, she should add activities slowly by working at an intensity and duration that does not produce discomfort or fatigue. Women who were fit during their pregnancies commonly return to exercise programs between 4 and 6 weeks postpartum. When discussing a return to previous exercise levels with a new mother, it is important to remember that perceived barriers pertaining to time, convenience, and access can be substantial.

During the perimenopausal transition, hormone changes that affect bone, muscle, brain, and cardiovascular and metabolic parameters enter onto a preset stage created by a combination of genetics, environment, and lifestyle behavior. As is true for all women, cardiovascular or aerobic conditioning extends its benefits to midlife women through positive changes in body composition, tolerance for oxidative stress, and muscle endurance.[43] Strength training, with its ability to increase muscle mass and bone density, improves metabolic functions that affect cardiovascular health and becomes increasingly more important as women age.

Whether a woman was previously active or not, a minimum of 30 minutes of moderate aerobic exercise five times a week or 20 to 30 minutes of vigorous exercise three times a week, or a combination of these programs, will be helpful to promote health of the woman in the perimenopausal period.[43] Specific benefits include reduction in risk of cardiovascular disease resulting from obesity, poor lipid profiles, insulin resistance, and high blood pressure; limits of bone loss and increases in balance and strength, contributing to the prevention of falls and fractures; some reduction in cancer risk and possible improvements in recovery outcomes; a degree of treatment for urinary incontinence; and improvements in cognition and mood. Of equal importance is the beneficial effect of exercise on quality of life (QOL). A 2009 randomized control trial among sedentary postmenopausal women examined the exercise dose effect and found that, compared to nonexercising controls, women expending 4, 8, or 12 kilocalories per kilogram of body weight per week experienced increasingly positive dose effects in eight mental and physical aspects of QOL at 6 months.[61] Gender-appropriate activities, an understanding that all movement is activity, time constraints, appropriate environment for exercise, health concerns as motivators, and the need for an exercise companion are themes appearing across all ethnic groups that affect midlife women's attitudes toward physical activity.[62]

The midwife plays a key role in implementing health enhancement in the form of physical activity by taking notes on exercise level, motivations, and health screening for exercise. To help women implement active lifestyles, the midwife will also need to identify resources available in the community and think creatively about what constitutes effective physical activity. Knowing which gyms or exercise studios have certified fitness professionals is another important resource for the midwife. Walking or running in one's neighborhood, along with participating in community, school, or workplace activity groups, may be among the most promising methods of increasing energy expenditure for women with limited resources, assuming they choose safe areas to engage in these activities. To help women with special needs such as acute or chronic health diseases, knowledge of group exercise programs designed for individuals for specific health conditions can be invaluable. Helping women begin, increase, or maintain health-enhancing physical activities can be integrated into the midwifery care model by following guidelines for assessment of motivations, as well as appropriate health screening. Through exercise counseling, support, and ongoing evaluation of women's activities, the midwife makes a substantial contribution to public health.

Sexual Health

Sexually transmitted infections (STIs) are a preventable cause of morbidity and mortality in the United States, with an estimated 19 million new STIs diagnosed each year, almost half of which are diagnosed among individuals age 15–24 years.[63] Recognizing that all sexually active adolescents are at risk for STIs, the USPSTF recommends high-intensity behavioral counseling for STI prevention for all sexually active adolescents.[63] It also recommends high-intensity behavioral counseling for all adults at increased risk for STIs. Adults at risk for STIs include women with a current STI or an infection within the past year, women who have multiple sexual partners, and women who live in communities with high prevalence rates for any STI.[63] The most effective counseling interventions are those that are delivered over the course of 3 to 9 hours, in group settings, and

in multiple sessions. The *Reproductive Tract and Sexually Transmitted Infections* chapter contains a detailed discussion of STIs and STI prevention.

The USPSTF has not made recommendations or addressed the prevention of unplanned pregnancy. However, most recent data indicate that 49% of pregnancies in the United States are unintended.[64] To meet the *Healthy People 2020* goal of decreasing the rate of unintended pregnancy to 44%,[64] it is likely that some form of intervention in the primary care setting will be necessary.

Skin Cancer Prevention

The most common form of cancer in the United States is skin cancer. Basal and squamous cell carcinomas, which are the two most common forms, are highly curable.[65] By comparison, melanomas, 65% to 90% of which are caused by ultraviolet (UV) light exposure,[65] result in approximately 8000 deaths in the United States each year.[66] The USPSTF recommends counseling fair-skinned adolescents and young adults through the age of 24 years about minimizing their risk for skin cancer by decreasing their exposure to UV light.[67] Because the lifetime risk for skin cancer is strongly linked to UV exposure early in life, the Task Force was unable to determine the net effect of counseling individuals older than 24 years about UV exposure. However, it found little harm associated with such counseling and recommends that decisions to provide counseling about UV exposure be made based on risk factors.[67]

Behavioral counseling interventions include reminding women about the risks for skin cancer associated with UV exposure and recommending that women avoid sun exposure between the hours of 10:00 A.M. and 3:00 P.M. When in the sun, the use of a broad-spectrum sunscreen with a sun-protection factor (SPF) of 15 or more and the use of protective clothing and sun glasses are recommended. Women should also be counseled to avoid using indoor tanning facilities.[67]

Tobacco Use

The top four leading causes of death in women—heart disease, cancer, stroke, and chronic respiratory disease—can all be linked to tobacco use.[12] Although tobacco use among both women and men has fallen over the past several decades, smoking remains the leading cause of preventable death in the United States.[68] Surpassing breast cancer in 1987, lung cancer is now the leading cause of cancer death in women in the United States.[68] In addition to lung and several other forms of cancer, the health risks associated with tobacco use include cardiovascular disease; diseases related to the endocrine system, including diabetes; menstrual dysfunction, including early menopause; osteopenia/osteoporosis; and premature death.[68]

Women who smoke during pregnancy are at increased risk for ectopic pregnancy and spontaneous abortion, preterm labor and birth, preterm premature rupture of membranes, placental abruption, placenta previa, and perinatal mortality.[68] Infants born to women who smoke during pregnancy are at increased risk for neonatal death, sudden infant death syndrome (SIDS), and low birth weight.[68] Finally, environmental exposure to cigarette smoke on the part of nonsmokers—a phenomenon characterized as secondhand or passive smoke—contributes to early death in almost 40,000 persons each year.[69] Some authorities are studying smoke retained in cars, rooms, and clothing, termed thirdhand smoking, to ascertain whether risks all exist in those situations. Smoking cessation at any age is associated with reductions in smoking-related disease and early death, and women who stop smoking before or during pregnancy can significantly reduce their risk for poor pregnancy outcomes.[68] Therefore, primary preventive strategies over the past several decades have focused on assisting current smokers to stop and reducing the number of individuals who have ever smoked.

The USPSTF strongly recommends that healthcare providers ask all patients, including pregnant women, about tobacco use and provide smoking cessation interventions for those who smoke.[69] The Task Force was unable to find sufficient evidence to recommend for or against routine screening and counseling of adolescents, although it recognizes that most adults who smoke start smoking during adolescence and encourages healthcare providers to offer screening and counseling to prevent tobacco use at their own discretion.

The most effective and efficient behavioral counseling intervention for women who smoke is based on the Five As construct (ask, advise, assess, assist, arrange), as shown in **Box 7-7**.[69] Convincing evidence indicates that even brief counseling interventions (of 3 to 10 minutes) in combination with pharmacotherapy can effectively increase the number of smokers who quit and remain abstinent for one year.[69] Pharmacotherapy to stop smoking includes nicotine replacement therapy (found in gums and lozenges) as well as treatment with bupropion (Wellbutrin) and varenicline (Chantix). The effectiveness of these agents in pregnancy is not well documented. Counseling interventions during pregnancy should be individualized for women and include information about health risks for both the woman and her baby.[69]

BOX 7-7 Modified Five As for Smoking Cessation

- **Ask** the woman about tobacco use.
- **Advise** the woman to stop smoking and provide information about the risks associated with continued use.
- **Assess** the woman's readiness and/or willingness stop smoking. This includes identifying barriers and motivating factors to stop smoking.
- **Assist** the woman to stop smoking. This includes setting goals to cut down/quit, providing support, identifying sources of social support, and dealing with motivational barriers.
- **Arrange** for regular follow-up visits with the midwife and/or refer to additional healthcare providers for more intensive treatment if necessary.

Source: U.S. Preventive Services Task Force. Counseling and interventions to prevent tobacco use and tobacco-caused disease in adults and pregnant women. 2009. Available at: http://www.uspreventiveservicestaskforce.org/uspstf09 /tobacco/tobaccors2.htm. Accessed October 17, 2012.

As is true for other sensitive topics, any discussion about tobacco use must be approached carefully, in a nonjudgmental way. Most women who smoke are fully aware of the health risks associated with smoking and experience feelings of guilt and shame about continuing the unhealthy behavior.[70] These feelings are especially prevalent among women who smoke during pregnancy[70] and among women who relapse after a cessation attempt.[70] Counseling interventions for women are most effective when the relationship between the midwife and the woman is based on mutual trust and respect and when the intervention is woman centered. Rather than attempting to manipulate pregnant women to stop smoking by instilling feelings of guilt and fear about the fetal effects of smoking, a more effective approach is to engage women in an open and respectful dialogue where the primary focus of the discussion is on maintaining and promoting the personal health of the woman.[70]

Immunizations

In addition to counseling interventions, immunization against several disease states is a primary preventive strategy for women across the lifespan. **Tables 7-5,**

7-6, and 7-7 summarize the immunization recommendations of the CDC[71-73] for adolescents, women of childbearing age, and women of perimenopausal/menopausal age, respectively. Midwives who administer immunizations are encouraged to consult the relevant Advisory Committee on Immunization Practices (ACIP) statements, available at http://www.cdc.gov/vaccines/pubs/acip-list.htm, for recommendation updates and special recommendations for women with immunocompromising conditions,

Table 7-5	Vaccination Recommendations for Adolescent Girls (11–18 Years)		
Vaccine	**Age at Administration**	**Dose/Series Timing**	**Contraindications and Other Considerations**
HPV vaccines: Gardasil (HPV4)[a] Cervarix (HPV2)	11 or 12 years 13–18 years if not previously immunized	Complete vaccination requires three-dose series: second dose given 1–2 months following the first dose; third dose given at least 24 weeks after the second dose.	
HepB (hepatitis B)	All adolescents not previously immunized	Complete vaccination requires three-dose series: second dose given 1–2 months following the first dose; third dose given at least 8 weeks after the second dose (no sooner than 16 weeks after the first dose).	Two-dose series (separated by 4 months) of adult formulation *Recombivax HB* may be used in girls age 11–15 years.
IIV (inactivated influenza) LAIV (live attenuated influenza)	Most nonpregnant girls age 9 years or older	Single dose administered each year, just prior to (or following) the start of the flu season.	LAIV is contraindicated in pregnant women and in girls with asthma or underlying conditions that predispose them to influenza complications.
MCV4 (meningococcal conjugate, quadrivalent)	11–12 years, with booster at age 16 years 13–18 years if not previously immunized	If first dose is received at age 13–15 years, administer booster at age 16–18 years (no sooner than 8 weeks after first dose). If first dose is received at 16 years or older, no booster is required.	Girls with compromised immune systems require different dosing (see CDC guidelines).
Tdap (tetanus and diphtheria toxoids and acellular pertussis)	11–18 years if not previously immunized	One dose, followed with Td booster every 10 years.	Can be given regardless of interval since last *Td* vaccine.
VAR (varicella)	Only girls without evidence of immunity[b]	Complete vaccination requires administration of two doses separated by at least 4 weeks for girls age 13 years and older. For girls age 7–12 years, the doses should be separated by 3 months.	Contraindicated in pregnancy.

Recommendations for Select Adolescent Populations

HepA (hepatitis A)	Recommended only for adolescents who live in areas with vaccination programs targeting older children, adolescents at increased risk for hepatitis A infection, or adolescents for whom immunity is desired (see CDC recommendations). Two-dose series; second dose given at least 6 months after the first dose.
IPV (inactivated poliovirus)	Recommended only for girls younger than age 18 if not previously immunized. Complete vaccination requires three-dose series: second dose given 2 months following the first dose; third dose given at least 6 months after the second dose.
MMR (measles, mumps, and rubella)	Recommended only for girls not previously immunized. Complete vaccination requires administration of two doses separated by at least 4 weeks. This vaccine is contraindicated in pregnancy.
PCV (pneumococcal conjugate) or PPSV (pneumococcal polysaccharide)	Recommended only for immunocompromised adolescents. See CDC guidelines for appropriate administration.

[a]Gardasil is also recommended for boys and men through age 21.

[b]Evidence of immunity = documented previous immunization or laboratory-confirmed evidence of immunity.

Source: Centers for Disease Control and Prevention. Recommended immunization schedules for persons aged 0 through 18 years—United States. 2012. Available at: http://www.cdc.gov/vaccines/schedules/downloads/child/mmwr-child-schedule.pdf. Accessed October 23, 2012.

Table 7-6	Vaccination Recommendations for Women of Childbearing Age (19–41 Years)		
Vaccine	**Age at Administration**	**Dose/Series Timing**	**Contraindications and Other Considerations**
HPV vaccines: Gardasil (HPV4)[a] Cervarix (HPV2)	Only women through age 26 years who have not been previously immunized	Complete vaccination requires three-dose series: second dose given 1–2 months following the first dose; third dose given at least 24 weeks after the second dose.	Ideally, women should be vaccinated prior to the onset of sexual activity; women through age 26 years who are already sexually active should still be vaccinated. Not recommended for use in pregnancy; women who become pregnant after starting the series should complete the series postpartum.
IIV (inactivated influenza vaccine) and LAIV (live attenuated influenza vaccine)	All women	Single-dose vaccination administered each year, just prior to (or following) the start of the flu season.	All adults, including pregnant women, can receive IIV. LAIV is contraindicated in pregnancy. Intradermally or intramuscularly administered IIV are both appropriate for women age 18–64 years. IIV is recommended for most adults; LAIV and FluMist may also be used for healthy, **nonpregnant** women younger than age 50 years. Healthcare workers who care for persons who are severely immunocompromised should receive IIV.
Tdap (tetanus, diphtheria, and pertussis vaccine)	Recommended to replace Td (tetanus, diphtheria) booster for all adults Recommended for all pregnant women at 27–36 weeks' gestation during each pregnancy (regardless of number of years since last Td or Tdap vaccination)	Nonpregnant adults should receive one dose of Tdap and boost with Td every 10 years. Three-dose series is recommended for all adults with unknown or incomplete vaccination history; first two doses administered at least 4 weeks apart; third dose administered 6–12 months after the second dose.	This vaccine can be given regardless of the interval since the last Td vaccine. Recommended in the immediate postpartum period for all women who were not vaccinated during pregnancy.

Recommendations for Select Populations

HepA (hepatitis A vaccine)	Only women at increased risk for infection	Two-dose series is given, with the doses administered 6–12 months apart.	Women at increased risk for infection include those who (1) use illicit drugs; (2) work with HAV-infected primates or HAV in laboratory settings; (3) have chronic liver disease; (4) receive clotting factor concentrates; (5) travel or work in countries with high or intermediated rates of hepatitis A; or (6) anticipate close contact with children from countries with high or intermediate rates of hepatitis A during the first 60 days after arrival in the United States (childcare providers or adoptive parents).
HepB (hepatitis B)	Only women at increased risk for infection (see CDC guidelines)	Complete vaccination requires administration of three doses. The second dose should be given 1 month after the first dose; third dose given at least 8 weeks after the second dose (no sooner than 16 weeks after the first dose).	

Table 7-6	Vaccination Recommendations for Women of Childbearing Age (19–41 Years) *(continued)*		
Vaccine	**Age at Administration**	**Dose/Series Timing**	**Contraindications and Other Considerations**
Recommendations for Select Populations *(continued)*			
MCV4 (meningococcal vaccine)	Only women who are first-year college students through age 21 years who live in residence halls and who were not previously vaccinated on or after their 16th birthday	One-time single dose; revaccination 5 years following first dose is necessary only for women who remain at increased risk for infection.	Also recommended for military recruits and women with select immunocompromising conditions (see CDC guidelines).
MMR (measles, mumps, and rubella)	Only women who are not considered immune	Second dose given at least 28 days after the first dose, and is necessary only for women who are college students, women who work in a healthcare facility, or women who plan to travel internationally. Women who received inactivated measles vaccine or vaccine of unknown type from 1963 to 1967 should be revaccinated with two doses of MMR. Women who received killed mumps vaccine or vaccine of unknown type before 1979 should be considered for revaccination with two doses of MMR.	**This vaccine is contraindicated in pregnancy.** Women who are not considered immune include those who have not received at least one documented dose of vaccine and women without laboratory confirmation of immunity to all three diseases. Regardless of birth year, women of childbearing age should have laboratory-confirmed rubella immunity. Vaccinate nonpregnant women during menses when nonpregnant status is certain. Pregnant women without evidence of laboratory-confirmed immunity should be vaccinated immediately postpartum or following pregnancy termination.
PPSV23 (pneumococcal polysaccharide)	Women younger than age 65 years only if they smoke, live in long-term care facilities, or have chronic lung disease, chronic cardiovascular disease, diabetes mellitus, chronic liver disease, alcoholism, cochlear implants, cerebrospinal fluid leaks, immunocompromising conditions, functional anatomic asplenia (including sickle cell)	Women vaccinated before age 65 years should be revaccinated one time at age 65 years (or later so that at least 5 years have passed since receipt of the first vaccine).	May be considered for American Indians/Alaska natives and other persons younger than age 65 if living in areas where the risk for invasive pneumococcal disease is increased. See CDC for additional recommendations for women with immunocompromising and other serious medical conditions.
VAR (varicella vaccine)	Only women without evidence of immunity	Complete vaccination requires administration of two doses, separated by at least 4 weeks.	**This vaccine is contraindicated in pregnancy.** Evidence of immunity includes documentation of previous vaccination with two doses at least 4 weeks apart, history of herpes zoster diagnosed by a healthcare provider, history of varicella diagnosed by a healthcare provider, or laboratory-confirmation of immunity. Laboratory confirmation should be obtained for women who report having had a mild or atypical case of varicella. Pregnant women should be evaluated for laboratory-confirmed varicella immunity. Those without evidence of immunity should begin the two-dose vaccination series **immediately postpartum** or following pregnancy termination.

[a]Gardasil is also recommended for men through age 21; men aged 22–26 may also be vaccinated.

Sources: Centers for Disease Control and Prevention. Recommended adult immunization schedule—United States. 2012. Available at: http://www.cdc.gov/vaccines/schedules/downloads/adult/mmwr-adult-schedule.pdf. Accessed October 24, 2012; Centers for Disease Control and Prevention. Recommended adult immunization schedule—United States. 2013. Available at: http://www.cdc.gov/vaccines/schedules/downloads/adult/adult-schedule.pdf. Accessed May 13, 2013.

Table 7-7	Vaccination Recommendations for Women of Perimenopausal and Menopausal Age (41–65 Years or Older)		
Vaccine	**Age at Administration**	**Dose/Series Timing**	**Contraindications and Other Considerations**
IIV (inactivated influenza vaccine)	All adults	Single dose administered each year, just prior to (or following) the start of the flu season.	IIV is recommended for most adults; LAIV and FluMist may also be used for healthy, **nonpregnant** women younger than age 50 years. Healthcare workers who care for persons who are severely immunocompromised should receive IIV. Women age 65 years and older may receive standard-dose IIV or Fluzone High-Dose.
PPSV (pneumococcal polysaccharide)	All women age 65 years and older who have not been previously immunized	Single, one-time dose; no need for revaccination.	See Table 7-6 for special considerations for women younger than 65 years.
Tdap (tetanus, diphtheria, and pertussis)	All adults—to replace Td booster	See Table 7-6.	See Table 7-6.
Zoster vaccine	60 years	Single, one-time dose; no need for revaccination.	Contraindicated in pregnancy and for persons with certain medical conditions (see CDC guidelines).

Recommendations for Select Populations

HepA (hepatitis A)	Identical to the recommendations for younger women (see Table 7-6).
HepB (hepatitis B)	Identical to the recommendations for younger women (see Table 7-6).
MCV4 and MPSV4 (meningococcal vaccines)	Recommended only for older women with functional asplenia or persistent complement component deficiencies (see CDC guidelines for vaccination and revaccination recommendations).
MMR (measles, mumps, and rubella)	Recommended only for women who are not considered immune; women born prior to 1957 are considered immune; see Table 7-6 for recommendations for women born after 1957.
VAR (varicella)	Recommended only for adults without evidence of immunity; women born in the United States prior to 1980 (except healthcare providers and pregnant women) are considered immune (see Table 7-6 for additional evidence of immunity).

Sources: Centers for Disease Control and Prevention. Recommended adult immunization schedule—United States. 2012. Available at: http://www .cdc.gov/vaccines/schedules/downloads/adult/mmwr-adult-schedule.pdf. Accessed October 24, 2012; Centers for Disease Control and Prevention. Recommended adult immunization schedule—United States. 2013. Available at: http://www.cdc.gov/vaccines/schedules/downloads/adult /adult-schedule.pdf. Accessed May 13, 2013.

healthcare workers, and travelers. Adverse events following vaccination should be reported to the Vaccine Adverse Event Reporting System at 800-822-7967.

Health Maintenance

In addition to primary preventive services to promote health and prevent the onset of disease in women, midwives provide secondary preventive services aimed at maintaining health through early detection and treatment of several disease states across the lifespan. Limiting morbidity and early death associated with chronic disease is a priority of the Patient Protection and Affordable Care Act. Under this law, by 2014, all U.S. citizens and permanent residents will be required to have some form of health insurance. Insurance policies will be available for purchase by small-business employers and by individuals on "exchanges" that are administered by government agencies or nonprofit groups.[74] Insurance policies sold on the exchange will be required to include an "essential health benefits package," with no cost sharing for certain preventive services. Although the specific components of the essential health benefits package have not yet been fully determined, it is likely that they will be congruent with screening recommendations from the USPSTF for recommended screening tests for which scientific evidence indicates that the benefits outweigh the potential harms.

Routine Screening Across the Lifespan

As has been discussed in this chapter, an important first step in the provision of secondary preventive services is the collection of a complete health history. The accompanying physical examination provides additional information to be included in the health screening of women across the lifespan. For example, the USPSTF has found insufficient evidence to recommend for or against screening women for several medical conditions and certain types of cancer, but suggests that healthcare providers remain alert for findings on history and physical exam that may indicate health problems in this area.

After completing the health history and physical exam, additional screening information is obtained with the collection of laboratory tests. Recommendations for these tests are made based on the existence of identified risk factors such as gender and age. Screening tests for asymptomatic women across the lifespan, for which the USPSTF found sufficient evidence to recommend, are presented in **Tables 7-8, 7-9, 7-10, and 7-11.**[75,76] Readers are encouraged to become familiar with and regularly access updated recommendations of the Task Force at the USPSTF website.

In addition to the recommendations of the USPSTF, it is important for midwives to remain

Table 7-8	Recommended Routine Screening for Adolescents (12–17 Years)	
Disorder	**Test Used**	**Screening Recommendation**
Chlamydia	Nucleic acid amplification tests	Screen all sexually active adolescents at least yearly with more frequent screening when adolescents have symptoms or concern about infection. Nucleic acid amplification tests can be used with urine and vaginal swabs if a pelvic examination is not performed.
Depression	Patient Health Questionnaire for Adolescents (PHQ-A) or Beck Depression Inventory—Primary Care Version (BDI-PC)	Recommended for all adolescents when systems are in place to ensure accurate diagnosis, treatment, and follow-up.
Gonorrhea	Vaginal culture or nucleic acid amplification tests	Screen all sexually active adolescents. Recommended screening frequency is unknown.
HIV	Enzyme immunoassay and confirmation with Western blot	Screen all adolescents at increased risk for infection; consider screening all adolescents, which is the current recommendation of the CDC.
Hypertension	Blood pressure measured with sphygmomanometer	Yearly screening of all adolescents is recommended. Updating the USPSTF recommendation is currently in process. These are the current recommendations of the JNC-7. Updating the JNC-7 is currently under way.
Obesity	BMI	Routine screening of all adolescents is recommended. See counseling interventions in this chapter.
Syphilis	VDRL or RPR—confirmed with FTA-ABS or TP-PA	Screen only adolescents at increased risk for infection. Women at risk include commercial sex workers, those who exchange sex for drugs, those in adult correctional facilities, and those who live in high-prevalence areas.
Tobacco use	Health history	See screening and counseling recommendations under counseling interventions in this chapter.

FTA-ABS: fluorescent treponemal antibody-absorption test; RPR: rapid plasma reagin; TP-PA: treponemal pallidum particle agglutination assay; VDRL: venereal disease research laboratory test.

Sources: Centers for Disease Control and Prevention. Recommended adult immunization schedule—United States. 2012. Available at: http://www.cdc.gov/vaccines/schedules/downloads/adult/mmwr-adult-schedule.pdf. Accessed October 24, 2012; Centers for Disease Control and Prevention. Recommended adult immunization schedule—United States. 2013. Available at: http://www.cdc.gov/vaccines/schedules/downloads/adult/adult-schedule.pdf. Accessed May 13, 2013; U.S. Preventive Services Task Force. USPSTF A–Z topic guide. Available at: http://www.uspreventiveservicestaskforce.org/uspstopics.htm. Accessed October 29, 2012; National Heart Lung and Blood Institute. Seventh report of the Joint National Committee on Prevention, Detection, Evaluation and Treatment of High Blood Pressure (JNC-7). Available at: http://www.nhlbi.nih.gov/guidelines/hypertension. Accessed January 10, 2013.

Table 7-9	Recommended Routine Screening for Adult Women (Age 18 and Older)[a]			
Disorder	**Test Used**	**Age at Initial Screen**	**Screening Frequency**	**Additional Considerations**
Breast cancer	Mammogram	50 years	Every 2 years until age 75	There is moderate evidence that the benefit of beginning biennial mammogram screening at age 40 years is small. The decision to begin screening at age 40 years should be made on an individual basis. Women with a family history of breast or ovarian cancer should be referred for genetic counseling and possible *BRCA* testing.
Cervical cancer	Pap smear	21 years	Every 3 years until age 65	See the *Gynecologic Disorders* chapter for detailed discussion of cervical cancer screening and management. Adolescents no longer are to be screened.
Chlamydia	Nucleic acid amplification tests	All sexually active women through age 24 years	At least yearly	Continued screening for women older than age 24 who are at increased risk for infection may be considered. See the *Reproductive Tract and Sexually Transmitted Infections* chapter for review of risk factors and management of STIs.
Depression	Any reliable screening tool	18 years	Unknown	Screening is recommended when clinical staff are available to provide some form of direct depression care. Asking women whether they have felt down, depressed, or hopeless during the past 2 weeks and whether they have lost interest or pleasure doing things over the past 2 weeks is an easy and reliable screen.
Gonorrhea	Vaginal culture or nucleic acid amplification tests	All sexually active women through age 24 years	Unknown	For women older than age 24, screen only those at increased risk for infection. See the *Reproductive Tract and Sexually Transmitted Infections* chapter for review of risk factors and management.
HIV	Enzyme immunoassay and confirmation with Western blot	All women at risk for infection	Unknown	Consider using CDC guidelines, which call for screening all adults regardless of risk factors.
Hypertension	Blood pressure measured with sphygmomanometer	18 years	Yearly	Systolic measurements of 140 mm Hg or higher or diastolic measurements of 90 mm Hg or higher—on two consecutive visits at least 1 week apart—is considered diagnostic for hypertension.
Lipid disorders	Nonfasting or fasting total cholesterol and HDL cholesterol	20 years	Every 5 years	Recommended for women at increased risk for coronary heart disease (CHD). Risk factors for CHD include diabetes, personal or family history of heart disease, tobacco use, hypertension, and obesity. Women with high-normal levels may benefit from more frequent screening. The USPSTF makes no recommendation for or against screening women not at increased risk.
Obesity	BMI	18 years	Regularly	See counseling interventions in this chapter.
Syphilis	VDRL or RPR—confirmed with FTA-ABS or TP-PA	Screen all adults at increased risk for infection. See the *Reproductive Tract and Sexually Transmitted Infections* chapter for review of risk factors and management.		The USPSTF recommends against screening asymptomatic adults who are not at increased risk for infection.
Type 2 diabetes	Fasting plasma glucose	Screen all adults with sustained blood pressure of greater than 135/80 mm Hg.	Every 5 years	Consider screening adults with symptoms of diabetes (polydipsia, polyphagia, and polyuria), established cardiovascular disease not previously diagnosed with type 2 diabetes, and ulcers or infections that do not heal.
Alcohol misuse	See screening and counseling recommendations under counseling interventions in this chapter.			
Tobacco use	See screening and counseling recommendations under counseling interventions in this chapter.			

FTA-ABS: fluorescent treponemal antibody-absorption test; RPR: rapid plasma reagin; TP-PA: treponemal pallidum particle agglutination assay; VDRL: venereal disease research laboratory test.

[a]These are the screening recommendations for healthy women who are not at increased risk for infection or disease. Women with risk factors may require more frequent screening or screening with the use of additional tests and/or procedures.

Source: U.S. Preventive Services Task Force. USPSTF A–Z topic guide. Available at: http://www.uspreventiveservicestaskforce.org/uspstopics.htm. Accessed October 29, 2012.

Table 7-10	Additional Screening Recommendations for Women Age 50 Years and Older			
Disorder	**Test Used**	**Age at Initial Screen**	**Screening Frequency**	**Additional Considerations**
Colorectal cancer	Fecal occult blood testing, sigmoidoscopy, or colonoscopy	50 years	Variable based on findings; recommended through age 75	Of the tests used, colonoscopy has the greatest sensitivity and specificity for colorectal cancer screening.
				The aim of screening is to reduce colon cancer–related death. Screening approaches vary in patient acceptance. Screening efforts should focus on improving screening of any sort. Thus screening decisions should be made on an individual basis with the midwife and the woman acting in partnership to determine the risk–benefit ratio, patient preference, and most appropriate screening tool.
				Earlier screening is recommended for women with Lynch syndrome and inflammatory bowel disease, and may be reasonable for women with a first-degree relative with early-onset (before age 50) colorectal disease.
				Recommendations for appropriate screening intervals are controversial and should be made based on clinical findings.
Osteoporosis	DXA scan of the hip and lumbar spine	65 years	Undetermined, but rescreening should not occur sooner than 2 years following initial screening	Earlier screening (age 50–64) is recommended for women with fracture risk equal to or greater than that of 65-year-old white women without risk factors.
				Risk factors include Caucasian race, smoking, daily alcohol use, BMI less than 21, and parental history of fracture.

DXA: dual-energy X-ray absorptiometry.

Source: U.S. Preventive Services Task Force. USPSTF A–Z topic guide. Available at: http://www.uspreventiveservicestaskforce.org/uspstopics.htm. Accessed October 29, 2012.

Table 7-11	Additional Screening Recommendations for Pregnant Women		
Disorder	**Test Used**	**Screening Recommendation**	**Additional Considerations**
Anemia	Hemoglobin and hematocrit	Screen all pregnant women.	
Bacteriuria	Urine culture	Screen all pregnant women at 12–16 weeks gestation.	
Chlamydia	Nucleic acid amplification tests	Screen all pregnant patients age 24 and younger at first prenatal visit and again in third trimester.	Screen pregnant women older than age 24 at increased risk for infection at first prenatal visit. Rescreen women older than age 24 who remain at increased risk in third trimester.
Gonorrhea	Vaginal culture or nucleic acid amplification tests	Screen pregnant women at increased risk for infection at first prenatal visit and again in third trimester if risk factors persist.	There is insufficient evidence to recommend for or against screening pregnant women not at risk for infection.
Hepatitis B	HBsAG	Screen all pregnant women at first prenatal visit. Rescreen women in labor who have unknown HBV status and who are at increased risk for STIs.	
HIV	Enzyme immunoassay and confirmation with Western blot	Screen all pregnant women at first prenatal visit	Rapid HIV antibody testing is accurate and may be considered for women with unknown HIV status who present in active labor.
Rh incompatibility	Blood type and antibody testing	Screen all pregnant women at first prenatal visit. Rescreen unsensitized Rh-negative women at 24–28 weeks gestation unless the biological father is known to be Rh negative.	
Rubella immunity	Serologic screen	Screen all pregnant women at first prenatal visit.	
Syphilis	VDRL or RPR—confirmed with FTA-ABS or TP-PA	Screen all pregnant women at first prenatal visit. Consider rescreening women at risk for STI in third trimester.	

FTA-ABS: fluorescent treponemal antibody-absorption test; HBsAg: hepatitis surface antigen; RPR: rapid plasma reagin; TP-PA: treponemal pallidum particle agglutination assay; VDRL: venereal disease research laboratory test.

Source: U.S. Preventive Services Task Force. USPSTF A–Z topic guide. Available at: http://www.uspreventiveservicestaskforce.org/uspstopics.htm. Accessed October 29, 2012.

aware of the recommendations of other groups (such as ACOG and the American Cancer Society). Healthcare facilities often look to these guidelines when establishing their institutional policies and procedures. Furthermore, individual communities may have "community standards" based on these recommendations. Recommendations of other groups *that differ from* the recommendations of the USPSTF are presented in **Table 7-12**. Online sources of

information regarding recommendations of professional organizations and other groups are presented in at the end of this chapter.

Early Intervention or Referral

The second step in the provision of secondary preventive services is early intervention, which may or may not require referral to another healthcare provider. Although most midwives practice independently, it

Table 7-12	Screening Recommendations That Differ from U.S. Preventive Services Task Force Recommendations[a]		
Disorder	**Cochrane**	**ACOG**	**American Cancer Society**
Breast cancer	2007: Recommend against screening with breast self-examination (BSE) and clinical breast exam alone. 2011: Although screening mammography will identify some women with breast cancer, it is not clear whether screening mammograms do more harm than good.	**Mammogram:** Yearly starting at age 40 years. **Clinical breast exam:** Every 1–3 years (age 20–39 years); yearly (starting at age 40 years). **BSE:** May be included in breast self-awareness, which should be taught to all women. Enhanced screening recommended for women who test positive for *BRCA1* and *BRCA2* mutations.	**Mammogram:** Yearly starting at age 40 years. **Clinical breast exam:** Every 3 years (age 20–39); yearly (starting at age 40). **BSE:** an option for women starting at age 20 years.
Cervical cancer	2012: Currently under review.	Begin screening at age 21. **Age 21–29 years:** Pap smear every 3 years. **Age 30–65 years:** Pap smear **plus** HPV test every 5 years *or* Pap smear alone every 3 years. Do not screen women younger than age 21 years. Do not screen women older than age 65 years with a history of negative screening. Discontinue screening following total hysterectomy for women who have never had cervical intraepithelial neoplasia-2 or higher.	Begin screening at age 21 years. **Age 21–29 years:** Pap smear every 3 years. **Age 30–65 years:** Pap smear **plus** HPV test every 5 years *or* Pap smear alone every 3 years. Do not screen women younger than age 21 years. Do not screen women older than age 65 years with a history of negative screening.
Colorectal cancer	2010: Fecal occult blood test (FOBT) can effectively detect colorectal cancer and will likely prevent 1 in 6 colorectal cancer deaths. 2012: Recommendations for colorectal cancer screening with sigmoidoscopy and colonoscopy are currently under review.	**Colonoscopy:** every 10 years beginning at age 50 years for women of low to average risk. Consider other forms of screening on an individual basis.	Begin screening at age 50 years with: • **Colonoscopy** every 10 years; *or* **flexible sigmoidoscopy** every 5 years;[b] *or* • **Barium enema** every 5 years;[b] *or* • **CT colonography** every 5 years;[b] *or* • Yearly **FOBT**;[b] *or* • Yearly **fecal immunochemical test (FIT)**[b]
Depression	2009: Depression screening/case-finding instruments used in primary care settings have little or no impact on recognition, management, or outcomes for depression.	Remain alert for symptoms in adolescents and older women during collection of the health history.	

(continues)

Table 7-12	**Screening Recommendations That Differ from U.S. Preventive Services Task Force Recommendations**[a] *(continued)*		
Disorder	**Cochrane**	**ACOG**	**American Cancer Society**
Gestational diabetes (GDM)	2010: Insufficient evidence to determine if screening for GDM (or which types of screening) improve maternal and neonatal outcomes. However, there is strong evidence that treating GDM leads to improved outcomes. More research on screening effectiveness is recommended.	Screen all pregnant women with history, identification of clinical risk factors, or 50-g 1-hour glucose challenge test (GCT) at 24–28 weeks gestation. Women with risk factors for GDM should be screened with 50-g 1-hour GCT. Diagnosis is confirmed with 100-g 3-hour glucose tolerance test.	
HIV		Routinely screen all women age 19–64 years, with targeted screening outside this age range.	
Intimate-partner violence (IPV)	2009: Review of evidence regarding screening for IPV in primary care settings is under way.	Periodically screen all women (including pregnant women) for IPV and/or sexual assault.	
Lipid disorders		Screen all women every 5 years beginning at age 45 years. Consider earlier screening based on risk factors.	
Type 2 diabetes mellitus (DM)	2009: Review of evidence regarding screening for type 2 DM is currently under way.	Screen all women age 45 years and older every 3 years. Consider screening younger women with risk factors for type 2 DM.	
Substance use		Universally screen all women, provide brief intervention, and refer for treatment when necessary.	
Suicide risk	2008: Review of evidence regarding prevention of suicide and suicidal behavior in adolescents is currently under way. 2011: Review of evidence regarding primary prevention of suicide in post-secondary educational settings is currently under way.	Screen adolescents with inquiry about suicidal ideation.	
Thyroid disease		Screen all women using thyroid-stimulating hormone (TSH) testing every 5 years beginning at age 50 years. Consider earlier screening for women with risk factors or symptoms.	

[a]These are the recommendations for low-risk women. Consider earlier/alternative screening for patients with risk factors.

[b]Follow up with colonoscopy if test is positive.

is important to remember that independent practice does not mean practicing alone. Independent practice includes working within a healthcare system that provides mechanisms for collaboration with other healthcare providers. Collaborative management is essential when a woman has health concerns that fall outside the midwife's scope of practice. When abnormal history, physical exam, or laboratory findings are identified, the midwife may need to seek the opinion of, or consult with, another healthcare provider to determine the most appropriate intervention. In some instances, it may be necessary for the midwife to work in collaboration with another healthcare provider to meet the woman's healthcare needs. In other cases, the midwife may need to refer the woman to another healthcare provider for her to receive the most appropriate care. Recommendations for these three types of collaborative management

(consultation, collaboration, and referral) can be found throughout this text.

Health Promotion and Health Maintenance in the Context of the Midwifery Management Process

The midwifery management process, as described in chapter titled *An Introduction to the Care of Women*, is a seven-step process that enables midwives to organize the delivery of health care in a logical manner. Although use of this management process is often associated with identification and management of problems related to pregnancy and women's health, it also provides a perfect framework for health promotion and health maintenance. **Box 7-8** provides an illustration of the delivery of preventive health services.

BOX 7-8 Health Promotion in Action

The following case illustrates the delivery of preventive health services.

Mandy is a 15-year-old girl who presents to the midwife's office on October 25 for her annual healthcare visit. Prior to Mandy's arrival, the midwife reviewed the medical record and noted that Mandy's hepatitis B, varicella, measles–mumps–rubella (MMR), and polio vaccines are up-to-date, and that Mandy received the Tdap vaccine 2 years ago after stepping on a nail. Her health record reveals no other concerns.

Upon her arrival, the midwife escorts Mandy to the exam room, where they are seated face-to-face. While Mandy is fully clothed, the midwife begins by asking Mandy if she has any questions or concerns about her health. Mandy says she doesn't have any questions. The midwife then collects a complete health history, including completion of the *Patient Health Questionnaire for Adolescents* (PHQ-A) to screen Mandy for depression. Mandy's health history is negative for risk factors for disease; findings of the PHQ-A are negative, there is no apparent family history of disease, she is not sexually active, and she does not use any drugs, alcohol, or tobacco.

The midwife steps out of the room while Mandy undresses from the waist down. The midwife returns to the room and conducts an age-appropriate physical exam. Upon completion of the exam, the midwife steps out of the room to allow Mandy privacy. The midwife evaluates all information that has been collected, including a blood pressure of 110/68 mm Hg and a calculated BMI of 21, and establishes a health promotion plan.

The midwife returns to the room and asks Mandy again if she has any questions. Hearing none, the midwife provides anticipatory counseling to Mandy regarding diet and exercise, dental health, automobile safety (including information about riding with impaired or distracted drivers), and skin cancer prevention. Anticipating that Mandy is at an age to consider experimenting with sexual activity and/or drug, alcohol, or tobacco use, the midwife praises Mandy for the healthy lifestyle choices she has made and provides brief counseling regarding continued avoidance of drug, alcohol, and tobacco use, as well as information about STI and pregnancy prevention.

Recognizing that Mandy lives in a state where 16-year-olds need parental consent for vaccination, the midwife asks Mandy if her mother can join them for a discussion about recommended vaccines. After providing information about the risks and benefits of recommended vaccines to Mandy and her mother, the midwife obtains informed consent from Mandy's mother and from Mandy, and then administers the first dose of Gardasil and the influenza vaccine. Mandy prefers to limit the "shots" at this visit and asks if she can return at a later date for the meningococcal vaccine. Mandy is also advised to contact the midwife if she has any adverse reaction to the vaccines. The midwife compliments Mandy for her active participation in maintaining her own health and schedules a return visit for vaccination completion in 4 weeks.

Step 1 (obtain all necessary data for complete evaluation of the woman) is completed with the conduct of a health history and physical examination, as well as the collection of appropriate laboratory tests. Based on correct interpretation of the data collected in Step 1, the midwife identifies problems, diagnoses, and the individual woman's healthcare needs (Step 2). Once the midwife identifies problems or diagnoses, it is important to anticipate potential problems or diagnoses that might emerge as a result of existing problems (Step 3).

Following data collection and problem identification, the midwife must evaluate the need for immediate midwife or physician intervention and for consultation or collaborative management with another member of the healthcare team (Step 4). Steps 5–7 are completed with the development of an individualized and comprehensive plan for evidence-based health promotion, implementation of the plan at current and future visits, and periodic evaluation of the effectiveness of the care provided. Evaluation of effectiveness includes rescreening at appropriate intervals and modifying the plan as necessary. Health promotion is an ongoing process that requires continual recycling of data collection, assessment, planning, implementation, and evaluation of the care provided for all women across the lifespan.

Conclusion

Health promotion is an essential component of care provided by midwives for women across the lifespan, which is accomplished through the delivery of primary and secondary preventive services. Primary preventive services, which include counseling/education and vaccination, are provided to healthy women as a means to prevent the onset of disease. Secondary preventive services, which include routine screening and early intervention, are provided to limit morbidity and mortality related to disease. As primary care providers who often see women at regular intervals across the lifespan, midwives are well positioned to provide the preventive services described in this chapter and to offer women the tools necessary for them to become active participants in their own health maintenance and to achieve optimal levels of wellness.

● ● ● References

1. International Confederation of Midwives. ICM international definition of the midwife. 2011. Available at: http://www.internationalmidwives.org/Portals/5/2011/Definition%20of%20the%20Midwife%20-%202011.pdf. Accessed September 2, 2012.

2. American College of Nurse-Midwives. Definition of midwifery and scope of practice of certified nurse-midwives and certified midwives. 2004. Available at: http://www.midwife.org/ACNM/files/ACNMLibraryData/UPLOADFILENAME/000000000266/Definition%20of%20Midwifery%20and%20Scope%20of%20Practice%20of%20CNMs%20and%20CMs%20Feb%202012.pdf. Accessed September 2, 2012.

3. American College of Nurse-Midwives. Core competencies for basic midwifery practice. 2012. Available at: http://www.midwife.org/ACNM/files/ACNMLibraryData/UPLOADFILENAME/000000000050/Core%20Competencies%20June%202012.pdf. Accessed September 2, 2012.

4. International Confederation of Midwives. Essential competencies for basic midwifery practice 2010. 2011. Available at: http://www.internationalmidwives.org/Portals/5/2011/DB%202011/Essential%20Competencies%20ENG.pdf. Accessed September 2, 2012.

5. World Health Organization. Reference and information services. 2002. Available at: http://www.paho.org/english/DD/IKM/LI/FAQ.htm. Accessed September 5, 2012.

6. Centers for Disease Control and Prevention. Physical activity: glossary of terms. 2011. Available at: http://www.cdc.gov/physicalactivity/everyone/glossary. Accessed September 5, 2012.

7. Agency for Healthcare Research and Quality. Putting prevention into practice. Available at: http://www.ahrq.gov/qual/kt/ppip/ppipslides/ppiplongsl1.htm. Accessed September 5, 2012.

8. Center for Public Health and Health Policy. The economic impact of prevention. 2008. Available at: http://publichealth.uconn.edu/images/reports/UCONN_EconomicImpactPrevention.pdf. Accessed September 5, 2012.

9. Henry J. Kaiser Family Foundation. Health care costs: a primer. 2012. Available at: http://www.kff.org/insurance/upload/7670-03.pdf. Accessed September 5, 2012.

10. American Public Health Association. The prevention and public health fund: a critical investment in our nation's physical and fiscal health. 2012. Available at: http://www.apha.org/NR/rdonlyres/8FA13774-AA47-43F2-838B-1B0757D111C6/0/APHA_PrevFundBrief_June2012.pdf. Accessed September 5, 2012.

11. Cawley J, Meyerhoefer C. The medical care costs of obesity: an instrumental variables approach. *J Health Econ.* 2012;31:219-230.

12. Centers for Disease Control and Prevention. Leading causes of death in females: United States 2008. 2012. Available at: http://www.cdc.gov/women/lcod/2008/index.htm. Accessed September 5, 2012.

13. Whitlock EP, Orleans T, Pender N, Allan J. Evaluating primary care behavioral counseling interventions: an evidence-based approach. *Am J Prev Med.* 2002;22(4):267-284.

14. Kennedy HP, Shannon M. Keeping birth normal: research findings on midwifery care during childbirth. *JOGNN.* 2004;33:554-560.

15. Knowles MS, Holton EF, Swanson RA. *The Adult Learner* (7th ed.). Burlington, MA: Elsevier; 2011.

16. Institute of Medicine. *Health Professions Education: A Bridge to Quality.* Washington, DC: National Academies Press; 2003.

17. Sackett DL, Rosenberg WM, Gray JA, Haynes RB, Richardson WS. Evidence based medicine: what it is and what it isn't. *Br Med J.* 1996;312(7023):71-72.

18. Melnyk B, Fineout-Overholt E. Consumer preferences and values as an integral key to evidence-based practice. *Nurs Admin Qtly.* 2006;30(2):123-127.

19. U.S. Preventive Services Task Force. Introduction. 2010. Available at: http://www.uspreventiveservicestaskforce.org/intro.htm. Accessed September 15, 2012.

20. U.S. Preventive Services Task Force. Screening for breast cancer: recommendation statement. 2009. Available at: http://www.uspreventiveservicestaskforce.org/uspstf09/breastcancer/brcanrs.htm. Accessed September 15, 2012.

21. Whitlock EP, Orleans CT, Pender N, Allan J. Evaluating primary care behavioral counseling interventions: an evidence-based approach. *Am J Prev Med.* 2002;22(4):267-284.

22. Centers for Disease Control and Prevention. Alcohol use and binge drinking among women of childbearing age—United States, 2006-2010. 2012. Available at: http://www.cdc.gov/mmwr/preview/mmwrhtml/mm6128a4.htm. Accessed October 2, 2012.

23. U.S. Preventive Services Task Force. Screening and behavioral counseling interventions in primary care to reduce alcohol misuse: recommendation statement. 2004. Available at: http://www.uspreventiveservicestaskforce.org/3rduspstf/alcohol/alcomisrs.htm#clinical. Accessed October 2, 2012.

24. National Institute on Alcohol Abuse and Alcoholism. Assessing alcohol problems: a guide for clinicians and researchers, second edition. 2003. Available at: http://pubs.niaaa.nih.gov/publications/AssessingAlcohol/index.pdf. Accessed October 2, 2012.

25. National Institute on Alcohol Abuse and Alcoholism. Screening tests. n.d. Available at: http://pubs.niaaa.nih.gov/publications/arh28-2/78-79.htm. Accessed October 2, 2012.

26. National Institute on Alcohol Abuse and Alcoholism. A pocket guide for alcohol screening and brief intervention. 2005. Available at: http://pubs.niaaa.nih.gov/publications/Practitioner/PocketGuide/pocket.pdf. Accessed October 3, 2012.

27. Centers for Disease Control and Prevention. Breastfeeding report card—United States. 2012. Available at: http://www.cdc.gov/breastfeeding/data/reportcard.htm. Accessed October 3, 2012.

28. U.S. Department of Health and Human Services. Healthy people 2020: maternal, infant, and child health. 2012. Available at: http://www.healthypeople.gov/2020/topicsobjectives2020/objectiveslist.aspx?topicId=26. Accessed October 3, 2012.

29. U.S. Preventive Services Task Force. Primary care interventions to promote breastfeeding. 2008. Available at: http://www.uspreventiveservicestaskforce.org/uspstf08/breastfeeding/brfeedrs.htm. Accessed October 3, 2012.

30. Woolf SH, Jonas S, Lawrence RS. *Health Promotion and Disease Prevention in Clinical Practice.* Baltimore, MD: Williams & Wilkins; 1996.

31. U.S. Preventive Services Task Force. Counseling for dental and periodontal disease. 1996. Available at: http://www.uspreventiveservicestaskforce.org/uspstf/uspsdent.htm. Accessed October 4, 2012.

32. Centers for Disease Control and Prevention. Healthy weight: it's not a diet, it's a lifestyle! 2011. Available at: http://www.cdc.gov/healthyweight/assessing/index.html. Accessed October 4, 2012.

33. U.S. Preventive Services Task Force. Behavioral counseling in primary care to promote a healthy diet. 2003. Available at: http://www.uspreventiveservicestaskforce.org/3rduspstf/diet/dietrr.htm. Accessed October 4, 2012.

34. U.S. Preventive Services Task Force. Screening for and management of obesity in adults. 2012. Available at: http://www.uspreventiveservicestaskforce.org/uspstf11/obeseadult/obesers.htm#summary. Accessed October 4, 2012.

35. U.S. Preventive Services Task Force. Behavioral counseling to promote a healthful diet and physical activity for cardiovascular disease prevention in adults. 2012. Available at: http://www.uspreventiveservicestaskforce.org/uspstf/uspsphys.htm. Accessed October 4, 2012.

36. U.S. Preventive Services Task Force. Counseling about proper use of motor vehicle occupant restraints and avoidance of alcohol use while driving. 2007. Available at: http://www.uspreventiveservicestaskforce.org/uspstf07/mvoi/mvoirs.htm. Accessed October 8, 2012.

37. U.S. Preventive Services Task Force. The guide to clinical preventive services 2010-2011: recommendations of the U.S. Preventive Services Task Force. 2011. Available at: http://www.ahrq.gov/clinic/pocketgd.htm. Accessed October 8, 2012.

38. National Highway Traffic Safety Administration. Occupant protection. 2012. Available at: http://www.nhtsa.gov/Driving+Safety/Occupant+Protection. Accessed October 8, 2012.

39. Centers for Disease Control and Prevention. Home and recreational safety. 2012. Available at: http://www.cdc.gov/homeandrecreationalsafety/Falls/adultfalls.html. Accessed October 8, 2012.

40. U.S. Preventive Services Task Force. Prevention of falls in community-dwelling older adults. 2012. Available at: http://www.uspreventiveservicestaskforce.org/uspstf11/fallsprevention/fallsprevrs.htm. Accessed October 8, 2012.

41. Vigen R, Ayers C, Willis B, DeFina L, Berry JD. Association of cardiorespiratory fitness with total, cardiovascular and non-cardiovascular mortality across 3 decades of follow-up in men and women. *Cir Cardiovasc Qual Outcomes.* 2012;5(3):358-354.

42. Stovitz SD. Contributions of fitness and physical activity to reducing mortality. *Clin J Sport Med.* 2012;22(4):380-381.

43. U.S. Department of Health and Human Services. 2008 physical activity guidelines for Americans. ODPHP Publication No. U0036. 2008. Available at: www.health.gov/paguidelines/pdf/paguide.pdf. Accessed January 13, 2010.

44. Meriwether RA, Lee JA, LaFleur AS, Wiseman P. Physical activity counseling. *Am Fam Physician.* 2008;77:1029-1136.

45. Ainsworth BE, Haskell WL, Whitt MC, et al. Compendium of physical activities: an update of activity codes and MET intensities. *Med Sci Sports Exerc.* 2000;32:S498-S504.

46. Fjorback LO, Arendt M, Ornbøl E, et al. Mindfulness-based stress reduction and mindfulness-based cognitive therapy: a systematic review of randomized controlled trials. *Acta Psychiatr Scand.* 2011;124(2):102-119.

47. Lee DC, Sui X, Ortega FB, et al. Comparisons of leisure-time physical at activity and cardiorespiratory fitness on predictors of all-cause mortality in men and women. *Br J Sports Med.* 2011;45(6):504-510.

48. Gulati M, Black HR, Amsdorf MF, Shaw LJ, Bakris GL. Kidney dysfunction, cardiorespiratory fitness and risk of death in women. *J Women's Health.* 2012;21(9):917-924.

49. Ekeland E, Heian F, Hagen KB, Abbott J, Nordheim L. Exercise to improve self-esteem in children and young people. *Cochrane Database Syst Rev.* 2004;1:CD003683.

50. Newman CL, Motta RW. The effects of aerobic exercise on childhood PTSD, anxiety, and depression. *Int J Merg Ment Health.* 2007;9(2):133-158.

51. Christo K, Cor J, Mendes N, et al. Acylated ghrelin and leptin in adolescent athletes with amenorrhea, eurmenorrheic athletes and controls: a cross-sectional study. *Clin Endocrinol.* 2008;69(4):628-633.

52. Dobbins M, De Coby K, Robeson P, Husson H, Tirilis D. School-based physical activity programs for promoting physical activity and fitness in children and adolescents aged 6-18. *Cochrane Database Syst Rev.* 2009;21(1):CD007651.

53. Kato T, Yamashita T, Mizutani S, Honda A, Matumoto M, Umemura Y. Adolescent exercise associated with long-term superior measures of bone geometry: a cross-sectional DXA and MRI study. *Br J Sports Med.* 2009;43(12):932-935.

54. U.S. Department of Health and Human Services, U.S. Department of Agriculture. *Dietary Guidelines for Americans.* Washington, DC: U.S. Department of Health and Human Services; 2005.

55. American Congress of Obstetricians and Gynecologists. Exercise during pregnancy and the postpartum period. ACOG Committee Opinion No. 267. *Obstet Gynecol.* 2002;99:171-173.

56. Sohnchen N, Melzer K, Teiada BM, et al. Maternal heart rate changes during labour. *Eur J Obstet Gynecol Reprod Biol.* 2011;158(2):173-178.

57. Clapp JF III. Exercise during pregnancy may improve perimenopausal fitness. *Am J Obstet Gynecol.* 2008;199:489.e1-489.e6.

58. Verhoef MJ, Love EJ. Women and exercise participation: the mixed blessings of motherhood. *Health Care Women Intl.* 1994;15:297-306.

59. Lewis B, Avery M, Jennings E, Sherwood N, Martinson B, Crain AL. The effect of exercise during pregnancy on maternal outcomes: practical implications for practice. *Am J Lifestyle Med.* 2008;2(5):441-455.

60. Blum JW, Beaudoin CM, Caton-Lemos L. Physical activity patterns and maternal well-being in postpartum women. *Matern Child Health J.* 2004;8(3):163-169.

61. Martin CK, Church TS, Thompson AM, Earnest CTP, Blair SN. Exercise dose and quality of life: a randomized controlled trial. *Arch Intern Med.* 2009;169(3):269-278.

62. Im E-O, Chee W, Lim H-J, Liu Y, Kim HK. Midlife women's attitudes toward physical activity. *J Obstet Gynecol Neonatal Nurs.* 2008;37(2):203-213.

63. U.S. Preventive Services Task Force. Behavioral counseling to prevent sexually transmitted infections. 2008. Available at: http://www.uspreventiveservicestaskforce.org/uspstf08/sti/stirs.htm. Accessed October 10, 2012.

64. U.S. Department of Health and Human Services. Healthy people 2020: family planning. 2012. Available at: http://www.healthypeople.gov/2020/topicsobjectives2020/objectiveslist.aspx?topicId=13. Accessed October 10, 2012.

65. Centers for Disease Control and Prevention. Cancer and women. 2012. Available at: http://www.cdc.gov/Features/WomenAndCancer. Accessed October 15, 2012.

66. Centers for Disease Control and Prevention. Melanoma surveillance in the United States. 2011. Available at:

http://www.cdc.gov/cancer/dcpc/research/articles/melanoma_supplement.htm. Accessed October 15, 2012.

67. U.S. Preventive Services Task Force. Behavioral counseling to prevent skin cancer. 2012. Available at: http://www.uspreventiveservicestaskforce.org/uspstf11/skincancouns/skincancounsrs.htm. Accessed October 15, 2012.

68. Department of Health and Human Services. Women and smoking: a report of the Surgeon General. 2012. Available at: http://www.cdc.gov/tobacco/data_statistics/sgr/2001/complete_report/index.htm. Accessed October 17, 2012.

69. U.S. Preventive Services Task Force. Counseling and interventions to prevent tobacco use and tobacco-caused disease in adults and pregnant women. 2009. Available at: http://www.uspreventiveservicestaskforce.org/uspstf09/tobacco/tobaccors2.htm. Accessed October 17, 2012.

70. Kirchner TR, Shiffman SW, Paul E. Relapse dynamics during smoking cessation: recurrent abstinence violation effects and lapse–relapse progression. *J Abnormal Psychol.* 2012;121(1):187-197.

71. Centers for Disease Control and Prevention. Recommended immunization schedules for persons aged 0 through 18 years—United States. 2012. Available at: http://www.cdc.gov/vaccines/schedules/downloads/child/mmwr-child-schedule.pdf. Accessed October 23, 2012.

72. Centers for Disease Control and Prevention. Recommended adult immunization schedule—United States. 2012. Available at: http://www.cdc.gov/vaccines/schedules/downloads/adult/mmwr-adult-schedule.pdf. Accessed October 24, 2012.

73. Centers for Disease Control and Prevention. Recommended adult immunization schedule—United States. 2013. Available at: http://www.cdc.gov/vaccines/schedules/downloads/adult/adult-schedule.pdf. Accessed May 13, 2013.

74. Henry J. Kaiser Family Foundation. Health reform source: implementation timeline. Available at: http://healthreform.kff.org/timeline.aspx?source=QL. Accessed November 1, 2012.

75. U.S. Preventive Services Task Force. USPSTF A-Z topic guide. Available at: http://www.uspreventiveservicestaskforce.org/uspstopics.htm. Accessed October 29, 2012.

76. National Heart Lung and Blood Institute. Seventh report of the Joint National Committee on Prevention, Detection, Evaluation and Treatment of High Blood Pressure (JNC-7). Available at: http://www.nhlbi.nih.gov/guidelines/hypertension. Accessed January 10, 2013.

● ● ● Additional Resources

Online Sources of Specialty Group Recommendations

Agency for Healthcare Quality and Research
    http://www.ahrq.gov

American Academy of Pediatrics
    http://www.aap.org

American Association of Clinical Endocrinologists
    http://www.aace.com

American Cancer Society
    http://www.cancer.org

American Congress of Obstetricians and Gynecologists
    http://www.acog.org

Centers for Disease Control and Prevention
    http://www.cdc.gov

Cochrane Collaboration
    http://www.cochrane.org

Endocrine Society
    http://www.endo-society.org/guidelines/index.cfm

Healthy People 2020
    http://www.healthypeople.gov/2020/default.aspx

International Osteoporosis Foundation
    http://www.iofbonehealth.org

National Heart Lung and Blood Institute
    http://www.nhlbi.nih.gov/guidelines/hypertension

U.S. Department of Agriculture
    http://www.usda.gov/wps/portal/usda/usdahome

U.S. Department of Health and Human Services
    http://www.hhs.gov

U.S Preventive Services Task Force
    http://www.uspreventiveservicestaskforce.org/index.html

CHAPTER

8

Common Conditions in Primary Care

JAN M. KRIEBS

Historically, midwives often were the healers in communities. In addition to attending births, a midwife was the herbalist, first responder, and health counselor. Thus midwives were among the original primary care providers. Today, midwives continue to be primary care providers, especially when they are the only healthcare providers for many women.[1] This chapter is an introduction to health problems commonly experienced by women that may be seen by midwives in practice.

Primary Care

No universally accepted definition of "primary care" exists. Variations exist among insurers, providers, professional organizations, and consumers. Perhaps the most widely accepted definition is the one issued in 1996 by the Institute of Medicine, which characterized primary care as follows:

> The provision of integrated, accessible health care services by clinicians who are accountable for addressing a large majority of personal health care needs, developing a sustained partnership with patients, and practicing in the context of family and community.[2]

For some, the "large majority" has been defined as provision of 80% of the care needed by a person annually. However, this definition of primary care fails to highlight the importance health maintenance, age-appropriate screening, and health education—all activities are that integral to the practice of midwifery and that are discussed in depth in the *Health Promotion and Health Maintenance* chapter.

Primary care services may be necessary when providing maternity care. Women who are pregnant also develop coughs, infections, and minor injuries, for example. Pregnancy does not provide protection from anemia or stomach pain, and in the course of a pregnancy, other healthcare specialists frequently defer to the clinician managing the pregnancy as being the most qualified to treat other conditions. Therefore, even midwives who care for women only during the maternity cycle have an obligation to be informed about primary care, to be able to identify and manage common minor illnesses, and to appropriately refer women to another clinician for more complex health problems. Women with medical disorders that significantly affect the course of pregnancy are the focus of the *Medical Complications in Pregnancy* chapter. The current chapter reviews care of women who are not pregnant, but who have disorders or conditions that can be characterized as in the realm of primary care rather than gynecologic care.

The first step when investigating healthcare problems is competency in basic physical assessment and history taking as discussed in the *An Introduction to the Care of Women* chapter. A comprehensive history and physical examination can lead to the identification of complex problems. All midwives should know the resources in their communities for referral to other providers. Any general health examination—including the gynecologic examination—requires complete assessment of a woman's condition through history and review of systems. For example, if after a comprehensive history has been taken, the woman reports no problems on a review of systems, and she then walks into the exam room and is able to undress and position herself for an examination without assistance or physical difficulty, the midwife will have a significant amount of information about her general well-being—including sight, hearing, cranial nerve function, memory and orientation, affect, and gait and range of motion. All the information gained through history, review of systems, and observation can be used to identify areas of concern during the physical exam and assessment.

Hematologic Conditions

Anemia

Among the most common reports from women seeking care is the familiar "I'm tired all the time." There are many causes of fatigue, ranging from anemia to thyroid disease to stress. Signs and symptoms associated with anemia are listed in **Table 8-1**.[3] In addition, if a woman has menstrual periods, the history and review of systems should include obtaining a history of how heavy her menstrual flow is, even though women's estimation of their flow has been demonstrated to be variable in accuracy. A prior diagnosis of anemia merits a description of the circumstances. For example, some women may have been treated for pregnancy-related anemia and believe that they will, therefore, always suffer from this condition.

A complete blood count (CBC) provides the first level of assessment and helps differentiate many of the underlying causes of anemia. Defined as a decrease in red blood cell mass, or more correctly as a decrease in total hemoglobin, the normal hemoglobin level for menstruating women is 12.2 g/dL.[4,5] However, adverse effects usually are not seen in a previously health woman unless the hemoglobin level is less than 10.0 g/dL. The U.S. Department of Health and Human Services does not recommend screening for anemia as part of routine health care for adults, except among pregnant women.[4]

A number of confounding factors should be considered when investigating the diagnosis of anemia. Lower economic status is associated with higher rates of poor nutrition and, therefore, a higher rate of iron-deficiency anemia. African American women average approximately 1 g/dL lower hemoglobin levels than whites regardless of socioeconomic level.[4] Women who smoke (because of competition for oxygen-binding sites on red blood cells) and women living at high altitudes (because of lower oxygen concentration in the atmosphere) often have higher hemoglobin and hematocrit levels as their bodies adapt to maintain adequate oxygenation (**Table 8-2** and **Table 8-3**).[6]

Identifying the cause of a low hemoglobin can lead to appropriate therapy and referral to a specialist if needed. One common categorization of anemia is by the size of the red blood cells. Microcytic anemia includes iron deficiency, the thalassemias, and anemia of inflammation, also called anemia of chronic disease. Macrocytic anemia includes folate and vitamin B_{12} deficiency, liver disease, increased reticulocyte production, and some medication effects. Normocytic anemias commonly reflect acute blood loss or conditions such as sickle cell disease, hemoglobin C disease, or glucose-6-phosphate dehydrogenase

Table 8-1	Signs and Symptoms Associated with Severe Anemia
Signs	**Symptoms**
Pallor	Fatigue, drowsiness
Jaundice	Weakness
Orthostatic hypotension	Dizziness
Peripheral edema	Headaches
Pale mucous membranes and nail beds	Malaise
	Pica
Smooth, sore tongue	
Splenomegaly	Poor appetite, changes in food preferences
Tachypnea, dyspnea on exertion	Changes in sleep habits
	Changes in mood
Tachycardia or flow murmur	

Source: Centers for Disease Control and Prevention. Recommendations to prevent and control iron deficiency in the United States. *MMWR Recomm Rep.* 1998;47(RR-3):1-29.

Table 8-2	Smoking Adjustments for Hemoglobin and Hematocrit Cutoff Points for Anemia	
Smoking Status	**Hemoglobin (g/dL)**	**Hematocrit (%)**
Nonsmoker	0.0	0.0
Smoker (all)	+0.3	+1.0
0.5 to < 1 ppd	+0.3	+1.0
1.0–2.0 ppd	+0.5	+1.5
> 2.0 ppd	+0.7	+2.0

ppd: packs per day.
Source: Centers for Disease Control and Prevention. Reference criteria for anemia screening. *MMWR.* 1989;38:400-404.

Table 8-3	Altitude Adjustments for Hemoglobin and Hematocrit Cutoff Points for Anemia	
Altitude (ft)	**Hemoglobin (g/dL)**	**Hematocrit (%)**
< 3000	0.0	0.0
3000–3999	+0.2	+0.5
4000–4999	+0.3	+1.0
5000–5999	+0.5	+1.5
6000–6999	+0.7	+2.0
7000–7999	+1.0	+3.0
8000–8999	+1.3	+4.0
9000–9999	+1.6	+5.0
> 10,000	+2.0	+6.0

Source: Centers for Disease Control and Prevention. Reference criteria for anemia screening. *MMWR.* 1989;38:400-404.

(G6PD) deficiency. Aplastic anemia, while normocytic, shows pancytopenia, or a reduction in the number of red blood cells (RBCs), white blood cells (WBCs), and platelets.

Table 8-4 lists the laboratory values associated with some common causes of anemia. For women with a hemoglobin below 10.0 g/dL, a laboratory panel including serum folate, and ferritin measurements should be ordered, and a hemoglobin electrophoresis performed. The ferritin level is the most

sensitive and specific predictor of iron stores and therefore true iron deficiency. A ferritin level below 10–15 mcg/L confirms the diagnosis of anemia and therefore ordering serum iron and total iron-binding capacity measurements is not necessary. Based on the severity of the anemia and its cause, consultation or referral may be indicated; when the hemoglobin indicates severe anemia (< 9.0 g/dL), consultation may be appropriate, even when the anemia is clearly caused by iron deficiency.

Iron-Deficiency Anemia

The most common anemia in the United States is due to iron deficiency, which usually is mild and easily reversible. The recommended daily reference intake (RDI) for iron for reproductive-age women is 15 mg for girls age 14–18 years and 18 mg for women age 19–50 years.[7] Following menopause, the RDI drops to 8 mg. The diets of most women in the United States include approximately 13–14 mg of iron daily.[8] Normal daily iron loss through excretion, sweat, and cellular shedding amounts to 1 mg; menses causes an additional monthly loss. Pregnancy-related demands increase the daily iron need among reproductive-age women by 2–3 mg/day.[9]

Occult blood loss, excessive menstrual loss, and inadequate nutritional intake, which is often encountered among vegetarians, are the most common causes of iron deficiency in adults. If nutritional deficiency is ruled out and in the absence of an identifiable source of bleeding such as heavy menses, assessment

Table 8-4	Laboratory Values in Common Anemias				
Laboratory Test	**Iron Deficiency**	**Vitamin B$_{12}$ Deficiency**	**Folate Deficiency**	**Thalassemia**	**Chronic Disease**
Red blood cells (RBCs)	Low	High	High	Normal	Normal
Hemoglobin	Low	Low	Low	Low	Low
Mean corpuscular volume (MCV)	Low	High	High	Low	Normal-low
Mean corpuscular hemoglobin (MCH)	Low	High	High	Low	Low
Mean corpuscular hemoglobin concentration (MCHC)	Low	Normal	Normal	Low	Normal-low
Ferritin	Low	High	High	High	Normal-high
Iron	Low	High	High	High	Low
Total iron-binding capacity (TIBC)	High	Normal	Normal	Normal	Low

for gastrointestinal bleeding is warranted, including inquiry about use of aspirin and nonsteroidal anti-inflammatory drugs (NSAIDs). Nutritional deficiencies causing significant iron depletion include restrictive vegetarian diets as well as pica, so a careful diet history is part of the work-up.

First-line treatment is to increase dietary intake of iron-rich foods, especially accompanied by consumption of vitamin C–enriched products to enhance absorption. Nutritional counseling should stress the importance of including iron-rich foods in the diet—such as green leafy vegetables, collard greens, egg yolks, raisins, prunes, liver, oysters, and some fortified cereals—as well as the elimination of picas, such as eating ice or nonfood starches.

Iron supplementation, either nutritional or with oral medications, should be initiated when the hemoglobin is less than 10.0 g/dL. Adding 1.0 mg of folic acid in cases where the serum folate is low or using a vitamin C–enriched product to facilitate iron absorption also may be useful.

When uncomplicated iron deficiency is the cause of the anemia and oral medications are used, any of several iron preparations, including ferrous sulfate (Feosol), ferrous fumarate (Feostat), and ferrous gluconate (Fergon), can be used. Each of these preparations is available under several different brand names. The equivalent of 325 mg of ferrous sulfate taken three times a day is standard. Taking iron preparations with meals will decrease absorption, but will also improve gastrointestinal side effects such as nausea and reflux. Certain drugs, such as antacids, should not be taken with iron supplements. After the hemoglobin level has returned to normal, continued supplementation for 3 months should adequately replenish iron stores in the body.

Hemoglobinopathies: Thalassemias

Normal adult hemoglobin is composed of four polypeptide subunits: two alpha-globin and two beta-globin chains. A hemoglobinopathy occurs when one or two of the subunits are replaced by a variant type of globin chain. Alpha- or beta-thalassemia occurs when deficient amounts of alpha or beta globin chains are made. Common hemoglobinopathies and thalassemias are listed in **Table 8-5.**

Thalassemias are Mendelian autosomal recessive inherited disorders of the globin chains that form normal adult hemoglobin (hemoglobin A). Worldwide, approximately 1.67% of the population is heterozygous for either alpha-thalassemia (α-thalassemia) or beta-thalassemia (β-thalassemia), and approximately 0.044% is affected by homozygous or multiple heterozygous mutations.[10] Among persons who have

alpha-thalassemias, decreased hemoglobin alpha production causes abnormal proportions of hemoglobins A, A_2, and F. The beta-thalassemias are associated with elevated levels of hemoglobin F and hemoglobin A_2 (higher than 3.5%). In both cases, the trait will appear as a microcytic anemia in which the mean cell volume (MCV) is markedly low relative to the hemoglobin level, usually less than 75 fl. The Metzer index is a calculation derived by dividing the MCV by number of RBCs. When the Metzer index is less than 13, a thalassemia is strongly suspected. Nonetheless, a complete anemia panel is justified to rule out a combination of iron deficiency and hemoglobinopathy. When the diagnosis is established, folic acid supplementation may be employed but iron therapy is inappropriate, as simple iron supplementation will not correct the anemia in persons who have beta-thalassemia or alpha thalassemia trait.

Alpha-thalassemia is most common among individuals of Chinese and Southeast Asian descent. Two genes on chromosome 16 control for alpha-globin chain production. Therefore, the number of mutations affects the severity of disease. A single deletion will create an asymptomatic carrier state; two deletions will cause a smaller MCV without anemia; and the three deletion state produces an increase in hemoglobin H with effects including splenomegaly and severe hemolytic anemia. The absence of all four alpha chains and the resultant increase in hemoglobin B produces non-immune fetal hydrops, which results in fetal demise.[11]

Beta-thalassemia is most common among women of Mediterranean origin and, to a lesser degree, among Chinese, Asian, and African women. Estimates of its frequency range from 3% to 10%.[12] More than 200 different point mutations can be involved in the beta-globin changes associated with thalassemia. Asymptomatic individuals with a mutation affecting a single beta-globin gene may be a silent carrier state or may present with only mild anemia (beta-thalassemia minor). For these women, the diagnosis in most likely made based on routine screening or incidental findings. Women with more severe disease—that is, beta-thalassemia intermediate and beta-thalassemia major—have mutations affecting multiple genes. The two conditions are differentiated by the age at diagnosis and degree of anemia, and both require lifelong therapy.[11,12]

Hemoglobinopathies: Sickle Cell Disease

Sickle cell disease (homozygous SS disease) is an autosomal recessive inherited disorder in which hemoglobin S is produced instead of hemoglobin A. Sickle cell trait (Hb AS) is found among approximately 8% of

Table 8-5	Disorders of Abnormal Hemoglobin	
Name	**Description**	**Clinical Significance**
Hemoglobinopathies		
Sickle cell disease	Hb SS	Severe illness with sickle cell crisis
Sickle cell trait	Hb SA	Mild anemia; increased risk for urinary tract infections; sickle cell crisis may occur at high altitudes, if dehydrated, or during extreme physical activity
Sickle cell hemoglobin C disease	Hb SC	Mild to moderate anemia and sickle cell crisis occur but less frequent than in Hb SS; increased risk for infection; risk for retinopathy and blindness in adulthood
Hemoglobin C disease	Hb CC	Generally benign mild hemolytic anemia; may not be diagnosed until adulthood; musculoskeletal pain, retinopathy, and cholestasis are associated with Hb CC; pregnancy complications are rare
Hemoglobin C trait	HB CA	Generally asymptomatic
Thalassemias		
Alpha-thalassemia silent carrier	1 of 4 genes deleted	Asymptomatic and difficult to detect
Alpha-thalassemia trait	2 of 4 genes deleted	Mild microcytic anemia; individual is asymptomatic
Hemoglobin H disease	3 of 4 genes deleted	Enlarged spleen; bone abnormalities; severe illness
	4 of 4 genes deleted	Incompatible with life; causes hydrops fetalis
Beta-thalassemia (Cooley's anemia)	Beta-thalassemia major, homozygous	Severe anemia; requires frequent blood transfusions
Thalassemia intermedia		Significant anemia but does not need blood transfusions
Thalassemia minor		Mild microcytic anemia; individual is asymptomatic

African Americans and generally is asymptomatic.[13] Although the trait itself does not cause severe health complications, identification of those persons carrying the sickle trait is important to enable couples planning to have children to obtain appropriate genetic counseling and testing. The primary complication for the nonpregnant woman is an increase in the development of urinary tract infections and hematuria.

The estimated incidence of sickle cell disease is 1 in 500 births for African Americans. However, midwives should not assume this disease is limited only to black women, as Hispanic infants accounted for more than 10% of newborns with the disease in a study in New York State of maternal ethnicity of individuals with sickle cell disease.[14] In the same study, a higher incidence of disease was found among immigrants rather than native-born individuals, even of the same race/ethnicity.

In sickle cell disease, repeatedly stressed RBCs form a permanent crescent moon or "sickle" shape; they may then clump together and block the microvasculature. Sickle cell crises involve acute episodes of severe pain from ischemia and infarction of tissue and organs. The disease has a multi-organ effect and is associated with a shortened lifespan as a consequence of renal damage, cardiac damage, infection, acute chest syndrome, and an increased risk for infection.

Hemoglobin S may also be present in heterozygous form as Hb SC disease or sickle thalassemia (HB S/B thal), conditions that are associated with somewhat milder forms of sickle crisis. In the face of these and other hemoglobinopathies, genetic counseling for couples planning a child is recommended.

G6PD Deficiency

Glucose-6-phosphate dehydrogenase (G6PD) deficiency is an X-linked genetic disease found among individuals of Mediterranean descent as well as African Americans. Because it is an X-linked condition, G6PD deficiency is rarely symptomatic among women. Even among individuals who have the condition, the clinical presentation ranges from being asymptomatic to presenting with severe acute or chronic hemolytic anemia. Hemolysis occurs when the individual has an infection or receives oxidative drugs. Among the medications commonly used in pregnancy and women's health care that must not be given to individuals with G6PD deficiency are sulfa drugs and sulfa derivatives, nitrofurantoin (Macrodantin, Macrobid), toluidine blue, and methylene blue. Eating fava beans also should be avoided because fava beans can produce hemolysis among individuals with the Mediterranean variant.

Because infection can cause hemolysis, prompt diagnosis and treatment of any infectious condition will minimize the risk. Surgery can also precipitate an episode of hemolysis. Therefore, the midwife should remind a woman to notify her surgical team prior to any surgical procedure.

Von Willebrand's Disease

Von Willebrand's disease is an autosomal dominant mutation causing defects in a protein necessary for platelet adhesion and affecting clotting factor VII.[15] This condition is the related to development of menorrhagia or heavy menses approximately 20% of the time, particularly among adolescents.[16] Von Willebrand's or another bleeding disorder should be suspected if the history includes heavy menstrual bleeding in association with prolonged bleeding after surgery or a family history of bleeding problems.[15] The initial assessment includes obtaining a platelet count, ferritin level, and bleeding time and coagulation studies. If the platelets are normal, the ferritin level is low, and the bleeding time is prolonged, von Willebrand's disease is a strong possibility. Referral for the woman to a hematologist for evaluation at this point is warranted, although the midwife may continue to provide general care. Women with this condition should avoid aspirin or other agents with anticoagulant properties.

Cardiovascular Conditions

Assessment of a woman's cardiovascular status begins with a history and review of systems that assess for hypertension, cardiac events, and vascular changes in the woman and her immediate family. The current surge in acute cardiac events among relatively young adults, associated with the national increases in cholesterol levels, poor dietary habits, sedentary lifestyles, and increased stress, underscores the importance of obtaining a complete database during history taking. Unfortunately, these factors all too often are not addressed during a reproductive health visit. Assessment of heart sounds and of the pulses during the physical examination is essential, as is an accurate blood pressure.

Cardiovascular disease is the leading cause of death among women and is the third most common cause of death for women of reproductive age.[17] Together, various forms of cardiovascular disease, including stroke, account for more than 30% of deaths among women. Risk factors for cardiovascular conditions include hypertension, dyslipidemia, diabetes, obesity, physical inactivity, smoking, and aging. Simple aging is noted as a risk because 20% of women age 65 years or older have some form of heart disease.

Hypertension

Hypertension is an arterial disease characterized by persistent high blood pressure and is the most frequent diagnosis associated with primary care visits in the United States.[18] Many clinicians take action based on blood pressure results that are not accurate because the technique of assessment is incorrect. Blood pressures should always be taken with the cuff at the level of the heart while using a properly sized cuff. The woman should have had several minutes to sit quietly and not have ingested tobacco or caffeine for at least 30 minutes prior to measuring the blood pressure.

Hypertension is more common among African Americans and among the elderly. More than 30% of all adults in the United States (66.9 million individuals) have high blood pressure, defined either as having a blood pressure of 140/90 mm Hg or as regularly taking antihypertensive medications.[19] Even though hypertension is more common among men, the lifetime risk of high blood pressure for women is in the range of approximately 90%.[20] It is estimated that 80% of women diagnosed with high blood pressure take medication, although only slightly more than half of those have well-controlled blood pressure.[21] Lack of awareness of a diagnosis of high blood pressure and/or failure to be treated effectively has been associated with lack of access to care and lack of health insurance.[22]

The classification of blood pressure as presented in the *Seventh Report of the Joint National Committee on Prevention, Detection, and Treatment of High Blood Pressure (JNC Report)* can be found in **Table 8-6**.[22] Prehypertension is not a disease category, but rather an alert that lifestyle changes may be necessary to reduce future risk. The JNC-7 report recommends that all individuals diagnosed with hypertension be treated.

Table 8-6	Classification of Blood Pressure for Adults			
Blood Pressure Classification	**SBP (mm Hg)**		**DBP (mm Hg)**	
Normal	< 120	and	< 80	
Prehypertension	120–139	or	80–89	
Stage 1 hypertension	140–159	or	90–99	
Stage 2 hypertension	> 160	or	> 100	

DBP: diastolic blood pressure; SBP: systolic blood pressure.

Source: Adapted from National High Blood Pressure Education Program. *The Seventh Report of the Joint National Committee on Prevention, Detection, Evaluation, and Treatment of High Blood Pressure: Complete Report.* Bethesda, MD: National Heart, Lung, and Blood Institute; August 2004.

Table 8-7	Recommendations for Follow-Up Based on Initial Blood Pressure Measurements for Adults Without Acute End-Organ Damage
Blood Pressure Classification	**Recommendation for Follow-Up**
Normal	Recheck in 2 years.
Prehypertension	Recheck in 1 year.
Stage 1 hypertension	Confirm within 2 months.
Stage 2 hypertension	Evaluate or refer for care within 1 month. If higher pressures (e.g., > 180/110 mm Hg), evaluate and treat immediately or within 1 week based on clinical situation.

Source: Adapted from National High Blood Pressure Education Program. *The Seventh Report of the Joint National Committee on Prevention, Detection, Evaluation, and Treatment of High Blood Pressure: Complete Report.* Bethesda, MD: National Heart, Lung, and Blood Institute; August 2004.

Reevaluation of blood pressure is a standard part of the general health examination. The frequency of monitoring recommended to ensure that lifestyle change and medication have achieved a normal blood pressure can be found in **Table 8-7**. When the systolic and diastolic measurements fall into different categories, the shorter interval for visits is the correct one to follow.[22]

Many cases of hypertension are directly related to lifestyle, rather than underlying disease. These causes are directly modifiable and include weight loss, nutritional counseling for a low-sodium diet, exercise, and moderation in alcohol consumption.[18,22]

A weight loss of as little as 10 pounds may have a salutary effect on blood pressure. Medication interactions that can provoke hypertension include estrogens, NSAIDs, steroids, ergotamine (Cafregot), St. John's wort, and numerous others. **Table 8-8** demonstrates the effect of lifestyle modification on blood pressure.[22] Achieving more than one modification has an independent effect on blood pressure.[23]

Table 8-8	Lifestyle Modifications to Prevent and Manage Hypertension[a]	
Modification	**Recommendation**	**Approximate SBP Reduction (Range)[b] [Source]**
Weight reduction	Maintain normal body weight (BMI: 18.5–24.9 kg/m²)	5–20 mm Hg/10 kg
Adopt DASH eating plan	Consume diet rich in fruits, vegetables, and low-fat dairy products with reduced saturated and total fat	8–14 mm Hg
Physical activity	Engage in regular aerobic physical activity such as brisk walking (at least 30 min per day, most days of the week)	4–9 mm Hg
Moderation of alcohol	Men: No more than 2 drinks per day Women (and lighter-weight men): No more than 1 drink per day 1 drink = 24 oz beer, 10 oz wine, or 3 oz 80-proof whiskey	2–4 mm Hg

BMI = body mass index; DASH = Dietary Approaches to Stop Hypertension; SBP = systolic blood pressure.

[a]For overall cardiovascular risk reduction, stop smoking.

[b]The effects of implementing these modifications are dose and time dependent, and could be greater for an individual.

Source: Adapted from National High Blood Pressure Education Program. *The Seventh Report of the Joint National Committee on Prevention, Detection, Evaluation, and Treatment of High Blood Pressure: Complete Report.* Bethesda, MD: National Heart, Lung, and Blood Institute; August 2004.

When evaluating a woman with hypertension, assessment of blood pressure in the other arm; checking for pulses; auscultation of bruits; a thorough heart, lung, and abdominal assessment; and assessment for edema and neurologic changes are key components of the physical examination. When the history and physical indicate further evaluation is warranted or when hypertension does not respond to medication therapy, other medical causes should be pursued, including thyroid disease, sleep apnea, chronic steroid use or Cushing's syndrome, mineralocorticoid excess states, kidney disease, coarctation of the aorta, and pheochromocytoma.[22]

Uncontrolled hypertension can be the cause of a variety of cardiovascular complications, including stroke, myocardial infarction, and other heart disease. In addition to lifestyle modifications, several categories of drugs can be prescribed for hypertension. Low-dose thiazide diuretics are an effective first-line choice; they have been demonstrated to reduce all-cause mortality, stroke, and coronary heart disease (CHD).[24] Angiotensin-converting enzyme (ACE) inhibitors, calcium-channel blockers, beta blockers, angiotensin II antagonists, and other drug categories are used either alone or in combination; ACE inhibitors have shown evidence of similar efficacy to thiazide diuretics, but are not superior and are more costly.[24] A meta-analysis of trials of antihypertensive drugs concluded that all classes of these medications were similar in preventing CHD.[25] Many women will require more than one medication to control blood pressure, and most midwives will refer nonpregnant women who need pharmaceutical therapies to a physician to initiate treatment and in some cases to alter medication regimens. However, many midwives will provide care for women at risk of or under treatment for hypertension, especially if current trends of obesity continue.

Dyslipidemia

Dyslipidemia—that is, elevated fat or cholesterol in the blood—is another major risk factor associated with cardiac disease, and often a preventable or modifiable one. Low-density lipoprotein (LDL) has been found to be a surrogate for cardiac disease and is the major component of cholesterol, accounting for approximately 65% to 70% of total cholesterol. An elevation in LDL level is directly associated with the development of atherosclerotic plaques.

Screening for dyslipidemia in women of reproductive age is not standardized in the same manner as screening for hypertension. The National Cholesterol Education Program Adult Treatment Panel III[26,27] recommends screening low-risk women

of reproductive age beginning at age 20 years, but other guidelines vary. However, the recommendation to screen all women with risk factors is more consistent.[28] **Box 8-1** identifies the National Heart, Lung, and Blood Institute's (NHLBI) classifications for cholesterol levels.[26] Available data suggest that among women age 20 to 45 years, 59% have either CHD, a CHD equivalent (stroke, diabetes, elevated fasting glucose), or one or more CHD risk factors, yet fewer than half receive screening.[29]

Specific risk factors for dyslipidemia include obesity, hypertension, diabetes, smoking, preexisting CHD, and a family history of early cardiovascular disease. Risk increases with age; for women, the clinically relevant increased risk is related to menopause, and age 55 years and older often is used as the surrogate for the point at which risk begins to spike upward. Medical conditions that increase the risk of dyslipidemia include diabetes; thyroid disease; kidney diseases including chronic renal failure and nephrotic syndrome; obstructive liver disease such as gallstones, hepatitis, and cirrhosis; and use of medications such as protease inhibitors, progestins, corticosteroids, and anabolic steroids. The appropriate screen includes a complete lipid profile obtained after

---

BOX 8-1 Classification of LDL, Total, and HDL Cholesterol (mg/dL)

LDL Cholesterol (mg/dL)

100–129 Near optimal/above optimal
130–159 Borderline high
160–189 High
> 190 Very high

Total Cholesterol (mg/dL)

< 200 Desirable
200–239 Borderline high
> 240 High

HDL Cholesterol (mg/dL)

> 240 High
< 40 Low
> 60 High

HDL = high-density lipoprotein; LDL = low-density lipoprotein.

Source: National Cholesterol Education Program. *Third Report of the National Cholesterol Education Program (NCEP) on Detection, Evaluation, and Treatment of High Blood Cholesterol in Adults (Adult Treatment Panel III Final Report).* Bethesda, MD: National Heart, Lung, and Blood Institute; May 2001.

an overnight fast of 9 to 12 hours. Women without risk factors should be screened every 5 years, whereas those with specific risk factors or borderline lipid levels should be rescreened more frequently.

When the midwife identifies high cholesterol levels, counseling always includes diet changes to decrease total and dietary fat to between 25% and 35% of total calories and add dietary fiber, stop smoking, and increase exercise levels. Medication therapy can be deferred while a trial of healthy behaviors is undertaken, as long as there is no family history suggestive of genetic predisposition to coronary artery disease and the LDL cholesterol level is less than 160 mg/dL for women without other cardiac risk factors. Determining the interplay of risk factors and laboratory results to determine which woman needs intervention and how her progress should be followed may be an indication for referral to a physician. Pharmacologic therapy is instituted based on LDL level and risk profile. Among the medications used for elevated cholesterol are statins (e.g., atorvastatin [Lipitor]), bile acid sequestrants (e.g., cholestyramine [Questran]), niacin (e.g., nicotinic acid [Niaspan]), fibric acids (e.g., gemfibrozil [Lopid]), and cholesterol absorption inhibitors (e.g., ezetimibe [Zetia]). Omega-3 fatty acids may be used as a complementary therapy. **Table 8-9** illustrates ways in which various classes of medication affect dyslipidemia.[30]

Conditions of the Respiratory System

Upper Respiratory Infections

Upper respiratory infections include the common cold, bronchitis, rhinosinusitis, otitis media, and pharyngitis. Commonly viral in nature, nonspecific upper respiratory infections (URIs) and influenza are a frequent reason for calls to healthcare providers, with individuals often asking for antibiotics that will

not cure the problem. Although rates of inappropriate prescribing have decreased, the overall rate of antibiotic prescribing for acute respiratory infections was higher than 50% in 2009, and the frequency of prescribing broad-spectrum antibiotics was noted to have increased in that year.[31] Overtreatment as well as inappropriate treatment has led to a rapid increase in the prevalence of drug-resistant *Streptococcus pneumoniae*, a problem with implications for the management of all respiratory disease because this microbe is the most common bacterial respiratory pathogen.[32]

Many URIs can be avoided through the use of simple hygiene techniques, most particularly the practice of hand washing. The use of antibacterial soaps and environmental sprays generally is not necessary in the home, but has not been linked to adverse ecological events. Hand sanitizers have become useful items in public areas, especially when respiratory infections are prevalent.

The diagnosis of nonspecific URI is made based on the presence of nasal congestion and a clear, white, or yellow/green discharge, as well as sore throat, muscle aches, headache, and cough. The symptoms of colds and influenza overlap, although high fever and dry cough are more typical of the "flu" than of a cold. Symptomatic management may reduce the severity of symptoms, although many interventions commonly attempted lack evidence of effectiveness. Treatments include rest, increased fluids, saline gargle or spray, and a variety of medications. Pharmaceuticals are best targeted to specific symptoms, such as dextromethorphan (Benylin) for coughs; therefore, combination drugs are not advised. Antibiotics are not indicated for treatment of nonspecific URI or influenza.[33]

Ipratropium bromide (Atrovent), an anticholinergic nasal spray, can be used if needed to relieve rhinorrhea, sneezing, and congestion. Initial use consists of two sprays in each nostril, three to four times daily.[34] Because kinins (a group of vasoactive peptides) are implicated in rhinitis symptoms, the use

Table 8-9	Effect of Drugs on Dyslipidemia		
Drugs	**LDL**	**HDL**	**Triglycerides**
Statins	Effective	Modest effect	Modest effect
Bile acid sequestrants	Modest effect	No effect	Minimal effect or increase
Fibrates	Minimal to no effect or increase	Modest effect	Effective
Niacin	Modest effect	Effective	Effective
Ezetimibe (Zetia)	Effective	Modest effect	No effect

HDL: high-density lipoprotein; LDL: low-density lipoprotein.

Source: King TL, Brucker MC. *Pharmacology for Women's Health.* Sudbury, MA: Jones and Bartlett; 2011:411.

of antihistamines has not been found to reduce cold symptoms significantly. Intranasal corticosteroids have not shown any benefit for URIs, but are not harmful and may be continued if being used for another condition.[35] Regardless of pharmaceutical treatments, resolution of symptoms should be complete within a week.

A bacterial cause for URI should be suspected when the symptoms persist or worsen after 8 to 10 days; when maxillo-facial pain is present (especially if only one side of the face is affected); when the symptoms over the first 3 to 4 days are severe; when symptoms are associated with a fever higher than 39°C (102.2°F), presence of purulent discharge; or when symptoms worsen after a viral infection had appeared to be resolving.[34] If antibiotic therapy is needed, the narrowest-spectrum drug effective against *S. pneumoniae* and *Haemophilus influenzae* should be used.

Common Cold

The common cold is a self-limited syndrome caused by many different viruses. The common cold is a mild URI and the most frequent illness experienced by adults and children in industrialized nations. Symptoms include varying patterns of nasal discharge, headache, sore throat, sore muscles, cough, or sneezing. The common cold is usually spread via droplets and hard surface contamination. The incubation period is 24 to 72 hours and the period of infectivity starts approximately on the second day of illness and peaks on the third day of illness but viruses that cause the common cold can be infective for several days. The initial differential diagnosis is allergic or bacterial rhinitis, bacterial pharyngitis, pertussis, and influenza. The complications associated with the common cold include rhinosinusitis, lower respiratory tract infections, exacerbation of asthma, and bronchitis.

Rhinosinusitis

When an acute URI has spread into the sinus cavities, the term *rhinosinusitis* generally is preferred to the older term *sinusitis*. A green or yellow discharge commonly is found in addition to pain and pressure over the affected sinus. Other symptoms may include a toothache near the affected sinus, fever, and a cough that worsens when lying down. More than 90% of these infections are viral.[36] Acute rhinosinusitis lasts less than 4 weeks, and more than 70% of cases will resolve spontaneously.[37] Although fewer than 10% of rhinosinusitis begin as bacterial infections, over-prescription of antibiotics is common, as one study found that these medications were prescribed in more

than 80% of rhinosinusitis epidodes.[38] Three clinical scenarios suggest a bacterial infection: (1) persistent symptoms for more than 10 days without improvement; (2) severe onset with a high fever of at least 39°C (102.2°F) and purulent nasal discharge 3 or more days beginning with the onset of symptoms; or (3) what has been called "double-sickening," when viral symptoms begin to improve but then suddenly worsen near the end of the first week.[33]

Therapy includes supportive management with over-the-counter decongestants, analgesics, and antipyretics. As with colds, antihistamines should not be used unless the congestion has an allergic component. When symptoms of a bacterial infection or super-infection are present, then antibiotics should be initiated. Ampicillin-clavulanate (Augmentin) or doxycycline (Vibramycin) is the preferred initial regimen. Fluoroquinolones can be used as an alternative; however, macrolides such as azithromycin (Zithromax), trimethoprim-sulfamethoxazole (TMP-SMX; Bactrim), and cephalosporins are not recommended due to the increased risk of resistance to these drugs.[33]

Influenza

The onset of viral influenza is abrupt, marked by fever, rhinitis, cough, sore throat, headache, muscle pain, and general malaise. Most symptoms will resolve in a week or less, although malaise and tiredness may persist. Influenza should be suspected as the cause of URI during the flu season that typically begins in October and lasts through April. Herd immunity achieved by widespread vaccination is the best protection against influenza outbreaks. Vaccines for the seasonal flu types anticipated by the Centers for Disease Control and Prevention (CDC) become available in early fall and should be recommended to all persons. The live attenuated influenza vaccine (LAIV) administered intranasally is available for immune-competent, nonpregnant adults younger than the age of 50 years. The trivalent inactivated vaccine (TIV) is administered intramuscularly or, in one preparation, intradermally. Persons older than 65 years should receive the high-dose vaccine, as most seniors have decreased immune response. Some individuals are at higher risk of severe complications of influenza and have a heightened need for vaccination; criteria pertaining to these persons are listed in **Box 8-2**.[39]

The CDC recommends the use of the neuraminidase inhibitors (oseltamivir [Tamiflu], zanamivir [Relenza]) to treat influenza.[40] Infections suspected of being influenza can be treated within 48 hours of the onset of symptoms to shorten the duration of

---

BOX 8-2 Individuals at Increased Risk of Complications of Influenza

Persons age 50 years and older

Persons with chronic disease:
- Pulmonary (including asthma)
- Cardiovascular (except hypertension)
- Renal
- Hepatic
- Neurologic
- Hematologic
- Metabolic disorders (including diabetes mellitus)

Persons who are immunosuppressed (caused by medications or HIV)

Women who are or may be pregnant during the influenza season

Children age 6 months to 18 years receiving long-term aspirin therapy who might be at risk for Reye's syndrome after influenza virus infection

Residents of nursing homes and other chronic care facilities

American Indians/Alaska natives

Persons with BMI > 40

Healthcare personnel

Household contacts and caregivers of the following:
- Children age younger than 5 years
- Adults age 50 years and older
- Children age younger than 6 months
- Persons with medical conditions that increase risk for severe complications of influenza

Source: Centers for Disease Control and Prevention. Seasonal influenza (flu): additional information about vaccination of specific populations. Available at: http://www.cdc.gov/flu /professionals/acip/specificpopulations.htm#personsat. Accessed January 20, 2013.

---

infection by approximately one day. Nevertheless, in healthy adults, influenza is a self-limiting disease and may be best treated with rest and supportive therapy.

Pharyngitis

Approximately 5% to 15% of sore throats are caused by group A beta-hemolytic *Streptococcus* (GAS); the remainder are primarily viral and require only supportive care while symptoms resolve. Testing for GAS is not necessary when symptoms clearly indicate a viral infection—cough, runny nose, oral sores, and hoarseness. In contrast, tonsillar exudate, tender anterior cervical lymph nodes, fever, and lack of a cough suggest a bacterial infection. Either a rapid antigen detection test or culture can be performed if symptoms do not exclude GAS. Follow-up culture after a negative rapid antigen detection test is no longer recommended in adults.[41]

Penicillin and amoxicillin regimens lasting 10 days are the most appropriate first-line treatments for GAS. A first-generation cephalosporin, clindamycin (Cleocin), and clarithromycin (Biaxin) for 10 days or azithromycin (Zithromax) for 5 days are all acceptable alternatives when penicillin allergy exists. An analgesic or antipyretic can be used for supportive therapy; corticosteroids are not recommended. It is not necessary to treat household contacts.[41]

Bronchitis

Infections of the lower respiratory tract limited to the trachea and bronchi are termed *bronchitis*; they can appear as an inflammatory response to an otherwise uncomplicated URI. In healthy women of reproductive age, acute bronchitis is typically a viral syndrome of low-grade fever, malaise, fatigue, sore throat, chest pain, and cough. The cough may be productive or nonproductive. The cough of bronchitis can be differentiated from the cough of the common cold when it persists more than 5 days. Smoking, exposure to irritating fumes in the environment, and gastric reflux that irritates the bronchi can also precipitate acute bronchitis. Long-term exposure to smoking or environmental pollutants can lead to chronic bronchitis. On auscultation, lung sounds other than over the bronchi should be clear; a chest X ray, if performed, should not show infiltrates. Worsening chest pain with shortness of breath or pain on inspiration suggests pneumonia.

In most cases, the infection and the cough will resolve within 1 to 2 weeks with supportive therapy. If cough is persistent after the primary infection has resolved and wheezing is noted, the use of an albuterol inhaler may provide relief.[42] If an inhaler is prescribed, the directions should be for two puffs every 4 to 6 hours as needed to relieve symptoms. Asthma should be considered as an alternative diagnosis.

Antibiotics are not useful in the case of viral bronchitis, but under certain circumstances suspected bacterial infections of the bronchi may require antibiotic therapy. Antibiotics should be avoided in healthy adults with moderate symptoms; their potential benefit is outweighed in most cases by the potential for increased resistance and the expense of therapy.[43] If the diagnosis is unclear, or if symptoms persist and worsen, both pneumonia and pertussis should be ruled out. Signs and symptoms that indicate the diagnosis is pneumonia include temperature higher than or equal to 38°C (100.4°F), tachypnea at more than 24 breaths per minute, tachycardia at more than 100 beats per minute, rales or decreased breast sounds, and symptoms that develop quickly.[44]

Community-Acquired Pneumonia

Influenza and pneumonia are the leading infectious cause of death in the United States and the eighth most frequent cause of death overall.[45] Predisposing factors for pneumonia include damage to the cilia of the respiratory tract from chronic cough, viral infections, or smoking. The common infecting organisms are *Streptococcus pneumoniae*, *Haemophilus influenzae*, *Mycoplasma pneumoniae*, *Chlamydia pneumoniae*, *Staphylococcus aureus*, and a variety of viruses, most commonly influenza. Because bacterial causes of community-acquired pneumonia (CAP) predominate, antibiotic therapy is instituted promptly when a diagnosis is made. Risk factors for CAP include age older than 65 years, underweight or BMI less than 19, smoking, excessive alcohol intake, decreased ciliary activity, prior episodes of pneumonia or chronic bronchitis, chronic obstructive pulmonary disease, use of H_2 blockers, immunosuppression, and chronic medical illnesses.[45,46] The onset of symptoms is usually abrupt, with fatigue, cough, difficulty breathing, chills/sweats, anorexia, headache, and chest pain being the most common. Fever of 38°C (100.4°F) or higher, tachycardia, tachypnea, rales, and lung consolidation can be found on examination. When the cause is bacterial, high fever and a productive cough are more likely, whereas viral causes produce a more generalized malaise. Chest X ray is indicated to confirm the diagnosis and to identify underlying complications. Microbiologic testing to confirm the pathogen is not routinely recommended before empiric therapy is initiated,[45] but at least one expert has recently argued that this practice runs counter to the need for better targeting of antibiotic therapy to reduce risk of resistance in common pathogens.[47]

Whether women with CAP are treated on an outpatient basis or are hospitalized is a decision with significant consequences in terms of treatment modalities, testing schemes, and costs. While uncomplicated pneumonia should be treated promptly with antibiotics and can safely be managed on an outpatient basis in healthy adults, the prudent midwife will consult with a physician if severe pneumonia is suspected.

Indications of severe disease include confusion, respiratory rate of 30 or more breaths per minute, systolic blood pressure less than 90 mm Hg or diastolic blood pressures less than 60 mm Hg, age 65 years or older, and urea level greater than 7 mmol/L. When none or only one of these factors is present, the risk of mortality is less than 2% and ambulatory treatment is safe. Two positive signs in this list indicate the need for hospital admission, and three or more indicate the need for intensive care unit admission. Other signs may increase risk and, therefore, the urgency of admission—for example, poor oxygenation, lack of a caregiver in the home, or comorbidities.

Initial therapy for mild CAP includes azithromycin (Zithromax) 500 mg daily for 3 days or another macrolide, or doxycycline (Vibramycin) 100 mg twice daily for 7 days.[45] If the individual has comorbidities or recent antibiotic use for other illnesses, collaboration with a physician is advised to select additional or alternative therapy, which should include a fluoroquinolone or a beta-lactam plus a macrolide.

Pertussis

Bordetella pertussis is an increasingly important respiratory pathogen; 27,550 cases of this infection were diagnosed in the United States in 2012, and the CDC suggests that many cases go unreported. **Figure 8-1** shows both the cyclic nature and the increasing incidence of pertussis in recent years.[48]

Pertussis affects the ability to clear the respiratory tract by paralyzing the cilia lining the respiratory tract and causing inflammation as well as directly invading the alveoli.[49] Incubation is approximately 7 to 10 days, but can occur as long as 6 weeks following exposure. Clinically, the first symptoms resemble a mild URI, with little temperature elevation. Although pertussis is milder in adults than in babies or young children, it can persist with an increasingly violent cough over several weeks. **Table 8-10** provides a description of the stages of the disease.[49]

Common complications of untreated pertussis in adults include rib fracture, pneumothorax, superimposed bacterial pneumonia, urinary incontinence,

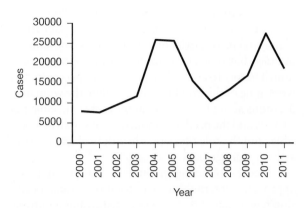

Figure 8-1 Reported pertussis incidence in the United States, 2000-2011.

Source: Adapted from Centers for Disease Control and Prevention. *The Pink Book: Epidemiology and Prevention of Vaccine-Preventable Diseases.* 12th ed. Atlanta, GA: Centers for Disease Control and Prevention; May 2012. Available at: http://www.cdc.gov/vaccines/pubs/pinkbook/index.html. Accessed April 10, 2013.

clarithromycin (Biaxin) that are better tolerated.[50] TMP-SMX (Bactrim) can also be used for therapy. Post-exposure prophylaxis with the same drugs is recommended for all close contacts. It is not known whether post-exposure vaccination has any benefit.[49]

Asthma

Asthma is a chronic inflammation of airways associated with intermittent worsening of symptoms; reversible obstruction from bronchospasm, edema, and mucus production; and hyper-responsiveness to stimuli. An individual's innate immunity, genetics, and environmental exposures all play roles in the development of chronic disease.[51] The prevalence of asthma in the United States is increasing, and this condition affects almost 10% of all women.[52] Among the almost 19 million women with asthma, those living in poverty have the highest risk.[52]

Box 8-3 identifies symptoms suggestive of asthma.[51] On examination, wheezing when breathing normally, prolonged expiratory phase, use of accessory muscles, increased nasal swelling, secretions or polyps, and evidence of atopy all increase the likelihood of an asthma diagnosis. Pulmonary function testing is required for diagnosis. The differential diagnosis in adults includes chronic obstructive pulmonary disease, vocal cord dysfunction, congestive heart failure, medication-related cough, pulmonary embolism, and gastroesophageal reflux disease, among others.[51] Midwives practicing in areas of high asthma frequency may keep flow meters in their offices either to assist in the presumptive diagnosis of asthma or to assess lung function when women with asthma present or are symptomatic. There are currently four classifications of asthma based on severity of disease as shown in **Table 8-11**.[51]

weight loss, and syncope. Other risks that are less common include dehydration, epistaxis, hernia, and—rarely—encephalopathy, pneumothorax, rectal prolapse, subdural hematoma, and seizure.[49]

Vaccination against pertussis with Tdap among adults is an effective measure to control the spread of pertussis, given that infants and young children have the highest rates and most severe infections. All adults who have close interaction with infants should have a recent Tdap vaccination.. Therapy for pertussis includes a macrolide antibiotic; the original recommendation for erythromycin was expanded to include azithromycin (Zithromax) and

Table 8-10	Stages of Pertussis (Whooping Cough)	
Stage	**Duration**	**Symptoms**
Catarrhal	1–2 weeks	Cough, runny nose, low-grade fever, sneezing
Paroxysmal	1–6 weeks	Episodes of rapid coughing 15 or more times per day, ending with a long inspiratory gasp and high-pitched "whooping" sound, occurring more often at night, accompanied by possible vomiting, exhaustion
Recovery	Weeks to months	Slowly resolving symptoms: cough disappears within 2–3 weeks, may return with subsequent respiratory illnesses

Source: Centers for Disease Control and Prevention. *The Pink Book: Epidemiology and Prevention of Vaccine-Preventable Diseases.* 12th ed. Atlanta, GA: Centers for Disease Control and Prevention; May 2012. Available at: http://www.cdc.gov/vaccines/pubs/pinkbook/index.html. Accessed April 10, 2013.

BOX 8-3 Characteristic Signs and Symptoms of Asthma

The presence of one or more of these symptoms is an indication for evaluation:

Wheezing (not required for diagnosis)

History of:
- Persistent cough
- Recurrent wheezing
- Recurrent difficulty in breathing
- Recurrent chest tightness

Symptoms provoked by:
- Exercise
- Viral infection
- Animals with fur
- Dust mites (in mattresses, pillows, upholstered furniture, or carpets)
- Mold
- Smoke (tobacco, wood)
- Pollen
- Changes in weather
- Strong emotional expression (laughing or crying hard)
- Airborne pollutants
- Menstrual cycles

Symptoms occur or worsen at night, awakening the individual

Source: National Asthma Education and Prevention Program. *Expert Panel Report: Guidelines for the Diagnosis and Management of Asthma (EPR-3).* Bethesda, MD: National Heart, Lung, and Blood Institute; 2007.

The National Asthma Education and Prevention Program guidelines for asthma[51] address education, management of environmental factors and comorbidities that worsen symptoms, and use of medication. The key to control of asthma and prevention of worsening of this condition is including the woman in decisions about her care, awareness of environmental triggers and the need to minimize exposure when possible, and the role that other health problems play in asthma management.

Medication management is based on a stepwise approach.[51] Intermittent symptoms of asthma (occurring fewer than 2 days a week, disturbing nighttime rest fewer than 2 days per month, not interfering with activities of daily living, and with one or fewer exacerbations per year) can be managed with short acting beta-agonists such as albuterol sulfate (Proventil) on an as-needed basis. Ipratropium bromide (Atrovent), an anticholinergic, can be used as an alternative. When a rescue inhaler is needed on more than 2 days per week, persistent asthma must be considered.

Anyone with persistent asthmatic symptoms needs to be on daily medication. Undertreatment limits physical activity, decreases pulmonary function, and increases the risk of recurrent attacks. The choice of medications is based on both the severity and the persistence of symptoms. The main categories of asthma drugs for long-term maintenance include inhaled corticosteroids, immunomodulators, leukotriene receptor antagonists, long-acting beta-agonists, 5-lipoxygenase inhibitors, mast cell mediators, methylxanthines, and combination drugs. In general, newly diagnosed asthma should be evaluated in consultation with or by referral to a physician experienced in respiratory care.

Table 8-11	Classification of Asthma				
Disease Severity	Daytime Symptoms	Nighttime Symptoms	PEF or FEV	Interference with Normal Activity	Use of Short-Acting Medication
Mild intermittent	≤ 2 days/week	≤ 2 nights/month	80	None	≤ 2 days/week
Mild persistent	> 2 days/week but < 1 time/day	> 2 nights/month	80	Minor	> 2 days/week but not daily and not more than 1 time/day
Moderate persistent	Daily	> 1 night/month	> 60 and < 80	Some	Daily
Severe persistent	Continual	Frequent	≤ 60	Extremely limited	Several times/day

FEV: Forced expiratory volume in 1 second; PEF: percentage of peak expiratory flow.

Source: Adapted from National Asthma Education and Prevention Program. *Expert panel report: guidelines for the diagnosis and management of asthma (EPR-3).* Bethesda, MD: National Heart, Lung, and Blood Institute; 2007.

Tuberculosis

Although the rate of tuberculosis (TB) infection has been declining in the United States for the last 20 years, more than 10,000 cases were reported in 2010.[52] Asians and Pacific Islander/Native Hawaiians are disproportionally affected by this infection, followed by African Americans. Additionally, tuberculosis among foreign-born individuals accounts for more than 60% of all diagnosed cases, with almost half of these persons having been in the United States for fewer than 5 years.[53] Poverty, lack of education, and HIV-positive status are associated with increased risk of acquiring the infection. Even though midwives may not provide first-line management for women with tuberculosis, because the higher risk occurs in populations for whom midwives often provide care, it is important that midwives have knowledge about this infection, including both acute and chronic care.

More than 11 million persons in the United States have latent tuberculosis, with the only evidence of that state being a positive tuberculin test.[54] Over time, 5% to 10% of those individuals with latent tuberculosis will develop active disease. For individuals with a damaged immune system—for example, persons with diabetes—the risk is as much as three times higher. For women who are HIV positive, without viral suppression, the risk of active TB may be as much as 100 times higher than the average rate.[55] Other factors as delineated in **Box 8-4** also influence the risk of progressive disease.[53]

Transmission

Because the tuberculosis bacterium is spread by droplet formation or aerosolization, casual contacts of individuals with active disease are at minimal risk of becoming infected; that is, close family members and those in close daily contact with the infected individual are most likely to have been exposed. The droplets are spread through the respiratory system before being neutralized by macrophage response. In some cases, the bacterium will also reach the lymph glands and spread through the body to other susceptible tissues. Because *Mycobacterium tuberculosis* does not produce toxins, infection with this pathogen does not induce an immediate host response. Cellular immune response and a positive tuberculin skin test occur 2 to 12 weeks after acquisition of the bacterium.

Even when an initial lesion in the lung develops, most immune-competent individuals will mount an adequate response and their bodies will encapsulate and calcify the inflammatory lesion, preventing further symptoms. On X ray, the lesion may be visible. Initial active clinical disease and reactivations of

---

BOX 8-4 Risk Factors for Active Tuberculosis

- Close contact of a person with active disease
- Immigration from areas with high rates of TB
- Persons who work or reside with people at high risk for TB
- Active substance abuse, especially IV drug use
- Tobacco or alcohol use
- Homelessness
- Malnutrition
- Body weight less than 90% ideal body weight
- Immune suppression: HIV/AIDS, diabetes mellitus, transplant recipients, chronic steroid treatment, renal disease, cancer of head, neck, and/or lung
- Intestinal bypass or gastrectomy procedures

TB = tuberculosis.

Sources: Centers for Disease Control and Prevention. *Reported Tuberculosis in the United States, 2011.* Atlanta, GA: CDC; October 2012; Centers for Disease Control and Prevention. *Core Curriculum on Tuberculosis: What the Clinician Should Know.* 5th ed. Atlanta, GA: CDC; 2011.

---

previously undiagnosed or inadequately treated disease may present as atypical pneumonia and patchy lung infiltrates, a generalized malaise and fatigue, night sweats, weight loss, fever, and a productive cough with or without hemoptysis. Pleuritic pain may develop, and on examination, crepitus and rales may be heard.[56]

Screening for Tuberculosis

The purpose of screening for tuberculosis is to detect those individuals who have inactive disease as well as those who have recently been infected. The most common test used is the intradermal tuberculin screening test (TST), formerly known as PPD (purified protein derivative).[56] This test is read 48 to 72 hours after being injected in the subcuticular area of the forearm. Results are assessed by the degree of the diameter of a palpable swelling (induration), measured in millimeters, excluding erythema. The amount of induration required for a positive reading is affected by several factors, as listed in **Table 8-12**.[56] When the TST is positive, the woman has disease that may or may not be currently active. The TST does not need to be repeated for anyone with a documented prior positive result.

The other tests that can be used to detect the presence of TB are the interferon-gamma release assays (IGRA): Quanti-FERON TB Gold in tube test

Table 8-12	Classification of the Tuberculin Skin Test Reaction[a]	
An **induration ≥ 5 mm** is considered positive in:	An **induration ≥ 10 mm** is considered positive in:	An **induration ≥ 15 mm** is considered positive in:
• HIV-infected persons • A recent contact of a person with TB disease • Persons with fibrotic changes on chest radiograph consistent with prior TB • Persons with organ transplants • Persons who are immuno-suppressed for other reasons	• Recent immigrants (< 5 years) from high-prevalence countries • Injection drug users • Residents and employees of high-risk congregate settings • Mycobacteriology laboratory personnel • Persons with clinical conditions that place them at high risk • Children < 4 years of age • Infants, children, and adolescents exposed to adults in high-risk categories	• Any person, including persons with no known risk factors for TB

[a]Targeted skin testing programs should be conducted only among high-risk groups.

TB: tuberculosis.

Source: Centers for Disease Control and Prevention. *Core Curriculum on Tuberculosis: What the Clinician Should Know.* 5th ed. Atlanta, GA: CDC; 2011.

(QFT-GIT), Quanti-FERON TB test (QFT-G), and the T-SPOT.TB test (T-Spot). These blood tests can be used in place of the TST for anyone who should be screened for TB. The IGRA tests measure the response to specific proteins in *M. tuberculosis*. They have been approved by the U.S. Food and Drug Administration (FDA) since 2005 and are now recommended by the CDC.

Many individuals from other countries may have received Bacillus Calmette-Guérin (BCG) vaccine in childhood to prevent tuberculosis infection, and this test may result in a permanent positive TST, necessitating other methods of screening. Although chest X ray will show abnormalities suggestive of TB, they are not by themselves diagnostic—although if normal, they help rule out disease.[56] The IGRA tests can be used when there is prior use of the BCG vaccine or when someone cannot return easily for test interpretation—for example, someone tested in an emergency room.

Sputum cultures should be performed when there is clinical suspicion of active tuberculosis. In many sites, a delay as long as 2 weeks may occur before results become available, but presumptive management should continue, even though diagnosis is not final without the confirmation of cultures. A smear from the sample can be evaluated for the presence of mycobacteria by acid-fast or fluorescent stain. Even when the stain is negative, the sputum sample should be sent for culture.[56] Any woman suspected of TB infection on screening should be promptly referred to a physician for ongoing care. In some settings,

it may be appropriate for the midwife to order the chest X ray or other testing to expedite treatment while the woman is waiting for an appointment with a physician.

Treatment

Women who have a positive skin test and in whom active tuberculosis has been ruled out by chest X ray are considered to have latent TB. They should receive treatment for 3 to 9 months with a regimen including isoniazid (Niazid), with or without the addition of rifapentine (Priftin) or rifampin (Rifadin). The latter agents may interfere with the effectiveness of hormonal contraceptives. The standard dosing remains 9 months of isoniazid 300 mg daily.[56] Active disease is treated with one of several multidrug combinations, which are administered over 6 to 9 months of uninterrupted therapy.

Prior to beginning therapy for tuberculosis, women should be screened for historic risk factors, for HIV or hepatitis, contraindications to the medications, and current medications. Teaching includes the benefits and risks of long-term therapy, the importance of adherence, and side effects. Baseline liver function studies should be obtained. At least monthly, the woman should be assessed for adherence to medication regimen, signs and symptoms of active disease, and symptoms of hepatitis.[57] Even though other providers will be responsible for prescribing and monitoring tuberculosis treatment regimens, midwives need to be cognizant of appropriate management to promote completion of therapy and monitoring.

Gastrointestinal Disorders and Abdominal Pain

Stomach aches and pains, diarrhea and constipation, and bloating are all common symptoms reported by women.[58] As part of the history for any woman of childbearing age, last menstrual period and potential pregnancy risk are routinely assessed. Ensuring that women of childbearing age are not pregnant is an essential first step whenever abdominal symptoms are present. This section focuses on general gastrointestinal health concerns common to all women. Obstetric complications producing abdominal symptoms are addressed in the *Obstetric Complications in Pregnancy* and *Medical Complications in Pregnancy* chapters. Similarly, gynecologic concerns are addressed in the *Menstrual Cycle Abnormalities* and *Gynecologic Disorders* chapters.

Gastroesophageal Reflux Disease

Gastroesophageal reflux disease (GERD) is the more severe and persistent form of gastroesophageal reflux, caused by involuntary relaxation of the sphincter muscle separating the esophagus and stomach. It is responsible for more than 8 million office visits annually, and is the most common gastrointestinal diagnosis.[58] When reflux occurs more than twice a week, GERD is diagnosed. GERD produces symptoms of heartburn that worsen with meals, bending over, and lying down. Other, less easily recognizable symptoms include an asthma-like wheeze, cough, laryngitis, and chest pain. Persistent severe disease may produce complications such as injury to the epithelium of the esophagus (Barrett's esophagus), stricture formation, and adenocarcinoma. Hiatal hernia—that is, separation of the diaphragm that allows the sphincter and upper portion of the stomach to penetrate into the chest cavity—is common in healthy older adults and can contribute to the symptoms of GERD. Obesity and smoking influence the development of GERD, as can pregnancy. *Helicobacter pylori* infection, the dominant cause of gastro-duodenal ulcers, does not appear to have an effect of the occurrence of GERD.[59]

Therapy for GERD includes weight reduction, consumption of a diet low in fat, and the avoidance of triggers such as caffeine, tobacco, and spicy or acidic foods. Eating small meals and remaining upright after meals may help prevent symptoms. If reflux occurs primarily at night, elevating the head while in bed will also help avoid discomfort. Certain medications, including beta-adrenergic agonists, tranquilizers, sedatives, progesterone, and calcium-channel blockers, may worsen symptoms. If these measures do not relieve symptoms, the use of antacids will bring short-term relief of intermittent symptoms. Step-up therapy for more severe symptoms begins with a trial of H_2 receptor antagonists such as cimetidine (Tagamet), famotidine (Pepcid), ranitidine (Zantac), and nizatidine (Axid). After 8 weeks, unresolved symptoms indicate the need to change to more powerful proton pump inhibitors, which include prescription drugs such as omeprazole (Prilosec), esomeprazole (Nexium), and lansoprazole (Prevacid).

A woman whose symptoms are unresolved following a trial of H_2 receptor antagonists should obtain consultation from a physician to assess the need for endoscopy or possible fundoplication of the stomach. Laparoscopic anti-reflux surgery appears to offer benefits for women with severe symptoms. Comparison of surgical outcomes with medical management has been shown to improve quality of life in severe cases, or when the woman is not satisfied with the results of medication therapy.[60,61]

Ulcers

Peptic ulcers are open lesions of the stomach or duodenum, penetrating through the mucosa into muscle. An estimated 15 million people, representing almost 7% of non-institutionalized adults in the United States, have these lesions.[61] Common etiologies include *H. pylori* infection, a condition responsible for 70% of gastric ulcers and 95% of duodenal ulcers,[62] and excessive use of NSAIDs, such as ibuprofen or aspirin.

Testing for *H. pylori* is indicated in adults younger than age 55 with a current or historical diagnosis of peptic ulcers, or undiagnosed dyspepsia. The exception is testing in individuals with "red flag" risk factors for gastric cancers such as bleeding, anemia, unexplained weight loss, changes in diet habits, or discomfort associated with eating or recurrent vomiting.[59] The American College of Gastroenterology does not recommend testing unless treatment is planned. Thus, for midwives, the decision to consult or refer for management of suspected *H. pylori* ulceration is made early in the evaluation process. Noninvasive testing methodologies include antibody screens, urea breath testing, and fecal antigen testing. Endoscopic testing offers excellent sensitivity and specificity, but is invasive and expensive.[59]

Counseling about avoiding aspirin and NSAIDs, stress reduction, and smoking cessation are all useful interventions in conjunction with medication for the management of ulcers. Alone, they will not resolve the disease; instead, antibiotic therapy to eliminate *H. pylori* from the gastrointestinal tract is essential for healing and reducing recurrent symptoms. Unless the ulceration has been caused solely by use of NSAIDs, no other therapy will provide lasting results. Recommended initial therapies include a proton pump inhibitor and clarithromycin (Biaxin) plus either amoxicillin (Amoxil) or metronidazole (Flagyl) for 10 to 14 days. Common side effects of these regimens include headache, altered taste, diarrhea, and stomach upset, and women should be aware that they will have gastrointestinal symptoms during therapy as a means to decrease nonadherence. Drugs that reduce the acid content of the stomach—including antacids, H_2 receptor antagonists, and proton pump inhibitors—are useful in promoting the healing of tissue, particularly in individuals with gastric ulcer.[62] The use of probiotics may offer some relief for side effects and assist in maintaining normal gastric flora.[63] Sucralfate (Carafate) is also often used to promote healing and reduce inflammation. Gastric ulcers that remain unresolved need to be evaluated to exclude cancerous lesions of the stomach.

Assessing Abdominal Pain

Abdominal pain has many causes, both gynecologic and nongynecologic. **Box 8-5** offers a partial listing of these etiologies. The diversity of this list reinforces the idea that midwives confronted with acute abdominal pain should not hesitate to seek consultation when the diagnosis is unclear. This section limits itself to consideration of two common nonreproductive causes of acute abdominal pain: cholecystitis and appendicitis. Either condition may present initially with more subtle symptoms.

When a woman presents with abdominal pain, assessment begins with a comprehensive history. The onset, description, duration, associated symptoms, and precipitating or relieving factors are determined, as well as identifying whether the pain is localized and, if so, to which quadrant.

Acute Abdomen

Characteristics that distinguish the acute abdomen include abdominal rigidity or distention, guarding, rebound pain, tachycardia, and decreased or absent bowel sounds. Fever may be present but is not essential to the diagnosis. Vomiting as well as urinary, bowel, or vaginal symptoms may be present. An acute abdomen is often a surgical emergency, and immediate referral to a physician is an appropriate plan.

Gallbladder Disease

Gallbladder disease affects approximately 20 million Americans. Cholecystitis is an inflammation of the gallbladder, an organ that collects, concentrates, and dispenses into the digestive tract the bile produced

---

BOX 8-5 Differential Diagnoses for Abdominal Pain[a]

- Ectopic pregnancy
- Ovarian torsion
- Ovarian cyst
- Endometriosis
- Mittelschmerz
- Pelvic inflammatory disease
- Endometritis
- Constipation
- Diarrhea
- Appendicitis
- Cholecystitis
- Gastroenteritis
- Diverticulitis
- Ulcer
- Inflammatory bowel disease
- Bowel obstruction
- Pyelonephritis
- Cystitis
- Hernia
- Pancreatitis
- Aortic dissection
- Lower lobe pneumonia

[a]This list is not exhaustive.

---

by the liver. Excess cholesterol triggers a crystallization process to form gallstones. Most gallstones are either asymptomatic or cause only mild biliary colic, a sharp pain after a fatty or large meal that may last a few hours and resolve. Acute cholecystitis presents with persistent, severe stabbing epigastric or right upper quadrant pain. In contrast, chronic cholecystitis occurs when repeated acute events have caused the wall of the gallbladder to thicken and the organ to shrink; symptoms will be milder and less easily distinguished from other causes of gastric upset. Choledocholithiasis is the term that describes blockage of the common bile duct by gallstones.

Risk factors for developing gallbladder disease include obesity followed by rapid weight loss, hypertriglyceridemia, female gender, pregnancy, older age, diabetes, and genetic predisposition. When cholecystitis develops, sharp epigastric pain may last for several hours or days and is often associated with nausea and vomiting. Women with acute attacks present with severe, persistent right upper quadrant pain, often radiating to the right shoulder blade or the central back opposite the epigastrium. Murphy's sign (**Figure 8-2**) is positive if the woman stops inspiration with deep palpation of the right upper quadrant of the abdomen. Leukocytosis, elevated liver function tests, and elevated bilirubin are common laboratory findings. Ultrasound is the most effective diagnostic tool.

Once a diagnosis of cholecystitis is considered, the midwife should refer the woman for physician care. Prompt surgical removal of the gallbladder is the usual treatment.[64,65] Despite the effectiveness of surgery, fewer than 75% of individuals with symptomatic gallbladder disease—cholecystitis, choledocholithiasis, or gallstone pancreatitis—undergo surgery immediately after diagnosis.[66] None of the nonsurgical approaches to treatment of gallstones has proved to be an effective alternative to surgery.

Appendicitis

When the appendix becomes obstructed, enlarged, and unable to drain, the subsequent bacterial response leads to appendicitis. After decades of decreases in its incidence. the rate of acute appendicitis is increasing in the United States.[66] Although the most common decade of life in which to develop appendicitis remains 10 to 20 years, this diagnosis is becoming more common among individuals older than age 40 years.[66] One suggested source of the relative increases in appendicitis incidence is improved diagnostic accuracy, particularly the accuracy of computerized tomography, which decreases missed diagnoses blamed on other, usually gynecologic, pelvic symptoms. One report hypothesizes that the combination of improved diagnostic testing, better access to health care, and longer lifespans are responsible for the observed increase in this diagnosis in different racial groups as well as in older adults.[67]

The classic descriptive symptoms for appendicitis are anorexia and generalized abdominal pain, resolving into acute right lower quadrant abdominal pain, vomiting, and fever. A complete blood count will show leukocytosis with an increased neutrophil ratio. Deep tenderness over McBurney's point in the lower right abdomen is an early sign of acute appendicitis. Rebound pain with release of pressure from the left lower abdomen is known as Rovsing's sign. **Figure 8-3** illustrates the locations of McBurney's point and Rovsing's sign.

When appendicitis is suspected, the woman should be referred for evaluation and possible surgery. Antibiotic therapy for nonsurgical management of appendicitis is being studied, but is not yet a standard practice.[68] Nonsurgical management is associated with risk of recurrent disease, but avoids the risk of surgical morbidity.[63]

Gastroenteritis and Acute Diarrhea

Some women report diarrhea when they have any change in bowel habits that produces soft, frequent, or less formed stools. When assessing history, true diarrhea has increased water content and may have increased mucus content. Associated symptoms of cramping, nausea or vomiting, or fever should be assessed. Careful examination of the abdomen, including auscultation of bowel sounds, palpation, and percussion, is necessary. Acute diarrhea is predominantly infectious; chronic diarrhea, lasting for more than 2 consecutive weeks, can result from diverse conditions, including infections such as malaria or cholera, medication, chronic illness, malabsorption syndromes, stress, and irritable bowel syndrome. Recent travelers, the elderly, members of an identified community outbreak, and those recently prescribed antibiotics require closer attention to a specific diagnosis. Most midwives will refer women with chronic watery diarrhea for further testing.

Viral gastroenteritis is a generally self-limiting disease, in which oral exposure to a pathogenic virus

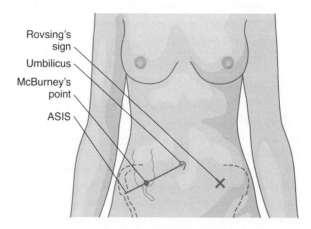

Rovsing's sign
Umbilicus
McBurney's point
ASIS

Figure 8-3 McBurney's point and Rovsing's sign. ASIS = anterior superior iliac spine. McBurney's point is on the abdominal wall that lies between the umbilicus and ASIS and is usually two-thirds the distance from the umbilicus toward the ASIS. Most common placement of the base of the appendix.

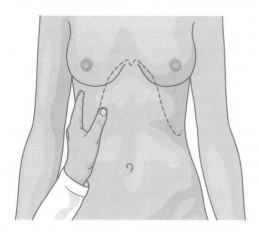

Figure 8-2 Murphy's sign.

such as norovirus or rotavirus leads to explosive onset of nausea, vomiting, and/or diarrhea, fever, and malaise within 1 to 3 days of exposure. The abdomen is tender; no guarding is present. Bowel sounds are increased. Norovirus alone accounts for 58% of acute foodborne illnesses.[69] Other causes of diarrhea-linked infections include *Escherichia coli* species, *Salmonella*, and a host of other bacteria, most of which are foodborne pathogens.

The majority of cases of diarrhea in healthy adults will clear spontaneously within 1 to 4 days. Rest and oral fluids are the basic components of care. Medications such as diphenoxylate (Lomotil) or loperamide (Imodium) can be offered to decrease the frequency of stools. Intravenous rehydration with electrolytes can be used for severe dehydration and for individuals at increased risk, such as the elderly and immunocompromised persons.

Investigation of acute diarrhea includes a stool sample to check for white blood cells or frank bleeding. Laboratory evaluation of electrolytes should be reserved for more severe or persistent cases when dehydration is suspected. If symptoms are not resolving or the woman becomes dehydrated, stool samples for culture or for ova and parasites (depending on the suspected pathogen) as well as a toxin assay for *Clostridium difficile* (with recent antimicrobial use) would be indicated.

Traveler's diarrhea, as distinguished from norovirus infections acquired in large travel groups such as cruises, is more likely to have a bacterial source—specifically, *E. coli* or another enterococcus. The CDC does not recommend prophylaxis for these pathogens, but infections associated with severe cramping or nausea, more than three stools in 8 hours, fever, and bloody stools can be treated with a fluoroquinolone.[70] When antibiotic treatment does not resolve symptoms, parasitic pathogens also have to be considered based on the location of travel. For example, parasitic infections have been reported as prominent among travelers from all regions except Southeast Asia.[71]

Constipation

Straining to produce hard stools, infrequent bowel movements (fewer than once in 3 days), and painful defecation are characteristic of constipation. Estimates of the frequency of constipation average almost 15% of the female U.S. population, with the elderly having a greater prevalence.[72] Initial questioning of women with these symptoms should include an assessment of their "usual" bowel function. Among healthy women, inadequate dietary fiber, possibly decreased fluid intake, and iron therapy for anemia, whether prescribed or self-initiated, are common causes of constipation. Other medications, such as tricyclic antidepressants (e.g., amitriptyline [Elavil]), anticholinergics (e.g., ipratropium bromide [Atrovent]), and calcium-channel blockers (e.g., diltiazem [Cardizem] and verapamil [Calan]), may slow peristalsis and increase stool transit time, leading to constipation. Misuse of laxatives leading to decreased natural stimulation of the bowel is also common, particularly among the elderly. Stress, anxiety, and depression may lead to changes in bowel habits, as may a history of sexual abuse. Other serious causes include hypothyroidism, cancer, strictures, and opioid abuse. A careful history and physical assessment of women with any chronic bowel changes is necessary to rule out serious underlying disease that would require a medical referral.

Management of chronic constipation in healthy women includes counseling about diet and exercise, and an increase in fluid intake. Avoidance of straining and recognizing the physical cues that indicate the need to defecate are included in teaching. Women should also be counseled to stop the overuse of laxatives, cathartics, and enemas. If any medication is necessary during early treatment, a bulk-forming over-the-counter drug such as Metamucil should be used; however, adding fiber to the diet is a better strategy because a pattern of healthy eating will help maintain normal function. If symptom relief is not obtained with the preceding measures, a trial of laxatives such as docusate sodium (Colace) is in order before referring the woman to a physician.

Irritable Bowel Syndrome

Irritable bowel syndrome (IBS) consists of lower gastrointestinal tract symptoms of increased bloating, diarrhea, or constipation in the absence of any structural or biochemical cause. This condition is chronic in nature, and one of the most common presentations in primary care practice. The current definition (Rome III) includes onset associated with changes in the frequency or composition of the stool and pain relief with defecation, persisting over 12 weeks within the last year. To meet the diagnostic criteria, the symptoms need not be continuous. Intermittent symptoms totaling 12 weeks are considered significant.[73] Increased or decreased stool frequency, abnormal stool formation (either hard or watery), bloating, difficulty in the passage of stool (straining, urgency, or failure to completely empty the bowel), and mucus in the stool are further confirmation of the diagnosis. Because the symptoms are unstable, the terms "IBS with diarrhea" and "IBS with constipation" are commonly used.[74]

The onset of IBS usually occurs during the young adult years; because organic causes of bowel changes are more frequent with increasing age, a new diagnosis should be made with care in adults older than age 40 years. Women are more often affected than men and are more likely to have alternating symptoms of diarrhea and constipation. Some women with IBS have chronic pelvic pain; making the correct diagnosis is essential to improve their treatment.

Assessment includes evaluation for bowel obstruction, including malignancies, and for gastrointestinal bleeding. Irritable bowel syndrome should not be confused with inflammatory bowel diseases such as Crohn's disease and ulcerative colitis, which are chronic, recurrent inflammations of the bowel. The relationship of symptom relief to having a bowel movement is strongly suggestive of IBS.

Some women will note food allergies or conditions such as lactose intolerance. Most food allergies present as acute upset, not as chronic bowel changes. If a woman has severely restricted her dietary intake, adding foods back into the diet may improve general health and nutrition as well as symptoms.

Although the symptoms of IBS are common among adults who do not seek care, those who do are more likely to be distressed by the condition. Thus an important step in managing care for individuals with this disorder is building a trusting relationship. Education about IBS, reassurance about the course and management possibilities, and dietary modification are important in helping women manage their symptoms effectively.[75] Evidence supports the benefits of tegaserod (Zelnorm), a 5HT$_4$ receptor agonist, to treat IBS associated with constipation, and alosetron, a 5HT$_3$ receptor agonist, in IBS with diarrhea. In contrast, there is little evidence of benefit from antidiarrheal agents, antispasmodic medications, and laxatives. Tricyclic antidepressants may help relieve abdominal pain.[74,75] Because of the strong likelihood of underlying psychological distress among women with IBS, a careful assessment for anxiety disorders and depression is warranted. Considerations in managing this aspect of the disease include the use of antidepressants, psychotherapy, and supportive behavioral therapy.

Hepatitis Infections

Viral hepatitis actually comprises a group of pathogenic viruses, identified by the letters A through G and linked to liver disease by the acute and chronic nature of the conditions. While hepatitis A and E are spread by the fecal–oral route, hepatitis B, C, and D are spread by contact with blood and body fluids and can be contracted sexually. Hepatitis B is discussed in the *Reproductive Tract and Sexually Transmitted Infections* chapter. Hepatitis A and B are the most common forms of hepatitis in the United States. Although there are fewer new cases per year of hepatitis C than hepatitis A and B, the C variant becomes chronic approximately 75% to 85% of the time among those who are infected. In contrast, hepatitis B develops as a chronic state in fewer than 6% of adult cases.[76] Together, the strains of A, B and C are responsible for 95% of all new viral hepatitis diagnoses in the United States.[76]

Hepatitis D occurs as a coinfection with hepatitis B or as a secondary infection, and requires the presence of hepatitis B for its transmission. Hepatitis D is uncommon in the general population of North America, although it may occur in intravenous drug users and persons with frequent exposure to blood products (e.g., persons with hemophilia) as well as their sexual contacts.[76] Hepatitis E is an enterically transmitted virus, often associated with contaminated water sources; it is most commonly found in Asia, the Middle East, South America, and Latin America. Hepatitis E has been diagnosed in the United States primarily in individuals traveling from developing countries, although it can be associated with food-borne transmission. Hepatitis E is frequently associated with only mild symptoms, and does not result in a carrier state.

Hepatitis can also result from generalized infection by other viruses, including cytomegalovirus, Epstein-Barr virus, herpes simplex virus, and measles virus. Nonviral causes of liver infection include bacterial sepsis and syphilis. Hepatitis can also be chemically induced by chronic alcohol ingestion or by medications such as acetylsalicylic acid (aspirin), acetaminophen (Tylenol), phenytoin (Dilantin), isoniazid (Niazid), and rifampin (Rifadin).

Hepatitis A

Hepatitis A (HAV) is an RNA virus transmitted through the fecal–oral route, and most cases are part of community-wide outbreaks. In the United States, vaccination has been successful and the rate of infection is estimated to be approximately 21,000 cases annually, of which 90% are asymptomatic.[77] Contaminated water and food (especially shellfish) are common sources of infection, with most cases being associated with close personal contact with an infected person, although blood-borne transmission has been documented in both infants and adults.[78]

Clinical Illness Hepatitis A has an incubation period of 28 days (range: 15–50 days), with the virus being shed through the feces approximately 2 weeks prior to the emergence of clinical symptoms. Hepatitis A has a short acute phase of 10 to 15 days, with symptoms resolving within 2 months, although as many as 15% of symptomatic persons have prolonged or relapsing disease lasting up to 6 months.[77,79] Viremia persists for at least 1 week following onset of symptoms, and may continue for several months in individuals with relapses.[80] However, there is no chronic state. The symptoms of acute vital hepatitis are similar to those observed with other viral hepatitis forms as well.

Diagnosis To diagnose acute hepatitis A, serologic testing with a finding of immunoglobulin M (IgM) antibody is required to confirm infection. IgM anti-HAV usually becomes detectable 5 to 10 days before the onset of symptoms and can persist for up to 6 months after infection. Immunoglobulin G (IgG) anti-HAV appears early in the course of the disease and will indicate lifelong protection against the disease.[80]

Prevention and Treatment Since 1995, two licensed inactivated hepatitis A vaccines have been available in the United States; they are recommended for individuals in specific high-risk groups, such as international travelers and individuals working in countries where hepatitis A is endemic.[81] In addition, routine vaccination is recommended for children.[80] When administered within 2 weeks of exposure, immune globulins provide passive immunity and decrease the risk of hepatitis A transmission by as much as 80% to 90%. Hepatitis A is managed with symptomatic treatment and monitoring for worsening liver disease. There is no cure for hepatitis A.

Hepatitis C

Hepatitis C virus (HCV) is rarely identified at the time of exposure. In 2007, the CDC estimated that it was likely that more than 15,000 cases occurred in the United States, but fewer than 1000 cases were reported.[82] Of the more than 3 million persons with chronic hepatitis C, the majority were probably exposed during the 1970s and 1980s, when rates of this infection reached their highest point. Risk factors include intravenous drug use, sexual contact, and being a healthcare worker who is exposed to blood. Women undergoing hemodialysis and those living with HIV are also at risk. Transfusion with unscreened blood is an uncommon risk today.[83]

Clinical Illness The period of incubation for hepatitis C ranges from 2 weeks to 6 months. Only approximately 30% of newly infected individuals will be symptomatic.[83] Chronic disease develops slowly. Excessive alcohol use and obesity have both been associated with progression.

Diagnosis Diagnosis of hepatitis C infection is made by serum enzyme immunoassay (EIA) detection of

antibody to the virus. Targeted screening for the hepatitis C virus is based on risk factors. Hepatitis C antibody testing is accurate 4 weeks to 6 months after exposure. If antibody to hepatitis C is positive, recombinant immunoblot assay (RIBA; also known as "Western blot") is used to confirm the result. If this test is positive for the antibody to HCV, then because of the high (70% to 85%) incidence of chronic disease, serum alanine aminotransferase (ALT) and quantification of HCV-RNA (viral load) should be performed.

Prevention and Treatment At this time, there is no vaccine for hepatitis C. Prevention counseling including use of barriers with sexual activity and avoiding sharing intravenous drug paraphernalia is essential. Treatment for acute hepatitis C is the same palliative care as for other viral hepatitis infections. Chronic hepatitis C can be treated with peg- interferon (Pegasys) and ribavirin (Rebetol). As with other infections managed with chronic medication, the individual's willingness to adhere to treatment must be identified.

Conditions of the Genitourinary System

The close proximity of the urinary tract to the reproductive organs means that women frequently call their gynecologic provider for management of urinary tract symptoms. Office evaluation and management of uncomplicated cystitis is an essential skill for midwives, as are prompt recognition and triage of more serious conditions.

Acute Cystitis

Uncomplicated acute cystitis is defined as the presence of 10^2 colony-forming units (CFU) per milliliter of urine in a culture from a catheter specimen for symptomatic women, or more traditionally, as 10^5 CFU or more per milliliter whether or not symptoms of a lower urinary tract infection (UTI) are present. "Asymptomatic bacteriuria" is the term applied when symptoms are absent and 10^5 or more CFU of a single organism grow in a urine culture. The predominant organism implicated in uncomplicated lower urinary tract infection is *E. coli*, with *Staphylococcus saprophyticus, Klebsiella pneumoniae, Proteus mirabilis, Enterobacter,* and *Enterococcus* species making up the majority of the other pathogens that are associated with UTI.[84]

Lower urinary tract infections are among the most common infections that a woman will have in her lifetime. In addition, once a woman has such an infection, she is at risk for reoccurrence, often within a few months. Symptoms of a lower urinary tract infection include pain on urination, increased voiding frequency, and persistent suprapubic or low back pain. Among healthy young women, those who are sexually active will have a higher risk. Lower urinary tract infection is frequently diagnosed in the midwife's office based on symptoms and urinalysis findings consistent with bacteriuria and pyuria.[85] When cystitis is suspected, a culture should be obtained on at least one occasion while the woman is symptomatic, to confirm that an infection is the cause of symptoms and ensure that an antibiotic is prescribed to which the pathogen is sensitive.

Recurrent lower urinary tract infection is diagnosed when the woman has three or more infections proven by culture within a year. Identifying characteristics of uncomplicated recurrences include frequent sexual activity, a prior history of pyelonephritis, and rapid symptom resolution after treatment. Nocturia, hematuria, dyspareunia, and persistent symptoms after antibiotic therapy are indicative of another source of irritation, such as interstitial cystitis or an association with urinary incontinence.[86] Among postmenopausal women, recurrent lower urinary tract infection is associated with urinary incontinence, cystocele, and prolapse. The use of vaginal estrogen creams or rings may assist in prevention of recurrent lower urinary tract infection in this population by restoring integrity to vaginal and urethral tissue affected by estrogen deprivation.[87]

Complicated urinary infections are associated with medical or physical conditions that impede bladder emptying. Diabetes mellitus, multiple sclerosis, immunosuppression, cystocele, obstruction of the urinary tract, and incontinence are all potential causes. These risk factors may warrant referral to a specialist, particularly if the initial treatment regimen is not successful in eradicating the infection.

Recommendations for treatment of lower urinary tract infection have become more complicated, as resistance to various antibiotics is rapidly increasing.[88] Nitrofurantoin (Macrodantin) or the combination of nitrofurantoin monohydrate with macrocrystals (Macrobid) is preferred if there is no suspicion of pyelonephritis, or TMP-SMX (Bactrim) if that regimen has not been used within 3 months. Amoxicillin or ampicillin should never be used as a sole agent; fluoroquinolones, amoxicillin-clavulanate (Augmentin), and beta-lactams should be reserved for more serious infections whenever possible or if the recommended drugs are contraindicated. Minimal evidence indicates that use of cranberry juice or cranberry tablets can assist in prevention of recurrent lower urinary

tract infection; however, no standardized dose has been tested. The most recent update of the Cochrane database no longer recommends cranberry juice as a means of preventing lower urinary tract infection.[89]

Interstitial Cystitis

Interstitial cystitis is a persistent inflammatory bladder condition that is associated with suprapubic or retropubic pain, dysuria, frequency and urgency, dyspareunia, and nocturia. The term "painful bladder system" is used as an alternative when symptoms do not meet all criteria for diagnosis but no other cause of inflammation and pain can be identified. Over time, the bladder wall can become irritated or scarred, leading to the development of submucosal bleeding. Diagnosis is often delayed because the symptoms are mistaken for lower urinary tract infection. No good evidence can be found for a microbial pathogen; however, a toxic factor is being investigated that inhibits epithelial cell growth and other growth factor abnormalities in the development of interstitial cystitis/painful bladder syndrome.[90] More than 3 million adult women are estimated to have pain and urinary symptoms of interstitial cystitis/painful bladder syndrome in the United States.[91]

Midwives can offer women with interstitial cystitis/painful bladder syndrome counseling on restricting alcohol and possible food triggers such as spicy or high-acid foods, caffeine, and chocolate; tobacco cessation; and bladder training. Referral for further evaluation, including a possible biopsy to rule out bladder cancer, and medication is warranted.[92]

Pyelonephritis

Acute pyelonephritis, an inflammation of the kidneys, should be included in the assessment of abdominal pain, as its characteristic presentation is severe flank pain and fever with associated chills, nausea or vomiting, and painful urination. Assessment of costovertebral angle tenderness (CVAT) by striking beneath the 12th rib in the acute angle formed with the spine can help to assess the location of the pain (**Figure 8-4**). The risk factors and pathogens associated with lower urinary tract infection are the same for pyelonephritis. The diagnosis should be confirmed by a urinalysis that is positive for white blood cells or the presence of pyuria and by urine culture. Physician consultation or referral is required when pyelonephritis is suspected, and treatment varies depending on whether it is delivered on an inpatient basis or at an outpatient site; a pending urine culture should not delay consultation. Commonly prescribed drugs include various combinations of ciprofloxacin (Cipro),

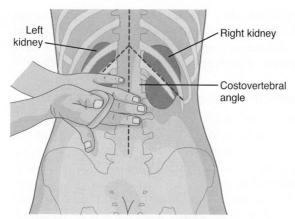

Left kidney

Right kidney

Costovertebral angle

Choose the technique that is most comfortable for both examiner and patient.

1. With the woman seated on the exam table, place the palm of one hand over her costovertebral angle on one side. Make a fist out of your other hand. Use the ulnar surface of your fist for striking. Strike the back of the hand that is over the costovertebral angle with the fist of your other hand.

OR

2. Put your hands around the woman's waist and locate, by palpation, the costovertebral angles with the flat part of your index and middle fingers on each hand. Alternately strike each costovertebral angle with your fingers by a sudden, upward motion of your hand.

Figure 8-4 Assessing for costovertebral tenderness.

cephalosporins, fluoroquinolones, aminoglycosides, and penicillins.[88]

Kidney Stones

Women have a 5% lifetime risk of developing nephrolithiasis (kidney stones), and the prevalence of this condition is increasing. Recurrence is common, and is estimated to be as high as 50% within 5 years.[93]

Kidney stones are of four major types. The most common, calcium oxalate or phosphate stones, account for approximately 70% to 93% of all stones. Causative factors for such stones include high dietary levels of protein and sodium, chronic dehydration, and inflammatory bowel disease, among others. Uric acid stones account for another 10% to 15% of stones; obesity and metabolic syndrome are among the factors in their development. Struvite (magnesium ammonium phosphate) stones represent another 10% to 15% of all kidney stones and are directly associated with urinary infections. Cysteine and medication-related stones can be involved, but are rarer.[93]

The usual symptoms of nephrolithiasis include severe renal colic caused by the stone passing into the ureter. As the stone enters the bladder, symptoms resemble those of a urinary tract infection. Hematuria is common but not required for diagnosis. Helical computerized tomography without contrast is the preferred confirmatory test.

When kidney stones are suspected, the midwife will need to refer the woman to a physician for management. However, NSAIDs can be initiated for pain management and are as effective as opioids for this purpose. Small stones, less than 0.5 to 1 centimeter in diameter, can be allowed to pass without surgery, using effective pain management and increasing fluids.[93] Calcium-channel blockers and alpha-adrenergic agonists have been shown to speed the passage of stones through the ureter, and are associated with decreased pain.[94] Counseling to increase fluid intake and recommending indicated dietary changes based on stone type may help to decrease recurrences.

Surgical management of kidney stones that are large, obstructive, or associated with infection now relies on extracorporeal shock-wave lithotripsy, ureteroscopy, and percutaneous nephrolithotomy to avoid open procedures. Stone type, size, and location affect the treatment recommendation, as does a high BMI that may prevent adequate treatment.[95]

Endocrine Conditions

Metabolic Syndrome

Obesity, especially central obesity, is associated with an increased risk of insulin resistance. The combination of elevation in blood insulin levels, blood glucose levels, and dyslipidemia sets the stage for the development of both diabetes mellitus and cardiac disease. One generally accepted definition of metabolic syndrome in women is found in **Box 8-6**.[96] Categorized

---

BOX 8-6 Characteristics of Metabolic Syndrome

Any three of the following:

- Waist circumference > 88 cm in women
- Serum triglycerides > 150 mg/dL or treatment to reduce triglyceride levels
- Serum HDL < 50 mg/dL or treatment for low HDL
- Blood pressure ≥ 130/85 mm Hg or treatment for hypertension
- Fasting plasma glucose ≥ 100 mg/dL or treatment for hyperglycemia

Source: Adapted from Grundy SM, Cleeman JI, Daniels SR, et al. Diagnosis and management of the metabolic syndrome: an American Heart Association/National Heart, Lung and Blood Institute scientific statement. *Circulation.* 2005;112(17):2735-2752.

on the basis of body mass index, obese women (BMI > 30) had a higher than 15 times the risk of a normal or underweight women of having three risk factors.[97]

Because of the close association between these risk factors and the development of serious medical conditions, women with one or more of these risk factors should be assessed with blood pressure measurement, waist circumference measurement, fasting glucose, and a full cholesterol panel. Counseling about lifestyle changes, including weight loss, increased exercise, and dietary changes, is essential.

Diabetes Mellitus

The definition of diabetes mellitus is based on the underlying cause of hyperglycemia. "Prediabetes" is the term used to describe women with abnormal blood glucose values that do not meet the measurement that defines diabetes. There are four classes of diabetes, as shown in **Box 8-7**.

Almost universally, type 1 diabetes is mediated by the immune system causing pancreatic B cell destruction; it is most commonly diagnosed in children or young adults and represents approximately 5% of all cases of diabetes overall. Type 2 diabetes, which is the most common form of diabetes, is the result of resistance to insulin and the inability of the pancreas to increase insulin production to compensate for this resistance. **Box 8-8** summarizes the criteria for the diagnosis of diabetes.[98] Together, types 1 and 2 diabetes affect more than 25 million persons in the United States, of whom approximately 7 million remain undiagnosed.[99] Rates rise with age and obesity. A first-degree family member with diabetes, poor diet choices, lack of physical activity, and smoking are other factors that increase risk.[99,100] Specifically, eating a Western diet high in red meat, high-fat dairy, and processed carbohydrates and sweets increases the risk for developing diabetes regardless of other characteristics.[101] Because of the interrelationship between hypertension lipid abnormalities and diabetes, these conditions also should be considered risk factors. Ethnic groups with an increased risk include non-Hispanic blacks, Mexican Americans and Puerto Ricans, Southwest American Indians, and Asian Americans.[99] Women with an obstetric history of giving birth to an infant with a high birthweight or large for gestational age and unexplained fetal losses should be considered at risk for diabetes as well.

Young women with type 1 diabetes generally present with symptoms of polyuria, including the need to urinate during the night, increased thirst, hunger with associated weight loss, and weakness or fatigue. Those women with type 2 diabetes also may notice thirst, frequent voiding, and weakness, but they are more likely to present with recurrent vaginal yeast infections, itching, skin infections, blurred vision, or even peripheral neuropathy. In many cases, particularly in women who are obese, diagnosis will occur only with laboratory screening.

Screening for diabetes mellitus should be performed for all women older than 45 years, and for anyone with a BMI of 25 or higher and one or more risk factors. Screening tests include the glycated hemoglobin (HBA1c), fasting blood glucose, and the 2-hour glucose tolerance test.[98] HBA1c measures the average plasma glucose level over the last month; its

---

BOX 8-7 Classification of Diabetes

Gestational diabetes: diabetes diagnosed during pregnancy that is not clearly overt (type 1 or type 2) diabetes

Type 1 diabetes: diabetes resulting from beta-cell destruction, usually leading to absolute insulin deficiency
- Without vascular complications
- With vascular complications (specify which)

Type 2 diabetes: diabetes resulting from inadequate insulin secretion in the face of increased insulin resistance
- Without vascular complications
- With vascular complications (specify which)

Other types of diabetes (e.g., genetic in origin, associated with pancreatic disease, drug-induced or chemically induced)

BOX 8-8 Diagnosis of Diabetes Mellitus

Hemoglobin A1c ≥ 6.5%

OR

Fasting plasma glucose ≥ 126 mg/dL

OR

2-hour plasma glucose ≥ 200 mg/dL after a 75-g glucose load

Source: Adapted from American Diabetes Association. Standards of medical care in diabetes—2013. *Diab Care.* 2013;36(suppl 1):S11–S66.

results are expressed as the percentage of total hemoglobin. This test can be used to assess either the degree of elevated blood glucose over time in persons with a new diagnosis of diabetes or the degree of glycemic control in persons who are being treated for diabetes. Because red blood cells have a turnover period of 120 days, the HBA1c levels will decline toward normal values as the woman blood sugar levels stabilize. A level at or below 6.5% is the primary goal.

Components of care for women with diabetes include diet education, promotion of moderate exercise, counseling for weight loss, and smoking cessation. It is in these areas that the midwife can play an important role. Women with diabetes continue to need regular gynecologic care and family planning, they have an increased need for preconception counseling, and will remain prone to vaginal symptoms if glucose control is not optimal. All women with diabetes should be encouraged to plan pregnancies carefully.

The American Diabetes Association recommends beginning lifestyle changes with the addition of the pharmaceutical agent metformin (Glucophage) as soon as type 2 diabetes is diagnosed.[98] Women newly diagnosed with diabetes should be referred to a provider skilled in this area.

Thyroid Disease

Women at the age of 60 years or older are at high risk for thyroid disease and should be screened for thyroid disorders, as these conditions are more common in women compared to men and more common as age increases. Thyroid conditions also are common among women of childbearing age, with an estimated incidence of more than 3%.[102]

Thyroid-releasing hormones from the hypothalamus stimulate pituitary release of thyroid-stimulating hormone (TSH). In turn, TSH stimulates the production and release of triiodothyronine (T_3) and thyroxine (T_4) from the thyroid gland. Although T_3 is the more active form of the thyroid hormones, little is produced in the thyroid itself. Instead, most T_3 is produced from circulating T_4 as it loses iodine.

In screening for or diagnosing thyroid disease, the first tests performed are generally measurements of TSH and free T_4. Because most circulating thyroid hormones are bound to thyroid-binding globulin (TBG) and other serum proteins, a total T_4 level is not as useful as the free T_4 level. Among the antibody tests, confirmation of thyroid peroxidase antibodies is associated with chronic autoimmune thyroiditis (Hashimoto's thyroiditis), the predominant cause of overt hypothyroidism. **Table 8-13** illustrates the changes in screening laboratory values associated with common thyroid disorders. Clinicians need to remember that, unlike the case for many other lab tests, TSH level varies *inversely* with thyroid conditions; for example, hypothyroidism is associated with high levels of TSH.

Hypothyroidism

Hypothyroid conditions result primarily from failure of the gland to produce adequate hormone and is more common than hyperthyroidism. The most common cause of hypothyroidism in the United States is the autoimmune disorder known as Hashimoto's thyroiditis. Other causes include treatment of Graves' disease, thyroidectomy, and medications. Secondary hypothyroidism, caused by pituitary or hypothalamic disorders, is uncommon. In primary hypothyroid states, the TSH level will be elevated. If the original problem is within the hypothalamic–pituitary axis, the TSH level will be low.

Uncomplicated primary hypothyroidism generally is treated with supplementation. For healthy young adults, a starting dose of 50 to 100 mcg/day of L-thyroxine can be titrated upward every 2 to 3 weeks until symptoms resolve and laboratory values are normal. Among older women, the increase in dose should be slower.

Subclinical hypothyroid disease occurs when the TSH level is abnormal but the free T_4 level remains

Table 8-13	Thyroid Hormone Values in Thyroid Disorders		
Condition	**Thyroid-Stimulating Hormone**	**Free T_4**	**Serum T_3**
Graves' disease	Absent	Elevated	Elevated
Subclinical hyperthyroid	< 0.1 mU/L	Normal	Normal
Hypothyroid	High with primary Low with secondary	Low	Low/normal
Subclinical hypothyroid	Mildly elevated (< 10.0 mU/L)	Low/normal	

normal. In pregnancy, thyroid screening treatment of asymptomatic women is controversial. Treatment to correct the TSH level among nonpregnant women generally is not recommended.[103] Measuring thyroid peroxidase (TPO) antibodies may help to identify women at risk of progression to overt hypothyroidism, and in women older than age 60 years or those with other risk factors, identification and treatment may be justified.[104] Women with menorrhagia should have TSH and free T_4 measurements done as part of the investigation, because even a TSH level in the range of 5–10 mU/L can be associated with excessive menstrual bleeding.[105]

Hyperthyroidism

The single most common cause of hyperthyroid state (also referred to as thyrotoxicosis) is Graves' disease, an autoimmune disease that is more common among women than men and the cause of more than 10% of all cases of thyrotoxicosis in young adults. The thyroid is typically enlarged and tender in hyperthyroidism. Many women will notice irritation of the conjunctiva, diplopia, or blurred vision, or present with proptosis (bulging of the eye or displacement forward of the eye in its orbit) and periorbital edema.

Box 8-9 lists the common signs and symptoms of thyroid disease.

Other causes of hyperthyroidism include toxic multinodular goiter, toxic adenomas, early stages of Hashimoto's thyroiditis, and postpartum thyroiditis. This disease has also been associated with very high levels of circulating human chorionic gonadotropin (hCG), such as those found in women who have a hydatidiform mole. Subclinical hyperthyroidism is most commonly associated with suppressive thyroid therapy, although mild Graves' disease is a possible cause. The midwife should refer for physician consultation any woman in whom hyperthyroidism is diagnosed or suspected.

Various therapies exist for treatment of hyperthyroid states. Thiourea drugs such as methimazole (Tapazole) and propylthiouracil, radioactive iodine, and surgical removal of the thyroid have all been used successfully. Beta blockers (e.g., atenolol [Tenormin]) may be given for symptomatic relief. None of these treatments is without risks, including the subsequent development of hypothyroidism. Thus the midwife who is caring for a woman with symptoms consistent with hypothyroidism after treatment for Graves' disease or other hyperthyroid states should screen for the presence of hypothyroidism.

BOX 8-9 Common Clinical Features of Thyroid Disease

Hypothyroid

- Fatigue, sleepiness
- Lethargy
- Muscle weakness
- Muscle cramping or pain
- Cold intolerance
- Constipation
- Dry skin, brittle nails, thinning hair
- Headaches
- Menorrhagia, amenorrhea (late)
- Delay in deep tendon reflex relaxation
- Depression
- Decreased sweating
- Edema (nonpitting)
- Hoarseness
- Pallor
- Loss of appetite
- Weight gain (occasionally weight loss)
- Slowed speech and body movements
- Bradycardia
- Goiter

Hyperthyroid

- Anxiety, nervousness
- Fatigue
- Weakness
- Increased sweating
- Heat intolerance
- Diarrhea
- Warm, moist skin
- Tremor
- Irregular menses
- Lid lag, stare
- Hyperreflexia
- Increased appetite with weight loss
- Palpitations with angina
- Goiter
- Ophthalmopathy

Neurologic Conditions

Headaches

Headaches have many causes and differing degrees of risk, and often are divided into two types: primary and secondary. Primary headaches include tension headaches, migraine, and cluster headaches, whereas secondary headaches are rarer and are related to an underlying disease such as a neoplasm. Symptoms related to each form should be covered in the history and included in the review of systems. A headache diary can be of help in diagnosis and treatment. Usual components of any assessment include frequency of severe headache, frequency of mild headache, level of interference with normal activities, and frequency of medication use to relieve symptoms. Additional questions can be asked about issues such as nausea, light sensitivity, and noise sensitivity, all of which suggest a migraine headache.[106]

The myriad other conditions that can provoke headache as a symptom, such as sinus infection or concussion, are not discussed here, nor are vascular emergencies such as aneurysm and arteriovenous (AV) malformation. Warning signs identified on history and examination that require immediate medical attention are summarized in **Box 8-10**.

Tension Headache

According to the International Headache Society (IHS), reported prevalence for the various tension headaches ranges from 30% to 78%.[107] At the high

---

> ### BOX 8-10 Warning Signs of Headache Emergencies
>
> Rapid onset of severe symptoms
>
> Alteration in consciousness or mental status
>
> High fever
>
> Severe vomiting
>
> Neck stiffness
>
> Neurologic symptoms:
> - Weakness
> - Loss of balance
> - Numbness
> - Paralysis
>
> Vision changes
>
> Pattern of worsening headache
>
> Increasing medication use to control headache
>
> Direct association with exercise or position change

---

end of that range, it is probable that missed diagnoses of migraine are included.

To diagnose tension headache, women must have two or more of the following criteria during at least 10 episodes: (1) mild to moderate intensity headache, (2) bilateral pain in head or neck, (3) nonpulsating character, (4) not associated with physical activity. Further, there cannot be light and sound sensitivity, nausea, or vomiting. Tension headaches are classified based on frequency: infrequent episodic (less than 1 day/month), frequent episodic (1–14 days/month), and chronic.[108] Most individuals with infrequent or moderate-frequency tension headaches do not seek treatment. Among persons with chronic tension headaches, it has been reported that most are able to continue working and managing daily activities, but they are more likely to have mood or anxiety disorders, decreased ability to function, disturbed sleep, and decreased emotional well-being.[109]

Respect for the woman's report of symptoms, assessment of the risk and need for treatment for anxiety or depression, and promotion of lifestyle changes that include relaxation and stress reduction are all part of providing care for episodic tension headaches. Symptomatic therapy with NSAIDs or acetaminophen should be used as initial therapy, especially in episodic tension headaches. Combination medications that include caffeine with aspirin (e.g., Excedrin), ibuprofen (Advil), or acetaminophen (Tylenol) are useful when a single medication is not adequate.[110,111] Prophylactic treatment is not effective or useful in managing episodic headache.[112]

Chronic tension headache is a more severe condition, often requiring prophylactic medication. The tricyclic antidepressants—most commonly, amitriptyline—can be used for this purpose; biofeedback, stress reduction, and other nonpharmacologic interventions to interrupt the cycle of headaches can be used as additional modalities.[111,113] When women report chronic headache over several months while using pain relievers, a medication overuse headache should be suspected, and a plan to stop or taper the drugs in question should be implemented. Women with chronic headache should be referred to a neurologist for management.

Migraine Headache

Migraine headache is both common and frequently underdiagnosed in primary care settings, with an estimated 25% of cases being missed, suggesting that a woman with episodic headaches should be assumed to have migraines unless otherwise diagnosed.[114] The majority of individuals with migraine report 1 to 4 days per month with symptoms, and the prevalence of migraine among women is estimated to be more than 20%.[108] Among all races, women are more likely than men to be diagnosed; the condition is more common among Caucasians. Incidence of new-onset migraine in women is highest in the decade after menarche, with the median age at new onset being 25 years.[115] Prevalence rises through the fourth decade of life, but then decline thereafter. Migraine is relatively rare among postmenopausal women, and new-onset headaches in this age group should be evaluated carefully for other causes. The prevalence of migraine also declines as income rises.[116] One group of researchers found that more than half the individuals included in their studies reported losing work time and limiting activities due to headaches.[116]

Both genetic predisposition and environmental triggers appear to be involved in the development of migraine headache. The underlying cause is an abnormally increased sensitization to neuronal stimuli, beginning in the cerebral cortex and affecting the trigeminovascular system. The diagnosis of migraine is subdivided based on the presence or absence of an aura, association with the menstrual cycle, and other characteristics.[117] The International Headache Society defines migraine without aura as a "recurrent headache disorder manifesting in attacks lasting 4 to 72 hours. Typical characteristics of the headache are unilateral location, pulsating quality, moderate or severe intensity, aggravation by routine physical activity and association with nausea and/or photophobia and phonophobia."[117] Migraine with aura adds "attacks of reversible focal neurological symptoms that usually develop gradually over 5–20 minutes and last for less than 60 minutes. Headache with the features of migraine without aura usually follows the aura symptoms."[117] Menstrual migraines are those that occur in relation to the menstrual cycle, arising "immediately 1–2 days before onset of menses or within first 3 days of the cycle in at least two out of three menstrual cycles and at no other times of the cycle,"[117]

Migraine is an intermittently recurring event, with well-defined stages: (1) the premonitory stage, sometimes called prodrome; (2) aura; (3) headache; and (4) postdrome. The premonitory stage is noted in approximately 30% of those with the condition and occurs up to 48 hours before onset of the actual headache; tiredness, fatigue, malaise, mood changes, and stomach upset are the most common symptoms.[118] Aura occurs up to an hour before headache onset in less than one-fourth of those with a migraine diagnosis. Visual, sensory, and speech symptoms associated with aura are reversible.[119] Following the headache, variable symptoms may persist for hours or days.

Over time, migraine may progress from an episodic to a persistent condition with almost daily symptoms. Chronic migraine (defined as occurring on 15 or more days per month) is accompanied in some individuals by both physiologic changes in pain perception and anatomic alterations within the brain.[118]

A number of lifestyle changes may improve the frequency of migraine. These modifications include the avoidance of substances that the individual can identify as headache triggers (such as cheese, alcohol, or chocolate), stress reduction, and stable patterns of eating and rest. Pharmacologic therapy depends on the severity and frequency of attacks. In mild, infrequent cases of migraine, NSAIDs taken in maximal doses, or acetaminophen 1000 mg, can be used as abortive therapy, especially if they can be taken during the warning prodrome. Either of these medications may be marketed in combination with caffeine in over-the-counter preparations. The most common abortive therapies include ergotamine preparations such as ergotamine tartrate/caffeine (Cafergot); the triptans, such as sumatriptan (Imitrex) and naratriptan (Amerge); and isometheptene/acetaminophen/dichloralphenazone (Midrin). A woman of childbearing age should be on an effective contraceptive method when using these medications, and those women planning a pregnancy may require a change in therapeutic management.

Prophylactic therapy for migraine includes a number of different drug classes, such as the tricyclic antidepressants, antiepileptics, beta blockers, calcium-channel blockers, ACE inhibitors, and angiotensin receptor blockers. Women requiring long-term migraine management should be under the care of a neurologist or another practitioner skilled in the management of headache.

Both pure menstrual migraines and menstrual-related migraines may benefit from long-cycle combined hormonal therapy or progesterone only contraception, particularly the levonorgestrel intrauterine system (IUS). Decreasing the frequency of estrogen withdrawal minimizes the headache response.[119] When estrogen is included in treatment, the woman must be monitored for possible increases in the frequency of headache, which would mandate the use of progesterone-only methods. Combined hormonal contraception is contraindicated in women who have migraine with aura, due to increased stroke risk.[119] Short-term use of a triptan in the days prior to the menses may also interrupt the headache cycle.

Epilepsy

The International League Against Epilepsy defines epileptic seizures as transient excessive aberrant or synchronous neuron activity causing physical signs or symptoms. As a disease condition, epilepsy requires at least one documented seizure, persistent changes within the brain that will lead to recurrences, and "associated neurobiologic, cognitive, psychological, and social disturbances."[120]

The classification of seizure disorders is based on whether they are generalized or partial, and are further subdivided by specific patterns of associated symptoms. Generalized seizures are caused by significant activity in both lobes of the brain, and almost always involve changes in consciousness. Tonic–clonic seizures (grand mal), absence (petit mal) seizures, and brief myoclonic seizures are all examples of generalized seizure activity. Partial seizures may or may not involve alteration in consciousness; if this symptom is present, they are referred to as complex partial seizures.

The midwife's role in caring for women diagnosed with a seizure disorder is primarily focused on the effect of epilepsy medications on reproductive health, the management of contraceptives, pregnancy concerns, and assessment for morbidity risks associated with epilepsy or medications used to treat epilepsy. Some epilepsy medications are associated with an increased risk for teratogenic effects and pregnant women on these medications should be referred to a physician for counseling. Seizure activity in women of childbearing age will peak around the times of ovulation and menstruation.[121] There is an increased risk of polycystic ovarian syndrome among women with seizures, especially those taking valproate (Depakote).[122] Although the timing of menarche does not appear to be affected by childhood epilepsy, persistent disease and ongoing therapy are associated with early menopause.[123] Decreased bone mineral density has also been linked to the use of antiepileptic drugs, although the contribution of seizure-associated falls to increased fracture rates is not clear.[124]

Contraceptive management is complicated by the interaction of estrogen-containing hormonal products with antiepileptic medications that affect the cytochrome P-450 metabolic pathway—for example, barbiturates, carbamazepine (Tegretol), lamotrigine (Lamictal), phenytoin (Dilantin), and topiramate (Topamax; in larger doses). The risk of unintended pregnancy is increased with this combination. The contraceptive implant etonogestrel (Nexplanon) has also been shown to have an increased risk of failure among women taking these types of antiepileptic agents.[125] Both depot medroxyprogesterone acetate (DMPA) and the levonorgestrel-containing IUS (Mirena) are safe for use, as is the copper intrauterine device (ParaGard); however, some authorities suggest DMPA may need

to be given at 10-week rather than 12-week intervals.[125] More information about contraception, including evidence-based criteria for eligibility, can be found later in this text. All women with epilepsy should receive counseling regarding risks associated with pregnancy, and referral to a maternal–fetal medicine specialist may prove valuable.

Another important concern among women with epilepsy is the increased risk of depression and suicide. Both the psychological and physical stress of living with the disease and the side effects of medication factor into these risks.[126] Regular screening for mood changes and suicidal ideation during routine gynecologic visits particularly is appropriate when caring for women with this disorder.

Carpal Tunnel Syndrome

The carpal tunnel carries the median nerve through the wrist, where compression from edema, inflammation of the tissue, or anatomic distortion can produce the classic symptoms of carpal tunnel syndrome—tingling, numbness, or altered sensation across the palmar surface of part of the thumb, the first two fingers, and part of the ring finger in the affected hand. Over time, carpal tunnel syndrome almost always becomes bilateral. The woman may report that pain and numbness are worse at night. **Figure 8-5** illustrates the area affected by carpal tunnel syndrome.

Female gender, pregnancy, increasing age, obesity, history of wrist injury or arthritis, diabetes, and hypothyroidism have all been associated with increased risk.[127] The relationship of workplace injury to carpal tunnel syndrome is disputed in the literature. When women engaged in a repetitive motion of the wrists at work or school report numbness or loss of sensation in this pattern, carpal tunnel syndrome is often assumed to be related to this cause, in part because of the increased insistence on ergonomics to reduce workplace injuries. Other forms of nerve damage can also present with similar symptoms. If additional symptoms unrelated to the median nerve are present, prompt referral is warranted.

Two simple tests can help to confirm that the woman's report is consistent with carpal tunnel syndrome. First, tapping over the wrist crease in the midline should produce tingling in the affected area; this is referred to as Tinel's sign. Second, holding the wrist flexed for 45 to 60 seconds and releasing should produce symptoms; this is referred to as the Phalen test (**Figure 8-6**). Electromyography and nerve conduction studies will confirm the diagnosis of carpal tunnel syndrome.

Initial treatment is conservative, and may begin with splinting at night to place the wrist in a neutral position. Only limited evidence supports the

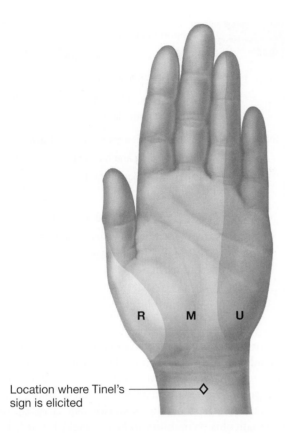

Figure 8-5 Distribution of sensation by the radial (R), median (M), and ulnar (U) nerves.

effectiveness of this technique.[128] Other conservative therapies, ranging from nerve gliding techniques to wrist manipulation to yoga and aerobic exercise, have been recommended, but there is little evidence of their effectiveness.[129] If symptoms are severe,

persist, or worsen with conservative management, the woman should be referred to an orthopedic surgeon or neurologist for further evaluation. Treatment may then include injections of steroids or surgical release of the nerve. If left untreated, the condition will worsen over time and eventually lead to permanent decrease in sensation.

Musculoskeletal Disorders

Sprains and Strains

Musculoskeletal complaints comprise approximately 10% to 15% of primary care visits. A systemic approach to any complaint of musculoskeletal pain will help the midwife evaluate for the multiple differential diagnoses that are possible.

When evaluating a woman for musculoskeletal pain, have her point to the pain and describe any associated injury. The initial assessment include determination of localized versus diffuse, acute versus chronic, and inflammatory versus non-inflammatory. Sprains are stretched or torn ligaments; strains are stretched or torn muscles or tendons. **Table 8-14** compares common signs and symptoms of the two conditions. Risk factors include active participation in sports with the related increase in accidental injury, obesity, poor balance, decreased flexibility, and a sedentary lifestyle leading to poor physical conditioning.

Sprains

The most commonly sprained joint is the ankle, with more than 600,000 ankle injuries occurring each year

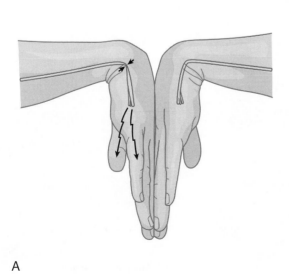

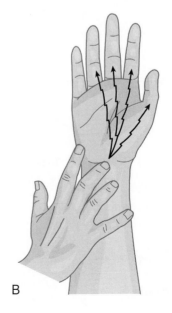

A   B

Figure 8-6 (A) Phalen's test. (B) Tinel's sign.

Table 8-14	Differential Diagnosis for Sprain or Strain
Type of Injury	**Symptoms**
Sprain	Swelling
	Pain
	Bruising over the joint
	Limited flexion/extension of joint
Strain	Swelling
	Pain
	Muscle spasm
	Limited contraction/release of muscle

Table 8-15	Sprain Grades
Grade	**Symptoms**
Grade 1	Ligament is stretched, may have micro-tears
	Minimal swelling, full weight bearing possible
	No instability in the joint
Grade 2	Macro-tears but ligament remains attached
	Moderate swelling and bruising
	Difficulty with weight bearing
	Joint is unstable
Grade 3	Complete tear through the ligament
	Extensive swelling, bruising, severe pain
	Unable to bear weight, significant joint instability

in the United States.[130] The knee, wrist, and thumb are other commonly injured sites. Twisting or over-stretching a joint can cause the ligaments securing the bones to be stretched or torn. Once injured, a joint is prone to re-injury, possibly from persistent laxity in the ligament, or damage to the nerves and muscles associated with the joint. Approximately 20% of ankle sprains will result in permanent instability.[131]

Sprains are graded based on degree of injury, as shown in **Table 8-15**.[132] Ankle stability can be evaluated using the talar tilt and anterior drawer tests (**Figure 8-7**). Normal inversion of the ankle is less than 35 degrees; normal plantar flexion is less than 50 degrees. Whenever evaluating the ankle, the opposite foot should also be assessed for comparison purposes, as there is significant individual variation

in normal joint flexion. Diagnosis of an ankle sprain includes ruling out a fracture. The Ottawa rules used to determine the need for X ray of the ankle include the presence of pain near the affected ankle, and either tenderness on the posterior aspect or tip of the malleolus or inability to bear weight for at least four steps both immediately after the event and in the examining room.[132]

The management of sprains is determined by the severity of the injury. NSAIDs and acetaminophen are generally sufficient pain medications for sprains. The use of opioids should be limited. The immediate implementation of a strategy to limit bruising

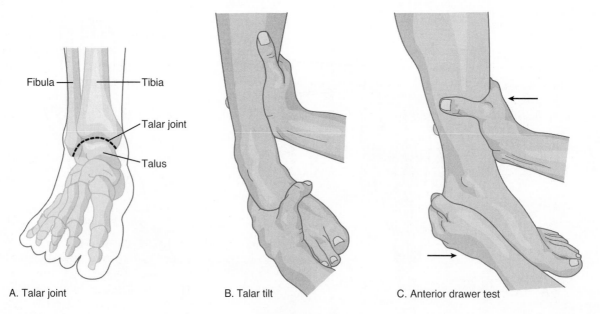

A. Talar joint   B. Talar tilt   C. Anterior drawer test

Figure 8-7 Talar tilt and anterior drawer tests to assess ankle sprain.

and swelling follows the mnemonic "PRICE" (**Table 8-16**). Progressive rehabilitation of the joint is appropriate in all cases. Long-term immobilization is less useful than an approach that encourages exercises to strengthen the joint after 2 to 3 days.[133] Only the most severe sprains require surgical repair, assuming physical therapy fails.[131]

Strains

Strains are the result of over-stretching a muscle or tendon causing a tear; the degree of risk of an injury is related to the strength and conditioning of the individual, the level of activity, and the direction and intensity of the movement involved. The actual degree of muscle tearing, the resultant bleeding into the tissue, and inflammation all are involved in determining the extent of injury. Clinical diagnosis is frequently all that is needed; ultrasound or magnetic resonance imaging (MRI) may be required for further evaluation.

Similar to treatment of sprains, management of the acute phase is with the PRICE therapies for the first 3 to 5 days, followed by gradual reintroduction of physical activity.[134] NSAIDs provide pain relief and decrease associated inflammation, and can be used as adjunctive treatment in the acute phase of tissue injury. Their long-term use may be associated with poorer tissue healing.[134,135]

Low Back Pain

Pain in the lower back, with or without sciatic nerve pain, is divided into acute pain lasting less than 7 weeks and chronic pain. In fact, many individuals with brief episodes do not seek medical care. Only 15% of women with acute low back pain have identifiable anatomic causes; the rest have nonspecific sources.[136] Approximately 25% of all individuals who experience

an episode of acute, nonspecific low back pain will have a recurrence within one year.[137] Lack of physical activity, obesity, genetics, and psychological issues are among the factors that may contribute to pain. The differential diagnosis ranges from sprain/strain to spinal conditions that include herniated discs, compression fractures, spinal stenosis; systemic diseases including cancer and connective tissue disease; and referred pain from pelvic or abdominal disease.[138]

Assessment of the woman presenting with symptoms consistent with acute lower back pain includes history and related symptoms, her subjective evaluation of the pain, associated psychological factors, ability to function normally, environmental or work-related risks, prior episodes, and questioning regarding red flag symptoms of more serious disorders. Red-flag signs and symptoms include history of trauma, parenteral drug use, unexplained weight loss, cancer history, long-term use of steroids, fever, incontinence, and intense localized pain on physical examination.

Clinical assessment does not require imaging for acute, episodic low back pain.[136,139] Imaging with MRI is required only for those individuals with progressive neurologic deficit. The assessment should allow differentiation of pain into nonspecific causes, possible radiculopathy or stenosis, and other medical risks including progressive neurologic disease.[139]

Initial management of acute low back pain includes education about exercise, encouragement to remain physically active, and pharmacologic management. Heat may offer relief from strains. Bed rest or prolonged immobilization is of no additional benefit in caring for women with acute low back pain.[136,139]

Pharmacologic therapy for acute low back pain begins with NSAIDs or acetaminophen (Tylenol). Short-term use (fewer than 4 days) of a muscle relaxant can assist when acute pain is severe. There is not strong evidence to recommend one agent over the others, although cyclobenzaprine (Flexeril) is commonly recommended.[140] While opiate medications can be effective pain relievers, their benefit in treating low back pain is often outweighed by their potential for abuse.[140,141] Prolonged use of opiates occurs frequently and is associated with higher rates of adverse outcomes including slower recovery, addiction, overdose, and accidental death.[141] Among women with chronic low back pain, tricyclic antidepressants have been shown to offer some benefit.[140] Nonpharmacologic therapies have also shown some benefit in the treatment of chronic low back pain. Cognitive-behavioral therapy, spinal manipulation, acupuncture, massage, and yoga, as well as interdisciplinary approaches, have all demonstrated moderate to significant benefit.[141]

Table 8-16	PRICE: A Conservative Strategy for Management of Sprains and Strains
Strategy	**Management**
Protection	Use of an air splint, fixed-joint, or adjustable walking cast
Rest	Limitation of activity involving weight bearing
Ice	Applied intermittently for up to 20 minutes each time
Compression	Elastic bandages that limit swelling and extravasation into damaged tissue
Elevation	To the level of the heart

Dermatologic Conditions

When assessing a skin lesion or rash, a history specific to the current concern, including the pattern of recurrence, timing and progression, and potential environmental exposures, will facilitate identification of the dermatologic condition. The physical examination includes the appearance, shape, and texture of the lesion; the pattern of multiple lesions; and distribution of lesions across the body. Knowing the terminology for common skin changes standardizes descriptions and facilitates identification; such terms are identified in **Table 8-17**.[142] Several of the more common or significant conditions found during the delivery of primary care are described in this section.

Atopic Dermatitis (Eczema)

The terms *atopic dermatitis* and *eczema* overlap, as atopic dermatitis requires an underlying predilection toward allergies and asthma. Several patterns of chronic skin rash can arise that include itchy, dry, scaling skin; blisters; cracked skin or sores; or papular rashes. Over time, chronic eczematous reactions can lead to thickening of the skin itself or lichenification. Joint flexures, the face and neck, hands, and feet are common locations of such lesions.

Initial signs of atopic dermatitis most often occur during infancy, and develop progressively throughout the years into adulthood. Much of the data on the prevalence of atopic dermatitis and eczema are based on pediatric data. However, a survey of adults found that more than 10% reported symptoms consistent with eczema and 6% met the more stringent definition of atopic dermatitis.[143] Living in urban areas, black race, and higher educational status among adults in the household all contribute to increased risk; higher family income is inversely associated with risk.[142,144]

Both genetic and environmental factors contribute to the development of symptomatic disease. Among the environmental triggers are aeroallergens such as pets and dust mites, and food sensitization, particularly to milk or eggs. Skin bacteria (such as *S. aureus*) and fungi (including *Malassezia* species) are also involved in atopic dermatitis.[145] Affected skin tends to be thinner and drier than normal, which makes it a less effective barrier. That defect, plus hypersensitivity to irritants including chemicals, rough fabrics such as wool, humidity, or temperature change, helps account for the pruritus associated with atopic dermatitis. Finally, increased stress is associated with worsening symptoms of atopic dermatitis.

Management of atopic dermatitis consists of the application of emollient creams, possibly use of moderate-strength topical corticosteroids, or topical calcineurin inhibitors (tacrolimus [Protopic], pimecrolimus [Elidel]). When secondary bacterial infections occur, topical treatment for short periods may be recommended; long-term use of topical antibiotics may lead to resistance and should be avoided. In addition to medication, education about maintenance use of emollients, avoidance of triggers, and stress reduction are important components of care. Referral to a dermatologist for development of a long-term plan of care often is indicated.

Psoriasis

Psoriasis is a chronic skin disorder caused by an underlying immune defect that produces thick pruritic, scaly plaques on the skin. Commonly the head and neck, elbow and knee joints, and lower back are affected; although lesions can occur anywhere on the body, the extremities are more often affected than the trunk. The prevalence of psoriasis in the United States is reported to be approximately 2% to 3% of the population, with the incidence of new cases peaking among young adults.[146] Among the various expressions of psoriasis, plaque psoriasis represents almost 90% of all cases. In this form, well-defined areas of thickened, erythematous skin with silvery, scaly patches are seen, usually with symmetric distribution.

Psoriasis is a complex condition that may remit, but rarely resolves. It has been associated with a number of medical and psychological comorbidities, including metabolic syndrome, cardiovascular disease, and autoimmune disorders. Associated psychological conditions include depression and suicidal ideation.[147] Assessment of depression status and stressors is an important part of the evaluation of women who have psoriasis. Counseling can include use of stress reduction techniques and comfort measures such as oatmeal baths.

Women for whom a diagnosis of psoriasis is made should be referred to a dermatologist for initial evaluation and plan of care. The majority of women have mild to moderate disease. For those whose plaques cover more than 5% of the body surface, topical therapy may sufficient, although this treatment rarely is associated with complete remission. Initial topical treatments include corticosteroids, salicylic acid (to soften keratinized skin), and moisturizers. Ultraviolet light therapy, retinoids, methotrexate (Trexall), cyclosporine-A (Neoral, Sandimmune), and biologic agents are used both for more severe cases and for more complete healing.[147]

Table 8-17	Terms and Descriptions for Common Skin Manifestations
Term	**Definition**
Acne	A dermatologic condition primarily of the sebaceous skin glands characterized by papules, pustules, or comedones. This condition is more properly termed acne vulgaris to differentiate it from other, less common types of acne.
Actinic keratosis (AK)	A premalignant skin condition with multiple crusty patches. Also termed solar keratosis.
Calcineurin inhibitors	Immunosuppressant agents that are theorized to act by selectively inhibiting inflammation through action on T-cell activation.
Carbuncle	A skin infection composed of a cluster of boils (furuncles). This infection is most frequently caused by *Staphylococcus aureas*.
Cellulitis	An acute spreading dermatologic bacterial infection characterized by significant edema, erythema, and pain.
Cosmeceutical	A word coined from the terms "cosmetic" and "pharmaceutical," which is used to describe agents that both have therapeutic effects and promote attractiveness.
Dermatophytes	Parasites that may infect the skin. An example is athlete's foot.
Eczema	Inflammatory dermatologic process that is characterized by pruritus, erythema, and lesions that may be encrusted and scaly.
Furuncle	Skin infection commonly involving a hair follicle. Also called a boil.
Humectant	Ingredient that absorbs water and promotes maintenance of moisture on the skin.
Intertrigo	Rash or inflammation of the body folds or intertriginous areas of the skin.
Keratinocyte	Epidermal cell that synthesizes keratin.
Langerhans cell	Dendritic skin cell that transports antigens to lymph nodes.
Melanin	Skin pigment produced by special cells (melanocytes).
Melanocyte	Cell located in the bottom layer (stratum basale) of the skin's epidermis that produces melanin.
Merkel cell	Cell found in the middle layers of the skin around hair follicles. Cancer originating among these cells—Merkel cell carcinoma—tends to be highly aggressive.
Onychomycosis	Fungal infection of the nails on either fingers or toes.
Psoriasis	Skin condition caused by overgrowth of keratinocytes, resulting in patchy thickened skin.
Pyoderma	Skin condition characterized by purulent filled lesions.
Retinoids	Natural or synthetic derivative of vitamin A that is widely used in pharmacotherapeutics in dermatology.
Seborrheic keratoses	Wart-like, benign skin lesions.
Solar lentigo	Flat pigmented lesions on sun-exposed skin. Also known as senile lentigo.
Sun protection factor (SPF)	A measure of how much ultraviolet radiation (sunlight) is required to produce a burn on skin that is protected with sunscreen. A sunscreen with an SPF factor of 15 or greater is recommended by the American Academy of Dermatology.
Telangiectasia	Dark red, elevated skin lesions caused by chronic dilation of capillaries.
Ultraviolet (UV) radiation	Rays from the sun that are invisible to the naked eye, but capable of skin damage and photoaging.
Xerosis	Dry skin.

Skin Cancers

Unprotected exposure to ultraviolet radiation is directly related to malignant melanomas and other skin cancers, as well as precursor lesions such as actinic keratosis, squamous cell carcinoma, and basal cell carcinoma. The exposure may occur via natural sun or a tanning facility. All of the skin cancers share the risk factors of fair skin with a tendency to freckle or burn, blond/red hair, blue or green eyes, history of severe sunburns, immunosuppression, and family history. More than 3 million persons in the United States are estimated to have a non-melanotic skin cancer.[148]

Counseling that focuses on the etiology of skin cancer and preventive measures, including using appropriate sunscreen, wearing protective clothing, limiting ultraviolet exposure, and having regular skin inspections, can act as a first-line prevention strategy for skin cancers. At every visit, the midwife should note the presence and number of moles or other skin lesions, ask about skin changes, document findings, and recommend dermatologic evaluation when appropriate.

Actinic Keratosis

Actinic keratoses are small, dry, rough textured papules or plaques caused by excess exposure to ultraviolet (UV) radiation. In the United States, as much as 25% of the population may develop actinic keratoses over a lifetime, with those older than the age of 40 years being at increased risk. Early actinic keratosis lesions are usually smaller than 2 cm; they may remain the color of the underlying skin, or be gray or pink. Over time, actinic keratoses may progress to a harder, warty texture. There is disagreement about whether actinic keratosis is itself a precancerous lesion or a squamous carcinoma in situ.[149]

The transformation rate for actinic keratosis into squamous cell carcinoma is unclear, but 60% to 80% of squamous cell carcinoma begin as actinic keratosis lesions. Signs associated with increased risk of progressive disease include induration/Inflammation, lesion diameter greater than 1 cm, rapid enlargement, bleeding, erythema, and ulceration. The observation of larger numbers of lesions also indicates an increased risk of progression.[150]

Treatment of actinic keratoses by a dermatologist may include removal of a lesion, potentially through excision, cryotherapy, or laser, and usually includes topical application of imiquimod (Aldara), diclofenac (Voltaren) or 5-fluorouracil (Efudex) to treat the area surrounding the lesion. The use of these "field agents" reduces the risk of progression in adjacent tissue with preclinical cellular changes.[151]

Basal Cell Carcinoma/ Squamous Cell Carcinoma

Basal cell carcinomas have a waxy or translucent appearance with a raised edge and central erosion. Risk factors for basal cell carcinoma include skin injuries such as old burns or scars, inflammation, radiation therapy, arsenic exposure, and skin ulcers.[150,151] Like actinic keratoses, squamous cell carcinoma is scaly, but the lesions will be thickened, poorly defined, occasionally hard (horn-like), on an erythematous base. In addition to the specific risk factors for basal cell carcinoma cited earlier, cutaneous human papillomavirus (HPV) infection and a history of actinic keratoses are factors that increase the risk of squamous cell carcinoma.

Similar to actinic keratoses, very early cases of skin cancer can occasionally be treated with imiquimod or another agent. Standard treatment includes surgery, electrodessication and curettage, or cryosurgery. Occasionally, radiation or chemotherapy is also required.

Melanoma

The incidence of melanoma has been steadily rising in the United States, such that the lifetime risk is now 1 in every 30 individuals. Currently, the incidence among younger women is rising at more than double the overall increase, and the use of tanning facilities has been implicated in this trend.[152] Ever-use of tanning facilities, early age at first use, and increased frequency are directly associated with increased risk.[153] Unlike the other skin cancers that are relatively easy to treat and have excellent prognoses, melanoma has an increased risk of metastasis. Disease-free survival depends on early diagnosis and prompt surgical excision. Five-year survival rates for individuals diagnosed with a localized tumor are greater than 90%; by comparison, metastatic disease has a 5-year survival rate of only 15%.[152]

Melanoma is more common among women with large numbers of moles, and those individuals with a dysplastic nevus. Dysplastic nevi are larger than common moles, with a rough texture, often irregular in outline, and of different colors.[152,153] Among women, melanomas are more common on the legs and trunk. Lesions also can appear on the genital area, and they should be carefully noted for follow-up. When in doubt, the midwife should initiate a referral to a dermatologist. Surgery is the basis of treatment for melanoma, followed by chemotherapy or immunotherapy.

Common Skin Infections

Herpes Zoster

Herpes zoster, also called shingles or zoster, is a reactivation of the varicella virus as immunity to it wanes. This virus lies dormant along one or more dermatomes, in the dorsal root of sensory nerve ganglia. Approximately 1 million cases of zoster occur in the United States annually. The incidence rises with age and in persons in whom cellular immunity is impaired. Other risk factors are unclear, but some—though not all—studies report female gender as a risk factor.[154] The incidence of zoster among whites is approximately twice that among African Americans.[155] Physical trauma at the affected dermatome and psychological stress may also play a role in the reactivation of varicella virus.

Clinically, zoster often presents with a prodrome of burning pain along the affected dermatome, accompanied by headache, fatigue, and malaise. The typical painful rash of papules on an erythematous base that progresses to vesicles, ruptures, and crusts over may take 7 days to develop. The entire cycle from initial rash to complete healing takes 2 to 3 weeks. When postherpetic neuralgia develops, severe pain may persist for months.

Management of acute herpes zoster includes antiviral drugs such as acyclovir (Zovirax) or valacyclovir (Valtrex), with the addition of analgesics to treat the pain. Initially, acetaminophen (Tylenol) or an NSAID should be given, with opioids being reserved for severe or intractable pain.[156]

The treatment of postherpetic neuralgia is more complicated and requires referral to a pain specialist. Tricyclic antidepressants, antiepileptic agents such as gabapentin (Neurontin) or pregabalin (Lyrica), and lidocaine patch are the first-line therapies. Opioids and tramadol (Ultram) are used as second-line therapies. While opioids are generally effective, the risk of misuse with these agents is higher than with other therapies.[156]

Transmission from direct contact with lesions is possible, but such contact will produce chickenpox, not herpes zoster. Only those persons without prior varicella exposure are at risk for chickenpox. Unlike with chickenpox, droplet transmission does not occur with zoster.

Vaccination against herpes zoster is now recommended for adults aged 60 years or older, and is FDA approved for persons older than 50 years.[155]

The vaccine should not be given to individuals with a history of anaphylactic reaction to its components, immune suppression, immunosuppressive therapy including high-dose corticosteroids, or anyone at risk of being pregnant. Vaccination reduces the likelihood of ever having an outbreak by more than 50%, and of having postherpetic neuralgia by approximately two-thirds.[155]

Herpes Simplex Labialis

Herpes simplex labialis (HSV-1) is most commonly transmitted nonsexually and during childhood. In 2006, Xu et al. reported the seroprevalence of HSV-1 infection to be 57.7% (95% confidence interval: 55.9–59.5%) in the United States, a 7% decrease from the last period surveyed.[156] Many cases are subclinical, diagnosed only by serology; many individuals do not realize that their cold sore is, in fact, a herpes lesion.[157]

Direct exposure of mucous membranes or abraded skin to viral shedding is required for transmission of HSV-1. However, the virus can be shed asymptomatically and can be transmitted by droplet or persist on skin or objects for brief periods of time.[158]

After initial exposure, the development of symptoms depends on the inoculum—that is, the amount of virus to which one was exposed—and may occur up to 3 weeks after exposure. The first HSV outbreak, which is typically the most widespread and painful, lasts for 10 to 14 days. Clusters of 1-mm to 2-mm painful vesicles develop on an erythematous base and open to create ulcerative lesions. Lymphadenopathy and flu-like symptoms accompany a primary outbreak. Pain may be severe enough to lead to avoidance of food and fluids, thereby producing dehydration.[159]

After the initial infection, herpes viruses enter a latent state in the nerve ganglia—usually the trigeminal nerve for HSV-1. Recurrent outbreaks are typically briefer and milder, moving through the stages of prodrome, lesion formation, ulceration, and crusting within 3 to 4 days. Complete skin healing can take an additional week.[160] In addition to causing oral lesions, HSV-1 can infect other locations including the eye (herpes keratitis) and the fingers (herpetic whitlow).

Management of primary oral lesions includes acyclovir (Zovirax), valacyclovir (Valtrex), or famciclovir (Famvir) for 7 days; the use of a topical anesthetic; and fluid/nutritional supplementation when needed.[161] Promptly providing oral antiviral treatment of recurrent lesions can reduce shedding and duration of lesions; topical products, however, have not been shown to have the same benefit. Single-day therapy can be prescribed in the form of either valacyclovir (2 g twice in 24 hours) or famciclovir (1500 mg once); acyclovir requires multiple doses over 5 days, but can be used if other medications are not accessible.[161] Suppression therapy with acyclovir 400 mg twice daily, valacyclovir 500 mg or 1 g daily, or famciclovir 500 mg twice daily can be provided when there are frequent recurrences.[161]

Tinea Versicolor (Pityriasis)

Tinea versicolor is a chronic infection, in which normal skin fungi that are present on the outer layer of the epidermis, in hair follicles and sebaceous glands, overgrow and become pathogenic. The fungi involved—*Pityrosporum orbiculare* and *Pityrosporum ovale*—also are referred to as *Malassezia*. Factors that increase the risk of outbreaks include heat and humidity; oily skin; medical conditions, including steroid therapy, immune suppression, malnutrition, burns, adrenalectomy, and Cushing's disease; and oral contraceptive use.

The associated rash consists of flat macules of discolored skin on the neck, upper back, or chest. Light-skinned individuals will notice hyperpigmented lesions, while those with darker skin may notice either hypopigmented or hyperpigmented lesions. The macules will spread to form large patches. Pruritus may be associated with the outbreaks.

Topical antifungals, including clotrimazole (Lotrimin, Mycelex) and ketoconazole (Nizoral), can be applied daily for 2 to 4 weeks. Ketoconazole shampoo (Nizoral) can also be used daily for 3 days as a body wash from the scalp to the hips. When the spread of the rash is extensive or treatment with topical medications proves ineffective, a course of oral antifungals can be prescribed. The affected woman should be advised that the presence of tinea versicolor is not secondary to poor hygiene; that she needs to continue the prescribed treatment even if lesions resolve during therapy; and that she may have areas of hypopigmentation when tanning until the melanocytes destroyed by the fungus have become reestablished.

Bacterial Skin Infections

Bacterial skin infections are a common reason for healthcare visits. Knowledge of the presentation of the most common bacterial skin infections informs proper management of these conditions.

Staphylococcus and Streptococcus

Among the normal skin flora, *Staphylococcus epidermis* and *Staphylococcus aureus* are the most common bacteria, along with the corynebacteria and mycobacteria; *Streptococcus pyogenes* is less common. The most significant pathogens within this group are *S. aureus* and *S. pyogenes* (group A beta-hemolytic *Streptococcus*). Risk factors for the development of cellulitis and other soft-tissue infections include trauma, bite injuries, prior cellulitis, diabetes, comorbidities that damage the venous or lymphatic systems, chronic renal disease, cirrhosis, or intravenous drug use.

Impetigo

Impetigo is a superficial infection that produces small vesicles on an erythematous base that open and crust; these vesicles are most often found on the mouth, nares, and arms. If left untreated, the infection may spread and can persist for weeks. Mupirocin (Bactroban) ointment applied three times daily is first-line therapy. Oral antibiotics can be used for resistant or widespread infection.

Erysipelas

S. pyogenes is the most likely source of erysipelas. This infection most often presents as a superficial infection of the skin producing a painful erythematous plaque with well-defined edges.

Cellulitis

Penetration of fluid into subcutaneous tissue, causing erythema, warmth, edema, pain, and possibly lymphadenopathy, is the hallmark of cellulitis. Elevated white blood cell count and fever may be present. When ulcers or other open lesions are present, *S. aureus* infection is the likely culprit. Diffuse infection occurs more commonly with *S. pyogenes*.[162] Both erysipelas and cellulitis are treated orally with penicillinase-resistant semi-synthetic penicillin (e.g., dicloxacillin [Dynapen]), cephalosporin (e.g., cephalexin [Keflex]), or clindamycin (Cleocin). More severe infections require parenteral therapy.[162]

Purulent Soft-Tissue Infections

Conditions such as furuncles and carbuncles are most commonly found in areas of the body where restrictive clothing or chafing occurs. A small, firm, red papule will enlarge and become painful as pus builds up inside, then may either resolve or open and drain spontaneously. When several furuncles coalesce into a carbuncle, the affected individual may experience systemic symptoms of fever or chills in addition to the local pain. Carbuncles will become fluctuant, thinning the skin above the site and drain, possibly from several openings. Treatment of sporadic lesions can be accomplished with warm soaks to help open and drain the site. More severe lesions may require incision and drainage. Once the carbuncle has become fluctuant, antibiotics are unlikely to affect the course of infection.[162]

Necrotizing Soft-Tissue Infection

Necrotizing fasciitis is a soft-tissue infection caused by secondary or polymicrobial extension of a surface infection, often mixed anaerobes or group A *Streptococcus*. The infection encompasses the subcutaneous tissue and extends to the muscle layer. In 80% of cases, there is a direct relationship to a skin lesion.[162] To distinguish cellulitis from a necrotizing infection, the following signs and symptoms can be identified: severe pain, development of bullae, skin bruising, rapid progression to systemic symptoms, edema, surface anesthesia, and a wooden or rigid texture to the underlying tissue.[162] Elevated white blood count, low serum sodium, and elevated C-reactive protein levels are associated with increased risk that what appears to be cellulitis is, in fact, a necrotizing infection.[162] Any suspicion of deep-tissue infection associated with a skin lesion should be referred emergently to a physician or emergency room care to be evaluated for antibiotic and possible surgical treatment.

Methicillin-Resistant Staphylococcus Aureus

S. aureus is one of a group of common bacteria—including *Enterococcus*, *E. coli*, and *Neisseria gonorrhea*—that have developed increasing resistance to the traditional antibiotic therapies. *Staphylococcus* colonization is common, with 2% of colonized individuals carrying methicillin-resistant *S. aureus* (MRSA).[163] Initially, MRSA was primarily associated with healthcare settings; invasive disease is associated with bacteremia, pneumonia, cellulitis, and endocarditis, among other infections.[164] In recent years, community-associated strains have become more common and are now invading healthcare settings as well. More than half of all serious skin and soft-tissue infections are now caused by MRSA.[164] In office settings, MRSA is most commonly seen as boils or carbuncles. The lesions begin with a "spider bite" appearance before enlarging and becoming painful.

The Infectious Disease Society of America's guidelines continue to recommend incision and drainage of boils as the most appropriate treatment. Its recommendation is to defer antibiotics unless the individual has cellulitis or severe disease with multiple locations. If MRSA is suspected, antibiotics that offer adequate coverage, including TMP-SMX (Bactrim), clindamycin (Cleocin), a tetracycline, or linezolid (Zyvox), should be prescribed for 5 to 10 days, and a culture taken prior to treatment.[164] Regardless of the midwife's choice to use supportive measures, incise the lesion for drainage, or prescribe antibiotics, women should be advised that signs of worsening infection or failure to begin healing are indications to seek further care.

Conclusion

Modern midwifery has been viewed as possessing a limited, albeit well-recognized scope of practice—that is, midwives take care of healthy pregnant women and help them give birth. Historically, however, midwives never limited their care exclusively to healthy pregnant women, if for no other reason than that many of the women traditionally served by midwives were at risk because of age, socioeconomic status, or lack of access to other healthcare resources. In addition, midwives have often provided first-line care for women and sometimes larger populations. As has always been true, the needs of the community and skills of the midwives help define midwifery scope of practice. Today midwifery is practiced in a healthcare system in which the only provider whom many women see is their "women's health" provider. While midwives still care for pregnant women, they are also obliged to correctly identify common conditions, minor and major, and facilitate treatment of conditions by themselves or through other strategies such as referral.

Midwives should describe abnormal or unusual symptoms or signs accurately, even when they cannot make a diagnosis with any certainty. They also must assess and triage women with these conditions, determining which can be managed autonomously by the midwife and which cannot. All midwives need to know to whom they will refer cases beyond their personal or professional scopes of practice. Referral can be to nurse practitioners or physician assistants, as well as to physicians, dieticians, social workers, and others. Creation of a large network of healthcare contacts serves both midwives and women well.

The astute reader may have noticed the frequency with which reference has been made to lifestyle changes that can help to prevent or treat diseases. One of the assets midwives bring to primary care for women is an understanding of the importance of health maintenance and disease prevention. Every midwife has the ability and responsibility to provide this aspect of primary care with all women.

Finally, the importance of combining an evidence-based approach with a holistic awareness of the various factors playing into the woman's life is increasingly recognized as positively influencing an individual's ability to adhere to treatment recommendations, whether these recommendations focus on lifestyle changes, medication, or other therapeutic interventions. Effective health care requires awareness and assessment of how poverty, insurance coverage, literacy, mental health, and other factors affect a woman's ability to achieve the goals she has set with the midwife from whom she obtains care.

• • • References

1. American College of Nurse-Midwives. *Position Statement: Midwives Are Primary Care Providers and Leaders of Maternity Care Homes.* June 2012.

2. Donaldson MS, Yordy K D, Lohr KN, Vanselow NA, eds. *Primary Care: America's Health in a New Era.* Washington DC: National Academy Press; 1996.

3. Centers for Disease Control and Prevention. Recommendations to prevent and control iron deficiency in the United States. *MMWR Recomm Rep.* 1998; 47(RR-3):1-29.

4. Beutler E, Waalen J. The definition of anemia: what is the lower limit of normal of the blood hemoglobin concentration? *Blood.* 2006;107(5):1747-1750.

5. Liu K, Kaffes AJ. Iron deficiency anemia: a review of diagnosis, investigation and management. *Euro J Gastroenterol Hepatol.* 2012;24:109-116.

6. Centers for Disease Control and Prevention. Reference criteria for anemia screening. *MMWR.* 1989;38: 400-404.

7. Institute of Medicine. Dietary Reference Intakes: tables and application. Available at: http://www.iom .edu/Activities/Nutrition/SummaryDRIs/~/media /Files/Activity%20Files/Nutrition/DRIs/New%20 Material/2_%20RDA%20and%20AI%20Values_ Vitamin%20and%20Elements.pdf. Accessed January 19, 2013.

8. Ervin RB, Wang CY, Wright JD, Kennedy-Stephenson J. Dietary intake of ten key nutrients for public health, United States: 1999-2000. Data from *Vital and Health Statistics,* no. 341. Hyattsville, Maryland: National Center for Health Statistics; 2004.

9. Scientific Advisory Committee on Nutrition. *Iron and Health.* London: TSO; 2010.

10. Rund D, Rachmielewitz E. β-Thalassemia. *N Engl J Med.* 2005;353:1135-1146.

11. Muncie HL, Campbell JS. Alpha and beta thalassemia. *Am Fam Physician.* 2009;80(4):339-344.

12. Olivieri NF. The β-thalassemias. *N Engl J Med.* 1999; 341:99-109.

13. Centers for Disease Control and Prevention. Sickle cell disease data and statistics. Available at: http://www .cdc.gov/NCBDDD/sicklecell/data.html. Accessed January 19, 2013.

14. Wang Y, Kennedy J, Caggana M, et al. Sickle cell disease incidence among newborns in New York State by maternal race/ethnicity and nativity. *Genet Med.* 2013;15(3):222-228.

15. National Heart, Lung, and Blood Institute. *The Diagnosis, Evaluation and Management of von Willebrand Disease.* NIH Publication No. 08-5832. Bethesda, MD: National Institutes of Health, December 2007.

16. Dilley A, Drews C, Miller C, et al. Von Willebrand disease and other inherited bleeding disorders in women with diagnosed menorrhagia. *Obstet Gynecol.* 2001;97:630-636.

17. Heron M. Deaths: leading causes for 2008. *National Vital Statistics Reports,* vol. 60, no. 6. Hyattsville, MD: National Center for Health Statistics; 2012.

18. Chobanian AV, Bakris GL, Black HR, et al. The seventh report of the Joint National Committee on Prevention, Detection, Evaluation, and Treatment of High Blood Pressure: the JNC 7 report. *JAMA.* 2003;289:2560-2572.

19. Centers for Disease Control and Prevention. Vital signs: awareness and treatment of uncontrolled hypertension among adults—United States, 2003-2010. *MMWR.* 2012;61(35);703-709.

20. Yoon SS, Burt V, Louis T, Carroll MD. Hypertension among adults in the United States, 2009-2010. *NCHS Data Brief,* no 107. Hyattsville, MD: National Center for Health Statistics; 2012.

21. Vasan RS, Beiser A, Seshadri S, et al. Residual lifetime risk for developing hypertension in middle-aged women and men: the Framingham Heart Study. *JAMA.* 2002;287:1003-1010.

22. National High Blood Pressure Education Program. *The Seventh Report of the Joint National Committee on Prevention, Detection, Evaluation, and Treatment of High Blood Pressure: Complete Report.* Bethesda, MD: National Heart, Lung, and Blood Institute; August 2004.

23. Appel LJ, Champagne CM, Harsha DW, et al. Effects of comprehensive lifestyle modification on blood pressure control: Main results of the PREMIER clinical trial. Writing Group of the PREMIER Collaborative Research Group. *JAMA.* 2003;289:2083-2093.

24. Wright JM, Musini VM. First-line drugs for hypertension. *Cochrane Database Syst Rev.* 2009;3:CD001841. doi: 10.1002/14651858.CD001841.pub2.

25. Law MR, Morris JK, Wald NJ. Use of blood pressure lowering drugs in the prevention of cardiovascular disease: meta-analysis of 147 randomised trials in the context of expectations from prospective epidemiological studies. *BMJ.* 2009;338:b1665.

26. National Cholesterol Education Program. *Third Report of the National Cholesterol Education Program (NCEP) on Detection, Evaluation, and Treatment of High Blood Cholesterol in Adults (Adult Treatment Panel III Final Report).* Bethesda, MD: National Heart, Lung, and Blood Institute; May 2001.

27. Grundy SM, Cleeman JI, Mertz CNB, et al. Implications of recent clinical trials for the National Cholesterol Education Program Adult Treatment Panel III guidelines. *Circulation.* 2004;110:227-239.

28. Robbins CL, Dietz PM, Bombard J, Tregear M, Schmidt SM, Tregear SJ. Lifestyle interventions for hypertension and dyslipidemia among women of reproductive age. *Prev Chronic Dis.* 2011;8(6):A123. Available at: http://www.cdc.gov/pcd/issues/2011/nov/11_0029.htm. Accessed January 20, 2013.

29. Kuklina EV, Yoon PW, Keenan NL. Prevalence of coronary heart disease risk factors and screening for high cholesterol levels among young adults, United States, 1999-2006. *Ann Fam Med.* 2010;8(4):327-333.

30. Mitchell AR, King TL. Cardiovascular conditions. In King TL, Brucker MC, eds. *Pharmacology for Women's Health.* Sudbury, MA: Jones and Bartlett Publishers; 2011:411.

31. Grijalva CG, Nuorti JP, Grigffin MR. Antibiotic prescription rates for acute respiratory tract infections in US ambulatory settings. *JAMA.* 2009;302(7):758-766.

32. Klugman KP, Lonks JR. Hidden epidemic of macrolide-resistant pneumococci. *Emerg Infect Dis.* 2005;11(6):802-807.

33. Chow AW, Benninger MS, Brook I, Brozek JL, Goldstein EJC, Hicks LA. IDSA clinical practice guideline for acute bacterial rhinosinusitis in children and adults. *Clin Infect Dis.* 2012;54 (8):1041-1045.

34. Graves BW. Respiratory conditions and cardiovascular conditions. In King TL, Brucker MC, eds. *Pharmacology for Women's Health.* Sudbury, MA: Jones and Bartlett Publishers; 2011:560.

35. Hayward G, Thompson MJ, Perera R, Del Mar CB, Glasziou PP, Heneghan CJ. Corticosteroids for the common cold. *Cochrane Database Syst Rev.* 2012;8:CD008116. doi: 10.1002/14651858.CD008116.pub2.

36. Gwaltney JM Jr, Wiesinger BA, Patrie JT. Acute community-acquired bacterial sinusitis: the value of antimicrobial treatment and the natural history. *Clin Infect Dis.* 2004;38:227-233.

37. Gill JM, Fleischut P, Haas S, Pellini B, Crawford A, Nash DB. Use of antibiotics for adult upper respiratory infections in outpatient settings: a national ambulatory network study. *Fam Med.* 2006;38:349-354.

38. Young J, De Sutter A, Merenstein D, et al. Antibiotics for adults with clinically diagnosed acute rhinosinusitis: a meta-analysis of individual patient data. *Lancet.* 2008;371:908-914.

39. Centers for Disease Control and Prevention. Seasonal influenza (flu): additional information about vaccination of specific populations. Available at: http://www.cdc.gov/flu/professionals/acip/specificpopulations.htm#personsat. Accessed January 20, 2013.

40. Fiore AE, Fry A, Shay D, Gubareva L, Bresee JS, Uyeki TM. Antiviral Agents for the treatment and chemoprophylaxis of influenza: recommendations of the Advisory Committee on Immunization Practices (ACIP). *Recommend Rep.* 2011;60(RR01):1-24.

41. Shulman ST, Bisno AL, Clegg HW, et al. Clinical practice guideline for the diagnosis and management of group A streptococcal pharyngitis: 2012 update by the Infectious Disease Society of America. *Clin Infect Dis.* 2012;55(10):e86-e102.

42. Braman SS. Chronic cough due to acute bronchitis: ACCP evidence-based clinical practice guidelines. *Chest.* 2006;129(1 suppl):95S-103S.

43. Smith SM, Fahey T, Smucny J, Becker LA. Antibiotics for acute bronchitis. *Cochrane Database Syst Rev.* 2004;4:CD000245. doi: 10.1002/14651858.CD000245.pub2.

44. Afshari A, Pagani L, Harbarth S. Year in review 2011: critical care—infection. *Crit Care.* 2012;16(6):242.

45. Mandell LA, Wunderink RG, Anzueto A, et al. Infectious Diseases Society of America/American Thoracic Society consensus guidelines on the management of community-acquired pneumonia in adults. *Clin Infect Dis.* 2007;44(suppl 2):S27-S72.

46. Almirall J, Bolibar I, Serra-Prat M, et al. New evidence of risk factors for community-based pneumonia: a population based study. *Euro Respir J.* 2008;31(6):1274-1284.

47. Bartlett JG. Diagnostic tests for agents of community-acquired pneumonia. *Clin Infect Dis.* 2011;52(suppl4):S296-S304.

48. Centers for Disease Control and Prevention. Pertussis (whooping cough) disease specifics. Available at: http://www.cdc.gov/pertussis/clinical/disease-specifics.html. Accessed January 20, 2013.

49. Centers for Disease Control and Prevention. *The Pink Book: Epidemiology and Prevention of Vaccine-Preventable Diseases.* 12th ed. Atlanta, GA: Centers for Disease Control and Prevention; May 2012. Available at: http://www.cdc.gov/vaccines/pubs/pinkbook/index.html. Accessed April 10, 2013.

50. Tiwari T, Murphy TV, Moran J. Recommended antimicrobial agents of the treatment and post-exposure

prophylaxis of pertussis: 2005 CDC guidelines. *MMWR Recomm Rep.* 2005;54(RR14):1-16.

51. National Asthma Education and Prevention Program. *Expert Panel Report: Guidelines for the Diagnosis and Management of Asthma (EPR-3).* Bethesda, MD: National Heart, Lung, and Blood Institute; 2007.

52. Akinbami LJ, Moorman JE, Bailey C, et al. *Trends in Asthma Prevalence, Health Care Use, and Mortality in the United States, 2001-2010.* Data Brief No. 94. Hyattsville, MD: National Center for Health Statistics, U.S. Department of Health and Human Services; May 2012.

53. Centers for Disease Control and Prevention. *Reported Tuberculosis in the United States, 2011.* Atlanta, GA: CDC; October 2012.

54. Bennett DE, Courval JM, Onorato I, et al. Prevalence of tuberculosis infection in the United States population: The National Health and Nutrition Examination Survey, 1999-2000. *Am J Respir Crit Care Med.* 2008; 177(3):348-355.

55. Rieder HL, Cauthen GM, Comstock GW, Snider DE. Epidemiology of tuberculosis in the United States. *Epidemiol Rev.* 1989;11:79-98.

56. Centers for Disease Control and Prevention. *Core Curriculum on Tuberculosis: What the Clinician Should Know.* 5th ed. Atlanta, GA: CDC; 2011.

57. Blumberg HM, Leonard MK Jr, Jasmer RM. Update on treatment of tuberculosis and latent tuberculosis infection. *JAMA.* 2005; 293:2776.

58. Peery AF, Dellon ES, Lund J, Crockett SD, McGowan CE, Bulsiewicz WJ. Burden of gastrointestinal disease in the United States: 2012 update. *Gastroenterology.* 2012;143(5):1179-1187, e3.

59. Chey WD, Wong BCY, Practice Parameters Committee of the American College of Gastroenterology. American College of Gastroenterology guideline on the management of *Helicobacter pylori* infection. *Am J Gastroenterol.* 2007;102;1808-1825.

60. Oelschlager BK, Ma KC, Soares RV, Montenovo MI, Munoz Oca JE, Pellegrini CA. A broad assessment of clinical outcomes after laparoscopic antireflux surgery. *Ann Surg.* 2012;256:87-94.

61. National Center for Health Statistics. *Summary Health Statistics for US Adults: National Health Interview Survey 2010.* Series 10, no. 252. Hyattsville, MD: U.S. Department of Health and Human Services. January 2012.

62. Ford AC, Delaney B, Forman D, Moayyedi P. Eradication therapy for peptic ulcer disease in Helicobacter pylori positive patients. Cochrane Database Syst Rev. 2006;2:CD003840. doi: 10.1002/14651858. CD003840.pub4.

63. Wilhelm SM, Johnson JL, Kale-Pradhan PB. Treating bugs with bugs: the role of probiotics as adjunctive therapy for *Helicobacter pylori. Ann Pharmacother.* 2011;45(7-8):960-966.

64. Gurusamy KS, Samraj K. Early versus delayed laparoscopic cholecystectomy for acute cholecystitis. *Cochrane Database Syst Rev.* 2006;4:CD005440.

65. Sheffield KM, Ramos KE, Djukom CD, et al. Implementation of a critical pathway for complicated gallstone disease: translation of population-based data into clinical practice. *J Am Coll Surg.* 2011;21(5): 835-843.

66. Buckius MT, McGrath B, Monk J, Grim R, Bell T, Ahuja V. Changing epidemiology of acute appendicitis in the United States: study period 1993-2008. *J Surg Res.* 2012;175(2):185-190.

67. Grover CA, Sternbach G. Charles McBurney: McBurney's point. *J Emerg Med.* May;42(5):578-581.

68. Wilms IMHA, de Hoog DENM, de Visser DC, Janzing HMJ. Appendectomy versus antibiotic treatment for acute appendicitis. *Cochrane Database Syst Rev.* 2011;11:CD008359. doi: 10.1002/14651858. CD008359.pub2.

69. Scallan E, Hoekstra RM, Angulo FJ, et al. Foodborne illness acquired in the United States—major pathogens. *Emerg Infect Dis.* 2011;17(1);7-16.

70. Centers for Disease Control and Prevention. Travelers diarrhea. Available at: http://www.cdc.gov/ncidod /dbmd/diseaseinfo/travelersdiarrhea_g.htm. Accessed January 20, 2013.

71. Freedman DO, Weld LH, Kozarsky PE, et al. Spectrum of disease and relation to place of exposure among ill returned travelers. *New Engl J Med.* 2006;354(2): 119-130.

72. Higgins DR, Johanson JF. Epidemiology of constipation in North America: a systematic review. *Am J Gastroenterol.* 2004;99:750-759.

73. Longstreth GF, Thompson WG, Chey WD, Houghton LA, Mearin F, Spiller RC. Functional bowel disorders. *Gastroenterology.* 2006;130:1480-1491.

74. American College of Gastroenterology, Functional Gastrointestinal Disorders Task Force. Evidence-based position statement on the management of irritable bowel syndrome in North America. *Am J Gastroenterol.* 2002;97(11 suppl):S1-S5.

75. Tack J, Fried M, Houghton LA, Spicak J, Fisher G. Systematic review: the efficacy of treatments for irritable bowel syndrome—a European perspective. *Aliment Pharmacol Ther.* 2006;24:183-205.

76. Centers for Disease Control and Prevention. Surveillance for viral hepatitis—United States, 2010. Available at: http://www.cdc.gov/hepatitis/Statistics /2010Surveillance/PDFs/2010HepSurveillanceRpt.pdf. Accessed January 19, 2013.

77. Centers for Disease Control and Prevention. Hepatitis A information for health professionals. Available at: http://www.cdc.gov/hepatitis/HAV/index.htm. Accessed January 19, 2013.

78. Fiore AE. Hepatitis A transmitted by food. *Clin Infect Dis.* 2004;38:705-715.

79. Klevens RM, Miller JT, Iqbal K, et al. The evolving epidemiology of hepatitis A in the United States: incidence and molecular epidemiology from population-based surveillance, 2005-2007. *Arch Intern Med.* 2010;170(20):1811-1818.

80. Centers for Disease Control and Prevention. Hepatitis A. In: *The Pink Book: Epidemiology and Prevention of Vaccine-Preventable Diseases.* 12th ed. May 2012. Available at: http://www.cdc.gov/vaccines/pubs/pinkbook/downloads/hepa.pdf. Accessed January 19, 2013.

81. Fiore AE, Wasley A, Bell BP. Prevention of hepatitis A through active or passive immunization: recommendations of the Advisory Committee on Immunization Practices (ACIP). *MMWR.* 2006;55(RR07):1-23.

82. Williams IT, Bell BP, Kuhnert W, Alter MJ. Incidence and transmission patterns of acute hepatitis C in the United States, 1982-2006. *Arch Intern Med.* 2011;171(3):242-248.

83. Ghany MG, Strader DB, Thomas DL, Seeff LB. Diagnosis, management, and treatment of hepatitis C: an update. *Hepatology.* 2009;49(4):1335-1374.

84. Ronald A. The etiology of urinary tract infection: traditional and emerging pathogens. *Am J Med.* 2002; 113(suppl 1A):145-195.

85. Griebling TS. Urinary tract infection in women. In: Litwin MS, Saigal CS, eds. *Urologic Diseases in America.* NIH Publication No. 07-5512. U.S. Department of Health and Human Services, Public Health Service, National Institutes of Health, National Institute of Diabetes and Digestive and Kidney Diseases. Washington, DC: U.S. Government Printing Office; 2007:587-620.

86. Gopal M, Northington G, Arya L. Clinical symptoms predictive of recurrent urinary tract infections. *Am J Obstet Gynecol.* 2007;197;74.e1-74.e4.

87. Perrotta C, Aznar M, Mejia R, Albert X, Ng CW. Oestrogens for preventing recurrent urinary tract infection in postmenopausal women. *Cochrane Database Syst Rev.* 2008;2:CD005131. doi: 10.1002/14651858.CD005131.pub2.

88. Gupta K, Hooton TM, Naber KG, Wullt B, Colgan R, Miller LG. International clinical practice guidelines for the treatment of acute uncomplicated cystitis and pyelonephritis in women: a 2010 update by the Infectious Diseases Society of America and the European Society for Microbiology and Infectious Diseases. *Clin Infect Dis.* 2011;52(5):e103-e120.

89. Jepson RG, Williams G, Craig JC. Cranberries for preventing urinary tract infections. *Cochrane Database Syst Rev.* 2012;10:CD001321. doi: 10.1002/14651858.CD001321.pub5.

90. Keay SK, Warren JW. Is interstitial cystitis an infectious disease? *Int J Antimicrob Agents.* 2002;19(6): 480-483.

91. Berry SH, Elliott MN, Suttorp M, et al. Prevalence of symptoms of bladder pain syndrome/interstitial cystitis among adult females in the United States. *J Urol.* 2011;186:540-544.

92. Nicolle LE. Uncomplicated urinary tract infection in adults including uncomplicated pyelonephritis. *Urol Clin North Am.* 2008;35(1):1-12.

93. Hall PM. Nephrolithiasis: treatment, causes, and prevention. *Cleveland Clin J Med.* 2009;76(10):583-591.

94. Hollingsworth JM, Rogers MAM, Kaufman SR, et al. Medical therapy to facilitate urinary stone passage: a meta-analysis. *Lancet.* 2006;368(9542): 1171-1179.

95. Samplaski MK, Irwin BH, Desai M. Less-invasive ways to remove stones from the kidneys and ureters. *Cleveland Clin J Med.* 2009;76(10):592-598.

96. Grundy SM, Cleeman JI, Daniels SR, et al. Diagnosis and management of the metabolic syndrome: an American Heart Association/National Heart, Lung and Blood Institute scientific statement. *Circulation.* 2005;112(17):2735-2752.

97. Ervin RB. Prevalence of metabolic syndrome among adults 20 years of age and over, by sex, age, race and ethnicity, and body mass index: United States, 2003-2006. *Natl Health Stat Report.* 2009;5(13):1-7

98. American Diabetes Association. Standards of medical care in diabetes—2013. *Diab Care.* 2013;36(suppl 1):S11-S66.

99. Centers for Disease Control and Prevention. *National Diabetes Fact Sheet: National Estimates and General Information on Diabetes and Prediabetes in the United States, 2011.* Atlanta, GA: U.S. Department of Health and Human Services, Centers for Disease Control and Prevention; 2011. Available at: http://www.cdc.gov/diabetes/pubs/factsheet11.htm#contents. Accessed January 19, 2013.

100. Reis JP, Loria CM, Sorlie PD, Park Y, Hollenbeck A, Schatzkin A. Lifestyle factors and risk for new-onset diabetes in a large population-based prospective cohort study. *Ann Intern Med.* 2011;155(5):292-299.

101. Fung TT, Schulze M, Manson JE, Willett WC, Hu FB. Dietary patterns, meat intake, and the risk of type 2 diabetes in women. *Arch Intern Med.* 2004; 164(20):2235-2240.

102. Aoli Y, Belin RM, Clickner R, Jeffries R, Phillips L, Mahaffey KR. Serum TSH and Total T4 in the United States population and their association with participant characteristics: National Health and Nutrition Examination Survey (NHANES 1999-2002). *Thyroid.* 2007;17(12):1211-1223.

103. Helfand M. Screening for subclinical thyroid dysfunction in nonpregnant adults: a summary of the evidence for the U.S. Preventive Services Task Force. *Ann Intern Med.* 2004;140(2):128-141.

104. Surks MI, Ortiz E, Daniels GH, et al. Subclinical thyroid disease: scientific review and guidelines for diagnosis and management. *JAMA.* 2004; 291(2): 228-238.

105. Weeks, WD. Menorrhagia and hypothyroidism. *BMJ.* 2000;320(7235):649.

106. Maizels M, Houle T. Results of screening with the brief headache screen compared with a modified ID-Migraine. *Headache J Head Face Pain.* 2008;48: 385-394.

107. International Headache Society. HIS Classification ICHD-II. Available at: http://ihs-classification.org /en/02_klassifikation/02_teil1/01.01.00_migraine .html. Accessed January 18, 2013.

108. Headache Classification Subcommittee of the International Headache Society. The international classification of headache disorders. 2nd edition. *Cephalalgia.* 2004;24(suppl 1):9.

109. Holroyd KA, Stensland M, Lipchik GL, et al. Psychosocial correlates and impact of chronic tension-type headaches. *Headache.* 2000;40:3-16.

110. Derry CJ, Derry S, Moore RA. Caffeine as an analgesic adjuvant for acute pain in adults. *Cochrane Database Syst Rev.* 2012;3:CD009281.

111. Diener HC, Pfaffenrath V, Pageler L, et al. The fixed combination of acetylsalicylic acid, paracetamol and caffeine is more effective than single substances and dual combination for the treatment of headache: a multicentre, randomized, double-blind, single-dose, placebo-controlled parallel group study. *Cephalalgia.* 2005;25(10):776-787.

112. Verhagena AP, Damena L, Bergera MY, Passchierb J, Koesa BW. Lack of benefit for prophylactic drugs of tension-type headache in adults: a systematic review. *Fam Pract.* 2010;27(2):151-165.

113. Fumal A, Schoenen J. Tension-type headache: current research and clinical management. *Lancet Neurol.* 2008;7(1):70-83.

114. Tepper SJ, Dahlöf CGH, Dowson A, et al. Prevalence and diagnosis of migraine in patients consulting their physician with a complaint of headache: data from the landmark study. *Headache J Head Face Pain.* 2004;44:856-864.

115. Stewart WF, Wood C, Reed ML, Roy J, Lipton RB. Cumulative lifetime migraine incidence in women and men. *Cephalalgia.* 20008;28(11):1170-1178.

116. Lipton RB, Bigal ME, Diamond M, Freitag F, Reed ML, Stewart WF. Migraine prevalence, disease burden, and the need for preventive therapy. *Neurology.* 2007;68:343-349.

117. Kelman L. The premonitory symptoms (prodrome): a tertiary care study of 893 migraineurs. *Headache.* 2004;44(9):865-872.

118. Bigal ME, Lipton RB. Clinical course in migraine: conceptualizing migraine transformation. *Neurology.* 2008;71(11):848-855.

119. MacGregor EA. Review: menstrual migraine: therapeutic approaches. *Ther Adv Neurol Dis.* 2009;2(5): 327-336.

120. Fisher RS, van Emde Boas W, Blume W, et al. Epileptic seizures and epilepsy: definitions proposed by the International League Against Epilepsy (ILAE) and the International Bureau for Epilepsy (IBE). *Epilepsia.* 2005;46(4):470-472.

121. Crawford PM. Managing epilepsy in women of childbearing age. *Drug Safety.* 2009;32(4):293-307.

122. Herzog A. Menstrual disorders in women with epilepsy. *Neurology.* 2006;66(suppl 3):S23-S28.

123. Vestergaard P. Epilepsy, osteoporosis and fracture risk: a meta-analysis. *Acta Neurol Scand.* 2005; 112(5):277.

124. Pack AM, Olarte LS, Morrell MJ, Flaster E, Resor SR, Shane E. Bone mineral density in an outpatient population receiving enzyme-inducing antiepileptic drugs. *Epilepsy Behav.* 2003;4(2):169.

125. Gaffield ME, Culwell KR, Lee CR. The use of hormonal contraception among women taking anticonvulsant therapy. *Contraception.* 2011;83(1):16-29.

126. Yuen AW, Thompson PJ, Flugel D, Bell GS, Sander JW. Mortality and morbidity rates are increased in people with epilepsy: is stress part of the equation? *Epilepsy Behav.* 2007;10(1):1-7. Epub October 27, 2006.

127. Becker J, Norab DB, Gomesa I, et al. An evaluation of gender, obesity, age and diabetes mellitus as risk factors for carpal tunnel syndrome. *Clin Neurophysiol.* 2002;113:1429-1434.

128. Page MJ, Massy-Westropp N, O'Connor D, Pitt V. Splinting for carpal tunnel syndrome. *Cochrane Database Syst Rev.* 2012;7:CD010003.

129. Page MJ, O'Connor D, Pitt V, Massy-Westropp N. Exercise and mobilisation interventions for carpal tunnel syndrome. *Cochrane Database Syst Rev.* 2012;6:CD009899.

130. Waterman BR, Owens BD, Davey S, Zacchilli MA, Belmont PJ Jr. The epidemiology of ankle sprains in the United States. *J Bone Joint Surg Am.* 2010;92(13):2279-2284.

131. Chan KW, Ding BC, Mrozeck KJ. Acute and chronic lateral ankle instability in the athlete. *Bull NYU Hospital for Joint Diseases.* 2011;69(1):17-26.

132. Stiell IG, Greenberg GH, McKnight RD, et al. Decision rules for the use of radiography in acute ankle injuries: refinement and prospective validation. *JAMA.* 1993;269(9):1127-1132.

133. Tiemstra JD. Update on acute ankle sprains. *Am Fam Physician.* 2012;85(12):1170-1176.

134. Smith C, Kruger MJ, Smith RM, Myburgh KH. The inflammatory response to skeletal muscle injury: illuminating complexities. *Sports Med.* 2008; 38(11):947-969.

135. Schoenfeld BJ. The use of nonsteroidal anti-inflammatory drugs for exercise-induced muscle damage implications for skeletal muscle development. *Sports Med.* 2012;42(12):1017-1028.

136. Goertz M, Thorson D, Bonsell J, et al. Institute for Clinical Systems Improvement. Adult acute and

subacute low back pain. Updated November 2012. Available at: https://www.icsi.org/_asset/gwss7d /LBP-Interactive1112b.pdf. Accessed January 20, 2013.

137. Stanton TR, Henschke N, Maher CG, Refshauge KM, Latimer J, McAuley JH. After an episode of acute low back pain, recurrence is unpredictable and not as common as previously thought. *Spine*. 2008; 33(26):2923-2928.

138. Casazza BA. Diagnosis and treatment of acute low back pain. *Am Fam Physician*. 2012;85(4):343-350.

139. Chou R, Qaseem A, Snow V, et al. Diagnosis and treatment of low back pain: a joint clinical practice guideline from the American College of Physicians and the American Pain Society. *Ann Intern Med*. 2007;147:478-491.

140. Chou R, Huffman LH. Medications for acute and chronic low back pain: a review of the evidence for an American Pain Society/American College of Physicians clinical practice guideline. *Ann Intern Med*. 2007;147:505-514.

141. Cifuentes M, Webster B, Genevay S, Pransky G. The course of opioid prescribing for a new episode of disabling low back pain: opioid features and dose escalation. *Pain*. 2010;151(1):22-29.

142. Kriebs J. Dermatology. In: King TL, Brucker MC, eds. *Pharmacology for Women's Health*. Sudbury, MA: Jones and Bartlett Publishers; 2011:794.

143. Hanifin JM, Reed ML, Eczema Prevalence and Impact Working Group. A population-based survey of eczema prevalence in the United States. *Dermatitis*. 2007;18(2):82-91.

144. Shaw TE, Currie GP, Koudelka CW, Simpson EL. Eczema prevalence in the United States: data from the 2003 National Survey of Children's Health. *J Invest Dermatol*. 2011;131(1):67-73.

145. Wollenberg A, Schnapp C. Evolution of conventional therapy in atopic dermatitis. *Immunol Allergy Clin North Am*. 2010;30(3):351-368.

146. Menter A, Gottlieb A, Feldman SR, et al. Guidelines for the management of psoriasis and psoriatic arthritis. Section 1. Overview of psoriasis and guidelines of care for the treatment of psoriasis with biologics. *J Am Acad Dermatol*. 2008;5:826-850.

147. Menter A, Korman NJ, Elmets CA, et al. American Academy of Dermatology guidelines of care for the management of psoriasis and psoriatic arthritis. Section 3. Guidelines of care for the management and treatment of psoriasis with topical therapies. *J Am Acad Dermatol*. 2009;60:643-659.

148. Rogers HW, Weinstock MA, Harris AR, et al. Incidence estimate of nonmelanoma skin cancer in the United States, 2006. *Arch Dermatol*. 2010; 146(3):283-287.

149. Rosen T, Lebwohl MG. Prevalence and awareness of actinic keratosis: barriers and opportunities. *J Am Acad Dermatol*. 2013;68:S2-S9.

150. Quaedvlieg PJ, Tirsi E, Thissen MR, Krekels GA. Actinic keratosis: how to differentiate the good from the bad ones? *Eur J Dermatol*. 2006;16(4):335-339.

151. Ceilley RI, Jorrizo JL. Current issues in the management of actinic keratosis. *J Am Acad Dermatol*. 2013;68:S28-S38.

152. Little EG, Eide MJ. Update on the current state of melanoma incidence. *Dermatol Clin*. 2012;30(3): 355-361.

153. Boniol M, Autier P, Boyle P, Gandini S. Cutaneous melanoma attributable to sunbed use: systematic review and meta-analysis. *BMJ*. 2012;345:e4757.

154. Thomas SL, Hall AJ. What does epidemiology tell us about risk factors for herpes zoster? *Lancet Infect Dis*. 2004;4(1):26-33.

155. Tseng HF, Smith N, Harpaz R, et al. Herpes zoster vaccine in older adults and the risk of subsequent herpes zoster disease. *JAMA*. 2011;305(2):160-166.

156. Xu F, Sternberg MR, Kottiri BJ, et al. Trends in herpes simplex virus type 1 and type 2 seroprevalence in the United States. *JAMA*. 2006;296(8):964-973.

157. Fatahzadeh M, Schwartz RA. Human herpes simplex virus infections: epidemiology, pathogenesis, symptomatology, diagnosis, and management. *J Am Acad Dermatol*. 2007;57:737-763.

158. Kolokotronis A, Doumas S. Herpes simplex virus infection, with particular reference to the progression and complications of primary herpetic gingivostomatitis. *Clin Microbiol Infect*. 2006;12(3):202-211.

159. Usatine RP, Tinitigan R. Nongenital herpes simplex virus. *Am Fam Physician*. 2010;82(9):1075-1082.

160. Cernik C, Gallina K, Brodell RT. The treatment of herpes simplex infections: an evidence-based review. *Arch Intern Med*. 2008;168(11):1137-1144.

161. Dworkin RH, O'Connor AB, Backonja M, et al. Pharmacologic management of neuropathic pain: evidence-based recommendations. *Pain*. 2007;132: 237-251.

162. Stevens DL, Bisno AL, Chambers HF, et al. Practice guidelines for the diagnosis and management of skin and soft-tissue infections. *Clin Infect Dis*. 2005;41(10):1373-1406.

163. Gorwitz RJ, Kruszon-Moran D, McAllister SK, et al. Changes in the prevalence of nasal colonization with *Staphylococcus aureus* in the United States, 2001-2004. *J Infect Dis*. 2008;197(9):1226-1234.

164. Liu C, Bayer A, Cosgrove SE, et al. Management of patients with infections caused by methicillin-resistant *Staphylococcus aureus*: clinical practice guidelines by the Infectious Diseases Society of America (IDSA). *Clin Infect Dis*. 2011;52:1-38.

CHAPTER

9

Mental Health Conditions

BARBARA W. GRAVES

RUTH JOHNSON

Mental health disorders affect millions of individuals and families in the United States. Primary care providers, including midwives, care for many women who are affected by mental health disorders, either as a sole disorder or comorbid with other illnesses. This chapter presents clinicians with an overview of mental health problems that commonly affect women, a framework for identification of common disorders, and screening to identify those who need urgent referral to a mental health provider. The authors also introduce the various treatment modalities used for many of these conditions.

Mental health disorders are the most common and costly cause of disability in the United States. Almost one-third of individuals older than age 19 years who reside in the United States will suffer from anxiety disorders, and between 15% and 20% will experience a major depressive episode.[1] Unfortunately, many persons with mental health disorders do not seek treatment, and of those who do, many are not able to access the mental health system due to widespread shortages of mental health providers. Members of uninsured, underinsured, low-income, and minority populations are the least likely to receive treatment.[1]

Mental health disorders affect more than just the individual with the disorder—they affect entire families. This is especially true when women have such disorders, as they are most often the primary care providers for children. In addition, women are at risk for serious hormonally associated mental health disorders such as premenstrual mood disorder and perinatal and postpartum mood disorders. **Figure 9-1** shows the lifetime prevalence of selected mental health disorders in men and women.[1] A cross-national

survey of 72,933 individuals in Africa, Asia, Europe, the Middle East, and the Americas found that in all cohorts in all countries, women had an odds ratio of 1.9 (95% confidence interval [CI], 1.8–2.0) for experiencing depression and an odds ratio of 1.7 (95% CI, 1.6–1.8) for experiencing an anxiety disorder as compared to men. No significant gender difference was seen for bipolar disorder, and the difference was less for social phobia (1.3; 95% CI, 1.2–1.4) than for other anxiety disorders.[2]

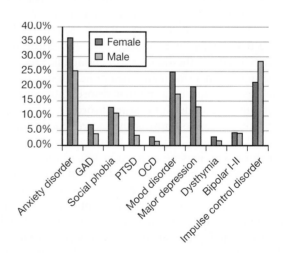

Figure 9-1 Lifetime prevalence of selected *DSM-IV* disorders from the World Mental Health Survey version of the Composite International Diagnostic Interview.

Source: Data from Kessler RC, Berglund P, Demler O, Jin R, Merikangas KR, Walters EE. Lifetime prevalence and age-of-onset distributions of *DSM-IV* disorders in the National Comorbidity Survey Replication. *Arch Gen Psychiatry.* 2005;62:593-602.

The etiology of mental health conditions is complex. The two most frequently encountered categories of mental health disorders in primary care are depression and anxiety, both of which are multifactorial in origin, with genetic, cultural, and environmental factors playing roles in their development. Studies of twins have found that genetic factors are a significant contributor to the development of both major depression and anxiety disorders, although perhaps more for depression than for anxiety. Genetics appears to have a greater influence in women than in men.

Attenuation appears to diminish the influence of genetics as individuals move from childhood to adulthood.[3,4] Environment and experiences are equally important in determining whether an individual will develop depression or anxiety. Culture plays a significant role in the meaning an individual assigns to mental illness and how symptoms are presented. Environmental risk factors include childhood adversity such as poor parental attachment, witnessing or experiencing trauma, and subsequent stressors such as relationship problems and poor social support.[5] Brain imaging studies demonstrate altered connectivity between the limbic system, including the amygdale, and the frontal cortex in individuals with generalized anxiety.[6,7]

The diagnostic standard used for psychiatric disorders is the *Diagnostic and Statistical Manual of Mental Disorders (DSM)*. The most recent revision of this work, *DSM-5*, was published in May 2013.[8] The *DSM* delineates specific diagnostic criteria for each distinct psychiatric diagnosis, and is the reference used for the tables throughout this chapter. The management of many mental health disorders, such as schizophrenia, bipolar disorder, obsessive–compulsive disorder, and eating disorders, is beyond the scope of care of most primary care practitioners; the role of the midwife as a primary care provider for those who may be affected by one of these diagnoses is to perform screening and referral. In contrast, midwives as primary care providers may diagnose, begin treatment for, and perhaps continue treatment for women with depression, including perinatal and postpartum depression, and some anxiety disorders. Although most primary care providers do not have the background or capacity to undertake mental health counseling or therapy, they often can prescribe psychopharmacologic medications, recommend lifestyle changes, and work in concert with psychiatric professionals. Proper education is necessary to prescribe psychotropic medications appropriately and safely.

Given the difficulty that many women have entering the mental health system, it often falls to the midwife in the role of primary care provider to screen for and manage common mental health disorders. Screening for depression has become widespread, but common depression screening tools may miss detection of individuals with other psychiatric disorders.

A recently developed tool, the M-3 Checklist, is a 23-item checklist that screens for depression, anxiety disorders, and bipolar disorder, and asks questions specific to functional impairment secondary to their symptoms. The study population in which this instrument was validated included 723 English-speaking individuals attending a family medicine clinic, 647 of whom completed all aspects of the study. Participants completed the M-3 Checklist while waiting to be seen by their clinician, and answered a brief exit questionnaire about the checklist. It took less than 5 minutes to complete the checklist. A master's-prepared diagnostic interviewer contacted each participant by phone within 30 days of the visit to administer the Mini Neuropsychiatric Interview (MINI). The mean time from the visit to the follow-up phone call was 8.8 days. The checklist was scored in a two-step method, beginning with assessment for functional impairment, which identified 53.9% of the participants who would be eliminated from further scoring because they had no impairment from psychiatric symptoms. This first step eliminated approximately 11% of the participants who actually met the MINI criteria for a psychiatric diagnosis. Of the participants who passed through this initial "gateway," 62.4% received a psychiatric diagnosis. Overall, 36.4% of the participants were diagnosed with one or more psychiatric disorders. Among the participants, 4.2% were identified with depression without anxiety, 12.1% with depression and anxiety, 9.1% with anxiety without depression, and 9.3% with bipolar disorder. The sensitivity, specificity, positive likelihood ratio, and negative likelihood ratios for depression, bipolar disorder, anxiety, and post-traumatic stress disorder were comparable to those obtained with single-disorder screening tools.[9]

The feasibility of using the M-3 Checklist should be included in the ongoing debate about the efficacy and cost-effectiveness of screening the general population for mental health disorders. An alternative would be to employ the Patient Health Questionnaire-2 (PHQ-2) and Generalized Anxiety Disorder-2 (GAD-2) as initial screens for anxiety and depression (both of these instruments are discussed in more detail later in this chapter), and then progress to more detailed tools for those individuals who have positive screening results.

Mood Disorders

Mood disorders include major depressive disorder (MDD), dysthymia (a mild, chronic depression), bipolar disorder, and premenstrual dysphoric disorder (discussed later in this chapter). MDD is the most common mental health diagnosis among adults in the United States, and is four times more prevalent than either dysthymia or bipolar I/II.[1] While dysthymia and bipolar disorders are less prevalent, each of these conditions is associated with significant suffering and financial cost to the individual, families, and society.

Depression

Depression is a widespread medical condition that affects millions of persons in the United States. Women are at an increased risk compared to men, as are ethnic minorities, persons living in poverty, and individuals who lack adequate medical insurance. Additional risk factors are listed in **Box 9-1**. Over a 12-month period, 6.6% of the U.S. population will experience MDD; at any given time, 9% of the population will be affected by a depressive disorder.[10] Approximately 16.6% of the population will have a major depressive disorder during their lifetime.[1]

BOX 9-1 Risk Factors for Major Depression

Divorce or other stressful life events
(job change, financial problems)

Recent death of a loved one or friend

Family members with depression

History of abuse or trauma

Exposure to traumatic event
(e.g., car accident, hurricane)

Intimate partner violence

A serious or chronic medical condition,

Alcohol or drug abuse

Prior episodes of depression.

Many medications may contribute to depression
or cause symptoms of depression

Depression has a major impact on quality of life and the ability to work. It is second only to back and neck pain as the cause of disability days.[11] Depressive disorders are often associated with other comorbid conditions such as chronic disease, and they may lead to decreased quality of life for persons whose medical conditions are aggravated by depression.[12] Depressed individuals may also be afflicted with other psychiatric disorders, including personality disorders, anxiety disorders such as obsessive–compulsive disorder, eating disorders, and substance abuse.[13] Individuals with combined diagnoses, including those exhibiting any psychotic features such as delusions or hallucinations, require specialist mental health services and should be referred appropriately.

Depression is the mental health disorder most frequently diagnosed by primary care providers. Even so, it is common for depression to be undiagnosed or treated suboptimally depending on the demands of the practice and attitudes of the provider. A 2008 systemic review of studies that looked at the diagnosis of depression by nonpsychiatric physicians found that the diagnosis of depression was missed more than half the time. Only 46% to 57% of those with major depression are being treated, with only 18% to 25% receiving adequate treatment.[14]

The diagnostic criteria for major depression and dysthymia are listed in **Box 9-2**. Individuals with mild major depression will present with the minimum of symptoms that meet the diagnostic criteria; those with moderate depression will exhibit more symptoms, but are generally able to carry out their usual activities; and those with major depression will often exhibit difficulty with normal activities.[15] The adverse effect of depression on health is worse in the presence of comorbidities.[16]

Individuals with bipolar disorders, which are defined in **Box 9-3**, may also present with depression. However, the depression associated with bipolar disorder is distinct from the more traditional depression syndromes. It is extremely important to screen for mania or hypomania when screening for depression because treating women who are bipolar with antidepressants can aggravate their condition. While management of women with depression may fall within the scope of primary care, individuals with symptoms of mania or hypomania should be referred to a mental health specialist.

Screening for Depression

A number of screening tools are available to assess for depression, ranging from a two-question instrument to a questionnaire with 21 items. The two-question

BOX 9-2 Common Depressive Disorders

Major Depression
Symptoms (SIGECAPS)

Symptoms must include either depressed mood or anhedonia (lack of interest) PLUS any of the following symptoms (to total five symptoms), which occur nearly every day for at least 2 weeks, and are severe enough to impede function:

1. **S**leep disorder (insomnia or hypersomnia)
2. **I**nterest deficit or a lack of feeling pleasure
3. **G**uilt (worthlessness, hopelessness, regret)
4. **E**nergy deficit (fatigue or loss of energy nearly every day)
5. **C**oncentration deficit
6. **A**ppetite disorder (increased or decreased), unplanned weight loss or gain
7. **P**sychomotor retardation or agitation
8. **S**uicidality (recurrent thoughts of death)

There has never been a manic or hypomanic episode.

Symptoms are not attributable to a medical condition or substance use.

Must be qualified as a single episode or recurrent.

Dysthymia
Symptoms

A. Depressed mood for most of the day, for more days than not, as indicated either by subjective account or observation by others, for at least 2 years.
B. Presence of two or more of the symptoms listed under major depression.
C. There has never been a manic or hypomanic episode.

Sources: Adapted from American Psychiatric Association. *Diagnostic and Statistical Manual of Mental Disorders.* 5th ed. Arlington, VA: APA; 2013; Hackley B, Sharma C, Kedzior A, Sreenivasan S. Managing mental health conditions in primary care settings. *J Midwifery Women's Health.* 2010;55:9-19.

BOX 9-3 Bipolar Disorder

Diagnosis includes major depression AND history of mania (Bipolar I) or hypomania (Bipolar II), leading to a marked impairment in occupational function, social activities, or relationships; may lead to hospitalization or psychotic features. The manic phase must last a minimum of 7 days.

Symptoms of Mania

- Inflated self-esteem or grandiosity
- Decreased need for sleep
- More talkative than usual or pressure to continue talking
- Flight of ideas or feels thoughts are racing, agitation
- High energy, irritability, or pleasure-seeking

Must have three symptoms (or four if only symptom is irritability) during the time of mood disturbance,

Symptoms of Hypomania

- Lasts a minimum of 4 days.
- Briefer duration and less severe symptoms.
- Associated with unequivocal change in functioning that differs from normal function for that individual.
- Is not severe enough to cause marked impairment in social or occupational functioning.
- Not associated with psychosis.

Sources: American Psychiatric Association. *Diagnostic and Statistical Manual of Mental Disorders.* 5th ed. Arlington, VA: APA; 2013; Hackley B, Sharma C, Kedzior A, Sreenivasan S. Managing mental health conditions in primary care settings. *J Midwifery Women's Health.* 2010;55:9-19.

screen, known as the Patient Health Questionnaire-2, is shown in **Table 9-1**; it was developed and validated in New Zealand, and has a sensitivity and specificity of 97% (95% CI, 83%– 99%) and 67% (95% CI, 62%–72%), respectively. The likelihood ratio for a positive test was 2.9 (95% CI, 2.5–3.4) and the likelihood ratio for a negative test was 0.05 (95% CI, 0.01–0.35).[17] Adding a third question as

to whether the individual desired help for his or her depression improved the specificity of the original 2 questions[18], but may decrease the sensitivity, and may result in some women who are depressed not being identified.[19]

The Center for Epidemiologic Studies—Depression Scale (CES-D) with 20 items, the Patient Health Questionnaire-2 (PHQ-2), the Patient Health Questionnaire (PHQ-9), the Beck Depression Inventory (BDI), and the Edinburgh Postnatal Depression Screen (EPDS) screening tools have all been validated, and have sensitivities ranging from 0.8 to 0.9 and specificities ranging from 0.7 to 0.85. All are written at the sixth-grade level and are easy to complete, and several can be completed and scored online. The accuracy levels of these tools appear to

Table 9-1	PHQ-2 Two-Question Screen for Depression				
Over the past month how often have you been bothered by any of the following problems?		Not at All	Several Days	More Than Half the Days	Nearly Every Day
Little interest or pleasure in doing things		0	1	2	3
Feeling down, depressed, or hopeless		0	1	2	3

Source: PHQ-2 Copyright © Pfizer Inc. All rights reserved.

be comparable for identifying individuals with depression.[20] While all have been widely employed for depression screening, each has some benefits and some detractors. In particular, the EPDS has been extensively validated for use in pregnancy and the postnatal time period;[21] it has not been validated for use outside of the perinatal period. The BDI is copyrighted, and requires a fee for each use. Having 20 items, the CES-D is the longest of the commonly used screening tools for depression. The PHQ-9, shown in **Table 9-2**, is available in the public domain, has 9 items, and is commonly used for monitoring response to treatment as well as screening for depression. An algorithm to for use in the differential diagnosis of mood disorders based on the PHQ-9 appears in **Figure 9-2**.[22]

Given the high prevalence of depression, incorporating routine screening into regular visits will help identify women with depression who might otherwise be missed. The U.S. Preventive Services Task Force (USPSTF), however, recommends screening for depression only in settings that have access to systems that provide accurate diagnosis, treatment, and follow-up. This organization found no benefits to screening in settings where these support resources were unavailable.[23] The 2010 guidelines from the United Kingdom's National Institute for Health and Clinical Excellence recommend that clinicians screen individuals who may have depression based on past history or chronic health conditions by employing the PHQ-2. Management for individuals who respond positively to either of the two questions depends on the expertise of the clinician and the resources available in the setting for managing mental health disorders. If either of these is lacking, the clinician should screen for immediate risk of harm to the individual or others; if a risk for harm is not present, the clinician should refer the individual to an appropriate mental health provider.[24]

Depression in women may have a significant effect on her fetus, infant, and family. Thus, while there is debate about the utility of generalized screening for depression, it may be prudent for the midwife

to incorporate the two-question screen, plus the question about whether help is needed, as part of the history of present illness taken during routine prenatal visits.

It is critical that the midwife assess for suicidal ideation in women who have screened positive for depression. Those at highest risk include individuals who have a specific plan or have access to the means to commit suicide, such as guns, prescription medications, or street drugs. Other risk factors for suicide include previous hospitalization or suicide attempt; family history of suicide; sense of hopelessness; experiencing family, romantic, or legal conflicts; social isolation; and insomnia.[24] Multiple screening instruments have been used to identify individuals at risk of suicide. Although no single instrument is considered the best or even most frequently used, they all address the same general concepts identified in **Table 9-3** and they are useful in assessing suicidal tendencies.[13] The midwife has a responsibility to refer any women with such a risk to emergency mental health services.

Depression screening can be conducted quickly using a using a two-step screening process. Each person is asked the two questions of the PHQ-2, which is then followed with the PHQ-9 if needed. This two-step screen provides a balance of sensitivity and specificity.[25] The midwife can then provide primary care or refer the woman to a mental health specialist as indicated and depending upon available resources.

Dysthymia

The term *dysthymia* comes from the Greek word meaning "bad state of mind" or "bad humor." Dysthymia is a chronic from of depression wherein the symptoms are neither as severe nor as numerous as they are in individuals who have major depression. This disorder has been identified in cultures worldwide, although its prevalence appears to be higher in high-income countries than in low- to middle-income countries.[26] Dysthymia can be just as disabling as major depression due to its chronic nature even though the symptoms are less severe.

Table 9-2	Patient Health Questionnaire (PHQ-9)				
Over the last 2 weeks, how often have you been bothered by any of the following problems?: (use "x" to indicate your answer)		**Not at All**	**Several Days**	**More Than Half the Days**	**Nearly Every Day**
1.	Little interest or pleasure in doing things	0	1	2	3
2.	Feeling down, depressed, or hopeless	0	1	2	3
3.	Trouble falling or staying asleep, or sleeping too much	0	1	2	3
4.	Feeling tired or having little energy	0	1	2	3
5.	Poor appetite or overeating	0	1	2	3
6.	Feeling bad about yourself or that you are a failure or have let yourself or your family down	0	1	2	3
7.	Trouble concentrating on things, such as reading the newspaper or watching television	0	1	2	3
8.	Moving or speaking so slowly that other people could have noticed; or the opposite—being so fidgety or restless that you have been moving around a lot more than usual	0	1	2	3
9.	Thoughts that you would be better off dead, or of hurting yourself in some way	0	1	2	3
		Add columns			
		TOTAL ____	____	____	
10.	If you checked off any problems, how difficult have those problems made it for you to do your work, take care of things at home, or get along with other people?	❑ Not difficult at all ❑ Somewhat difficult ❑ Very difficult ❑ Extremely difficult			

Interpretation of Total Score

Total Score	*Depression Severity*
1–4	Minimal depression
5–9	Mild depression
10–14	Moderate depression
15–19	Moderately severe depression
20–27	Severe depression

Consider a depressive disorder if there are at least four "x" marks in the shaded section (including Questions 1 and 2). Add up the score to determine severity.

Consider a major depressive disorder if there are at least five "x" marks in the shaded section (one of which corresponds to Question 1 or 2).

Consider another depressive disorder if there are two to four "x" marks in the shaded section (one of which corresponds to Question 1 or 2).

Question 10 Note: All responses should be verified by the clinician. Diagnoses of major depressive disorder or other depressive disorder also require impairment of social, occupational, or other important areas of functioning (Question #10) and ruling out normal bereavement, a history of a manic episode (bipolar disorder), and a physical disorder, medication, or other drug as the biological cause of the depressive symptoms.

Source: PHQ-9 Copyright © Pfizer Inc. All rights reserved.

Like major depression, dysthymia occurs more commonly in women, and is often underdiagnosed except when complicated by comorbid major depressive episodes.[27] The lifetime community prevalence is between 3% and 6%, although a higher prevalence—between 5% and 15%—has been noted in primary care settings.[28] While the specific depressive symptoms may be less severe, dysthymia may be associated with slower and less complete recovery than major depression.[29,30] It is not uncommon for an individual with dysthymia to experience a major depressive disorder, a phenomenon known as "double depression."[30]

Treatment for Depression

There are many treatment modalities for depression, including cognitive-behavioral therapy, counseling,

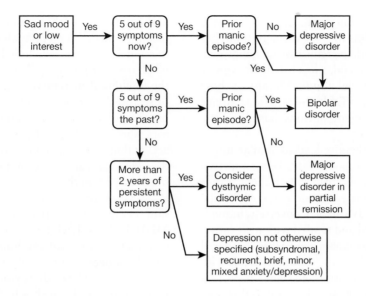

Figure 9-2 Differential diagnoses of mood disorders.

Source: U.S. Department of Health and Human Services. *Depression in Primary Care: Volume 1. Detection and Diagnosis.* AHCPR Publication No. 93-0550. Rockville, MD: Agency for Health Care Policy and Research; 1993:20.

Table 9-3	Questions That Assess for Suicidality (Thoughts, Plans, Behaviors, Intent)[a,b,c]	
Purpose	**Possible Questions**	**Clinical Notes**
1. Suicidal ideation	Have you lost hope? Have you thought that life is not worth living? Have you wished you were dead or wished you could go to sleep and not wake up?	Consider additional questions that assess frequency, intensity, and duration of suicidal ideation
2. Suicidal thoughts	Have you had thoughts about hurting yourself? Have you had thoughts about killing yourself?	Consider additional questions that assess frequency of suicidal thoughts
3. Suicidal thoughts with method	Have you thought about how you might kill yourself?	Consider additional questions that assess frequency of suicidal thoughts about a possible method of suicide
4. Suicidal intent with specific plan	Have you worked out the details of how to kill yourself? Do you intend to act on these thoughts?	Consider additional questions that assess availability of method (e.g., guns in house), or any preparatory acts
6. Suicidal behavior	6a. Have you ever done anything that moved you toward killing yourself? 6b. Have you ever actively tried to kill yourself? If so when? 6c. What has prevented you from acting on this plan?	Consider additional questions that assess: Preparatory acts (e.g., collected pills, wrote a suicide note, obtained a gun) or Rehearsals for suicide (e.g., loading gun) vs. nonsuicidal self-injurious acts
7. Suicidal intent	Do you expect to carry out this plan?	Consider additional questions that assess how much the individual believes the act will be lethal versus self-injurious.

[a]Use a direct communication style that is also empathic but nonjudgmental.

[b]Whenever possible ask open-ended questions and use follow-up questions to encourage elaboration.

[c]Women may require time to answer each of these questions so patient waiting can encourage a response.

faith-based therapy, group work, and psychotropic medications. Regardless of the treatment modality selected, the goal should be remission of symptoms. Education and recommendations for sleep hygiene and exercise are beneficial adjuncts to any of these treatment modalities.[31] **Table 9-4** provides advice on appropriate treatment options based on the PHQ-9 score.

Medication and therapy lead to similar initial improvement,[32] with response rates being approximately 58%. Individuals treated with medications tend to achieve slightly higher rates of remission—46% as opposed to 40%. Conversely, individuals who are depressed and treated with medication alone are more likely to experience relapse compared to those treated with therapy.[32] For individuals with moderate to severe depression who have persistent symptoms or have not responded to initial single-modality treatment, a combination of medication and counseling with a mental health specialist is recommended.[31] A meta-analysis that focused on remission and relapse concluded that the combination of pharmacotherapy and psychotherapy improves the likelihood of remission and decreases the risk of relapse.[33] The decision to initiate treatment with psychotherapy or medication is based on many factors, such as individual preferences, access to and acceptability of counseling, insurance coverage, and the individual's ability to commit to the time involved to participate in therapy.

Several studies have suggested that antidepressant therapy is more effective for dysthymia than for MDD. In 2011, Levkovitz et al. published the results of a meta-analysis of randomized trials that compared antidepressants to placebo in subjects with a diagnosis of MDD or dysthymia. Those with dysthymia who received placebos had lower response rates than those with MDD who received placebo (37.9%

Table 9-4	Translating PHQ-9 Depression Scores into Practice	
PHQ-9 Score	**Likely Diagnosis**	**Primary Care Midwifery Management**[a,b,c]
5–9	Mild or minimal depressive symptoms	If no improvement after 1 or more months with education, behavioral activation, and physical therapy, consider referral to behavioral health for evaluation
10–14	Mild major depression	Screen for suicidal ideation
		Refer to a clinician who can prescribe pharmacotherapy and/or clinician who can perform psychotherapy following discussion with the woman
		Consider weekly contact to ensure continuity of support for an initial period, then at least monthly
15–19	Moderate major depression	Screen for suicidal ideation
		Refer to a clinician who can prescribe pharmacotherapy
		Refer to a clinician who can perform psychotherapy
		Consider weekly contact to ensure continuity of support for an initial period, then at least twice monthly
≥ 20	Severe major depression	Screen for suicidal ideation
		Urgently refer to a clinician who can prescribe pharmacotherapy
		Consider beginning psychopharmacology if appointment with psychiatric provider delayed
		Offer referral to a clinician who can perform psychotherapy
		Plan weekly contact to ensure continuity of support until symptoms are less severe

Every woman who has a score that is higher than 5 should be counseled about the following:

a. Education about depression including possible diagnosis, how to monitor symptoms, treatment options, and warning signs of progression

b. Behavioral activation: Increase daily involvement in pleasant activities and positive interactions with their environment. Examples include: regular visits with a supportive friend, daily meditation, or daily gardening

c. Appropriate physical activity: focus on feasible, easily attainable regular exercise that can be adhered to

versus 29.9%; $P = 0.42$).[34] While interpersonal psychotherapy may be useful,[35,36] it is not believed to be as effective as pharmacotherapy.[37] In the end, the individual will choose among the options for care depending on her own perceptions of her disorder, use of psychotropic medication and therapy, insurance coverage, and her time available for counseling.

Evidence-based guidelines are available to the primary care provider for the management of depression on the Internet. These include the Depression Management Tool Kit,[38] the Institute for Clinical Systems Improvement's Guidelines for Major Depression in Adults and Primary Care,[13] and the IMPACT evidence-based depression care guidelines.[39] All three of these resources incorporate the PHQ-9 as the tool used both to diagnose depression and to track improvement with treatment. They also recommend collaboration with a mental health provider.

The University of Washington's AIMS Center/Advancing Integrated Mental Health Solutions has developed the IMPACT model, which recommends a team approach to follow persons who are diagnosed with depression.[40] Implementation of collaborative care using this model, which involves a case manager (either a specially trained nurse or a social worker) and a psychiatrist, has been found to improve outcomes when compared to usual care.[41,42] The case manager educates the woman about depression, monitors depression symptoms, coaches her in behavioral activation and pleasant-event scheduling, encourages physical activity, and supports the mutually agreed-upon plan of care with close follow-up; in addition, the case manager may provide initial adjustments to medication dosages. The case manager also helps coordinate referrals and reinforces follow-through. The psychiatric consultant regularly reviews the all cases in which patients are not improving as expected and is available for consultation for any specific concerns. Two key processes in this model are the systematic diagnosis and tracking of individual outcomes and stepped care that changes the treatment regimen if the woman is not improving as expected. The goal is to have a 50% reduction in symptoms within 10 to 12 weeks. Inadequate treatment has been a continuing concern,[14] and stepped care for depression—similar to stepped care for asthma management—is a strategy to assess ongoing improvement and adjust the treatment regimen as needed.[12]

Complementary treatments that have been found to be efficacious as adjuncts to psychotherapy or medication include yoga and acupuncture.[13] While some evidence suggests that the herb known as St. John's wort may benefit those persons with mild or moderate depression, it is not regulated for purity or consistent dosing, and it is known to adversely interact with many medications including other antidepressants, HIV protease inhibitors, and oral contraceptives.[43]

Whether or not the midwife practices within a collaborative care model, any clinician who opts to care for individuals with depression has the responsibility to continue to follow the response to complete remission, as adequate treatment decreases the risk of relapse.[44] Tamburrino and Nagel followed 94 participants with diagnoses of dysthymic disorder or major depression, or both, who were taking antidepressant medication prescribed by their primary care providers. They found that approximately 75% of participants did not have any medication adjustments during the 12-week study period despite having scores on the Beck Depression Inventory-II that indicated moderate depression.[44] Repeating the PHQ-9 or other tool that was used for the initial diagnosis is an effective means to assess the individual's ongoing symptoms. Close follow-up is essential, and increases or adjustments to medication are often necessary. If the woman's depression does not improve despite changes in medication, a referral to a mental health provider is indicated.

Most midwives' practices are not structured to provide ongoing psychotherapy for the women for whom they care. Nevertheless, the midwife's responsibility for follow-up continues even after referral to a mental health specialist to ensure that the woman who has depression has not stopped therapy prior to achieving remission. The midwife may also be in unique position to provide targeted time-limited counseling as a result of having developed an ongoing therapeutic relationship with the woman. This relationship provides an opportunity to advise the woman on behaviors that improve depression, such as engaging in a realistic exercise program[13] and engaging in pleasurable activities. Bright light therapy has been shown to be effective in treating depression that has a seasonal component, and has benefits as an adjunct for individuals with nonseasonal depression as well.[13,45]

When discussing psychotherapy, reassure the woman that for most persons with depression, therapy is short term in nature, rather than an endless process. Cognitive-behavioral therapy, problem-solving therapy, short-term psychodynamic therapy, and interpersonal therapy have comparable outcomes.[13] Early studies of Internet-delivered psychotherapy with guidance from a therapist have been promising. Self-guided Internet-delivered psychotherapy has been shown to have fewer, albeit some tangible benefits.[46]

Pharmacotherapy

Due to the many challenges of entering into psychotherapy, many depressed individuals will opt to initiate pharmacologic treatment for depression rather than counseling. Prior to beginning pharmacotherapy for depression, it is critical that the clinician has ruled out bipolar disorder, as treatment with an antidepressant may trigger mania,[13] suicidal ideation, or psychosis.[47] Important signs to screen for to rule out bipolar disorders include a history of taking multiple antidepressants without improvement, a history of suicide attempts, and a history of agitation or irritability while taking antidepressants in the past.[47]

Psychotropic medications affect the three neurotransmitters that modulate mood—that is, dopamine, serotonin, and norepinephrine. **Figure 9-3** illustrates the effects and interactions of these neurotransmitters.[47] Second-generation antidepressants, which include selective serotonin reuptake inhibitors (SSRIs), norepinephrine-dopamine reuptake inhibitors (NDRIs), and serotonin-norepinephrine reuptake inhibitors (SNRIs) are the first-line medications for treating depression.[15,48,49] Some providers may also opt to prescribe bupropion (Wellbutrin, Zyban), an NRDI that has fewer adverse effects on sexual function, but lowers the threshold for seizures. Bupropion should not be used with other medications that also lower the seizure threshold or by individuals with risk factors for seizures. Bupropion typically has no effect on anxiety, though in some cases it may actually aggravate anxiety.[49] Classes of drugs that have been used for depression in the past, and may be prescribed by psychiatric clinicians in specific situations, include monoamine oxidase inhibitors and tricyclics. These medications have a narrow therapeutic range, potential for high toxicity, and serious interactions with many foods and other medications.

The SSRIs are metabolized through the CPY450 enzyme system. As such, they interact with a wide variety of other medications that are metabolized by the same systems. Some of the specific medications that are known to interact with the second-generation antidepressants include older antidepressants such as tricyclic antidepressants, digoxin (Lanoxin), warfarin (Coumadin), anticonvulsants, and theophylline (Theo-Dur).[47] Prior to prescribing any psychotropic medication, the clinician is responsible for reviewing all medications the individual is taking to avoid potentially serious interactions.

Serotonin syndrome is a rare but potentially life-threatening reaction that results from excess serotonergic activity. In 2005, there were 8585 cases of serotonin syndrome reported in the United States with moderate to major, but not life-threatening, effects, and 118 deaths due to serotonin syndrome.[50] The incidence is suspected to be rising due to the more frequent prescribing of serotonergic medications. Serotonin syndrome may potentially occur in response to therapeutic dosing of an SSRI or SNRI, but more often is a complication of either drug–drug interactions or overdose. Combination treatment consisting of more than one SSRI or SRNI, MAO inhibitors, lithium, or concurrent use of St. John's wort may precititate serotonin syndrome. Some other classes of drugs, such as triptans, anticonvulsants, and some opioids, also have serotonergic activity. Many recreational drugs, including amphetamines, cocaine, and ecstasy, can trigger serotonin syndrome as well. Signs and symptoms include agitation, diaphoresis, fever, hyperreflexia, confusion or hypomania, myoclonus, tremor, and diarrhea.[51,52] The clinical manifestations can be highly variable, and referral of persons who are suspected of experiencing serotonin syndrome to the emergency room is indicated.[52]

Research has failed to demonstrate any significant difference in efficacy among the various SSRIs, SNRIs, and NDRIs.[48,49] Individual medications in these classes do, however, have different side-effect profiles, as summarized in **Table 9-5**. The choice of which medication is used to initiate therapy is made based on the individual's preference, past successful treatment with a given medication, and predominant symptoms that accompany the depression. For example, all of the SSRIs may be associated with weight gain, but fluoxetine (Prozac) is more stimulating and

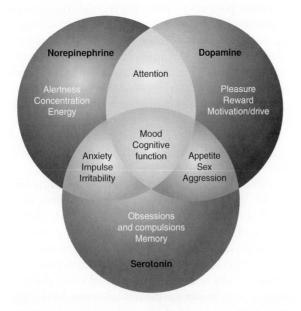

Figure 9-3 Role of dopamine, norepinephrine, and serotonin.
Source: King TL, Brucker MC. *Pharmacology for Women's Health.* Sudbury, MA: Jones and Bartlett; 2011:757.

Table 9-5	Antidepressant Medications for Use by Primary Care Providers			
Generic Agent (Brand Name)	Starting Dose (mg)	Range (mg/day)	Side-Effect Profile	Pharmacokinetic Half-life
SSRIs				
Fluoxetine (Prozac)	10–20	20–80	Maintain at 20 mg/day for 4–6 weeks, then 30 mg for 2–4 weeks before additional increases. Weight gain is common, more likely after 6 months of use; sexual side effects, may be too stimulating.	Longer half-life of 3–4 days and long elimination of active metabolites, making withdrawal symptoms the least likely to occur among all the SSRIs.
Sertraline (Zoloft)	50	50–200	Maintain 50 mg for 4 weeks, then may increase in 25-mg increments weekly. Weight gain is common, more likely after 6 months of use; sexual side effects.	Half-life of 2–4 days and some minimally active metabolites, so withdrawal symptoms are less likely to occur.
Paroxetine (Paxil)	20	20–50	Maintain at 20 mg before dose increase, then may increase dose by 10 mg every week to a maximum of 50 mg/day. Weight gain is more likely than with other SSRIs; sexual side effects may be more common in the short term; may be sedating.	Short half-life and no active metabolites, so patients are more likely to experience serotonin withdrawal symptoms.
Fluvoxamine (Luvox)	100	100–300	Weight gain is common, more likely after 6 months of use.	Short half-life and no active metabolites, so patients are more likely to experience withdrawal symptoms.
Citalopram (Celexa)	10–20	20–40	May have fewer sexual side effects than other SSRIs; weight gain is common, more likely after 6 months of use. Maintain initial dose for 4 weeks before increase. Few drug interactions.	35-hour half-life and few metabolites, so missing a dose can cause serotonin withdrawal symptoms.
Escitalopram (Lexapro)	10	10–20	Increase to 20 mg if partial response after 4 weeks. More sexual side effects compared to citalopram in the short term, no long-term difference; weight gain is common, more likely after 6 months of use.	Short half-life of 27–32 hours, so missing a dose can cause serotonin withdrawal symptoms.
NDRIs				
Bupropion (Wellbutrin, Zyban)	200 (in two divided doses)	100–150 three times per day	May increase to 100 mg three times per day after 7 days. May be stimulating. No sexual side effects; weight neutral or minor weight loss; lowers seizure threshold.	Half-life is 29 hours for sustained release; withdrawal symptoms have not been reported.
Bupropion SR 12 hr	100	150–200 twice daily	Increase to 150 mg twice daily after 7 days.	
SNRIs				
Venlafaxine (Effexor)	37.5	75–300 in two to three divided doses	Weight neutral; fewer sexual side effects than SSRIs; increases blood pressure in a dose-dependent fashion.	Withdrawal symptoms have been reported, but their frequency is unknown.
Venlafaxine XR (Effexor XR)	37.5	37.5–300 once daily		

NDRI: norepinephrine-dopamine reuptake inhibitor; SNRI: serotonin-norepinephrine reuptake inhibitor; SSRI: selective serotonin reuptake inhibitor.

Source: Adapted from Hackley B, Sharma C, Kedzior A, Sreenivasan S. Managing mental health conditions in primary care settings. *J Midwifery Women's Health.* 2010;55:9-19; MacArthur Initiative on Depression and Primary Care. *Depression Management Tool Kit.* 2009.

sertraline (Zoloft) is more sedating.[38,53] Thus fluoxetine would be a better choice for a woman with hypersomnia and low energy. As a group, the SNRIs are less frequently associated with weight gain than the SSRIs.[15] The woman's ability and motivation to comply with therapy is another consideration in selecting which SSRI or SNRI to use when initiating treatment. Abrupt discontinuation of SSRIs or SNRIs usually leads to serotonin withdrawal (or discontinuation) syndrome. Symptoms include dizziness, ataxia, agitation, headache, tremor, and confusion.[15,47] Fluoxetine has the longest half-life of the second-generation antidepressants, and it may be the most appropriate medication for those women who are less able to take their pills consistently.

Initiating Treatment

Once the clinician has made the diagnosis of major depression and ruled out bipolar disorder, the decision to begin psychotropic medication is made jointly with the woman. All of the SSRIs and SNRIs may cause gastrointestinal upset, jitteriness, and headache after initiation, as the body adapts to the higher levels of neurotransmitters. Within approximately 2 weeks, the receptors are desensitized and downregulated, leading to the disappearance or significant decrease in these side effects.[47] Unfortunately, these adverse side effects often recur prior to attaining therapeutic effect, and may lead the woman to discontinue the medication. Psychotropic drugs should be initiated at a low dose for the first 2 weeks to minimize these symptoms. The lower dose, when accompanied by anticipatory guidance, will improve the likelihood of continuing the medication.

The risk of suicide and suicide attempts has been found to increase during the first 1 to 2 months after beginning treatment with SSRIs, especially in adolescents and young adults. Close monitoring is indicated during this time.[53] Response to and side effects from the many SSRIs, SNRIs, and NDRIs vary greatly, and most persons using these medications will require adjustments to the initial dose. The American College of Physicians recommends monitoring to begin within 1 to 2 weeks after initiating therapy, which can be accomplished either by phone or via a face-to-face visit.[48] This encounter is an important time during which to discuss whether the woman has filled the prescription, begun taking it, and is continuing the medication, and if not, what are her barriers or reasons. This first follow-up visit also allows for assessment of side effects and possible increases in suicidal thoughts or behaviors.

Follow-up

Some depressed persons may experience an improvement in their depression by their 1- to 2-week follow-up visit, although many will not appreciate a response until as late as 6 weeks after beginning medication. It is recommended that a reassessment of depressive symptoms be repeated 4 to 8 weeks after initiating therapy. Repeat use of the screening tool employed during the initial diagnosis allows the provider and the woman to see an objective, quantifiable response to the therapy. The goal of therapy is complete remission from depression, which would mean a score of less than 5 on the PHQ-9. **Table 9-6** provides guidance for alterations in management based on the woman's response to the PHQ-9.[38,39]

An assessment of compliance, barriers to compliance, and side effects is completed at this time. The undertreatment of individuals being treated for depression[14] may be evidence of failure to provide the necessary follow-up. A partial response to treatment may be an indication to increase the dose of the antidepressant. If the woman has less than a 25% decrease in symptoms, either an increase in the dose or a switch to a different antidepressant is appropriate. Referral for concurrent psychotherapy may be useful as well. Ongoing monitoring is recommended at least

Table 9-6	Using the PHQ-9 to Assess Clinical Response to Treatment	
Initial Response After Four Weeks of Antidepressant Treatment		
PHQ-9	**Treatment Response**	**Treatment Plan**
Drop of 5 points from baseline	Adequate	No treatment change needed. Follow up in 4 weeks.
Drop of 2–4 points from baseline	Possibly inadequate	May warrant an increase in antidepressant dose.
Drop of 1 point or no change or increase	Inadequate	Increase dose; augmentation; switch; informal or formal psychiatric consultation; add psychological counseling.

Source: Adapted from Unutzer J, Oisha S. *Impact Intervention Manual.* Los Angeles, CA: UCLA NPI, Center for Health Services Research; 2004.

monthly until full remission is achieved, and then every 2 to 3 months. Further treatment of individuals who fail to respond to therapy is best managed either through referral to or in consultation with a psychiatric provider.

Relapse is common in persons suffering from depression, with 20% to 85% of depressed individuals experiencing a second episode of depression within 2 years of the initial episode.[49] The risk of relapse is lower when antidepressant therapy is continued for 4 to 9 months after remission has been achieved, for a total duration of 6 to 12 months.[13,15,38] Individuals who have had or who are at high risk for relapses will benefit from long-term maintenance therapy. Characteristics of women for whom maintenance therapy should be considered are listed in **Box 9-4**. These women should be encouraged to continue therapy for at least 2 years, during which time provider–patient interactions may take place every 3 to 12 months as long as the woman's mental health status remains stable.[13,49] Due to the chronic nature of dysthymia and risk of episodes of double depression, many women suffering from this disorder will benefit from ongoing, or even lifelong, treatment.[54]

When a decision is made to discontinue psychotropic medications, the dose should be tapered over several weeks to months to avoid serotonin withdrawal syndrome.[13] It is beneficial to provide women with information regarding discontinuation when initiating therapy, as individuals may decide to stop the medication without consulting their providers. This information should be reinforced at each follow-up encounter.

Anxiety, Stress, and Obsessive-Compulsive Disorders

As can be seen in Figure 9-1, anxiety disorders as a group are more prevalent than mood disorders in the United States, yet they are less often screened for or detected in primary care practices.[55] Seedat et al.,[2] working under the aegis of the World Health Organization, administered World Mental Health surveys to 72,933 participants from 5 developing countries and 10 developed countries and found that in all cohorts women were almost twice as likely as men to experience both anxiety and mood disorders. Anxiety disorders are distinct from common anxiety. Anxiety disorders cause significant stress; lead to impairment of social, family, or occupational functioning; and are out of proportion to any actual threat. For example, many persons dread having an injection. Those with a needle phobia would consciously avoid having blood drawn or receiving an injection, even when the benefit of doing so is clear. While much public effort has been made to identify individuals with major depression, less attention has been directed at screening for individuals with anxiety disorders. Phobias are the largest subcategory of anxiety disorders. Stress disorders and obsessive-compulsive disorders were previuosly categorized as subcategories of anxiety disorders. The *DSM-5* has creeated separate new categories for "Obsessive–Compulsive and Related Disorders" and "Trauma and Stressor-Related Disorders," which now includes PTSD.[8] A suggested scheme for exploration of a suspected anxiety disorder is presented in **Figure 9-4**.

Phobias and obsessive–compulsive disorder (OCD) typically develop during childhood, adolescence, or early adulthood. Panic disorders and generalized anxiety disorder (GAD) have significant variation in age of onset, as does post-traumatic stress disorder (PTSD), due to the fact that trauma may occur at any age.[56] Neuroimaging data suggest a significant neurobiological contribution to the development of anxiety disorders.[57]

All anxiety disorders, including OCD and PTSD, are frequently compounded by other anxiety or mood disorders—more so than other psychiatric disorders.[56,58] It is also common to have a three-way interaction among anxiety disorders, depression, and

---

BOX 9-4 Indicators for Possible Maintenance Antidepressant Therapy

- Residual symptoms after adequate treatment
- Persistent sleep disturbance
- Family history of mood disorders
- Ongoing psychosocial stressors
- Three or more previous episodes of major depression
- Two or more closely spaced episodes
- Dysthymia
- Dysthymia with an episode of major depression (double depression)

Sources: Adapted from MacArthur Initiative on Depression and Primary Care. *Depression Management Tool Kit.* 2009; Gilbody S, Bower P, Fletcher J, Richards D, Sutton AJ. Collaborative care for depression: a cumulative meta-analysis and review of longer-term outcomes. *Arch Intern Med.* 2006;166:2314-2321; American Psychiatric Association. *Practice Guideline for the Treatment of Patients with Major Depressive Disorder.* 3rd ed. Arlington, VA: APA; 2010.

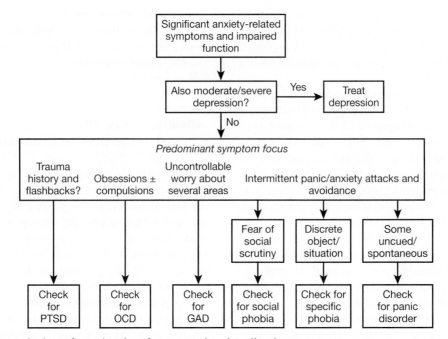

Figure 9-4 Suggested scheme for exploration of a suspected anxiety disorder.
Source: Baldwin DS, Anderson IM, Nutt DJ, et al. Evidence-based guidelines for the pharmacological treatment of anxiety disorders: recommendations from the British Association for Psychopharmacology. *J Psychopharm.* 2005;19:567-596. Reprinted by permission of SAGE.

somatic symptoms,[55] including irritable bowel syndrome, chronic pain or malaise, fatigue, atopic disorders,[59] and even heart disease.[60] Anxiety disorders are highly internalizing, which contributes to the associated somatic complaints.[58] Individuals suffering from anxiety disorders may experience somatic symptoms such as palpitations, chest pain, shortness of breath, and dizziness that mimic symptoms of medical conditions and lead to increased healthcare utilization and reduced quality of life.[56,58]

The lifetime prevalence of phobias is approximately 6% to 12%; social anxiety disorder has a lifetime prevalence as high as 10%; PTSD has a prevalence of between 6% and 9%[55,56,60]; and GAD, occurs in approximately 3% to 7.6% of the population.[51,53,54] Panic disorders and other anxiety disorders have a lower prevalence. The prevalence of OCD is 2% to3%, and that of panic disorder is 2% to 7%.[55,56,59]

Phobias

Phobias involve fear or anxiety about a specific object or situation, which provokes immediate fear or anxiety that is out of proportion to any actual danger. This fear or anxiety is persistent, lasting more than 6 months.[8] Social anxiety disorder, also referred to as social phobia, is a specific phobia related to social situations where the individual is exposed to

potential scrutiny by others.[8] Studies suggest that maternal stress, overprotection, hypercriticism, abuse, and neglect may contribute to the development of social phobia. Social phobias are more common in the United States than in Western Europe.[56]

Generalized Anxiety Disorder

Generalized anxiety disorder is characterized by excessive worry or anxiety related to family, health, finances, and work or school. A majority of women with GAD also experience other mental health disorders—most commonly depression or dysthymia, but also panic disorder and agoraphobia. As with all anxiety disorders, women are at greater risk for GAD than men.[60] Generalized anxiety disorder is associated with numerous somatic symptoms, leading to frequent primary care, specialist, and emergency room visits, and absences from work.[60]

Generalized anxiety is characterized by: (1) Excessive anxiety and worry (apprehensive expectation) about of activities or events (e.g., family, health, finances, and school/work difficulties), occurring on more days than not, for 6 months or more, (2) The anxiety and worry are difficult to control and (3) The anxiety and worry are associated with three (or more) of the following behaviors: restlessness, muscle tension, difficulty with concentration, sleep disturbance, fatigue, or irritability.[8]

Panic Attack

Panic attacks are a period of intense anxiety or fear that has a sudden onset. They can be expected to occur in the presence of a particular trigger or they can be unexpected. The symptoms of a panic attack are dramatic and usually frightening to the person who experiences one. A panic attack usually peaks at about 10 minutes but can full recovery can take days. Symptoms include sweating, trembling, or shaking, sensation of shortness of breath or smothering, nausea, abdominal pain, or chest discomfort, chest pain or discomfort, dizziness, lightheadedness, unsteadiness, or fainting, fear of losing control or going crazy; fear of dying, paresthesias, and chills or hot flashes. Individual attacks may occur with any of the anxiety disorders, although the presence of recurrent attacks is formally characterized as panic disorder.[8]

Agoraphobia is marked fear or anxiety about being outside the home, being in a crowd, or at times open places, or using public transportation. Individuals with agoraphobia actively avoid being in one of the triggering situations, and, if forced to do so, may experience panic attacks or disproportionate anxiety. Agoraphobia often, but not always, coexists with panic disorder.[8]

Panic Disorder

A panic disorder involved recurrent unexpected panic attacks, followed by: (1) Persistent concern or worry about additional panic attacks or their consequences (e.g., losing control, having a heart attack, or "going crazy"), or (2) Significant maladaptive change in behavior related to the attacks (e.g., behaviors designed to avoid having panic attacks, such as avoidance of exercise or unfamiliar situations).[8]

Screening for Anxiety Disorders

Anxiety disorders are underdetected, and therefore undertreated. Similar to the PHQ-2 and PHQ-9 screening tools, the GAD-2 and GAD-7 instruments (Table 9-7) have been developed and validated to screen for anxiety disorders. While the GAD-7 was initially developed specifically to screen for GAD,[61] it has since been validated as a screen for not only GAD, but also panic, social anxiety, and post-traumatic stress disorders.[62] It has been found to be equally effective in screening four racial/ethinc groups of undergraduate students: African American, Caucasian, Hispanic/Latino, and Asian.[63]

Both psychotherapy and pharmacotherapy play important roles in the treatment of anxiety disorders. The same benefits seen with collaborative care models that employ a specially trained case manager for the treatment of depression are observed when this kind of model is applied to the treatment of anxiety.[64] The efficacy of pharmacotherapy and the efficacy of psychotherapy are similar for anxiety disorders,[65] and combined treatment has higher response rates than monotherapy.[66] Using a collaborative model, the specially trained case manager provides cognitive-behavioral therapy and education, monitors medications, and evaluates response to treatment. Individuals with anxiety disorders are

Table 9-7	Generalized Anxiety Disorder Screening Tool (GAD-7)				
Over the last 2 weeks, how often have you been bothered by the following problems?	**Not at All**	**Several Days**	**More Than Half the Days**	**Nearly Every Day**
Feeling nervous, anxious, or on edge	0	1	2	3
Not being able to stop or control worrying	0	1	2	3
Worrying too much about different things	0	1	2	3
Trouble relaxing	0	1	2	3
Being so restless that it is hard to sit still	0	1	2	3
Becoming easily annoyed or irritable	0	1	2	3
Feeling afraid as if something awful might happen	0	1	2	3
Total Score _____ =	_____ +	_____ +	_____ +	_____

Scores of 5, 10, and 15 are cut-off points for mild, moderate, and severe anxiety, respectively.

Further evaluation is recommended for a score ≥ 10.

The GAD-2 uses the first two questions of the GAD-7 and a score ≥ 3 suggests the presence of an anxiety disorder.

Source: Developed by Drs. Robert L. Spitzer, Janet B.W. Williams, Kurt Kroenke, and colleagues, with an educational grant from Pfizer Inc.

more likely to prefer cognitive-behavioral therapy over medication alone.[64]

Cognitive-behavioral therapy—a time-limited therapy that aims to change maladaptive patterns of thinking and behaviors—has been demonstrated to be efficacious in the treatment of anxiety disorders.[67] Topics, or "lessons," for sessions often include psychoeducation, behavioral activation, cognitive restructuring, problem solving, graded exposure, relapse prevention, and assertiveness skills.[68] While this therapy has traditionally been delivered by mental health specialists, the scarcity of such providers has limited its impact. More recently, cognitive-behavioral therapy has been delivered or supported by primary care providers, specially trained nurses, and social workers. In this model, cognitive-behavioral therapy may be Internet or computer based, or delivered on a face-to-face basis.[69] Andrews et al. performed a meta-analysis of 22 randomized controlled trials (RCTs) of computer therapy for both anxiety and depression, and concluded that it was an effective and acceptable alternative to face-to-face therapy, with the advantage of providing an alternative for those individuals who might otherwise be unable to access mental health specialists.[70]

Stress Disorders

PTSD is distinct from the other anxiety disorders in that psychotherapy utilizing exposure therapy and cognitive-behavioral therapy has been found to be more effective than pharmacotherapy. Eye movement desensitization and reprocessing (EMDR) may also be useful in the tretment of PTSD.[76] Treatment with an SSRI or SNRI may be used for individuals with PTSD who prefer medication rather than psychotherapy.[71]

Post-traumatic Stress Disorder

The diagnostic criteria for PTSD includes the following five criteria. All of these criteria include significant distress or impairment in social, occupational, or other areas of function, and are not attributed to the direct physiological effects of a substance such as medication, drugs, or alcohol. Nor can they be ascribed to another medical condition.[8]

1. Exposure to actual or threatened (a) death, (b) serious injury, or (c) sexual violation, by either directly experiencing the traumatic event(s), witnessing or learning of the event occurring to a significant other, or experiencing repeated exposure to traumatic events.[8]

2. Presence of one or more of the following intrusion symptoms associated with the traumatic event(s), beginning after the traumatic event(s) occurred: such as intrusive, disturbing memories; distressing dreams; dissociative reactions; intense psychological distress in response to cues related to the event(s); marked physiological reactions to reminders of the event(s).[8]

3. Persistent avoidance of stimuli associated with the traumatic event(s), beginning after the traumatic event(s) occurred, as evidenced by avoidance or efforts to avoid one or more of the following: (a) Distressing memories of the event, (b) Thoughts or feelings associated with the event, (c) External reminders of the event.[8]

4. Negative alterations in cognitions and mood associated with the traumatic event(s), beginning or worsening after the traumatic event(s) occurred), as evidenced by two or more of the following: (a) Inability to remember an important aspect of the traumatic event(s) (typically due to dissociative amnesia that is not due to head injury, alcohol, or drugs), (b) Persistent and exaggerated negative beliefs or expectations about oneself, others, or the world, (c) Persistent, distorted blame of self or others about the cause or consequences of the traumatic event(s), (d) Persistent negative emotional state, (e) Markedly diminished interest or participation in significant activities, (f) Feelings of detachment or estrangement from others, (g) Persistent inability to experience positive emotions (e.g., unable to have loving feelings, psychic numbing).[8]

5. Marked alterations in arousal and reactivity associated with the traumatic event(s), beginning or worsening after the traumatic event(s) occurred, as evidenced by aggressive or destructive behaviors, hypervigilance, difficulty concentrating and sleep disturbances.[8]

The common inciting event in individuals with PTSD is exposure to a traumatic event. Precipitating events may include mass conflict, population displacement, combat, or life-threatening accidents or illness. Some subgroups in the United States have significantly higher prevalence of PTSD than the general population. For example, in one study, Cambodian refugees who had relocated to the United States 20 years earlier were found to have a 62% prevalence of PTSD.[72] Women are two to four times more likely than men to develop PTSD.[60] Sexual assault is the most frequent trauma leading to PTSD in women. A study of college-age women in 2000 found that approximately 20% to 25% of these women were subjected to sexual assault or attempted sexual assault,[73] leading to a large pool of women at risk for developing PTSD.

Childbirth, which is often thought of as a joyous occasion, can also lead to post-traumatic stress, and approximately 2% of women will develop full-blown PTSD postpartum.[74] Verreault et al. found that 7.6% of a cohort of women living in Canada (n = 308) met the criteria for PTSD according to the Modified PTSD Symptom Scale Self-Report, and 16.6% had symptoms of partial PTSD at one month postpartum. A correlation was seen between a history of sexual trauma or anxiety and PTSD.[75]

Many individuals are exposed to traumatic events, yet only a minority of them develop PTSD. Resilience allows the majority of individuals who experience a traumatic event to recover without any long-lasting mental health disorder.[76] Further research is needed to explore factors that might improve resilience.

Pharmacotherapy

SSRIs are the recommended first-line pharmacotherapy for GAD, generalized social anxiety, and PTSD.[77-79] The benefits of the SSRIs in the treatment of anxiety disorders are the same as described for the treatment of depression. These agents have been well studied, and are safe, efficacious, and well tolerated. As with use of SSRIs for depression, it may take as long as 4 weeks for an individual to have a response; if no clinical response is apparent by 6 weeks of treatment, there is a low likelihood of eventual response.[77] The same cautions that were described regarding the initiation of SSRIs for the treatment of depression apply for anxiety. The midwife should counsel the woman that there may be a transient increased nervousness in the first few days for treatment, but that this effect usually resolves within 2 weeks. The doses for the treatment of anxiety disorders are similar to those for depression. Treatment should begin with a low dose for the first 2 weeks to minimize adverse symptoms, with the dose then being increased no more frequently than every 1 to 2 weeks. Counseling includes the importance of tapering the medication when it is discontinued. Treatment should continue for at least 12 months if the response to the medication has been adequate. If the response is inadequate, the midwife may increase the same medication, switch to a different SSRI, recommend cognitive-behavioral therapy, and/or refer the woman to a prescibing mental health specialist who has experience with other

pharmacotherapy, such as anticonvulsants including gabapentin (Neurontin) or pregabalin (Lyrica).[71,80] Management will depend on the midwife's individual scope of practice and practice guidelines.

Benzodiazepines, usually clonazepam (Klonopin) or lorazepam (Ativan), may also be useful in the short term for individuals with significant impairment while waiting for the therapeutic effect of an SSRI to become evident. These medications may also be useful for the episodic treatment of panic disorder.[71] Benzodiazepines can be highly addictive, cause drowsiness, and may aggravate depression. The risk of dependence is higher in individuals who have dependences on other substances.[47,70]

Mental Health Disturbances Related to the Menstrual Cycle

Many women report emotional and physical discomforts that appear around the time of their menses. Approximately 80% of women will experience cyclic fluctuations in mood, sleep, and sense of well-being during their fertile years. Approximately 50% of women will have symptoms severe enough to impair daily function during premenstrual days; perhaps 5% of women are severely disabled for several days per month by disturbances in mood, energy, and sleep.[81]

The terms "premenstrual syndrome" (PMS) and "premenstrual tension" (PMT) have been used since the 1950s to describe the discomforts that some women experience during the luteal phase of the menstrual cycle. Diagnostic criteria for PMS and PMT varied over the years until 2008, when the International Society for Premenstrual Disorders issued consensus standards for premenstrual disorders (PMD) to guide diagnosis and research.[82,83] These definitions and criteria are summarized in **Table 9-8**.[83] The American Psychiatric Association published diagnostic criteria for premenstrual dysphoric disorder (PMDD) in 1994 to encourage study of the most severe mental disturbances that are associated with the menstrual cycle. That research now allows PMDD to appear in the *DSM-5* as a subtype of "Mood Disorder Not Otherwise Specified."[84]

Premenstrual Dysphoric Disorder

Premenstrual dysphoric disorder is a psychiatric illness that affects approximately 5% of women during their fertile years. It is the most severe but

Table 9-8	Classification of Premenstrual Disorders Consensus[a] Criteria of the International Society for Premenstrual Disorders, 2008
Definition	**Characteristics**
Core Premenstrual Disorders	
Premenstrual syndrome	Multiple symptoms appear only during the luteal phase; must not be an exacerbation of another condition; symptoms are severe enough to interfere with daily functioning and cause significant distress
Premenstrual dysphoric disorder	Classified separately from PMS based on severe psychological symptoms during the luteal phase and remit entirely during the rest of the menstrual cycle
Variant Premenstrual Disorders	
Premenstrual exacerbation	Luteal phase exacerbation of another condition, e.g.: depression, diabetes, migraine, epilepsy, asthma
Nonovulatory premenstrual disorders	Cyclic follicular activity may not result in ovulation; limited evidence supports the existence of this phenomenon
Progesterone-induced premenstrual disorders	Women receiving exogenous progestogens may develop PMS symptoms as a form of progestin sensitivity
Premenstrual disorders without menstruation	Many women continue to experience PMS following medically or surgically induced amenorrhea if ovarian function is preserved

[a] Consensus on diagnostic criteria:
1. There is currently no imaging or biochemical test that is pathognomonic for PMD.
2. Diagnosis is based on structured interview, self-report, and prospective recording of at least two menstrual cycles.

Source: Adapted from O'Brien PM, Backstrom T, Brown C, et al. Towards a consensus on diagnostic criteria, measurement and trial design of the premenstrual disorders: the ISPMD Montreal consensus. *Arch Women's Ment Health.* 2011;14:13-21.

least common of the menstrual disorders, however diagnosis and treatment of PMDD informs the management of the less severe and more common menstrual disturbances. The most frequent and disabling symptoms of PMDD are extreme irritability and mood lability. Disordered sleep—either insomnia or hypersomnia—and extreme changes in tension or energy are also reported. Confusion and alterations in mental status are prominent in PMDD, which results in women being to be unable to work. They may have difficulties in their personal relationships on the days that they are ill. The burden of illness for PMDD has less to do with the expense of treating it than with the lost productivity among otherwise high-functioning women.[85]

The diagnosis of PMDD requires that symptoms occur in the majority of menstrual cycles in the past year in which five or more of the following symptoms occured in the week prior to menses. These symptoms start to improve within a few days after menses begin and they are minimal or resolve in the week following menses. The five symptoms must include one of the following: (1) marked affective lability (e.g. mood swings, feeling suddenly sad or tearful or

increased sensitivity to rejection; (2) marked irritability or anger or increased interpersonal conflicts; (3) markedly depressed mood, feelings of hopelessness, or self deprecating thoughts; (4) marked anxiety, tension, feelings of being "keyed up" or "on edge.[8]" In addition to one of the previous 4 symptoms, one of the following symptoms must be present: (1) decreased interest in usual activities (e.g., work, school, friends, hobbies), (2) subjective sense of difficulty in concentration; (3) lethargy, easy fatigability, or marked lack of energy, (4) marked change in appetite, overeating, or specific food cravings; (5) hypersomnia or insomnia; (6) a subjective sense of being overwhelmed or out of control; or (7) other physical symptoms such as breast tenderness or swelling, joint or muscle pain, a sensation of "bloating," weight gain.[8] The symptoms of PMDD are associated with clinically significant distress or interference with activities of daily living or relationships with others. The disturbance is not an exacerbation of another disorder, such as major depressive disorder or other mental disorder, however one of these disorder may co-occur with PMDD.[8,86] Finally the symptoms are not due to the physiological effects of a substance such as a drug of abuse or medication and they are not due to treatment of another medical condition such as hyperthyroidism.[8]

Women who suffer from PMDD may also experience comorbidity with other mood or anxiety disorders such as MDD, bipolar disorder, or OCD.[86] It is also possible for a woman to have PMDD or PMS in addition to another psychiatric diagnosis. For example, a woman with schizophrenia may experience mood or sleep disturbances only during the days before her menses.[81]

PMDD does not have a clearly identified etiology. Historically, PMS was attributed to abnormalities in gonadal hormone function, but more recent research points to extreme neurologic sensitivity to normal hormone variations. Genetic vulnerability also probably plays a role in determining which women suffer from PMDD.[87,88] The clearest evidence for effective treatment of PMDD involves suppressing ovulation or boosting neurotransmitter function. The first strategy aims to create a steady hormonal state, without the cyclic fluctuations that appear to trigger the neurologic cascade resulting in PMDD. Hormonal contraceptives can suppress ovulation and are widely acceptable to women during their fertile years. Oral contraceptives containing drospirenone have been the most-studied agents for their effectiveness in treating PMDD and PMS.[89,90] Fluctuation of hormone levels can be further minimized by using long-cycle or continuous-dosing regimens.[91]

The SSRIs are the most-studied antidepressants for treating PMDD. All of the SSRIs appear to be equally effective for this indication, and both continuous and intermittent dosing regimens are used. A moderate dose may be effective and well tolerated.[92,93] Two basic differences in the action of SSRIs for PMDD and for other psychiatric conditions are as follows:

- Relief of symptoms occurs in the first cycle of use. Ordinarily, SSRIs require up to 2 months before reaching full effectiveness.

- The SSRI is effective when taken used intermittently, rather than every day. Withdrawal symptoms do not appear when the medication is discontinued after several days or a week of use.

When treatment with oral contraceptives and/or SSRIs has failed to relieve PMDD, long-term suppression of ovulation using leuprolide acetate (Lupron, Lupron Depot) plus add-back estrogen may be effective.[94] The most extreme effective treatment is oophorectomy with or without hysterectomy.[95]

Premenstrual Exacerbation of Psychiatric Conditions

Much more common than PMDD is the cyclic worsening of other psychiatric conditions during the menstrual cycle. Mood and anxiety disorders are more prevalent in menstruating women than is PMDD. Because women themselves often feel confused about the causes of their distress, it is important to carefully identify menstrual-related symptoms to correctly diagnose and treat the underlying condition.

Most women who report significant emotional distress around the time of menses do not meet the stringent diagnostic criteria for PMDD. Given the prevalence of mood and anxiety disorders during the childbearing years and the rarity of pure PMDD, it is more likely that these women are suffering from an underlying mental illness that worsens at some point in the menstrual cycle. Reviewing the woman's daily symptom diary can help the midwife distinguish between PMDD or another psychiatric diagnosis.

If the woman already knows that she has a psychiatric diagnosis, the management is fairly straightforward: to prevent hormonal fluctuations that trigger cyclic destabilization of the mental illness. Gonadotropin hormones interact with the metabolism of psychotropic medications, so a close collaboration with the psychiatric prescriber is important prior to prescribing hormonal agents.

Fortunately, PMDD treatment strategies can help women with other conditions. Hormonal contraceptives have been used as an adjunct treatment for underlying depression that worsens premenstrually,[96] and the midwife who is familiar with the range of products and dosing regimens can fine-tune treatment to an individual woman's needs. The SSRIs that are part of the primary care treatment armamentarium can also be prescribed for "premenstrual" distress.

Women with psychiatric illness may have difficulty making sound decisions in their own best interest. Depression, for example, can interfere with cognition and impair memory; anxiety can cause confusion and distraction. Women with bipolar illness may have difficulty with impulse control and irritability. In working with these women to minimize their symptoms across the menstrual cycle, midwives need to remain mindful of the impaired decision making that mental illness can cause. It may be necessary to consult with the woman's mental health clinicians in determining the most effective plan of care. Inclusion of significant others or family members in making a diagnostic plan can be helpful as well.[97]

Perinatal Mental Health Disorders

Childbearing is a time of profound change. While having a child is usually a joyous and positive time, it can also be fraught with situational stresses and emotional vulnerability. An increasingly robust body of literature has found strong associations between the mental health of women and optimal outcomes of pregnancy and birth, as well as the cognitive and social development of the offspring. Women with mental disorders may struggle to negotiate the demands of parenthood, and when they falter, their children—and other family members—may suffer as well.[98]

Longstanding cultural traditions hold that pregnancy protects a woman from dark thoughts and negative emotions. Historically, women whose experiences differed from these expected norms endured their distress quietly and in shame. However, recent longitudinal studies have shown that pregnancy does not protect women from mental illness. In fact, just the opposite is true—women are *more* likely to be diagnosed with a psychiatric disorder during their childbearing years than at any other time in their lives. In addition, women are most vulnerable to psychiatric illness while they are pregnant or during the postpartum period.[99]

Mental Illness In Pregnancy

The prevalence of various psychiatric conditions during pregnancy mirrors their prevalence in the general population. Approximately 10% to 20% of women will experience major or minor depression during pregnancy. Mood and anxiety disorders predominate in women across all sociodemographic and age groups; they are also the most commonly diagnosed psychiatric conditions during pregnancy.[1]

Untreated major depression and anxiety disorders can adversely affect the course and outcome of pregnancy[100]; these risks are described in **Box 9-5**. The strongest predictors for postpartum depression can all be identified during pregnancy, including depression or anxiety during pregnancy, stressful life effects and poor social support, or a history of depression at any other time in the woman's life.[101,102]

Screening for Depression and Anxiety During Pregnancy

Although universal depression screening for all pregnant women has not been formally recommended, the American College of Obstetricians and Gynecologists (ACOG) states that universal screening should be

---

BOX 9-5 Risks of Untreated Depression and Anxiety During Pregnancy

1. Burden of disability directly due to the mental illness: Poor self-care; impaired judgment; self-medication with harmful drugs; insomnia; poor appetite and inadequate weight gain.
2. Possible adverse effects of the illness on pregnancy: Increased risk for premature birth and fetal growth restriction. The specific etiology and epidemiology of these risks have not been well characterized.
3. Antepartum mental illness predicts the worsening of illness postpartum: Increased risk for postpartum depression, postpartum psychosis, postpartum obsessive–compulsive disorder, and suicide or infanticide.

Sources: Adapted from Meltzer-Brody S. New insights into perinatal depression: pathogenesis and treatment during pregnancy and postpartum. *Dialogues Clin Neurosci.* 2011;13:89-100; Yonkers KA, Gotman N, Smith MV, et al. Does antidepressant use attenuate the risk of a major depressive episode in pregnancy? *Epidemiology.* 2011;22:848-854; Hackley B. Antidepressant medication use in pregnancy. *J Midwifery Women's Health.* 2010;55:90-100.

---

considered, and the U.S. Preventive Services Task Force recommends routine screening in settings that have staff-assisted depression care in place.[22] Regardless of the choice to do routine screening or targeted screening, any woman who has risks for depression or symptoms of depression should be screened at least once, and preferably two or three times, during pregnancy.

Symptoms of prenatal depression include crying, weepiness, sleep problems, fatigue, appetite disturbance, anhedonia, anxiety, poor fetal attachment, and irritability. Because many of these symptoms can also be normal transient problems in pregnancy, formal screening to differentiate normal symptoms from major or minor depression is essential.

General screening for mental disorders should also include assessment for thyroid and other endocrine abnormalities that can trigger psychiatric symptoms. Elevations in levels of thyroid-stimulating hormone (TSH), free T_4, and thyroid autoantibodies have been associated with depression during pregnancy and postpartum.[103] A recent study by Sylven et al. found that an abnormal TSH level at the time of birth was associated with a significant elevated risk for postpartum depression at 6 months following birth (OR 11.30; 95% CI: 1.93–66.11).[104] Thus it is reasonable to include TSH measurement in the evaluation of women for depression during pregnancy.

Although many screening tools are available for screening during pregnancy, the PHQ-2[105] and/or the GAD-2[67] may represent a quick, cost-effective method for identifying those women at risk for depression. Both the Edinburgh Postnatal Depression Scale (**Table 9-9**) and the Pregnancy Depression Scale have been validated for use during pregnancy and postpartum.[23,106] Use of the M-3 Checklist will screen for both depression and bipolar disorder. As stated previously in this chapter, it is extremely important to distinguish unipolar depressive illness from bipolar depression, as the treatment and prognosis for each condition is quite different, and because treatment of bipolar disorder with antidepressant medications may exacerbate this illness.[103]

Overview of Mental Disorders During Pregnancy

A thorough history should reveal previous episodes of mental illness experienced by the pregnant woman or members of her family.[107] Whenever possible, contact the mental health professionals who cared for the woman in the past to confirm her account, as mental disorders may cloud memory. Women who have discontinued their psychotropic medication before becoming pregnant should be counseled that approximately 86% of women who discontinue antidepressant medication will relapse during pregnancy.[99] Similarly, approximately 85% of women who discontinue mood-stabilizing medication for bipolar disorder prior to pregnancy will have a relapse in pregnancy.[108]

Risk factors such as onset of depression before age 18 years, individual or family history of suicide attempts, and multiple unsuccessful trials of antidepressant medications often predict a bipolar origin of depression.[109] Aggressive treatment of bipolar illness and protection of sleep are key elements in preventing mania and psychosis postpartum; such measures can reduce, but not eliminate, these risks.[110]

Anxiety disorders can also develop de novo or relapse during pregnancy, and it can be difficult to differentiate the normal parental anxieties from disabling illness. GAD appears to have a prevalence of approximately 7% among pregnant women, but the risk may be higher for women with a history of abuse, poor social support, or previous episodes of anxiety.[111] Obsessive–compulsive symptoms can be present during pregnancy, and tend to become worse postpartum and be highly comorbid with depressive illness.[112]

Psychiatric illnesses have a frequent comorbidity with each other; therefore when one disorder is identified in a pregnant woman, the possibility that more than one condition is present should be considered. For example, recent studies of pregnant women who screened positive for depression found that anxiety disorders were also present in about one-third of these women.[113]

Treatment of Depression During Pregnancy

Depression during pregnancy requires collaborative management between the woman, her midwife, and mental health clinicians. The choice of treatment is dictated by the severity of the illness and the likelihood of morbidity if the condition is not treated. Women who have a history of major mental illness, such as bipolar disorder, eating disorders, and PTSD, need to be co-managed with a mental health clinician who develops the plan of care. Therapy plus psychotropic medication has been shown to have higher remission and lower relapse rates than either type of treatment alone.

Midwives who are knowledgeable about both depression and the pharmacology of medications used to treat depression may prescribe these medications. Safe practice requires that the midwife has access to mental health resources, is able to provide continuity of care, and that the woman does not have symptoms that indicate a need for mental health referral such as suicidal ideation or a history of hospitalization. Many of the common SSRIs have drug–drug interactions of clinical import, so it is imperative that a prescribing midwife obtain a history of all medications and other products the woman is taking, and be aware of all potential interactions. Women who have multiple comorbidities are best managed by a mental health specialist.

The choice to use medication during pregnancy is complex. The risks of not treating depression must be balanced with the risks associated with medications. Untreated depression is associated with some adverse pregnancy outcomes, including preterm birth and low birth weight.[103,114,115] Similarly, SSRIs have been linked to some potential teratogenic, fetal, and newborn complications, although the absolute risks are very small. Studies that have evaluated adverse outcomes of antidepressant use in pregnancy have produced conflicting results, and methodology limitations of the studies preclude knowledge of real etiologic relationships. Several of the adverse effects associated with untreated depression are the same as those associated with antidepressants, which makes this cost-benefit calculation difficult

Table 9-9	The Edinburgh Postnatal Depression Scale

1. I have been able to laugh and see the funny side of things.
   - 0 As much as I always could
   - 1 Not quite so much now
   - 2 Definitely not so much now
   - 3 Not at all

2. I have looked forward with enjoyment to things.
   - 0 As much as I ever did
   - 1 Rather less than I used to
   - 2 Definitely less than I used to
   - 3 Hardly at all

3. I have blamed myself unnecessarily when things went wrong.
   - 3 Yes, Most of the time
   - 2 Yes, some of the time
   - 1 Not very often
   - 0 No, never

4. I have been anxious or worried for no good reason.
   - 0 No, not at all
   - 1 Hardly ever
   - 2 Yes, sometimes
   - 3 Yes, very often

5. I have felt scared or panicky for no good reason.
   - 3 Yes, quite a lot
   - 2 Yes, sometimes
   - 1 No, not much
   - 0 No, not at all

6. Things have been getting on top of me.
   - 3 Yes, most of the time I haven't been able to cope at all
   - 2 Yes, sometimes I haven't been coping as well as usual
   - 1 No, most of the time I have coped quite well
   - 0 No, I have been coping as well as ever

7. I have been so unhappy that I have had difficulty sleeping.
   - 3 Yes, most of the time
   - 2 Yes, quite often
   - 1 Not very often
   - 0 No, not at all

8. I have felt sad or miserable.
   - 3 Yes, most of the time
   - 2 Yes, quite often
   - 1 Not very often
   - 0 No, not at all

9. I have been so unhappy that I have been crying.
   - 3 Yes, most of the time
   - 2 Yes, quite often
   - 1 Only occasionally
   - 0 No, never

10. The thought of harming myself has occurred to me.
    - 3 Yes, quite often
    - 2 Sometimes
    - 1 Hardly ever
    - 0 Never

The scores for each item are totaled. Scores above 12 require evaluation and possible referral to a mental health specialist. Scores between 10-12 indicate the presence of symptoms of distress. The test should be repeated in 1-2 weeks and referral considered. Scores between 0-9 indicate that any symptoms of distress may be short-lived and not likely to interfere with day to day function. If they persist more than 1-2 weeks, further evaluation is recommended.

Source: Cox JL, Holden JM, Sagovsky R. Detection of postnatal depression: development of the 10-item Edinburgh Postnatal Depression Scale. *Br J Psychiatry.* 1987;150:782-786.

to conduct. RCTs are impossible to conduct with pregnant women as participants, leaving clinicians to consider the conflicting findings of many observational, anecdotal, retrospective, and open trials. In addition, these studies may conflate possible medication side effects. Thus, to date, no hard-and-fast rules for prescribing medications to treat mental health conditions during pregnancy have emerged despite a great deal of research. Each woman needs to make an individual choice based on her diagnosis, her likely prognosis, and the results of a thorough informed consent. The components of informed consent prior to starting antidepressant medication should include possible adverse effects over the course of pregnancy, including risks of no treatment, teratogenicity, fetal effects such as preterm birth or small-for-gestational-age neonates, newborn effects, and neurobehavioral effects on the child.

Reputable, evidence-based online resources are available that can help guide decisions about medication use during pregnancy and breastfeeding. The Massachusetts General Hospital Center for Women's Mental Health offers online resources for both clinicians and women that may help allay concerns regarding the potential effects of the transfer of antidepressants through breastmilk.[116] The Organization of Teratology Information Specialists (OTIS) is a network of teratology information services throughout the United States and Canada that provides information about exposure to medications during pregnancy and lactation.[117] Motherisk, an affiliate of OTIS based out of the Hospital for Sick Children in Toronto, is yet another online resource.[118] Both OTIS and Motherisk provide telephone consultations free of charge.

Benefits and Risks Associated with Medications for Depression Used in Pregnancy

The use of antidepressants in pregnancy has increased dramatically in recent years, with the rate of use rising from fewer than 1% of pregnant women in 1988–1990 to 7.5% of pregnant women in 2004–2008.[119] A wealth of studies have evaluated possible adverse effects of SSRIs in this population. Although no consistent, replicable pattern of harm to pregnant women or their offspring has emerged, the information in **Box 9-6** represents our current understanding of the various risks.[120–123]

There is no evidence that some medications work better during pregnancy than others. Unless a woman's usual psychotropic regimen includes agents that are known to be harmful in pregnancy, the best medication for a pregnant woman is the one that keeps her well. When treating a relapse of depression during pregnancy, it is recommended that the medication that has worked well for the woman in the past be initiated first. For new-onset illness, the choice of medication is based on the same criteria as for nonpregnant women.

In general, dosing regimens for pregnant women are similar to those for nonpregnant women, albeit with several unique considerations:

- Blood volume expansion begins early in pregnancy, and hemodilution may necessitate progressively higher doses of medication as pregnancy progresses to achieve a stable clinical effect.[124]
- As a result of changes in gestational hormones, metabolism and excretion of medications can vary over the course of pregnancy. This can alter the effectiveness of a medication, and is another reason why monitoring psychiatric symptoms frequently throughout the pregnancy is important.

Postpartum Mood Disorders

A description and diagnostic criteria of the common postpartum mood disorders appears in **Table 9-10**. Changes in mood are experienced by a majority of women who give birth. Estrogen levels, which have a significant influence in neurotransmitter systems, decrease postpartum. In addition, lower serotonergic activity following birth has been noted. Downregulation of the hypothalamic–pituitary–adrenal axis following birth may also contribute to a woman's vulnerability to depression.[103] While these physiologic changes do not lead to depression in all postpartum women, when coupled with a history of prior depression or bipolar disorder, a genetic predisposition, inadequate social support, and multiple stressors, it is not surprising that childbirth can present a challenge to a woman's mental health and well-being. Disturbances in sleep patterns and circadian rhythms are also universal in new mothers. Melatonin release is suppressed by exposure to light when a person would normally be sleeping.[125] Postpartum insomnia may both contribute to and be aggravated by MDD.[126]

Postpartum Blues

Postpartum blues, also known as baby or maternity blues, is the most common mood change, occurring in between 50% and 75% of women after giving birth.[127] The symptoms of crying, anxiety, emotional lability, irritability, and fatigue develop within the

BOX 9-6 Risks Associated with Use of Selective Serotonin Reuptake Inhibitors in Pregnancy[a]

Teratogenic Risks

- There is no evidence to date that SSRIs are associated with major congenital anomalies as a group.

- Citalopram (Celexa): Some studies have found a small association between citalopram and septal defects.

- Fluoxetine (Prozac): There is no apparent risk of teratogenicity secondary to use of fluoxetine in multiple studies. This is the SSRI most studied to date.

- Paroxetine (Paxil): Paroxetine has been associated with an increased risk for congenital heart defects in some studies but not others. The product label for paroxetine warns that it may be associated with cardiac anomalies, and the manufacturer has changed the FDA pregnancy Category from C to D.

- Sertraline (Zoloft): Some studies have found a small association between sertraline use in early pregnancy and an increased risk for omphalocele and septal defects.

- Venlafaxine (Effexor): One small study with inconclusive data.

Fetal Risks

- There is a small association between SSRIs and preterm labor, and between SSRIs and small-for-gestational-age births, but the studies done have not been able to determine whether these findings are secondary to medication use or the underlying condition.

Newborn Risks

- *Persistent pulmonary hypertension*: SSRIs are associated with an increased risk of persistent pulmonary hypotension. The absolute risk is 3 per 1000 live-born infants. compared to a background incidence of 1.2 per 1000 live-born infants. The FDA has indicated that these findings are inconclusive and healthcare professionals should not alter their practice on the basis of a concern about persistent pulmonary hypertension.

- *Neonatal abstinence syndrome*: Approximately 30% of newborns exposed to SSRIs in utero will have mild withdrawal symptoms such as tremors, jitteriness, increased muscle tone, and feeding difficulty. These symptoms typically peak at 3 to 4 days after birth and resolve spontaneously. They rarely need treatment. The two SSRIs most associated with this syndrome are fluoxetine (Prozac) and paroxetine (Paxil). There have been no reports of severe withdrawal symptoms.

Neurobehavioral Risks

- There is no conclusive evidence for adverse long-term neurodevelopment effects from fetal exposure to SSRIs.

- Prospective, blinded newborn neurobehavioral assessments do not show significant differences between infants of depressed mothers who took SSRI medications versus depressed women who did not take medication during pregnancy.

Additional Clinical Considerations

- Sertraline (Zoloft) has the lowest serum levels and least placental transfer of drug among the various SSRIs, and some authors suggest it be considered the first choice for initial therapy.

- Fluoxetine (Prozac) has the longest half-life, which may predispose it to accumulation in the newborn.

[a]It is not recommended that SSRI medications be discontinued in the first or third trimesters given that the absolute risks of these complications are small. In addition, there is no evidence that lowering the dose is safe or effective.

Sources: Adapted from Jimenez-Solem E, Andersen JT, Petersen M, et al. Exposure to selective serotonin reuptake inhibitors and the risk of congenital malformations: a nationwide cohort study. *BMJ Open.* 2012;2:e001148; Diav-Citrin O, Ornoy A. Selective serotonin reuptake inhibitors in human pregnancy: to treat or not to treat? *Obstet Gynecol Int.* 2012;2012:698947; Kieler H, Artama M, Engeland A, et al. Selective serotonin reuptake inhibitors during pregnancy and risk of persistent pulmonary hypertension in the newborn: population based cohort study from the five Nordic countries. *BMJ.* 2011;344:d8012; Moses-Kolko EL, Bogen D, Perel J, et al. Neonatal signs after late in utero exposure to serotonin reuptake inhibitors: literature review and implications for clinical applications. *JAMA.* 2005;293:2372-2383; Alwan S, Reefhuis J, Rasmussen SA, Olney RS, Friedman JM, National Birth Defects Prevention Society. Use of selective serotonin-reuptake inhibitors in pregnancy and the risk of birth defects. *N Engl J Med.* 2007;356:2684-2692.

Table 9-10	Description and Diagnostic Criteria of Postpartum Depression Disorders and Related Conditions	
Type	**Onset and Prevalence**	**Diagnostic Criteria**
Postpartum blues	The first 7–10 days after birth. Peak prevalence is usually postpartum days 4–6.	No specific diagnostic criteria. Most common symptom is weepiness. Other symptoms include mood lability, feeling overwhelmed, sadness and frustration, fatigue/exhaustion

Postpartum depression	Onset is first 2 to 3 months postpartum. Peak prevalence is 2–6 months postpartum.	Must include depressed mood or anhedonia and any of the following symptoms which occur nearly every day for at least 2 weeks are severe enough to impede function:
		
		1. Sleep disorder (Insomnia or hypersomnia)
		  a. Has to be evaluated in context on expected sleep pattern with newborn
		  b. Can she sleep when her infant is asleep?
		2. Interest deficit or a lack of feeling pleasure
		  a. Inability to appreciate infant, not bonding
		  b. Persistent sadness
		3. Guilt (worthlessness, hopelessness, regret)
		  a. More common than feeling sad
		  b. Feeling inadequate as a mother
		4. Fatigue or loss of energy nearly every day
		  a. Feeling of being overwhelmed, unable to cope
		5. Concentration deficit
		  a. Persistent difficulty with normal daily tasks
		  b. Difficulty remembering things
		6. Appetite disorder (increased or decreased)
		  a. Is she drinking enough and urinating regularly based on normal postpartum physiology?
		7. Psychomotor retardation or agitation
		  a. Unable to get out of bed or go to sleep
		  b. Loss of interest in caring for oneself
		  c. Obsessive thoughts of harm to the infant
		8. Suicidality (Recurrent thoughts of death)
		  a. Thoughts of harming oneself
		  b. Do you wish you could go to sleep and not wake up? (passive suicidal ideation)
		  c. Do you think about ways to kill yourself? (active suicidal ideation)

Postpartum psychosis	Usually starts within 2 to 4 weeks of birth, but can start as early as 2 to 3 days after birth and often progresses rapidly)	Emergency psychiatric condition characterized by delusional beliefs, hallucinations, and disordered thinking. Women often report everything is black or dark Feeling of hopelessness Delusions about the infant Auditory hallucinations, which can be instructions to harm the infant Visual hallucinations

Source: Modified from National Institute for Health Care Management Foundation. *Identifying and Treating Maternal Depression: Strategies and Considerations for Health Plans.* Issue Brief June 2010. Available at: http://nihcm.org/pdf/FINAL_MaternalDepression6-7.pdf. Accessed May 19, 2013. Reprinted with permission of National Institute for Health Care Management Foundation.

first 10 days after birth, with a peak onset of approximately 5 days.[127,128] Although postpartum blues is usually benign and self-limited, these mood changes can be frightening to a woman. If a woman in the early postpartum period calls with concerns about her emotional symptoms, it is prudent to ask the two questions of the PHQ-2 about having pleasure and interest in things, or feeling predominately down, depressed, or hopeless. If she reports anhedonia, a more thorough screen for postpartum depression is warranted. Some practices routinely use the Edinburgh Postpartum Depression Scale to screen any postpartum women who reports emotional distress

The primary difference among postpartum blues, postpartum depression, and postpartum psychosis is duration and severity. Selected differing characteristics are presented in **Table 9-11** to help the clinician distinguish between the two conditions when assessing a woman who reports disordered mood during the postpartum period.

Once postpartum blues are determined to be the likely cause of symptoms, anticipatory guidance that these mood swings are commonly experienced and usually resolve spontaneously within 10 to 14 days can reassure women that they are not "going crazy." Women should also be counseled to seek further evaluation if the symptoms do not resolve within 2 weeks, as 1 in 5 women with postpartum blues may develop postpartum depression.

Postpartum Depression

Postpartum depression (PPD) is a major depressive disorder. PPD affects women of all cultures, ages, incomes, races, and ethnicities.[129,130] The peak onset

for this form of depression is in the second month postpartum, and there remains an elevated risk up to 6 months or even 1 year following birth.[127,131,132] The point prevalence of MDD and minor depression ranges from 6.5% to 12.9% through the first postpartum year, and as many as 19.2% of women will have a major depressive episode at some time during the first three months postpartum.[133]

Risk factors for PPD are listed in **Box 9-7**. Adolescents are at almost twice the risk for PPD compared to adult women.[134] They are still achieving their normal development tasks, and often have unrealistic expectations of motherhood or the demands of parenting. In addition, adolescents tend to be more socially isolated from their peers compared to adult women.[134] Immigrant women may also have a higher risk for developing PPD, depending on the circumstances of their immigration, social and language isolation, and the unavailability of traditional childbirth rituals.[134] When assessing a woman for PPD, it is critical to rule out postpartum bipolar disorder, which can be severe and possibly lead to postpartum psychosis.[135] One way to screen for bipolar disorder is to ask one of the following two questions:

- Have you ever had 4 continuous days when you felt so good, high, excited, or hyper that other people thought you were not your normal self or that you got into trouble?

- Have you ever had 4 continuous days when you were so irritable that you found yourself shouting at people or starting fights?

Even women who do not meet the criteria for MDD in the postpartum period often experience negative

Table 9-11	Common Clinical Features That Distinguish Postpartum Blues and Postpartum Depression[a]				
			Characteristics		
Disorder	**Onset**	**Duration**	**Characteristic Symptoms**	**Degree of Disability**	**Suicidal Ideation**
Postpartum blues	7-10 days after birth	Less than 2 weeks	Crying, sad, labile mood	Minimal, cares for infant without problem	Unlikely
Postpartum depression	2 months to 1 year after birth	More than 2 weeks	Anhedonia, sleep disturbance, guilt, feeling of isolation and loneliness	Severe, may have difficulty caring for infant without help	Possibly present
Postpartum psychosis symptoms	Anytime in the first 2-4 weeks	Mean duration is approximately 40 days	Acute onset of psychosis and delusional thoughts	Severe, psychiatric emergency	Likely, may also have thoughts that infant is being harmed

[a] This list is a selected list of symptoms that can aid a clinician during the initial evaluation of a woman on the phone or in a triage setting.

BOX 9-7 Risk Factors for Postpartum Depression

Strong Risk Factors

Anxiety during pregnancy

Depression during pregnancy

Stressful life events during pregnancy

Low level of social support: single marital status

History of depression

Postpartum depression after a prior pregnancy

Additional Risk Factors

Biologic vulnerability

Family history of depression or postpartum depression

Unplanned pregnancy

Young maternal age

Lower socioeconomic status, financial insecurity

History of interpersonal violence

Thyroid dysfunction

thoughts that are associated with depression symptomatology. Hall and Wittkowski[136] in the United Kingdom developed a questionnaire of postpartum negative thoughts through qualitative interviews with 10 postpartum women who were suffering from postpartum depression. They then distributed 354 questionnaires, along with the Edinburgh Postnatal Depression Scale (EPDS), to potential participants at 42 baby-weight clinics. Of the 185 women who returned the questionnaires, 22 who scored 12 or higher on the EPDS were excluded from the analysis, as the purpose of the study was to assess negative thoughts in women who did not screen positive for depression. Items on the Negative Thoughts questionnaire were scored as "not at all," "occasionally," "frequently," or "almost always." Three of the items on the questionnaire were experienced either frequently or almost always by more than 15% of participants: 26.6% for "Everything in my life should revolve around my baby"; 19.8% for "I must show everyone that I am coping"; and 15.9% for "As a mother, everything must be perfect." The feeling that "My baby could die" was experienced either frequently or almost always by 9.5% of participants, and 9.8% indicated having thoughts similar to "If there is something wrong with my baby, it's my fault."

In 2005, Childbirth Connection conducted a two-stage national survey of women giving birth in the United States. This survey collected data from women between 18 and 45 years who had given birth to live infants during 2005. The majority of the sample (n = 1373) completed the survey online, but an additional 200 minority women were interviewed by phone to ensure a sample that was representative of the U.S. population. The first stage of the survey was administered to women at a mean of 7.3 months postpartum, and covered characteristics, behaviors, and knowledge prior to and during pregnancy, labor and birth, and early postpartum. Participants in the first stage completed variables assessing physical symptoms, health behaviors, and postpartum depression. Postpartum depression was assessed via the Postpartum Depression Screening Scale-Short form (PDSS—Short Form). The second stage was administered 6 months following the first stage. This follow-up study included 859 of the original 1373 women via an online survey, and 44 of the original 200 women were evaluated by telephone interview. The same instrument was used to assess physical symptoms and health behavior, and the PHQ-2 was used to assess depressive symptoms. In addition, participants completed the Posttraumatic Stress Disorder Symptom Scale Self-Report, which had been adapted for use postpartum.[137]

A majority (63%) of the women reported depressive symptoms on the first survey, with the most frequent dimension being emotional lability. At the 6-month follow-up study, 42% of the stage 2 participants reported symptoms of depression. In total, 305 (22.2% of the initial cohort) women reported depressive symptoms at both times. Public or self-insurance and unplanned pregnancy were associated with higher scores on the PDSS—Short Form. Variables associated with higher depressive symptom scores on the PHQ-2 at the 6-month follow-up visit included lack of private insurance, as well as being pregnant at the time of the survey, not returning to work, and multiparity. Higher scores on the PTSD scale were also associated with more depressive symptoms. Exclusive breastfeeding at 1 month and being able to breastfeed as long as desired were associated with lower scores, as was engaging in more health-promoting behaviors.[137] Clearly, depressive symptoms exist in many more women than meet the diagnostic threshold for "postpartum depression."

Effects of Postpartum Depression on the Family

Partners of women with postpartum depression are also at risk for depression, having up to 2.5 times the risk of developing depression when compared to individuals whose partners are not depressed.[138]

Depressed women may be less responsive to their infants. They are less likely to engage in face-to-face interactions that would otherwise contribute to infant communication skills, such as vocalizing, smiling, imitation, and gameplaying, than mothers who are not depressed. They also display less synchrony in their mother–baby interactions. Less time is spent reading, telling stories, touching and stroking, or singing to their infants.[130] In turn, untreated depression has been associated with impaired child development. Tactile contact with the infants influences the infants' sensitivity to pain, affect, and growth.[139,140] Animal research has shown that tactile stimulation in infancy can have epigenetic effects on brain architecture and function that can persist into adolescence and childhood. Similar effects can also be seen, again in animal studies, from childhood abuse and neglect. Infants appear to have neuroplasticity such that either maternal or early infant/childhood intervention may attenuate the long-term effects of infant neglect of abuse.

In addition to epigenetic studies with animals, human studies have found consistent evidence for the long-term effects of PPD on subsequent childhood development and behavior.[128,141] Many women with PPD were also depressed during the pregnancy, so in some cases it is difficult to separate the contribution of prenatal depression from that of postpartum depression.

Screening for Postpartum Depression

There is a lack of consensus about the benefits of routine screening for PPD. The American College of Obstetricians and Gynecologists' Committee on Obstetric Practice states that although screening for PPD should be "strongly considered," there is insufficient evidence to support a firm recommendation for universal postpartum screening.[142] Hewitt et al.[143] reviewed the existing literature on the benefits of screening for PPD, and concluded that there was inadequate evidence of clinical and cost effectiveness to recommend universal screening, but suggested that using the two-question screen (PHQ-2) deserves study. The U.S. Preventive Services Task Force does not make specific recommendations regarding screening for depression in the postpartum period, but recommends screening when staff-assisted supports to ensure accurate diagnosis, effective treatment, and appropriate follow-up are in place. While there are varied opinions regarding universal screening for PPD, performing screening in women with any of the

risk factors described in Box 9-7 will identify many women with PPD who would otherwise remain unrecognized and untreated.

Several tools ar available to screen for PPD. Whereas the PHQ-9 is gaining favor for screening for depression in the general population, it does not include items that are specific to childbirth. The EPDS, which was developed in the mid-1980s specifically for use in the postpartum period, consists of a 10-item self-report scale. It is available for use free of charge, and has been well validated for use both during pregnancy and postpartum.[134] The scale may be completed by the mother while waiting to be seen for a postpartum appointment, and reviewed with her by her provider. The Postpartum Depression Screening Scale (PDSS) is another tool developed for use in the postpartum period. It is self-administered, and is available as a long form of 35 items or the previously mentioned abbreviated "short" form of 7 items.[144] The PDSS also is well validated, and it may be used to evaluate response to treatment in a depressed woman. Both the EDPS and the PDSS appear to be more accurate in identifying postpartum depression than generic screening tools for depression such as the CES-D or BDI.[145] A major advantage of the EPDS over the PDSS is the ability to employ the tool free of charge, whereas a charge is levied for the PDSS manual and forms.[144]

All of the screening tools are just that—screens. A positive result on any screen should be followed up with a diagnostic evaluation by a qualified clinician to establish an accurate diagnosis. The screening tools also do not differentiate between unipolar or bipolar depression, so women identified as being depressed should be evaluated for a history or symptoms of mania or hypomania. A positive response to the questions that assess suicidality—question number 9 on the PHQ-9 or question number 10 on the EPDS—requires immediate attention by the clinician. The diagnosis of postpartum thyroiditis should be considered for depressed women with a history of autoimmune disorders.[146]

The optimal time to screen for PPD is between 2 weeks to 6 months postpartum,[128] as the point prevalence of postpartum depression has bimodal peaks at 2 and 6 months postpartum.[145] Following a 6-week postpartum visit, women are less likely to be in contact with their obstetric provider, so many women who develop PPD will go unrecognized if screening depends on self-recognition or recognition by family or friends. For this reason, it has been recommended that screening for PPD be incorporated in the the infant's well-child visits to the pediatric care provider. The American Academy of Pediatrics suggests that pediatricians should have a low threshold of suspicion for parental depression and consider, at a minimum, asking parents the two questions in the PHQ-2. Gjerdingen et al. studied the value of administering the PHQ-2 to women during well-child visits, followed by the PHQ-9 if the initial screen was positive. They found that the PHQ-2 was highly sensitive (100%) but had a specificity of only 44%. By comparison, the PHQ-9 had a sensitivity of only 82%, with higher specificity of 84%. These researchers concluded that a two-stage screening procedure, beginning with the two-question screen and followed by the PHQ-9 if indicated, is a worthwhile and easily implemented strategy.[147]

Prevention of Postpartum Depression

Primary prevention and secondary prevention addressing early detection and intervention are always preferable to dealing with the sequelae of an illness. Identifying a vulnerability to PPD may allow an opportunity to recommend interventions that may decrease the risk for PPD. Interventions that may help prevent postpartum depression include interpersonal psychotherapy, regular physical activity, improving or developing a social support system, and arranging to obtain sufficient sleep postpartum.[148,149] Many of these behaviors can be fostered prior to or during pregnancy. For example, counseling regarding exercise (especially outdoors), healthy eating, and good sleep habits can be reinforced at each prenatal visit, not only to ensure the physical well-being of the pregnancy, but also to promote the mother's mental well-being.

CenteringPregnancy has been shown to improve social support and be associated with less depression at 1 year postpartum.[150,151] Joining other support groups may also help women to develop coping skills.

Psychotherapy may help a woman learn to identify and access sources of support from family and friends, thereby avoiding the development of postpartum depression. Women who are at risk for PPD who have a desire to avoid medication may be especially receptive to this advice. If a woman has experienced depression prior to the pregnancy, but opted to discontinue the medication during the pregnancy, her plan of care may be to restart the medication immediately postpartum, and continue it for at least 6 months.[149]

Placing the newly born infant in skin-to-skin contact with the mother has been documented to provide many maternal and infant benefits, including a more stable physiologic transition, less crying, and more restful sleep.[148] These neonatal adaptations in and of themselves may allow for less maternal stress. In a quasi-experimental study, Bigelow et al.[148] evaluated the effects of continuing daily skin-to-skin contact throughout the first month. Women giving birth in one of two hospitals were initially assigned to the skin-to-skin contact group, whereas those giving birth at the second hospital received routine counseling. Halfway through the study, the assignments of the hospitals were switched. Participants completed self-report depression scales at 1 week and 1, 2, and 3 months postpartum. Women in the skin-to-skin contact group reported significantly lower scores on both the EPDS and CES-D scales at the 1-week and 1-month visits. This benefit attenuated over time, and no clinically or statistically significant differences were noted at 2 or 3 months postpartum.

Management of Postpartum Depression

Identifying women with PPD is only half the battle. Helping women to obtain appropriate treatment is also necessary to have the desired impact on the health of mothers and their families. Unfortunately, only a minority of women who screened positive for depression are referred for treatment or follow through with their care.[138] The primary care provider is in the best position to maintain ongoing contact with the woman to reinforce ongoing treatment. Such follow-up will decrease the chance that the woman discontinues treatment before attaining a satisfactory response.

Accumulated data from many studies indicate that psychotherapy is helpful for women with mild to moderate PPD, and women who are breastfeeding may opt to begin treatment with psychotherapy.[103,152] The evidence most strongly supports the benefits of interpersonal psychotherapy and cognitive-behavioral therapy for PPD.[103]

Pharmacotherapy

After excluding the diagnosis of bipolar disorder, a midwife may recommend or prescribe antidepressants for the woman with PPD. The same considerations that make SSRIs the first-line antidepressants for MDD unrelated to childbirth makes them the mainstay for pharmacologic treatment for PPD. Any of the SSRIs listed in Table 9-5 can be considered for use postpartum. Guidelines for postpartum antidepressant management are presented in **Figure 9-5**. There is no evidence that one medication is better than any other in the SSRI category,[153] and the choice of which SSRI to prescribe is based on similar considerations as when starting an SSRI at another time. These factors include patient preference and

Pharmacologic Treatment of Postpartum Major Depression

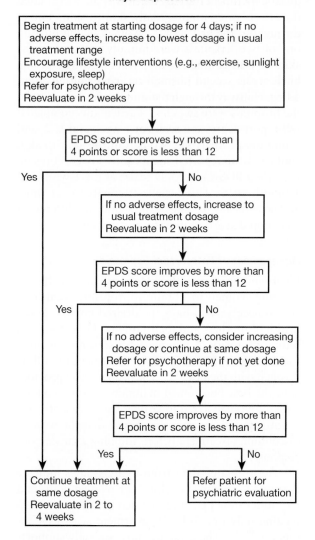

Figure 9-5 Pharmacologic treatment algorithm for postpartum major depression.

Source: Reprinted with permission from Postpartum Major Depression, October 15, 2010, Vol 82, No 8, *American Family Physician* Copyright © 2010 American Academy of Family Physicians. All Rights Reserved.

Many nursing women, pediatricians, and obstetric care providers have concerns about the effects of antidepressants on breastfed infants. Fortunately, research findings have been reassuring about the safety of breastfeeding while taking many of the antidepressants. Breastfed infants' serum levels of sertraline (Zoloft), paroxetine (Paxil), and nortriptyline (a tricyclic antidepressant) have been undetectable, and levels of fluoxetine (Prozac) and citalopram (Celexa) in such infants are detectable, but extremely low.[153] A variety of reputable, evidence-based online resources can help guide decisions about medication use during pregnancy and breastfeeding.

The approach to starting pharmacotherapy for PPD is to begin at a low dose for 4 to 7 days, then titrate the dose upward until remission is achieved. Whichever tool was used to initially screen for PPD, whether the EPDS or the PHQ-9, should also be used to monitor the response to treatment. Antidepressant therapy should be continued for 6 to 9 months after achieving remission. Counsel the woman that if the medication is stopped abruptly, she may experience unpleasant symptoms; thus the agent should be tapered over a period of at least 2 weeks.

Postpartum Bipolar Disorder and Postpartum Psychosis

Although the prevalence of bipolar disorder (BPD) is low,[1] there is a significant risk of relapse following birth. Women who were diagnosed with BPD prior to pregnancy are best cared for by a multidisciplinary team including a psychiatrist to manage medications and decrease the chance of a relapse. Between 80% and 100% of women who discontinue their mood stabilizer medication during pregnancy experience a relapse. While the discontinuation of medication is the most important risk factor for relapse, the hormonal and circadian rhythm alterations that occur postpartum are also important factors. Women experiencing a bipolar episode postpartum often appear overly euphoric, talkative, and less in need for sleep. Conversely, they may present with the depressive symptoms associated with the disorder. BPD may also present as postpartum psychosis. Any woman with a history of BPD, or exhibiting signs of either mania or hypomania, should be assessed by a psychiatric clinician.

Postpartum psychosis is a rare and life-threatening emergency condition that requires immediate psychiatric evaluation. It is seen among 0.1% to 0.2% of women, and may occur anytime in the first year postpartum. The peak incidence occurs during the first 2 weeks postpartum.[155] Women with BPD

past response to any given medication. A decision to begin an antidepressant is made jointly by the mother and her care provider after a thorough discussion of risks and benefits, including the potential effects of postpartum depression on her infant and any other children. Women who feel that a treatment decision has been imposed on them are less likely to follow through with the treatment regimen. Most postpartum women will need higher than the starting doses to achieve a therapeutic effect; Wisner et al., found that 50% of women needed 100 mg/day of sertraline (Zoloft) to achieve remission.[154]

are at a much higher risk for developing postpartum psychosis than other women, and many women who present with postpartum psychosis are ultimately diagnosed with BPD. Autoimmune thyroid disease may also contribute to the development of postpartum psychosis. Bergink et al. recommend checking thyroperoxidase antibodies in women with BPD or a history of postpartum psychosis.[110] Women suffering from postpartum psychosis have a 4% to 5% risk of either suicide or infanticide.[138]

Postpartum Post-traumatic Stress Disorder

Post-traumatic stress disorder is a response to a traumatic event, followed by reexperiencing the event with nightmares, flashbacks, or other intrusive thoughts; avoidance of anything associated with the traumatic event and/or emotional numbing; and alterations in arousal such as sleep disturbance, difficulty concentrating, or aggressive behavior.[8,63] The reported incidence of postpartum PTSD ranges from 1% to more than 7%, with the higher incidence based on the Modified PTSD Symptom Scale Self-Report (MPSS-SR) and the lower incidence based on the structured Clinical Interview for *DSM-IV* (SCID-I).[63,64,156] Culture plays a large role in the risk of exposure to trauma and the resulting prevalence of PTSD. Many more women suffer from "partial" PTSD, reporting reexperiencing as well as arousal and/or avoidance symptoms. Some consider partial PTSD to be a normal response following a highly stressful experience,[156] whereas others approach it as potentially impairing function and increasing the risk for full-blown PTSD in the future.

Women who have experienced childhood trauma, sexual abuse, depression, or PTSD preceding the pregnancy are at increased risk for postpartum PTSD.[64,156,157] Anxiety sensitivity, which is a tendency to respond fearfully to anxiety itself as opposed to just responding to stressors, has also been found to increase vulnerability to PTSD.[64] Depression, anxiety, or a fear of childbirth during the pregnancy are other predictors of postpartum PTSD. The traumatic stressor for postpartum PTSD is birth trauma, "an event occurring during the labor and delivery process that involves actual or threatened serious injury or death to the mother or her infant."[158] It is the subjective perception of risk that predisposes women to PTSD rather than the absolute risk. In fact, many women perceive their births as traumatic despite the perception by the clinician that everything was routine.[158] Not surprisingly, emergency cesarean delivery and and instrumental delivery are associated with PTSD—but so are negative emotions such as a negative experience of labor and birth and a loss of

control. A sense of not receiving adequate support—especially from care providers, but also from a partner—contributes to the risk for postpartum PTSD.[156]

Being alert to risk factors for postpartum PTSD and signs of crisis, such as withdrawal, signs of acute distress during labor, or dissociative behaviors, may allow midwives to identify women at high risk for postpartum PTSD, and provides the opportunity to offer more intensive support and communication during labor and make an early referral if indicated. Limited research has addressed treatment for PTSD specifically following childbirth; those studies that have been conducted suggest that many of the same therapies that are employed for PTSD in general have a benefit for postpartum PTSD. These measures include debriefing and counseling, cognitive-behavioral therapy, and eye movement desensitization and reprocessing.[63]

Conclusion

Millions of women are afflicted by mental health disorders in the United States, which are likely to affect the well-being of families and individuals. For some of these women, the midwife may be the first—and in some cases, the only—healthcare provider available. As primary care providers, midwives are, at a minimum, responsible for appropriate screening and referral for women at risk for mental health conditions. A system of universal screening will help identify those individuals with mental health concerns, and determine who can be treated safely within a primary care setting and who should be referred for more specialized treatment. With psychiatric consultation and collaboration, midwives can provide first-line treatment for many women.

Psychopharmacology is an important component of treatment for mental health disorders. With careful screening, counseling, follow-up, and potential referral, this treatment strategy can be within the scope of midwifery practice. As when prescribing any medication regimen, it is essential that the midwife be familiar with psychotropic medications.

Women's susceptibility to mental health disorders is influenced by their life stage and hormonal status. Pregnancy and the puerperium are times characterized by dramatic hormonal shifts, which when compounded with the stresses of becoming a parent can place a woman at increased risk for mood and anxiety disorders. Early identification and treatment can decrease long-term morbidity, but at the same time potential effects of medications on the fetus and the nursing newborn must be considered.

• • • **References**

1. Kessler RC, Berglund P, Demler O, Jin R, Merikangas KR, Walters EE. Lifetime prevalence and age-of-onset distributions of *DSM-IV* disorders in the National Comorbidity Survey Replication. *Arch Gen Psychiatry*. 2005;62:593-602.

2. Seedat S, Scott KM, Angermeyer MC, et al. Cross-national associations between gender and mental disorders in the World Health Organization World Mental Health Surveys. *Arch Gen Psychiatry*. 2009;66:785-795.

3. Kendler KS, Gardner CO. A longitudinal etiologic model for symptoms of anxiety and depression in women. *Psychol Med*. 2011;41:2035-2045.

4. Kendler KS, Gardner CO, Gatz M, Pedersen NL. The sources of co-morbidity between major depression and generalized anxiety disorder in a Swedish national twin sample. *Psychol Med*. 2007;37:453-462.

5. Hettema JM. The nosologic relationship between generalized anxiety disorder and major depression. *Depress Anxiety*. 2008;25:300-316.

6. Etkin A, Prater KE, Schatzberg AF, et al. Disrupted amygdalar subregion functional connectivity and evidence of a compensatory network in generalized anxiety disorder. *Arch Gen Psychiatry*. 2009;66: 1361-1372.

7. Price JL, Drevets WC. Neurocircuitry of mood disorders. *Neuropsychopharmacology*. 2010;35:192-216.

8. American Psychiatric Association. *Diagnostic and Statistical Manual of Mental Disorders*. 5th ed. Arlington, VA: APA; 2013.

9. Gaynes BN, DeVeaugh-Geiss J, Weir S, et al. Feasibility and diagnostic validity of the M-3 Checklist: a brief, self-rated screen for depressive, bipolar, anxiety, and post-traumatic stress disorders in primary care. *Ann Fam Med*. 2010;8:160-169.

10. Strine TW, Mokdad AH, Balluz LS, et al. Depression and anxiety in the United States: findings from the 2006 behavioral risk factor surveillance system. *Psychiatr Serv*. 2008;59:1383-1390.

11. Merikangas KR, Ames M, Cui L, et al. The impact of comorbidity of mental and physical conditions on role disability in the US adult household population. *Arch Gen Psychiatry*. 2007;64:1180-1188.

12. Unutzer J, Park M. Strategies to improve the management of depression in primary care. *Primary Care*. 2012;39:415-431.

13. Trangle M, Dieperink B, Gabert T, et al. *Major Depression in Adults in Primary Care*. Bloomington, MN: Institute for Clinical Systems Improvement (ICSI); 2012.

14. Kessler RC, Berglund P, Demler O, et al. The epidemiology of major depressive disorder: results from the National Comorbidity Survey Replication (NCS-R). *JAMA*. 2003;289:3095-3105.

15. Hackley B, Sharma C, Kedzior A, Sreenivasan S. Managing mental health conditions in primary care settings. *J Midwifery Women's Health*. 2010;55:9-19.

16. Moussavi S, Chatterji S, Verdes E, Tandon A, Patel V, Ustun B. Depression, chronic diseases, and decrements in health: results from the World Health Surveys. *Lancet*. 2007;370:851-858.

17. Arroll B, Khin N, Kerse N. Screening for depression in primary care with two verbally asked questions: cross sectional study. *BMK+J*. 2003;327:1144-1146.

18. Arroll B, Goodyear-Smith F, Kerse N, Fishman T, Gunn J. Effect of the addition of a "help" question to two screening questions on specificity for diagnosis of depression in general practice: diagnostic validity study. *BMJ*. 2005;331:884.

19. Lombardo P, Vaucher P, Haftgoli N, et al. The "help" question doesn't help when screening for major depression: external validation of the three-question screening test for primary care patients managed for physical complaints. *BMC Med*. 2011;9:114.

20. Sharp LK, Lipsky MS. Screening for depression across the lifespan: a review of measures for use in primary care settings. *Am Fam Phys*. 2002;66:1001-1008.

21. Berginik V, Kooistra L, Lambregtse-van den Berg MP, et al. Validation of the Edinburgh Depression Scale during pregnancy. *J Psychiatr Res*. 2011;70:385-389.

22. U.S. Department of Health and Human Services. *Depression in Primary Care: Volume 1. Detection and Diagnosis*. AHCPR Publication No. 93-0550. Rockville, MD: Agency for Health Care Policy and Research; 1993:20.

23. U.S. Preventive Services Task Force. Screening for depression in adults: U.S. Preventive Services Task Force recommendation statement. *Ann Intern Med*. 2009;151:784-792.

24. Breedlove G, Fryzelka D. Depression screening during pregnancy. *J Midwifery Women's Health*. 2011;56: 18-25.

25. Maurer DM. Screening for depression. *Am Fam Phys*. 2012;85:139-144.

26. Gureje O. Dysthymia in a cross-cultural perspective. *Curr Opin Psychiatry*. 2011;24:67-71.

27. Dunner DL. Dysthymia and double depression. *Int Rev Psychiatry*. 2005;17:3-8.

28. Spitzer RL, Williams JB, Kroenke K, et al. Utility of a new procedure for diagnosing mental disorders in primary care: the PRIME-MD 1000 study. *JAMA*. 1994;272:1749-1756.

29. Klein DN, Shankman SA, Rose S. Ten-year prospective follow-up study of the naturalistic course of dysthymic disorder and double depression. *Am J Psychiatry*. 2006;163:872-880.

30. Rhebergen D, Beekman AT, de Graaf R, et al. Trajectories of recovery of social and physical functioning in major depression, dysthymic disorder and

double depression: a 3-year follow-up. *J Affect Disord.* 2010;124:148-156.

31. National Collaborating Centre for Mental Health. *The NICE Guideline on the Management and Treatment of Depression in Adults* (updated edition). London, UK: National Institute for Health and Clinical Excellence; 2010.

32. DeRubeis RJ, Siegle GJ, Hollon SD. Cognitive therapy versus medication for depression: treatment outcomes and neural mechanisms. *Nat Rev Neurosci.* 2008;9:788-796.

33. Oestergaard S, Moldrup C. Optimal duration of combined psychotherapy and pharmacotherapy for patients with moderate and severe depression: a meta-analysis. *J Affect Disord.* 2011;131:24-36.

34. Levkovitz Y, Tedeschini E, Papakostas GI. Efficacy of antidepressants for dysthymia: a meta-analysis of placebo-controlled randomized trials. *J Clin Psychiatry.* 2011;72(4):509-514. doi: 10.4088/JCP.09m05949blu.

35. Cuijpers P, van Straten A, Schuurmans J, van Oppen P, Hollon SD, Andersson G. Psychotherapy for chronic major depression and dysthymia: a meta-analysis. *Clin Psychol Rev.* 2010;30:51-62.

36. Hollon SD, Ponniah K. A review of empirically supported psychological therapies for mood disorders in adults. *Depress Anxiety.* 2010;27:891-932.

37. Markowitz JC, Kocsis JH, Bleiberg KL, Christos PJ, Sacks M. A comparative trial of psychotherapy and pharmacotherapy for "pure" dysthymic patients. *J Affect Disord.* 2005;89:167-175.

38. MacArthur Initiative on Depression and Primary Care. *Depression Management Tool Kit.* 2009.

39. Unutzer J, Oisha S. *Impact Intervention Manual.* Los Angeles, CA: UCLA NPI, Center for Health Services Research; 2004.

40. AIMS Center. Advancing integrated mental health solutions. 2012. Available at: http://uwaims.org/index .html. Accessed October 15, 2012.

41. Gilbody S, Bower P, Fletcher J, Richards D, Sutton AJ. Collaborative care for depression: a cumulative meta-analysis and review of longer-term outcomes. *Arch Intern Med.* 2006;166:2314-2321.

42. Williams JW Jr, Gerrity M, Holsinger T, Dobscha S, Gaynes B, Dietrich A. Systematic review of multifaceted interventions to improve depression care. *Gen Hosp Psychiatry.* 2007;29:91-116.

43. Barbui C, Cipriani A, Patel V, Ayuso-Mateos JL, van Ommeren M. Efficacy of antidepressants and benzodiazepines in minor depression: systematic review and meta-analysis. *Br J Psychiatry.* 2011;198(1):11-16.

44. Tamburrino MB, Nagel RW, Lynch DJ. Managing antidepressants in primary care: physicians' treatment modifications. *Psychol Rep.* 2011;108:799-804.

45. Freeman MP, Fava M, Lake J, Trivedi MH, Wisner KL, Mischoulon D. Complementary and alternative medicine in major depressive disorder: the American Psychiatric Association Task Force report. *J Clin Psychiatry.* 2010;71:669-681.

46. Titov N. Internet-delivered psychotherapy for depression in adults. *Curr Opin Psychiatry.* 2011;24:18-23.

47. King T, Johnson R, Gamblian V. Mental health. In: King TL, Brucker MC, eds. *Pharmacology for Women's Health.* Sudbury, MA: Jones and Bartlett; 2011:750-791.

48. Qaseem A, Snow V, Denberg TD, Forciea MA, Owens DK, Clinical Efficacy Assessment Subcommittee of American College of Physicians. Using second-generation antidepressants to treat depressive disorders: a clinical practice guideline from the American College of Physicians. *Ann Intern Med.* 2008;149: 725-733.

49. American Psychiatric Association. *Practice Guideline for the Treatment of Patients with Major Depressive Disorder.* 3rd ed. Arlington, VA: APA; 2010.

50. Lai MW, Klein-Schwartz W, Rodgers GC, et al. 2005 annual report of the American Association of Poison Control Centers' national poisoning and exposure database. *Clin Toxicol.* 2006;44:803-932.

51. Iqbal MM, Basil MJ, Kaplan J, Iqbal MT. Overview of serotonin syndrome. *Ann Clin Psychiatry.* 2012; 24(4):310-318.

52. Ables AZ, Nagubilli R. Prevention, recognition, and management of serotonin syndrome. *Am Fam Phys.* 2010;81:1139-1142.

53. Demyttenaere K. Bupropion and SSRI-induced side effects. *J Psychopharmacol.* 2008;22(7):792-804.

54. Sansone RA, Sansone LA. Dysthymic disorder: forlorn and overlooked? *Psychiatry.* 2009;6:46-51.

55. Kroenke K, Spitzer RL, Williams JB, Monahan PO, Lowe B. Anxiety disorders in primary care: prevalence, impairment, comorbidity, and detection. *Ann Intern Med.* 2007;146:317-325.

56. Kessler RC, Ruscio AM, Shear K, Wittchen HU. Epidemiology of anxiety disorders. *Curr Top Behav Neurosci.* 2010;2:21-35.

57. Damsa C, Kosel M, Moussally J. Current status of brain imaging in anxiety disorders. *Curr Opin Psychiatry.* 2009;22:96-110.

58. Simms LJ, Prisciandaro JJ, Krueger RF, Goldberg DP. The structure of depression, anxiety and somatic symptoms in primary care. *Psychological Med.* 2012;42:15-28.

59. Simon NM, Herlands NN, Marks EH, et al. Childhood maltreatment linked to greater symptom severity and poorer quality of life and function in social anxiety disorder. *Depress Anxiety.* 2009;26: 1027-1032.

60. Karsnitz DB, Ward S. Spectrum of anxiety disorders: diagnosis and pharmacologic treatment. *J Midwifery Women's Health.* 2011;56:266-281.

61. Marshall GN, Schell TL, Elliott MN, Berthold SM, Chun CA. Mental health of Cambodian refugees 2 decades after resettlement in the United States. *JAMA*. 2005;294:571-579.

62. Fisher BS, Cullen FT, Turner MG. *The Sexual Victimization of Women*. Washington, DC: U.S. Department of Justice, Office of Justice Programs; 2000.

63. Lapp LK, Agbokou C, Peretti CS, Ferreri F. Management of post traumatic stress disorder after childbirth: a review. *J Psychosom Obstet Gynecol*. 2010; 31:113-122.

64. Verreault N, Da Costa D, Marchand A, et al. PTSD following childbirth: a prospective study of incidence and risk factors in Canadian women. *J Psychosomat Res*. 2012;73:257-263.

65. Lukaschek K, Kruse J, Emeny RT, Lacruz ME, von Eisenhart Rothe A, Ladwig KH. Lifetime traumatic experiences and their impact on PTSD: a general population study. *Soc Psyciatry Psychiat Epidem*. September 25, 2012 [Epub ahead of print].

66. Spitzer RL, Kroenke K, Williams JB, Lowe B. A brief measure for assessing generalized anxiety disorder: the GAD-7. *Arch Intern Med*. 2006;166:1092-1097.

67. Kroenke K, Spitzer RL, Williams JB, Lowe B. The Patient Health Questionnaire Somatic, Anxiety, and Depressive Symptom Scales: a systematic review. *Gen Hosp Psychiatry*. 2010;32:345-359.

68. Robinson CM, Klenck SC, Norton PJ. Psychometric properties of the Generalized Anxiety Disorder Questionnaire for *DSM-IV* among four racial groups. *Cogn Behav Ther*. 2010;39:251-261.

69. Roy-Byrne P, Craske MG, Sullivan G, et al. Delivery of evidence-based treatment for multiple anxiety disorders primary care: a randomized controlled trial. *JAMA*. 2010;303:1921-1928.

70. Baldwin DS, Anderson IM, Nutt DJ, et al. Evidence-based guidelines for the pharmacological treatment of anxiety disorders: recommendations from the British Association for Psychopharmacology. *J Psychopharm*. 2005;19:567-596.

71. Baldwin DS, Ajel KI, Garner M. Pharmacological treatment of generalized anxiety disorder. *Curr Top Behav Neurosci*. 2010;2:453-467.

72. Hofmann SG, Smits JA. Cognitive-behavioral therapy for adult anxiety disorders: a meta-analysis of randomized placebo-controlled trials. *J Clin Psychiatry*. 2008;69:621-632.

73. Mewton L, Wong N, Andrews G. The effectiveness of Internet cognitive behavioural therapy for generalized anxiety disorder in clinical practice. *Depress Anxiety*. 2012;29:843-849.

74. Hoifodt RS, Strom C, Kolstrup N, Eisemann M, Waterloo K. Effectiveness of cognitive behavioural therapy in primary health care: a review. *Fam Pract*. 2011;28:489-504.

75. Andrews G, Cuijpers P, Craske MG, McEvoy P, Titov N. Computer therapy for the anxiety and depressive disorders is effective, acceptable and practical health care: a meta-analysis. *PloS One*. 2010;5:e13196.

76. Bandelow B, Sher , Bunevicius R, et al.; WFSBP Task Force on Mental Disorders in Primary Care; WFSBP Task Force on Anxiety Disorders, OCD and PTSD. Guidelines for the pharmacological treatment of anxiety disorders, obsessive–compulsive disorder and post-traumatic stress disorder in primary care. *J Psychiatry Clin Pract*. 2012;16(2):77-84.

77. Baldwin DS, Waldman S, Allgulander C. Evidence-based pharmacological treatment of generalized anxiety disorder. *Int J Neuropsychopharmacol*. 2011;14: 697-710.

78. Batelaan NM, Van Balkom AJ, Stein DJ. Evidence-based pharmacotherapy of panic disorder: an update. *Int J Neuropsychopharmacol*. 2011:1-13.

79. Ravindran LN, Stein MB. The pharmacologic treatment of anxiety disorders: a review of progress. *J Clin Psychiatry*. 2010;71:839-854.

80. Huh J, Goebert D, Takeshita J, Lu BY, Kang M. Treatment of generalized anxiety disorder: a comprehensive review of the literature for psychopharmacologic alternatives to newer antidepressants and benzodiazepines. *Prim Car Companion CNS Disord*. 2011;3(2):PCC.08r00709.

81. American Psychiatric Association. *Diagnostic and Statistical Manual of Mental Disorders*. 4th ed., text revision. Washington, DC: American Psychiatric Association; 2000.

82. Kadian S, O'Brien S. Classification of premenstrual disorders as proposed by the International Society for Premenstrual Disorders. *Menopause Int*. 2012;18: 43-47.

83. O'Brien PM, Backstrom T, Brown C, et al. Towards a consensus on diagnostic criteria, measurement and trial design of the premenstrual disorders: the ISPMD Montreal consensus. *Arch Women's Ment Health*. 2011;14:13-21.

84. Epperson CN, Steiner M, Hartlage SA, et al. Premenstrual dysphoric disorder: evidence for a new category for *DSM-5*. *Am J Psychiatry*. 2012;169: 465-475.

85. Pearlstein T, Steiner M. Premenstrual dysphoric disorder: burden of illness and treatment update. *J Psychiatry Neurosci*. 2008;33:291-301.

86. Fornaro M, Perugi G. The impact of premenstrual dysphoric disorder among 92 bipolar patients. *Euro Psychiatry: J Assoc Euro Psychiatrists*. 2010;25: 450-454.

87. Schmidt PJ, Nieman LK, Danaceau MA, Adams LF, Rubinow DR. Differential behavioral effects of gonadal steroids in women with and in those without premenstrual syndrome. *N Engl J Med*. 1998;338:209-216.

88. Rubinow DR, Schmidt PJ. Gonadal steroid regulation of mood: the lessons of premenstrual syndrome. *Frontiers Neuroendocrinol.* 2006;27:210-216.

89. Pearlstein TB, Bachmann GA, Zacur HA, Yonkers KA. Treatment of premenstrual dysphoric disorder with a new drospirenone-containing oral contraceptive formulation. *Contraception.* 2005;72:414-421.

90. Yonkers KA, Brown C, Pearlstein TB, Foegh M, Sampson-Landers C, Rapkin A. Efficacy of a new low-dose oral contraceptive with drospirenone in premenstrual dysphoric disorder. *Obstet Gynecol.* 2005;106:492-501.

91. Coffee AL, Kuehl TJ, Willis S, Sulak PJ. Oral contraceptives and premenstrual symptoms: comparison of a 21/7 and extended regimen. *Am J Obstet Gynecol.* 2006;195:1311-1319.

92. Shah NR, Jones JB, Aperi J, Shemtov R, Karne A, Borenstein J. Selective serotonin reuptake inhibitors for premenstrual syndrome and premenstrual dysphoric disorder: a meta-analysis. *Obstet Gynecol.* 2008;111:1175-1182.

93. Kornstein SG, Pearlstein TB, Fayyad R, Farfel GM, Gillespie JA. Low-dose sertraline in the treatment of moderate-to-severe premenstrual syndrome: efficacy of 3 dosing strategies. *J Clin Psychiatry.* 2006;67:1624-132.

94. Di Carlo C, Palomba S, Tommaselli GA, Guida M, Di Spiezio Sardo A, Nappi C. Use of leuprolide acetate plus tibolone in the treatment of severe premenstrual syndrome. *Fert Steril.* 2001;75:380-384.

95. Cronje WH, Vashisht A, Studd JW. Hysterectomy and bilateral oophorectomy for severe premenstrual syndrome. *Hum Reprod.* 2004;19:2152-55.

96. Joffe H, Petrillo LF, Viguera AC, et al. Treatment of premenstrual worsening of depression with adjunctive oral contraceptive pills: a preliminary report. *J Clin Psychiatry.* 2007;68:1954-1962.

97. Pinkerton JV, Guico-Pabia CJ, Taylor HS. Menstrual cycle–related exacerbation of disease. *Am J Obstet Gynecol.* 2010;202:221-231.

98. Davalos DB, Yadon CA, Tregellas HC. Untreated prenatal maternal depression and the potential risks to offspring: a review. *Arch Women's Ment Health.* 2012;15:1-14.

99. Cohen LS, Altshuler LL, Harlow BL, et al. Relapse of major depression during pregnancy in women who maintain or discontinue antidepressant treatment. *JAMA.* 2006;295:499-507.

100. Meltzer-Brody S. New insights into perinatal depression: pathogenesis and treatment during pregnancy and postpartum. *Dialogues Clin Neurosci.* 2011;13:89-100.

101. Robertson E, Grace S, Wallington T, Stewart DE. Antenatal risk factors for postpartum depression: a synthesis of recent literature. *Gen Hosp Psychiatry.* 2004;26:289-295.

102. Chojenta C, Loxton D, Lucke J. How do previous mental health, social support, and stressful life events contribute to postnatal depression in a representative sample of Australian women? *J Midwifery Women's Health.* 2012;57:145-150.

103. Yonkers KA, Vigod S, Ross LE. Diagnosis, pathophysiology, and management of mood disorders in pregnant and postpartum women. *Obstet Gynecol.* 2011;117:961-977.

104. Sylven SM, Elenis E, Michelakos T, et al. Thyroid function tests at delivery and risk for postpartum depressive symptoms. *Psychoneuroendocrinology.* 2012;38(7):1007-1013.

105. Cox JL, Holden JM, Sagovsky R. Detection of postnatal depression: development of the 10-item Edinburgh Postnatal Depression Scale. *Br J Psychiatry.* 1987;150:782-786.

106. Altshuler LL, Cohen LS, Vitonis AF, et al. The Pregnancy Depression Scale (PDS): a screening tool for depression in pregnancy. *Arch Women's Ment Health.* 2008;11:277-285.

107. Yonkers KA, Gotman N, Smith MV, et al. Does antidepressant use attenuate the risk of a major depressive episode in pregnancy? *Epidemiology.* 2011;22:848-854.

108. Viguera AC, Whitfield T, Baldessarini RJ, et al. Risk of recurrence in women with bipolar disorder during pregnancy: prospective study of mood stabilizer discontinuation. *Am J Psychiatry.* 2007;164:1817-1824.

109. Doyle K, Heron J, Berrisford G, et al. The management of bipolar disorder in the perinatal period and risk factors for postpartum relapse. *Euro Psychiatry: J Assoc Euro Psychiatrists.* 2012;27:563-569.

110. Bergink V, Bouvy PF, Vervoort JS, Koorengevel KM, Steegers EA, Kushner SA. Prevention of postpartum psychosis and mania in women at high risk. *Am J Psychiatry.* 2012;169:609-615.

111. Buist A, Gotman N, Yonkers KA. Generalized anxiety disorder: course and risk factors in pregnancy. *J Affect Disord.* 2011;131:277-283.

112. Chaudron LH, Nirodi N. The obsessive–compulsive spectrum in the perinatal period: a prospective pilot study. *Arch Women's Ment Health.* 2010;13:403-410.

113. Grigoriadis S, de Camps Meschino D, Barrons E, et al. Mood and anxiety disorders in a sample of Canadian perinatal women referred for psychiatric care. *Arch Women's Ment Health.* 2011;14:325-333.

114. Hackley B. Antidepressant medication use in pregnancy. *J Midwifery Women's Health.* 2010;55:90-100.

115. Latendresse G, Ruiz RJ. Maternal corticotropin-releasing hormone and the use of selective serotonin

reuptake inhibitors independently predict the occurrence of preterm birth. *J Midwifery Women's Health.* 2011;56:118-126.

116. Massachussetts General Hospital. 2012. Available at: http://www.womensmentalhealth.org. Accessed December 6, 2012.

117. Organization of Teratology Specialists. 2012. Available at: http://www.otispregnancy.org. Accessed January 12, 2013.

118. Motherisk. Hospital for Sick Children. 2012. Available at: http://www.motherisk.org/women/index.jsp. Accessed January 12, 2013.

119. Mitchell AA, Gilboa SM, Werler MM, et al. Medication use during pregnancy, with particular focus on prescription drugs: 1976-2008. *Am J Obstet Gynecol.* 2011;205(51):e1-e8.

120. Jimenez-Solem E, Andersen JT, Petersen M, et al. Exposure to selective serotonin reuptake inhibitors and the risk of congenital malformations: a nationwide cohort study. *BMJ Open.* 2012;2:e001148.

121. Diav-Citrin O, Ornoy A. Selective serotonin reuptake inhibitors in human pregnancy: to treat or not to treat? *Obstet Gynecol Int.* 2012;2012:698947.

122. Kieler H, Artama M, Engeland A, et al. Selective serotonin reuptake inhibitors during pregnancy and risk of persistent pulmonary hypertension in the newborn: population based cohort study from the five Nordic countries. *BMJ.* 2011;344:d8012.

123. Moses-Kolko EL, Bogen D, Perel J, et al. Neonatal signs after late in utero exposure to serotonin reuptake inhibitors: literature review and implications for clinical applications. *JAMA.* 2005;293: 2372-2383.

124. Sit DK, Perel JM, Helsel JC, Wisner KL. Changes in antidepressant metabolism and dosing across pregnancy and early postpartum. *J Clin Psychiatry.* 2008; 69:652-658.

125. Breese McCoy SJ. Postpartum depression: an essential overview for the practitioner. *Soc Med J.* 2011;104:128-132.

126. Bernstein IH, Rush AJ, Yonkers K, et al. Symptom features of postpartum depression: are they distinct? *Depress Anxiety.* 2008;25:20-26.

127. Beck CT. Postpartum depression: it isn't just the blues. *Am J Nurs.* 2006;106:40-50.

128. Pearlstein T, Howard M, Salisbury A, Zlotnick C. Postpartum depression. *Am J Obstet Gynecol.* 2009; 200:357-364.

129. Callister LC, Beckstrand RL, Corbett C. Postpartum depression and culture: Pesado Corazon. *MCN Am J Mat Child Nurs.* 2010;35:254-261; quiz 61-63.

130. Field T. Postpartum depression effects on early interactions, parenting, and safety practices: a review. *Infant Behav Develop.* 2010;33:1-6.

131. Forty L, Jones L, Macgregor S, et al. Familiality of postpartum depression in unipolar disorder: results of a family study. *Am J Psychiatry.* 2006;163: 1549-1553.

132. Munk-Olsen T, Laursen TM, Pedersen CB, Mors O, Mortensen PB. New parents and mental disorders: a population-based register study. *JAMA.* 2006;296:2582-2589.

133. Gavin NI, Gaynes BN, Lohr KN, Meltzer-Brody S, Gartlehner G, Swinson T. Perinatal depression: a systematic review of prevalence and incidence. *Obstet Gynecol.* 2005;106:1071-1083.

134. Clare CA, Yeh J. Postpartum depression in special populations: a review. *Obstet Gynecol Surv.* 2012; 67:313-323.

135. Toohey J. Depression during pregnancy and postpartum. *Clin Obstet Gynecol.* 2012;55:788-797.

136. Hall PL, Wittkowski A. An exploration of negative thoughts as a normal phenomenon after childbirth. *J Midwifery Women's Health.* 2006;51:321-330.

137. Beck CT, Gable RK, Sakala C, Declercq ER. Postpartum depressive symptomatology: results from a two-stage US national survey. *J Midwifery Women's Health.* 2011;56:427-435.

138. National Institute for Health Care Management Foundation. *Identifying and Treating Maternal Depression: Strategies and Considerations for Health Plans.* Issue Brief June 2010. Available at: http://nihcm .org/pdf/FINAL_MaternalDepression6-7.pdf. Accessed May 19, 2013.

139. Field T. Touch for socioemotional and physical wellbeing: a review. *Develop Rev.* 2010;30:367-383.

140. Alwan S, Reefhuis J, Rasmussen SA, Olney RS, Friedman JM, National Birth Defects Prevention Society. Use of selective serotonin-reuptake inhibitors in pregnancy and the risk of birth defects. *N Engl J Med.* 2007;356:2684-2692.

141. Cuijpers P, Brannmark JG, van Straten A. Psychological treatment of postpartum depression: a meta-analysis. *J Clin Psychol.* 2008;64:103-118.

142. American College of Obstetricians and Gynecologists, Committee on Obstetric Practice. Committee opinion no. 453: Screening for depression during and after pregnancy. *Obstet Gynecol.* 2010;115:394-395.

143. Hewitt C, Gilbody S, Brealey S, et al. Methods to identify postnatal depression in primary care: an integrated evidence synthesis and value of information analysis. *Health Technol Assess.* 2009;13:1-145, 7-230.

144. Postpartum Depression Screening Scale. Available at: http://portal.wpspublish.com/portal/page ?_pageid=53,70428&_dad=portal&_schema= PORTAL. Accessed December 1, 2012.

145. Gaynes BN, Gavin N, Meltzer-Brody S, et al. Perinatal depression: prevalence, screening accuracy, and

screening outcomes. *Evidence Rep Technol Assess.* 2005 Feb;(119):1-8

146. Stagnaro-Green A. Approach to the patient with postpartum thyroiditis. *J Clin Endocrinol Metab.* 2012;97:334-342.

147. Gjerdingen D, Crow S, McGovern P, Miner M, Center B. Postpartum depression screening at well-child visits: validity of a 2-question screen and the PHQ-9. *Ann Fam Med.* 2009;7:63-70.

148. Bigelow A, Power M, MacLellan-Peters J, Alex M, McDonald C. Effect of mother/infant skin-to-skin contact on postpartum depressive symptoms and maternal physiological stress. *JOGNN.* 2012;41: 369-382.

149. Miller LJ, LaRusso EM. Preventing postpartum depression. *Psychiatr Clin North Am.* 2011;34: 53-65.

150. Ickovics JR, Reed E, Magriples U, Westdahl C, Schindler Rising S, Kershaw TS. Effects of group prenatal care on psychosocial risk in pregnancy: results from a randomised controlled trial. *Psychol Health.* 2011;26:235-250.

151. McNeil DA, Vekved M, Dolan SM, Siever J, Horn S, Tough SC. Getting more than they realized they needed: a qualitative study of women's experience of group prenatal care. *BMC Pregn Childbirth.* 2012;12:17.

152. National Collaborating Centre for Mental Health. *NICE Clinical Guideline 45: Antenatal and Postnatal Mental Health.* London: National Institute for Health and Clinical Excellence; 2007.

153. Hirst KP, Moutier CY. Postpartum major depression. *Am Fam Phys.* 2010;82:926-933.

154. Wisner KL, Hanusa BH, Perel JM, et al. Postpartum depression: a randomized trial of sertraline versus nortriptyline. *J Clin Psychopharm.* 2006;26: 353-360.

155. Valdimarsdottir U, Hultman CM, Harlow B, Cnattingius S, Sparen P. Psychotic illness in first-time mothers with no previous psychiatric hospitalizations: a population-based study. *PLoS Med.* 2009;6:e13.

156. Andersen LB, Melvaer LB, Videbech P, Lamont RF, Joergensen JS. Risk factors for developing post-traumatic stress disorder following childbirth: a systematic review. *Acta Obstet Gynecol Scand.* 2012;91(11):1261-1272.

157. Seng TS, Sperlich M, Low LK, Ronis DL, Muzik M, Liberzon I. Childhood abuse history, posttraumatic stress disorder, postpartum mental health and bonding: a prospective cohort study. *J Midwifery Women's Health.* 2013;58(1):57-68.

158. Beck CT. Birth trauma: in the eye of the beholder. *Nurs Res.* 2004;53:28-35.

C H A P T E R

10

Preconception Care

MARY ANN FAUCHER

Introduction

Preconception care is the healthcare services a woman or man receives that focus on the components of health that have been shown to increase the chance of having a healthy baby. Preconception care may differ for each person depending upon individual needs. The purpose of preconception care is to identify reducible or reversible risks, maximize maternal health, and intervene to achieve optimal maternal and newborn outcomes. Most importantly, preconception care is a strategy of care, not an isolated visit. Readiness for pregnancy often involves increasing knowledge, changing attitudes, and developing skills that decrease risks and promote health.[1]

For women, individual components of preconception care include a risk assessment of the woman's health history and her psychological, financial, and environmental risks; health promotion counseling, such as providing diet and lifestyle recommendations; and medical and psychosocial interventions as indicated. For some women, risks can be eliminated; for others, measures can be taken to ameliorate the effect of certain risks for a developing fetus. For the majority of women and their partners, preconception care will help identify methods to make positive lifestyle changes to improve their overall health and to promote the potential for a healthy pregnancy and baby. Preconception care provides the woman and the couple with information to make informed decisions about their childbearing.[2]

It is imperative that preconception care includes both women and men whenever possible. Although the focus on preconception care needs to be strengthened for both genders, men in particular are under-recognized for the way in which their health may influence reproductive outcomes. In this chapter, where women are solely mentioned, the reader should intuitively apply the content to men when appropriate. Similarly, this content can be applied to lesbian or transgender couples as appropriate. For example, readiness for pregnancy, screening for sexually transmitted infections, and assessment of genetic risks are all applicable to men as well as to women.

"Every Woman, Every Visit"

A good slogan to adopt in practice regarding preconception care is "Every woman, every visit." Dedication to health promotion, education, and preventive care positions midwives as ideal providers of preconception care. Every visit—from family planning, regular Pap smears, or pregnancy tests and sexually transmitted infection screenings, to postpartum or post-abortion visits—provides opportunities for counseling.

A few couples will come to a midwife seeking a preconception health assessment and anticipatory guidance. The majority, however, will present for midwifery care for many reasons, and it is left to the midwife to be proactive in providing relevant preconception information. This chapter reviews a wide range of possible topics to be considered for preconception care. The goals of preconception health are best met, however, when the focus of the health visit centers on a single risk behavior and planned intervention rather than addressing multiple concerns in one visit.[2]

Because addressing the full scope of preconception care is not realistic for each encounter, the midwife must use clinical acumen to perform individualized preconception risk assessment and target teaching/counseling regarding effective interventions. For example, at an annual visit, a woman may be encouraged to stop smoking for general health benefits; by doing so, she also avoids smoking-related problems in a future pregnancy. A negative pregnancy test visit provides an opportune time to question the woman about whether pregnancy is being attempted. Based on the answer, either contraception can be discussed based on the woman's or couple's reproductive plan or a full assessment of pregnancy-related risk factors can be undertaken.

Individualizing the preconception assessment does not necessarily prolong the time allocated during a clinical visit. Midwives and all primary care providers can bill for preconception care with a separate and distinct code from other services provided during a visit (i.e., V26.49). However, the amount paid based on that billing code varies according to commercial insurer as well as from state to state for Medicaid coverage.[3] In addition, payment for specific components of a preconception care assessment (e.g., HIV screening, vaccinations) also varies.

Why Is Preconception Care Important?

In an ideal world, all pregnancies would be planned and every infant would be conceived in a healthy environment. However, in 2006 (the latest year for which data are available), 49% of pregnancies in the United States were unintended and chronic diseases that are known to have adverse pregnancy effects remained common among reproductive-age women.[3] Among women age 19 years and younger, four of five pregnancies were not planned.[4]

The Centers for Disease Control and Prevention's (CDC's) Pregnancy Risk Assessment Monitoring System (PRAMS)—a surveillance program that collects state-specific, population-based data on maternal attitudes and experiences before, during, and shortly after pregnancy—has identified some important healthcare concerns related to preconception care. More than half of the women in the PRAMS data reported not using contraception, even though they also stated that they were not seeking pregnancy. The majority of women said they consumed alcohol, although the quantity was not identified; almost 25% of women reported tobacco use; and only 35% said they took a multivitamin four times a week, the latter being an important surrogate for folic acid ingestion to prevent fetal neural tube defects.[5] The preconception and interconception periods are clearly the optimal times to help women identify behaviors that have adverse effects for a fetus and the best time to support them in making desired changes.

History of Preconception Care

During the 1980s and 1990s, the pregnancy-related national emphasis in the United States was on preventing poor pregnancy outcomes by providing quality prenatal care. However, as prenatal care has been critically evaluated, it has become more obvious that the time to prevent complications of pregnancy often is before a woman conceives.

Preconception care was first emphasized in a 1985 Institute of Medicine document that highlighted the significant impact that preconception care can have on preventing low birth weight.[6] In 1989, the U.S. Public Health Service Expert Panel on the Content of Prenatal Care declared that preconception care "should be standard care,"[7] and among the goals outlined in the Public Health Service's 1991 publication *Healthy People 2000* was the provision of age-appropriate preconception care and counseling by a majority of primary care providers.[8] These goals have been restated and strengthened in all subsequent *Healthy People* guidelines including the 2020 document, which emphasizes increasing the proportion of women who receive preconception care and who practice key recommendations that promote healthy pregnancy.[9]

In 2005, the CDC and 35 partner organizations convened a workgroup that identified components of a preconception visit and issued recommendations for implementation.[1] Preconception care was broadly defined as a set of services, targeting both reproductive-age women and men, that identify conditions that could affect a future pregnancy or fetus, with initiation of health promotion counseling and recommendations and interventions to reduce risk. A focus on increasing readiness for pregnancy also was articulated.[1] There is widespread recognition that more research is needed to elucidate a clearer understanding of factors associated with both planned and unplanned pregnancies.[10]

Preconception Care Successes and Barriers

Preconception care has enjoyed some notable successes, particularly in reducing the incidence of neural tube defects in all women and the incidence of congenital anomalies associated with hyperglycemia in women who have diabetes.

Folic Acid Supplementation

Evidence collected from both randomized controlled trials (RCTs) and cohort studies has consistently demonstrated that the chance of having a fetus with a neural tube defect is decreased in women who take folate supplements in the preconception period as compared to women who do not take folate supplements (odds ratio [OR], 0.52; 95% confidence interval [CI], 0.39–0.69).[11,12] The benefit of folate can be fully realized only when women take folate supplementation prior to and in the early weeks of a pregnancy because organogenesis begins early in the course of embryonic development, with the neural tube closing by 28 days after conception. Informing women of the risk for neural tube defects and the benefits of folate supplementation is one hallmark of preconception care. Yet, despite this evidence and success in increasing the number of women who consume folate supplements, few women actually take 400 micrograms of folate per day for primary prevention of neural tube defects prior to conception.[13]

Women in a focus group looking at barriers and enablers of preconception care noted that they did not think about preparing for pregnancy unless they were actually considering becoming pregnant.[13] In addition, they did not think they were at risk for pregnancy complications if they were not pregnant. In contrast, the women in this group noted that once they were pregnant, seeking health care was important.[13] In other studies, women also have noted that healthcare providers do not initiate conversations about preparation for pregnancy or specific risks that have perinatal implications.[11]

Low Birth Weight and Prematurity

Preconception care also has the potential to decrease prematurity rates and the number of infants who are born at a low birth weight. For example, adolescents have approximately 11% of all births worldwide, and they have disproportionally higher rates of preterm births.[14] Adolescent women are also at increased risk for eating disorders, substance abuse, and physical violence, which can have adverse effects on the fetus.[14] Increasing dissemination of information and counseling about effective contraceptive methods in this population has the potential to decrease prematurity by effectively delaying pregnancy until women mature and assume healthier diets and lifestyles. Both prematurity and low birth weight are influenced by modifiable risk factors that are potentially responsive to preconception care.

Barriers to Preconception Care

A survey of both family planning providers (*n* = 459) and their patients (*n* = 1991) published in 2012 documented barriers to effective preconception care in low-income women.[15] The providers cited lack of familiarity with referral sources for low-income women as a major barrier to delivering effective preconception care. For their part, the women noted that lack of access to healthcare providers was a barrier to preconception care. Fifty-nine percent of the women reported not having a provider other than for family planning, and 71% reported not having any health insurance to pay for medical care.[15] Oral health, HIV-positive status, and mental health status were the conditions least likely to be treated by family planning providers,[15] even though these conditions are directly linked to perinatal health and outcomes.

Many women of childbearing age in the United States do not have health insurance, and frequently women in the reproductive-age group do not access care until they become pregnant.[16] For those women with insurance, only one in six obstetricians or family physicians reports providing preconception care to women to whom they subsequently provided prenatal care.[2] In a recent survey of focus groups of women in Georgia, women planning to become pregnant stated they did not like the term "preconception care" because it was too clinical and could be off-putting to women.[17] Those who were not planning pregnancy advised that health messages integral to preconception care should be framed as messages on how to improve one's health rather than on how to prepare for pregnancy, as the latter message was not likely to be heard by these women if they were not actively planning for pregnancy.[17]

The concept of preconception care has been widely criticized for a number of other reasons, including the perception that it should not be solely a clinical initiative.[18] This criticism stems from recognition that health behaviors result from an interplay of various influences between the woman and her cultural norms, environment, her interpersonal networks, and institutional influences.[18] Over time, a broad and more inclusive partnership with other health professionals, organizations, social marketing initiatives, and policy is needed to improve the adoption of preconception care and its ultimate impact on perinatal health.[18]

National Guidelines: A "Life-Course Perspective"

Several professional organizations publish goals and guidelines for preconception care, including *Healthy People 2020* and the CDC (**Table 10-1** and **Box 10-1**).[2,7] The goals for preconception care as stated in the *Healthy People 2020* guidelines[7] acknowledge the importance of maternal and child health as a "life-course" perspective for the woman. This "life-course" perspective includes health promotion

Table 10-1	*Healthy People 2020* Goals for Preconception Health and Behaviors
Maternal/Infant Child Health Goal (MICH)	**Goal**
MICH-14	Increase the proportion of women of childbearing potential with intake of at least 400 mcg of folic acid from fortified foods or dietary supplements
MICH-15	Reduce the proportion of women of childbearing potential who have low red blood cell folate concentrations
MICH-16	Increase the proportion of women delivering a live birth who received preconception care services and practiced key recommended preconception health behaviors
	MICH 16.1: Increase the proportion of women delivering a live birth who discussed preconception health with a healthcare worker prior to pregnancy
	MICH 16-2: Increase the proportion of women delivering a live birth who took multivitamins/folic acid prior to pregnancy; benchmark is to increase from 30.1% of women to 33.1%
	MICH 16-3: Increase the proportion of women delivering a live birth who did not smoke prior to pregnancy; benchmark is an increase from 77.6% to 85.4%
	MICH 16-4: Increase the proportion of women delivering a live birth who did not drink alcohol prior to pregnancy; benchmark is an increase from 51.3% to 56.4%—a 10% improvement
	MICH 16-5: Increase the proportion of women delivering a live birth who had a healthy weight prior to pregnancy; benchmark is an increase from 48.5% to 53.4%
	MICH 16-6: Increase the proportion of women delivering a live birth who used contraception to plan pregnancy
MICH-17	Reduce the proportion of persons age 18–44 years who have impaired fecundity (i.e., a physical barrier preventing pregnancy or carrying a pregnancy to term)
	MICH-17.1: Reduce the proportion of women age 18–44 years who have impaired fecundity; benchmark is a decrease from 12% to 10.8%
	MICH-17.2: Reduce the proportion of men age 18–44 years who have impaired fecundity

Source: Healthy People 2020: 2020 topic and objectives, maternal, infant and child health: national health promotion and disease prevention objectives. Available at: http://www.healthypeople.gov/2020/topicsobjectives2020/objectiveslist.aspx?topicId=26. Accessed November 15, 2012.

activities to modify knowledge, attitudes, and behaviors with a focus on reproduction, and encourages women and men to articulate the number of children desired and the timing of pregnancies in the context of their life goals.

Creation of a reproductive life plan is suggested as one way to motivate reproductive-age women and men to adopt healthier lifestyles and develop a consciousness about preparing for pregnancy. In addition to a life-course perspective and a reproductive life plan, *Healthy People 2020* supports the examination of "quality of life" regarding maternal and child health.[7] A "quality of life" perspective acknowledges social determinants of health (e.g., income, environment, race and ethnicity) as important in addressing the numerous healthcare disparities reported in perinatal data.[7] Healthcare providers can access up-to-date information and resources for promoting preconception care by accessing the CDCs website "Before, Between and Beyond Pregnancy."[19]

The American Congress of Obstetricians and Gynecologists (ACOG) includes four interventions

in its framework for preconception care—namely, physical assessment, risk screening, vaccinations, and counseling.[20] The ACOG guidelines also include eight areas of risk screening: (1) reproductive awareness; (2) environmental toxins and teratogens; (3) nutrition and folic acid; (4) genetics; (5) substance use; (6) medical conditions and medications; (7) infectious diseases and vaccinations; and (8) psychosocial concerns (e.g., depression or violence).

The March of Dimes also has a variety of resources and initiatives for both reproductive-age women and men and health professionals that intended to foster the adoption of preconception care by both women and men and by health professionals.[21]

Components of Preconception Care

The three overarching components of preconception counseling are (1) identification or risks related to pregnancy; (2) education about pregnancy risks, management options, and reproductive alternatives;

and (3) initiation of interventions to ensure optimal pregnancy outcomes. Box 10-2 lists the specific components of preconception care that are reviewed in this chapter.

Reproductive Life Plan

Preconception care entails a deliberate focus on reproductive health that covers the reproductive life span of both men and women. For example, weight, change of medications, and management of substance abuse are all conditions that adversely affect pregnancy and that require time to correct prior to conception. In addition, counseling about behavior change takes time and may include many healthcare visits once a woman has an intentional plan.

When integrating preconception care into primary care visits, assessment of emotional readiness, financial readiness, and maximization of personal health can be determined. A midwife may open the discussion by asking a woman about her thoughts about pregnancy: Does she envision never getting pregnant, or does she envision getting pregnant within 1 year, or 5 years, or 10 years? The woman's answer will dictate which focused components of preconception care are appropriate for discussion. Examples include topics such as whether there is room in the relationship for children, the woman's rationale for childbearing, the stability of the woman and/or the couple emotionally and financially, and/or expectations of the experience of childbearing and parenting.

A "Contraceptive Vital Sign"

A recent study suggested the "contraceptive vital sign" might be used as a method to improve routine

---

BOX 10-1 Centers for Disease Control and Prevention's Goals to Improve Preconception Health

Goals to Improve Preconception Health Before Conception of a First or Subsequent Pregnancy

1. Improve knowledge attitudes and behaviors of men and women related to preconception health.

2. Ensure that all women of childbearing age in the United States receive preconception care services that enable them to enter pregnancy in optimal health.

3. Reduce risks indicated by a previous adverse pregnancy outcome through interventions during the interconception period that can prevent or minimize health problems for a mother and her future children.

4. Reduce disparities in adverse pregnancy outcomes.

Recommendations to Improve Health Before Conception of a First or Subsequent Pregnancy

1. Individual responsibility across the lifespan: Each woman, man, and couple should be encouraged to have a reproductive health plan.

2. Consumer awareness: Increase the number of prompts (e.g., commercials, billboards, smart phone apps) to increase public knowledge about importance of preconception care.

3. Preventive visits: Visits that address health promotion and health behaviors, aimed at reducing risks related to pregnancy.

4. Interventions for identified risks.

5. Interconception care: Care between pregnancies that focuses on decreasing adverse outcomes that occurred in previous pregnancies.

6. Prepregnancy check-up.

7. Health insurance for women with low incomes: Advocates for coverage, including expanded Medicaid coverage.

8. Public health programs and strategies.

9. Research: Expanded research related to preconception care.

10. Monitor improvements by maximizing public health surveillance and related research mechanisms to monitor preconception health.

Source: Adapted from Johnson K, Posner SF, Biermann J, et al. Recommendations to improve preconception health and health care—United States. *MMWR.* 2006;55(RR06):1-23.

BOX 10-2 Major Components of the Preconception Visit

Components of Preconception Care

1. Reproductive life plan
2. Risk identification
3. Health promotion
4. Health history and medical conditions
5. Medication assessment
6. Environment and workplace exposures
7. Laboratory evaluation (dictated by individual risks)

assessment of a woman's use of a contraceptive method and intentions regarding a future pregnancy. In this study, women presenting to care were routinely asked on an intake questionnaire, "Are you currently pregnant, or trying to become pregnant?" Women were also asked whether they were using a contraceptive method and if so, which kind. This information was then available to the healthcare provider during the current encounter. Results showed a significant change in provider documentation related to contraceptive counseling from a baseline of 23% to 57% ($P < .001$) by using this "contraceptive vital sign."[22]

Preparing for Pregnancy

When a woman is intentionally seeking pregnancy, a formal preconception care visit should begin with an assessment of risks based on maternal age, race and ethnicity, maternal and paternal health conditions, reproductive history, and family history, ideally including three generations as a basis to assess genetic risk.[23] Collectively, these components of preconception care are too expansive to be accomplished in one visit; thus the provider may want to consider using some type of a check-off sheet as a reminder or tally record of the content areas of preconception care that have been discussed with the woman.

The preconception period is an ideal time for women/couples to consider their access to and availability of health care. Do they wish to see a midwife, general obstetrician, family practice physician, or a maternal–fetal medicine specialist? The choice of birth place is important, but is often not considered until pregnancy is established. This factor, as well as the payment for the provider, may be controlled by the insurance carrier and subject to certain limitations. If couples investigate these options early, they may be able to make the arrangements for the birth provider and environment they need and prefer.

When to Discontinue Contraceptive Methods

Many women question how long they should wait after discontinuing a contraceptive method before attempting to conceive. Although many providers recommend using a barrier method for a set period of time before discontinuing contraception completely, such recommendations often are not evidence-based but rather based on the convenience of having a normal menstrual period that can be used as the basis of determining an estimated date for birth. After using a hormonal method of contraception, the first menses may be anovulatory or ovulation may occur quickly. When ovulation does occur quickly, a woman may conceive prior to having a menstrual period, which makes gestational dating more difficult, but the woman should be reassured that there is no association with an increased risk of spontaneous abortion or congenital anomalies.

The most common length of time prior to resumption of normal menses after use of hormonal contraceptives varies from method to method, as described in the chapters of this text that review contraceptive methods. Women who used oral contraceptives may resume menses within a month or two after discontinuation of contraception, whereas women who used injectables or implants may not menstruate regularly for several months after they stop contraception. The importance of maintaining a menstrual calendar should be emphasized, as it validates normalcy of menses and ultimately is the basis for determining the estimated date of birth once pregnancy occurs.

For women who have irregular menses, predicting ovulation timing and, therefore, dating of a pregnancy may be difficult. For these women, basal body temperature charting or ovulation predictor kits may be useful.

As a general guideline, a woman who is seeking pregnancy, engaging in regular intercourse, and not using any contraceptive method will usually become pregnant within a year. If pregnancy does not ensue after 12 months, an infertility evaluation for the woman and her partner should be initiated. The exception is when the woman has stopped use of a long-acting reversible contraceptive agent; in that case, the timing may be longer. Alternatively, in some practices women age 35 years or older may seek infertility care after only 6 months of failing to become pregnant because fertility wanes with increasing age.

Risk Identification

Table 10-2 summarizes fertility and pregnancy complications that are more common in women and men who are older than 35 years.[23] Although older women have no increased risk for genetic disorders, they are more likely to have a fetus with a chromosomal abnormality as compared to women who are younger than age 35 years. In addition, as women age, their risks for diabetes, hypertension, and other chronic diseases increase. These chronic conditions, in turn, can have adverse effects on pregnancy. Thus it is difficult to distinguish the risks that are secondary to age, age and a chronic condition, or multiparity, which also increases with age. In addition, even though most of these risks increase incrementally over time, many women see the age of 35 years as marking a sudden transition from a "low risk" to a "high risk" category—a misconception that can be eased during preconception counseling.

Major changes in an established lifestyle, such as giving up the benefits of a disposable income or unencumbered schedules, also occur for couples of advanced age who become pregnant—a topic that may be important to consider for some couples.

Preconception Genetic Screening

Genetic screening done during the preconception period has the potential to positively impact pregnancy outcomes. A woman's personal and family history should reveal any specific need for genetic screening/counseling based on race, ethnicity, and family history. Genetic counseling based on race/ethnicity is summarized in **Table 10-3**, and risk factors noted based in family history and personal reproductive history are listed in **Box 10-3**.[24]

A three-generation history is recommended to identify recessive inheritance of problematic genes.[23] If a specific risk factor is identified or if the future parents have concerns, referral to a genetic counselor is recommended.[25] Reproductive autonomy—not prevention of pregnancy—should be the focus of the conversation when genetics risks are identified.[24] A 2012 survey of nurse-midwives found that the midwives felt genetic-related activities are very important or essential in clinical practice, yet the level of importance subscribed to genetics was higher than the respondents' self-confidence in providing genetic services.[26] Midwives may need to seek expanded education related to clinical genetics to become more confident in their ability to counsel women and their partners about genetic inheritance.[26]

Table 10-2	Increased Risk for Congenital Conditions Related to Gender and Age
Demographic Characteristics	**Congenital Conditions**
Maternal age ≥ 35 years[a]	Miscarriage
	Ectopic pregnancy
	Chromosomal abnormalities
	Congenital malformations
	Multiple gestation
	Hypertension
	Diabetes mellitus
	Placental problems (placenta previa and placenta abruption)
	Low birth weight
	Preterm delivery
	Stillbirth
	Dysfunctional labor
	Cesarean section
Paternal age ≥ 35 years[b]	Miscarriage (although this risk is lower than the increased risk for miscarriage associated with maternal age ≥ 35 years)
	Autosomal dominant disorders
	Schizophrenia
	Autism spectrum disorder
	X-linked genetic mutations

[a]Many of the pregnancy complications in this list are secondary to the development of chronic conditions that increase pregnancy risks. Thus it is not easy to determine the effect of multiparity alone.

[b]Most increased risks associated with paternal age are statistically significant in retrospective analyses but very small in absolute numbers. For example, the risk for autosomal dominant disorders is approximately 0.5% or less.

Table 10-3	Congenital Conditions Associated with Race/Ethnicity
Ethnicity (At Least One Member of a Couple)	**Associated Congenital Condition**
Asian	Thalassemia
Asian: Southeast Asian or Chinese	Alpha thalassemia
Asian: Indian	Beta thalassemia
African	Sickle cell disease or trait, thalassemia
Ashkenazi Jewish	Canavan disease, cystic fibrosis,[a] familial dysautonomia, Tay-Sachs disease, Gaucher's disease, Niemann-Pick disease, Bloom syndrome, mucolipidosis IV, Fanconi anemia group C
Cajun	Tay-Sachs disease
European	Cystic fibrosis[a]
French Canadian	Tay-Sachs disease
Mediterranean	Thalassemia
White	Cystic fibrosis[a]

[a]Although some race/ethnicities are at increased risk for cystic fibrosis, this disorder and testing should be discussed with all persons of all races.

Source: Adapted from Solomon BD, Jack BW, Ferro WG. The clinical content of preconception care: genetics and genomics. *Am J Obstet Gynecol.* 2008:199(6 suppl 2):S340-S344.

BOX 10-3 Congenital Conditions Associated with Family and Reproductive History

Family History

Chromosomal disorders or genetic disorders
- Cystic fibrosis
- Clotting disorders
- Marfan syndrome
- Phenylketonuria
- Sickle cell trait
- Thrombophilia or hemophilia
- Trisomy 21 (Down syndrome)

Deafness

Developmental delay or mental retardation, especially in males

Early infant death, sudden infant death syndrome, or stillbirth

Heart defects

Neural tube defects

Orofacial clefts such as cleft lip or cleft palate

Reproductive History

Multiple miscarriages (two or more)

Stillbirth

Abnormal chromosomal or congenital cognition in previous pregnancy

---

Health Promotion

The need for greater emphasis on health promotion is evidenced by recent statistics. More than 50% of childbearing women are overweight or obese,[23] more than 30% report current smoking, and 50% report drinking alcohol.[2] Healthcare providers can increase their influence on health promotion by individualizing recommendations and by familiarizing themselves with resources and models to promote behavior change, as discussed in the *Health Promotion and Health Maintenance* chapter.

Assessment for Abuse

Assessment of existing or potential physical, sexual, or emotional abuse should always be performed. Physical and/or emotional abuse in pregnancy is associated with poor weight gain, infection, sexually transmitted infections, anemia, low birth weight, preterm birth, and bleeding in pregnancy. Abuse is widespread; it does not have any correlation with ethnicity, socioeconomic status, or education, and it often begins or escalates during pregnancy.[21]

Standard screening techniques are reviewed in more detail in the *Health Promotion and Health Maintenance* chapter.

Safe Sex

The important discussion of safe sex should occur during most health visits. Safe sex discussions include a review of methods for the prevention of sexually transmitted infections. Risk assessment includes questions regarding number of sexual partners, types of sexual practices (e.g., oral or anal sex; same-sex partner), and use of barrier methods (e.g., male or female condoms). When a risk is identified, recommendations for specific interventions should follow. These interventions may include immunizations (e.g., human papillomavirus [HPV] immunization) and additional screening (e.g., HIV testing; syphilis, gonorrhea, and chlamydia screening). Risky sexual practices may be accompanied by other risk behaviors (e.g., substance abuse) and lead the midwife to further questioning.

Nutrition and Exercise

Nutrition and exercise recommendations for healthy nonpregnant women are also emphasized when providing preconception care. Achieving ideal body weight of a body mass index [BMI] in the range of 18.5 kg/m^2 to 24.99 kg/m^2, controlling eating disorders or pica, and developing nutritionally balanced dietary habits are all important for general health.

Prepregnant obesity (BMI > 25 kg/m^2) has been associated with an increased risk for neural tube defects, preterm delivery, diabetes, large-for-gestational-age infants, cesarean birth, hypertension, and thromboembolic disease. Weight loss prior to pregnancy reduces these risks.[27] A BMI less than 18.5 kg/m^2 is associated with subfertility, anemia, and fetal growth restriction.[28]

Referral to a dietician may be necessary for women who have significant nutritional deficits or obesity. Women with eating disorders have higher rates of miscarriage, low birth weight, obstetric complications, and postpartum depression. If a woman has or may have an eating disorder, counseling about these risks and referral for psychological treatment are recommended. Women with phenylketonuria should be counseled about the importance of maintaining a diet low in phenylalanine during their childbearing years, especially when planning to become pregnant.

Additional components of nutritional counseling include screening for iron deficiency and risk factors for anemia such as short spacing between births, pica, and vegetarian-type diets.[2] Anemia in pregnancy is associated with fetal growth restriction. Iron-deficiency anemia is easily corrected once identified, with both supplement and food sources rich in iron.

Food Safety

Food safety is an important nutrition-related topic for the health of women in general and for preconception counseling in particular. Avoidance of uncooked foods such as raw meat or fish, raw sprouts, unpasteurized cheeses, milk, and juice and avoidance of fish high in mercury are the primary recommendations for pregnant women. These precautions also help to prevent infection with the parasite *Toxoplasma gondii*, which may be transmitted from raw meats, and the bacterium *Listeria monocytogenes*, which is commonly transmitted from spoiled lunch meats or cheese.[29] However, women should not be discouraged from eating up to 12 ounces of fish per week. The website for the Food and Drug Administration (FDA) has several resources for professionals and women that provide detailed information about food safety in pregnancy.

Dietary Supplements

Dietary supplements include vitamins, herbal products, nutritional supplements such as weight-loss products, folk medicines, and traditional remedies. Because dietary supplements are not subject to rigorous standards for purity in the same way that prescription medications are, the quality of these products can vary widely. Women should be counseled to avoid vitamins or multivitamin preparations that exceed the current recommended daily allowances. For example, vitamin A is associated with fetal malformations if very high doses are consumed in the first trimester. In addition, because nutritional supplements can adversely interact with absorption of foods or medications, a complete accounting of dietary supplements that are used is important to review and document.

Folic Acid

Some dietary supplements may be beneficial. All women of childbearing age are recommended to take folic acid supplements to ensure a consumption of at least 400 micrograms per day, thereby reducing the risk of having a fetus with spina bifida or another neural tube defect.[30] Most over-the-counter multivitamins contain 400 micrograms (0.4 milligrams) of folic acid, and generic preparations are sufficient. Prescriptive prenatal vitamins usually are formulated with 1.0 mg of folic acid, although the need for a prescription may be a barrier that prevents some women from taking these supplements.

For some women, the idea of taking a prenatal vitamin when they are not yet pregnant is perceived as intruding into their privacy. Others may eschew the use of artificial supplementation in general. However, folic acid supplements are recommended to meet the folate requirements because supplements have high bioavailability compared to food sources of folate and they ensure ingestion of a constant, adequate level. If a woman is highly motivated to consume folic acid from natural sources and does not want to take supplements, then a detailed discussion about absorption of folate from foods and dietary sources of folate should be provided. For example, some foods and food products have good levels of folic acid and others are fortified with folic acid.[31]

Women who have an increased risk for having a child with a neural tube defect relative to the general population include women who had a previous infant with a neural tube defect, women who have a first-degree relative with a neural tube defect, and women who take specific anticonvulsants (folate antagonists).[30] In addition, women who have diabetes or who are obese have an increased risk for neural tube defects, as do Hispanics and non-Hispanic white persons when compared to black and Asians. For women who previously had an infant with a neural tube defect and women taking anticonvulsants, the recommended dosage of folic acid is 4.0 mg daily for at least one month prior to conception and through the first 12 weeks of pregnancy.[30] Some authors also suggest that women with pre-gestational diabetes take 4.0 mg of folic acid preconceptionally to reduce the incidence of neural tube defects; this recommendation is not yet universal, however, as human studies linking diabetes to neural tube defects have not yet definitely found an association between folic acid supplementation and fewer neural tube defects in this population.

Vitamin D

Vitamin D deficiency is widespread, and healthcare providers should be attuned to emerging data and changing recommendations. Many reproductive-age women may already be taking a vitamin D supplement. At present, universal routine supplementation of maternal vitamin D is not a public health recommendation. However, ingestion of 1000 IU/day is considered a reasonable amount if the woman chooses to take a vitamin D supplement.[32] Calcium supplementation may also be recommended if dietary sources of calcium are low.

Immunizations

During pregnancy, a woman's immune system is altered in ways that put her at increased risk for some infections. Communicable diseases often are more severe in pregnant women, and influenza vaccine is recommended for all women planning pregnancy.

Evidence exists that several vaccines are effective interventions to promote healthy pregnancies when delivered prior to pregnancy in the absence of prior immunity. All women of reproductive age should have their immunization status for tetanus–diphtheria toxoid (Tdap); measles, mumps, and rubella (MMR); hepatitis B; and varicella reviewed annually, including inquiring about the date of last Tdap immunization.[32] If immunity is lacking, these immunizations should be offered.

Rubella is a known teratogen, causing congenital rubella syndrome when nonimmune women are infected during the first 16 weeks of pregnancy. Women who receive the rubella immunization should be counseled to avoid pregnancy for 1 month, based on a theoretical risk of passing rubella to a developing embryo. However, there are no reports of teratogenicity secondary to receiving rubella vaccine in early pregnancy; thus pregnancy termination is not recommended for women who are inadvertently vaccinated for rubella within 4 weeks of becoming pregnant or when they are pregnant.

Infections

Infections that should be screened for in the preconception period include tuberculosis, HIV, and possibly hepatitis C. Healthy childbearing women are not at high risk for cytomegalovirus (CMV) infection. Women at risk for tuberculosis may be screened with the PPD (tuberculin) test. If they have previously had a positive PPD test or received the bacillus Calmette-Guérin (BCG) vaccine, a chest X ray can be done if indicated.

The U.S. Preventive Services Task Force (USPSTF) has updated the recommendation concerning hepatitis C screening in adults. The 2013 statement recommends screening for hepatitis C virus (HCV) infection in adults at high risk, including those with any history of intravenous drug use or blood transfusions prior to 1992. Additionally, the USPSTF recommends that clinicians offering screening for HCV infection to adults born between 1945 and 1965.[33]

The USPSTF statement for HIV screening, with a Grade A recommendation, recommends that clinicians screen adolescents and adults age 15 to 65 years for HIV infection. Younger adolescents and older adults who are at increased risk also should be screened.[34] Individuals who have a positive result on one of the screening tests should be referred for a diagnostic test and medical care if a diagnosis of HIV is made. Telling a woman that she is HIV positive is a highly emotional event and should be conducted with sensitivity, in person; it is best done with an interdisciplinary group of providers who can help the woman plan her care. Antiretroviral therapy can minimize mother-to-child transmission of the HIV pathogen.

Some infections that can adversely affect a fetus are not on the list of those that should be screened for in pregnant women. Toxoplasmosis, for example, has a low prevalence in the United States. This infection is transmitted through raw meats and via contact with infected cat litter. Therefore, although there are no vaccines or tests that are recommended, women should be asked about their exposure to domestic cats and provided with counseling about prevention of toxoplasmosis, such as asking someone else to clean the litter box or using gloves when doing so.

There is no vaccine for CMV, and there are no data suggesting that preconception screening for parvovirus would be beneficial. Women who are at increased risk for CMV include daycare workers and registered nurses who work in specific settings. Preconception care involves counseling about this risk and recommending protections such as hand washing and universal precautions.

Risks for sexually transmitted infections should be included in this assessment and testing done based on individual risk. For women with a history of genital herpes, counseling can be done about managing genital herpes infections during pregnancy. Candidacy for the HPV vaccine should be assessed.

Dental Care

More than 80% of women have dental caries or poor oral health.[2] Women should be advised to obtain any needed dental work that requires radiation exposure, sedation, anesthesia, or gum surgery prior to pregnancy. Oral health is an important preconception topic, as research has demonstrated an increased risk of preterm birth when women have significant periodontal disease during pregnancy.[35] This increase in the incidence of preterm birth in conjunction with periodontal disease is linked to the inflammatory process.[35] Ideally, dental work should be completed prior to pregnancy. The increased blood volume during pregnancy and resulting hyperemia in the gums will cause excessive bleeding if gum surgery is required when a woman is pregnant.

Health History and Medical Conditions

Detection and optimal control of chronic diseases are important goals of preconception care. Women with chronic diseases should be informed about maternal and newborn morbidity risks associated with these diseases prior to becoming pregnant. This discussion should include current and potential treatment options based on the woman's health and the potential embryonic/fetal health.

Diabetes

Almost two-thirds of pregnancies in women with diabetes are unplanned.[36] When blood glucose levels are consistently elevated (i.e., HBA1c > 7.5%) at the time of conception and early organogenesis, there is a significantly increased risk for development of multiple adverse pregnancy outcomes, as identified in **Table 10-4**.[37] However, these risks can be reduced up to threefold by ensuring adequate glycemic control prior to conception.[38] All women with preexisting diabetes should receive preconception care and be counseled about the importance of blood glucose control prior to pregnancy. Studies in women with either type 1 or type 2 diabetes have found that preconception care is associated with a significant reduction in the incidence of congenital malformations.[38] Other preconception topics for women with preexisting diabetes include the importance of self-monitoring of blood glucose; achieving an ideal prepregnant weight; engaging in regular exercise; avoidance of tobacco, alcohol, and other dangerous substances; folic acid supplementation, given that women with diabetes have a higher risk for having a child with a neural tube defect; and effective methods of contraception that can be used until blood glucose levels are normalized.[39]

It is recommended that a multidisciplinary team see women with diabetes who are contemplating pregnancy. Evaluation for diabetic retinopathy, nephropathy, coronary artery disease, and hypertension is a key component of preconception care for women with pre-gestational diabetes. Use of angiotensin-converting enzyme (ACE) inhibitors should be discontinued and another antihypertensive agent substituted in women who have both diabetes and elevated blood pressure, although there is no consensus on the best antihypertensive agent to prescribe. Women should be counseled that statins are not to be used in pregnancy. Metformin (Glucophage) and acarbose (Precose) are considered safe for use in pregnancy, as is insulin.[36]

The prevalence of type 2 diabetes is increasing and is currently 21 per 1000 women between 18 and 44 years of age in the United States.[40] Screening for prediabetes and preexisting diabetes during the preconception and interconception periods should be offered to all women of childbearing age who are overweight or obese and have one additional risk factor for diabetes, such as a history of gestational diabetes.[39] Women with a history of gestational diabetes should be informed that they are at increased risk for abnormal carbohydrate metabolism during future pregnancies. Preconception diabetic control has the potential to minimize the risk of pregnancy loss and congenital malformations in approximately 113,000 births per year.[40]

Hypertension

Preexisting hypertension imparts several risks to pregnancy for both the woman and her unborn child. These risks increase in frequency with the severity of the hypertension (**Table 10-5**).[41] Pregnancy outcomes are partially dependent upon the presence or absence of superimposed preeclampsia. Women who develop preeclampsia have worse pregnancy outcomes. The primary goals in the preconception period are blood pressure control without use of ACE inhibitors or angiotensin II receptor antagonists.[39,41] Members of these two antihypertensive drug families are associated with an increased risk of fetal malformation, oligohydramnios, fetal growth restriction, and fetal death. Women with long-standing hypertension should have an evaluation for ventricular hypertrophy, retinopathy, and renal disease prior to becoming pregnant.[39]

Cardiac Disease

The woman with known or suspected cardiac disease should be strongly counseled to plan the timing

Table 10-4	Pregnancy Risks That Are More Likely in Women with Type 1 Diabetes
Pregnancy Complication	**Risk (Diabetes Versus No Diabetes)**
Miscarriage	Slightly elevated relative to women without diabetes overall. Rates vary widely depending on degree of glycemic control.
Congenital anomalies, major malformations	4.7% versus 1.8%
Preterm birth	21% versus 5.1% before 37 weeks' gestation
Preeclampsia	9.7% versus 2.0% for mild preeclampsia
Large for gestational age infant	12.6% versus 3.9% for birth weight ≥ 4500 g
Cesarean delivery	46% versus 12%
Shoulder dystocia	13.7% versus 0.2%
Stillbirth	1.5% versus 0.3%

Source: Adapted from Persson M, Norman M, Hanson U. Obstetric and perinatal outcomes in type 1 diabetic pregnancies: a large, population-based study. *Diab Care.* 2009;32:2005.

Table 10-5	Pregnancy Risks That Are More Likely in Women with Pregestational Hypertension[a]
Pregnancy Complication	**Risk**
Preterm delivery	12–33%
Fetal growth restriction	8–11%
Preeclampsia	10–25%
Eclampsia[b]	2–3%
Placenta abruption	0.7–1.5%

[a]Risks increase with severity of progestational hypertension.

[b]The risk of eclampsia is approximately 0% to 0.6% for women with mild preeclampsia and 2% to 3% for women with severe preeclampsia who are not treated with seizure prophylaxis medications.

Source: Adapted from Sibai BM. Chronic hypertension: chronic hypertension in pregnancy. *Obstet Gynecol.* 2002;100;369-373.

of pregnancy with advice from a cardiologist and a perinatologist. Cardiac disease may represent a minimal risk, as in the case of mitral valve prolapse, or it may confer a life-threatening risk, as is possible for women who have pulmonary hypertension. During the preconception period, the woman's cardiac status must be assessed, and she and her family apprised of the implications that pregnancy may carry. Perinatal outcomes are closely associated with the severity of the heart disease.

Embryopathy is associated with warfarin (Coumadin) use in pregnancy; heparin may be an acceptable alternative in women who desire to become pregnant.[39] The American Heart Association is a good resource to consult when women who are seeking pregnancy report use of oral anticoagulants. For many women with cardiac disease, the possibility of multiple office and hospital visits as well as close medical scrutiny should be anticipated. Therefore, advance planning for workplace concerns, health insurance, and childcare for other children as well as for medical care is essential. Genetic counseling may also be indicated, as some cardiac disorders can be inherited.[22]

Thyroid Disorders

Uncontrolled hypothyroidism and hyperthyroidism are a significant cause of maternal and newborn morbidity. Complications associated with uncontrolled hyperthyroidism include a higher risk for congenital malformations, hypertension, preeclampsia, low birth weight, fetal growth restriction, preterm birth, placental abruption, and stillbirth.[39] Similarly, overt hypothyroidism during a woman's first trimester of

pregnancy is associated with dwarfism and intellectual impairment.[42] Additional pregnancy complications associated with hypothyroidism include miscarriage, preterm birth, preeclampsia, placental abnormalities, and low birth weight. For both hypothyroidism and hyperthyroidism, the goal is for the woman to be euthyroid prior to pregnancy.

For women who have either hypothyroidism or hyperthyroidism, medical consultation and follow-up are indicated to establish a plan for assessment of thyroid levels and medications that are safe to use during pregnancy. Of the two conditions, hypothyroidism is more common and use of thyroid supplementation should be discussed, including alerting the woman about the possibility of needing to titrate doses during pregnancy.

Hyperthyroidism, although less common, is more challenging. The medications currently prescribed for this condition have some controversial effects. Propylthiouracil (PTU) is the medication of choice for pregnant women with hyperthyroidism. Available evidence suggests that methimazole (Tapazole) may be associated with congenital anomalies; however, methimazole may be prescribed if propylthiouracil is not available, or if a woman cannot tolerate or has an adverse response to propylthiouracil.[42] The general recommendation is to avoid pregnancy for 6 months after receiving radioactive treatment.[39]

Screening women for subclinical hypothyroidism is controversial.[43] Maternal subclinical hypothyroidism has been linked to an increased risk for miscarriage, placental abruption, preterm birth, low birth weight, and gestational hypertension, although the risks are less than with overt thyroid disease.[43] Moreover, the benefits of levothyroxine replacement for the treatment of subclinical hypothyroidism in reducing the incidence of these complications remain unclear.[43] Currently, there are no recommendations to routinely screen for subclinical thyroid disease in nonpregnant women.

Asthma

Approximately one-third of women with asthma will have worsening of their condition when they become pregnant. Those women with uncontrolled asthma are more likely to experience an exacerbation of symptoms when pregnant. Women with uncontrolled asthma are at risk for both maternal and fetal complications of pregnancy, including preeclampsia and hyperemesis gravidarum. Fetal risks include stillbirth, fetal growth restriction, preterm birth, and low birth weight.[39] In contrast, these risks are significantly diminished in children born to women with controlled asthma. All women with asthma, but especially women who do not regularly use medications, should be counseled about the risk of impaired oxygenation to the fetus when the asthma is uncontrolled.

Inhaled medications—including inhaled glucocorticosteroids, which are a mainstay of asthma therapy—are recommended for use while a woman is pregnant given the known adverse effects of uncontrolled asthma. Oral glucocorticosteroid use in the first trimester has been associated with cleft anomalies,[44] but no association has been found between use of inhaled glucocorticosteroids and an increased risk for orofacial clefts (OR, 1.05; 95% CI, 0.80–1.38; for cleft lip with or without cleft palate).[44]

Autoimmune Conditions

Rheumatoid arthritis is more common in women than men. The most important component of preconception care for women with rheumatoid arthritis is a review of current medications. Some agents commonly prescribed for this autoimmune disease, such as methotrexate (Trexall) and leflunomide (Arava), are teratogenic. Use of nonsteroidal anti-inflammatory drugs (NSAIDs) in the first trimester does not appear to be associated with fetal anomalies; however, because NSAIDs are contraindicated later in pregnancy, women with rheumatoid arthritis will need to plan medication use carefully with their primary care provider.[39]

As many as 80% of women with rheumatoid arthritis can expect their disease to improve during pregnancy. Nevertheless, 20% to 30% of women may experience worsening of their symptoms in pregnancy, and the majority of women will have a flare during the first three months postpartum.[39]

Systemic lupus erythematosus (SLE) is a multisystem autoimmune disorder characterized by the presence of autoantibodies directed at one or more components of cell nuclei (DNA, RNA, nuclear proteins, and protein–nucleic acid complexes). SLE is one of several disease entities classified within the lupus family of disorders. It is the most common autoimmune disease in reproductive-age women, with more African American women being affected compared to women in other racial/ethnic groups.

Women with SLE have many perinatal risks, and severity of outcomes is associated with stability of the disease. Perinatal outcomes are improved when SLE is latent for at least 6 months prior to a pregnancy. Women with SLE have an increased risk of miscarriage, preeclampsia, fetal growth retardation, and preterm birth.[45] In addition, the fetus can develop neonatal lupus erythematosus (NLE) or heart block. Both conditions are treatable and, if mild, usually resolve after birth.

A review of medications is an important component of preconception care for women with SLE. Women taking cytotoxic medications should be informed of the teratogenicity of these medications and referred for a medical consultation, as care from a collaborative healthcare team is essential for maximizing preconception health in these women. The antimalarial drug hydroxychloroquine (Plaquenil) is considered safe for use in pregnancy.[39]

Seizure Disorders

Preconception care for a woman with a seizure disorder includes obtaining a detailed history regarding the frequency of seizures and the medications she takes to control seizures. Consultation or referral to a physician who is an expert in care of women with seizure disorders will enable the woman to be appropriately assessed, especially with regard to pharmacologic management. Women who take anticonvulsant medications should take folate supplementation at a level of 4 mg/day for at least 1 month prior to pregnancy.[12]

Women affected by a seizure disorder impart a risk to their offspring both by virtue of the disease itself and through the effect of medications used to treat the condition.[46] The incidence of seizures does not increase during pregnancy, but seizures do cause transient fetal hypoxia. However the overall effect of seizures on fetal well-being has not been determined.

Although phenytoin (Dilantin), carbamazepine (Tegretol), barbiturates, and valproate (Depakote) are known teratogens, their use may be recommended depending on the woman's condition. Preconception care focuses on tapering medication doses to the lowest effective level with monotherapy and maintaining effective contraception until the condition is stabilized and the best medication profile for pregnancy is achieved. Some women may tolerate withdrawal from seizure medications, especially if they have not experienced any seizures in several years. A successful withdrawal is considered 2 years without a seizure and not on medication.[39] Most women with a seizure disorder have to consider that amelioration of all risks to the newborn are unlikely, but attenuation of risk is certainly possible.

Mental Health and Major Stressors

Women should be screened for depression, anxiety, domestic violence, and major life stressors at any healthcare encounter and offered counseling and referral when indicated. The pregnancy risks associated with untreated or treated mental disorders are described in more detail in the *Mental Health Conditions* chapter.

Women who experience chronic stress may be at risk for perinatal complications including preterm birth, although the physiologic mechanisms have not been fully elucidated.[47] However, discussion of life stressors such as financial or food insecurity should be explored and resources for assistance offered.

Previous Obstetric History

Care provided after a pregnancy and before another pregnancy is termed interconception care. A woman's previous obstetric history provides a risk assessment litmus test. Women who have experienced preeclampsia or gestational diabetes in a prior pregnancy, for example, should be followed closely during the interconception period. Efforts should be made to decrease a woman's modifiable risks that can either promote or deter both of these medical conditions.

Previous preterm birth is a strong predictor for preterm birth. Moreover, complications such as an incompetent cervix, large uterine fibroids, or previous eclampsia may indicate a need to plan an intervention during the subsequent pregnancy to facilitate the best outcome. Women with excessive blood loss at delivery or postpartum anemia will benefit from having a discussion related to iron replacement.

In addition to medical/obstetric risk factors, women may have concerns from previous birth experiences regarding vaginal versus cesarean birth, use of analgesia, positions for giving birth, support of care providers, or other aspects of the previous birth that were traumatic. It is important to help her determine if there are ways to increase her satisfaction with the birth process. Conversely, she may have had an excellent experience and want assistance in ensuring a similarly positive outcome in future pregnancies.

Medication Assessment

As the section on health history and medical conditions indicated, women should be asked about which medications—both prescription and over the counter—they are taking at every healthcare encounter. Other pharmaceutical agents including recreational substances, herbal remedies, and botanicals should be included in the questioning as well. Medications should be evaluated for potential teratogenic effects, and the continuing need for the medication should be assessed. Women should not be automatically counseled to discontinue medication because they are pregnant, as this may negatively affect their medical or mental health. Ideally, a plan

should be in place for use of any specific medication in the preconception period and during the early stages of organogenesis. When a medication that has identified risks in pregnancy is one a woman reports taking, then the midwife should discuss the pregnancy implications with the woman and recommend a safer alternative medication if available.

Environment and Workplace Risks

For many years, little was known or studied about the influence of the environment on reproductive health for both women and men. Today, more studies are revealing the importance of this area. Preconception care includes identifying potential environmental toxin exposures in women and men and providing instructions on avoiding such exposures.

Pesticides that are common in our environment have been associated with increased risks for miscarriage, preterm birth, birth defects, and learning disabilities.[48] The strongest evidence supporting a link between pesticide exposure and reproductive risk comes from studies of cohorts of women who live and work in agricultural settings.[48] Home pesticide use should be limited. When pest elimination measures are necessary, trapping of pests is recommended over use of aerosol agents.[48] When aerosols are required, then food and utensils should be removed or covered during the treatment and children and pets removed from the area. If possible, someone not at reproductive risk should perform the treatment. When exposed to pesticides in the soil—for example, when gardening—rubber gloves should be worn. Everyone should wash all food and vegetables before consumption to minimize pesticide exposure.

Although not backed by consistent evidence, some women may want to consider buying organic produce, especially in regard to the "dirty dozen"—that is, the most pesticide-contaminated fruits and vegetables. A list of these foods is published by the Environmental Working Group and is available on the group's website.

Exposure to phthalates, a type of plasticizer, should also be avoided. Phthalates are found in food storage containers and food can liners. Many products are now available that are described as being phthalate free (e.g., water bottles). Phthalates can be avoided by not microwaving foods in plastic containers and by avoiding containers that are labeled with the letters "PC," meaning they contain polycarbonate.[46]

Exposure to lead poisoning from lead paint in the home or in the community should be investigated (**Box 10-4**; **Table 10-6**).[49,50] Although no level of lead exposure is safe, the blood level of lead associated with toxicity generally is considered to be more than 10 mcg/dL.[49] Ways to avoid lead exposure, especially when residing in an older home, include running water for 15–20 seconds before using it for consumption or cooking and using only cold water. A water filter that is certified to eliminate lead could be considered.

Mercury is another teratogen, and exposure to this metal should ideally be addressed in the preconception care visit. Women should be made aware that significant mercury exposure results from eating large fish (e.g., swordfish, king mackerel) on a frequent basis. The FDA website has extensive material on the mercury content of fish, both nationally and for specific locales.

Arsenic is not a common exposure, but women living near incinerators that burn garbage may increase their risk for exposure through inhalation.[46]

Occupational Risks

The workplace may be the route of exposure to harmful chemicals, irradiation, or biologic risks such as viruses. These agents may directly affect the worker, and they can be secondarily transmitted to other members of their family. For instance, lead and pesticides in the workplace may be carried on one's clothing, skin, or hair. If possible, contaminated clothing should be left in the workplace, such as scrub uniforms in a hospital. If this is not possible, then clothes should be removed prior to exposing others in the home environment. The March of Dimes provides an excellent online resource for both women and men that identifies potential environmental toxins and ways to avoid exposure.

Preconception Counseling for Men

The overall health of a man can influence perinatal outcomes and preconception care recommendations advocate assessing men's health in a comparable manner as women's health. Nevertheless, preconception guidelines specific to men are generally lacking. Similar to women, men should be encouraged to have a reproductive life plan. This includes engaging men in efforts to control fertility and assessing the man's maturity and readiness for parenting.[51] For men, the preconception period is an ideal time for routine screening for HIV and other sexually transmitted

---

BOX 10-4 Environmental Risk Assessment Survey for Lead Exposure

1. Do you or others in your household have an occupation that involves lead exposure? Examples include: lead production, battery, ammunition, plastic or paint manufacturing, ship building.
2. Sometimes pregnant women have the urge to eat things other than food, such as clay, soil, plaster, or paint chips. Do you ever eat any of these things?
3. Do you live in an old house with ongoing renovations that generate a lot of dust? Does your house have lead pipes for drinking water? To your knowledge, has your home been tested for lead in the water and, if so, were you told that the level was high?
4. Do you live near a source of lead such as a lead mine, smelter, hazardous waste site, or battery recycling plant?
5. Do you use any traditional foods, remedies, or cosmetics that are not sold in a regular drug store or are homemade, which may contain lead? Examples of cosmetics that may have lead include kohl or surma.
6. Do you or others in your household have any hobbies or activities likely to cause lead exposure? Examples include stained glass or pottery making.
7. Have any of your children had a history of elevated blood lead levels?
8. Do you use noncommercially prepared pottery or leaded crystal?
9. Have you recently emigrated from an area where the ambient lead contamination is high? Examples include countries where leaded gasoline is used or where industrial emissions are not well controlled.

Source: Adapted from Hackley B, Katz-Jacobson A. Lead poisoning in pregnancy: a case study with implications for midwives. *J Midwifery Women's Health.* 2003;48: 30-38; Agency for Toxic Substances and Disease Registry. Public health statement: lead. CAS #7439-92-1. Available at: http://www.atsdr.cdc.gov/ToxProfiles/tp13-c1-b.pdf. Accessed May 13, 2013.

---

infections as well as screening for unhealthy habits, genetic risk factors such as sickle cell trait/disease, and other known inheritable diseases.

Damaged sperm can cause infertility, miscarriage, birth defects, and childhood cancers.[50] For example, sperm DNA can be damaged by smoking,

Table 10-6	Sources of Lead Exposure	
Occupation Related	**Hobbies and Other Activities**	**Folk Remedies**
Lead abatement and home renovation/restoration	Making stained glass	*Alkohl*: black powder used as eye cosmetic and on umbilical stump (Middle Eastern, African, Asian cultures)
Recycling operations	Copper enameling	
Manufacturing/installation of plumbing	Bronze casting	*Azarcon*: bright orange powder used by Hispanic cultures for gastrointestinal upset and diarrhea
	Pottery with lead glaze and paint	
Foundry work	Hunting and target shooting	*Bali Goli*: a black bean dissolved in "gripe water" in Asian Indian cultures for stomachache
Firing range work	Jewelry making with lead solder	
Production/use of chemicals	Electronics with lead solder	*Ghazard*: brown powder used within Asian Indian cultures to aid digestion
Bridge, tunnel, construction	Glassblowing with leaded glass	*Greta*: yellow-orange powder used within Hispanic cultures to treat digestive problems
Auto repair shop	Print making and other fine arts	
Battery manufacture/repair	Liquor distillation	*Pay-loo-ah*: orange-red powder used within Southeast Asian cultures to treat rash or fever
Manufacture of industrial machinery		*Koo Sar*: pills used by Cambodian women for the treatment of menstrual cramps

Source: Hackley B, Katz-Jacobson A. Lead poisoning in pregnancy: a case study with implications for midwives. *J Midwifery Women's Health*. 2003;48:30-38. Reprinted with permission of Wiley.

alcohol, drugs (e.g., marijuana, anabolic steroids), caffeine, poor diet, radiation, chemotherapy, and testicular hyperthermia.[50] A number of environmental toxins, including polycyclic aromatic hydrocarbons (PAHs), polychlorinated biphenyls (PCBs), dioxins, phthalates, and acrylamide, can damage sperm DNA. Men have an opportunity to change behaviors and exposures to maximize sperm health when provided with knowledge about the consequences of these factors, particularly given that new sperm are produced every 3 months. Moreover, men have an important role in fostering healthy behaviors in their partner.[51]

Older men have age-related declines in sperm and decreased sperm quality. Down syndrome and increased risk of offspring developing schizophrenia have been reported as paternal age-related outcomes.[51] A cohort study reported that the hazard ratio (HR) of having a child with schizophrenia was 1.47 for each 10-year increase in paternal age, after adjusting for familial history of schizophrenia and a variety of other covariates.[52] Another study reported a significant increase in relative risk for schizophrenia with every 5-year increase in paternal age, culminating with the highest risk at age 50.[53]

The immunization status of men also should be assessed as part of preconception care. Consideration should be given to offering immunization for HPV if risk factors are identified and candidacy is confirmed, and Tdap if indicated.

Workplace, hobbies, or environmental exposures may be of concern to some men.[51] Refinishing furniture, car repairs, painting, and model building, for example, increase exposure to organic solvents.

Psychosocial issues also are important but often overlooked in men. Any history of depressive symptoms, anxiety, or other mental health issues should be considered when planning for a family.[51] Men often bear responsibility for financial stability in families and find the anticipation of the birth of a child to be stressful. An opportunity for open discussion of responsibilities, feelings, and relationship changes may reveal a need for assistance prior to conception.

Conclusion

Preconception care provides a strategy to improve the knowledge, attitudes, and behaviors concerning health for both women and men of childbearing age. Healthy parents are most likely to have healthy pregnancies. Preconception care includes risk assessment, health promotion, and specialized care to meet individual needs in preparation for a healthy and planned pregnancy. The midwife needs to be knowledgeable about and have established contacts with a variety of treatment and counseling resources (primary care providers, mental health centers, genetic counseling centers, drug treatment centers, smoking cessation programs, outreach programs, support groups, fitness and exercise centers, nutritional counseling services, and women's shelters, to name a few) and be ready to make the necessary referrals and consultations. Widespread implementation of preconception care has the potential to elevate maternal and child health in the United States into the top 10 among developed nations. Midwives should remember the slogan "Every Woman, Every Visit"—it is a call to action.

• • • References

1. Centers for Disease Control and Prevention (CDC), Agency for Toxic Substances and Disease Registry (ATSDR). *Recommendations to Improve Preconception Health and Health Care—United States: A Report of the CDC/ATSDR Preconception Care Work Group and the Select Panel on Preconception Care.* Atlanta: CDC; 2006.

2. Johnson K, Posner SF, Biermann J, et al. Recommendations to improve preconception health and health care—United States. *MMWR.* 2006;55(RR06):1-23.

3. Finer LB, Zolna MR. Unintended pregnancy in the United States: incidence and disparities 2006. *Contraception.* 2011;84(5):478-485.

4. Centers for Disease Control and Prevention (CDC). Prepregnancy contraceptive use among teens with unintended pregnancies resulting in live births: Pregnancy Risk Assessment Monitoring System (PRAMS), 2004-2008. *MMWR.* 2012;61:25.

5. D'Angelo D, Williams L, Morrow B, et al. Preconception and interconception health status of women who recently gave birth to a live-born infant: Pregnancy Risk Assessment Monitoring System (PRAMS), United States, 26 reporting areas, 2004. *MMWR.* 2007;56(10):1-35.

6. Comerford Freda M, Moos MK, Curtis M. The history of preconception care: evolving guidelines and standards. *Matern Child Health J.* 2006;10:S43-S52.

7. Public Health Service Expert Panel on the Content of Prenatal Care. *Caring for Our Future: The Content of Prenatal Care.* Washington, DC: US Public Health Service; 1989:25.

8. *Healthy People 2000: National Health Promotion and Disease Prevention Objectives.* Washington, DC: U.S. Public Health Service; 1991.

9. Healthy People 2020: 2020 topic and objectives, maternal, infant and child health: national health promotion and disease prevention objectives. Available at: http://www.healthypeople.gov/2020/topicsobjectives2020/objectiveslist.aspx?topicId=26. Accessed November 15, 2012.

10. Hood JR, Parker C, Atrash HK. Recommendations to improve preconception health and health care: strategies for implementation. *J Women's Health.* 2007;16(4):454-457.

11. U.S. Preventive Services Task Force. Folic acid for prevention of neural tube defects. Available at: http://www.uspreventiveservicestaskforce.org/uspstf09/folicacide/folicacidrs.htm. Accessed November 8, 2012.

12. De-Regil LM, Fernandez-Gaxioloa AC, Dowswell T, Pena-Rosas JP. Effects and safety of periconceptional folate supplementation for preventing birth defects [review]. *Cochrane Database Syst Rev.* 2010;10:CD007950. doi: 10.1002/14651858. CD007950pub2.

13. Mazza D, Chapman A. Improving the uptake of preconception care and periconceptional folate supplementation: what do women think? *BioMed Central.* 2010;10:786. Available at: http://www.biomedcentral.com/1471-2458/10/786. Accessed November 8, 2012.

14. Dean S, Bhutta Z, Mason EM, et al. Care before and between pregnancy. In: *Born Too Soon: The Global Action Report on Preterm Birth.* Geneva, Switzerland: World Health Organization; 2012.

15. Bronstein JM, Felix HC, Bursac Z, Steward MK, Foushee HR, Klapow J. Providing general and preconception health care to low income women in family planning settings: perception of providers and clients. *Matern Child Health J.* 2012;16:346-354.

16. DeVoe JE, Fryerm GE, Phillips R, Green L. Receipt of preventive care among adults: insurance status and usual source of care. *Am J Public Health.* 2003; 93:786-791.

17. Squires L, Mitchell EW, Levis DM, et al. Consumers' perceptions of preconception health. *Am J Health Promot.* 2013;27(3):S10-S19.

18. Moos MK. From conception to practice: reflections on the preconception health agenda. *J Women's Health.* 2010;19(3):561-567.

19. Centers for Disease Control and Prevention (CDC). Before, between, and beyond pregnancy. Available at: http://www.beforeandbeyond.org. Accessed November 8, 2012.

20. American College of Obstetricians and Gynecologists, Preconception Work Group. The importance of preconception care in the continuum of women's health care. *Obstet Gynecol.* 2005;106:665-666.

21. March of Dimes, PMNCH, Save the Children, World Health Organization. *Born Too Soon: The Global Action Report on Preterm Birth*, ed. CP Howson, MV Kinney, JE Lawn. Geneva, Switzerland: World Health Organization; 2012.

22. Schwarz EB, Parisis SM, Williams SL, Shevchik GJ, Hess R. Promoting safe prescribing in primary care with contraceptive vital sign: a cluster-randomized controlled trial. *Ann Fam Med.* 2012;10:516-522.

23. Luke B, Brown MB. Contemporary risks of maternal morbidity and adverse outcomes with increasing maternal age and plurality. *Fertil Steril.* 2007;88:283.

24. Solomon BD, Jack BW, Ferro WG. The clinical content of preconception care: genetics and genomics. *Am J Obstet Gynecol*. 2008:199(6 suppl 2):S340-S344.

25. De Wert G, Dondorp WJ, Knoppers BM. Preconception care and genetic risk: ethical issues. *J Community Genet*. 2012; 3:221-228.

26. Crane MJ, Quinn Griffin MT, Andrews CM, Fitzpatrick JJ. The level of importance and level of confidence that midwives in the United States attach to using genetics in practice. *J Midwifery Women's Health*. 2012;57:114-119.

27. Schrauwers C, Dekker G. Maternal and perinatal outcome in obese pregnant patients. *J Matern Fetal Neonat Med*. 2009;22(3):218-226.

28. Verma A, Shrimali L. Maternal body mass index and pregnancy outcome. *J Clin Diagn Res*. 2012;6(9): 1531-1533.

29. Lamont RF, Sobel J, Mazaki-Tovi S, et al. Listeriosis in human pregnancy: a systematic review. *J Perinat Med*. 2011;39(3):227-236.

30. Centers for Disease Control and Prevention (CDC). Recommendations for the use of folic acid to reduce the number of cases of spina bifida and other neural tube defects. *MMWR*. 1992;41(RR-14):l-5.

31. Simpson J, Bailey L, Pietrzik K, Shane B, Holzgreve W. Micronutrients and women of reproductive potential: required intake and consequences of dietary deficiency or excess. Part I: folate, vitamin B$_{12}$, vitamin B$_6$. *J Matern Fetal Neonatal Med*. 2010;23(12): 1323-1343.

32. American College of Obstetricians and Gynecologists. *Vitamin D: Screening and Supplementation During Pregnancy*. Committee Opinion 495. July 2011.

33. U.S. Preventive Services Task Force. Screening for hepatitis C virus infection in adults: US Preventive Services Task Force recommendation statement. Release date June 2013. Available at: http://www.uspreventive servicestaskforce.org/uspstf/uspshepc.htm. Accessed July 15, 2013.

34. U.S. Preventive Services Task Force. Screening for HIV: US Preventive Services Task Force. Available at: http://www.uspreventiveservicestaskforce.org/uspstf /uspshivi.htm. Accessed July 15, 2013.

35. Boggess KA, Edelstein BL. Oral health in women during preconception and pregnancy: implications for birth outcomes and infant oral health. *Matern Child Health J*. 2006;10:S169-S174.

36. American Diabetes Association. (2008). Standards of medical care in diabetes: 2008 position statement. Available at: http://care.diabetesjournals.org/content /31/Supplement_1/S12.full.pdf. Accessed January 22, 2011.

37. Persson M, Norman M, Hanson U. Obstetric and perinatal outcomes in type 1 diabetic pregnancies: a large, population-based study. *Diab Care*. 2009;32:2005.

38. Temple R. Preconception care for women with diabetes: is it effective and who should provide it? *Best Pract Res Clin Obstet Gynecol*. 2011;25:3-14.

39. Dunlop AL, Jack BW, Bottalico JN, et al. The clinical content of preconception care: women with chronic medical conditions. *Am J Obstet Gynecol*. 2008;199(6 suppl 2):S310-S327.

40. National Center for Health Statistics. *Ambulatory Health Care Data: NAMCS Description*. Washington, DC: U.S. Department of Health and Human Services, Centers for Disease and Control and Prevention, National Center for Health Statistics; 2004. Available at: http://www.cdc.gov/nchs/about/major/ahcd /namcsdes.htm. Accessed November 17, 2012.

41. Sibai BM. Chronic hypertension: chronic hypertension in pregnancy. *Obstet Gynecol*. 2002;100;369-373.

42. Endocrine Society. *Management of Thyroid Dysfunction During Pregnancy and Postpartum: An Endocrine Society Clinical Practice Guideline*. Chevy Chase, MD: Endocrine Society; 2007.

43. Cooper DS, Blondi B. Subclinical thyroid disease. *Lancet*. 2012;379:1142-1154.

44. Hviid A, Molgaard-Nielsen D. Corticosteroid use during pregnancy and risk of orofacial clefts. *CMAJ*. 2011. doi: 10:1503/cmaj.101063.

45. Ostensen M. Rheumatological disorders. *Best Pract Res Clin Obstet Gynecol*. 2001;15(6):953-969.

46. Pennell PB. Using current evidence in selecting antiepileptic drugs for use during pregnancy. *Epilepsy Curr*. 2005;5(2):45-51.

47. Wadwha PD, Entringer S, Buss C, Lu MC. The contribution of maternal stress to preterm birth: issues and considerations. *Clin Perinatol*. 2011;38(3):351-384.

48. Sathyanarayana S, Focareta J, Dailey T, Buchanan S. Environmental exposures: how to counsel preconception and prenatal patients in the clinical setting. *Am J Obstet Gynecol*. 2012;207(6):463-470.

49. Hackley B, Katz-Jacobson A. Lead poisoning in pregnancy: a case study with implications for midwives. *J Midwifery Women's Health*. 2003;48:30-38.

50. Agency for Toxic Substances and Disease Registry. Public health statement: lead. CAS #7439-92-1. Available at: http://www.atsdr.cdc.gov/ToxProfiles /tp13-c1-b.pdf Accessed May 13, 2013.

51. Frey KA, Navarro SM, Kotelchuck M, Lu MC. The clinical content of preconception care for men. *Am J Obstet Gynecol*. 2008;199(6 suppl 2):S389-S392.

52. Sipos A, Rasmussen F, Harrison G, et al. Paternal age and schizophrenia: a population based cohort study. *BMJ*. 2004;329:1070.

53. Malaspina D, Harlap S, Fennig S, et al. Advancing paternal age and the risk of schizophrenia. *Arch Gen Psychiatry*. 2001;58:361-367.

• • • Additional Resources

Websites That Provide Information About Preconception Care

Centers for Disease Control and Prevention:
http://www.cdc.gov/preconception/index.html
A general website that provides links to different content areas relevant to preconception care.

Before, Between, and Beyond Pregnancy:
http://www.beforeandbeyond.org
A national preconception healthcare curriculum for health professionals.

March of Dimes

The March of Dimes offers a variety of resources and initiatives for reproductive-age women and men as well as health professionals.

For consumers:
http://www.marchofdimes.com/pregnancy/getready_indepth.html
"Get Ready for Pregnancy"

For professionals:
http://www.marchofdimes.com/professionals/professionals.html
A resource page that provides links to different content areas relevant to preconception care.

U.S. Department of Health and Human Services, Office of Women's Health:
http://www.womenshealth.gov/pregnancy/before-you-get-pregnant/preconception-health.cfm
A general website that provides the major talking points related to preconception care.

Food Contaminants

American Pregnancy Association:
http://www.americanpregnancy.org/pregnancyhealth/fishmercury.htm

U.S. Food and Drug Administration:
http://www.fda.gov/food/foodsafety/product-specificinformation/seafood/foodbornepathogenscontaminants/methylmercury/ucm115644.htm

Environmental Protection Agency

EPA's Roadmap for Mercury, 2009:
http://www.epa.gov/mercury/executivesummary.htm

What You Need to Know About Mercury in Fish and Shellfish:
http://www.epa.gov/waterscience/fish/advice

Environmental Working Group, "Food Guide":
http://www.ewg.org/foodnews/

Physicians for Social Responsibility, "Healthy Fish, Healthy Families":
http://www.psr.org/resources/healthy-fish-healthy.html

Pesticides and Environmental Toxins

Making our Milk Safe (MOMS):
http://www.safemilk.org/wp-content/uploads/2012/09/Preconception_080612_vf_b.pdf

Natural Resources Defense Council, "Chemicals in Plastic Bottles: How to Know What's Safe for Your Family":
http://www.nrdc.org/health/bpa.pdf

III

Gynecology

Midwives as Providers of Gynecologic Care

Today, the average life expectancy at birth for a woman who resides in the United States is nearly 81 years.[1] Within this lifespan, the average woman wants two children, and thus spends about five years pregnant, postpartum, breastfeeding, or trying to become pregnant. She will spend six times that long (approximately 30 years) trying to avoid pregnancy. This represents more than more than three-fourths of her reproductive life.[2] Moreover, given modern life expectancy, this woman will enjoy 3 or more decades of life after her reproductive years have ended.

Ideally, most of this woman's life will be spent in good health, where health as defined by the World Health Organization (WHO), is a state of complete physical, mental, and social well-being, and not merely the absence of disease or infirmity.[3] Ideally, she will also enjoy reproductive health at all stages of her life, defined by WHO as the ability to have a responsible, satisfying, and safe sex life; the capability to reproduce; and the freedom to decide if, when, and how often to do so.[4] Making these hopes for good health a reality requires health promotion, disease prevention, health education, and empowering women to make the choices that are meaningful to them and choices that will optimize their health.

Fortunately, these are skills in which midwives excel. Add the recognition that life stages, normal physiology, and developmental processes are not diseases; that continuity of care is a value to be promoted; that informed choice, shared decision making, and the right to self-determination are important to health; and that evidence-based decision-making should underlie the health care of women, and we have several of the hallmarks of midwifery important for providing gynecologic, sexual, and reproductive health care.[5] While midwifery is often associated with pregnancy and birth, women have healthcare needs at all stages of their lives that are not related to pregnancy. Thus gynecologic, sexual, and reproductive care are, and should be, essential aspects of midwifery practice that are well established in the American College of Nurse-Midwives (ACNM) Core Competencies,[5] where specific knowledge and skills of midwifery responsibilities beyond perinatal care are detailed in several sections.

Caring for women in the area of gynecologic, sexual, and reproductive health gives midwives the opportunity to truly be with women for a lifetime, from adolescence through old age. Most women spend only a few years of their lives needing maternity care services, but they need healthcare services that midwives can provide for many more years. Gynecologic, sexual, and reproductive health care provided by midwives is particularly timely given the new regulations associated with the 2012 Patient Protection and Affordable Care Act and the changing face of U.S. health care. Women can now receive annual well-woman visits, human papillomavirus testing, counseling for sexually transmitted infections, HIV screening, and contraceptive methods and counseling without a co-payment, coinsurance, or a deductible.[6] As women's access to these services increases, midwives must be poised to provide them. The knowledge found in the chapters in this section will provide the foundation for being "with women for a lifetime."[7]

Patricia Aikins Murphy
Frances E. Likis

● ● ● References

1. National Center for Health Statistics. *Health, United States, 2011: With Special Feature on Socioeconomic Status and Health*. Hyattsville, MD: National Center for Health Statistics; 2012. Available at: http://www.cdc.gov/nchs/data/hus/hus11.pdf#022. Accessed March 5, 2013.

2. Guttmacher Institute. *Facts on Publicly Funded Contraceptive Services in the United States*. New York, NY: Guttmacher Institute; 2012. Available at: http://www.guttmacher.org/pubs/fb_contraceptive_serv.html. Accessed March 5, 2013.

3. World Health Organization. *WHO Definition of Health*. Geneva, Switzerland: World Health Organization; 1948. Available at: http://www.who.int/about/definition/en/print.html. Accessed March 5, 2013.

4. World Health Organization. Reproductive health. Available at: http://www.who.int/topics/reproductive_health/en. Accessed March 5, 2013.

5. American College of Nurse-Midwives. *Core Competencies for Basic Midwifery Practice*. Silver Spring, MD: American College of Nurse-Midwives; 2012.

6. Health Resources and Services Administration. Women's preventive services: required health plan coverage guidelines. Available at: http://www.hrsa.gov/womensguidelines. Accessed March 5, 2013.

7. Williams DR. Unveiling an evidence-based image for ACNM: "with women for a lifetime." *J Midwifery Women's Health*. 2001;46(3):vi.

CHAPTER

11

Anatomy and Physiology of the Female Reproductive System

JENIFER O. FAHEY

MARY C. BRUCKER

Introduction

Midwives' expertise in "normal" begins with an understanding of the reproductive anatomy and physiology that is essential to nearly all aspects of midwifery care. To perform an accurate bimanual exam, the midwife must know the normal position and shape of the uterus and ovaries. To comprehend how oral contraceptives work to suppress ovulation, the midwife must understand how ovulation occurs. To correctly repair a perineal laceration, the midwife must be familiar with the musculature of the perineum and pelvic floor in order to identify the tissues that have been lacerated and determine how they must be approximated.

This understanding of the normal structure and function of a woman's body at various stages of her life also enables a midwife to identify variations in normal as well as abnormalities. Only by truly understanding how a woman's body develops and works through the life course is a midwife able to articulate this knowledge in a way that women can understand and use.

Four chapters in this text specifically focus on the anatomy and physiology underpinning clinical practice. This chapter provides a general overview of the anatomy of the female reproductive system, including the breast, and describes basic reproductive physiology, including menstrual physiology. The *Anatomy and Physiology of Pregnancy: Placental, Fetal, and Maternal Adaptations* chapter reviews maternal anatomic and physiologic adaptations to pregnancy, and fetal and placental development and function. The *Anatomy and Physiology During Labor and Birth* chapter focuses on the processes involved in labor and birth, and the chapter titled *The Anatomy and*

Physiology of Postpartum describes the physiology of the puerperium. Other chapters also include information on important physiologic processes. The physiology of lactation, for example, is described in the *Breastfeeding and the Mother–Newborn Dyad* chapter, while the transition of the newborn to extrauterine life is covered in the *Anatomy and Physiology of the Newborn* chapter.

The Breast

Breast Anatomy

The mature female breast extends vertically from approximately the second rib to the sixth rib, and horizontally from the edge of the sternum to the mid-axillary line with an extension of tissue into the axilla known as the tail of Spence (**Figure 11-1**). The breast tissue is composed of epithelial (glandular or secretory) tissue, between which is interspersed stromal (adipose and connective) tissue. These two types of tissue are present in roughly equal amounts in the breasts of women who are not pregnant or lactating.[1] During pregnancy and lactation, however, the glandular tissue proliferates and becomes the predominant breast tissue.[2] The glandular tissue in each breast is organized into 15 to 20 lobes made up of clusters of 10 to 100 alveoli referred to as lobules (**Figure 11-2**). The lobes, as well as the ducts that drain the lobules, are interconnected; they are not the distinct, independent structures that terminate in a lactiferous sinus as has historically been described.[1] The shape of the breast is maintained primarily by suspensory ligaments, known as Cooper's ligaments that connect the dermis of the breast to the deep pectoral fascia, which

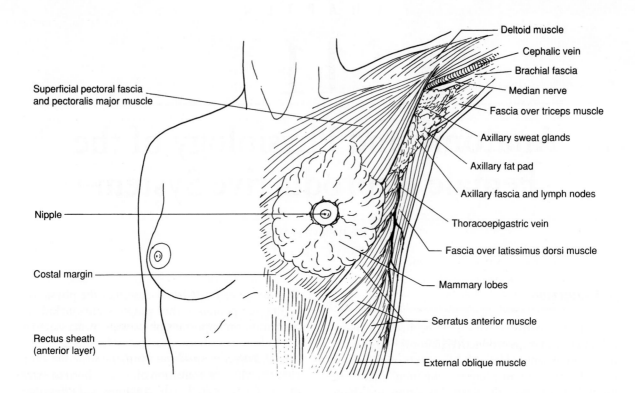

Figure 11-1 Anterior pectoral dissection.
Source: Adapted from Carmine D. Clemente, *Anatomy: a regional atlas of the human body*, 6th ed., 2010 (Figure 4.1). Reprinted by permission of the author.

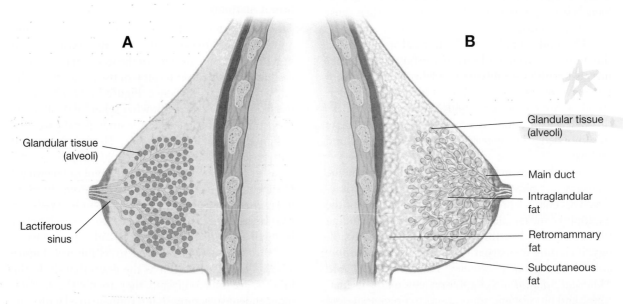

Figure 11-2 (A) Traditional schematic diagram of the anatomy of the breast. The main milk ducts below the nipple are depicted as dilated portions or lactiferous sinuses and the glandular tissue is deeper within the breast. (B) Schematic diagram of the ductal anatomy of the breast based on the findings of Ramsay et al. (2005). Milk ducts are shown to be small and branch a short distance from the base of the nipple. The ductal system is erratic and glandular tissue is situated directly beneath the nipple.

Source: © 2008 Medela AG. Reprinted by permission.

overlays the pectoralis major and serratus anterior muscles of the chest.

The alveoli are dilated sac-like structures composed of two layers of cells. The inner luminal cells are responsible for synthesis and secretion of breast milk. They are surrounded by myoepithelial cells that eject milk during lactation (Figure 11-2). During pregnancy, the alveoli gain the capacity to produce and excrete milk. These differentiated alveoli are referred to as acini. The secretory cells in these acinar units are stimulated by prolactin to secrete milk into the lumen of the alveolus, whereas the myoepithelial cells are stimulated by oxytocin to contract, which compresses the alveolar sacs so that milk is ejected into the milk ductules. The ductules are connected to larger lactiferous ducts, which merge to form a smaller number of ducts that lead to openings at the nipple, through which milk exits the breast. The exact number of these openings is not known and has been reported to vary from 4 to 18, but the most recent evidence seems to suggest that there are, on average, 5 to 9 patent ducts in each nipple of a lactating woman.[2]

The nipple, which is located slightly below the center of each breast, is surrounded by a circular area of pigmented skin known as the areola. The tissue under the nipple and areola contains smooth muscle fibers that, when they contract, cause the nipple to become erect. Toward the outer edges of the areola are the openings of coalesced sebaceous and mammary glands known as Montgomery glands. These glands become enlarged in pregnancy and will produce secretions that may assist in the initiation of lactation by providing olfactory cues to the newborn.[3] A more detailed description of lactogenesis can be found in the *Breastfeeding and the Mother–Newborn Dyad* chapter.

Blood is supplied to the breast primarily by the mammary artery and by the lateral thoracic arteries. Venous flow from the breast drains into the internal thoracic, axillary, and cephalic veins. The lymphatic vessels of the breast serve an important function during lactation by draining milk molecules that are too large to move into blood vessels. Lymphatic flow is also significant because it determines the location of metastasis of cancer cells from the breast to other parts of the body. The majority of breast lymph flows to the axillary lymph nodes, which is, therefore, the main route of cancer metastasis from the breast. The intermammary lymph nodes are the other main group of lymph nodes that drain the breast, but they receive only a small fraction of the lymph flow from the breast.

The breast is innervated by the lateral and anterior cutaneous branches of the second to the sixth intercostal nerves and from the supraclavicular nerves. The nipple and areola are innervated primarily by the cutaneous branch of the fourth intercostal nerve.

Breast Development

Human breast development begins during the embryologic period and is believed to originate with the appearance of the primitive milk streaks bilaterally from the axilla to the groin of the embryo. This ridge regresses except for the region that eventually becomes the mammary gland. On occasion, additional areas of this ridge may not regress; these areas then develop into accessory nipples and sometimes even into glandular mammary tissue capable of milk production and excretion. Such auxiliary nipples may be noted on a physical examination.

At birth, all newborns have an opening of a primitive ductal system to the surface, a protruding nipple, and a circular area of skin that has proliferated into what is the areola. Varying degrees of development of the glandular breast tissue occur during the fetal period, however, so that at birth, the structures present can range from simple blunt-ended tubular structures to well-developed branching ductal systems with lobular–alveolar structures.[4] Under the influence of maternal and neonatal pro-lactation hormones, these structures are capable of producing milk shortly after birth. In some cases, this milk is excreted and exits via the neonate's nipple (sometimes referred to as "witch's milk"). Once the maternal hormones are removed, however, the infant breast tissue undergoes a period of involution so that by 2 years of age there remains only a small ductal system. Some growth in this tissue is noted during childhood, but no development occurs until puberty, at which point the female breast undergoes a period of extensive development.

With the onset of puberty, a process of elongation and branching of the ductal system begins, along with formation of lobules through development of some of the ductal endings into clusters of ductules and alveolar buds. This gradual process of branching and lobule formation occurs primarily under the influence of estrogen, but actually involves multiple hormones, including growth hormone. In the adult woman, some of these lobules will undergo further branching and glandular development with each menstrual cycle. However, full glandular differentiation and formation of the secretory acini capable of producing and secreting milk do not occur until pregnancy. The changes in breast structure that take place in pregnancy and lactation are detailed in the *Anatomy and Physiology of Pregnancy: Placental, Fetal, and Maternal Adaptations* and *Breastfeeding and the Mother–Newborn Dyad* chapters, respectively.

The External Female Genitalia

The external female genitalia, which can also be referred to as the vulva, are those structures located between the pubis and the perineum. They include the mons pubis, the labia minora, the labia majora, the clitoris, the hymen, the vestibule, and the urinary meatus or urethral opening. Although they cannot be seen externally, Bartholin glands and Skene's glands and ducts as well as the vestibular bulbs are also considered part of the external genitalia.

The mons pubis is the layer of fatty tissue that overlays the pubic bone. In the postpubertal woman, the skin of the mons is covered with coarse, curly hair. The labia majora are folds of connective and adipose tissue that extend inferiorly from the mons and merge posteriorly into the perineal body to form the posterior commissure. Medial to the labia majora are the labia minora, which are two thin folds of connective tissue. The area between the labia minora that extends from the clitoris to the fourchette is referred to as the vestibule and is the area into which the urethra, the ducts of the Bartholin glands, the vagina, and, sometimes, the Skene's ducts open. The labia minora merge superiorly to form the prepuce and frenulum of the clitoris and inferiorly to form the fourchette. Prior to a vaginal birth, both the labia majora and the labia minora assist in keeping the vaginal introitus closed and in protecting the urethral opening. In multiparous women, the labia minora may project beyond the labia majora; in contrast, in nulliparous women, the labia minora are usually not visible unless the labia majora are separated.

The clitoris is a highly innervated, erectile organ located in the superior portion of the vestibule where the labia minora fuse. The clitoris is often described as the homologue of the penis. Unlike the penis, however, the function of the clitoris is purely erogenous. The clitoris, which is approximately 1.5 to 2.0 centimeters in total length,[5] has a glans, a corpus, and two crura composed of erectile tissue that create an inverted V structure attached to the pubic arch and extending along the pubic rami. Adjacent to the crura and flanking the vaginal orifice are the vestibular bulbs, which are also composed of vascular, erectile tissue. These structures become engorged with blood during sexual arousal.

The Bartholin glands, which are also known as the major or greater vestibular glands, are located beneath the fascia of the vestibule on either side of the vaginal opening at about 4 o'clock and 8 o'clock. Each gland has a duct that opens into the inferior part of the vestibule between the labia minora and the hymen. These glands secrete mucus during sexual arousal. The Skene's glands, which are also known as the lesser vestibular glands or the periurethral glands, usually open onto the vestibule on either side of the urethra, but sometimes open on the posterior wall of the urethra. These glands also secrete mucus during sexual stimulation and/or arousal.

The Internal Female Genitalia

Figure 11-3 shows a midsagittal view of the internal organs and associated structures that make up the female reproductive system. These include the vagina, the uterus, the fallopian tubes, and the ovaries. A detailed description of each component follows.

The Vagina

The vagina is a muscular structure that extends from the vulva to the cervix. It is a potential space, in that the walls are usually in opposition, but can be separated as occurs during intercourse or childbirth. Anteriorly, the vagina is separated from the bladder by connective tissue known as the vesicovaginal septum; posteriorly, it is separated from the rectum by the rectovaginal septum (in the lower segment) and by the rectouterine pouch or cul-de-sac of Douglas (in the upper segment). The walls of the vagina, which are referred to as the anterior, posterior, and lateral vaginal walls, run from the vaginal opening at the vestibule to the cervix posteriorly, where they create a "dead end." The spaces created between the cervix and the ends of the vaginal walls are called the fornices. There are four fornices: the anterior fornix, the posterior fornix, and two lateral fornices.

The vaginal walls are lined with a layer of stratified squamous epithelium, which in premenopausal women is folded into ridges known as rugae that can stretch and provide distensibility to the vagina. Beneath this lining is a layer of smooth muscle as well as a layer of connective tissue referred to as the adventitia. These layers maintain vaginal tone. The blood supply to the vagina comes from the vaginal artery, which branches from the uterine artery, or directly from the internal iliac artery, the inferior vesical arteries, and the middle rectal and internal pudendal arteries. Blood is drained from the vaginal area by a venous plexus that follows the arteries, and lymph is drained primarily via the inguinal lymph nodes.

The vagina is innervated mostly by the uterovaginal plexus, which arises from the inferior hypogastric or pelvic plexus; this latter structure contains

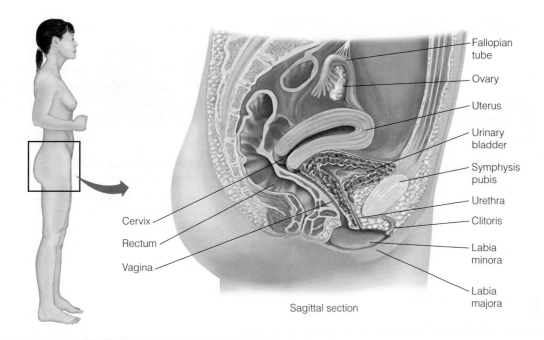

Sagittal section

Figure 11-3 Midsaggital view of a woman's pelvis.
Source: Schuiling KD, Likis FE. *Women's Gynecologic Health.* 2nd ed. Burlington, MA; 2013.

sympathetic efferent fibers from the second, third, and fourth sacral nerves. In addition, the vagina is innervated by a few filaments from the first two sacral ganglia. The lower two-thirds of the vagina is primarily innervated by the pudendal nerve.

The Uterus

The uterus is a pear-shaped, muscular organ that, in the nonpregnant state, is situated in the pelvic cavity superior to the urinary bladder. The uterus is anchored in place, usually—but not always—in an anteverted position, by the uterine ligaments. The adult nulliparous uterus measures approximately 6 to 8 centimeters in length, 5 centimeters across, and 4 centimeters in thickness, and it weighs approximately 50 grams.[6] The functions of the uterus include receiving a fertilized ovum, providing the environment for the embryo and the fetus, and contracting to help in the expulsion of the fetus and placenta. The uterus has two main parts: the body and the cervix. During pregnancy, the body of the uterus differentiates into an upper segment called the fundus and lower segment called the isthmus (Figure 11-4).

The Cervix

The cervix is the cylindrical, fibromuscular lower portion of the uterus that is sometimes referred to as the neck of the uterus. It is composed of dense, collagenous connective tissue, which contains blood vessels, nerves, and glands that secrete thick mucus. The cervix has two areas of constriction at each end: the internal os, which is found at the junction of the cervix and uterine body, and the external os, which opens into the vagina. The role of the cervix and the cervical ora in pregnancy and birth are detailed in the *Anatomy and Physiology of Pregnancy: Placental, Fetal, and Maternal Adaptations* and *Anatomy and Physiology During Labor and Birth* chapters. The tunnel-like area between the internal and external os is called the cervical canal. The external surface of the cervix, known as the ectocervix, is lined with squamous epithelial cells like those that line the vagina, while the inner part of the cervix, known as the endocervix, is lined with glandular epithelial cells. The area where the endocervix and exocervix meet is the transformation zone; metaplastic cells are found here. It is in this region where most cervical cancers originate, which is why obtaining a sample of these cells during a Pap test is important.

The Uterine Body

The body of the uterus is made up of external serosal layer formed by the peritoneum, a muscular (myometrial) layer, and a mucosal (endometrial) layer (Figure 11-4).

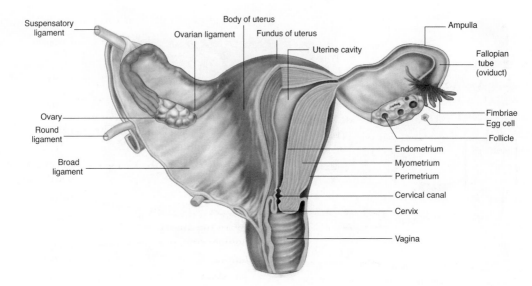

Figure 11-4 Anterior view of uterus.

Endometrium

The endometrium is the mucosal lining of the uterine cavity. It is composed of (1) ciliated columnar epithelial cells; (2) glands that secrete a thin alkaline mucus rich in proteins, sugars, and secretions that allows survival of the zygote and blastocyst before implantation; and (3) the mesenchymal stroma, a layer of connective and vascular tissue that lies between the epithelial layer and the myometrium. This stroma can be subdivided into two layers: the stratum basalis, which is closest to the myometrium and is not shed during menstruation, and the stratum functionalis, the layer of the endometrium that proliferates and degenerates cyclically in menstruating women.

The endometrium receives blood from two different sets of arteries: a "straight" set of arteries that supply the stratum basalis and a set of "coiled" spiral arterioles that supply the stratum functionalis (**Figure 11-5**). During the menstrual cycle, these vessels and the rest of the endometrium undergo marked changes. As part of the proliferative phase of the menstrual cycle, under the effects of rising levels of estrogen and progesterone, the endometrium becomes increasingly vascularized and the glands of the endometrium become longer and increasingly convoluted and fill with secretions. As a result, there is a 10-fold increase in thickness of the myometrium, from 0.5 to 5 millimeters.[6]

If fertilization and implantation do not occur, the subsequent drop in estrogen and progesterone levels leads to atrophy of the functional layer of the endometrium, which in turn leads to increased coiling of the spiral arterioles and a regression of the glandular

development. The excessive coiling of the spiral arterioles diminishes the blood flow to the endometrial layer, which in turn produces tissue ischemia and necrosis and endometrial bleeding.[7] Menstrual flow is, therefore, the result of this bleeding and shedding of necrotic endometrial tissue. A more detailed description of the menstrual cycle can be found later in this chapter. Once a woman has reached menopause, the endometrium becomes atrophic: The epithelium flattens, the glands gradually disappear, and the endometrial stroma becomes increasingly fibrous. In some cases, however, it may retain a weak proliferative capacity, which may contribute to the development of endometrial cancer.[8]

Myometrium

The bulk of the uterus is made up of the myometrium, which is composed of bundles of smooth muscle fibers separated by connective tissue made primarily of collagen and elastin. The muscle fibers of the myometrium are arranged in three distinct patterns that contribute to this tissue's ability to contract effectively. In the inner layer of the myometrium, the fibers run in a circular pattern that spirals in a perpendicular orientation to the long axis of the uterus. In the middle layer, the muscle fibers are interlaced and form figure-eight patterns running diagonally along the long axis of the uterus.[9, 10] The outermost layer of the myometrium contains an arrangement of fibers in both longitudinal and spiral patterns. These layers become more differentiated in pregnancy with the hypertrophy of the myometrial cells that occurs in pregnancy. Changes

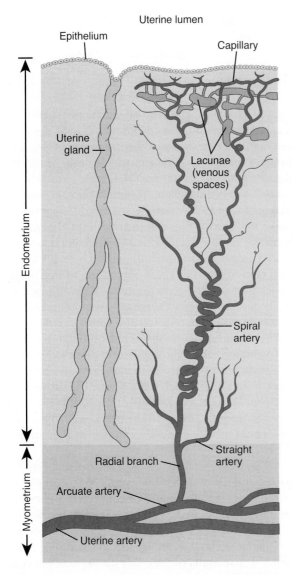

Uterine lumen

Epithelium

Capillary

Uterine gland

Lacunae (venous spaces)

Endometrium

Spiral artery

Radial branch

Straight artery

Myometrium

Arcuate artery

Uterine artery

Figure 11-5 Anatomy and circulation of the endometrium.
Source: This figure was published in Moore, KL, and Persaud, TVN. *The Developing Human: Clinically Oriented Embryology,* 7th ed., Copyright Saunders 2003. Reprinted by permission of Elsevier.

in the uterus during pregnancy are discussed in the *Anatomy and Physiology of Pregnancy: Placental, Fetal, and Maternal Adaptations* chapter, and the *Anatomy and Physiology During Labor and Birth* chapter contains a detailed description of the physiology of uterine contractions.

A gradient in the amount of muscle tissue found throughout the uterus is apparent, such that at the fundus, the myometrium contains mostly muscle fibers, whereas only 10% to 15% of the tissue mass in the cervix is composed of muscle fibers.[9] The proportion of muscle fibers present determines the

contractile strength of the uterine muscle, so this distribution of muscle creates a contraction strength gradient along the length of the uterus.

Uterine Ligaments, Blood Supply, and Innervation

The broad ligaments of the uterus are composed of folds in the peritoneum. These two wing-like structures extend from the sides of the uterus to the pelvic sidewalls. The superior part of the broad ligaments forms the suspensory ligament of the ovary and the mesosalpinx (to which the fallopian tubes are attached). The round ligaments also extend from the side of the uterus, but course downward through the inguinal ring, into the inguinal canal and to the labia majora. These ligaments maintain the anteversion of the uterus. The peritoneal ligaments (uterosacral, cardinal, and pubocervical) extend from the cervix to different parts of the pelvis and help stabilize the uterus.

The vessels that supply the uterus are derived primarily from the uterine and ovarian arteries. The uterine artery is a branch of the anterior branch of the internal iliac arteries (also referred to as the hypogastric arteries). The uterine artery enters the side of the uterus through the broad ligament and divides into several branches to supply the lower cervix and upper vagina, the upper portion of the cervix, and the body of the uterus. One large branch of the uterine artery travels along the margin of the uterus toward the fundus. At approximately the height of the round ligament, this branch of the uterine artery furcates into three vessels. One vessel joins the terminal branch of the ovarian artery, one supplies part of the fallopian tube, and one supplies the uterine fundus. The vessels that supply and drain blood from the uterus are collectively referred to as the arcuate vessels of the uterus.

The ovarian artery is a direct branch of the aorta that enters the broad ligament. The main stem of the ovarian artery travels near the mesosalpinx (the part of the broad ligament that encloses the fallopian tubes) all the way to the upper, lateral portion of the uterus to join with the ovarian branch of the uterine artery. Branches from this main stem perfuse the ovaries and fallopian tubes.

The arcuate uterine veins that make up the uterine venous plexus join to form the uterine vein, which empties into the internal iliac vein. The blood from the upper and outer parts of the uterus and ovaries is collected by multiple veins that form the pampiniform plexus that drains into the ovarian vein. The right ovarian vein empties into the vena cava, while the left ovarian vein empties into the left renal vein.

The lymph from the body of the uterus is drained by lymph vessels that carry their contents to either the internal iliac nodes or the periaortic nodes. The periaortic nodes also receive lymphatic drainage from the ovaries.

The uterus is innervated primarily by the parasympathetic system by branches arising from the second, third, and fourth sacral nerves. In addition, it receives some innervation from the sympathetic nervous system via the presacral nerve and lumbar sympathetic chain.

The Fallopian Tubes

The fallopian tubes (also referred to as oviducts and salpinges) are the 8- to 14-centimeter-long, narrow, muscular tubes that extend from the uterine horns or cornua. The oviducts, as their name would imply, transport the ovum from the ovary to the uterus. It is also in the fallopian tubes that fertilization normally takes place. The fallopian tubes have three layers: (1) the mucosa, a single-layer lining of ciliated or secretory columnar cells; (2) the muscularis layer; and (3) the serosa, the outer covering of the tubes, which is derived from the visceral peritoneum.

The fallopian tubes can be divided into four sections:

- The pars interstitialis is the portion of the tube that penetrates the muscular wall of the uterus and connects the cavity of the oviduct with the uterine cavity.
- The isthmus is the narrow segment that extends from the uterus.
- The ampulla is a wider segment of the oviduct and is where fertilization of the ovum most commonly occurs.
- The infundibulum is the fimbriated, open distal end of the fallopian tube.

The fimbriae are fine, fingerlike mucosal projections at the end of the fallopian tube that sweep near the ovaries, but that are not connected to the ovaries. As a consequence, the oviducts open directly into the abdominal cavity. The fallopian tubes vary in diameter at the different segments, with the isthmus measuring approximately 2 to 3 millimeters in thickness while the ampulla reaches a diameter of 5 to 8 millimeters.[6]

The structure of the oviducts promotes movement of the ovum from the ovary into the tubes and down toward the uterine cavity. The cilia of the mucosa move in waves to assist with transport of the ovum, and the fibers of the muscularis layer are arranged in a way that allows the oviducts to move and contract in a way that promotes transport of the ovum.

The Ovaries

The ovaries are the organs of gamete production in the female. In addition to producing ova, the ovaries manufacture the steroid hormones estrogen and progesterone and, therefore, are also part of the endocrine system. The two ovaries, which are almond shaped, vary in size from one another, from woman to woman, and in the same woman in different stages of her life. During the reproductive years, the ovaries measure, on average, 2.5 to 5 centimeters in length, 1.5 to 3 centimeters in width, and 0.6 to 1.5 centimeters in thickness.[5] These organs are located in the upper part of the pelvic cavity and are attached to the broad ligament by the mesovarium; to the uterus by the utero-ovarian ligaments, which extend from below the insertion points of the fallopian tubes in the posterior part of the uterus; and to the pelvic wall by the suspensory ligament of the ovary (also referred to as the infundibulopelvic ligament). The suspensory ligament of the uterus is a fold of the peritoneum that extends from the ovary to the pelvic wall. This fold also contains blood vessels and nerves that supply the ovary.

The ovary is made up of two main parts: the cortex and the medulla. The cortex—the outer layer of the ovary—is composed of connective tissue and contains follicles in different stages of development. It is lined with germinal epithelium, and its dull and whitish outer layer is referred to as the tunica albuginea. The medulla of the ovary also consists of connective tissue and contains arteries, veins, and some smooth muscle fibers.

Two primary glandular cells within the ovarian follicles are involved in the synthesis of steroids: the thecal cells and the luteal or granulosa cells. Theca cells differentiate from the interfollicular stroma of ripening follicles in response to proteins secreted by growing follicles.[11] They produce the androgen substrate required for ovarian estrogen biosynthesis.

Ovarian Development

The human gonads are derived from three types of embryonic tissues: (1) the coelomic epithelium, (2) mesenchyme, and (3) primordial germ cells. The primordial germ cells, which eventually will produce the gametes, originate in the yolk sac of the developing embryo. Until approximately 4 weeks' gestation, no sexual differentiation occurs in the development of the gonads.[12] Once the sex-determining region of the Y gene becomes activated, however, the process of sex differentiation begins. Whereas development of the male reproductive system relies on activation of this gene and the effects of specific hormones, the development of the ovaries and female genitals follows the "default" process that happens in the absence of these hormones. For example, in the absence of testosterone, the Wolffian structures (which in the male embryo will become the male internal genitalia) will regress. Similarly, the Müllerian ducts, without suppression from Müllerian-inhibiting hormone from the fetal testes, will continue to develop and become the uterus, the oviducts, and the upper part of the vagina.

The ovaries develop from the coelomic epithelium, which proliferates to form the medulla and the cortex by the third month of gestation. The primordial germ cells in these fetal ovaries undergo rapid division and then differentiate into primary oocytes. By the fourth month of gestation, each ovary contains approximately 10 million primary oocytes and some primordial follicles (oocytes surrounded by follicular cells). Most of the oocytes degenerate so that by birth the neonate has approximately 250,000 to 500,000

oocytes; by puberty, only about 200,000 oocytes are left.[13] The oocytes stop developing and will remain in a state of arrested meiosis until puberty.

The Bony Pelvis

The bony pelvis has multiple functions. First, it provides an attachment site for the muscles and connective tissue of the pelvis, thereby providing support and stability to the pelvic organs. Second, it provides the site of attachment and articulation for the lower limbs. Third, it supports the weight of the upper trunk and distributes it to the lower extremities. Finally, in the female, the fetus passes through the bony pelvis during childbirth.

Pelvic Bones

The pelvis comprises four bones: two innominate bones, the sacrum, and the coccyx (**Figure 11-6**).

Each innominate bone has three parts: the pubis, the ischium, and the ilium. The ilium is the posterior and upper portion of the innominate bone; the two ilia join the sacrum along the sides at the sacroiliac

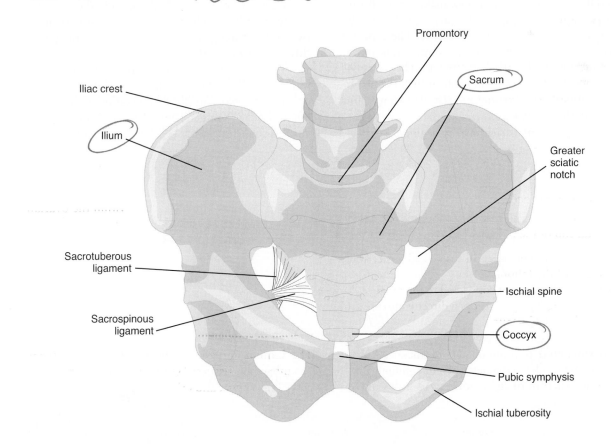

Figure 11-6 The bony pelvis with ligaments (front view).

synchondroses. The ischium is the medial and lower portion of the innominate bone. Important bony landmarks of the ischium include the ischial spine, the ischial tuberosity, and the pelvic sidewall. The pubis is the anterior portion of the innominate bone. The two pubic bones join at the symphysis pubis, where they are attached to an avascular fibrocartilage disc. The inferior margin of the symphysis pubis and the descending rami create the pubic arch, another important bony landmark of the pelvis.

The longitudinal axis of the symphysis pubis is normally parallel to the longitudinal axis of the sacrum. If the symphysis pubis is not at least approximately parallel to the sacrum, the anteroposterior diameters of two of the three pelvic planes that the fetus passes through during birth, the pelvic inlet and the pelvic outlet, can be changed significantly. Tilting of the superior margin of the symphysis pubis toward the sacral promontory and of the inferior margin away from the sacrum is called anterior inclination. Tilting of the inferior margin of the symphysis pubis toward the sacrum and the superior margin away from the sacral promontory is called posterior inclination (**Figure 11-7**).

The sacrum and the coccyx make up the posterior portion of the pelvis. The sacrum is formed by the fusion of the five sacral vertebrae. The superior part of the sacrum, the sacral promontory, is an important bony landmark of the pelvic. The coccyx is formed by the fusion of four (but sometimes three or five) rudimentary vertebrae and is itself an important bony landmark. The sacrum and the coccyx join at the sacrococcygeal symphysis.

Pelvic Joints

There are four joints within the bony pelvis: the symphysis pubis, the two sacroiliac synchondroses (or sacroiliac articulations), and the sacrococcygeal symphysis. These joints are made of a network of cartilage and/or ligaments that join the bones of the pelvis. During pregnancy, the joints of the pelvis soften under the influence of the hormones of pregnancy, such as relaxin. This softening allows for movement and widening of the pelvis, which increases its potential size to facilitate birth.

The pubic symphysis is composed of fibrocartilaginous tissue. During pregnancy, it widens slightly. Although this widening usually does not exceed 10 millimeters, it may cause tenderness, particularly with motion.[14] Rarely, the symphysis pubis may separate traumatically (or surgically) during labor.

The sacroiliac joints are primarily weight-bearing joints that take the weight of the upper body and distribute it to the lower limbs. They are synovial joints, meaning that the surfaces of the articulating bones are covered by a thin membrane of cartilage and are separated by a joint cavity lined by a synovial membrane that produces a lubricating fluid. The resulting hinge-type movement gives the sacrum the ability to rotate slightly, which enlarges the measurements of two of the three pelvic planes that the fetus passes through during birth.

The sacrococcygeal joint is also a synovial hinge joint that allows flexion and extension of the coccyx. Extension occurs during relaxation of the levator ani and rectal sphincter muscles—an event that occurs normally during defecation and during the birth

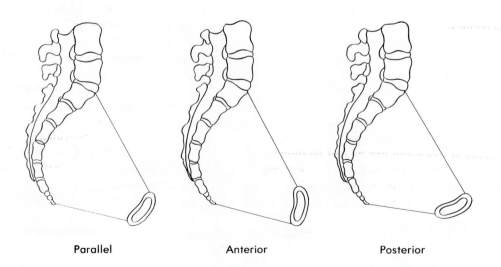

Parallel   Anterior   Posterior

Figure 11-7 Inclination of symphysis pubis.

process. Extension of the coccyx increases the antero-posterior diameter of the plane at the pelvic outlet.

Pelvic Ligaments

The term "ligament" is generally used to describe connective tissue that joins two bones. However, in the pelvis, in addition to indicating a connection between bones, the term "ligament" is used to describe a variety of tissues that connect pelvic organs to bones. The sacrospinous and sacrotuberous ligaments of the sacrum, however, are "true" ligaments in the bony pelvis that help provide stability to the pelvis in part by supporting the sacrum and restricting its ability to tilt.

The sacrospinous ligaments are triangular with a broad base that attaches to the lateral margins of the sacrum and coccyx and insertion at the apex of the ischial spine. The coccygeus muscle lies along the pelvic aspect of this ligament, and the pudendal nerve, which innervates the skin and muscles of the perineum, lies just posterior to it where it attaches to the ischial spine. The sacrotuberous ligaments attach to the sacrum at the level of the S3 through S5 vertebrae and extend to the inferior spine of the illium where it becomes the ischial tuberosity extending inferior and lateral to the sacrospinous ligament.

The Pelvic Floor

The pelvic floor is made up of major muscle groups as well as ligaments and fascia that together support the abdominal and pelvic organs, maintain continence, control urination and elimination, and facilitate passage of the fetus during birth. From the most superior to the most inferior, the major components of the pelvic floor are (1) the endopelvic fascia, (2) the pelvic diaphragm, (3) the urogenital diaphragm, and (4) the superficial perineal muscles. The muscles of the pelvic floor are described in **Table 11-1**.

The endopelvic fascia is a layer of connective tissue that surrounds the vagina and provides support to it and to the visceral organs. This fascia also plays a role in urinary continence by providing support to the urethra and neck of the bladder.[15]

The pelvic diaphragm separates the pelvic cavity from the perineal space and can be can be thought of as a diamond-shaped hammock that supports the viscera, abdominal, and pelvic organs. The pelvic diaphragm consists of the levator ani muscles, which is made up of the puborectalis, pubococcygeus, and iliococcygeus, the coccygeus muscle, and their associated fascia (**Figure 11-8**). Insertions of the muscles of the levator ani group around the vagina, urethra, and rectum allow passage of these openings and create

functional sphincters that contribute to fecal and urinary continence. The levator ani maintains the position of the pelvic organs. This muscle originates at the posterior surface of the superior ramus of the pubis then runs along the arcus tendineus, a line of fascia on the internal surface of the ischium. The muscle inserts into the last segments of the coccyx laterally and into tendons on the rectum, vagina, and urethra medially so that they make up part of the sphincters for these organs.

The urogenital diaphragm has often been described as being composed of multiple layers, including the deep transverse perineal muscles and its associated inferior and superior fascia. However, newer studies suggest that this urogenital diaphragm is really a single layer of muscle and fascial tissue that should be referred to as the perineal membrane.[16] The urethra and the vagina pass through this membrane.

Superficial to the perineal membrane are the bulbocavernosus, ischiocavernosus, and superficial transverse perineal muscles (**Figure 11-9**). The central tendinous point of the perineum, which crosses the midline of the perineum between the vaginal and anal openings, anchors the superficial transverse perineal muscle, the urogenital sphincter, the bulbocavernosus muscles, and the external anal sphincter.

An understanding of how the pelvic floor anatomy promotes urinary and fecal continence is necessary to understand how the changes related to pregnancy, childbirth, and aging results in some women developing pelvic floor dysfunction, including stress urinary incontinence.

In the female, the urethra is approximately 4 centimeters long and runs posteriorly along the pubic symphysis from the external opening (i.e., the urethral meatus) to the bladder. The urethra is made up of an inner layer of epithelium surrounded by a layer of vascular tissue and a layer of muscular tissue that help maintain the urethra closed during rest. It is stabilized by the pubourethral ligaments, which attach the anterior portion of the urethra to the symphysis pubis. To maintain urinary continence, urethral closing pressure must be greater than bladder pressure. This pressure balance is achieved in part by the constriction provided by the urethral muscles and sphincters and in part by the support/compression provided by the pelvic floor muscles and their associated structures. Two sphincter structures are involved in urinary continence: the inner sphincter at the neck of the bladder, and the external urethral rhabdosphincter/urethrovaginal sphincter complex. The inner sphincter is an extension of the detrusor smooth muscle of the bladder that is under autonomic control, whereas the urethral

Table 11-1	Muscles of the Perineum	
Muscle	**Description**	**Function**
Pubococcygeus	Primary portion of the levator ani. Originates at posterior border of the symphysis pubis and sweeps back to insert on lateral margins of the coccyx. Divided into three bands:	
	• **Pubovaginalis**: origin is the posterior aspect of the pubis and insertion is the fascia of the vagina and perineal body. The muscle is in a U shape around the vagina.	• Acts as a sling for the vagina and vaginal sphincter (muscle that causes spasm during vaginismus).
	• **Puborectalis**: intermediate fibers that form a U loop around the anal rectal junction and insert into the posterior wall of the rectum, blending with the anal sphincter.	• Sling and accessory sphincter for the rectum.
	• **Pubococcygeus proper**: lateral fibers go directly back to form a Y and insert on the lateral margins of the coccyx.	• Flexes the coccyx to increase anal–rectal flexure and control defecation.
Iliococcygeus	Arises from a facial line on the obturator internus muscle along the pelvic wall of the obturator foramen and extends to insert on the lateral margins of the coccyx and anococcygeal raphe.	Pelvic organ support and urinary continence.
Bulbocavernosus	Two bulbocavernosus muscles: posteriorly, they attach to the central tendinous point of the perineum; anteriorly, they insert into the corpus cavernosus of the clitoris; laterally, they surround the orifice of the vagina, covering the vestibular bulbs and Bartholin glands on either side.	Known as the sphincter vaginae, their contraction reduces the size of the vaginal orifice; the anterior muscle fibers and contribute to clitoral erection.
Ischiocavernosus	Two ischiocavernosus muscles, one on either lateral boundary of the perineum: posteriorly, they arise from the inner surface of the ischial tuberosities; anteriorly, they cover and insert into the sides and posterior surface of the crus clitoris; laterally, they extend from the clitoris to the ischial tuberosities along the ischial ramus, from which they derive some of their fibers.	Maintain clitoral erection.
Superficial transverse perineal (transversus perinei superficialis)	Two superficial transverse perineal muscles: arise from the inner and anterior surfaces of the ischial tuberosity of the superior ramus of the ischium by a small tendon; insert into the central tendinous point of the perineum.	Fix the location of the central tendinous point of the perineum.
Perineal membrane	Arises from the inferior ramus of the ischium and spans the anterior pelvic outlet and is attached to the lateral vaginal walls. The urethra passes through this membrane.	Helps to stabilize the vagina.
Central tendinous point of the perineum	A fibromuscular structure in the midline between the vagina and the anus and at the base of the urogenital diaphragm; the tissue is fibrous because it is the point of fusion of both the superior and inferior fascia of the urogenital diaphragm and the external perineal and Colles' fascia; it has muscular fibers because it is a common point of attachment for a number of muscles whose fibers blend together into the central tendinous point of the perineum, among them the bulbocavernosus, superficial transverse perineal, some fibers of the deep transverse perineal, external anal sphincter, and the levator ani–pubococcygeus.	Common point of attachment for a number of layers of fascia and muscles.

rhabdosphincter/urethrovaginal sphincter complex is composed of skeletal muscle and is under voluntary control. Support by the pelvic floor musculature is also critical to maintaining urinary continence. The major components of this supportive structure are the vaginal wall, the endopelvic fascia, the arcus tendineus fasciae pelvis, and the levator ani muscles. The endopelvic fascia surrounds the vagina and attaches to the arcus tendineus fascia, which serves to suspend and support the urethra.

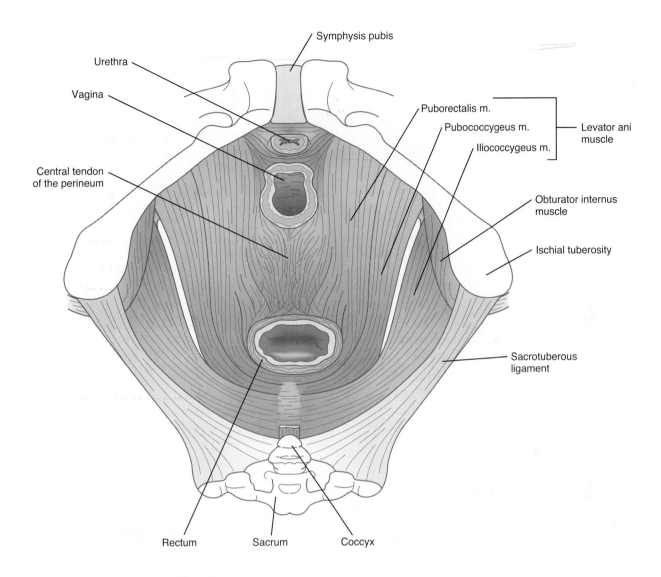

Figure 11-8 Structures of the pelvic diaphragm.

The urethra exits the pelvis via the urogenital hiatus of the levator ani, through which the vagina also passes. The baseline muscle tone of the levator ani, therefore, is critical in maintaining urinary continence by keeping the urethra compressed. When the muscles of the pelvic floor become damaged, which can occur during childbirth, support of the urethra and other pelvic structures becomes increasingly dependent on the ligaments and fascia, which under the strain of continuous or prolonged stretching can fail and become unable to prevent organ prolapse and/or stress incontinence.

Similarly, the perineal body, which is the attachment site of the two sides of the perineal membrane, provides support to the posterior vaginal wall and helps prevent rectal prolapse. The levator ani muscles of the pelvic diaphragm are also critical in

preventing rectal prolapse. Damage to the perineal body or stretch of the levator ani muscles that can happen during the second stage of labor can result in rectal prolapse.

Damage can occur to the anal sphincter during childbirth, especially when a midline episiotomy is employed, which can lead to incontinence of flatus and feces. The anal sphincter is a multilayer structure that includes the anal mucosal lining, the internal sphincter, and the external sphincter. The internal anal sphincter comprises a layer of muscle that is a continuation of the muscular layer of the rectum that ends approximately 1 centimeter from the anal opening. The external anal sphincter is a cylindrical muscular structure like the internal sphincter; it extends all the way to the anal opening. The external anal sphincter is composed of striated muscle under voluntary control.

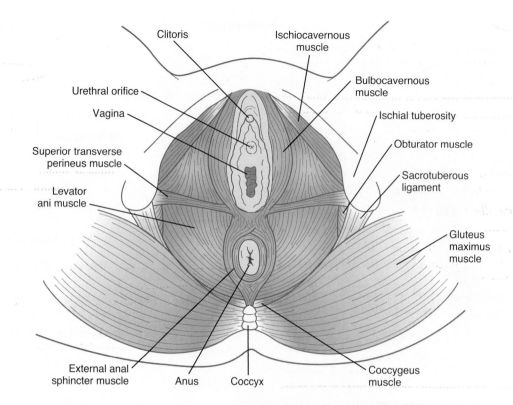

Figure 11-9 Structures of the perineum.

The perineum is perfused by the internal puden-dal artery and branches of the pudendal artery including the inferior rectal artery. These vessels are branches of the anterior division of the internal iliac (hypogastric) artery. Perineal innervation occurs via the pudendal nerve and its branches, which originate from S2, S3, and S4. The pudendal nerve also innervates the levator ani, rectal sphincter, skin of the vulva and lower portion of the birth canal, and muscles of the urogenital diaphragm.

The Obstetric Pelvis

The pelvis is divided into the "false pelvis" and the "true pelvis" by the linea terminalis, an imaginary line that runs along the pelvic brim from the superior part of the symphysis pubis around to the sacral promontory (**Figure 11-10**). The false pelvis, which includes the iliac fossa and iliac crest, receives that name because it has little obstetric significance yet defines the lower border of the abdominal cavity. The true pelvis constitutes the bony passageway through which the fetus must maneuver to be born vaginally. This bony passage is actually a curved canal with a

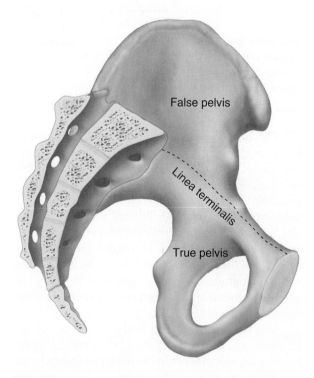

Figure 11-10 True and false pelvis.

shallow anterior wall that is approximately 5 centimeters long, and a deep concave posterior wall that is approximately 10 centimeters long.

The true pelvis has five boundaries:

1. *Superiorly:* the sacral promontory, linea terminalis, the upper margins of the pubic bones
2. *Inferiorly:* the inferior margins of the ischial tuberosities and the tip of the coccyx
3. *Posteriorly:* the anterior surface of the sacrum and coccyx
4. *Laterally:* the sacroiliac notches and ligaments and the inner surface of the ischial bones
5. *Anteriorly:* the obturator foramina and the posterior surfaces of the symphysis pubis, pubic bones, and ascending rami of the ischial bones

Clinically Important Aspects of the True Pelvis

The birth canal shape is determined by the architecture of the sacrum, sacrosciatic notch, sidewalls, ischial spines, and subpubic arch. Therefore the shape of the true pelvis has several clinically relevant aspects including the following.

Pelvic Planes and Pelvic Diameters

The true pelvis has three planes of obstetric significance: the inlet, the midplane, and the outlet. **Table 11-2** describes these planes. Each plane has anteroposterior and transverse diameters of import that are critical for evaluation of pelvic adequacy for vaginal birth.

Angle of the Pubic Arch

The descending rami of the pubic bones and the inferior margin of the symphysis pubis form what is known as the *pubic arch*. The angle of this arch should be at least 90° as determined just below the symphysis pubis. An arch that is 90° a few centimeters below the symphysis pubis but narrow above that (just below the symphysis pubis) decreases the available space in the anteroposterior diameter of the pelvic outlet.

General Structure of the Forepelvis

The inner aspect of the forepelvis (the anterior portion of the pelvis) should be rounded. A forepelvis that is not rounded but instead angles sharply toward the lateral portion of the pelvis decreases the oblique diameters of the inlet.

Angle of the Pelvic Sidewalls

The pelvic sidewalls extend from the upper anterior angle of the sacrosciatic notch at the point of the widest transverse diameter of the pelvic inlet in a downward and forward line to the ischial tuberosities at the point of the widest transverse diameter of the pelvic outlet. They are normally slightly convergent in that, if the lines of their angles were extended beyond the pelvis, the two lines would meet at about the level of the knees. However, when felt on pelvic examination they feel generally straight. The obstetric import of the pelvic sidewalls is whether the width of the pelvis at the inlet remains the same throughout the pelvis. Divergence or convergence is based on whether the point of origin at the inlet and the ending point at the ischial tuberosities are essentially equidistant from the anteroposterior diameter of the pelvis. Convergent sidewalls usually decrease the angle of the pubic arch and may be accompanied by more prominent ischial spines. Divergent sidewalls always indicate a very wide angle of the pubic arch.

Sacrosciatic Notch

The shape and width of the sacrosciatic notch are important because they affect the posterior sagittal diameter of the inlet, which combines with the shape and rotation of the sacrum to determine the amount of room in the posterior portion of the pelvis for passage of the fetus.

Pelvic Types

Each plane of the pelvis has a shape, which is defined by the anterior–posterior and transverse diameters. These shapes have been classified into four basic pelvic types by Caldwell and Moloy in X-ray studies done in the 1920s.[17]: (1) gynecoid, (2) android, (3) anthropoid, and (4) platypelloid (**Table 11-3**). The pelvic types are determined by the shape of the pelvic inlet and the posterior characteristics of the pelvis, including the posterior sagittal diameter, which is the distance from the midpoint of the transverse diameter to the sacral promontory. Anatomic portions of the pelvis used in evaluation of pelvic types are the inlet, sacrum, sacrosciatic notch, sidewalls, ischial spines, and pubic arch. Characteristics of these structures affect the obstetric capacity of the pelvis. Caldwell and Moloy went on to characterize the labor outcomes associated with each type of pelvis. They reviewed and improved our knowledge of the mechanisms of labor and added information about how the position and diameter of the fetal head affects the progress of labor. In the aggregate, this knowledge is invaluable in the assessment of labor progress.

Table 11-2	Pelvic Planes and Obstetric Diameters	
Plane	**Boundaries of Plane**	**Significant Obstetric Diameters of Plane**
Pelvic *inlet* (superior strait): upper entry into the true pelvis	**Posterior:** sacral promontory **Lateral:** linea terminalis **Anterior:** upper portion of the symphysis pubis and horizontal rami of the pubic bones	**Anteroposterior diameters:** 1. *Conjugata vera:* true conjugate of the inlet; extends from the middle of the sacral promontory to the middle of the upper posterior margin of the symphysis pubis; this diameter is normally 11 cm or more. 2. *Obstetric conjugate of the inlet:* extends from the middle of the sacral promontory to the middle of the posterior symphysis pubis. The pelvis is considered contracted if the obstetric conjugate measures less than 10 cm. 3. *Diagonal conjugate of the inlet:* extends from the middle of the sacral promontory to the middle of the inferior (lower) margin of the symphysis pubis. This is the only diameter of the pelvic inlet that can be measured clinically. A normal clinical measurement is considered to be 11.5 cm or more. **Transverse diameter:** greatest distance between the linea terminalis on either side of the pelvis; this distance is approximately 13.5 cm. **Oblique diameters:** distance between the sacroiliac synchondrosis on one side of the pelvis and the iliopectineal eminence on the opposite side of the pelvis. The oblique diameters average slightly less than 13 cm (12.75 cm) each.
Pelvic *midplane*: plane of least dimensions	**Posterior:** sacrum at the junction of the fourth and fifth sacral vertebrae **Lateral:** ischial spines **Anterior:** inferior border of pubic symphysis	**Transverse diameter (*interspinous diameter*):** distance between the ischial spines. Normally measures approximately 10 cm. Smallest diameter of the pelvis that the fetal presenting part has to accommodate to during the process of labor and birth. **Anteroposterior diameter:** extends from the middle of the inferior margin of the symphysis pubis through the middle of the transverse diameter and to the sacrum. This diameter is normally 11.5 cm or more.
Pelvic *outlet*: can be thought of as composed of two triangles, with the transverse diameter of the outlet serving as the common base of these two triangles	**Posterior:** sacrococcygeal joint **Lateral:** inner surface of ischial tuberosities **Anterior:** lower border of pubic symphysis	**Anteroposterior diameter:** extends from the middle of the inferior margin of the symphysis pubis to the sacrococcygeal joint. This measurement is normally 11.5 cm or more. **Transverse diameter (*intertuberous*, or *biischial*, *diameter*):** distance between the inner aspect of the lowermost part of ischial tuberosities. This diameter has a measurement of approximately 10 cm.

The pelves of most women are not pure types, but rather a mixture of types. By convention, the pelvis is named for the posterior characteristics with a *tendency* for the anterior characteristics. For example, a pelvis with a curved sacrum and wide sacrosciatic notch may have slightly convergent sidewalls that narrow the anterior segment of the midpelvis and outlet. Such a pelvis would be described as a gynecoid pelvis with android tendencies.

The Menstrual Cycle: An Introduction

"Menstruation" is a term derived from the Latin word *mensis*, meaning "month." In several cultures, if not most cultures, this single biological event engenders negative connotations. According to the *British Medical Journal* in 1878, "it is undoubtedly the fact, that meat will be tainted if cured by women at the catamenial [*sic* menstrual] period."[18] In today's

Table 11-3	Pelvic Types and Their Identifying Characteristics	
Pelvic Type and Description	**Identifying Characteristics**	**Image**
Gynecoid Commonly known as the "female pelvis" because it is the type that occurs most frequently in women; 41–42% of women's pelves are gynecoid. This shape is ideal for childbearing.	*Inlet:* rounded. Transverse diameter approximately greater than or equal to the anteroposterior diameter. Posterior sagittal diameter only a little shorter than the anterior sagittal diameter. *Sacrum:* parallel with the symphysis pubis. *Sacrosciatic notch:* rounded with an approximate distance of 2½ to 3 fingerbreadths along the sacrospinous ligament. *Sidewalls:* straight pelvic sidewalls. *Ischial spines:* blunt and neither prominent nor encroaching. *Pubic arch:* a wide arch ($\geq$ 90 degrees).	
Android Commonly known as the "male pelvis" because it occurs more frequently in men. Occurs in 32.5% of white women and in 15.7% of nonwhite women. The android pelvis is a heavy pelvis, which poses difficulty for vaginal birth and increases the incidence of posterior position and forceps-assisted delivery. The midplane and outlet contracture of the android pelvis increases the incidence of fetopelvic disproportion and cesarean sections.	*Inlet:* heart shaped. Posterior segment is wedge shaped and the anterior segment (forepelvis) is narrow and triangular. The posterior sagittal diameter is short in comparison to the anterior sagittal diameter. Limited space in the posterior portion of the pelvis for accommodating the fetal head. *Sacrum:* anteriorly inclined and flat. *Sacrosciatic notch:* highly arched and narrow, with an approximate distance of 1½ to 2 fingerbreadths along the sacrospinous ligament. *Sidewalls:* pelvic sidewalls usually convergent. *Ischial spines:* prominent and frequently encroaching, thereby decreasing the transverse (interspinous) diameter of the midplane. *Pubic arch:* narrow, with an acute angle of much less than 90 degrees.	
Anthropoid The anthropoid pelvis is most common in the nonwhite races, occurring in 40.5% of nonwhite women as compared to 23.5% of white women. The anthropoid pelvis had the longest sacrum of the four types of pelves and, therefore, is the deepest pelvis. The potential problem of outlet contracture because of a narrow pubic arch is counterbalanced by the lengthy anteroposterior diameter, thus providing room in the posterior portion of the pelvis for the fetus. The shape of the anthropoid pelvis favors a posterior position of the fetus. It is adequate for vaginal birth if it is on the large size.	*Inlet:* oval. The anteroposterior diameter is much larger than the transverse diameter. The anterior segment of the pelvis (forepelvis) is pointed and narrower than the posterior segment. *Sacrum:* posteriorly inclined, so the posterior sagittal diameters are long throughout the pelvis. More space in the posterior portion of the pelvis for accommodating the fetal head. *Sacrosciatic notch:* of average height but quite wide; has an approximate distance of 4 fingerbreadths along the sacrospinous ligament between the ischial spine and the sacrum. *Sidewalls:* somewhat convergent. *Ischial spines:* usually prominent but not encroaching. Transverse (interspinous) diameter of the midplane is generally less than that of the gynecoid pelvis but not as contracted as the android pelvis. *Pubic arch:* somewhat narrow.	

(continues)

Table 11-3	Pelvic Types and Their Identifying Characteristics *(continued)*	
Pelvic Type and Description	**Identifying Characteristics**	**Image**

Platypelloid

Platypelloid pelvis is rare and not particularly conducive to vaginal birth. It is the widest of all pelvic types and also shallow. These characteristics make rotation and descent of the fetal head difficult. This shape occurs in less than 3% of women in both white and nonwhite races.	*Inlet:* flat. Short anteroposterior diameter and a wide transverse diameter. The anterior segment of the pelvis (forepelvis) is quite wide. *Sacrum:* inclined posteriorly and quite hollow. *Sacrosciatic notch:* wide and flat with an acute angle between the ischial spines and the sacrum. *Sidewalls:* slightly convergent. *Ischial spines:* somewhat prominent but, because of wide transverse diameters throughout the pelvis, this prominence has no effect. *Pubic arch:* quite wide; this pelvis is the widest of all the pelvic types.	

English language, euphemisms for the event abound, including "the curse" and "being sick this month." In the Polynesian language, the word "taboo" is synonymous with "menstruation."[19] Even today, national advertisements for sanitary products continue to avoid using the term.

Much still remains unknown about the menstrual cycle, including the basic question of whether menses is an essential healthy physiologic event. Although human females usually menstruate monthly, some other primates do not; many other mammals have an estrus cycle that includes ovulation and reabsorption instead of menstruation. Some scientists, such as the evolutionary biologist Profit, have postulated that menstruation is useful to a woman because it expels bacteria from the body.[20] Others question whether menstruation has any benefits and instead should be considered obsolete. These scientists are among those who advocate that the average woman who wants contraception should use regular hormonal suppression.[21]

Today it is known that the physiology of the menstrual cycle is a sophisticated process. Over the last few decades, scientific discoveries have revealed more information about the interplay between functions of the female organs and the hormonal milieu. As additional discoveries have been made, understanding the process has become more complicated. Clearly, however, knowledge of the menstrual cycle is needed throughout the practice of midwifery.

As part of understanding the menstrual cycle, a few assumptions are made. Predominant among them is that every woman has a 28-day cycle and

is ovulatory. In real life, neither of these "facts" is necessarily true. In addition, for the purpose of explanation, menstrual cycle events are initially separated and presented in a set time sequence. Once again, however, it must be recognized this type of presentation is an artificial convention.

The discussion of the menstrual cycle presented here divides the physiology into several sections, beginning with a discussion of the steroidogenesis and hypothalamus–pituitary–ovarian axis. Next the anatomy of the ovarian cycle with associated physiology and anatomic developments is reviewed, and finally the endometrial cycle is presented.

Steroidogenesis and the Hypothalamus–Pituitary–Ovarian Axis

Steroidogenesis

In the human body, a number of hormones exist, which generally are one of three different types: amines, prostaglandins, or steroid hormones. Sex hormones, also termed gonadocorticoids, are steroid hormones; all of them are synthesized from cholesterol through a series of chemical reactions known as steroidogenesis. The sex steroids commonly are identified as estrogen, progesterone, and androgen.

The major site of biosynthesis for all sex steroid hormones in the healthy ovulating women is the ovary. Other peripheral sites, including adiposity and skeletal muscle, produce small amounts of these hormones.

All of the sex hormones are derived from the 27-carbon-chained cholesterol. From the 27 carbons, a mitochondrial enzyme called P450 scc (scc signifies cholesterol side-chain cleavage) catalyzes conversion of cholesterol to pregnenolone. Pregnenolone is the precursor from which 21-carbon-chained progestogens and corticoids emerge. Further chemical reactions reduce the carbons from hydroxypregnenolone to 19-carbon-chained androstenedione, the precursor from which androgens, including testosterone, are derived. Aromatization further reduces the 19 carbons to the 18-carbon-chained estranes, which include all of the estrogens[22] (**Figure 11-11**). In summary, steroidogenesis is an exquisitely efficient method by which all sex hormones are derived in a few chemical steps by starting with cholesterol and reducing the carbons in cholesterol from 27 to 18 in number.

Steroidogenesis does not occur without interaction with the gonadotropins, follicle-stimulating hormone (FSH), luteinizing hormone (LH), and normal reproductive organs. Production of FSH and LH is part of the hypothalamus–pituitary–ovarian axis, as illustrated in **Figure 11-12**.

Hypothalamus–Pituitary–Ovarian Axis

The hypothalamus–pituitary–ovarian axis is the term used when referring to the effects created by these individual endocrine organs when they work in concert as if they were a single endocrine organ. As will be described, the interplay between the hypothalamus, pituitary, and ovary is controlled through feedback loops.

The hypothalamus controls the reproductive system by secreting either releasing or inhibitory factors in a pulsatile fashion into the hypothalamic–pituitary portal system. These factors then act on the anterior pituitary gland. The hypothalamus releasing factors that control reproduction include follicle-stimulating releasing factor (FRF), luteinizing hormone releasing factor (LRF), and prolactin-inhibiting factor (PIF). The releasing factors FRF and LRF also are collectively referred to as gonadotropin-hormone releasing factors (GnRH).

The pituitary gland is composed of two main lobes: the adenohypophysis and the neurohypophysis. When stimulated by the hypothalamic releasing hormones, the cells of the adenohypophysis secrete the gonadotropins FSH and LH, as well as prolactin. After their release, LH and FSH travel via the circulation to the ovary. A woman's ovaries are the site of production of estrogen and progesterone from either the ovarian theca or granulosa cells.

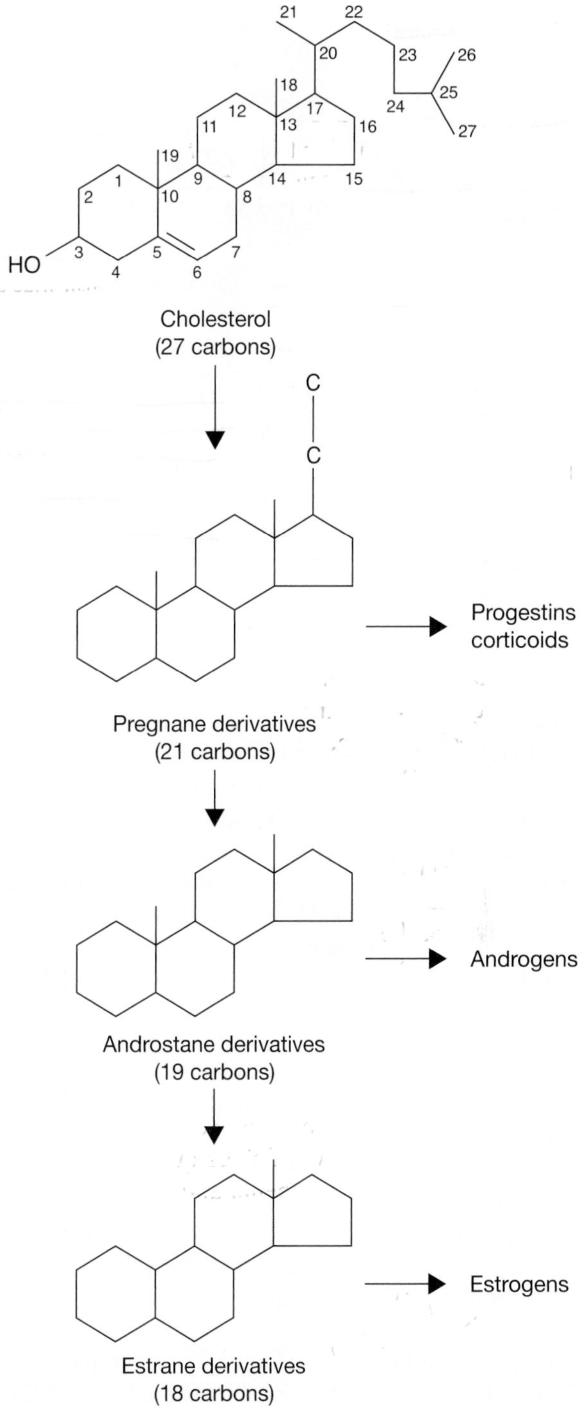

Figure 11-11 Biosynthesis of sex steroids.

Source: King TL, Brucker MC. *Pharmacology for Women's Health.* Sudbury, MA: Jones and Bartlett; 2011.

Control of the Hypothalamus–Pituitary–Ovarian Axis Through Feedback Loops

A feedback system, whether it is in biology or informatics, is a method in which factors either inhibit

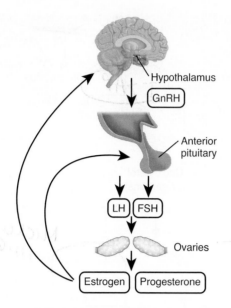

Figure 11-12 The hypothalamus–pituitary–ovarian axis.

or stimulate production of a specific agent. Positive feedback indicates stimulation, whereas negative feedback is inhibitory. It was not long ago that the feedback system for the hypothalamus–pituitary–ovarian axis was depicted as a simple graph, which was then used as the universal prototype to illustrate negative feedback in basic science classes. However, this simple diagram failed to account for several factors found in a woman's body. For example, GnRH is not static but rather pulsatile, with its release amplitude changing as the result of feedback modulation of steroids and peptides that originate in the dominant follicle and act directly on the hypothalamus and anterior pituitary.

Also, although the hypothalamus–pituitary–ovarian axis sometimes does have a negative feedback system, it does not exclusively fill this function, nor are estrogen and progesterone the only agents of note. Some agents stimulate the hypothalamus *and* the pituitary, others stimulate neither, and still others stimulate one but not the other. For example, low levels of estrogen inhibit LH, while high levels of the same hormone stimulate LH.

Among the factors that influence feedback are three specific peptides—inhibin, activin, and follistatin—that are synthesized by ovarian granulosa cells in response to FSH stimulation and secreted into the follicular fluid. Inhibin, as its name implies, inhibits FSH secretion. This peptide also augments LH stimulation of theca cells to accelerate production of androgens, and it diminishes actions of GnRH. In contrast, activin simulates FSH and diminishes

progesterone production from the granulosa cells. It is hypothesized that follistatin, the third major peptide, may inactivate activin by binding it, thereby decreasing FSH activity.

Other factors are also known to have important actions on ovarian function. For example, the ovary is a site of production for insulin-like growth factor 1 (IGF-1), which acts independently of most other factors. The growth factor also amplifies androgen production in theca cells and FSH action in granulosa cells. In general, FSH has multiple activities in the granulosa cells, with all being influenced by growth factors—of which IGF-II is theorized to be the most important.[23]

In summary, no simple feedback loop exists that describes the entire menstrual cycle. The menstrual cycle is known to have a potent negative feedback system, although at different times of the cycle, a positive feedback process may be seen as well. In general, as more factors of influence are being discovered, more is being acknowledged to be unknown.

The Ovarian Cycle

Intrauterine Development to Puberty

Some midwives like to remind a woman that if she is pregnant with a daughter, she also is carrying the eggs for her grandchildren. The intrauterine daughter, like all women, has the most number of primary oocytes when she is a fetus at approximately 20 to 28 weeks' gestational age. The number of primary oocytes decreases from millions to thousands by the time of puberty via atresia, although the mechanism of atresia itself is not well understood. After establishment of menses, meiosis occurs monthly as part ovum maturation. During this process the primary oocytes which originally had 46 chromosomes, splits into a secondary oocyte consisting of 23 chromosomes and a polar body. The latter usually disappears and is reabsorbed.

Granulosa cells are the type of cells that surround each secondary oocyte. The surrounded oocyte is called a primordial follicle (**Figure 11-13**). Follicles are scattered throughout the cortical zone of the ovary.

Menarche to Menopause

During her reproductive life, a woman's ovaries tend to be in a constant state of change. These changes are characterized by the ovarian cycle within the menstrual cycle. The ovarian cycle is subdivided into two

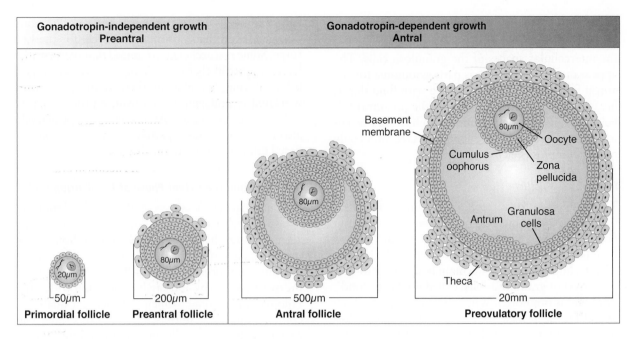

Figure 11-13 Follicular development.

major phases—follicular and luteal phases—with events such as ovulation and menstruation identified separately. Because hormones are receptor specific, the cells within the ovary contain receptor sites that are essential to normal ovarian function and a normal menstrual cycle. As the various ovarian changes occur, receptors on ovarian cells appear and interface with the feedback system.

Follicular Phase of Ovarian Cycle

Overview

The follicular phase varies in length, but averages 10 to 14 days. The goal of this phase of the ovarian cycle is to produce an ovum for fertilization. Follicles can be found in an ovary in different levels of maturation. Groups of immature ovarian follicles develop over time. Taking more than a year on average, these primordial follicles grow until one major follicle matures and the others regress. As early as menstrual cycle day 5, one follicle out of a group begins to emerge as a dominant one. It remains unknown why one follicle is chosen and others regress to stromal tissue, but local growth factors are theorized to be involved. During its development, the dominant follicle has an increased number of FSH receptors compared to other follicles and then is able to produce its own estrogenic environment. As estrogen levels in the circulation increase secondary to follicular production, there is a concomitant decrease in FSH secretion—an action that may seal the fate of those

follicles that are unable to produce an estrogenic milieu. Simultaneously, theca cells grow rapidly in the ovary. Perhaps in response to the high estrogen level, the granulosa cells of the dominant follicles begin to develop LH receptors.

Preantral Follicle

As a primordial follicle grows, a layer of theca cells forms around the granulosa cells, with a basement membrane separating the two groups. This follicle then is known as a preantral follicle. Under the influence of FSH, the granulosa cells surrounding the maturing follicle proliferate and begin to produce androgens and estrogens, especially the latter. FSH receptors appear on the preantral granulosa cells so that using energy from cyclic AMP (cAMP), the cell is able to convert, though aromatization, androgens into estrogens as described in steroidogenesis; meanwhile, the theca cells, which have LH receptors, use cAMP to produce the androgens. In the preantral follicle, FSH and estrogen promote the development of more FSH receptors.

Although the follicular cycle usually progresses normally, in some women large amounts of androgens are produced and the granulosa cells cannot compensate and convert them into estrogen. In such a case, eventually the follicle regresses secondarily to atresia. This phenomenon is noted to occur among women with polycystic ovary syndrome, a topic discussed in more detail in the *Gynecologic Disorders* chapter.

Antral Follicle

Eventually a cavity, called the antrum, is formed in the intercellular spaces of the granulosa cells. The appearance of the antrum is pathognomonic for the antral follicle. The antrum is filled with fluid that is heavily estrogenic in nature. Like the preantral follicle, the antral follicle continues to have LH receptors exclusively on theca cells and FSH receptors only on the granulosa cells.

Preovulatory Follicle

The outer layer of the follicle becomes somewhat translucent, at which point it is termed the zona pellucida. The zona pellucida then is surrounded by more granulosa cells, also known as the corona radiate, and attached to the main body of the follicle by a mass of granulosa cells, called the "egg cloud" or cumulus oophorus. When these changes become apparent, this follicle is called the preovulatory follicle or the Graafian follicle. By day 12 or 13 of a menstrual cycle, the oocyte is floating in the antrum; by cycle day 14, the mature or Graafian follicle is protruding from the ovary. Even before ovulation occurs, the granulosa cells begin to increase in size and assume a yellow shading of lutein as the LH receptors appear on the cells.

As illustrated in **Figure 11-14**, the hormones estrogen and LH are intimately related to each other.

Approximately 24 to 36 hours before ovulation, estrogen levels peak, priming the cycle for the LH surge. Some researchers have found that women athletes are more likely to sustain injuries when estrogen is high during this time and theorize this propensity is related to collagen metabolism, a process that is influenced by estrogen.[24] At this time, androgen levels also begin to increase, perhaps in an evolutionary-based effort to stimulate the libido.

Ovulation and the Luteal Phase of the Ovarian Cycle

No one single event causes ovulation. Ovulation, as defined by release of the ovum, usually occurs 10 to 12 hours after the LH peak and 24 to 36 hours after the estrogen surge. The oocyte is released with the cumulus oophorus and antral fluid. The fimbria of the ovary sweeps by and catches the ovum within the fallopian tube. Some women experience a small discomfort, known as mittelschmerz, at this time. The remaining follicular cells (granulosa and theca cells) in the ovary are transformed into a structure called the corpus luteum (yellow body), which grows for at least a week and forms a mature corpus luteum. If fertilization does not occur, the corpus luteum begins to degenerate into the corpus albicans.

The LH surge is the most reliable single indicator of ovulation.[25] Likely to last for 48 hours or longer, it promotes luteinization of the granulosa cells in the

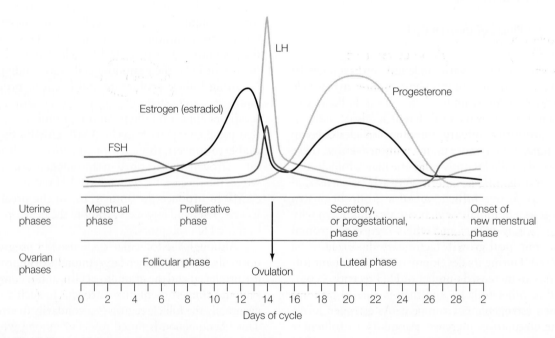

Figure 11-14 Hormonal changes throughout the menstrual cycle.

follicle and the synthesis of prostaglandins and other eicosanoids needed for follicle rupture. Progesterone levels continue to rise with the LH surge and may be part of the termination of the event as well as the FSH peak that accompanies the peak of LH. Low levels of progesterone contribute to LH and FSH peaks, whereas high levels can prevent LH surge. Progesterone works with prostaglandins to enhance digestion of the follicle's wall, thereby promoting ovulation. High levels of intrafollicular prostaglandins may cause the oocyte to be retained, which forms the basis for some of the theories regarding the decrease in ovarian cancer associated with use of oral contraceptives. Appropriate surges mean nothing if the dominant follicle is not present; and without the mature preovulatory follicle, it is likely that the surges may not occur.

Other physiologic events accompany ovulation. For example, under the influence of estrogen in the mid- to late follicular phase, the cervical mucus becomes clear, thin, and more profuse; the cervix softens; and the external os opens slightly. The changes in cervical mucus facilitate sperm transport. After ovulation, the higher progesterone levels lead to production of thick cervical mucus that sperm cannot penetrate.

Luteal Phase

A luteinized granulosa cell is able to produce both estradiol and progesterone. The old "simple" description of the menstrual cycle implied that progesterone was produced only after ovulation. Increases in progesterone levels may be noted as early as day 10 of the cycle, although progesterone production rises sharply after ovulation and peaks at 8 days after the LH surge. Progesterone suppresses new follicular growth.

Whereas the length of the follicular phase of the ovarian cycle may vary, the duration of the luteal phase essentially remains constant at 14 days. This length of time is directly related to the life of corpus luteum, assuming no interference by conception. In the luteal phase, estrogen is still produced and may facilitate destruction of the corpus luteum. Because progesterone is associated with an elevation in basal body temperature (BBT), a daily measurement of BBT will demonstrate a rise *after* ovulation has occurred—which makes the thermal activity useful as a post hoc measure and has been the basis of some of the natural family planning methods. A variety of other factors, including oxytocin, are likely to be involved in this period.

Luteal–Follicular Transition Period

During the luteal–follicular transition, the corpus luteum dies and estrogen, progesterone, and inhibin levels decrease such that there is transitional time between one cycle and the next. Because production of inhibin A drops, FSH levels begin to increase; conversely, because estrogen and progesterone levels are low, GnRH pulses increase, which in turn facilitates production and release of FSH and LH from the hypothalamus and pituitary. FSH helps a group of follicles to be rescued from atresia and the cycle to begin anew.

The Endometrial Cycle

Most sources subdivide the endometrial cycle into two periods: proliferative and secretory. Other authorities note that ischemic changes occur at the end of the secretory phase, with this ischemic period being designated as a separate phase. Similarly, other sources identify menses as a first phase of the endometrial menstrual cycle (**Figure 11-15**).

Proliferative Phase

The proliferative phase of the endometrial cycle corresponds to the follicular phase of the ovarian cycle. During this time the endometrial tissue develops under the increasing influence of estrogen. Endometrial glands change from being narrow and tubular to being enlarged to an extent that they link to each other, forming a continuous lining.

In rare situations, such as during unopposed treatment with exogenous estrogen or among women with anovulation, a proliferative endometrium becomes persistent. When this occurs, there is a higher risk that endometrial hyperplasia will ensue; this state is associated with endometrial cancer. These conditions are discussed in more detail in the *Menstrual Cycle Abnormalities* chapter.

Secretory Phase

The rising progesterone levels that occur with ovulation have a major influence on the endometrium, turning a proliferative endometrium into a secretory one. The length of the endometrium does not regress, but the appearance of the tissue does. Notably, the coiling of spiral vessels and tortuosity of the glands increase. The stroma become edematous and at the time of implantation, approximately days 21–27 of the cycle, three distinct zones have appeared: the

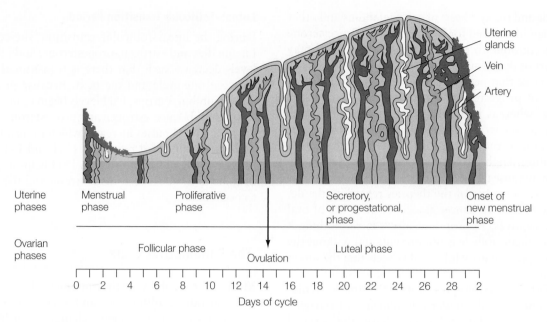

Uterine glands
Vein
Artery

Uterine phases | Menstrual phase | Proliferative phase | Secretory, or progestational, phase | Onset of new menstrual phase

Ovarian phases | Follicular phase | Ovulation | Luteal phase

Days of cycle
0 2 4 6 8 10 12 14 16 18 20 22 24 26 28 2

Figure 11-15 Endometrial cycle.

stratum spongiosum (the most superficial layer), the stratum compactum (midportion), and the stratum basale (the innermost layer).

Once an endometrium becomes secretory, the risks associated with persistent proliferative endometrium are diminished. Since the discovery that exogenous progesterone facilitates development of a secretory endometrium, it has become standard practice for women on perimenopausal hormone therapy to also take progesterone as an adjunctive treatment with the estrogen.

Ischemic Period

By approximately cycle day 25, if implantation does not occur, the decreasing levels of estrogen and progesterone result in disorganization of the endometrium. The tissue shrinks, venous drainage diminishes, and blood flow within the spiral arteries is compromised, resulting in rhythmic constriction and relaxation. The process of apoptosis transpires and the uterus is ready for the next step—menses.

Menstruation

As the lining of the uterus weakens, blood escapes into the endometrial cavity. The appearance of blood for the woman marks the first day of her next menstrual period. The consistency of bleeding after the

withdrawal of estrogen and progesterone is indicative of a normal menstrual cycle with functional organs and endocrine system.

Investigation of amenorrhea often involves a challenge test in which women are given progesterone to ascertain if, after completion of the dose, withdrawal bleeding occurs. If so, the assumption is made that there is no end organ disorder and there is adequate endogenous estrogen. More information about this testing is found in the *Menstrual Cycle Abnormalities* chapter.

Conclusion

Considering that menstruation is a normal event experienced by millions of women every day in the world, it is somewhat surprising that much remains unknown about the physiology of this event. However, perhaps the greatest surprise is that for the average woman, in spite of the complexity of the menstrual cycle, menses occurs on a regular basis without major mishap. **Figure 11-16** depicts the full menstrual cycle, including ovarian cycle, hormonal cycle, and uterine cycle, in one illustration. **Table 11-4** provides an overview of the menstrual cycle, including sequencing of the major events.

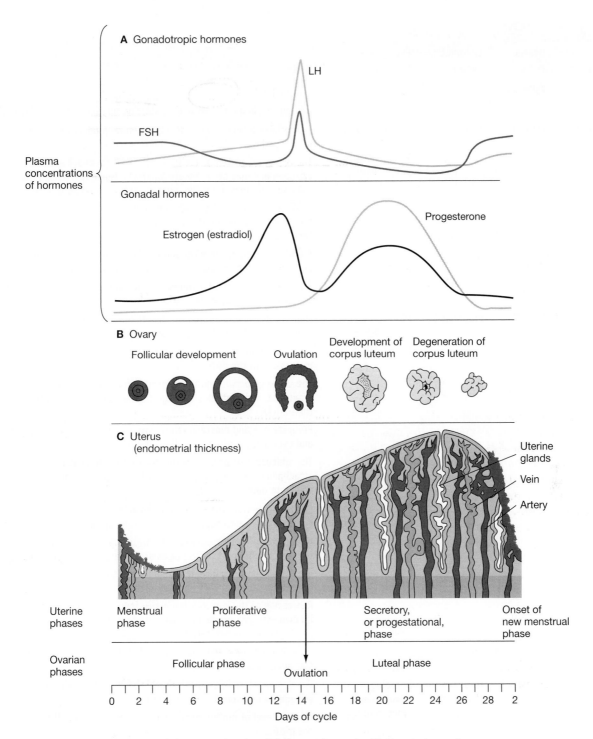

Figure 11-16 The menstrual cycle. (A) Hormonal cycles. (B) The ovarian cycle. (C) The uterine cycle.

Source: Source: Chiras DD. *Human Biology.* 7th ed. Sudbury, MA: Jones & Bartlett; 2012.

			Table 11-4	Overview of the Menstrual Cycle

Days	Ovarian Cycle	Endometrial Cycle	Estrogen and Progesterone	Actions
1–5	Follicular	Menstrual	Low estrogen and progesterone	Inhibin falls.
				LH and FSH begin to slowly rise, starting on approximately day 27.
6–14	Follicular	Proliferative	Building estrogen (and, to a lesser extent, progesterone)	LH initiates luteinization and progesterone production in the granulosa layer.
				The rise of progesterone facilitates positive feedback action of estrogen and may be necessary for the midcycle FSH peak, although the complete reason for the midcycle FSH peak remains unclear.
				Estrogen production becomes sufficient to achieve and maintain the threshold concentration of estradiol that is required to induce the LH surge.
				A midcycle increase in local and peripheral androgens occurs, derived from the thecal tissue of unsuccessful follicles.
				A few hours after the LH surge, changes in hormone levels release suppression of oocyte maturation.
14	Ovulation	Proliferative	High estrogen and building progesterone	High levels of estrogen induce the LH surge at midcycle and lead to sustained elevated LH secretion.
				Suppression of inhibition of oocyte maturation allows final maturation of the oocyte.
				The LH surge occurs and is responsible for luteinization of the granulosa, and synthesis of progesterones and prostaglandins in the follicle.
				Progesterone and prostaglandins work together to digest, weaken, and eventually rupture the follicular wall.
				The midcycle FSH peak frees the oocyte from follicular attachments, and ensures sufficient LH receptors to allow an adequate normal luteal phase.
15–26	Luteal	Secretory (implantation phase)	Progesterone most dominant, but estrogen present	Progesterone from the corpus luteum acts both centrally and within the ovary to suppress new follicular growth.
				High levels of progesterone inhibit pituitary secretion of gonadotropins by inhibiting GnRH pulses at the level of the hypothalamus.
				High levels of progesterone antagonize the pituitary response to GnRH by interfering with estrogen action.
				Regression of the corpus luteum may involve luteolytic action of its own estrogen production, mediated by an alteration in local prostaglandin concentration.
				In early pregnancy, hCG maintains luteal function until placental steroidogenesis is established.
27–28	Luteal	Late secretory (ischemic)	Dropping estrogen and progesterone	The degeneration of corpus luteum results in low levels of estrogen, progesterone, and inhibin.
				The low level of inhibin removes the suppression of FSH on the pituitary.
				The low level of estrogen and progesterone allows an increase in GnRH pulsatile secretion and the removal of the pituitary from the negative feedback suppression.
				The removal of inhibin and estradiol and increased GnRH pulses allow an increase in FSH (and to lesser extent LH).
				The increasing FSH is instrumental in the maturation of a dominant follicle.

FSH = follicle stimulating hormone; GnRH= gonadotropin-releasing hormone; hCG = human chorionic gonadotropin; LH = leutinizing hormone.

Source: King TL, Brucker MC. *Pharmacology for Women's Health*. Sudbury, MA: Jones and Bartlett; 2011.

● ● ● **References**

1. Geddes DT. Inside the lactating breast: the latest anatomy research. *J Midwifery Women's Health.* 2007;52: 556-563.

2. Ramsey DT, Kent JC, Hartmann RA, Hartman PE. Anatomy of the human breast redefined with ultrasound imaging. *J Anat.* 2005;206:525-534.

3. Doucet S, Soussignan R, Sagot P, Schaal B. The secretion of areolar (Montgomery's) glands from lactating women elicits selective, unconditional responses in neonates. *PLoS One.* 2009;4(10):e7579.

4. Howard BA, Gusterson BA. Human breast development. *J Mammary Gland Biol Neoplasia.* 2000;5(2): 120-137.

5. Katz V. Reproductive anatomy. In: Katz V, Lentz G, Lobo G, Gershenson D, eds. *Comprehensive Gynecology.* 5th ed. Philadelphia: Mosby Elsevier; 2007:43-71.

6. Cunningham F, Leveno K, Bloom S, et al. *Williams Obstetrics.* 23rd ed. New York: McGraw-Hill Medical; 2010:17-35.

7. Abberton KM, Taylor NH, Healy DL, Rogers PAW. Vascular smooth muscle cell proliferation in arterioles of the human endometrium. *Hum Reprod.* 1999;14(4):1072-1079.

8. Sivridis E, Giatromanolaki A. Proliferative activity in the postmenopausal endometrium: the lurking potential for giving rise to an endometrial carcinoma. *J Clin Pathol.* 2004;57(8):840–844.

9. Blackburn ST. *Maternal, Fetal, and Neonatal Physiology.* 4th ed. New York: Elsevier; 2013:119.

10. Deveduex D, Marque C, Masour S, Germain G, Duchêne J. Uterine electromyography: a critical review. *Am J Obstet Gynecol.* 1993;169(6):1636-1653.

11. Magoffin DA. Ovarian theca cell. *Int J Biochem Cell Biol.* 2005;37(7):1344-1349.

12. Coad J, Dunstall M. *Anatomy and Physiology for Midwives.* 3rd ed. New York: Elsevier; 2011:69-98.

13. Gilbert SF. *Developmental Biology.* 6th ed. Sunderland, MA: Sinaur Associates; 2000: Chapter 19, The saga of the germ line. Available at: http://www.ncbi.nlm.nih.gov/books/NBK10008. Accessed October 1, 2012.

14. Ritchie JR. Orthopedic considerations during pregnancy. *Clin Obstet Gynecol.* 2003;46(2);456-466.

15. Ashton-Miller JA, DeLancey JOL. Functional anatomy of the female pelvic floor. *Ann NY Acad Sci.* 2007;1101:266-296.

16. Stoker J. Anorectal and pelvic floor anatomy. *Best Pract Res Clin Gastroenterol.* 2009;23:463-475.

17. Caldwell WE, Moloy HC. Anatomical variations in the female pelvis: their classification and obstetrical significance. *Proc R Soc Med.* 1938;32(1):1-30.

18. Story W. Menstruation and the curing of meat. *Br Med J.* 1878;1(904):633.

19. Mills J. *Womanwords,* New York: Holt; 1989.

20. Profit M. Menstruation as a defense against pathogens transported by sperm. *Qtly Rev Biol.* 1993;68(3): 335-386.

21. Hitchcock CL. Elements of the menstrual suppression debate. *Health Care Women Int.* 2008;29(7):702-719.

22. Miller WL, Auchus RJ. The molecular biology, biochemistry, and physiology of human steroidogenesis and its disorders. *Endocr Rev.* 2011;32(1):81-151.

23. Fritz MA, Speroff L. *Clinical Gynecologic Endocrinology and Infertility,* 8th ed. Philadelphia: Wolters Kluwer/Lippincott Williams and Wilkins; 2011.

24. Vescovi JD. The menstrual cycle and anterior cruciate ligament injury risk: implications of menstrual cycle variability. *Sports Med.* 2011;41(2):91-101.

25. Sherman JJ, LeResche L. Does experimental pain response vary across the menstrual cycle? A methodological review. *Am J Physiol Regul Integr Comp Physiol.* 2006;291(2):R245-R256.

Additional Resources

Hoffman B, Schorge J, Schaffer J, Halvorson L, Bradshaw K, Cunningham F. *Williams Gynecology.* 2nd ed. New York: McGraw-Hill Medical; 2012.

Schuiling KD, Likis FE. *Women's Gynecologic Health.* 2nd ed. Burlington, MA: Jones & Bartlett Learning; 2013.

CHAPTER

12

Menstrual Cycle Abnormalities

DAWN C. DURAIN

WILLIAM F. MCCOOL

Introduction

At some point in adolescence, most healthy girls experience their first menses. This universal experience may be met with any of a wide variety of reactions, including expressions of joy, sadness, fear, or excitement. Regardless of the significance or insignificance of this overt manifestation of a change in a girl's hormonal status, the fact remains that a very particular physiologic bridge has been crossed. From this point forward, and most often for many years to come, this cyclic "bleed" will continue to have an impact on the life of each individual girl or woman. Later, as a woman's cycle changes and begins to diminish during normal aging, this transition may likewise be met with a variety of emotions and reactions. The potential impact of a woman's cycle on her complete physical and emotional health must always be considered as one cares for women in a holistic and meaningful clinical relationship.

While minor variations in the cyclic nature of this experience may not be deemed important by clinicians, providers must realize that the particular personal, cultural, or family context of each woman's life must be considered in her report of her menses. Menstruation, and changes in menstrual characteristics, may have deep meaning to a woman in terms of her sense of femaleness, her fertility, and even perhaps her worth as a woman. Additionally, what is "normal" for a particular woman may be limited by her own experience and must always be verified by careful history taking and sensitive exploration. The *Anatomy and Physiology of the Female Reproductive System* chapter addressed the physiology of the monthly menstrual cycle; the present chapter reviews common variations and abnormalities of the menstrual cycle.

Amenorrhea

Throughout an individual's life, the absence of menses—that is, amenorrhea—can be due to routine events such as pregnancy, menopause, or the use of contraceptive methods. At the same, a number of events or conditions may be related to abnormal amenorrhea. The challenge for the practitioner is to differentiate between normal and abnormal, and to discover the cause of the latter. The term *amenorrhea* is traditionally thought to be applicable to one of several clinical situations. *Primary amenorrhea* refers to a female younger than 14 or 16 years old who has never experienced menses and does not exhibit physical signs of secondary sex characteristics. *Secondary amenorrhea* refers to either a menstruating female with the absence of menses from 3 intervals typical of her previous menstrual cycles or a menstruating female with the absence of menses for 6 calendar months.

While a number of different approaches to understanding, diagnosing, and treating amenorrhea are possible, one that has proved helpful to many clinicians is to think of the causes as occurring in one of four anatomic areas: the (1) outflow area of the genitalia (uterus and vagina); (2) the ovaries; (3) the pituitary gland; or (4) the central nervous system (CNS).[1] Generally, outflow area problems are obstructive in nature, whereas ovarian, pituitary, and CNS problems involve disruptions in the hypothalamic–pituitary–ovarian (HPO) axis that controls the neuroendocrine processes required for a normal menstrual cycle. Obstructions can generally be found on physical examination or with the aid of ultrasonography or other imaging modalities; other causes usually are assessed via laboratory analyses and/or the use of hormone therapy.

Assessment of a Woman with Amenorrhea

The first step in diagnosing amenorrhea is to rule out pregnancy. While this may seem obvious, the woman's sexual and social history, as well as preconceived assumptions on the part of the clinician, can lull the practitioner into thinking that pregnancy is not a possible or likely determinant of the amenorrheic state (e.g., an adolescent who states she is not sexually active, but is actually living in a sexually abusive environment). Discounting the possibility of pregnancy can lead to an expensive and anxiety-provoking amenorrheic work-up that could have been avoided with clear and thorough history taking followed by a simple urine human chorionic gonadotropin (hCG) test. Situations such as abuse or sexual activity need to be broached using honest and sensitive approaches before deciding pregnancy is not a possibility.

Episodes of amenorrhea are also part of the normal transition during perimenopause. Often, a woman will begin to experience heavier and more frequent menses during perimenopause, or will eventually have fewer and lighter menses as menopause itself nears. These occurrences of amenorrhea are normal and usually do not require any intervention beyond a thorough history and discussion with the woman about contraception and concurrent physiologic changes associated with menopause. This woman also may benefit from a discussion of the potential emotional impact of nearing menopause and changes in her fertility. Cessation of menses may be an event that is welcomed or, alternatively, may evoke fears of aging and loss of "femininity." Further guidance in assisting women through this transition may be found in the *Midlife, Menopause, and Beyond* chapter.

In addition to assessing the woman with amenorrhea for pregnancy and perimenopause, querying her about her overall health, nutritional and exercise status, recent weight changes, use of medications and herbs, and emotional state can provide important information. These subjective findings are usually followed by calculation of the woman's current body mass index (BMI) and a confirmatory physical examination (PE) as appropriate. Chronic

illness; malnutrition; disordered eating patterns such as anorexia nervosa, bulimia, crash dieting, or other extreme methods of rapid weight loss; and obesity have all been found to result in amenorrhea, as have certain degrees of physical activity or athleticism that inhibit the development of sufficient levels of body fat and normal estrogen metabolism. The use of some medications and herbal preparations, as well as increased overall emotional stress, also may contribute to a cessation of menses.[1] A need to explore disordered eating patterns or emotional distress may ultimately be the outcome of visits for women whose presenting concern is absent or irregular menses.

In the majority of women with amenorrhea, cessation of menses occurs secondary to different types of disruptions that affect the HPO axis. Successfully addressing or removing the underlying diseases or conditions often can resolve the amenorrhea. However, this is not always a simple task. For example, with a diagnosis of disordered eating or depression, a healthcare team consisting of the woman, midwife, and other specialists may provide the best care.

The link between low BMI or weight loss and amenorrhea has historically been a focus of exploration; more recently, the increase in obesity among the general population, both nationally and internationally, has emerged as a contemporary gynecologic concern.[2,3] Recent reports have pointed to a possible relationship between childhood obesity or high BMI and early menarche.[4] Periods of amenorrhea are common in the initial period after menses first start. Likewise, societal emphasis on and concern with weight and appearance may be manifested in disordered eating, unhealthy exercise patterns, dramatic weight loss, or weight gain that can be associated with menstrual cycle abnormalities among women of any age.

Once potential etiologies such as anatomic abnormalities, pregnancy, breastfeeding-induced amenorrhea, perimenopausal changes, use of hormonal contraception, general ill health, and nutritional, physical, medicinal/herbal, and emotional causes of menstrual disruption have been ruled out, a comprehensive investigation is initiated. The initial step usually is to measure levels of thyroid-stimulating hormone (TSH) and prolactin. An elevated TSH level, often accompanied by an increased prolactin level, is indicative of hypothyroidism, which is readily treated with thyroid hormone replacement therapy. In addition, any type of hyperthyroidism (e.g., Graves' disease) can be the underlying cause of amenorrhea; depending on the method of treatment for such disease, regular menstrual cycles will return upon control of thyroid function.

When amenorrhea is accompanied by galactorrhea, increased levels of prolactin and normal levels of TSH are often identified by the initial laboratory tests. Multiple causes of hyperprolactinemia and galactorrhea exist related to endocrine deviations or a pituitary tumor. Thus women with an elevated prolactin level require a more extensive work-up, including referral to a practitioner specializing in endocrinology.

Progesterone Challenge Testing

If thyroid and pituitary function appear normal, the next step in diagnosing and treating amenorrhea is a progesterone challenge test. The purpose of this test is twofold: to assess the presence of endogenous estrogen, which is required for healthy buildup of endometrial tissue, and to examine the patency of the genital outflow tract (uterus and vagina).

Medroxyprogesterone acetate (Provera), 5–10 mg for 5–10 days, or progesterone (Prometrium), as a single daily dose of 400 mg taken in the evening for 10 days, can be prescribed and administered. Prometrium contains peanut oil and should not be taken by women with a peanut allergy; it should be taken at bedtime as it may cause dizziness or sleepiness.[5] As early as 2 days after the medication regimen is completed (withdrawn), and usually within a week, vaginal bleeding may occur, thereby establishing the presence of endogenous estrogen and the patency of the outflow tract. The woman should stop taking progesterone when the bleeding occurs, as the *challenge* has succeeded. The vaginal bleeding indicates that the woman is not ovulating and the next steps of the evaluation will focus on function of the ovaries, pituitary, or CNS.

If the progesterone challenge fails to result in withdrawal bleeding and the amenorrhea continues, then the midwife needs to pursue assessment for a hormonal dysfunction or outflow tract obstructions. At this point, a question arises regarding whether the progesterone withdrawal would have been successful if there had been adequate estrogen-influenced endometrium. Thus the woman is given exogenous estrogen before a progesterone withdrawal. A commonly used method is to administer estrogen and progesterone (estradiol [e.g., Estrace] 4.0 mg, or conjugated equine estrogen [e.g., Premarin] 2.5 mg., given orally for 21 days, with medroxyprogesterone acetate [e.g., Provera] 10 mg orally per day added for the last 5 days) or to use a monophasic combination oral contraceptive for one cycle. If progesterone withdrawal bleeding occurs after cessation of this medication regimen, then the patency of the outflow tract is confirmed. If withdrawal bleeding does not occur, then the healthcare provider should strongly suspect an obstruction of the outflow tract. Investigation includes obtaining an ultrasound, and referring the woman appropriately based on the results. Such obstructions are rare, and if present, are often found on physical examination. If an adolescent has secondary sexual characteristics but no established menstrual flow, then obstruction should be considered. Most frequently, amenorrhea will be secondary to physiologic causes at the ovarian, pituitary, or CNS level.

If the patency of the outflow tract has been established by the presence of withdrawal following the estrogen/progesterone challenge, then the midwife can assume that the woman's body is not producing enough estrogen to enable menstruation to occur. According to the previously described approach of diagnosing the cause of amenorrhea from one of four anatomic areas, the disruption of estrogen production is now known to be occurring at either the ovarian, pituitary, or CNS level. Therefore, the next part of the evaluation is to assess the level of gonadotropins to determine whether the lack of estrogen originates in the follicle of the ovary or along the pituitary–CNS axis. Gonadotropin testing is accomplished by obtaining serum samples to assay follicle-stimulating hormone (FSH) and luteinizing hormone (LH) levels. Normal levels range from 5 to 30 IU/L for FSH and from 5 to 20 IU/L for LH. Any levels outside of these ranges can indicate one of a number of possible diagnoses **Figure 12-1**).

Several factors are important to consider at this point. First, both FSH and LH surge to levels approximately two to three times their baseline during a normal midcycle. Also, if the woman had been undergoing an estrogen/progesterone challenge, a delay of 2 weeks before drawing a gonadotropin assay is advisable to avoid finding artificially elevated values. Depending on the midwife's scope of practice with regard to gynecologic care, the practitioner may choose to refer the individual to a provider specializing in female endocrine disorders or to personally continue to investigate the situation. While gonadotropin assays can better isolate the source of amenorrhea (high FSH and LH point to ovarian problems; low or normal FSH and LH indicate either pituitary or CNS problems), further differential diagnosis and subsequent treatment are indicated with these results.

The experience of an evaluation for amenorrhea can be frightening, and the lack of definitive testing can be frustrating for everyone. Educating the woman about the potential causes and the likelihood of each etiology can help alleviate her anxiety.

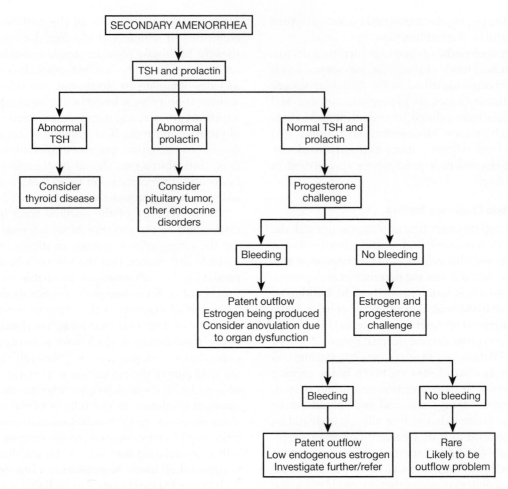

Figure 12-1 Algorithm for assessment of woman with secondary amenorrhea.

Other remedies for amenorrhea have been suggested that are not traditionally prescribed by practitioners of allopathic medicine. For example, herbalists may recommend blessed thistle or blue cohosh for the relief of amenorrhea, while acupuncture and homeopathic remedies have been suggested as other treatment modalities.[6,7] To date, no published, evidence-based investigations have addressed the efficacy or safety of using these herbs for this condition.

Polycystic Ovary Syndrome and Amenorrhea

Polycystic ovary syndrome (PCOS) affects approximately 4% to 6% of women, and has a slightly higher incidence among certain ethnic groups.[1] PCOS is the most common diagnosis implicated in ovarian dysfunction related to infertility.[1] This condition was first identified in 1935 by two physicians, Irving Stein and Michael Leventhal, and for some time was termed Stein-Leventhal syndrome, only to later be renamed polycystic ovary syndrome.

The early recognition of this condition focused on enlarged ovaries and the often resultant infertility. In current practice, PCOS is more correctly viewed as a constellation of signs and symptoms that may include hyperandrogenism, with menstrual abnormalities ranging from amenorrhea to oligomenorrhea. The exact diagnostic criteria continue to be debated by international experts.[8] Women with PCOS are more likely than their unaffected counterparts to have obesity, acne, alopecia, and hirsutism. Women with PCOS are often insulin resistant and may exhibit signs of diabetes, including acanthosis nigricans, a brown velvety appearance to the skin in various folds, such as the back of the neck, in the axillae, under the breasts, or in the groin.[8] The cause of PCOS remains unknown, but a finer recognition of the possible long-term medical sequelae is emerging, resulting in greater attention to diagnosis and treatment.[1,9]

In addition to targeted diagnosis, the diagnosis of PCOS may be made coincidentally in other situations, such as during diagnostic surgery for a woman with infertility, during routine pelvic examination, or by laboratory studies that reveal elevated levels of serum androgens. On ultrasound, one or both ovaries may be significantly enlarged and contain multiple, immature follicles. The enlarged, polycystic ovary is actually a consequence of the anovulatory state and not a cause of anovulation. Even among women with chronic amenorrhea, individuals with PCOS are not always anovulatory, and some may experience a spontaneous conception and pregnancy.

Due to the associated obesity in some women with PCOS, enlarged ovaries may be difficult to palpate on pelvic examination. Laboratory studies that may aid in diagnosis include serum levels of LH and FSH, testosterone, TSH, prolactin, and 17-hydroxyprogesterone (17-OHP).[1] If the diagnosis is confirmed, assessment of a woman's risk of diabetes or cardiovascular disease is warranted, including measurement of glucose, insulin, and lipid levels. On examination, an assessment of woman's BMI, blood pressure, waist-to-hip circumference, and hirsutism should also be made. A waist-to-hip ratio of 0.85 or more indicates abdominal obesity and an increased risk for metabolic and cardiovascular conditions in women.[10]

Immediate treatment of PCOS varies and often depends on the degree of infertility or desire for conception. PCOS among obese women has been treated with weight-loss programs alone. Obese women who experience weight loss have been observed to resume more normal ovulatory and menstrual patterns and have conceived spontaneously.[11] The use of the anti-hyperglycemic drug metformin (Glucophage) has increased in popularity in recent years, although the effectiveness of this medication is not clear.[11,12] Because there is an association between obesity and depression, a screen for depression may be warranted when caring for a woman who has a high BMI.[13]

If conception is not immediately desired, ovarian function (and continued physical enlargement of the ovaries) may be suppressed with the use of combination hormonal contraceptives. This temporary ovarian suppression optimally will result in the initiation of normal ovarian function for a short time upon discontinuation of the hormonal contraceptive. Use of a hormonal contraceptive method will also protect the woman from the potential risks of unopposed estrogen stimulation of the endometrium, which might otherwise result in endometrial hyperplasia and endometrial cancer. A variety of other medications, such as gonadotropin-releasing hormone (GnRH) agonists and the diuretic spironolactone (Aldactone), have also been employed as antiandrogens. Induction of ovulation, with the use of clomiphene citrate (Clomid), is a common strategy for the prompt treatment of infertility in women with PCOS.[1]

Several important theories have emerged regarding the long-term health of women with PCOS. The first is founded on the knowledge that women with PCOS—even those who are not obese—may have significant insulin resistance and, therefore, are at a higher lifetime risk for the development of both type 2 diabetes and cardiovascular disease.[1] The second theory suggests that due to the potential of lifelong adverse effects, it is especially important to diagnose and treat PCOS in adolescent girls presenting with amenorrhea, irregular menses, obesity, or hirsutism.[14] This information has offered greater support for the continued research about the use of metformin (Glucophage) for PCOS, because in addition to its antihyperglycemic action, this medication increases insulin sensitivity.[8] Lastly, unopposed stimulation of the endometrium, as found in chronic anovulation, poses a risk for endometrial hyperplasia, which is a precursor for endometrial cancer. Therefore, interruption of these cycles is another important goal of treatment.

A woman with amenorrhea also may have evidence of hirsutism (which may not be readily apparent if the woman regularly uses hair removal techniques). Although idiopathic hirsutism may represent a racial or ethnic variation, occurring in women with normal menstrual cycles and ovulatory patterns, it also may be a sign of PCOS in a woman with normal menses and a normal BMI. A cautionary note to providers here is to remember that a dramatic short-term increase in hirsutism is not likely to be the result of PCOS, but rather may indicate the presence of a rapidly progressing adrenal tumor, which must be ruled out.

In conclusion, early diagnosis and intervention for PCOS, with respect to the physical health risks of hyperglycemia, abnormal cholesterol and lipid profiles, and reproductive cancer risk, may positively influence a woman's overall health. In addition, a woman's long-term mental health as regards a potential diminished sense of femaleness or self-esteem due to physical appearance and perceived or actual inability to conceive require the midwife's attention.[15]

Dysmenorrhea

Painful menstruation, particularly in the lower abdomen and back and usually of a cramping nature, is known as *dysmenorrhea*. It has been reported in the United States to be experienced by anywhere from

60% to 91% of women.[1] Dysmenorrhea is most prevalent in the first 3 years after menarche (*primary dysmenorrhea*), although it can arise later in any woman's reproductive life (*secondary dysmenorrhea*). Prior to the 1970s, many practitioners viewed dysmenorrhea as being psychosomatic in origin, and few resources were offered for relief.[16] More recent research has presented a clearer picture of the nature and treatment of this potentially debilitating condition. In distinguishing dysmenorrhea from other causes of pelvic pain, it is important to establish this pain as cyclic in nature, coinciding with the onset of menses and resolving after cessation of the menstrual flow. As with any other characteristic of menses, women with significant dysmenorrhea may regard severe pain as "normal" and may not seek or discuss relief modalities. Additionally, the variety of responses to pain and to pain relief strategies must be considered.

Primary Dysmenorrhea

The principal cause of primary dysmenorrhea is the presence prostaglandin F2alpha (PGF2a), which originates in the endometrium.[1] This prostaglandin is necessary for stimulating uterine contractions during menstruation. For adolescents with dysmenorrhea, the amount of PGF2a produced is more than normal, so decreasing the amount of available PGF2a is the primary method of relief (**Figure 12-2**).

Because combined hormonal contraceptives decrease prostaglandin synthesis and menstrual flow, these drugs are frequently used on an off-label basis for the treatment of women with dysmenorrhea.[1,17] In addition, the various progestin-only methods of contraception—injectable depot medroxyprogesterone acetate (DPMA; Depo-Provera), progestin-only oral contraceptives, the progestin-containing intrauterine system Mirena, and the etonogestrel-containing implants Implanon and Nexplanon—often result in temporary states of amenorrhea due to decreased endometrial stimulation. In turn, these methods can result in less dysmenorrhea. As with any other use of hormonal contraception, attention must be paid to medical eligibility criteria[18,19] as well as the woman's desire for the drug or device.

For individuals who are unable or unwilling to use hormonal contraceptives, dysmenorrhea can be treated with nonsteroidal anti-inflammatory drugs (NSAIDs), as shown in **Table 12-1**. These medications should be taken for 2 to 3 days beginning on the first day of symptoms. Contrary to earlier beliefs, there is no evidence that initiation of medication a few days prior to menstruation is more effective.[1] The benefits of NSAID therapy may require up to 6 months to become evident, so women need education and counseling to prevent early self-discontinuation. Long-term therapy with NSAIDs can have some adverse effects, so a look at alternative therapies if dysmenorrhea continues for an extended period of time may become necessary. Although aspirin (ASA)—another NSAID—has also been shown to offer some relief from dysmenorrhea, there is no evidence that the non-NSAID analgesic acetaminophen is beneficial in eliminating menstrual pain.[20]

Several nonpharmaceutical approaches to treatment of women with dysmenorrhea have been widely advocated. Among them are the application of local heat in the form of small heat packs continuously applied to the abdomen,[21] homeopathy (e.g., belladonna

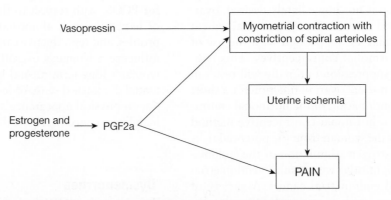

The prostaglandin PGF2a stimulates myometrial contraction and sensitizes the afferent nerves to pain, thereby contributing to dysmenorrhea in two ways.

Figure 12-2 Pathophysiology of primary dysmenorrhea.
Source: Modified from King TL, Brucker MC. *Pharmacology for Women's Health.* Sudbury, MA: Jones and Bartlett; 2011.

and chamomilla), acupuncture, biofeedback, relaxation techniques, massage, exercise, aromatherapy (e.g., rose oil), and the use of certain herbs (e.g., black cohosh, raspberry leaf, shakuyaku-kanzo-to, semen coicus, and chaste berry).[22–27] With the exception of the use of local heat application, there is limited scientific evidence of effectiveness for these various nonpharmaceutical modalities.[28]

Secondary Dysmenorrhea

Secondary dysmenorrhea has been described as painful menstruation that arises later in a woman's life, after she has experienced menstrual cycles not associated with significant pain. However, in its current use the term has come to signify dysmenorrhea caused not by prostaglandins, but rather by anatomic or pathologic factors.[1] These factors include endometriosis, uterine myomas, endometrial polyps, uterine cancer, and the presence of pelvic inflammatory disease (PID). The presence of an intrauterine device (IUD) can also contribute to dysmenorrhea.

A tubal ligation has been suggested to be associated with subsequent painful menstruation, theoretically due to postsurgical reduction in blood supply to the ovaries, resulting in hormonal changes that affect menstruation. However, this notion of post-tubal ligation dysmenorrhea has been questioned in the literature.[1]

Assessment of a woman with secondary dysmenorrhea is accomplished through physical examination, ultrasound or other imaging techniques, and additional testing dependent on the suspected diagnosis. A potential diagnosis of pelvic inflammatory disease requires the collection of specimens for sexually transmitted infection (STI) testing and is discussed in more detail in the *Reproductive Tract and Sexually Transmitted Infections* chapter. If endometrial cancer is suspected, an endometrial biopsy, uterine imaging, and referral are warranted. A suspicion of endometriosis may require referral for further investigation based upon the midwife's scope of practice and practice guidelines.

Treatment of endometrial cancers, benign tumors (myomas), and endometriosis are discussed in the *Gynecologic Disorders* chapter. If the IUD is thought to be the source of dysmenorrhea, the midwife should discuss the use of NSAIDs or even the removal of the IUD. IUD removal should be accompanied with exploration of alternative contraceptive methods. As with primary dysmenorrhea, the use of NSAIDs or the nonpharmacologic approaches mentioned earlier often serve as the initial therapy.

Table 12-1	Nonsteroidal Anti-inflammatory Drugs Commonly Used to Treat Primary Dysmenorrhea[a]			
Drug Name Generic (Brand)	**Dose/Route**	**Frequency**	**Onset/Peak**	**Duration**
Diclofenac potassium (Cataflam)	50 mg orally	Three times per day	30 minutes/2–3 hours	8 hours
Ibuprofen (Advil, Motrin, Midol IB)	400 mg orally 600–800 mg	Every 4–6 hours Every 6–8 hours	Varies/1–2 hours	4–6 hours
Ketoprofen (Orudis, Orudis KT)	25–50 mg orally	Every 6–8 hours Maximum dose 300 mg/daily	2–3 hours/6–7 hours	Unknown
Naproxen (Naprosyn)	500 mg orally initial dose, then 250 mg orally	250 mg orally every 6–8 hours up to 1.25 g/daily	1 hour/2–4 hours	6–8 hours
Naproxen sodium (Aleve)	550 mg orally initial dose, then 275 mg	275 mg orally every 6–8 hours up to 1375 mg/daily	1 hour/2–4 hours	7 hours
Naproxen sodium (Naprelan)	Sustained-release formulation 375 mg or 500 mg tablets; dose is 1000 mg orally	Once daily	Unknown	Unknown
Acetylsalicylic acid (aspirin)	325–650 mg orally 500 mg orally	Every 3–4 hours Maximum dose 4 g/day	15–20 minutes/ 1–3 hours	3–6 hours

[a]Medications should be initiated on the first day of symptoms and continued for 2 to 3 days.

Source: King TL, Brucker MC. *Pharmacology for Women's Health.* Sudbury, MA: Jones and Bartlett; 2011.

Abnormal Uterine Bleeding

A menstrual cycle may vary from the woman's "typical" cycle characteristics in terms of interval, duration, or flow at any time in her life; while the cycle may be "irregular," it should not necessarily be a cause for alarm or an indication of pathology. The exception to this is the onset of vaginal bleeding after a woman has experienced menopause. This bleeding pattern always warrants prompt investigation. Outside of this postmenopausal circumstance, as long as the cycle returns to the usual characteristics within a short time (e.g., within a cycle or two), there is little reason for alarm or clinical evaluation. These occasional variations are normal and may be due to a change in routine such as travel and/or time zone change, nutrition, exercise, emotional stress, or an unexplained cause.

Providers have struggled with accurate nomenclature to describe unusual menstrual bleeding. The International Federation of Gynecology and Obstetrics[29,30] has proposed a system, PALM-COEIN, that advocates replacing the term "dysfunctional uterine bleeding" (DUB) with "abnormal uterine bleeding" (AUB), and then adding a suffix to identify the proposed etiology. For example, AUB-P designates bleeding secondary to polyps. In this system, other terms associated with DUB also are recommended to be retired from use. These terms include "menorrhagia," which traditionally has been used to describe heavy menses, usually lasting for more days than considered normal by the woman. The PALM-COEIN system promotes use of a descriptor such as "heavy menstrual bleeding" (HMB), which it defines as a monthly flow in excess of 80 mL with each menses, and "prolonged menses," which is defined as 8 or more days of bleeding.[30] The American College of Obstetricians and Gynecologists has proposed that all clinicians use the PALM-COEIN lexicon[31] (Table 12-2). The widespread use of more precise language ultimately may facilitate both diagnostic efforts and health education/communication with women. Because the PALM-COEIN nomenclature has not been accepted universally yet, this chapter uses both the traditional and newer terms together at this time of transition.

Many pharmacologic and surgical approaches to abnormal bleeding exist in practice. Some of these

Table 12-2	Abnormal Menstrual Bleeding Assessment Framework: PALM-COEIN	
	Etiologies	**Investigation**
PALM (structural causes)	**P**olyp	History:
	Adenomyosis	Risk factors
	Leiomyoma	Physical exam
	Malignancy and hyperplasia	Imaging studies:
		Ultrasound
		MRI
		Endometrial biopsy
COEIN (nonstructural causes)	**C**oagulopathy	History:
	Ovulatory dysfunction	Risk factors
	Endometrial	Hormonal contraceptive (i.e., use, misusing, or discontinued)
	Iatrogenic	Intrauterine contraceptive (history of use)
	Not yet classified	Laboratory studies:
		Endocrine: TSH, prolactin
		Hormones: FSH, LH
		Coagulation indices
		Pregnancy test
		Endometrial biopsy

FSH = follicle-stimulating hormone; LH = luteinizing hormone; MRI = magnetic resonance imaging; TSH = thyroid-stimulating hormone.

Source: Adapted from Munro MG, Critchley HO, Broder MS, Fraser IS; FIGO Working Group on Menstrual Disorders. FIGO classification system (PALM-COEIN) for causes of abnormal uterine bleeding in nongravid women of reproductive age. *Int J Gynaecol Obstet.* 2011;113(1):3-13

medical treatments can be managed by the midwife; others require referral to other providers. When referrals are required, the midwife can provide anticipatory guidance for the woman and encourage her to express any anxieties or doubts about this possible step in managing her problem.

Heavy Menstrual Bleeding/Menorrhagia

Heavy menstrual bleeding, or menorrhagia (also sometimes referred to as hypermenorrhea), is defined as excessive bleeding, either in amount or in duration, at the regular interval of normal menstruation. A thorough history will provide the woman with the opportunity to describe her normal flow and to compare the recent flow to what she has ascertained as normal for her.

Objectively determining what is excessive bleeding can be a difficult task. A common perception has been that the saturation of three to four pads/tampons over a 4-hour period at the time of menstruation is excessive. Yet, for some women this can be part of their normal pattern, especially on the first 2 to 3 days of flow, and one individual's definition of a saturated pad/tampon can be different from that of another woman.[32] The amount of blood loss considered normal during menses has been described as approximately 30 mL based on research conducted in the 1960s, with anything more than 80 mL deemed abnormal.[1] However, many women either overestimate or underestimate the amount of menstrual bleeding that occurs on a monthly basis.[32] Newer, more accurate methods of measuring blood loss during menstruation, such as the alkaline hematin laboratory procedure that measures blood loss found on tampons or pads, and the Pictorial Blood Loss Assessment Chart (PBLAC), which estimates blood loss using diagrammatic prompts, have been shown to be effective. However, due to their cost, inconvenience, or lack of exposure, their use has been limited to research endeavors.

Perhaps the best method to determine whether a woman's heavy bleeding is of clinical significance is to obtain laboratory values of hemoglobin and/or hematocrit to rule out anemia. No matter what the etiology, if the woman believes that her menses is excessive, then the clinician must address this issue from a psychosocial perspective to promote the woman's well-being. Evaluation of menstrual flow by way of history or diagnostic measures is especially important for the adolescent woman. Some clinicians propose that menses should regarded as a "fifth vital sign" in young women, as it provides evidence of hormonal status as well as bleeding patterns in general.[32]

When collecting evidence to determine whether the woman's menstrual flow is excessive, other descriptors such as duration, color, presence of clots, and character of bleeding can be helpful. The next step in investigation is to discover the origin of the condition. Differential diagnoses associated with HMB are listed in **Table 12-3**. Any accompanying physical changes associated with the heavier menstrual flow warrant further inquiry, but particularly if there are potential contraceptive causes such as the presence of an IUD. Additional etiologies to be considered include stress, illicit drug use, sexual correlates (e.g., STIs, sexual practices), obesity, and gynecologic factors (e.g., past surgery, a history of unusual menstrual patterns). Finally, inheritable coagulation disorders can be assessed by asking the woman if any close relatives have a history of hematologic disorders, especially related to clotting.

Physical and pelvic examination includes assessment for signs of anemia and bleeding (e.g., bruising or petechiae). The vagina and cervix need to be assessed for masses, lesions, infections, or foreign bodies (e.g., IUD) that could contribute to heavier menses. If a Pap test has not been performed within the recommended schedule for this woman, it should be obtained. Bimanual examination includes assessing for ovarian or uterine masses or pelvic pain.

A pregnancy test is appropriate at this time, although the woman presenting with a report of abnormally heavy menstrual bleeding/menorrhagia usually has experienced this symptom for several cycles, and typically will not describe signs or symptoms of pregnancy. Screening for STIs and chronic vaginitis or cervicitis should be considered. If endometrial hyperplasia or cancer is suspected, an endometrial biopsy should be performed. This brief, ambulatory care procedure allows for laboratory histologic analysis of endometrial tissue. Any nondefinitive or positive results should lead to a referral for additional investigation or treatment.

In addition to the hemoglobin and/or hematocrit and the pregnancy test, obtaining a complete blood count (CBC) can enable the healthcare provider to detect an abnormally low platelet count (thrombocytopenia) that can accompany a bleeding disorder. However, several bleeding disorders (e.g., von Willebrand's disease) do not result in lowered platelet counts, and will require additional laboratory testing to ascertain their presence. Other useful tests may include a thyroid-stimulating hormone (TSH) level, to rule out thyroid disease; prothrombin time (PT) and partial thromboplastin time (PTT), to assess for certain bleeding disorders; and liver function tests (LFTs), to rule out liver disease.

Table 12-3	Common Etiologies for Heavy Menstrual Bleeding or Menorrhagia	
Etiology	**Example**
Typically Presents as a One-Time Event	
Pregnancy	Intrauterine
	Ectopic
	Gestational trophoblastic neoplasm (e.g., hydatidiform mole)
Infections	Endometritis
	Salpingitis
	(Usually related to PID or following instrument-based intrauterine procedure)
Typically Presents as an Ongoing, Cyclic Pattern	
Neoplasia	Ovarian cysts
	Uterine fibroids (myoma)
	Adenomyosis: endometrial tissue located within the myometrium
	Endometrial hyperplasia
	Polyps
	Carcinoma
Coagulation disorders	Inherited (e.g., von Willebrand's disease)
	Acquired (e.g., idiopathic thrombocytopenic purpura [ITP])
	Pharmacologic (e.g., use of heparin or aspirin)
Liver disorder	Cirrhosis
Endocrine	Hypothyroidism
Intrauterine contraceptive	Inert and mineral-based intrauterine contraceptives

Pelvic ultrasound, or other imaging techniques, also can be effective diagnostic tools given that a common cause of chronic heavy menstrual flow is the presence of uterine myomata (fibroids). While a myomata may be palpated during a physical examination, the least distinctive of these masses on bimanual exam—the submucosal fibroids—are those closest to the endometrium. These fibroids are considered the most likely to cause menorrhagia. Imaging studies will detect myomata as well as endometrial polyps (benign growths that can cause menorrhagia), and will report on the "endometrial stripe," or thickness of the endometrium. Normally, during the follicular (preovulatory) phase of the menstrual cycle, the endometrium grows from a postmenstrual thickness of 1.0 to 2.0 mm to a preovulation thickness of 3.5 to 5.0 mm. Although the endometrium can reach a normal thickness of 5.0 to 7.0 mm during the luteal phase of the menstrual cycle, any evidence of an endometrial stripe larger than 5.0 mm on ultrasound suggests the possibility of endometrial hyperplasia or carcinoma, and points to the need for continued investigation and possible surgical treatment such as endometrial curettage.[1,34]

Treatment of Heavy Menstrual Bleeding

If excessive bleeding is reported as a single, acute event, the likely diagnosis is either pregnancy or infection, and immediate action is generally required. Appropriate steps must be taken depending on the type of pregnancy (e.g., intrauterine versus ectopic) or infection and the desires of the woman. Management of bleeding during pregnancy or of ectopic pregnancy is covered in the *Obstetric Complications in Pregnancy* chapter, while caring for the woman with endometritis or salpingitis is discussed in the *Reproductive Tract and Sexually Transmitted Infections* chapter.

If the bleeding is found to be chronic and cyclic, management still depends on the specific cause deemed responsible for the excessive bleeding. If an IUD is in place, the midwife should consider its removal, after discussing the woman's desire for alternative contraception. One IUD, the Mirena, is indicated not only for birth control, but also for treatment of abnormal menstrual bleeding,[35] and may be considered as a method of resolving menorrhagia while continuing with an intrauterine form of contraception.

Abnormally heavy menstrual bleeding found to be caused by a coagulation disorder or liver disease requires referral to a specialist, who will usually first treat the woman pharmacologically, followed by surgery if drug therapy is not successful. Heavy menstrual bleeding caused by endocrine dysfunction is manageable, at least initially, by the primary care practitioner, and usually begins with placing the woman on monophasic low-dose combination oral contraceptives (COCs). While the typical treatment prescribes COCs in the same manner as for women using the pills for contraception, evidence suggests that a regimen in which active COCs are taken continuously for some time before the inert pills are taken may be a more effective approach for the woman with menorrhagia. This approach facilitates the stabilization of the endometrium and offers a brief respite from the previously experienced excessive bleeding.[1] Use of other combined hormonal contraceptive methods, such as the combined hormonal contraceptive patch and ring, also are being evaluated for efficacy as treatment modalities for heavy menstrual bleeding.[1,35]

Additional pharmacologic approaches to treating the woman with heavy menstrual bleeding include the use of progestins, GnRH agonists, NSAIDs, and danazol (Danocrine), a synthetic steroid that suppresses HPO axis activity (**Table 12-4**). Progestins specifically can be helpful because they change the endometrium from proliferative to secretory in nature, limit endometrial growth, and simultaneously enrich any existing endometrial structure, resulting in reduced and less uneven menstrual flow.[5] For individuals who have difficulty with a daily pill schedule, injectable DMPA (either 104 mg subcutaneous or 150 mg intramuscular) can also be used to reduce menstrual flow. Additionally, the long-term progestin-containing contraceptives—the levonorgestrel intrauterine system (Mirena intrauterine contraceptive) and Implanon and Nexplanon (implant)—can be employed should the woman desire to include her contraceptive as a modality in the treatment of her bleeding.[4,35–38] With each of these methods, irregular bleeding frequently occurs until the woman develops amenorrhea.[4,39]

GnRH agonists (e.g., leuprolide [Lupron]) affect the HPO axis, retarding the ovaries' ability to release hormones required for normal function of the menstrual cycle. Interfering with cyclic menstruation causes the woman to enter a physiologic state most

Table 12-4	Common Pharmaceutical Management for Woman with Heavy Menstrual Bleeding/Menorrhagia	
Drug Generic (Brand)	**Dose**	**Schedule**
Aqueous progesterone (progesterone in oil)	5–10 mg/day IM × 6–8 days	Must take on consecutive days
Contraceptive implant (Implanon, Nexplanon)	Implant (contains 68 mg of etonogestrel at the time of insertion)	Effective for contraception for up to 3 years
Depot medroxyprogesterone acetate (Depo-Provera)	150 mg IM	Administered every 12 weeks
Levonorgestrel-releasing intrauterine contraceptive (Mirena)	Contains 52 mg levonorgestrel at time of insertion	Effective for contraception for up to 5 years
Medroxyprogesterone acetate (Provera)	5–10 mg PO/day × 5–10 days	Start on day 16 or 21 of the menstrual cycle
Nonsteroidal anti-inflammatory drugs (Table 12-2)	Various	First three days of bleeding
Norethindrone acetate (Aygestin)	2.5–10 mg PO	Start on day 5 of the menstrual cycle and end on day 25
Oral micronized progesterone (Prometrium Crinone)*	400 mg PO × 10 days	Take in the evening; may cause drowsiness

Abbreviations: PO = oral; IM = intramuscular; IUS = intrauterine system.

*Contraindicated for persons who are allergic to peanuts.

Source: Adapted from Schuiling KD, Brucker MC. Pelvic and menstrual disorders. In King TL, Brucker MC. *Pharmacology for Women's Health.* Sudbury, MA: Jones and Bartlett; 2011.

resembling menopause. Not only is menstrual blood loss decreased, but in many cases amenorrhea occurs. However, because of bone mass loss associated with the drop in estrogen levels, use of these medications tends to be limited to women for whom other therapies have been unsuccessful, and may be best managed by the practitioner specializing in gynecologic disorders.[1] At a minimum, any prolonged treatment using GnRH agonists requires regularly monitoring the woman's bone density status.

Reduction in heavy menstrual bleeding also has been demonstrated in women who are taking NSAIDs due to the ability of these medications to block the synthesis of prostaglandins necessary for cyclic endometrial sloughing.[1] However, NSAID therapy does not work for all women, can cause gastrointestinal bleeding with long-term use, and for some individuals can result in an increase in vaginal bleeding due to inhibition of platelet aggregation and prolongation of bleeding time. Women on COCs also may take NSAIDs at the time of menstruation, and may benefit from the combination of these medications.

Danazol (Danocrine), a synthetic steroid, often is indicated for treatment of endometriosis. It has been successful in controlling heavy menstrual bleeding in some women, although it requires daily dosage for 3 to 6 months, given as 100 mg orally twice a day, during which time a state of amenorrhea is likely to occur. The medication should then be discontinued for a period of time to assess whether the menorrhagia has returned; it may be restarted after a hiatus if necessary. Significant androgenic side effects, including weight gain, acne, and seborrhea, are common with this medication, and the availability of other treatments has resulted in danazol no longer being the first choice of treatment for menorrhagia. As is true with GnRH agonists, this therapy may be best managed by the practitioner specializing in gynecologic disorders.

While some evidence supports the treatment of heavy menstrual bleeding with traditional Chinese medicines and acupuncture,[40–43] and the use of herbal, homeopathic, and aromatherapy remedies, the overall body of evidence supporting these nonpharmacologic methods is limited at this time. Based on evidence derived from clinical practice reports, three herbs have been suggested to lessen menstrual bleeding: nettles, shepherd's purse, and yarrow. Likewise, the homeopathic solutions chamomilla, Lachesis, and veratrum album are sometimes recommended for relief of a variety of menstrual disorders, including heavy bleeding. In the field of aromatherapy, rose oil has been recommended for the relief of menorrhagia. Unfortunately, there is limited scientific evidence to support these treatments' use, and the midwife should consult first with a knowledgeable practitioner regarding amounts and contraindications if women desire the use of such modalities.

Nutritionally, lack of vitamin K has been suspected as a contributor to heavy bleeding in general. Improving vitamin K intake, through ingesting green, leafy vegetables and cereals, could help reduce menorrhagia if this vitamin deficiency is the root cause of heavy bleeding. Finally, it should be noted that the use of ergot derivatives, either naturally occurring or as a synthetic pharmaceutical, which have a longstanding history of usefulness in controlling postpartum bleeding, appear to have little or no effect in alleviating menstrual bleeding.

In addition to, or in lieu of, the pharmacologic and therapeutic remedies described here, surgery may be a necessity for a woman to obtain relief from heavy menstrual bleeding. The surgeon to whom the woman is referred may first perform a hysteroscopic examination to identify the source of excessive bleeding. Surgical interventions include dilatation and curettage (D & C); various endometrial ablation techniques, using hysteroscopic visualization; and hysterectomy.[1] Of the procedures available, D & C is the one least likely to result in long-term resolution of the excessive bleeding.

Irregular Menses/Metrorrhagia

When menstruation occurs at irregular intervals, or incidents of spotting or bleeding occur between periods, the term "intermenstrual bleeding" or "metrorrhagia" has been used to describe the abnormality. Of the various forms of abnormal bleeding patterns, this can be one of the most disconcerting because of the unpredictable timing at which spotting or bleeding occurs.

Discovering the origin of erratic bleeding begins with a thorough history. Use of the PALM-COEIN framework will also be useful in this investigation, as outlined in Table 12-2. An attempt should be made to have the woman describe, in as much detail as possible, how the bleeding she presents with differs from what has been her normal menstruation pattern. For example, could it be a shortened menstrual cycle resulting in more frequent menses rather than intermenstrual bleeding? Can she identify whether the amount is inconsistent as well as the timing? Do any factors aggravate or relieve the situation? Is the woman taking any new medication? At the first visit for irregular bleeding the midwife can recommend that the woman keep a daily log of her bleeding. This log may be helpful in identifying any patterns that will help elucidate an etiology.

Many etiologies have been associated with irregular bleeding (**Table 12-5**). As with heavy regularly occurring menses, the midwife should first always consider the possibility of pregnancy as irregular pattern of spotting or bleeding may suggest a threatened spontaneous abortion, an ectopic pregnancy, or a gestational trophoblastic neoplasm, such as a hydatidiform mole. If the woman is not pregnant and the spotting typically occurs monthly between her menses, the clinician should explore spotting with monthly ovulation as the underlying cause of the metrorrhagia state.

Once the diagnosis of pregnancy or regular spotting at the time of ovulation has been ruled out, other causes such as sexually transmitted infections or vaginal infections can be considered. A severe cervicitis or vaginitis, as well as an ascending infection such as pelvic inflammatory disease, can result in vaginal, cervical, or uterine bleeding related to the inflammation. In addition to infection, trauma to the genitals as a result of sexual activity or abuse needs to be considered. This can usually be ascertained with a thorough sexual history. Intimate-partner violence or sexual assault requires a more extensive assessment, and should involve consultation or referral to a community center or medical professional experienced in working with victims of assault or abuse (e.g., a rape crisis center or a sexual assault nurse examiner [SANE]).[44] Depending on local laws governing such cases, the midwife may also be legally required to report suspicion of abuse. Most importantly, the midwife should initiate safety and support mechanisms for the woman. Referral to a surgeon may be necessary if any anatomic damage from the trauma, such as a laceration, appears to require surgery or extensive treatment.

Aside from pregnancy, ovulation, infection, or trauma, the most likely causes of irregularly occurring bleeding are hormonal in nature, including the use of contraceptives, pharmaceuticals, or hormone therapy (HT); side effects of medications or herbal preparations; and HPO axis disorders. With regard to contraception, each woman reacts differently to the standardized doses contained in hormonal

Table 12-5	Possible Causes of Irregular/Intermenstrual Bleeding or Metrorrhagia	
Etiology	**Examples**
Pregnancy	Intrauterine Ectopic Gestational trophoblastic neoplasm (e.g., hydatidiform mole)
Infections	Endometritis Salpingitis (Usually related to PID or following instrument-based intrauterine procedure)
Hormonal causes/contraception	Ovulation Hormonal therapy Combination oral contraceptives Contraceptive injectables Contraceptive implants Intrauterine contraceptives Perimenopausal hormone therapy Medications, herbs Thyroid disorder Polycystic ovary syndrome
Neoplasia	Ovarian cysts Uterine myoma (fibroids) Adenomyosis: endometrial tissue located within the myometrium Endometrial hyperplasia Polyps Carcinoma
Coagulation disorders	Inherited (e.g., von Willebrand's disease) Acquired (e.g., idiopathic thrombocytopenic purpura) Pharmacologic (e.g., use of heparin or aspirin)
Organ disease	Liver or renal failure

contraceptive agents. Irregular bleeding in this instance is usually secondary to an endometrium that is not well supported with the exogenous estrogen being used. Even the copper IUD ParaGard, while containing a mineral rather than a hormone, can contribute to irregular bleeding.[45] Likewise, for menopausal women on HT, some spotting is possible. As previously mentioned, any postmenopausal genital bleeding, even if the individual is on HT, requires the practitioner to assess for malignancies. Many prescriptive medications and herbs (e.g., ginseng) have irregular menstrual bleeding as a side effect. As with all healthcare assessments, it is vital to know which medications and substances the woman regularly takes.

Any disease or interruption along the HPO axis can lead to menstrual bleeding disorders, although most endocrine disruptions involving the hypothalamus or pituitary gland result in amenorrhea. The exception is hypothyroidism, which can lead to heavy menses.[46] As discussed earlier in this chapter, PCOS may result in a range of menstrual disruption due to anovulation. Therefore PCOS should be considered as a cause of menorrhagia or the combination of heavy and irregular menses that some professionals term "menometrorrhagia." The presentation of irregular bleeding should also suggest the possibility that the woman has a bleeding disorder (e.g., von Willebrand's disease). Organic causes include polycystic ovaries, cervical polyps or erosion, uterine myomas, adenomyosis, endometriosis, endometrial polyps, and cancer, as detailed in the PALM-COEIN system. The diagnostic process for many of these conditions was described earlier in the discussion of heavy menstrual bleeding.

In addition to a thorough history, the work-up for irregular menstrual bleeding includes a complete physical and pelvic examination, with possible endometrial tissue sampling (**Appendix 12A**); laboratory studies usually include a complete blood count, TSH level, liver function tests, platelet studies, and possibly coagulation testing; and in many cases, a pelvic ultrasound.

Treatment of Irregular Bleeding

Management of bleeding due to pregnancy, infection, or abuse matches that discussed earlier in this chapter. If the bleeding is caused by oral contraceptives, the midwife may change the pill to one with a different hormonal structure or dose. It has been noted that menstrual irregularities are the most frequently stated reasons by women for the discontinuation of COCs.[47] If the individual has recently initiated COC use, reassurance and education may be the best

treatment. First check whether the woman is taking the pill in the correct manner, as erratic use or missed pills will contribute to untimely spotting. If the pill is being taken correctly, irregular bleeding is most often resolved by the start of the fourth cycle after its initiation. Switching the woman to a COC that stimulates and supports the endometrium better will often resolve this hormone-induced irregular bleeding. Alternatively, a woman may benefit from the switch to another combined hormonal contraceptive method (NuvaRing or the Ortho Evra patch) or the use of any of these methods in a continuous fashion by eliminating or reducing the hormone-free interval.

The levonorgestrel IUD (Mirena) is associated with lighter periods and over time can cause amenorrhea. However, irregular light spotting is a common side effect in the first several months of use. If a woman is adequately counseled and comfortable that irregular bleeding may continue for awhile, this IUD can ultimately correct irregular bleeding.[35] If the woman decides against continued intrauterine contraception use, the midwife needs to discuss with her an alternative form of contraception unless she is seeking pregnancy.

Knowing which medications or herbal preparations a woman may be taking, especially on a routine basis, often can lead the clinician to discover the source of, and remedy, irregular bleeding. Simple removal or change of the medication(s) or herb(s) is often the solution to the abnormal bleeding. However, this seemingly easy step may not always be feasible, depending on the original reason for the woman's taking these agents. In that case, working in conjunction with the professional or other practitioner who has been caring for the woman can lead to development of a plan in which the bleeding is resolved and optimal health is maintained.

As with heavy menstrual bleeding, if the cause of a woman's irregular bleeding is thought to be a neoplasm, coagulation disorder, or chronic disease, referral to a specialist is indicated. The woman should be informed of these possible diagnoses and their treatment as preparation for her visit with the specialist.

If the etiology of the abnormal bleeding is thought to be hormonal in nature, then exogenous hormones are usually the treatment of choice. Whether to initiate treatment with progestin, estrogen, or a combination of the two has historically depended on the type of bleeding with which the woman presents. In general, amenorrhea or infrequent menses has been treated first with progestin, while irregular bleeding has been treated initially with estrogen.[1] However, combination hormonal contraceptives are very effective in controlling a number of menstrual disorders. Thus many clinicians use COCs or another combined hormonal method as the first line of treatment, especially if the woman is interested in, or has no objection to the use of, contraception. With each monthly withdrawal cycle while on the combined hormonal methods, the individual should experience decreased amounts of bleeding and cramping.

If contraception is not necessary or the hormonal method is not her preferred option, then discontinuing use of the method usually results in the return of regular ovulation and the healthy buildup of endometrium by endogenous estrogen.[4]

If spontaneous menses does not occur when expected following discontinuation of the contraceptive method, then an anovulatory state should be suspected. After pregnancy is ruled out, progestin therapy is recommended to help facilitate the shedding of estrogen-driven endometrial proliferation. This can be accomplished by prescribing medroxyprogesterone acetate (Provera) tablets, 10 mg orally, once daily for 10 days, beginning approximately midcycle each month. Menstrual flow will occur anywhere from 2 to 7 days after the woman takes the last pill.[1] This therapy can be continued monthly to help maintain a cyclic balance between endometrial buildup and shedding. Each woman will need to be assessed for contraindications to exogenous hormone use before initiating this therapy, especially with regard to the use of estrogen and its association with cardiovascular risks. If combined hormones or progestin therapy do not result in a regular menstrual flow, or metrorrhagia continues, referral for a more extensive evaluation must be considered.

For the woman who is not using a hormonal contraception or estrogen preparation, the midwife should suspect low levels of cyclic endogenous estrogen, or higher amounts of progesterone than are normally required to balance with estrogen for a healthy menstrual cycle. This results in poor endometrial buildup that leads to a less than optimal, intermittent shedding of tissue and irregular bleeding in this instance can normally be resolved with the use of estrogen therapy. While this condition can be found in women who are not using hormonal forms of contraception, spotting is more likely to be reported by individuals using injectable medroxyprogesterone acetate (DMPA), etonogestrel implants (Implanon or Nexplanon), or combined hormonal contraceptives.

Oral estrogen can be prescribed in the form of conjugated estrogen (e.g., Premarin), 1.25 mg, or estradiol (e.g., Estrace), 2.0 mg, given once daily for 7 to 10 days.[1] For the individual not taking any other form of hormonal medication, this course of estrogen will need to be followed with exogenous progesterone to initiate a withdrawal bleed and protect the woman from the potential harm of endometrial hyperplasia due to prolonged unopposed estrogen. The protection is most often accomplished through the use of a COC, initiated at the same time as the estrogen therapy. Gynecologic endocrinologists, such as Speroff et al.,[1] then recommend continuing the woman on a COC or other combined hormonal therapy.

Discussions in the literature regarding other therapeutic approaches to irregular bleeding are limited. Most information about the use of traditional Chinese medicines, acupuncture, herbs, homeopathy, aromatherapy, and other modalities have not been associated with treatment of irregular bleeding, and further evidence is needed before specific recommendations can be made. Thus the midwife should work with a practitioner knowledgeable in the particular modality being suggested and keep abreast of the scientific literature regarding evidence-based studies that support or caution against use of various alternative modalities.

Any continued bleeding after therapy has been attempted, or any acute bleeding putting the individual at risk of systemic illness or compromise, requires prompt evaluation and referral to the appropriate specialist. Providing anticipatory education to the woman about the type of evaluation and possible treatment to expect from the specialist can do much to relieve her anxiety in this situation.

Scant Menses or Oligomenorrhea/Hypomenorrhea

The term "oligomenorrhea" usually refers to scanty menstrual flow, although in some clinical sites it also is used to designate irregular menses. Some professionals label only infrequent flow, or decreased number of periods, as oligomenorrhea, and refer to scanty, but regular menses as "hypomenorrhea."[1] Both conditions are approached similarly, however, because the term "oligomenorrhea" is frequently used clinically to refer to either form of diminished menstrual flow, use of these terms may potentially result in confusion. Thus describing the menstrual pattern more accurately as "infrequent in occurrence" or "light flow" is advisable. Light or scant menses and infrequent menses are often a reflection of normal development or physiologic processes, and neither is necessarily a sign of disease or pathology.

The most common occasions that infrequent menses occur are in the first few years following menarche and in the decade before menopause. Scant bleeding during these two periods of time seldom requires intervention, except in the form of reassurance and anticipatory guidance. The most likely cause of infrequent menses is anovulation—for the adolescent because a regular pattern of ovulation has yet to occur, and for the perimenopausal woman because she is moving toward a menopausal state, in which ovulation no longer occurs. If the midwife is able to rule out other potential states, such as pregnancy or thyroid disease, then the key management tool is education. The adolescent needs to be made aware that a regular menstrual pattern should eventually develop, and if it does not, a thorough assessment will most likely lead to a definitive diagnosis. The perimenopausal woman benefits from understanding the normalcy of this time of her life. Options for long-term health maintenance will need to be reviewed, with a candid discussion required about lifestyle, diet, and healthful aging. In both cases, a discussion of the ongoing need for contraception in spite of occasional anovulation is in order if the woman is engaging in heterosexual sexual activity.

Another nonpathologic cause of infrequent menses or scant flow is the use of, or withdrawal from, hormonal contraception. Using combined hormonal contraceptives, DMPA, Implanon or Nexplanon, or a hormone-based IUD often reduces the flow or frequency of menstruation, and the discontinuation of one of these contraceptive methods can result in a delay in the return of a regular menstrual pattern (secondary amenorrhea). Following discontinuation of DMPA, Implanon, or Nexplanon, normal menses can take close to a year to resume.[38,40] Also, if the midwife is caring for a woman who has recently come to the United States from another country, the clinician must inquire about the woman's possible use of a hormonal contraceptive that may not be available in this country and that may have influenced her menstrual pattern. In general, no harm is associated with these cases of oligomenorrhea, and the clinician must simply reassure the woman. In contrast, if underlying pathology is suspected, an appropriate assessment and possibly referral are warranted. Even though oligomenorrhea is often not a sign of ill health, the woman's fears and anxieties must still be acknowledged, and she must be supported in adjusting to any physical and lifestyle changes. Finally, for the woman who is experiencing secondary amenorrhea after discontinuing hormonal contraception, she may believe incorrectly that reduced menstrual flow is an indication that she cannot become pregnant.

Other factors that can contribute to infrequent menses or secondary amenorrhea oligomenorrhea include anxiety and stress, chronic disease, certain medications, disease states, poor nutrition, a change in exercise patterns that alter body fat, and significant weight gain or loss. In addition, any malfunction along the HPO axis can result in decreased menstrual flow. Potential diseases and conditions of this regulatory axis include hyperprolactinemia, Cushing's syndrome, and PCOS.

The clinical evaluation required to find the cause of infrequent or scant menses resembles those actions taken to discover the reasons for amenorrhea. The initial step in assessment is to rule out pregnancy. Depending on the timing of the visit in relation to the last normal menses and last sexual contact, a serum or urine hCG test usually will enable the clinician to make this diagnosis.

An elevated TSH level suggests primary hypothyroidism and is an indication for treatment with a synthetic thyroid hormone preparation. Abnormally low levels of TSH could indicate secondary hypothyroidism or hyperthyroidism (e.g., Graves' disease), and will require further testing that typically indicates the need for consultation with or referral to an endocrinology practitioner. Treatment of any of these potential thyroid conditions should contribute to alleviation of the oligomenorrhea state.

If the woman is not pregnant, the midwife should ask her about her overall health, nutritional and exercise status, use of medicines and herbs, and emotional state. Combining this exploration with a complete physical examination will enable the midwife to rule out most chronic illnesses, disordered eating patterns, obesity, physically demanding activities, medicinal/herbal side effects, and overall emotional stress as potential causes of the individual's decreased or scant menstrual flow.[1] Typically, resolving an underlying illness or condition will result in more regular menses and flow.

Once pregnancy, normal developmental changes, general ill health, and nutritional, physical, medicinal/herbal, and emotional problems have been ruled out, the next step is to measure levels of prolactin. Again, as with the assessment of amenorrhea, the midwife attempts to rule out hypothyroidism, hyperthyroidism, hyperprolactinemia, and galactorrhea, and seeks to implement those specific treatments that should contribute to the resumption of regular menstrual flow.

Menstrual Cycle Abnormalities and Galactorrhea

As addressed in the section discussing amenorrhea, galactorrhea may accompany cessation of menses and often is identified either on clinical examination by the woman or by an abnormal prolactin level. In assessing a woman's report of galactorrhea. the midwife must be vigilant to rule out pregnancy, breastfeeding, medication-induced lactation (e.g., owing to certain antipsychotic medications), and unilateral breast discharge due to breast cancer. The assessment may be accomplished by a careful history and breast examination.

Elevated prolactin levels are an indication of hyperprolactinemia, the causes of which are usually prolactinomas, secretory tumors of the pituitary. Hyperprolactinemia is generally an indication for referral to a practitioner who has expertise in evaluating endocrine abnormalities. Bromocriptine (Parlodel) or a dopamine agonist can be prescribed, resulting in more consistent ovulation and subsequent menses.

Conclusion

With any menstrual irregularity evaluation, the midwife must offer the woman knowledge and support throughout the process. Depending on her age and desired fertility, a number of potentially anxiety-provoking concerns need to be addressed, such as fears of infertility or cancer. Consistent communication between the midwife and the woman's other healthcare providers and/or specialists can do much to support her during the assessment and treatment phases of the disrupted menses work-up.

A variation in menstruation is a common concern for women and girls of all ages, and its assessment requires a sensitive and thorough approach. Exploring a woman's sense of reproductive or hormonal well-being or normalcy can often be achieved by taking a comprehensive history of the woman's menstrual pattern and examining her attitudes and beliefs about the significance of, and even need for, cyclic bleeding. Treatment of the woman with menstrual abnormalities may have an impact on a woman's long-term physical and mental health well beyond that appreciated by the woman herself. This aspect of women's health care calls upon midwives' expertise as primary and gynecologic care clinicians who are concerned with the entirety of women's health.

• • • References

1. Speroff L, Fritz MA. *Clinical Gynecologic Endocrinology and Infertility.* Philadelphia, PA: Lippincott Williams and Wilkins; 2011.

2. De Pergola G, Tartagni M, d'Angelo F, et al. Abdominal fat accumulation, and not insulin resistance, is associated to oligomenorrhea in non-hyperandrogenic overweight/obese women. *J Endocrinol Invest.* 2009; 32:98-101.

3. Yilmaz W, Kilic S, Kanat-Pektas M, et al. The relationship between obesity and fecundity. *J Women's Health.* 2009;18:633-636.

4. Himes JH, Park K, Styne D. Menarche and assessment of body mass index in adolescent girls. *J Pediatr.* 2009;155:393-397.

5. Schuiling K, Brucker MC. Pelvic and menstrual disorders. In: King TL, Brucker MC. *Pharmacology for Women's Health.* Sudbury, MA: Jones and Bartlett; 2011;916-949.

6. Cardigno P. Homeopathy for the treatment of menstrual irregularities: a case series. *Homeopathy.* 2009;98:97-106.

7. Yan H. Treatment of secondary amenorrhea with abdomen acupuncture. *J Trad Chin Med.* 2004;24(1): 42-43.

8. Tang T, Lord JM Norman RJ, et al. Insulin-sensitizing drugs (metformin, rosiglitazone, pioglitazone, D-chiro-inositol) for women with polycystic ovary syndrome, oligo amenorrhea and subfertility (review). *Cochrane Rev.* 2010;4:1-134.

9. Wang ET, Calderon-Margalit R, Cedars MI, et al. Polycystic ovary syndrome and risk for long-term diabetes and dyslipidemia. *Obstet Gynecol.* 2011;117: 6-13.

10. Klein S, Allison DB, Heymsfield SB, et al. Waist circumference and cardiometabolic risk: a consensus statement from Shaping America's Health: Association for Weight Management and Obesity Prevention; NAASO, the Obesity Society; the American Society for Nutrition; and the American Diabetes Association. *Obesity.* 2007;15(5):1061-1067.

11. Katsiki N, Georgiadou E, Hatzitolios AI. The role of insulin-sensitizing agents in the treatment of polycystic ovary syndrome. *Drugs.* 2009;69:1417-1431.

12. Legro RS, Barnhart HX, Schlaff WD, et al. Clomiphene, metformin, or both for infertility in the polycystic ovary syndrome. *N Engl J Med.* 2007;356:551-566.

13. Luppino FS, de Wit LM, Bouvy PF, et al. Overweight, obesity, and depression; a systematic review and meta-analysis of longitudinal studies. *Arch Gen Psychiatry.* 2010;67(3):220-229.

14. Berlan ED, Emans SJ. Managing polycystic ovary syndrome in adolescent patients. *J Pediatr Adolesc Gynecol.* 2009;22:137-140.

15. Kitzenger C, Willmott J. "The thief of womanhood": women's experience of polycystic ovarian syndrome. *Soc Sci Med.* 2002;54:349-361.

16. Bettendorf B, Shay S, Tu F. Dysmenorrhea: contemporary perspectives. *Obstet Gynecol Surv.* 2008;63: 597-603.

17. ACOG Practice Bulletin #110. Noncontraceptive uses of hormonal contraceptives. *Obstet Gynecol.* 2010;115:206-218.

18. U.S. medical eligibility criteria for contraceptive use, 2010: adapted from the World Health Organization medical eligibility criteria for contraceptive use, 4th edition. *MMWR*. 2010;59(RR04):1-6.

19. *Medical Eligibility Criteria for Contraceptive Use: 2008 Update*. Geneva, Switzerland: World Health Organization; 2008.

20. Zahradnick H, Hanjalic-Beck A, Groth K. Non-steroidal anti-inflammatory drugs and hormonal contraceptives for pain relief from dysmenorrhea: a review. *Contraception*. 2010;81:185-196.

21. Akin M, Price W, Rodriguez G, et al. Continuous, low-level, topical heat wrap therapy as compared to acetaminophen for primary dysmenorrhea. *J Reprod Med*. 2004;49:739-745.

22. Dennehy CE. The use of herbs and dietary supplements in gynecology: an evidence-based review. *J Midwifery Women's Health*. 2006;51(6):402-409.

23. Zhu X, Proctor M, Bensoussan A, et al. Chinese herbal medicine for primary dysmenorrhoea. *Cochrane Database System Rev*. 2008;2:CD005288. doi: 10.1002/14651858.CD005288.pub3.

24. Jia W, Wang X, Xu D, et al. Common traditional Chinese medicinal herbs for dysmenorrhea. *Phytother Res*. 2006;20:819-824.

25. Kennedy S, Jin X, Yu H. Randomized controlled trial assessing a traditional Chinese medicine remedy in the treatment of primary dysmenorrhea. *Fertil Steril*. 2006;86:762-764.

26. Han S, Hur M, Buckle J, et al. Effect of aromatherapy on symptoms of dysmenorrhea in college students: a randomized placebo-controlled clinical trial. *J Altern Complement Med*. 2006;12:535-541.

27. Ostad SN, Soodi M, Shariffzadeh M, et al. The effect of fennel essential oil on uterine contraction as a model for dysmenorrhea, pharmacology, and toxicology study. *J Ethnopharmacol*. 2001;76:299-304.

28. Cochrane update: exercise for dysmenorrhea. *Cochrane Database System Rev*. 2001;16:186-187.

29. Fraser IS, Critchely HOD. A process designed to lead to international agreement of terminologies and definitions used to describe abnormalities of menstrual bleeding. *Fertil Steril*. 2007;87:466-476.

30. Munro MG, Critchley HO, Broder MS, Fraser IS; FIGO Working Group on Menstrual Disorders. FIGO classification system (PALM-COEIN) for causes of abnormal uterine bleeding in nongravid women of reproductive age. *Int J Gynaecol Obstet*. 2011;113(1):3-13.

31. American College of Obstetricians and Gynecologists. Diagnosis of abnormal uterine bleeding in reproductive-aged women. Practice Bulletin No. 128. *Obstet Gynecol*. 2012;120:197-206.

32. American Academy of Pediatrics, Committee on Adolescence, American College of Obstetricians and Gynecologists, and Committee on Adolescent Health Care. Menstruation in girls and adolescents: using the menstrual cycle as a vital sign. *Pediatrics*. 2006;118:2245-2250.

33. James AH, Kouides PA, Abdul-Kadir R, et al. Von Willebrand disease and other bleeding disorders in women: consensus on diagnosis and management from an international expert panel. *Am J Obstet Gynecol*. 2009;201:12.e1-e8.

34. Goldstein SR. Modern evaluation of the endometrium. *Obstet Gynecol*. 2010;116:168-176.

35. Kaunitz AM, Meredith M, Inki P, et al. Levonorgestrel-releasing intrauterine system and endometrial ablation in heavy menstrual bleeding: a systematic review and meta-analysis. *Obstet Gynecol*. 2009;113:1104-1116.

36. Hohmann HL, Reeves MF, Chena BA, et al. Immediate versus delayed insertion of the levonorgestrel-releasing intrauterine device following dilation and evacuation: a randomized controlled trial. *Contraception*. 2012;85:240-245.

37. Barreirosa FA, Guazzellia CAF, Barbosab R, et al. Extended regimens of the contraceptive vaginal ring: evaluation of clinical aspects. *Contraception*. 2010;81:223-225.

38. Pillai M, O'Brien K, Hill E. The levonorgestrel intrauterine system (Mirena) for the treatment of menstrual problems in adolescents with medical disorders, or physical or learning disabilities. *Br J Obstet Gynecol*. 2010;117:216-221.

39. Adams K, Beal MW. Implanon: a review of the literature with recommendations for clinical management. *J Midwifery Women's Health*. 2009;54:142-149.

40. Zhang Y, Wang X. Fifty cases of dysfunctional uterine bleeding treated by puncturing the effective points: a new system of acupuncture. *J Trad Chin Med*. 1994;15:287-291.

41. Wang Z. Differential TCM treatment of anovulatory dysfunctional uterine bleeding. *J Trad Chin Med*. 1995;15(4):270-272.

42. Tiran D. *Aromatherapy in Midwifery Practice*. London: Bailliere Tindall; 1996.

43. Romm A. *Botanical Medicine for Women's Health*. Amsterdam: Elsevier; 2010.

44. Hatmaker D, Pinholster L, Saye J. A community-based approach to sexual assault. *Public Health Nurs*. 2002;19:124-127.

45. Hubacher D, Chen P, Park S. Side effects from the copper IUD: do they decrease over time? *Contraception*. 2009;79:356-362.

46. Poppe K, Velkeniers B, Glinoert D. Thyroid disease and female reproduction. *Clin Endocrinol*. 2009;66:309-321.

47. Westhoff CL, Heartwell S, Edwards S, et al. Oral contraceptive discontinuation: do side effects matter? *Am J Obstet Gynecol*. 2007;196:412.e1-412.e7.

12A

Endometrial Biopsy

WENDY GRUBE

WILLIAM F. MCCOOL

Endometrial biopsy (EMB) is a cost-effective, safe, and simple method of collecting a histologic sample of the uterine endometrium. A variety of clinical circumstances require investigation of the endometrium, especially among women who experience unusual vaginal bleeding as well as those undergoing analysis of infertility. The diagnostic dilatation and curettage (D & C) is no longer considered the "gold standard" for this purpose,[1] and the evolution of sampling devices has allowed EMB to be easily accomplished in an office setting by midwives.[2]

The sensitivity and specificity of EMB have been noted to be in the range of 95% to 100% for detection of endometrial carcinoma, but sensitivity for detection of other uterine pathology, such as polyps or submucosal fibroids, has been found to be relatively weak, at 28% to 44.6%.[3–5] This limitation is primarily due to the small surface area of the uterine lining (4.5% to 15%) that is capable of being sampled via EMB devices.[1] Combining transvaginal ultrasonography and sonohysterography with EMB can assist with the identification of such structural abnormalities. However, EMB remains an effective method of sampling the uterine endometrium for evidence of pathology.

Indications[1,2,6–9]

1. Identify endometrial cancer or its precursors.
2. Examine thickened endometrium (≥ 5 mm) noted on transvaginal ultrasound to rule out hyperplasia.
3. Evaluate abnormal or dysfunctional uterine bleeding.
4. Identify luteal-phase defects or other uterine pathology during infertility investigation.
5. Assist in evaluation of atypical glandular cells or endometrial cells found in cervical cytology sampling.
6. Assess the effect of hormone therapy or tamoxifen (Nolvadex) on the endometrium. (This indication is not considered necessary by some researchers and clinicians.)

Contraindications[2,6–9]

1. Pregnancy
2. Known or suspected cervical cancer
3. Infection of the vagina, cervix, or uterus (requires evaluation and treatment prior to procedure)

Precautions[2,6–9]

1. Blood dyscrasias, coagulation disorders, or the use of medications that may alter clotting (require consultation with a provider who is knowledgeable in hematological disorders)
2. History of prosthetic heart valve (requires cardiologist consultation, and probable antibiotic prophylaxis)
3. Fever (temperature > 38°C [100.4°F]) at the time of the procedure
4. Severe cervical stenosis or atypical uterine anatomy (requires consultation with or referral to a gynecologist)

Potential Side Effects/Complications and Preventive Measures[2,6–9]

1. Cramping, uterine spasm, and vasovagal response; can be prevented by

   a. Prophylactic analgesia with 600–800 mg ibuprofen (Advil) 60 minutes prior to the procedure

   b. Eating prior to the procedure, thus avoiding a hypoglycemic state

2. Uterine perforation; can be prevented by

   a. Making certain the woman is not pregnant or has a well-involuted postpartum uterus

   b. Performing a thorough pelvic exam prior to the procedure to note the uterine and cervical size, position, and angulation, as well as any structural abnormalities

   c. Use of a tenaculum to straighten the utero-cervical angle if unable to easily insert the device into the uterine cavity

3. Uterine infection, which can be prevented by identification and treatment of any existing genital infections

Procedure and Rationale

1. If the purpose of the sample is confirmation of ovulation/diagnosis of luteal-phase defects, schedule the procedure for day 22 or 23 of the menstrual cycle. Timing is not important if the sampling is to be performed to detect cancer or its precursors.

2. Gather equipment needed for the procedure:

   • Informed consent form
   • Nonsterile and sterile gloves
   • Vaginal speculum of appropriate size
   • Ring forceps and cotton balls or large cotton swabs
   • Antiseptic solution (such as Betadine or Hibiclens)
   • Topical anesthetic such as Benzocaine gel 20% (Hurricaine)
   • Scissors
   • Labeled specimen containers with 10% formalin
   • Endometrial sampling devices (make certain there are at least two available)
   • Tenaculum

3. Thoroughly review the health history, including the date of last menses, contraception and possibility of pregnancy, risk of sexually transmitted infection, known bleeding disorder, medication or supplement use, and allergies. Based on this information, contraindications may emerge that preclude performance of the procedure, or additional testing prior to the EMB may be necessary such as a pregnancy test, STI diagnostic testing, wet prep, or complete blood count.

4. Provide education and instruction regarding EMB. Because this is an invasive procedure, the midwife should spend time with the woman explaining what she should expect, facilitating an informed decision. An informed consent must be obtained before proceeding.

5. Offer an NSAID oral agent, as these agents decrease cramping and uterine spasm associated with the procedure.

6. Place the woman in a lithotomy position and, using nonsterile gloves, perform a bimanual and rectovaginal exam (if needed) to verify uterine and cervical position and structure in order to be able to place the curette in the appropriate direction and minimize the risk of uterine perforation.

7. Insert the appropriately sized speculum.

8. Apply antiseptic solution to the cervix with a large cotton swab or cotton ball.

9. If desired, apply topical anesthetic (e.g., Benzocaine gel 20%) to the anterior lip of the cervix and also into the os with a small cotton swab to lessen the pain associated with the curette or tenaculum.

10. Place a tenaculum on the anterior lip of the cervix, and gently pull the device to straighten the utero-cervical angle.

11. After changing to sterile gloves, remove the curette (the outer sheath and inner piston) from the sterile package as instructed on the package insert.

12. With the piston fully inserted into the sheath, gently introduce the curette through the cervical os and into the uterine cavity until resistance is felt (**Figure 12A-1**). (If strong resistance is encountered prior to reaching the fundus, stop the procedure.)

13. If there is difficulty advancing the device through the inner os while using steady, moderate pressure, small cervical dilators can be helpful. Another option is the use of a 3-mm osmotic laminaria, which can be placed in the cervix on the morning of the day of the EMB

and removed that afternoon prior to the actual procedure.

14. Once resistance is felt, note the distance the curette has entered the uterus, using the markings located on the sheath. On average, the length of the cervix from external to internal os is 2.5 cm, and the total distance from the external os to the wall of the fundus is approximately 6 to 9 cm.[10-12] This information can be recorded in any written note that follows the procedure.

15. With the tip of the device at the fundus, hold the curette securely and withdraw the inner piston as far as possible. Withdrawal of the piston creates the suction, or negative pressure, at the tip needed to collect the tissue sample.

16. Move the sheath of the device back and forth, with the tip moving from fundus to internal os, while simultaneously rolling it between the thumb and fingers to allow collection of cells from different levels of the endometrium as well as different locations. Avoid allowing the tip of the device to slip back out of the internal os into the cervical canal, as this will result in the loss of suction.

17. Complete the simultaneous moving and rolling of the sheath maneuver until the sheath is filled. Both tissue and some blood should be visible.

18. Remove the device. If only blood can be visibly identified within the sheath, after removing the entire curette, place the contents in formalin, and another curette can be used to

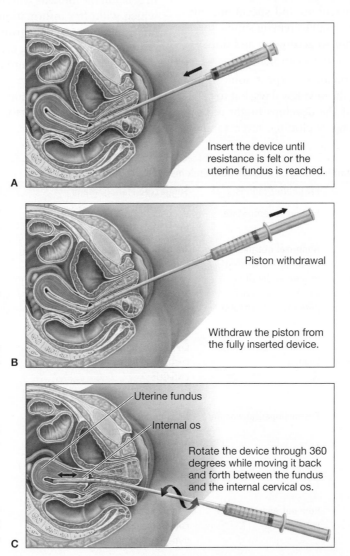

Figure 12A-1 Endometrial biopsy technique. (A) Insert the device until resistance is felt or the uterine fundus is reached (Step 12). (B) Withdraw the piston from the fully inserted device (Step 15). (C) Rotate the device through 360 degrees while moving it back and forth between the fundus and the internal cervical os.

attempt the procedure once or twice more depending on the woman's consent and how she tolerates the procedure.

19. Once the tissue has been adequately collected, cut the distal tip from the device and place the tip in the labeled formalin container. Cutting the tip from the device allows the sample to be removed intact, without causing the cell breakup that can occur when tissue is forced through the tip. Placing the tip of the catheter in the specimen container ensures that any tissue collected in this portion of the device will be analyzed with the remainder of the specimen.

20. Gently press the piston back into the sheath to expel the remaining specimen into the same labeled container.

21. Remove the tenaculum and speculum, but encourage the woman to remain supine for a few minutes prior to getting up and dressed to reduce the risk of a vasovagal response.

22. Instruct the woman to expect some light spotting during the next few days, but to contact the office if she develops bright red or excessive bleeding or clotting, fever, vaginal discharge with a foul odor, pelvic cramping, or pain. She should abstain from sexual intercourse for 2 to 3 days after the procedure.

23. Document the procedure, including any analgesic or anesthetic given, any abnormal findings during examination or procedure, the sampling device used, the depth of insertion of the curette, adequacy of the specimen obtained, and the woman's toleration of the procedure.

Results and Management

Laboratory findings can vary in language and presentation depending on the laboratory reporting system. In general, the midwife will receive a histology report, which will offer information that can contribute to making a diagnosis regarding the woman's uterine lining. In communicating the findings to the woman, the midwife should ensure that the woman understands the results and the possible courses of action to follow. The most common histologic reports received, with suggestions for follow-up, are listed in **Table 12A-1**.

Table 12A-1	**Common Histologic Findings from Endometrial Biopsy Samples**		
Histology	**Probable Diagnosis**	**Suggested Management**	**Need for Referral**
Inactive endometrium	Hypoestrogenic state	Dependent on clinical indication for EMB	Dependent upon specific clinical indication
Proliferative (estrogen influenced preovulation) or secretory (progesterone influenced postovulation)	Abnormal uterine bleeding—discussed in greater detail in the *Menstrual Cycle Abnormalities* chapter	Transvaginal ultrasonography (TVUS) to rule out structural pathology Hormonal therapy such as combined oral contraceptives, or cycling with progestins or the levonorgestrel intrauterine system (LNG-IUS)	Women with an abnormal TVUS or those who do not respond to hormonal therapies
Simple or complex nonatypical hyperplasia	Pre- or perimenopausal woman	Combined oral contraceptives or cycling with pro-gestins or the LNG-IUS Repeat EMB in 6 months	No response to hormonal therapy
	Postmenopausal woman	No therapy, or hormonal therapy depending on amount of bleeding, age, and time lapsed from menopause—discussed in more detail in the *Midlife, Menopause, and Beyond* chapter	Continued irregular bleeding, or no response to hormonal therapy
Atypical hyperplasia (simple or complex)—suspicion of cancer	Rule out endometrial carcinoma	Refer to specialist (e.g., collaborating physician or gynecologic oncologist)	Continued irregular bleeding, or no response to hormonal therapy

EMB = endometrial biopsy; TVUS = transvaginal ultrasound.

● ● ● References

1. Association of Professors of Gynecology and Obstetrics. *Clinical Management of Abnormal Uterine Bleeding.* APGO Educational Series on Women's Health Issues. Crofton, MD: APGO; May 2002.

2. American College of Nurse-Midwives. Endometrial biopsy. Clinical Bulletin No. 5. *J Midwifery Women's Health.* 2001;46:321-326.

3. Apgar BS, Newkirk GR. Office procedures: endometrial biopsy. *Primary Care.* 1997;24:303-326.

4. Van den Bosch T, Vandendael A, Van Schoubroeck D, et al. Combining vaginal ultrasonography and office endometrial sampling in the diagnosis of endometrial disease in post-menopausal women. Available at: www.gyncph.suite.dk/procedur/ref/gyn/p ust2 v~1.htm. Accessed December 16, 2002.

5. van Hoeven KH, Zanian SS, Deger RB, Artymyshyn RL. Efficacy of the Endo-pap sampler in detecting endometrial lesions. *Acta Cytologica.* 1996;40:900-906.

6. Endometrial biopsy. *Family Practice Notebook.com.* Available at: http://aroundrtp.com/GYN129.html. Accessed December 11, 2002.

7. Mayeaux EJ. Performing an endometrial aspiration biopsy (EMB). Louisiana State University Health Sciences Center Family Medicine. Available at: http://lib-sh.lsumc.edu/fammed/atlases/emb/emb.htnil. Accessed December 11, 2002.

8. Schnare S. *Endometrial biopsy (EMB).* Paper presented at the Contraceptive Technology Conference; Washington, DC; March 2001.

9. Zuber T. Endometrial biopsy. *Am Earn Phys.* March 15, 2001. Available at: www.aafp.org/afp/20010315/1131.html. Accessed December 11, 2002.

10. Moore KL, Dalley A. *Clinically Oriented Anatomy,* 4th ed. Philadelphia, PA: Lippincott Williams and Wilkins; 1999.

11. Hasson H. Clinical studies of the Wing Sound II metrology device. In: Zatuchni G, Goldsmith A, Sciarra J, eds. *Intrauterine Contraception: Advances and Future Prospects.* Philadelphia, PA: Harper and Row; 1985:126-141.

12. Hasson H. Differential uterine measurements recorded in vivo. *Obstet Gynecol.* 1974;43:400-412.

● ● ● Bibliography

Ash SJ, Farrell SA, Flowerdew G. Endometrial biopsy in DUB. *J Reprod Med.* 1996;41:892-896.

Mihm LM, Quick V, Brumfield J, et al. The accuracy of endometrial biopsy and saline sono-hysterography in the determination of the cause of abnormal uterine bleeding. *Am J Obstet Gynecol.* 2002;186:858-860.

National Cancer Institute. Screening for endometrial cancer, (n.d.). Available at: www.nci.nih.gov/cancerinfo/pdq/ screening/endometrial/healthprofessional. Accessed December 11, 2002.

O'Connell LP, Fries MH, Zeringue E, Brehm W. Triage of abnormal postmenopausal bleeding: a comparison of endometrial biopsy and transvaginal sonohysterography versus fractional curettage with hysteroscopy. *Am J Obstet Gynecol.* 1998;178:956-961.

Weber AM, Belinson JL, Bradley LD, Piedmonte MR. Vaginal ultrasonography versus endometrial biopsy in women with post-menopausal bleeding. *Am J Obstet Gynecol.* 1977;177:924-929.

CHAPTER

13

Gynecologic Disorders

WILLIAM F. MCCOOL

DAWN C. DURAIN

Introduction

The American College of Nurse-Midwives (ACNM) has a motto, "With women, for a lifetime™," that speaks simply to the scope of midwifery care. While the name "midwife" conjures up images of pregnancy care and attendance at birth, for centuries midwives have been called upon to assist women in healthcare matters that have extended beyond childbearing. Historically, midwives have helped women with menarche, menstruation, and menopause. This ancient role has expanded further with healthcare practices for the health needs of women of all ages in the twenty-first century.

The average number of children born to women in the United States over a lifetime today is 2.1.[1] Yet, many women never experience pregnancy or birth at all. In a national survey of women in the United States between the ages of 15 and 44 years, 43% reported being childless, either by choice or due to infertility conditions.[1] Therefore, most women spend most of their lives in a state where gynecologic health plays a large role in their well-being, a fact recognized by most midwives in practice. Recent surveys of certified nurse-midwives (CNMs) and certified midwives (CMs) have reported that more than half of those midwives in clinical practice offer gynecologic care, and a third offer primary care.[2] As noted by the ACNM "Midwifery as practiced by certified nurse-midwives (CNMs) and certified midwives (CMs) encompasses a full range of primary health care services for women from adolescence beyond menopause. These services include primary care, gynecologic and family planning services, [and] preconception care."[3]

Gynecology textbooks are thick with diagnoses ranging from difficulties with the brain to malformations of the genitalia. Fortunately, most of these conditions are rare and better left with specialists who focus on caring for individuals with rare maladies. For most women, and for the practitioners who work with them, the majority of gynecologic health concerns are limited to a few general categories. This chapter focuses on some of the more common diagnoses found in gynecologic care, as well as knowledge needed for screening women for gynecologic cancers. Other matters of adult women's health, including gynecology and primary care, are addressed in other chapters of this text.

Abdominal and Pelvic Pain

Overview

Reports of abdominal and pelvic pain account for a significant number of visits from women for gynecologic care. Entire volumes are dedicated to the evaluation and treatment of pelvic pain, and interested midwives will find many opportunities to read more on this topic. This section addresses the most relevant issues in the evaluation of pelvic pain and the most common causes of the pain.

Chronic pain often is an underlying reason for a woman to seek care from a midwife. This pain may have a significant impact on a woman's quality of life, producing fatigue, tension, or depression, yet she may be reluctant to discuss it for a variety of reasons. Perhaps previous providers may have overtly or inadvertently discounted her pain, or perhaps the woman is uncomfortable discussing her pain completely. Pelvic pain often triggers many emotions centered on the individual's sense of self as a woman, her ability to conceive and bear children, or her feelings pertaining to her sexuality.

On other occasions, a woman may present with abdominal or pelvic pain after having been seen by one or more other practitioners who have reached the limits of their skills and have recommended a gynecologic consult. This woman, and perhaps her family members as well, may be angry and frustrated, and have ever-mounting concerns regarding the source of the woman's pain and what she (they) may see as a lack of an easy treatment.

Acute abdominal or pelvic pain also commonly presents as a problem visit in the office or on the phone. Careful screening must accompany the evaluation of acute pain to ensure appropriate management. If the situation is not an obvious emergency, one or more visits often are needed for this assessment. The current emphasis in some practices is on short, focused visits that are seemingly incompatible with a high-quality, comprehensive approach to a problem; however, as with the assessment of many ambulatory problems, the midwife must be able to adapt the visit structure and time to allow for flexibility in the appropriation of office time and resources.

The most comprehensive and efficient manner in which to assess pelvic pain is to take a biopsychosocial approach, which assesses the physical, psychological, and sociocultural realities of the person experiencing the pain.[4] To establish a trusting, mutually satisfying clinical relationship, the midwife must validate the woman's experience and communicate a commitment to a comprehensive exploration of the problem as it is perceived by the woman. The midwife also should explain that the cause may be elusive and not lend itself to a simple explanation or solution. It is useful to share that relief may result from dietary changes, activity changes, or a variety of other approaches to the woman's life and lifestyle, and does not necessarily depend on a particular medical or surgical intervention.[5]

The often unspoken knowledge that each woman holds as her own reference point for "normal"—her own social, cultural, or religious influences on her sense of self as a woman and her unique perception of the various aspects of reproductive function—should be recognized. A woman's personal beliefs with regard to what is or is not normal will have an inevitable impact on her interpretation of her menstrual cycle, vaginal secretions, and emotional response to any perceived variation in function related to the pain or discomfort.

Historically, many women were told that their gynecology-based problems were "all in your head."[6] Conversely, some women might react negatively to the notion that an emotional issue could contribute to physical distress. The midwife often can overtly reinforce the notion that the body and the mind are interrelated, and that comprehensively addressing a problem often necessitates a multifaceted approach. For example, some mind-body therapies such as mindfulness training have been shown to be effective in helping individuals manage chronic pain.

Types of Abdominal/Pelvic Pain

Acute Pain

The ability to safely care for individuals experiencing an emergency such as acute pain necessitates the establishment of a preexisting relationship with surgical and nongynecologic referral systems and providers. It is often the case that for women of childbearing age, an ectopic pregnancy or other serious gynecologic problem must be ruled out before the woman receives care from other medical or surgical providers. Other possible causes of acute pain that necessitate prompt diagnosis include appendicitis, pelvic inflammatory disease (PID), and ovarian torsion.

In an emergency situation, the midwife may need to enlist support services to address a lack of health insurance, childcare needs, or other issues. If a diagnosis of pregnancy has been made, the midwife must consider issues of confidentiality.

Chronic Pain

The woman with chronic pelvic pain may have had a long series of encounters with healthcare providers. Both she and the significant others in her life may have found their contacts with providers less than satisfying or may be seeking care from several different providers in hopes of receiving a diagnosis or treatment. The inability of the woman's system of care to meet her perceived needs can lead to inappropriate or overuse of healthcare resources, including diagnostics and treatment interventions.[7] It is crucial to be clear about her motivations for this visit and her expectations for midwifery involvement in her care. The woman's history of her previous care is just as important as the history of her pain. Conversely, she may have chronic pain that has never been fully articulated or fully explored with a care provider.

Evaluation of Pelvic Pain

The collection of data in the evaluation of pain must be particularly thorough to reach an accurate conclusion. A helpful tool in the evaluation of any complaint, including pain, is the "OLD CARTS" acronym (**Table 13-1**).[8] The "OLD CARTS" system is useful to start several lines of inquiry. All of the information described in Table 13-1 should be obtained.

Several instruments are available for use in the evaluation of chronic pain.[9] Should the midwife be in a practice where caring for women with chronic pain is common, the use of such questionnaires is advisable. Many women will answer these questionnaires in detail and provide a wealth of information; however, other women who have not considered their pain in a comprehensive manner may need to return for a future visit with a pain diary or history. Finally,

it is always important to ask perhaps the most obvious question: What does the woman think the cause of the pain is?

History

A thorough history, including menstrual cycle characteristics and sexual activities, includes the woman's assessment of how her pain has affected her quality of life. She may have adapted many of her daily activities, including her work, school, athletics, and sexual activities, in response to her pain. If her pain has affected her quality of life or her relationships, it may also have negative effects on her emotional well-being. In the case of long-standing pain, evaluation and treatment by a mental health professional to complement the evaluation and care being offered by the midwife is recommended.

If further screening or diagnostic studies or referral for treatment is indicated, it is useful to determine whether the woman's ability to obtain further care is influenced by her socioeconomic or health insurance status. A midwife should be familiar with the payment options and eligibility criteria of institutions available

Table 13-1	"OLD CARTS" Acronym for Obtaining a History of Reported Pain
Desired Information	**Questions to Be Asked**
Onset	When did the pain begin? Can the individual identify a particular event or point in time related to the initial recognition of the pain?
Location/radiation	Specifically identify the location of the pain. Does the pain move or radiate or have a different quality in varying locations?
Duration	Is the pain cyclic or noncyclic? Is it related to other health factors (e.g., bowel function, physical activity, sexual activity, menstrual cycle)? Is the onset of the pain related to diet or diet changes? Is it related to work activities? Is it related to the individual's emotional state of being or to the onset of emotional stress?
Character	Ask the individual to describe the pain. Offer a wide variety of descriptors used for pain, such as sharp/dull, gnawing, burning, and achy.
Aggravating/**a**ssociated factors	What makes the pain worse (e.g., exercise, diet, constipation, diarrhea, urination, physical activity, sexual activity, menses)?
Relieving factors	What relieves the pain (e.g., rest, diet change, bowel movement,), and to what degree? Which treatments have been used to help alleviate the pain? Were they recommended by other providers or suggested by a family member, friend, book, or website? Were medications used (over-the-counter and/or prescription)? Were any alternative treatment modalities used? What was the success or failure of any treatments that were used?
Temporal/timing factors	How often is the pain occurring? Was there a single incident, or is the pain intermittent or chronic in nature? Have the symptoms improved or worsened over time? Is there a specific time of day when the pain is felt more often?
Severity of symptoms	How severe is the pain on a scale of 0 to 10, with 10 being the worse pain the woman can imagine? Has the pain had an effect on the individual's lifestyle? On her ability to work?

Source: Adapted from Seidel H, Ball J, Dains J, et al. *Mosby's Guide to Physical Examination.* 7th ed. St. Louis, MO: Mosby Elsevier; 2010.

for referral and laboratories, such as the availability of a sliding payment scale based on income. Additionally, low-income women may be eligible for free or low-cost gynecologic cancer screening or treatment via federal, state, or private-sponsored programs.

General Physical Examination

Examination of a woman presenting with abdominal or pelvic pain may require a complete exam or may be narrowly focused, depending on the level of previous care and the acuity of the pain. Immediate consultation/referral is indicated for the woman with acute pain, especially when such pain is accompanied by fever, tachycardia, significant change in blood pressure, signs of shock, vomiting, or evidence of significant blood loss. Diagnoses of ectopic pregnancy, appendicitis, bowel obstruction, sepsis, and ovarian torsion all require immediate physician consultation and referral for care.

In the absence of an acute presentation, a complete examination can be performed. The woman's demeanor and presentation should be included in the evaluation. Is she relaxed or tense in her stance or posture? Is her stance or posture asymmetrical, indicating guarding of an area or long-term discomfort? Evaluation of the back and lower extremities is often useful to rule out a musculoskeletal injury, such as a muscle strain or stress fracture, or an anatomic variation, such as scoliosis.

Abdominal Examination

A standard abdominal exam should be performed. The goal in palpation is to note organ enlargement or displacement, identify masses or enlarged lymph nodes, and determine whether the pain can be reproduced. It is often useful to first ask the woman if she herself can reproduce the pain. If not, proceed with care and attention to the unaffected side or area first. Communicating findings and letting the woman know which part of the examination is next can help maintain an atmosphere of trust and caring. Special attention should be paid to any area of tension or guarding, and knowledge of patterns of referred pain points is useful.

Pelvic Examination

The ability to perform a thorough examination can be facilitated by an environment of trust, although inordinate discomfort can limit the ability of the midwife to obtain needed information.

At the time of visual inspection of the vulva and vagina, the midwife should check for any signs of swelling, lesions, trauma, or other skin changes. The woman's tolerance of the insertion of a vaginal speculum is an important observation, especially if she reports pain with sexual activity. After insertion of the speculum, a sample of any discharge for a wet prep examination and subsequent sexually transmitted infection (STI) testing is indicated. Visual inspection of the cervix may reveal a protruding intrauterine device (IUD), color change indicative of pregnancy, cervicitis, or the presence of a polyp or other mass.

After the speculum has been withdrawn, a slow bimanual examination allows the midwife to observe whether the woman exhibits discomfort at the introitus versus deep in the vagina. Any cervical, adnexal, or uterine motion tenderness elicited may provide more information. Organ dislocation or the inability to completely palpate the uterus or adnexa, which indicates dislocation, is another important finding. Palpation for any masses, uterine fibroids (myomata), or uterine or adnexal enlargement indicative of pregnancy is the next step, with muscle tone and the presence of any cystocele or rectocele or of uterine prolapse to be assessed. Confirmation of findings can be accomplished with a rectal exam as well as assessment for constipation, polyps, or masses. A fecal occult blood test (FOBT) may aid in the management of any abdominal mass. Any woman with a positive FOBT should be referred to a specialist for an examination and possible colonoscopy or sigmoidoscopy.

Findings should be shared with the woman and as many of her fears allayed as possible. Descriptions of a mass or enlarged organ should include the size, shape, location, consistency, mobility, and relation of the mass to other organs. Additionally, if pain is elicited, the intensity and location of the pain should be described.

Laboratory/Screening/Diagnostic Tests

It is important to perform only those tests for which the results will directly inform management plans. A pregnancy test is indicated if there is any suspicion of pregnancy, missed menses, or other unexplained vaginal bleeding in a woman who is heterosexually active and of childbearing potential. A complete blood count (CBC) is often ordered as a standard test; however, in the absence of an infectious process or concerns related to anemia, a CBC may not be particularly useful. If concerns exist that the cause of the pain is urologic in nature, a urinalysis or urine culture may be useful. Tests for STIs or a wet prep for vaginitis may be useful if these diagnoses are suggested by history and examination.

A pelvic or abdominal ultrasound is a common test to aid in the diagnosis of uterine or adnexal abnormalities. If an ultrasound is ordered, a vaginal probe will most likely be recommended as part of the examination. For women who have never had vaginal penetration, or who have cultural prohibitions with regard to pelvic procedures, this part of the test may be distressing. Anticipatory guidance for this portion of the examination includes an explanation of its purpose. If the midwife will not personally perform the ultrasound, a note should be placed on the order form stating that this is an initial pelvic ultrasound for the individual to alert the ultrasound staff that additional patience and time should be afforded this woman.

Consultation and referral for further evaluation by a specialist are indicated upon diagnosis of a condition requiring treatment or management beyond the midwife's scope of practice. In such circumstances, the woman should be provided with as much information as possible about what to expect and a report of the woman's care by the consultant physician be sent to the midwife.

If the evaluation does not reveal the cause of the woman's pain, a variety of plans may be made. If the woman wishes to continue investigation of her pain with the midwife, a more detailed "history" of her pain should be suggested. Assessment modalities might include anatomic drawings used to locate her pain, the use of a pain diary with a pain severity scale, or the use of a journal to chart her pain in relation to her daily activities, menstrual cycle, bowel habits, sexual activity, and diet.

If all abnormal processes are definitively ruled out, the midwife may review normal anatomy and physical sensations related to gynecologic and menstrual function, including the wide range of normal variations. Education and support may provide the woman with a new perspective on her relationship to her "gynecologic self."

Referrals to specialists may be appropriate, including mental health specialists, if it is felt that an exploration of the woman's psychological well-being might be useful. Many support groups exist for women who experience a variety of conditions, such as endometriosis, as well as for those women who have been abused or sexually traumatized (see the "Additional References" section for a list of support groups and websites related to abdominal and pelvic pain).

Causes of Acute Abdominal/Pelvic Pain

Ectopic Pregnancy

Ectopic pregnancy is any pregnancy implanted outside the endometrial cavity. In the past, ectopic pregnancies were considered to be emergency situations that necessitated surgical intervention and loss of the affected fallopian tube. While still considered an emergency, an ectopic pregnancy currently may be treated using a medical approach (e.g., methotrexate [Rheumatrex; Trexall]), and in the event of surgical intervention, efforts often are made to preserve the integrity of the fallopian tube. Regardless of the therapeutic regimen chosen, ectopic pregnancy must be viewed as a life-threatening condition.

The woman with an ectopic pregnancy may report an absence of her normal menses followed by intermittent, light bleeding. This bleeding often is accompanied by cramp-like abdominal or pelvic pain, which can be unilateral or diffuse, and may be described as mild or severe in nature.[10] Any combination of these symptoms must trigger an evaluation for an ectopic pregnancy when a woman has a risk of pregnancy, even it it seems to be remote. Additionally, women who present with any of these symptoms plus shoulder pain (referred pain that occurs secondary to the presence of blood in the abdominal cavity), fever, tachycardia, or low blood pressure must be evaluated for shock and emergency referral even in the absence of overt vaginal bleeding. Adnexal enlargement or tenderness on pelvic examination, a pregnancy test, and ultrasound will likely confirm the diagnosis of ectopic pregnancy.

Sharing the diagnosis of an ectopic pregnancy with the woman must be done in a manner that conveys the serious nature of the problem and the need for referral to a provider capable of a potential surgical intervention. The woman with an ectopic pregnancy may have not suspected a pregnancy at this time and might need to integrate a great deal of information at a very stressful moment.

Appendicitis

Appendicitis is another common abdominal emergency. The classic symptoms of this condition—right lower quadrant pain accompanied by a fever and an elevated white blood count (WBC)—are not always present, however. Appendicitis may present with left lower quadrant pain, fever may or may not be present, and changes in the WBC do not always initially occur. Other presentations of appendicitis include right-sided pain, bilateral pain, nausea, vomiting, diarrhea, constipation, referred shoulder pain, fever, and a loss of appetite.[11] The management of appendicitis includes surgery and inpatient observation, or possibly outpatient observation.

Ovarian Torsion

An uncommon cause of acute pelvic pain is ovarian torsion, also referred to as adnexal torsion.[12] While causes of torsion include previous adnexal surgical manipulation, especially tubal ligation, an adnexal structural anomaly, and pregnancy, as many as 95% of cases are related to ovarian enlargement caused by either an ovarian cyst or neoplasm.[13] The woman may present with point-specific pain or with more generalized unilateral pelvic or flank pain, as well as nausea and vomiting. This diagnosis may be confused with gastrointestinal disorders.

The treatment for ovarian torsion is surgery during which the ovary is repositioned and fixed in place or removed depending on the etiology, if evident, and any presence of tissue damage or necrosis. It is not uncommon to make a false-positive diagnosis of ovarian torsion at surgery, with the pain actually being due to endometriosis, ovarian enlargement without torsion, or unknown causes not readily apparent.[13]

Additional Causal Considerations

Acute/abdominal pain also can be a manifestation of any of several gynecologic, gastrointestinal, urologic, and circulatory conditions. These potential etiologies include ovarian mass, pelvic inflammatory disease, bowel obstruction, gastroenteritis, irritable bowel syndrome (IBS), hernia, pyelonephritis, urinary tract infection (UTI), and abdominal aortic aneurysm.[11] Often, referral to the nearest emergency department is the best course of action for individuals with severe acute abdominal pain.

Causes of Chronic Abdominal/Pelvic Pain

Urologic Conditions

Urinary tract infections can present as acutely painful conditions or as more chronic lower abdominal pain that occurs either alone or in concert with the common symptoms of dysuria, urinary frequency, hematuria, and changes in the appearance or odor of the urine. Either type of infection can present with increasingly intense pain, fever, and a feeling of malaise. Women with pyelonephritis may also have back or flank pain and tenderness at the costovertebral angle.

Pelvic Inflammatory Disease/Salpingitis

Women with pelvic inflammatory disease can present with either acute or chronic pelvic pain. Diagnosis and management of women with PID is discussed in the *Reproductive Tract and Sexually Transmitted Infections* chapter.

Interstitial Cystitis

Interstitial cystitis (IC) is a chronic urinary irritation that manifests as a chronic pain or achiness in a woman's pelvic region.[14] Sometimes referred to as "painful bladder syndrome," its etiology remains theoretical. It is postulated that the bladder lining may be permeable to unusual toxins and irritants, which results in inflammation and symptoms of IC.[14] The affected woman may experience urinary frequency, urgency, nocturia (urination more than two to three times in a night), and relief upon emptying her bladder. Dysuria, although not always present, can be a symptom of IC. Because these symptoms are the same ones that arise with urinary tract infections, many women are treated initially with a variety of medications with little or no relief. Women with a frequent history of UTIs or unsuccessfully treated UTIs may benefit from an evaluation for IC. The urine cultures of individuals with IC usually are negative, with the exception of the presence of small to numerous white blood cells. The physical examination of a woman with IC is not particularly remarkable, although in some cases she may have pain in the pelvic floor. The diagnosis of IC essentially is one of exclusion.

Spicy foods, alcohol, stress, or sexual activity may aggravate the IC symptoms. Vaginal penetrative sexual activity may be so painful as to render this activity impossible for some women. Because the cause of IC has not yet been identified successfully, a wide variety of pharmacologic and surgical treatments have been used for this condition, with varying degrees of success. Some women with IC experience relief from a change in diet, bladder training exercises, or long-term pain medication; others do not. The most commonly discussed pharmaceutical treatment is pentosan polysulfate sodium (PPS; Elmiron); however, the success achieved with this approach has been limited at best. Intravesical and surgical treatments can be useful for some women but not others, and the greatest relief appears to be achieved with the use of multiple-modality treatments.[14] If a midwife suspects the woman she is seeing has IC, referral to a practitioner with expertise in treating IC is indicated.

Dyspareunia and Vulvar Pain

The woman with vulvar pain or pain associated with sexual activity may have difficulty articulating her discomfort due to embarrassment, a lack of anatomic information, or reluctance to discuss sexual activity.[15] The use of anatomic drawings can be helpful in obtaining an accurate history of her pain. A frank discussion of her sexual activities and habits is important, including the use of douches, tampons and pads, sex toys, lubricants, moisturizers, condoms, and contraceptives.

Fear of pain, as well as pain during sexual activity, can produce a distressing cycle of sexual frustration and tension in relationships. The woman's partner may be present during a visit intended to discuss dyspareunia, and it is important to first clarify the woman's desire to have her sexual partner present. Common causes of tension resulting in painful or difficult sexual activity include a fear of pregnancy, a history of assault or sexual trauma, a history of infertility, a lack of trust in the contraceptive method used, a latex allergy if latex condoms are used, and a lack of vaginal lubrication, hormonal status, medications, sexual arousal, or lack of partner patience. A disinterest in sex or an interest that does not match that of the woman's partner may also be present.

Potential physical causes of vulvar pain, irrespective of pain during sexual activity, include herpes simplex virus (HSV) lesions; vaginal tears as a result of trauma, vaginal scarring, history of urogenital surgery, or childbirth; vaginitis; Skene's or Bartholin's gland infections; and vulvodynia. An inquiry into, and appropriate follow-up of, the source of the trauma is required. A referral to a practitioner specializing in treatment of women with dyspareunia and vulvar pain or a gynecologic surgeon may be required.

Vulvodynia

Vulvodynia has been defined by the International Society for the Study of Vulvovaginal Disease as "vulvar discomfort, most often described as burning pain, occurring in the absence of relevant visible findings or a specific, clinically identifiable, neurologic disorder."[16] The cause of vulvodynia is not yet well understood, and consequently the expectations for treatment must be realistic. Practitioners may distinguish between two types of vulvodynia: (1) vulvar vestibulitis syndrome, or "provoked vulvodynia," which means that the discomfort is the result of some form of physical contact (e.g., intercourse, tampon use, clothing, bicycle riding) and is generally limited to the vestibule of the vulva; and (2) dysesthetic vulvodynia, or "unprovoked vulvodynia," which entails discomfort more diffuse than just the vestibule and not necessarily of a tactile nature, although touch can worsen the pain.[17,18] The presentation of vulvodynia may include vulvar symptoms that are chronic and unrelenting, or those that are cyclic in nature. The diagnosis of this condition can be difficult, although various algorithms have been written to facilitate ruling out other conditions (**Figure 13-1**).[19]

The evaluation for vulvodynia starts with obtaining a comprehensive history of the onset and duration of symptoms; aggravating activities; sexual activities; use of topical preparations; a history of vaginitis or other STIs; use of contraceptives consisting of latex, including condoms, diaphragms, and cervical caps;

use of feminine "hygiene" products, such as tampons or menstrual pads/panty liners; and any treatments attempted to date. A woman experiencing vulvar pain frequently has tried numerous over-the-counter treatments, including antifungal medications and topical steroid preparations. These treatments in themselves may have caused a dermatitis that must be minimized before further evaluation can occur.[20]

Examination of the vulva includes evaluation of skin changes, vaginal secretions, presence of lesions, and changes in the vulvar architecture.[17] It is useful to perform an evaluation of point-specific pain and sensitivity by using a cotton swab and gently proceeding in a clockwise fashion on the vulva. Particular areas of sensitivity may be noted, especially at the 11 to 1 o'clock points and the 5 to 7 o'clock points (**Figure 13-2**).[13,21]

Dermatologic conditions such as lichens sclerosus, lichens planus, and lichen simplex are treated with topical steroids.[22] Relief measures include avoidance of potential irritants by using white unscented toilet tissue, loose cotton clothing, unscented soaps, and showers instead of baths, as well as avoiding the use of feminine hygiene products, bath additives, baby/personal wipes, over-the-counter anti-itch products, detergent additives, fabric softeners, dryer sheets, and latex products.[22] Antidepressants—either tricyclic antidepressants (TCAs), selective serotonin reuptake inhibitors (SSRIs), or serotonin and noradrenalin reuptake inhibitors (SNRIs)—also have been used in the treatment of this condition, and appear to have some value in the relief of pelvic neuropathies.[21]

A variety of alternative or complementary therapies have been used for the treatment of vulvodynia with some success. These treatments include biofeedback, pelvic floor exercises, cognitive-behavioral therapy (CBT), acupuncture, hypnotherapy, and physical therapy.[19,21,23]

When all or most of the aforementioned modalities prove unsuccessful in relieving the pain, specialists who care for women with these discomforts may recommend surgery. Such procedures can include efforts to excise nerve pathways or nerve injuries associated with specific locations of pain; a vestibulectomy, which is a complete resection of the vestibule; or perineoplasty, which involves resection of the vestibule and perineum.[18]

Endometriosis

Endometriosis is the presence of endometrial tissue outside of the uterine cavity. It has proved difficult to gauge the prevalence of this condition, but endometriosis is believed to affect 6% to 10% of all

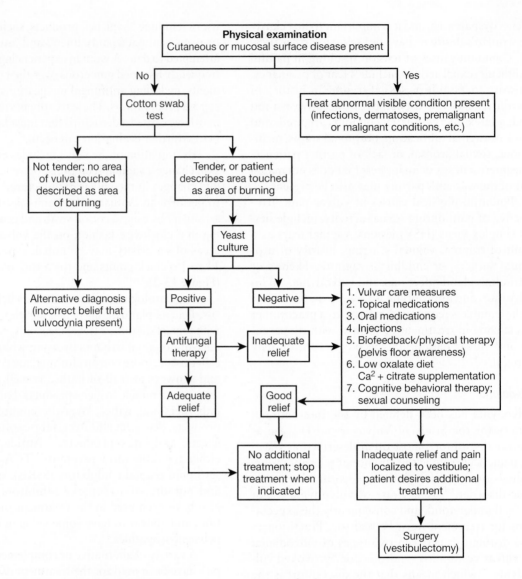

Figure 13-1 Algorithm for the diagnosis of vulvodynia.
Source: J. Schorge, et al., *Williams Gynecology,* 2008, p. 98 (Fig. 4.10). Reproduced with permission of The McGraw-Hill Companies, Inc.

childbearing-age women.[24] Among women with pelvic pain, 40% to 50% have been found to have endometriosis. The degree of symptoms can range from none to major pelvic pain or infertility. The presence of endometriosis is rare before menarche and after menopause, and this condition is less commonly found in women who experienced late menarche. Although the mean age at diagnosis is between 25 and 35 years, as many as two-thirds of women with endometriosis have stated that their symptoms initially appeared during adolescence.[25]

Endometriosis is typically classified as one of four stages depending on its location(s), depth of the endometrial implants, extent, presence of adhesions, and presence of ovarian endometriomas: stage I is minimal; stage II is mild; stage III, which is characterized

by the presence of adhesions, is termed moderate; and stage IV, which is associated with infertility, is termed severe. However, the severity of symptoms does not correlate with the stage.

The cause of endometriosis remains elusive, and multiple etiologic theories have been proposed.[24] Retrograde menstruation followed by extrauterine implantation remains the oldest and most commonly supported theory for explaining this condition. Findings during laparoscopy have revealed that during menses the endometrial tissue migrates into the peritoneal cavity via the fallopian tubes, attaching itself to the pelvic organs.[24] However, this theory does not explain all of the cases of endometriosis that have been documented. Other theories are listed in **Table 13-2.**[24]

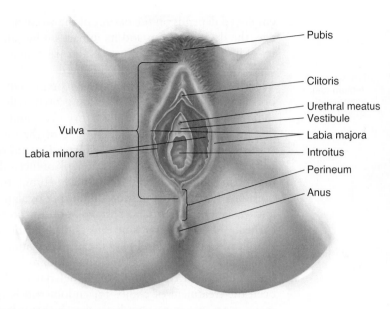

Pubis

Clitoris

Urethral meatus

Vestibule

Labia majora

Introitus

Perineum

Anus

Vulva

Labia minora

• Apply gentle pressure with cotton swab to sites surrounding the introitus (1 o'clock thru 12 o'clock positions). Ask patient to rate the severity of pain she experiences at each site.

• Pain is typically most severe in the anterior vestibule (between 11 and 1 o'clock positions) and the posterior vestibule (between 5 and 7 o'clock positions).

Figure 13-2 Cotton swab test for specific location of vulvodynia.
Source: Godena-Stone T. Vulvar pain syndromes: vestibulodynia. *J Midwifery Women's Health.* 2006;51:502-509. Reprinted with permission of Wiley.

The presentation of endometriosis can include a number of symptoms, the most common of which are pelvic pain (particularly dysmenorrhea), dyspareunia, and infertility. However, because endometrial tissue can be found in or around at least 12 extrauterine sites (**Figure 13-3**), symptoms can also include lower back pain, menorrhagia, irregular menses, pain between menstrual cycles, dysuria, constipation or diarrhea, postcoital bleeding, lower abdominal pain associated with ovarian cysts, and chronic fatigue.

Conversely, surgeons may discover incidental findings of endometriosis in a significant number of asymptomatic women during the course of pelvic surgery or procedure.

Pelvic or lower abdominal pain due to endometriosis may be related to the menstrual cycle, typically appearing at ovulation or intermittently from ovulation to menses. This pain may continue throughout the menses. Endometriosis pain may also occur in patterns unrelated to the menstrual cycle.

Table 13-2	Proposed Etiologies of Endometriosis
Proposed Etiology	**Rationale**
Retrograde menstruation	During menses, endometrial tissue migrates into the peritoneal cavity via the fallopian tubes, attaching itself to pelvic organs.
Deviations in cellular physiology	Peritoneal tissue can spontaneously transform into endometrial tissue.
Deviations in the lymphatic system	Endometrial tissue is transported to other organs via the lymphatic pathways.
Deviations in the immune system	Menstrual tissue found outside the uterus is normally cleared by the immune system, which appears unable to do so in women found to have endometriosis.
Deviations in the hormonal system	Unlike intrauterine endometrial tissue, the estrogenic effects of extrauterine endometrial tissue are unaffected by the antagonistic action of progesterone.
Genetics	A 6 to 7 times increased incidence is found among first-degree relatives of affected women (i.e., mothers or siblings) compared to the incidence in the general population.
Environmental influences	Dioxin-like compounds discovered in industrial waste by-products can alter gene development or estrogen–progesterone balance in a manner that leads to extrauterine development of endometrial tissue.

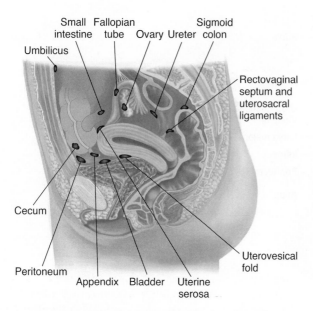

Umbilicus

Small intestine | Fallopian tube | Ovary | Ureter | Sigmoid colon

Rectovaginal septum and uterosacral ligaments

Cecum

Peritoneum | Appendix | Bladder | Uterine serosa

Uterovesical fold

Figure 13-3 Possible locations of the presence of extrauterine endometrial tissue.

Pain during or after coitus may be so severe as to preclude sexual activities. Endometriosis can confound a diagnosis of appendicitis or ectopic pregnancy, as acute onset of severe, unilateral, pelvic pain is a classic symptom of these conditions as well.

Physical examination findings may be normal, with no significant tenderness associated with organ palpation or movement. In other women, significant cervical motion tenderness, bilateral or unilateral adnexal tenderness, tender nodules on the uterosacral ligaments, ovarian enlargement, or a fixed, retroverted uterus may be noted. Definitive diagnosis requires visualization during surgery. Biopsies typically are taken to confirm the diagnosis and assist in future treatment. The use of imaging modalities such as magnetic resonance imaging (MRI) and transvaginal ultrasonography (TVU) may provide diagnostic information when the woman has advanced endometriosis; however, these imaging techniques are not helpful is discovering small or early lesions associated with this condition.

The treatments for endometriosis have had variable success. Treatments may include pain relief measures such as the use of nonsteroidal anti-inflammatory drugs (NSAIDs), medications that suppress hormonal stimulation of the endometrial tissue such as combined or progestin-only hormonal contraceptives, surgical removal of the lesions, a combination of medical and surgical means, or complete surgical removal of endometriotic tissue, including hysterectomy and oophorectomy.[26–30] The treatment

employed depends on the desires of the woman, her age, the degree of pain and its impact on her quality of life, her desire for future childbearing, and the degree to which her fertility is impaired.

Medical treatment for endometriosis centers on the premise that pain and lesion growth will be diminished by altering the ovulatory cycle and inducing a hypoestrogenic state.[25] One of the more traditionally pharmaceutical approaches entails use of danazol (Danocrine). Danazol reduces the luteinizing hormone (LH) and follicle-stimulating hormone (FSH) surge that occurs during ovulation and at higher doses produces anovulation and amenorrhea. The androgenic side effects of danazol are significant, however, and may include deepening of the voice, weight gain, and lowering of high-density lipoprotein (HDL) cholesterol. Although danazol has been the treatment of choice for endometriosis for many years, recent reviews have shown that it is no more or less effective than other, newer pharmacologic approaches.[28]

Various progestins and antiprogestins have also been employed, such as depot medroxyprogesterone acetate (DMPA; Depo-Provera), and mifepristone (Mifeprex). Common side effects of these medications include irregular vaginal bleeding.

Combination oral contraceptives (COCs) are other options for treatment of endometriosis as well.[27] If adequate relief is not obtained with routine COC use, a continuous regimen (i.e., omitting the use of any hormone-free pills in the COC pack and taking the hormone-containing pills continuously) may be employed to produce amenorrhea.

Gonadotropin-releasing hormone (GnRH) agonists may be used to reduce ovarian stimulation and produce a low estrogen hormonal state similar to menopause.[31] Side effects of GnRH agonists include hot flashes, irregular vaginal bleeding, vaginal dryness, decreased libido, breast tenderness, depression, and sleep disturbances. Additionally, the GnRH agonists may have an adverse effect on bone mineral density. This side effect is sometimes treated by the use of hormonal "add-back" therapy, which comprises the concurrent use of an estrogen and/or progestin with the GnRH. Norethindrone acetate (Aygestin), COCs, a levonorgestrel-based intrauterine device (Mirena), or DMPA are typical "add-back" approaches.[31]

The goals of surgical treatment for endometriosis may include the attempt to restore normal reproductive function in addition to the reduction of pain by removing the lesions. Medical and surgical treatments are commonly combined when treating women experiencing infertility, although there is limited evidence regarding the effectiveness of this approach.[32] Definitive surgical treatment, consisting of the removal of the uterus and, depending on the age of the woman, her ovaries as well—is the management option of last resort.

Some evidence exists that auricular (ear) acupuncture has been effective in reducing pain associated with endometriosis.[33] However, current recommendations for women with endometriosis published by major Western medicine professional societies advocate beginning with NSAIDs and hormonal therapy, while recognizing that no single drug has proved more effective than any other.[34] The choice of which regimen to follow must include a discussion with the woman of the potential side effects and the costs associated with individual drugs. Although laparoscopic surgery remains the most definitive mechanism for diagnosing endometriosis, surgery itself is viewed as a last resort for actually treating most cases of this condition.

Pelvic Masses

Fibroids

Fibroids, also known as leiomyomas or fibromyomas, are benign tumors that develop from uterine smooth muscle. They are the most common type of gynecologic masses among women. Estimations of occurrence range from 20% to 40% in women reporting symptoms, while sonographic or postmortem examinations have increased the estimate to 70% to 80% of the female population.[12, 35] Fibroids are also known to have a higher prevalence in some racial and ethnic groups, such as among African American women.[35,36] Estrogen and progesterone promote fibroid growth. Thus these benign tumors may grow in size during pregnancy, and they tend to degenerate after menopause. Fibroids can usually be visualized on ultrasound.[36]

Fibroids are described based on their location. *Subserous fibroids* exist just under the uterine serosa and are located outside of the uterus. They are attached to the uterus by a large or small base, stalk, or peduncle. This type of fibroid usually is palpated on abdominal exam (**Figure 13-4**). *Intramural fibroids* are located within the uterine myometrium and may give the uterus an irregular contour. *Submucosal fibroids* are located in the uterine endometrium and are usually palpable only as an enlarged uterus.

On bimanual examination, the fibroid will be firm and the uterus will be irregular in shape. Upon noting a fibroid during an examination, the midwife should share this information with the woman and discuss any appropriate follow-up or pertinent information.

Fibroids usually are asymptomatic. Women with large, bulky fibroids may grow accustomed to feelings of pelvic fullness and report few symptoms or little pain. Other women may have chronic pelvic

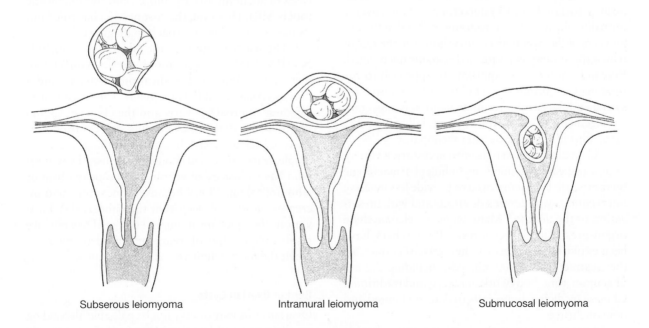

Subserous leiomyoma   Intramural leiomyoma   Submucosal leiomyoma

Figure 13-4 Classification of fbroids (leiomyomas) by location in relation to the uterus.

pain, lower abdominal "pressure," or abnormal uterine bleeding. Fibroids can cause urinary frequency, rectal pressure, or interference with sexual activity. Depending on their location, they may also interfere with pregnancy and can cause infertility, spontaneous abortion, premature labor, malpresentation of a fetus during pregnancy or labor, or abnormal labor progress.[36] Fibroids may also be implicated in abnormal uterine bleeding, especially in the perimenopausal phase of a woman's life. This bleeding can be significant enough to cause anemia.

Large fibroids may cause pain during pregnancy. Although the etiology of such masses is not well understood, it appears that their rapid growth results in torsion or degeneration secondary to insufficient blood supply. Treatment of pain from degenerating fibroids during pregnancy depends on the gestational age and severity of pain. Midwives may collaborate in the care of women who are experiencing fibroid pain in pregnancy following consultation and determination of a treatment plan.

Fibroids in women without physical symptoms may be observed indefinitely. For asymptomatic women, a careful documentation of fibroid size and shape at each annual examination, along with a thorough history of any change in symptoms, is an acceptable management plan.

Hysterectomy remains the most common non-pregnancy-related surgical procedure for women in the United States, with the rate of this surgery being 5.4 per 1000 women of 15 years of age or older in the United States.[37] Fibroids are the most common diagnosis associated with hysterectomy.[38] Controversy regarding the use of hysterectomy surfaced in the latter years of the twentieth century; however, the rate at which the surgery is performed remains unchanged. Research on the most appropriate approach to the treatment of fibroids has yet to provide definitive answers, and the current recommendation is expectant management for most women, especially given that many fibroids degenerate after menopause.[12,35,36]

When intervention is deemed necessary, a variety of nonsurgical procedures, including pharmacologic therapies, are being employed to provide less invasive interventions with fewer side effects and with preservation of the uterus.[36] Many women welcome these organ-preserving procedures.[35] Researchers have been exploring a variety of alternative therapies for the treatment of uterine fibroids, including the use of acupuncture, bodywork, imagery, and traditional Chinese medicine, but results to date are limited and nonconclusive.[39]

Pharmacologic methods of treating fibroids include the traditional use of GnRH agonists (e.g., leuprolide acetate [Lupron]), as well as the levonorgestrel-based IUD (Mirena). Success rates in diminishing the size or symptoms of fibroids vary considerably with these methods. While the most success has been obtained with the use of GnRH agonists, significant side effects preclude their use by many women.[12] However, if surgical intervention is deemed appropriate, a GnRH agonist may be used to shrink the masses prior to myomectomy. A reduction in size prior to surgery may provide the physician the option of a vaginal versus an abdominal surgery.[40]

Adenomyosis

Unlike fibroids, which are made up of uterine smooth muscle, adenomyosis results from the growth of endometrial tissue in the myometrium layer of the uterus, typically causing uterine enlargement. Two forms of adenomyosis have been identified: (1) diffuse adenomyosis, in which endometrial tissue is found throughout the myometrium, and (2) focal, in which one or more nodular lesions, known as adenomyomas, are located in specific locations of the uterine myometrium.[12,35,41]

The incidence of adenomyomas ranges anywhere from 5% to 70%.[12,42,43] While many women with this condition are asymptomatic, one-third of individuals report menorrhagia, dysmenorrhea, and, at times, dyspareunia. In general, women with adenomyosis have borne children, and they typically develop the condition in their fourth or fifth decade of life.[12,41] While ultrasound can be helpful in diagnosing many cases of adenomyosis, the more definitive diagnostic tool is MRI. However, the cost of MRI has ruled out its use as a first-line approach to diagnosis.[12,42,43]

The usual treatments for adenomyosis include NSAIDs, COCs, progestin-only agents, GnRH agonists, tranexamic acid medication (Lysteda), and a progesterone-based IUD (Mirena). The success rates for these approaches vary, and the clinician should be familiar with the risks, benefits, and contraindications of each approach before prescribing it. For example, tranexamic acid should not be used by women who have a history of venous thromboembolism or who are taking COCs because tranexamic acid increases the risk of deep vein thrombosis (DVT). If various therapies are attempted but yield few positive results, the last line of treatment for adenomyosis—albeit the most definitive—is hysterectomy.[12,41]

Benign Ovarian Cysts

Ovarian cysts may or may not be palpable, depending on their size and location. Due to their commonly asymptomatic nature, most ovarian cysts are found incidentally after an ultrasound examination that was performed for some other reason. Except for dermoid cysts or large cysts causing acute pain, most ovarian cysts do not require intervention and may be managed via careful monitoring for changes in size or in the individual's perception of pain or discomfort. It is vital to reassure women that most ovarian cysts are not associated with malignancy and that watchful waiting is preferable to the risks of surgery.

Large ovarian cysts can cause adnexal motion tenderness or pelvic pain and may grow to such a size that they cause ovarian torsion. The differential diagnosis of the pelvic pain in women with these types of cysts can be difficult, as adnexal motion tenderness is nondiagnostic and can result from PID, ectopic pregnancy, endometriosis, or adhesions from prior surgical procedures.

Follicular Cysts

If a normal ovarian follicle does not rupture or an immature follicle does not undergo normal atresia, a functional ovarian cyst known as a "follicular cyst" may form. Follicular cysts—the most common type of ovarian masses—are generally asymptomatic and require no specific treatment unless the woman notes symptomatic changes. The most common management approach is to reassess the cyst periodically with ultrasound to confirm that it is not growing or to document regression. Historically, oral contraceptives have been used as a method of hastening resolution of follicular cysts; however, a review of the available evidence has shown no value to the use of COCs for treatment of ovarian cysts.[44] If the cyst increases in size, further evaluation must be made to rule out an ovarian neoplasm or other mass.

Corpus Luteum Cysts

A corpus luteum cyst develops following hemorrhage of the corpus luteum, most often during days 20–26 of the menstrual cycle. Ultrasound may confirm the diagnosis. In the absence of a large amount of continued bleeding, no intervention is necessary, as the cyst will regress spontaneously. In the event of significant bleeding or acute pain secondary to the bleeding, a negative pregnancy test may assist in differentiating the ruptured corpus luteum cyst from an ectopic pregnancy. If bleeding continues, surgical intervention may become necessary.

Dermoid/Cystic Teratomas

Dermoid cysts or cystic teratomas are asymptomatic, unilateral ovarian cysts that arise from all three germ cell layers (ectoderm, endoderm, and mesoderm) and,

therefore, may contain skin, bone, hair, and teeth. Dermoid cysts are generally found on pelvic examination and diagnosed via ultrasound. Such cysts do not regress and have a small chance of becoming malignant; therefore, the recommended treatment is surgical removal.[12] At the time of surgery, a thorough examination of the ovary, surrounding tissues, and the other ovary for any signs of abnormality or cancer is indicated.

Polycystic Ovary Syndrome

Ovarian enlargement can be a sign of polycystic ovary syndrome (PCOS), which is discussed in more detail in the *Common Menstrual Cycle Abnormalities* chapter.

Congenital Uterine Anomalies

Congenital uterine anomalies, also referred to as Müllerian anomalies, are present in as many as 7% of the female population.[45–47] These variations are often undiagnosed until a woman presents for evaluation due to infertility, recurrent miscarriages, pelvic pain, difficulty with vaginal penetrative sexual activity, or ectopic pregnancy.[45,46] The diagnosis may be made by pelvic examination, by ultrasound, or during a surgical procedure.

In the embryo, the two Müllerian ducts differentiate to form the uterus, cervix, superior portion of the vaginal, and fallopian tubes. Abnormal development can result in a wide range of anatomic malformations. The current classification of congenital uterine anomalies follows a system first proposed by the American Fertility Society (**Table 13-3**).[48]

The American Society for Reproductive Medicine's classification of congenital uterine anomalies includes those changes due to the use of diethylstilbestrol (DES), a nonsteroidal estrogen that was widely used from 1948 to 1971 in an effort to prevent a number of complications of pregnancy. Initially prescribed as a treatment for threatened spontaneous/recurrent abortions, DES came to be used extensively for this purpose, despite evidence that it was not effective. It has been estimated that several million pregnant women received the drug.[49] In 1971, the Food and Drug Administration withdrew its approval for DES, as reports began to appear of younger women with clear-cell adenocarcinoma who had been exposed to DES in utero. Since that time, a number of structural and functional abnormalities have been identified as effects of in utero exposure to DES, including changes to the uterus,

Table 13-3	Classification of Congenital Uterine Anomalies	
	Description	**Figure**
Class I Hypoplasia/Agenesis		
I-A	Vaginal agenesis or hypoplasia. Uterus may be normal or have malformations.	
I-B	Cervical agenesis or hypoplasia.	
I-C	Fundal agenesis or hypoplasia.	
I-D	Fallopian tube agenesis or hypoplasia.	
I-E	Combined agenesis or hypoplasia.	
Class II Unicornuate		
II-A	Communicating unicornuate: rudimentary horn with an endometrial cavity that communicates with the single-horned uterus. The chances of infertility, endometriosis, and dysmenorrhea are increased with this anatomic condition.	
II-B	Noncommunicating: rudimentary horn with an endometrial cavity that does not communicate with the single-horned uterus.	
II-C	Rudimentary horn with no endometrial cavity.	
II-D	No rudimentary horn.	

Table 13-3	Classification of Congenital Uterine Anomalies *(continued)*	
	Description	**Figure**
Class III Didelphus		
III	Two separate cavities, each with its own cervix.	
Class IV Bicornuate Uterus		
IV-A	IV-A: complete bicornuate uterus has two separate uterine cavities separated by myometrial tissue and one cervix. It is estimated that 60% of women with a bicornuate uterus can maintain a pregnancy, although prior reconstructive surgery may be required to do so, and the risks of a spontaneous abortion or a preterm delivery are higher than those in women without this anatomic condition.	
IV-B	Partial bicornuate uterus: the septum is confined to the fundus.	
Class V Septate Uterus		
V-A	Complete septate: The septum extends into the internal cervical os. The septate uterus has two cavities separated by avascular tissue and one cervix. While individuals with a septate uterus can become pregnant, the outcome is often a spontaneous abortion or a fetus with growth malformations.	
V-B	Partial septate: The septum does not reach the internal os.	
Class VI Arcuate Uterus		
VI	The uterine fundus is concave instead of convex or straight. It is considered to be a mild deviation from a normal anatomic uterus, and may have no impact on the ability to conceive, although second-trimester spontaneous abortions and preterm labor are possible.	
Class VII DES-Related Anomalies		
VII-A	T-shaped uterus.	
VII-B	T-shaped uterus with dilated horns.	
VII-C	Uterine hypoplasia.	

Source: Adapted from American Fertility Society. The American Fertility Society classifications of adnexal adhesions, distal tubal occlusion, tubal occlusion secondary to tubal ligation, tubal pregnancies, Müllerian anomalies and intrauterine adhesions. *Fertil Steril.* 1988;49:944-955.

vagina, and cervix. Reproductive health risks to the daughters of women who took DES include infertility, ectopic pregnancy, spontaneous abortion, and premature delivery. In addition, these women are at greater risk for cervical and uterine carcinomas at ages of 30 years or younger, and of breast cancer after the age of 40 years.[50]

Suggestions have been made that the offspring of women who were exposed to DES in utero might themselves suffer consequences of their grandmothers taking the drug. To date, data on the outcomes of granddaughters of women who took DES are inconclusive.[51]

The contraceptive choices of a woman with any anomalous uterus may be somewhat complicated. If the woman does not desire to become pregnant, the most effective choices might involve hormonal methods or condoms as opposed to other female-based barrier methods or an IUD.

Concerns related to fertility and childbearing may be uppermost in the mind of the woman of childbearing age and must be addressed promptly. Regardless of her age or childbearing plans, information pertaining to an organ anomaly, especially one so closely associated with one's "womanhood," may have a significant emotional impact. Continued support and referral to any local resources or national organizations with web-based information are essential for the midwife offering care. Selected resources are listed in the additional references for this chapter.

Pelvic Floor Conditions

Urinary incontinence and pelvic organ prolapse can occur secondary to a number of anatomic or physiologic conditions. Risk factors include pregnancy (regardless of the mode of birth), older age, family history, obesity, smoking, constipation, a history of heavy lifting, prior lower abdominal or pelvic surgeries, a lower abdominal or pelvic mass, a history of chronic lung disease, and a history of a connective tissue disorder (e.g., Marfan syndrome).[52,53] The two most common findings related to pelvic floor changes are pelvic organ prolapse and urinary incontinence.

Pelvic Organ Prolapse

Approximately 50% of parous women suffer from some degree of pelvic organ prolapse, and 40% of all women between the ages of 45 and 85 years experience this condition.[54] Due to pelvic floor relaxation, a *cystocele* (bladder descent into the vagina), *rectocele*

(protrusion of the rectum into the vagina), or *uterine prolapse* (descent of the uterus into the vagina) may occur. Each of these conditions, or a combination of them, can cause abnormal bladder or rectal function, pelvic or lower back pain, and decreased pleasure with sexual activity.[53,55]

The extent to which pelvic organ prolapse occurs is concordant with three described levels of vaginal support:

- Level I, involving the proximal area of the vagina
- Level II, referring to support in the middle region of the vagina
- Level III, describing the vaginal ligaments and muscles that connect the distal area of the vagina to adjacent tissues and muscles

Lax support at Level I can lead to apical prolapse of organs, such as the small bowel, into the vaginal wall. A relaxed vaginal wall at Level II potentially leads to anterior and/or lateral prolapse of organs, such as the bladder. A woman lacking in Level III vaginal support will typically present with both anterior and posterior prolapse of organs into the vagina, which are usually visible at the introitus.[53]

Evaluation of pelvic floor disorders includes obtaining a comprehensive history and visualizing the women's external genitalia, vagina, and cervix for any signs of urinary leakage or organ displacement/prolapse. Asking the woman to perform a Valsalva maneuver or cough allows the midwife to visually assess the level of vaginal wall support. Uterine prolapse may also be observed with the woman in an upright position, as the cervix may protrude through the vulva simply by the pull of gravity in severe cases. The visual examination is followed by a speculum examination that can offer additional visual signs of the nature and degree of any prolapse.[53] A follow-up bimanual examination, during which the woman is asked to tighten her vaginal muscles around the fingers of the clinician, will allow the midwife to gauge the strength of the woman's pelvic muscles, and presents the opportunity to teach the woman the correct manner in which to perform muscle-tightening exercises. In addition, a variety of short survey instruments are freely available to help clinicians determine the nature and extent of the condition, including the Pelvic Floor Impact Questionnaire and the Pelvic Floor Distress Inventory.[56,57]

In the absence of pelvic masses, treatment for pelvic floor relaxation may include the initiation of pelvic floor muscle training (PFMT), more commonly known as Kegel exercises. While evidence suggests that PFMT alone can improve pelvic organ prolapse, many women require specific instruction and feedback during a vaginal examination to learn how to perform PFMT correctly, and referral of the individual to a physiotherapist specializing in PFMT may be warranted.[58] Additional therapies that have proved useful to varying degrees include the use of vaginal cones during PFMT, biofeedback, and vaginal electrical stimulation.[52,59]

A variety of support devices or pessaries can be employed in the case of significant uterine prolapse.[53,60] In general, midwives can fit either of two types of pessaries: those that offer support (e.g., ring pessary) and those that fill space in the vagina (e.g., cube pessary) (**Figure 13-5**). The former are suited for the women with Level I or II vaginal support, while the latter are designed for individuals with Level II or III support. After the initial exam and placement of the pessary, the woman often returns for a follow-up visit in 1 to 2 weeks to assess comfort and normal urinary function. The woman then returns in 3 to 6 months, and semi-annually thereafter, to assess proper use and effectiveness of the pessary. The woman with a pessary in place in her vagina must be visually inspected at least annually, if not every 6 months, to assess for any lesions or bleeding due to tissue erosion from the pessary. The pessary should be removed and cleaned weekly with soap and warm water. A woman with a pessary in place should be cautioned to report any vaginal bleeding promptly, as this may be a sign of tissue damage or may be intrauterine bleeding indicative of the growth of a malignancy.

Several surgical procedures have been used in attempts to repair or restore lost muscle tone associated with pelvic organ prolapse. The long-term success rates of different surgical approaches vary, however, and such procedures may result in complications such as urinary incontinence.[60]

Urinary Incontinence

Urinary incontinence (UI) is underreported for a variety of reasons, including embarrassment, denial, and the prevailing notion that the only treatment option is surgical.[51] This phenomenon of underreporting has made it difficult to identify how many women experience UI, but reviews of investigations of UI estimate that between 25% and 45% of adult women experience UI at some point in their lives, with occurrence increasing with age.[61] This condition is often associated with significant diminishment of a woman's quality of life. The results of UI include impaired sleep, limitations on the ability to travel far from home or have social engagements, and inability

to maintain good hygiene and avoid skin irritation or breakdown. In general, the role of the midwife in assessing and treating urinary incontinence is most often accomplished in consultation with other midwives or colleagues who specialize in this area of urogynecologic care.

The causes of UI are varied and require a detailed history and thorough work-up by a primary care provider, urologist, or urogynecologist. Incontinence may be temporary if it is the result of a side effect of a pharmaceutical agent, change in mental status, change in mobility, or constipation. Structural and functional abnormalities such as a small bladder capacity; an unexpected contraction of the detrusor (bladder) muscle during the filling of the bladder, known as idiopathic detrusor overactivity; or a urethral abnormality (e.g., urethral diverticulum) can also cause UI. In addition, obesity has been shown to contribute to UI.[62] Certain disease states have the effect of increased urination and incontinence, such as diabetes, a urinary tract infection or other renal disease, a bladder mass, or pelvic masses such as fibroids or ovarian cancer. Neuropathies may result in a variety of incontinent presentations. Surgery, childbirth, and pelvic trauma may also result in some degree of involuntary loss of urine.[52,63] However, having a vaginal delivery does not appear to increase the chances of experiencing UI when compared to experiencing a cesarean section birth. There may be a familial disposition that increases the risk of UI even if the woman has never been pregnant.[64]

The types of urinary incontinence are defined based on their presenting symptoms and signs (**Table 13-4**). It is not uncommon for stress incontinence to occur with detrusor overactivity, which is defined as involuntary bladder contractions during the filling phase of the bladder. A less common type of incontinence is urge incontinence, which can be due to a variety of neuropathies. The combination of stress and urge incontinence is termed mixed urinary incontinence.[65]

When a report of incontinence is made, a detailed history and physical examination are performed, including assessment of the woman's voiding habits, pattern of incontinence, and intake of fluids is needed. Several clinical assessment tools are also available to aid making a diagnosis of urinary incontinence (**Table 13-5**).[66]

In the absence of a urinary tract infection, a pelvic mass, or some other extrinsic cause of incontinence, the diagnosis of incontinence is made using a combination of the woman's history and a variety of urinary function tests. Urinary function tests can range from the simple—such as the "cough stress

SPACE-OCCUPYING
PESSARIES

SUPPORT
PESSARIES

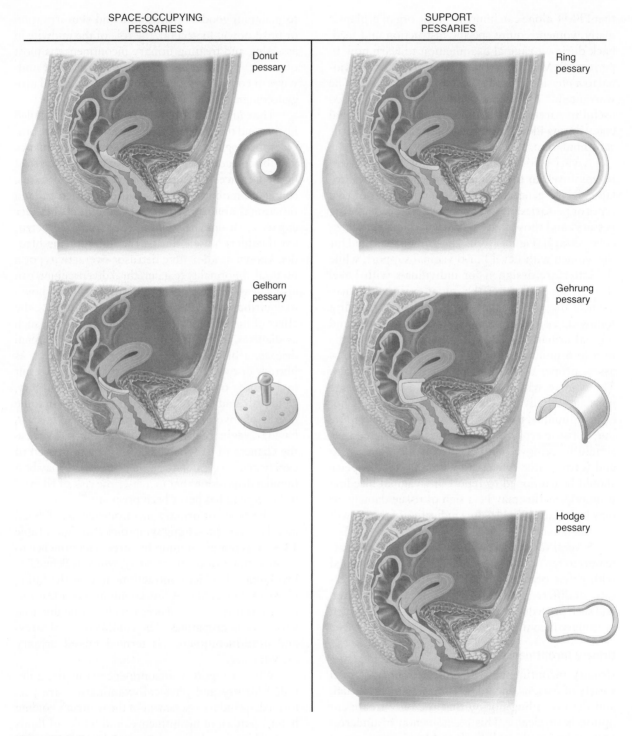

Donut
pessary

Gelhorn
pessary

Ring
pessary

Gehrung
pessary

Hodge
pessary

Figure 13-5 Types of pessaries.

test," which can be performed in the office by asking the woman to cough with a full bladder and subsequently observing for leaking from the urethra—to the complex—such as urodynamic testing, which involves the use of equipment that can evaluate urethral function, bladder capacity, bladder stability, and the ability of the individual to control voiding. The latter form of assessment can be expensive and is usually reserved as a second line of testing, typically performed in the office of a urologist or urogynecologist.[67]

Reassurance that having to void once or twice during the night is not necessarily indicative of urinary dysfunction, or that an occasional episode of "leaking urine" does not meet the criteria for

Table 13-4 Types of Urinary Incontinence

Type of Incontinence	Definition
Stress urinary incontinence	Involuntary leakage caused by effort or exertion (e.g., sneezing or coughing)
Urgency urinary incontinence	Urge to urinate comes suddenly, associated with involuntary leakage
Mixed urinary incontinence	Involuntary leakage associated with both urgency and stress incontinence
Nocturnal enuresis	Involuntary leakage occurring during sleep
Continuous urinary leakage	Continuous leakage of urine
Idiopathic detrusor overactivity	Involuntary bladder contractions during the filling phase of the bladder, with no clear cause
Neurogenic detrusor overactivity	Involuntary bladder contractions during the filling phase of the bladder, due to a defined neurologic condition
Urodynamic stress incontinence	Involuntary leakage associated with increased abdominal pressure
Overflow incontinence	Frequent or constant dribbling or stress incontinence, typically caused by underactive detrusor muscle or outlet obstruction; urinary retention can also occur secondary to drug therapy

Table 13-5 Questionnaire for Urinary Incontinence Diagnosis (QUID)

Question	None of the Time (score 0)	Rarely (score 1)	Once in a While (score 2)	Often (score 3)	Most of the Time (score 4)	All of the Time (score 5)
Do you leak urine (even small drops), wet yourself, or wet your pads or undergarments...						
1. When you cough or sneeze?	❑	❑	❑	❑	❑	❑
2. When you bend down or lift something up?	❑	❑	❑	❑	❑	❑
3. When you walk quickly, jog, or exercise?	❑	❑	❑	❑	❑	❑
4. While you are undressing to use the toilet?	❑	❑	❑	❑	❑	❑
5. Do you get such a strong and uncomfortable need to urinate that you leak urine (even small drops) or wet yourself before reaching the toilet?	❑	❑	❑	❑	❑	❑
6. Do you have to rush to the bathroom because you get a sudden, strong need to urinate?	❑	❑	❑	❑	❑	❑

For scoring purposes, each item's responses range from 0 to 5 points.

Items 1, 2, and 3 contribute to the stress score; a diagnosis of stress incontinence is made if the woman's total score for items 1, 2, and 3 ≥ 4.

Items 4, 5, and 6 contribute to the urge score; a diagnosis of urge incontinence is made if the woman's total score for items 4, 5, and 6 ≥ 6.

Women are diagnosed with both stress and urge urinary incontinence if the stress score ≥ 4 and the urge score ≥ 6.

Source: Reprinted with permission from Bradley C, Rovner E, Morgan M, et al. A new questionnaire for urinary incontinence diagnosis in women: development and testing. *Am J Obstet Gynecol.* 2005;192:66-73.

incontinence treatment, can help the woman. She may, however, benefit from an evaluation of her fluid intake and voiding frequency.

The treatment for urinary incontinence depends on the type and degree of incontinence identified. For women with stress incontinence, initial treatment includes pelvic floor muscle exercises, behavioral modifications, and dietary changes. Some clinicians advocate use of Knack exercises, which are similar to Kegel exercises but focus more on strengthening urethral muscles. Knack exercises involve contracting the pelvic muscles as deep into the vagina as possible and holding the contraction while doing other activities during which the woman usually experiences incontinence, such as coughing or exercising in general.

The successful use of PFMT can be enhanced using provider *feedback* (giving the woman instructions while performing a bimanual examination) or *biofeedback* (using a vaginal insertion device that offers feedback on the success of the woman's attempt at the exercises).[61] Similarly, the promotion of healthy weight can help to reduce incontinence related to obesity.[62]

Pharmaceutical treatments for women with stress incontinence are unavailable in the United States. Some success has been reported with the off-label use of duloxetine hydrochloride (Cymbalta), a selective serotonin and norepinephrine reuptake inhibitor (SSNRI) that is used to treat depression,[67] and of pseudoephedrine (e.g., Sudafed), but either the side effects of these medications or their ineffectiveness in treating individuals with moderate to severe conditions often outweigh their efficacy in stemming urinary incontinence.

If an individual is assessed as having urgency or detrusor overactivity incontinence, bladder training can be promoted. This involves either encouraging the woman to delay any initial urges she has to void by using the Knack technique and by distracting herself with mental exercises, or teaching her to empty her bladder before an urge occurs. Medications used to treat detrusor overactivity are listed in **Table 13-6** and the least expensive are oral generic forms.

Several anticholinergic drugs have been approved in the United States to treat women with urge incontinence, all of which have demonstrated some effectiveness.[68] Oxybutynin has been available for the longest time, but the newer regimens are noted as producing fewer side effects, especially dry mouth (Table 13-6).

Estrogen use for urinary incontinence was once thought to be a promising therapy, especially for postmenopausal women. While some evidence indicates that vaginal application of estrogen can improve incontinence, systemic use of this hormone has been shown to worsen symptoms. In the face of the evidence linking long-term estrogen use to the development of endometrial and breast cancer, this pharmaceutical approach is limited in its application.[52]

Mechanical devices for control of urinary incontinence have been prescribed with varying success. These interventions include vaginal cones and pessaries. However, their use has not been shown to make a significant difference in bladder control in population studies,[69] and should be limited to individual customization.

The last-resort approach to treatment of urinary incontinence usually is surgery, which is limited to treatment of stress incontinence and is not applicable to urge incontinence. A variety of procedures, both through the abdominal wall and the vaginal wall, have been employed to correct anatomic defects or dysfunctions resulting in incontinence, with varying degrees of success. It appears that abdominal approaches are more successful than vaginal procedures.[70] although both techniques are associated with the risk of adhesion formations and a potentially greater loss of urinary function. However, for women who have not achieved relief with nonsurgical approaches to stress incontinence, surgery may be the most effective method for alleviating their condition. It should be noted that the injection of bulking agents, including collagen-based agents and Botox, around the urethra is another approach that appears to offer short-term relief, but its effects diminish over time.[71]

Special Considerations in Providing Gynecologic Care

For care of women with any gynecologic condition, several key factors can influence her health, as well as the follow-up care required. These special conditions include age, culture, fertility status, sexual well-being, and past history of sexual abuse.

Age

Children

Children experiencing gynecologic problems, including pelvic pain, present a unique challenge. Pediatric providers typically assume care for children with gynecologic issues. However, in the absence of pediatric gynecologists, the midwife may be called upon to consult with the pediatrician. The use of pictures or dolls may be useful in obtaining an accurate description or history of a problem. One must always assess for abuse in children presenting with pelvic pain and proceed according to the practice guidelines

Table 13-6	Food and Drug Administration–Approved Medications Used to Treat Overactive Bladder[a]		
Medication **Generic (Brand)**	**Action**	**Dose**	**Comments**
Oxybutynin (Ditropan IR)	Targets M1–M3 Mild antispasmodic Peak action: 1 hour Duration: 6–10 hours	2.5 mg or 5 mg daily, up to 5 mg 4 times a day	Has an active metabolite. GI absorption/liver metabolism related to increased potential for side effects and drug interactions. Available in liquid formula (5 mg/5 mL). Women with cardiac conditions should take with caution due to tachycardic side effects. Crosses blood–brain barrier. Excretion in breast milk is unstudied; lactation suppression has been reported. Use with osteoporosis medications like alendronate (Fosamax) with caution.
Oxybutynin (Ditropan) XL	Targets M1–M3 Mild antispasmodic Peak action: 4–6 hours Duration: > 24 hours	5, 10, and 15 mg daily, up to 30 mg daily	Start with 10 mg and titrate; can increase to 30 mg or decrease to 5 mg. GI absorption; similar efficacy and side-effect profile as IR. Cannot be chewed or crushed due to internal dispensing mechanism.
Oxybutynin transdermal (Oxytrol Patch)	Targets M1–M3 Mild antispasmodic Steady dose	Change biweekly	Avoids liver first-pass effect and active metabolite production to decrease side effects. Discontinuation may occur due to skin site reaction.
Tolterodine IR (Detrol)	Nonspecific anti-M Peak: 1–3 hours	2 mg twice a day (1 mg and 2 mg tablets)	GI absorption/liver metabolism. Less lipophilic, so it decreases CNS effects, though they are reported. Pill form only. Start with 4 mg daily, decrease to 2 mg as needed
Tolterodine (Detrol LA)	Nonspecific anti-M Peak: 2–6 hours	2–44 mg daily (2 mg and 4 mg tablets)	GI absorption/liver metabolism. Less lipophilic, so it decreases CNS effects, though they have been reported. Pill form only. Start with 4 mg daily, decrease to 2 mg as needed
Trospium (Sanctura IR)	Quaternary amine, nonselective peripheral effect Peak: 4–6 hours	20 mg bid	Minimal liver metabolism with decreased drug–drug interaction possible. Water-soluble, larger molecule for possible decreased crossing of lipid blood–brain barrier. Cognitive side-effect profile in elderly may be improved, but is not eliminated. Due to water solubility, take on empty stomach. In elderly, start with one dose daily.
Solifenacin (VESIcare ER)	Targets M2, M3 antispasmodic	5–10 mg daily	Metabolized in liver. Long half-life (approximately 50 hours); no head-to-head comparisons relating to effect. Can be taken with food.
Darifenacin (Enablex ER)	Targets M3	7.5–15 mg daily	Metabolized in liver. Advantages and disadvantages of M3 selectivity unknown due to no head-to-head trials. Can be taken with food. Half-life is 12 hours.

CNS = central nervous system; IR = immediate release; LA, ER, and XL = long acting or extended release; M, M1, M2, and M3 refer to parasympathetic muscarinic receptors.

[a]Food and Drug Administration (FDA) assigned risk factors for pregnancy and lactation vary for these medications.

Source: Adapted from O'Dell KK, Labin LC. Common problems of urination in nonpregnant women: causes, current management and prevention strategies. *J Midwifery Women's Health.* 2006;51:159-173. Reprinted with permission of Wiley.

of the practice or institution, as well as the laws of the jurisdiction in which the midwife practices, including those that dictate to which authority the midwife must report any suspicion or evidence of abuse. Obviously, any pelvic examination of children must be done sensitively and demands the use of appropriate-sized specula.

Adolescents

The need for confidentiality must always be balanced with the legal requirements for parental notification and involvement in care when caring for an adolescent. In cases when the parent and the adolescent have a conflicting view of management, it is important to try and sort out the best course of action for both the young woman and her family. The midwife must respect the autonomy of the adolescent and her ability to make safe decisions, as well as the adolescent's unique perspective on her health and her life choices. One must be cognizant of the legal ramifications of providing care to an adolescent in the absence of her parents and must be familiar with the relevant state or local laws pertaining to the care of minors. For example, in some states, adolescents are "emancipated" for the purposes of seeking care for pregnancy, family planning, or treatment for sexually transmitted infections. In the evaluation of pelvic pain, pelvic masses, or menstrual cycle dysfunction, it is important to include assessment of sexual activity, previous or current pregnancy, past or current sexually transmitted infections, past or current substance abuse, and eating disorders.

Adolescents may present for gynecologic evaluation based on their perceptions and possible misinformation regarding normal menstrual and gastrointestinal function. Body image often has a direct impact on how a young woman perceives her physical sensations and developmental changes. Misuse of laxatives or a restricted diet might lead to gastrointestinal distress or constipation, either of which might be interpreted as a gynecologic problem. The activity level of adolescents, especially young athletes, might also contribute to a musculoskeletal injury presenting as pelvic pain. Any contact with adolescents provides a special opportunity to evaluate their needs for information regarding sexual well-being, contraceptives, and substance abuse, including cigarette smoking and diet. Performing an initial pelvic exam also affords the midwife a unique opportunity to introduce the adolescent to nontraumatic, respectful, empowering care and information concerning the menstrual cycle, achieving and/or avoiding pregnancy, and the risks of pregnancy at an early age.

Older Women

Postmenopausal priorities often include disease prevention, disease detection, and preservation of function. Consequently, the role of the midwife includes addressing these health concerns in a comprehensive fashion. Relationship issues and family demands should continue to be discussed, as the care of children may have been replaced by the care of aged parents or ill partners. Health education includes anticipatory guidance about physiologic changes related to aging in addition to preventive and screening measures for disease. Fear of cancer, or other terminal illness diagnoses, may cause a woman to delay evaluation. The clinician must also continue to direct efforts to assess safety in the home with regard to both intimate-partner violence and violence stemming from other family members, especially if the woman is frail and requires assistance with personal needs.

Women with Disabilities

The care of women with physical or mental disabilities must be individualized and often requires some planning prior to the visit itself. These elements might include being certain that accessible exam tables or other equipment are available and being cognizant of the use of alternative examination positions to minimize pain or muscle spasm. Caring for hearing-impaired women, for example, requires access to staff or equipment that can address the preferred communication modality of the woman herself, whether that is sign language, lip reading, writing on paper, or typing on an electronic device.

Care for women with mental disabilities typically requires longer time for office interaction, examination, and health education, depending on the actual capabilities of the woman herself and whoever might be involved in her care. Special sensitivity to potential issues of sexual coercion, decision making with regard to contraception or medications use, and the ability to recognize gynecologic problems or abnormalities is required. The avoidance of assumptions with regard to sexual activity, desire for childbearing, and the ability of the woman to self-direct her care are critical considerations to keep in mind.

Culture

The evaluation of gynecologic concerns requires addressing the role of culture in a woman's view of her body and her ability to address her health needs in an autonomous fashion. Trained language interpreters are especially crucial in the evaluation and treatment of any gynecologic issue. Using family members, especially children, is never appropriate when dealing with sensitive and potentially embarrassing information. Permission to limit the presence of her partner or male relative might be a difficult, but important negotiation for the midwife to accomplish.

The ability to learn what the woman believes about her body and her identified problem are of primary importance. Additionally, the woman's beliefs and influences with regard to sexual activities, fertility, and pain are crucial. Pertinent questions might also include the following:

- What is this pain/problem called in your community? What is the meaning of this pain/problem?
- Do other family members or friends experience this condition as well? What do they do about it?
- How is this treated? How has the woman treated it so far?
- Are there other family or community members who must be consulted before treatment in this healthcare system can occur?

Fertility

The desire for or fear of pregnancy can have an enormous impact on how a woman perceives pelvic pain or menstrual irregularity. Feelings of depression, sadness, or worry about gynecologic function may contribute to or manifest as physical pain. An exploration of the nature of these events and their significance for the woman often proves useful.

Sexual Well-being

Despite the fact that all humans are sexual beings, it remains difficult for many women and the midwives who provide their care to articulate sexual concerns or to perceive sexual health as an important element of general health care. Overtly encouraging an atmosphere of safety and acceptance can result in the disclosure of significant concerns regarding pain with, or as a result of, sexual activity. Further exploration may reveal that the emotional overlay of guilt or fear related to sexual activity has exacerbated any physical problem that might exist. A nonjudgmental atmosphere established by the midwife will enable the woman to honestly discuss her sexual activities and concerns.

Sexual Abuse and Assault

Any woman who has experienced sexual abuse presents with a unique perspective on her gynecologic needs, especially that of pelvic pain. It must be the primary goal of the midwife providing her care to address her health needs in a manner that does not add to her physical or emotional distress. A detailed explanation of the nature of the exam and a discussion of the cycle of "tension–fear–pain" might be of use in these circumstances. Patience and use of skills in facilitating relaxation are essential in this situation. The nature of the gynecologic examination may retraumatize the woman if her abuser and the healthcare provider are of the same gender. If abuse is known to the midwife or revealed during the visit, the midwife should offer the presence of another staff member or a support person for the examination, thereby giving the woman control of the exam. If it is difficult for the woman to proceed with an exam, the visit may be conducted in smaller steps and encounters unless an acute, emergent problem is apparent. If the problem appears to be acute, the midwife should assess which type of examination other providers (e.g., Sexual Assault Nurse Examiners [SANEs]) may need to do and limit the current examination to only those elements that are absolutely necessary for consultation or referral.

Regardless of the reason for the visit, the midwife should acknowledge the woman's experience and offer the office as a safe haven for exploration and healing. Any suspicion or evidence of abuse in a woman of any age will require following practice and institutional guidelines, as well as the laws of the jurisdiction in which the midwife practices, including those that dictate to which authority the midwife legally must report any suspicion or evidence of abuse.

Cancer Screening/Diagnoses

It is estimated that one-third of all women in the United States and one-half of all men will be diagnosed with cancer over their lifetimes.[72] Only heart disease exceeds cancer as the leading cause of death in both women and men. For women in the United States, malignant neoplasms are the primary cause of death between 35 and 74 years of age.[73] Today, screening for cancer remains the best defense against this potentially lethal disease.

Because most persons fear cancer, screening for any health problems related to a cancerous process can challenging. Helping women understand the importance of breast self-awareness, cervical cancer screening via Pap tests, or other regular cancer screening modalities without raising excessive fears requires skilled communication. A regular healthcare visit offers several opportunities to assess for signs or symptoms of a cancerous or precancerous process, teach individuals about screening that can be accomplished at home, and introduce preventive measures for reducing the risks of ever experiencing cancer.

While cancer can occur in a number of body sites, including the lungs and the circulatory system, the following discussion focuses on those organs/areas most closely associated with gynecologic health—namely, the cervix, endometrium/uterus, ovaries, vulva, and vagina. Breast health, including breast cancer, is discussed in depth in the *Breast Conditions* chapter.

Cancer of the Cervix

One of the greatest success stories in U.S. public health in the twentieth century was the dramatic decrease in mortality due to cervical cancer. This success was due primarily to the invention and promotion of the cervical cytology smear (Pap smear) by a physician, George Papanicolaou, in the 1940s. With its effectiveness being enhanced by more recently improved technologies, the Pap smear reduced death by cervical cancer in the United States by more than 70% by the year 2003.[74] The Pap smear, now more accurately referred to as the "Pap test" due to advances in techniques for gathering cervical cells, continues today to be the first-line screening tool for detecting cervical cancer.[75] The American Cancer Society (ACS) estimated that in the United States in 2012 more than 12,000 new cases of cervical cancer would be diagnosed and more than 4000 women would die from this cause.[76]

Screening for Cervical Cancer

Pap Test A variety of organizations, including the ACS, the National Cancer Institute (NCI), and the United States Preventive Services Task Force (USPSTF), have published recommendations for cancer screening. With regard to Pap testing, changes in the schedule for screening of women who are at low risk of acquiring cervical cancer occurred as recently as 2012 (**Table 13-7**).[77–79]

All organizations discourage doing a Pap test for a woman who has undergone a hysterectomy that included removal of the cervix unless the woman had a history of a high-grade lesion (cervical intraepithelial neoplasia [CIN] 2 or 3) or cervical cancer itself prior to her hysterectomy. Women who are at risk, and thus require more frequent screening, include those individuals with a history of immunosuppressed conditions (e.g., HIV); those who were exposed to DES while in utero; and those who have a history of prior treatment for a high-grade precancerous cervical lesion or cervical cancer itself.[77,78] If this testing had occurred inadvertently in someone younger than age

21, and the result was either atypical squamous cells of undetermined significance (ASC-US) or low-grade squamous intraepithelial lesion (LSIL), a repeat cytology can be performed in 1 year. If the result of the original Pap test was high-grade squamous intraepithelial lesion (HSIL), a colposcopy is warranted.[75]

The cervical cytologic screening recommendations for women who have received the human papillomavirus (HPV) vaccination have not changed. This vaccine has been shown to protect against cancers caused by HPV strains 6, 11, 16, and 18. However, because 30% of cervical cancers are not preventable by current HPV vaccination methods, and because it is unclear at this time how many women actually receive the three injections necessary to complete the protective regimen of the vaccination, routine cytologic screening should continue for all women, based on the age and health history parameters discussed previously.[77–79]

Significant changes in screening techniques for cervical cancer have occurred over the last two decades. With the introduction of liquid-based cytology (e.g., ThinPrep, SurePath, and MonoPrep) and the advent of testing for specific HPV DNA types, the ability to screen for cervical cancer in asymptomatic women has improved considerably. Although the traditional technique of collecting endocervical cells using a spatula, a glass slide, and a fixative is just as sensitive and specific as the use of the newer liquid-based cytology[80] and remains less costly to process, the newer technique of collecting cells using a spatula, cytobrush, or a cervibroom, or a combination of two of these tools, and then transferring them into a vial containing the fixative has allowed for follow-up HPV testing when indicated. No matter which technique is used, the primary goal of collecting a Pap sample has always been to obtain cells from the endocervical/transformation zone region of the cervix.[81] Despite the potentially increased amount of bleeding caused by using two devices in combination, their use is still the recommended Pap test collection method for both nonpregnant *and* pregnant women.

HPV DNA Testing Two additional beneficial developments in cervical cancer screening have been the recognition that almost all cervical cancers are caused by exposure to specific strains of HPV and the ability through endocervical sampling to identify HPV according to type. More than 150 genotypes of HPV have been identified,[82] yet to date only approximately 15 of these types have been linked to the development of cervical cancer; notably, types 16 and 18 are related to approximately 70% of carcinoma cases.[77]

Table 13-7	Cervical Cancer Screening Guidelines for Women Who Are at Low Risk for Cervical Cancer[a]		
	ACS, ASCCP, ASCP	**UPSTF**	**ACOG**
< 21 years	No screening	No screening	No screening
21–29 years[b]	Every 3 years conventional cytology without HPV co-test	Every 3 years conventional cytology without HPV co-test	Every 3 years conventional cytology without HPV co-test
30–65 years	Every 3 years conventional cytology or every 5 years with HPV co-test	Every 5 years with HPV co-testing preferred or every 3 years conventional cytology	Every 5 years conventional cytology with HPV co-testing preferred or every 3 years with conventional cytology
> 65 years	No further screening if prior screening was negative and no other high risk for cervical cancer exists	No further screening if prior screening was negative and no other high risk for cervical cancer exists	No further screening if no abnormal tests in past 10 years
> 65 years with history of CIN II, CIN3, or AIS	Continue screening for 20 years after regression or management		Continue screening for 20 years after regression or management
After hysterectomy with removal of cervix	No screening unless positive history of high-grade precancerous lesion or cervical cancer	No screening unless positive history of high-grade precancerous lesion or cervical cancer	No screening unless positive history of high-grade precancerous lesion or cervical cancer
HPV-vaccinated	Regular age-specific screening	Regular age-specific screening	Regular age-specific screening

ACOG = American College of Obstetricians and Gynecologists; ACS = American Cancer Society; ASCCP = American Society for Colposcopy and Cervical Pathology; ASCP = American Society for Clinical Pathology; CIN = cervical intraepithelial neoplasia; HPV = human papillomavirus; USPSTF = U.S. Preventative Services Task Force.

[a]These guidelines do not apply to women who were exposed in utero to DES, women who have had a diagnosis of a high-grade precancerous cervical lesion or cervical cancer, women who are HIV positive, or women who are immunosuppressed.

[b]Women older than 21 years who have never had sex are at very low risk for developing cervical cancer, and screening in this population is dependent on individual clinician's judgment.

Sources: Adapted from Saslow D, Solomon D, Lawson H, et al. American Cancer Society, American Society for Colposcopy and Cervical Pathology, and American Society for Clinical Pathology screening guidelines for the prevention and early detection of cervical cancer. *J Low Genit Tract Dis.* 2012;16:175-204; Moyer V. Screening for cervical cancer: U.S. Preventive Services Task Force recommendation statement. *Ann Intern Med.* 2012;156:880-891.

While HPV testing is increasingly being conducted automatically when an abnormal Pap test has been identified, a major prohibitive factor to conducting HPV typing routinely as a screening test has been the cost of this approach. There is increasing evidence that testing for HPV alone, without the use of the cytologic Pap test, may generate more accurate findings,[83] thus eventually reducing the overall cost of routine screening. However, current guidelines continue to recommend HPV DNA testing only as an adjunct to Pap test screening in women 30 years and older, and HPV testing is not recommended during routine screening in women younger than 30 years.[77,84] Infection with most HPV types, including 16 and 18, regresses in younger women and does not contribute to the development of cervical cancer later in life unless there is repetitive exposure to the virus over time.[84]

HPV can be contracted without heterosexual intercourse, and even without any history of sexual contact.[75,85] Thus the midwife should take a thorough approach to screening and resist any temptation to avoid doing a Pap test based on presumptive lifestyle factors (e.g., a woman with a same-sex partner or a non-sexually active individual).

Management of Abnormal Pap Test Results Interpretation of cytology findings, as reported by a properly accredited external laboratory, is accomplished best by using the internationally accepted Bethesda Classification System of cervical cytologic reporting (**Box 13-1**).[86] This classification is a "cytologic" one, and not a "histologic" report. Cytologic testing involves examination of individual cells, and the results serve as a screening tool that addresses the absence or presence of precancerous or cancerous

---

BOX 13-1 The 2001 Bethesda System

Specimen Adequacy
- Satisfactory for evaluation (presence/absence of endocervical/transformation zone component noted with any other quality indicators such as partially obscuring blood or inflammation)
- Unsatisfactory for evaluation (reason specified)
- Specimen rejected/not processed (reason specified)
- Specimen processed and examined, but unsatisfactory for evaluation of epithelial abnormality because of (reason specified)

General Categorization (Optional)
- Negative for intraepithelial lesion or malignancy
- Epithelial cell abnormality
- Other

Interpretation/Result
- Negative for intraepithelial lesion or malignancy:
  - Organisms:
    Trichomonas vaginalis
    Fungal organisms morphologically consistent with *Candida* species
    Shift in flora suggestive of bacterial vaginosis
    Bacteria morphologically consistent with Actinomyces species
    Cellular changes consistent with herpes simplex virus
  - Other non-neoplastic findings (optional to report)
    Reactive cellular changes associated with:
       Inflammation (includes typical repair)
       Radiation
       Intrauterine contraceptive device
  - Glandular cells status post hysterectomy
  - Atrophy
- Epithelial cell abnormalities
  - Squamous cell
    Atypical squamous cells (ASC)[a]:
       Of undetermined significance (ASC-US)
       Cannot exclude HSIL (ASC-H)
    Low-grade squamous intraepithelial lesion (LSIL)
    High-grade squamous intraepithelial lesion (HSIL)
       [Encompassing old terminology of moderate and severe dysplasia, carcinoma in situ, CIN 2 and CIN 3]
    Squamous cell carcinoma
       Glandular cell
    Atypical glandular cells (AGC) (endocervical or endometrial or not otherwise specified); formerly known as
       AGUS (atypical glandular cells of undetermined significance)
    Atypical glandular cells, favor neoplastic (endocervical or not otherwise specified)
    Endocervical adenocarcinoma in situ (AIS)
    Adenocarcinoma
- Other malignant neoplasms

Automated Review and Ancillary Testing (Included as Appropriate)
For example, if a slide has been scanned by an automated computer system, the instrumentation used and the automated review result should be included in the cervical cytology report.

Educational Notes and Suggestions (Optional)
Although not required, there has been evidence reported in the literature that laboratory staff suggestions included on a Pap report regarding further evaluation improve the likelihood that appropriate follow-up actually will occur.

[a]It has been suggested by the American Society for Colposcopy and Cervical Pathology (ASCCP) that laboratory personnel conduct HPV DNA typing for high-risk viruses, if the clinician requested "reflex to HPV hybrid capture" on the original laboratory request form when a report of "ASC" is given." If "reflex" was not specifically requested by the clinician, some laboratories' staff will inquire on the written report if the clinician desires follow-up typing. Reflex HPV DNA typing is only available if cervical cells were collected originally using liquid-based cytology.

Source: Adapted from Saslow D, Solomon D, Lawson H, et al. American Cancer Society, American Society for Colposcopy and Cervical Pathology, and American Society for Clinical Pathology screening guidelines for the prevention and early detection of cervical cancer. *J Low Genit Tract Dis.* 2012;16:175-204.

cells. Histology, in contrast, involves the examination of both cells and larger tissue samples, and involves the use of a tissue biopsy. The staging of any cervical cancer findings is performed histologically, and necessitates testing beyond that of a Pap screen—most often a biopsy obtained during a follow-up colposcopic examination.

Despite the use of the Bethesda Classification System by most laboratories, follow-up actions based on report findings may vary. In general, if the test result reflects the presence of atypical squamous cells of undetermined significance, it is recommended that HPV DNA testing be implemented. If this further testing is negative for high-risk HPV (HR-HPV; e.g., HPV-16 or HPV-18), then repeat Pap testing at 12 months is recommended. If HPV testing does reveal high-risk DNA, then the follow-up to an ASC-US finding should be a colposcopy. A colposcopy also is warranted if a woman has recurrent cytology results of ASC-US, no matter what the HPV DNA testing reveals, or if she has atypical squamous cells for which high-grade lesions cannot be ruled out (ASC-H). Likewise, if a high-grade squamous intraepithelial lesion is reported, then a colposcopic evaluation is warranted.

If a low-grade squamous intraepithelial lesion is found, and the woman is 21 years of age or older but premenopausal, then a colposcopy is recommended. If the woman is younger than the age of 21, she can have a repeat Pap test 1 year later, and then would need a follow-up colposcopy only if the latest results showed evidence of HSIL or greater changes in the condition of the woman's cervix since her prior Pap test. It is important to repeat, however, that routine cytologic examinations for women younger than the age of 21 are no longer recommended. If the woman with an LSIL result is postmenopausal, the recommendation is for HPV DNA testing, repeat Pap testing at 6 and 12 months, or colposcopy. If the HPV testing for high-risk strains is negative or if colposcopy findings are negative, then a repeat Pap test in 12 months is recommended. Once two consecutive negative cytologic results are obtained, then the woman can return to the recommendation for women older than the age of 65 who have had prior positive results, which is to obtain screening every 3 years or once every 5 years with accompanying HPV testing.[87] If a woman with an LSIL result is pregnant, she should obtain a colposcopic examination, either during the pregnancy or after 6 weeks postpartum.

The presence of abnormal glandular cells (AGC) on a Pap sample requires a follow-up colposcopy, HPV DNA testing, and endometrial sampling. If atypical endometrial cells are the only result noted on the Pap report, it is recommended that endometrial and endocervical sampling occur next. If no endometrial abnormality is found, then a colposcopy is warranted.[88]

The role of the midwife in this testing can range from immediate referral to the actual performance of these tests, depending on the individual practitioner's experience and skill level. If the results of a Pap test involve any finding of advanced disease, such as squamous cell carcinoma or adenocarcinoma, immediate referral to a specialist working with gynecologic carcinomas is necessary.

Visual Inspection with Acetic Acid While not commonly found in the more populated regions of developed nations, an alternative screening tool to the Pap test for assessing potential lesions of the cervix is the use of visual inspection with acetic acid (VIA). This approach involves "painting" the cervix with acetic acid (5%) during a speculum examination and then visually inspecting the cervix for acetowhite lesions. The discovery of any such lesions results in referral for further testing, usually involving a colposcopic examination.[89] Because the sensitivity and specificity of the VIA do not differ dramatically from the sensitivity and specificity of a Pap test,[90] and because the VIA's cost in terms of equipment and laboratory personnel is much less, this tool's use in low-resource regions of developed nations and in low-resource developing nations is recommended for cervical cancer screening.

Diagnosis of Cervical Cancer
Pap Test Interpretation The clinical action taken in response to Pap report findings that indicate the presence of an organism depends on the organism named. The Pap test has been found to be a highly *specific* tool for identifying *Trichomonas*, meaning that if "trich" is found on a Pap slide, the woman almost certainly has the organism present in her vagina and, therefore, should be treated.[91] However, the Pap test is not a very *sensitive* mechanism for diagnosing *Trichomonas*. Only approximately half of women with this parasite will have it detected by a Pap test. Therefore, diagnosis is still best accomplished in symptomatic women using a wet prep microscopic examination. If the Pap report states that the sample was difficult to interpret due to inflammation of the captured cells, then treatment is warranted, and should be followed by a repeat Pap test for a more accurate reading.

Candida found on a Pap test most likely does not require treatment. Almost all women have *Candida* colonized intravaginally as a part of their normal flora, and this organism's presence on a Pap report gives no indication of the amount of *Candida* present, nor does the result indicate the actual clinical presentation of the individual woman.[93] If the woman has symptoms of vaginal candidiasis, treatment is warranted, especially if the condition is confirmed with a positive wet mount. As with the presence of *Trichomonas*, inflammation causing difficulty in interpreting the Pap test suggests that treatment of the candidiasis should occur, followed by a repeat Pap test.

Similarly, Pap test results that report HSV are highly *specific* but not very *sensitive*. Thus a Pap test should not be used to screen for or diagnose HSV on the cervix.[91] If the woman is symptomatic, obtaining HSV cultures remains the most accurate method of identifying this organism. In the asymptomatic individual, a serology test for HSV will determine if the woman have ever experienced an HSV infection, but a positive result does not give any information about the current outbreak or the timing of exposure to the virus. Nonetheless, if a Pap result indicates the presence of HSV, the woman should be notified and discussion regarding potential symptoms and diagnostic testing should occur.

Many laboratories still report a predominance of coccobacilli when greater numbers of these organisms are present than are normally found in vaginal flora. This finding suggests the presence of bacterial vaginosis (BV). However, the sensitivity and specificity of the Pap test in diagnosing BV have been reported as both low and high, and the use of the Pap test as an accurate method of diagnosing BV is debatable.[91] As with the presence of other organisms noted on a Pap result, the midwife should inquire whether the woman is symptomatic and offer her a vaginal examination to assess for BV.

The woman with an IUD or intrauterine system (IUS) in place and a finding of *Actinomyces* on a Pap report needs to be examined for any signs and symptoms of PID. *Actinomyces* is a strain of bacteria that can be found in the normal female genital tract, but in rare cases it has been found to cause PID in women using IUDs, especially if they have been long-term users, in which case the IUD may be removed and antibiotics initiated. If the woman is asymptomatic, the device can be left in place, and the woman should be taught the signs and symptoms of PID so that she can receive immediate treatment if needed.

To summarize, the main purpose of the Pap test is to categorize and describe epithelial cell abnormalities; consequently, the Pap test is primarily a screening mechanism, not a diagnostic tool. Certainly, if the clinician discovers an unusual lesion or mass on the cervix, a Pap test will be performed. However, in current practice, a colposcopy should be the main diagnostic tool used in this situation.

Colposcopy The primary tool for determining the presence of cervical cancer or precancerous cells is colposcopy. This technique of illuminating and magnifying the cervix to search for premalignant or cancerous cells was first used in Germany in the 1920s, but did not enter into widespread use in the United States until the 1980s. Today, an increasing number of midwives are receiving formal training in performing colposcopy and have incorporated the procedure into their clinical practices.

Diagnostic and follow-up indications for a colposcopy are found in **Box 13-2**.[92,93] For the woman undergoing colposcopy, the experience is similar to that of Pap test, in that a speculum examination is performed. However, individuals need to be made aware that the procedure lasts longer than a Pap test does, and pain or discomfort, as well as post-examination bleeding, can result from any biopsy procedures accompanying a colposcopy.

If any lesions of the cervix are found during the magnified inspection of the colposcopic procedure, sampling of the region is required. This is accomplished through the use of biopsy for suspicious

---

BOX 13-2 Common Indications for Colposcopic Examination of the Cervix

- Grossly visible or palpable abnormality of the cervix
- Abnormal cervical cytology
- Positive screening test for cervical neoplasia (e.g., high-risk HPV-DNA strain)
- Persistent unsatisfactory cervical cytology
- History of in utero diethylstilbestrol (DES) exposure
- Unexplained cervico-vaginal discharge
- Unexplained abnormal lower genital tract bleeding
- Surveillance for lower genital tract neoplasia (cervical, vaginal, vulvar)
- Post-lower genital tract cancer treatment surveillance

Source: Adapted from American Society for Colposcopy and Cervical Pathology (ASCCP). *Colposcopy: Indications.* Hagerstown, MD: ASCCP; 2012. Available at: http://www.asccp.org /PracticeManagement/Cervix/Colposcopy/tabid/7506 /Default.aspx.

lesions on the ectocervical region. Endocervical curettage (ECC) is recommended in certain situations (e.g., no lesion is found during an adequate colposcopy) to evaluate tissue not easily visible during a colposcopic examination. The purpose of a tissue biopsy or an ECC is to rule out cancer or precancerous lesions, and subsequently provide treatment for the woman. Depending on the clinician's level of experience and preference, treatment can occur during an initial colposcopic examination, prior to laboratory confirmation of diagnosis, if any lesion is found to be suspicious of cancer. This approach avoids the need for follow-up surgery and a delay in treatment, yet runs the risk of unnecessary surgery being performed based on visual inspection without laboratory confirmation.

As with any procedure, the possible actions to be taken during a colposcopy need to be discussed with the individual *before* the examination begins. No matter which procedures were performed during the initial colposcopic examination, positive results on any tissue analysis require follow-up with a practitioner experienced in the treatment of cervical cancer, usually a gynecologic oncologist.

Cervicography Due to the high cost of colposcopy, or the lack of equipment and training in low-resource countries or areas, alternative methods to colposcopy have been proposed and tested for accuracy in diagnosing cervical lesions found on Pap tests, or have been suggested as first-line screening tools in lieu of cervical cytology. One example of these alternative methods is cervicography, also known as a cervigram. Introduced in the United States in the 1980s, this method involves the use of low-magnification photographs of the cervix, which are then read by a cytopathologist, often at a different site and later in time—an approach similar to the process by which Pap tests are read. While cervicography is not as sensitive or specific as colposcopy, there is sufficient evidence to show that this technique can serve an important role in cervical cancer screening, especially in locations where access and cost are issues with which to contend.[94]

As previously mentioned, the principal diagnostic tool for cervical cancer or precancerous lesions remains the colposcopy. With regard to the potential reported findings of colposcopic examinations, it is beyond the scope of this chapter to review them. However, understanding of colposcopic findings and the potential treatments that could follow positive results will benefit the midwife in supporting any women who undergo the experience of being told about positive colposcopic results.

Cancer of the Endometrium

Almost four times more women in the United States are diagnosed each year with uterine cancer than with cervical cancer.[82] While a variety of carcinomas may potentially be found in the uterus, including sarcomas and gestational trophoblastic tumors (e.g., hydatidiform mole), the endometrium is the source of most cancers involving the corpus of the uterus. The cure rate for endometrial cancer, when detected early in the disease process, is high because tumors tend to be localized and well defined. Nevertheless, the high incidence of this form of cancer results in more than 8000 deaths per year; the ratio of deaths to new diagnoses (1 to 5.9) for endometrial cancer is, therefore, comparable to the ratio for breast cancer (1 to 5.7).[82]

Classification of endometrial cancer historically organizes cases into two types. Type I, which is estrogen dependent and is the variant most commonly encountered, usually occurs in the premenopausal or perimenopausal years; if discovered in early stages, it is treatable. Type II, which is not related to the presence of estrogen, is rarer than Type I. This cancer occurs among women who are more likely to be postmenopausal and has a less optimal prognosis than its counterpart. Some oncologists recognize a third type of endometrial cancer, which is known to be hereditary in nature and is less commonly found than Type I or II. The most common cause of this tumor is hereditary nonpolyposis colorectal cancer (HNPCC), also known as Lynch syndrome, which is caused by a genetic mutation and is more closely identified with cancer of the digestive tract.[95]

Screening for Endometrial Cancer

The primary diagnostic tool for endometrial cancer today is the endometrial curettage or biopsy (EMB).[96] For many years, the standard of care in diagnosing endometrial hyperplasia—an overgrowth of the endometrium that often leads to the development of cancer—has been dilatation and curettage (D & C). However, this invasive procedure has always been considered too involved and costly to justify its use as a screening tool for endometrial cancer.

Other tools that have been proposed as possible mechanisms for routine screening of endometrial cancer include the Pap test and transvaginal ultrasound. However, the effectiveness of these methods led to the conclusion that routine screening of asymptomatic women for endometrial cancer, no matter which method is used, is currently of no proven benefit.[97] The primary use of these tools is in diagnosing women who are at high risk for endometrial cancer (**Box 13-3**) or who display signs of endometrial

> **BOX 13-3 Risk Factors Associated with Endometrial Cancer**
>
> - Age > 50 years
> - Early menarche or late menopause
> - Polycystic ovary syndrome; anovulation
> - Nulliparity; infertility
> - Obesity; high-fat diet
> - Family history
> - White race
> - Residency in northern European or North American countries
> - Use of unopposed exogenous estrogen (estrogen therapy [ET])
> - History of breast or ovarian cancer
> - Use of tamoxifen (Nolvadex) for treatment of breast cancer
> - History of hereditary nonpolyposis colorectal cancer (HNPCC; also known as Lynch syndrome)
> - Estrogen-secreting ovarian tumors
> - Diabetes
> - Gallbladder disease
> - Hypertension
> - Prior history of pelvic radiotherapy
>
> *Source:* Adapted from National Cancer Institute. Endometrial cancer screening. Available at: http://www.cancer.gov/cancer topics/pdq/screening/endometrial/HealthProfessional. Accessed September 7, 2012.

hyperplasia or cancer.[97] The most common sign of endometrial cancer, which always requires diagnostic follow-up, is unexplained vaginal bleeding, especially in a postmenopausal woman.

Diagnosis of Endometrial Cancer

Endometrial hyperplasia, and the possible subsequent development of endometrial cancer, occurs most often in women older than the age of 50, with the average age of diagnosis being approximately 61 years.[98] However, other risk factors besides age exist, and the midwife should not make a decision to assess for endometrial cancer based on age alone.

Clinically, the most significant sign of endometrial cancer is bleeding. For a postmenopausal woman, *any* bleeding, except that experienced in a regular pattern while on hormone therapy, is considered to be a sign of potential cancer. Prior to menopause, irregular bleeding could be a sign of cancer. However, because most endometrial cancers occur among postmenopausal women, any irregular bleeding prior to menopause should be assessed with that as part of the differential diagnosis. Other signs or symptoms of endometrial cancer, such as pain, usually occur only during late-stage disease, when the cancer has spread beyond the uterus.

Endometrial Biopsy Today, EMB is the most frequently used method for diagnosing disorders of the endometrium. This procedure has been reported to be safe and cost-effective, and can easily be performed during an ambulatory setting visit.[98] However, the rather wide range of evidence regarding EMB's sensitivity and specificity for diagnosing endometrial abnormalities has inspired objections to this test being the sole diagnostic tool used to assess for carcinoma.[97] Yet, EMB serves an important role when used in conjunction with other assessment tools. Thus the midwife should consider the use of EMB in ruling out endometrial hyperplasia or cancer, but not rely solely on the information that is obtained from EMB.

Transvaginal Ultrasound Often accompanying EMB as an assessment of endometrial abnormality is transvaginal ultrasound, which, in addition to detecting possible intrauterine masses, measures the thickness of the endometrium (the "endometrial stripe") as a gauge of intrauterine health. Depending on the study reviewed, a thickness of more than 4 to 6 mm is thought to be associated with pathology.[97] While not yet sophisticated enough or sufficiently cost-effective to be used as a routine screening tool for endometrial cancer, transvaginal ultrasound has been suggested as an initial method for diagnosing endometrial cancer.[99] When combined with EMB, the use of transvaginal ultrasound further increases the sensitivity in ruling out carcinoma of the endometrium.

Dilatation and Curettage The traditional method for ruling out suspected endometrial cancer was the use of D & C. Not only did this procedure give the practitioner a more than adequate sample of endometrial tissue for analysis, but it also initiated treatment of any anomalies by removing potentially harmful tissue. However, in the 1980s the value of this diagnostic procedure, which requires considerable time and money, began to be questioned, especially given that its sensitivity and specificity in ruling out endometrial cancer were unclear. Today, there is disagreement about whether D & C remains the "gold standard" for diagnosing endometrial cancer.[99] Nevertheless, when less invasive diagnostic measures have been unable to identify a cause of suspected bleeding, a D & C procedure can be a useful tool for reaching a diagnosis.

Advanced Techniques The two most common advanced assessment tools are hysteroscopy and sonohysterography. These techniques are not covered in basic midwifery education, but any midwife referring a woman for further uterine assessment should understand them so that the woman can be prepared.

Hysteroscopy involves direct visualization of the uterine cavity using an endoscope that is inserted through the cervix, and can be performed in the ambulatory setting. During the examination, visible masses (e.g., polyps) or suspicious areas of endometrial lining can be biopsied or completely removed. Due to this ability to directly visualize the endometrium, the hysteroscopy is effective in discovering the source of uterine bleeding. While the combination of EMB and transvaginal ultrasound is more commonly used in diagnosing endometrial cancer, there have been recommendations that hysteroscopy be considered as the initial tool in diagnosing not only endometrial cancer, but any suspected intrauterine abnormalities.[100]

Sonohysterography involves inserting sterile saline into the uterine cavity through the cervix, and then imaging the uterus with a transvaginal ultrasound. This technique separates the two walls of the endometrium, allowing for a more detailed examination of endometrial thickness and possible polyp growths. In addition, submucosal myomas are more readily visible in sonohysterography than they are in transvaginal ultrasound, allowing for a better assessment of their site and size. Sonohysterography is used for diagnosis only, and any sampling of endometrium or removal of polyps requires additional interventions. As with all medical procedures, the woman undergoing sonohysterography should be aware of these advantages and disadvantages, and make an informed decision regarding whether to have this procedure performed.

In summary, several mechanisms are used for *diagnosing* endometrial cancer. However, an accurate and cost-effective *screening* method for endometrial cancer remains elusive. Midwives are encouraged to keep abreast of new developments in endometrial assessment techniques; seek training in advanced, postgraduate skills so that women can be offered a variety of assessment procedures without the need for seeing additional practitioners; and inform and support individuals in their choices regarding the ruling out of endometrial cancer.

Additional Uterine Cancers

While endometrial cancer is by far the most common form of uterine cancer, two additional forms of abnormal growth are important to note: gestational trophoblastic tumors (e.g., hydatidiform mole) and uterine sarcoma.

The most common of these tumors is the hydatidiform mole, which in its beginning stages is a benign but abnormal growth of placental tissue. The woman presents with a positive pregnancy test, usually accompanied by excessively elevated human chorionic gonadotropin (hCG) levels and abnormal bleeding. Her uterus commonly will be larger than expected given her gestational dates, and confirmation of diagnosis is accomplished through ultrasonography. Treatment most frequently involves the use of suction curettage with the goal of preventing the development of metastatic disease.[101]

Uterine sarcomas are a rare form of gynecologic cancer (incidence is less than 1%) that accounts for approximately 3% to 8% of all uterine carcinomas.[102] Generally occurring after menopause, these anomalies originate in the uterine muscle or the endometrial epithelium. Risk factors include prior therapeutic radiation to the pelvic region, generally used in the past to curtail benign uterine bleeding; prolonged use of tamoxifen; an excess of lifetime estrogen exposure; and African American race. There is no recommended form of routine screening for these sarcomas, other than the assessment of uterine size and shape that occurs with annual examination. The most common symptom/sign of this form of cancer is abnormal uterine bleeding. Initial diagnosis requires a bimanual examination to discover any unusual growth or shape to the uterus. While sarcomas cannot be easily distinguished on physical examination from benign leiomyomas, sarcomas usually are found post menopause, whereas leiomyomas more commonly manifest themselves prior to menopause, but then begin to shrink in size after menopause when estrogen stimulation diminishes.

If sarcoma is suspected after a careful history and thorough physical examination, further assessment may involve an endometrial biopsy or D & C. Unfortunately, these diagnostic tools are less sensitive for sarcomas than for endometrial carcinomas. More sensitive assessment is achieved with imaging studies, such as computed tomographic (CT) scans or MRI. Employing ultrasound for the diagnosis of sarcoma is not considered a very useful approach.

A midwife usually will refer the woman in whom uterine sarcoma is suspected to an appropriate specialist. Prognosis depends on the extent of the disease when diagnosis is made. If the cancer is confined to the uterine corpus upon discovery, the 5-year survival rate is 50%. Survival rates at 5 years for sarcoma that has metastasized ranges from 0% to 20%.[103] Early discovery is vital to curtailing the spread of this disease. As with efforts to successfully diagnose endometrial cancer in beginning stages, it is important to stress the significance of uterine bleeding in postmenopausal women.

Ovarian Cancer

Perhaps the most troubling of gynecologic cancers faced by both women and the clinicians who care for them is ovarian cancer, which accounts for an estimated 25% of new cases of genital forms of cancer diagnosed each year, yet is responsible for more than half of all deaths of women who suffer from carcinoma of the genital organs.[76] Even more troubling is the fact that the 5-year survival rate for ovarian cancer is estimated to be only 44%—markedly less than comparable rates for other cancers experienced exclusively or predominately by women. For example, the 5-year survival rate for breast cancer now stands at 90%.[76,104] Women and clinicians perhaps can take some comfort in realizing that in comparison to the 1 in 8 lifetime risk of being diagnosed with breast cancer, the comparable lifetime risk of being diagnosed with ovarian cancer is 1 in 72.[104] As with most cancers, the risk of contracting the disease rises with age. It is most prevalent after the age of 45 years, and the median age of diagnosis is 63 years.[104]

There exists an almost total absence of reliably specific signs and symptoms for the earlier stages of this disease, and its presence often goes undetected until the cancer is advanced, which partly accounts for the high rate of mortality. The difficulty in diagnosing ovarian cancer also is a result of minimal understanding of its etiology. While several types of ovarian cancer exist, including germ cell and sex cord-stromal tumors, 90% to 95% of ovarian malignancies are of epithelial origin.[105] Because nulliparity, early menarche, and late menopause are all associated with an increased risk of ovarian cancer, repetitive stimulation of the epithelium of the ovary is theorized to result in the development of a malignant state. However, the exact physiologic cause of the disease remains unknown.

Known and possible risk factors for ovarian cancer are listed in **Box 13-4**.[104–107] Increased parity, the use of oral contraceptives, breastfeeding, a history of hysterectomy or tubal ligation, and a history of prophylactic oophorectomy are all associated with a decreased risk of developing ovarian cancer.[105,107]

Screening for Ovarian Cancer

The lack of evidence regarding the etiology of ovarian cancer, definitive risk factors, and means of early detection make screening for this disease difficult for both women and practitioners. Currently, there

---

BOX 13-4 Risk Factors Associated with Ovarian Cancer

Known Risk Factors

- Age: ≥ 50 years
- Strong family history of ovarian or breast cancer (first-degree relative [e.g., mother or sister] or multiple second-degree relatives)
- Evidence of mutations in the BRCA1 or BRCA2 gene
- Presence of hereditary nonpolyposis colorectal cancer (HNPCC; also known as Lynch syndrome)
- More than 40 years of active ovulation (e.g., nulliparous never-user of oral contraceptives)
- Early menarche
- Nulliparity
- Late menopause (> 56 years of age)
- Obesity (body mass index [BMI] ≥ 30)
- Use of hormone therapy (HT) that contains an estrogen component

Possible Risk Factors

- Smoking
- Possible exposure to asbestos or talcum powder
- Exposure to asbestos
- Use of infertility drugs particularly if no pregnancy ensues
- High-fat diet
- White race

Sources: Adapted from Hoffman B, Schorge J, Schaffer J. Epithelial ovarian cancer. In: Hoffman B, Schorge J, Schaffer J, et al., eds. *Williams Gynecology.* 2nd ed. New York: McGraw-Hill; 2012:853-878; National Cancer Institute. BRCA1 and BRCA2: cancer risk and genetic testing. Available at: http://www.cancer.gov/cancertopics/factsheet/Risk/BRCA. Accessed September 18, 2012; McLemore M, Miaskowski C, Aouizerat B, Chen L, Dodd M. Epidemiological and genetic factors associated with ovarian cancer. *Cancer Nurs.* 2009;32:281-288.

---

are no effective routine screening tools for detecting ovarian cancer.

Reminders for women about the signs and symptoms of ovarian cancer may potentially aid in detecting this carcinoma. These indicators include abdominal distension or bloating; flatulence, difficulty eating or easily feeling full when eating, and other persistent gastrointestinal disturbances; abdominal or pelvic pain; fatigue; urinary complaints, including urgency or frequency; and irregular vaginal bleeding.[107] It is essential that possibility of ovarian cancer be considered by the midwife as the woman's clinical examination is performed. However, the fact that a majority of individuals afflicted with this malignancy do not become symptomatic until late in the disease process means that the sensitivity of screening through education and history taking is low. Bimanual examinations during regular well-woman visits had long been the only ovarian cancer screening tool not dependent on self-report. However, there is no evidence on the sensitivity or specificity of these examinations with regard to detecting ovarian cancer.[105]

Because history taking and physical examination have not been very predictive in the detection of ovarian cancer, particularly in its earlier stages, other more technological assessment tools have been suggested as screening mechanisms for this disease. For example, detection of increased blood levels of the CA-125 tumor antigen in women with early onset of ovarian cancer, or even in nonaffected individuals at risk for later developing this form of cancer, has been suggested as a screening option. However, early optimism about this potential screening method has been tempered for several reasons: Individuals already in early stages of ovarian cancer often have normal serum levels of CA-125; elevated levels of CA-125 have been found in women diagnosed with nongynecologic cancers; levels of CA-125 can be elevated in women with benign conditions, such as endometriosis or the presence of uterine fibroids or benign ovarian masses; and healthy women can have positive results for the CA-125 marker for a number of reasons, including menstruation and pregnancy.[107,108]

Even less specific than CA-125 in screening for ovarian cancer is the presence of mutations of the BRCA1 and BRCA2 genes. Originally linked to breast cancer, these mutations have also been discovered in some women found to have ovarian cancer—a finding that had led to hope that screening for the BRCA1 and BRCA2 mutations, especially in families with a history of ovarian cancer, would aid in the early diagnosis of this disease. However, only 10% of ovarian cancer cases are due to these mutations[76] and additional genetic mutations associated with ovarian cancer continue to be discovered.[108] Thus the notion of screening the general female population for BRCA1 and BRCA2 mutations as a means to identify the subclinical presence of ovarian cancer currently is not recommended.

Some ethnic groups of women, such as those whose family's heritage includes Ashkenazi (Eastern European) Jewish, Norwegian, Dutch, and Icelandic peoples, have a higher incidence of inheriting BRCA 1 or BRCA 2 mutations. Women with these backgrounds will often ask if they should be tested for these mutations to screen for ovarian cancer. Currently, there is not sufficient evidence, due to the low specificity and sensitivity rates of this screening approach, to make this recommendation. Current recommendations from the NCI call for testing only if a family member has been diagnosed with ovarian cancer *and* the woman has had a positive test for BRCA1 or BRCA2.

Transvaginal ultrasound is able to detect greater details of ovarian structure and physiologic changes as compared to the use of abdominal ultrasound. In turn, transvaginal ultrasound has been suggested as a possible screening tool for ovarian cancer within the general population. However, findings regarding the use of transvaginal ultrasound as a screening tool have been varied at best, with some investigations demonstrating a positive predictive value, or the ability of the transvaginal ultrasound to accurately diagnose a woman with ovarian cancer, as low at 1.0%.[109] The financial and emotional costs, involving further testing and even the possibility of surgery, that would result from the large number of false-positive results associated with transvaginal ultrasound screening for ovarian cancer would be very high when weighed against the number of ovarian cancer cases that would actually be discovered.

The difficulty of screening for ovarian cancer has led some researchers to explore the use of a combination of CA-125 and transvaginal ultrasound testing to see if results in diagnosing the presence of this disease could be improved. However, to date this combination screening approach has not proved successful enough to recommend its use for the general population.[105,109]

Diagnosis of Ovarian Cancer

The limitations in screening for ovarian cancer and the fact that the diagnosis of the disease often occurs only late in the pathologic process make it imperative for the clinician to pay close attention to women's physical signs and symptoms that could signal the presence of ovarian cancer.

Although not very sensitive in diagnosing ovarian cancer, the earliest symptoms reported by women later discovered to have this disease tend to be gastrointestinal in nature. There is no evidence that screening *any* woman with these GI symptoms will either improve the rate of discovery of ovarian cancer or improve overall outcomes. Yet, it behooves the midwife who hears of these symptoms from an individual with risk factors for ovarian cancer[105–107,110] (Box 13-4) to proceed toward investigating this disease. Attention to this change in a woman's lifestyle could help the clinician move forward with diagnostic testing or referral to an oncology specialist for further evaluation.

Additional symptoms of ovarian cancer—such as abdominal or pelvic pain; fatigue; urinary problems, including urgency or frequency; and irregular vaginal bleeding—tend to appear later in the course of the disease.[107] The presence of these symptoms in any woman should lead to the midwife to consider ovarian cancer in the differential diagnosis.

The initial step in ruling out this disease is to conduct a thorough history, including family history and social history, as well as a discussion with the woman regarding any potential environmental exposures (e.g., asbestos) that may be associated with ovarian cancer. The history should be followed by a physical examination, with emphasis on the bimanual pelvic examination to explore for a possible mass. Even if no distinct mass is palpated, a transvaginal ultrasound may be ordered if the midwife suspects ovarian tumors, although the use of technological diagnostic tools usually is initiated by an oncologist to whom the midwife has referred the woman.

To date, the only manner in which to clearly diagnose ovarian cancer is through surgery, usually involving laparoscopy with appropriate biopsy. Midwifery care for the woman diagnosed with ovarian cancer should include assisting the woman in reducing risky behaviors, such as smoking and consumption of a high-fat diet, as well as encouraging her to educate her female relatives about the possible familial link involved with ovarian cancer.

Cancer of the Vulva or Vagina

The forms of genital cancer that affect mortality but are the least frequent in occurrence are those involving the vulva and the vagina. Together, these diseases account for approximately 6% to 7% of all forms of gynecologic malignancies.[111] It was estimated that in 2012 there would be approximately 7100 new cases of these forms of cancer found in the United States, with vulvar incidences accounting for almost two-thirds of these genital forms of cancer. The estimated number of deaths in 2012 from vulvar and vaginal cancers was predicted to be close to 1800.[76] The relative 5-year survival rates for vulvar and vaginal cancers are approximately 72% and 50%, respectively.[112] The lower survival rate for vaginal cancer is in part due to the fact that this malignancy usually presents as a result of metastatic spreading of a cancer whose primary source of development was in another gynecologic organ, such as the vulva or the cervix.[113,114] When vaginal cancer is discovered prior to nodal involvement, the 5-year survival rate is approximately 90%.[114]

The majority of both forms of cancer are squamous cell in nature, and the incidence increases with age; most cases are found in women older than the age of 50.[113] A rarer form of vaginal cancer, found primarily in daughters of women who took DES during pregnancy, is clear cell adenocarcinoma (CCA); it typically affects women in their late adolescence and early twenties.[115] Both vulvar and vaginal cancer can be related to HPV infection, with approximately 50% of vulvar cancers now being linked to exposure to high-risk HPV types.[116] Consequently, the Centers for Disease Control and Prevention (CDC) now emphasizes that receiving the HPV vaccine will protect against not only cervical cancer, but vulvar and vaginal cancer as well. Additionally, any individual with a history of having contracted a high-risk HPV type, most likely identified on a Pap test, should be considered at risk for vulvar or vaginal cancer.

Other risk factors for vulvar or vaginal malignancies include smoking; a history of other gynecologic cancers; a history of lichen sclerosus, a dermatologic condition characterized by a lightening of tissue, particularly in the genital area, accompanied with severe itching and scratching; and a history of HIV, which results in immunosuppression that can contribute to the growth of cancerous cells.[21,117]

Both screening and diagnosis of vulvar and vaginal cancers involve taking a history of a growth in the genital area noted by the woman, followed by pelvic examination, with visualization and palpation playing major roles. The most common site of vulvar involvement is the labia majora, while the most common location of vaginal cancer is the upper third of the vaginal wall.[113] Early symptoms of vulvar cancer may include persistent pruritus and the presence of condylomata, whereas vaginal disease may be accompanied by bleeding, unusual discharge, and pelvic discomfort. Depending on the extent of the latter disease process, pelvic examination can reveal a mass at the site of involvement, and possible lymphadenopathy. Any suspicious lesion should be biopsied, either by a midwife with experience in collecting such samples or by the specialist to whom the woman has been referred. Referral should occur if any of the following exist: unexplained lymphadenopathy, an HPV lesion that does not improve with topical treatment, or a lesion with an unusual presentation or with continued growth over time. As is the case with other gynecologic malignancies, early detection of a vulvar or vaginal cancer can result in a high rate of survival.

Nongynecologic Cancer Screening and Teaching

During a well-woman examination, teaching regarding healthy habits and lifestyle can be included to help thwart the development of cancer. As always, individual and cultural differences need to be acknowledged when counseling women about cancer prevention. Knowledgeable recommendations to women depend on the midwife staying apprised of the latest scientific literature, as well as each individual's health and cultural background, and then assisting the individual in making optimal choices for preventing cancer and the ill health that accompanies it.

Conclusion

The phrase "With women, for a lifetime" speaks well to the role of the midwife. The majority of most women's well-being over the lifespan focuses on gynecologic health. Both historically and currently, the care offered by midwives has included the diagnosis and management of gynecologic health and disorders. This chapter has summarized some of the more common of gynecologic problems, as well as advanced diseases such as pelvic organ prolapse and gynecologic cancers, and has presented the diagnostic/management steps associated with these various conditions. As with all midwifery care, the essential element of practice in each of these situations is to listen to the woman and what she has to say about her condition and the effect it has on her life. Not only will this approach to care validate that which the woman is feeling and experiencing, but it will also reveal the most essential information needed for making an accurate diagnosis and subsequent plan of care.

• • • References

1. Martinez G, Daniels K, Chandra A. Fertility of men and women aged 15-44 years in the United States: national survey of family growth, 2006-2010. *Natl Health Stat Rep*. 2012;51:1-29.

2. Schuiling K, Sipe T, Fullerton J. Findings from the analysis of the American College of Nurse-Midwives' Membership Surveys: 2006-2008. *J Midwifery Women's Health*. 2010;55:299-307.

3. American College of Nurse-Midwives (ACNM). *Definition of Midwifery and Scope of Practice of Certified Nurse-Midwives and Certified Midwives*. Silver Spring, MD: ACNM; 2011.

4. Daniels J, Khan K. Chronic pelvic pain in women. *BMJ*. 2010;341(c4834):772-775.

5. Stones W, Cheong YC, Howard FM, Singh S. Interventions for treating chronic pelvic pain in women. *Cochrane Database Syst Rev*. 2005;2:CD000387. doi: 10.1002/14651858.CD000387.

6. Ehrenreich B, English D. *Witches, Midwives, and Nurses: A History of Women Healers*. 2nd ed. New York: Feminist Press; 2010.

7. Dalpiaz O, Kerschbaumer A, Mitterberger M, et al. Chronic pelvic pain in women: Still a challenge. *BJU Int*. 2008;102:1061-1065.

8. Seidel H, Ball J, Dains J, et al. *Mosby's Guide to Physical Examination*. 7th ed. St. Louis, MO: Mosby Elsevier; 2010.

9. Fauconnier A, Dallongeville E, Huchon C, Ville, Y, Falissard B. Measurement of acute pelvic pain intensity in gynecology: a comparison of five methods. *Obstet Gynecol*. 2009;113:260-269.

10. Barnhart, K. Ectopic pregnancy. *N Engl J Med*. 2009; 361:379-387.

11. Flasar MH, Goldberg E. Acute abdominal pain. *Med Clin North Am*. 2006;90:481-503.

12. Hoffman B, Schorge J, Schaffer J, et al. Pelvic mass. In: Hoffman B, Schorge J, Schaffer J, et al., eds. *Williams Gynecology*. 2nd ed. New York: McGraw-Hill; 2012: 246-280.

13. Varras M, Tsikini A, Polyzos D, Samara CH, Hadjopoulos G, Akrivis CH. Uterine adnexal torsion: pathologic and gray-scale ultrasonographic findings. *Clin Exp Obstet Gynecol*. 2004;31:34-38.

14. Dell J, Mokrzycki M, Jayne C. Differentiating interstitial cystitis from similar conditions commonly seen in gynecologic practice. *Eur J Obstet Gynecol Reprod Biol*. 2009;144:105-109.

15. Groysman V. Vulvodynia: new concepts and review of the literature. *Dermatol Clin*. 2012;28:681-696.

16. Moyal-Barracco M, Lynch PJ. 2003 ISSVD terminology and classification of vulvodynia: a historical perspective. *J Reprod Med*. 2004;49:772-777.

17. Stone-Godena T. Vulvar pain syndromes: vestibulodynia. *J Midwifery Women's Health*. 2006;51:502-509.

18. Cox K, Neville C. Assessment and management options for women with vulvodynia. *J Midwifery Women's Health*. 2010;57,231-240.

19. Haefner H, Collins M, Davis G, et al. The vulvodynia guideline. *J Low Genit Tract Dis*. 2005;9(1):40-51.

20. O'Hare PM, Shetetz EF. Vulvodynia: a dermatologist's perspective with emphasis on an irritant contact dermatitis component. *J Women Health Gender-Based Med*. 2000;9(5):565-569.

21. Petersen C, Lundvall L, Kristensen E, Giraldi, A. Vulvodynia: definition, diagnosis and treatment. *Acta Obstet Gynecol*. 2008;87:893-901.

22. Thorstensen K, Birenbaum D. Recognition and management of vulvar dermatologic conditions: lichen sclerosus, lichen planus, and lichen simplex chronicus. *J Midwifery Women's Health*. 2010;57;260-275.

23. Bergeron S, Brown C, Lord M, et al. Physical therapy for vulvar vestibulitis syndrome: a retrospective study. *J Sex Marital Ther*. 2002;28:183-192.

24. Burney RO, Giudice L. Pathogenesis and pathophysiology of endometriosis. *Fertil Steril*. 2012;98:511-519.

25. Treloar S, Bell A, Nagle C, Purdie D, Green A. Early menstrual characteristics associated with subsequent diagnosis of endometriosis. *Am J Obstet Gynecol.* 2010;202:534.e1-534.e6.

26. Brown J, Pan A, Hart RJ. Gonadotrophin-releasing hormone analogues for pain associated with endometriosis. *Cochrane Database Syst Rev.* 2010;12:CD008475. doi: 10.1002/14651858.CD008475.pub2.

27. Davis LJ, Kennedy SS, Moore J, Prentice A. Oral contraceptives for pain associated with endometriosis. *Cochrane Database Syst Rev.* 2007;3:CD001019. doi: 10.1002/14651858.CD001019.pub2.

28. Farquhar C, Prentice A, Singla AA, Selak V. Danazol for pelvic pain associated with endometriosis. *Cochrane Database Syst Rev.* 2007;4:CD000068. doi: 10.1002/14651858.CD000068.pub2.

29. Jacobson TZ, Duffy JMN, Barlow D, Koninckx PR, Garry R. Laparoscopic surgery for pelvic pain associated with endometriosis. *Cochrane Database Syst Rev.* 2009;4:CD001300. doi: 10.1002/14651858.CD001300.pub2.

30. Brown J, Kives S, Akhtar M. Progestagens and antiprogestagens for pain associated with endometriosis. *Cochrane Database Syst Rev.* 2012;3:CD002122. doi: 10.1002/14651858.CD002122.pub2.

31. Olive D. Gonadotropin-releasing hormone agonists for endometriosis. *N Engl J Med.* 2008;359:1136-1142.

32. Furness S, Yap C, Farquhar C, Cheong YC. Pre and post-operative medical therapy for endometriosis surgery. *Cochrane Database Syst Rev.* 2004;3:CD003678. doi: 10.1002/14651858.CD003678.pub2.

33. Zhu X, Hamilton KD, McNicol ED. Acupuncture for pain in endometriosis. *Cochrane Database Syst Rev.* 2011;9:CD007864. doi: 10.1002/14651858.CD007864.pub2.

34. Giudice L. Endometriosis. *N Engl J Med.* 2010;362:2389-2398.

35. Verga C. Benign gynecologic conditions. In: Schuiling K, Likis F, eds. *Women's Gynecologic Health.* Burlington, MA: Jones & Bartlett Learning; 2012:669-699.

36. Rice K, Secrist J, Woodrow E, Hallock L, Neal J. Etiology, diagnosis, and management of uterine leiomyomas. *J Midwifery Women's Health.* 2012;57:241-247.

37. Whiteman M, Hillis S, Jamieson D, et al. Inpatient hysterectomy surveillance in the United States, 2000-2004. *Am J Obstet Gynecol.* 2008;198:34.e1-34.e7.

38. American College of Obstetricians and Gynecologists. Alternatives to hysterectomy in the management of leiomyomas. Practice Bulletin No. 96, *Obstet Gynecol.* 2008;112:387-400; reaffirmed 2010.

39. Liu JP, Yang H, Xia Y, Cardini F. Herbal preparations for uterine fibroids. *Cochrane Database Syst Rev.* 2009;2:CD005292. doi: 10.1002/14651858.CD005292.pub.

40. Sardo A, Mazzon I, Bramante, S et al. Hysteroscopic myomectomy: a comprehensive review of surgical techniques. *Hum Reprod Update.* 2008;14(2):101-119.

41. Cockerham A. Adenomyosis: a challenge in clinical gynecology. *J Midwifery Women's Health.* 2012;57:212-220.

42. Fritz M, Speroff L. Abnormal uterine bleeding. In: *Clinical Gynecologic Endocrinology and Infertility.* 8th ed. Baltimore: Lippincott Williams & Wilkins; 2011:591-620.

43. Garcia L, Isaacson K. Adenomyosis: review of the literature. *J Min Invas Gynecol.* 2011;18:428-437.

44. Grimes DA, Jones LB, Lopez LM, Schulz KF. Oral contraceptives for functional ovarian cysts. *Cochrane Database Syst Rev.* 2011;9:CD006134. doi: 10.1002/14651858.CD006134.pub4.

45. Fritz M, Speroff L. The uterus. In: *Clinical Gynecologic Endocrinology and Infertility.* 8th ed. Baltimore: Lippincott Williams & Wilkins; 2011:121-156.

46. Hoffman B, Schorge J, Schaffer J, et al. Anatomic disorders. In: Hoffman B, Schorge J, Schaffer J, Halvorson L, Bradshaw K, Cunningham F, eds. *Williams Gynecology.* 2nd ed. New York: McGraw-Hill; 2012:481-505.

47. Grimbizis G, Campo R. Congenital malformations of the female genital tract: the need for a new classification system. *Fertil Steril.* 2010;94:401-407.

48. American Fertility Society. The American Fertility Society classifications of adnexal adhesions, distal tubal occlusion, tubal occlusion secondary to tubal ligation, tubal pregnancies, Müllerian anomalies and intrauterine adhesions. *Fertil Steril.* 1988;49:944-955.

49. Goodman A, Schorge J, Greene M. The long-term effects of in utero exposures: the DES story. *N Engl J Med.* 2011;364:2083-2084.

50. Titus-Ernstoff L, Hatch EE, Hoover RN, et al. Long-term cancer risk in women given diethylstilbestrol (DES) during pregnancy. *Br J Cancer.* 2001;84(1):126-133.

51. Titus-Ernstoff L, Troisi R, Hatch E, et al. Offspring of women exposed in utero to diethylstilbestrol (DES): a preliminary report of benign and malignant pathology in the third generation. *Epidemiol.* 2008;19:251-257.

52. Hoffman B, Schorge J, Schaffer J, et al. Urinary incontinence. In: Hoffman B, Schorge J, Schaffer J, et al., eds. *Williams Gynecology.* 2nd ed. New York: McGraw-Hill; 2012:606-632.

53. Hoffman B, Schorge J, Schaffer J, et al. Pelvic organ prolapse. In: Hoffman B, Schorge J, Schaffer J, Halvorson L, Bradshaw K, Cunningham F, eds. *Williams Gynecology.* 2nd ed. New York: McGraw-Hill; 2012:633-658.

54. Hagen S, Stark D. Conservative prevention and management of pelvic organ prolapse in women. *Cochrane Database Syst Rev.* 2011;12:CD003882. doi: 10.1002/14651858.CD003882.pub4.

55. Novi J, Jeronis S, Morgan M, Arya, L. Sexual function in women with pelvic organ prolapse compared to women without pelvic organ prolapse. *J Urol.* 2005;173:1669-1672.

56. Barber M, Walters M, Bump R. Short forms of two condition-specific quality-of-life questionnaires for women with pelvic floor disorders (PFDI-20 and PFIQ-7). *Am J Obstet Gynecol.* 2005;193:103-113.

57. Flynn M, Amundsen C. Diagnosis of pelvic organ prolapse. In: Chapple C, Zimmern P, Brubaker L, Smith R, Bo K, eds. *Multidisciplinary Management of Female Pelvic Floor Disorders.* Philadelphia: Churchill Livingstone Elsevier; 2006:115-124.

58. Brækken I, Majida M, Ellström Engh M, Bø K. Can pelvic floor muscle training reverse pelvic organ prolapse and reduce prolapse symptoms? An assessor-blinded, randomized, controlled trial. *Am J Obstet Gynecol.* 2010;203:170.e1-170.e7.

59. Boyle R, Hay-Smith EJC, Cody JD, Mørkved S. Pelvic floor muscle training for prevention and treatment of urinary and faecal incontinence in antenatal and postnatal women. *Cochrane Database Syst Rev.* 2012;10:CD007471. doi: 10.1002/14651858.CD007471.pub2.

60. Kuhn A, Bapst D, Stadlmayr W, Vits K, Mueller M. Sexual and organ function in patients with symptomatic prolapse: are pessaries helpful? *Fertil Steril.* 2009;91:1914-1918.

61. Herderschee R, Hay-Smith EJC, Herbison GP, Roovers JP, Heineman MJ. Feedback or biofeedback to augment pelvic floor muscle training for urinary incontinence in women. *Cochrane Database Syst Rev.* 2011;7:CD009252. doi: 10.1002/14651858.CD009252.

62. Subak L, Wing R, Smith West D, et al. Weight loss to treat urinary incontinence in overweight and obese women. *N Engl J Med.* 2009;360:481-490.

63. Kaya S, Akbayrak T, Beksac S. Comparison of different treatment protocols in the treatment of idiopathic detrusor overactivity: a randomized controlled trial. *Clin Rehab.* 2011;25:327-338.

64. Buchsbaum G, Duecy E, Kerr L, Huang L, Guzick D. Urinary incontinence in nulliparous women and their parous sisters. *Obstet Gynecol.* 2005;106:1253-1258.

65. O'Dell KK, Labin LC. Common problems of urination in nonpregnant women: causes, current management and prevention strategies. *J Midwifery Women's Health.* 2006;51:159-173.

66. Bradley C, Rovner E, Morgan M, et al. A new questionnaire for urinary incontinence diagnosis in women: development and testing. *Am J Obstet Gynecol.* 2005;192:66-73.

67. Rogers R. Urinary stress incontinence in women. *N Engl J Med.* 2009;358:1029-1036.

68. Nabi G, Cody JD, Ellis G, Hay-Smith J, Herbison GP. Anticholinergic drugs versus placebo for overactive bladder syndrome in adults. *Cochrane Database Syst Rev.* 2006;4:CD003781. doi: 10.1002/14651858.CD003781.pub.

69. Lipp A, Shaw C, Glavind K. Mechanical devices for urinary incontinence in women. *Cochrane Database Syst Rev.* 2011;7:CD001756. doi: 10.1002/14651858.CD001756.pub5.

70. Glazener CMA, Cooper K. Anterior vaginal repair for urinary incontinence in women. *Cochrane Database Syst Rev.* 2001;1:CD001755. doi: 10.1002/14651858.CD001755.

71. Appell R. Urethral and bladder injections for incontinence including Botox. *Urol Clin North Am.* 2011; 38:1-6.

72. American Cancer Society. Learn about cancer. n.d. Available at: http://www.cancer.org/index. Accessed May 12, 2012.

73. Heron M. *Deaths: Leading Causes for 2007. National Vital Statistics Report, 59(8).* Hyattsville, MD: National Center for Health Statistics; 2011.

74. American Cancer Society. Cervical cancer: prevention and early detection. n. d. Available at: http://www.cancer.org/Cancer/CervicalCancer/MoreInformation/CervicalCancerPreventionandEarlyDetection/cervical-cancer-prevention-and-early-detection-toc. Accessed June 22, 2012.

75. Wallace M, Barlow A. Gynecologic cancers. In: Schuiling K, Likis F. *Women's Gynecologic Health.* 2nd ed. Burlington, MA: Jones & Bartlett Learning; 2012:701-748.

76. American Cancer Society. *Cancer Facts and Figures 2012.* Atlanta, GA: American Cancer Society; 2012.

77. Saslow D, Solomon D, Lawson H, et al. American Cancer Society, American Society for Colposcopy and Cervical Pathology, and American Society for Clinical Pathology screening guidelines for the prevention and early detection of cervical cancer. *J Low Genit Tract Dis.* 2012;16:175-204.

78. Moyer V. Screening for cervical cancer: U.S. Preventive Services Task Force recommendation statement. *Ann Intern Med.* 2012;156:880-891.

79. Screening for cervical cancer. Practice Bulletin No. 131. American College of Obstetricians and Gynecologists. *Obstet Gynecol.* 2012;120:1222-1238.

80. Siebers A, Klinkhamer P, Grefte J, et al. Comparison of liquid-based cytology with conventional cytology for detection of cervical cancer precursors: a randomized controlled trial. *JAMA.* 2009;302:1757-1764.

81. Mashburn J. Evolution of the evidence-based Papanicolaou smear. *J Midwifery Women's Health.* 2001;46:181-189.

82. Schiffman M, Wentzensen N, Wacholder S. Human papillomavirus testing in the prevention of cervical cancer. *J Natl Cancer Inst.* 2011;103:368-383.

83. Mayrand M, Duarte-Franco E, Rodrigues I, et al. Human papillomavirus DNA versus Papanicolaou screening tests for cervical cancer. *N Engl J Med.* 2007;357:1579-1588.

84. ACOG Practice Bulletin. Management of abnormal cervical cytology and histology. *Obstet Gynecol.* 2008; 112:1419-1444.

85. Eaton L, Kalichman S, Cain D. Perceived prevalence and risks for human papillomavirus infection among women who have sex with women. *J Women's Health.* 2008;17:75-83.

86. Solomon D, Davey D, Kurman R, et al. The 2001 Bethesda System: terminology for reporting results of cervical cytology. *JAMA.* 2002;287:2114-2119.

87. Wright T, Massad S, Dunton C, et al. 2006 consensus guidelines for the management of women with abnormal cervical cancer screening tests. *Am J Obstet Gynecol.* 2007;197:346-355.

88. Warren J, Gullett H, King V. Cervical cancer screening and updated Pap guidelines. *Prim Care Clin Office Pract.* 2009;36:131-149.

89. Abdel-Hady E, Emam M, Al-Gohary A, et al. Screening for cervical carcinoma using visual inspection with acetic acid. *Int J Gynecol Obstet.* 2006;93:118-122.

90. Sangwa-Lugoma G, Mahmud S, Nasr S, et al. Visual inspection as a cervical cancer screening method in a primary health care setting in Africa. *Int J Cancer.* 2006;119:1389-1395.

91. Fitzhugh V, Heller D. Significance of a diagnosis of microorganisms on Pap smear. *J Low Gen Tract Dis.* 2008;12:40-51.

92. Jeronimo J, Schiffman M. Colposcopy at a crossroads. *Am J Obstet Gynecol.* 2006;195:349-353.

93. American Society for Colposcopy and Cervical Pathology (ASCCP). *Colposcopy: Indications.* Hagerstown, MD: ASCCP; 2012. Available at: http://www .asccp.org/PracticeManagement/Cervix/Colposcopy /tabid/7506/Default.aspx.

94. Bomfim-Hyppolito S, Franco E, Franco R, et al. Cervicography as an adjunctive test to visual inspection with acetic acid in cervical cancer detection screening. *Int J Gynaecol Obstet.* 2006;92:58-63.

95. Smith R, Cokkinides V, Brawley O. Cancer screening in the United States, 2009: a review of current American Cancer Society guidelines and issues in cancer screening. *CA Cancer J Clin.* 2009;59:27-41.

96. American College of Nurse-Midwives. Endometrial biopsy. Clinical bulletin no. 5. *J Midwifery Women's Health.* 2001;46:321-326.

97. National Cancer Institute. Endometrial cancer screening. Available at: http://www.cancer.gov/cancertopics /pdq/screening/endometrial/HealthProfessional. Accessed September 7, 2012.

98. National Cancer Institute. SEER stat fact sheets: corpus and uterus, NOS. 2012. Available at: http ://seer.cancer.gov/statfacts/html/corp.html. Accessed September 7, 2012.

99. McFarlin B. Ultrasound assessment of the endometrium for irregular vaginal bleeding. *J Midwifery Women's Health.* 2006;51:440-449.

100. van Dongen H, de Kroon C, Jacobi C, Trimbos J, Jansen F. Diagnostic hysteroscopy in abnormal uterine bleeding: a systematic review and meta-analysis. *BJOG.* 2007;114:664-675.

101. Monchek R, Wiedaseck S. Gestational trophoblastic disease: an overview. *J Midwifery Women's Health.* 2012;57:255-259.

102. Amant F, Coosemans A, Debiec-Rychter M, et al. Clinical management of uterine sarcomas. *Lancet Oncol.* 2009;10:1188-1198.

103. National Cancer Institute. Uterine sarcoma treatment. Available at: htwww.cancer.gov/cancertopics /pdq/treatment/uterinesarcoma/HealthProfessional. Accessed September 18, 2012.

104. National Cancer Institute. Ovary. Surveillance Epidemiology and End Results (SEER). Available at: http://seer.cancer.gov/statfacts/html/ovary.html. Accessed May 18, 2012.

105. Hoffman B, Schorge J, Schaffer J. Epithelial ovarian cancer. In: Hoffman B, Schorge J, Schaffer J, et al., eds. *Williams Gynecology.* 2nd ed. New York: McGraw-Hill; 2012:853-878.

106. National Cancer Institute. BRCA1 and BRCA2: cancer risk and genetic testing. Available at: http ://www.cancer.gov/cancertopics/factsheet/Risk /BRCA. Accessed September 18, 2012.

107. McLemore M, Miaskowski C, Aouizerat B, Chen L, Dodd M. Epidemiological and genetic factors associated with ovarian cancer. *Cancer Nurs.* 2009; 32:281-288.

108. Nossov V, Amneus M, Su F, et al. The early detection of ovarian cancer: from traditional methods to proteomics. Can we really do better than serum CA-125? *Am J Obstet Gynecol.* 2008;199(3):215-223.

109. Clarke-Pearson D. Screening for ovarian cancer. *N Engl J Med.* 2009;361:170-177.

110. Bankhead C, Collins C, Stokes-Lampard H, et al. Identifying symptoms of ovarian cancer: a qualitative and quantitative study. *BJOG.* 2008;115: 1008-1014.

111. Centers for Disease Control and Prevention. Vaginal and vulvar cancers. Available at: http://www.cdc .gov/cancer/vagvulv. Accessed September 20, 2012.

112. National Cancer Institute. SEER survival monograph: cancer survival among adults: US SEER program, 1988-2001: patient and tumor characteristics. Available at: http://seer.cancer.gov/publications/survival. Accessed February 19, 2013.

113. Hoffman B, Schorge J, Schaffer J, et al. Vaginal cancer. In: Hoffman B, Schorge J, Schaffer J, et al., eds. *Williams Gynecology.* 2nd ed. New York: McGraw-Hill; 2012:808-816.

114. National Cancer Institute. Vulvar cancer treatment. Available at: http://www.cancer.gov/cancertopics/pdq/treatment/vulvar/HealthProfessional. Accessed September 30, 2012.

115. Centers for Disease Control and Prevention. Information to identify and manage DES patients. Available at: http://www.cdc.gov/DES/hcp/information/daughters/risks_daughters.html#cca. Accessed September 30, 2012.

116. American Cancer Society. Vulvar cancer. Available at: http://www.cancer.org/Cancer/VulvarCancer/DetailedGuide/vulvar-cancer-risk-factors. Accessed September 30, 2012.

117. Centers for Disease Control and Prevention. Vaginal and vulvar cancer. Available at: http://www.cdc.gov/cancer/vagvulv/pdf/vagvulv_facts.pdf. Accessed September 30, 2012.

• • • Additional Resources

Abdominal and Pelvic Pain—General

National Guideline Clearinghouse. Chronic pelvic pain. Available at: http://guideline.gov/content.aspx?id=10940. Accessed November 16, 2012.

Causes of Acute Abdominal/Pelvic Pain

Ectopic Pregnancy

Lozeau AM, Potter B. Diagnosis and management of ectopic pregnancy. Available at: http://www.aafp.org/afp/2005/1101/p1707.html. Accessed November 13, 2012.

National Guideline Clearinghouse. Medical management of ectopic pregnancy. Available at: http://guideline.gov/content.aspx?id=12625 . Accessed November 12, 2012.

Appendicitis

National Guideline Clearinghouse. ACR appropriateness criteria right lower quadrant pain — suspected appendicitis. Available at: http://guideline.gov/content.aspx?id=23816. Accessed November 13, 2012.

Ovarian Torsion

Chang HC, Bhatt S, Dogra VS. Perals and pitfalls in diagnosis of ovarian torsion. Available at: http://www.ncbi.nlm.nih.gov/pubmed/18794312. Accessed November 14, 2012.

Causes of Chronic Abdominal/Pelvic Pain

Pelvic Inflammatory Disease/Salpingitis

Elsevier Clinical Key. Pelvic inflammatory disease. Available at: https://www.clinicalkey.com/topics/radiology/pelvic-inflammatory-disease.html. Accessed November 15, 2012.

Interstitial Cystitis

Harvard Women's Health Watch. Diagnosing and treating interstitial cystitis. Available at: http://www.health.harvard.edu/newsletters/Harvard_Womens_Health_Watch/2011/August/diagnosing-and-treating-interstitial-cystitis. Accessed November 15, 2012.

National Kidney and Urologic Diseases Information Clearinghouse (NKUDIC). Interstitial cystitis/painful bladder syndrome. Available at: http://kidney.niddk.nih.gov/kudiseases/pubs/interstitialcystitis. Accessed November 15, 2012.

Dyspareunia and Vulvar Pain

Heim LJ. Evaluation and differential diagnosis of dyspareunia. Available at: http://www.aafp.org/afp/2001/0415/p1535.html. Accessed November 15, 2012.

Vulvodynia

National Vulvodynia Association. Vulvodynia: integrating current knowledge into clinical practice. Available at: http://learnprovider.nva.org. Accessed November 16, 2012

Endometriosis

National Guideline Clearinghouse. Endometriosis: diagnosis and management. Available at: http://guideline.gov/content.aspx?id=23864&search=endometriosis. Accessed November 16, 2012.

Medscape Reference. Endometriosis. Available at: http://emedicine.medscape.com/article/271899-overview. Accessed November 16, 2012.

Pelvic Masses

Fibroids

National Guideline Clearinghouse. ACR appropriateness criteria treatment of uterine leiomyomas. Available at: http://guideline.gov/content.aspx?id=23820&search=uterine+fibroids. Accessed November 16, 2012.

Adenomyosis

Medscape Reference. Endometriosis. Available at: http://emedicine.medscape.com/article/271899-overview. Accessed November 16, 2012.

Benign Ovarian Cysts

National Guideline Clearinghouse. Management of suspected ovarian masses in premenopausal women. Available at: http://guideline.gov/content.aspx?id=36084&search=benign+ovarian+cyst. Accessed November 18, 2012.

Pelvic Organ Prolapse

Bordman R, Telner D, Jackson B, Little D. Step-by-step approach to managing pelvic organ prolapse. Available at: http://www.ncbi.nlm.nih.gov/pmc/articles/PMC1949085. Accessed November 18, 2012.

Urinary Incontinence

Culligan PJ, Heit M. Urinary incontinence in women: evaluation and management. Available at: http://www.aafp.org/afp/2000/1201/p2433.html. Accessed November 18, 2012.

National Guideline Clearinghouse. Urinary incontinence in women. Available at: http://guideline.gov/content.aspx?id=13195. Accessed November 18, 2012.

Cervical Cancer

PubMed Health. Cervical cancer. Available at: http://www.ncbi.nlm.nih.gov/pubmedhealth/PMH0001895. Accessed November 18, 2012.

National Cancer Institute. Cervical cancer. Available at: http://www.cancer.gov/cancertopics/types/cervical. Accessed November 18, 2012.

Endometrial Cancer

PubMed Health. Endometrial cancer. Available at: http://www.ncbi.nlm.nih.gov/pubmedhealth/PMH0001908. Accessed November 19, 2012.

National Guideline Clearinghouse. Management of endometrial cancer. Available at: http://www.guideline.gov/content.aspx?id=10930&search=maintaining+and+progestin+the+patient. Accessed November 19, 2012.

Ovarian Cancer

National Guideline Clearinghouse. Ovarian cancer: the recognition and initial management of ovarian cancer. Available at: http://guideline.gov/content.aspx?id=34829&search=ovarian+cancer. Accessed November 19, 2012.

Vulvar and Vaginal Cancer

National Cancer Institute. Vaginal cancer. Available at: http://www.cancer.gov/cancertopics/types/vaginal. Accessed November 19, 2012.

National Cancer Institute. Vulvar cancer. Available at: www.cancer.gov/cancertopics/types/vulvar. Accessed November 19, 2012.

CHAPTER

14

Breast Conditions

JOYCE L. KING

Culturally, the female breast is frequently linked to our concept of womanhood. Even though the primary function of breasts is lactation, the size and shape of the breasts capture our attention and breasts are often considered to be erotic. The loss or injury of the breast can be devastating to a woman.

Diseases of the breast encompass a broad range of pathology, from benign disorders such as fibroadenomas to breast malignancies. According to American Cancer Society statistics, breast cancer is the most frequently diagnosed cancer in women and ranks second as a cause of cancer deaths in women exceeded only by lung cancer.[1] In fact, there are more deaths due to breast cancer each year than due to ovarian, uterine, fallopian tube, cervical, and vulvar cancers combined.[2] This chapter reviews normal growth and development of the breast, including normal breast anatomy and physiology, current recommendations for breast examination, common benign breast disorders, and an overview of the risk factors, diagnosis and staging, treatments, and prognosis of breast cancer.

Breast Development

The process of development of secondary sexual characteristics takes place in an orderly and predictable sequence. Tanner's classification of sexual maturity is a scale used to evaluate breast and pubic hair growth as a way of assessing normal growth and development. Often the first sign of puberty is thelarche, or the onset of breast development. On average, breast development is initiated at 10 years of age in white girls and 8.9 years of age in African American girls.[3] Both estrogen and progesterone influence the development of the breast, with estrogen stimulating the ductal portion of the glandular system and progesterone stimulating the alveolar or milk-producing components of the system.[4] To achieve optimal growth and development, the breast also requires the stimulation of insulin, cortisol, thyroxine, prolactin, and insulin-like growth factor I. It is not uncommon for the breasts to develop asymmetrically, but usually by the end of puberty the breasts are approximately the same size in most women—although as many as 25% of women have persistent visible breast asymmetry. Significant asymmetry is correctable by surgery; hormone therapy is ineffective at treating this condition. The complete development of the alveolus into a mature milk-producing gland is accomplished with the increase in estrogen and progesterone levels that occur during pregnancy.[4]

Breast tissue changes with aging. The adolescent breast has increased density, as it consists predominantly of glandular tissue. Over time, breasts become less dense as they progressively acquire more fat tissue that gradually replaces the glandular tissue.[4]

Gynecomastia, or breast enlargement in males, can be physiologic, may be associated with specific diseases (e.g., Klinefelter syndrome, hyperthyroidism, liver failure), may be a side effect of certain medications (e.g., spironolactone, digoxin), or may result from the decrease in testosterone production as men age. Fifty percent of adolescent males will experience physiologic gynecomastia during early puberty, which should resolve within 6 months to 2 years after onset. If symptoms persist after 2 years or continue past 17 years of age, further evaluation is needed.[5]

Anatomy and Physiology

The breast is composed of a superficial subcutaneous layer of fascia and a deep layer of facia next to the chest wall, lobules (the glandular tissue), milk ducts, connective tissue, and fat. The breast glandular tissue is organized into 15 to 20 lobes, with the majority of tissue located in the upper outer quadrant of each breast. The lobules drain into a series of milk ducts that lead to the nipple.

The amount of fat present determines the size of the breast. The fatty tissue in the dependent lower breast can become a discrete inframammary ridge secondary to the effects of gravity. The Cooper's ligaments are the connective tissue of the breast that run from the fascia that overlies the pectoralis muscle to the dermis of the skin overlying the breast. These ligaments help to support the breast in its normal position and maintain the shape. Adipose tissue, or fat, is interspersed through the lobules. The nipple is surrounded by the areola, a pigmented area where sebaceous glands (Montgomery's tubercles) are located. Most lymphatic vessels within the breast drain toward the axillary lymph nodes, making them a prime location for breast cancer metastasis.

The major physiologic role of the breasts is milk secretion during lactation. Two primary hormones—prolactin and oxytocin—are involved in the regulation of milk secretion, with prolactin being responsible for milk synthesis and oxytocin being responsible for milk ejection. The release of both of these hormones is stimulated by a neuroendocrine reflex triggered by suckling. Cortisol, insulin, parathyroid hormone, and growth hormone are also essential for the ongoing maintenance of milk production.[4,6] The breast also undergoes cyclic changes in the nonpregnant state due to the influence of estrogen and progesterone that may include increased size of breasts, fluid secretion, and premenstrual tenderness.

Breast Screening

Widespread use of screening for breast cancer as well as the advances in treatment have significantly reduced mortality due to breast cancer.[7] The current recommendations for routine breast screening include clinical breast examination, mammography, and ultrasound with self-breast examination as another option. Magnetic resonance imaging may be indicated for women who are at high risk for developing breast cancer (e.g., carriers of *BRCA1* or *BRCA2* mutations).

Breast Self-Examination

In the past, all women beyond menarche have been encouraged to perform monthly breast self-examination (BSE) as a tool for early diagnosis of cancerous tumors and, therefore, as a means to ensure early treatment and decrease the mortality associated with breast cancer. Controversy now surrounds the recommendations regarding BSE, as several randomized trials conducted in the 1990s found no reduction in breast cancer mortality in women who practiced monthly BSE.[8,9] This is a complex problem in that studies with differing methodologies have several different findings.

In a case-control study within the Canadian National Breast Screening Study, Harvey et al. observed that proficiency in the practice of BSE may reduce the risk of death from breast cancer, especially if abnormal findings are discussed with a healthcare provider in a timely fashion.[10] A study conducted by the Mayo Clinic observed that while the majority of women with breast cancer presented with image-detected breast cancer, 36% of women presented with palpable disease that was found on either BSE or clinical breast examination (CBE). Those with palpable disease tended to present symptomatically between screening mammograms. Such women also tended to be younger and have more aggressive tumor characteristics (e.g., larger tumor size, axillary node involvement, high grade, and estrogen receptor negative tumors) compared to women whose tumors are detected via mamogram. The researchers concluded that BSE and CBE remain important components in breast cancer diagnosis.[11]

A prospective study found that 43% of new breast cancers were detected by BSE in 147 high-risk women undergoing intensive breast cancer screening (e.g., yearly mammograms and yearly magnetic resonance imaging), and who are more likely to present with screening-interval cancers.[12] These results provide evidence that BSE is an important surveillance tool for women who have a high risk for developing breast cancer and that BSE education should be a component of the follow-up of this population.[12]

Nevertheless, based on the earlier studies, several organizations—including the Canadian Task Force on Preventive Health Care, the U.S. Preventive Services Task Force, and the World Health Organization—recommend against teaching women how to perform BSE, stating that BSE may actually be harmful because it increases both the number of imaging procedures and the number of breast biopsies.[7] The American Cancer Society (ACS) no longer recommends monthly BSE, but does state that BSE can be an option for women starting after age 20 years. The ACS recommends that women should be told about the benefits, the limitations, and the potential harms (the possibility of a false-positive result) of this examination technique.[13]

Today, "breast awareness" is recommended in place of BSE for women who do not want to perform BSE regularly or formally. Women should be taught to be aware of the normal shape and consistency of their breasts and taught to report any changes in how their breasts feel or look. Women who have breast implants should probably do BSE.

The BSE technique that is recognized by the ACS includes both inspection and palpation using the vertical stripe technique described in the *Breast Examination* appendix in the chapter titled *An Introduction to the Care of Women*. Some evidence indicates that the up-and-down pattern of examining the breast decreases the likelihood that breast tissue will be missed.[13]

Clinical Breast Examination

Routine examination of the breasts by a healthcare professional has also been recommended as an important part of breast cancer screening, although there have been no randomized trials that have evaluated the benefits of clinical breast examination as a sole screening modality. The Canadian National Breast Screening Study compared CBE/BSE plus mammography to CBE alone in women between the ages of 40 and 49 years and between ages 50 and 59 years. CBE was performed by healthcare professionals who were trained in the techniques of CBE and who also had periodic evaluations of performance quality. The frequency of cancer diagnosis, stage, and breast cancer mortality noted 11 to 16 years after entry into the study was similar in the two groups.[14] A study that screened women who had a positive family history of breast cancer observed that after a normal initial evaluation, BSE and/or CBE found more cancer than mammography.[15] Miller et al., in a review of the literature, found that poorly performed CBE (e.g., clinicians who fail to use a systematic search pattern) is widely prevalent.[14]

Mammography

Mammography, which utilizes X rays to study breast tissue, can be done as either a screening modality or a diagnostic test. A standard screening mammogram involves four images that are evaluated for changes that are suspicious of cancer, microcalcifications, distortions of the normal architecture of the breast, and any nonpalpable lesions. A diagnostic mammogram is utilized to further examine areas of concern that are seen on the screening mammogram. Mammography can often detect early-stage breast cancers for which treatment may be more effective and there is an increased likelihood of a cure. Numerous studies have shown that routine mammography reduces breast cancer mortality by 30% overall and by 20% in women age 40 to 49 years. It is estimated that mammography detects between 80% and 90% of breast cancers in asymptomatic women.[1,16,17]

There is debate regarding the point at which to initiate mammography screening and the frequency of such screening. Studies have indicated that the sensitivity of mammography is highest among women age 50 years and older who have reduced breast density due to increased fatty tissue within the breast and is lowest among women younger than 50 years due to increased breast density and possibly because of rapid tumor growth in women in this age group.[18] Based on this information, the U.S. Preventive Services Task Force issued new guidelines in 2009 recommending against routine mammography screening in women age 40 and 49 years and for biennial mammography screening for women between the ages of 50 and 74 years.[7] This is in contradiction to the current recommendations of the American College of Obstetricians and Gynecologists, the ACS, and other groups that recommend mammography be performed every 1 to 2 years between ages 40 and 49 years, and annually thereafter.[19]

Ultrasonography

Ultrasonography is used to examine breast tissue in younger women, to differentiate between solid and cystic breast masses, and to guide core-needle biopsies. The performance of this test is not affected by breast density. The American College of Radiology Imaging Network's randomized trial showed that adding ultrasound to mammography screening in high-risk women with dense breasts improved the sensitivity of the screening, but also increased the rate of false-positive examinations.[20] Women who are at high risk for breast cancer most likely are more fearful of a delayed diagnosis of breast cancer than of a false-positive result.[4]

Magnetic Resonance Imaging

Magnetic resonance imaging (MRI) is the most sensitive test for breast cancer. Nevertheless, due to its high expense, it is recommended only for testing of women who are at very high risk for breast cancer such as those who are positive for the *BRCA* gene mutation. MRI is recommended for use in conjunction with mammography as indicated.

Evaluation of Breast Symptoms

The missed diagnosis of breast cancer is a frequent cause of malpractice claims. A systematic approach to breast examination is important to evaluate breast-related complaints.

History

The purpose of the history when evaluating a woman with breast symptoms is to both learn about the symptoms and assess her risk factors for breast cancer.[21] A number of factors have been identified that increase the risk for breast cancer (**Table 14-1**). The majority of women who develop breast cancer (85%), however, have no identifiable risk factors other than their gender and their age.[4] When evaluating a woman for any breast symptoms or pain, risk factors that increase her risk for breast cancer as well as factors that decrease her risk for breast cancer should be reviewed and documented in her medical record.

In addition to risks for breast cancer, the history of presenting symptoms should always include the items noted in **Box 14-1**. Each of the answers to these items should also be documented in the record of the woman's visit.

Physical Examination

The clinical examination should include examination of the neck, breasts, chest wall and axillae. The technique for examination of the breast is detailed in the *Breast Examination* appendix in the chapter titled *An Introduction to the Care of Women*. A full physical examination may also be indicated.

Breast findings characteristic of nonmalignant breast disorders include painful or tender, firm, mobile, well-defined masses that may fluctuate in size and tenderness with menstrual cycle changes. A breast mass is considered a dominant mass if it is a three-dimensional lesion that cannot be replicated in the same location on the other breast. The classic sign of a breast lesion suspicious for breast cancer is a hard, rocky, immobile mass with irregular or ill-defined borders.

Management

Physical examination findings do not distinguish well between malignant and non-malignant masses. A palpable mass should be evaluated with a diagnostic mammogram, ultrasound, or fine needle biopsy. One can find several different algorithms for evaluation of dominant breast masses.[20–22] Some recommend a fine needle biopsy as the first step and others recommend ultrasound or mammography first. Variations depend

Table 14-1	Risk Factors for Breast Cancer
Risk Factor	**Increases Risk for Breast Cancer**
Age	Older than 65 years
Gender	Female
Family history	First-degree relative with breast cancer at an early age
	Male breast cancer
	First-degree relative with ovarian cancer
	Multiple relatives with cancer
Reproductive history	Early menarche before age 12 years
	Nulliparity
	Older than 30 years when first gave birth
	Late onset of menopause after age 55 years
Prior biopsies	Increased number of biopsies is associated with an increased risk
	Prior biopsies showing atypical ductal hyperplasia, atypical lobular hyperplasia, or lobular carcinoma in situ
Past medical history	High-dose radiation to chest
	Never breastfed
	Previous cancer of the endometrium, ovary, or colon
	High bone density if postmenopausal
	Inherited mutations
Medications	Hormone replacement therapy with estrogen and progesterone for 5 to 9 years of use[a]
Lifestyle factors	Alcohol consumption 2–5 drinks per day
Physical examination	High breast density if postmenopausal
	Postmenopausal obesity

[a]The increased risk of breast cancer is no longer present if there has been more than 5 years since discontinuation of hormone replacement therapy.

on local radiology, pathology and surgical resources, the woman's age, and her preferences. Ultrasound is generally recommended for women younger than age 30 years and diagnostic mammography for women older than 30 years because the increased density of breast tissue in younger women tends to obscure abnormal findings from mammography.

Documentation

The location of the woman's breast symptoms should be documented. Any masses should described as dominant or nondominant and measured in centimeters when possible. The location, consistency, symmetry, and mobility should be recorded. The location may be recorded as distance in centimeters from the areola and by comparing the breast to a clock so that the "o'clock" location can also be noted (e.g., a 2 × 3 cm firm, discrete, smooth, mobile, nontender mass 3 cm from the areola at the 4 o'clock position). Negative findings should also be documented in the medical record.

Benign Breast Disorders

Benign breast disorders are a common diagnosis in women's health and encompass all nonmalignant conditions of the breast, including benign tumors, breast pain (i.e., mastalgia), and nipple discharge. Benign breast disorders are classified as nonproliferative, proliferative without atypia, or atypical hyperplasias. The risk of malignancy is related to the classification. Nonproliferative disorders, which include fibrocystic changes and breast cysts, are not associated with a risk of malignancy. Proliferative without atypia disorders, which include fibroadenomas and intraductal papillomas, are associated with a modest increase in risk for malignancy. Atypical ductal hyperplasia and atypical lobular hyperplasia are associated with a significant increased risk for malignancy.[21] The most common benign disorders are fibrocystic changes, breast cysts, and fibroadenomas.

Fibrocystic Changes

Fibrocystic changes (previously called fibrocystic disease) are commonly seen in the breast and are associated with hormonal stimulation. Fibrocystic changes are rare in postmenopausal women. These changes may be asymptomatic or associated with pain, tenderness, and lumpy areas throughout the breast tissue that fluctuate with the menstrual cycle. Clinical findings include symmetrical nodularity, with nodularity being more prominent in the upper outer region of the breast, and consistency described as like a "bag of beans." The fibrous tissue may feel firm or rubbery but not rock hard. The cystic portion may feel like grapes. Management can include aspiration of large or painful cysts and combined oral contraceptives to decrease the risk of developing fibrocystic breast changes. There is minimal evidence to suggest that change in dietary practices, the use of vitamins (e.g., vitamin E) or herbal preparations (e.g., evening primrose), or avoidance of methylxanthines decreases the symptomology associated with fibrocystic changes. There is no evidence that fibrocystic changes increase the risk for developing breast cancer.[21,22]

Breast Cysts

Breast cysts are smooth, round or oval, mobile, fluid filled masses with well-described borders that are derived from terminal breast lobules. Breast cysts may be single or a multiple cluster of small cysts and painful, tender, or painless. They are hormonally influenced and typically appear during menstrual changes in premenopausal or perimenopausal women.

Breast cysts are classified as simple, complex, or complicated depending on ultrasonographic findings of the thickness of the cyst wall and presence of echogenic material within the cyst. The risk of malignancy in simple and complicated cysts is rare, but there is a risk of malignancy in complex cysts that ranges from 1% to 23%. The wide range is presumed to be secondary to variation in interpretation of ultrasound findings and difficulties in the ability of the ultrasound technology to identify breast cancer.

Simple cysts can be diagnosed via ultrasound or fine needle biopsy that reveals non-bloody fluid and results in disappearance of the cyst. Because the risk of malignancy is very low, a simple cyst generally does not need additional evaluation or follow-up, although it can be aspirated if it is very large or painful. Some authors recommend a follow-up clinical examination or ultrasound in 2 to 4 months to document that the cyst has not changed.

The differential diagnosis for complex and complicated cysts is more extensive and includes abscess, breast cancer, hematoma, fat necrosis, and galacto-cele. These cysts need a fine needle biopsy, core bi-opsy, or excisional biopsy to establish the diagnosis.

Fibroadenoma

Fibroadenomas are common breast masses that are seen most frequently in adolescent and young women, although they may occur until menopause. These masses tend to be solitary, although multiple fibroadenomas occur in 10% to 15% of women who have fibroadenomas. On examination, the tumors are nontender, firm or rubbery consistency, mobile, and well circumscribed. The majority are solitary masses. Mammogram or ultrasound will determine whether the mass is solid or fluid-filled (cystic), al-though the diagnosis is confirmed through either core needle or open biopsy. It is not appropriate to make a diagnosis on the basis of the clinical examination only. If the biopsy indicates that the tumor is a fibro-adenoma, it does not need to be removed. The tumor can be followed clinically and only removed if it be-comes enlarged or visibly distorts the breast. If the pathology is unclear, the tumor should be surgically excised.[22] Fibroadenomas can increase rapidly during pregnancy or estrogen therapy and may regress after menopause. Fibroadenomas are not associated with an increased risk of breast cancer.

Atypical Hyperplasia and Lobular Carcinoma In Situ

Atypical hyperplasia includes atypical ductal hyper-plasia and atypical lobular hyperplasia. Both are often incidental findings from a core needle biopsy that is performed as part of the evaluation of another breast mass. Atypical hyperplasia is a pathologic diagnosis that describes abnormal cells of the breast that are associated with an increased risk of breast cancer. This condition is generally treated with surgery (e.g., wide-excision biopsy or lumpectomy) to remove all the affected tissue. More frequent screening for breast cancer (e.g., mammograms) and strategies to reduce breast cancer risk (e.g., preventive medications such as tamoxifen [Nolvadex] or raloxifene [Evista]; **Table 14-2**) may be recommended as well.[25]

Table 14-2	Selected Adjuvant/Preventive Therapies		
Agent	**Brand Name**	**Route**	**Side Effects and Toxicities**
Antiestrogens			
Tamoxifen	Nolvadex	Oral	The most common side effects are hot flashes, fluid retention, vaginal discharge, nausea, vomiting, and irregular vaginal bleeding. Increased risk of thromboembolic events (e.g., deep vein thrombosis, pulmonary embolism, and stroke) also exists. Tamoxifen acts as an estrogen agonist in the uterus, increasing the risk for endometrial cancer.
Raloxifene	Evista	Oral	Side effects are similar to tamoxifen, although raloxifene does not increase the risk for endometrial cancer.
Aromatase Inhibitors			These drugs have a low incidence of serious short-term side effects. They are not associated with an increased risk of endometrial cancer or thromboembolism.
Anastrozole	Arimidex	Oral	The most common side effects associated with anastrozole are hot flashes, vaginal dryness, musculoskeletal pain, and headache, but they are usually mild.
Letrozole	Femara	Oral	Most common side effects are musculoskeletal pain and nausea.
Exemestane	Aromasin	Oral	Most common side effects are fatigue, nausea, hot flushes, depression, and weight gain.
Monoclonal Antibody			
Trastuzumab	Herceptin	Intravenous	The major concern with this drug is cardiac damage that can lead to ventricular dysfunction and congestive heart failure. Many persons experience flu-like symptoms during the first infusion. Infrequently, patients may have a serious hypersensitivity reaction. Trastuzumab does not cause bone marrow suppression or hair loss.

Lobular carcinoma in situ (LCIS) is also a histologic finding diagnosed when a biopsy is conducted for another breast condition associated with an increased risk for breast cancer. There are no breast masses associated with LCIS and because it is not a precursor lesion for breast cancer, complete excision is not indicated. Increased surveillance for breast cancer and the medication tamoxifen (Nolvadex) is generally recommended.

Nipple Discharge

Nipple discharge is common in reproductive age women and generally benign, although 10% to 15% of women with nipple discharge do have breast cancer.[24] The primary differential diagnosis of nipple discharge is to differentiate that which is benign versus that which is pathologic. Benign discharge is generally bilateral, milky or green in color, and occurs with breast manipulation. Bilateral milky nipple discharge may occur with both pregnancy and lactation and may continue for as long as 1 year after giving birth or cessation of breastfeeding. Discharge that is unilateral, clear, serous, or bloody, and occurs spontaneously is more likely to be associated with cancer especially when it occurs in conjunction with a breast mass and in women who are older than 40 years.

Galactorrhea is defined as bilateral discharge that occurs in women who have not been pregnant or lactating within the last 12 months and is not caused by breast disease. Most often galactorrhea is idiopathic, but it can be associated with prolactin-secreting pituitary adenomas, medications that inhibit dopamine (e.g., some psychotropic medications, combined oral contraceptives, metoclopramide [Reglan], phenothiazines), hypothyroidism, breast stimulation, trauma, and herpes zoster.

Uniductal, bloody discharge may be associated with intraductal papilloma, a benign tumor of the lactiferous ducts that is generally managed with surgical excision. With unilateral, uniductal, spontaneous, and clear, serous, or bloody discharge, a diagnostic mammogram and ultrasound and indicated.[21]

Mastalgia

Mastalgia (breast pain) can be either cyclic or noncyclic. Cyclic breast pain generally occurs bilaterally during the luteal phase of the menstrual cycle and resolves after the onset of menses. It is often described as sharp, shooting, or deep aching and throbbing pain. Noncyclic breast pain may be caused by mastitis, cysts, tumors, history of breast surgery, or medications, or it may be idiopathic. Noncyclic mastalgia tends to be localized, sub-areolar or medial and characterized as tender, burning, stabbing, pulling, or pinching.

Approximately 15% of women with mastalgia require some pain-relieving therapy. Well-fitting bras may relieve some cyclical and noncyclical mastalgia. Both evening primrose oil and flaxseed have been evaluated for treatment of mastalgia. Evening primrose oil has not been shown to be effective but flaxseed is recommended as a first-line treatment for cyclical mastalgia. Reduction of caffeine has not been shown to be of value in several randomized trials and therefore, women should not be counseled to decrease caffeine for this purpose. Vitamin E, 600 units/day, has been associated with significant improvement with minimal side effects.

Danazol (Danocrine) 100–200 mg/day has been shown to relieve breast pain but is associated with significant side effects such as depression, acne, and hirsutism. Danazol can also interfere with oral contraceptive effectiveness so that women using combined oral contraceptives should also use another form of birth control if taking danazol. Bromocriptine (Parlodel) at 2.5 mg/day and low-dose tamoxifen (Nolvadex) at 10 or 20 mg/daily are also effective for treating breast pain. Low-dose tamoxifen is associated with fewer side effects and should be considered the drug of first choice if non-pharmacologic approaches are not sufficient, although tamoxifen is not FDA approved for treatment of mastalgia.[4,25] Tamoxifen is associated with an increase in endometrial cancer if taken for longer than 5 years by women who have had breast cancer. This adverse effect has not been found in women taking low-dose tamoxifen for up to 6 months.

Breast Cancer

The American Cancer Society estimated that 226,870 new cases of invasive breast cancer and 63,300 new cases of in situ breast cancer would occur in the United States during 2012, with an estimated 39,920 breast cancer deaths occurring during this same time period. The good news is that between 2004 and 2008 there was a 3.1% per year decrease in the death rate for breast cancer in women younger than 50 years and a 2.1% per year decrease in women 50 years and older. These improvements in the death rates are attributed to earlier detection and improved treatment modalities.[1]

Factors That Increase or Decrease Breast Cancer Risk

The National Cancer Institute has an Internet site that can be used to calculate the risk for an individual woman (see the Additional Resources list at the end of this chapter). The variables that are used to calculate this risk include a history of ductal carcinoma in situ or lobular carcinoma in situ, current age, age at menarche, age at first live birth, number of previous breast biopsies, number of first-degree relatives with breast cancer, and the woman's race/ethnicity.[26,27]

Although most women with breast cancer do not have a family history of the disease, approximately 5% to 10% have inherited gene mutations that place them at increased risk for developing this disease. Most of these mutations are located on the *BRCA1* and *BRCA2* genes (genes that are associated with tumor suppression). These gene mutations also place the individual at increased risk for ovarian cancer. Women who have a strong family history of breast cancer or ovarian cancer should consider genetic counseling to decide whether genetic testing is indicated. Knowing her genetic status may allow the woman to seek out preventive measures such as prophylactic removal of the breasts and/or ovaries or the use of medications (e.g., tamoxifen, raloxifene, aromatase inhibitors) to lower her risk for breast cancer.

According to the National Cancer Institute's Surveillance, Epidemiology, and End Results (SEER) survey, African American women have a lower incidence of breast cancer but have a higher risk of breast cancer recurrence as well as increased mortality from breast cancer when compared to white women.[28]

A meta-analysis of prospective studies regarding soy isoflavones consumption and risk of breast cancer suggests that soy isoflavones intake is associated with a significant reduction in the risk of breast cancer in Asian populations, but not in Western populations—although further studies are needed to confirm this finding.[29]

Other factors that may be associated with lowering the risk of breast cancer include breastfeeding, 3 to 5 hours of moderate to vigorous physical exercise per week,[30] limiting alcohol intake, and maintaining a healthy body weight.[31–33]

Diagnosis/Staging

The definitive diagnosis of breast cancer is generally made through tissue sampling. This can be accomplished through fine-needle aspiration, mammography- or ultrasound-guided core needle biopsy, or excisional breast biopsy. The tissue is then sent for histologic examination. If cancer is present, the report will state whether the tumor is ductal or lobular in origin. The physical examination, while not definitive, can identify suspicious lesions. Suspicious lesions are usually firm or hard to palpation, have irregular borders, are painless, tend to be fixed to

surrounding tissue, and may be associated with enlarged axillary or supraclavicular lymph nodes, or skin changes.

Once the diagnosis of cancer has been made, it is also necessary to assess the lungs, abdomen, brain, and bone for metastasis. Once breast cancer has been diagnosed, the malignancy is staged using the TNM system (**Table 14-3** and **Table 14-4**), which describes characteristics of the tumor, involvement of regional lymph nodes, and presence or absence of distant metastasis. Staging is helpful as a guide to determine appropriate therapy options.

An essential component of staging is investigation of the axillary nodes. In women with Stage I or II breast cancer, sentinel lymph node biopsy is performed. This is accomplished by injection of radioisotope dye into the breast tissue surrounding the cancer site in order to locate the axillary node to which the dye initially spreads. The tissue from this node is then examined intraoperatively for cancer cells. If the sentinel node is positive for breast

Table 14-3	Breast Cancer Staging Terminology: TNM System[a]
	The T category describes the original (primary) tumor.
TX	Primary tumor cannot be evaluated
T0	No evidence of primary tumor
Tis	Carcinoma in situ (early cancer that has not spread to neighboring tissue)
T1–T4	Size and/or extent of the primary tumor

The N category describes whether the cancer has reached nearby lymph nodes.

NX	Regional lymph nodes cannot be evaluated
N0	No regional lymph node involvement (no cancer found in the lymph nodes)
N1-N3	Involvement of regional lymph nodes (number and/or extent of spread)

The M category tells whether there are distant metastases (spread of cancer to other parts of the body).

M0	No distant metastasis (cancer has not spread to other parts of the body)
M1	Distant metastasis (cancer has spread to distant parts of the body)

[a]Each cancer type has its own classification system, so letters and numbers do not always mean the same thing for every type of cancer.

Source: Edge, SB, Byrd DR, Compton CC, eds. *AJCC Cancer Staging Manual.* 7th ed. New York, NY.: Springer, 2010. Used with permission of the American Joint Committee on Cancer (AJCC), Chicago, Illinois. The original source for this material is the *AJCC Cancer Staging Manual, Seventh Edition* (2010) published by Springer Science and Business Media LLL, www.springer.com.

Table 14-4	Breast Cancer Staging		
Stage	**Primary Tumor**	**Nodes**	**Metastases**
Noninvasive			
Stage 0 (DCIS and LCIS)	In situ (Tis)	No regional node metastasis (N0)	No distant metastases
Early Invasive			
Stage IA	Tumor ≤ 20 mm in greatest dimension (T1)	No regional node metastasis (N0)	No distant metastases
Stage IB	No primary tumor (T0) or T1	Micrometastasis (none greater than 2.0 mm) (N1 mi)	
Stage IIA	T0 or T1 or tumor > 20 mm but ≤ 50 mm (T2)	Metastasis in up to 1–3 axillary or internal mammary lymph nodes (N1)	
Stage IIB	T2 or tumor > 50 mm (T3)	N0 or N1	
Locally Advanced Invasive			
Stage IIIA	T0–T3 (tumor of any size)	N0, N1, or metastasis in 4–9 axillary or internal mammary lymph nodes (N2)	No distant metastases
Stage IIIB	Tumor of any size with direct extension to chest wall and/or to skin (T4)	N0–N2	
Metastatic stage IV	Any size tumor	Any configuration of local node metastasis	Distant metastasis present

Abbreviations: T describes the original primary tumor, N describes whether the cancer has reached nearby lymph nodes, and M tells whether there is distant metastasis.

Source: Edge, SB, Byrd DR, Compton CC, eds. *AJCC Cancer Staging Manual.* 7th ed. New York, NY.: Springer, 2010. Used with permission of the American Joint Committee on Cancer (AJCC), Chicago, Illinois. The original source for this material is the *AJCC Cancer Staging Manual, Seventh Edition* (2010) published by Springer Science and Business Media LLL, www.springer.com.

cancer, additional axillary nodes will be removed for evaluation. If the staging indicates greater than Stage II cancer, an axillary node dissection of at least 10 nodes from the first two levels of lymph drainage in the breast is indicated.

In addition to staging, receptor status of the tumor is assessed. This evaluation provides information for treatment options and serves an indicator of breast cancer prognosis. For example, the presence of estrogen and progesterone receptors improves prognosis, whereas over-expression of the growth factor receptor coded by the oncogene *Her2/neu* confers a poorer prognosis.[34,35]

Treatment

Breast cancer treatment usually involves surgery that may be followed with radiation therapy, chemotherapy, hormonal therapy, or immunotherapy. Radiation therapy or systemic therapies can be administered prior to surgery (neoadjuvant) with the goal of shrinking the tumor size, or they may be administered after surgery (adjuvant) with the goal of preventing cancer recurrence. Systemic therapy for breast cancer can also be used for palliation of symptoms.

Most women with Stage I and Stage II breast cancers can be managed with breast-conserving surgery (lumpectomy) and sentinel node dissection, generally followed by radiation therapy. Breast-conserving surgery is contraindicated for women who have more advanced disease, those who have received previous radiation therapy, women who are pregnant (radiation is contraindicated), and women who have two or more primary tumors in separate quadrants of the breast or diffuse malignant-appearing microcalcifications. A history of collagen vascular disease (e.g., scleroderma or lupus) is a relative contraindication for breast conservation treatment, as reports indicate that women with these diseases do not tolerate radiation.[36]

Mastectomy involves removal of the breast tissue and the nipple–areolar complex, with conservation of the pectoralis muscle, as well as sentinel lymph node dissection. Many women who are diagnosed with breast cancer are concerned about developing cancer in the contralateral breast and, therefore, request contralateral prophylactic mastectomy. The actual risk of developing contralateral breast cancer in the general population is extremely low (annual risk is 0.1% to 0.75%), so current breast cancer treatment guidelines strongly discourage this practice. However, women who are carriers of the *BRCA1/BRCA2* gene mutations have a 40% estimated 10-year risk of contralateral breast cancer; thus contralateral prophylactic mastectomy may be recommended for these women, although the benefit of contralateral prophylactic mastectomy when compared to conventional annual screening in this population is currently unclear.[37]

According to the Early Breast Cancer Trialists' Collaborative Group (EBCTCG), radiation therapy after breast-conserving surgery reduces the recurrence rate for breast cancer by 50% and the breast cancer death rate by 16.7%.[38] Radiation is used with mastectomy only for late-stage breast cancers. In women with breast cancer who have axillary lymph node involvement, studies have shown that irradiation of the regional lymph nodes increases both disease-free years and survival years. Women need to be educated regarding both the short-term (skin rashes and redness) and long-term side effects of radiation therapy (damage to the heart, lungs, or blood vessels in the chest; development of lung cancer; and osteoradionecrosis).

Adjuvant (systemic) therapy is used to treat all stages of breast cancer and includes chemotherapeutic agents, hormonal therapies that are estrogen antagonists (e.g., tamoxifen, aromatase inhibitors) for cancer that is estrogen receptor positive, and immunotherapy (e.g., trastuzumab, a monoclonal antibody) for cancer that is found to overexpress the Her2/neu protein. All of these therapies are associated with a number of side effects. When considering the use of chemotherapeutic agents, it is important that the woman understands the associated side effects as well as her treatment options (**Table 14-5**). Approximately 4% of women who take trastuzumab (Herceptin) will develop ventricular dysfunction and congestive heart failure.[4]

Breast reconstruction should be an option for all women. Several methods of reconstruction include insertion of an implant under the pectoralis muscle, accompanied by tissue flap procedures where tissue from the lower abdomen, back, buttocks, or thighs (e.g., transverse rectus abdominis muscle [TRAM]; latissimus dorsi) is used to rebuild the breast. The reconstruction can be performed immediately post mastectomy or at a later time. It is important for

Table 14-5	Management of Common Side Effects of Chemotherapy
Side Effect	**Management**
Fatigue	Methylphenidate (Ritalin)
	Erythropoietin
Anemia	Iron supplementation
	Blood transfusion
	Erythropoiesis-stimulating drug (Procrit, Epogen)[a]
Neutropenia	Avoiding contact with individuals who are sick or who are at risk for infection (e.g., school children)
	Agents that stimulate the production of neutrophils (Neupogen, Neulasta)
Nausea and vomiting	Small, frequent meals
	Stay well hydrated
	Avoid nausea triggers (unpleasant smell)
	Rest after eating
	Relaxation techniques
	Antiemetic drugs (e.g., ondansetron [Zofran], metoclopramide [Reglan], dexamethasone [Decadron])
Mucositis	Cold liquids and ice chips
	2% viscous lidocaine
	50/50 attapulgite/diphenhydramine (Kaopectate/Benadryl)
	Systemic analgesics
Diarrhea	Loperamide (Imodium)
	Octreotide (Sandostatin)
Constipation	Psyllium (Metamucil)
	Senna (SenoKot)
	Docusate sodium (Colace)
	Bisacodyl (Dulcolax)

[a]The FDA has issued a black-box warning that states recent studies have found that these drugs increase the risk of thromboembolic disease and may promote tumor growth.

Source: Adapted from Carlson N, King J. Overview of breast cancer treatment and reconstruction for primary care providers. *J Midwifery Women's Health.* 2012;57(6):558-568. Reprinted with permission of Wiley.

the woman to understand that reconstructive surgery does not impact recurrence of the breast cancer or overall survival.

Treatment During Pregnancy

Treatment options for breast cancer during pregnancy are the same as for nonpregnant women, except for radiation therapy, which is considered to be unsafe for the embryo/fetus throughout all stages of gestation. It is also recommended that chemotherapy be delayed until after the first trimester of pregnancy due to an increase in spontaneous miscarriages as well as a possible increase in the risk for major fetal malformations secondary to exposure to chemotherapeutic agents. Chemotherapy in the second and third trimesters, while not associated with major malformations, may cause fetal growth restriction. Termination of pregnancy does not improve survival rates and is generally not recommended.[35]

Follow-up

For the first 2 years after breast cancer treatment is completed, follow-up appointments generally occur after 3 to 6 months and include physical examination and mammography. Routine laboratory evaluation for metastasis (e.g., liver function tests, bone scans) is not recommended unless specifically indicated clinically.[39] Ovarian dysfunction is common in women of reproductive age and reflects their age, ovarian function at the time of treatment, and the specific chemotherapy agents that used. One study observed that 83.1% of women between the ages of 18 and 34 years resumed menstruating, on average, 3.5 months following breast cancer treatment; therefore a discussion regarding contraception is merited.[40]

Contraception Following Breast Cancer

According to the U.S. Medical Eligibility Criteria, hormonal contraception is contraindicated for women with current or a past history of breast cancer. Copper-containing intrauterine devices, tubal ligation, or vasectomy are considered to be better contraceptive options for women with a history of breast cancer.[41]

The safety of estrogen-containing hormone therapy for menopausal symptoms in women with a history of breast cancer is not well established. Nonhormonal treatments, such as selective serotonin reuptake inhibitors or gabapentin (Neurontin), are effective alternative options for the treatment of vasomotor symptoms. Vaginal estrogens are effective for the treatment of atrophic vaginitis, although few data have been published on the safety of these medications in women with a history of breast cancer.[42]

Breast Masses During Pregnancy and Lactation

The same breast disorders that occur in nonpregnant women can also be present during pregnancy. However the breast examination can be more difficult when examining a pregnant woman secondary to engorgement and proliferation of breast tissue. Thus, small breast masses are more difficult to detect. Fibroadenomas can grow during pregnancy and occasionally they infarct and become painful. In addition, there are a few benign lesions that are unique in pregnancy and lactating women. The most common of these are lactational adenomas, galactoceles, mastitis and breast abscess. The diagnosis and management of mastitis and breast abscess is reviewed in the *Breastfeeding and the Mother–Newborn Dyad* chapter.

Lactational adenomas usually occur during the third trimester or during lactation.[43] These breast masses are similar to fibroadenomas in that they are painless, soft mobile masses. A lactational adenoma may appear as a fibroadenoma on ultrasound. These masses are not associated with an increased risk for malignancy.

A galactocele is a distended mammary duct with milk retention (milk retention cyst). Galactoceles usually present after cessation of breastfeeding.[43] They are usually round, soft, painless mass that may be associated with nipple discharge. Risk factors for galactocele include poor latch and abrupt cessation of breastfeeding. They usually regress spontaneously and do not require aspiration.

Conclusion

Midwives are in the unique position to ensure appropriate breast cancer screening for all women. The midwife may be the first person whom a woman consults for breast-related concerns. The midwife is also an important member of the multidisciplinary team caring for a woman with the diagnosis of breast cancer, and fulfills this role by providing accurate information and support as the woman is making decisions regarding breast cancer treatment, including reconstructive surgical options.

• • • References

1. American Cancer Society. *Cancer Facts and Figures 2012*. Atlanta, GA: American Cancer Society; 2012.

2. Jemal A, Siegel R, Ward E, et al. Cancer statistics, 2009. *CA Cancer J Clin*. 2009;59(4):225-249.

3. Carswell JM, Stafford DEJ. Normal physical growth and development. In: Neinstein LS, ed. *Adolescent Health Care*. 5th ed. Philadelphia: Wolters Kluwer/Lippincott Williams & Wilkins; 2008:3.

4. Fritz MA, Speroff L. The breast. In: Fritz MA, Speroff L, eds. *Clinical Gynecologic Endocrinology and Infertility*. 8th ed. Philadelphia: Wolters Kluwer/Lippincott Williams & Wilkins; 2011:621-673.

5. Dickson, G. Gynecomastia. *Am Fam Physician*. 2012; 85(7):716-722.

6. Beckmann CRB, Ling FW, Barzansky BM, Herbert WNP, Lube DW, Smith RP. Postpartum care. In Beckmann CRB, Ling FW, Barzansky BM, Herbert WNP, Laube DW, Smith RP, eds. *Obstetrics and Gynecology*. 6th ed. Philadelphia: Wolters Kluwer/ Lippincott Williams & Wilkins; 2010:129.

7. U.S. Preventive Services Task Force. Screening for breast cancer: U.S. Preventive Services Task Force Recommendation Statement. *Ann Intern Med*. 2009; 151(10):716-726.

8. Semiglazov VF, Sagaidak VN, Moiseyenko VM, Mikhailov EA. Study of the role of breast self-examination in the reduction of mortality from breast cancer. *Eur J Cancer*. 1993;29A:2039-2046.

9. Thomas DB, Gao DL, Self SG, et al. Randomized trial of breast self-examination in Shanghai: methodology and preliminary results. *J Natl Cancer Inst*. 1997;89:355-365.

10. Harvey BJ, Miller AB, Baines CJ, Corey, PN. Effect of breast self-examination techniques on the risk of death from breast cancer. *Can Med Assoc J*. 1997; 157(9):1205-1212.

11. Ma I, Dueck A, Gray R, et al. Clinical and self breast examination remain important in the era of modern screening. *Ann Surg Oncol*. 2012;19:1484-1490.

12. Wilke LG, Broadwater G, Rabiner S, et al. Breast self-examination: defining a cohort still in need. *Am J Surg*. 2009;198(4):575-579.

13. American Cancer Society. Breast cancer: early detection. Available at: http://www.cancer.org/cancer/breast cancer/moreinformation/breastcancerearlydetection /breast-cancer-early-detection-toc. Accessed October 14, 2012.

14. Miller AB, Baines CJ. The role of clinical breast examination and breast self-examination. *Prevent Med*. 2011;3:118-120.

15. Gui GPH, Hogben RKF, Walsh G, A'Hern R, Eeles R. The incidence of breast cancer from screening women according to predicted family history risk: does annual clinical examination add to mammography? *Eur J Cancer*. 2001;37:1668-1673.

16. Humphrey LL, Helfand M, Chan BK, Woolfe SH. Breast cancer screening: a summary of the evidence for the US Preventive Services Task Force. *Ann Intern Med*. 2002;137(5 part1):347-360.

17. Berry DA, Cronin KA, Plevritis SK, et al. Effect of screening and adjuvant therapy on mortality from breast cancer. *N Engl J Med*. 2005;353:1784-1792.

18. Kerlkiowske K, Grady D, Barclay J, Sickles EA, Ernster V. Effect of age, breast density, and family history on the sensitivity of first screening mammography. *JAMA*. 1996;276(1):33-38.

19. Gemignani ML. The new mammographic screening guidelines: what were they thinking? *Obstet Gynecol*. 2010;115(3):484-486.

20. Berg WA, Blume JD, Cormack JB, et al. Combined screening with ultrasound and mammography vs mammography alone in women at elevated risk of breast cancer. *JAMA*. 2008;299(18):2151-2163.

21. Pearlman MD, Griffin JL. Benign breast disease. *Obstet Gynecol*. 2010;116(3):747-758.

22. Milten DM, Speights VO. Benign breast disease. *Obstet Gynecol Clin North Am*. 2008;5(2):285-300.

23. Srivastava A, Mansel RE, Arvind N, Prasad K, Dhar A, Chabra A. Evidence-based management of mastalgia: a meta-analysis of randomized trials. *Breast*. 2007;16:503-512.

24. Degnim AC, Visscher DW, Berman HK, et al. Stratification of breast cancer risk in women with atypia: a Mayo cohort study. *J Clin Oncol*. 2007; 25(10):2671-2677.

25. Hussain AN, Policarpio C, Vincent MT. Evaluating nipple discharge. *Obstet Gynecol Surv*. 2006;61(4): 278-283.

26. Gail MH, Brinton LA, Byar DP, et al. Projecting individualized probabilities of developing breast cancer for white females who are being examined annually. *J Natl Cancer Inst*. 1989;81:1879-1886.

27. Gail MH, Costantino JP, Pee D, et al. Projecting individualized absolute invasive breast cancer risk in African American women. *J Natl Cancer Inst*. 2007; 99(23):1782-1791.

28. Christiansen N, Chen L, Gilmore J, Pechar D, Szabo S. Association between African American race and outcomes in patients with nonmetastatic triple-negative breast cancer: a retrospective analysis by using results from the Georgia Cancer Specialist Database. *Clin Breast Cancer*. 2012;12(4):270-275.

29. Dong JY, Qin L. Soy isoflavones consumption and risk of breast cancer incidence or recurrence: a meta-analysis of prospective studies. *Breast Cancer Res Treat*. 2011;25:315-323.

30. Magne N, Melis A, Chargari C, et al. Recommendations for a lifestyle which could prevent breast cancer and its relapse: physical activity and dietetic aspects. *Crit Rev Oncol Hematol*. 2011;80:450-459.

31. Patterson RE, Cadmus LA, Emond JA, Pierce JP. Physical activity, diet, adiposity and female breast cancer prognosis: a review of the epidemiologic literature. *Maturitas*. 2010;66:5-15.

32. Chen WY, Rosner B, Hankinson SE, Colditz GA, Willett WC. Moderate alcohol consumption during

adult life, drinking patterns, and breast cancer risk. *JAMA*. 2011;306(17):1884-1890.

33. Kabat GC, Kim M, Phipps AI, et al. Smoking and alcohol consumption in relation to risk of triple-negative breast cancer in a cohort of postmenopausal women. *Cancer Causes Control*. 2011;22:775-783.

34. Yaziji H, Goldstein LC, Barry TS, et al. *HER-2* testing in breast cancer using parallel tissue-based methods. *JAMA*. 2004;291(16):1972-1977.

35. Carlson N, King J. Overview of breast cancer treatment and reconstruction for primary care providers. *J Midwifery Women's Health*. 2012;57(6):558-568.

36. Reszko A, Aasi SZ, Wilson LD, Leffett DJ. Cancers of the skin. In: DeVita VT, Lawrence TS, Rosenberg SA, eds. *Cancer: Principles and Practice of Oncology*. 8th ed. Philadelphia: Wolters Kluwer/Lippincott Williams & Wilkins; 2008:1624-1625.

37. Barry M, Sacchini V. When is contralateral mastectomy warranted in unilateral breast cancer? *Expert Rev Anticancer Ther*. 2011;11(8):1209-1214.

38. Darby S, McGale P, Correa C, et al. Effect of radiotherapy after breast-conserving surgery on 10-year recurrence and 15-year breast cancer death: meta-analysis of individual patient data for 10,801 women in 17 randomised trials. *Lancet*. 2011;378(9804): 1707-1716.

39. Rojas MP, Telaro E, Moschetti I, et al. Follow-up strategies for women treated for early breast cancer. *Cochrane Database Syst Rev*. 2005;CD001768.

40. Hickey M, Peate M, Saunders CM, et al. Breast cancer in young women and its impact on reproductive function. *Human Reprod Update*. 2009;15(3) 323-339.

41. Centers for Disease Control and Prevention. U.S. medical eligibility criteria for contraceptive use, 2010. *MMWR*. 2010;59:15, 39, 56.

42. King J, Smith L. Cancer. In: King TL, Brucker MC, eds. *Pharmacology for Women's Health*. Sudbury, MA: Jones and Bartlett; 2011:854-878.

43. Vashi R, Hooley R, Butler R, Geisel J, Phipotts L. Breast imaging of the pregnant and lactating patient: Physiologic changes and common benign entities. *AJR*. 2013;200:329-336

● ● ● **Additional Resources**

National Cancer Institute Breast Cancer Risk Tool
http://www.cancer.gov/bcrisktool

CHAPTER

15

Reproductive Tract and Sexually Transmitted Infections

JULIA C. PHILLIPPI

Introduction

A woman's overall well-being includes sexual and reproductive components. The healthy expression of sexuality and the ability to safely engage in sexual and reproductive behaviors is supported by national and international organizations such as the United Nations,[1] the World Health Organization (WHO),[2] and the *Healthy People* initiative in the United States.[3] Unfortunately, women across the globe continue to struggle to obtain services to improve their sexual and reproductive health. Midwives are ideal care providers for women's sexual health needs, which include screening, diagnosis, and treatment of infections in women and their partners.[4] This chapter reviews midwifery care for women with reproductive tract and sexually transmitted infections.

A broad range of terms have been used to describe conditions that are transmitted through sexual contact. Many of these terms, including *venereal disease*, may have connotations of judgment or shame related to their use with public health campaigns designed to decrease infections. To avoid these negative stereotypes, the term *sexually transmitted disease* became more commonly used, and is the current term of choice of the Centers for Disease Control and Prevention (CDC). However, the term *sexually transmitted infection* (STI) is more precise, as not all sexually transmitted pathogens have immediate disease manifestations. The term "sexually transmitted infections" will be used throughout this chapter for precision and clarity.

STIs impact health across the lifespan with both wide-ranging and persistent effects. According to WHO, more than 448 million cases of curable STIs occur annually.[5] The CDC reports that 19 million new STI infections occur each year in the United States, with an immediate cost of more than $17 billion. While immediate costs are easy to calculate, the long-term costs of STIs may be much higher, as STI infection is linked with pelvic inflammatory disease, infertility, ectopic pregnancy, and lifelong malformations and blindness in infants born to women who have an STI during pregnancy or at the time of birth.[6]

Women have a disproportionate health burden from STIs.[6] Compared to men, women are more likely to contract an STI from a single sexual encounter and are more likely to have long-term sequelae. In addition, women are often disproportionately stigmatized for STIs due to taboos surrounding female sexuality. Furthermore, accessing appropriate and affordable services related to STI care and prevention may be difficult for some women.

The prevalence of STIs varies by location and personal risk factors. The CDC monitors reportable diseases, such as chlamydia, gonorrhea, and syphilis. Current information on these conditions is maintained on the agency's website and is also available through its state-by-state interactive atlas.[7] The CDC also periodically publishes guidelines for diagnosis and treatment of STIs, which are useful for clinical practice in the United States. These guidelines can be downloaded to computers and mobile electronic devices; paper copies can also be ordered. In addition, the CDC makes available free mobile electronic device applications to assist clinicians in accessing guidelines quickly at the point of care.

The U.S. Preventive Services Task Force (USPSTF) also releases guidelines on STI screening based on current evidence. The USPSTF clinical practice guidelines are specific to individual STIs and can be accessed through the organization's website. In addition, the Agency for Healthcare Research and Quality (AHRQ) has a mobile electronic device application that displays the USPSTF-recommended STI screenings based on patient age and risk factors. It can be useful in translating the guidelines into practice.

Most states require healthcare providers to notify the local health department when a person is diagnosed with certain sexually transmitted diseases, as shown in **Box 15-1**. Notifiable diseases are those for which obtaining information regarding individual cases is important for prevention and control of that disease. Reporting usually involves revealing the patient name to the local health department and denoting whether the sexual partner was treated. The woman should be told that this report will take place. This information is used to notify and treat sexual partners and to monitor prevalence of STIs on local, state, and national levels.[8] While reporting infection is a requirement for clinicians, accessing partner services should be voluntary for the woman unless state or federal law specifically stipulates otherwise.[9] Partner services are a collection of services that include partner notification, prevention counseling, testing, and treatment. Federal law requires that the spouse (current or within the past 10 years) of a person who is positive for human immunodeficiency virus (HIV) be notified and the health department can assist in this endeavor. Midwives should be aware of laws concerning partner notification in their state or legal jurisdiction.

History and Physical Examination for Vaginal Symptoms and Sexually Transmitted Infections

Sexual History

An in-depth sexual history is important during well-woman care and problem-based visits, as it helps determine the woman's risk for infections and her need for screening and prevention. The woman is an essential partner in her health care, and listening to her concerns and history is one of the first steps in establishing a trusting relationship with her. It is important to be respectful when obtaining a sexual history. Likewise, it is important to obtain a thorough history. While striving to put the woman at ease, the clinician should not shy away from asking highly personal questions. It is crucial to know the extent of sexual contact with her partner and previous partners. For example, a vaginal test for gonorrhea would be useless if the woman has engaged in only anal or oral intercourse.

There are a variety of ways to approach a thorough sexual history. Some midwives begin with a paper form for the woman to complete as a guide for discussion and clarification, while others talk through the history with the woman. It is important to provide privacy to complete the forms and a private space for discussion. A woman may be less forthcoming when others are with her, especially parents or children. While she may want her family or friends nearby for support, it is ideal to speak with her alone at some point during her visit. When discussing sensitive topics, it helps if the clinician and the woman are seated on equal levels without anything blocking their vision. While taking note of key items that are discussed, the focus should be on the woman, rather than the chart or computer, during this conversation.

A guide for obtaining a sexual history can be found in **Box 15-2** and additional questions can be found in the *Collecting a Medical History* appendix to the *Introduction to the Care of Women* chapter. Ask about needed information without making assumptions about the woman's sexuality or beliefs. Remain open and engaged no matter what the woman reveals, using open- and closed-ended questions as needed. This is not the time for teaching or correction of poor health behaviors. Instead, focus on building rapport and obtaining the needed information to guide your assessment. Teaching will take place later in the visit.

BOX 15-1 Sexually Transmitted Infections Reportable for National Surveillance

- Chancroid
- Gonorrhea
- Hepatitis B
- Hepatitis B, perinatal infection
- Hepatitis C
- Human immunodeficiency virus (HIV)
- Syphilis
- Syphilis, congenital

Source: Centers for Disease Control and Prevention (CDC). List of notifiable conditions, historically by year 1993–2011. Available at: http://wwwn.cdc.gov/nndss /document/NNDSS_history_spreadsheet_2011_for_web _v3.pdf. Accessed November 11, 2012.

BOX 15-2 Obtaining a Sexual History: The Five Ps

---

1. Partners

- Do you have sex with men, women, or both?
- In the past 2 months, how many people have you had sexual contact with?
- Is it possible that any of your partners in the past 12 months had sex with someone else?

2. Prevention of Pregnancy

- What are you doing to prevent pregnancy?

3. Protection from STIs

- What do you use to protect yourself from STIs like HIV?

4. Practices

To understand your risk of STIs, I need to know the kind of sex you have had recently.

- Have you ever had oral sex, meaning mouth on penis or vagina sex? Do you use condoms never, sometimes, or always?
- Have you ever had vaginal sex, meaning penis in vagina sex? Do you use condoms never, sometimes, or always?
- Have you ever had anal sex, meaning penis in rectum/anus sex? Do you use condoms never, sometimes, or always?

5. Past History of STIs

- Have you ever had an STI?
- Has any of your partners ever had an STI?

Additional Questions

- Have you or any of your partners ever injected drugs?
- Have you or any of your partners ever exchanged money or drugs for sex, including oral sex?
- Is there anything else about your sexual practices that I need to know?

Source: Centers for Disease Control and Prevention (CDC). Sexually transmitted diseases treatment guidelines. *MMWR.* 2010;59(RR-12). Available at: http://www.cdc.gov/mmwr/pdf/rr/rr5912.pdf. Accessed November 11, 2012.

Problem-Focused Visit

Women may come to see the midwife with concerns about vaginitis or STIs. Ideally, these women will have already participated in a more comprehensive visit that included a complete history and physical exam. In these cases, a targeted but thorough history of the symptoms is important. Begin by asking the woman in an open and inviting tone the reason for her clinic visit. If a woman is embarrassed about her concern, she may have not been completely forthcoming with previous staff. Give her a chance to talk without interruption, as listening patiently establishes rapport and provides important information.

The chief concern should be used to generate a list of differential diagnoses. It is helpful to use a systematic method to assess the problem. Many clinicians use the OLDCARTS method to assess to Onset, Location, Duration, Character, Aggravating and Alleviating factors, Radiation, Timing, and Severity

of symptoms.[10] After exploring the woman's chief concern for the visit, query her about additional STI-related symptoms such as fever, sore throat, enlarged lymph nodes, sores in the mouth or genital area, dysuria, discharge, and dyspareunia.[11]

Physical Exam for Vaginitis and STIs

The physical exam for STIs includes evaluation of all systems that may be affected. These systems are included in a complete well-woman exam but are examined individually during a targeted physical exam. **Table 15-1** provides a list of important systems to include in a targeted examination if the woman or midwife has concerns about STIs. While looking closely for STIs, take a holistic approach to the examination and avoid ruling out non-STI-related diagnoses too soon. A comprehensive and gentle physical exam can reveal many non-infection-related abnormalities that may be causing symptoms. Although laboratory

Table 15-1	Physical Exam for Sexually Transmitted Infections	
Organ/System	**Abnormal Findings Related to STIs**
Mouth	Lesions, pharyngitis
Cervical lymph nodes/chains	Palpable lymph nodes, possibly painful
Abdominal palpation	Abdominal tenderness
Inguinal lymph nodes	Palpable lymph nodes, which may be fluctuant or draining
Inspection of the pubis	Parasites, lesions, excoriations
Vulva, vagina, and perineum	Lesions, warts, excoriations, edema, discharge
• Paraurethral (Skene's) glands	Enlarged glands, discharge on palpation
• Greater vestibular (Bartholin's) glands	Enlarged glands, discharge on palpation
• Urethra	Inflammation, swelling, discharge
Rectal area and anus	Lesions, warts, excoriations, signs of trauma
Speculum exam	
• Vaginal mucosa	Lesions, discharge, color, and character of vaginal walls
• Cervix	Overall appearance, lesions, discharge
• Obtain needed specimens	Wet mount, gonorrhea and chlamydia tests, cultures/testing of lesions
Bimanual exam	
• Uterus	Enlarged uterus could indicate pregnancy; tenderness is a symptom of PID
• Cervix	Cervical motion tenderness is a sign of PID
• Adnexa	Adnexal tenderness is a sign of PID and ectopic pregnancy
Urine testing as indicated (nitrites, leukocytes, NAAT for gonorrhea and chlamydia)	Urinary tract infection signs include nitrites, leukocytes
	Urine screening for chlamydia and gonorrhea is appropriate for screening and testing
Blood work as indicated (HIV, VDRL, RPR, HSV)	Blood testing can confirm or enhance physical exam findings

HIV = human immunodeficiency virus; HSV = herpes simplex virus; NAAT = nucleic acid amplification test; PID = pelvic inflammatory disease; RPR = rapid plasma reagin; VDRL = Venereal Disease Research Laboratory test.

data are very valuable in the diagnosis of an STI, the physical exam is important to help determine which lab tests are indicated. In addition, treatment may be initiated on the basis of physical findings without waiting for laboratory confirmation.

Indications for STI Screening

If a woman is concerned that she has been exposed to a STI, offer her tests for all STIs common in the geographical area.[12] Use local and regional prevalence rates to determine which infections are prevalent in your region or in the woman's or her partner's area of origin.[7] The woman should be informed of all recommended tests and their results when available.[12]

Anyone with symptoms of an STI, including urethritis, abnormal vaginal discharge, dysuria, cervicitis, or cervical motion tenderness, should be evaluated with a thorough history, targeted physical exam, and indicated lab tests. If a woman has one STI, such as trichomoniasis, she is at risk for having another and should be offered testing for HIV and all common STIs.[6]

Sexually Active Women 25 Years or Younger

Half of all STIs occur in persons younger than 25 years.[6] The CDC recommends all sexually active women 25 years old or younger be screened for chlamydia and gonorrhea annually.[12] In addition, they should be offered HIV screening. Pap smears with human papillomavirus (HPV) testing should begin at 21 years of age, regardless of the number of sexual partners or age at first intercourse.

Adolescents can receive STI testing without parental notification or consent in all 50 states and the

District of Columbia.[12] However, if a woman uses health insurance for payment, the services provided will be included on the insurance explanation of benefits, which could breech patient confidentiality.[12] Young women, especially those using parental insurance, should be informed about insurance reports. If this practice is not acceptable to the client, refer her to local resources for free or low-cost STI testing; if it is acceptable, it may help to discuss with her parent(s) that all women younger than 25 years old are screened for STIs, regardless of whether they are sexually active.

Pregnant Women

Sexually transmitted infections can adversely affect the embryo or fetus, causing a wide range of complications, including lifelong morbidity and intrauterine death. Early screening and treatment for STIs can prevent maternal and fetal/neonatal complications. For this reason, comprehensive STI testing should be performed during the first visit for pregnancy or as soon as possible. States often mandate the provision of these services within a set time frame. As a consequence, STI tests should not be delayed to coincide with other testing, such as second-trimester fetal screening. The STI tests that are recommended by the CDC for pregnant women are shown in **Table 15-2**.[12] Women who have multiple sexual partners or who are diagnosed with an STI during pregnancy should be rescreened in the third trimester or in labor if needed. Women should be rescreened with each pregnancy, regardless of interconceptional spacing.[12]

Opt-Out versus Opt-In Screening Strategies

Women should be informed of recommended tests and allowed to "opt out" of routine testing.[12] While women can decline screening, the information provided by such tests is valuable; moreover, all pregnant women have had exposure to bodily fluids, so they should be encouraged to accept testing. An opt-out approach to STI testing decreases barriers to screening and presents this screening as a routine procedure. The CDC advises clinicians to use an opt-out approach that presents women with a consent form listing all of common tests, which allows them to opt out of any tests if they wish.

An "opt-in" approach to screening asks women about STI tests individually and obtains consent to screen for each infection. This approach presents STI screening as routine, thereby decreasing stigma and normalizing testing, but it results in much lower rates of STI screening, as women are more likely to decline testing. By comparison, the opt-out approach greatly increases screening rates for HIV both in pregnancy and when people enter the hospital for medical care.[12]

Pregnant women who are considered to be at risk for gonorrhea and hepatitis C should be routinely screened for these STIs. At-risk groups for gonorrhea include individuals who have the following characteristics: living in an area with a high prevalence of gonorrhea, such as the southern United States; age younger than 25 years old; a history of STIs; new or multiple sex partners; sex work, drug use; and irregular condom use, which is common among pregnant women. Women who are at continued risk and those who acquire a risk factor over the course of pregnancy should be rescreened in the third trimester. High-risk categories for hepatitis C include persons engaging in current or previous use of injected drugs, and history of blood transfusion or organ transplantation prior to 1992.

While all pregnant women should be offered first-trimester testing for chlamydia and HIV using

Table 15-2	Centers for Disease Control and Prevention's Recommended Screening for Sexually Transmitted Infections in Pregnancy		
Routine Screening with Opt-Out Approach		**Screen Women at Risk**	**Screen Only Symptomatic Women**
Human immunodeficiency virus		Gonorrhea[a]	Bacterial vaginosis
Hepatitis B surface antigen		Hepatitis C[b]	Trichomoniasis
Syphilis			Herpes simplex virus (if no previous history)
Chlamydia			

[a] Risk factors for gonorrhea: age < 25 years, new or multiple sex partners, inconsistent condom use, drug use, sex work, a history of a previous STI, or living in a geographic area with a high prevalence of gonorrhea (which includes the southeastern United States).

[b] Risk factors for hepatitis C that warrant screening in pregnancy: history of injection-drug use or blood transfusion/organ transplantation before 1992.

Source: Centers for Disease Control and Prevention (CDC). Sexually transmitted diseases treatment guidelines. *MMWR.* 2010;59(RR-12). Available at: http://www.cdc.gov/mmwr/pdf/rr/rr5912.pdf. Accessed November 11, 2012.

an opt-out approach, women at high risk need repeat screening in the third trimester. High-risk groups for chlamydia include women who have tested positive for chlamydia during this pregnancy, are younger than 25 years old, or those who have a new or multiple sexual partners. High-risk status for HIV is conferred by the following factors: living in a high-prevalence area, drug use, diagnosis of an STI during pregnancy, and new, multiple, or HIV-positive sexual partner(s). Even if screened earlier in pregnancy, women at risk for STIs should be rescreened in the third trimester or at the time of admission in labor. Some states mandate third-trimester testing for STIs unless the woman specifically declines such screening.[12]

Regardless of their risk status, women do not need to be routinely screened for trichomoniasis or bacterial vaginosis in pregnancy. Identification and treatment of women with these conditions does not decrease adverse health outcomes and may increase the risk of preterm birth. However, women should be tested for these two disorders if they have symptoms of these conditions, and they should be offered treatment with informed consent about the increased risk of preterm birth.[12]

Women Who Have Sex with Women

Sex and sexual contact with female partners presents a risk for STI transmission related to contact with skin, genitals, and oral and vaginal mucosa. While the prevalence of infections is different in women who have sex with women, the guidelines for STI and cervical cancer testing do not change with the sex/gender of the partner.[12]

Women Not at Risk for Pregnancy

Women who are unable to conceive due to known infertility, menopause, or sterilization may neglect to take precautions against STIs. Women may have new sexual partners after divorce or death of a long-term partner and not consider the risk of STIs. *Any* woman with a new or non-monogamous sexual partner is at risk for STIs and should be offered testing. Guard against age bias in the decision to offer STI testing; rates of STIs among people older than 50 years have been increasing over the past decade.[7]

Incarcerated Women

Women entering correctional facilities are a vulnerable group who are more likely than women not in correctional facilities to have been abused or to have exchanged sexual contact for food, housing, or money. The CDC recommends that all juvenile and adult women younger than 35 years be routinely screened for gonorrhea and chlamydia on intake to a correctional facility. Routine syphilis screening should be based on local prevalence rates.[12] Testing can allow for treatment and prevention of lifelong morbidity.

Vaginitis

Vaginitis, which is inflammation of the vagina, is a disruption of the normal healthy microbial environment within the vagina. Vaginitis can have many causes and origins that are not fully understood. It can be a symptom of an STI, a disruption in the normal vaginal flora, or simple vaginal irritation. Recurrent vaginitis can have many causes and warrants a thorough sexual and lifestyle history that includes the woman's overall health and stress level. In addition, the role of the sexual partner should be explored. While partner transmission of noninfectious vaginitis is not common, female and uncircumcised male partners may act as a bacterial reservoir, reinoculating susceptible women. Vaginitis is a common problem for women from menarche through menopause. The most common causes of vaginitis are reviewed here and initial treatments outlined.

Bacterial Vaginosis

Bacterial vaginosis (BV) is the most common cause of vaginal infections in childbearing women[6] (**Figure 15-1**). Formerly known as *Gardnerella vaginalis*, *Haemophilus vaginalis*, or *Corynebacterium vaginitis*, BV is a dysbiosis of vaginal bacteria.[13] In essence, this infection represents a disturbance in the vaginal microflora characterized by diminished or absent *Lactobacillus* species, which allows for overgrowth of anaerobic and facultative bacteria. A healthy vaginal flora involves a predominance of *Lactobacillus* species. During episodes of BV, the vaginal flora is shifted toward a preponderance of anaerobic bacteria. The bacterial imbalance is associated with sexual contact but is not usually spread through sex.

Although the exact cause of bacterial vaginosis is not known, many risk factors are associated with BV, including smoking, menstruation, douching, sexual contact without a condom, low level of education, and engaging in oral or anal sex. Menopausal women have an increased risk for BV as a consequence of loss of healthy vaginal flora. Women who have sex with women have increased prevalence of BV, which has been attributed to oral sex and partner inoculation.[13] Women of African descent also have increased prevalence of BV than women of other races, for unknown reasons.

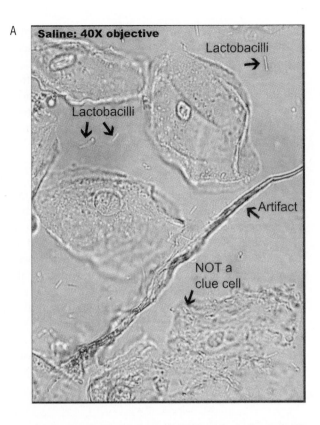

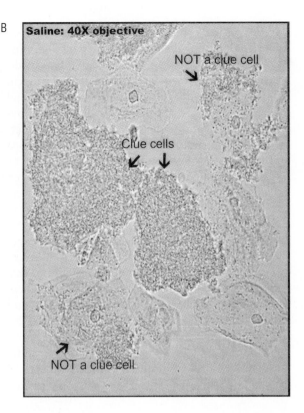

Figure 15-1 Microscopic diagnosis of bacterial vaginosis (BV). (A) No BV; note normal epithelial cells and presence of lactobacilli. (B) BV; note clue cells and lack of lactobacilli.

Source: Used with permission from Seattle STD/HIV Prevention Training Center and Cindy Fennell, MS, MT, ASCP.

Bacterial vaginosis is associated with many adverse health outcomes, including preterm birth, postoperative infections, endometritis following pregnancy, and acquisition of other STIs. However, treatment of BV does not decrease most of these risks and, in fact, may increase the risk of preterm birth.[12] This conundrum is explored in more detail in the later section on management of BV during pregnancy.

Although BV is not usually sexually transmitted, new studies show that the anaerobic bacteria involved in this infection can be passed between partners.[13] Symptoms include vaginal irritation and itching, dyspareunia, and a "fishy" odor after unprotected sex with men; alternatively, the condition may be asymptomatic.

Physical Examination and Laboratory Findings

On speculum exam, BV is usually evident as a thin white/gray homogenous discharge, irritated vaginal mucosa, and introitus, possible cervicitis. To make the diagnosis via clinical microscopy, a sample of the vaginal discharge is collected with a swab. The sample is first tested to determine the pH, and then a sample of the discharge is placed on two slides. Normal saline is added to one slide, which is covered with a slide cover and then set aside for microscopy. Finally, KOH is added to the other slide, which is used immediately for the "whiff test." Clinically, BV is diagnosed when three of four of Amsel's criteria are present:

1. Presence of a thin homogenous discharge that adheres to vaginal walls

2. Presence of clue cells on the normal saline prepared slide

3. pH of the vagina or vaginal discharge > 4.5 (90% of women with BV will have a pH > 4.5)

4. Positive "whiff test," which signals the release of an amine "fishy" odor when vaginal discharge contacts alkaline KOH (70% of women with BV will have a positive whiff test)

Treatment and Nonpharmacologic Support

Table 15-3 outlines pharmacologic treatments for BV.[12] The choices for treatment include oral medications such as metronidazole (Flagyl), clindamycin (Cleocin), and tinidazole (Tindamax), and vaginal medications such as metronidazole gel or clindamycin cream or ovules. Drinking alcohol during treatment with metronidazole can cause severe nausea and vomiting. Vaginal creams may be perceived as messy, and those containing clindamycin can weaken latex condoms. Taking these medication side effects into consideration, the plan of care is developed in partnership with the affected woman.

Some studies have shown that probiotics, especially *Lactobacillus crispatus*, can be helpful in establishing a normal vaginal flora and reducing BV recurrence.[14] However, the safety and efficacy of these therapies have not been conclusively established, and they may not be eligible for reimbursement by health insurance plans. Health education includes abstaining from intercourse during treatment and washing all objects before they touch the vagina. Receptive oral and anal sex may increase risk for BV related

to microbial inoculation. Condoms may reduce the risk of BV by preventing contact with alkaline semen.

Relapses are common, especially after menses, until a normal vaginal flora is reestablished.[13] After initial treatment, follow up with another evaluation only if symptoms persist or reoccur. Chronic reinfection warrants further investigation and more intense treatments as outlined by the CDC.

Vulvovaginal Candidiasis

Candidiasis is an overgrowth *Candida* (yeast) species that affects the vagina, vulva, groin, and other moist areas of the body. The most common cause is *Candida albicans*, but other species are found as well. While candidiasis can be found in many locations, this section focuses on infections of the female genitals. Ninety percent of women will have vulvovaginal candidiasis (VVC), commonly known as a yeast infection, at some point in their lives.[12] VVC can be classified as uncomplicated or complicated. Uncomplicated VVC, the most common form, is associated with mild to moderate symptoms and manifestations. Uncomplicated VVC is a common condition

Table 15-3	Treatment for Bacterial Vaginosis		
Recommended Treatments for Nonpregnant Women Generic (Brand)	**Alternative Treatments for Nonpregnant Women Generic (Brand)**	**Recommended Treatments for Pregnant Women Generic (Brand)**	**Recommended Treatments for Breastfeeding Women Generic (Brand)**
Metronidazole (Flagyl) 500 mg orally twice a day for 7 days	Tinidazole (Tindamax) 2 g orally for 2 days	Metronidazole (Flagyl) 500 mg orally twice a day for 7 days	Vaginal administration of metronidazole (Flagyl) is preferred for breastfeeding women.
Metronidazole gel (MetroGel) 0.75%, one applicator full per vagina at bedtime for 5 days	Tinidazole (Tindamax) 1g orally for 5 days	Metronidazole (Flagyl) 250 mg orally three times a day for 7 days	Metronidazole (Flagyl) taken orally by nursing women is excreted in breast milk and has active metabolites, increasing infants' exposure, but has not been demonstrated to be harmful.
			Timing the dose after nursing may decrease infant exposure.
Clindamycin (Cleocin) cream 2%, one applicator full per vagina at bedtime for 7 days	Clindamycin (Cleocin) 300 mg orally for 7 days	Clindamycin (Cleocin) 300 mg orally for 7 days	
	Clindamycin (Cleocin) ovules 100 mg intravaginally at bedtime for 3 days		

Sources: Centers for Disease Control and Prevention (CDC). Sexually transmitted diseases treatment guidelines. *MMWR.* 2010;59(RR-12). Available at: http://www.cdc.gov/mmwr/pdf/rr/rr5912.pdf. Accessed November 11, 2012; U.S. National Library of Medicine. Drugs and lactation database (LactMed). 2012. Available at: http://toxnet.nlm.nih.gov/cgi-bin/sis/htmlgen?LACT. Accessed January 19, 2013.

that occurs sporadically throughout a woman's life. If infections occur more than four times per year, produce severe symptoms, or occur in women who are immunocompromised, the VVC is classified as complicated and requires more intensive treatment.[12]

Several factors can make conditions favorable for *Candida* growth and increase the chance of candidiasis. When the vulva is kept moist because of nonbreathable clothes or very humid or warm living conditions, the risk of candidiasis is increased. The hormonal changes that occur in pregnancy and while on oral contraceptive pills also increase risk. In addition, diabetes is associated with increased incidence of candidiasis. Antibiotics alter the vaginal flora, allowing *Candida* proliferation. Immunosuppressed states, such as that seen with HIV and corticosteroid use, can also increase the risk of candidiasis in the vulvovaginal region and other moist areas of the body.

Although species of *Candida* can be passed between sexual partners, candidiasis involves an overgrowth of normal flora and is not contagious. Symptoms include vaginal itching, burning, irritation, dyspareunia, and increased vaginal discharge.

Diagnosis of Candidiasis

The vulva may be erythematous and slightly swollen, and have areas of redness with 1- to 2-mm "satellite"

lesions extending from the affected area on external examination. The vagina is often red and slightly edematous. The vaginal discharge is usually thick, white, and curd-like, but it can also be thin and watery, or adherent to the vaginal walls. Recent douching can complicate the physical exam by washing away discharge. Manifestations of severe candidiasis include widespread and severe erythema, skin fissures, edema, and excoriations.

A wet mount may reveal a lack of lactobacillus on a saline preparation or the presence of hyphae and pseudo-hyphae with a saline or KOH preparation (**Figure 15-2**). However, lack of hyphae does not rule out candidiasis, especially for women experiencing recurrent or severe symptoms, as the species of *Candida* implicated in recurrent and infection— *C. glabrata*—does not form hyphae. A culture can be performed in the absence of hyphae to check for non-*albicans* varieties of yeast.[12] Treatment can begin without culture results.

Treatment and Nonpharmacologic Support

Treatment options for VVC are listed in **Table 15-4**. Many treatments are available without a prescription, and women may use these medications prior to a clinical diagnosis of candidiasis. There is no standard recommendation about the need to be seen in the office prior to treatment. Use of over-the-counter

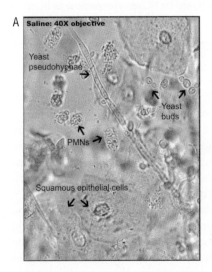 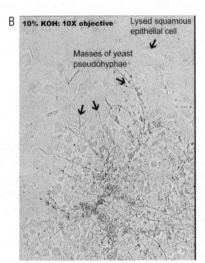 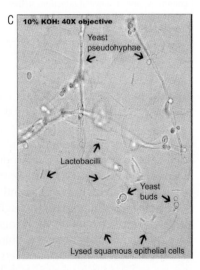

Figure 15-2 Candida pseudohyphae and budding spores under microscopic examination. (A) Saline, 40×. (B) KOH, 10×. (C) KOH, 40×, PMNs = polymorphonuclear cells.
Source: Used with permission from Seattle STD/HIV Prevention Training Center and Cindy Fennell, MS, MT, ASCP

Table 15-4	Recommended Treatment for Vulvovaginal Candidiasis			
Intravaginal Agents	**Over-the-Counter or Prescription**	**Brand Name**	**Dose**	**Duration**
Butoconazole 2% cream	Rx	Gynazole-1	5 g intravaginally once at night	Single dose[a]
Clotrimazole 1% cream	OTC	Gyne-Lotrimin-7	5 g intravaginally once at night	7–14 days[a]
Clotrimazole 2% cream	OTC		5 g intravaginally	3 days
Miconazole 2% cream	OTC	Monistat-7	5 g intravaginally once at night	7 days[a]
Miconazole 4% cream	OTC		5 g intravaginally	3 days
Miconazole 100 mg suppository	OTC	Monistat-7	1 suppository intravaginally once at night	7 days
Miconazole 200 mg suppository	OTC	Monistat-3	1 suppository intravaginally once at night	3 days
Miconazole 1200 mg suppository	OTC		1 suppository	Single dose
Nystatin 100,000 unit vaginal tablet	Rx	Mycostatin	1 tablet intravaginally once at night	14 days
Terconazole 0.4% cream (45 g)	Rx	Terazol-7	5 g intravaginally once at night	7 days
Terconazole 0.8% cream (30 g)	Rx	Terazol-3	5 g intravaginally once at night	3 days
Terconazole 80 mg suppository	Rx	Terazol-3	1 suppository intravaginally once at night	3 days
Oral Agents				
Fluconazole	Rx	Diflucan	150 mg oral tablet once at night	Single dose

OTC = over-the-counter; Rx = prescription.

[a] Recommended during pregnancy.

Sources: Adapted from Centers for Disease Control and Prevention (CDC). Recomendations for partner services programs for HIV infection, syphilis, gonorrhea, and chlamydial infection. *MMWR.* 2008;57(RR-9):1-64; Mashburn J. Vaginitis. In: King TL, Brucker MC, eds. *Pharmacology for Women's Health.* Sudbury, MA: Jones and Bartlett; 2011:950.

medications can decrease costs for women if they have VVC, but can also mean that women delay seeking treatment for harder-to-treat or more serious vaginal infections. Options include oral treatments, vaginal creams and tablets, and topical preparations. The costs and side effects of these therapies vary. All locations of infection (vaginal and/or vulva) should be treated. The creams require vaginal insertion and they may weaken condoms. The oral medication fluconazole (Diflucan) does not require handling of the genitals but has systemic side effects including alterations in hepatic function and several drug–drug interactions.[15] Complicated VVC in nonpregnant women, which includes skin fissures, should be treated with a longer treatment course of either 7 to 14 days of a topical "azole" or two doses of 150 mg fluconazole,

72 hours apart.[12] Involve the woman in the choice of route and medication.

Probiotics, especially oral *Lactobacillus*, may help to restore normal vaginal flora. Topical tea-tree oil and garlic may also be beneficial, but no conclusive research supports the use of these products. Douching is not a recommended treatment.[16]

Health education includes methods to decrease yeast growth by reducing vulvar moisture, including wearing only cotton underwear, avoiding tight-fitting clothing, avoiding plastic-backed panty liners and pads unless necessary, drying the vulva thoroughly after bathing without causing abrasions (a hair dryer is ideal), and not wearing underwear at night if possible. Some complementary medicine sources call for lifestyle changes, including decreasing consumption of refined sugars and yeast products. While these strategies have minimal potential for harm, they have not been substantiated as beneficial in otherwise healthy women. There is no need for a test of cure if symptoms resolve; rescreen women only if they are symptomatic.

Recurrent Candidiasis

Recurrent candidiasis is defined as four or more occurrences of candidiasis within one year.[12] If a woman has recurrent candidiasis, assess for contributing lifestyle factors and perform a culture to test for non-*albicans Candida* strains. Pharmaceutical-grade boric acid (600 mg once daily for 2 weeks) can be useful in treating recurrent, non-*albicans* yeast.[12] For recurrence of C. *albicans* strains, consider longer topical treatment combined with sequential oral treatment, following CDC guidelines. Suppressive therapy of weekly fluconazole (Diflucan) can be considered once the infection is controlled.[12] Testing for underlying diabetes or HIV infection may be appropriate depending on the woman's history and risk factors.

Atrophic Vaginitis

Atrophic vaginitis is a collection of vaginal symptoms related to low estrogen levels. Lower estrogen levels can cause vaginal changes, including decreased collagen and adipose tissue, and increased pH.[17] These changes make the vagina more friable and prone to irritation, and increase the risk of vaginal infections. Low estrogen levels can occur with natural menopause or cycle cessation during breastfeeding, chemotherapy, or treatment with gonadotropin-releasing hormone (GnRH) agonists such as leuprolide (Lupron). While not an infection, these changes place women at increased risk for other infections such as BV, candidiasis, and STIs.

Vaginal changes in menopause are normal and do not require intervention unless they adversely impact the woman's functioning or quality of life. However, some women may be reluctant to disclose problems. Questions about vaginal dryness, irritation, and dyspareunia are important history components in menopausal or noncycling women. Potential symptoms of atrophic vaginitis include vaginal irritation and dryness, frequent vaginal infections, dyspareunia, and lack of lubrication with sexual activity.

Diagnosis of Atrophic Vaginitis

Diagnosis of atrophic vaginitis is made via physical examination. Factors that suggest diagnosis include thinning vulvar skin, decreasing prominence of the inner labia, small, nonelastic vaginal introitus, few vaginal rugae, pale pink vaginal walls, shortening of the vagina, and a lack of vaginal moisture. The woman's vaginal pH may be higher than 4.5.[17]

Treatment and Nonpharmacologic Support

Over-the-counter vaginal moisturizers for daily use can decrease symptoms. Women should select a water-based moisturizer that helps maintain a slightly acidic vaginal pH. Use of water-based lubricant products such as Astroglide, K-Y Jelly, or K-Y Liquibeads during sexual activity can decrease discomfort. Nonpharmacologic recommendations for decreasing symptoms of vaginitis can be found in **Box 15-3**.

Estrogen can also be used to alleviate symptoms. Topical estrogen administration is preferable to oral administration as a first-line pharmacologic treatment.[18] When used topically, estrogen does not need to be paired with progesterone in women with an intact uterus.[18] However, long-term data on the safety of topical estrogens are not available.[18] Some research supports the hypothesis that endometrial hyperplasia can occur with topical estrogen administration.[19] A Cochrane review of 19 randomized trials that assessed the effects of topical estrogen preparations (*n* = 4162) identified one randomized trial that found estrogen cream (conjugated equine

---

BOX 15-3 Health Education for Prevention of Vaginal Irritation and Vaginitis

- Clean only the outside of the vagina with gentle, unscented soap.
- Stop douching, as it eliminates helpful bacteria and increases risk of infection.
- Use unscented and dye-free soaps and detergents for skin and clothes.
- Double-rinse underwear to eliminate contact with soap.
- Avoid pads and panty liners unless needed.
- Try a variety of pads, especially those without a plastic covering against the skin.
- Use a lubricant to prevent chafing during sexual activities.
- Try a variety of pH-balanced lubricants to determine which is least irritating.
- Sexual contact should be gentle and nonpainful.
- Spermicides may irritate the vagina; consider changing birth control methods.
- Only clean objects should touch or enter the vagina (e.g., fingers, penis, sex toys).

estrogen) was associated with side effects of endometrial hyperplasia and bleeding. A ring preparation of estrogen was found to have fewer side effects and lead to greater user satisfaction.[19]

If topical treatments are not sufficient to relieve severe symptoms, systemic estrogen or estrogen/progesterone can be used by menopausal or postmenopausal women, often in combination with topical estrogen.[18] However, oral estrogens have more side effects, including increased risk of ischemic stroke and venous thromboembolism. Breastfeeding women and women who are not cycling related to medical treatment should not be given systemic estrogens.

Other Causes of Vaginitis

The skin of the vulva and vagina can become inflamed in response to many substances. For example, exposure to urine or stool, such as occurs with even mild incontinence, can cause chronic irritation and vaginitis. Perfumes and chemicals found in soaps, laundry detergents, and feminine hygiene products can also cause irritation. Personal lubricants can disrupt vaginal pH and normal flora, resulting in vaginitis. Spermicides may irritate the vagina as well. Douching washes away beneficial bacteria and irritates the vaginal mucosa, increasing the risk for vaginitis. A thorough exploration of all substances that contact the vulva and vagina is warranted for women who have unexplained or recurrent vaginitis. Women with incontinence should strive to keep the vulva dry and free of urine or stool, cleaning as needed with water and soft, nonabrasive wipes.

Vaginal irritation can also occur during intercourse if the woman is not well lubricated or the contact is rough or damaging; this finding may be indicative of greater relationship problems and needs further exploration. Chronic vaginitis can also be a marker for larger life stressors, which can be gently explored with the woman in a holistic and helpful way. Continuity of care and a trusting partnership between the woman and midwife make it more likely that she will disclose her needs.

Anything left within the vagina can cause vaginitis. This includes tampons, pessaries, or any other foreign body. Odor and irritation are usually presenting symptoms. A speculum exam is helpful to determine the cause of the odor. On speculum exam, a tampon may at first appear to be a fleshy mass as it blends in with surrounding tissue. Forgotten tampons have an extreme odor; prepare a plastic bag or container with water before removal. Tampons can be removed with ring forceps or digitally. Pessaries, which are left in the vagina for long time periods, can become irritating, especially if the woman has atrophic vaginal changes. While an increase in vaginal discharge is normal with pessary use, check for vaginal infections and skin erosions if the woman reports problems.

Sexually Transmitted Infections

Because sexual contact involves close bodily proximity, many microbes are shared between partners, most of which are nonpathogenic. This section focuses on infections that are predominately transmitted through sexual contact. The close contact of mucous membranes and the sharing of bodily fluids during such contact allow several pathogenic organisms the opportunity to find a new host. STIs may be caused by bacterial, viral, protozoal, or parasitic organisms, as shown in **Table 15-5**. Some clinicians, however, prefer to organize their list of differential diagnoses according to the woman's chief concern, as shown in **Table 15-6**. Many STIs are asymptomatic even while causing bodily damage. Anyone at risk for STIs should be screened according to CDC guidelines to prevent health sequelae and transmission to others.

Table 15-5	Causes of Sexually Transmitted Infections	
Bacterial Disease (Organism)	**Virus (Abbreviation)**	**Protozoal and Parasitic Disease (Organism)**
Chlamydia (*Chlamydia trachomatis*)	Human papillomavirus (HPV)	Trichomoniasis (*Trichomonas vaginalis*)
Gonorrhea (*Neisseria gonorrhoeae*)		Pubic lice/crabs (*Phthirus pubis*)
Syphilis (*Treponema pallidum*)	Herpes simplex virus (HSV-1 and HSV-2)	Scabies (*Sarcoptes scabiei*)
Chancroid (*Haemophilus ducreyi*)		
Lymphogranuloma venereum (*Chlamydia trachomatis* serovars L1, L2, and L3)	Human immunodeficiency virus (HIV)	
Granuloma inguinale (*Klebsiella granulomatis*)		

Table 15-6	Common Presenting Concerns for Sexually Transmitted Infections	
Discharge Disease (Organism)	**Sores (Organism or Virus)**	**Warts Disease (Organism or Virus)**
Chlamydia (*Chlamydia trachomatis*)	Herpes (herpes simplex virus [HSV-1 and HSV-2])	Genital warts (human papillomavirus)
Gonorrhea (*Neisseria gonorrhoeae*)	Syphilis (*Treponema pallidum*)	Condyloma acuminata (human papillomavirus)
Trichomoniasis (*Trichomonas vaginalis*)	Chancroid (*Haemophilus ducreyi*)	Condylomata lata (*Treponema pallidum*)
	Lymphogranuloma venereum (*Chlamydia trachomatis* serovars L1, L2, and L3)	
	Granuloma inguinale (*Klebsiella granulomatis*)	

Chlamydia

Chlamydia trachomatis is a small gram-negative bacterium that is an obligate intracellular organism. Chlamydia is the most common reportable STI, with more than 1.3 million new cases occurring each year in the United States.[6] The majority of these cases occur in individuals age 25 years or younger, although any sexually active person is at risk.[6] Because the majority of cases of chlamydia are asymptomatic, the CDC recommends screening all women with a new sexual partner and annual screening for women 25 years and younger.[12]

When left untreated, chlamydia can ascend into the upper reproductive tract and cause pelvic inflammatory disease (PID). Ascending infections increase the risk of subsequent ectopic pregnancy and infertility. Vertical transmission during birth can cause conjunctivitis or pneumonia in affected neonates. Urogenital transmission is the most common form of spread of this infection, but sexual transmission to the oropharynx and rectum is possible as well. Vertical transmission can occur during vaginal birth.

Most women infected with chlamydia are asymptomatic. However, increased vaginal discharge, dysuria, or Bartholin gland infection can be presenting symptoms, and some women are initially diagnosed when they present with salpingitis (infection in the fallopian tubes) or PID.

Diagnosis of Chlamydia

On exam, cervicitis, mucopurulent discharge or cervical motion tenderness may be present. Wet prep may show an increased number of white blood cells. Diagnosis of chlamydia is based on laboratory tests. Nucleic acid amplification test (NAAT) is the most common diagnostic test for chlamydia; it can be performed on urine, cervical, vaginal, or liquid cytology specimens. The CDC states women can self-collect their own vaginal sample.[12] NAAT detects small amounts of gene sequences in bacterial DNA and replicates those sequences so a large amount is present. Most samples sent to the laboratory for STI diagnosis are tested with NAAT technology. Such tests may also be used with rectal samples depending on the manufacturer and laboratory. Urine testing is the least invasive and has high sensitivity rates.[20] NAAT on liquid cytology (liquid Pap smear) may have a lower sensitivity for detecting infection. Diagnosis of PID resulting from chlamydia is based on the findings of a physical examination (see "Pelvic Inflammatory Disease" later in this chapter.)

Treatment and Nonpharmacologic Support

Pharmacologic treatment is listed in **Table 15-7**.[20] Single-dose treatment is preferable if the woman is not able to remember multiple doses. Ensure treatment of all sexual partner(s) from the last 60 days.[12] The woman with chlamydia should abstain from intercourse until her partner(s) are treated and for 7 days after single-dose treatment or until she completes her multidose treatment.[12]

Follow-up

Women who test positive for chlamydia should be tested for all common STIs, as coinfections frequently occur.[12] Nonpregnant women do not need a test-of-cure unless they are reexposed to the bacterium or have a new sexual partner. Pregnant women should be retested no sooner than 3 weeks after treatment and then should be rescreened again 3 months later and/or in the third trimester.

Management of Chlamydia in Pregnancy

Women with a history of chlamydial infection are at increased risk for ectopic pregnancy. The CDC recommends routine screening for chlamydia for all

Table 15-7	Treatments for Chlamydia			
Recommended Treatments for Nonpregnant Women and Males Generic (Brand)	**Alternative Treatments for Nonpregnant Women and Males Generic (Brand)**	**Recommended Treatments for Pregnant Women Generic (Brand)**	**Breastfeeding Considerations**
Azithromycin (Zithromax, Z-Pak) 1 g orally once	Erythromycin base 500 mg orally four times a day for 7 days	Azithromycin (Zithromax, Z-Pak) 1 g orally once	Azithromycin is compatible with breastfeeding.
Doxycycline (Vibramycin) 100 mg orally twice a day for 7 days	Erythromycin ethylsuccinate (E-Mycin) 800 mg orally four times a day for 7 days	Amoxicillin (Amoxil) 500 mg orally three times a day for 7 days	There is controversy about the use of doxycycline in nursing mothers, as there is the theoretical potential for staining of forming teeth. However, its levels in breast milk are low. If doxycycline must be used, consider strategies to minimize its transfer to the milk.
	Levofloxacin (Levaquin) 500 mg orally for 7 days	Alternative treatments for pregnant women are the same as for nonpregnant women and males	
	Ofloxacin (Floxin) 300 mg orally twice a day for 7 days		

Sources: Centers for Disease Control and Prevention (CDC). Sexually transmitted diseases treatment guidelines. *MMWR.* 2010;59(RR-12). Available at: http://www.cdc.gov/mmwr/pdf/rr/rr5912.pdf. Accessed November 11, 2012; U.S. National Library of Medicine. Drugs and lactation database (LactMed). 2012. Available at: http://toxnet.nlm.nih.gov/cgi-bin/sis/htmlgen?LACT. Accessed January 19, 2013.

pregnant women as early as possible during pregnancy. Pregnant women at increased risk for this infection (e.g., those younger than 25 years, those with a new sexual partner during pregnancy) should be rescreened in the third trimester.[12] Treatment should occur as soon as possible after diagnosis, using a treatment regimen compatible with pregnancy.

Fetal/Neonatal Considerations

Chlamydial ophthalmia can cause scarring and blindness in the fetus and/or pneumonia that is life threatening in the neonate.[12] Because routine neonatal ocular prophylaxis is not effective against chlamydia, infants born to infected mothers should be closely observed for symptoms but not routinely treated.[12] Additional information about eye prophylaxis for newborns to prevent chalmydial and gonorrheal ophthalmia can be found in the *Neonatal Care* chapter.

Gonorrhea

Neisseria gonorrhoeae is a gram-negative intracellular diplococcus that exclusively affects humans. This bacterium primarily infects the mucocutaneous surfaces of the genitourinary tract, pharynx,

conjunctiva, and anus. Gonorrhea is the second most common reportable disease in the United States and is experiencing a surge in antibiotic resistance, with the potential to become resistant to all currently available antibiotics. The CDC monitors infectious disease resistance patterns and releases updates as needed.[21] Refer to the guidelines on the CDC website for the most current information on recommended treatments. Women with gonorrhea are also frequently coinfected with chlamydia, so all CDC-approved treatments for gonorrhea include treatment for chlamydia; this strategy is intended both to the reduce the incidence of PID and to combat increasing antibiotic resistance.[21] Thus women with gonorrhea should be treated with azithromycin (Zithromax) or doxycycline (Vibramycin) in addition to a cephalosporin, even if they test negative for chlamydia.

Transmission of gonorrhea occurs through oral, anal, and vaginal sex and contact with secretions from the urogenital tract. Vertical infection is possible, resulting in ocular infections in neonates. Individuals infected with gonorrhea can be asymptomatic or may experience a variety of symptoms. Women may have dysuria, abnormal vaginal discharge, or bleeding if infected vaginally. Oral infection can result in a sore throat. Anal infection can cause anal itching, soreness, bleeding, discharge, or painful bowel movements. Disseminated gonorrhea is a rare life-threatening condition characterized by symptoms of joint pain and a rash. Women with PID from gonorrhea can have symptoms of fever, vaginal discharge, and abdominal pain. Gonorrhea can increase the risk of HIV acquisition and is associated with PID, infertility, and ectopic pregnancy.[6]

Diagnosis of Gonorrhea

The physical examination may be unremarkable in persons with gonorrhea. Conversely, lymph nodes surrounding the affected area may be enlarged. Urethritis and inflammation and discharge from the periurethral (Skene's) and greater vestibular (Bartholin) glands may be present. Cervicitis is common. If the woman has mucopurulent discharge from her cervix and uterus, adnexal tenderness, or cervical motion tenderness, PID is a likely diagnosis.

NAAT performed on endocervical, vaginal, or urine samples is acceptable for initial screening and diagnosis of gonorrhea. If rectal, oropharyngeal, or ophthalmic testing is needed, ensure that the laboratory has tests that are specific to *N. gonorrhoeae*, as common bacteria present in these areas may cause false-positive results. While NAAT is useful in diagnosis, culture should be performed to determine whether treatment has been successful—an approach known as a test-of-cure. Persistent infections should also be cultured, as a culture is able to provide information about antibiotic susceptibility while NAAT assessment does not. However, if the lab does not have the capability to perform gonorrhea cultures, the CDC provides information on alternative options for a test-of-cure.[21]

Diagnosis of gonorrhea is based on laboratory tests. However, if this infection is a likely diagnosis based on clinical findings, treatment can begin prior to knowing the results of testing.

Treatment and Nonpharmacologic Support

Table 15-8 describes treatment of uncomplicated gonorrhea infection. Dual drug therapy is recommended to prevent drug resistance, and is also effective against chlamydia. Use alternative regimens only if ceftriaxone is not available or the patient is severely allergic. The CDC website provides further guidance for unusual or complicated cases, such as treatment failure or disseminated gonorrhea.

Otherwise healthy nonpregnant adults do not need a test-of-cure if treated with the ceftriaxone (Rocephin) and azithromycin/doxycycline regimen. If treatment with ceftriaxone (Rocephin) was not possible, the woman will need a test-of-cure, with a

Table 15-8	Treatments for Uncomplicated Gonorrhea		
Recommended Treatments for Nonpregnant Women and Males **Generic (Brand)**	**Alternative Treatments for Nonpregnant Women and Males** **Generic (Brand)**	**Recommended Treatments for Pregnant Women** **Generic (Brand)**	**Recommended Treatments for Breastfeeding Women**
Ceftriaxone (Rocephin) 250 mg orally in one intramuscular dose AND Azithromycin (Zithromax, Z-Pak) 1 g orally twice a day for 7 days or doxycyline (Vibramycin) 100 mg orally twice a day for 7 days	Use alternative only if unable to give ceftriaxone (Rocephin): Cefixime (Suprax) 400 mg orally in a single dose PLUS Azithromycin (Zithromax, Z-Pak) 1 g orally in a single dose (preferred) or doxycycline (Vibramycin) 100 mg orally twice a day for 7 days Use only if person has a severe cephalosporin allergy: Azithromycin (Zithromax, Z-Pak) 2g orally once	Same as for nonpregnant women **except** alternative treatment must use azithromycin (Zithromax, Z-Pak), NOT doxycycline	Treatments are the same as for nonpregnant women

Sources: Centers for Disease Control and Prevention (CDC). Sexually transmitted diseases treatment guidelines. *MMWR*. 2010;59(RR-12). Available at: http://www.cdc.gov/mmwr/pdf/rr/rr5912.pdf. Accessed November 11, 2012; U.S. National Library of Medicine. Drugs and lactation database (LactMed). 2012. Available at: http://toxnet.nlm.nih.gov/cgi-bin/sis/htmlgen?LACT. Accessed January 19, 2013.

culture, 1 week after finishing treatment. The CDC recommends rescreening for gonorrhea 3 months after treatment to test for reinfection.[21]

Management of Gonorrhea in Pregnancy

Screen women at risk for gonorrhea, and treat them as soon as possible after diagnosis. Pregnant women should receive a test-of-cure following treatment and should be retested in 3 months or during the third trimester.[21]

Fetal/Neonatal Considerations

Gonorrhea can be transmitted during birth and cause ophthalmia, localized infections of mucosa, abscesses at fetal monitoring sites, or disseminated infection. Because gonococcal ophthalmia can result in permanent blindness, the CDC advises ophthalmia neonatorum prophylaxis using erythromycin ophthalmic ointment for *all* newborns, regardless of maternal testing status or route of birth.[12] Many state laws mandate such treatment, and a parent must sign a waiver to opt out of treatment. Infants born to women with untreated gonorrhea should also receive parental antibiotics to prevent more severe infections.[12]

Pelvic Inflammatory Disease

PID results from a variety of causative organisms that ascend from the vagina into the upper urogenital tract, causing an inflammatory response.[12] *N. gonorrhoeae* and *C. trachomatis* are the most common causative organisms, and the presence of BV may increase the risk of PID in conjunction with these infections. There is a slight increase in the risk of PID in the first few weeks following insertion of an intrauterine device (IUD) as pathogenic bacteria may be deposited in the uterus during placement.[22] While many risk factors for PID have been identified, including young age and multiple or new sexual partners, any sexually active woman is at risk for this disease. Potential symptoms include abnormal vaginal bleeding or discharge, dyspareunia, abdominal pain or tenderness, and fever higher than 38.3°C (101°F). Any woman with PID-type symptoms that cannot be attributed to another cause should be treated for PID promptly.[12]

PID has several adverse short- and long-term sequelae for women. Perihepatitis and tubo-ovarian abscess are immediate risks of untreated PID and occur in as many as 30% of women with advanced PID. Both of these conditions cause severe abdominal pain and warrant further testing and hospitalization.[23] The inflammation from even mild cases of PID can cause scaring and permanent damage to

tubal cilia, impairing fertility and increasing the risk of ectopic pregnancy throughout the reproductive years. Women may also develop chronic pelvic pain related to adhesions caused by PID.[23]

Diagnosis of PID

To make the diagnosis of PID, the woman must have pelvic or lower abdominal pain and at least one of the following symptoms: cervical motion tenderness, uterine tenderness, or adnexal tenderness. Additional symptoms, such as fever and mucopurulent vaginal or cervical discharge, increase the specificity of the diagnosis. Invasive tests are rarely warranted, as definitive diagnosis is not needed for treatment of PID. **Box 15-4** provides the full diagnostic criteria for PID.[12] A complete physical exam is needed to rule out other causes of abdominal pain, including gastrointestinal problems, ovarian cysts, and appendicitis or other surgical emergencies.

A wide range of tests for PID may be performed depending on the woman's presentation and the

---

BOX 15-4 Diagnostic Criteria for Pelvic Inflammatory Disease

Minimum Criteria
(1 or more needed for diagnosis)

- Cervical motion tenderness OR
- Uterine tenderness OR
- Adnexal tenderness

Additional Criteria
(increase specificity of diagnosis)

- Fever > 38.3°C (101°F)
- Mucopurulent cervical or vaginal discharge
- Numerous white blood cells on saline wet prep
- Elevated C-reactive protein
- Elevated erythrocyte sedimentation rate
- Documented infection with *C. trachomatis* or *N. gonorrhoea*

Definitive Criteria

- Transvaginal ultrasound, magnetic resonance imaging, or Doppler studies showing thickened and fluid-filled tubes
- Laparoscopic visualization of PID-related abnormalities

Source: Centers for Disease Control and Prevention (CDC). Sexually transmitted diseases treatment guidelines. *MMWR.* 2010;59(RR-12). Available at: http://www.cdc.gov /mmwr/pdf/rr/rr5912.pdf. Accessed November 11, 2012.

likelihood of other diagnoses. A wet mount showing many white blood cells is suggestive of PID. Clue cells, positive whiff test, and altered pH may be present. Blood tests may reveal an elevated white blood cell count and erythrocyte sedimentation rate. NAAT should be performed for gonorrhea and chlamydia. A urine or blood test for human chorionic gonadotropin (hCG) might be needed to rule out ectopic pregnancy. HIV testing is also appropriate.

Diagnosis is based on clinical presentation alone. Laboratory tests for gonorrhea and chlamydia should be performed, but treatment should not be delayed while awaiting their results. The CDC advises a low threshold for diagnosis, as PID may have minimal symptoms but still cause tubal damage.[12]

Treatment and Nonpharmacologic Support

Treat women with PID presumptively for both gonorrhea and chlamydia (**Table 15-9**). Strongly consider metronidazole (Flagyl) to cover potential anaerobic causes of PID.[12] Oral treatment is acceptable unless the woman has not responded to oral treatment or is acutely ill. If a woman has an IUD in place, treat her as usual; the IUD does not need to be removed.[22] Symptoms should improve dramatically with 72 hours. If no improvement is evident within 3 days, the woman should be reevaluated and hospitalization is indicated. Hospitalization should also be considered when oral treatment is not possible; when the PID appears to be severe, with the woman experiencing a high fever or nausea and vomiting; and when emergencies such as appendicitis, tubo-ovarian abscess, or conditions cannot be excluded.[12]

The CDC recommends HIV testing for all women diagnosed with PID.[12] Sexual partners should be treated presumptively for gonorrhea and chlamydia.[12] Health teaching includes recommending use of condoms and other practices to decrease STI transmission. Follow-up and test-of-cure depend on the infections identified through laboratory screening.

Table 15-9	Outpatient Treatments for Pelvic Inflammatory Disease		
Recommended Treatments for Nonpregnant Women and Males Generic (Brand)	**Alternative Treatments for Nonpregnant Women and Males Generic (Brand)**	**Recommended Treatments for Pregnant Women Generic (Brand)**	**Recommended Treatments for Breastfeeding Women**
Ceftriaxone (Rocephin) 250 mg orally in one intramuscular dose AND Azithromycin (Zithromax, Z-Pak) 1 g orally twice a day for 7 days WITH or WITHOUT Metronidazole (Flagyl) 500 mg orally for 14 days (for parenteral or inpatient treatment, refer to CDC guidelines)	Use alternative only if unable to give ceftriaxone: Cefixime (Suprax) 400 mg orally in a single dose PLUS Azithromycin (Zithromax, Z-Pak) 1 g orally in a single dose (preferred) or doxycycline (Vibramycin) 100 mg orally twice a day for 7 days WITH or WITHOUT Metronidazole (Flagyl) 500 mg twice a day for 14 days If woman has a severe cephalosporin allergy: Azithromycin (Zithromax, Z-Pak) 2 g orally once WITH or WITHOUT Metronidazole (Flagyl) 500 mg twice daily for 14 days	Pregnant patients with suspected PID should be hospitalized for evaluation according to CDC guidelines.	Same as non-nursing women, except that metronidazole administered orally to the mother is excreted in breast milk and has active metabolites in the infant. While no harm has been shown in nursing infants, the potential amount ingested by the infant should be considered.

Sources: Centers for Disease Control and Prevention (CDC). Sexually transmitted diseases treatment guidelines. *MMWR.* 2010;59(RR-12). Available at: http://www.cdc.gov/mmwr/pdf/rr/rr5912.pdf. Accessed November 11, 2012; U.S. National Library of Medicine. Drugs and lactation database (LactMed). 2012. Available at: http://toxnet.nlm.nih.gov/cgi-bin/sis/htmlgen?LACT. Accessed January 19, 2013.

PID and Pregnancy

Women with a history of PID are at increased risk for ectopic pregnancy. Though rare in pregnancy related to the protective effect of the cervical mucus plug, pregnant women with PID should be hospitalized for evaluation and treatment.[12]

Syphilis

Syphilis is a sexually transmitted infection with a long documented history. Caused by the spirochete *Treponema pallidum*, syphilis is known as the "Great Pretender" because it may be asymptomatic or present with a variety of symptoms mimicking other conditions. In the United States, more 45,000 new syphilis cases were identified in 2010.[6] Globally, 12 million people acquire syphilis each year.[5] Transmission occurs through oral, anal, or vaginal sexual contact. Condoms do not fully protect against syphilis if the lesion is not covered.

Approximately 50% of exposed individuals will develop infection if not treated. The progression of syphilis can be divided into three overlapping phases known as primary, secondary, and tertiary syphilis. In addition, a latent form of syphilis can develop between the secondary and tertiary phases. Neurologic manifestations of syphilis can occur at any time in the disease process.

Primary syphilis is characterized by a chancre that appears at the site of inoculation approximately 21 days after exposure. The chancre is a nontender indurated ulcerous lesion. It is usually a single lesion, filled with spirochete-laden purulent discharge, and is highly infectious. The chancre begins as a papule that erodes into a well-demarcated area with induration of the base and circumference. Because the chancre is usually painless and heals spontaneously in 2 to 8 weeks, it may not be noticed. The chancre is an open wound, however, so its presence increases the risk that other infections can get established, including other STIs such as HIV and herpes. In addition, other secondary infections may occur within the chancre, resulting in purulent discharge.

The manifestations of secondary syphilis usually appear 4 to 10 weeks after infection and can reappear following periods of latency. Secondary syphilis marks the change from local to systemic infection. The most characteristic symptom of this stage of syphilis is a rash that appears on the palms of the hands, soles of the feet, and trunk; this rash can be macular, papular, or psoriasiform.[24] Other symptoms include patchy alopecia, condylomata lata, lesions of the mucous membranes, and symptoms of a systemic illness such as low-grade fever, sore throat, hoarseness, malaise, headache, anorexia, and generalized lymphadenopathy. Condylomata lata are highly contagious, flat, moist, wart-like lesions that usually occur in body folds such as the vulva and perianal area.

After the symptoms of secondary syphilis resolve, some affected individuals convert to early or late latent syphilis before the symptoms of tertiary syphilis appear. Persons with latent syphilis have no clinical manifestations, but their infection can be detected with blood tests. Individuals with latent syphilis who have been infected within the past year are classified as having early latent syphilis. Individuals infected for a year or more are classified as having late latent syphilis and will need a longer course of treatment.

Tertiary syphilis can appear anywhere from 1 to 2 years after infection to 30 years or more later, and is rare in the developed world. Associated with high morbidity and mortality, it takes two forms: gumma and cardiovascular syphilis. Gumma are soft-tissue granuloma tumors, which occur in tissues throughout the body. These masses cause extensive damage within the body and are difficult to distinguish from carcinomas. Cardiovascular syphilis may result in aortic valve disease, aortic aneurysm, and coronary artery disease.

Neurosyphilis can occur during any stage of syphilis. Clinical symptoms of central nervous system disease in the presence of positive serologic evidence of syphilis warrant examination of the cerebrospinal fluid. The disease may also present as acute syphilitic meningitis, syphilis of the spinal cord, vascular neurosyphilis, or syphilitic eye disease.

Syphilis can cross the placenta as early as 9 weeks' gestation and cause fetal malformations and death, so early screening of all pregnant women is important; women at risk should be rescreened in the third trimester.[25] Although syphilis is less commonly diagnosed in the United States than HIV, the number of documented congenital syphilis infections is more than double the number of perinatally acquired HIV infections, suggesting a need for more diligent screening and treatment of pregnant women.[6]

Screening for syphilis is done with one of two tests that look for nonspecific antibodies caused by the disease. The most common non-treponemal tests, known as VDRL (Venereal Disease Research Laboratory) and RPR (rapid plasma reagent), can be falsely positive. Pregnancy, autoimmune disorders, and acute bacterial or viral infections, for example, can cause a false-positive result. All positive non-treponemal tests are confirmed with a treponemal test (fluorescent treponemal antibody absorption test [FTA-ABS], passive particle agglutination [TP-PA] assay, various enzyme immunoassays (EIAs), or chemiluminescence immunoassays), which detect antibodies that are specific for *T. pallidum*.

Diagnosis of Syphilis

Laboratory testing for syphilis requires several steps, and different protocols can be followed. If a woman presents with a chancre, positive results on dark-field microscopy of exudate from a chancre lesion provide the definitive diagnosis; dark-field microscopy is not available everywhere, however.[12,24]

The usual first step if no chancre is present is to screen with a non-treponemal test (VDRL or RPR) and, if positive, to confirm the results with a treponemal test. If there is no chancre present, the VDRL and RPR may not be positive for the first few weeks or infection (false-negative); in 1% to 2% of the population, they will have positive results secondary to other conditions (false-positive).[24] Although diagnosis is based on a positive treponemal test, because this test remains positive for life after infection, it cannot be used to determine the presence of active infection or response to treatment. Therefore, after treatment, serial quantitative non-treponemal titers of immunoglobulin antibodies are used to determine the response to treatment and to detect reinfection. The protocol for diagnosis and treatment of syphilis is more complex if the woman has a previous history of syphilis or she is HIV positive; one can consult the CDC guidelines for testing strategies for current syphilis in such clients.

Treatment and Nonpharmacologic Support

Parenteral penicillin G is the best treatment for syphilis. Other forms of penicillin are not as effective. **Table 15-10** identifies the recommended doses and routes of treatment. Treatment of early syphilis can

Table 15-10	Outpatient Treatments for Syphilis			
Stage of Syphilis	Recommended Treatments for Nonpregnant Women and Males Generic (Brand)	Alternative Treatments for Nonpregnant Women and Males Generic (Brand)	Recommended Treatments for Pregnant Women Generic (Brand)	Recommended Treatment for Breastfeeding Women
Primary, secondary, and early latent syphilis	Benzathine penicillin G (Bicillin LA) 2.4 million units IM in a single dose	Doxycycline (Vibramycin) 100 mg orally twice a day for 14 days OR Tetracycline (Sumycin) 500 mg four times a day for 14 days	Benzathine penicillin G (Bicillin LA) 2.4 million units IM in a single dose If the woman is penicillin allergic, desensitize per CDC guidelines. Jarish-Herxheimer reaction may cause preterm labor or fetal distress in the first 24 hours of treatment; consider additional monitoring.	Benzathine penicillin is safe during breastfeeding. Doxycycline and tetracycline (Sumycin) have the theoretical risk of staining forming teeth. Longer courses of therapy with these drugs are not recommended for nursing mothers. However, if alternative therapies are not available, consider strategies to minimize drug transfer to the breast milk.
Late latent syphilis or syphilis of an unknown duration	Benzathine penicillin G (Bicillin LA) 2.4 million units IM once a week for three doses			

IM = intramuscular.

Sources: Centers for Disease Control and Prevention (CDC). Sexually transmitted diseases treatment guidelines. *MMWR.* 2010;59(RR-12). Available at: http://www.cdc.gov/mmwr/pdf/rr/rr5912.pdf. Accessed November 11, 2012; U.S. National Library of Medicine. Drugs and lactation database (LactMed). 2012. Available at: http://toxnet.nlm.nih.gov/cgi-bin/sis/htmlgen?LACT. Accessed January 19, 2013.

be accomplished with one injection, while late latent syphilis requires three doses given 1 week apart.

To test for treatment effectiveness, clinical assessment and a non-treponemal test (VDRL or RPR) should be performed at 6 months and 1 year following treatment. With adequate treatment, titers usually decline fourfold, but in 15% of treated cases, the titer does not decline. An increase in titers by fourfold following treatment is indicative of treatment failure or reinfection.[12] All women who test positive for syphilis should be offered HIV screening. Also, all sexual partners from within the past 90 days should be treated presumptively for syphilis.

Management of Syphilis in Pregnancy

Syphilis readily crosses the placenta after 9 weeks' gestation. Transmission of the pathogen to the fetus usually occurs between the 16th and 28th weeks of pregnancy.[25] As many as 40% of women with untreated syphilis during pregnancy will miscarriage. Syphilis is also associated with preterm birth, low birth weight, and congenital malformations as described in the "Fetal/Neonatal Considerations" subsection.

Penicillin G is the only acceptable treatment for syphilis in pregnancy. If a woman is allergic to penicillin, she should be desensitized prior to treatment. The Jarisch-Herxheimer reaction, which can appear approximately 2 hours after initiation of treatment, manifests as fever, chills, rigor, hypotension, and tachycardia. This reaction can cause preterm labor or fetal distress, so additional monitoring during the first 24 hours of treatment may be indicated. If the woman is treated for syphilis less than 4 weeks before birth, the newborn will need additional testing and treatment as outlined by the CDC. Women without documented syphilis testing should be screened in labor.

Fetal/Neonatal Considerations

Congenital malformations are common in infants born to women with untreated syphilis during pregnancy, and include deafness, hepatomegaly, and bone abnormalities. Syphilis can cause intrauterine fetal demise, and maternal screening is recommended following stillbirth at any gestation. Syphilis can cause the placenta to be large and pale. Infants born to women with positive serologic tests need in-depth evaluation including testing of the placenta, serologic tests on the newborn's blood (cord blood is not acceptable), and dark-field microscopy testing of suspicious body lesions. Abnormal results

warrant treatment and more invasive testing per CDC guidelines.[12]

Chancroid

Chancroid ulcers are nonindurated painful lesions caused by a gram-negative anaerobic bacillus, *Haemophilus ducreyi*. The infection is transmitted through sexual contact with mucous membranes. These lesions are usually found on the vulva, cervix, or perineum, and approximately 50% of affected women have associated unilateral adenitis that can develop into buboes—that is, abscesses of the local lymph nodes. The buboe can rupture and drain, spreading infection and leading to permanent scarring. While the incidence of chancroid has declined around the world, outbreaks continue to occur, often associated with the sale or exchange of sex. In the United States, there were 24 total reported cases of chancroid distributed across 9 states in 2010.[6]

Diagnosis of Chancroid

Diagnosis is based on the physical examination. The presence of a painful ulcer on the genitals combined with tender inguinal lymphadenopathy suggests chancroid. Lymph nodes may be fluctuant and drain when pressed.[26] Given that many infections can cause genital lesions (**Table 15-11**), it is important to perform several tests directly on the genital lesion, including cultures for herpes simplex virus (HSV) and secondary infections, and dark-field microscopy for syphilis. If possible, obtain a culture for *H. ducreyi*; however, the culture medium is not widely available and has a low specificity. The woman should also be evaluated for chlamydia and gonorrhea. If it has been more than 7 days since the lesion appeared, perform a non-treponemal test for syphilis.[12] Negative serologic tests for syphilis and wound tests that are negative for HSV and syphilis

Table 15-11	Differentiation of Genital Lesions by Symptoms	
Typically Painless	**Typically Painful**
Genital warts	Herpetic vesicles and open lesions
Condyloma acuminata	
	Chancroid
Syphilis chancre	
Condylomata lata	Lymphogranuloma venereum lymphadenopathy and lesions

are needed as further confirmation for the chancroid diagnosis.[12]

Treatment and Nonpharmacologic Support

Table 15-12 outlines pharmacologic treatment for chancroid. Single-dose therapy is preferred for ease of use. There have been reports of *H. ducreyi* resistance to ciprofloxacin (Cipro) and erythromycin (E-mycin) outside the United States. All of the woman's sexual partners within the last 10 days preceding onset of symptoms should be treated presumptively for this STI.

A clinical exam is recommended 3 to 7 days following treatment. The pain of the lesion and the lymphadenopathy should improve by day 3, and the lesion should be healing by day 7 of treatment. All women with chancroid should be screened for HIV. Slow healing can be indicative of underlying HIV infection.

Lymphogranuloma Venereum

Lymphogranuloma venereum (LGV) is caused by *C. trachomatis* that is transmitted via genital or rectal mucosal contact. LGV is primarily an infection of the lymphatics and lymph nodes; although LGV is caused by *C. trachomatis*, it involves different serovars, or subtypes, of the bacterium than the subtypes that cause chlamydial infection of the vagina or upper reproductive tract. Thus LGV is a distinct disorder that differs from the more common manifestations of chlamydial infection. Women with LGV most commonly present with unilateral, painful inguinal lymphadenopathy or pelvic pain. Approximately one-third of infected individuals remember having a nontender genital lesion.[26] Constipation, anal pain, tenesmus, and bloody and mucoid anal discharge are common symptoms with rectal infection. Left untreated, LGV can lead to fistulas and permanent tissue damage as lymph nodes rupture and spread

Table 15-12	**Treatments for Nonsyphilitic Genital Ulcer Diseases**			
Genital Ulcer Disease	**Recommended Treatments for Nonpregnant Women and Males Generic (Brand)**	**Alternative Treatments for Nonpregnant Women and Males Generic (Brand)**	**Recommended Treatments for Pregnant Women Generic (Brand)**	**Recommended Treatments for Breastfeeding Women**
Chancroid	Azithromycin (Zithromax, Z-Pak) 1 g orally once OR Ceftriaxone (Rocephin) 250 mg IM once OR Ciprofloxacin (Cipro) 500 mg orally twice a day for 3 days OR Erythromycin base 500 mg orally three times a day for 7 days	None	Azithromycin (Zithromax, Z-Pak) 1 g orally once OR Ceftriaxone (Rocephin) 250 mg IM once OR Erythromycin base 500 mg orally three times a day for 7 days	Same as for pregnant women
Lymphogranuloma venereum	Doxycycline (Vibramycin) 100 mg orally twice a day for 21 days	Erythromycin base 500 mg orally four times a day for 21 days	Erythromycin base 500 mg orally four times a day for 21 days Azithromycin (Zithromax, Z-Pak) 1 g orally once a week for 3 weeks may be effective but is not currently a recommended treatment by the CDC.	Same as for pregnant women Doxycycline (Vibramycin) is not recommended but may be used if risks to the infant can be minimized.

IM = intramuscular.

Sources: Centers for Disease Control and Prevention (CDC). Sexually transmitted diseases treatment guidelines. *MMWR.* 2010;59(RR-12). Available at: http://www.cdc.gov/mmwr/pdf/rr/rr5912.pdf. Accessed November 11, 2012; U.S. National Library of Medicine. Drugs and lactation database (LactMed). 2012. Available at: http://toxnet.nlm.nih.gov/cgi-bin/sis/htmlgen?LACT. Accessed January 19, 2013.

infection. LGV was previously rare in developed countries, but since 2000 there have been outbreaks in Europe and the United States.[26]

Diagnosis of Lymphogranuloma Venereum

The physical exam will be remarkable for unilateral, painful, inguinal lymphadenopathy. Lymph nodes may be fluctuant and rupture on compression. The skin over the affected area may be darkened. Rectal exam reveals symptoms of proctocolitis, including inflammation of the rectal mucosa if the rectum is infected.

Laboratory tests include NAAT for *C. trachomatis* performed vaginally or from lymph node or lesion exudate. Even though laboratory tests should be performed, clinical symptoms alone can be used for diagnosis to begin treatment.

Treatment and Nonpharmacologic Support

Pharmacologic treatment for LGV is listed in Table 15-12. Very large and fluctuant lymph nodes may require needle aspiration and drainage to prevent ulcerations. Nonsteroidal anti-inflammatory drugs (NSAIDs) may help mitigate pain and inflammation. All sexual partners within the past 2 months should be evaluated, tested, and treated if needed.[12]

Granuloma Inguinale

Granuloma inguinale is rare in the United States, but is more common in less-developed tropical areas around the world. This infection is predominately transmitted through sexual contact, though non-sexual transmission may be possible.[26] Caused by a gram-negative bacteria, *Klebsiella granulomatis*, granuloma inguinale infection begins with painless beefy-red lesions that bleed on contact. These genital lesions are progressive, spreading across the anogenital and inguinal area. While local lymphadenopathy does not occur, subcutaneous granulomas (pseudo-boboes) may form under the skin of the inguinal area. Direct testing for *K. granulomatis* is difficult even in well-supplied laboratories. Thus diagnosis relies heavily on clinical assessment.

Diagnosis of Granuloma Inguinale

Physical exam reveals ulcerative lesions that are red and bleed easily. Lesions may also be hypertrophic or have necrotic wound portions. Local or regional lymphadenopathy and subcutaneous granulomas may be present as well. Secondary infections may cause a purulent exudate. Laboratory tests for the differential diagnosis include HSV culture, culture for secondary bacterial infection, and dark-field microscopy

for *T. pallidum*. Consider non-treponemal testing for syphilis. Because direct culture is difficult, diagnosis relies on clinical presentation and presence of risk factors for the disease (e.g., tropical location, local prevalence).

Treatment and Nonpharmacologic Support

Table 15-12 summarizes pharmacologic treatment for granuloma inguinale. Treatment also includes basic wound management to treat or prevent secondary infections. Sexual partners within the past 60 days should be evaluated and offered treatment, but the value of treatment for asymptomatic individuals has not been established.[12]

Viral Sexually Transmitted Infections

Human Papillomavirus

HPV is estimated to be the most common sexually transmitted disease; as many as half of all sexually active adults will contract one or more subtypes of HPV in their lifetime.[12] More than 100 subtypes of HPV have been identified to date, of which more than 40 subtypes infect the genital area.[12] Papilloma viruses infect the surface epithelia and mucous membranes and cause varying cellular changes, depending on the subtype of the HPV virus. Most HPV infections are asymptomatic, and 90% are eliminated by the immune system within 2 years following infection. However, certain subtypes are associated with persistent infection, leading to symptoms such as genital warts or cancers of the genital area, cervix, and rectum. HPV subtypes 6 and 11 cause 90% of genital warts, although subtypes 18, 31, and 33 are also found in warts.[12] HPV subtypes 16 and 18 cause 70% to 80% of anogenital cancers, but subtype 31 is associated with anogenital cancers as well.[28]

Screening for cervical HPV infection and cancer is part of routine health promotion, as noted in the *Health Promotion and Maintenance* chapter. This section focuses on HPV infection manifesting as growths or warts on the vulva, perineum, or anus, or within the vagina. Warts caused by HPV subtypes 6 and 11 can also be found on mucous membranes of the mouth, nose, and eyes. Symptoms can occur years after exposure.[12]

Genital warts are common in the United States, accounting for hundreds of millions of dollars in healthcare expenditures annually.[6] However, the prevalence of HPV may decrease dramatically in the next 10 to 15 years due to administration of the HPV vaccine to females and males younger than 26 years. This vaccine is expected to decrease transmission of HPV subtypes, 6, 11, 16, and 18.

The virus that causes genital warts is transmitted through contact with genitals, vulva, perineum, or rectum. Condoms do not thoroughly protect from HPV; female condoms offer some additional protection for the vulva when compared with male condoms, but do not completely eliminate the risk of HPV infection.[27]

Diagnosis of Genital Warts

Diagnosis of genital warts caused by HPV occurs via physical examination, which will reveal fleshy papules or pedunculated warty lesions on the vulva, introitus, perineum, anus, cervix, and vaginal walls. Large warts, known as condylomata acuminata, may take on a cauliflower-like appearance and may bleed when abraded. These lesions may appear similar to the condylomata lata associated with syphilis; however, the condylomata lata usually has a flat appearance. Warts caused by HPV will turn white when exposed to acetic acid, although this test is not specific enough for diagnosis and is not recommended by the CDC as a diagnostic test.[12] Non-treponemal tests can be useful to differentiate condylomata acuminata from condylomata lata if needed. A biopsy is indicated if lesions have not responded to 3 months of initial treatment or are unevenly pigmented, ulcerated, or fixed.

Treatment and Nonpharmacologic Support

Many genital warts will resolve spontaneously and may not need treatment. The number, size, and location of warts and the cost and availability of treatments are important considerations.[12] All treatments for warts have localized side effects, including irritation, pain, and burning. While treatment may diminish the size and number of genital warts, it may not decrease transmission rates. The woman or provider can apply treatment; self-applied medications may facilitate prolonged treatment if it is needed. Decisions about treatment should be made in partnership with the woman.

Treatments recommended by the CDC for nonpregnant women are presented in **Table 15-13**.[12] Sinecatechins are derived from green tea and allow women a botanically based option. Sexual partners should be treated only if they are symptomatic and desire treatment. While HPV is an STI, it is impossible to determine the time of acquisition. The growth of genital warts is not a reliable indicator of recent infection.

The need for follow-up visits is influenced by the size of lesions and their responsiveness to treatment. Warts may return following treatment and can be (re)treated the same way as the initial infection was treated. Regular Pap screening according to current guidelines is important to evaluate affected women for cervical cancer, but a diagnosis of genital warts does not change regular screening frequency. Women should be offered screening for common STIs.

Genital Warts in Pregnancy:

Warts may initially appear or increase in size during pregnancy. Treatment with trichloracetic acid (TCA) or bichloroacetic acid (BCA) is safe during pregnancy, but other medications used to treat HPV such as podophyllin are not recommended for use in pregnant women. It may be difficult to fully eliminate warts during pregnancy, but they may regress spontaneously postpartum. Surgical treatment is indicated if the warts might complicate vaginal birth.

Intrapartum Considerations

Genital warts are highly vascularized and may bleed excessively if torn or cut during birth. Care should be taken to avoid warts during suturing or if an episiotomy is needed. Cesarean section is indicated only if extensive warts obstruct the vaginal opening or are expected to bleed uncontrollably during birth.[12]

Fetal/Neonatal Considerations

Infants born to women with genital warts attributable to HPV subtypes 6 and 11 may develop respiratory papillomatosis—that is, warts within their airway—during the neonatal period or beyond. The mode of transmission to the fetus or neonate is not clear, and cesarean birth may not decrease the incidence of papillomatosis.[12] The infant's healthcare provider should be alerted about the potential for respiratory papillomatosis.

Herpes Simplex Virus

A variety of herpes viruses affect humans. Sexually transmitted herpes infection is a result of one of two subtypes of herpes simplex virus: HSV-1 or HSV-2. These viruses are not completely cleared from the infected tissues after the initial infection and can cause recurrent symptoms throughout life, especially during periods of high stress. HSV-1 and HSV-2 can lead to painful ulcerations of the anogenital region and the mucous membranes of the mouth and nose.

HSV-1 is commonly acquired in childhood but can be sexually transmitted, especially through

Table 15-13	Treatments for Genital Warts Caused by Human Papillomavirus for Nonpregnant Women		
	Treatments Generic (Brand)	**Clinical Considerations**	**Patient Instructions**
External	**Podofilox 0.5% solution or gel (Condylox, Podofilox)** Applied by the woman twice a day for 3 days	Useful when warts are smaller than 10 cm × 10 cm Maximum dose of 0.5 mL of the solution per day Demonstrate application in office for instruction	Apply to warts with a cotton swab or finger twice a day for 3 days, then no treatment for 4 days.
	Imiquimod 5% cream (Aldara) Applied by the woman		Apply at bedtime three times a week for up to 16 weeks. Wash off cream with soap and water after 6–10 hours. The cream may weaken latex condoms and diaphragms.
	Sinecatechins 15% ointment (Veregen) Applied by the woman	Contraindicated for individuals who have herpes or HIV, or who are immunocompromised	Apply a thin film over the affected area using a finger three times a day for up to 16 weeks. Do not wash the film off the affected area. Ointment will weaken latex condoms and diaphragms.
	Trichloroacetic acid (TCA) or bichloroacetic acid (BCA) 80–90%[a] Applied by the provider	Protect areas surrounding the wart with petroleum jelly Apply acid sparingly and allow to dry, forming a white frosting Excessive acid can be neutralized with sodium bicarbonate or liquid soap Treatment can be repeated once a week	
	Podophyllin resin 10–25% in compound tincture of benzoin Applied by the provider	Maximum dose of 0.5 mL of solution per application Treat only a 10 cm by 10 cm area per treatment Cannot be used if the skin of the lesion of surrounding area is not intact	The resin should be washed off in 1–4 hours to decrease irritation.
	Cryotherapy with liquid nitrogen or cytoprobe Performed by the provider	Requires specialized training Can be repeated every 1–2 weeks Not appropriate for vaginal warts	
	Surgical removal Performed by the provider	Requires specialized training	Useful for extensive or hard-to-treat lesions.
Vaginal	**Trichloroacetic acid (TCA) or bichloroacetic acid (BCA) 80–90%**[a] Applied by the provider	Protect areas surrounding the wart with petroleum jelly Apply acid sparingly and allow to dry, forming a white frosting Excessive acid can be neutralized with sodium bicarbonate or liquid soap Treatment can be repeated once a week	

Table 15-13	Treatments for Genital Warts Caused by Human Papillomavirus for Nonpregnant Women *(continued)*		
	Treatments **Generic (Brand)**	**Clinical Considerations**	**Patient Instructions**
Vaginal *(continued)*	**Cryotherapy with liquid nitrogen or cytoprobe** Performed by the provider	Requires specialized training Can be repeated every 1–2 weeks Not appropriate for vaginal warts	
Urethral Meatus	**Podophyllin resin 10–25% in compound tincture of benzoin** Applied by the provider	Ensure all surfaces are dry prior to application Cannot be used if the skin of the lesion of surrounding area is not intact Maximum dose of 0.5 mL of solution per application Treat only a 10 cm × 10 cm area per treatment	The resin should be washed off in 1–4 hours to decrease irritation.
	Cryotherapy with liquid nitrogen or cytoprobe Performed by the provider	Requires specialized training Can be repeated every 1–2 weeks Not appropriate for vaginal warts	
Anal	***Trichloroacetic acid (TCA) or bichloroacetic acid (BCA) 80–90%** Applied by the provider	Protect areas surrounding the wart with petroleum jelly Apply acid sparingly and allow to dry, forming a white frosting Excessive acid can be neutralized with sodium bicarbonate or liquid soap Treatment can be repeated once a week	
	Cryotherapy with liquid nitrogen or cytoprobe Performed by the provider	Requires specialized training Can be repeated every 1–2 weeks Not appropriate for vaginal warts	
	Surgical removal Performed by the provider	Requires specialized training	Useful for extensive or hard-to-treat lesions.

[a] Acceptable pharmacologic treatment in pregnancy.

Sources: Centers for Disease Control and Prevention (CDC). Sexually transmitted diseases treatment guidelines. *MMWR.* 2010;59(RR-12). Available at: http://www.cdc.gov/mmwr/pdf/rr/rr5912.pdf. Accessed November 11, 2012; U.S. National Library of Medicine. Drugs and lactation database (LactMed). 2012. Available at: http://toxnet.nlm.nih.gov/cgi-bin/sis/htmlgen?LACT. Accessed January 19, 2013.

orogenital contact. In some populations, this virus is the major cause of genital herpes.[6] HSV-1 usually has a more mild clinical presentation than HSV-2, both with the first infection and subsequent outbreaks. In addition, it is associated with lower rates of asymptomatic viral shedding.[12]

HSV-2 is nearly always sexually transmitted and is associated with more severe symptoms and more frequent reoccurrences.[12] This virus is more commonly associated with genital herpes than is HSV-1 in most of the United States. While the clinical presentation of the two subtypes is indistinguishable, the CDC recommends typing via blood testing to guide teaching and treatment decisions, as HSV-2

has more virulent reoccurrences and a higher rate of transmission.[12]

It is estimated that approximately 16% of adults in the United States are infected with HSV-2, with some demographic groups having a nearly 48% seropositive rate.[6] Both HSV-1 and HSV-2 are contracted through mucous membrane contact with infected secretions. Anogenital and oral infections are common in part because HSV is shed into bodily secretions. Female and male condoms and dental dams reduce the risk of HSV transmission but do not completely eliminate this risk .[27]

Women are especially vulnerable to HSV-2 infection and have higher baseline rates of infection when compared to men, in part due to prolonged contact with semen during vaginal intercourse. Herpes is a lifelong infection that has the potential for transmission throughout the lifespan. In addition, individuals can have HSV for many years before becoming symptomatic. An outbreak, while caused by a sexually transmitted virus, does not mean that either partner recently acquired the infection. This factor can complicate health education and partner counseling. Genital herpes infection increases the risk of acquiring HIV by fourfold, in part due to skin breaks and open lesions.[6] Safer sex precautions throughout life are important for women who have HSV infection.

Most herpes infections are asymptomatic or unreported. The first episode of herpes is usually worse than subsequent outbreaks. Prodromal symptoms may occur before the appearance of lesions and include tingling and burning. Constitutional symptoms include fever, malaise, headache, and myalgia. The main symptom of the outbreak is painful sores on the affected area. Initial outbreaks may include lesions in a wide swath or in multiple body locations; in contrast, subsequent outbreaks are usually more localized. Women may also have dysuria as urine touches the open lesions.

Diagnosis of Herpes

The woman having an HSV outbreak usually presents with small, very painful vesicles or open lesions on the mouth, vulva, perineum, or anus. The lesions usually appear in small groups and are disproportionately painful in comparison to their size and depth. They may be fluid-filled vesicles—that is, small skin splits that are covered, oozing, crusted, or nearly healed. Edema, diffuse inflammation, and vaginal or urethral discharge may be present as well. A speculum exam may be excessively painful and is not required for diagnosis. Tender inguinal lymphadenopathy may also be present.

Diagnosis of herpes is based on physical exam and confirmed with viral and serologic testing. Viral culture or polymerase chain reaction (PCR) testing of exudate from the lesion is the standard for confirmation of viral lesions. However, viral culture has low sensitivity, especially if the area is crusted over or healing.[12] Type-specific immunoglobulin G (IgG)–based assay blood testing can diagnose herpes and reveal the subtype, which is recommended by the CDC to assist in treatment decisions. The woman should also be tested for all common STIs, especially if she has a new partner.

Treatment and Nonpharmacologic Support

Serologic and viral test results are not needed to begin treatment for herpes with antiviral therapy.

Treatments for initial and episodic outbreaks are shown in **Table 15-14**, along with suppression regimens. For episodic outbreaks, medication should be started at the first prodromal symptom for best efficacy; nevertheless, treatment is beneficial even if delayed until the outbreak of lesions.12 Suppressive treatment should be considered if recurrences are frequent or disruptive for the woman. Suppression also decreases the risk of asymptomatic shedding and transmission.12 The woman's physical and psychological need for suppressive therapy may change over time and should be reevaluated yearly.12

Cost and frequency of dosing are considerations when choosing a treatment with the woman. Famciclovir (Famvir) and valacyclovir (Valtrex) have greater oral bioavailability than acyclovir (Zovirax), but are more expensive. Topical treatments are not effective for management of initial or subsequent outbreaks. Support includes non-narcotic pain management. If experiencing dysuria, the woman can use a peri-bottle or urinate while sitting in water in a bowl or the bathtub to decrease symptoms. Limited definitive research has focused on the efficacy of complementary suppressive therapies, such as L-lysine and bee pollen, and the woman can decide if the costs and side effects of such treatments are worth the personal benefit.

Partner treatment is not needed for herpes. Ideally, the woman will have an open conversation with her sexual partners about the risk of asymptomatic transmission and the need for safer sexual practices. The woman should avoid sexual contact with uninfected partners while having prodromal or outbreak symptoms, as condoms do not provide full protection from transmission of the virus. A well-placed follow-up visit is best for teaching about prevention when compared to a problem visit for the initial outbreak, because when the woman is feeling better she will be more prepared to hear and understand the information.

Prenatal Considerations

All women should be asked if they have a history of herpes or genital lesions as part of their initial visit for pregnancy.[12] Recurrent infections during pregnancy pose little to no risk during the prenatal period and produce immunoglobulins against HSV for the fetus. In contrast, primary outbreaks during pregnancy have been associated with a small increase in fetal abnormalities and a larger risk for intrapartum transmission.[29] Women can be treated for herpes infections during pregnancy, as shown in Table 15-14. Severe outbreaks with dissemination in pregnancy warrant hospitalization and treatment with intravenous acyclovir.[30] Prophylactic administration of acyclovir

Table 15-14	Pharmacologic Treatments for Herpes Simplex Virus		
Diagnosis	**Recommended Treatments for Nonpregnant Women[12] and Males Generic (Brand)**	**Recommended Treatments for Pregnant Women Generic (Brand)**	**Recommended Treatment for Breastfeeding Women[15]**
Initial outbreak of HSV in an adult	Acyclovir (Zovirax) 400 mg by mouth three times a day for 7–10 days OR Acyclovir (Zovirax) 200 mg by mouth five times a day for 7–10 days OR Famciclovir (Famvir) 250 mg by mouth three times a day for 7–10 days OR Valacyclovir (Valtrex) 1 g by mouth twice a day for 7–10 days	Acyclovir has more data supporting benefit without risks to fetus and is preferred by the CDC.[12] ACOG supports the use of acyclovir (Zovirax) or valacyclovir (Valtrex).[30] Severe infections should be treated with intravenous acyclovir. Acyclovir (Zovirax) 400 mg by mouth three times a day for 7–10 days OR Acyclovir (Zovirax) 200 mg orally five times a day for 7–10 days OR Valacyclovir (Valtrex) 1 g by mouth twice a day for 7–10 days	Acyclovir (Zovirax) is considered safe in breastfeeding, with drug passage to the infant being much less than newborn therapeutic doses.[15] Lower dosages may lead to lower maternal serum levels, allowing less transfer to the milk. Alternatively, the mother can time administration to breastfeed at times of low serum levels to minimize transfer. Valacyclovir (Valtrex) is acceptable for use during lactation, as it is converted to acyclovir in the mother and excreted in very low amounts into breast milk.[15] Famciclovir (Famvir) is not recommended during lactation.
Recurrent outbreak in an HIV-positive adult	Acyclovir (Zovirax) 400 mg by mouth three times a day for 5 days OR Acyclovir (Zovirax) 800 mg twice by mouth three times a day for 2 days OR Famciclovir (Famvir) 125 mg by mouth two times a day for 5 days OR Famciclovir (Famvir) 1000 mg by mouth two times one day OR Famciclovir (Famvir) 500 mg by mouth once, then 250 mg twice a day for 2 days OR Valacyclovir (Valtrex) 500 mg by mouth twice a day for 3 days OR Valacyclovir (Valtrex) 1 g by mouth once a day for 5 days	The CDC states that acyclovir has a higher safety profile in pregnancy.[12] ACOG supports the use of valacyclovir (Valtrex) if needed.[30] Acyclovir (Zovirax) 400 mg by mouth three times a day for 5 days OR Acyclovir (Zovirax) 800 mg twice OR three times a day for 2 days OR Famciclovir (Famvir) 125 mg by mouth two times a day for 5 days OR Famciclovir (Famvir) 1000 mg by mouth two times one day OR Famciclovir (Famvir) 500 mg by mouth once, then 250 mg twice a day for 2 days	Acyclovir (Zovirax) is considered safe in breastfeeding, with drug passage to the infant being much less than newborn therapeutic doses. Lower dosages may lead to lower maternal serum levels, allowing for less transfer to the milk. Alternatively, the mother can time drug administration to breastfeeding at times of low serum levels to minimize transfer. Valacyclovir (Valtrex) is acceptable for use during lactation as it is converted to acyclovir in the mother and excreted in very low amounts into breast milk.[15] Famciclovir (Famvir) is not recommended during lactation.[15]

(continues)

Table 15-14	**Pharmacologic Treatments for Herpes Simplex Virus** (continued)		
Diagnosis	**Recommended Treatments for Nonpregnant Women[12] and Males Generic (Brand)**	**Recommended Treatments for Pregnant Women Generic (Brand)**	**Recommended Treatment for Breastfeeding Women[15]**
Suppression of HSV outbreaks	Acyclovir (Zovirax) 400 mg orally two times a day OR Famciclovir (Famvir) 250 mg orally two times a day OR Valacyclovir (Valtrex) 500 mg orally once a day OR Valacyclovir (Valtrex) 1 g orally once a day	The CDC does not have recommendations specific to pregnant women but states that acyclovir has a better safety profile.[12] ACOG recommends: Acyclovir (Zovirax) 400 mg by mouth three times a day beginning at 36 weeks OR Valacyclovir (Valtrex) 500 mg orally twice a day beginning at 36 weeks[30]	See above.

ACOG = American Congress of Obstetricians and Gynecologists.

Sources: Centers for Disease Control and Prevention (CDC). Sexually transmitted diseases treatment guidelines. *MMWR.* 2010;59(RR-12). Available at: http://www.cdc.gov/mmwr/pdf/rr/rr5912.pdf. Accessed November 11, 2012; Mashburn J. Vaginitis. In: King TL, Brucker MC, eds. *Pharmacology for Women's Health.* Sudbury, MA: Jones and Bartlett; 2011:950; U.S. National Library of Medicine. Drugs and lactation database (LactMed). 2012. Available at: http://toxnet.nlm.nih.gov/cgi-bin/sis/htmlgen?LACT. Accessed January 19, 2013; American College of Obstetricians and Gynecologists. Management of herpes in pregnancy. *Obstet Gynecol.* 2007;109(6):1489-1498.

(Zovirax) beginning at 36 gestational weeks has been shown to decrease the incidence of asymptomatic shedding and outbreaks at term, the rate of cesarean section for HSV lesions, and the neonatal incidence of HSV.[12,31] Routine administration of antiviral drugs beginning at 36 weeks' gestation for women with a previous history of HSV-2 confirmed by serologic testing is currently recommended.[30] HSV-1 infection does not require prophylaxis unless genital outbreaks occur during pregnancy.[12,30]

Pregnant women without a history of herpes whose sexual partners have herpes should be encouraged to use safer sex practices and avoid sexual contact when the partners have prodromal or outbreak symptoms. This consideration is especially important when pregnant women are close to term. In addition, women should not have orogenital contact near their estimated date of delivery if their partner has a history of oral herpes sores.[12]

Intrapartum Considerations

If a woman has a history of genital herpes, a careful perianal assessment is important at the first labor examination or prior to induction to rule out active infection. The greatest risk of intrapartum transmission to the infant is during the woman's initial outbreak. Vaginal birth during a primary outbreak can have vertical transmission rates as high as 60%.[30] Vaginal birth during recurrent infections has a lower transmission rate of 3%, due in part to passage of maternal immunoglobulin across the placenta to the fetal circulation.[30] However, because neonatal morbidity and mortality are high following infection, a cesarean section may be offered if the woman has *any* active genital lesions or prodromal symptoms at the onset of labor in an area that could come in contact with the fetus during vaginal birth.[30]

If a woman has nongenital lesions when she begins labor, vaginal birth may proceed normally. All nongenital lesions should be covered with an occlusive dressing to decrease risk of transmission.[30] Occasionally a woman will have a precipitous labor and give birth vaginally during a herpetic outbreak. In these cases, viral cultures of the newborn and prophylactic treatment with acyclovir may be considered, especially if this is the mother's first outbreak.[6]

Fetal/Neonatal Considerations

Though such transmission is rare (accounting for only 5% of all neonatal cases), herpes can be transmitted across the placenta. Manifestations of this condition are similar to intrauterine varicella infection and include skin lesions, malformations of the eyes, and central nervous system dysfunction.[29] The majority of infants in the United States who develop neonatal herpes are born to women with no known history of the disease; this is due in part to increased monitoring of women with a history of herpes.[30] Approximately 85% of neonatal cases of HSV are contracted during birth through contact with maternal secretions, whereas 10% are contracted after birth via contact with infected individuals.[31] In addition, ritual circumcision with suction of the baby's blood using the adult's mouth has been shown to transmit HSV.[32]

Regardless of the route of transmission or subtype, HSV infection is very risky for the newborn. Symptoms of neonatal herpes usually appear on days 5 to 9 of life and include respiratory distress, irritability, jaundice, and vesicular lesions around the site of infection. Late symptoms include seizures and shock. Although 45% of cases of neonatal herpes remain localized to one area, there is a large risk of disseminated infection and central nervous system involvement. The mortality rate for untreated disseminated disease is 85%. Early treatment with antiviral agents can improve chances of survival.

Breastfeeding Considerations

HSV is communicable only through contact with infected secretions from mucous membranes of the mouth or genitals. Women with HSV should be encouraged to breastfeed unless there is a herpetic lesion directly on the nipple.

Hepatitis B

More than 2 billion people worldwide have been infected with hepatitis B virus (HBV) at some point in their lives.[33] Hepatitis B is transmitted via contact with infected blood and bodily secretions including infected semen or (rarely) saliva. Such transmission may occur during sexual contact (genital and oral), birth, needle-sticks or sharing of needles, and use of nonsterilized medical instruments. HBV can remain infectious outside the body for several days, even if dry, and is able to establish infection with very few initial organisms, making it highly infectious.[33]

HBV infection is often asymptomatic or symptoms are vague enough to go unnoticed. Commonly noted symptoms include fatigue, nausea, and diffuse epigastric or right upper quadrant pain. Later symptoms include jaundice, dark urine, and gray stools. Women with fulminant hepatitis may have bleeding problems and altered mental status.[12]

Hepatitis B can become a chronic infection. Approximately 25% of all persons who become chronically infected develop liver cancer or other liver disease. The chances of chronic infection vary by age at the time of initial infection.[33]

The overall rate of HBV infection has declined more than 80% since 1991, when the CDC began a campaign to reduce the prevalence of HBV infections.[6] The HBV vaccine is produced from derivatives of yeast, without the use of blood products, so it cannot cause hepatitis.[12] Vaccination is recommended for several at-risk groups, as described in **Box 15-5**.[34] Routine screening of pregnant women and immunoprophylaxis of all newborns of infected mothers has also been useful in decreasing the prevalence of chronic hepatitis in the United States.[12] Other preventive strategies include universal precautions, careful medical instrument sterilization, safer sex practices, and not sharing toothbrushes and razors with infected individuals.[6,12]

Diagnosis of Hepatitis B

Physical examination findings during acute HBV infection include upper abdominal tenderness,

---

BOX 15-5 Indications for Hepatitis B Vaccination

- All newborn infants and children and adolescents not yet vaccinated for hepatitis B
- Sexually active adults not within a long-term mutually monogamous relationship
- Individuals exposed to blood and bodily fluids at work (healthcare, daycare, and public-safety workers)
- Individuals with diabetes who are younger than age 60 years
- Adults with chronic conditions including HIV, renal, and liver disease
- Persons who live in group institutions (prisons, facilities for care of people with developmental delays)
- Sexual partners and household contacts of HBV-infected individuals
- International travelers to areas of high HBV prevalence
- Anyone seeking care at an STI clinic or drug treatment program
- Men who have sex with both male and female partners

Source: Centers for Disease Control and Prevention (CDC). Sexually transmitted diseases treatment guidelines. *MMWR.* 2010;59(RR-12). Available at: http://www.cdc.gov/mmwr/pdf/rr/rr5912.pdf. Accessed November 11, 2012.

hepatomegaly, and, occasionally, jaundice. Women should be screened for hepatitis B via serologic testing for hepatitis B surface antigen (HBsAg). If the woman is HBsAg positive, a complete hepatitis panel can be obtained, which includes the following data: hepatitis B "e" antigen (HBeAg), which is a marker of a high degree of infectivity; IgM anti-core antibody (IgM anti-HBc), which is a marker of recent infection within the last 6 months and indicates acute infection; IgG anticore antibody (IgG anti-HBc), which is a marker of past or current infection; anti-hepatitis B surface antibody (anti-HBs), which is a marker of an immune response to HBV; antihepatitis B "e" antigen (anti-HBe), which may be present in a person who is either infected or immune; and "viral load," which reveals the concentration of the hepatitis B virus DNA within the blood. Women with hepatitis may also exhibit other abnormal serum tests, including elevated aspartate aminotransferase (AST), elevated alanine amino-trasferase (ALT), elevated bilirubin, and a prolonged prothrombin time.[33] Diagnosis is based on interpretation of hepatitis serology, as shown in **Table 15-15** and **Figure 15-3**.

Treatment and Nonpharmacologic Support

There is no specific treatment for adults with acute hepatitis other than a supportive lifestyle to assist the body in healing.[12] Postexposure prophylaxis may decrease rates of acute and chronic infection but is most useful if prophylaxis is administered within 24 hours of exposure, as is possible following needle-stick, rape, or birth to an infected mother. Information about postexposure prophylaxis resources for viral blood-borne infections can be found in **Box 15-6**. Chronically infected individuals can receive treatment to decrease the risk of liver disease,[12] and should be referred to providers knowledgeable in the management of hepatitis and chronic liver disease.[12] All cases of newly diagnosed hepatitis B should be reported to the local health department.

Prenatal Considerations

Serologic screening for HBsAg is a routine component of the initial laboratory test panel for pregnant women. Women who are acutely infected with hepatitis may need additional care if they have severe symptoms or show signs of coagulopathy or encephalopathy. However, there is no change in prenatal care for women with mild acute or chronic hepatitis infection other than supportive care and avoidance of abdominal trauma.[35] Pregnancy does not change the course of HBV infection. Women who are HBsAg and HBeAg positive are at the greatest risk for vertically transmitting the virus. The woman's chart should note her HBsAg status, and this information

Table 15-15	Interpretation of Hepatitis B Serology						
Interpretation	HBsAg	HBeAg	IgM Anti-HBc	Total Anti-HBc	HepB Serum Titer	Anti-HBe	Anti-HBs
Never infected (susceptible)	–	–	–	–	–	–	–
Early acute[a]	+	+	+	+	High	–	–
Resolving acute	+	–	+	+	Low	+ or –	–
Chronic	+	+ or –	–	+	High or low	+ or –	--
Resolved (immune)	–	–	–	+	–	+ or –	+
Vaccinated (immune)	–	–	–	–	–	–	+
False positive[b]	–	–	–	+	–	–	–

Anti-HBc = IgM antibody to Hepatitis B core antigen; anti-HBe = anti-hepatitis Be antibody; anti-HBs = anti-hepatitis B surface antibody; HBeAg = hepatitis B "e" antigen; HBsAg = hepatitis B surface antigen.

+ = positive; – = negative.

[a]The HBsAg test can be falsely positive because it can react to other viral antigens. To ensure that a positive HBsAg is not falsely positive, samples that are positive should be tested with an FDA-cleared test that will look specifically for HBsAg only.

[b]If the anti-HBc is positive and other hepatitis serologies are negative, there are four possible interpretations: (1) distant resolved infection, (2) false-positive test and the person is susceptible, (3) low level chronic infection, (4) passive transfer to infant born to HBsAg-positive mother.

Sources: Centers for Disease Control and Prevention (CDC). Sexually transmitted diseases treatment guidelines. *MMWR.* 2010;59(RR-12). Available at: http://www.cdc.gov/mmwr/pdf/rr/rr5912.pdf. Accessed November 11, 2012; Brook MG, Mutimer D. Viral hepatitis: screening and vaccination strategies. In: Zenilman JM, Shahmanesh M, eds. *Sexually Transmitted Infections.* Sudbury, MA: Jones & Bartlett Learning; 2012:241-250.

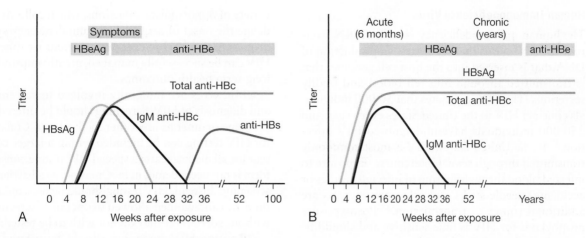

Figure 15-3 (A) Acute hepatitis B virus infection with recovery types—serological course. (B) Chronic hepatitis B virus infection—serological course.

Source: Centers for Disease Control and Prevention (CDC). Recommendations for identification and public health management of persons with chronic hepatitis B virus infection. MMWR. 2008;57(No. RR-8):3-4.

should be conveyed to the woman's chosen birth location to allow preparation for hepatitis B immunoglobulin (HBIG) administration to the newborn following birth.

Hepatitis B vaccination is safe in pregnancy and appropriate for women at risk. Pregnancy is a good time for vaccination of at-risk women, as they are already in the clinic at the appropriate intervals.

Intrapartum Management with Hepatitis B Infection

Intrapartum management of HBV-infected women is the same as that of noninfected women. Hepatitis status should not influence the preferred route of birth (vaginal or cesarean section). However, because fetal scalp electrodes may increase the risk of neonatal infection, an electrode should be applied only if the benefits outweigh the potential risks.

Neonatal Considerations

The CDC advises routine HBV vaccination of all infants weighing more than 2000 g, regardless of the mother's HBV status.[36] Newborns of women infected with HBV should be given HBIG and their first hepatitis vaccine within 12 hours of birth.[36] Without treatment, 90% of newborns infected at birth will become chronic carriers, resulting in a 25% lifetime risk of hepatitis-related mortality. The CDC is an excellent resource for comprehensive information about prevention of perinatal transmission of hepatitis B and provides patient education information in a variety of languages.

Breastfeeding

Hepatitis B is *not* transmitted through breast milk, and women should be encouraged to breastfed regardless of their hepatitis B status. While there have been concerns about transmission of HBV from women with cracked or bleeding nipples, there is no conclusive evidence of transmission by this route. Breastfeeding should not be interrupted for this reason, although women will be counseled about ways to protect their nipples from damage.[36–38]

BOX 15-6 Resources for Information on Postexposure Prophylaxis: Evidence-Based Resources

National Clinicians' Post-Exposure Prophylaxis Hotline (PEPline) and Website:
http://www.nccc.ucsf.edu/about_nccc/pepline

Centers for Disease Control and Prevention Guidelines for Occupational Post-Exposure Prophylaxis:
http://www.cdc.gov/hiv/resources/guidelines/#occupational

Centers for Disease Control and Prevention STD Treatment Guidelines:
http://www.cdc.gov/std/treatment/2010/default.htm

Human Immunodeficiency Virus

The human immunodeficiency virus is an RNA retrovirus (RNA virus that replicates via production of DNA that is inserted into the host cell genome) that is transmitted through infected blood and bodily secretions. The CDC estimates that 50,000 individuals contract HIV in the United States every year, and 250,000 individuals have undiagnosed HIV infection.[39] In the United States, HIV is most commonly transmitted through sexual intercourse. Exposure to infected blood through sharing of infected needles or accidental needle-sticks and other mechanisms are additional routes of transmission.[39] Postexposure prophylaxis for HIV is time sensitive and should be administered as soon as possible after exposure up to 72 hours after contact with the virus.[39]

The risk of acquisition of HIV during sex is greatly increased if a woman has other sexually transmitted diseases such as herpes, gonorrhea, or STIs causing genital ulcers. Sexual acts that are more damaging to the vaginal and rectal mucosa also increase the risk of contracting HIV.[40]

HIV infection proceeds through several stages after infecting the immune system CD4 cells, which are a type of T-cell. The first stage is called acute retroviral syndrome. This stage occurs within the first few weeks after infection and includes fever, malaise, a skin rash, nausea or diarrhea, headache, sore throat, and lymphadenopathy; symptoms that are much like mononucleosis.[12] The symptoms of acute retroviral syndrome can be mild or severe. The infection then becomes asymptomatic during a period of clinical latency that can last a short time or up to 8 years or longer, depending on the individual. During this time, HIV reproduces at very low levels, although it is still active. When the CD4 cell count falls below 200 cells/mm^3, symptoms of advanced infection or acquired immunodeficiency syndrome (AIDS) appear. Symptoms of AIDS include fever, weight loss, diarrhea, cough, shortness of breath, and possibly opportunistic infections, and more intense illnesses and infections. Infections and illness are more severe than would be expected for the woman's age or health status.

In late stages of untreated HIV, the number of functioning CD4 cells decrease as viral replication kills the host cells, rendering the woman susceptible to a wide variety of opportunistic infections. Presenting symptoms may include vulvovaginal or oral candidiasis, shingles, abnormal Pap smears, and other STIs. In addition, HIV makes women more susceptible to cancer. Once the CD4 count falls below 200 cells/mm^3, the woman is likely to develop a variety of opportunistic infections, which collectively define the onset of acquired immunodeficiency syndrome (AIDS).[12] However, with current treatment, HIV can be successfully managed, greatly improving long-term health outcomes.

Midwives are integrally involved in screening and diagnosis of HIV. Screening should be offered in the same manner as any other medical test. Consent for HIV testing can be included within a larger consent for all medical care; a special HIV testing consent form is not needed and, in fact, may act as a barrier to screening. Instead, HIV testing should be presented as the norm and women allowed to opt out of screening without coercion if they do not wish to be tested.[40]

Routine HIV screening should be offered to all women at risk for STIs and annual screening to women at high risk, as outlined in **Box 15-7**. In addition, all pregnant women should be screened at least once in pregnancy using an opt-out approach, and another HIV test should be considered in the third trimester for all women.[40] Many states require third-trimester testing for all pregnant women, unless

---

BOX 15-7 Recommendations for HIV Testing

Screening for HIV Infection

- Individuals 13–64 years old who are seen in a healthcare setting
- Anyone seeking evaluation for or treatment of a sexually transmitted infection
- Individuals initiating treatment for tuberculosis
- Individuals who have had sex with more than one partner (or their partner has had more than one partner) since their last HIV test
- Anyone whose blood or bodily fluids were a source of an occupational exposure for a healthcare worker (e.g., needle-stick injury)
- All pregnant women
- Intravenous drug users and their sexual partners
- Anyone who exchanges sex for money or drugs
- Sexual partners of HIV-positive individuals
- Anyone considering having a new sexual partner
- Heterosexual persons or men who have sex with men who themselves or whose sex partners have had more than one partner since their most recent HIV test

Source: Centers for Disease Control and Prevention (CDC). Revised recommendations for HIV testing of adults, adolescents, and pregnant women in health-care settings. *MMWR.* 2006;55(RR14):1-17.

they opt out of screening.[40] State requirements can be found on state health websites and in CDC's HIV web resources.

Two types of HIV viruses exist: HIV-1 and HIV-2. The vast majority of HIV infections in the United States and worldwide are caused by the HIV-1 virus. HIV-2 is predominately found in West Africa; owing to its transmission on a wider scale, this subtype is now becoming more common throughout the world.[41] Both types of HIV have similar symptoms and effects within the body, though their infectivity and immune system impact vary slightly.[41]

While initial screening tests for HIV are able to detect antibodies to both HIV-1 and HIV-2, the screening tests cannot distinguish between the viruses. In contrast, the supplementary, or diagnostic, tests for HIV are type specific and can detect only one of the viruses. Therefore, if a woman is at risk for HIV-2 and has two positive screening tests, her blood should be tested using confirmatory tests for both HIV-1 and HIV-2 to rule out both infections. Risks for HIV-2 infection involve contact or travel to endemic areas such as West Africa or Portugal. If a woman or her sexual or needle-sharing partners have recently traveled to an endemic area, then confirmatory testing for HIV-2 is warranted if initial screening tests are positive.

Diagnosis of HIV

Often the physical exam in an HIV-infected person is unremarkable. Lymphadenopathy and the presence of opportunistic infections uncharacteristic for the woman's age or health status, such as oral candidiasis in a nondiabetic woman, are suggestive of advanced HIV infection. An algorithm for screening and testing of HIV is found in **Figure 15-4**.

Most common screening tools detect antibodies to HIV, not the presence of the virus itself, and are appropriate first tests for most individuals. Antibodies

appear 2 to 12 weeks after infection occurs. Routine screening can be performed with in-office test kits using oral fluids, blood, or serum or with laboratory testing on blood. In-office rapid testing allows provision of results in 20 minutes. The most commonly used laboratory screening test is a conventional/rapid enzyme immunoassay (EIA) or, rarely, a chemiluminescent immunoassay (CIA).

There is a risk of false-positive results with all the screening tests for HIV. Therefore, if the screening test is positive, it is repeated. If both the first and repeat tests are positive, a supplemental diagnostic test is performed to ensure the person has HIV infection.

Appropriate supplemental tests for confirmation of HIV-1 status include the Western blot, an indirect immunofluorescence assay, or an HIV-1 RNA assay. A positive supplementary test, such as Western blot, indirect immunofluorescence assay, or HIV RNA assay, provides the definitive diagnosis of HIV-1. If a person is suspected of having HIV-2, additional HIV-2 specific tests are warranted.

If a woman has had a recent exposure to HIV and is experiencing symptoms of acute retroviral syndrome, she should be tested using an HIV-1 RNA assay even if her screening tests were negative, as antibody-based testing may not be effective for up to 3 months after exposure.[12]

Negative HIV test results can be conveyed by phone, but positive results should be given to the individual in person. It may be best to have a physician or healthcare team who can offer ongoing care present when a woman is told she has HIV. Some experts recommend that the woman be told when she is alone and others recommend that she have a family member present.[40] Although an HIV diagnosis used to be widely perceived as a death sentence, due to advances in medical treatment, HIV can be considered more like a chronic condition needing ongoing treatment

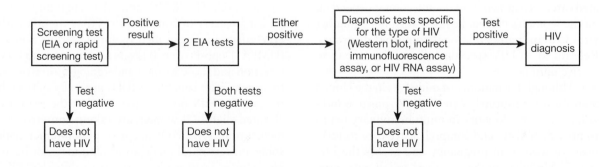

Figure 15-4 HIV screening and testing algorithm.

and care. Even so, a diagnosis of HIV still carries significant stigma and fear. Telling a woman she has HIV is difficult even for experienced clinicians. Proper preparation prior to the visit can be helpful. There are often local or regional organizations that provide specific behavioral and psychological services for HIV-positive individuals, and these organizations can be contacted to provide needed information. The midwife should gather needed written materials to supplement the conversation and provide the woman with reference materials in case she cannot remember the full conversation. Midwifery presence and therapeutic communication skills are useful in providing an honest diagnosis while remaining compassionate and adjusting the information to be sensitive to the woman's needs. Similar to providing information about other STIs, provide the woman with the diagnosis and allow her time to react and formulate questions.

The CDC recommends that a diagnosis of HIV infection be provided in conjunction with key health education points, as listed in **Box 15-8**.[12] Essential health teaching should be discussed verbally and reinforced with written materials. All persons with a new diagnosis of HIV should also be screened for intimate partner violence and a discussion of how to disclose HIV status to a sexual partner should be explored. If the person is at risk for intimate partner violence, resources and ways to assure safety are a priority for this visit. The other information is important but can wait until subsequent visits if the woman is overwhelmed or uninterested. The information provided should be adjusted to be compatible with the woman's educational level, culture, and desire for knowledge.

Treatment, Contraception, and Support

Midwives should refer all women with a positive supplementary HIV test to appropriate local or regional specialists and verify that these individuals have initiated care.[12] Treatment for HIV infection is dependent on the woman's current health status, including her viral load and any additional comorbid disorders. Referral to an HIV specialist allows the woman to receive optimal care.

Although the majority of midwives in the United States do not routinely care for HIV-positive individuals,[42] some do work in multidisciplinary teams to provide holistic and comprehensive care to HIV-positive women in pregnancy and across the lifespan.[43] Midwives in these settings collaborate with, consult with, or refer to a variety of healthcare providers to ensure women with HIV infection receive

---

BOX 15-8 Health Education for HIV Diagnosis

Essential Teaching at Time of Diagnosis (Verbally and Written Handouts)

- Effectiveness of HIV treatments
- Potential for transmission to others and safer sexual practices
- Importance of early and ongoing medical care
- Where to get medical care for HIV (referral name and phone number)
- What to expect with HIV care (regular medications, frequent preventive visits)
- Referrals to behavioral and psychosocial services for HIV-positive individuals

Additional Needed Teaching When the Woman Is Ready

- Information on health insurance and health-care provision for HIV-positive individuals
- Reproductive choices with HIV diagnosis, including need for birth control until ready to conceive
- Substance abuse screening and counseling if indicated

Source: Centers for Disease Control and Prevention (CDC). Recomendations for partner services programs for HIV infection, syphilis, gonorrhea, and chlamydial infection. *MMWR.* 2008;57(RR-9):1-64.

---

care at facilities that are accessible, are acceptable, and provide evidence-based care.

Women who are HIV positive, who are sexually active, and who do not desire pregnancy need contraception. While condoms are an essential part of safer sex practices, their effectiveness in prevention of pregnancy may not be adequate for the woman's needs. HIV affects the woman's choice of birth control method. The WHO and CDC eligibility criteria list a variety of contraceptives that are safe with HIV infection. Depot medroxyprogesterone acetate (DMPA [Depo-Provera]) is safe for women with HIV infection and those women undergoing antiretroviral treatment. The benefits of IUDs generally outweigh the risk for HIV-positive women, but the risks are elevated slightly if women are taking antiretroviral medication. Oral contraceptive pills interact with some antiretroviral medications and may not be an ideal choice. Spermicides can increase the risk of HIV transmission, so their use is not advised.[44] If an HIV-positive woman wants to conceive, preconception planning is essential to optimize her own health, avoid birth defects from teratogenic medications, and prevent transmission of HIV to her partner and her fetus.

Women with HIV face a wide range of potential sequelae from infection. Because HIV cannot be eradicated from the body, infection is lifelong. Treatment to prevent immune system depletion and opportunistic infections is ongoing and requires close collaboration between the women and her healthcare team. Recommended preventive care, including Pap smears and physical exams, is more frequent for HIV-positive women due to increased susceptibility to infections and cancer.[45]

Prenatal Considerations

Women should be screened for HIV early in pregnancy and, ideally, again in the third trimester. Women who are HIV positive should receive antiretroviral drugs throughout pregnancy to protect their own health and decrease the risk of vertical transmission of HIV to the fetus.[46] Some antiretroviral agents, such as efavirenz (Sustiva), have been linked with neural tube disorders and other fetal anomalies. Ideally, an HIV-positive woman can work with her infectious disease specialist prior to pregnancy to adjust her medications to avoid such problems.

Women who are HIV positive should receive enhanced prenatal care. They can benefit from ancillary counseling and services in addition to traditional prenatal care. While pregnancy does not affect HIV progression to AIDS, HIV has been associated with poor perinatal outcomes, especially in the developing world.

Women with HIV infection need an early ultrasound to confirm their due date because a scheduled cesarean section before labor is an option for decreasing vertical transmission to the fetus. Noninvasive testing for fetal anomalies is appropriate at the same intervals as for women who are HIV negative. Invasive fetal testing, such as amniocentesis, carries a risk of HIV transmission to the fetus and is reserved for situations where noninvasive testing has shown abnormalities.[47]

Prenatal care for women with HIV infection should also involve practitioners skilled in HIV management and pregnancy care. Ideal care involves multidisciplinary collaboration between clinicians and behavioral and psychological health professionals. Midwives can be a component of this care, but the knowledge needed for HIV management is beyond the American College of Nurse-Midwives Core Competencies. If advanced skills are practiced, they should be added to practice guidelines using the procedures outlined in the Standards for the Practice of Midwifery.[48]

Assessment of viral load at term is indicated to determine the ideal route of birth. Cesarean section prior to the start of labor for all women with a viral load of 1000 copies/mL is recommended. The combination of antiretroviral medications and cesarean birth for women with a high viral load has reduced vertical transmission from rates as high as 25% to 2% or less in the United States.[47]

Intrapartum Considerations

Women who have not been screened in pregnancy or women at risk for HIV infection without a third-trimester screening should be screened while in labor. A rapid test is appropriate, as it will yield results in time to begin intrapartum interventions to decrease transmission. While a positive rapid test warrants intrapartum treatment, a set of full screening and diagnostic tests should be performed for definitive diagnosis.

If a laboring woman is HIV positive, or suspected to be HIV positive, antiretroviral medications should be begun. If the woman's viral load is known to be greater than 1000 copies/mL, a cesarean birth following several hours of antiretroviral treatment has been shown to decrease vertical transmission.[49] If a vaginal birth is planned, it is appropriate to minimize risk to the infant by facilitating a physiologic birth. Rupture of membranes, placement of a fetal scalp electrode, and cutting an episiotomy increase the risk of virus transmission to the fetus and should be avoided.[50]

Fetal/Neonatal Considerations

Newborns should be treated with antiretroviral therapy as soon as possible after birth, preferably within 6 to 12 hours of birth.[50] Oral zidovudine (AZT, Retrovir) is the drug of choice for term infants whose mother received prenatal prophylaxis with antiretroviral agents. Guidelines call for zidovudine treatment to continue for as long as 6 weeks. Newborns of mothers treated with antiretroviral medications can have a variety of problems, including anemia, jaundice, and birth defects, and need evaluation by clinicians experienced in HIV care.

Breastfeeding Considerations

Breastfeeding exposes the infant to HIV through breast milk and has been demonstrated to increase maternal–child transmission of the virus. In areas where safe breast milk substitutes are consistently available, breastfeeding is not recommended due to risk of infection.[51] This is the case in the United States and throughout the developed world, and the CDC recommends that HIV-positive women in the United States do not breastfed their infants.[12]

Worldwide, however, the majority of cases of HIV/AIDs occur in areas where safe breast milk substitutes are not reliably available. Infants and children fed breast milk substitutes in these areas may have higher rates of morbidity and mortality when compared with their breastfed peers. In these circumstances, the risk of death from other infections, especially diarrheal illness, is higher than the risk of HIV acquisition from breastfeeding.[51] Therefore, in these cases, the benefit of breastfeeding outweighs the risk. If the child is already known to be HIV positive, the benefits of breastfeeding have been established and the infant should be breastfed as long as the mother and infant desire. However, if the infant is HIV negative or has an unknown HIV status, the risk of HIV acquisition through breastfeeding accumulates as the infant ages. The mother's viral load and CD4 count play a role in maternal–child transmission of the virus, and antiretroviral therapy may be beneficial in decreasing transmission through breast milk. The mother's personal health, her environment, the child's HIV status, and the availability of safe feeding alternatives all influence the decision of when to wean the infant.[51]

Protozoal and Parasitic Infections

Trichomoniasis

Trichomoniasis, commonly known as "trich," is a vaginal or urethral infection with the protozoa *Trichomonas vaginalis* (**Figure 15-5**). The pear-shaped protozoa have five flagella and are highly motile. They are transmitted through sexual contact, which transfers infected secretions to the urethra and vagina. Fomites are a possible, but unlikely, mechanism of infection, as trichomonads must be kept moist and warm.

Trichomoniasis is often asymptomatic, with half of all infected women not having any symptoms. Symptoms include vaginal itching, irritation, and malodorous vaginal discharge. Abdominal discomfort may also be present.

Diagnosis of Trichomoniasis

While the woman may be asymptomatic, common physical examination findings include an inflamed and irritated vulva with minor excoriations, and possibly a frothy, thin, yellow-green vaginal discharge.

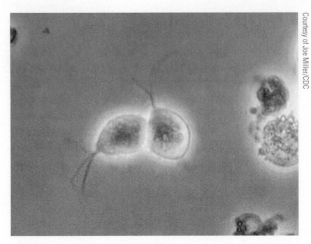

Figure 15-5 Trichomonas.

The vagina and cervix may be a deep red or pink, known as "strawberry cervix."

Criteria for diagnosis include vaginal discharge pH > 4.5, positive whiff test, and saline wet-mount microscopic evaluation that identifies motile trichomoniasis. The absence of these criteria, however, does not rule out infection.[52] Trichomonads can be visualized under the microscope in a saline wet prep but are very sensitive to salinity and temperature, resulting in a detection rate of only 60% to 70%. If the saline has been left open and become more concentrated, the trichomonads will be lysed. If the sample becomes cold, the trichomonads will not be mobile and will be difficult to distinguish from other cells.

Other tests, such as the OSOM Trichomonas Rapid Test and the Affirm VP III, have improved specificity but require special kits and are more expensive. The OSOM Trichomonas Rapid Test has a sensitivity of better than 80% and can be performed in many clinic laboratories within 10 minutes. The Affirm VP III is a nucleic acid probe that tests for trichomoniasis, bacterial vaginosis, and candidiasis. While it has a high sensitivity, it requires 45 minutes to obtain results. A liquid cytology Pap smear can also be used for diagnosis but will delay treatment as compared with in-office testing. Culture of *Trichomonas* is highly sensitive and specific, and this technique should be used when trichomoniasis is suspected but unable to be confirmed with microscopy.[53]

Treatment and Nonpharmacologic Support

Treatment options for trichomoniasis are shown in **Table 15-16**. Oral therapies are required, as topical treatment with metronidazole is not effective in eradicating infection. Counseling includes avoidance of alcohol for 24 hours after treatment with

Table 15-16	Treatments for Trichomoniasis		
Recommended Treatments for Nonpregnant Women and Males Generic (Brand)	**Alternative Treatments for Nonpregnant Women and Males Generic (Brand)**	**Recommended Treatments for Pregnant Women Generic (Brand)**	**Recommended Treatments for Breastfeeding Women**
Metronidazole (Flagyl) 2 g orally once	Metronidazole (Flagyl) 500 mg orally twice a day for 7 days	Metronidazole (Flagyl) 2 g orally once	Oral metronidazole (Flagyl) taken in high doses during breastfeeding is not recommended due to active metabolites transferred to the infant via breast milk. The woman should not breastfeed for 12–24 hours after taking the large dose of metronidazole.
			Women can choose the alternative of 500 mg twice a day for 7 days treatment and time breastfeeding to coincide with low plasma levels of the drug.
Tinidazole (Tindamax) 2 g orally in a single dose			Women should not breastfeed for 72 hours after taking tinidazole (Tindamax). Metronidazole is preferred secondary to the higher maternal plasma levels that occur with the tinidazole 2 g single dose.

Sources: Centers for Disease Control and Prevention (CDC). Sexually transmitted diseases treatment guidelines. *MMWR.* 2010;59(RR-12). Available at: http://www.cdc.gov/mmwr/pdf/rr/rr5912.pdf. Accessed November 11, 2012; U.S. National Library of Medicine. Drugs and lactation database (LactMed). 2012. Available at: http://toxnet.nlm.nih.gov/cgi-bin/sis/htmlgen?LACT. Accessed January 19, 2013.

metronidazole (Flagyl) and 72 hours after treatment with tinidazole (Tindamax). Current sexual partner(s) should be treated, even if they are asymptomatic. Both partners should abstain from sexual contact until after treatment is completed and symptoms have resolved.[12] If the initial treatment fails to eliminate the symptoms and trichomonads, consider tinidazole or the longer course of metronidazole. For strains resistant to both these drugs, contact the CDC for susceptibility tests and additional treatments.[12] Rescreen women 3 months after treatment, if possible, to test for reinfection. Trichomoniasis can increase the risk of HIV acquisition.

Prenatal Considerations

Only women with symptoms of trichomoniasis need to be screened for this infection during pregnancy. Infection with *Trichomonas* has been associated with an increased risk for prelabor rupture of membranes, preterm birth, and low birth weight. However, treatment with metronidazole (Flagyl) does not appear to decrease preterm birth rates[54] and, in fact, may increase the risk of this outcome.[55] Pregnant women should be given the option of immediate treatment, at any gestation, for symptom relief, or waiting until 37 weeks to be treated if symptoms are not

bothersome.[12] Until treated, the woman can still transmit the infection. Partner treatment can occur at any time but may need to be repeated when the woman is treated to prevent reinfection.[55] Vertical transmission can occur during vaginal birth.

Fetal/Neonatal Considerations

Transfer of trichomoniasis to a fetus or newborn during vaginal birth is rare but can happen. The newborn may present with fever and either respiratory or genital infection.

Pubic Lice (Pthiriasis)

Pubic lice (*Pthirus pubis*; **Figure 15-6**), also known as "crabs," are found on course body hairs including pubic, axillary, and occasionally facial hair (eyebrows, eyelashes, or beard). Women usually present with itching and report of visible lice or nits. Sexual transmission is most common, as parasites are pushed onto a new host's hair. However, pubic lice can live for as long as 44 hours off the body, so transmission via fomites such as towels, linens, and other objects is possible.[56] Scalp infestations are not common but can occur, especially in advanced cases. While rare, head lice can occasionally be found in the genital area, especially if pubic hair is fine. Head lice (*Pediculus*

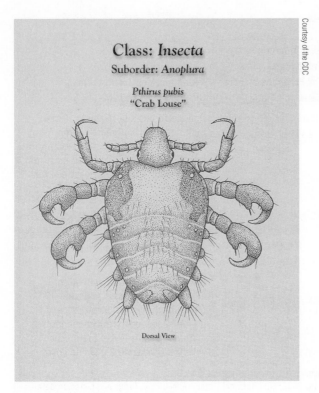

Figure 15-6 Pubic lice.

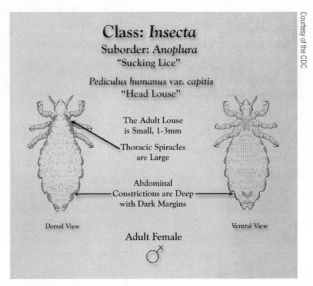

Figure 15-7 Head lice.

humanus capitis; **Figure 15-7**) and pubic lice can be differentiated by their appearance, as pubic lice have a characteristic crab-like appearance and have a lower length-to-width ratio than head lice.

Diagnosis of Pubic Lice

Inspect all hairy areas of the body to differentiate the type of infection. Lice and nits are visible on hairs in one or more body area(s), with coarse hairs being more frequently infested than scalp hairs. Small punctuate lesions and bluish macules may also be seen.[56] Lice can be viewed under the microscopic for confirmation if needed, but the physical exam is all that is needed for diagnosis.

Treatment and Nonpharmacologic Support

Table 15-17 lists recommended treatments for all body areas except the eyes. Pubic lice infestation of the eyelashes should be treated with occlusive ophthalmic ointment twice a day for 10 days. All clothing and bedding should be washed and dried on a hot setting, dry cleaned, or kept from body contact for 72 hours. Bagging items is more affordable for women without washer/dryers. The CDC advises treatment for all sexual partners from the last month. Household contacts should be examined

and treated as needed.[12] Screen women with pubic lice for all common STIs. Retreatment is necessary if no improvement occurs in 1 week. Resistance to treatment is common, and malathion (Ovide) is recommended for retreatment of nonpregnant women in cases where resistance is suspected.[12] Pregnant women infected with pubic lice should receive third-trimester rescreening for STIs.

Other Infectious Conditions Spread by Sexual Contact

Because sex involves the transmission of body fluids and skin contact, a wide variety of infections and parasites can be spread by this means. For example, viruses such as cytomegalovirus and Epstein-Barr virus can be transmitted through sharing of bodily fluids. *Molluscum contagiosum* is spread through skin-to-skin contact and, in adults, is most often seen on the genitals, upper thighs, and abdomen with sexual transmission.[57] These infections are summarized in **Table 15-18**. Intestinal infections, such as shigellosis and *Giardia* infection, can be transmitted sexually, especially when there is contact with the anus or mouth.

Other Conditions Spread by Sexual Contact

Many primary care conditions may result in symptoms in the groin region that can mimic STIs. A few of these commonly encountered conditions are listed

Table 15-17	Treatments for Pthiriasis		
Recommended Treatments for Nonpregnant Women and Males Generic (Brand)	**Alternative Treatments for Nonpregnant Women and Males Generic (Brand)**	**Recommended Treatments for Pregnant Women Generic (Brand)**	**Recommended Treatments for Breastfeeding Women**
Permethrin 1% cream (Nix) rinse applied to affected area and washed off after 10 minutes Pyrethrins with piperonyl butoxide (RID) applied to area and then washed off after 10 minutes	Malathion 0.5% (Ovide) lotion applied for 8–12 hours and washed off (has a strong odor but is useful for resistant cases) Ivermectin (Stromectol) 250 µg/kg orally, repeated in 2 weeks (limited data on this treatment are available)	Permethrin 1% cream (Nix) rinse applied to affected area and washed off after 10 minutes Pyrethrins with piperonyl butoxide (RID) applied to area and then washed off after 10 minutes Malathion (Ovide) is contraindicated in pregnancy	Permethrin 1% cream (Nix) rinse applied to affected area and washed off after 10 minutes Pyrethrins with piperonyl butoxide (RID) applied to area and then washed off after 10 minutes Malathion (Ovide) is contraindicated during lactation

Sources: Centers for Disease Control and Prevention (CDC). Sexually transmitted diseases treatment guidelines. *MMWR.* 2010;59(RR-12). Available at: http://www.cdc.gov/mmwr/pdf/rr/rr5912.pdf. Accessed November 11, 2012; U.S. National Library of Medicine. Drugs and lactation database (LactMed). 2012. Available at: http://toxnet.nlm.nih.gov/cgi-bin/sis/htmlgen?LACT. Accessed January 19, 2013.

in **Table 15-19.** Other conditions, such as tinea cruris and other forms of dermatitis, can manifest on and around the vulva, complicating diagnosis. While targeting the exam to the woman's chief concern, the clinician should not prematurely rule out primary care diagnosis that may have genital manifestations.

Communicating Information about Sexually Transmitted Infections

Telling a woman she has an STI is often difficult for both novice and experienced practitioners. The CDC advises clinicians to discuss positive HIV testing in person.[40] However, for STIs other than HIV, discussion of the diagnosis and planning for treatment may occur via the phone. Phone consultations are acceptable, but not ideal, as it is more difficult for the midwife to gauge how the woman is responding to the diagnosis. However, phone visits can facilitate prompt treatment and decrease the chance the woman is unable to receive treatment. Prior to phoning a woman with STI results, make sure she consented to be contacted by phone; once she answers, ask if she is in an acceptable location for the discussion before beginning the conversation.

Maintaining a normal tone of voice without judgment is helpful in being present for the woman. It may take time for the woman to adjust to the news that she has an STI. Openly discuss the fact that the infection is sexually transmitted and address whether it is possible for the infection to be transmitted in other ways,

such as through common contact. While nonsexual transmission is possible with some infections, such as scabies, it is very unlikely for others, such as gonorrhea. Some infections produce symptoms soon after initial infection, whereas others, such as HPV, may not manifest for months or years. Avoid assumptions about the origin of the STI, and use open- and closed-ended questions to further explore the woman's feelings and needs. Always assess for the possibility of intimate partner violence if the diagnosis is shared with a sexual partner. While health promotion teaching to avoid future infections is needed, it can be difficult for a woman to concentrate on health promotion immediately after receiving an STI diagnosis. Written materials that the woman can take home will allow her to review the information when she is more receptive to it. A well-placed follow-up visit in person or by phone may be a better time for additional teaching and promotion of lifestyle change if the woman seems overwhelmed at the time of diagnosis.

Relationship Stressors and Violence

STIs can be a clue to intimate-partner relationship problems. Although many STIs are acquired from a new partner who was previously infected, a new STI diagnosis may reveal infidelity of a long-term sexual partner. A diagnosis of an STI can spark or enhance relationship tension that may lead to cessation of the relationship or even violence.[9] However, partner notification and treatment has not been shown to greatly increase the rate of violence or relationship dissolution.[9]

Table 15-18	Selected Primary Care Conditions Also Spread by Sexual Contact			
	Symptoms	Physical Exam	Treatment	Follow-up
Hepatitis C	Asymptomatic until late in chronic infection when liver problems manifest.	The CDC recommends screening people at risk and all adults born between 1945 and 1964.[63]	Antiretroviral treatment can reduce liver damage and achieve clearance of the virus. Lifestyle changes include decreasing alcohol consumption, maintenance of a normal weight, and careful consideration of all prescription, over-the-counter, and herbal medications to decrease interactions and liver stress. If positive for current or previous hepatitis C infection, the CDC recommends an immediate brief counseling session about reducing alcohol consumption.[63]	Women should be referred to a clinician experienced in monitoring and management of hepatitis and chronic liver disease.
Scabies (*Sarcoptes scabiei*)	Severe itching of the groin, between fingers, and in body folds. Itching is bilateral and often occurs more at night.[64]	Excoriations surrounding papules, consisting of small linear or curved burrows, may be present. Definitive diagnosis is based on microscopic visualization of the mite obtained from skin scrapings. Secondary infections are common.	Permethrin 5% applied to the body from the neck down and washed off after 8–14 hours (safe in pregnancy and lactation) OR Ivermectin (Stromectol) 200 mcg/kg orally, repeated in 14 days (This treatment is preferred for outbreaks at residential facilities.) Household linens need to be dried on hot or isolated for 72 hours.[12]	Itching may persist for 2–4 weeks.[64] If treatment fails, lindane is recommended as a second treatment in otherwise well, nonpregnant and nonlactating women.[12]
Molluscum contagiosum	Lesions can be found on any part of the body. With sexual transmission, they are more common on the legs, abdomen, and genital area.	Multiple 2- to 5-mm, shiny white or flesh-colored papules with an indented (umbilicated) center. A thick white discharge can be expressed from the center of the lesion. Large and extensive lesions are more common in HIV-positive adults.	Symptoms are usually self-limiting and resolve without scarring in more than 90% of otherwise healthy adults. Treatments are not usually recommended but can decrease the spread of the infection. Treatments include cryotherapy, excision, oral cimetidine, and topical creams. Transmission can be decreased by covering lesions and not sharing towels or clothing.	None needed; lesions usually heal within a year.

Table 15-19	Diagnoses That May Mimic Sexually Transmitted Infections That Are Not Sexually Transmitted		
	Presenting Concerns and History	Physical Exam	Treatment Generic (Brand)
Chiggers (*Trombicula* mite bites)	Severe itching usually 3–24 hours after outdoor activity in hot, humid weather.	Small, grouped, excoriated papules along panty-line or in fold of groin, often found along a line of clothing constriction.	Irritation is self-limiting. Topical antihistamines and corticosteroids may provide relief. Oral antihistamines can be used in severe cases.
Herpes zoster ("shingles")	Open lesions that are painful superficially and have a deeper nerve pain component. Often occurs in elderly or immuno-suppressed women. 10–15% of affected individuals will have postherpetic neuralgia following an initial outbreak.	Painful papules, or vesicles that rupture and crust over. Lesions may be in various stages of forming and healing. Found on L5 and S1 dermatomes. Indistinguishable from herpes by exam. Serologic tests will be negative for HSV infection.	Treatment within 72 hours is ideal to decrease incidence of postherpetic neuralgia: <ul><li>Acyclovir (Zovirax) 800 mg five times a day</li><li>Famciclovir (Famvir) 500 mg three times a day</li><li>Valacyclovir (Valtrex) 100 mg three times a day</li><li>Patient-appropriate pain control medications</li></ul> Lesions are contagious via the air and physical contact, and can cause varicella in previously uninfected individuals. Covering the lesions reduces transmission risk.[65]

Psychosocial Needs

Women with STIs are more likely to be from vulnerable social groups. Being young, poor, and/or drug using are all risks for STI acquisition.[6] Sometimes sexual activity is one of many risk-taking behaviors. In other cases, women did not have a choice about engaging in sexual contact. Women who are abused or forced into sexual encounters may not be able to advocate for condom use. Negotiating for safer sexual practices requires self-confidence and power within the relationship. Obtaining condoms requires money or access to social services, which may be difficult to obtain for women of low socioeconomic status or those who do not have a strong support network. Women who trade sex for food, housing, drugs, or money are more likely to acquire STIs, as they often have multiple sexual partners who have little concern for the woman's health.[6] Women often enter care for one reason but have other needs besides the chief concern and can benefit from a holistic approach that provides them with needed information or referrals beyond their presenting diagnosis.

Contraception

Women who are sexually active with men are at risk for pregnancy. The diagnosis of an STI is an excellent opportunity to discuss birth control and ensure a woman is preventing unintended pregnancy as well as protecting herself from STIs. Whereas both male and female condoms offer some STI protection, other birth control methods offer little protection from STI acquisition. However, condoms have a fairly high failure rate for pregnancy prevention and may be an inadequate primary method for women wishing to prevent conception. In contrast, a woman may need to use condoms in addition to other contraceptive methods to prevent STIs and may need to be reminded of the importance of safer sexual practices even when she is not concerned about pregnancy prevention. Women may need guidance on how to negotiate for safer sexual practices even if they are protected from pregnancy.

Evaluation of the Need for Immediate Intervention, Consultation, or Collaboration

The treatment of STIs often involves interprofessional collaboration. Local pharmacists, physicians, and health department staff may be involved in this process. While consultation may involve disclosing the woman's name and diagnosis, this should be done in ways that respect her rights and maintain her confidentiality. Proper communication among care providers can allow for quick and effective treatment of women and newborns, thereby preventing morbidity and mortality, and is consistent with the Institute of Medicine's call for improvement in the quality of patient care.[58]

If the woman has a disseminated or advanced STI, hospitalization and consultation with physicians, pharmacists, and infectious disease specialists may be appropriate. Multiple treatment failures may necessitate consultation with regional health departments or the CDC. Pediatric care providers need to know about any STIs in the pregnant or laboring woman that may affect her newborn or infant. Judicious use of other members of the interprofessional healthcare team can improve the quality of the care received while protecting a woman's rights and dignity.

Reporting of STIs to local health departments is a responsibility that does not violate confidentiality. While local health departments should not reveal the name of the "index patient," there is always the chance that someone could guess which partner had an STI, and this recognition could have wide-ranging implications for the woman, including violence.[9] Therefore, the CDC advises all health departments to ask women, without coercion, to provide information about previous sexual partners so they can be notified and treated.[9] Partner treatment is within the scope of midwifery practice as long as it permissible by state laws.

Development of a Comprehensive Plan of Care That Is Supported by a Valid Rationale

It is important to ensure that women are treated with the appropriate medications for STIs to prevent short- and long-term morbidity and to reduce the spread of infections. Treatment options can be presented to the woman and a plan of care developed to meet her needs. Cost and convenience are chief considerations in choosing a treatment method. Dosing frequency, privacy, and ability to apply or wash off the medicine may also be important in the decision-making process.

Assumption of Responsibility for Safe and Efficient Implementation of Care

Midwives are prepared to provide excellent, evidence-based care to women and men experiencing STIs.[59] While other practitioners may be involved in care, the diagnosing clinician should assume responsibility for ensuring the woman and her partner receive adequate and prompt treatment and health counseling to prevent future infections and long-term health sequelae.

Partner Treatment

Treatment of the woman's sexual partner for STIs is within the scope of midwifery practice.[60] Partner treatment may involve examination and testing of the sexual partner or presumptive treatment without a clinic visit depending on the diagnosed STI. It is acceptable to treat sexual partners for STIs without a physical exam, a practice known as expedited partner therapy (EPT).[61] EPT allows for rapid treatment of sexual partners, thereby reducing the risk of reinfection and decreasing healthcare costs. EPT has demonstrated positive outcomes for male sexual partners of women who have gonorrhea and/or chlamydia. There is inadequate research to support use of this approach for trichomoniasis, however, and it is not well supported for use with partners of women younger than 19 years.[61] EPT should not be used to treat syphilis or long-term chronic STIs such as herpes or HIV. To prevent adverse outcomes from drug allergies, provide information with the prescription about potential side effects and an allergy warning.[61]

EPT has legal protection for some prescribers in 32 states, has uncertain legal status in 11 states, and is expressly prohibited in 7 states.[62] However, while a state may legally allow expedited partner treatment, some state licensure boards, such as boards of nursing, prohibit writing prescriptions for individuals who have not been evaluated or do not have a chart within the clinic of the prescribing provider. The CDC maintains an interactive database of state statutes concerning EPT that can provide guidance on pertinent state regulations.[62]

Evaluation and Follow-Up

Follow-up after STI diagnosis and treatment differs by infection. The appropriate follow-up care and intervals are discussed for each infection in the specific section covering that STI. Performing a test-of-cure too early can result in a falsely positive test, while delayed follow-up can result in increased morbidity and STI transmission.[12] While it can be difficult for women to find time to return to the clinic and for providers to find time for repeat testing, appropriate and well-timed follow-up is important to decrease infection-related morbidity, prevent transmission, and detect drug-resistant strains early.

● ● ● References

1. United Nations. Millennium Project: goals, targets and indicators. 2006. Available at: http://www.unmillenniumproject.org/goals/gti.htm. Accessed November 11, 2011.

2. World Health Organization (WHO). *Sexual and Reproductive Health Core Competencies in Primary Care: Attitudes, Knowledge, Ethics, Human Rights, Leadership, Management, Teamwork, Community Work, Education, Counselling, Clinical Settings, Service, Provision.* Geneva, Switzerland: WHO; 2011. Available at: http://whqlibdoc.who.int/publications /2011/9789241501002_eng.pdf. Accessed November 11, 2012.

3. U.S. Department of Health and Human Services. Healthy people 2020. Available at: http://www .healthypeople.gov/2020/topicsobjectives2020 /default.aspx. Accessed November 11, 2012.

4. American College of Nurse-Midwives. Core competencies for basic midwifery practice. 2007. Available at: http://www.acnm.org/siteFiles/descriptive/Core_ Competencies_6_07_3.pdf. Accessed March 21, 2008.

5. World Health Organization (WHO). Sexually transmitted infections. 2011. Available at: http://www .who.int/mediacentre/factsheets/fs110/en.index.html . Accessed November 11, 2012.

6. Centers for Disease Control and Prevention (CDC). *Sexually Transmitted Disease Surveillance 2010.* Atlanta, GA: Department of Health and Human Services; 2011. Available at: http://www.cdc.gov/std /stats10/surv2010.pdf. Accessed November 11, 2012.

7. Centers for Disease Control and Prevention (CDC). NCHHSTP Atlas. 2012. Available at: http://gis.cdc .gov/GRASP/NCHHSTPAtlas/main.html. Accessed August 31, 2012.

8. Centers for Disease Control and Prevention (CDC). List of notifiable conditions, historically by year 1993–2011. Available at: http://wwwn.cdc.gov/nndss /document/NNDSS_history_spreadsheet_2011_for_ web_v3.pdf. Accessed November 11, 2012.

9. Centers for Disease Control and Prevention (CDC). Recommendations for partner services programs for HIV infection, syphilis, gonorrhea, and chlamydial infection. *MMWR.* 2008;57(RR-9):1-64.

10. Bates B. *Bates Guide to Physical Examination and History-Taking.* 11th ed. Philadelphia: Lippincott, Williams & Wilkins; 2012.

11. Chandeying V. The sexual history. In: Zenilman JM, Shahmanesh M, eds. *Sexually Transmitted Infections.* Sudbury, MA: Jones & Bartlett Learning; 2012:3-12.

12. Centers for Disease Control and Prevention (CDC). Sexually transmitted diseases treatment guidelines. *MMWR.* 2010;59(RR-12). Available at: http://www .cdc.gov/mmwr/pdf/rr/rr5912.pdf. Accessed November 11, 2012.

13. Marrazzo J. It's not just the pathogen anymore: the genital microbiome and implications for sexually transmitted infections. *STD Prevention Science Series 2012* [Webinar]. 2012.

14. Ngugi BM, Hemmerling A, Bukusi EA, et al. Effects of bacterial vaginosis-associated bacteria and sexual intercourse on vaginal colonization with the probiotic *Lactobacillus crispatus* CTV-05. *Sex Trans Dis.* 2011;38(11):1020-1027.

15. Mashburn J. Vaginitis. In: King TL, Brucker MC, eds. *Pharmacology for Women's Health.* Sudbury, MA: Jones and Bartlett; 2011:950.

16. Van Kessel K, Assefi N, Marrazzo J, Eckert L. Common complementary and alternative therapies for yeast vaginitis and bacterial vaginosis: a systematic review. *Obstet Gynecol Surv.* 2003;58(5):351-358.

17. Fritz MA, Speroff L. *Clinical Gynecologic Endocrinology and Infertility.* 8th ed. Philadelphia: Lippincott, Williams & Wilkins; 2012.

18. North American Menopause Society. The 2012 hormone therapy position statement of the North American Menopause Society. *Menopause.* 2012; 19(3):257-271.

19. Suckling J, Lethaby A, Kennedy R. Local oestrogen for vaginal atrophy in postmenopausal women. *Cochrane Database System Rev.* 2003;4:CD001500. doi: 10.1002/14651858.CD001500.

20. U.S. National Library of Medicine. Drugs and lactation database (LactMed). 2012. Available at: http ://toxnet.nlm.nih.gov/cgi-bin/sis/htmlgen?LACT. Accessed January 19, 2013.

21. Centers for Disease Control and Prevention (CDC). Update to CDC's sexually transmitted diseases treatment guidelines, 2012: oral cephalosporins no longer recommended treatment for gonococcal infections. *MMWR.* 2012;61(31):590-594.

22. Dean G, Schwarz EB. Intrauterine contraceptives. In: Hatcher RA, Trussel J, Nelson AL, et al., eds. *Contraceptive Technology.* 20th ed. Atlanta, GA: Ardent Media; 2011:147.

23. Sweet RL. Treatment of acute pelvic inflammatory disease. *Infect Dis Obstet Gynecol.* 2011;561909. doi: 10.1155/2011/561909.

24. Golden MR, Marra CM, Homes KK. Update on syphilis: resurgence of an old problem. *JAMA.* 2003; 29(11):1510-1514.

25. World Health Organization (WHO). *The Global Elimination of Congenital Syphilis: Rationale and Strategy for Action.* Geneva: WHO; 2007.

26. Roett MA, Mayor MT, Uduhiri KA. Diagnosis and management of genital ulcers. *Am Fam Physician.* 2012;85(3):254-262.

27. Cates W, Harwood B. Vaginal barriers and spermicides. In: Hatcher RA, Trussel J, Nelson AL, et al., eds. *Contraceptive Technology.* Atlanta, GA: Ardent; 2011:391-408.

28. Murphy J, Marks H. Cervical cancer screening in the era of human papiloma virus testing and vaccination. *J Midwifery Womens Health.* 2012;57(6):1-8.

29. Marquez L, Levy ML, Munoz FM, Palazzi DL. Report of three cases and review of intrauterine herpes simplex virus infection. *Pediatr Infect Dis J.* 2011;30(2):153-157.

30. American College of Obstetricians and Gynecologists. Management of herpes in pregnancy. *Obstet Gynecol.* 2007;109(6):1489-1498.

31. Knezevic A, Martic J, Stanojevic M, et al. Disseminated neonatal herpes caused by herpes simplex virus types 1 and 2. *Emerg Infect Dis.* 2007;13(2):302-304.

32. Centers for Disease Control and Prevention (CDC). Neonatal herpes simplex virus infection following Jewish ritual circumcisions that included direct orogenital suction—New York City, 2000–2011. *MMWR.* 2012;61(22):405-409.

33. Brook MG, Mutimer D. Viral hepatitis: screening and vaccination strategies. In: Zenilman JM, Shahmanesh M, eds. *Sexually Transmitted Infections.* Sudbury, MA: Jones & Bartlett Learning; 2012:241-250.

34. Centers for Disease Control and Prevention (CDC). Recommended adult immunization schedule—United States, 2012. *MMWR.* 2012;61(4):1-7.

35. American College of Obstetricians and Gynecologists. ACOG Practice Bulletin No. 86: viral hepatitis in pregnancy. *Obstet Gynecol.* 2007;110(4):941-956.

36. Mast EE, Margolis HS, Fiore AE, et al. Advisory Committee on Immunization Practices (ACIP). A comprehensive immunization strategy to eliminate transmission of hepatitis B virus infection in the United States: recommendations of the Advisory Committee on Immunization Practices (ACIP). Part 1: immunization of infants, children, and adolescents. *MMWR Recomm Rep.* 2005 Dec 23;54(RR-16):1-31. Erratum in: *MMWR.* 2007 Dec 7;56(48):1267. *MMWR.* 2006 Feb 17;55(6):158-159.

37. Shi Z, Yang Y, Wang H, et al. Breastfeeding of newborns by mothers carrying hepatitis B virus: a meta-analysis and systematic review. *Arch Pediatr Adolesc Med.* 2011;165(9):837-846.

38. World Health Organization (WHO). *Hepatitis B and Breastfeeding.* Global Programme for Vaccines and Immunization (GPV), Divisions of Child Health and Development (CHD), Reproductive Health (RHT), eds. Geneva: WHO; 1996.

39. Centers for Disease Control and Prevention (CDC). *HIV Surveillance Report, 2010, vol. 22.* Atlanta, GA: CDC; 2012.

40. Centers for Disease Control and Prevention (CDC). Revised recommendations for HIV testing of adults, adolescents, and pregnant women in health-care settings. *MMWR.* 2006;55(RR-14):2-13.

41. Centers for Disease Control and Prevention (CDC). HIV-2 infection surveillance—United States, 1987–2009. *MMWR.* 2011;60:985-988.

42. Hastings-Tolsma M, Emeis C, McFarlin B, Schmiege S. *2012 Task Analysis: A Report of Midwifery Practice.* Linthicum, MD: American Midwifery Certification Board; 2012.

43. De Ferrari E, Paine LL, Gegor CL, et al. Midwifery care for women with human immunodeficiency virus disease in pregnancy: a demonstration project at the Johns Hopkins Hospital. *J Nurs Midwifery.* 1993;38(2):97-102.

44. Centers for Disease Control and Prevention (CDC). Update to the CDC's US medical eligibility criteria for contraceptive use, 2010: revised recomendations for the use of hormonal contraception among women at high risk for HIV infection or infected with HIV. *MMWR.* 2010;61(24):449-452.

45. U.S. Department of Health and Human Services. Clinical guide: testing and assessment interim history and physical examination. 2011. Available at: http://hab.hrsa.gov/deliverhivaidscare/clinicalguide11/. Accessed October 4, 2011.

46. Siegfried N, van der Merwe L, Brocklehurst P, Sint TT. Antiretrovirals for reducing the risk of mother-to-child transmission of HIV infection. *Cochrane Database Syst Rev.* 2011;7:CD003510. doi: 10.1002/14651858. CD003510.pub3

47. Recommendations for use of antiretroviral drugs in pregnant HIV-1-infected women for maternal health and interventions to reduce perinatal HIV transmission in the United States. 2012. Available at: http://aidsinfo.nih.gov/contentfiles/lvguidelines/PerinatalGL.pdf. Accessed October 4, 2012.

48. American College of Nurse-Midwives. Standards for the practice of midwifery. 2009. Available at: http://www.midwife.org/siteFiles/descriptive/Standards_for_Practice_of_Midwifery_12_09_001.pdf. Accessed January 19, 2013.

49. Mother-to-child (perinatal) HIV transmission and prevention. 2007. Available at: http://www.cdc.gov/hiv/topics/perinatal/resources/factsheets/pdf/perinatal.pdf. Accessed January 19, 2013.

50. Office of AIDS Research Advisory Council (OARAC). Recomendations for use of antiretroviral drugs in pregnant HIV-1 infected women for maternal health and interventions to reduce perinatal HIV transmission in the United States. 2012. Available at: http://aidsinfo.nih.gov/contentfiles/lvguidelines/PerinatalGL.pdf. Accessed October 4, 2012.

51. World Health Organization (WHO). *HIV Transmission through Breast-Feeding: A Review of Available Evidence.* Geneva: WHO; 2008.

52. Schwebke JR. Vaginitis. In: Zenilman JM, Shahmanesh M, eds. *Sexually Transmitted Infections*. Sudbury, MA: Jones & Bartlett Learning; 2012:57-66.

53. Pattullo L, Griffeth S, Ding L, et al. Stepwise diagnosis of *Trichomonas vaginalis* infection in adolescent women. *J Clin Microbiol*. 2012;50(10):59-63.

54. Okun N, Gronau KA, Hannah ME. Antibiotics for bacterial vaginosis or *Trichomonas vaginalis* in pregnancy: a systematic review. *Obstet Gynecol*. 2005; 105(4):857-868.

55. Gülmezoglu AM, Azhar M. Interventions for trichomoniasis in pregnancy. *Cochrane Database Syst Rev*. 2011;5:CD000220. doi: 10.1002/14651858. CD000220.pub2.

56. Kumar DH. Rashes and genital dermatoses. In: Zenilman JM, Shahmanesh M, eds. *Sexually Transmitted Infections*. Sudbury, MA: Jones & Bartlett Learning; 2012:97-112.

57. Centers for Disease Control and Prevention (CDC), National Center for Emerging and Zoonotic Infectious Diseases, Division of High-Consequence Pathogens and Pathology. Clinical information: *Molluscum contagiosum*. 2011. Available at: http://www.cdc.gov/ncidod/dvrd/molluscum/clinical_overview.htm. Accessed September 12, 2012.

58. Institute of Medicine. *Crossing the Quality Chasm: A New Health System for the 21st Century*. Washington DC: National Academy Press; 2001.

59. American College of Nurse-Midwives. Definition of midwifery and scope of practice of certified nurse-midwives and certified midwives. Available at: http://www.midwife.org/ACNM/files/ACNMLibraryData/UPLOADFILENAME/000000000266/Definition%20of%20Midwifery%20and%20Scope%20of%20Practice%20of%20CNMs%20and%20CMs%20Feb%202012.pdf. Accessed January 19, 2013.

60. American College of Nurse-Midwives. Core competencies for basic midwifery practice. 2012. Available at: http://www.midwife.org/ACNM/files/ACNMLibraryData/UPLOADFILENAME/000000000050/Core%20Competencies%20June%202012.pdf. Accessed January 19, 2013.

61. Centers for Disease Control and Prevention (CDC). Expedited partner therapy in the management of sexually transmitted diseases. 2006. Available at: http://www.cdc.gov/std/treatment/EPTFinalReport2006.pdf. Accessed November 12, 2012.

62. Legal status of expedited partner therapy. 2012. Available at: http://www.cdc.gov/std/ept/legal/default.htm. Accessed September 30, 2012.

63. Smith BD, Morgan RL, Beckett GA, et al. Recommendations for the identification of chronic hepatitis C virus infection among persons born during 1945–1965. *MMWR*. 2012;61(RR04):1-18.

64. Chosidow O. Clinical practice: scabies. *N Engl J Med*. 2006;354(16):1718-1727.

65. Sampathkumar P, Drage LA, Martin DP. Herpes zoster (shingles) and postherpetic neuralgia. *Mayo Clin Proc*. 2009;84(3):274-280.

CHAPTER

16

Family Planning

MICHELLE R. COLLINS

SHARON L. HOLLEY

TONIA L. MOORE-DAVIS

DEBORAH L. NARRIGAN

History of Contraception

Throughout history, women and men have used a wide variety of methods to prevent unintended pregnancy. For example, ancient Egyptians designed the first contraceptive sponge and the first diaphragm. Chinese women reportedly ingested mercury, which resulted in a decrease of their fertility, and unfortunately for many, their deaths.[1] Beginning in the twentieth century, the impact on society of maternal death was publically acknowledged, leading to public health interventions that included avoiding unintended pregnancy as a strategy to decrease maternal mortality.

Margaret Sanger (1879–1966), a nurse, advocated for the right of families to limit their size and specifically worked with impoverished families in New York. The term "birth control" has been attributed to Sanger, who in 1916 founded the Planned Parenthood Federation of America. However, contraceptive methods were limited primarily to barrier methods until the mid-twentieth century. At that time, scientific developments produced the first modern hormonal contraception, and several clinical sites provided testing of the "pill." One of these clinical sites was the Frontier Nursing Service, where over a 3-year period in the late 1950s, not only was oral contraceptive safety investigated, but research also demonstrated the advantages of the midwife as the primary provider of contraceptive care.[2] Based on the clinical trials, in 1960 the Food and Drug Administration (FDA) approved the first oral contraceptive for use by women in the United States. A new era of contraception had dawned.

This chapter presents an overview of family planning, including an explanation of terminology pertinent to efficacy, effectiveness, contraceptive counseling, unintended pregnancy options, pregnancy termination services, emergency contraception, and emerging trends in contraception. The *Nonhormonal Contraception* and *Hormonal Contraception* chapters provide detailed discussion of the various types of contraceptive methods.

Definitions

Though the terms "birth control," "contraception," and "family planning" are often used interchangeably, they are not analogous in meaning, nor are they always used accurately. *Family planning* has the broadest connotation; this term refers to the process whereby women plan the number and timing of births, which may include the use of contraceptive methods or treatment of infertility. The term *birth control* is defined as voluntary limitation of the number of children who are conceived, or ways to control reproduction via use of methods that improve or diminish fertility. *Contraception* refers to the voluntary prevention of pregnancy through use of specific contraceptive methods. The term "family planning" was chosen as the title of this chapter because of its comprehensive nature.

Unintended pregnancy is a pregnancy that is mistimed, unwanted, or unplanned at the time of conception. More than 3 million pregnancies in the United States are unintended each year.[3,4] Although many of these pregnancies result in offspring who become loved members of a family, an estimated 40% of unintended pregnancies are voluntarily terminated.[3]

The Enigma of Establishing Efficacy and Effectiveness

The concepts of efficacy and effectiveness are used to describe how well a form of contraception works and often are thought to be synonymous, though they are distinctly different. *Efficacy* is the chance that conception will occur despite consistent and correct ("perfect") use of a given method. *Effectiveness* describes the success of a method preventing pregnancy when used "typically," including pregnancies that occur because of incorrect or inconsistent use of a given contraceptive method. To clarify, efficacy can be thought of in terms of true method failure, while effectiveness corresponds to user error and true method failure.[4]

A basic principle in counseling women is providing factual education about contraceptive methods. However seemingly easy, calculation of the risk of unintended pregnancy associated with a particular contraceptive method is not simple in that problems with estimates of efficacy and effectiveness have long been recognized.[5,6] The Pearl index, also called the Pearl rate, has been used for more than 7 decades in clinical trials to report the effectiveness of a contraceptive method. This calculation is defined as the number of method failures per 100 woman-years of exposure to the method.[7] The number of pregnancies that occur are divided by the number of months of contraceptive exposure and then multiplied by 1200 or 1300. Based on the statistical formula used, a woman-year is defined by either the number 12 (1200 for the index) to designate months or the number 13 (1300 for the index) to designate average number of menstrual cycles based on 28 days within a year. A lower Pearl index indicates a lower risk of unintended pregnancy.

Some studies report two Pearl indices, one labeled as typical or actual use for a contraceptive method. This Pearl index illustrates effectiveness and the data from which these indices are calculated include all pregnancies, regardless of whether they involved user error or method failure. Other reports use a "perfect use" Pearl index and include studies that are limited to cycles in which there is assurance that the method was correctly and consistently used.[4]

Major problems have been noted with using the Pearl index to assess a contraceptive method. Some assumptions on which the method is based may not be valid. Because of the statistical calculations, if all of the women became pregnant in the first year, the rate would not be a logical 100% or an index of 1000, but rather either 1200 or 1300 because of the definition of woman-year used in the calculation. Another problem is the mistaken assumption that a failure rate for a method is constant over time. In a large sample of individuals, the most fertile women will get pregnant earlier, and those with lower fertility will take longer to get pregnant, regardless of which type of contraceptive method is employed. For some methods such as the diaphragm, the longer the method is used, the more likely women are to become experienced with using it correctly. Conversely, some contraceptive methods are time limited, such as implants, and are associated with more pregnancies if they are used for prolonged periods beyond the recommended length.

In addition, the Pearl index does not recognize other confounding factors. For instance, the Pearl index is not able to provide reasons for self-discontinuation, such as side effects, dissatisfaction or change in desire to attempt pregnancy, and loss of women to follow-up who may continue to use the method correctly and successfully avoid pregnancy.

To compensate for some of the problems with the Pearl index, some researchers use life tables for statistical calculations of unintended pregnancies rates. These tables present separate effectiveness rates for each month of study among a group of individuals using a specific contraceptive method over a set period of time (e.g., 12 months). When results are subdivided by months, the assumption that contraceptive failure rates remain static is corrected. Other statistical analyses using life tables can differentiate between net effectiveness, which promotes comparison of reasons for dropping out of a study, and gross effectiveness, which enables comparison of one study to another. Studies today tend to use both the Pearl index and life table analysis, although many do not clearly designate which approach they use.

In addition to the statistical quagmire, research studies reporting data often are part of clinical trials undertaken for FDA approval. Trials involving contraceptives differ from the more traditional drug trials. Usual Phase 2 and 3 clinical trials are randomized, are often double blinded, and compare an agent to a placebo. In Phase 3 trials, the participants are individuals with a health condition that the new drug is likely to treat. Obvious ethical and methodological issues prohibit the use of this approach for investigation of new contraceptives. Therefore, most clinical trials are composed of "typical" women who are healthy and seeking a method to use for family planning. The concept of the "typical" participant in trials is problematic because females younger than the age of 18 are considered under pediatric policies and are not included in contraceptive trials. In addition to eliminating most adolescents, clinical trials of contraceptives tend to enroll participants of average weight/body mass index (BMI), even though obesity is epidemic in the United States. Exempting women from both of these populations is a limitation for generalizing the findings to all U.S. women.

Another problem is apparent in the manner in which contraceptive methods are compared to one another. Effectiveness of one method can usually be compared to effectiveness of another method only by using results from already conducted studies, not a head-to-head study. For example, assume a new oral contraceptive was found to be associated with a 20% rate of amenorrhea in users. Previously published research about an older contraceptive will most likely be used for the comparison with this new contraceptive. Therefore, the assumption is made that both of the studies in question, old and new, have similar methodological approaches and populations. In reality, that similarity cannot be guaranteed.

Because of the challenges in determining exact risk of unintended pregnancies associated with a method, quoting statistics to women about the effectiveness of contraceptive methods is an imperfect science. Many midwives use generally agreed-upon ranges of effectiveness. Others present the information by ranking which methods are more effective than others without resorting to exact, and perhaps somewhat inaccurate, numbers. In any case, although efficacy and effectiveness of methods are critical pieces of information, a woman's choice of a contraceptive method will take into account other factors, such as her past history of contraceptive use, her interpretation of the personal consequences of contraceptive failure, and the simple consideration of whether she will use a method correctly and consistently. Fortunately, most studies provide relatively similar results regarding effectiveness and efficacy, and rates found in this chapter are generally agreed upon by several references. **Table 16-1** provides a widely used list of effectiveness rates for typical and perfect use of contraceptives.[6]

Family Planning Counseling

Role of the Midwife

Hallmarks of midwifery care include concepts integral in family planning and contraception counseling, such as promotion of family-centered care, empowerment of women as partners in health care, promotion of public health, advocacy for informed choice, and the right to self-determination.[8] Responsibilities of the midwife in this area include identification of needs, health education, assisting in decision making, and provision of contraceptive methods. In some settings, midwives may also provide abortion services. To effectively provide family planning care, midwives must be aware of their own feelings and attitudes about sexuality, gender roles, contraception, religious beliefs, and other beliefs that could affect family planning counseling. Counseling is one of the most important aspects of family planning care, which has different components depending on the type of counseling provided.

The Essential Component of Choice

When a woman presents for family planning care, it is important to solicit information and then acknowledge the woman's attitudes, beliefs, and plans for family size, pregnancy spacing, and relationship status. In addition, the midwife must conduct several assessments.

An initial essential step is to perform a comprehensive health history, while simultaneously assessing for risk factors that preclude use of certain contraceptive methods. In addition, the midwife must consider the noncontraceptive advantages of certain methods. For example, barrier methods prevent transmission of sexually transmitted infections (STIs) in addition to their contraceptive action, and combined oral contraception (COC) can decrease a woman's lifetime risk for ovarian cancer.

Desired family size and choices about contraceptive methods are strongly influenced by culture and religion. A woman's preference for a specific method can be influenced by a variety of individual factors, including past contraceptive experiences, the woman's comfort with her body, the level of control desired, the ease of use, and the desire for either a short-acting or long-acting method. Privacy of the contraceptive method also may be a major consideration for some women. The choice of a particular contraceptive method may be further tailored based on the woman's occupation as well as her partnership status.

The cost of the method, both for initiation and for long-term maintenance, must be considered and should be discussed with the woman. For example, some methods may be covered by health insurance, whereas other methods may result in more out-of-pocket costs, precluding their use by some women who have lower incomes or lack insurance to defray the cost. Other methods have an expensive initial use,

Table 16-1	Percentage of Women Experiencing an Unintended Pregnancy During the First Year of Typical Use and the First Year of Perfect Use of Contraceptives and the Percentage Continuing Use at the End of the First Year, United States		
Method **Column (1)**	**Women Experiencing Unintended Pregnancy Within the First Year of Use (%)**		**Women Continuing Use at 1 Year (%)[a]**
	Typical Use[b] **Column (2)**	**Perfect Use[c]** **Column (3)**	**Column (4)**
No method[d]	85	85	
Spermicides[e]	28	18	42
Fertility awareness–based methods	24		47
StandardDays method[f]		5	
TwoDay method[f]		4	
Ovulation method[f]		3	
Symptothermal method[f]		0.4	
Withdrawal	22	4	46
Sponge			
Parous women	24	20	46
Nulliparous women	12	9	36
Condom[g] (without spermicide)			
Female	21	5	41
Male	18	2	43
Diaphragm[e] (with spermicide)	12	6	57
Combined pill and progestin-only pill	9	0.3	67
Evra patch	9	0.3	67
NuvaRing	9	0.3	67
Depo-Provera	6	0.2	56
Intrauterine contraceptives			
ParaGard (copper T)	0.8	0.6	78
Mirena (LNG)	0.2	0.2	80
Implanon	0.05	0.05	84
Female sterilization	0.5	0.5	100
Male sterilization	0.15	0.10	100
The lactational amenorrhea method (LAM) is a highly effective, temporary method of contraception[i]			

[a]Among couples attempting to avoid pregnancy, the percentage of who continue to use a method for 1 year.

[b]Among typical couples who initiate use of a method (not necessarily for the first time), the percentage who experience an accidental pregnancy during the first year if they do not stop use for any other reason. Estimates of the probability of pregnancy during the first year of typical use for spermicides and the diaphragm are taken from the 1995 NSFG corrected for underreporting of abortion; estimates for fertility awareness–based methods, withdrawal, the male condom, the pill, and Depo-Provera are taken from the 1995 and 2002 NSFG corrected for underreporting of abortion. See the source text for the derivation of estimates for other methods.

(continues)

Table 16-1	Percentage of Women Experiencing an Unintended Pregnancy During the First Year of Typical Use and the First Year of Perfect Use of Contraceptives and the Percentage Continuing Use at the End of the First Year, United States (continued)

[c]Among typical couples who initiate use of a method (not necessarily for the first time) and who use it perfectly (both consistently and correctly), the percentage who experience an accidental pregnancy during the first year if they do not stop use for any other reason. See the source text for the derivation of the estimate for each other method.

[d]The percentages becoming pregnant in columns 2 and 3 are based on data from populations in which contraception is not used and from women who cease using contraception so as to become pregnant. Among such populations, about 89% become pregnant within 1 year. This estimate was lowered slightly (to 85%) to represent the percentage who would become pregnant within 1 year among women now relying on reversible methods of contraception if they abandoned contraception altogether.

[e]Foams, creams, gels, vaginal suppositories, and vaginal creams.

[f]The ovulation and TwoDay methods are based on evaluation of cervical mucus. The StandardDays method avoids intercourse on cycle days 8 through 19. The symptothermal method is a double-check method based on evaluation of cervical mucus to determine the first fertile day and evaluation of cervical mucus and temperature to determine the last fertile day.

[g]Without spermicides.

[h]With spermicidal cream or jelly.

[i]To maintain effective protection against pregnancy, another method of contraception must be used as soon as menstruation resumes, the frequency or duration of breastfeeding is reduced, bottle feeding is introduced, or the baby reaches 6 months of age.

Source: Trussell J. Contraceptive failure in the United States. *Contraception.* 2011;83(5):397-404. *Contraception* by ELSEVIER INC. Copyright 2011 by Elsevier. Reproduced with permission of ELSEVIER INC. in the format reuse in a book/textbook via Copyright Clearance Center.

such as insertion of an intrauterine contraceptive device, but over a period of several years are less costly than use of oral contraceptives, even though the latter has a stable, less expensive monthly expenditure. The age of the woman can factor into the choice of method. For example, a nonsmoking woman who has completed childbearing may choose oral contraceptives based on the noncontraceptive benefits of relief of perimenopausal symptoms.

The presence of or potential for transmitting genetic disorders to offspring may be an additional consideration, and for some women is a factor in choosing permanent sterilization. Of note, personal genetic risk factors may influence a woman's physiologic response to a contraceptive method as well as her personal risk factors. A woman with a strong family history of coagulation disorders may choose an intrauterine device as opposed to a contraceptive patch because of the former's lower risk of triggering a thrombotic event, recognizing the inheritable nature of the disorder even if she does not know her personal risk.

A number of other factors can influence a woman's selection of a contraceptive method including: needed length of time planned for contraception; rapidity of reversibility after discontinuation; efficacy/effectiveness; influence of popular media, including direct-to-consumer advertising; side effects and questions of safety; noncontraceptive health benefits; and frequency of intercourse.

Not all women who are sexually active are at risk of pregnancy. Some have a partner of the same gender; other women are engaged in a mutually monogamous relationship with a man who has had a vasectomy. Some women prefer not to share information about the contraceptive method with their partners because of personal privacy concerns. Women may seek contraceptives because they are anticipating exposure to pregnancy, voluntarily or not. For example, today's women in the military may be placed in positions where they are vulnerable to sexual violence, or where a contraceptive-associated amenorrhea may be preferable because of deployment to areas with lack of hygienic conditions.[9] Women who have physical or intellectual disabilities also have unique needs in the area of contraception and menstruation.[10,11] These needs may be related to or separate from voluntary sexual activity.

Incorporation of a partner into the process of choosing the method is a decision made by the woman. In some cases midwives may provide education to couples, whereas in other situations the woman alone consults with the professional. Throughout this chapter, content regarding education and care may be extrapolated to include significant others when their inclusion is preferred by the woman.

Any one factor may be of more importance to a woman than another. For some women, the major concern is effectiveness of the contraceptive method, and they are willing to deal with additional side effects to gain greater effectiveness. For other women, unintended pregnancies would be ill timed but not devastating, so other factors such as cost, ease of use, and acceptability to their partner may contribute more to the decision about which contraceptive method to use.

A woman should be informed of the risks and benefits of the various contraceptive methods, as well as the risks and benefits of a specific contraceptive method for the individual. Practice varies as to how the informed consent process is acknowledged and documented. Some practices require that women sign consent forms. Informed decision making is essential, and written consent must always be obtained prior to initiation of any invasive method, such as an implant or intrauterine device.

Medical Eligibility Criteria

Today all healthcare providers involved in family planning can benefit from the publication of evidence-based guidelines regarding the safety of contraceptive methods for individuals with specific medical conditions or some characteristics such as age. In 1996, the first edition of *Medical Eligibility Criteria for Contraceptive Use* (WHO MEC) was published by the World Health Organization; it is regularly updated based on new evidence.[12] The WHO MEC currently is in its fourth edition and is useful especially for midwives working internationally. The WHO has encouraged countries to modify the MEC as needed.

In recognition that practice in United States may differ in some aspects from international care, the Centers for Disease Control and Prevention (CDC) has published nationally focused guidelines. Known as the *U.S. Medical Eligibility Criteria for Contraceptive Use, 2010* (U.S. MEC), this publication can be downloaded for free and is closely related to the fourth edition of the WHO MEC[13] (**Box 16-1**). Modifications of the WHO MEC for women in the United States includes exclusion of methods not available in the United States and inclusion of several more health conditions of note within the country.[14] In particular, modifications in the areas of breastfeeding, intrauterine device use, valvular heart disease, ovarian cancer, uterine fibroids, and venous thromboembolism were made to reflect the U.S. population and practice. The U.S. MEC also added information about care of women with inflammatory bowel disease, history of bariatric surgery, rheumatoid arthritis, endometrial hyperplasia, history of peripartum cardiomyopathy, and history of solid-organ transplant that is not found in the WHO MEC.

BOX 16-1 Categories of Medical Eligibility Criteria for Contraceptive Use

1 = A condition for which there is no restriction for the use of the contraceptive method

2 = A condition for which the advantages of using the method generally outweigh the theoretical or proven risks

3 = A condition for which the theoretical or proven risks usually outweigh the advantages of using the method

4 = A condition that represents an unacceptable health risk if the contraceptive method is used

Sources: World Health Organization. *Medical Eligibility Criteria for Contraceptive Use.* 4th ed. Geneva, Switzerland: WHO; 2009; Centers for Disease Control and Prevention. The U.S. medical eligibility criteria for contraceptive use, 2010. *MMWR.* 2010;59(RR04):1-85.

The U.S. MEC, as shown in **Figure 16-1**, is a guide to be used when counseling women and men about contraceptive choices. This document focuses primarily on safety of use of various contraceptives, especially for both initiation and continuation. The midwife and woman can quickly verify recommendations for use of a specific method by referring to multiple tables in the publication. Eligibility is described in terms of the four categories listed in Box 16-1, ranging from suggesting no restriction in use to other considerations based on risks.[12,13] The U.S. MEC is a set of guidelines—it is not mandatory. Thus deviations from its recommendation may occur in consideration of an individual woman's situation. Nevertheless, variation in practice is rare and the U.S. MEC guidelines are used widely throughout the United States.

Options Counseling

Options counseling is the process by which women who are undecided about their choices are provided with information about all available options.[15] When faced with an unintended pregnancy, a woman generally has the following options: She can continue the pregnancy and keep the baby; continue the pregnancy and surrender the infant for adoption; or electively terminate the pregnancy. One of the American College of Nurse-Midwives (ACNM) Hallmarks of Midwifery addresses advocacy for informed choice, shared decision making, and the right to self-determination.[8]

Key:	
1 No restriction (method can be used).	
2 Advantages generally outweigh theoretical or proven risks.	
3 Theoretical or proven risks usually outweigh the advantages.	
4 Unacceptable health risk (method not to be used).	

Updated July 2011. This summary sheet only contains a subset of the recommendations from the U.S. MEC. For complete, see: http://www.cdc.gov/reproductivehealth/unintendedpregnancy/USMEC.htm

Most contraceptive methods do not protect against sexually transmitted infections (STIs). Consistent and correct use of the male latex condom reduces the risk of STIs and HIV.

Condition	Subcondition	Combined pill, patch, ring		Progestin-only pill		Injection		Implant		LNG-IUD		Copper IUD	
		I	C	I	C	I	C	I	C	I	C	I	C
Age		Menarche to < 40 = 1		Menarche to < 18 = 1		Menarche to < 18 = 2		Menarche to < 18 = 1		Menarche to < 20 = 2		Menarche to < 20 = 2	
		≥ 40 = 2		18–45 = 1		18–45 = 1		18–45 = 1		≥ 20 = 1		≥ 20 = 1	
				> 45 = 1		> 45 = 2		> 45 = 1					
Anatomic abnormalities	a) Distorted uterine cavity									4		4	
	b) Other abnormalities									2		2	
Anemias	a) Thalassemia	1		1		1		1		1		2	
	b) Sickle cell disease‡	2		1		1		1		1		2	
	c) Iron-deficiency anemia	1		1		1		1		1		2	
Benign ovarian tumors	(including cysts)	1		1		1		1		1		1	
Breast disease	a) Undiagnosed mass	2*		2*		2*		2*		2		1	
	b) Benign breast disease	1		1		1		1		1		1	
	c) Family history of cancer	1		1		1		1		1		1	
	d) Breast cancer‡												
	i) Current	4		4		4		4		4		1	
	ii) Past and no evidence of current disease for 5 years	3		3		3		3		3		1	
Breastfeeding (see also postpartum)	a) < 1 month postpartum	3*		2*		2*		2*					
	b) 1 month or more postpartum	2*		1*		1*		1*					
Cervical cancer	Awaiting treatment	2		1		2		2		4	2	4	2
Cervical ectropion		1		1		1		1		1		1	
Cervical intraepithelial neoplasia (CIN)		2		1		2		2		2		1	
Cirrhosis	a) Mild (compensated)	1		1		1		1		1		1	
	b) Severe‡ (decompensated)	4		3		3		3		3		1	
Deep venous thrombosis (DVT)/pulmonary embolism (PE)	a) History of DVT/PE, not on anticoagulant therapy												
	i) Higher risk for recurrent DVT/PE	4		2		2		2		2		1	
	ii) Lower risk for recurrent DVT/PE	3		2		2		2		2		1	
	b) Acute DVT/PE	4		2		2		2		2		2	
	c) DVT/PE and established on anticoagulant therapy for at least 3 months												
	i) Higher risk for recurrent DVT/PE	4*		2		2		2		2		2	
	ii) Lower risk for recurrent DVT/PE	3*		2		2		2		2		2	
	d) Family history (first-degree relatives)	2		1		1		1		1		1	
	e) Major surgery												
	i) With prolonged immobilization	4		2		2		2		2		1	
	ii) Without prolonged immobilization	2		1		1		1		1		1	
	f) Minor surgery without immobilization	1		1		1		1		1		1	

Figure 16-1 Summary chart of U.S. medical eligibility criteria for contraceptive use.
Source: Centers for Disease Control and Prevention. The U.S. medical eligibility criteria for contraceptive use, 2010. *MMWR.* 2010;59(RR04):1-85.

Condition	Subcondition	Combined pill, patch, ring		Progestin-only pill		Injection		Implant		LNG-IUD		Copper IUD	
		I	C	I	C	I	C	I	C	I	C	I	C
Depressive disorders		1*		1*		1*		1*		1*		1*	
Diabetes mellitus (DM)	a) History of gestational DM only	1		1		1		1		1		1	
	b) Non-vascular disease												
	i) Non-insulin dependent	2		2		2		2		2		1	
	ii) Insulin dependent‡	2		2		2		2		2		1	
	c) Nephropathy/retinopathy/neuropathy‡	3/4*		2		3		2		2		1	
	d) Other vascular disease or diabetes of > 20 years' duration‡	3/4*		2		3		2		2		1	
Endometrial cancer‡		1		1		1		1		4	2	4	2
Endometrial hyperplasia		1		1		1		1		1		1	
Endometriosis		1		1		1		1		1		2	
Epilepsy‡§	See drug interactions	1*		1*		1*		1*		1		1	
Gall-bladder disease	a) Symptomatic												
	i) Treated by cholecystectomy	2		2		2		2		2		1	
	ii) Medically treated	3		2		2		2		2		1	
	iii) Current	3		2		2		2		2		1	
	b) Asymptomatic	2		2		2		2		2		1	
Gestational trophoblastic disease	a) Decreasing or undetectable β-hCG levels	1		1		1		1		3		3	
	b) Persistently elevated β-hCG levels or malignant disease‡	1		1		1		1		4		4	
Headaches	a) Non-migrainous	1*	2*	1*	1*	1*	1*	1*	1*	1*	1*	1*	
	b) Migraine												
	i) Without aura, age < 35	2*	3*	1*	2*	2*	2*	2*	2*	2*	2*	1*	
	ii) Without aura, age ≥ 35	3*	4*	1*	2*	2*	2*	2*	2*	2*	2*	1*	
	iii) With aura, any age	4*	4*	2*	3*	2*	3*	2*	3*	2*	3*	1*	
History of bariatric surgery‡	a) Restrictive procedures	1		1		1		1		1		1	
	b) Malabsorptive procedures	COCs: 3 P/R: 1		3		1		1		1		1	
History of cholestasis	a) Pregnancy-related	2		1		1		1		1		1	
	b) Past COC-related	3		2		2		2		2		1	
History of high blood pressure during pregnancy		2		1		1		1		1		1	
History of pelvic surgery		1		1		1		1		1		1	
HIV	High risk or HIV infected‡	1		1		1		1		2	2	2	2
	AIDs (see drug interactions)‡§	1*		1*		1*		1*		3	2*	3	2*
	Clinically well on ARV therapy§	If on treatment see drug interactions								2	2	2	2
Hyperlipidemias		2/3*		2*		2*		2*		2*		1*	
Hypertension	a) Adequately controlled hypertension	3*		1*		2*		1*		1		1	
	b) Elevated blood pressure levels (properly taken measurements)												
	i) Systolic 140–159 or diastolic 90–99	3		1		2		1		1		1	
	ii) Systolic ≥ 160 or diastolic ≥ 100‡	4		2		3		2		2		1	
	c) Vascular disease	4		2		3		2		2		1	

Figure 16-1 Summary chart of U.S. medical eligibility criteria for contraceptive use.

Source: Centers for Disease Control and Prevention. The U.S. medical eligibility criteria for contraceptive use, 2010. *MMWR.* 2010;59(RR04):1-85.

Condition	Subcondition	Combined pill, patch, ring		Progestin-only pill		Injection		Implant		LNG-IUD		Copper IUD	
		I	C	I	C	I	C	I	C	I	C	I	C
Inflammatory bowel disease	(Ulcerative colitis, Crohn's disease)	2/3*		2		2		1		1		1	
Ischemic heart disease‡	Current and history of	4		2	3	3		2	3	2	3	1	
Liver tumors	a) Benign												
	i) Focal nodular hyperplasia	2		2		2		2		2		1	
	ii) Hepatocellular adenoma‡	4		3		3		3		3		1	
	b) Malignant‡	4		3		3		3		3		1	
Malaria		1		1		1		1		1		1	
Multiple risk factors for arterial cardiovascular disease	(Such as older age, smoking, diabetes, and hypertension)	3/4*		2*		3*		2*		2		1	
Obesity	a) ≥ 30 kg/m² body mass index (BMI)	2		1		1		1		1		1	
	b) Menarche to < 18 years and ≥ 30 kg/m² BMI	2		1		2		1		1		1	
Ovarian cancer‡		1		1		1		1		1		1	
Parity	a) Nulliparous	1		1		1		1		2		2	
	b) Parous	1		1		1		1		1		1	
Past ectopic pregnancy		1		2		1		1		1		1	
Pelvic inflammatory disease	a) Past (assuming no current risk factors of STIs)												
	i) With subsequent pregnancy	1		1		1		1		1	1	1	1
	ii) Without subsequent pregnancy	1		1		1		1		2	2	2	2
	b) Current	1		1		1		1		4	2*	4	2*
Peripartum cardiomyopathy‡	a) Normal or mildly impaired cardiac function												
	i) < 6 months	4		1		1		1		2		2	
	ii) ≥ 6 months	3		1		1		1		2		2	
	b) Moderately or severely impaired cardiac function	4		2		2		2		2		2	
Postabortion	a) First trimester	1*		1*		1*		1*		1*		1*	
	b) Second trimester	1*		1*		1*		1*		2		2	
	c) Immediately post septic abortion	1*		1*		1*		1*		4		4	
Postpartum (see also breastfeeding)	a) < 21 days	4		1		1		1					
	b) 21 days to 42 days												
	i) With other risk factors for VTE	3*		1		1		1					
	ii) Without other risk factors for VTE	2		1		1		1					
	c) > 42 days	1		1		1		1					
Postpartum (in breastfeeding or nonbreastfeeding women, including postcaesarean section)	a) < 10 minutes after delivery of the placenta									2		1	
	b) 10 minutes after delivery of the placenta to < 4 weeks									2		2	
	c) ≥ 4 weeks									1		1	
	d) Puerperal sepsis									4		4	
Pregnancy		NA*		NA**		NA*		NA*		4*		4*	
Rheumatoid arthritis	a) On immunosuppressive therapy	2		1		2/3*		1		2	1	2	1
	b) Not on immunosuppressive therapy	2		1		2		1		1		1	
Schistosomiasis	a) Uncomplicated	1		1		1		1		1		1	
	b) Fibrosis of the liver‡	1		1		1		1		1		1	

Figure 16-1 Summary chart of U.S. medical eligibility criteria for contraceptive use.
Source: Centers for Disease Control and Prevention. The U.S. medical eligibility criteria for contraceptive use, 2010. *MMWR.* 2010;59(RR04):1-85.

Condition	Subcondition	Combined pill, patch, ring		Progestin-only pill		Injection		Implant		LNG-IUD		Copper IUD	
		I	C	I	C	I	C	I	C	I	C	I	C
Severe dysmenorrhea		1		1		1		1		1		2	
Sexually transmitted infections	a) Current purulent cervicitis or chlamydial infections or gonorrhea	1		1		1		1		4	2*	4	2*
	b) Other STIs (excluding HIV and hepatitis)	1		1		1		1		2	2	2	2
	c) Vaginitis (including *Trichomonas vaginalis* and bacterial vaginosis)	1		1		1		1		2	2	2	2
	d) Increased risk of STIs	1		1		1		1		2/3*		2/3*	2
Smoking	a) Age < 35	2		1		1		1		1		1	
	b) Age ≥ 35, < 15 cigarettes/day	3		1		1		1		1		1	
	c) Age ≥ 35, ≥ 15 cigarettes/day	4		1		1		1		1		1	
Solid organ transplantation‡	a) Complicated	4		2		2		2		3	2	3	2
	b) Uncomplicated	2*		2		2		2		2		2	
Stroke‡	History of cerebrovascular accident	4		2	3	3		2	3	2		1	
Superficial venous thrombosis	a) Varicose veins	1		1		1		1		1		1	
	b) Superficial thrombophlebitis	2		1		1		1		1		1	
Systemic lupus erythematosus‡	a) Positive (or unknown) antiphospholipid antibodies	4		3		3	3	3		3		1	1
	b) Severe thrombocytopenia	2		2		3	2	2		2*		3*	2*
	c) Immunosuppressive treatment	2		2		2	2	2		2		2	1
	d) None of the above	2		2		2	2	2		2		1	1
Thrombogenic mutations‡		4*		2*		2*		2*		2*		1*	
Thyroid disorders	Simple goiter/hyperthyroid/hypothyroid	1		1		1		1		1		1	
Tuberculosis‡	a) Nonpelvic	1*		1*		1*		1*		1		1	
	b) Pelvic	1*		1*		1*		1*		4	3	4	3
Unexplained vaginal bleeding	(Suspicious for serious condition) before evaluation	2*		2*		3*		3*		4*	2*	4*	2*
Uterine fibroids		1		1		1		1		2		2	
Valvular heart disease	a) Uncomplicated	2		1		1		1		1		1	
	b) Complicated‡	4		1		1		1		1		1	
Vaginal bleeding patterns	a) Irregular pattern without heavy bleeding	1		2		2		2		1	1	1	
	b) Heavy or prolonged bleeding	1*		2*		2*		2*		1*	2*	2*	
Viral hepatitis	a) Acute or flare	3/4*	2	1		1		1		1		1	
	b) Carrier/chronic	1	1	1		1		1		1		1	
Drug interactions													
Antiretroviral therapy (ARV)	a) Nucleoside reverse transcriptase inhibitors	1*		1		1		1		2/3*	2*	2/3*	2*
	b) Non-nucleoside reverse transcriptase inhibitors	2*		2*		1		2*		2/3*	2*	2/3*	2*
	c) Ritonavir-boosted protease inhibitors	3*		3*		1		2*		2/3*	2*	2/3*	2*
Anticonvulsant therapy	a) Certain anticonvulsants (phenytoin, carbamazepine, barbiturates, primidone, topiramate, oxcarbazepine)	3*		3*		1		2*		1		1	
	b) Lamotrigine	3*		1		1		1		1		1	
Antimicrobial therapy	a) Broad spectrum antibiotics	1		1		1		1		1		1	
	b) Antifungals	1		1		1		1		1		1	
	c) Antiparasitics	1		1		1		1		1		1	
	d) Rifampicin or rifabutin therapy	3*		3*		1		2*		1		1	

I = initiation of contraceptive method; C = continuation of contraceptive method
* Please see the complete guidance for a clarification to this classification. http://www.cdc.gov/reproductivehealth/usmec
‡ Condition that exposes woman to increased risk as a result of unintended pregnancy
§ Please refer to the U.S. MEC guidance related to drug interactions at the end of this chart

Figure 16-1 Summary chart of U.S. medical eligibility criteria for contraceptive use.
Source: Centers for Disease Control and Prevention. The U.S. medical eligibility criteria for contraceptive use, 2010. *MMWR.* 2010;59(RR04):1-85.

This underscores the midwife's role in counseling, advising, and informing the woman of her options.

Options counseling is distinctly different from abortion counseling, which is important for practitioners who choose not to offer abortion counseling or abortion services. Options counseling is a nonjudgmental description of the three options that may be intertwined with values clarification exercises that can help the woman decide what is right for her.

To effectively provide options counseling, the midwife must be able to personally detach from the decision that the woman may make, acknowledging that her decision may conflict with the midwife's personal beliefs. Principles of options counseling include the ability to actively listen to the woman, provide to her all necessary information from which to make her decision, and support her in evaluating her options.[15]

Via the use of nonjudgmental verbal and nonverbal communication, as well as the use of open-ended questions, the midwife can therapeutically discuss options with the woman. It is imperative that the woman is guided through exploration of her own feelings and beliefs in regard to all appropriate options. Assisting her to understand the outcome of each option is important not only to her decision-making process, but also to her ability to accept the decision she will eventually have to make.

Adoption Counseling

If a pregnant woman chooses to place a baby for adoption, the primary role of the midwife is to connect the woman with the appropriate resources to assist her in creating an adoption plan. Ideally this would occur in collaboration with a social worker who has knowledge of the full range of services available in the area, though in some communities the midwife may need to personally provide these referrals. Thus it is incumbent upon the midwife to become familiar with locally available adoption services.

The midwife should have an awareness of all adoption options available to provide initial counseling to a woman considering this option. Adoption choices include open, closed, or semi-open adoption.

- *Open adoption* occurs when the birth mother and adoptive family are known to each other and have varying levels of communication, ranging from visits to letters or phone calls, although the birth mother does not necessarily have any input about the way the child is parented. Women should understand that in most cases of open adoption, there is no legal requirement for the adoptive family to follow the terms of such an agreement and legal restrictions will vary by state.
- *Closed adoption* is the term that describes an adoption in which birth records are sealed, and all identities are concealed.
- *Semi-open adoption* is the term used when some identifying information is shared, and communication occurs at prearranged intervals, usually through an intermediary such as an attorney or adoption agency. The degree of communication and "openness" may change with time.

Making the decision to place a baby for adoption can be a difficult one, and the woman will need emotional support, both during prenatal care and during the birth and the early postpartum period.

Abortion Counseling

When a woman learns that she has conceived, she can have an array of reactions, ranging from delight to despair. There never should be an assumption that confirmation of pregnancy will be positively received news for all women. The midwife should, therefore, be prepared to listen and respond appropriately. The ACNM has emphasized that there is a wide range of diversity among certified nurse-midwives (CNMs)/certified midwives (CMs) and the women they serve, who may make a variety of personal and professional choices related to reproductive health care. Nevertheless, all women have the right to have access to unbiased, factual information about available reproductive health choices from which they can then make informed decisions about their reproductive health.[8]

The legalization of abortion means that every woman, upon becoming pregnant, has a choice to carry the pregnancy to its natural conclusion or abort the pregnancy. Annually, 2% of U.S. women age 15–44 have an abortion.[16] Women age 20–29 have more than half of all abortions performed in the United States. Approximately 61% of pregnancy terminations are obtained by women who have had at least one or more previous children.

A woman's decision to have an abortion is not lightly made. In many cases she will turn to the midwife for counsel, advice, and information. Some midwives may decide that they cannot provide abortion counseling due to personal, religious, or moral conflicts. A delicate balance is involved between respecting the autonomy of the individual midwife who is morally opposed to providing termination counseling, while at the same time respecting the woman's right to be informed about all of her family planning options. Any midwife whose conscience will not allow her to provide abortion counseling needs to inform the woman of that fact, and facilitate the woman in finding another provider who will offer this type of counseling. Midwives who desire to provide abortion counseling need be knowledgeable about local resources, the methods used, and ways to make appropriate referrals as needed.

When abortion counseling is performed, components of such counseling include discussion of method-specific risks, benefits, informed consent, and gestational age limits. Gestational age limits will vary by setting, state regulations, and local availability of trained providers.

Types of Pregnancy Termination

More than 90% of planned abortions occur in the first trimester. A small percentage (7.3%) are performed between 14 and 20 weeks' gestation, and 1.3% are performed at 21 weeks' gestation or greater.[17] For women whose blood is Rh negative, Rho(D) immunoglobulin (anti-D serum; RhoGAM) is indicated prior to start of either medical or surgical termination.

In the first trimester, abortions may be performed using pharmacologic agents or surgical interventions such as vacuum aspiration or dilation and curettage. After the first trimester, surgical dilation and evacuation is used, potentially requiring a 2-day procedure, with the insertion of osmotic dilators at least 24 hours before the termination of pregnancy.

Surgical Abortion

Manual vacuum aspiration (MVA) may be used for pregnancies that are up to approximately 12 gestational weeks. This method involves using a handheld syringe as the suction source for emptying the uterine contents.[18] MVA has been found to be equally effective as suction curretage for abortion during the first trimester.[18] The procedure takes 5 to 15 minutes, and can be performed in the office setting, resulting in removal of the intact gestational sac, thus enabling confirmation of pregnancy termination.[19]

Termination using suction dilation and curettage (D & C) is accomplished by dilation of the cervix, followed by curettage to empty the uterine contents. This technique can be used up to 13 gestational weeks. The overall risk of complications is less than 1% for surgical termination.[17] The main complications of surgical abortion are continued intrauterine pregnancy; heavy bleeding; infection, including endometritis; uterine perforation or injury to organs; and risk of retained products of conception, requiring further surgical intervention.[20,21]

Abortion Using Pharmacologic Agents (Medical Abortion)

Three agents currently are used for medical abortion: mifepristone (Mifeprex, RU-486), methotrexate (Rheumatrex), and misoprostol (Cytotec). A combination of mifepristone and misoprostol was FDA approved in 2000 for women seeking a medical abortion. According to that approval, oral mifepristone is administered in the dosage of 600 mg. Two days later, 400 mcg of oral misoprostol is administered. At 2 weeks post treatment, the woman should be evaluated to confirm that a complete termination has occurred. However, 200 mg of mifepristone has been found in studies to be as effective as the higher dose and often is used due to the cost saving and decrease in side effects. Because studies found that 800 mcg of vaginal misoprostol is superior to 400 mcg administered orally, the higher vaginal dose often is substituted for the oral agent.[22]

Mifepristone inhibits progesterone, which is necessary for normal placental attachment, thereby preventing fertilization and sensitizing the uterus to the effects of prostaglandin.[23] Maximal sensitization occurs at approximately 24 to 48 hours following administration of mifepristone.[24] Misoprostol, a prostaglandin E_1 analogue, causes expulsion of uterine contents.[23] The two-medication regimen of mifepristone followed by misoprostol has a 95% to 98% effectiveness rate when used by women whose gestations are 63 days or less after their last menstrual period.[25] When used alone, mifepristone is approximately 76% effective; hence it is rarely used as a sole agent.[25] The effectiveness of misoprostol alone varies widely, from 68% to 94%,[26] depending on whether it is used vaginally, it is inserted dry or moistened (most effective), or it is taken orally.[27] When used alone, misoprostol is associated with significantly higher rates of nausea, vomiting, fever, chills, and diarrhea. It has also been found to be a teratogen, being associated with the rare congenital neurological disorder called Mobius syndrome if the pregnancy continues.[28]

Although methotrexate has been used for pregnancy termination, its effectiveness as an abortifacient is not as high as the effectiveness of the other methods. Methotrexate works by inhibiting dihydrofolate reductase, an enzyme necessary for DNA synthesis, and often is categorized as an antimetabolite or an antifolate agent.[29] Rapidly dividing cells are not able to undergo normal mitosis when exposed to methotrexate. When used alone, this agent's effectiveness is between 60% and 84%.[30]

Women who plan a medical abortion are counseled to expect heavy bleeding and significant painful cramping. The bleeding will be heaviest in the first 6 hours after misoprostol administration. Approximately 50% of women report nausea following use of mifepristone. Nonsteroidal anti-inflammatory drugs (NSAIDs) can be effective in mitigating pain, and they do not interfere with the effect of misoprostol. Because there is a risk of teratogenicity if pregnancy is not aborted, women should be counseled about a possible need for surgical abortion in the event of failure of the medical approach.

The contraindications to medical abortion are listed in **Table 16-2**.[30] Women who are breastfeeding should avoid nursing their infant for 2 days after using mifepristone and for 4 hours after taking misoprostol. Complications of medical abortion methods may include incomplete expulsion of uterine contents and subsequent need for surgical procedure; uterine infection (less than 1%); and heavy bleeding that requires hemostatic curettage (0.3% to 1.3%).[24] Some providers counsel women that if they are saturating more than two maxi-pads per hour for 2 hours or longer following a medical abortion, they should notify a healthcare provider.

Post-termination Care

Regardless of whether a midwife is involved in the termination procedure, it is common for a midwife to care for women who have recently had a pregnancy termination. Women who have undergone either a surgical or medical abortion should be seen for a follow-up visit within 2 weeks. The follow-up visit assessment includes the following elements: assessment for complications including incomplete abortion, evaluation of emotional status, and discussion of ongoing contraceptive needs.

A pelvic ultrasound, urine pregnancy test, or qualitative serum beta–human chorionic gonadotropin (beta-hCG) measurement may be used to confirm expulsion of the products of conception. A systematic review of the literature has revealed controversy

Table 16-2	Contraindications to Medical Abortion	
General Contraindications	**Contraindications to Misoprostol or Mifepristone**	**Contraindications Based on Individual Factors**
Gestational age > 63 days of gestation[a]	Allergy to mifepristone	Desire for rapid termination of pregnancy
Confirmed or suspected ectopic pregnancy	Seizure disorder	Inability to access emergency care quickly (no telephone, lack of transportation)
Undiagnosed adnexal mass	Allergy or adverse reactions to prostaglandins	
Intrauterine device in place		Inability to care for oneself
Chronic adrenal failure		Inability to comprehend instructions
Current long-term systemic corticosteroid therapy		
Severe anemia		
Known coagulopathy or anticoagulant therapy		
Inherited porphyrias		
Upper genital tract infection		
Cardiovascular disease		
Severe asthma not controlled by therapy[b]		

[a]The upper limit of gestation for medical abortion depends somewhat on the drugs used and the doses of those drugs that are used. The mifepristone-misoprostol combination is highly effective up to 63 days of gestation. Regimens with misoprostol only have a lower success rate. It is also important to consider the woman's experience. The experience is more painful and difficult when there is more material in the uterus that will be expelled. Therefore, it is important to counsel women about what to expect based on the gestational age and size of gestational sac.

[b]Severe asthma not controlled by therapy is a recommended contraindication by some organizations and not listed by others. Per the American College of Obstetricians and Gynecologists, asthma is not a contraindications because misoprostol is a weak bronchodilator. However, if the woman has severe asthma, a consultation is recommended before proceeding with a medical abortion.

Sources: Adapted from American College of Obstetricians and Gynecologists (ACOG). *Medical Management of Abortion.* (ACOG Practice Bulletin No. 67). Washington, DC: ACOG; October 12, 2005; World Health Organization (WHO). *Medical Eligibility Criteria for Contraceptive Use.* 4th ed. Geneva, Switzerland: WHO; 2009; National Abortion Federation (NAF). Medical abortion history and overview. Available at: http://www.prochoice.org/education/resources/med_history_overview.html. Accessed June 11, 2013.

about routine use of ultrasound to rule out retained products of conception. Although ultrasound has high sensitivity and specificity for this indication, it is expensive and not always available. The use of alternative modalities, such as standardized questioning of a woman's symptoms, telephone consultations, and urine hCG measurement, are effective strategies for follow-up. However, if there is a strong suspicion of an abortion failure, ultrasound remains the most common intervention.[31]

Role of Midwives in Performing Abortions

In 1971, ACNM issued a practice statement that prohibited CNMs from performing abortions. This statement preceded the 1973 the U.S. Supreme Court's ruling in *Roe v. Wade*, which legalized abortion nationwide. The 1971 statement was the only prohibitive statement ever issued by the ACNM and, after discussion within the membership, it was retracted in 1992.[32]

Today, midwives are being sought as providers to meet the demand for abortions. The abortion care provided by midwives and other nonphysician providers has been demonstrated to be equal to that provided by physicians.[33] The University of California San Francisco, in 2005, was granted a waiver from the Office of State Health Planning and Development to provide education for CNMs, physician assistants (PAs), and nurse practitioners (NPs) in the procedure of uterine aspiration evacuation.[34] Privileging NPs, PAs, and CNMs/CMs who desire to perform aspiration evacuations would increase access to this service, particularly in those areas of the United States where there are no physician providers currently providing this care.

Emergency Contraception

Misnamed as postcoital or "morning after" contraception, this family planning method is more appropriately termed *emergency contraception* (EC). EC is not intended for use as a regular method of birth control. Rather, it is recommended either when there has been a method failure, such as condom breakage, or after unintended unprotected intercourse. EC may be used anytime in the first 3 to 5 days after unprotected intercourse.[34] All women seeking contraceptive services should be counseled about the availability and correct use of EC.

Access to EC has been the subject of controversy, especially for minors. For several years, EC

pills were available by prescription only and even when approved for nonprescription status access were restricted based on age. In mid-2013, several judicial courts ruled in favor of nonprescription access to EC by women regardless of age. At the time of this writing, the federal administration has decided not to block or appeal these rulings. However, many states have different regulations regarding EC, some mandating access and others restricting it. Thus, midwives are advised to be aware of current national rules and state laws but also realize that changes may continue to occur in this area.

Although greater use of EC has been proposed to decrease the number of unintended pregnancies by as many as 1.7 million pregnancies per year, EC has not yet been used widely enough to significantly decrease the number of unintended pregnancies that occur in the United States.[35] Various reasons contribute to the low use of EC, including misinformation related to EC availability, indications, and use.[36] Additionally, some healthcare organizations do not endorse its use, while some providers choose not to discuss EC for reasons that include personal, moral, or religious objections, as well as time constraints.

Four methods of EC currently are available in the United States: the Yuzpe method; levonorgestrel (LNG) formulations (Plan B One Step, Next Choice, Next Choice One Dose); selective progesterone receptor modulators (ulipristal acetate [UPA; ella]); and the copper intrauterine contraceptive device (IUD). The dose, use, and effectiveness of these methods are presented in **Table 16-3**.[12,13,19,22,29,37,38]

Hormonal EC: Mechanisms of Action

The mechanism of action of hormonal EC methods is inhibition and/or delay of ovulation secondary to suppression, delaying, or blunting of the luteinizing hormone (LH) surge depending on when in the menstrual cycle the contraceptive pill is ingested.[30] Oral contraceptive and LNG formulations of pregnancy prevention do not effectively prevent follicular rupture if used in the late preovulatory stage; thus these two are most effective if used prior to ovulation and as soon as possible after unprotected intercourse.[39] UPA does prevent follicular rupture if taken before the onset of the LH surge and reduces endometrial thickness, thereby making the endometrium less hospitable for implantation of an embryo. Hormonal EC methods do not interfere with a conceptus that has already implanted and presents no risk to a conceptus that has already implanted in the uterus.[23,38,40-43]

Calculating effectiveness rates for EC is complex because accurately estimating when ovulation

Table 16-3   Comparison of Emergency Contraceptive Methods

Emergency Contraceptive Method (Brand Name)	Dose	Pregnancy Rate After Use	Maximum Time for Use	US MEC Category[a]	Clinical Considerations
Levonorgestrel (Next Choice)	.75 mg per tablet. Taken as two pills 12 hours apart[b]	.7–2.6%[c]	Up to 5 days (120 hours) after unprotected intercourse, may be somewhat less effective from 72 to 120 hours	1 or 2	May be less effective for women with BMI ≥ 30
Levonorgestrel (Plan B One Step)	1.5 mg per tablet administered orally in 1 dose	1.7–2.6%[c]	Up to 5 days (120 hours) after unprotected intercourse, may be somewhat less effective from 72 to 120 hours	1 or 2	May be less effective for women with BMI ≥ 30
Levonorgestrel (Next Choice One Dose)	1.5 mg per tablet administered orally in 1 dose	.7–2.6%	Up to 5 days (120 hours) after unprotected intercourse, may be somewhat less effective from 72 to 120 hours	1 or 2	May be less effective for women with BMI ≥ 30
Ulipristal acetate (ella)	30 mg administered orally, 1 dose	0.9–1.8%[c] 2.6% from 48 to 72 hours[d]	Up to 5 days, effectiveness does not wane between 72 and 120 hours	Not evaluated	May reduce the contraceptive action of progestin-containing hormonal contraceptive methods because of its affinity for binding to the progesterone receptor; reliable barrier contraception should be used until next menses. U.S. MEC has not evaluated contraindications for use of ella. Package insert lists pregnancy, poorly controlled asthma, and hepatic dysfunction as contraindications.
Ethinyl estradiol and levonorgestrel hormonal contraceptives (Yuzpe regimen)	One oral contraceptive pill administered orally in various combinations[e]	2–3%	Up to 72 hours[f] after unprotected intercourse	1 or 2	Higher rates of nausea and vomiting compared to other oral regimens. Consider prescribing an antiemetic.

(continues)

Table 16-3	Comparison of Emergency Contraceptive Methods (continued)			
Emergency Contraceptive Method (Brand Name)	Dose	Pregnancy Rate After Use	Maximum Time for Use	US MEC Category[a]	Clinical Considerations
Copper T 380A (ParaGard)	Intrauterine	0.1–0.2%	Up to 5 days after unprotected intercourse Up to day 12 of a regular menstrual cycle At other times of cycle if not more than 5 days after ovulation	1 or 2 except sexual assault victims at high risk for STI is category 3 and pregnancy is category 4	Candidates for the copper IUD must meet standard criteria for IUD insertion. Contraindications to use of the copper T IUD are listed in the *Nonhormonal Contraception* chapter.

IUD = intrauterine device; STI = sexually transmitted infection.

[a]U.S. MEC cCategories:

Category 1: a condition for which there is no restriction

Category 2: a condition for which the advantages of using the method generally outweigh the theoretical or proven risks

Category 3: a condition for which the theoretical or proven risks usually outweigh the advantages of using the method

Category 4: a condition that represents an unacceptable health risk if the contraceptive method is used

[b]A single dose has been shown to be as effective as two doses, although some package labeling continues to state it should be taken in two doses 12 hours apart.

[c]Rates taken from clinical trials that compared levonorgestrel and ulipristal acetate calculated actual risk, not relative risk.

[d]This rate was taken from a single-arm trial that evaluated the effectiveness of ulipristal acetate beyond 72 hours.

[e]The Yuzpe regimen is not the first choice, due to associated rates of nausea and vomiting. If they are the only option available for a woman, the number of pills and dosing from 19 different branded combined oral contraceptive products is available from the Princeton University Office of Population Research and Association of Reproductive Health Professionals and can be accessed at http://ec.princeton.edu/questions/dose.html.

[f]No studies have evaluated effectiveness beyond 72 hours.

Source: Adapted from Murphy P. Update on emergency contraception. *J Midwifery Women's Health.* 2012;57(6):593-602.

occurs relative to the timing of sexual intercourse is difficult.[44] In general, EC is most effective when the interval between intercourse and use is short. Longer intervals result in decreased effectiveness.[38]

The Yuzpe Method

The Yuzpe method is the oldest of the EC methods, and involves the ingestion of a high dose of estrogen and progestin, which is accomplished by administering several combined oral contraceptive pills in a single dose so that ovulation is inhibited. **Table 16-4** lists combined oral contraceptive formulations used for this purpose.[45]

The pregnancy rate following use of the Yuzpe method is approximately 2% to 3%. This contraceptive method frequently causes nausea, vomiting, headache, vertigo, and breast tenderness. The woman may also experience irregular bleeding or spotting in the 3 to 4 weeks following treatment.[38,46] If the Yuzpe method is used, an over-the-counter antiemetic, such as meclizine (Antivert, Bonine, Dramamine II) in a dose of 25–50 mg, can be recommended for use 1 hour prior to taking the EC dose. There is conflicting information on whether either dose should be repeated if the woman vomits within 1 hour of ingesting the medication.[46]

Levonorgestrel: Plan B One Step and Next Choice

Although still available, the Yuzpe method has been largely replaced by the progestin-only formulations made of LNG. The LNG formulations are more effective and have fewer side effects than those that contain both estrogen and progestins.[38,46] LNG primarily inhibits or delays ovulation by preventing the LH surge if taken before the LH surge occurs.[47] If taken close to or during the LH surge, it blunts and delays the surge and makes the ovum resistant to fertilization.[34]

LNG for EC use is formulated under the brand name Plan B One Step; a generic version is also marketed as Next Choice. When using Plan B One Step, a single dose of 1.5 mg LNG is taken within 72 hours following unprotected intercourse.[34,48] If vomiting occurs within 2 hours of taking a single-dose LNG, a repeat dose should be considered. Next Choice contains two doses of 0.75 mg LNG that can be taken 12 hours apart; alternatively, they can be taken as one single dose. The convenience of taking one dose rather than two may improve use and, therefore, effectiveness.[49]

Studies that have evaluated LNG agents ingested within 72 hours following intercourse found the effectiveness is approximately 79% for the two-dose

Table 16-4	Oral Formulations Approved for Emergency Contraception in the United States
Brand	**Pills per Dose**
Dedicated Emergency Contraception: One Dose-Regimen	
Plan B One Step	1 white pill
Next Choice	2 peach pills
Next Choice One Dose	1 peach pill
ella	1 white pill
Combined Progesterone and Estrogen Pills: Two-Dose Regimen, Second Dose Taken 12 Hours After First Dose	
Aviane	5 orange pills per dose
Cryselle	4 white pills per dose
Enpresse	4 orange pills per dose
Jolessa	4 pink pills per dose
Lessina	5 pink pills per dose
Levora	4 white pills per dose
Lo/Ovral	4 white pills per dose
Lutera	5 white pills per dose
Lybrel	6 yellow pills per dose
Nordette	4 light orange pills
Ogestrel	2 white pills
Portia	4 pink pills
Quasense	4 white pills
Seasonale	4 pink pills
Seasonique	4 light blue-green pills
Sronyx	5 white pills
Trivora	4 pink pills

Sources: Adapted from the Emergency Contraception website not-2-late.com; Association of Reproductive Health Professionals. Update on emergency contraception. March 2011. Available at: http://www.arhp.org/uploadDocs/CPECUpdate.pdf. Accessed November 22, 2012.

regimen and 84% for the single-dose regimen.[49] Pregnancy rates are approximately 2% and generally lower than the pregnancy rates following use of the Yuzpe method.[34]

Ulipristal Acetate (ella)

In 2010, UPA, a selective progesterone receptor modulator (SPRM) marketed under the brand name "ella," received FDA approval for use as EC; thus ella is the first—and to date only—SPRM agent available for EC. SPRMs bind to progesterone receptors and inhibit or delay ovulation, depending on when the agent is taken during the menstrual cycle. If used during the midfollicular phase, UPA prevents follicular rupture.[39,41,50,51] When UPA is taken in the late follicular phase, it delays the normal LH surge, thereby delaying ovulation.[42,51]

UPA appears to be more effective than either the Yuzpe method or LNG, and can be effective up to 120 hours after unprotected intercourse, an effect attributed to it's ability to prevent follicular rupture, although its effectiveness does decrease with time.[34,50,52] Pregnancy rates following use of UPA are in the range of 1%. Side effects are the same as those reported for the Yuzpe method and LNG, but occur less frequently. Because most of these side effects are also symptoms of pregnancy, it is not clear exactly which ones occur secondary to administration of the drug. While some evidence indicates that there may be continued benefit in terms of preventing pregnancy even when UPA is given more than 120 hours following intercourse, the data are severely limited on delayed use and no effectiveness rates have been published.[53]

Contraindications to EC

The only contraindication to the use of any method of EC is known pregnancy as defined as implantation. Oral formulations of EC are contraindicated in pregnancy because they are ineffective; the contraindication is not related to concerns about teratogenicity. Because these hormones are given in low doses for a short period of time, women with medical conditions for which oral contraceptives are contraindicated can use EC safely.[34] UPA is new and has not been evaluated in the U.S. MEC.

Although adverse drug–drug interactions have not been reported by women using oral EC, adverse drug interactions are possible. Anticonvulsants such as phenobarbital (Luminal), carbamazepine (Tegretol), and phenytoin (Dilantin) induce the CYP450 system and could decrease effectiveness of the contraceptive. Other drugs that interfere with the metabolism of oral contraceptive agents include rifampin (Rifadin), topiramate (Topamax), and St. John's Wort.[34]

Copper Intrauterine Device

The copper IUD (ParaGard) can be used as EC when inserted within 120 hours (5 days) following intercourse and is the most effective EC method currently available.[34] The IUD is not effective for EC if inserted after the fertilized egg has implanted in the uterus, which normally occurs 6 to 12 days after ovulation.[34] The technique for insertion is described in the appendix to the *Nonhormonal Contraception* chapter titled *Procedure for IUD Insertion.*

Pregnancy rates following insertion of a copper IUD are approximately 0.1%.[54] The copper IUD alters tubal transport, is toxic to ovum, and incapacitates sperm, so that fertilization is prevented.[34] Unlike oral formulations of EC, the copper IUD also creates an inhospitable uterine environment for implantation.[29] If a woman is a candidate for intrauterine contraception, placement of a copper IUD for EC offers the additional advantage of establishing an ongoing contraceptive method. The levonorgestrel-releasing intrauterine system IUD is not effective for EC.

Contraindications to Copper IUD for EC

General contraindications to use of a copper IUD are reviewed in detail in the *Nonhormonal Contraception* chapter. Insertion of a copper IUD for EC after rape is an important topic to review. The U.S. MEC category for insertion of a copper IUD for EC is 3 if the woman has a high risk for being exposed to an STI and it is 1 if she has a low risk for being exposed to an STI. There are no agreed-upon definitions for what constitutes "high-risk" versus "low-risk" for STI. In addition, the U.S. MEC category 3 means that the theoretical risks generally outweigh the advantages. Thus clinician judgment is needed to assess the history and circumstances for each individual who has been raped and is a good candidate for a copper IUD.

Special Considerations for Dispensing EC

Some pharmacies may opt out of dispensing EC methods.[55,56] In such cases, the midwife can prescribe a single package of combined oral contraceptive pills, and instruct the woman about the specific type and number of pills to take, thereby creating a Yuzpe regimen.

Most national women's health organizations recommend that all women who are victims of sexual assault be offered EC.[46] As of 2012, approximately 12 states mandated that emergency departments dispense EC to women post assault upon request.[35] The midwife who may have occasion to care for a woman post assault should discuss whether she has either received appropriate information or been treated with EC.

Midwifery Management Plan

Women using EC may be counseled to return for evaluation 1 to 3 weeks following EC use, specifically to assess the result of EC and discuss ongoing contraceptive needs, although this follow-up visit is not considered a necessary component of EC care by all professional organizations. Whenever possible, a suitable method of contraception should be started immediately after the woman has used an EC method.[36] Women who need EC also should be offered screening for STIs including HIV.

Health Education

Women using EC should be advised that the next menses may be delayed after using oral regimens. It is important to be evaluated for pregnancy if menses does not occur within 3 weeks after EC use. Women should also be counseled regarding signs of ectopic pregnancy and advised to contact a healthcare provider as soon as possible if experiencing severe abdominal pain at any time. In addition, women using EC should avoid unprotected intercourse until a method of contraception has been initiated.

Emerging Trends/Future Contraceptive Methods

There is no "one size fits all" method of contraception. Therefore, the greater the variety of options, the more likely that women will be able to find a method that they can consistently and correctly use in concert with their lifestyles. Development of new contraceptives often takes long periods of time, and sometimes these agents never are introduced to the U.S. market. This section discusses some potential new methods of contraception for women and men. Some of these options are variations of current methods, such as oral contraceptives; others, if FDA approved, could be the first of their kind to reach the market, such as injection of polymer gels in the vas deferens.

Female Methods

Levonorgestrel-Releasing Intrauterine Systems

At the time of this text's writing, a global Phase 3 study including 2884 women was comparing two levonorgestrel-releasing intrauterine systems (IUSs): the LNG-IUS12 and LNG-IUS16. This type of IUD is anticipated to be effective for as long as 3 years. The LNG-IUS12 is a low-dose version of the current Mirena and Skyla intrauterine systems, which are discussed in the *Nonhormonal Contraception* chapter. LNG-IUS12 is currently awaiting FDA approval.[57,58]

Combination Oral Contraceptives

Several new formulations of COCs currently are in development. One new oral COC containing tablets of estradiol valerate alone and tablets with estradiol valerate/dienogest combined (Natazia) was approved by the FDA in 2010 but is not yet in common use.

In several studies, the bleeding profiles of the estradiol valerate/dienogest COC and levonorgestrel- and ethinyl estradiol–containing COCs were compared, and the estradiol valerate and estradiol valerate/dienogest pill was found to be superior.[59,60] Another COC that contains estradiol and nomegestrol acetate is in clinical development and has been available for several years in Europe. An oral contraceptive that combines estrogen, progesterone, and androgen (Pill Plus) in an attempt to support sexual arousal and responsiveness is under consideration. This COC is the first of its type, called an androgen restored contraceptive (ARC). In addition to these drugs, two extended-cycle formulations are in development: an ethinyl estradiol/drospirenone pill and an ethinyl estradiol/levonorgestrel pill.

Patches

To date, only one contraceptive patch has reached the U.S. market, but two new combined contraceptive patches are in development. Twirla contains low-dose ethinyl estradiol and levonorgestrel, whereas Bay86-5016 contains ethinyl estradiol and gestodene. Both patches have been found to suppress follicle growth with a dose that would be less than that of the currently available Evra patch, which contains 6.00 mg norelgestromin (NGMN) and 0.75 mg ethinyl estradiol (EE).[61] A progestin-only patch currently is in Phase 2 trials and could be useful for women in whom estrogen is contraindicated.[62]

Vaginal Ring

Two large Phase 3 clinical trials have evaluated a vaginal ring that released 150 mcg/day of nestorone and 15 mcg/day of ethinyl estradiol. The same ring is used for 21 continuous days, followed by 7 days without use. A new ring is reinserted every month for 12 months. Another vaginal ring that is effective for 3 months contains a natural progesterone, which is released at a rate of 10 mg/day. This product is available in other parts of the world, but clinical trials have not been yet conducted for it in the United States.[63]

Injectable Methods

An injectable contraceptive that contains levonorgestrel butanoate (LNG-B) is in development. In the past, 50 mg of this agent has been found to suppress ovulation for up to 6 months. This injection has been hypothesized to have fewer progestin-related side effects than the depot medroxyprogesterone acetate (DMPA) injection.[62]

A vaccine using human chorionic gonadotropin that stimulates development of antibodies in women and inhibits fertility is being investigated. However, to date the clinical trial difficulties have included issues with unexpected complex production and the need for frequent booster immunizations.[63]

Barrier Methods

A single-sized diaphragm is in development. In addition, new types of female condoms are under development. A new soft, thin, and easy-to-use female condom that can be inserted like a tampon is being tested in Phase 3 clinical trials.[62]

Spermicides

Vaginal gels that have both microbicidal and spermicidal properties are being investigated.[62] The advantage of these products is that they may provide contraceptive action as well as protection against STIs. Those products in development now will be available in both contraceptive and noncontraceptive formulations, to accommodate the varied needs of women. Several different compounds are currently under development.

Permanent Contraception

New nonsurgical female sterilization procedures are under development. For example, quinacrine pellets, which have been used in the past for this purpose, are being reevaluated. These pellets are placed transcervically into the uterine fundus to ultimately produce tubal occlusion. The World Health Organization has stopped recommending this method until its long-term safety can be established.

Polidocanol, a non-ionic surfactant currently used to cosmetically sclerose veins, has been suggested as an infection to cause endothelial disruption.[64] Primate studies using the liquid formulation have not found any effect; the foam formulation is currently under study.[62]

Male Methods

Hormonal Methods

Currently, there are no male hormonal contraceptives on the market for use.[65] However, research focused on exogenously administered sex steroids to suppress pituitary secretion of luteinizing hormone (LH) and follicle-stimulating hormone (FSH) that inhibits spermatogenesis is ongoing. Androgen preparations also are being researched and some appear promising, such as injections, implants, and transdermal gels.[66] A 500 mg monthly testosterone undecanoate injection is being evaluated. In a study in China, the injection showed a failure rate of 6.1%, without any serious adverse events being reported.[67]

Vas Injection

Injectable silicone plugs that block the vas deferens, do not damage the vas, and are considered reversible have been studied as male contraceptive options. The procedure known as reversible inhibition of sperm under guidance (RISUG) involves injecting the vas deferens with a polymer gel that kills sperm. If reversal is desired, the polymer can be flushed out with an injection of dimethyl sulfoxide. RISUG has been in Phase 3 clinical trials in India since 2002, with several delays experienced mid-trial. In 2010, a technology transfer agreement was completed for the use of RISUG in the United States. The plan was to manufacture RISUG in the United States and conduct preclinical safety tests. It is expected that RISUG will begin clinical trials in U.S. men soon.[63]

Barrier Methods

New male condom designs are being evaluated. Spiral-shaped and loose-fitting designs, purportedly for increased friction and sexual pleasure, are being developed. A female condom, proposed to be inserted like a tampon, is currently in Phase 3 clinical trials.[62]

Conclusion

The midwife's role in assessing a woman's needs, preexisting knowledge, and desire in regard to family planning is paramount so that a woman can choose her best options. Such choice is individualized based on a myriad of factors, including age, health, culture, desire, and response should a method fail. Despite the correct use of appropriate contraception, unintended pregnancies will occur, and when they do, the midwife must be prepared to inform and support women through the difficult decision-making process. Counseling women about the options of parenting, adopting out, and pregnancy termination are important functions of the midwife as part of providing reproductive services. It is imperative that personal values do not adversely affect the provision of needed counseling.

● ● ● References

1. Riddle JM. *Contraception and Abortion from the Ancient World to the Renaissance.* Cambridge, MA: Harvard University Press, 1992.

2. Beasley WBR. After office hours, coping with family planning in a rural area. *Obstet Gynecol.* 1973;41: 155-159.

3. Finer LB, Zolna MR. Unintended pregnancy in the United States: incidence and disparities 2006. *Contraception*. 2011;84(5):478-485.

4. Murphy P, Morgan K, Likis FE. Contraception. In Schuiling K, Likis F, eds. *Women's Gynecologic Health*, 2nd ed. Burlington, MA: Jones & Bartlett Learning; 2013:170.

5. Trussell J. Contraceptive failure in the United States. *Contraception*. 2011;83(5):397-404.

6. Trussell J. Understanding contraceptive failure. *Best Pract Res Clin Obstet Gynaecol*. 2009 Apr;23(2):199-209. doi: 10.1016/j.bpobgyn.2008.11.008. Epub February 14, 2009.

7. Pearl R. Factors in human fertility and their statistical evaluation. *Lancet*. 1993;222:607.

8. American College of Nurse-Midwives. *Core Competencies for Basic Midwifery Practice*. Silver Spring MD: ACNM; 2012.

9. Doherty ME, Scannell-Desch E. Women's health and hygiene experiences during deployment to the Iraq and Afghanistan wars, 2003 through 2010. *J Midwifery Women's Health*. 2012;57(2):172-177.

10. Grover SR. Gynaecological issues in adolescents with disability. *J Paediatr Child Health*. 2011 Sep;47(9):610-613.

11. FIGO Committee for Ethical Aspects of Human Reproduction and Women's Health. Ethical issues in the management of severely disabled women with gynecologic problems. *Int J Gynaecol Obstet*. 2011;115(1):86-87. doi: 10.1016/j.ijgo.2011.07.003. Epub August 11, 2011.

12. World Health Organization (WHO). *Medical Eligibility Criteria for Contraceptive Use*. 4th ed. Geneva, Switzerland: WHO; 2009.

13. Centers for Disease Control and Prevention. The U.S. medical eligibility criteria for contraceptive use, 2010. *MMWR*. 2010;59(RR04):1-85.

14. Jacobson JC, Aikins Murphy P. United States medical eligibility criteria for contraceptive use 2010: a review of changes. *J Midwifery Women's Health*. 2011;56(6):598-607. doi: 10.1111/j.1542-2011.2011.

15. Singer J. Options counseling: techniques for caring for women with unintended pregnancies. *J Midwifery Women's Health*. 2004;49(3):235-242.

16. Jones R, Kooistra K. Abortion incidence and access to services in the United States, 2008. *Perspect Sex Reprod Health*. 2011;43(1):41-50.

17. Pazol K, Zane S, Parker W, Hall L, Berg C, Cook D. Abortion Surveillance—United States 2008: Centers for Disease Control and Prevention. *MMWR*. 2011;60(15):1-12. Available at: http://www.cdc.gov/mmwr/pdf/ss/ss6015.pdf. Accessed January 3, 2013.

18. Stubblefield PG, Carr-Ellis S, Borgatta L. Methods for induced abortion. *Obstet Gynecol*. 2004;101(1):174-178.

19. Edelman A, Nichols MD, Jensen J, Comparison of pain and time of procedures with two first-trimester abortion techniques performed by residents and faculty. *Am J Obstet Gynecol*. 2001;184(7):1564-1567.

20. Cleland K, Creinin MD, Nucatola D, Nshom M, Trussell J. Significant adverse events and outcomes after medical abortion. *Obstet Gynecol*. 2013;121(1):166-171.

21. Niinimäki M, Pouta A, Bloigu A, et al. Immediate complications after medical compared with surgical termination of pregnancy. *Obstet Gynecol*. 2009;114(4):795-804.

22. Kapp N, Whyte P, Tang J, Jackson E, Brahmi D. A review of the evidence for safe abortion care. *Contraception*. December 19, 2012. Epub ahead of print. doi: 10.1016/j.contraception.2012.10.027

23. Hatcher R, Trussell J, Nelson A, Cates Jr. W, Kowal D, Policar M, eds. *Contraceptive Technology*. 20th ed. New York, NY: Ardent Media; 2011:705.

24. Bartz D, Goldberg A. Medication abortion. *Clin Obstet Gynecol*. 2009;52(2):140-150.

25. Nguyen T, Blum J, Raghavan S, et al. Comparing two early medical abortion regimens: mifepristone + misoprostol vs. misoprostol alone. *Contraception*. 2011;83:410-417.

26. Nkansah-Amankra S, Luchok KJ, Hussey JR, Watkins K, Liu X. Effects of maternal stress on low birth weight and preterm birth outcomes across neighborhoods of South Carolina, 2000-2003. *Matern Child Health J*. 2010;14(2):215-226.

27. Ngai S, Tang O, Chan Y, Ho P. Vaginal misoprostol alone for medical abortion up to 9 weeks of gestation: efficacy and acceptability. *Hum Reprod*. 2000;15(5):1159-1162.

28. Bos-Thompson MA, Hillaire-Buys D, Roux C, Faillie JL, Amram D. Möbius syndrome in a neonate after mifepristone and misoprostol elective abortion failure. *Ann Pharmacother*. 2008;42(6):888-892. doi: 10.1345/aph.1K550.

29. Murphy PA. Contraception and reproductive health. In King TL, Brucker MC. *Pharmacology for Women's Health*. Sudbury, MA: Jones and Barlett; 2011:909.

30. American College of Obstetricians and Gynecologists (ACOG). *Medical Management of Abortion*. (ACOG Practice Bulletin No. 67). Washington, DC: ACOG; October 12, 2005.

31. Grossman D, Grindlay K. Alternatives to ultrasound for follow-up after medication abortion: a systematic review. *Contraception*. 2011;83(6):504-510.

32. Levi A, James E, Taylor D. Midwives and abortion care: a model for achieving competency. *J Midwifery Women's Health*. 2012;57:285-289.

33. Renner RM, Brahmi D, Kapp N. Who can provide effective and safe termination of pregnancy care? A systematic review. *BJOG*. 2013;120(1):23-31.

34. Murphy P. Update on emergency contraception. *J Midwifery Women's Health.* 2012;57(6):593-602.

35. Raymond E, Stewart F, Weaver M, Monteith C, Van Der Pol B. Impact of increased access to emergency contraceptive pills: a randomized controlled trial. *Obstet Gynecol.* 2006;108(1098):2006.

36. Dalby J, Hayon R, Paddock E, Schrager S. Emergency contraception: an underutilized source. *J Fam Pract.* 2012;61(7):392-397.

37. Trussell J, Ellertson C, von Hertzen H, et al. Estimating the effectiveness of emergency contraceptive pills. *Contraception.* 2003;67(4):259-265.

38. Trussell J, Ellertson C, Dorflinger L. Effectiveness of the Yuzpe regimen of emergency contraception by cycle day of intercourse: implications for mechanism of action. *Contraception.* 2003;67(3):167-171.

39. Gemzell-Danielsson K, Berger C, PGL L. Emergency contraception: mechanisms of action. *Contraception.* 2013;87(3):300-308

40. Novikova N, Wesiberh E, Stanczyk F, Croxatto H, Fraser I. Effectiveness of levonorgestrel emergency contraception given before or after ovulation: a pilot study. *Contraception.* 2007;75(112):2007.

41. Stratton P, Hartog B, Hajizadeh N, et al. A single mid-follicular dose of CDB-2914, a new antiprogestin, inhibits folliculogenesis and endometrial differentiation in normally cycling women. *Hum Reprod.* 2000;15(5):1092-1099.

42. Brache V, Cochon L, Jesam C, et al. Immediate pre-ovulatory administration of 30 mg ulipristal acetate significantly delays follicular rupture. *Hum Reprod.* 2010;25(9):2256-2263.

43. Marions L, Hultenby K, Lindell I, et al. Emergency contraception with mifepristone and levonorgestrel: mechanism of action. *Obstet Gynecol.* 2002;100(65):2002.

44. Von Hertzen H, Piaggio G, Ding J, et al. Low dose mifepristone and two regimens of levonorgestrel for emergency contraception: a WHO multicentre randomized trial. *Lancet.* 2002;360(9438):1803-1810.

45. Association of Reproductive Health Professionals. Update on emergency contraception. March 2011. Available at: http://www.arhp.org/uploadDocs/CPECUpdate.pdf. Accessed November 22, 2012.

46. American College of Obstetricians and Gynecologists (ACOG). ACOG practice bulletin no. 112: emergency contraception. *Obstet Gynecol.* 2010;115:1100-1109.

47. Rodriguez M, Godfrey E, Warden M, Curtis K. Prevention and management of nausea and vomiting with emergency contraception: a systematic review. *Contraception.* October 31, 2012. Epub ahead of print.

48. Fine PM. Update on emergency contraception. *Adv Ther.* 2011 Feb;28(2):87-90.

49. Sambol N, Harper C, Kim L, et al. Pharmacokinetics of single-dose levonorgestrel in adolescents. *Contraception.* 2006;74(104).

50. Glasier A, Cameron S, Fine P, et al. Ulipristal acetate versus levonorgestrel for emergency contraception: a randomised non-inferiority trial and meta-analysis. *Lancet.* 2010;375(9714):555-562.

51. Fine P, Mathe H, Ginde S, et al. Ulipristal acette taken 48-120 hours after intercourse for emergency contraception. *Obstet Gynecol.* 2010;115:257-263.

52. Creinin M, Schlaff W, Archer D, et al. Progesterone receptor modulator for emergency contraception: a randomized controlled trial. *Obstet Gynecol.* 2006; 108:1089-1097.

53. Cheng L, Che Y, Gülmezoglu AM. Interventions for emergency contraception. *Cochrane Database Syst Rev.* 2012;8:CD001324. doi: 10.1002/14651858. CD001324.pub4.

54. Cleland K, Zhu H, Goldstuck N, et al. The efficacy of intrauterine devices for emergency contraception: a systematic review of 35 years of experience. *Hum Reprod.* 2012;27(7):1994-2000.

55. American College of Clinical Pharmacy. Prerogative of a pharmacist to decline to provide professional services based on conscience. August 2005. Available at: http://www.accp.com/docs/positions/positionStatements/pos31_200508.pdf. Accessed October 22, 2012.

56. Wernow JR, Grant DG. Dispensing with conscience: a legal and ethical assessment. *Med Law Ethics.* 2008;42(11):1669-1678.

57. Apter D, Gemzell Danielsson K, Hauck B, Rosen K, Zurth C, Nelson A. Pharmacokinetics (PK) and effect on ovarian and cervical function of two low-dose levonorgestrel-releasing intrauterine systems (LNG-IUSS): results of randomized, Phase II and III studies. *Fertil Steril.* 2012;98(3):S5.

58. Nelson A, Apter D, Hauck B, Rybowski S, Rosen K, Gemzell Danielsson K. A global randomized, Phase III, Pearl index study comparing the efficacy and safety of two low-dose levonorgestrel-releasing intrauterine systems (LNG-IUSS) in nulliparous and parous women. *Fertil Steril.* 2012;98(3):S5.

59. Borgelt L, Martell C. Estradiol valerate/dienogest: a novel combined oral contraceptive. *Clin Ther.* 2012; 34(1):37-55.

60. Ahrendt H, Makalova D, Parke S, Mellinger U, Mansour D. Bleeding pattern and cycle control with an estradiol-based oral contraceptive: A seven-cycle, randomized comparative trial of estradiol valerate/

dienogest and ethinyl estradiol/levonorgestrel. *Contraception.* 2009;80:436-444.

61. Heger-Mahn D, Warlimont C, Faustmann T, Gerlinger C, Klipping C. Combined ethinylestradiol/gestodene contraceptive patch: two center, open-lanel study of ovulation inhibition, acceptability and safety over two cycles in female volunteers. *Eur J Contracept Reprod Health Care.* 2004;9:173-178.

62. Jensen J. The future of contraception: innovations in contraceptive agents: tomorrow's hormonal contraceptive agents and their clinical implications. *Am J Obstet Gynecol.* 2011;205(4):S21-S25.

63. Stevens V. Progress in the development of human chorionic gonadotropin antifertility vaccines. *Am J Reprod Immunol.* 1996;35:148-155.

64. Jensen J, Rodriguez M, Liechtenstein-Zabrak J, Zalanyi S. Transcervical polidocanol as a nonsurgical method of female sterilization: a pilot study. *Contraception.* 2004;70:111-115.

65. Grimes DA, Lopez LM, Gallo MF, Halpern V, Nanda K, Schulz KF. Steroid hormones for contraception in men. *Cochrane Database Syst Rev.* 2012;3:CD004316. doi: 10.1002/14651858.CD004316.pub4.

66. Page S, Amory J, Anawalt B, et al. Testosterone gel combined with depomedroxyprogesterone acetate is an effective male hormonal contraceptive regimen and is not enhanced by the addition of a GnRH antagonist. *J Clin Endocrinol Metab.* 2006;91(11):4374.

67. Li J, Gu Y. Predictors for partial suppression of spermatogenesis of hormonal male contraception. *Asian J Androl.* 2008;10:723-730.

68. Chaudhury K, Bhattacharyya A, Guha S. Studies on the membrane integrity of human sperm treated with a new injectable male contraceptive. *Hum Reprod.* 2004;19(8):1826-1830.

● ● ● **Additional Resources**

Association of Reproductive Health Professionals (AHRP)
Emergency Contraception Update
http://www.arhp.org/uploadDocs/CPECUpdate.pdf

Centers for Disease Control and Prevention (CDC)
U.S. Medical Eligibility for Contraceptive Use
http://www.cdc.gov/mmwr/pdf/rr/rr59e0528.pdf
(US MEC)

Unintended Pregnancy and Updates on U.S. MEC
http://www.cdc.gov/reproductivehealth
/unintendedpregnancy/usmec.htm

Guttmacher Institute
http://www.guttmacher.org

World Health Organization (WHO)
WHO Medical Eligibility for Contraceptive Use
http://www.who.int/reproductivehealth/publications
/family_planning/9789241563888/en/index.html

CHAPTER

17

Nonhormonal Contraception

MICHELLE R. COLLINS

SHARON L. HOLLEY

TONIA L. MOORE-DAVIS

DEBORAH L. NARRIGAN

MARY C. BRUCKER

Introduction

Prior to the scientific breakthroughs that allowed the development of oral contraceptives, contraceptive methods were limited to abstinence, breastfeeding, coitus interruptus, and barrier devices that blocked the sperm's path to the cervix. Today, however, women have an array of both hormonal and nonhormonal contraceptive methods available to them. This chapter reviews all contraceptive methods that do not contain or use hormones. These methods include coitus interruptus, barriers and spermicides, and one intrauterine device (IUD).

The IUD is unique in this group as it is highly effective, is long acting, and requires clinical evaluation and sterile procedure for insertion. In contrast, the remaining nonhormonal methods or "behavioral methods" share several characteristics. They are user controlled, are relatively inexpensive, and have few or relatively minor side effects. Many do not require a prescription (e.g., foam, condoms), and most are used only when coitus is anticipated. Some behavioral methods use no device at all, relying instead on biologic processes such as breastfeeding or observing changes during the menstrual cycle to avoid pregnancy.

Most of the nonhormonal contraceptive methods have no unacceptable health risks—that is, category 4 conditions—based on the U.S. medical eligibility criteria.[1] The IUD, spermicidal agents, and diaphragms (when used with spermicides) are exceptions. Unacceptable health risks, where relevant, are detailed in the section specific to each method in this chapter.

The effectiveness of these methods relies on the user for correct, consistent use. This characteristic can be considered as either an advantage or a disadvantage. If a woman or couple use no contraceptive method, approximately 85 of 100 of them will have an unintended pregnancy in the first year of no contraceptive use.[2] Effectiveness rates for typical use of the nonhormonal methods vary widely, ranging from less than 1 unintended pregnancy per 100 women who use the ParaGard IUD to 28 unintended pregnancies per 100 women who use spermicide only.

Nonhormonal Contraceptive Methods

Abstinence

Although personal definitions of abstinence vary, for the purpose of avoiding pregnancy, abstinence is defined as refraining from penile–vaginal intercourse. If, however, abstinence is defined to include prevention of sexually transmitted infections (STIs), then abstinence includes not engaging in sexual contact that has a risk of STI transmission. For example, anal intercourse with an infected partner confers a higher risk of transmission of human immunodeficiency virus (HIV) than vaginal penetration. Oral intercourse confers a higher risk of transmission of human papillomavirus (HPV) and herpes simplex virus (HSV).

Abstinence is free and available at any time. Complete abstinence is 100% effective and prevents exposure to STIs. Planned abstinence, however, can be unrealistic for some couples and may be difficult to achieve in high-pressure situations.

Coitus Interruptus/Withdrawal Method

With the coitus interruptus (withdrawal) method, the penis is completely removed from the vagina and away from the female external genitalia before ejaculation. In a survey of contraceptive usage of women from 2006 to 2008, approximately 5% of women reported current use of this method, but more than half reported they had used this method at a prior time.[2] In addition, some couples use this method interchangeably or in combination with other methods, such as fertility awareness or condoms.[3] Coitus interruptus is free, requires no contact with healthcare services, has no side effects, and is a contraceptive method that is always available. With typical use, 12 of 100 women will experience an unintended pregnancy within the first year of use.[2]

For coitus interruptus to be effective, the couple must use it at each act of intercourse. Couples with beliefs that prohibit use of other contraceptive methods may use this method. Using coitus interruptus relies to a great extent on both the male partner's awareness of the sensation of imminent ejaculation and his ability to withdraw completely from the vagina consistently in time to avoid semen coming in contact with the vagina. Of note, pre-ejaculate fluid may contain sperm, and could possibly result in pregnancy.[4] Interrupting the sexual response cycle also may diminish pleasure for either or both partners. In addition, women may not be comfortable relinquishing control of contraception to their male partners. Coitus interruptus should be included in a discussion of birth control methods, as rates of its use have been reported as high as 25% to 60% among adolescents.[5] Additionally, coitus interruptus does not protect against STIs, nor does it have any noncontraceptive benefits.

Lactational Amenorrhea Method

The lactational amenorrhea method (LAM) relies on physiologic changes associated with breastfeeding for contraception. Breastfeeding confers a natural method of contraception in the initial postpartum period because the high levels of prolactin that occur during breastfeeding inhibit secretion of gonadotropin-releasing hormone from the hypothalamus, thereby preventing ovulation. LAM requires that the following conditions be met:

- The infant receives all nutrition from suckling, with no more than 5% from food or formula supplementation, and is nursing on demand, with no more than 4 hours between feeds in the daytime and no more than 6 hours between feeds in the night.
- The infant is younger than 6 months of age.
- Maternal menses has not resumed.[6]

The major advantages of LAM include that it is immediately available and free, and its effectiveness rates are as high as 98% to 99.5% during the first 6 months postpartum when the three essential conditions are operational.[2,7] Pumping or manual expression of breast milk may reduce the effectiveness of LAM.[8]

Male Condom

The male condom is a strong, thin, elastic sheath that is unrolled over the erect penis to catch the seminal fluid during ejaculation and prevent it from being deposited in the vagina. Most male condoms available in the United States are made of natural rubber latex. Condoms made of polyurethane, a synthetic material, provide an option for men who are allergic to latex. Five types are currently available. Compared to latex condoms, the polyurethane condoms are odorless and colorless, fit more loosely, have a longer shelf life, and can be used with any lubricant.[9] Latex condoms are effective in preventing transmission of HIV and STIs; however, the effectiveness of nonlatex condoms in protection against HIV and STIs has not been established.[9] Condoms are widely available over the counter and come in a variety of colors, textures, transparencies, sizes, and shapes. Latex condoms are less expensive than polyurethane condoms. Both types can be used either dry or with lubricants.

Male condoms remain the most widely available and commonly used barrier method in the United States. Approximately 16% of women using a contraceptive report that their male partners use condoms, making it a popular method for preventing pregnancy.[2] When used correctly and consistently with each coitus, during the first year of use among typical users, approximately 12% will have an unintended pregnancy.[2] Most condom failures result from breakage or slippage during intercourse or while removing the condom. In a meta-analysis of 11 randomized trials that compared latex and synthetic condoms, failure rates were comparable for all latex and synthetic condoms, although synthetic condoms had higher reported rates of breakage and slippage.[9] The one exception was the eZ-on polyurethane condom, which was less likely to prevent pregnancy and had a higher rate of breakage and slippage (7%) when compared to latex condoms (2%).

Condoms can cause vaginal irritation or discomfort, with synthetic condoms reported to cause less vaginal irritation and discomfort than the latex versions.[10] Latex condoms should not be used by a couple when either partner has an allergy to latex. Disadvantages include perceived reduced sensitivity and lack of spontaneity, especially during foreplay, when the condom should be worn. Some men have difficulty maintaining erections while the condom is on, and some individuals may be embarrassed to use a condom or ask that one be used. Lastly, male condoms are male controlled. Women in relationships where they cannot negotiate condom use by their partner may be exposed to risks of unwanted pregnancy.

Condoms can be used as an adjunct to other contraceptives. For example, if a woman using combined oral contraceptives (COCs) misses one or more pills, using a condom for the duration of the pill cycle usually is advisable. Dual use of condoms with a second contraceptive for STI risk reduction should also be advocated for women with multiple partners, women with new partners, and for women seeking added protection against unintended pregnancy.[11]

Reviewing correct use is best done by demonstration, using a penile model or simple substitute such as a banana. Several excellent teaching videos are available on the Internet that offer straightforward, step-by-step instructions. In the event of condom breakage or slippage, emergency contraception is available as an option, as described in the *Family Planning* chapter.

Female Condom

The female condom is a soft, loosely fitting, thin sheath of synthetic latex (**Figure 17-1**). It has two flexible rings—one on the closed end of the sheath that is inserted into the vagina, and a larger ring on the open end that remains outside the vagina and covers the introitus. The female condom is available in only one size and does not need to be fitted by a healthcare professional. Although the product is prelubricated with a silicone-based, nonspermicidal agent, additional lubricants or spermicidal preparations may be used with it. Only one company manufactures this device, and each condom is intended for one-time use.

The effectiveness of the female condom is slightly less than that of male condoms, with 79% of users in the first year of typical use avoiding unintended pregnancy, while the male condom effectiveness rate is 82%.[2] There is a large discrepancy in failure rates between perfect use and typical use, perhaps reflecting problems mastering insertion as well as inconsistent

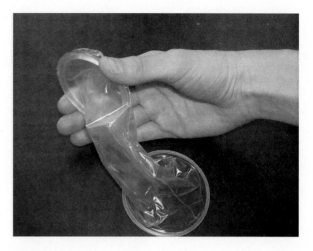

Figure 17-1 Female condom.
Source: Reprinted with permission from The Cervical Barrier Advancement Society and Ibis Reproductive Health.

use.[12] The female condom protects as effectively as male condoms against STIs and HIV transmission when used correctly, in part because the external portion provides a barrier between the labia and the base of the penis during intercourse.[2,13]

The female condom can be inserted as long as 8 hours before sexual intercourse, but must be in place before the penis enters vagina. Some men prefer the freedom of movement and looseness of the female condom compared to the male condom. Some women have reported that the edge of the outer ring provides clitoral stimulation. Both partners may experience uncomfortable sensations, including feeling the inner ring, having the condom adhere to the penis, and feeling the outer ring press against the vulva during intercourse. Checking for correct placement and adding more lubricant may alleviate these problems. Learning the correct steps for insertion may be challenging, but can be achieved with close instruction. Most women need to practice two to three times to successfully place the condom.[12] Several excellent short videos, available on the Internet, offer clear instruction.

Spermicidal Agents

Spermicides are chemical agents that kill sperm. Spermicidal agents are formulated as gels, creams, aerosol foam, suppositories, vaginal film, and sponges (**Figure 17-2**). The active agent in all spermicidal preparations available in the United States is nonoxynol-9, a surfactant that destroys the sperm cell membrane. This agent is combined with an inert base that creates the specific formulation such as cream or gel. The inert base material serves as a mechanical

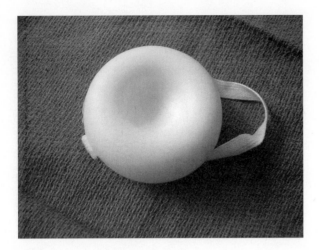

Figure 17-2 Today sponge.
Source: Courtesy of Tekoa King

barrier to the cervical os and facilitates vaginal distribution and formation of a surface film that withstands coital activity. The active spermicide in all formulations is nonoxynol-9, which is present in dose ranges from 52 mg to 150 mg, depending on the actual product used. Effectiveness of this contraceptive method is directly related to the nonoxynol-9 dose: Products with at least 100 mg of nonoxynol-9 are more effective than preparations with lower doses.[14] **Table 17-1** provides detailed information on spermicidal products. Spermicidal preparations are relatively easy to use, are "woman controlled," and are immediately effective. They are available in drug stores and online without prescription.

For this contraceptive method to be effective, women must be motivated to use spermicides consistently with each intercourse. Also, for some preparations, as noted in Table 17-1, timing of initiating use is critical to effectiveness. For example, the contraceptive film and suppositories need 10 to 15 minutes in the vagina to become effective prior to being exposed to sperm. The film and sponge may not be good choices for women who object to inserting a finger into the vagina. Some postcoital leakage is common to all of the spermicidal preparations except film.

The most important disadvantage of spermicidal preparations is the low effectiveness rate for typical use. Spermicides used alone are among the least effective contraceptive methods. For typical users during the first year of use, approximately 28% will have an unintended pregnancy—a rate similar to those for the fertility awareness and withdrawal methods.[2] The one exception is the sponge, for which effectiveness rates differ according to women's parity: The rates of unintended pregnancy in the first year of use are 12% and 24% for nulliparous and multiparous women, respectively. Even given this limited effectiveness, using this contraceptive method is much more effective than using no method.

Side effects and adverse effects of nonoxynol-9 include a contact dermatitis local irritation of the vulva, vagina, or penis, which is sometimes referred to as an allergic reaction. Nonoxynol-9 is a surfactant with the potential to damage the vaginal epithelium, increasing risks of infection. If women at low risk for STIs report vaginal irritation or inflammation,

Table 17-1	Spermicidal Preparations			
Preparation	Nonoxynol-9 (mg/dose)	Timing of Application	Duration of Action	Comments
Gels, creams	52–100	Up to 1 hour before coitus		Use alone or with diaphragm
Foam	100	Insert immediately before coitus	1 hour	Aerosol, under pressure in container; apply with applicator
Suppository	100–125	Insert 10–15 min prior to coitus	1 hour	Activated when melted; spermicide is embedded in cocoa butter or glycerin
Sponge	100	Any time up to 24 hours before coitus	Leave in place for 6 hours after coitus but not longer than 30 hours	Polyurethane "pillow"; moistening prior to use activates nonoxynol-9; remove 6 hours after coitus; do not leave in place > 30 hours total to avoid rare risk of toxic shock syndrome

decreasing frequency of use or changing to a formulation with less nonoxynol-9 should be considered.

Spermicides are contraindicated (U.S. Medical Eligibility Criteria [MEC] category 4) for women at high risk for exposure to HIV.[15] The risk of microabrasions to vaginal epithelium increases with use more than twice a day, and thereby increases the risk of HIV infection.[15] In addition, women who are HIV positive or who have AIDS should not use spermicides because the microabrasions caused by the spermicide also increase viral shedding and thereby increase the risk of HIV transmission to an uninfected partner (U.S. MEC category 3).

A rare but serious side effect of sponge use is toxic shock syndrome (TSS). TSS is an immunologic-mediated, potentially fatal, septic reaction to bacterial toxins of the species *Staphylococcus aureus* and/or *Streptococcus pyogenes*.[16] When the contraceptive sponge was introduced in the mid-1980s, a few cases of TSS occurred. All were associated with either recent childbirth, leaving the device in place for more than 24 hours, difficult removal, or fragmentation of the sponge.[17] TSS associated with sponge or diaphragm use is extremely rare.[18] TSS usually presents as 2 to 3 days of mild symptoms, such as low-grade fever, muscle aches, chills, and malaise. The symptoms worsen rapidly, and include fever higher than 38°C (101.4°F), with diffuse macular erythema and hypotension. Women using any barrier method should be educated about the symptoms of TSS, and can avoid this rare disorder by removing the device within 24 hours of its insertion.

Diaphragm

The diaphragm is a dome-shaped silicone or latex cup with a flexible rim to permit compression of the device for insertion while allowing the diaphragm to regain its shape and fit snugly against the vaginal walls (**Figure 17-3**). When properly positioned, the diaphragm rim rests against the anterior and lateral vaginal walls, and extends posteriorly to completely cover the cervix. A diaphragm is used with a spermicidal gel or cream that is spread around the rim and inside the dome of the diaphragm for maximum effectiveness. The diaphragm therefore provides both a physical and chemical barrier to sperm.[19] Diaphragms come in three types based on the presence or absence of a spring in the rim and each type has several sizes. Diaphragms require a prescription. Advantages of diaphragm use include that this method is controlled by the woman herself and is effective. It is not necessarily coital dependent, and insertion and removal can be done privately.

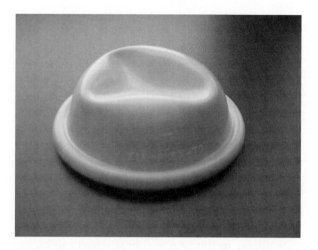

Figure 17-3 All-Flex diaphragm.
Source: Reprinted with permission from The Cervical Barrier Advancement Society and Ibis Reproductive Health.

While the diaphragm has been available in the United States since the 1930s, few women today choose this contraceptive method. Approximately 12% of typical users will have an unintended pregnancy in the first year of use, making the diaphragm more effective than male condoms and all other female barrier methods.[2] Effectiveness appears to be inversely related to frequency of intercourse. Studies have shown that among consistent diaphragm users, those who have intercourse at least three times weekly are almost three times as likely to have an unintended pregnancy.[20] Male condoms can be used at the same time a woman uses a diaphragm, enhancing contraceptive effectiveness and adding protection against STI transmission.

The size of the diaphragm must be determined for each individual because the distance from the posterior fornix to the posterior aspect of the symphysis pubis varies among women. The appendix to this chapter titled *Fitting Diaphragms* describes the procedure for determining the right size diaphragm for a woman. After the proper size is determined, the woman should demonstrate the ability to insert and remove the device. The midwife will complete the visit by reinforcing the points of routine and safe use and care for the diaphragm. The diaphragm can be inserted up to 6 hours at most before intercourse and should remain in the vagina at least 6 hours after intercourse (so that the spermicide remains effective), but no more than 24 hours.

Side effects of diaphragm use include an increased risk for urinary tract infections as compared to other contraceptive methods, perhaps due to pressure on the urethra exerted by the diaphragm's rim, causing incomplete bladder emptying, or from the spermicide altering the vaginal flora that may increase *Escherichia coli* bacteriuria.[21] If the woman experiences recurrent urinary tract infections, the diaphragm may be too large or the rim too rigid, and refitting is indicated. If refitting does not help, the woman can be counseled to select another contraceptive method.

Local irritation from the spermicidal agent used may occur. If the diaphragm was improperly fitted or is left in place longer than 24 hours after having intercourse, vaginal wall abrasions can occur. If recurrent vaginal or vulvar irritation occurs without evidence of an infection, these symptoms may indicate allergy to the latex diaphragm itself; in such a case, the woman should be advised to discontinue use. In addition, the risk of toxic shock syndrome may increase if the diaphragm is left in place for more than 24 hours.

Contraindications for use of a diaphragm are the same as those for use of spermicide and are related to the spermicide component of this contraceptive method. Diaphragms are U.S. MEC category 3 for women with a history of TSS because TSS has been associated with use of a diaphragm. Latex diaphragms should not be prescribed for women who have an allergy to latex and occasionally a diaphragm cannot be fitted for a woman who had an anatomic abnormality such as pelvic organ prolapse. Diaphragms may increase the risk for urinary tract infection and therefore the benefit needs to outweigh the risk for women who have a history of frequent urinary tract infections.[22]

The diaphragm should be refitted if the woman experiences weight change of more than 15 pounds, or has had a second trimester abortion or vaginal birth within 6 weeks. The diaphragm should not be used after birth until uterine involution is complete. All women using a diaphragm should be instructed about the symptoms of toxic shock syndrome.

Cervical Cap

The cervical cap is a dome-shaped silicone cap that resembles a sailor's hat (**Figure 17-4**). The concave dome fits snugly over the cervix and is held in place by the muscular walls of the vagina. The brim is slightly wider on the side that fits into the posterior fornix. The cap has a strap that stretches over the diameter of the dome, which facilitates removal. Spermicide should be applied inside the dome, around the brim, and in the groove between the dome and the brim.[23]

The only cervical cap currently available in the United States is marketed with the brand name

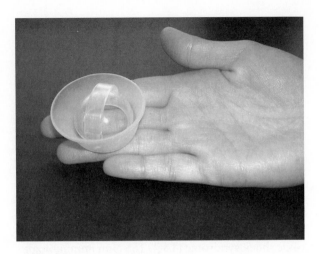

Figure 17-4 Cervical cap (FemCap).
Source: Reprinted with permission from The Cervical Barrier Advancement Society and Ibis Reproductive Health.

FemCap. It was approved by the Food and Drug Administration (FDA) in 2003, and is available in three sizes, with size determined by obstetric history: 22 mm if nulligravida, 26 mm if ever pregnant (nullipara), and 30 mm if the woman has had a full-term vaginal birth. A prescription is needed, and the device is available only at selected pharmacies in California, at all Planned Parenthood affiliates nationwide, or by ordering it directly from the manufacturer. The advantage of the cervical cap is that it is immediately available, is effective, and can be inserted up to 42 hours before intercourse, thereby avoiding interruption of foreplay; it should be left in place for 6 hours after intercourse.[23,24]

In a clinical trial reported to the FDA prior to approval of the originally designed cap, the 6-month effectiveness rate was 77% overall, but 86% for nulliparous women. That first-generation device was not approved by the FDA. The current FDA-approved FemCap is a different design, and limited data about its effectiveness are available. The first-generation FemCap was compared to the diaphragm in one randomized clinical trial and found not to be as effective as the diaphragm.[25,26]

Contraindications to use of a cervical cap are the same as the contraindications to use of spermicides and diaphragms with a few additions. Women who have cervical cancer, cervical intraepithelial neoplasia, and those with an marked abnormally shaped cervix should be advised to use another form of contraception.[23]

Using the cervical cap during menstruation may increase the risk of toxic shock syndrome and, therefore, should be avoided.[24] The cap does not protect against STI transmission, so using a male condom in combination with the cap adds this protection. While a pelvic examination is not needed to select the correct size, a clinician should insert and remove the device to illustrate proper technique for the woman, and then have the woman perform a return demonstration. Urinary tract infections occur less often than with the diaphragm, and vaginitis at rates similar to diaphragm users.[23] The cap should be replaced after each year of use.[26] The size should not need to be changed unless the woman was nulligravid and has had an abortion or given birth vaginally.[23]

Fertility Awareness–Based Methods

Fertility awareness–based methods of contraception are sometimes referred to as "natural family planning." Both of these approaches are based on identifying the fertile days in the menstrual cycle when an ovum can be fertilized, and then abstaining from intercourse during that interval. Natural family planning, however, refers specifically to practices approved by the Roman Catholic Church.

Currently, five fertility awareness–based methods are in use. **Table 17-2** summarizes the techniques for use for each method.[27–29] Fewer than 1% of women[2] in the United States who use contraception employ these methods. Reasons that may account for the limited use of these strategies include the complexity of the methods, the need for both providers and women to obtain education, and providers' personal views that these methods are not effective.[30]

Abstaining from intercourse at specified times during each menstrual cycle is the basic mechanism of action in each of these methods. All fertility awareness–based methods require abstinence or use of a second contraceptive method when the chance of pregnancy is the greatest. Fertility awareness–based methods are based on three regularly occurring biologic events during the menstrual cycle: (1) ovulation occurs once, about 14 days before menses begins; (2) the lifespan of the ovum is at most 12 to 24 hours[31]; and (3) sperm are viable after ejaculation for approximately 3 to 5 days. The most likely time for pregnancy to occur is during the fertile window, which spans from approximately 5 days prior to ovulation until the day after ovulation, for a total of 6 days each month.[32]

Overall, fertility awareness–based methods are among the least effective type of contraceptive for typical use. Approximately 24 in 100 women who use these contraceptive methods will have an unintended pregnancy in the first year of use.[33] Reliable effectiveness data for many of these methods is hampered by a lack of randomized controlled trials comparing the fertility awareness–based methods to each other or to other methods. The studies that are available have yielded inconclusive results due to protocol violations and high rates of participant dropout.[34]

Fertility awareness–based methods are low-cost, user-controlled contraceptive methods. To use any of these methods, two behaviors are requisite: (1) being willing and able to abstain from coitus for several days a month, and (2) being willing to learn and then use techniques to observe signs of biologic change during the menstrual cycle consistently, month after month. In addition, these methods rely heavily on both partners' participation. Moreover, fertility awareness–based methods do not protect against transmission of STIs.

Relative contraindications to fertility awareness–based methods include conditions that result in irregular menstrual cycles, including recent childbirth, onset of menarche, perimenopause, breastfeeding, frequent anovulatory cycles, and recent discontinuation of hormonal contraceptives. Women with the following conditions also may have difficulty using fertility awareness–based methods: persistent vaginitis or other infections that may disrupt signs of fertility; not being comfortable examining vaginal secretions (for some methods); intermenstrual bleeding; and inability to correctly interpret the signs of fertility.

Calendar Methods

Two calendar fertility awareness–based methods are available. The "rhythm" method, also known as the calendar method, is the oldest fertility awareness–based methods method, and was developed in the 1930s. A new calendar method, the StandardDays method, has recently been developed.

Rhythm Method

The rhythm method attempts to predict the days in a menstrual cycle during which a woman is most likely to become pregnant based on the projected time of ovulation. This interval is determined by calculations made from recording the length of the last 8 to 12 menstrual cycles. To use this method, a woman keeps a record of her menstrual cycles to identify the longest and shortest cycles so that all possible fertile days may be projected. The couple then abstains from sexual intercourse during the calculated fertile period. Although extremely popular many years ago, the rhythm method is the least used of the fertility awareness–based methods available today.

Table 17-2	Techniques for Fertility Awareness–Based Methods				
Method	Signs or Symptoms Used by Method	Observations	Days to Avoid Unprotected Intercourse	Efficacy, First Year of Typical Use[a]	Unintended Pregnancy in First Year of Use with Perfect Use
StandardDays method	Day of cycle	Track cycle days beginning with first day of menses Note days 8–19 of cycle	Days 8–19 of cycle Total: 12 days per cycle	88%	5
Calendar method	Day of cycle	Record cycle lengths for 6–12 cycles Identify shortest and longest cycles Shortest number of cycle days minus 18 = beginning of fertile window Longest number of cycle days minus 11 = end of fertile window	Days identified as fertile by calculations (repeat calculations every cycle) Total: Depends on cycle length variability	87%[b]	3–5
TwoDay method	Cervical secretions	Note presence or absence of cervical secretion Record on chart	All days with secretions One day following days with secretions Total: Approximately 10–14 days each cycle	86%	4
Ovulation method	Cervical secretions	Monitor cervical secretions daily Assess quality and quantity of secretions Record observations on chart	Menses Preovulatory days following days with intercourse All days with fertile-type secretions Until 4 days past "peak" day Total: Approximately 14–17 days each cycle	80%	3–5
Symptothermal method	Cervical secretions Vaginal mucus BBT	Monitor cervical secretions daily Assess quantity and quality of secretions Take BBT daily Record observations on chart	Menses Preovulatory days following days with intercourse All days with fertile-type secretions Until 3 days of higher temperatures, or 4 days past peak Total: Approximately 14–17 days each cycle	80%	2–5

BBT = basal body temperature.

[a]Number of pregnancies per 100 women per year of use with perfect use.

Sources: Data from *Family Planning: A Global Handbook for Providers.* WHO Press; 2011. Available at: http://whqlibdoc.who.int/publications /2011/9780978856373_eng.pdf. Accessed February 14, 2013; Kambric R, Lamprecht V. Calendar rhythm efficacy: a review. *Adv Contracept.* 1996;12:123-128; Arevalo M. Expanding the availability of and improving delivery of natural family planning services and fertility awareness education providers' perspectives. *Adv Contracept.* 1997;13:275-281.

StandardDays Method

This relatively new method is also based entirely on tracking the days of the menstrual cycle. Women using this method must have regular cycles that range from 26 to 32 days.[35] The user notes the first day of menstruation and abstains from intercourse between days 8 and 19 of each menstrual cycle.[36] The use of a simple device, known as CycleBeads, helps in tracking the days of the cycle. CycleBeads consists of a circle of beads in several colors that a woman uses to determine whether she should be considered fertile or infertile on a particular day (**Figure 17-5**).[37]

Ovulation Methods

The three ovulation methods focus on identifying the days of fertility and infertility in every cycle that occur because of changes in hormonal blood levels. These include changes in amount and characteristics of cervical mucus and vulvar wetness, basal body temperature (BBT), and the position and consistency of the cervix (**Figure 17-6**).[38,39]

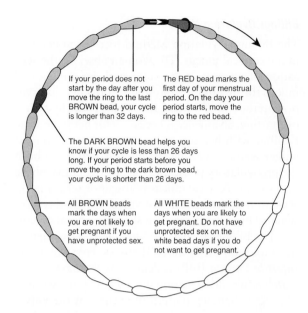

If your period does not start by the day after you move the ring to the last BROWN bead, your cycle is longer than 32 days.

The RED bead marks the first day of your menstrual period. On the day your period starts, move the ring to the red bead.

The DARK BROWN bead helps you know if your cycle is less than 26 days long. If your period starts before you move the ring to the dark brown bead, your cycle is shorter than 26 days.

All BROWN beads mark the days when you are not likely to get pregnant if you have unprotected sex.

All WHITE beads mark the days when you are likely to get pregnant. Do not have unprotected sex on the white bead days if you do not want to get pregnant.

Figure 17-5 How to use CycleBeads.
Source: Reprinted with permission of Institute for Reproductive Health, Georgetown University.

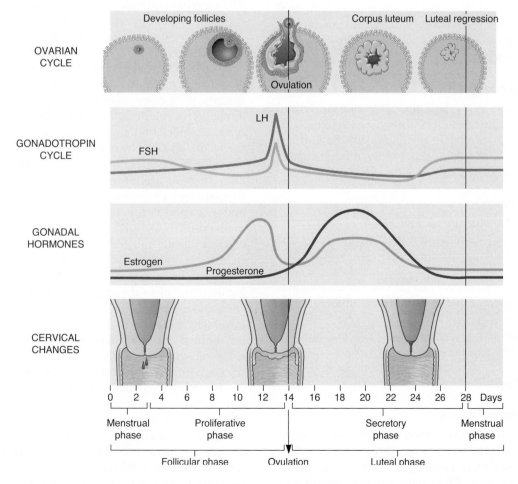

Figure 17-6 Hormonal, follicular, temperature, secretions, and cervical changes during the menstrual cycle.

Billings Ovulation Method

The Billings Ovulation Method focuses on changes in the cervical mucus. The woman observes the sensation of wetness at the vulva and the presence of mucus throughout the day and records her observations at the end of the day. During the entire first cycle of charting, abstinence is necessary for her to become familiar with her cervical mucus and sensations of vulvar wetness. During the *infertile pattern* in both the preovulatory phase and the postovulatory phase of the cycle, cervical mucus is absent or results in no sensation of wetness at the vulva. Fertile days are signaled by vulvar wetness or slippery cervical mucus.

The Billings Ovulation Method uses two definitions for monitoring cervical mucus. First, the *Basic Infertile Pattern* (BIP) is defined as the days immediately after menstruation during which the woman has an unchanging pattern of dryness at the vulva. Second, *Peak* is defined as the change in vulvar sensation from wet to slippery. Under the influence of estrogen, the mucus increases in volume and becomes clear and stretchy, with an egg-white consistency (spinnbarkeit). The last day this slippery sensation occurs is called the *Peak Day*. Intercourse is avoided during all days with fertile pattern secretions and for 4 days after the Peak Day for a total of 14 to 17 abstinent days in a cycle.

Creighton Model FertilityCare System

A modification of the Billings Ovulation Method is the Creighton Model FertilityCare System. This model uses the same principles as the Billings Ovulation Method, but has a standardized teaching plan and a code system for charting.

TwoDay Method

The TwoDay method simplifies observation of cervical mucus.[40] It does not require distinguishing the quality of the mucus. Instead, a woman using this method asks herself two specific questions: (1) Did I note secretions today? and (2) Did I note secretions yesterday? She should abstain from intercourse if the answer to either of these questions is "yes." The usual number of days in a cycle requiring abstinence is 10 to 14. Women with irregular cycles can use this method because it relies entirely on observing one physical sign of fertility.

Symptothermal Method

The symptothermal method combines three observations: basal body temperature, cervical mucus observation, and changes in the cervix itself (**Figure 17-7**). The rise in BBT occurs as more progesterone is released by the corpus luteum, signaling that ovulation has occurred. A BBT shift is defined as ovulatory when the BBT rises at least 0.4°F above the previous six daily BBT measurements.

Several patterns of ovulatory temperature rise occur. These include an abrupt rise over 1 to 2 days or a slow rise over several days, consisting of either a staircase pattern with slight temperature increases (0.2°F) every 2 to 3 days, or a saw-tooth pattern (e.g., increase of 0.4°F, decrease of 0.2°F, increase of 0.4°F, and so on). Occasionally a sharp dip in temperature precedes the rise in BBT occurring with ovulation. The pattern of the rise in temperature may vary both from woman to woman and from cycle to cycle for the same woman.

The fertile days begin with the sharp temperature rise and continue either until there has been a sustained elevation or a plateau of the temperature for 3 days, or until there have been 5 days of progressive increase (e.g., the saw-tooth, staircase, or slow rise pattern). The infertile days are marked by a decline in BBT and continue until the next menstruation.

Observing cervical mucus changes augments the BBT pattern to help identify fertile and infertile days. As with the Billings Ovulation Method, this method also includes observing changes in the fertile days when the cervical mucus has an egg-white consistency and can be stretched between the fingers.

In addition to BBT and cervical mucus observation, the third component of this method is changes in the cervix itself that can be felt by palpating the cervix. As ovulation approaches, the cervix softens, the os dilates slightly, and the cervix is positioned higher in the vaginal canal. After ovulation, the cervix returns to being firm, closed, and lower in the vaginal canal. Detection of the cervical position is an optional sign. A woman using this method records observation of the three parts of the method—BBT, cervical mucus, and cervical characteristics—using specifically designed tracking charts.

All of the fertility awareness–based methods are highly personal to the couple's motivation and desires; consequently, it is difficult to recommend one method over the others. The symptothermal method has the highest efficacy in perfect-use studies, but the true typical-use effectiveness of the various methods has not been determined through large rigorous studies. Emerging technology may be used in combination with these methods, thereby increasing their effectiveness. For example, Internet hormonal urine monitoring and electronic hormonal fertility monitors are becoming available and have been tested in research studies.[41] All require intensive education, so it may be best to refer couples to counselors who

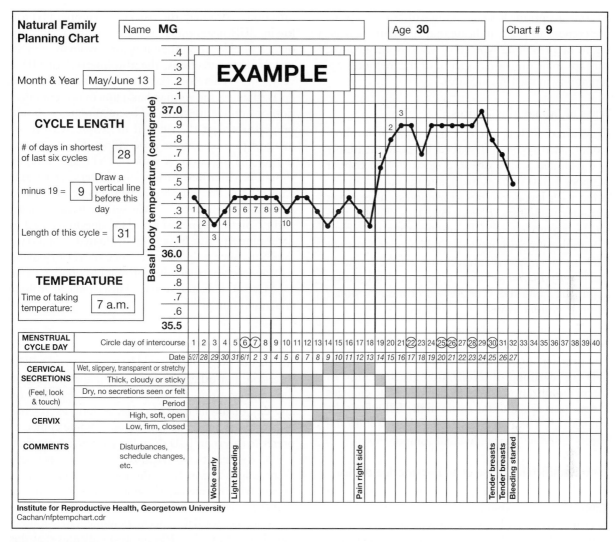

Figure 17-7 Symptothermal method.
Source: Reprinted by permission of Institute for Reproductive Health, Georgetown University.

specialize in these methods. Additional resources for fertility awareness–based methods are listed at the end of this chapter.

The Intrauterine Device

Several synonyms are used interchangeably to describe intrauterine devices, including intrauterine contraceptives (IUCs, IUCDs) and intrauterine systems (IUSs). By standard convention, the term IUD is used in this chapter. IUDs and contraceptive implants are the two types of long-acting reversible contraceptive devices (LARC) available in the United States. Pregnancy rates are lower and continuation rates are higher for women who use LARCs versus women who use oral contraceptives.

IUDs are the most commonly used reversible contraceptive in the world. In the United States, however, they are used by only 7.7% of women in the United States who use some form of contraception. Multiple factors have contributed to the lower prevalence of IUD use in the United States, including a lack of widespread marketing, especially compared to oral contraceptives; common misconceptions about IUDs' mechanism of action; misinformation about associated risks; and a history of negative publicity. Rates of IUD use reached as high as 10% in the United States during the 1970s,[28] but use decreased significantly following highly publicized pelvic inflammatory disease (PID) episodes linked to the Dalkon Shield before this device's eventual removal from the market. Thus the current generation of reproductive-age women has been underexposed to IUDs as a method of contraception. Recent surveys of contraceptive preference, however, indicate that IUDs are increasing in favor among women of various age groups, perhaps indicating a resurgence of the method's acceptability in the United States.[42]

Types of Intrauterine Devices

IUDs are classified as either hormonal or nonhormonal. Two types of T-shaped IUDs are available in the United States: one impregnated with copper (Copper T 380A [ParaGard]), and the other impregnated with levonorgestrel (levonorgestrel-releasing intrauterine system [LNG-IUS]). This chapter presents an overview of IUDs and information about the nonhormonal copper IUD. Use of the copper IUD for emergency contraception can be found in the *Family Planning* chapter. Specific information about the LNG-IUS is addressed in the *Hormonal Contraception* chapter.

Mechanism of Action of Intrauterine Devices

The primary mechanism of action of both types of IUD is prevention of fertilization via inhibition of sperm mobilization and sperm viability and changes in transport speed of the ovum in the fallopian tube transport.[21] The two types of IUD have additional effects based on their individual components.

Contraindications to Use of an Intrauterine Device

The medical contraindications to IUD use are listed in **Table 17-3**.[1] Any abnormal uterine bleeding should be evaluated for pathologic causes prior to IUD insertion. An IUD should not be used if the woman has a known hypersensitivity to any device component. The copper IUD is contraindicated for women with Wilson's disease because Wilson's disease causes an impairment of copper metabolism.

Midwifery Management

The procedure for inserting an IUD is in the appendix to this chapter titled *Procedure for IUD Insertion*.

Pre-insertion Screening for Sexually Transmitted Infections

Routine pre-insertion STI screening is not recommended for women are at low risk for acquiring an STI.[48] IUD insertion in women who are at high risk for STIs requires additional information and clinician judgment. The U.S. MEC category for women who are at high risk for gonorrhea or chlamydia is Category 2/3 and the text states that the MEC category 3 applies only to women who have a very high individual risk of exposure to one of these two infections. Although the risk of developing PID following IUD insertion is higher if a woman has gonorrhea or chlamydia than it is for a woman without one of these infections, the absolute risk of PID is very low.[42] Therefore IUD insertion should not be delayed unless the woman has a mucopurulent infection or known infection. STI screening tests should be performed at the time of insertion, with treatment of positive results proceeding after confirmation of the infection. A woman's STI risk category should be determined using the Centers for Disease Control and Prevention (CDC) risk assessment and screening parameters.[43,44] The sensitivity, specificity, and predictive values of standard questions used to determine STI risk have been evaluated.[44] Standard questions such as positive history of STI or having two or more partners do not reliably predict a risk for STI; thus screening and IUD insertion can be done concomitantly.[44]

Timing of IUD Placement

Absence of pregnancy should be verified prior to IUD insertion, but otherwise there are few pre-insertion recommendations. IUD insertion can take place on any day of the menstrual cycle, as long as absence of pregnancy has been confirmed.[45] Some clinicians prefer to insert an IUD during a woman's menstrual period because the cervical os is slightly open and there is lubrication from the menses. Additionally, insertion during menses provides further reassurance that the woman is not pregnant.

Evidence for IUD placement immediately following birth (i.e., within 10 minutes) indicates that this procedure is both safe and feasible.[46,47] Nevertheless, immediate postpartum insertion is not performed widely in the United States. Because uterine involution occurs in the postpartum period, there is also a higher rate of expulsion of an IUD following immediate postpartum insertion. The insertion procedure when performed immediately postpartum is the same as that when performed in a woman with a nonpregnant uterus, but the midwife should use caution because the uterine isthmus is much softer and more prone to perforation at this time.[46] Some evidence supports IUD placement following spontaneous or elective abortion. Both immediate and interval insertion at 4 to 8 weeks post abortion have been studied and shown to be safe.[48,49]

Premedication Prior to Insertion

Before IUD insertion, some clinicians offer the woman premedication for pain or anxiety. Such medication may include a nonsteroidal anti-inflammatory

Table 17-3	Contraindications for Use of an Intrauterine Device: United States Medical Eligibility Criteria Categories 3 or 4[a]
Contraindications	**Medical Eligibility Criteria**
Contraindications for Any IUD	
Cervical cancer awaiting treatment	4 for initiation and 2 for continuation
Distorted uterine cavity	4
Endometrial cancer	4 for initiation and 2 for continuation
Gestational trophoblastic disease with decreasing or undetectable beta-hCG levels	3
Gestational trophoblastic disease with persistently elevated beta-hCG levels or malignant disease	4
Immediately post septic abortion	4
Pelvic inflammatory disease (PID)	4
Pelvic tuberculosis	4 for initiation and 3 for continuation
Pregnancy	4
Puerperal sepsis	4
Sexually transmitted infections	
Chlamydia	4 for initiation and 2 for continuation
Gonorrhea	4 for initiation and 2 for continuation
Purulent cervicitis	4 for initiation and 2 for continuation
Increased risk for STI	2 or 3; if a woman has a very high risk of chlamydia or gonorrhea, the category is 3
Solid organ transplant	3 for initiation and 2 for continuation
Unexplained vaginal bleeding that is suspicious for a serious condition	4
Contraindications for Use of Copper IUD	
Allergy to copper	Listed in product label
Use for EC in case of rape	High risk for STI is category 3 and low risk for STI is category 1
Systemic lupus erythematosus with severe thrombocytopenia	3 for initiation and 2 for continuation
Wilson's disease	Listed in product label
Contraindications for Use of LNG-IUD	
Current breast cancer	4
Breast cancer history with no evidence of current disease for 5 years	3
Current and history of ischemic heart disease	2 for initiation and 3 for continuation of IUD
Theoretic risk related to effect of LNG on lipids	
Liver disease: severe cirrhosis, hepatocellular adenoma, malignant hematoma	3
Systemic lupus erythematosus with positive antiphospholipid antibodies	3

[a]U.S. MEC Categories:

   Category 1: a condition for which there is no restriction
   Category 2: a condition for which the advantages of using the method generally outweigh the theoretical or proven risks
   Category 3: a condition for which the theoretical or proven risks usually outweigh the advantages of using the method
   Category 4: a condition that represents an unacceptable health risk if the contraceptive method is used

Source: Centers for Disease Control and Prevention. U.S. medical eligibility criteria for contraceptive use. *MMWR.* 2010;59(RR04):1–6. Available at: http://www.cdc.gov/mmwr/preview/mmwrhtml/rr5904a1.htm?s_cid=rr5904a1_e. Accessed February 14, 2013.

drug (NSAID) or an oral analgesic given 30 minutes to 1 hour prior to the procedure. Evidence is conflicting about the actual benefits of NSAIDs for IUD insertion pain.[50] Another option is to use a local anesthetic at the tenaculum insertion sites or a paracervical block. Research has failed to demonstrate significant differences in perceived pain with either lidocaine injection or topical gel application at the time of IUD insertion.[50-52]

In recent years, several research reports have touted a potential benefit of using preprocedure misoprostol to facilitate IUD insertion, especially in nulliparous women.[53,54] While clear evidence shows that misoprostol does not decrease the pain experienced by women,[50] there is conflicting evidence as to the ease of insertion being facilitated with preprocedure misoprostol.[55] Several studies have demonstrated an increase in procedural side effects with the use of misoprostol.[54]

Several randomized controlled trials have been conducted that evaluated the use of prophylactic antibiotics given before IUD insertion to decrease the incidence of PID. Infection rates in women who have an IUD are very low overall but arise most frequently in the first 20 days following IUD placement.[56] However, the overall rate of PID following IUD insertion is only 0.54%.[57] In addition, a Cochrane meta-analysis of randomized controlled trials found that prophylactic antibiotics do not lower PID rates.[58] Therefore antibiotics are not indicated for IUD insertion.

Side Effects and Adverse Effects

Occasionally a woman will have a vasovagal response when the tenaculum is placed on the cervix or during insertion of an IUD. When this occurs, symptomatic treatment and waiting for a short time before proceeding is usually all that is required. Women should be counseled that IUDs may be associated with changes in menstrual bleeding patterns. The copper IUD may increase menstrual bleeding and the LNG-IUS often decreases menstrual bleeding.

Some inherent risks are related to the minimally invasive procedures of IUD insertion and removal. Bleeding, infection, perforation of the uterus, and pain can occur, although serious complications are rare.

Missing IUD strings can be attributed to four possible causes: pregnancy, uterine perforation, spontaneous expulsion, and strings cut too short.[59] It is important to rule out pregnancy whenever strings are not visible. Often strings may have simply receded into the cervix, out of view. Gentle cervical exploration with a cytobrush or cotton swab may elicit the hidden strings. If unable to locate strings with gentle exploration, follow-up ultrasound is necessary. If no IUD is noted on ultrasound, consultation with a gynecologist is indicated.

Pregnancy with an Intrauterine Device In Situ

A woman who becomes pregnant with an IUD in place should be informed of the risks involved if the pregnancy is continued—namely, chorioamnionitis, spontaneous abortion, septic abortion, and preterm labor.[60] Although the risk of pregnancy is small with an IUD in place, those women who become pregnant in this scenario should also be evaluated for ectopic pregnancy, as the risk of any pregnancy being ectopic is higher with an IUD in situ. If pregnancy is confirmed and the IUD strings are visible, the IUD should be removed to decrease the risk of spontaneous abortion. The incidence of spontaneous abortion is approximately 50% for women whose IUDs are left in place—a higher rate than if the device is removed.[61] The IUD should be removed even if the woman wishes to terminate the pregnancy in order to reduce her risk of septic abortion.[60] If pregnancy is confirmed and the strings of the IUD are not visible, ultrasound should be performed; if the IUD cannot be located by ultrasound, consultation with a physician is warranted.

Copper T 380A (ParaGard)

The current nonhormonal IUD, known as ParaGard, is composed of polyethylene and an inert plastic material that is flexible, non-inflammatory, and resumes its original shape easily after being flexed for insertion (**Figure 17-8**). The vertical stem of ParaGard's polyethylene body is wrapped with 176 mg of copper wire, while each of its horizontal arms has a 68.7-mg copper collar attached. The copper components of ParaGard release ions into the endometrial cavity that affect tubal and endometrial fluids, and subsequently incapacitate sperm. The ParaGard has a length of plastic thread attached to the lower segment that facilitates removal and enables both the midwife and the woman to confirm the presence of the device. Embedded within the IUD's polyethylene body is a small amount of barium sulfate that provides for localization of the device with standard X-ray imaging. ParaGard provides contraception for as long as 10 years after insertion. Other types of nonhormonal IUDs are available in countries outside the United States.

The effectiveness rate for ParaGard is high, in that less than 1 woman in 100 using it will experience an unintended pregnancy in the first year of use.[1] The copper in the IUD alters tubal transport, has toxic effects on ovum, and impairs normal sperm activity by slowing motility, reducing sperm capacitation, and

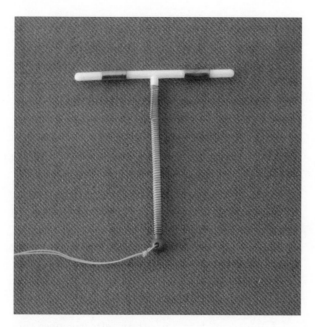

Figure 17-8 Paragard IUD.
Source: © Jones and Bartlett Publishers. Photographed by Kimberly Potvin

increasing sperm destruction. In addition, the copper creates a localized reaction[62] in the endometrial tissue that is unfavorable for implantation.[63]

The copper IUD is associated with menstrual changes such as 1 to 3 more days of bleeding per cycle, increased severity of dysmenorrhea, and potential increase in blood loss, which can exacerbate iron-deficiency anemia. Consequently, ParaGard is not a good form of contraception for women with menorrhagia.

Copper-bearing IUDs appear to convey protection against endometrial cancer (OR = 0.54 (95% CI, 0.47–0.63), although the mechanism of action has not been elucidated.[64,65] Use of an IUD is noncoital dependent, does not require further consideration of cost after the initial insertion, and is effective for as long as 10 years. Some women find the IUD-associated side effects such as bleeding too discomfiting, and others do not like the idea of having a foreign object inside their body. Conversely, for women who do not desire any hormones for contraception, ParaGard may be a good choice.

Permanent Contraception: Sterilization

Sterilization is the surgical interruption or closure of pathways for sperm or ova to unite that prevents fertilization. Since the 1970s, female sterilization has become an increasingly available and acceptable contraceptive choice.[66]

This form of contraception is considered safe, highly effective, and permanent. Overall, both female and male sterilization (vasectomy) are more than 99% effective in preventing pregnancy.[1] Sterilization is an elective procedure.

Methods of female sterilization include tubal ligation and transcervical sterilization. Male sterilization, or vasectomy, is safer, simpler, and approximately half the cost of female sterilization, although female sterilization is more common in the United States.[67]

The term "tying tubes" is a common phrase, but should be avoided as it may incorrectly indicate to a woman that the fallopian tubes could later be easily untied, when in fact reversal of a tubal ligation is a complicated and costly procedure with a high failure rate. In the United States, sterilization is second only to oral contraceptives as the most frequently chosen method of contraception and is one of the most frequently performed surgeries. Female sterilization procedures can be performed soon after a vaginal birth, in conjunction with a cesarean section, immediately following an uncomplicated first-trimester abortion, or independent of pregnancy.

Female Surgical Sterilization (Tubal Ligation)

Fallopian tubes may be surgically cut and ligated with or without a section of tube being removed, mechanically blocked using clips or rings, electrically coagulated, or blocked by a fibrotic reaction induced by chemicals or microinserts. There are three basic approaches to female surgical sterilization: transabdominal, via mini-laparotomy or laparoscopy, and transcervical.

The percentage of women experiencing an unintended pregnancy within the first year following surgical sterilization is 0.5%, which translates into a 99.5% effectiveness rate.[1] This number includes those women with an unsuspected pregnancy at the time when the procedure is performed. Failure can also happen many years after the procedure is performed. However, because spontaneous pregnancy after tubal ligation is rare, the overall risk of ectopic pregnancy is lower in women who undergo surgical sterilization than in the general population. If pregnancy occurs after tubal sterilization, there is a high risk that it will be an ectopic pregnancy. Overall, there are few, if any, medical contraindications to sterilization for the individual who desires this form of contraception.

Sterilization is not coital dependent, nor does it require partner compliance or purchasing of supplies. Some studies show a positive effect on sexuality, likely related to reduced worry about unintended pregnancy.[28] Complications are those associated with any surgery.

Regret that the procedure was performed has been reported.[69] Various studies indicate that the percentage of women who regret the decision ranges from 1% to 26%.[1] Higher rates of regret are found in women who were younger than age 30 at the time of sterilization,[68] who are in an unstable relationship or have experienced the death of a child,[69] and who are low parity.[67]

The midwife must be aware of applicable federal and state regulations about sterilization. Because of abuses in the past, strict criteria must be met to verify informed consent, including that the consenting woman must be an adult. Consent must be obtained within a specified time period before giving birth, and the time interval may differ by state, facility, and payer. The Affordable Care Act (the health insurance reform legislation signed into law in 2010) requires health insurance coverage for female sterilization. The midwife should provide information that is at the appropriate health literacy level, and in the woman's native language, to facilitate informed decision making. The woman should be informed of her ability to decline the sterilization even after the consent form has been signed. In addition, a surgical consent will be obtained just prior to performing the procedure, no matter when the procedure is performed. Women should also be informed that sterilization does not prevent transmission of STIs or HIV. In addition, information should be given regarding alternative contraceptive methods as well as the risks and benefits of the procedure and anesthesia.

Sterilization is not a recommended choice for birth control for any woman uncertain of her desire regarding future fertility. Restoring fertility after sterilization is difficult, and not always possible. Reversal of sterilization is expensive, requiring either costly assisted reproductive technology or highly technical microsurgery, and results cannot be guaranteed. Successful pregnancy following sterilization reversal may vary with the type of tubal occlusive method used and with the age of the woman. Rates of successful reanastomosis following reversal procedures vary between 30% and 70%. The long-term effects of tubal sterilization on menstrual pattern (post-tubal ligation syndrome) appear to be negligible. Most recent studies found no difference in menstrual patterns between women before and after sterilization.[66]

Female Transcervical Sterilization (Essure)

The transcervical female sterilization method involves gaining access to the fallopian tubes hysteroscopically via the cervix. Currently the only available transcervical method is marketed under the brand name Essure (**Figure 17-9**). Its mechanism of action involves irritation and growth of new tissue that results in permanent occlusion of the fallopian tubes as the fallopian tubes respond to the polyester fibers within the Essure coil microinserts. Tubal occlusion occurs approximately 3 months after the procedure is done. The tissue response has been found to be reliable and localized to the insert. Small metal springs (microinserts) are placed into the proximal end of each fallopian tube. Upon release, they expand and anchor to the tube. Over time, scar tissue is created, which then occludes the fallopian tube.[66]

Female transcervical sterilization is generally a safe, well-tolerated office procedure, with highly successful bilateral placement rates and high patient satisfaction.[68] The procedure is performed via hysteroscopy under local anesthesia.[68]

Long-term data on safety, effectiveness, effectiveness, and pregnancy rates for Essure remain unavailable. Of note, many of the existing studies were funded by the manufacturer.[68,70] In the two clinical trials on which the FDA approval for Essure was primarily based, no pregnancies were reported in more than 600 women using the microinserts up to 5 years.[68] U.S. and worldwide literature indicates that this sterilization technique has 99.8% effectiveness.[68] However, other clinical trials and reviews have reported unintended pregnancies that appear to be related to failure to strictly comply with the follow-up protocol, not performing a urinary pregnancy test on the day of the procedure, or failure to instruct the woman to return for the hysterosalpingogram (HSG) follow-up visit to confirm bilateral occlusion via the injection of radiopaque contrast material into the uterus to detect fallopian tube patency.[71]

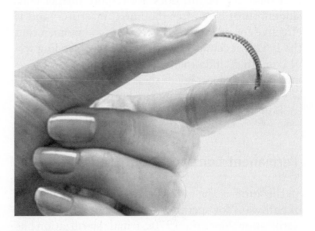

Figure 17-9 Essure.
Source: Image courtesy of Conceptus, Inc.

Because the Essure coil contains nickel, a known hypersensitivity to nickel confirmed by skin test is a contraindication to placement of the microinserts.[68] Transcervical sterilization may be an ideal procedure for women who have comorbidities, such as obesity, cardiorespiratory disease, or complex abdominal issues.[72] Like all permanent sterilization options, this procedure is not coital dependent, it does not require partner compliance, and there is no need to buy further supplies, enhancing the factor of convenience. There may also be a positive effect on sexuality, likely related to reduced worry about unintended pregnancy.

Sterilization does not occur immediately after the procedure, so women must be educated to use additional contraception for 3 months until permanent tubal occlusion is verified by HSG. If the confirmation HSG, conducted at 3 months post procedure, reveals there is still tubal patency, the woman needs to be instructed to use an alternative contraceptive method. Other methods for verification of tubal occlusion have been suggested, such as ultrasound, but the gold standard for confirmation remains the HSG. Currently there are no data on the safety or effectiveness of a reversal procedure.

Female Chemical Sterilization (Quinacrine)

Quinacrine, which was originally approved as an antimalarial drug, is the best-studied chemical agent used for female sterilization. It is most commonly used in developing countries because it is inexpensive and does not require expensive equipment for placement. However, at the time of this text's writing, the World Health Organization (WHO) recommended that until totality of the safety, effectiveness, and epidemiologic data has been reviewed, quinacrine should not be used for nonsurgical sterilization in women.[73]

Male Surgical Sterilization (Vasectomy)

Vasectomy is one of the few contraceptive options currently available for men. Sterilization is achieved by cutting or occluding the vas deferens so that sperm can no longer pass out of the body in the ejaculate. The technique can be done in an outpatient setting under local anesthetic by a trained provider. Advantages of this method include the short procedure time and the reduced risk of hematoma, infection, and postoperative discomfort when compared to female tubal ligation.[68]

Vasectomy is a highly effective and relatively low-cost permanent method of sterilization with a low morbidity rate and extremely low mortality rate. The incidence of pregnancy 5 years after the procedure was performed is 1.1%.[67] Vasectomy is not immediately effective, however: it may take 12 weeks or more, or between 12 and 20 ejaculations, before the ejaculate is sperm free. Alternative contraception needs to be used until azoospermia is confirmed.

Both the man and the woman should be informed that recanalization infrequently does occur. Regret among men about vasectomy has been reported in approximately 5% of men who have the procedure done.[68] The majority of men who report regret had the procedure when they were younger than age 30, were in an unstable marriage, had no or very young children, or made the decision to have a vasectomy during a time of financial crisis or for reasons related to a pregnancy.[74]

Conclusion

This chapter reviewed all currently available nonhormonal methods of contraception for both for women and men. It is important to conduct appropriate screening relative to each method, and offer health education about risks, benefits, effectiveness, and relative advantages prior to use of the selected contraceptive method. Options for contraception change frequently; therefore it is imperative for midwives to remain informed of the latest options so that women for whom they provide care can make informed decisions. Each woman has individual needs and a different lifestyle, which make decision making unique.

● ● ● References

1. Centers for Disease Control and Prevention. U.S. medical eligibility criteria for contraceptive use. *MMWR.* 2010;59(RR04):1-6. Available at: http://www.cdc.gov/mmwr/preview/mmwrhtml/rr5904a1.htm?s_cid=rr5904a1_e. Accessed February 14, 2013.

2. Mosher WD, Jones J. Use of contraception in the United States: 1982-2008. National Center for Health Statistics. *Vital Health Stat.* 2010;23(29). Available at: http://www.cdc.gov/nchs/data/series/sr_23/sr23_029.pdf. Accessed February 14, 2013.

3. Ortayli N, Bulut A, Ozugurlu M, Cokar M. Why withdrawal? Why not withdrawal? Men's perspectives. *Reprod Health Matt.* 2005;13(25):164-173.

4. Killick S, Leary C, Trussell J, Guthrie K. Sperm content of pre-ejaculatory fluid. *Hum Fertil.* 2011;14(1):48-52.

5. Sznitman S, Romer D, Brown L, et al. Prevalence, correlates, and sexually transmitted infection risk related to coitus interruptus among African-American adolescents. *Sex Transm Dis.* 2009;36(4):218-220.

6. Labbock M, Hight-Laukaran V, Peterson A, Fletcher V, von Hertzen H, Van Look P. Multicenter study of the lactational amenorrhea method (LAM): I. efficacy, duration, and implications for clinical application. *Contraception.* 1997;55(6):327-336.

7. Kramer MS, Kakuma R. Optimal duration of exclusive breastfeeding. *Cochrane Database Syst Rev.* 2012; 8:CD003517. doi: 10.1002/14651858.CD003517.pub2.

8. Valdes V, Labbok M, Pugin E, Perez A. The efficacy of the lactational amenorrhea method (LAM) among working women. *Contraception.* 2000;62(5):217-219.

9. Gallo MF, Grimes DA, Lopez LM, Schulz KF. Non-latex versus latex male condoms for contraception. *Cochrane Database Syst Rev.* 2006;1:CD003550. doi: 10.1002/14651858.CD003550.pub2.

10. Steiner M, Dominik R, Rountree R, Nanda K, Dorflinger L. Contraceptive effectiveness of a polyurethane condom and a latex condom: a randomized controlled trial. *Obstet Gynecol.* 2003;101(3):539-547.

11. Higgins J, Cooper A. Dual use of condoms and contraceptives in the US. *Sex Health.* 2012;9(1):73-80.

12. Beksinska M, Smit J, Joanis C, Hart C. Practice makes perfect: reduction in female condom failures and user problems with short-term experience in a randomized trial. *Contraception.* 2012;86(2):127-131.

13. Hoffman S, Mantell J, Exner T, Stein Z. The future of the female condom. *Perspect Sex Reprod Health.* 2004;36:120-126.

14. Raymond E, Dominik R. Contraceptive effectiveness of two spermicides: a randomized trial. *Obstet Gynecol.* 1999;93:896-903.

15. Van Damme L, Ramjee G, Alary M, Vuylsteke B, Chandeying V, Rees H. Effectiveness of COL-1492, a nonoxynol-9 vaginal gel, on HIV-1 transmission in female sex workers: a randomized controlled trial. *Lancet.* 2002;360:971-977.

16. Eckert L, Lentz G. Chapter 23 Infections of the lower genital tract: vulva, vagina, cervix, toxic shock syndrome, endometritis, and salpingitis. In: Lentz G, Lobo R, Gershenson D, Katz V, eds. *Comprehensive Gynecology,* 6th ed. Philadelphia, PA: Mosby Elsevier; 2012:519-561.

17. Schwartz B, Brome C. Nonmenstrual toxic shock syndrome associated with barrier contraceptives: report of a case-control study. *Rev Infect Dis.* 1989;suppl 1(S43-S48):S48-S49.

18. Faich G, Pearson K, Fleming D, Sobel S, Anello C. Toxic shock syndrome and the vaginal contraceptive sponge. *JAMA.* 1986;255:216-218.

19. Woodhams EJ, Gilliam M. Contraception. *Ann Intern Med.* 2012;157(7):ITC4-1-ITC4-15.

20. Trussell J, Strickler J, Vaughn B. Contraceptive efficacy of the diaphragm, the sponge, and the cervical cap. *Fam Plann Perspect.* 1993;25:100-105, 35.

21. Murphy P, Morgan K, Likis F. Contraception. In: Schuiling K, Likis F, eds. *Women's Gynecologic Health.* 2nd ed. Burlington, MA: Jones & Bartlett Learning; 2013:161.

22. Allen RE. Diaphragm fitting. *Am Fam Physician.* 2004; 69(1):97-100.

23. Koeniger-Donohue R. The FemCap: a non-hormonal contraceptive. *Women's Health Care.* 2006;5(4):79-91.

24. Gallo MF, Grimes DA, Schulz KF, Lopez LM. Cervical cap versus diaphragm for contraception. *Cochrane Database Syst Rev.* 2002;4:CD003551.

25. Peipert JF, Madden T, Allsworth JE, Secura GM. Preventing unintended pregnancies by providing no-cost contraception. *Obstet Gynecol.* 2012;120(6): 1291-1297.

26. Mauck C, Callahan M, Weiner D, Dominick R. A comparative study of the safety and efficacy of the FemCap, a new vaginal barrier contraceptive and the Ortho All-Flex diaphragm. The FemCap Investigator's Group. *Contraception.* 1999;60:71-80.

27. Jennings VH, Burke AE. Fertility awareness–based methods. In Hatcher RA, Trussell J, Nelson A, et al., eds. *Contraceptive Technology.* 20th ed. New York, NY: Ardent Media; 2011:432.

28. *Family Planning: A Global Handbook for Providers.* WHO Press; 2011. Available at: http://whqlibdoc .who.int/publications/2011/9780978856373_eng.pdf. Accessed February 14, 2013.

29. Kambric R, Lamprecht V. Calendar rhythm efficacy: a review. *Adv Contracept.* 1996;12:123-128.

30. Arevalo M. Expanding the availability of and improving delivery of natural family planning services and fertility awareness education providers' perspectives. *Adv Contracept.* 1997;13:275-281.

31. Pyper C. Fertility awareness and natural family planning. *Eur J Contracept Reprod Health Care.* 1997; 2:131-146.

32. Arevalo M, Sinai I, Jennings V. A fixed formula to define the fertile window of the menstrual cycle as the basis of a simple method of natural family planning. *Contraception.* 1999;60(6):357-360.

33. Mansour D, Inki P, Gemzell Danielsson K. Efficacy of contraceptive methods: a review of the literature. *Eur J Contracept Reprod Health Care.* 2010;15:14-16.

34. Grimes D, Gallo M, Grigorieva V, et al. Fertility awareness–based methods for contraception systematic review of randomized controlled trials. *Contraception.* 2005;72:85-90.

35. Pallone SR, Bergus GR. Fertility awareness–based methods: another option for family planning. *J Am Board Fam Med.* 2009;22(2):147-157.

36. Arevalo M, Jennings V, Sinai I. The Standard Days method. *Contraception.* 2002;65:333-338.

37. University of Georgetown. *CycleBeads*. Washington, DC: Cycle Technologies; October 12, 2012. Available at: http://www.cyclebeads.com.

38. *About CycleBeads*. Washington, DC: Institute for Reproductive Health; 2012 [updated 2009; cited October 22, 2012]. Available at: http://www.irh.org/?q=content/how-use-cyclebeads.

39. Germano E, Jennings V. New approaches to fertility awareness–based methods: incorporating the Standard Days and TwoDay methods into practice. *J Midwifery Women's Health*. 2006;51:471-477.

40. Dunson D, Sinai I, Colombo B. The relationship between cervical secretions and the daily provabilities of pregnancy: effectiveness of the TwoDay algorithm. *Hum Reprod*. 2001;16:2278-2282.

41. Fehring R, Schneider M, Raviele K, Rodriquez D, Pruszynski J. Randomized comparison of two Internet-supported fertility awareness–based methods of family planning. *J Contraception*. 2012 [Epub ahead of print].

42. Mohllajee A, Curtis K, Peterson H. Does insertion and use of an intrauterine device increase the risk of pelvic inflammatory disease among women with sexually transmitted infection? A systematic review. *Contraception*. 2006;73:145-153.

43. Workowski K, Berman S. Sexually transmitted diseases treatment guidelines 2010. Centers for Disease Control and Prevention. *MMWR*. 2010;59(RR-12):1-56.

44. Murphy PA, Jacobson J, Turok DK. Criterion-based screening for sexually transmitted infection: sensitivity, specificity, and predictive values of commonly used questions. *J Midwifery Women's Health*. 2012;57(6):622-628.

45. American College of Obstetricians and Gynecologists. ACOG practice bulletin no. 121: long-acting reversible contraception: implants and intrauterine devices. *Obstet Gynecol*. 2011;118(1):184-196.

46. Grimes D, Lopez L, Schulz K, Stanwood N. Immediate post-partum insertion of intrauterine devices. *Cochrane Database Syst Rev*. 2010;CD003036.

47. Celen S, Sucak A, Yildiz Y, Danisman N. Immediate postplacental insertion of an intrauterine contraceptive device during cesarean section. *Contraception*. 2011;84(3):240-243.

48. Fox M, Oat-Judge J, Severson K, et al. Immediate placement of intrauterine devices after first and second trimester pregnancy termination. *Contraception*. 2011;83(1):34-40.

49. Grimes D, Lopez L, Schulz K, Stanwood N. Immediate postabortal insertion of intrauterine devices. *Cochrane Database Syst Rev*. 2010;CD001777.

50. Allen RH, Bartz D, Grimes DA, Hubacher D, O'Brien P. Interventions for pain with intrauterine device insertion. *Cochrane Database Syst Rev*. 2009;3:CD007373. doi: 10.1002/14651858.CD007373.pub2.v.

51. Mody S, Kiley J, Rademaker A, Gawron L, Stika C, Hammond C. Pain control for intrauterine device insertion: a randomized trial of 1% lidocaine paracervical block. *Contraception*. 2012;86(6):704-709.

52. McNicholas C, Madden T, Zhao Q, Secura G, Allsworth JE, Peipert JF. Cervical lidocaine for IUD insertional pain: a randomized controlled trial. *Am J Obstet Gynecol*. 2012;207(5):384.

53. Dijkhuizen K, Dekkers O, Holleboom C, et al. Vaginal misoprostol prior to insertion of an intrauterine device: an RCT. *Hum Reprod Update*. 2011;26(2): 323-329.

54. Edelman A, Schaefer E, Olson A, et al. Effects of prophylactic misoprostol administration prior to intrauterine device insertion in nulliparous women. *Contraception*. 2011;84(3):234-239.

55. Swenson C, Turok D, Ward K, Jacobson JC, Dermish A. Self-administered misoprostol or placebo before intrauterine device insertion in nulliparous women: a randomized controlled trial. *Obstet Gynecol*. 2012; 120(2):341-347.

56. Farley T, Rosenberg M, Rowe P, Chen JH, Meirik O. Intrauterine devices and pelvic inflammatory disease: an international perspective. *Lancet*. 1992; 339(8796):785-788.

57. Sufrin CB, Postlethwaite D, Armstrong MA, Merchant M, Wendt JM, Steinauer JE. *Neisseria gonorrhea* and *Chlamydia trachomatis* screening at intrauterine device insertion and pelvic inflammatory disease. *Obstet Gynecol*. 2012 Dec;120(6):1314-21.

58. Grimes DA, Lopez LM, Schulz KF. Antibiotic prophylaxis for intrauterine contraceptive device insertion. *Cochrane Database Syst Rev*. 1999;3:CD001327. doi: 10.1002/14651858.CD001327

59. Moschos E, Twickler DM. Intrauterine devices in early pregnancy: findings on ultrasound and clinical outcomes. *Am J Obstet Gynecol*. 2011 May;204(5):427. e1-e6. doi: 10.1016/j.ajog.2010.12.058.

60. Brahmi D, Steenland M, Renner R-M, Gaffield ME, Curtis KM. Pregnancy outcomes with an IUD in situ: a systematic review. *Contraception*. 2012;85(2): 131-139.

61. Treiman K, Liskin L, Kols A, Rinehart W. *IUDs: An Update*. Contract No. 6. Baltimore, MD: Johns Hopkins School of Public Health, Population Information Program CfCP; 1995.

62. Shimoni N. Intrauterine contraceptives: a review of uses, side effects and candidates. *Semin Reprod Med*. 2010;28(2):118-125.

63. Gemzell-Danielsson K, Berger C, Lalitkumar PGL. Emergency contraception—mechanisms of action. *Contraception*. 2013 Mar;87(3):300-308.

64. Guleria K, Agarwal N, Mishra K, Gulati R, Mehendiratta A. Evaluation of endometrial steroid receptors and cell mitotic activity in women using

copper intrauterine device: can Cu-T prevent endometrial cancer? *J Obstet Gynecol Res.* 2004;30:181-187.

65. Beining RM, Dennis LK, Smith EM, Dokras A. Meta-analysis of intrauterine device use and risk of endometrial cancer. Ann Epidemiol. 2008 Jun;18(6): 492-499.

66. Peterson B. Sterilization. *Obstet Gynecol.* 2008;111(1): 189-203.

67. American College of Obstetricians and Gynecologists. Benefits and risks of sterilization. Practice Bulletin No. 133. *Obstet Gynecol.* 2013;121:392-404.

68. Curtis K, Mohllajee A, Peterson H. Regret following female sterilization at a young age: a systematic review. *Contraception.* 2006;73(2):205-210.

69. Chi I, Jones D. Incidence, risk factors, and prevention of poststerilization regret in women: an updated international review from on epidemiological perspective. *Obstet Gynecol Surv.* 1994;49(10):722-732.

70. Hurskainen R, Hovi S-L, Gissler M, et al. Hysteroscopic tubal sterilization: a systematic review of the Essure system. *Fertil Steril.* 2010;94(1):16-19.

71. Veersema S, Vleugel M, Moolenaar L, Janssen C, Brölmann H. Unintended pregnancies after Essure sterilization in the Netherlands. *Fertil Steril.* 2010;93(1):35-38.

72. Gebbie A, Hardman S. Contraception in the perimenopause: old and new. *Menopause Int.* 2010;16:33-37.

73. The safety of quinacrine when used as a method of non-surgical sterilization in women: interim statement. World Health Organization; 2009 [October 1, 2012]. Available at: http://www.who.int/reproductivehealth /publications/family_planning/WHO_RHR_09_21 /en/index.html.

74. Potts J, Pasqualotto F, Nelson D, Thomas AJ, Agarwal A. Patient characteristics associated with vasectomy reversal. *J Urol.* 1999;161:1835-1839.

17A

Fitting Diaphragms

A diaphragm is a soft latex or silicone dome that covers the cervix during intercourse. The rim has a spring inside that ensures the diaphragm fits between the posterior symphysis and the posterior vagina, covering the cervix.

The diaphragm is always used with a spermicide. The spermicide is placed in the dome designed directly to face the cervix and spread upwards to around the rim of the diaphragm.

The mechanism of action is twofold: (1) The spring in the rim forms a seal against the vaginal wall, providing a physical barrier to prevent sperm from entering the cervix, and (2) during vaginal intercourse, the diaphragm moves slightly and coats the cervix and vaginal wall with spermicide. The types of diaphragms are listed in **Table 17A-1**.

Contraindications (U.S. MEC Category 3 or 4)

- Allergy to latex
- History of toxic shock syndrome
- High risk for HIV
- HIV infection or AIDS

Timing of Diaphragm Fitting

1. Postpartum: 6 weeks or more postpartum
2. Post-miscarriage or abortion: 2 weeks or more
3. Lactation: Refit after weaning
4. Weight change: Refit after 15 lb or more

Table 17A-1	Types of Diaphragms	
Type	**Description**	**Indications**
Arcing spring	The rim is firmer than the coil spring and the diaphragm folds into an arc when compressed	Strongest type of rim May be used by women who have cystocele, rectocele, uterine prolapse, retroverted uterus, or an anteverted or retroverted cervix May be easier than flat spring to insert as the arc naturally curves into the posterior vaginal fornix
Wide-seal rim	Has a flexible 1½ cm wide "skirt" extending from the inner edge of the rim	Latex-free, arcing spring design The small skirt is designed to hold gel in place and improve the seal
Flat spring	Thinnest rim Made by only one manufacturer in the United States	For women with firm vaginal tone and shallow pubic arch behind symphysis May be difficult to find Can be used with an introducer

Equipment and Supplies

- A complete set of fitting rings or fitting diaphragms, from 50 mm to 95 mm
- Nonsterile gloves
- Lubricant

Diaphragm Fitting Procedure

Preparation

1. Encourage the woman to empty her bladder prior to examination.
2. Gather all needed equipment and arrange it so it is in easy reach.
3. Perform a regular pelvic examination to rule out any infections or abnormalities.
4. Initial choice of a fitting diaphragm or fitting ring usually begins with a size in the center of the probable range for the woman's parity. Generally a nulliparous woman will be fitted with size 65, 70, or 75, and a multiparous woman with size 75, 80, or 85.

Procedure

1. Insert a gloved index and middle finger into the vagina until the middle finger reaches the posterior wall of the vagina, to determine the distance between the posterior symphysis and the posterior vagina behind the cervix.
2. Mark the point at which the index finger touches the inferior pubic arch.

3. Remove the fingers and place a diaphragm rim on the tip of the middle finger. The opposite rim of the correct size of diaphragm should lie approximately in front of the mark.
4. Lubricate or moisten the diaphragm or fitting ring, compress the sides together with the fingers and thumb of one hand, and introduce it into the vagina (**Figure 17A-1**). Be certain to direct the diaphragm or fitting ring downward and inward, thereby applying pressure against the posterior vaginal wall and avoiding the more sensitive anterior structures.
5. Once the diaphragm is inserted, check its placement with a gloved finger. It is the correct size if:
   a. The rim is behind the cervix in the posterior fornix.
   b. The circumference is against the lateral vaginal walls.
   c. A fingertip can be inserted between the diaphragm and the posterior surface of the pubis.
   d. The cervix is covered.
6. The diaphragm is *too small* if:
   a. There is more than enough space for the flat portion of a fingertip to be inserted between the rim of the diaphragm and the posterior surface of the pubis.
   b. It moves about freely in the vagina.
   c. It dislodges when the woman coughs or bears down.

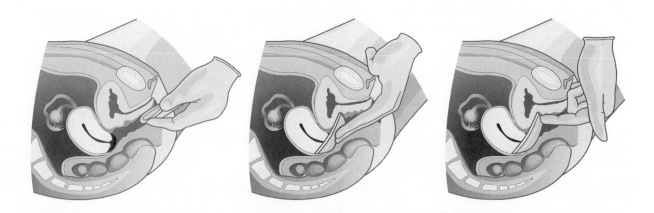

Figure 17A-1 Diaphragm fitting.

7. The diaphragm is *too large* if:
   a. It fits tightly against the symphysis pubis.
   b. The rim buckles forward against the lateral vaginal walls.
   c. If it dislodges or protrudes out the vagina when the woman performs the Valsalva maneuver.
   d. The woman feels discomfort when the diaphragm is in place.

8. Many midwives will verify the appropriate size by inserting diaphragms of successive size until the correct size is ascertained and then inserting one size larger for confirmation.

9. Return demonstration:
   a. Have the woman wash her hands and then assume a comfortable position that will allow her to insert two fingers into her vagina and reach her cervix. Optional positions include the following:
      i. Lying on the exam table with the head of the table elevated, knees flexed
      ii. Standing with one leg on a stool, bending forward
   b. As she inserts her fingers into her vagina, verbally guide the woman to locate and feel the symphysis pubis and then her cervix.
   c. Have her hold the lightly lubricated diaphragm in one hand, dome side down. Then have her compress the sides of the diaphragm between her thumb and fingers, with her hand on top of the diaphragm, and spread her labia with her other hand and introduce the end of the folded diaphragm into her vagina in a downward and backward direction.
   d. Once the diaphragm has been introduced into the vagina, the woman can use the hand that has been separating the labia to complete insertion until the rim is under the pubis. Instruct her to then use a finger to tuck the rim upward, behind the pubis.
   e. Have the woman check the placement, feeling the rim behind the pubis and the cervix covered by the diaphragm.
   f. The midwife may ask the woman to walk around the room to note any sensation or discomfort. When correctly fitted, the diaphragm will not be felt.
   g. Have the woman lie down in modified lithotomy position; insert a gloved finger into the vagina and check that the diaphragm is fitted correctly.
   h. To remove the diaphragm, have the woman resume the position she chose for insertion. She inserts a finger into her vagina, bears down, grasps the rim behind the pubis with two fingers or thumb and index finger, and gently slides the diaphragm down and out.
   i. Have her repeat this practice insertion and removal until she is confident she can insert the diaphragm, check its correct placement, and remove it.
   j. Demonstrate use of the spermicide. Squeeze 1 to 2 teaspoons of the gel from the tube into the dome, spreading it evenly over the inside and around the rim of the diaphragm.

Health Education: Key Points

1. The diaphragm ensures the best protection when inserted correctly and used with spermicide.

2. The diaphragm can be inserted up to a maximum of 6 hours prior to intercourse.

3. It is recommended that the diaphragm be left in place a minimum of 6 hours after intercourse, although there are no studies that document the optimal time needed for full contraceptive protection.

4. Do not leave the diaphragm in situ for more than 24 hours after intercourse secondary to the theoretical risk of toxic shock syndrome.

5. When a diaphragm fits correctly, the woman will not feel it inside her vagina.

6. Do not use oil-based lubricants with a latex diaphragm as they can degrade the latex.

7. Symptoms of toxic shock syndrome are sudden very high fever, muscle aches, chills, malaise.

17B

Procedure for IUD Insertion

MARY C. BRUCKER

MICHELLE R. COLLINS

SHARON HOLLEY

TONIA L. MOORE-DAVIS

DEBORAH NARRIGAN

Intrauterine devices can be referred to by several different terms and abbreviations: intrauterine device (IUD), intrauterine contraceptive device (IUCD), intrauterine contraception (UC), intrauterine system (IUS). For the purposes of this appendix, the terms "intrauterine device" and "IUD" will be used throughout.

Three different brands of IUDs currently are available in the United States, which are either impregnated with copper (copper IUD) or with levonorgestrel (LNG IUD). Therefore, more information about use of these devices is found in both the *Nonhormonal Contraception* and *Hormonal Contraception* chapters. In addition to use as a contraceptive, the LNG IUD can be used in the treatment of menorrhagia because it decreases uterine bleeding. Although this appendix appears in the *Nonhormonal Contraception* chapter, it can be used as a guide for insertion of any of the current IUDs discussed in the *Family Planning* and *Hormonal Contraception* chapters.

Preparation for IUD Insertion

As with all interventions, health education and informed decision making should precede any procedure. A host of myths and misconceptions exist regarding IUDs and should be addressed. Intrauterine devices are long-acting reversible contraceptive (LARC) agents that require little, if any action, by the woman after they are inserted, making them very effective contraceptives. Menstrual changes are the most common side effect and vary based on the IUD type. The copper IUD is associated with an increase in menstrual flow, whereas the LNG IUD is associated with irregular bleeding and amenorrhea. It has been proposed that women who are aware of these menstrual changes and accept them prior to insertion may be able to tolerate them better than women for whom these effects occur unexpectedly. A written consent form granting permission to the clinician for IUD insertion, signed by the woman either on paper or by electronic means, is part of the informed consent.

Health education should include the costs involved with IUD insertion. Although more expensive than several other contraceptive methods, once an IUD is in situ for approximately 2 years or more, it is likely to be more cost-effective than methods requiring regular replacements and visits such as combination oral contraceptives (COCs), patches, and injections. Some financial support may be available for women who are in need from the pharmaceutical companies or their associated philanthropic programs.

Timing of the IUD Insertion

IUDs may be inserted postpartum, after an abortion, or in nonpregnant women. Immediate postpartum insertion is not commonly performed in the United States, largely because of an increased expulsion rate—more than six times higher than the rate observed following IUD insertion after the first several postpartum weeks.[1] Post abortion is a common time for insertion and has been found to be safe and effective.[2] The copper IUD also can be used as a type of emergency contraception and is discussed for that indication in the *Family Planning* chapter.

In years past, IUDs for interconceptional use were almost exclusively inserted during a woman's menses. This timing was designed to provide additional assurance that the woman was not pregnant as well as the belief that insertion would be easier during menses. It was thought that the cervix might be slightly open and softer at this time. However, little evidence exists to support this timing.[3] Currently, insertion can occur at any time for a woman without preexisting contraindications to the method, given there is reliable evidence that she is not currently pregnant.

Screening for Sexually Transmitted Infections

Some practice sites continue to require an office visit prior to IUD insertion to screen for sexually transmitted infections (STIs) and allow time for results to be available before the device is placed. However, if the woman has a low risk of being exposed to an STI based on her sexual history, evidence suggests that this two-visit policy imposes an unnecessary barrier to the use of IUDs and serves to make access to an IUD more difficult.[4] Similarly, the requirement that the woman have a normal Pap test at a prior visit is considered by many to be unnecessary because it is questionable whether Pap test variations would be affected by an IUD in situ.[5] Today many midwives obtain STI cultures or testing at the time of insertion and treat or remove the IUD based on the STI test results and clinical symptoms.

For women who already are using a hormonal contraceptive method such as COCs, the IUD can be inserted at any time during the cycle and no secondary method of contraception is needed. This seamless transition also can occur when a woman has one IUD removed, which is then replaced with another IUD.

Choice of an IUD

The three available IUDs are compared and contrasted in **Table 17B-1**. All three provide effective contraception and all three can be identified on ultrasound if needed. However, the Mirena IUD has received approval from the Food and Drug Administration (FDA) for both contraception and for treatment of heavy menses among women desiring an IUD. The Skyla is the newest IUD available and is being marketed especially for nulliparous women because it is slightly smaller than the other two. Long-term costs vary for the three IUDs but the ParaGard IUD may be the most cost-effective as it has a duration of action of at least twice as many years as the others.

Day of IUD Insertion

This section discusses the steps involved in insertion of an IUD. Insertion of copper IUDs and LNG IUDs differs based on the configuration of both the inserter and the device. In all cases, the intention is to place the IUD in the fundus of the uterus. If the IUD placement is not fundal, there is a higher likelihood of unintended pregnancy as well as expulsion of the IUD.

Several training programs exist for clinicians desiring to insert an IUD. Most of these programs are sponsored by manufacturers of the devices, and they may restrict use of their products until such education is completed. Multiple resources for IUD insertion procedures exist on the Internet, including video recordings that help the clinician review the process. In addition, the FDA-approved prescribing information for each device includes insertion instructions. These resources are particularly valuable if the procedure is not performed regularly. The following steps for insertion are general guidelines and cannot replace hands-on experiences.

Premedication

Prior to insertion, it is common practice to administer a prophylactic nonsteroidal anti-inflammatory agent such as ibuprofen to the woman. These drugs are an effective means to treat the pain associated with IUD use, such as copper IUD–associated dysmenorrhea, but there is no evidence suggesting that they diminish discomfort at time of insertion. Similarly, using misoprostol (Cytotec) as a cervical softening agent may facilitate insertion, but no significant decrease in women's pain has been found compared to women who are not given misoprostol prior to insertion. Thus, misoprostol is not recommended for routine use as part of the insertion procedure.[6,7] Anesthesia such as topical lidocaine may or may not decrease pain, but published studies on this topic lack enough rigor to draw any conclusion.[8] Paracervical nerve blocks may be of use for women who have had previous difficult insertions or require cervical dilatation. Nitrous oxide also has been suggested as a possible analgesia option for women during an IUD insertion.

The use of antimicrobial agents as prophylaxis against infection remains controversial. A systematic review found a small, but significant reduction in infections among women receiving such treatment, but cautioned that the number of women in the studies was small and routine use was likely not to be cost-effective. In the published studies on use of antimicrobials, the risk of IUD-associated infection was small in both the treated and control groups.[9]

Equipment Required for IUD Insertion

General equipment includes the following items:

- Clean, nonsterile gloves for a bimanual examination
- Adequate lighting for visualization

Table 17B-1	Types of IUDs						
Type of IUD	Brand Name	Size	Active Components	Release Rate	FDA Indications	Length of Effectiveness[*]	Comments Specific to the Method
Copper T 380A	ParaGard	36 mm × 32 mm	380 mm^2 sleeves of copper on arms of device	NA	Contraception	10 years	Associated with irregular bleeding, dysmenorrhea, heavier menses rarely leading to anemia
Levonorgestrel (LNG) IUD	Mirena	32 mm × 32 mm	52 mg LNG	20 mcg/day	Contraception Treatment of heavy menses for women choosing intrauterine contraception	5 years	Associated with irregular bleeding, but lighter and then marked decrease or amenorrhea after the first few months Often used as an alternative to hysterectomy for women who have heavy bleeding
	Skyla	28 mm × 30 mm	13.5 mg LNG	14 mcg/day	Contraception	3 years	Introduced in 2013 Based on trials, menstrual irregularities expected to be similar to those associated with Mirena Not FDA indicated as a treatment for women with heavy menses

[*]Original length of time of effectiveness for newly marketed IUDs may be changed to longer durations as additional data emerge.

- Speculum of appropriate shape and size for the woman
- Sharp scissors to cut the IUD threads after insertion
- IUD insertion requires a sterile field that contains the following sterile items:
  - Uterine sound to verify the size of the uterine cavity and the appropriateness of a specific IUD
  - Tenaculum (single tooth) to grasp the cervix, straighten the cervical canal, and stabilize the uterus during insertion
  - Sterile gloves

The IUD of choice may be placed on the field or handed to the clinician by an assistant. In some areas, a secondary IUD may be available should contamination occur with the first one. In other sites, the woman must obtain a prescription and purchase her own IUD. In those situations, it is likely that only one IUD will be available.

Optional equipment may include the following items:

- Antiseptic solution (e.g., povidone-iodine or chlorhexidine) and applicator for washing the cervix and vagina (although there is no evidence such action decreases infection)
- Equipment for anesthesia (e.g., for paracervical block or instillation of lidocaine)

Key Points for Insertion of Any IUD

1. A bimanual pelvic examination should be carefully performed to ascertain position of the uterus and rule out any gross abnormalities. Note that a retroflexed uterus or the

softer uterus of a breastfeeding woman may have a higher risk of perforation, but these conditions are not contraindications to the procedure.

2. The woman should have signed an informed consent for documentation and verification of understanding of the procedure.

3. The woman should be positioned such that she is comfortable for the procedure and the examiner has good visualization of the vagina and cervix. Optimally the clinician should have another individual to assist with the procedure.

4. The clinician should reassure the woman that the procedure can be stopped at any time should she make this request.

5. The insertion is begun using sterile technique.

6. The cervix and vagina can be swabbed with the antiseptic if desired; similarly, anesthesia can be administered as appropriate.

7. The tenaculum grasps the anterior lip of the cervix with the teeth placed parallel to the plane of the speculum blades. If the uterus is retroverted, it may be more effective to place the tenaculum on the posterior lip. Gentle traction is exerted toward the clinician to straighten the cervical canal in alignment with the uterine cavity. Usually the clinician uses the nondominant hand to hold the tenaculum.

8. While performing these actions, the clinician should also be observing the woman because manipulation of the cervix can result in a vasovagal response. If the woman is faint or very nauseated, the clinician should stop the procedure and wait. Usually the second attempt at insertion is successful if several minutes have elapsed.

9. While the nondominant hand holds the tenaculum in place, the dominant hand slides the uterine sound into the uterus to measure the depth of the uterine cavity (**Figure 17B-1**). Caution must be taken not to aggressively force the sound. All three of the currently available IUDs are designed for a uterine cavity that sounds between 6 and 9 centimeters. The depth of the uterus in centimeters should be noted. If the sound does not confirm a depth within that range, the insertion

procedure should be aborted and an alternative method of contraception discussed with the woman.

10. At this point, the steps for the insertion vary based on the device. However, for all IUDs, the professional must maintain scrupulous sterile technique.

Insertion of an LNG IUD

Both the Mirena and Skylar IUDs are inserted in a similar manner.

1. The IUD package is opened, usually by the assistant, and the clinician reaches for the device in a sterile manner. Alternatively, the entire package can be opened by the clinician, who then dons sterile gloves and proceeds with the insertion. **Figure 17B-2** provides a view of the device in the packaging. The anatomy of an LNG device can be seen in **Figure 17B-3**.

2. Threads will be secured on the handle of the inserter and are to be released from the groove so they can hang freely.

3. Placement of a thumb or forefinger on the slider will stabilize it. The slider should *not* be moved downward at this time, as this

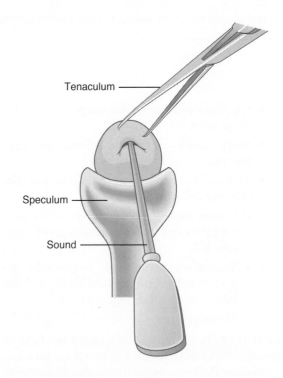

Figure 17B-1 Cervix with tenaculum and uterine sound.

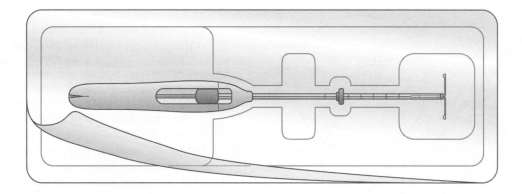

Figure 17B-2 LNG IUD packaging.

action may prematurely release the threads of the IUD. Once the slider is moved below the mark, the IUD cannot be reloaded. The clinician should keep the thumb or forefinger on the slider until the insertion is complete.

4. The arms of the device should be in a horizontal position. If they are not, they can be re-aligned on a flat sterile area such as the inside of the sterile package (**Figure 17B-4**).

5. The slider is gently pushed toward the insertion tubing while the threads are pulled. This two-handed action retracts the IUD arms in the tubing (**Figure 17B-5**).

6. Care should be taken to load the LNG IUD into the insertion tubing with correct orientation of knobs at the end of the arms. After

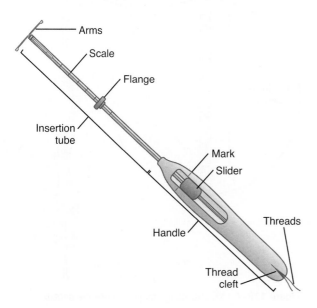

Figure 17B-3 Anatomy of an LNG IUD.

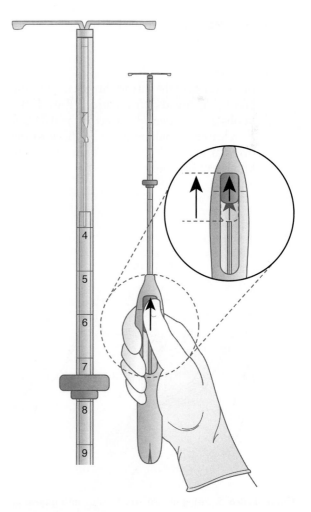

Figure 17B-4 Stabilization of slider and verification of position of IUD.

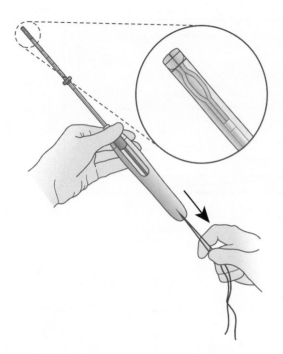

Figure 17B-5 Retraction of LNG IUD into tubing.

7. Based on the uterine size determined by the sound, the flange on the insertion device is set at that number by sliding the flange over the marked increments on the IUD insertion tube (**Figure 17B-7**).

8. The nondominant hand exerts gentle traction on the tenaculum. Simultaneously, continued pressure is applied to the slider on the IUD handle. By performing these actions, the insertion tubing is placed into the vagina at the level of the external cervical os.

9. The insertion tubing is gently advanced until the flange is approximately 1.5 to 2 cm from the external cervical os. The IUD will be into the uterus but should not be in the fundus at this time (**Figure 17B-8**).

10. The slider on the handle is pulled back toward the clinician until the level of the raised mark on the insertion handle is reached.

this is verified, the threads are secured in the groove or thread cleft (**Figure 17B-6**). If the knobs are not aligned correctly, the IUD can be released by pulling the slider back to the original mark on the handle and then the knobs can be repositioned.

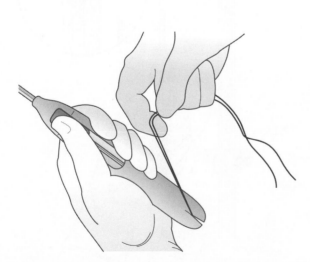

Figure 17B-6 Securing of LNG IUD threads into groove or cleft.

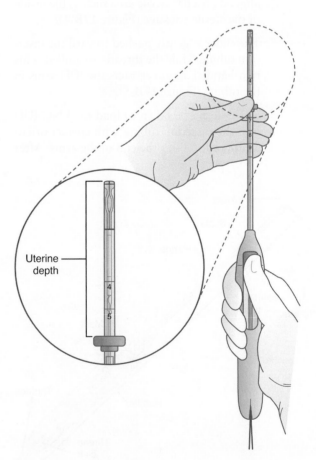

Uterine depth

Figure 17B-7 LNG IUD flange moved to uterine depth.

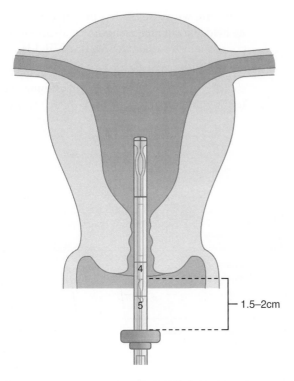

Figure 17B-8 LNG IUD Inserter guided through cervix.

At that time, the IUD arms are expelled from the insertion tubing (**Figure 17B-9**). The clinician must wait 10 seconds to allow the arms to open completely.

11. The insertion tubing is advanced until the flange is at the external cervical os. At that point, the IUD is in the uterine fundus (**Figure 17B-10**).

12. The slider is moved toward the clinician to release the IUD (**Figure 17B-11**).

13. The IUD handle and insertion tubing are gently removed from the uterus and cervix and appropriately discarded.

14. The threads will remain in place.

Insertion of a Copper IUD (CU 380A IUD)

1. The IUD package (**Figure 17B-12**) is opened, usually by the assistant, and handed to the

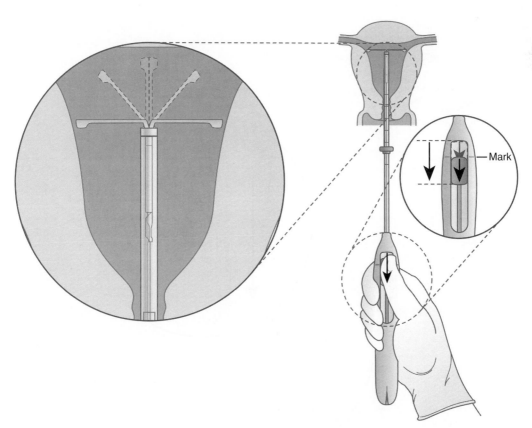

Figure 17B-9 Opening of LNG IUD arms via moving slider to preset mark.

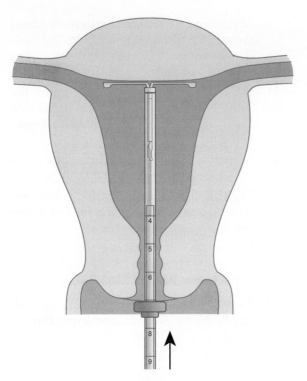

Figure 17B-10 IUD in fundus and flange at level of external cervical os.

clinician, who already has prepared the sterile field. The clinician should be aware of the components of this IUD (**Figure 17B-13**).

2. The IUD is loaded into the insertion tubing by slightly withdrawing the insertion tubing and folding the horizontal arms of the IUD down

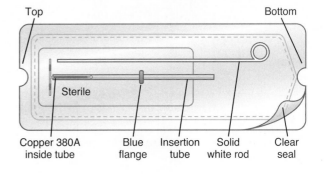

Figure 17B-12 Packaging of copper IUD.

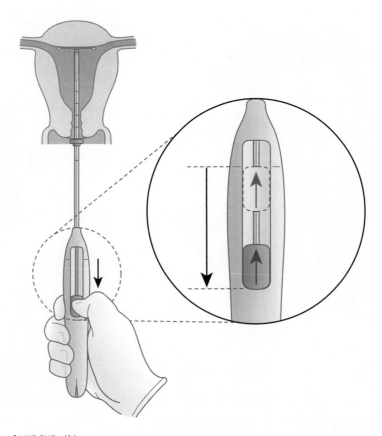

Figure 17B-11 Release of LNG IUD slider.

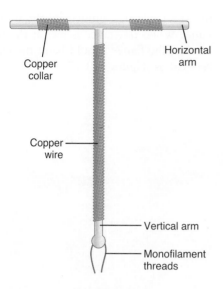

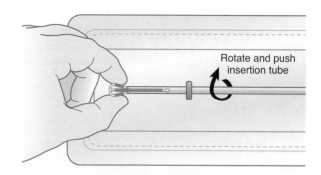

Figure 17B-15 Placement of arms of copper IUD into tubing by open sterile technique.

Figure 17B-13 Anatomy of a copper IUD.

along the vertical arm using the thumb and forefinger. This can be accomplished through the packaging (**Figure 17B-14**) or by an open sterile technique (**Figure 17B-15**). Precautions must be taken to ensure that the arms are not bent into the tubing until immediately before insertion. If the arms are folded for more than 5 minutes, they may not completely unfold in the uterus.

3. The insertion tubing is advanced so that the horizontal arms sit securely within the insertion tubing.

4. The solid white rod is placed into the bottom of the insertion tubing. It is advanced until it touches the bottom of the IUD (**Figure 17B-16**).

5. The insertion tube is grasped at the open end, and the flange is set to the centimeter level predetermined by sounding the uterus.

6. The insertion tubing is rotated so that the horizontal arms of the IUD are parallel to the long axis of the flange.

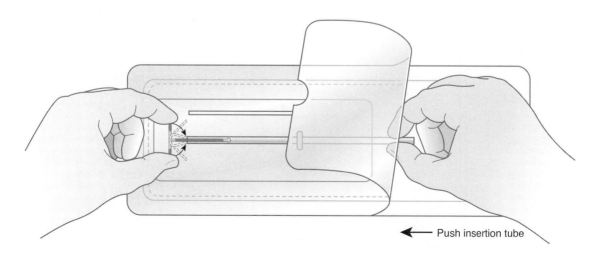

Figure 17B-14 Placement of arms of copper IUD into tubing through packaging.

7. The tenaculum stabilizes the cervix. This stabilization usually is accomplished by the nondominant hand holding the tenaculum as the loaded insertion tube is passed through the cervical canal guided by the dominant hand. When resistance is met at the uterine fundus, the flange should be at the external cervical os (**Figure 17B-17**).

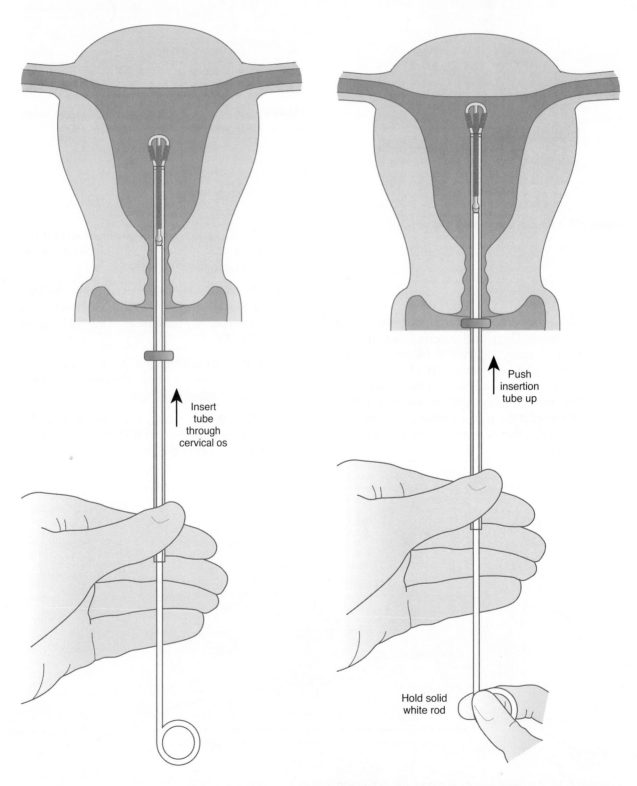

Figure 17B-16 Insertion of copper IUD and inserter through cervical os.

Figure 17B-17 Placement of copper IUD through inserter to fundus.

8. While the nondominant hand stabilizes the solid white rod, the insertion tubing is withdrawn with the clinician's other hand for a distance of approximately 1 cm. At this time the IUD is released from the inserter.

9. The insertion tube is gently advanced to ensure that the IUD is placed in the fundus (**Figure 17B-18**).

10. Gently, the insertion tubing is withdrawn (**Figure 17B-19**), and both the rod and the tubing are appropriately discarded.

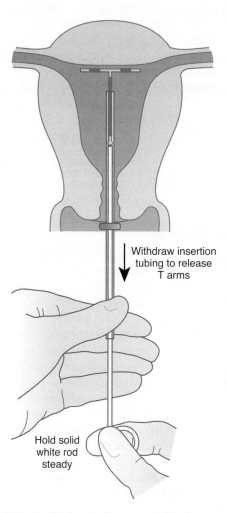

Figure 17B-18 Withdrawal of insertion tubing to release arms for copper IUD.

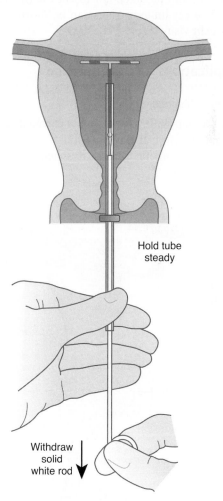

Figure 17B-19 Withdrawal of rod and insertion tubing for copper IUD.

Postinsertion Care for Any IUD

IUD threads or strings should be able to be visualized in the vagina after insertion is complete and the inserter materials removed. Threads are trimmed to a length of approximately 3 cm from the external os by the use of sharp scissors. If the woman is overweight or obese, she may need a longer length than 3 cm to assure that she can easily feel the strings. Caution should be taken not to cut the threads too short, whereas longer strings can be shortened at a subsequent visit (**Figure 17B-20**).

Complications of IUD Insertion

Vasovagal Response

A few women will experience a vasovagal reaction secondary to cervical manipulation. Common symptoms include syncope, vertigo, dyspnea, nausea, and

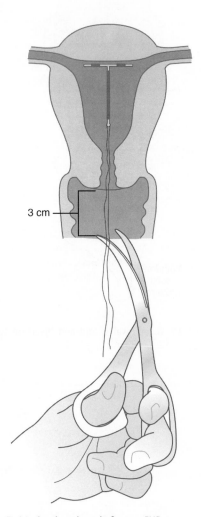

3 cm

Figure 17B-20 Cutting threads for any IUD.

diaphoresis. This response usually resolves spontaneously if the clinician stops any manipulation and waits for the resolution, colloquially termed "treatment with tincture of time." Usually insertion can be resumed without incident. It is rare that an IUD cannot be inserted due to a vasovagal reaction.

Uterine Perforation

Perforation of the uterus at the time of IUD insertion is always a risk, but it is rare with an incidence estimated at 0.4 per 1000 insertions. If uterine perforation occurs during placement of the IUD, the clinician may find that during fundal placement, the IUD continues to travel beyond the original uterine depth and the threads begin to travel upward. More often perforation is suspected within the first 6 months after insertion. When perforation is suspected, the IUD should be removed and the woman should be evaluated closely. Most perforations are small and require little treatment.[10,11] Any woman demonstrating symptoms of bleeding or shock should be transferred to an appropriate care facility for prompt treatment.

Missing IUD Strings

A woman who reports being unable to feel the threads should be advised to go to an ambulatory facility. In some cases, the threads may have curled behind the cervix and become difficult to palpate. A cotton-tipped applicator may be able to gently guide and straighten the strings—a technique often is called "fishing" for the strings. Care should be taken not to pull on the threads and dislodge the device. If the strings are not apparent to the clinician, it is possible that the device was spontaneously expelled and the woman was unaware of its loss. An ultrasound can identify whether the IUD is in situ. In the unusual situation of the IUD being in the fundus but the threads being unable to be felt, the woman needs to make an informed decision regarding whether she wishes to have the IUD removed and replaced or to continue as is. She should be reassured that contraceptive effectiveness is not dependent upon the threads extending from the uterus into the vagina.

Ectopic Pregnancy and the IUD

Although the rate of ectopic pregnancy is lower for women who use an IUD than for those who do not use any contraceptive method because of the overall contraceptive effectiveness of the device, IUDs are more effective in preventing intrauterine pregnancies than ectopic pregnancies. Therefore, a woman who is pregnant with an IUD in situ should be carefully assessed for the presence of an ectopic pregnancy.

Pregnancy with an IUD in Situ

When a woman using an IUD has an intrauterine pregnancy and wishes to continue the pregnancy, evidence suggests that removal of the IUD decreases the risk of adverse events, including miscarriage, when compared to retaining the device. This benefit is most apparent when the IUD is removed during the first 12 gestational weeks. The IUD is removed in the usual fashion as described later in this appendix.

Health Education

After insertion of an IUD, health education should include teaching the woman how to feel for and identify the threads in her vagina (**Figure 17B-21**). A sample IUD with strings she can feel may be used as a teaching aid. The woman can be cautioned to report any significant variations such as unusual lengthening of the strings, which may indicate non-fundal placement, or feeling any part of the plastic of the device, which suggests partial expulsion.

For the woman who is contraceptive naïve, most clinicians advise use of a secondary contraceptive method for a week after insertion while the IUD is becoming effective unless it is placed within the first week after menses. For women using a method such as an injectable contraceptive agent or COCs, those methods can be used until the usual timing of discontinuation. All women should be reminded that IUDs do not provide any protection from sexually transmitted infections.

An acronym, PAINS, often is shared with a woman as an easy reminder of potentially significant deviations that should be reported (**Table 17B-2**). In all cases, women should be encouraged to contact their provider with questions or concerns, although most women using an IUD do not have major side effects.

Among the most common side effects of all IUDs are menstrual irregularities. In some women, especially those using a copper IUD, dysmenorrhea or heavy bleeding may occur; the use of NSAIDs provides relief from either or both of these symptoms. Conversely, women using a LNG IUD may experience decreased menstrual flow or amenorrhea. However, sudden amenorrhea for any woman with an IUD suggests pregnancy, and she should be evaluated for this condition.

Follow-Up Care

Usually a subsequent visit is scheduled for a woman in 4 to 6 weeks after the IUD is inserted. At that time, any concerns she has can be addressed and a

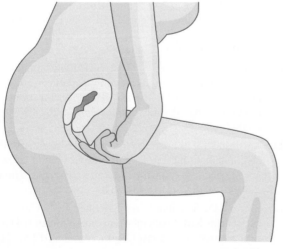

Figure 17B-21 How a woman feels for her IUD threads or strings.

Table 17B-2	PAINS Acronym for IUD Adverse Effects
	Comments
Period	Amenorrhea, especially sudden onset; with the copper IUD, may be associated with pregnancy. Light bleeding and amenorrhea are side effects of LNG IUDs.
Abdominal pain	General abdominal pain can suggest an ectopic pregnancy, sexually transmitted infection, or intolerance of copper.
Infection	Vaginal discharge, pelvic pain, history of exposure or any suspicion of sexually transmitted infections.
Not feeling well	Malaise, fever, nausea and vomiting suggesting infection or sepsis.
Strings	Strings or threads of the IUD changing in length or missing entirely.

speculum exam can be performed to confirm that the threads are visible. After the initial postinsertion visit, future appointments should be made based on other reasons such as the need for cervical cancer screening. The only other IUD-related visit should be at the time when the duration of the IUD expires (e.g., Skyla at 3 years); at that point, a new device can be inserted if desired by the woman.

Removal of an IUD

Common reasons expressed by women who request removal of their IUDs include desire for a pregnancy, unnecessary troublesome side effects of menstrual irregularities, establishment of menopause, or end of duration of effectiveness. Removal of an IUD is the same for any of the three IUDs.

Procedure for Removing an IUD

1. Removal of an IUD requires clean, but not sterile technique.

2. Removal is a rapid procedure. A visit in the office takes approximately the same amount of time as a visit for a Pap test.

3. Constant communication should occur between the clinician and the woman during the removal.

4. A woman is placed in a lithotomy or dorsal position of comfort and bimanual examination is performed to determine the position of the uterus. Then a speculum is inserted.

5. The IUD threads are visualized, and an instrument (e.g., sponge forceps) grasps the threads.

6. The IUD threads are guided downward toward the clinician until the IUD emerges through the cervix and vagina. Some women may feel a sharp cramp as the device passes the cervix, whereas others report no discomfort/ little sensation.

7. Most clinicians show the device to the woman to reassure her it has been removed.

8. The removal is now completed. If the woman wishes a new device, it can be immediately placed by following the procedure presented earlier in this appendix.

References

1. Grimes DA, Lopez LM, Schulz KF, Van Vliet HAAM, Stanwood NL. Immediate post-partum insertion of intrauterine devices. *Cochrane Database Syst Rev.* 2010;5:CD003036. doi: 10.1002/14651858. CD003036.pub2.

2. Grimes DA, Lopez LM, Schulz KF, Stanwood NL. Immediate postabortal insertion of intrauterine devices. *Cochrane Database Syst Rev.* 2010;6:CD001777. doi: 10.1002/14651858.CD001777.pub3.

3. Whiteman MK, Tyler CP, Folger SG, Gaffield ME, Curtis KM. When can a woman have an intrauterine device inserted? A systematic review. *Contraception.* 2013;87(5):666-673.

4. Sufrin CB, Postlethwaite D, Armstrong MA, Merchant M, Wendt JM, Steinauer JE. Neisseria gonorrhea and Chlamydia trachomatis screening at intrauterine device insertion and pelvic inflammatory disease. *Obstet Gynecol.* 2012;120(6):1314-1321.

5. Tepper NK, Steenland MW, Marchbanks PA, Curtis KM. Laboratory screening prior to initiating contraception: a systematic review. *Contraception.* 2013; 87(5):645-649.

6. Sääv I, Aronsson A, Marions L, Stephansson O, Gemzell-Danielsson K. Cervical priming with sublingual misoprostol prior to insertion of an intrauterine device in nulliparous women: a randomized controlled trial. *Hum Reprod.* 2007;22(10):2647-2652.

7. Edelman A, Schaefer E, Olson A, et al. Effects of prophylactic misoprostol administration prior to intrauterine device insertion in nulliparous women. *Contraception.* 2011;84(3):234-239.

8. Allen RH, Bartz D, Grimes DA, Hubacher D, O'Brien P. Interventions for pain with intrauterine device insertion. *Cochrane Database Syst Rev.* 2009;3:CD007373. doi: 10.1002/14651858.CD007373.pub2.

9. Grimes DA, Lopez LM, Schulz KF. Antibiotic prophylaxis for intrauterine contraceptive device insertion. *Cochrane Database Syst Rev.* 1999;3:CD001327. doi: 10.1002/14651858.CD001327.

10. Kaislasuo J, Suhonen S, Gissler M, Lähteenmäki P, Heikinheimo O. Intrauterine contraception: incidence and factors associated with uterine perforation: a population-based study. *Hum Reprod.* 2012;27(9): 2658-2663.

11. Kaislasuo J, Suhonen S, Gissler M, Lähteenmäki P, Heikinheimo O. Uterine perforation caused by intrauterine devices: clinical course and treatment. *Hum Reprod.* 2013;28(6):1546-1551.

12. Brahmi D, Steenland MW, Renner RM, Gaffield ME, Curtis KM. Pregnancy outcomes with an IUD in situ: a systematic review. *Contraception.* 2012;85(2): 131-139.

CHAPTER

18

Hormonal Contraception

MICHELLE R. COLLINS

SHARON L. HOLLEY

TONIA L. MOORE-DAVIS

DEBORAH L. NARRIGAN

MARY C. BRUCKER

Introduction

In 1960, Enovid, an agent combining estrogen and progesterone, became the first FDA-approved oral contraceptive—and thus began the story of modern hormonal contraception in the United States.[1] The "pill," as it came to be known colloquially, enabled women to make their own choices regarding pregnancy, when and if they desired.

Today's hormonal methods of contraception contain synthetic steroidal hormones, which act centrally, altering the functions of the pituitary gland and hypothalamus. Although it may seem counterintuitive that supplementing natural progesterone and estrogen with synthetic analogues of the same hormones can prevent ovulation and sperm transport, this remains the most common mechanism of action for these contraceptives.

Enovid was removed from the market several decades ago and replaced with agents with less hormones and have fewer side effects. Today, combination oral contraceptives (COCs) and progestin-only pills (POPs) remain a popular method of contraception. Non-oral hormonal formulations, including rings, patches, and subdermal implants, are also available. Currently intrauterine contraceptive devices impregnated with progesterone are available; they will also be discussed in this chapter. One of these agents, Mirena, is advertised as an intrauterine system (IUS) by its manufacturer; the other one, Skyla, uses the term intrauterine device (IUD) in its description. For clarity, IUD will be the abbreviation used throughout this chapter for both devices.

Evolution of Hormonal Methods

All current oral contraceptives are composed of either a combination of estrogen and progestin or a progestin alone. Most of the hormone-containing active pills are accompanied by inert pills for the last few days of a 28-day cycle, although in some packaging the non-active pills contain supplements such as iron or folic acid. For the last several decades, modifications of the types of the hormones and doses have been made in attempts to decrease risks while maintaining contraceptive effectiveness. Implants, because they are not user dependent, are more effective than oral agents and are gaining in popularity.

The Role of Estrogen

The primary action of estrogen in hormonal contraception is to stabilize the endometrium, thereby providing cycle control and minimizing breakthrough bleeding.[2] Estrogen also suppresses follicle-stimulating hormone (FSH) and inhibits development of a dominant follicle. Several pharmacologic formulations of estrogen exist. The major estrogen used in hormonal contraception is ethinyl estradiol (EE). Although popular in years past, mestranol is a less potent type of estrogen and now is found only in the few 50-microgram COCs that remain available in the United States.[3]

Metabolism of EE varies markedly among women; in turn, EE's side effects range from being nonexistent to a major discomfort. The most common side effects are headaches and nausea. More than 150 drugs have been suggested as agents having drug interactions with EE. Prominent among interacting drugs are the drugs metabolized by cytochrome P pathways. The drug interactions range from potentiating or inhibiting either estrogen or the other drug. Concomitant use of any pharmacologic agent should be individually evaluated. Nevertheless, drug interactions do not necessarily indicate that the contraceptive effect related to estrogen is diminished. Clinically relevant drug interactions are discussed later in the chapter.

Estrogen use does increase the risk for a few severe adverse effects. Notably, it is associated with an increased risk for deep vein thrombosis (DVT) and other thromboembolic events. Women who both smoke and are older than age 35 and who use estrogen are at a higher risk for myocardial infarction. Breast cancer is rare among premenopausal women; use of estrogen is associated with a slight increase in the risk of breast cancer in this group, especially among women already at higher than average risk. Because estrogen is not used alone for contraception purposes, it often is difficult to ascribe specific actions to the single agent. For example, some of the risks associated with contraceptives may be attributed to an undetermined synergy between estrogen and progestins.

The Role of Progestins

Progestins include both synthetic and natural progesterone. In contraceptive methods, progestins inhibit the release of luteinizing hormone (LH), preventing the LH surge necessary for ovulation. Additional mechanisms of action are theorized to include thickening of the cervical mucus and delayed sperm transport. Progestin-only agents lack the endometrial stabilization from estrogen, which increases irregular vaginal bleeding. Unlike estrogen, in which a single type (EE) is used almost exclusively for contraception, several types of progestins are prescribed. Progestins include estranes and gonanes that are derived from 19-nortestosterone as well as the first non-testosterone agent drospirenone, as illustrated in **Figure 18-1**.

Common side effects of progestins include acne and premenstrual-type symptoms such as edema, breast tenderness, and transient depression, which is usually mild. An increased risk of DVT may be associated with certain progestins. The incidence of DVT is increased among women who take COCs containing desogestrel, norgestimate, or gestodene as compared to women who take COCs with levonorgestrel or any of the estranes. Some studies have suggested that progestins also are associated with increasing

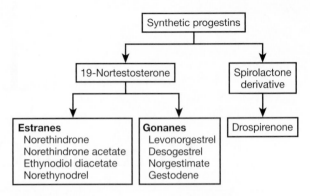

Figure 18-1 Progestins used for contraception.

the risk of breast cancer, although these studies were primarily conducted among perimenopausal/postmenopausal women. Relationships between progestins and cardiovascular risk and bone health continue to be studied.

The Search for New Methods

It has been estimated that 1 million pregnancies occur annually among women who say they are taking oral contraceptives, many because of inconsistent use. More than 50% of women using COCs miss two or more pills during the second month they use them.[4] This statistic illustrates how difficult it may be for women consistently to take a daily pill. Methods that are less dependent upon daily user action are more effective contraceptives. Therefore, the focus in contraception recently has shifted to development of alternative routes for delivery of hormones. Newer novel approaches include hormonal transdermal patches, IUDs, subdermal implants, and injectable options. Contraceptive options beyond the oral formulations offer women a wider variety of choices in hormone delivery method and duration of action. Non-oral methods are also lower maintenance. This chapter reviews hormonal methods and will classify each method as either a short-acting reversible contraceptive (SARC) or a long-acting reversible contraceptive (LARC).

Hormonal Contraceptives: General Considerations

LARCs and SARCs

Hormonal contraceptives are among the most commonly used forms of birth control in the United States. In contrast to nonhormonal contraceptives, which tend to be both coital and user dependent, hormonal contraceptives are remote from sexual activity. Nevertheless, the effectiveness of some of the hormonal methods such as oral contraceptives, rings, and patches does depend on a woman using them consistently and correctly. These methods are categorized as short-acting reversible contraceptives. Most failures with these hormonal methods are associated with user error, and the perfect use rate is considerably higher than the typical use rate. Depot medroxyprogesterone acetate (DMPA), a contraceptive injection, is considered a SARC because the user must regularly return to a provider for injections. By comparison, long-acting reversible contraceptives, such as IUDs and implants, require a visit for placement, but are neither coital nor user dependent; thus their typical use rates are similar to their perfect use rates.

Effectiveness

Hormonal contraceptives are the most effective method of reversible contraception. **Table 18-1** summarizes the effectiveness of the hormonal methods, with the most effective one listed first.[5] Because of their lack of dependency upon user actions, it is not surprising that LARCs are more effective than SARCs.

Return to Fertility

For most hormonal methods, including LARCs, return to fertility is relatively rapid, rarely taking more than a few months.[6] The exception is DMPA, for which an average of 9 months usually passes after the last injection before normal fertility resumes. **Table 18-2** lists the length of time for the average woman to attain fertility after discontinuation of specific hormonal methods.[5,7]

Table 18-2	Average Length of Time for Return to Fertility After Discontinuation of Contraceptive Method
Contraceptive Method	**Average Length of Time for Return to Fertility**
Combination oral contraceptives	1–3 months
Progestin-only pills	1–3 months
Transdermal patch	1–3 months
Contraceptive ring	1 week–1 month
Contraceptive injections	9 months after last injection
Levonorgestrel IUD	Immediately upon removal
Subdermal implants*	1–3 weeks after removal

*Based on studies of Implanon. It is anticipated that Nexplanon will have similar effectiveness.

Sources: Adapted from Trussell J, Guthrie KA. Choosing a contraceptive: efficacy, safety and personal considerations. In: Hatcher RA, Trussell J, Nelson AL, Cates W, Kowal D, Policar MS. *Contraceptive Technology.* New York: Ardent Media; 2011:45-75; Sibai B, Odlind V, Meador M, Shangold G, Fisher A, Creasy G. A comparative and pooled analysis of the safety and tolerability of the contraceptive patch (Ortho Evra/Evra). *Fertil Steril.* 2002;77(2):S19-S26.

Noncontraceptive Benefits

Discussion of hormonal contraceptives often focuses on side effects and adverse effects associated with their use. Most of the side effects are minor, and the adverse effects are rare. However, a number of noncontraceptive benefits also are associated with these agents, as described in **Box 18-1**. Women should be equally counseled about the noncontraceptive

Table 18-1	Effectiveness of Hormonal Contraceptive Methods	
Contraceptive Method	**Type of Method**	**Percentage of Women Experiencing an Unintentional Pregnancy During the First Year of Use**
Combination oral contraceptives Progestin-only pills	SARC	9
Transdermal patch	SARC	9
Contraceptive ring	SARC	9
Contraceptive injections	SARC	6
Levonorgestrel IUD	LARC	0.2
Subdermal implants*	LARC	0.05

SARC = short-acting reversible contraceptive; LARC = long-acting reversible contraceptive.

*Based on studies of Implanon. It is anticipated that Nexplanon will have similar effectiveness.

Source: Adapted from Trussell J, Guthrie KA. Choosing a contraceptive: efficacy, safety and personal considerations. In: Hatcher RA, Trussell J, Nelson AL, Cates W, Kowal D, Policar MS. *Contraceptive Technology.* New York: Ardent Media; 2011:45-75.

BOX 18-1 Noncontraceptive Benefits of Hormonal Contraceptives

- Reduction of menstrual-associated conditions
  - Dysmenorrhea
  - Heavy menstrual flow
  - Irregularity
  - Menstrual migraines
  - Perimenopausal symptoms
    (e.g., hot flashes)
  - Premenstrual syndrome
- Treatment of bleeding associated with fibroids
- Treatment of pelvic pain associated
  with endometriosis
- Treatment of acne
- Decrease in the risk of the following conditions:
  - Colorectal cancer
  - Endometrial cancer
  - Hirsutism
  - Osteoporosis
  - Ovarian cancer
- Lifestyle (drug-induced) amenorrhea

Source: Adapted from American College of Obstetricians and Gynecologists (ACOG). Noncontraceptive uses of hormonal contraceptives. Practice Bulletin No. 110. *Obstet Gynecol.* 2010;115:206-218.

---

benefits of these products, just as they are counseled about their untoward effects.[8]

Drug Interactions

Millions of women in the United States use hormonal methods to prevent pregnancy. When one drug is used at the same time as another, several phenomena can occur. The effect of one or both of the agents can be potentiated; one or both can be inhibited; one can be inhibited and the other potentiated; or nothing clinically relevant can occur. Most of these effects occur because the same liver enzymes metabolize the two drugs and one or the other drug alters function of enzymes that metabolize one of the drugs. Many drug interactions are associated with pharmacologic agents that are liver enzyme inducers (i.e., they potentiate the effect of the liver enzyme, which leads to rapid metabolism of the other drug). Even so, several agents have been found to be liver enzyme inducers that have no known effect on contraceptive effectiveness.

Fortunately, most of the drugs that decrease contraceptive effectiveness are not commonly used by healthy women, and the majority of drug interactions

occur with oral (rather than non-oral) contraceptives. Nevertheless, the midwife should be particularly alert for potential interactions if a woman is taking medications to treat tuberculosis, a seizure disorder, a clotting disorder, HIV, or mild depression. Among the drugs that have been suggested to decrease the effectiveness of contraceptives are anti-infectives (specifically rifampin [Rifadin]), anticonvulsants (e.g., carbamazepine [Tegretol], phenytoin [Dilantin], phenobarbital [Luminal]), antifungals (specifically griseofulvin [Fulvicin]), protease inhibitors (e.g., saquinavir [Invirase], ritonavir [Norvir]), and non-nucleoside reverse transcriptase inhibitors (e.g., efavirenz [Sustiva], nevirapine [Viramune]).[9] St. John's wort—a nutritional supplement used to treat individuals with mild depression—also has been found to decrease hormonal contraceptive effectiveness. Women should be advised that taking oral contraceptives at the same time they use an over-the-counter antacid (e.g., Maalox, Mylanta) can decrease contraceptive effectiveness due to impaired absorption of the hormones.

Several of these agents also have been suggested to affect the effectiveness of POPs—specifically, rifampin, anticoagulants, antiretrovirals, and St. John's wort. It is noteworthy that the majority of these drug interactions are associated with breakthrough bleeding and not necessarily pregnancies, but a secondary method should be recommended for women using any of the aforementioned agents. Finally, anticoagulants may impair steroid metabolism and increase the side effects of oral contraceptives.

Pharmacogenomics also may be involved in drug interactions with contraceptives, and more information is needed in this area. A good practice is always to obtain a complete history from a woman regarding medications (both prescribed and over-the-counter agents), botanicals, and nutritional supplements and to verify whether any potential drug interaction exists, especially because this information can change rapidly. Several electronic resources exist to quickly provide this information to the provider in clinical practice.

Contraindications to Use of Hormonal Contraceptives

Although most women can use hormonal contraceptives, there are some situations in which the agents are not recommended or are even contraindicated. Contraindications to hormonal contraceptive use are primarily contraindications to estrogen, progestins, or both, and include—most notably—breast cancer and pregnancy. The list of contraindications to estrogen is longer than the list of contraindications to use of progestins. For example, women with a history of cardiovascular disease or coagulopathies should not use estrogen-containing products. Women seeking to use hormonal contraceptives should always be screened for the presence of any contraindications first; if any are present, alternative contraceptive methods should be discussed and recommended. The United States Medical Eligibility Criteria for Contraceptive Use (U.S. MEC), which is summarized in the *Family Planning* chapter, includes specific contraceptive eligibility guidelines for women who have many disorders and medical conditions.[10] The U.S. MEC is also available as an application for smartphones, and on the Centers for Disease Control and Prevention (CDC) website.

Midwifery Management for Women Using Hormonal Contraceptives

It should be clear to the reader that hormonal contraceptives have significant benefits and rare, but serious, complications. Thus shared decision-making and a careful cost/benefit assessment is the essential first step prior to prescribing any hormonal contraception. This section reviews clinical considerations and midwifery management steps that apply to all hormonal contraceptives. **Box 18-2** summarizes the components of midwifery management for any woman initiating or changing a contraceptive method.

Limitations of Clinical Trials

In general, most clinical trials of contraceptive methods are placebo controlled; that is, these studies explore the risk of use of an agent compared to any risk with use of a placebo. One of the challenges in the study of hormonal contraceptives is that ethics precludes such experimentation. Therefore, the majority of studies lack the rigor of randomized controlled trials. In addition, contraceptive clinical trials generally focus on healthy women and usually exclude adolescents, women with preexisting conditions, and even women who are outside the normal parameters for weight. As a result, application of data from studies

---

BOX 18-2 Midwifery Management When Caring for Women Initiating or Changing a Hormonal Contraceptive Method

- Obtain reasonable assurance that the woman is not pregnant:
  - Negative pregnancy test/no unprotected sexual intercourse in last 2 weeks
  - Current reliable use of other hormonal method or discontinuation within last 7 days
  - Last normal menstrual period within last 5 days
- Verify that the method to be initiated is one she desires and is likely to be used correctly. Because hormonal methods influence menstrual flow, it is wise to explore her feelings about decreased flow, irregular bleeding, and amenorrhea.
- Assure that no contraindications exist for the chosen method.
  - If the method is Category 3 according to the U.S. Medical Eligibility Criteria, discuss both risks and benefits with the woman so she can make an informed choice.
- Verify she is not taking drugs likely to interact with hormonal contraceptives.
- Review the following points:
  - For all women using hormonal contraceptives:
    - Signs or symptoms indicating serious complications (danger or warning signs)
    - Common side effects
    - Effect on menstrual flow

- Noncontraceptive benefits
- Average time for return to fertility
- Lack of protection from sexually transmitted infections
- Date and time for follow-up appointment
- Health promotion or screening activities as appropriate, separate from contraceptive needs
  - For women using a short-acting reversible contraceptive (e.g., daily pills, weekly patch) that are woman dependent, also include:
    - When and how to initiate the method
    - Back-up or secondary protection for 1 week (and additional supplies for occasional use if needed)
    - How to use the method correctly and continuously
    - Common mistakes to avoid
    - What to do if she fails to use the method correctly (e.g., missed pills)
    - Safe disposal of used contraceptives and packages
    - Specific information regarding prescriptions, including when to be renewed and general cost
- Provide opportunities for the woman to ask questions.

to everyday clinical practice becomes challenging. Because the participants in clinical trials are healthy women, some risks may not become apparent until large postmarketing populations adopt the methods. The U.S. MEC, as found in the *Family Planning* chapter, provide guidelines for use of the different hormonal methods based on clinical trials as well as national and international studies.[10] In 2013, the Centers for Disease Control and Prevention published a set of recommendations on a select of common issues regarding use of contraceptives as a companion to the U.S. MEC.[11]

The first step is assisting the woman to put her personal risk into context. For example, a woman may decide that the benefits in terms of the reliability and effectiveness of a hormonal method for preventing pregnancy outweigh a relatively minor increase in risk for a specific condition. Consideration of risk of a condition also should be viewed in light of risk of pregnancy with a less reliable method. For example, even when the risk of DVT is known to increase with a specific hormonal method, that risk remains less than the risk of developing DVT during pregnancy.

Initiation of Method

For decades, midwives and other providers delayed initiation of a hormonal contraceptive method until after a woman's next menstrual period to reassure both the provider and the woman that the woman was not pregnant. Timing in tandem with a menstrual period also represented an attempt to minimize breakthrough bleeding, although this has not been proven. Some providers advocated starting a method on the first day of menses, others within 5 days of a menses, and yet others within a week of menses. For years, many clinicians advised women to start oral contraceptives on the Sunday after a menses started. This method was promoted as a strategy to prevent subsequent menses beginning on a weekend. Although all these methods of initiation were based on opinion and not evidence, they continue to be used in some practices today.

Quick Start or Same-Day Start

In 2002, a study was published advocating a new initiation method called *Quick Start*. Quick Start is the term used to describe an initiation method wherein the woman begins taking oral contraceptives as soon as she gets them, regardless of where she is in her menstrual cycle. A pregnancy test is done at the time the contraceptive is prescribed to ensure that she is not pregnant. The original Quick Start technique had the woman take the first pill in the office when the pills were prescribed.

Quick Start was developed in response to consumer desires. As many as 25% of women who were provided with a prescription for contraceptive pills never had it filled, often using another, less reliable method or no method of contraception at all.[12,13] Women were found to be more satisfied when they were able to obtain the contraceptive method they desired in a timely manner. In addition, waiting for a menses is a questionable practice often deemed unnecessary because of the improved reliability of pregnancy tests. Even in the rare event that a woman is pregnant and is inadvertently exposed to contraceptive hormones, there is no evidence of an increase in the risk of miscarriage or any teratogenic effects from hormonal contraceptives. Quick Start was also initially promoted as a way to ensure longer continuation rates when compared to traditional approaches, although this was not shown to be a significant advantage in typical use.[14]

The Quick Start practice has since expanded from its first use at the time oral contraceptives are dispensed.[15] Studies suggest it can be used for initiation of patches, rings, and injections as well as pills.[16,17] **Figure 18-2** provides an algorithm for Quick Start and various other hormonal methods.[18]

In general, regardless of when a woman begins a hormonal method, there should be some reasonable

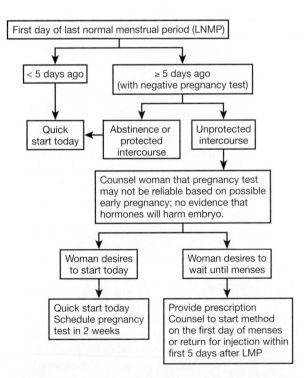

Figure 18-2 Quick start for pills, patches, rings, and injections.
Source: Adapted from Quick Start Algorithm, www.rhedi.org. Used by permission of RHEDI/Center for Reproductive Health Education in Family Medicine, Montefiore Medical Center, New York City, 2007.

assurance that she is not pregnant. This assurance can take the form of a normal menses within the last 5 days, a negative pregnancy test, or history indicating that she has not had sexual intercourse since her last menses. Upon initiation of a hormone-based contraceptive method, most women are advised to use a back-up or secondary method until the plasma level of hormone is such that ovulation is suppressed.

Use of Back-up Methods

Evidence regarding the optimal duration of use of back-up contraception is lacking, and most guidelines are empirical. Years ago, it was not uncommon to recommend back-up use for a full month after initiation of COCs. Today, a week is more common. Similarly, back-up recommendations for missed pills or patches are not based on scientific studies, but instead represent common clinical practice with extrapolation from some pharmacologic studies.

The suggested back-up method also varies. Some midwives recommend condoms as the back-up, whereas others recommend condoms combined with another spermicidal methods such as foam or film. Women who are comfortable with a diaphragm may choose to use that method. As usual, the choice should be based on considerations outlined in the *Family Planning* chapter and individualized to the woman's needs and desires.

Side Effects

Menstrual Irregularities

Managing the care of a woman experiencing the side effects of any contraceptive is a key role that a midwife can assume to help women optimally use the method.[9] Studies regarding contraceptive use reveal that side effects are the primary reason that the majority of women discontinue their hormonal contraceptive.[5] These studies indicate that in addition to counseling women about potential side effects, it is important to include in health education the caveats that not all women will experience these side effects, and that not all discomforts or health concerns experienced while using hormonal contraception will be related to the contraceptive method being used.

Unusual menstrual bleeding may be viewed as either an advantage or a disadvantage. Lighter menses generally are well received by most women. Many women are comfortable with amenorrhea, while others are not.[19] The majority of women find unpredictable or breakthrough bleeding at least a nuisance.

Originally women were counseled that breakthrough bleeding might occur during the first 3 months of use of a hormonal method. However, especially with use of modern low-dose pills, such bleeding may continue for as long as 6 months. Progestin-only methods are more likely than COCs to be associated with irregular bleeding and even amenorrhea. Strong evidence has not yet emerged regarding how to manage hormone-associated bleeding. Most individuals base their practice in this area on observation or expert opinions. **Figure 18-3** provides a sample algorithm for basic management of a woman with problematic irregular bleeding.[20] The pharmacologic treatments included in the algorithm are based on common clinical practices and should not be accepted as evidence based, and most medications provide temporary relief at best.

Headaches

Many women have mild occasional headaches, usually associated with tension or allergies. However, for some women, headaches can be disabling and may even herald a severe adverse effect such as a cerebral vascular accident. Some contraceptive methods are associated with an increase in the incidence of headaches, such that the midwife is faced with the perplexing problem of identifying whether the headache is minor or signals a significant medical problem. If a woman presents with neurovascular symptoms such as flashing lights, loss of vision, muscle weakness, slurred speech, dizziness, or abnormal cranial nerve changes as well as a headache, these symptoms are a medical emergency and the woman requires immediate care to rule out a stroke. She also should discontinue the hormonal contraceptive method as quickly as possible and be counseled to use a nonhormonal method until the neurologic condition is resolved. For women who have headaches but no neurologic symptoms, and for whom no abnormalities are found upon examination, the midwife may consider alternative hormonal therapies. For example, often women using COCs have mild headaches during the withdrawal period and might benefit from an extended-cycle method.

Nausea

Nausea is a common side effect reported by women using any medication, but is more likely with oral agents and patch contraceptives. There is no simple remedy. No one type of COCs or POPs is superior to another for mitigating nausea. Ultimately, if the nausea and vomiting prove onerous for her, the woman may be forced to seek another contraceptive method, especially the ring or a LARC.[21]

If the nausea is mild but problematic, several suggestions for its management may be made, although evidence is lacking regarding effectiveness. Among

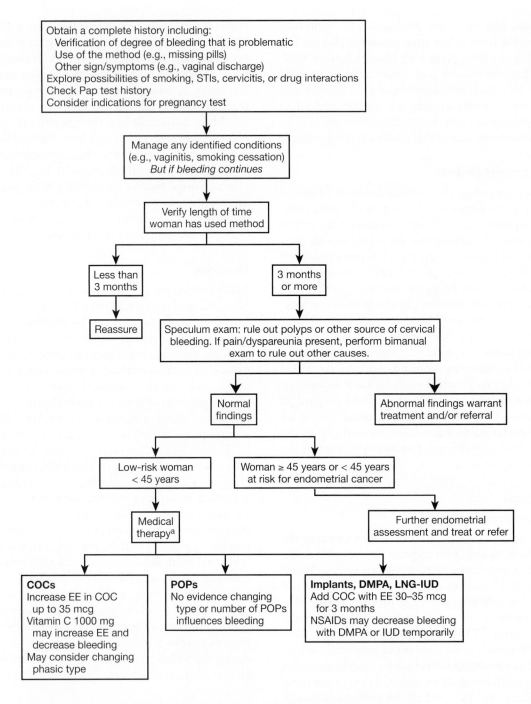

COCs = combination oral contraceptives; DMPA = depot medroxyprogesterone acetate;
LNG-IUD = levonorgestrel intrauterine device; POPs = progestin-only contraceptives.

aMedical therapy is primarily based on expert opinion and common practice. Little strong
    evidence exists in this area.

Figure 18-3 Sample algorithm for management of women with hormone-associated breakthrough bleeding.
Source: Reproduced from Faculty of Sexual and Reproductive Healthcare Clinical Effectiveness Unit in collaboration with RCOG. *Management of Unscheduled Bleeding in Women using Hormonal Contraception.* London: RCOG; 2009, with the permission of the Royal College of Obstetricians and Gynaecologists on the behalf of the FSRH.

the most common empirical management strategies for women experiencing nausea with oral contraceptives are to take the pill before sleep and to avoid ingesting it on an empty stomach. Ginger often is suggested as a food with antinausea effects.

Weight Gain

No evidence exists that hormonal contraceptive methods cause consistent weight gain in general.[22,23] Certain groups of women, such as adolescents, especially if they are overweight prior to DMPA use, may be more likely to gain weight while using the progestin-only DMPA, as are adult women who are either of normal weight or overweight. Conversely, adult women who are obese are less likely to gain weight when using DMPA.[24] Adolescents who experience a weight gain of more than 5% of total body weight after 6 months of DMPA use are at risk for continued excessive weight gain; therefore counseling about food intake and regular exercise should be performed. For any woman, if the weight gain becomes excessive, she should consider alternative methods of contraception if she is unable to control her weight through diet and exercise.

Clinical Challenges

Caring for the Woman Who Is Obese

Obesity currently has been characterized as an epidemic. Some evidence has been published suggesting that hormonal contraception—particularly pills, patches, and implants—may be less effective among women who are obese compared to their thinner counterparts. However, conflicting study findings exist. Body weight may be more important than body mass index (BMI) calculations, perhaps indicating a metabolic effect associated with the amount of adiposity, circulating volume of blood, or increased metabolic rate found among women who are obese. Additional research is needed in this area.

Studies of women using oral contraceptives suggest that women weighing more than 70 kg (154 pounds) may be at an increased risk of contraceptive failure, although this is not a current contraindication for use.[25] Women who desire to use the patch should be informed that a body weight of 90 kg (198 pounds) or more is considered a concern with the method, because premarket clinical trials found a higher risk of pregnancy in women in this weight group, even though they were not obese according to their BMI.[26]

Based on studies of serum concentration of etonogestrel, women who are 130% of ideal body weight may be at risk for decreased contraceptive effectiveness when using subdermal implants, although studies have not found such a decrease in clinical practice.[27] Even if hormonal methods are less effective for this population of women, they remain, along with the copper IUD (ParaGard), the most effective reversible methods of contraception. Prevention of pregnancy is a major consideration for women who are obese, as an emerging body of literature has demonstrated the hazards for both the woman and her fetus/newborn when a woman becomes pregnant while obese.[28] Contraception can provide these women with time to lose weight and become healthier in anticipation of a planned pregnancy if and when they desire one.

Caring for the Woman Who Is in Perimenopause

Age is not a contraindication for use of hormonal methods. The exception is prescription of estrogen-containing pills for the woman who smokes and is 35 years of age or older. This woman has a risk of myocardial infarction far greater than her nonsmoking counterpart.

Healthy women in their 40s continue to be sexually active and fertile, even if the degree of fertility is less than when they were younger.[29] An early perimenopausal symptom is irregular menses, often lulling women into the assumption that they are not ovulating and, therefore, not at risk of pregnancy. Yet escape ovulation and a subsequent pregnancy can occur unpredictably. Women who are older than 40 years account for a large percentage of the elective abortions performed following unintentional pregnancies. Therefore, these women need effective contraception. Many of them may opt for permanent sterilization, but others could benefit from hormonal methods. COCs can provide relief from many perimenopausal discomforts such as irregular bleeding, hot flashes, and dyspareunia. The levonorgestrel IUD (LNG-IUD) has an FDA indication as a therapy for menorrhagia or heavy menses. Other contraceptive methods associated with amenorrhea also may be of value for perimenopausal women, although there is some controversy regarding use of DMPA for this population because of a potential decrease in bone mass density immediately prior to entering the postmenopausal period, a time during which bone loss is more likely.

For the woman who is in the perimenopausal period, hormonal methods usually mask menopause because of the changes in bleeding patterns. There is no evidence to guide the midwife when it is best to discontinue a hormonal method; however, many clinicians discontinue the hormone contraceptive method when a woman is 55 years old.[30] At that time, essentially all woman naturally are postmenopausal. If desired, a woman at that time may consider hormone therapy. It is important to note that the hormone therapy used to treat perimenopausal symptoms, albeit usually the same steroid hormones of estrogen and progesterone, is not of sufficient potency to provide contraceptive effectiveness.

Short-Acting Reversible Contraceptives

Short-acting reversible hormonal methods include tablets (pills), injectable agents, transdermal patches, and intravaginal rings that contain either estrogen and a progestin or only a progestin.[31] Once initiated, the duration of action of these methods can range from a single day to as long as 12 weeks. The primary mechanism of action for all combined hormonal methods is similar. Advantages of these methods include high rates of effectiveness, relative ease of use, and reduction in dysmenorrhea. Disadvantages include the woman's need to take a daily pill/weekly patch or ring, a continued expense, and lack of protection against STI transmission. Hormonal methods also can cause side effects and have risks of serious adverse reactions, as noted earlier in this chapter.

Combination Oral Contraceptives

The main variations among the formulations of the combination pill relate to the hormonal dose, the relative proportions of estrogen and progestin, and the particular progestin component used. The result is a wide variety of pills, each with a different side-effect profile. COCs often are identified according to one of three regimens: monophasic, multiphasic, or extended cycle.

Monophasic

The pills in the monophasic regimen come in packs of either 21 or 24 pills that are identical every day in terms of the amount and type of estrogen and progestin. The packs also include either 7 or 4 placebo pills, respectively. One pill is taken each day for a total of 28 days, and then a new pack is begun. Although monophasic COCs have been marketed for decades, the newer regimen of 24 active pills and 4 placebo tablets shortens the duration of withdrawal bleeding and increases effectiveness.[32,33]

Multiphasic

The hormone-containing pills in this pack vary in amount of estrogen and/or progestin provided during particular weeks of the cycle of pills and also include either 4 or 7 days of placebo pills. Multiphasic regimens often are referred to as biphasic when two different combinations of estrogen and progestin are provided, or triphasic when the pack has three different combinations or doses.

Extended Cycle

The newest regimen also includes hormone and placebo pills, but the hormone pills are taken daily for three consecutive months instead of monthly. For example, in one type of extended-cycle COC, known as Seasonale, the pack includes 84 active hormone pills and 7 placebos. This extended regimen results in menstrual suppression as evidenced by a decreased frequency of withdrawal bleeding and potential amenorrhea. Some of the extended-cycle regimens use pills that contain a reduced dose of ethinyl estradiol instead of placebos, in an attempt to decrease dysmenorrhea and other menstrual-related symptoms.[34]

Dynamics of the Oral Contraceptive Method

COCs produce a pharmacologic, rather than a physiologic, cycle. When the placebo pills are taken, the exogenous estrogen and progestin are "withdrawn" and endometrial wall shedding takes place. This bleeding is sometimes called a "pseudo-menstruation," but the more common term is "withdrawal bleeding," although most women will characterize it as a "period." Typically this bleeding is scant and of shorter duration when compared to a woman's menses associated with normal physiologic events.

Special Considerations

Adolescents can safely use COCs but often discontinue their use if they experience side effects such as nausea; adolescents may also find taking a daily pill more challenging than older women.[35] Counseling about common side effects, strategies to enhance regular use of the agents such as taking the pill before sleep, and emergency contraception generally are included in care.

For women who recently have given birth, use of COCs postpartum should be delayed until at least 4 weeks after the birth because of the increased risk for venous thrombosis resulting from the hypercoagulable state during pregnancy and the early postpartum period. In addition, according to the U.S. Medical Eligibility Criteria for Contraceptive Use, breastfeeding women need to postpone initiating use of COCs until 4 weeks postpartum to allow lactation to be established.[10] For women who are perimenopausal, COCs can safely be used by nonsmokers.

Midwifery Management Plan

Midwifery management for women requesting to use COCs begins with a thorough health history (family, medical, and reproductive) to determine any contraindications to use of this method. If the woman is a candidate for COCs, the next steps include reviewing previous contraceptive methods used, explaining how COCs work, outlining their health benefits, and reviewing self-administration guidelines, side effects, steps to take if a pill is missed, and signs of adverse conditions (colloquially known as warning signs or danger signs). It is also common to advise a new user about use of a secondary contraceptive method such as condoms as a back-up during the first week of COC use, and to consider prescribing emergency contraception in case the COCs are discontinued and emergency contraception is needed. Physical examination, at a minimum, should include blood pressure and weight.

When selecting the specific COC, the lowest dose of estrogen possible should be chosen to minimize risks and side effects. A woman's past experience with oral contraceptives and the cost of the regimen also should be considered. As a practical matter, some midwives attempt to prescribe the same COC for sisters or women in the same family as long as there are no contraindications. Prescribing four to six cycles for a new user with a return visit to assess the woman's concerns with the method is recommended but may not be needed for all users. **Figure 18-4** provides a guide that can be used to counsel women about missed pills. The majority of women, even when using an extended-cycle regimen, will resume normal ovulatory function within 90 days or 3 months of taking the last COC. For years, women have been advised to postpone pregnancy until after 3 months to ensure credible dating of a pregnancy. However, there is no evidence that earlier conception is associated with untoward perinatal outcomes. **Box 18-3** lists content that specifically should be emphasized when counseling women using COCs in addition to the health education reviewed for any hormonal contraception (Box 18-2).

Progestin-Only Pills

Progestin-only pills contain a low dose of a single progestin and, therefore, can be used by women who want to use hormone-containing contraceptive pills but for whom estrogen is contraindicated. Originally FDA approved in the early 1970s, these agents tend to occupy a niche market for women who are breastfeeding or unable to use estrogen. Although some individuals have called these agents "mini-pills," use of that term can be confusing for women and providers alike because of the number of low-dose COCs available. Therefore, "progestin-only pills" is the

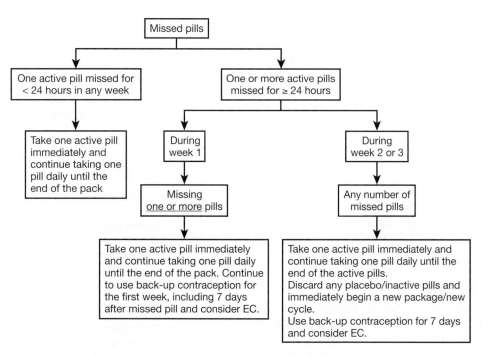

EC = emergency contraception.

Figure 18-4 Algorithm for counseling women who have missed pills (COCs or POPs).

preferred term. Currently three POPs are available; two contain 0.35 mcg of norethindrone (Micronor, Nor-QD and generics) in each of the active pills, and the other contains 0.075 mcg of norgestrel (Ovrette).

Mechanism of Action

In addition to the other mechanisms of action of progestins, POPs cause thinning of the endometrium, resulting in an inhospitable environment for implantation of a fertilized ovum. Because the progesterone dose is low, risk of pregnancy is higher for the average woman using POPs as compared to COCs. To minimize risk of pregnancy, the daily dose must be taken at the same time each day to maintain a steady state plasma level of the progestin. If more than 24 hours elapses between doses, the plasma level falls and escape ovulation can occur, allowing possible pregnancy if sexual intercourse takes place during that interval.

Special Considerations

Although women who are breastfeeding often use POPs, there is conflicting information regarding the amount of progesterone transmitted to breast milk. POPs have not been associated with an increased risk of DVT.

Midwifery Management Plan

While the management plan for women choosing to initiate progestin-only pills is the same as that for women using COCs, two points should be emphasized. The regularity of the daily dose is unforgiving with POPs; that is, women must take the pills at 24-hour intervals with no more than 3 hours of

variation. Second, irregular spotting and bleeding are expected, not simply possible.

Box 18-4 lists education topics to be emphasized for the woman regarding progestin-only pill use in addition to the health education required for women using any type of hormonal contraception (Box 18-2). Prescribing 4 months of POPs with a follow-up appointment with the woman in 3 months allows assessment of method satisfaction and review of her experience with side effects, including bleeding irregularities, and her willingness to cope with them. Similar to using COCs, the majority of women using POPs resume ovulatory function within 90 days or 3 months after discontinuing this contraceptive method.

While it is not unusual for women using POPs to have irregular bleeding and amenorrhea, if more than 45 days elapse without any vaginal withdrawal bleeding, the woman should be evaluated for possible pregnancy. If the woman experiences severe abdominal pain, she will need to be evaluated emergently for possible ovarian cyst, ectopic pregnancy, or pelvic inflammatory disease.

Transdermal Contraception (The Patch)

Currently, only one transdermal delivery system for contraception is available in the United States. Ortho Evra was FDA approved in 2002 and is a medicated, adhesive patch with a surface contact area os 20 cm². The patch is composed of a thin, lightweight polyester material and constructed in three layers. The outer surface of the patch, called a backing layer, consists of a flexible, beige polyester film and serves as a protective covering. The patch's middle layer contains both the adhesive component and active drug compounds. A third layer of clear polyethylene film protects the adhesive layer during storage and is removed prior to use.

The contraceptive patch is a combined hormonal method of contraception containing 6 mg norelgestromin and 0.75 mg ethinyl estradiol. Norelgestromin is the primary active metabolite of norgestimate, a progestin commonly used in formulations of some oral contraceptives.

Mechanism of Action

The primary mechanism of action for the contraceptive patch is similar to that of COCs. The transdermal absorption of exogenous estrogen and progestin inhibits ovulation by suppression of gonadotropins within the hypothalamic–pituitary–ovarian axis. Alterations in cervical mucus and endometrial lining are secondary mechanisms of contraceptive action. The active drug is absorbed through the skin, thereby avoiding a first-pass effect through the liver. This route therefore can decrease the total dose of exogenous hormones delivered as compared to oral contraceptive methods.

The contraceptive patch is self-applied by the woman. Each patch is impregnated with hormones that are adequate for approximately 1 week. To mimic the normal 28-day menstrual cycle, a single contraceptive patch is applied for 7 days and then immediately replaced with a new patch. Three patches are used in a month, resulting in 21 consecutive days of hormone exposure. The fourth week is a patch-free week, and a withdrawal bleed is expected following that interval. The contraceptive cycle is restarted with the application of a new patch immediately following the 7-day patch-free week.

Four application sites have been approved for use with Ortho Evra and studied for their therapeutic effectiveness: the buttocks, the upper outer arm, the abdomen, and the upper torso. The area of the breasts is to be excluded, not because of known problems, but because of general concerns about breast tissue being exposed to hormones. Application of the patch to each of these sites has demonstrated therapeutic equivalence by releasing 150 mcg of norelgestromin and 20 mcg of ethinyl estradiol into the bloodstream daily. To avoid problems with adherence/effectiveness, patches should be applied to clean, dry skin and women should be counseled

to avoid areas that have been recently exposed to perfumes, gels, lotions, shampoos, and other topical products unless they clean and dry the skin first. In clinical trials, increased body weight was associated with higher rates of unintended pregnancy, especially among women who weighed 90 kg (198 pounds) or more, leading the FDA to issue a statement that the patch may be less effective for women who weigh 198 pounds or more.[36]

Situations in which the transdermal delivery of the active drugs is disrupted (e.g., partial detachment) can result in decreased effectiveness. However, the adhesive component of the contraceptive patch is not affected by heat, humidity, or exercise.

Special Considerations

Contraindications to the use of the contraceptive patch are the same as for any combination hormonal contraceptive method and include, most notably, a history of cardiovascular disease, coagulopathies, and breast cancer. Side effects include headaches and breast discomfort. There also have been reports of application-site reactions, a non-hormonal-related side effect.

Unlike oral contraceptives, the patch does not require daily maintenance. When dispensed from a pharmacy as a single-month supply, the contraceptive patch is packaged as a set of three individual patches. Even though the patch is marketed for 7 days of use, studies have found that after the second week, a single patch will continue to deliver a sufficient amount of hormones for an additional 2 days, providing some forgiveness at that time should the woman be delayed in making the patch change after week 2 or 3.[37]

A significant amount of media attention has been given to the contraceptive patch and its association with venous thromboembolism (VTE). A Cochrane review estimated that the risk of VTE with patch use is 53 per 100,000 women.[38] Other studies have yielded conflicting evidence related to VTE risk in women with contraceptive patch use, with some studies reporting an observed doubling of risk.[39,40] The general consensus is that the risk of VTE with the patch is higher than the risk associated with levonorgestrel-containing COCs, but still less than the risk of VTE during pregnancy.

Midwifery Management Plan

The midwife should screen the woman for previous skin allergies such as reactions to bandages or other medicated patches. The woman's current weight must also be considered. If it exceeds 90 kg (198 pounds), the woman should be advised of the potentially decreased effectiveness of the patch.

It is reasonable for the midwife to initially prescribe 4 months of contraceptive patch therapy and schedule a follow-up appointment with the woman in 3 months. The follow-up visit should include assessment of the woman's satisfaction with the method and experience of any side effects or problems with method use. **Box 18-5** discusses health education specifically related to use of a transdermal contraceptive patch.

A patch should not be used if it is touched or becomes stuck to itself or to something else before being applied to skin. Additionally, no adhesive devices—such as tape or a wrap—should be used to try to keep the patch in place. Used patches should be discarded in areas away from children or pets, as they may contain residual hormones. The midwife may provide two prescriptions: one for ongoing monthly supply and a second for a single replacement patch in case one is detached.

If the woman forgets to apply her second or third patch of the cycle and no more than 9 days has elapsed since the application of her current patch, she should apply a new patch as soon as possible (**Figure 18-5**). The original patch change schedule remains unaltered. If more than 9 days has elapsed since the application of the current patch, she should understand that she is not protected from pregnancy and that she should start a new 21-day cycle by applying a new patch and using a back-up contraceptive method for the first week.[9]

If the woman forgets to take off the patch at the beginning of the patch-free week, she should remove it as soon as she remembers. If more than 9 days has elapsed since placement of the third patch, she should replace the patch according to the original schedule. Depending on how far into the patch-free week she removes the third patch, she may or may not experience a withdrawal bleed, although contraceptive protection is maintained.

If the woman forgets to restart a new patch following the patch-free week, she needs to understand that she is not protected from pregnancy and that she should put on a new patch and use a secondary method for pregnancy prevention for the first week of this new cycle.

BOX 18-5 Education Content to Be Emphasized When Counseling Women Using the Contraceptive Patch[a]

- When removing the patch from packaging, the woman should not touch the medicated side. Instead, she should remove only half of the release liner, apply it to skin, and then remove the remaining half, following with gentle pressure to ensure adhesion.
- Only one patch at a time should be used. Use of multiple patches is more likely to increase side/adverse effects than effectiveness.
- Verify attachment daily. If there is indication that the patch may be detaching, gently press on the patch for approximately 10 seconds. If that effort is unsuccessful, remove the patch and replace it with a new one.
- Patches should not be reused or relocated.
- Patches should not be secured by other tape or wrapping.
- Do not attempt to reapply a patch that has adhered to clothing, as this may decrease effectiveness.
- Used patches can be discarded in the trash, away from pets and children. They should never be flushed down a toilet.

[a]In addition to the information in Box 18-2.

Intravaginal Contraceptives (The Contraceptive Ring)

Currently, only one intravaginal delivery system for contraception is available in the United States. NuvaRing, manufactured by Merck Pharmaceuticals, was introduced in the U.S. market in 2001. It is a flexible, vinyl ring measuring approximately 4 mm thick and 54 mm in diameter. The ring is composed of ethylene vinyl acetate, which encases the active components and controls the daily release of the drugs. The ring is a combined hormonal method of contraception containing both estrogen and progestin components. The active drugs in the contraceptive ring consist of 11.7 mg etonogestrel and 2.7 mg ethinyl estradiol.

Mechanism of Action

The primary mechanism of action for the contraceptive ring is similar to that of combination oral contraceptives. The vaginal mucosa absorbs the exogenous estrogen and progestin compounds, inhibiting ovulation via suppression of gonadotropins within the hypothalamic–pituitary–ovarian axis. Alterations in cervical mucus and endometrial lining are secondary mechanisms of contraceptive action. Because the hormones are released directly into the vagina, a lower dose per day of hormones is required in comparison to COCs.

The contraceptive ring is self-administered by the woman, who inserts a ring once per month. Each ring

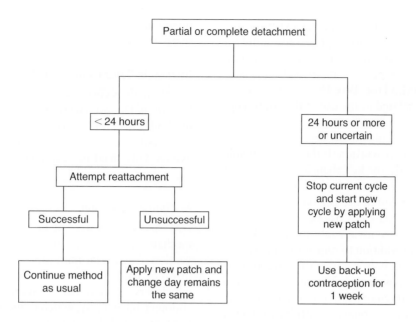

Figure 18-5 Algorithm for management of women with a partial or completely detached transdermal contraceptive patch.

is impregnated with sufficient hormones to last for approximately 21 days. To mimic the normal 28-day menstrual cycle, a single contraceptive ring is inserted and left in place for 21 days. It is then removed for 7 days, thereby inducing a withdrawal bleed. The contraceptive cycle restarts with the insertion of a new ring immediately following the 7-day ring-free week.

The vaginal ring comes in only one size, does not require fitting, and is not position dependent. That is, as long as the ring is in contact with vaginal mucosa, the hormones will be absorbed. The contraceptive ring releases 0.015 mcg of ethinyl estradiol and 0.120 mcg of etonogestrel into the bloodstream daily. The contraceptive ring is intended to be left in the vagina for a continuous period of 21 days; however, if it is out of the vagina for less than 3 hours, contraceptive effectiveness has not been found to be reduced.[41,42]

Special Considerations

The most prevalent side effects with the vaginal ring include headache, dysmenorrhea, and breast discomfort. Additionally, a method-specific, nonhormonal side effect is vaginal irritation. When dispensed from a pharmacy, the contraceptive ring comes individually packaged in a resealable foil pouch. NuvaRing is available to be dispensed in boxes of one or three foil pouches. Prior to dispensing, NuvaRing is stored refrigerated, but it can be stored for up to 4 months at room temperature afterward. Temperature extremes should be avoided when storing the contraceptive

ring, as there is potential for decreased effectiveness in those situations.

Response to the contraceptive ring has been positive from both women and their partners.[43] The contraceptive ring is convenient because it does not require daily or weekly maintenance, and its insertion and removal are not difficult. The ring usually is not perceived by the woman and only occasionally felt by her partner during sexual intercourse. If the woman desires, the contraceptive ring can be removed from the vagina for intercourse; it has been shown to maintain its effectiveness as long as it is replaced within 3 hours. The contraceptive ring should be rinsed only with cool water. Soap, hot water, or other cleansers should not be used on the ring, as they can affect this method's effectiveness.

Midwifery Management Plan

The management plan for women using the contraceptive ring is similar to that of other combination hormonal contraceptive methods. The midwife should screen for contraindications to combination hormonal contraception.[10] A prescription for emergency contraception should be considered, and women should be encouraged to have spermicide and condoms available in the event that the ring is expelled or an error occurs in removing or starting a new ring on schedule.

It is reasonable for the midwife to initially prescribe 4 months of rings and schedule a follow-up appointment with the woman in 3 months. The follow-up visit is the same as the return visit for any combination hormonal contraceptive and should include assessment of the woman's satisfaction with the method and her experience of any side effects or problems with method use. **Box 18-6** outlines health education points related to the use of the contraceptive ring.

Spontaneous expulsion occurs in fewer than 3% of women using NuvaRing. If the ring is outside of the woman's body for less than 3 hours, then it should simply be rinsed with tepid water and reinserted. If it has been out of her vagina for more than 3 hours, then the woman may not be protected from pregnancy and needs to use a back-up method for 7 consecutive days in addition to reinserting the ring.[42]

If the woman fails to remove the ring and no more than 28 days has passed since she first inserted this ring, she should remove it and insert a new ring. She may or may not experience a withdrawal bleed, but contraceptive protection is maintained. As with the patch, the ring may retain some residual active agent and should be carefully discarded away from children and pets. If more than 28 days has passed since the ring's initial insertion, the woman may not be protected from pregnancy. She should perform a

---

BOX 18-6 Education Content to Be Emphasized When Counseling Women Using the Contraceptive Ring[a]

- The contraceptive ring should be removed from its packaging and inserted into the vagina by compressing the sides.
- The ring must be completely inserted into the vagina.
- Only one ring should be inserted at any time. Use of multiple rings is likely to increase side/adverse effects but not effectiveness.
- Rings usually are best removed by the woman slipping her index finger under the rim of the ring and guiding it down and out of the vagina.
- Because rings should be removed every 21 days, a woman may benefit from using a paper or electronic calendar as a reminder.
- A used ring can be replaced inside its foil pouch and discarded in the trash, away from pets and children. Rings should never be flushed down a toilet.

[a]In addition to the information in Box 18-2.

---

pregnancy test. If the test is negative, she should insert a new ring and use a back-up method for 7 days.

Injectable Contraceptives (DMPA)

Depot medroxyprogesterone acetate (DMPA), also known as Depo-Provera, is an injectable hormonal method. Injectable contraception is highly effective, is reversible, does not require partner participation, avoids daily need for compliance, and is not coital dependent.

Mechanism of Action

DMPA is a derivative of progesterone. Its primary mechanism of action is inhibition of ovulation by prevention of follicular maturation.[44] Secondary mechanisms of action include thickening of cervical mucus, which serves as a barrier to sperm, and induction of endometrial atrophy, which reduces the likelihood of implantation. Like other steroidal hormones, DMPA is metabolized by the liver and excreted in the urine.[45]

Two formulations of DMPA are available, both of which require a prescription. The first is Depo-Provera, or DMPA-IM 150 mg/mL, which is contained in a 1-mL vial or prefilled syringe and administered every 12 weeks intramuscularly. DMPA is detected in the serum levels within 30 minutes after an injection of 150 mg of this formulation. Serum concentrations vary, but gradually plateau for approximately 3 months, after which the serum concentration gradually declines. The second formulation is Depo-subQ Provera 104, an agent administered subcutaneously every 12 weeks that has been found to be equally effective in inhibiting ovulation. The Depo-subQ Provera 104-mg dose and serum levels are approximately 30% lower than that of the standard DMPA-IM 150-mg dose. This formulation has been shown to have equal, if not improved, tolerability, as side effects of DMPA are dose dependent.

Special Considerations

Allergic reactions are possible with DMPA-IM 150 and DMPA-SC 104, but rare. The two major and common side effects of DMPA are menstrual changes and delayed return of fertility. The overall incidence of irregular bleeding experienced by women on DMPA can be as high as 70% in the first year of use.[46] Variations usually begin as episodes of unpredictable irregular bleeding and spotting that may last as long as 7 days or more or may be heavy during the first few months. These episodes gradually become less frequent and of shorter duration until the woman has amenorrhea. Approximately 10% to 30% of women experience amenorrhea after one injection, and 40%

to 50% do so by the fourth injection. The rates of irregular bleeding and amenorrhea are similar for the subcutaneous and intramuscular formulations.

Weight gain often is noted as a concern among women using DMPA. However, as mentioned earlier in this chapter, the largest systematic review failed to find a consistent association of DMPA with significant increase in weight among users. However, women who already are obese have been reported to gain additional weight according to anecdotal reports, suggesting special attention should be given to counseling for these women in the areas of diet and exercise.

Headaches have been reported among DMPA users. Women who develop migraines with aura should stop using DMPA (U.S. Medical Eligibility Criteria Category 3) because aura is a specific risk for stroke. However, studies examining use of natural progesterone or progestin use have found these agents to be associated with a decrease in frequency of migraines.[47] Therefore, a history of headaches is not a contraindication to initiation of DMPA, but women should be counseled to report the development of headaches to their healthcare provider. If a woman develops severe headaches while using DMPA, she should have a thorough evaluation to diagnose the type of headache she experiences.

Long-term DMPA users may develop temporary, but usually reversible, decreased bone density, with declines ranging from 5% to 7% in the hip and spine.[48] DMPA suppresses gonadotropin secretion, which in turn suppresses ovarian estradiol production. In this hypoestrogenic state, bone resorption outpaces bone formation, resulting in a decline in bone mineral density (BMD). Based on studies of adolescents, bone loss is greatest during the first 2 years of use, but then slows dramatically.[49] Bone density has been shown to return to baseline following discontinuation of DMPA in women of all ages, with this effect being seen as early as 24 weeks after stopping therapy.[50 51] As the effects of DMPA on BMD are reversible, the lifetime risk of fracture is small.[52] This finding is similar to that of lactational hypoestrogenism, which also has not been associated with an increased risk of fracture. However, women with conditions that place them at high risk for osteoporosis and fracture, such as chronic corticosteroid use, disorders of bone metabolism, a strong family history of osteoporosis, or anorexia nervosa, may not be well suited for long-term DMPA use. Women who have other risk factors that may contribute to lower BMD, such as low calcium intake, alcohol abuse, and lower body mass index, also should be evaluated carefully to assess suitability of

DMPA use.[53] Inadequate vitamin D levels may also contribute to more substantial BMD loss, particularly among adolescents.[54]

Studies have been inconsistent regarding the effects of DMPA on mood changes. Administration of DMPA in the immediate postpartum period does not appear to predispose women to postpartum depression. If depression occurs or worsens in a woman given DMPA, her symptoms may persist for the 3-month duration of the drug's effects.

DMPA may cause changes within the vaginal environment and cervical ectopy that can increase susceptibility to STIs, although evidence of such changes is inconclusive. Other potential side effects include nervousness, decreased libido, breast discomfort, dizziness, hair loss, and bloating.[55] Among those women using the subcutaneous formulation, some report an indentation or induration at the injection site (granuloma or atrophy) or other minor skin reactions.[56]

Return to fertility for women using DMPA tends to take longer than for women who have used other hormonal methods. Ovulation suppression following DMPA discontinuation is not related to the duration of use, but rather to the weight of the woman. Women with lower body weights may conceive sooner after discontinuation of DMPA than women with higher body weights. If inadvertently used during pregnancy, DMPA is not associated with increased risk of birth defects.

The use of progestins may cause fluid retention. Certain conditions may, in turn, be exacerbated by this fluid retention, such as headache, asthma, and cardiac or renal dysfunction. A decrease in glucose tolerance has been observed in some women on DMPA. Detectable amounts of the drug have been found in the breast milk of women receiving DMPA; however, no adverse changes in milk composition, quality, or amount have been identified. Likewise, neonates and infants receiving breast milk containing medroxyprogesterone appear to have no adverse developmental and behavioral effects through puberty. Nevertheless, based on theoretical concern for neonatal exposure to exogenous steroids, many providers reserve use of progestin-only contraceptive methods for new mothers until after the first 6 weeks postpartum.

Midwifery Management Plan

DMPA can be administered at any time in a menstrual cycle if the woman can be reasonably certain that she is not pregnant. However, if it is given later than the seventh day in the menstrual cycle, the woman should use back-up contraception for 7 days and receive a follow-up pregnancy test several weeks later to diagnose an early pregnancy prior to a second dose of DMPA. If DMPA is initiated within the first 5 to 7 days of the menstrual cycle, a pregnancy test is unnecessary. A pregnancy test is warranted if DMPA is initiated outside of this period.

When a woman currently is using a hormonal contraceptive method, DMPA can be initiated while the woman is protected by that method or within 7 days of the last day of active hormone use. A pregnancy test is unnecessary when transitioning from another reliable method. If switching from intrauterine contraception, the injection should be given before removal of the intrauterine device. A secondary contraceptive method should be used if the first injection is not given within 7 days of menses onset. For women who have had an abortion or miscarriage, DMPA should be given within 5 days. A woman who is postpartum and not breastfeeding can receive a DMPA injection at any time, optimally prior to resumption of sexual activity.

A woman transitioning from DMPA to another form of hormonal or intrauterine contraception should start the new method no later than 12 to 14 weeks after the last injection. This spacing ensures that she is not pregnant at the time she starts a new contraceptive method. Women can safely continue to use DMPA until menopause.

DMPA is injected either subcutaneously or intramuscularly, depending on the formulation. Massaging the injection site can lower the effectiveness of the DMPA. Ovulation does not occur for at least 14 weeks post injection. If the woman is more than 2 weeks late for her subsequent dose, a pregnancy test is recommended prior to administration to assure she is not pregnant. Various methods of appointment reminder are available. Starting at 13 weeks post injection, a secondary contraceptive method is recommended until the next dose is given. Conversely, subsequent injections may be administered up to 2 weeks early (10 weeks after the previous DMPA injection) without adverse effects. **Box 18-7** contains important information for women regarding DMPA injections.

Long-Acting Reversible Contraceptives

Long-acting reversible contraceptives tend to be more effective than their short-acting counterparts because they are not user dependent. LARCs include implants and IUDs.[57] Once inserted, these methods convey contraceptive protection for years.

> ### BOX 18-7 Educational Content to Be Emphasized When Counseling Women Using DMPA[a,b]
>
> - Women should eat a diet high in calcium and vitamin D. If not, a woman should consider taking a daily multi-vitamin supplement.
> - Although rare, a woman should be aware of and report any signs or symptoms of infection at the injection site, such as a fever, or changes at the insertion site, including drainage, redness, and warmth.
> - Other conditions that should be reported to a healthcare provider:
>   - Significant headaches
>   - Menorrhagia
>   - Depression
>   - Severe lower abnormal pain or any other signs or symptoms that may suggest pregnancy
>
> [a]In addition to the information in Box 18-2.
>
> [b]Education counseling is primarily based on expert opinion and common practice. Little strong evidence exists in this area.

Subdermal Implants

Implantable contraceptives consist of one or more matchstick-sized rods or tubes containing progestin. These implants are inserted beneath the top layers of skin, on the inner aspect of the upper arm. Depending on the model of implant, subdermal devices can provide contraception for up to 7 years. The first subdermal implant available in the United States was Norplant. It consisted of six plastic tubes containing levonorgestrel, a progestin. In 2002, the manufacturer removed Norplant from the U.S. market, citing limited availability of product components. Although Norplant is not currently available in the United States, it continues to be used internationally and a woman may have it inserted outside the country and desire to retain it for 7 years.

Although more implants may be available in the future, the only subdermal implant currently available in the United States is an etonogestrel-containing, single-rod device. Nexplanon entered the U.S. market in 2012, replacing its predecessor Implanon.

Mechanism of Action

Nexplanon is a polyethylene vinyl rod, 4 cm in length and 2 mm in diameter. The device is impregnated with 68 mg of etonogestrel, a progestin analogue, as well as 12 mg of barium sulfate. This latter substance makes the device detectable by X ray. Nexplanon works by continuous release of etonogestrel to suppress ovulation. A single Nexplanon implant provides contraception for up to 3 years.

Special Considerations

As with most long-acting contraceptive devices, initial costs are significantly higher when compared to SARCs. However, when averaged over 3 years of use, the total costs of subdermal implants usually are less expensive than COCs, POPs, or DMPA. At the time of implant removal, a new device can be re-inserted in the same site, thereby providing continuing contraception.

Midwifery Management Plan

Timing of insertion of implants must take into consideration the phase of the menstrual cycle, the possibility of current pregnancy, and the need for secondary contraception if recent ovulation cannot be excluded. At the time of this book's writing, all providers were required to complete a manufacturer-sponsored training program prior to providing Nexplanon. During this method-specific training, explanations for insertion and removal procedures are taught in detail. Implants can be obtained and inserted only by midwives and other professionals who have completed the educational process.

Monitoring for detrimental side effects, menstrual pattern, blood pressure, and user satisfaction can be done at a follow-up visit approximately 3 months following insertion. Limited data are available regarding the use of the implants by breastfeeding women, but small amounts of etonogestrel have been observed in breast milk. As with other progesterone-only methods, it is generally acceptable to initiate this method after the sixth postpartum week. No changes in infant behavior or breast milk production have been documented. **Box 18-8** lists health education topics for women using Nexplanon.

Hormonal Intrauterine Devices (Mirena, Skyla)

Mechanism of Action

The LNG-IUD is a T-shaped, flexible polyethylene device widely marketed in the United States. The body of the device includes a reservoir that contains 52 mg of the progestin levonorgestrel. The LNG-IUD provides a continuous release of levonorgestrel, which is absorbed locally by the endometrium and results in increased viscosity of cervical mucus, remodeling of

---

> **BOX 18-8 Educational Content to Be Emphasized When Counseling Women Using Contraceptive Implants[a]**
>
> Although rare, a woman should be aware of and report any signs or symptoms of infection at the insertion site, such as a fever, or changes at the insertion site, including drainage, redness, and warmth.
>
> [a]In addition to the information in Box 18-2.

---

the endometrial lining, and impaired tubal motility. As a result of these localized effects, sperm motility is impaired, thereby inhibiting fertilization of the ovum. A possible secondary mechanism of action is suppression of ovulation.

The LNG is not coital dependent, nor does it require major user action. It is a long-term contraceptive method, which makes it cost-effective when used over a period of years. Women who have an aversion to checking for the device strings after each menstrual period may not choose this method. A few women are intolerant of IUD-associated side effects, and others simply do not like the idea of having a foreign object inside their body.

In 2000, the FDA approved the first LNG-IUD, which was marketed with the brand name Mirena. The Mirena IUD releases an average of 20 mcg levonorgestrel per day and provides contraception for up to 5 years. This device measures 33 mm by 32 mm wide. Nine years after initial approval, the FDA approved an additional indication for this device—namely, its use as a therapeutic agent for women with menorrhagia.

In 2013, another LNG-IUD received FDA approval. Named Skyla, this device is slightly smaller than the Mirena IUD, measuring 28 mm by 30 mm. It has been approved for prevention of pregnancy for as long as 3 years.

Special Considerations

There are risks related to the IUD insertion and removal procedures, even though they are only minimally invasive. Bleeding, infection, perforation of the uterus, and pain can occur, although serious complications are rare. While IUDs do not cause ectopic pregnancy, if fertilization occurs with an IUD in place, there is a greater risk of ectopic implantation.

It is important to underscore, however, that the overall risk of ectopic pregnancy for a woman with any IUD is lower than the risk of ectopic pregnancy for a woman not using contraception.

Midwifery Management Plan

Most women, including adolescents and nulliparas, are good candidates for intrauterine contraception.[58] Absence of pregnancy should be verified prior to IUD insertion, but otherwise there are few pre-insertion recommendations. IUD insertion can take place on any day of the menstrual cycle, if absence of pregnancy has been confirmed. Many clinicians prefer to insert an IUD during a woman's menstrual period because the cervical os is slightly open and there is lubrication from the menses. Additionally, insertion during menses offers further reassurance that the woman is not pregnant.

Routine pre-insertion STI screening is not recommended for low-risk women.[59] IUD insertion in women who are at high risk for STIs should not be delayed; rather, STI screening should be performed at the time of insertion and treatment of positive results can proceed after confirmation. This recommendation is based on the low risk of pelvic inflammatory disease (PID) if such treatment is prompt. A woman's STI risk category should be determined using the CDC's risk assessment and screening parameters.[60]

Evidence collected regarding IUD placement immediately following birth (i.e., within 10 minutes) has shown the safety and feasibility of this procedure, although it is associated with a higher rate of expulsion.[61,62] Immediate postpartum insertion, however, is not performed widely in the United States. The insertion procedure immediately postpartum is the same as that used with a nonpregnant uterus, although the midwife should use caution as the uterine isthmus is much softer and more prone to perforation at this time. IUDs also may be placed following spontaneous or elective abortion, either immediately or at 4 to 8 weeks post abortion.[63]

Some clinicians offer the woman a nonsteroidal anti-inflammatory drug (NSAID) as premedication for pain approximately 30 minutes prior to IUD insertion, although there is no clear evidence as to the utility of such medications. Other midwives apply a local anesthetic at the tenaculum insertion sites or a paracervical block, although research has failed to demonstrate significant differences in perceived pain.[64,65] In recent years, several research reports have touted a potential benefit of using preprocedure

misoprostol (Cytotec) to facilitate IUD insertion, especially in nulliparous women.[66] Studies are conflicting regarding the use of misoprostol. Although it is infrequent, a vasovagal response may occur during or immediately following insertion of an IUD. When such a reaction occurs, the midwife should stop the procedure and allow the women to recover. In most cases insertion may be attempted again and usually is successful.

A woman who becomes pregnant with an IUD in place should be informed of the risks involved if the pregnancy is continued. These risks include chorioamnionitis, spontaneous abortion, septic abortion, and preterm labor.[67] Women who become pregnant with their IUD in place should also be evaluated for ectopic pregnancy, as the risk of ectopic pregnancy is higher. If pregnancy is confirmed and the IUD strings are visible, the IUD should be removed to decrease the risk of spontaneous abortion. The incidence of spontaneous abortion is less for a woman whose IUD is left in place than if the device is removed. The IUD should be removed even if the woman wishes to terminate the pregnancy, as septic abortion is a risk. If pregnancy is confirmed and the strings of the IUD cannot be identified, ultrasound and obstetric consultation are warranted.

Post-insertion pelvic infections occur most frequently in the first 20 days following IUD placement, suggesting that contamination of the upper genital tract with pathogens at the time of insertion is the cause, rather than the IUD itself or exposure to a STI. Therefore, it is important for the midwife to assess the woman's risk for infection prior to IUD placement and to maintain asepsis during the insertion procedure. If a woman shows any signs and symptoms of pelvic infection, antibiotic therapy should be started immediately. Although IUD removal is not necessary, the woman's appropriateness for continued use of an IUD should be reassessed.

Missing IUD threads or strings can be attributed to four possible causes: pregnancy, uterine perforation, spontaneous expulsion, and strings cut too short. It is important to rule out pregnancy whenever strings are not visible. Often strings may have simply receded into the cervix, out of view. Gentle cervical exploration with a cytobrush or cotton swab may elicit the hidden strings. If the midwife is unable to locate strings with gentle exploration, follow-up ultrasound is necessary. If no IUD is noted on ultrasound, consultation with a gynecologist is indicated. **Box 18-9** lists educational content to be included when counseling women using an LNG-IUD.

BOX 18-9 Educational Content to Be Emphasized When Counseling Women Using an LNG-IUD[a]

- Women should verify that the device is in situ by feeling for strings at least monthly.
- Use of the mnemonic PAINS can provide a reminder for women regarding conditions that should be reported to the midwife:
  - **P**eriod is late/abnormal bleeding (although this is relatively common for these women)
  - **A**bdominal pain or dyspareunia
  - **I**nfection, especially associated with exposure to STI or an abnormal vaginal discharge
  - **N**ot feeling well, especially if woman experiences fever, chills, or generalized malaise
  - **S**trings missing or inability to feel the plastic thread of the device

[a]In addition to the information in Box 18-2.

Conclusion

The availability of hormonal contraception caused a revolution among both women and the larger society. Over the last half-century, hormonal contraceptives have expanded from a drug category that included only combined pills to an armamentarium of effective methods such as progestin-only pills, transdermal patches, intrauterine devices, vaginal rings, and implants. Hormonal contraception, like nonhormonal methods, is not a *one size fits all* situation: Women should choose the option that represents the best fit for their unique personal circumstances. A woman's decision should consider her own eligibility, the conceptive method's effectiveness, noncontraceptive benefits, and her ability to use the method correctly and consistently.

● ● ● References

1. Christin-Maitre S. History of oral contraceptive drugs and their use worldwide. *Best Pract Res Clin Endocrinol Metab.* 2013;27(1):3-12.

2. Likis FE. Contraceptive applications of estrogen. *J Midwifery Women's Health.* 2002;47(3):139-156.

3. Brucker MC, Likis FE. Steroid hormones. In: King TL, Brucker MC. *Pharmacology for Women's Health.* Sudbury MA: Jones and Bartlett; 2011:362-378.

4. Potter L, Oakley D, deLeon-Wong E, Canamar R. Measuring compliance among oral contraceptive users. *Fam Plann Perspect.* 1996:28:154-158.

5. Trussell J, Guthrie KA. Choosing a contraceptive: efficacy, safety and personal considerations. In: Hatcher RA, Trussell J, Nelson AL, Cates W, Kowal D, Policar MS. *Contraceptive Technology.* New York: Ardent Media; 2011:45-75.

6. Speroff L, Darney P. *A Clinical Guide for Contraception.* 5th ed. Philadelphia, PA: Lippincott Williams & Wilkins; 2010.

7. Sibai B, Odlind V, Meador M, Shangold G, Fisher A, Creasy G. A comparative and pooled analysis of the safety and tolerability of the contraceptive patch (Ortho Evra/Evra). *Fertil Steril.* 2002;77(2):S19-S26.

8. American College of Obstetricians and Gynecologists (ACOG). Noncontraceptive uses of hormonal contraceptives. Practice Bulletin No. 110. *Obstet Gynecol.* 2010;115:206-218.

9. Murphy PA. Contraception and reproductive health. In: King TL, Brucker MC. *Pharmacology for Women's Health.* Sudbury MA: Jones and Bartlett; 2011: 881-910.

10. Centers for Disease Control and Prevention. *U.S. Medical Eligibility Criteria for Contraceptive Use.* Atlanta, GA: Division of Reproductive Health, Centers for Disease Control; 2010.

11. Centers for Disease Control and Prevention (CDC). U.S. selected practice recommendations for contraceptive use, 2013: Adapted from the World Health Organization Selected Practice Recommendations for Contraceptive Use, 2nd ed. *MMWR.* 2013;62(RR05):1-46.

12. Westhoff C, Kerns J, Morroni C, Cushman LF, Tiezzi L, Murphy PA. Quick Start: novel oral contraceptive initiation method. *Contraception.* 2002;66(3):141-145.

13. Westhoff C, Morroni C, Kerns J, et al. Bleeding patterns after immediate vs conventional oral contraceptive initiation: a randomized, controlled trial. *Fertil Steril.* 2003;79:322-329.

14. Brahmi D, Curtis KM. When can a woman start combined hormonal contraceptives (CHCs)? A systematic review. *Contraception.* 2013;87(5):535-538.

15. Sneed R, Westhoff C, Morroni C, Tiezzi L. A prospective study of immediate initiation of depo medroxyprogesterone acetate contraceptive injection. *Contraception.* 2005;71(2):99.

16. Nelson A, Katz T. Initiation and continuation rates seen in 2-year experience with Same Day injections of DMPA. *Contraception.* 2007;75(2):84.

17. Lopez LM, Newmann SJ, Grimes DA, Nanda K, Schulz KF. Immediate start of hormonal contraceptives for contraception. *Cochrane Database Syst Rev.* 2012;12:CD006260. doi: 10.1002/14651858. CD006260.pub3.

18. RHEDI/Center for Reproductive Health Education in Family Medicine, Montefiore Medical Center, New York City, 2007.

19. Jacobson JC, Likis FE, Murphy PA. Extended and continuous combined contraceptive regimens for menstrual suppression. *J Midwifery Women's Health.* 2012;57(6):585-592.

20. Clinical Effectiveness Unit. *Management of Unscheduled Bleeding in Women Using Hormonal Contraception.* London, UK: Faculty of Sexual and Reproductive Healthcare; 2009.

21. Grossman Barr N. Managing adverse effects of hormonal contraceptives. *Am Fam Physician.* 2010;82(12): 1499-1506.

22. Gallo MF, Lopez LM, Grimes DA, Schulz KF, Helmerhorst FM. Combination contraceptives: effects on weight. *Cochrane Database Syst Rev.* 2011;9: CD003987. doi: 10.1002/14651858.CD003987.pub4.

23. Lopez LM, Edelman A, Chen-Mok M, Trussell J, Helmerhorst FM. Progestin-only contraceptives: effects on weight. *Cochrane Database Syst Rev.* 2011;4:CD008815. doi: 10.1002/14651858. CD008815.pub2.

24. Bonny A, Secic M, Cromer B. Early weight gain related to later weight gain in adolescents on depot medroxyprogesterone acetate. *Obstet Gynecol.* 2011; 117(4):793-797.

25. Holt VL, Scholes D, Wicklund KG, Cushing-Haugen KL, Daling JR. Body mass index, weight, and oral contraceptive failure risk. *Obstet Gynecol.* 2005;105(1):46-52.

26. Audet MC, Moreau M, Koltun WD, et al. Evaluation of contraceptive efficacy and cycle control of a transdermal contraceptive patch vs an oral contraceptive: a randomized controlled trial. *JAMA.* 2001;285(18): 2347-2354.

27. Xu H, Wade JA, Peipert JF, Zhao Q, Madden T, Secura GM. Contraceptive failure rates of etonogestrel subdermal implants in overweight and obese women. *Obstet Gynecol.* 2012;120(1):21-26.

28. Shaw KA, Edelman AB. Obesity and oral contraceptives: a clinician's guide. *Best Pract Res Clin Endocrinol Metab.* 2013;27(1):55-65.

29. Cochrane RA, Gebbie AE, Loudon JC. Contraception in obese older women. *Maturitas.* 2012;71(3): 240-247.

30. ESHRE Capri Workshop Group. Female contraception over 40. *Hum Reprod Update.* 2009;15(6): 599-612.

31. Freeman S. Nondaily hormonal contraception: considerations in contraceptive choice and patient counseling. *J Am Acad Nurse Pract.* 2004;16(6):226-238.

32. Willis S, Kuehl T, Spiekerman A, Sulak P. Greater inhibition of the pituitary–ovarian axis in oral contraceptive pill users: the effect on follicular suppression. *Contraception.* 2006;74:100-103.

33. Schlaff W, Lynch A, Hughes H, Cedars M, Smith D. Manipulation of the hormone-free interval in oral contraceptive pill users: the effect on follicular suppression. *Am J Obstet Gynecol.* 2004;190:943-951.

34. Kroll R, Reape K, Margolis M. The effectiveness and safety of a low-dose, 91-day, extended-regimen oral contraceptive with continuous ethinyl estradiol. *Contraception.* 2010;81:41-48.

35. Westhoff C, Heartwell S, Edwards S, Zieman M, Stuart G, Cwiak C. Oral contraceptive discontinuation: do side effects matter? *Am J Obstet Gynecol.* 2007;196:412.e1-412.e6.

36. Zieman M, Guillebaud J, Weisberg E, Shangold G, Fisher A, Creasy G. Contraceptive effectiveness and cycle control with the Ortho Evra/Evra transdermal system: the analysis of pooled data. *Fertil Steril.* 2002;77:S13-S18.

37. Smallwood G, Meador M, Lenihan JJ. Effectiveness and safety of a transdermal contraceptive system. *Obstet Gynecol.* 2001;98(5):799-805.

38. Lopez LM, Grimes DA, Gallo MF, Schulz KF. Skin patch and vaginal ring versus combined oral contraceptives for contraception. *Cochrane Database Syst Rev.* 2010;3:CD003552. doi: 10.1002/14651858. CD003552.pub3.

39. Cole J, Norman H, Doherty M, Walker A. Venous thromboembolism, myocardial infarction, and stroke among transdermal contraceptive system users. *Obstet Gynecol.* 2007;109:339-346.

40. Dore D, Norman H, Loughlin J, Seeger J. Extended case-control study results on thromboembolic outcomes among transdermal contraceptive users. *Contraception.* 2010;81(5):408-413.

41. Duijkers IJM, Klipping C, Verhoeven CHJ, Dieben TOM. Ovarian function with the contraceptive vaginal ring or an oral contraceptive: a randomized study. *Hum Reprod.* 2004;19:2668-2673.

42. Mulders TMT, Dieben TOM. Use of the novel combined contraceptive vaginal ring NuvaRing for ovulation inhibition. *Fertil Steril.* 2001;75:865-870.

43. Roumen FJ, Mishell DR. The contraceptive vaginal ring, NuvaRing®, a decade after its introduction. *Eur J Contracep Reprod Health Care.* 2012;17(6):415-427.

44. Petta C, Faundes A, Dunson T, et al. Timing of onset of contraceptive effectiveness in Depo-Provera users. II. Effects on ovarian function. *Fertil Steril.* 1998;70(5): 817-820.

45. Jain J, Jakimiuk A, Bode F, Ross D, Kaunitz A. Contraceptive efficacy and safety of DMPA-SC. *Contraception.* 2004;70:269-275.

46. Haider S, Darney P. Injectable contraception. *Clin Obstet Gynecol.* 2007;50:898-906.

47. Kaunitz A. Injectable depot medroxyprogesterone acetate contraception: an update for U.S. clinicians. *Int J Fertil Women's Med.* 1998;43(2):73.

48. World Health Organization. *Hormonal Contraception and Bone Health: Provider Brief.* Geneva, Switzerland: World Health Organization, Department of Reproductive Health and Research; 2007.

49. Scholes D, Lacroix A, Ichikawa L, Barlow W, Ott S. Change in bone mineral density among adolescent women using and discontinuing depot medroxyprogesterone acetate contraception. *Arch Pediatr Adolesc Med.* 2005;159:139-144.

50. Kaunitz A, Arias R, McClung M. Bone density recovery after depot medroxyprogesterone acetate injectable contraception use. *Contraception.* 2008;77(2):67-76.

51. Harel Z, Johnson C, Gold M. Recovery of bone mineral density in adolescents following the use of depot medroxyprogesterone acetate contraceptive injections. *Contraception.* 2010;81(4):281-291.

52. World Health Organization. WHO statement on hormonal contraception and bone health. *Wkly Epidemiol Rec.* 2005;80:297-304.

53. Harel Z, Wolter K, Gold M, Cromer B. Biopsychosocial variables associated with substantial bone mineral density loss during the use of depot medroxyprogesterone acetate in adolescents: adolescents who lost 5% or more from baseline vs. those who lost less than 5%. *Contraception.* 2010;82(6):503.

54. Harel Z, Wolter K, Gold M. Inadequate vitamin D status in adolescents with substantial bone mineral density loss during the use of depot medroxyprogesterone acetate injectable contraceptive: a pilot study. *J Pediatr Adolesc Gynecol.* 2010;23(4):209-214.

55. Chern-Hughes B, Archer B, Irwin D, Jensen K, Johnson M, Rorie J. Depot medroxyprogesterone: management of side-effects commonly associated with its contraceptive use. *J Midwifery Women's Health.* 1997;42(2):104-111.

56. Prabhakaran S, Sweet A. Self-administration of subcutaneous depot medroxyprogesterone acetate for contraception: feasibility and acceptability. *Contraception.* 2012;85(5):453-457.

57. Winner B, Peipert JF, Zhao Q, et al. Effectiveness of long-acting reversible contraception. *N Engl J Med.* 2012;366(21):1998-2007.

58. Tang JH, Lopez LM, Mody S, Grimes DA. Hormonal and intrauterine methods for contraception for women aged 25 years and younger. *Cochrane Database Syst Rev.* 2012;11:CD009805. doi: 10.1002/14651858. CD009805.pub2.

59. Mohllajee A, Curtis K, Peterson H. Does insertion and use of an intrauterine device increase the risk of pelvic inflammatory disease among women with sexually transmitted infection? A systematic review. *Contraception.* 2006;73:145-153.

60. Workowski KA, Berman S. Sexually transmitted diseases treatment guidelines, 2010. *MMWR Recomm Rep.* 2010;59(RR-12):1-110.

61. Chen B, Reeves M, Hayes J, Hohmann H, Perriera L, Cerinin M. Postplacental or delayed insertion of the levonorgestrel intrauterine device after vaginal delivery: a randomized controlled trial. *Obstet Gynecol.* 2010;116(5):1079-1087.

62. Grimes DA, Lopez LM, Schulz KF, Van Vliet HAAM, Stanwood NL. Immediate post-partum insertion of intrauterine devices. *Cochrane Database Syst Rev.* 2010;5:CD003036. doi: 10.1002/14651858. CD003036.pub2.

63. Grimes DA, Lopez LM, Schulz KF, Stanwood NL. Immediate postabortal insertion of intrauterine devices. *Cochrane Database Syst Rev.* 2010;6:CD001777. doi: 10.1002/14651858.CD001777.pub3.

64. Mody S, Kiley J, Rademaker A, Gawron L, Stika C, Hammon C. Pain control for intrauterine device insertion: a randomized trial of 1% lidocaine paracervical block. *Contraception.* 2012;86(6):704-709.

65. Allen RH, Bartz D, Grimes DA, Hubacher D, O'Brien P. Interventions for pain with intrauterine device insertion. *Cochrane Database Syst Rev.* 2009;3:CD007373. doi: 10.1002/14651858.CD007373.pub2.

66. Swenson C, Turok D, Ward K, Jacobson J, Dermish A. Self-administered misoprostol or placebo before intrauterine device insertion in nulliparous women: a randomized controlled trial. *Obstet Gynecol.* 2012; 120(2):341-347.

67. Brahmi D, Steenland M, Renner R-M, Gaffield M, Curtis K. Pregnancy outcomes with an IUD in situ: a systematic review. *Contraception.* 2012;85(2):131-139.

19

Midlife, Menopause, and Beyond

ANNE Z. COCKERHAM

Menopause is a process that involves the whole woman—body, mind, and spirit—and is inclusive of physical, mental, emotional, and spiritual aspects. At the same time, the phenomenon also presents within the context of her life situation, time, place, and space. Therefore, women have connections with and are affected by external factors/variables. It is a phenomenon of multidimensionality and complexity, and it includes both negative and positive aspects of a normal life-course transition process toward aging.[1]

Menopause is a normal life event, not a disease. Furthermore, when considering care of women who are of a perimenopausal or postmenopausal age, the midwife should consider caring for the entire woman within a holistic framework. Indeed, caring for women during the menopausal transition presents a rich and rewarding practice opportunity for midwives. There is no such thing as a "typical" menopausal woman presenting for care and advice, because women's experiences with, and perceptions of, menopause vary tremendously based on lifestyle, economic and demographic factors, family and cultural influences, access to health care, and views about femininity and aging.[2] Regardless of whether a woman experiences menopause as a smooth transition from her reproductive to nonreproductive years, or if menopause is a time of physical or emotional crisis, midwives are well positioned to reinforce a healthy attitude toward menopause and to assist women in optimizing their health. Midwives should partner with women to provide accurate and easily understood information regarding the changes surrounding menopause, nonpharmacologic and pharmacologic options to manage bothersome symptoms if needed, and lifestyle modifications to optimize health during the many years that most women live after menopause. As noted in **Table 19-1**, menopause is a retrospective diagnosis, which is only accurate 12 months after a woman's last menstrual period. Table 19-1 also includes other terms frequently used to describe aspects of this period of time.[2–6]

Menopause: Normal Life Process Versus Medical Event

Menopause symbolizes two separate processes: aging and the change from being able to reproduce to not being able to do so. Focusing only on loss of youth and the ability to bear children, however, overlooks the normal developmental context and positive aspects of midlife. The older approach of conceptualizing menopause as a deficiency disease creates a mindset that a woman's worth is equivalent to her reproductive capacity.[7] Broadening the concept of the role of menopause to include positive changes in family interrelationships, growth in the capacity to work, and physical and psychological changes can lead to a deeper, more nuanced, and more functional view of menopause.[1]

What is normal and what is considered a disease process, as well as the way individuals experience and report symptoms, have varied over time, and continue to vary even today in different settings.[8]

Table 19-1	Menopause Definitions
Term	**Definition**
Climacteric	Process of age-related change from reproductive to nonreproductive state. Sometimes used interchangeably with *perimenopause*. This imprecise term has fallen out of favor.
Early menopause	Natural or induced menopause that occurs long before the average age of spontaneous menopause. This somewhat vague umbrella term encompasses premature menopause. Frequently used cutoff is 40 years.
Final menstrual period (FMP)	Last menstrual period of a woman's life; recognized as her FMP after 12 months of amenorrhea have passed after the FMP. Average age at FMP in the Western world is 51 years; range: 40–58 years.
Induced menopause	Cessation of menstruation due to surgical removal of a woman's ovaries or ablation of ovarian function from chemotherapy or pelvic radiation therapy.
Menopause	One-time event that marks permanent cessation of ovulation and menstruation. Diagnosed when a woman has had 12 months of amenorrhea with no other identified cause.
Menopause transition	Time of menstrual and endocrine changes, beginning with variation in cycle length and ending with the FMP. Average age at onset is 46 years; range: 39–51 years. Average duration is 5 years; range: 2–8 years.
Perimenopause	Symptomatic years of menopausal transition, encompassing the time from early menopausal transition to 12 months after the FMP. Menopause experts disagree about whether this term should be reserved for use with a lay audience or if it is suitable for use in scientific literature.
Postmenopause	Time after a woman's FMP.
Premature menopause	Any menopause that occurs in women younger than 2 standard deviations (SD) below the mean estimated age for the reference population. Frequently used cutoff is 40 years.
Premenopause	Time approaching the FMP. Some menopause experts do not recommend using this somewhat imprecise term.
Primary ovarian insufficiency	Ovarian failure leading to amenorrhea in women younger than 40 years; sometimes used synonymously with *premature ovarian failure*. Some authorities prefer premature ovarian *insufficiency* rather than premature ovarian *failure*, because cessation of ovarian function is not always permanent.
Progesterone	A steroid hormone secreted by the corpus luteum and by the placenta. This term is most commonly used to describe women's naturally occurring hormone.
Progestin	A natural or synthetic substance that mimics the actions of progesterone. This term is most commonly used to describe the therapies women use for contraception and menopausal hormone therapy.

Sources: Adapted from North American Menopause Society. *Menopause Practice: A Clinician's Guide*, 4th ed. Mayfield Heights, OH: North American Menopause Society; 2010; Hale GE, Burger HG. Hormonal changes and biomarkers in late reproductive age, menopausal transition and menopause. *Best Pract Res Clin Obstet Gynaecol.* 2009;23:7-23; Harlow SD, Gass M, Hall JE, et al. Executive summary of the Stages of Reproductive Aging Workshop + 10: addressing the unfinished agenda of staging reproductive aging. *Fert Steril.* 2012;97:843-851; NIH state-of-the-science conference statement on management of menopause-related symptoms. *NIH Consens State Sci Statements.* March 21–23, 2005;22:1-38; Fritz MA, Speroff L. *Clinical Gynecologic Endocrinology and Infertility*, 8th ed. Philadelphia, PA: Lippincott Williams & Wilkins; 2011.

Nineteenth-century Americans, including physicians, viewed menopause as a crisis that resulted in physical and psychological diseases such as tumors, depression, hysteria, and insanity.[9] Menopause indicated that a woman was unable to comply with her prescribed social role.[10]

It was not until the twentieth century that the average lifespan of women began to gradually reach the age of 50, implying that half the female population lived long enough to experience menopause. Yet several events of the twentieth century reinforced negative views of menopause. The development of synthetic estrogen in 1938 led to the concept that care of menopausal women required medical management. Influential writings after mid-century emphasized this philosophy: in 1966, Robert A. Wilson, author of *Feminine Forever*, suggested that readers "think of menopause as a deficiency disease…similar to diabetes: caused by a lack of insulin or estrogen."[11] In 1975, articles in the *New England Journal of Medicine* emerged questioning the safety of such treatments by linking estrogen use with endometrial cancer.[12] When the etiology of this cancer was found to be associated with estrogen's proliferative effects on the endometrium, medical researchers and pharmaceutical companies began a campaign to "rehabilitate" estrogen therapy by demonstrating that the benefits of use outweighed the risks,[13] particularly with the addition of progestin to counteract estrogen's proliferative effects on the endometrium. Observational studies helped buttress the positive claims about hormone therapy, and health researchers and physicians argued that hormone therapy also was an effective prevention strategy for heart disease and osteoporosis, among other conditions. Most recently, in the first years of the twenty-first century, the landmark study known as the Women's Health Initiative (WHI) shed new light on ways to evaluate the risks and benefits of hormone therapy; this study is discussed in more detail later in this chapter.

The essential questions remain: Is menopause a disease to be treated? Is menopause a negative experience to be feared? Fortunately, sociologists and others have begun to examine why and how societies have defined common human experiences such as pregnancy, homosexuality, alcoholism, and social anxiety as "medical problems." This evaluation is particularly meaningful when considering menopause because, while there is often room for improvement in any woman's health, most women entering midlife are healthy. The normal midlife changes often are not a negative transition[14] but rather signify a time of changing hormones, relationships, and roles during a transition managed well by most women. The only universal "change" is the cessation of menstruation; other aspects of the menopausal experience are highly individualized. The meaning of menopausal symptoms is culturally determined to a great degree; however, so generalizing from the experiences of one group of women to other groups can lead to misunderstandings and suboptimal care.[8]

Today, medical institutions, pharmaceutical companies, and the mass media provide an abundance of information on menopause, both to healthcare providers and to women encountering this transition. This blitz of input from scientific, technological, and medical sources may leave women more vulnerable to messages from medical institutions or pharmaceutical companies that often—albeit not always—have a major economic stake in "medicalizing" menopause. Many midlife women can benefit

from a knowledgeable guide who can assist them in navigating the opportunities and challenges of the menopausal transition and beyond. Midwives are ideally suited to this task.

Physiology and Stages of Reproductive Aging

Menopause is not a sudden event for most women, but rather the cumulative result of many events. During the menopausal transition, physiologic changes occur, including in the ovary, the endocrine milieu, receptor tissues throughout the body (e.g., cardiovascular and skeletal systems), and the way in which a woman and her family perceive physical and emotional changes.

The ovaries and the endocrine system change over time. During fetal life, the ovaries contain approximately 1 to 2 million follicles—the maximum number of follicles a woman will ever have.[2] The loss of follicles eventually leading to menopause occurs primarily due to atresia, not ovulation, because most women will ovulate fewer than 500 times during their reproductive years.[15] As a woman ages, the rate of follicular loss increases; as the number of follicles diminishes, the ovaries become more resistant to the action of follicle-stimulating hormone (FSH).[2] The ovaries also produce decreased quantities of estrogen, androgen, and progesterone. Loss of the negative feedback from ovarian estrogen production indicates that gonadotropin production is no longer inhibited; hence levels of FSH and luteinizing hormone (LH) rise markedly, so that the FSH level exceeds the LH level. Secretion of the ovarian glycoprotein inhibin, which selectively inhibits FSH, also decreases. The decreased release of inhibin eventually results in sustained elevation of FSH. Elevated FSH levels stabilize approximately 24 months after the final menstrual period.[4] Although these hormones generally trend upward over time throughout this process, hormone levels can be unexpectedly erratic. This instability is one reason why testing hormone levels generally is unreliable for diagnosing menopausal stages.

After menopause, the ovary changes considerably both in physical appearance and in function. In spite of the absence of functional follicles, both the remaining corticostromal cells and the hilar cells are steroidogenic; as such, they contribute to androgen production and continue to provide significant amounts of androstenedione and testosterone for several years. These hormones influence a woman's muscle strength and sexual drive, making them important to the quality of life for postmenopausal women.[6]

The three main human estrogens are estrone (E_1), estradiol (E_2), and estriol (E_3). Postmenopausally, estrone accounts for the majority of circulating estrogen; it is derived principally from the metabolism of estradiol and from the conversion of androstenedione in adipose tissue. Conversely, estradiol—the most potent of the three estrogens—accounts for 95% of the circulatory estrogen in premenopausal women. The dominant follicle and the corpus luteum both excrete large amounts of estradiol in reproductive-age women.[2] Estriol, a weak estrogen, is secreted from the placenta and also is metabolized from estrone.[2]

Postmenopausal women have serum estradiol levels lower than 37 pg/mL (picograms/milliliter) and mean estrone levels between 6 and 63 pg/mL. In contrast, premenopausal women have estradiol levels in the range of 10–100 pg/mL in the early follicular phase, 200–800 pg/mL at midcycle, and 200–340 pg/mL during the luteal phase, as well as premenopausal estrone levels in the range of 30–180 pg/mL. Although 95% of postmenopausal androstenedione production occurs in the adrenal gland and 5% in the ovaries, the ovarian stroma continues to produce androstenedione and testosterone under the influence of LH. These hormones, along with androstenedione produced by the adrenal glands, are converted to estrone in peripheral adipose tissue. Thus the body weight of the postmenopausal woman contributes to her postmenopausal estrogen level, such that increased conversion occurs with increasing weight.[2] Some estradiol continues to be produced, but the amount is significantly less than that produced in reproductive-age women.

Stages of Reproductive Aging Workshop

Because chronological age often is not an accurate predictor of a woman's path to menopause, leading menopause researchers developed an alternative system for assessing women's stages of life at the Stages of Reproductive Aging Workshop (STRAW). Investigators published the initial system in 2001, research continued during the next 10 years, and the updated STRAW + 10 system was published in 2012. This system has become the gold standard for describing reproductive aging through menopause.[4] **Figure 19-1** provides a graphic representation of the STRAW + 10 stages.

Use of the STRAW + 10 stages can aid clinicians and women in understanding expected physiologic changes during the menopausal transition. The stages progress from a woman's reproductive years toward her final menstrual period and then beyond.[4]

Late Reproductive Stage (Stage–3b)

During this stage, women begin to notice changes in the amount of menstrual flow and in cycle length, and they often have shorter cycles. FSH levels usually increase, but can vary from one cycle to the next. Importantly, even irregular or long cycles can still be ovulatory. In as many as 25% of these cycles, women may ovulate;[6] thus women still need to protect themselves from pregnancy in this stage.

Early Menopausal Transition (Stage–2)

As women move closer to their final menstrual period, menstrual cycle length becomes even more variable. In this stage, there is often a difference of 7 days or more in the length of consecutive cycles, and these variations persist for at least 10 cycles after the first variable-length cycle. FSH level remains elevated but this level, once again, is variable. Estradiol levels remain in the normal range and are even slightly elevated until approximately 1 year before the cessation of follicular development. This finding is contrary to earlier research that indicated estradiol levels gradually waned in the years before menopause.[6]

Late Menopausal Transition (Stage–1)

During this stage, women generally are amenorrheic for episodes of 60 days or longer, have wide variations in cycle length and marked fluctuations in hormone levels, and are increasingly anovulatory. This stage usually lasts 1 to 3 years, and women frequently experience vasomotor symptoms during this stage. The conclusion of the late menopausal transition phase is the final menstrual period (FMP).

Early Postmenopause (Divided into Stages +1a, +1b, and +1c)

FSH level continues to increase and estradiol levels continues to decrease until approximately 2 years after the FMP. Early menopause is subdivided into three distinct stages. **Stage +1a** usually lasts 1 year, and its end marks the 12-month period required to make the retrospective diagnosis of spontaneous menopause. Similarly, **Stage +1b** lasts approximately 1 year and is characterized by rapid changes in FSH and estradiol levels. Symptoms such as hot flashes are most likely to occur in stage +1b. **Stage +1c** lasts approximately 3 to 6 years, during which women experience a period of stabilization with high FSH and low estradiol levels.

Late Postmenopause (Stage +2)

This stage encompasses a woman's remaining lifespan and today may comprise another one-third of

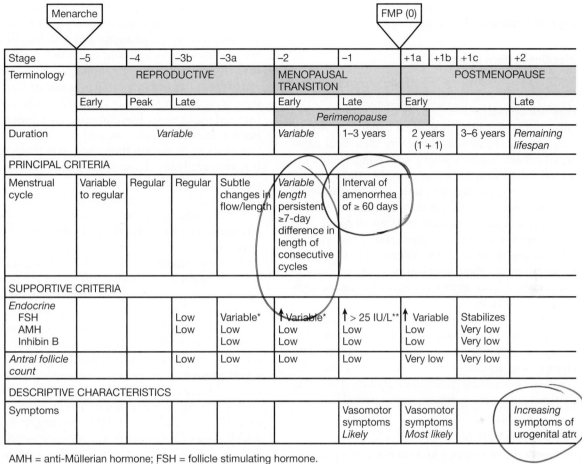

Stage	−5	−4	−3b	−3a	−2	−1	+1a	+1b	+1c	+2
Terminology	REPRODUCTIVE				MENOPAUSAL TRANSITION		POSTMENOPAUSE			
	Early	Peak	Late		Early	Late	Early			Late
					Perimenopause					
Duration	Variable				Variable	1–3 years	2 years (1 + 1)	3–6 years		Remaining lifespan
PRINCIPAL CRITERIA										
Menstrual cycle	Variable to regular	Regular	Regular	Subtle changes in flow/length	Variable length persistent ≥7-day difference in length of consecutive cycles	Interval of amenorrhea of ≥ 60 days				
SUPPORTIVE CRITERIA										
Endocrine FSH AMH Inhibin B			Low Low	Variable* Low Low	↑ Variable* Low Low	↑ > 25 IU/L** Low Low	↑ Variable Low Low	Stabilizes Very low Very low		
Antral follicle count			Low	Low	Low	Low	Very low	Very low		
DESCRIPTIVE CHARACTERISTICS										
Symptoms						Vasomotor symptoms Likely	Vasomotor symptoms Most likely		Increasing symptoms of urogenital atr	

AMH = anti-Müllerian hormone; FSH = follicle stimulating hormone.
*Blood draw on cycle days 2–5 ↑ = elevated
**Approximate expected level based on assays using current international pituitary standard[67–69]

Figure 19-1 The Stages of Reproductive Aging Workshop + 10 Staging System.
Source: Reprinted with permission from Harlow SD, Gass M, Hall JE, et al. Executive summary of the Stages of Reproductive Aging Workshop + 10: addressing the unfinished agenda of staging reproductive aging. *Fert Steril.* 2012;97:843-851. Used with permission of Elsevier, Ltd.

her life or more. Hormone levels stabilize during this stage, and symptoms associated with low estrogen levels, such as vulvovaginal atrophy, can become increasingly apparent.

Smoking, lower body weight, nulliparity, never-use of oral contraceptives, and lower socioeconomic status are factors that have been found to be associated with spontaneous menopause occurring earlier than the average age of 51 years.[16] Some experts consider higher body weight to be associated with later age at menopause,[5,16] but others argue that this association is not clear.[17] Family history can also affect a woman's age at her final menstrual period.[16]

Although study findings have implicated these factors to varying degrees in the timing of menopause, the midwife must primarily consider the individual woman's presentation. A woman's menstrual and medical histories and her reported bodily changes are

far more important in making a menopause diagnosis than any statistical associations with factors such as body weight, family history, or smoking.

Presentation of Perimenopause and Menopause

Following is a discussion of the most commonly reported physical changes experienced by women during perimenopause and menopause, as well as a more comprehensive list of possible symptoms. Potential therapies for each symptom, including lifestyle measures and pharmacologic therapies, are summarized in the treatment section of this chapter. In keeping with holistic, woman-centered care, it is important to assess the degree to which particular bodily changes are bothersome to the woman herself before assuming that treatment should be undertaken.

Bleeding Pattern Changes

Changes in menstrual cycle length and menstrual flow amount and duration are so common that they are considered hallmarks of perimenopause. Approximately 90% of women experience 4 to 8 years of menstrual changes before their final menstrual period.[2] Exactly what those changes entail for an individual woman is unpredictable and variable. Consequently, women may have little idea of what to expect as they approach menopause, and this uncertainty can create anxiety for some women. The most common pattern is a gradual decrease in both amount and duration of the menstrual flow, leading to spotting and then to cessation. However, some women experience more frequent or heavier periods in perimenopause.

Although bleeding changes are common during perimenopause, the clinician should not ignore the possibility of a pathologic cause for uterine bleeding changes such as endometrial carcinoma. **Table 19-2** compares normal and potentially abnormal bleeding patterns during the perimenopausal period.

Vasomotor Symptoms

Although the physiology of vasomotor symptoms is poorly understood,[6] the terms *vasomotor symptoms*, *hot flashes*, *hot flushes*, and *night sweats* all refer to the same experience: recurrent, transient periods of flushing, sweating, and a sensation of heat, often accompanied by palpitations and a feeling of anxiety, and sometimes followed by chills.[2] A single hot flash usually lasts 1 to 5 minutes, during which time a woman experiences a sudden wave of heat that soon spreads over her body and particularly over her face and upper torso. Elevations in skin temperature, heart rate, skin blood flow, and metabolic rate follow quickly. As the hot flash ends, skin temperature begins to gradually return to normal and the woman sometimes feels chilled, often due to heat loss from sweating and continued peripheral vasodilation.[18]

Vasomotor symptoms are extremely common, although the exact prevalence is difficult to determine and the reasons for the variations are poorly understood. Studies provide widely varying statistics on this phenomenon, with estimates of the percentage of women reporting hot flashes ranging from 8% to 80%.[19] Regardless of the precise number, hot flashes, like bleeding changes, are so common that they are hallmarks of perimenopause.[18] Ethnicity, diet, climate, lifestyle factors, and women's attitudes about aging may all influence women's perceptions of vasomotor changes. In North America, African American women report hot flashes more frequently than Hispanic, white, or Asian women.[18] Women who have undergone surgically induced menopause have a higher incidence of hot flashes, at least for the first year, compared to women having naturally occurring menopause; moreover, the former group's

Table 19-2	Normal Versus Potentially Abnormal Bleeding Patterns in Perimenopausal Women
Common Perimenopausal Menstrual Changes	**Potentially Abnormal Perimenopausal Bleeding Patterns**[a]
Shorter intervals between periods (but at least 21 days)	Very heavy bleeding, especially with clots
Longer intervals between periods	Long bleeding duration: > 7 days or ≥ 2 days longer than usual
Lighter bleeding	Very short cycles: < 21 days from beginning of one period to beginning of next period
Heavier bleeding than normal (difficult to quantify; consider evaluation if significant change)	Irregular bleeding: spotting or bleeding between periods
Shorter duration of bleeding	Bleeding after sex
Longer duration of bleeding (up to 1–2 days longer than usual)	
Skipped periods	
No changes	

[a] The clinician must evaluate any bleeding that occurs after menopause (i.e., after 12 months of amenorrhea) for pathologic cause.

Source: Adapted from North American Menopause Society. *Menopause Practice: A Clinician's Guide*, 4th ed. Mayfield Heights, OH: North American Menopause Society; 2010.

hot flashes tend to be more severe.[2] Women who are younger at menopause tend to have more vasomotor symptoms.[5] Recently, new information has emerged about the relationship between body weight and hot flashes. Previous theory and research indicated that women with low body mass index (BMI) and minimal adipose tissue suffered from more hot flashes because of a lowered amount of endogenous estrogen production. However, today's evidence indicates that women with higher BMI—at least heavy premenopausal and perimenopausal women—have more hot flashes, perhaps because of the role of adipose tissue as an insulator, which promotes a higher core body temperature.[2]

The length of time an individual woman will have hot flashes and her personal degree of distress are unpredictable. Some women may experience hot flashes for short periods of time; others do so for many years. The highest prevalence of this symptom is in the first 1 to 2 years post menopause. Approximately 50% of women have hot flashes for 4 to 5 years after their final menstrual period, 25% have hot flashes for more than 5 years, and 10% for as long as 15 years.[6] A small number of women report hot flashes for decades after menopause. Some women have relatively few hot flashes, as few as several per month, whereas other women have very frequent hot flashes, as many as several per hour. Moreover, some women experience their vasomotor symptoms as easily managed, while hot flashes disrupt the lives of others.

Sleep Disturbances

Midlife women frequently report problematic sleep patterns, defined as an inadequate number of hours of sleep, sleep of poor quality, or an inability to function in an alert state during desired waking hours. Women might experience insomnia as a prolonged time needed to fall asleep, as inability to stay asleep all night, or as early awakening without being able to get back to sleep. These sleep difficulties can be either short term or persistent. Estimates of sleep difficulties vary widely, but as many as 48% of women in the United States age 40 to 64 years report sleep difficulties, including fewer hours of sleep than desired, more frequent insomnia, and more frequent use of prescription sleep aids as compared to premenopausal women.[2,5,20]

Midlife sleep difficulties are complex and multifactorial, and can have significant effects on quality of life. Primary sleep disorders such as restless legs syndrome are common in midlife women, as are other causes of perceived poor sleep such as hot flashes and anxiety from stressful life events that can interrupt sleep. Additionally, clinicians must be alert to the presence of chronic conditions that have the potential to disrupt sleep and diminish sleep quality in perimenopausal women. Women who report sleep problems in addition to diminished enthusiasm and capacity to enjoy life, energy loss, appetite disturbance, or increased somatic complaints, or who have poorly diagnosable physical problems may be experiencing major depression. Thyroid dysfunction, autoimmune disorders, illnesses causing chronic pain, and medication effects are also worthy of consideration when providing care to women reporting sleep difficulties.[2]

Genitourinary Changes

After menopause, women experience an overall decreased amount of estrogen and a predominance of estrone, a relatively low-potency estrogen. Together, these changes have significant effects on the vagina, cervix, uterus, ovaries, and urinary tract. Unlike bothersome vasomotor symptoms that usually subside after a period of time, genitourinary changes—particularly vulvovaginal effects—tend to become worse over time for susceptible women.[21]

At least half, and perhaps as many as 90%, of postmenopausal women experience some atrophic changes of the genitourinary tract that affect their quality of life and sexual function.[22,23] The term *atrophy* refers to vaginal and cervical epithelium that is thin, dry, and pale in a diminished-estrogen environment. This tissue sometimes becomes inflamed, and a more visible capillary bed may lead to a diffusely red appearance or one characterized by small petechial hemorrhages. Diminished estrogen levels also may cause a woman's vagina to change from the normal, healthy, acidic environment dominated by lactobacilli to an alkaline environment with more diverse flora that can include pathogenic organisms.[2,22] Women bothered by atrophic symptoms sometimes report dryness or itching of the vulva and vagina and pain with vaginal penetration. Upon vaginal exam, the clinician might find microabrasions and few or absent vaginal rugae—that is, pleat-like folds of vaginal tissue that enable comfortable expansion of the tissue when the vaginal walls are stretched.

A woman's cervix, uterus, and ovaries also change at menopause and in the years following menopause. The cervix usually decreases in size and produces less mucus; this change can contribute to painful intercourse. Progressive atrophy of the cervical epithelium creates an increasingly sparse capillary bed and makes the surface of the cervix appear smooth, shiny, and pale.[2] After ovarian follicular activity ceases, hormonal stimulation of the endometrium and myometrium also stops. Endometrial tissue inside the uterus as well as outside the uterus (endometriosis implants) becomes atrophic and inactive. Although atrophic endometrial tissue occasionally bleeds, the clinician should never assume normalcy if a menopausal woman reports vaginal bleeding—any vaginal bleeding in a menopausal woman requires evaluation. Small to moderate-size fibroids, which are highly sensitive to estrogen stimulation, usually shrink after menopause, as do the cyst-like invasions of the myometrium characteristic of adenomyosis.[24] A postmenopausal woman's ovaries become small and are normally nonpalpable on bimanual exam. Thus, if a clinician palpates a postmenopausal woman's ovary, an ovarian neoplasm must be ruled out.[2]

Women may report urinary tract discomfort after menopause, and problems such as urinary incontinence and overactive bladder become increasingly common in women at midlife and beyond. Although the urinary tract does exhibit some normal age-related atrophic changes, incontinence and overactive bladder are not inevitable with aging and clinicians should not regard them as normal.[2]

Sexuality

Unfortunately, many myths about sex and aging exist, including the myth that midlife and older women are not interested in sex. According to findings of the National Social Life, Health, and Aging Project published in 2011, many women are sexually active at midlife and beyond: 62% of women ages 57 to 64 years reported partnered sexual activity in the previous year, as did 39% of women ages 65 to 74 years, and 17% of women ages 75 to 85 years.[25] More than 50% of sexually active women in all age groups reported having sexual activity 2 or 3 times per month.

Midlife and older women enjoy sex for a variety of reasons, including feeling more feminine, reducing tension, improving sleep, enhancing feelings of intimacy with their partner, and for sheer pleasure. For many couples, sex continues to improve with aging and lifestyle changes for both men and women. With more leisure time, more privacy with their children out of the house, and fewer responsibilities, sex can become a wonderful adventure.

However, some midlife women report difficulties with sexual functioning. Each woman's experience will be different, but the three main sexual health concerns that midlife women report are decreased sexual desire, decreased vaginal lubrication, and inability to have an orgasm.

For some women, the most problematic aspect of the menopausal transition is a lack of knowledge.

Many clinicians do not routinely ask about sexual health, perhaps mistakenly assuming that women would find it intrusive. Because some women do not feel comfortable broaching the topic, begin by using open-ended questions to ask about changes in a woman's sexual health, vaginal changes, including moisture or dryness, itching, or pain, as well as more direct questions about anything she wants to ask or discuss about her sex life or sexuality. For example, the question, "Is there anything about your sexual life that you would like to change?" is a good opening for this discussion.

Certain situations might require even more time to evaluate in depth. If a woman has undergone a hysterectomy or mastectomy, she may have questions about sexual adjustment in relation to the surgery. Anxiety or depression can cause problems with arousal phase disorders. Medications such as antidepressants and antihypertensives also can contribute to sexual dysfunction. Some women experience an unwelcome lack of available sexual partners due to divorce or death, which might lead them explore other relationships with new partners or satisfy their sexual needs alone with masturbation or fantasy.

Emotional and Psychological Changes

Experts disagree about whether changing hormone levels actually *cause* mood symptoms. The interactions between estrogen and mood are complex, as are the interactions between "symptom clusters," including pain, vasomotor symptoms, and sleep disruption that women face around the time of the menopause.[26] Moreover, many women experience coexisting stressors[6] such as career or education challenges, socioeconomic difficulties, changes in self-concept and body image, relationship difficulties, perhaps exacerbated by a newly empty nest, and the "sandwich generation" phenomenon of caring for both children and elderly family members.[2] In spite of the controversies surrounding this topic, several risk factors for mood problems are certain: women with a history of depression or premenstrual syndrome seem to be particularly vulnerable to depression around menopause[5] and women who undergo bilateral oophorectomy, especially when younger than 48 years, are at increased risk of experiencing anxiety symptoms.[2,27]

Weight Changes

Midlife women frequently report weight gain, with the average weight gain during the menopause transition being approximately 5 pounds. However, evidence does not support a causal relationship: neither menopause nor hormone therapy appears to *cause* weight gain.[2,17,28] Instead, aging and lifestyle factors are more likely to cause an increase in weight. Lean muscle mass decreases with age, lowering a woman's metabolic rate. This reduced metabolic rate, combined with a more sedentary lifestyle, causes women to burn fewer calories and gain weight if they do not lower their caloric intake.[28]

Regardless of cause, it is clear that many midlife women in the United States are overweight or obese and are likely to suffer significant and negative health consequences stemming from this condition including cardiovascular disease, hypertension, type 2 diabetes, certain cancers, and premature death. Thus diagnosis and management of obesity and overweight, including counseling about lifestyle management strategies, are vitally important roles for midwives.

Hair and Skin Changes

Sun damage, redistributed or decreased subcutaneous fat, skin laxity from weight changes, and decreased underlying muscle tissue cause most of the skin changes that women notice at menopause. Other potential midlife skin changes include dryness, acne, hair loss, brittle and slow-growing nails, and decreased wound healing, all of which may contribute to psychological distress or altered body image.[2,29]

The midwife is likely to find a great variety of benign skin lesions when examining the skin of midlife women. Some examples are skin tags (fibroepitheliomas)—benign, soft, brown, pedunculated polyps usually found on eyelids and the neck; seborrheic keratosis—sharply defined, flat, light or dark brown papules usually found on the trunk; and Campbell de Morgan spots (cherry angiomas)— red dome-shaped papules that are found primarily on the trunk. Acne rosacea, an inflammatory condition of the sebaceous glands, also has an increased incidence with age.

Although the great majority of skin lesions are not worrisome, the clinician should always consider the possibility of a skin malignancy and consult or refer the client as appropriate. This vigilance is particularly important when a woman has a lesion that has asymmetry, border irregularities, color variations, a diameter greater than 6 mm, or a sudden increase in size.[2] It is important to be particularly vigilant for vulvar cancer if any vulvar lesions have an atypical appearance.

Changes in Thyroid Function

Thyroid dysfunction becomes more common as women age, making thyroid dysfunction screening more cost-effective for perimenopausal and postmenopausal women than it is in younger women. In a large multiethnic study of women age 42 to 52 years, approximately 10% of women had thyroid dysfunction.[2] Relying on classic symptoms of thyroid disease to prompt screening is problematic in this age group because other usual perimenopausal symptoms overlap with symptoms of thyroid dysfunction. These symptoms include changes in menstrual bleeding characteristics, sleep difficulties, fatigue, mood changes, heat intolerance, and palpitations. Thus the healthcare provider must have a higher index of suspicion to diagnose and treat thyroid disease early in the older woman compared to her younger counterpart.[2,30] **Table 19-3** provides a summary of a variety of symptoms that women report during perimenopause and postmenopause.

Diagnosing Menopause

No single laboratory test can predict or confirm menopause. Instead, the diagnosis of menopause is based on a woman's menstrual and medical histories and on her report of symptoms.[2] Thus a diagnosis of menopause is generally assured if a woman has been amenorrheic for 12 months and has had hot flashes, vaginal dryness, or other typical menopausal symptoms, and if there is no reason to suspect an underlying alternative cause of the woman's symptoms.

Women sometimes request "hormone testing" to confirm menopause, to predict its course, or to help manage symptoms. However, testing hormones is seldom necessary or helpful. Although there are occasionally reasonable clinical uses for testing of hormones, many problems are associated with hormone testing. **Table 19-4** identifies potential reasons to order hormone levels as well as recognized problems associated with hormone testing.[2,6,31,32] As with any test, prior to ordering the test, ask first how the result might affect management. If the result is unlikely to change management, the test is unnecessary.

Lifestyle Strategies for Management of Women with Perimenopausal or Menopausal Symptoms

An array of healthy lifestyle strategies can be offered to women who request relief from menopausal symptoms such as hot flashes, sleep difficulties, sexual concerns, and vulvovaginal discomfort. Some of these strategies, such as maintenance of a healthy weight,

Table 19-3	Summary of Symptoms Women Report During Perimenopause and After Menopause
System or Body Area	**Symptom**
Constitutional	Vasomotor symptoms: hot flashes, night sweats[a]
	Insomnia
	Weight gain
	Muscle and joint aches
	Dizziness
	Fatigue
	Anxiety, nervousness, irritability, mood swings
	Inability to concentrate, forgetfulness
Head	Headache
	Hair thinning/hair loss
	Unwanted hair growth
Eyes	Blurred vision
	Dry or tired eyes
	Swollen and reddened eyelids
	Increased tear production
	Presbyopia (inability to see close objects)
Dental and oral cavity	Tooth loss
	Gum inflammation
Skin	Laxity, sagging
	Dryness
	Acne
Breasts	Mastalgia
Cardiac	Palpitations
Uterus	Menstrual irregularity[a]
	Heavy or light menses
Urinary	Recurrent urinary tract infection
	Urinary frequency, urgency, nocturia
Vulvovaginal	Vaginal and vulvar irritation, burning, itching
	Vaginal dryness, difficulty with lubrication with sexual activity
	Recurrent vaginitis

[a] Extremely common; considered hallmarks of perimenopause/menopause.

Sources: Adapted from North American Menopause Society. *Menopause Practice: A Clinician's Guide,* 4th ed. Mayfield Heights, OH: North American Menopause Society; 2010; NIH state-of-the-science conference statement on management of menopause-related symptoms. *NIH Consens State Sci Statements.* March 21–23, 2005;22:1-38.

smoking cessation, and increased exercise, have additional benefits for cardiovascular and bone health.

Vasomotor Symptoms

Women who have mild hot flashes often find relief with common-sense and relatively easily instituted lifestyle changes. Women who prefer to avoid medications for treatment of their symptoms should also try the following lifestyle changes.[2,18]

Recognition and Avoidance of Hot Flash Triggers

Keeping a symptom diary can help women identify connections between their hot flashes and common precipitating factors so they can work to decrease or eliminate those triggers if desired. Commonly reported triggers include hot drinks or meals, spicy food, alcohol, and emotional upset. Importantly, these factors are triggers for some women but not for others, and evidence is mixed, so midwives should

Table 19-4	Hormone Testing During Perimenopause and Menopause	
Hormone	**Problems Associated with Use**	**Possible Reasons to Order**
Estrogen levels	Estradiol and estrone levels are erratic; isolated levels unlikely to give meaningful information	To assess absorption of estrogen in women with persistent vasomotor symptoms in spite of hormone therapy
Progesterone	Levels likely to be low in anovulatory cycles; isolated levels unlikely to give meaningful information	To document ovulation in perimenopausal women who are trying to conceive
Follicle-stimulating hormone (FSH)	Highly variable during perimenopause: even elevated FSH levels(> 30 mIU/mL) can return to premenopausal range days, weeks, or months later	Multiple FSH levels demonstrating sustained elevation > 30 mIU/mL, or months of amenorrhea and FSH > 40 mIU/mL, can provide a reasonably sound diagnosis of menopause; sometimes useful in women with unclear or unusual clinical presentations
Luteinizing hormone (LH)	LH elevation occurs late in perimenopause, much later than FSH elevation; minimal or no utility in confirming perimenopause or menopause	If a woman taking hormonal contraceptives needs laboratory confirmation of menopause, a serum FSH:LH ratio greater than 1 on the seventh pill-free day can provide a reasonably sound diagnosis of menopause
Prolactin	N/A	To rule out a pituitary cause for oligomenorrhea or amenorrhea, particularly in the presence of galactorrhea
Thyroid-stimulating hormone (TSH)	N/A	To rule out thyroid dysfunction as a cause for symptoms otherwise attributed to perimenopause and menopause (e.g., oligomenorrhea, hot flashes, sleep difficulties, fatigue, weight gain)
Testosterone	Levels change little from 4 years before to 2 years after menopause; little value in diagnosing testosterone insufficiency because testosterone levels are only one part of total androgen status	To rule out testosterone excess state from testosterone treatment or endogenous excess

Sources: Data from North American Menopause Society. *Menopause Practice: A Clinician's Guide,* 4th ed. Mayfield Heights, OH: North American Menopause Society; 2010; Fritz MA, Speroff L. *Clinical Gynecologic Endocrinology and Infertility,* 8th ed. Philadelphia, PA: Lippincott Williams & Wilkins; 2011; Santoro N, Randolph JF. Reproductive hormones and the menopause transition. *Obstet Gynecol Clin North Am.* 2011;38:455-466; Butler L, Santoro N. The reproductive endocrinology of the menopausal transition. *Steroids.* 2011;76:627-635.

advise women of the possibility but encourage each woman to evaluate possible associations for herself. A benefit to a woman's identification and avoidance of her triggers is an enhanced sense of control, a factor that one recent study identified as having an especially powerful effect in diminishing vasomotor symptoms.[33]

Regular Physical Exercise and Maintenance of Healthy Weight

Evidence is mixed regarding whether poor exercise habits and obesity have a causal relationship with hot flashes. However, women who maintain a regular exercise pattern—and particularly women with higher fitness levels[34]—and a stable, healthy weight have fewer problematic hot flashes.[35,36] Because these

strategies have positive effects on overall health, including them in recommendations has potential benefit beyond mitigating the frequency of hot flashes.

Avoidance or Cessation of Smoking

Women who smoke tend to have more hot flashes than women who do not; in addition, the more a woman smokes, the greater her risk for more severe vasomotor symptoms.[18] Considering the long list of real and possible benefits of smoking cessation, strongly advising women to cut down or quit smoking is an important recommendation.

Use of Relaxation Techniques

Women can consider modalities such as yoga, meditation, deep breathing, muscle relaxation, guided imagery, mindful stretching, massage, aromatherapy, and prayer. These techniques, many of which diminish the anxiety that can lead to hot flashes, are promising.[18] Methodological challenges have thus far limited researchers' abilities to fully document the evidence, but there is little likelihood of harm and most of these techniques have little cost.

Maintaining a Cool Environment

Women can sleep with a fan, keep the thermostat down, and dress in layers of breathable clothing such as cotton to aid in staying cool.

Sleep Difficulties

Women with mild sleep problems or women who are motivated to avoid medication therapy are often successful in improving the quality and quantity of their sleep with the following lifestyle measures.

Avoidance of Substances and Activities Prior to Bedtime That Can Interfere with Sleep

Most women understand the relationship between wakefulness and caffeine, but they might not realize that they are ingesting caffeine in substances other than coffee, tea, and cola drinks. Caffeine can also be found in energy drinks, some nonprescription pain relievers, premenstrual syndrome symptom-relief remedies, weight-control products, alertness aids, cold medications, and diuretics. Moreover, a susceptible woman might feel the effects of caffeine longer than she realizes: it might take 7 hours for the caffeine to clear her system and she could feel the cumulative effects for as long as 20 hours.[2]

Alcohol can initially assist in falling asleep (and, therefore, may be used inappropriately as a sleep aid), but alcohol's effects can also include fragmented sleep and early awakening. Nicotine also disrupts sleep, as do drugs such as marijuana, heroin, and prescription narcotics.

A large, heavy meal before bedtime can disrupt sleep, whereas a light snack with protein and complex carbohydrates, or a source of tryptophan such as milk or chamomile tea, can be helpful. Vigorous exercise or stressful activities close to bedtime can cause difficulties in relaxing and falling asleep, but regular, moderate exercise earlier in the day can promote healthy sleep habits.[2]

Maintenance of Nightly Rituals and a Regular Sleep Schedule

Women should maintain a regular bedtime every night of the week, regardless of other commitments. Midlife and older women who do not work or whose children are grown may not be obligated to get out of bed at a particular time. However, erratic sleep hours, as well as naps, can negatively affect sleep quality. A regular schedule also capitalizes on the light/dark cycle. A warm bath or other pleasant ritual, as well as reserving the bedroom for only sleep and sex, can condition better sleep patterns.[2]

Vulvovaginal and Sexuality Concerns
Enhancement and Protection of Moisture

To promote adequate moisture throughout the body as well as in the reproductive system, women can humidify their homes and drink adequate amounts of fluids each day. A variety of over-the-counter products, including vaginal moisturizers and lubricants, can reduce vaginal and vulvar irritation. Women can use water-based *lubricants* (e.g., Astroglide, K-Y Jelly, K-Y Liquibeads) during sexual activity. Lubricants work at the surface of the skin to reduce friction, and their effects are immediate and short term. In contrast, *moisturizers* (e.g., Replens, K-Y Long Lasting, K-Y Silk-E) are not used at the time of sexual activity, but rather are longer-lasting products that can maintain moisture and beneficially lower vaginal pH.[37] Products that are *not* helpful include oil-based products (such as baby oil or Vaseline), which can coat the vaginal lining, thereby preventing the release of natural secretions, or cause condom breakage. Women should avoid antihistamines and other over-the-counter drugs that might have drying effects, including douches, sprays, and colored or perfumed toilet paper and soaps.

Promotion of Adequate Time for Arousal and Sexual Activity as Possible

Arousal time slows with aging for both women and men, so allowing more time for foreplay is advisable. However, sexual activity itself improves blood supply to the pelvis and the vaginal tissues. Consequently, sexually active older women often have less atrophy than older women who are not sexually active.[2]

Recognition That Information Is Power

According to a survey of approximately 3500 women in the United States and six other countries, the vast majority of women experiencing atrophic symptoms did not recognize the cause or know that ongoing treatment of the underlying cause is needed.[22] Indeed, caring for women with sexual concerns should include explaining the physiology of aging as it relates to sexuality and correcting problems when possible. It is helpful to explain the psychology of aging and to note that some midlife and older women experience improved sexuality. Women should consider alternative, noncoital activities either with or without a partner. Midwives should consider referring women of any age for sex therapy, especially when there is long-standing sexual dysfunction, current or past abuse, or an acute psychological event.

Nonhormonal Prescription Options for Vasomotor Symptoms

Some women attempt lifestyle strategies to manage their vasomotor symptoms but do not experience sufficient relief; many of these women do not desire hormone therapy or are not candidates to take hormones. In those situations, discussion of off-label use of certain nonhormonal medications, as listed in **Table 19-5**, may be warranted.[2,6,38–41] Although some of these medications have evidence to support their effectiveness, none is as effective as systemic hormone therapy in treating hot flashes. These medications have varying side-effect profiles.

Hormonal Prescription Options for Treatment of Menopausal Symptoms

Some midlife women have significant menopausal symptoms and desire hormone therapy (HT), in the form of either estrogen therapy (ET) or estrogen–progestin therapy (EPT). **Tables 19-6, 19-7,** and **19-8** list compositions, brand names, doses, and routes of administration for commonly used HT products.[21,42–44] Note that the terms "hormone replacement therapy" (HRT) and "estrogen replacement therapy" (ERT) have fallen out of favor because "replacement" implies that the pharmacologic agent provides premenopausal hormonal levels. This implication is untrue: HT provides only a small fraction of the hormone levels produced by premenopausal ovaries. Moreover, replacement connotes an unnatural deficiency state when, in fact, the changed endogenous hormone levels a menopausal woman experiences are natural and expected.

For a midlife woman considering hormone therapy, consider the following questions, in partnership with the woman.

Does She Need Pregnancy Prevention Instead of Perimenopausal Therapy?

Until a woman is menopausal (i.e., has reached 12 months since her final menstrual period), pregnancy

is possible. Any perimenopausal woman who wants to avoid pregnancy should use contraception and not rely on hormone therapy to prevent pregnancy. Although both HT and combined hormonal contraceptives contain estrogen and progestin, the dose and formulation of HT will not prevent pregnancy. Moreover, a woman whose ovaries are still functioning in a reproductive capacity is not likely to benefit from the doses of hormones found in HT because they are low in comparison to a reproductive-age woman's hormone levels. Therefore, women generally do not begin taking HT until they have reached menopause. For healthy women who experience perimenopausal symptom relief with hormonal contraception use, many clinicians recommend making the transition to HT, if needed, when the woman has reached age 55 years—an age at which 90% of women will have reached menopause.[2]

Should She Have ET or EPT?

A woman with a uterus needs a progestin in addition to (systemic-level) estrogen to protect her from the endometrium-building effects of estrogen and predisposition to endometrial hyperplasia. Conversely, a woman who has undergone a hysterectomy does not need a progestin, with rare exceptions. Note that most menopause experts agree that women with a uterus who use estrogen in *nonsystemic* doses (i.e., local vaginal therapy) do not need a progestin, although Fritz and Speroff[6] advocate endometrial surveillance with an ultrasonographic measurement of endometrial thickness when women use a local vaginal therapy for more than 6 to 12 months. If a woman is using a progestin therapy that is separate from the estrogen component, inquire about the woman's continued adherence to the progestin therapy. Some women experience side effects from progestin therapy and discontinue its use without understanding the importance of the agent or without notifying the midwife.

Which Route of Administration Is Best?

ET is available in oral, transdermal, topical, and vaginal therapies. EPT is available in oral and transdermal formulations. Clinicians can also add a progestin to ET via a levonorgestrel-releasing intrauterine system (Mirena IUS). When considering the optimal route of administration, an important first consideration is whether the woman needs *systemic* or *local* vaginal therapy. If a woman needs relief from systemic symptoms (e.g., hot flashes), she needs systemic-level dosing; this can be achieved with oral, transdermal, or

Table 19-5	Nonhormonal Prescription Options for Vasomotor Symptoms	
Medication and Starting Dose **Generic (Brand)**	**Class**	**Comments**
Fluoxetine (Prozac) 20 mg/day Paroxetine (Paxil) 12.5–25 mg/day Venlafaxine (Effexor) 37.5–75 mg/day Desvenlafaxine (Prisiq) 50–100 mg/day	SSRI/SNRI antidepressants	Moderate effectiveness for hot flashes Especially useful for women with coexisting mood disorders Rapid response Taper to discontinue Decreased libido can be problematic
Gabapentin (Neurontin) 300 mg/day at bedtime	Anticonvulsant	Moderate effectiveness for hot flashes Somnolence is possible side effect but can be helpful to promote sleep Taper to discontinue May be used in combination with antidepressant therapy
Clonidine (Catapres) 0.05–0.1 mg twice a day	Antihypertensive	Less effective than SSRI/SNRIs and gabapentin Available as patch Significant side-effect profile Taper to discontinue
Pregabalin (Lyrica) 50 mg orally once a day	Anticonvulsant	Approved to treat fibromyalgia and neurologic conditions NAMS considers early results promising but advises more research before recommending
Methyldopa (Aldomet)	Antihypertensive	NAMS does not recommend this product because of its limited effectiveness and high potential for adverse effects

NAMS = North American Menopause Society; SNRI = serotonin–norepinephrine reuptake inhibitor; SSRI = selective serotonin reuptake inhibitor.

Sources: Data from North American Menopause Society. *Menopause Practice: A Clinician's Guide*, 4th ed. Mayfield Heights, OH: North American Menopause Society; 2010; Fritz MA, Speroff L. *Clinical Gynecologic Endocrinology and Infertility*, 8th ed. Philadelphia, PA: Lippincott Williams & Wilkins; 2011; Guttuso T. Effective and clinically meaningful non-hormonal hot flash therapies. *Maturitas.* 2012;72:6-12; Umland EM, Falconieri L. Treatment options for vasomotor symptoms in menopause: focus on desvenlafaxine. *Int J Women's Health.* 2012;4:305-319; Andrews JC. Vasomotor symptoms: an evidence-based approach to medical management. *J Clin Outcome Manage.* 2011;18:112-128; Villaseca P. Non-estrogen conventional and phytochemical treatments for vasomotor symptoms: what needs to be known for practice. *Climacteric.* 2012;15:115-124.

topical therapy or one of the vaginal rings (Femring). The decision to chose oral administration versus another route can be guided by individual preference or other factors such as avoidance of first-pass effect with transdermal products. If a woman needs relief only from vaginal symptoms (e.g., atrophy, vaginal dryness), she is best served by local therapy that does not result in systemic levels of hormone. Local therapy is formulated in vaginal creams, the vaginal tablet Vagifem, and the vaginal ring Estring. Clinicians should be aware that systemic HT is associated with worsening of preexisting stress and urge urinary incontinence and increased incidence of new urinary incontinence.[45] In contrast, local vaginal estrogen therapy appears to improve continence.[46]

Does She Have Any Contraindications to HT?

ET and EPT package inserts list the same contraindications regardless of whether their effects are local or systemic. However, some menopause experts question this practice and feel comfortable with considering local ET for women with an HT contraindication. Package insert contraindications for ET/EPT include undiagnosed abnormal vaginal bleeding; known, suspected, or history of breast cancer; known or suspected estrogen-dependent cancer; current or history of deep vein thrombosis or pulmonary embolism; current or recent (within the last year) stroke or myocardial infarction; liver disease; known or suspected pregnancy; and known hypersensitivity to

Table 19-6	Estrogen Plus Progestin Combination Therapies	
Composition	**Brand Names**	**Dose**
CEE (14 tabs) then CEE + MPA (14 tabs)	Premphase	Sequential, once daily: 0.625 mg E then 0.625 mg E + 5.0 mg P
CEE + MPA	Prempro	Continuous, once daily: 0.3 mg E + 1.5 mg P 0.45 mg E + 1.5 mg P 0.625 mg E + 2.5 mg P 0.625 mg E + 5 mg P
EE + NETA	Femhrt	Continuous, once daily: 2.5 mcg E + 0.5 mg P 5.0 mcg E + 1 mg P
17ß-e + NETA	Activella	Continuous, once daily: 0.5 mg E + 0.1 mg P
17ß-e + DRSP	Angeliq	Continuous, once daily: 1 mg E + 0.5 mg P 1 mg E + 1 mg P
17ß-e (3 tabs) then 17ß-e + NGM (3 tabs), repeated continuously	Prefest	Intermittent/sequential, once daily: 1 mg E + 0.09 mg P
17ß-e + NETA	Combipatch	Apply twice weekly: 0.05 mg E + 0.14 mg P 0.05 mg E + 0.25 mg P
17ß-e + LNG	Climara Pro	Apply once weekly: 0.045 mg E + 0.015 mg P

17ß-e = 17ß-estradiol; CEE = conjugated equine estrogen; DRSP = drospirenone; E = estrogen; EE = ethinyl estradiol; LNG = levonorgestrel; MPA = medroxyprogesterone acetate; NETA = norethindrone acetate; NGM = norgestimate; P = progestogen.

Sources: Reprinted by permission of The North American Menopause Society from http://www.menopause.org/docs/professional/htcharts .pdf?sfvrsn=6, Table 4. Copyright © The North American Menopause Society. 2012. All rights reserved.

ET/EPT. Note that smoking is not a contraindication to ET/EPT, unlike for combined hormonal contraceptive users older than the age of 35 years.

Should the EPT Be Cyclic or Continuous?

A variety of dosing options have been used and are available for the estrogen and progestin dosages. One of the oldest EPT regimens is *cyclic EPT*, in which a woman takes estrogen from calendar day 1 to day 25 and adds progestin during the last 10 to 14 days of the cycle. This regimen is seldom used now because women tend to experience withdrawal bleeding and hot flashes on the hormone-free days. Another regimen not commonly used today is *cyclic-combined EPT*, in which a woman takes both estrogen and progestin on days 1 through 25.

With *continuous-cyclic (sequential) EPT*, women take estrogen every day and add progestin for 10 to 14 days each month, providing predictable withdrawal bleeding but no hot flash–inducing estrogen-free days. Premphase is one brand-name product that uses this formulation; it is sometimes prescribed for women in the menopausal transition during which HT-induced endometrial growth is likely. Premphase creates a predictable pattern of bleeding during this transitional period.

Continuous-combined EPT, in which women take estrogen and progestin every day, is currently the most commonly used formulation of HT. Within a few months of using this dosing option, a woman's endometrium becomes thin and most women are amenorrheic.

Intermittent-combined EPT (also called *pulsed progestin* or *continuous-pulsed EPT*) is also in common use now. In this regimen, women take estrogen every day plus progestin taken intermittently for 3 days on, 3 days off, repeated without interruption. Only one product, Prefest, uses this regimen.

Table 19-7	Estrogen-Only Preparations		
Composition	**Brand Names**	**Route**	**Available Doses**
CEE	Premarin	Oral	0.3; 0.45; 0.625; 0.9; 1.25 (mg/day)
CE	Cenestin	Oral	0.3; 0.45; 0.625; 0.9; 1.25 (mg/day)
CE	Enjuvia	Oral	0.3; 0.45; 0.625; 0.9; 1.25 (mg/day)
Est E	Menest	Oral	0.3; 0.625; 1.25; 2.5 (mg/day)
Estropipate	Ortho-Est	Oral	0.625 (0.75 estropipate, calculated as sodium estrone sulfate 0.625); 1.25 (1.5); 2.5 (3.0); 5.0 (6.0) (mg/day)
17ß-e	Estrace	Oral	0.5; 1.0; 2.0 (mg/day)
Estradiol acetate	Femtrace	Oral	0.45; 0.9; 1.8 (mg/day)
17ß-e	Esclim, Vivelle, Vivelle-Dot	Patch (matrix)	Replace patch twice weekly: 0.025; 0.0375; 0.05; 0.075; 0.1 (delivery in mg/day)
17ß-e	Alora	Patch (matrix)	Replace patch twice weekly: 0.025; 0.05; 0.075; 0.1 (delivery in mg/day)
17ß-e	Climara	Patch (matrix)	Replace patch once weekly: 0.025; 0.0375; 0.05; 0.075; 0.1 (delivery in mg/day)
17ß-e	Fempatch	Patch (matrix)	Replace patch once weekly: 0.025 (delivery in mg/day)
17ß-e	Menostar	Patch (matrix)	Replace patch once weekly: 0.014 mg (delivery in mg/day)
17ß-e	Estraderm	Patch (reservoir— cannot be cut)	Replace patch twice weekly: 0.05; 0.1 (delivery in mg/day)
17ß-e	EstroGel	Transdermal gel	Apply daily, 1 metered pump: delivers 1.25 g gel containing 0.75 mg 17ß-e
17ß-e	Elestrin	Transdermal gel	Apply daily, 1–2 metered pumps: 1 metered pump delivers 0.87 g gel containing 0.52 mg 17ß-e
17ß-e	Divigel	Transdermal gel	Apply daily, 3 strengths of packets (0.25, 0.5, or 1 g): 0.003; 0.009; or 0.027 mg dose
17ß-e	Estrasorb	Topical emulsion	Apply 2 packets daily: 1 packet delivers 1.74 g emulsion
17ß-e	Evamist	Transdermal spray	Initial: 1 spray/day of 1.7% solution; increase to 2–3 sprays/day if needed
17ß-e	Estrace	Vaginal cream	Initial: 2–4 g/day × 1–2 weeks, then 1 g/day (0.1 mg active ingredients/g)
Conjugated estrogens	Premarin	Vaginal cream	0.5–2 g/day (0.625 mg active ingredients/g)
17ß-e	Estring	Vaginal ring	Replace every 90 days 1 strength, releases 7.5 mcg/day (Minimal systemic amount)
Estradiol acetate	Femring	Vaginal ring	Replace every 90 days 2 strengths, releases 0.05 mg/day; 0.10 mg/day (Systemic level—progestogen needed if intact uterus)
Estradiol hemihydrate	Vagifem	Vaginal tablet	Initial: 1 tablet/day × 2 weeks; then 1 tablet twice/week Tablet contains equivalent of 10 mcg estradiol

17ß-e = 17ß-estradiol; CE = conjugated estrogen; CEE = conjugated equine estrogen; E = estrogen; Est E = esterified estrogen.

Sources: Data from Krychman ML. Vaginal estrogens for the treatment of dyspareunia. *J Sex Med.* 2011;8:666-674; North American Menopause Society. *Hormone Products for Postmenopausal Use in the United States and Canada.* Mayfield Heights, OH: North American Menopause Society; October 25, 2011.

Table 19-8	Progestin-Only Preparations		
Composition	**Brand Names**	**Route**	**Dose per Day**
Medroxyprogesterone acetate	Provera	Oral tablet	2.5 mg, 5 mg, 10 mg
Norethindrone acetate	Aygestin	Oral tablet	5 mg
Micronized progesterone (in peanut oil)	Prometrium	Oral capsule	100 mg, 200 mg
Levonorgestrel	Mirena	Intrauterine system	Releases approximately 20 mcg/day

Sources: Data from North American Menopause Society. *Hormone Products for Postmenopausal Use in the United States and Canada.* Mayfield Heights, OH: North American Menopause Society; October 25, 2011; Hitchcock CL, Prior JC. Oral micronized progesterone for vasomotor symptoms: a placebo-controlled randomized trial in healthy postmenopausal women. *Menopause.* 2012;19:886-893; Spark MJ, Willis J. Systematic review of progesterone use by midlife and menopausal women. *Maturitas.* 2012;72:192-202.

Which Dose Is Best?

Most HT products are available in a variety of doses. The effective dose for symptom relief varies from woman to woman, so a certain amount of trial and error is often needed to determine the correct dose. The guiding principle should be to start with a low dose and titrate upward, eventually selecting the lowest dose that accomplishes the goal for using the product.[47]

What About Timing of Initiation?

Current evaluation of scientific evidence indicates that the ideal time to initiate HT for symptom relief is as early as possible. Initiation generally is thought to be best within the first 10 years after menopause or between ages 50 and 59 years, rather than initiating HT far removed from the time of menopause. Because HT usually is indicated for treatment of women with symptoms, the early time frame best corresponds to the time of a woman's most bothersome vasomotor symptoms.[48]

When and How Should Women Discontinue Systemic HT?

Women should be counseled to use systemic HT for the shortest duration necessary for symptom relief. Substantial individual variations are evident in the length of time women have bothersome hot flashes, but it is generally a relatively short period of time. However, one should also respect women's decision making when they are fully apprised of the risks and benefits of extended HT use and decide to continue it for longer periods of time. The midwife and the woman should discuss the risks and benefits of HT use at each visit and strongly consider discontinuation at 5 years of use. When women discontinue HT, intuition would indicate that gradual tapering would result in a less unpleasant experience than abrupt discontinuation. In reality, evidence does not support this theory: women's experiences seem to be no better with gradual tapering of HT than with sudden discontinuation.[2,6]

Androgen Therapy

Androgen therapy is controversial. Some clinicians argue that it is beneficial for menopausal women because even a slight and gradual decrease in a postmenopausal woman's total testosterone is associated with decreased libido and other negative changes that can be managed with androgen therapy.[2,6] Others argue that women often require supraphysiologic dosing to appreciate any improvement in sexuality, women's serum androgen levels do not accurately predict sexual function,[2] and exogenous androgen use is not associated with an actual increase in sexual behavior.[6]

Currently there are no Food and Drug Administration (FDA)–approved androgen-containing hormone therapy products, although some clinicians prescribe custom compounded micronized testosterone or various other androgen-containing products on an off-label basis. A product formerly available in the United States, Estratest, composed of ethinyl estradiol and methyltestosterone, often was used off-label for the treatment of moderate to severe hot flashes that did not respond to estrogen therapy. Estratest is no longer available but several "quasi-generic" products such as Covaryx are available by prescription.[2]

If a postmenopausal woman with decreased sexual desire wants to try androgen therapy, the clinician should advise her of the potential adverse effects of androgen therapy and explain that the risks increase when androgen levels exceed women's normal physiologic levels. Side effects associated with such therapy include acne, growth of facial and body hair, clitoral enlargement, permanent voice deepening, emotional volatility, and deleterious effects on lipids and liver function.[2] Effects on cardiovascular disease or breast cancer, as well as long-term consequences of androgen therapy, are poorly understood. In addition, androgens do not protect the endometrium from estrogen's hyperplasia effects and women with an intact uterus who receive estrogen–androgen therapy must also use a progestin.[6]

Bioidentical Hormone Therapy

Bioidentical hormones are exogenous hormones that are chemically identical to endogenous hormones (e.g., estrogen, progesterone) that a woman's ovaries produce during her reproductive years.[2,49] Many bioidentical hormone therapies are available in FDA-approved, well-tested formulations. Although the list is long, a few examples include 17ß-estradiol products such as Estrace, Climara, Divigel, Evamist, and Estring; estradiol acetate products such as Femring; and oral micronized progesterone (Prometrium).[2]

Unfortunately, some consumers, healthcare providers, and pharmacists use the term "bioidentical hormone" to describe formulations that are more accurately described as "custom-compounded." Custom-compounded products were initially intended for use by the rare women for whom standard FDA-approved products were ineffective, but post-WHI safety concerns caused an increasing number of women and clinicians to explore options other than the commercial products used in the WHI.[2] Custom compounding of hormone therapy involves individual mixing of preparations, usually by a compounding pharmacist. Custom-compounded therapy may use one or more hormones, sometimes delivered via nonstandard dosing routes such as subdermal implants, sublingual tablets, rectal suppositories, or nasal sprays, in an attempt to individualize therapy for a particular woman.[44]

Menopause experts have raised a number of concerns about custom-compounded hormone therapy. Clinicians who prescribe custom-compounded hormones often base the dosing on salivary hormone testing, even though there is no scientific evidence to support the claim that salivary hormone testing can accurately dictate hormone therapy doses.[2,44,49,50] Moreover, there is no evidence that custom-compounded hormones are safer than traditional HT. Safety concerns stem from the lack of batch-to-batch testing for consistency, purity, or dose.[51] The FDA does not regulate compounded products. Instead, individual state agencies regulate compounding pharmacies, and this regulation process varies widely from state to state.

Topical progesterone, in the gels, creams, and lotions that custom-compounded hormone therapy typically includes, does not adequately raise serum levels to protect the endometrium against estrogen's stimulatory effects, which may ultimately lead to endometrial hyperplasia and endometrial cancer in some women.[2,49,50] Custom-compounded hormones also may be substantially more expensive to women because they are often considered experimental and are not covered by insurance.[50]

A number of organizations—including the North American Menopause Society (NAMS), the FDA, the American Congress of Obstetricians and Gynecologists (ACOG), the Endocrine Society, the American Medical Association, and the American Cancer Society—agree that custom-compounded therapy is no safer than traditional, commercially prepared and FDA-approved therapies and that compounding may impart additional risks.[2]

Complementary and Alternative Therapies During Menopause

Complementary and alternative medicine (CAM) encompasses a variety of healthcare practices and products that are not generally considered part of mainstream medicine in the United States. Complementary therapies are used *in addition to* and alternative therapies are used *instead of* conventional approaches. American midlife women are robust users of CAM, particularly after the WHI raised new questions about the safety of conventional hormone therapy, especially with regard to increased risk of breast cancer and cardiovascular disease.

In spite of the extensive use of CAM, few of these therapies have solid evidence to support their safety and effectiveness. Thus it can be challenging for clinicians to maintain current knowledge about CAM in order to provide accurate and useful counseling for women. A valuable resource for clinicians and the public about the safety and effectiveness of CAM is the National Center for Complementary and Alternative Medicine (NCCAM), part of the National Institutes of Health (NIH).

NCCAM divides CAM into five categories. These categories and examples of each are outlined in **Table 19-9**, and the CAM therapies that menopausal women use most often are discussed next.

Acupuncture

Practitioners of acupuncture stimulate precise points of the body, usually by inserting fine needles into the skin. Studies show inconsistent results for the

Table 19-9	Complementary and Alternative Medicine Categories and Examples
CAM Category	**Examples**
Alternative medical systems	Homeopathy, naturopathic medicine, traditional Chinese medicine, Ayurveda
Mind–body medicine	Cognitive-behavioral therapy, support groups, meditation, clinical hypnosis
Biologically based treatment	Herbs, foods, vitamins
Manipulative and body-based methods	Chiropractic, osteopathic manipulation, massage
Energy medicine	Biofield therapies, bioelectromagnetic therapies

Source: Adapted from North American Menopause Society. *Menopause Practice: A Clinician's Guide,* 4th ed. Mayfield Heights, OH: North American Menopause Society; 2010.

effectiveness of acupuncture for relieving menopausal symptoms. Methodological limitations, such as challenges in creating double-blind study designs for acupuncture, limit researchers' ability to more definitively answer questions about effectiveness. Thus many experts agree that acupuncture is a promising therapy but requires more study to determine its effectiveness.[2,52,53]

Homeopathy

Homeopathy is based on the principle of "like cures like," in which practitioners use highly diluted preparations of plant extracts and minerals to promote an individual's innate healing processes. As yet, the precise mechanisms of action of homeopathy are poorly understood. The homeopathic remedies that menopausal women use most to relieve symptoms are Lachesis (derived from South American Bushmaster snake venom), Pulsatilla (derived from the wildflower *Anemone pulsatilla*), and Sepia (derived from cuttlefish ink). Although some trials show promising results with such therapies,[54] most homeopathy research has failed to show robust results of effectiveness in improving menopausal symptoms. Further study using high-quality study designs is needed. Nevertheless, although its effectiveness may be unproven, homeopathy is thought to be quite safe.[2,52,55]

Phytoestrogens

A large number of botanically based phytoestrogen supplements and foods are purported to ease menopausal symptoms. In addition to conflicting research findings about these substances, there is also a great deal of confusion about the terminology associated with them. *Phytoestrogens* is a broad term for plant-derived compounds that have estrogenic and antiestrogenic effects. The three major classes of phytoestrogens are isoflavones, lignans, and coumestans.[52]

Isoflavones are plant-derived compounds with estrogen-like activity and a similar chemical structure to estradiol. Soy and red clover are the two most commonly used isoflavones for the relief of menopausal symptoms. Soy is usually derived from whole soybeans and is the most widely consumed isoflavone-containing food. The amount of isoflavones in soy-containing foods varies widely, from 151.17 mg isoflavones per 100 g of raw green soybeans to 9.65 mg isoflavones per 100 g of soymilk . Moreover, the manufacturing process used for each food can have significant negative effects on the amount of isoflavones found in the final product. Although research evidence about soy is complex, it is likely that soy has modest benefits in the short-term (e.g., 3 months) treatment of hot flashes but not for longer periods. Moreover, a trial of 3 months is sufficient to evaluate whether a woman is likely to respond to therapy. Women during menopausal transition can be reassured that soy does not appear to have harmful effects on the endometrium or on the breast, even in women at increased risk for breast cancer and breast cancer survivors.[2,41,56]

Red clover contains different types of isoflavones and has different affinities for various steroid receptors when compared to soy. Evidence is mixed about its effectiveness, with a few studies demonstrating small beneficial effects on hot flash reduction but most evidence pointing to a lack of effectiveness.[2,41,57–60]

Lignans are another type of phytoestrogen. They are thought to have a much lower hormonal affinity than isoflavones and therefore are not very useful in decreasing menopausal symptoms. Lignans are found in flaxseed oil and whole grains.

Coumestans, another type of phytoestrogen, are also thought to have much lower hormonal affinity than isoflavones and therefore are not very effective in decreasing menopausal symptoms. Coumestans are found in alfalfa sprouts and certain beans and peas.[2,53,56,57]

Herbal Therapies

Menopausal women frequently use herbal remedies in an attempt to relieve symptoms such as hot flashes, mood instability, and irregular bleeding, and to promote overall feelings of well-being. Demand for herbal treatment of menopausal symptoms has increased even further since the release of the Women's Health Initiative results.

In spite of widespread consumer interest in herbal therapies, midwives face significant challenges when counseling women about the safety and effectiveness of such remedies. These challenges include the ever-increasing number and variety of products on the market, a lack of standardization of doses, and too few high-quality, large studies to evaluate herbs' safety and effectiveness. Additionally, clinicians are sometimes unaware that their patients are using herbal remedies because there is a mistaken belief that anything "natural" is safe and unworthy of mentioning to a clinician. Herbal therapies can cause adverse events and are associated with herb–drug interactions, although the extent of each is difficult to determine.[2,52]

The herbal remedies that women most often use to relieve menopausal symptoms are black cohosh, chastetree berry, dong quai, evening primrose oil, gingko, ginseng, kava, licorice root, St. John's wort, valerian, and wild yam. **Table 19-10** identifies each herb's proposed effects on menopausal symptoms, dosages, and summary of safety and effectiveness.[2,38,40,52,53,57,60–64]

Other CAM Therapies

Among other therapies that have been advocated for treatment of women with vasomotor symptoms is clinical hypnosis. A multiyear, NIH-funded project on this topic has included small randomized clinical trials that demonstrate women undergoing clinical hypnosis have a decreased number of hot flashes compared to a placebo group.[65] Additional research is needed in this area, although these results are promising.

The Women's Health Initiative: A Dramatic Change in Menopause Practice

The Women's Health Initiative had extensive and wide-reaching effects on the care of menopausal women. This research created a vast shift in women's and clinicians' attitudes, the tone and content of menopause symptom management counseling options, and clinicians' prescribing habits. For decades prior to the termination of the WHI in 2002, clinicians and experts used the best available, albeit largely observational, evidence to conclude that hormone therapy was effective and safe for treating several important menopausal problems. Not only was HT thought to be the optimal therapy for menopausal symptoms, but it was also believed to be cardioprotective. Indeed, HT was considered to be effective for primary prevention and, before the Heart and Estrogen Progestin Replacement Study (HERS), for secondary prevention of cardiovascular disease.[66] Many clinicians encouraged all midlife and older women—including women without specific menopausal symptoms—to take systemic HT as a prophylactic measure.[67]

This landscape changed drastically and quickly in 2002, when investigators announced that they had prematurely terminated what was intended to be a 15-year clinical trial. Media reports emphasized that HT users faced increased risks of breast cancer and cardiovascular disease.[68] Women became frightened, and many stopped taking HT overnight. Many clinicians immediately changed their prescribing and counseling habits, encouraging use of non-HT remedies, writing fewer standard-dose HT prescriptions, and prescribing proportionately more transdermal and low-dose HT.[67,69,70] **Table 19-11** summarizes the findings from the WHI that prompted this sea change in practitioner behavior.[48,71]

Following the discontinuation of the WHI, analyses of the vast amounts of data that the trial had generated were untaken. As WHI was the only large, long-term, randomized controlled trial for certain study outcomes, findings about the care of menopausal women have been considered extremely important. However, several factors related to the study design have given researchers and clinicians pause in extrapolating the WHI findings to all menopausal women. WHI study participants used only oral hormone therapy, only one type of estrogen (conjugated estrogens), and only one progestin (medroxyprogesterone acetate). Moreover, the WHI included women age 50 to 79 years and participants were, on average, 63 years of age at entry to the study. Age is a critical factor to consider because these women were much older than the recently menopausal women who are most likely to request HT for symptom relief,[45] which led to questions about the effects of timing of HT initiation on study outcomes.[44] Due to these questions and others, analysis of the WHI findings has been complex and many controversies remain. However, as of 2012, experts from the North American Menopause Society, as well as those from

Table 19-10	Herbal Remedies Used Most Often for Relief of Menopausal Symptoms		
Herb	**Proposed Effects on Menopausal Symptoms**	**Provision of Therapy**	**Clinical Summary**
Black cohosh (*Cimicifuga racemosa*)	Diminishes hot flashes	20 mg twice/day of proprietary standardized extract; recommended dose of Remifemin supplement is 40–80 mg/day	Possible evidence of benefit for hot flash relief. Most widely studied herb for menopausal symptoms, but recent studies have many methodological limitations. Much variation in brands and preparations.
Chastetree berry (*Vitex agnus castus*)	Diminishes PMS symptoms; regulates menses	250 mg of crude herb or 20 mg/day of 12:1 ratio of standardized extract	Evidence of benefit for PMS symptoms. Possible benefits for regulating irregular perimenopausal bleeding. Popular in Europe and approved therapy in Germany for PMS, mastalgia, and menopause symptoms.
Dong quai (*Angelica sinensis*)	Treats various gynecologic conditions; diminishes hot flashes	2 capsules 2–3×/day	No data indicating effectiveness. Usually used in conjunction with other herbs. Can trigger heavy uterine bleeding; avoid in women with fibroids or coagulation problems.
Evening primrose oil (*Oenothera biennis*)	Diminishes hot flashes and breast tenderness	1500–4000 mg/day in divided doses	No data indicating effectiveness.
Gingko (*Gingko biloba*)	Promotes good memory	40–80 mg of standardized extract taken 3×/day	No data indicating effectiveness. Potential safety concerns regarding increased bleeding, including subdural hematoma.
Ginseng (*Panax ginseng*)	Improves mood, minimizes fatigue	100–600 mg/day of standardized extract in divided doses	No data indicating effectiveness for hot flashes. Possible effectiveness for overall feelings of well-being. Significant problems with purity of preparations.
Kava (*Piper methysticum*)	Minimizes irritability, promotes sleep	150–300 mg of root extract per day in divided doses	Effective for treating anxiety but effect is small. Possible hepatotoxicity; some experts recommend avoiding completely.
Licorice root (*Glycyrrhiza glabra*)	Diminish hot flashes	5–15 mg/day of root equivalent in divided doses	No data indicating effectiveness. High doses or long-term use can cause HTN and kidney, liver, or cardiac dysfunction.
St. John's wort (*Hypericum perforatum*)	Diminishes hot flashes, decreases irritability, treats depression	300 mg of standardized extract taken 3×/day	Evidence of benefit for mood stabilization. Mixed evidence for hot flash relief. Sometimes used in conjunction with black cohosh. Do not use with SSRIs and certain other medications.
Valerian (*Valeriana officinalis*)	Promotes sleep; decreases anxiety	Insomnia: 300–600 mg aqueous extract 30–60 min before bed Anxiety: 150–300 mg aqueous extract each morning and 300–400 mg each evening	Evidence of benefit for insomnia and anxiety. Few side effects at recommended dosages and with relatively short-term use.

(continues)

Table 19-10	Herbal Remedies Used Most Often for Relief of Menopausal Symptoms *(continued)*		
Herb	**Proposed Effects on Menopausal Symptoms**	**Provision of Therapy**	**Clinical Summary**
Wild yam (*Dioscorea villosa*)	Diminishes hot flashes	Unknown	No demonstrated benefits. Wild yam cream does not convert to progesterone in the body as product manufacturers claim.

HTN = hypertension; PMS = premenstrual syndrome; SSRI = selective serotonin reuptake inhibitor.

Sources: Data from North American Menopause Society. *Menopause Practice: A Clinician's Guide*, 4th ed. Mayfield Heights, OH: North American Menopause Society; 2010; Guttuso T. Effective and clinically meaningful non-hormonal hot flash therapies. *Maturitas.* 2012;72:6-12; Andrews JC. Vasomotor symptoms: an evidence-based approach to medical management. *J Clin Outcome Manage.* 2011;18:112-128; Borrelli F, Ernst E. Alternative and complementary therapies for the menopause. *Maturitas.* 2010;66:333-343; Hall E, Frey BN, Soares CN. Non-hormonal treatment strategies for vasomotor symptoms: a critical review. *Drugs.* 2011;71:287-304; Panay N. Taking an integrated approach: managing women with phytoestrogens. *Climacteric.* 2011;14:2-7; Geller SE, Shulman LP, van Breemen RB, et al. Safety and efficacy of black cohosh and red clover for the management of vasomotor symptoms: a randomized controlled trial. *Menopause.* 2009;16:1156-1166; Darsareh F, Taavoni S, Joolaee S, Haghani H. Effect of aromatherapy massage on menopausal symptoms: a randomized placebo-controlled clinical trial. *Menopause.* 2012;19:995-999; Regestein QR. Is there anything special about valerian? *Menopause.* 2011;18:937-939; Taavoni S, Ekbatani N, Kashaniayn M, Haghani H. Effect of valerian on sleep quality in postmenopausal women: a randomized, placebo-controlled clinical trial. *Menopause.* 2011;18:951-955; Leach MJ, Moore V. Black cohosh (*Cimicifuga* spp.) for menopausal symptoms. *Cochrane Database Syst Rev.* 2012;9:CD007244. doi: 10.1002/14651858.CD007244.pub2.

12 other major medical organizations, agreed on the following conclusions from the WHI, which can guide clinical practice.[72]

Is HT Still a Viable Option?

Systemic HT is a reasonable option for women with moderate to severe menopausal symptoms, particularly healthy women who are younger than the age of 60 years or within 10 years of the date of their menopause.

What Are the Risks of HT?

The risks of venous thromboembolism and ischemic stroke increase with the use of ET and EPT, but these events are rare in women younger than age 60 years. A small but real risk of breast cancer occurs after 5 years or more of EPT, and possibly earlier with continuous use since menopause. This risk decreases after HT is discontinued. Estrogen alone used for an average of 7 years in the WHI did not increase the risk for breast cancer. Because of the media exposure accorded to the

Table 19-11	Summary of Outcomes from Estrogen-Progestin Arm of the Women's Health Initiative		
Outcome Measure	**Women Using HT: Events per 10,000 Person-Year**	**Women on Placebo: Events per 10,000 Person-Year**	**Absolute Risk: HT vs. No HT in 10,000 Women over 1 Year**
Invasive breast cancer	38	30	8 more women affected
Coronary heart disease	37	30	7 more women affected
Stroke	29	21	8 more women affected
Venous thromboembolism, including deep vein thrombosis and pulmonary embolism	34	16	18 more women affected
Hip fracture	10	15	5 fewer women affected
Colorectal cancer	10	16	6 fewer women affected

Sources: Data from Langer RD, Manson JE, Allison MA. Have we come full circle—or moved forward? The Women's Health Initiative 10 years on. *Climacteric.* 2012;15:206-212; Writing Group for the Women's Health Initiative. Risks and benefits of estrogen plus progestin in healthy postmenopausal women: principal results from the Women's Health Initiative randomized controlled trial. *JAMA.* 2002;288:321-333.

WHI results, many women now are inappropriately frightened that use of any hormone therapy is associated with an extremely high risk for breast cancer; providers need to clarify the actual risks, including absolute risks associated with age and gender.

Who Should Use HT?

HT should be used solely for menopausal symptom relief, rather than for prevention. Therapy decisions should be made with the individual woman, considering the quality of life she desires, her age and time since menopause, and her personal risk factors for cardiovascular disease and breast cancer. **Table 19-12** identifies cardiovascular and breast cancer risk factors to consider when counseling a woman about risks and benefits of HT.

Which Type of Therapy Should Clinicians and Women Choose?

Systemic HT is the most effective therapy for hot flashes. For women who have only vulvovaginal conditions, the preference is local vaginal therapy.[73] Women who have an intact uterus and take systemic estrogen therapy must take a progestin to minimize the risk of endometrial cancer. Women who have undergone a hysterectomy do not need a progestin. Although comparison randomized clinical trial data are not available, some evidence indicates that transdermal estrogen therapy confers less risk of venous thromboembolism and stroke when compared to standard-dose oral estrogen preparations.

Which Dose and for How Long?

Clinicians should prescribe the lowest dose of HT that effectively manages symptoms and encourage women to use it for the shortest time possible. Optimally, combined estrogen plus progestin therapy should be taken for no longer than 5 years, but a decision to discontinue therapy should be individualized. For estrogen therapy, longer duration may be safer. **Box 19-1** contains for a brief case study illustrating midwifery care for a perimenopausal woman.

Menopause researchers Pal and Manson eloquently describe the post-WHI landscape in which clinicians care for women:

> In the wake of WHI, as clinicians, we stand enhanced, having become more familiar with concepts of individualized care. As clinical researchers, we stand educated, being more aware of the strengths and limitations of different types of research and more cautious about extrapolation of findings. As a community, we stand strengthened, as women have become more active participants in decision-making regarding their own well-being.[67]

Table 19-12	Cardiovascular and Breast Cancer Risk Factors to Guide Risk–Benefit Decisions
Cardiovascular Risk Factors	**Breast Cancer Risk Factors**
Postmenopausal/older age	Personal history of breast, endometrial, ovarian, or (possibly) colon cancer
Cigarette smoking	Family history of breast cancer in a mother, sister, or daughter, particularly if premenopausal
Sedentary lifestyle	
Hypertension	Menarche before age 12 years
Diabetes mellitus	Menopause after age 55 years
Abnormal lipids	Nulliparity or first child born after age 30 years
Obesity, especially central adiposity	Obesity after menopause
Unhealthy diet	Alcohol consumption of ≥ 2 drinks/day
Family history of premature cardiovascular disease	Minimal exercise, < 4 hours/week
	Low levels of vitamin D
Metabolic syndrome	Diet low in fruits and vegetables
	Radiation exposure
	Long-term(> 5 years) use of estrogen–progestogen therapy

Source: Adapted from North American Menopause Society. *Menopause Practice: A Clinician's Guide*, 4th ed. Mayfield Heights, OH: North American Menopause Society; 2010.

Bone Health, Osteopenia, and Osteoporosis

Osteoporosis is a deceptively silent disease with significant medical and economic implications. In this disorder, bone mass and strength are lost and bone quality deteriorates—changes that increase the risk that the bone will fracture.[74,75] **Table 19-13** defines key terms related to osteoporosis. There usually are no symptoms until a fracture occurs. Approximately 2 million osteoporosis-related fractures occur annually in the United States, which lead to significant morbidity among women and cost the healthcare system approximately $17 billion each year.[74,76]

Hip fracture is the most costly and dramatic type of fracture; 24% of persons age 50 years and older die within the year after a hip fracture.[77-78] That problem is on the rise: the U.S. Surgeon General estimates that the economic and medical costs of hip fractures could triple by the year 2040.[74] Thus preventing fracture—particularly hip fracture—is a pressing task.

Humans build bone throughout childhood, adolescence, and young adulthood, with bone mass peaking by ages 18 to 25 years. Genetic factors, and to a lesser extent nutrition, physical activity, and general health, determine the amount and quality of bone that an individual has at her peak. Throughout the bone formation process, osteoclasts help to

---

BOX 19-1 Case Study: Midwifery Management of a Perimenopausal Woman

Case

M.M. is a 50-year-old woman who is being seen by a midwife to discuss a number of personal symptoms as well as her treatment options. Her periods have always been regular until approximately 5 years ago, when they became heavier and irregular, with some months without menses occurring within the last 2 years. Her last period was 3 months ago. M.M. has four or five hot flashes per day that are moderately bothersome to her. She has difficulty getting to sleep at night and often wakes at 3:30 a.m., unable to get back to sleep. M.M. cries often and has some "very blue" periods, although she is able to function normally and still reports a generally contented life. She has dry skin and reports a 10-pound weight gain in the last 2 years. She smokes one pack of cigarettes a day. Her medical history is uncomplicated. A pelvic exam reveals pale vaginal tissue with few rugae; the remainder of her exam is normal.

Assessments

M.M. is likely in the late menopausal transition stage, which has an average length of 1 to 3 years. Although there can be substantial individual variation, based on her age, symptom constellation, and menstrual history, it is likely that she is nearing her final menstrual period.

It is also reasonable to consider thyroid dysfunction because it is so common in midlife women and because M.M. reports weight gain and dry skin.

Plan

Offer thyroid testing. Educate M.M. about dressing in layers, keeping a hot flash symptom record to recognize

and avoid hot flash triggers, and maintaining a regular sleep schedule. Discuss the types of interventions that M.M. has already considered or attempted. Clarify if M.M. is sexually active.

If M.M. is interested in CAM, offer and discuss the evidence for black cohosh for hot flashes, St. John's wort to regulate her mood, and valerian to promote sleep. If she is interested in prescriptive therapy, offer and discuss use of a selective serotonin reuptake inhibitor (SSRI) or serotonin-norepinephrine reuptake inhibitor (SNRI) to help with mood and hot flashes, as well as the use of gabapentin to decrease hot flashes and potentially help her sleep better. The midwife should also further assess M.M.'s mood issues and consider whether a referral for counseling is indicated.

Assuming that M.M., like most women her age, is sexually active, discuss her fertility status. Given that M.M. is a smoker, the midwife should assess her readiness for smoking cessation. M.M. is not eligible for *combined hormonal contraceptives* to regulate her bleeding or hormonal fluctuations during the perimenopause, but other options such as the levonorgestrel IUS or depot medroxyprogesterone acetate (DMPA) may provide pregnancy prevention as well as treatment for abnormal uterine bleeding.

Introduce information about *hormone therapy* (oral, transdermal, or vaginal estrogen plus a progestogen because M.M. has not had a hysterectomy) for use after her final menstrual period should she desire. This visit is a good time to clarify misinformation and misconceptions.

Note: This case is limited to menopause. The reader should refer to chapters about breast health, cervical cytology, and preventive care for details of other aspects of complete health care of a woman of this age.

remove old bone and osteoblasts help to build new bone. With increasing age and as women become postmenopausal, more bone is removed than is built; the result can be weakened bone structure and decreased bone mass. As a result, bone becomes more fragile and is more prone to fracture even without significant trauma.[74,75,77] Certain risk factors predispose individuals to experience an even greater extent of bone loss and/or an even higher risk of fracture. **Table 19-14** summarizes risk factors for osteoporosis and osteoporosis-related fractures.

Clinicians usually diagnose and manage low bone mass by measuring bone mineral density (BMD) through dual-energy X-ray absorptiometry (DXA), an enhanced type of X ray (**Table 19-15**). Although BMD is not a perfect surrogate for fracture, a person's BMD is more predictive of fracture than cholesterol level is predictive of myocardial infarction.[76] If bone mass is placed on a continuum in which normal bone mass is 1 standard deviation (SD) above and below 0, *osteopenia* represents the next finding on the continuum. Osteopenia is defined as decreased bone mass

Table 19-13	Osteoporosis Definitions
Term	**Definition**
Bone mineral density (BMD)	Surrogate marker for bone strength and resistance to fracture
	Measured by dual-energy X-ray absorptiometry
	Usually measured and reported for hip, femoral neck, and spine
	Results reported as standard deviations from the mean of a reference population
Dual-energy X-ray absorptiometry (DEXA or DXA)	Gold standard diagnostic technology for measuring BMD
FRAX	Online fracture risk assessment tool to assist in clinical decision making for screening and treatment decisions
	Calculates absolute fracture risk/estimate of risk for fracture in next 10 years
	Calculations include age, bone density, and risk factors
Osteoblasts	Bone-building cells
	Remember: "Blasts build"
Osteoclasts	Bone-breakdown cells
	Remember: "Clasts cut down"
Osteopenia	Low bone mass
	T-score between −1.0 and −2.5
Osteoporosis	Skeletal disease of low bone mass and deterioration of bone micro-architecture
	Resulting bone fragility increases risk that bone will fracture
	BMD T-score < −2.5 constitutes osteoporosis
T-score	Comparison with mean peak BMD of a normal, young, same-sex population
	Number of standard deviations that a person's BMD differs from the mean peak BMD of a normal young adult of the same sex
	Most commonly used measurement when making clinical decisions about midlife and older women
Z-score	Comparison with a reference population of the same age, gender, and ethnicity
	Not commonly used when evaluating midlife and older women; can be misleading because bone density is often low in older adults
	Used mostly for children, teens, and young adults

Sources: Data from National Osteoporosis Foundation. *Clinician's Guide to Prevention and Treatment of Osteoporosis.* Washington, DC: National Osteoporosis Foundation; 2010; Osteoporosis. Practice Bulletin No. 129. American College of Obstetricians and Gynecologists. *Obstet Gynecol.* 2012;120:718-734; Pollycove R, Simon JA. Osteoporosis: screening and treatment in women. *Clin Obstet Gynecol.* 2012;55:681-691; North American Menopause Society. Management of osteoporosis in postmenopausal women: 2012 position statement of the North American Menopause Society. *Menopause.* 2012;17:25-54.

Table 19-14	Considerations for Ordering Bone Mineral Density Testing	
Women Who Generally Should Have BMD Testing	**Women Who Generally Should Not Have BMD Testing**	
All women 65 years and older	As a "baseline" or routine screen of newly menopausal women who do not have significant risk factors	
At menopause: women with a history of fracture or with a parent who had a hip fracture or multiple vertebral or nonvertebral fragility fractures	To monitor effects of depot medroxyprogesterone acetate (DMPA; Depo-Provera) on bone density	
Before menopause or during menopausal transition: women with specific risk factors for increased fracture risk such as anorexia, long-term glucocorticoid use, metabolic bone disease, hyperthyroidism, low body weight, prior low-trauma fracture, or high-risk medication		
For treatment decisions: to monitor effects of osteoporosis therapy, if being considered for medications, or if evidence of bone loss would lead to treatment		
As indicated by FRAX: clinicians can use FRAX to determine which women younger than 65 years should have BMD testing; if FRAX indicates that a woman has a 9.3% or higher 10-year risk of major osteoporotic fracture, it is reasonable for that woman to have a DXA		

BMD = bone mineral density; FRAX= World Health Organization's Fracture Risk Assessment Tool.

Sources: Data from National Osteoporosis Foundation. *Clinician's Guide to Prevention and Treatment of Osteoporosis.* Washington, DC: National Osteoporosis Foundation; 2010; Osteoporosis. Practice Bulletin No. 129. American College of Obstetricians and Gynecologists. *Obstet Gynecol.* 2012;120:718-734; Pollycove R, Simon JA. Osteoporosis: screening and treatment in women. *Clin Obstet Gynecol.* 2012;55:681-691

Table 19-15	Risk Factors for Osteoporosis and Osteoporotic Fractures in Women	
Nonmodifiable Risk Factors	**Potentially Modifiable Risk Factors**	
Age > 65 years	Smoking	
Personal history of fracture without substantial trauma as an adult	BMI < 20 or weight < 127 lb	
Family history of osteoporosis	Eating disorder or excessive exercise-induced amenorrhea	
Hip, spine, or wrist fracture without substantial trauma in first-degree relative	Chronic glucocorticoid use (e.g., prednisone > 5 mg/day for > 3–6 months)	
Race: white and Asian women are at greatest risk, followed by Hispanic and African American women	Multiple risk factors for falling (e.g., decreased leg or arm muscle strength, diminished vision, environmental hazards, impaired cognition)	
Female gender	Chronic illnesses: rheumatoid arthritis, hyperparathyroidism, impaired absorption syndromes	
Late menarche(> 15 years) or early menopause (< 45 years)	Heavy alcohol use (≥ 3 drinks/day)	

Sources: Data from National Osteoporosis Foundation. *Clinician's Guide to Prevention and Treatment of Osteoporosis.* Washington, DC: National Osteoporosis Foundation; 2010; Osteoporosis. Practice Bulletin No. 129. American College of Obstetricians and Gynecologists. *Obstet Gynecol.* 2012;120:718-734; North American Menopause Society. Management of osteoporosis in postmenopausal women: 2012 position statement of the North American Menopause Society. *Menopause.* 2012;17:25-54.

ranging from 1 SD below 0 to 2.5 SD below 0. This condition is three times more prevalent than osteoporosis. Moving even farther away from normal bone mass on the continuum, *osteoporosis* represents even more significantly decreased bone mass, 2.5 SD below 0 and lower (**Figure 19-2**). A T-score is the most commonly used reporting method for the results of BMD evaluation.[76] Generally, DXA measurements are taken at the femoral neck, at the posterior–anterior lumbar spine, and as a total hip measurement; the lowest of the three values determines the diagnostic category to which the individual assigned.[76]

FRAX: The Fracture Risk Assessment Tool

Clinically, the important goal related to bone health is *fracture prevention*, rather than simply promoting a specific bone mineral density score. BMD is just one aspect of a person's bone health, as other factors also influence fracture risk. To assist clinicians in making optimal decisions about who is at risk for fracture and when to intervene, in 2008, osteoporosis experts from the World Health Organization (WHO) introduced the Fracture Risk Assessment Tool, known as FRAX. FRAX is an algorithm-based, computerized risk assessment tool that provides an estimate of the likelihood of a major (e.g., hip, spine, forearm) fracture in the next 10 years.[74,79] Economic modeling for cost-effectiveness determines the cutoffs for treatment recommendations. For the U.S. population, the National Osteoporosis Foundation recommends treatment for persons with a 3% or higher chance of breaking a hip in the next 10 years or a 20% or greater chance of breaking any major bone in the next 10 years.[79]

Risk factors in the FRAX algorithm include age, gender, smoking, three or more alcoholic drinks per day, rheumatoid arthritis, low BMI, prolonged corticosteroid use, secondary osteoporosis, parent with a hip fracture, and BMD.[79,80] The algorithm does not take into account certain aspects of these risk factors,

such as the amount of tobacco use or corticosteroid use, and does not consider some other risk factors at all (e.g., activity level, risk for falling, and intake of calcium, vitamin D, and caffeine).[79]

Clinicians can assess an individual's FRAX score from WHO's Collaborating Centre for Metabolic Diseases by accessing http://www.shef.ac.uk/FRAX/. Several other clinical point-of-care options are available, including desktop or laptop applications that do not require Internet access as well as an iPhone application. Midwives can find more information about these tools by visiting the main FRAX website. Imaging centers that use updated DXA machines also include FRAX scores in their DXA reports.[79]

The National Osteoporosis Foundation provides several clinical caveats to consider when using FRAX. When caring for women in the United States, for example, clinicians should consider that FRAX is intended for postmenopausal women and not for younger adults or children. For individuals currently or previously taking osteoporosis medications, the midwife should exercise caution in interpreting FRAX scores because FRAX has not been validated in this population. Moreover, while the intent of FRAX is to make clinical decisions more straightforward, all treatment decisions require careful clinical judgment of individual patient characteristics. FRAX does not capture all risk factors; conversely, its recommendations do not mandate treatment.[74]

Lifestyle and Nonmedication Strategies to Promote Bone Health

Several lifestyle and nonmedication strategies can promote bone health to all women. Robust scientific evidence indicates these strategies are effective in improving bone mineral density and reducing fracture risk. Moreover, these strategies are generally inexpensive, have minimal inherent risks, and can confer benefits for other aspects of a person's health. These strategies include consuming a healthy diet with an adequate amount of certain nutrients, participating in regular weight-bearing exercise, maintaining a healthy weight, and avoiding tobacco use and excessive alcohol intake.

Consume a Healthy Diet and Adequate Calcium and Vitamin D

Although a balanced diet is key for healthy bones, some populations—such as the elderly, women with eating disorders, or impoverished women—may not consume adequate vitamins, minerals, fruits, vegetables, and grains. Of the various dietary nutrients, calcium and vitamin D are the most vital for

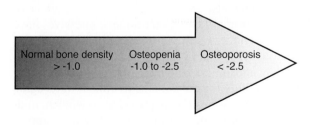

Normal bone density
> -1.0

Osteopenia
-1.0 to -2.5

Osteoporosis
< -2.5

Figure 19-2 Bone mineral density continuum.

Source: Data from National Osteoporosis Foundation. *Clinician's Guide to Prevention and Treatment of Osteoporosis.* Washington, DC: National Osteoporosis Foundation; 2010.

bone health, and consumption of a diet rich in these nutrients and/or supplement intake of them lowers fracture risk.[74,76] Major organizations such as the National Osteoporosis Foundation, the National Academy of Sciences, and the Institute of Medicine recommend that women older than age 50 years consume 1200 mg of calcium per day and 600–1000 IU of vitamin D per day.[74,75,78] The best sources of vitamin D and calcium are in foods. Vitamin D and calcium supplements for the purpose of improving bone health have not been shown to be effective and are not recommended for healthy adults.

Engage in Regular Exercise

Muscle-strengthening and weight-bearing exercise has multiple benefits for the bone health (and overall well-being) of midlife and older women. Improved strength, balance, agility, and posture can reduce the risk of falling; falling has the potential for significant negative sequelae such as fractures, pain, disability, and death. Exercise also has modest effects on bone density by virtue of increased bone mass in response to activities that place stress on bones.[78] Women should weigh the risk of falling against the benefits of particular exercises. Examples of exercises that are usually beneficial are walking, jogging, stair climbing, dancing, tennis, tai chi, and reasonable weight-lifting regimens.[74,78]

Maintain a Healthy Weight

Body weight less than 127 pounds or a BMI less than 21 are risk factors for low bone mass and increased fracture risk. The benefits of gaining weight should be discussed with very thin women so their weight is in a healthful range.[78]

Avoid Smoking and Excessive Alcohol Intake

In addition to the many other deleterious health effects of smoking and excessive alcohol intake, these lifestyle choices have significantly negative effects on women's bones. Women smokers have lower bone mass, lose bone more quickly, and have significantly higher fracture risk than nonsmokers.[78] While moderate alcohol intake does not have any recognized detrimental effects on bones, consuming three or more alcoholic drinks per day increases the risk of osteoporotic fracture and falling.[74,78]

Pharmacologic Options for Osteoporosis Management

A focus on lifestyle strategies may be all that is needed to promote bone health and minimize fracture risk for midlife and older women at low risk for fracture. However, midwives should consider pharmacologic therapy for women with any of the following: osteoporosis (T-score of –2.5 or lower), history of a low-trauma hip or vertebral fracture, or osteopenia (T-score between –1 and –2.5) *if* FRAX indicates a 10-year probability of 3% or greater of a hip fracture or a 10-year probability of 20% or greater of a major osteoporosis-related fracture.[74,75,78]

A variety of FDA-approved medications are available to prevent and/or treat osteoporosis, including bisphosphonates, estrogen, raloxifene, calcitonin, and teriparatide. A summary of the medications in each category, dose, and basic prescribing issues can be found in **Table 19-16**. Adherence to pharmacologic osteoporosis treatment is poor, however, with adherence rates in 6- to 12-month studies ranging from less than 25% to 81%.[78] Thus, if the midwife and the woman decide that medications are necessary, it is vitally important the woman be educated about her fracture risk and the purpose of therapy, and then identify and eliminate barriers to adherence.[78] Dosing frequency seems to affect adherence; weekly dosing enhances adherence for many women when compared to daily dosing.[81] **Box 19-2** contains a brief case study illustrating midwifery care of a menopausal woman.

Conclusion

Additional resources related to menopause and osteoporosis are listed at the end of this chapter. Menopause, similar to pregnancy, is a time when women often present to the healthcare system for help with changes, to gain knowledge of the processes occurring, and for regular health care. Midwives who care for women at midlife have the opportunity to develop an individualized preventive health program, health screening, disease identification and treatment, maintenance of continuity of care, appropriate referrals, and supervision of cost-effective care. As primary care practitioners, midwives have an opportunity to provide leadership in the delivery of holistic, woman-centered health care to women as they age and to influence society to accept more responsibility for the humane treatment of its aging population. As healthcare providers to women, midwives can offer support to, and hold genuine appreciation of, the journey that women traverse from the menopausal transition through old age and celebrate each woman's strengths, struggles, decisions, and accomplishments.

Table 19-16	Medications for Osteoporosis Management	
Medication **Generic (Brand)**	**Dose**	**Comments**
Bisphosphonates		
Alendronate (Fosamax)	Prevention: 5 mg daily or 35 mg weekly tablet or oral solution Treatment: 10 mg daily or 70 mg weekly tablet or oral solution	Bisphosphonates are considered by many experts to be first-line therapy for osteoporosis Choice of bisphosphonate is often made based on the desired dosing regimen
Ibandronate (Boniva)	Prevention: 2.5 mg daily or 150 mg monthly tablet Treatment: 2.5 mg daily or 150 mg monthly tablet or 3 mg every 3 months IV	Must take 30–60 min before eating in the morning, with 8 oz water; must sit/stand upright for 30–60 min
Risedronate (Actonel)	Prevention and treatment: 5 mg daily; 35 mg weekly; 35 mg weekly packaged with 6 tablets of 500 mg calcium carbonate; 75 mg on two consecutive days every month; and 150 mg monthly tablet	Side effects for all oral bisphosphonates: difficulty swallowing, esophageal inflammation, gastric ulcers
Zoledronic acid (Reclast)	Prevention: 5 mg IV every 2 years Treatment: 5 mg IV annually	
Calcitonin		
Salmon calcitonin (Miacalcin; Fortical)	Treatment (> 5 years postmenopause): 200 IU daily nasal spray	FDA approved for treatment of vertebral osteoporosis but not at nonvertebral sites (e.g., hip) Other agents are more reliable at both vertebral and nonvertebral sites; calcitonin is not a first-tier therapy
Hormone Therapy		
Various ET/HT preparations	See Tables 19-6, 19-7, and 19-8	Protects against bone loss and reduces risk of fractures FDA approved for osteoporosis prevention but not treatment Useful in women who need osteoporosis prevention *and* menopausal symptom treatment
Estrogen Agonist/Antagonist (Selective Estrogen Receptor Modulator [SERM])		
Raloxifene (Evista)	Prevention and treatment: 60 mg daily	Not only inhibits bone resorption, but also decreases risk of breast and uterine cancers Effective at reducing the risk of vertebral fractures but not hip or other nonvertebral fractures Can cause hot flashes Contraindicated in women with venous thromboembolism history
Parathyroid Hormone		
Teriparatide (Forteo)	Treatment (postmenopausal women at very high fracture risk): 20 mcg daily SQ	Indicated for patients with established osteoporosis at very high risk of primary fracture or patients with continued fractures in spite of other antiresorptive therapies

Sources: Data from National Osteoporosis Foundation. *Clinician's Guide to Prevention and Treatment of Osteoporosis.* Washington, DC: National Osteoporosis Foundation; 2010; North American Menopause Society. Management of osteoporosis in postmenopausal women: 2012 position statement of the North American Menopause Society. *Menopause.* 2012;17:25-54; Agency for Healthcare Research and Policy (AHRQ). *Treatment to Prevent Osteoporotic Fractures: An Update.* May 2012.

BOX 19-2 Case Study: Midwifery Management of a Postmenopausal Woman

Case

V.A. is 62-year-old white woman who is seeing her midwife for a regular gynecologic visit. V.A. is healthy, takes no medications, and has no active medical problems. She is 11 years past menopause and is doing well but has a few questions and concerns. Her primary concern is that she is bothered by vaginal dryness and pain with penetration when she has sexual intercourse. Lubricant and moisturizers have not been useful. V.A. never took hormone therapy because she never had very severe hot flashes but she wonders if she should start it now to help with her vaginal symptoms. V.A.'s aunt had breast cancer at the age of 58 and her mother died of a myocardial infarction at the age of 70. V.A. is a nonsmoker and drinks 1 glass of wine per day.

V.A. brought the results of the DXA scan she had last week. Her T-scores are −2.6 at the femoral neck, −2.7 at the lumbar spine, and −2.9 total hip score. V.A. weighs 121 pounds and is 63 inches tall. Her physical exam is unremarkable, with the exception of extensive atrophic changes in her vulvovaginal tissue.

Assessment

V.A. has significant vulvovaginal atrophy that is unlikely to improve with anything other than estrogen therapy.

V.A. is an ideal candidate for local vaginal estrogen, but not for systemic estrogen. She does not have systemic symptoms such as hot flashes. Also, she has an unfavorable risk–benefit ratio for systemic hormone therapy because she is 11 years post menopause and has a family history of breast cancer and cardiovascular disease.

V.A. has osteoporosis and her T-score indicates that the midwife should offer V.A. treatment.

Plan

The midwife should discuss vaginal estrogen products such as a vaginal cream, tablet, and the vaginal ring Estring for V.A.'s vaginal atrophy. These therapies provide local, vaginal effects only and do not require a progestogen for endometrial protection. (Contrast this with the systemic dosing that would come from oral or transdermal therapies or the vaginal ring Femring; all of these options require a progestogen for endometrial protection. These systemic-level products are not necessary for V.A. because she does not have systemic-level symptoms such as hot flashes.) Note that estrogen is not indicated for treatment of osteoporosis.

To build or maintain bone health, the midwife should encourage V.A. to have daily intake of 1200 mg of calcium and 600–1000 IU of vitamin D, through diet and/or supplements; to make a slow and steady weight gain of approximately 5–10 pounds through adding healthy calories each day; and to walk each day with a gradual increase in distance.

V.A. is also a candidate for osteoporosis pharmacologic therapy. The midwife should offer and discuss the risks and benefits of each therapy type. The initial drug therapy would be a bisphosphonate with the dosing regimen that V.A. thinks would be most convenient for her. The midwife should plan to order a repeat DXA in 1 to 2 years to monitor the response to therapy.

Note: This case is limited to menopause and osteoporosis issues. The reader should refer to chapters about breast health, cervical cytology, and preventive care for other details of other aspects of complete health care of a woman of this age.

● ● ● References

1. Harris MTC. Aging women's journey toward wholeness: new visions and directions. *Health Care Women Int.* 2008;29:962-979.

2. North American Menopause Society. *Menopause Practice: A Clinician's Guide.* 4th ed. Mayfield Heights, OH: North American Menopause Society; 2010.

3. Hale GE, Burger HG. Hormonal changes and biomarkers in late reproductive age, menopausal transition and menopause. *Best Pract Res Clin Obstet Gynaecol.* 2009;23:7-23.

4. Harlow SD, Gass M, Hall JE, et al. Executive summary of the Stages of Reproductive Aging Workshop + 10: addressing the unfinished agenda of staging reproductive aging. *Fert Steril.* 2012;97:843-851.

5. NIH state-of-the-science conference statement on management of menopause-related symptoms. *NIH Consens State Sci Statements.* March 21-23, 2005; 22:1-38.

6. Fritz MA, Speroff L. *Clinical Gynecologic Endocrinology and Infertility.* 8th ed. Philadelphia, PA: Lippincott Williams & Wilkins; 2011.

7. Notman MT. Menopause and adult development. In: Flint M, Kronenberg F, Utian W, eds. *Annals of the New York Academy of Sciences.* New York: New York Academy of Sciences; 1990:149.

8. Lock M. Menopause: lessons from anthropology. *Psychosom Med.* 1998;60:410.

9. Smith-Rosenberg C. Puberty to menopause: the cycle of femininity in nineteenth-century America. *Feminist Stud.* 1973;1:58.

10. Bell SE. Sociological perspectives on the medicalization of menopause. *Ann NY Acad Sci.* 1990;592:173-178.

11. Wilson RA. *Feminine Forever.* New York: J. B. Lippincott; 1966.

12. Ziel HK, Finkle WD. Increased risk of endometrial carcinoma among users of conjugated estrogens. *N Engl J Med.* 1975;293:1167-1170.

13. Kaufert P, McKinlay S. Estrogen replacement therapy: the production of medical knowledge and the emergence of policy. In: *Women, Health, and Healing.* New York: Tavistock; 1985;113.

14. Flint M. The menopause: reward or punishment? *Psychomatics.* 1975;16:161.

15. Broekmans FJ, Soules MR, Fauser BC. Ovarian aging mechanisms and clinical consequences. *Endocr Rev.* 2009;30:465-493.

16. Nelson HD. Menopause. *Lancet.* 2008;371:760-770.

17. Wildman RP, Sowers MR. Adiposity and the menopausal transition. *Obstet Gynecol Clin North Am.* 2011;38:441-454.

18. Fisher TE, Chervenak JL. Lifestyle alterations for the amelioration of hot flashes. *Maturitas.* 2012;71:217-220.

19. Freeman EW, Sherif K. Prevalence of hot flushes and night sweats around the world: a systematic review. *Climacteric.* 2007;10:197-214.

20. Blümel JE, Cano A, Mezones-Holguín E. A multinational study of sleep disorders during female mid-life. *Maturitas.* 2012;72:359-366.

21. Krychman ML. Vaginal estrogens for the treatment of dyspareunia. *J Sex Med.* 2011;8:666-674.

22. Nappi RE, Kokot-Kierepa M. Vaginal Health: Insights, Views & Attitudes (VIVA): results from an international survey. *Climacteric.* 2012;15:36-44.

23. Sturdee DW, Panay N. Recommendations for the management of postmenopausal vaginal atrophy. *Climacteric.* 2010;13:509-522.

24. Cockerham A. Adenomyosis: a challenge in clinical gynecology. *J Midwifery Women's Health.* 2012;57:212-220.

25. Shifren JL. Increasing our understanding of women's sexuality at midlife and beyond. *Menopause.* 2011;18:1149-1151.

26. Cray LA, Woods NF, Herting JR, Mitchell ES. Symptom clusters during the late reproductive stage through the early postmenopause: observations from the Seattle Midlife Women's Health Study. *Menopause.* 2012;19:864-869.

27. Bryant C, Judd FK, Hickey M. Anxiety during the menopausal transition: a systematic review. *J Affect Disord* 2012;139:141-148.

28. Hirschberg AL. Sex hormones, appetite and eating behaviour in women. *Maturitas.* 2012;71:248-256.

29. Calleja-Agius J, Brincat M. The effect of menopause on the skin and other connective tissues. *Gynecol Endocrinol.* 2012;28:273-277.

30. Bailey Spitzer TL. What the obstetrician/gynecologist should know about thyroid disorders. *Obstet Gynecol Surv.* 2010;65:779-785.

31. Santoro N, Randolph JF. Reproductive hormones and the menopause transition. *Obstet Gynecol Clin North Am.* 2011;38:455-466.

32. Butler L, Santoro N. The reproductive endocrinology of the menopausal transition. *Steroids.* 2011;76:627-635.

33. Pimenta F, Leal I, Maroco J, Ramos C. Perceived control, lifestyle, health, socio-demographic factors and menopause: impact on hot flashes and night sweats. *Maturitas.* 2011;69:338-342.

34. Elavsky S, Gonzales JU, Proctor DN, et al. Effects of physical activity on vasomotor symptoms: examination using objective and subjective measures. *Menopause.* 2012;19(10):1095-1103.

35. Daley A, Stokes-Lampard H, MacArthur C. Exercise for vasomotor menopausal symptoms. *Cochrane Database Syst Rev.* 2011;5:CD006108. doi: 10.1002/14651858.CD006108.pub3.

36. Kroenke CH, Caan BJ, Stefanick ML, et al. Effects of a dietary intervention and weight change on vasomotor symptoms in the Women's Health Initiative. *Menopause.* 2012;19:980-988.

37. Tan O, Bradshaw K, Carr BR. Management of vulvovaginal atrophy-related sexual dysfunction in postmenopausal women: an up-to-date review. *Menopause.* 2012;19:109-117.

38. Guttuso T. Effective and clinically meaningful non-hormonal hot flash therapies. *Maturitas.* 2012;72:6-12.

39. Umland EM, Falconieri L. Treatment options for vasomotor symptoms in menopause: focus on desvenlafaxine. *Int J Women's Health.* 2012;4:305-319.

40. Andrews JC. Vasomotor symptoms: an evidence-based approach to medical management. *J Clin Outcome Manage.* 2011;18:112-128.

41. Villaseca P. Non-estrogen conventional and phytochemical treatments for vasomotor symptoms: what needs to be known for practice. *Climacteric.* 2012;15:115-124.

42. North American Menopause Society. *Hormone Products for Postmenopausal Use in the United States and Canada.* Mayfield Heights, OH: North American Menopause Society; October 25, 2011.

43. Hitchcock CL, Prior JC. Oral micronized progesterone for vasomotor symptoms: a placebo-controlled randomized trial in healthy postmenopausal women. *Menopause.* 2012;19:886-893.

44. Spark MJ, Willis J. Systematic review of progesterone use by midlife and menopausal women. *Maturitas.* 2012;72:192-202.

45. Nelson HD, Walker M, Zakher B, Mitchell J. Menopausal hormone therapy for the primary prevention of chronic conditions: a systematic review to update the U.S. Preventive Services Task Force Recommendations. *Ann Intern Med.* 2012;157:104-113.

46. Weinstein MM. Hormone therapy and urinary incontinence. *Menopause.* 2012;19:255-256.

47. North American Menopause Society. The 2012 hormone therapy position statement of the North American Menopause Society. *Menopause.* 2012;19:257-271.

48. Langer RD, Manson JE, Allison MA. Have we come full circle—or moved forward? The Women's Health Initiative 10 years on. *Climacteric.* 2012;15:206-212.

49. Pinkerton JV. The truth about bioidentical hormone therapy. *Female Patient.* 2012;37:16-20.

50. Pattimakiel L, Thacker HL. Bioidentical hormone therapy: clarifying the misconceptions. *Cleve Clin J Med.* 2011;78:829-836.

51. Bhavnani BR, Stanczyk FZ. Misconception and concerns about bioidentical hormones used for custom-compounded hormone therapy. *J Clin Endocrin Metab.* 2012;97:756-759.

52. Borrelli F, Ernst E. Alternative and complementary therapies for the menopause. *Maturitas.* 2010;66:333-343.

53. Hall E, Frey BN, Soares CN. Non-hormonal treatment strategies for vasomotor symptoms: a critical review. *Drugs.* 2011;71:287-304.

54. Nayak C, Singh V, Singh K, et al. Management of distress during climacteric years by homeopathic therapy. *J Altern Complement Med.* 2011;17:1037-1042.

55. Thompson EA. Alternative and complementary therapies for the menopause: a homeopathic approach. *Maturitas.* 2012;66:350-354.

56. North American Menopause Society. NAMS 2011 isoflavones report: the role of soy isoflavones in menopausal health: report of the North American Menopause Society/Wulf H. Utian Translational Science Symposium in Chicago, IL (October 2010). *Menopause.* 2011;18:732-753.

57. Panay N. Taking an integrated approach: managing women with phytoestrogens. *Climacteric.* 2011;14:2-7.

58. van Die MD. Phytoestrogens in menopause. *Austr J Medic Herb.* 2011;23:11-17.

59. Hudson T. Botanicals for managing menopause-related symptoms: state of the science. *Integr Med.* 2009/2010;8:30-37.

60. Geller SE, Shulman LP, van Breemen RB, et al. Safety and efficacy of black cohosh and red clover for the management of vasomotor symptoms: a randomized controlled trial. *Menopause.* 2009;16:1156-1166.

61. Darsareh F, Taavoni S, Joolaee S, Haghani H. Effect of aromatherapy massage on menopausal symptoms: a randomized placebo-controlled clinical trial. *Menopause.* 2012;19:995-999.

62. Regestein QR. Is there anything special about valerian? *Menopause.* 2011;18:937-939.

63. Taavoni S, Ekbatani N, Kashaniayn M, Haghani H. Effect of valerian on sleep quality in postmenopausal women: a randomized, placebo-controlled clinical trial. *Menopause.* 2011;18:951-955.

64. Leach MJ, Moore V. Black cohosh (*Cimicifuga* spp.) for menopausal symptoms. *Cochrane Database Syst Rev.* 2012;9:CD007244. doi: 10.1002/14651858.CD007244.pub2.

65. Elkins GR, Fisher WI, Johnson AK, et al. Clinical hypnosis in the treatment of postmenopausal hot flashes: a randomized controlled trial. *Menopause.* 2013;20(3):291-298.

66. Corbelli JA, Hess R. Hormone therapy prescribing trends in the decade after the Women's Health Initiative: how patients and providers have found a way to sleep better at night. *Menopause.* 2012;19:600-601.

67. Pal L, Manson JE. The Women's Health Initiative: an unforgettable decade. *Menopause.* 2012;19:597-599.

68. Brown S. Shock, terror and controversy: how the media reacted to the Women's Health Initiative. *Climacteric.* 2012;15:275-280.

69. Ettinger B, Wang SM, Leslie RS, et al. Evolution of postmenopausal hormone therapy between 2002 and 2009. *Menopause.* 2012;19:610-615.

70. Steinkellner AR, Denison SE, Eldridge SL, et al. A decade of postmenopausal hormone therapy prescribing in the United States: long-term effects of the Women's Health Initiative. *Menopause.* 2012;19:616-621.

71. Writing Group for the Women's Health Initiative. Risks and benefits of estrogen plus progestin in healthy postmenopausal women: principal results from the Women's Health Initiative randomized controlled trial. *JAMA.* 2002;288:321-333.

72. Stuenkel CA, Gass MLS, Manson JE, et al. A decade after the Women's Health Initiative: the experts do agree. *Menopause.* 2012;19:846-847.

73. Hansen KA, Eyster KM. What happened to WHI: menopausal hormonal therapy in 2012. *Clinical Obstet Gynecol.* 2012;55:706-712.

74. National Osteoporosis Foundation. *Clinician's Guide to Prevention and Treatment of Osteoporosis.*

Washington, DC: National Osteoporosis Foundation; 2010.

75. Osteoporosis. Practice Bulletin No. 129. American College of Obstetricians and Gynecologists. *Obstet Gynecol.* 2012;120:718-734.

76. Pollycove R, Simon JA. Osteoporosis: screening and treatment in women. *Clin Obstet Gynecol.* 2012; 55:681-691.

77. Tufts G. New treatment approach for osteopenia. *J Midwifery Women's Health.* 2011;56:61-67.

78. North American Menopause Society. Management of osteoporosis in postmenopausal women: 2012 position statement of the North American Menopause Society. *Menopause.* 2012;17:25-54.

79. Dunniway DL, Camune B, Baldwin K, Crane JK. FRAX counseling for bone health behavior change in women 50 years of age and older. *J Am Acad Nurse Pract.* 2012;24:382-389.

80. McCloskey E, Kanis JA. FRAX updates 2012. *Curr Opin Rheumatol.* 2012;24:554-560.

81. Agency for Healthcare Research and Policy (AHRQ). *Treatment to Prevent Osteoporotic Fractures: An Update.* May 2012.

● ● ● **Additional Resources for Further Information About Menopause and Osteoporosis**

FRAX: World Health Organization's Fracture Risk Assessment Tool: http://www.shef.ac.uk/FRAX

International Society for Clinical Densitometry (ISCD): http://www.iscd.org

National Center for Complementary and Alternative Medicine (NCCAM) at the National Institutes of Health (NIH): http://nccam.nih.gov

National Osteoporosis Foundation (NOF): http://www.nof.org

North American Menopause Society (NAMS): http://www.menopause.org

North American Menopause Society. *Menopause Practice: A Clinician's Guide.* 4th ed. Mayfield Heights, OH: North American Menopause Society; 2010.

Women's Health Initiative (WHI; on the National Heart, Lung and Blood Institute website): http://www.nhlbi.nih.gov/whi

IV

Antepartum

Promotion of Health During Pregnancy

It is generally accepted that prenatal care is essential for achieving the best outcomes of pregnancy. However, the quality of prenatal care, when it is initiated, the number of "visits," the qualifications and expertise of the caregiver, the context of the care (birth center, clinic, hospital based, private or public), as well as the accessibility of secondary, consultative care are all important to achieve positive health outcomes. It is ideal for prenatal care to occur within a collaborative, multidisciplinary, context wherein various health professionals are available to contribute to timely and accurate diagnosis of problems and offer appropriate intervention(s). Ultrasonography, genetic diagnosis, and prenatal educational resources are especially important.

The chapters in this section on prenatal care include guidelines for the assessment of pregnancy status, the use and interpretation of screening tests and various diagnostic strategies, and decisions on when to seek consultation and how to transact collaborative care when the woman's needs merit midwifery care, along with medical management of complications.

The general health and reproductive history of a pregnant woman are critical antecedents to the healthy progression of a pregnancy and positive birth outcome. It would be ideal if prenatal care was preceded by preconceptional care, but often this is not the case. Lack of preconceptional care makes prenatal care especially important in achieving optimal pregnancy outcomes, as well as an occasion to influence the future health of the woman—indeed, the health of her children and family and, ultimately, society—through timely recognition of health problems and the promotion of health practices. This type of care is especially important for recognition of chronic diseases and health behaviors that might be modified or addressed during the course of prenatal care. Key behaviors to be considered include nutritional practices, substance use, and exercise. The chapters in this section provide specific information regarding the interpretation of pregnancy status, including the assessment of key physical parameters, and guidance regarding the recognition of health problems and complications unique to pregnancy.

A key initial consideration is the gestational age of the pregnancy—that is, the age of the fetus. Assessment and determination of gestational age are included in the organization of the topics addressed in this section and incorporated in the accompanying boxes and tables that summarize key information. Gestational age is an essential "lens" through which the midwife should "hear" and "view" the information acquired in conversation with the woman and in clinical observation. Gestational age is a key parameter that helps the midwife achieve the purposes of prenatal care—namely, accurately assessing the status of pregnancy during a prenatal visit, recognizing problems through the interpretation of the woman's symptoms and the results of diagnostic tests, and offering timely interventions to achieve healthy pregnancy outcomes and a satisfying pregnancy and birth experience for the expectant mother.

Two basic dimensions of pregnancy must be considered in providing prenatal care. One is the physical health of the pregnant woman, the status of her pregnancy, and the growth and well-being of the fetus. The second is the experiential aspects of pregnancy and the woman's responses to her pregnancy. The chapters in this section provide essential content about the scope and content of prenatal care with consideration of the woman's emotional status, as well as the physical dimensions of pregnancy and fetal growth. This content includes the assessment of pregnancy status, the genetic basis for fetal condition, the critical features of diagnostic tests, and the screening, recognition, and management of health problems and complications of pregnancy within a care setting that allows for consultation and multidisciplinary care. This information is presented in a systematic fashion that will enable the reader to interpret the objective data related to prenatal assessment and care and to use it in a way that reflects the following principles used in providing prenatal care.

The first principle is to initially consider, and ask about, the woman's concerns and "how she is doing" with an "ear" that hears her expression of symptoms within her social situation and her gestational age—that is, what is common and expected at this point in her pregnancy. These concerns can be addressed initially or incorporated in the rest of the visit.

The second principle is assessment of the physical, objective features of the pregnancy and the laboratory data that pertain to the gestational age and the potential for the development of any problems, such as the recognition of anemia, multiple pregnancy, or excessive amniotic fluid. Careful listening and thoughtful interpretation of the available data, using the epidemiologic principles for understanding test outcomes that are included in these chapters, can lead to accurate interpretation and purposeful dialogue with the expectant mother about how to use the information, get further data, get consultation, or offer helpful education.

The third principle is the provision of appropriate information and education based on the gestational age and the woman's needs and interests. This education includes anticipatory information that can be offered to minimize anxiety (e.g., when the baby usually "moves"), prevent problems (such as constipation with advancing pregnancy), or lead to the recognition of problems (e.g., preeclampsia or preterm labor). Recognizing the limited accuracy of diagnostic testing and the uncertainty of the outcomes of interventions, it is essential that the midwife deliberately engage the woman in her own assessment of her situation, take care that information and alternatives are understood, and ensure that the woman considers interventions in accordance with her beliefs and values.

These chapters will enable midwives to address the challenges of providing prenatal care—specifically, obtaining and interpreting information about the ongoing pregnancy, knowledgably recognizing health problems and complications of pregnancy, and using a deliberative approach within the interactive context of ongoing prenatal visits with pregnant women and their support persons. In addition, the midwife is oriented toward facilitating the woman's "readiness" for labor and for the dealing with the challenges of early parenting, including breastfeeding.

Joyce E. Roberts

20

Anatomy and Physiology of Pregnancy: Placental, Fetal, and Maternal Adaptations

TEKOA L. KING

MICHELE R. DAVIDSON

MELISSA D. AVERY

CINDY M. ANDERSON

Introduction

Pregnancy is a time of profound anatomic and physiologic changes in a woman's body. In addition to the reproductive organs, all maternal physiologic systems make adaptions needed to support the developing fetus and, at the same time, maintain maternal homeostasis. A thorough understanding of these changes is an essential foundation for all healthcare providers—including midwives—who care for women during pregnancy. This chapter provides an overview of changes in the reproductive organs, the effect of the major hormones of pregnancy, fetal development, maternal adaptations that take place during pregnancy, and finally a review of fetal–pelvic relationships during pregnancy necessary for clinical prenatal care. This chapter is just the beginning. The reader is encouraged to expand the knowledge presented in these pages to have the thorough understanding needed to care for women.

The Reproductive Organs During Pregnancy

Pregnancy lasts approximately 266 days or 38 weeks from ovulation. This translates into 10 lunar months or 9 calendar months (because some months have 5 weeks). Over the course of pregnancy, a woman's breasts grow and prepare for lactation. The uterus increases to approximately 5 times its normal size so that at 38 gestational weeks, the uterus measures approximately 32 centimeters long, 22 centimeters across, and 24 centimeters wide. The cervix must first act as a barrier maintaining the uterine contents. However, at the end of pregnancy, the cervix becomes soft and short, and it opens to allow for passage of the fetus during birth. These remarkable changes are the result of a complex interplay of hormonal stimulation that has important clinical implications for all women and especially those who experience miscarriage, preterm labor, preeclampsia, and other pregnancy complications.

The Breast

Under the direction of several different pregnancy hormones, the breast undergoes two distinct developmental changes in pregnancy to prepare for lactation. Both stages—mammogenesis and lactogenesis I—include hyperplasia and hypertrophy.[1] Hyperplasia refers to an increase in the number of cells, or cellular proliferation. Hypertrophy refers to enlarging cells; that is, cells grow in size.

Mammogenesis begins early in pregnancy. The breasts enlarge via cellular hyperplasia, and the breast lobules increase in size. The nipples become erectile, the areola becomes proportionately bigger and darker, and superficial veins can be visible. During this process, the breasts can be very tender or painful. Alveoli expand and proliferate at the end of breast lobules as the lobules also proliferate.

Toward the middle of pregnancy, the alveoli epithelial cells change into secretory epithelium, which is the first stage of lactogenesis. Toward the end of pregnancy, the alveoli secrete colostrum but are primarily quiescent secondary to inhibition by progesterone, one of the primary pregnancy hormones. After birth, the influence of progesterone abruptly ceases and lactogenesis II—that is, the onset of milk production—begins. A more detailed description of lactogenesis II is presented in the *Breastfeeding and Maternal–Infant Dyad* chapter.

The Uterus

The uterus grows at a steady, predictable rate during pregnancy, with its expansion first becoming detectable at approximately 5 weeks' gestation. Uterine growth is due to estrogen- and progesterone-induced hyperplasia of uterine smooth muscle cells within the myometrium during early pregnancy and due to hypertrophy later in pregnancy. The muscles increase their content of actin, myosin, sarcoplasmic reticulum, and mitochondria, which serve as the machinery used to contract the muscle, as described in the *Anatomy and Physiology During Labor and Birth* chapter. The myometrium's primary purposes are contractility and elasticity. Contractility allows for lengthening and shortening, whereas elasticity is the ability to stretch. The three layers of the uterus (endometrium, myometrium, and perimetrium) become clearly defined over the course of pregnancy.

The initial uterine growth occurs in the anteroposterior diameter, while the isthmus or lower segment of the uterus can become very soft. This softening results in marked compressibility in the lower uterine segment, which is the basis of Hegar's sign. The uterine shape changes from the nonpregnant pear shape to a ball or sphere in the first trimester, and then expands to an elongated cylinder. The anatomic location of the uterus in relation to maternal anatomy is shown in **Figure 20-1**.

The Endometrium Becomes the Decidua

The secretory endometrium contains columnar epithelium, epithelial cells, and nonresident or migratory immune cells. The basal arteries that supply the myometrium branch into spiral arteries that supply part of the myometrium and the endometrium.[2]

When conception occurs, the endometrial changes that allow and facilitate implantation are collectively termed the decidual reaction. The name "decidua" was chosen because, like the leaves on

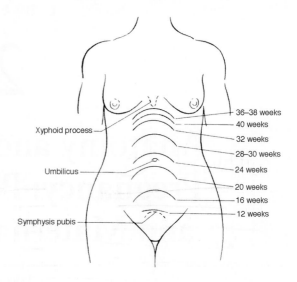

Figure 20-1 Approximate normal fundal heights during pregnancy.
Source: Schuiling KD, Likis FE. *Women's Gynecologic Health.* 2nd ed. Burlington, MA: Jones & Bartlett Learning; 2013.

deciduous trees, this tissue is shed after birth.[3] The decidual reaction occurs in response to estrogen, progesterone, and a complex dance or "cross-talk" of locally produced chemicals generated by the blastocyst and maternal endometrium.

Approximately 8 days after ovulation, the secretory endometrium provides a 4- to 5-day "window of opportunity" for blastocyst implantation.[4] During this short period, immune cells congregate, the endometrial glands become more secretory, and the epithelial surface develops small protrusions called pinopods. The pinopods absorb fluid from the uterine cavity and probably attract the blastocyst. Once the blastocyst is in contact with the endometrium, the pinopods and trophoblastic protrusions interact to support implantation (**Figure 20-2**).[5] It is thought that physiologic variations in the development of the endometrial "window of opportunity" could result in failure of implantation; this hypothesis is currently the subject of infertility research.

The decidual reaction starts once the blastocyst is present at the endometrial site of implantation. The stromal cells become larger, round, decidual cells that have a membrane to which the trophoblast can anchor itself, and another surge of chemical "cross-talk" occurs.[6] As the blastocyst becomes implanted in the endometrium, the spiral arteries are markedly altered by trophoblastic tissue so that the endothelial and smooth muscle portion of the vessel walls are destroyed, which renders them smooth and

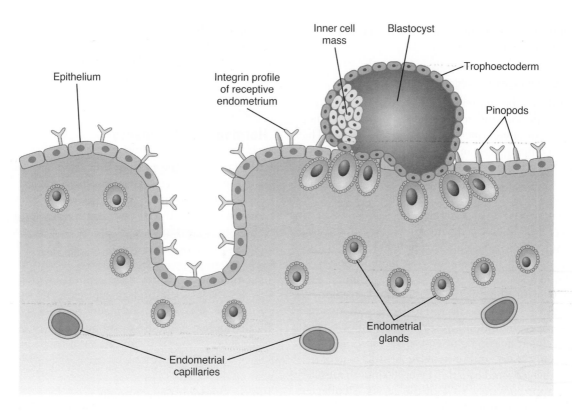

Figure 20-2 Implantation.

unable to constrict or expand in response to vaso-active agents. This step is a critical determinant of fetal and maternal health. When the spiral arteries do not remodel appropriately, fetal growth restriction, altered placental growth, or preeclampsia may develop. This process is discussed in more detail later in this chapter.

The decidual reaction remodels the extracellular matrix, resulting in changed levels of collagen, proteoglycans, and glycoproteins. The decidua fulfills multiple roles, including nutrition of the embryo in the early stages of embryology and protection of the uterus from invasion by the invasive trophoblastic cells.

The entire maternal decidua is divided into three regions: the decidua basalis, the decidua capsularis, and the decidua parietalis. These three regions are named for their positional relationship to the conceptus. The decidua basalis is the site where implantation occurs and is the future site of the maternal potion of the placenta. The basalis can be subdivided into a zona compacta and a zona spongiosa (where the detachment of the placenta takes place following birth). The decidua capsularis lies like a capsule

around the chorion, whereas the decidua parietalis is found on the opposite uterus wall. Around the fourth month of gestation, the decidua capsularis comes into contact with the decidua parietalis. The merging of these two causes the uterine cavity to become obliterated.

Uterine Innervation

Uterine innervation is one of the more interesting physiologic changes that occurs in pregnancy. The uterus is primarily innervated by the sympathetic nervous system, with some fibers coming from the parasympathetic nervous system and cerebrospinal tract. Innervation is not even throughout the uterus, however; more nerve fibers are found near the cervix as compared to the fundus. The nerve fibers in the uterine fundus virtually disappear during pregnancy, whereas those in the cervix remain.[7,8] Although the reasons for these changes are not clear, it is postulated that the lack of sympathetic innervation protects the uterus from sympathetic stimulation via catecholamines and resultant contraction activity. Uterine contractions during pregnancy and labor occur secondary to endocrine stimulation rather than nerve stimulation of muscle fibers.

Cervical Changes in Pregnancy

Over the course of pregnancy, labor, birth, and postpartum period, the cervix undergoes four distinct phases: softening, ripening, dilation, and repair. The cervix comprises two major structures: the ectocervix and the endocervix. The ectocervix, which is visible from the vagina, consists of a layer of columnar epithelial cells and a layer of squamous epithelial cells. The endocervix is the internal, canal-like portion of the cervix, which opens into the uterus. It consists of a single layer of columnar epithelial cells. In nulliparous women, the opening of the endocervix is pinpoint and circular in size; in contrast, in multiparous women, the cervix has a slit-like appearance. The cervix is composed primarily of connective tissue covered by a thin layer of smooth muscle. The extracellular matrix tissue within the cervix contains collagen, elastin, and proteoglycans; this matrix tissue is then covered by a thin layer of smooth muscle. Thus approximately 80% of the cervix is collagen and 15% is smooth muscle.[9]

Under the influence of estrogen in pregnancy, the cervix begins to soften in the first trimester (Goodell's sign).[10] As vascularization increases, a cyanosis or bluish purple discoloration occurs (Chadwick's sign). Following the initial relatively rapid softening, the cervix continues to soften throughout the pregnancy, albeit at a slower rate. Glandular tissue in the cervix produces a thick, tenacious mucus, which forms the mucous plug that seals the endocervical canal, thereby preventing ascending bacteria or pathogens from entering the uterine cavity during pregnancy.

Cervical Ripening Prior to Labor

Cervical ripening begins weeks prior to the onset of labor and results from a series of interactions between hormonal and mechanical factors that have not been fully elucidated. As progesterone levels fall and estrogen levels rise, the water content and vascularization of the cervix increase and the collagen cells become disorganized, which results in a marked reduction in the mechanical strength of the collagen bundles.

The local paracrine activity of prostaglandins PGE2 and PGF2a also influence the cervical ripening and the onset of labor. Fetal production of corticotropin-releasing hormone and cortisol causes an upregulation of prostaglandin receptors in the cervix and uterus PGE2 facilitates cervical vasodilatation. Finally, production of pro-inflammatory cytokines leads to infiltration of the cervix by leukocytes

and macrophages. These cells release enzymes that facilitate alterations in extracellular matrix proteins, loosening of collagen fibers, and a reduction in collagen content.

Hormones of Pregnancy

The placenta is the primary interface between the maternal and fetal compartments physiologically and is in a central position to mediate chemical messages between the fetus and mother. The primary hormones of pregnancy produced by the placenta are estrogen, progesterone, human chorionic gonadotropin (hCG), and human placental lactogen (hPL). Each of these hormones has a major role in supporting pregnancy (**Table 20-1**). In addition, the placenta and the fetus synthesize other chemical mediators that act both locally and systemically to support growth and development of the fetus and placenta itself, many of which are still being discovered.

Human Chorionic Gonadotropin

Human chorionic gonadotropin is secreted by the syncytiotrophoblast tissue within the blastocyst before implantation occurs and then later by the placenta. The main role of hCG is to sustain estrogen and progesterone production in early pregnancy by preventing degeneration of the corpus luteum. hCG levels rise in early pregnancy and are first detectable approximately 8 to 10 days after ovulation, which coincides with implantation of the fertilized ovum.[11] The level of this hormone doubles approximately every 48 to 72 hours in 85% of normal pregnancies and continues to do so until it reaches a peak of approximately 100,000 mIU/mL at 8 to 11 gestational weeks (weeks after the last menstrual period); at that point, plasma levels of hCG slowly to decrease to a stable level of approximately 20,000 mIU/mL (**Figure 20-3**).[11] The characteristic doubling time of hCG has been used in serial measurements of blood values to assess the viability of pregnancy. Because there is wide individual variability in hCG levels, however, some patterns of serial hCG levels (e.g., slower than expected increases) can be difficult to interpret and although it is common to obtain an hCG level every 2 days if clinically indicated, assessing these values every 48 hours can sometimes be too soon to see a full doubling of the hCG plasma level.

hCG is a glycoprotein with both alpha and beta subunits. The alpha subunit is structurally the same as luteinizing hormone (LH), follicle-stimulating hormone (FSH), and thyroid-stimulating hormone

Table 20-1	Major Hormones and Functions During Pregnancy	
Hormone	**Source**	**Selected Functions During Pregnancy**
Human chorionic gonadotropin (hCG)	Syncytiotrophoblast Placenta	Prevents degeneration of the corpus luteum, thereby ensuring ongoing estrogen and progesterone production
		Stimulates thyroid production of thyroxine in the first trimester
Human placental lactogen (hPL)	Placenta	Increases insulin resistance
		Stimulates production of growth hormones
Estrogen	Ovaries	Soften collagen fibers in cervix and ligaments
	Corpus luteum	Increases uterine blood flow
	Placenta	Promotes growth of the uterus and breast glandular tissue
	Fetus	Increases production of insulin-like growth factors
		Enhances myometrial contractility
		Increases myometrial sensitivity to oxytocin, may upregulate oxytocin receptors
Progesterone	Corpus luteum	Systemic vasodilation
	Placenta	Anti-inflammatory actions protect trophoblast from being rejected
		Decidualization within the endometrium
		Prevents myometrial contractility
		Inhibits uterine production of prostaglandins
		Mammary growth for lactation
		Withdrawal at term leads to uterine contractions

(TSH). Plasma levels (or the presence in urine) of the beta subunit are the basis of tests for pregnancy verification. Serial quantitative measures of the beta subunit are used to determine the viability of a pregnancy, as described more in the *Obstetric Complications in Pregnancy* chapter. Plasma levels

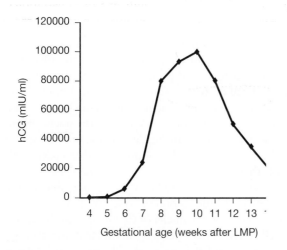

Figure 20-3 Human chorionic gonadotropin values in the first trimester of pregnancy.

of the beta subunit are also used as a tumor marker for tumors that have an embryologic origin, such as choriocarcinomas and hydatiform mole.

The natural rise and fall of hCG levels corresponds to the natural history of nausea and vomiting in the first trimester.[12] Although the direct etiology of nausea and vomiting in pregnancy is not known, it has been postulated that hCG may play a role. Nevertheless, studies that have linked hCG levels to nausea symptoms have not shown a direct correlation between the two. It is interesting to note that women who have severe nausea and vomiting or hyperemesis may also have subclinical hyperthyroidism; in such women, the alpha subunit of hCG is able to stimulate the thyroid gland as though it were TSH.[13]

Human Placental Lactogen

Human placental lactogen ensures adequate fetal nutrition by altering maternal glucose metabolism so that glucose is available for fetal uptake. hPL is secreted by the placental syncytiotrophoblast and is detectable in maternal circulation at 6 to 8 gestational weeks, with levels increasing in direct proportion to placental growth. This hormone initiates increases in the plasma levels of free fatty acids and triglycerides, which become available as an additional energy substrate for the pregnant woman. hPL also increases maternal insulin resistance, thereby assuring consistent blood levels of glucose for fetal use. Glucose is transported across the placenta via facilitated diffusion. The fetus relies primarily on glucose for nutritional needs; fetal production of glucose either does not occur or is undetectable.[14] It appears that the fetal liver does not develop the mechanism necessary for gluconeogenesis until just before birth. The hPL-induced insulin resistance results in an increase in maternal insulin levels. This, in turn, stimulates amino acid production, thereby ensuring that amino acids are also available for fetal growth and development.

Progesterone

Progesterone and estrogen—both steroid hormones—act as intracellular chemical messengers by binding to intracellular receptors. They influence many aspects of DNA transcription and cellular activities.

Progesterone is essential for maintenance of pregnancy in all mammals, and its name is derived from this function: "pro-gestational steroidal ketone." This hormone maintains the uterus in a quiescent state and helps suppress the maternal immune response to fetal antigens so that the fetal tissue is not rejected. Progesterone is produced by the corpus luteum in early pregnancy until the placenta takes over progesterone production between 7 to 9 gestational weeks, an event called the "luteal-placental shift." Additional functions are listed in Table 20-1.

Administration of mifepristone, a progesterone receptor antagonist, will cause miscarriage. Low levels of progesterone in pregnancy are associated with an increased risk of spontaneous abortion. Women with luteal-phase defects can have progesterone levels that drop in early pregnancy, leading to spontaneous abortions. Progesterone supplementation has been shown to be effective in for treating threatened miscarriage.[15] Progesterone is also beginning to be used to prevent preterm birth in women who had a previous preterm birth.[16]

Estrogen

Three types of naturally occurring estrogens have been identified: estrone, estradiol, and estriol. Estriol (E3) is the primary estrogen of pregnancy. Estrogen production during pregnancy entails a three-part interplay between the woman, fetus, and placenta, in that each is able to complete part of estrogen synthesis but not all of it. Estrogen is initially synthesized in the corpus luteum until the eighth or ninth week of gestation, when the fetal adrenal glands are

able to produce the necessary estrogen precursors and the placenta is able to produce and excrete the active forms of estrogen. Placental estrogen production depends on input from both the fetal and maternal adrenal cortex because the placenta is unable to produce the androgenic C19 steroid dehydroepiandrosterone [DHEA], and its sulfoconjugate, DHEA-S, which are essential substrates of estriol.

The effects of estrogen during pregnancy are listed in Table 20-1. Estrogen encourages growth of breast tissue, stimulates uterine contractility, and increases uterine receptiveness to oxytocin. For most of pregnancy, however, the uterus remains refractory to the effects of estrogen because under the influence of progesterone, the uterine myometrium has very few estrogen receptors.

Fertilization and Implantation

The processes that make it possible for the single cell that results from the fusion of the maternal ovum and the paternal sperm to become a human being within the course of months are the subject of many fields of study, including genetics, embryology, and fetology. It is beyond the scope of this chapter and this text to cover these topics in detail. Instead, this chapter reviews the minimal knowledge needed by a practicing midwife to understand in general terms the milestones of embryologic and fetal development and the intricate and vulnerable steps that create organs and organ systems. This understanding will help the midwife discuss embryonic and fetal development with the woman and her family, and also have a general understanding of the causes of congenital malformations.

Fertilization

Fertilization is the process of fusion of two haploid (containing 23 chromosomes) cells—a sperm and an ovum—to form a diploid (containing 46 chromosomes) cell or zygote. Once a sperm cell binds to receptors on the oocyte membrane, its nucleus is pulled into the cytoplasm of the oocyte and the oocyte membrane depolarizes, causing destruction of other sperm cells. This prevents the binding of other sperm cells and, therefore, polyspermy. Once the sperm enters the ovum, the oocyte, which was arrested in the metaphase of the second meiotic division, completes metaphase. As the nuclei of the ovum and the sperm swell, fertilization occurs, the nuclear membranes disappear, and pairing of the chromosomes occurs to create the diploid zygote (**Figure 20-4**).

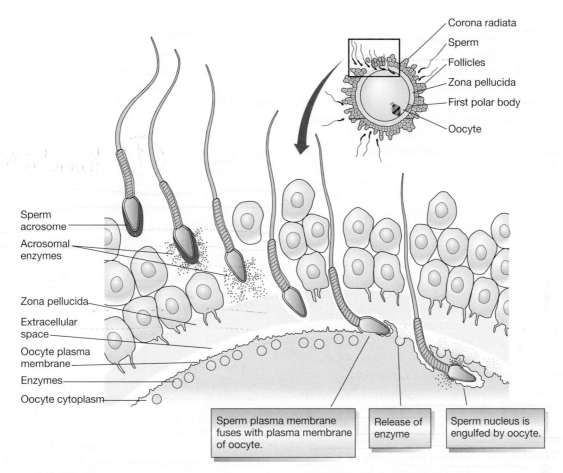

Figure 20-4 Fertilization.

The process of fertilization usually occurs in the fallopian tube and takes 18 to 24 hours. The fertilized oocyte becomes known as a zygote. The zygote begins as a single cell that contains 46 chromosomes: 23 from the ovum and 23 from the sperm. At this stage, the genetic code for that individual is formed. The 23rd pair of chromosomes determines the fetus's sex. The ovum contains only an X chromosome, so the X or Y chromosome that pairs with the maternal X chromosome is donated by the sperm.

Blastocyst

As the zygote moves through the fallopian tube into the uterine cavity, the cells divide (rapid mitotic activity) and create additional cells. These cells, known as blastomeres, are held together by the zona pellucida (an extracellular glycoprotein matrix) and form a solid ball of 12 to 16 cells known as the morula. As the morula enters the uterus, which occurs approximately 4 days after fertilization, intracellular fluid increases and a central cavity forms. The zygote is now called a blastocyst. The blastocyst is composed of four components: (1) the zona pellucida, (2) an inner cell mass, (3) an outer layer of cells called the trophoblast, and (4) a fluid-filled cavity. The trophoblast eventually forms the placenta and chorion, while the inner cell mass develops into the embryo and amnion.

The blastocyst is said to "hatch" when it sheds the zona pellucida. The blastocyst then encounters the uterine endometrium and selects a receptive area, usually in the fundus, for implantation. It orients itself so that the embryonic pole is closest to the endometrium, and the process of implantation begins.

The Trophoblast and Implantation

The trophoblast is a unique tissue that plays a clinically important role in pregnancy. The trophoblast, in contact with the endometrium, first differentiates into two distinct tissues: the syncytiotrophoblast and the cytotrophoblast. The syncytiotrophoblast is a syncytium or multinucleate protoplasmic mass formed by the fusion of cells, some of which were endometrial decidual cells. The syncytiotrophoblast burrows into the endometrium and becomes the primary source of hCG.[17] This implantation process can be associated with light vaginal bleeding or spotting. It is referred to as "implantation bleeding" but can be mistaken for a light menses by women who are not expecting to be pregnant or those who normally have irregular menses.

As the syncytiotrophoblast invades the endometrium, it disrupts maternal endometrial capillaries, portions of which are engulfed and become the lacunae. This process initiates the lacunar stage, which is marked by growth of small vacuoles in the syncytiotrophoblast that multiply and eventually fuse to form a system of lacunae. Initially, these lacunae fill with a substance derived from glandular secretions of the endometrium and a filtrate of maternal blood that diffuses through the trophoblastic tissue and serves to nourish the embryo. The lacunar networks continue to grow larger and communicate with each other as they evolve into the intervillous space (IVS). The intervillous space will fill with maternal blood and bathe placental villi as they form into this space (**Figure 20-5**).

The cytotrophoblast tissue is the point of contact between fetal and maternal tissue. It forms into columns of cells that become the anchoring villi of the placenta (**Figure 20-6**). The cytotrophoblast cells also invade the uterine spiral arteries, replace their endothelial layer, and begin the process of remodeling those arteries into low-pressure, high-volume, deinnervated open vessels needed to sustain the developing fetus. This cytotrophoblastic invasion of the spiral arteries occurs in two waves. The first wave takes place in the first weeks following implantation, as cytotrophoblast cells invade the spiral arteries in the decidua. The second wave occurs between 12 and 20 weeks of gestation. During this period, the cytotrophoblast extends into the myometrial portion of the spiral arteries (**Figure 20-7**).[18] The changed spiral artery architecture accommodates a remarkable change in uterine blood flow. Prior to pregnancy, uterine blood flow is approximately 50 mL per minute; in contrast, at the end of pregnancy, uterine blood flow is approximately 750 mL per minute.

Both superficial and extended invasion of the spiral arteries by cytotrophoblast cells can lead to pregnancy complications. The genesis of preeclampsia is cytotrophoblast invasion, wherein the second wave does not occur and the maternal spiral arteries remain small, high-resistance vessels. The effects of preeclampsia become evident when the nutritional needs of the fetus are no longer met by the small placenta owing to the limited maternal blood flow.[19,20] Abnormal placentation can also cause fetal growth restriction and has more recently been associated with preterm premature rupture of membranes and preterm labor.[21] In contrast, when the trophoblastic tissue invades indiscriminately without the normal complex immunologic checks and balances that occur between the maternal and trophoblastic tissues, placenta accreta can develop.

The Placenta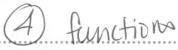

The placenta is a vital endocrine, hemochorial, villous organ with four well-known functions: (1) it is an endocrine organ that produces hormones and other bioactive substances; (2) it transports substances between the maternal and fetal circulations, including acting as the respiratory organ for gas exchange; (3) it metabolizes and synthesizes agents necessary for sustaining pregnancy; and (4) it provides an immunologic barrier between the maternal and fetal systems. Many of these functions overlap. But that is just the beginning.

The placenta has been an organ of import for centuries and has been imbued with many different meanings. In some cultures, the placenta is considered the alter ego or "secondary self."[22] In early Egypt, the placenta was described as the "External Soul."

Interestingly, current scientific study of placental function may substantiate some of these beliefs. Instead of being simply a passive filter or barrier, which has been the perceived role of the placenta, this amazing organ integrates a wide range of chemical messages produced by the fetus and maternal systems and actively adapts to different conditions. In short, the placenta plays an active and possibly independent role in fetal growth and development. More importantly, it is instrumental in making epigenetic changes to the fetal genome that will affect postnatal life.[23] This developmental plasticity in placental function is an area of current research interest.

Development of the Placenta

The cytotrophoblast lines the decidua and firmly anchors the placenta ,as the extraembryonic mesoderm—another tissue from the original blastocyst—grows into the cytotrophoblastic columns to form villi that float freely in the intervillous space. The fetal vessels that form within the villi are separated from maternal blood by three layers of cells: fetal endothelial cells, connective tissue, and cytotrophoblastic cells that are eventually called the chorionic villi epithelium.

Blood flow begins in the placenta when intervillous spaces become filled with maternal blood.

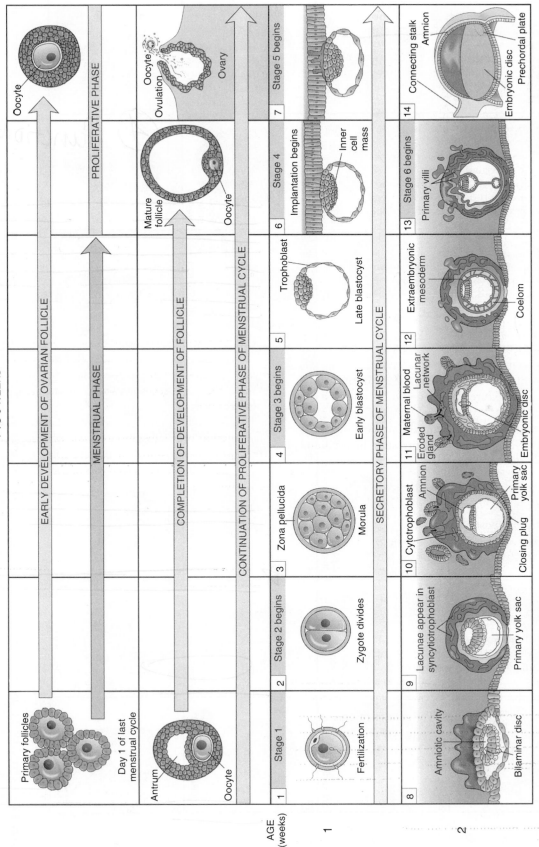

Figure 20-5 Development of an ovarian follicle containing the oocyte, ovulation, and phases of the menstrual cycle are illustrated. Human development begins at fertilization, about 14 days after the onset of the last menstruation. Cleavage of the zygote in the uterine tube, implantation of the blastocyst, and early development of the embryo are shown. *(continues)*

Source: Moore KL, Persaud TVN. *The Developing Human: Clinically Oriented Embryology.* 6th ed. Philadelphia, PA: W. B. Saunders; 1998.

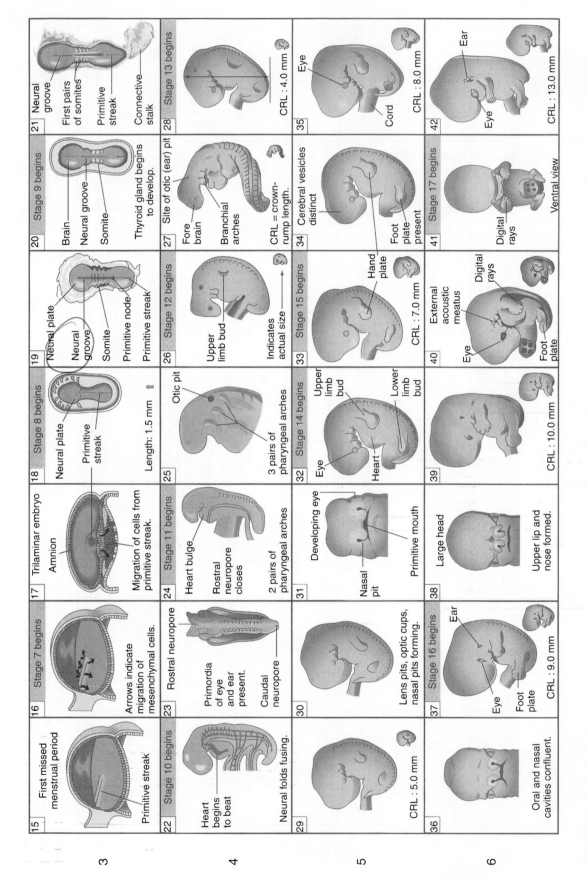

Figure 20-5 Development of an ovarian follicle containing the oocyte, ovulation, and phases of the menstrual cycle are illustrated. Human development begins at fertilization, about 14 days after the onset of the last menstruation. Cleavage of the zygote in the uterine tube, implantation of the blastocyst, and early development of the embryo are shown. (*continues*)

Source: Moore KL, Persaud TVN. *The Developing Human: Clinically Oriented Embryology.* 6th ed. Philadelphia, PA: W. B. Saunders; 1998.

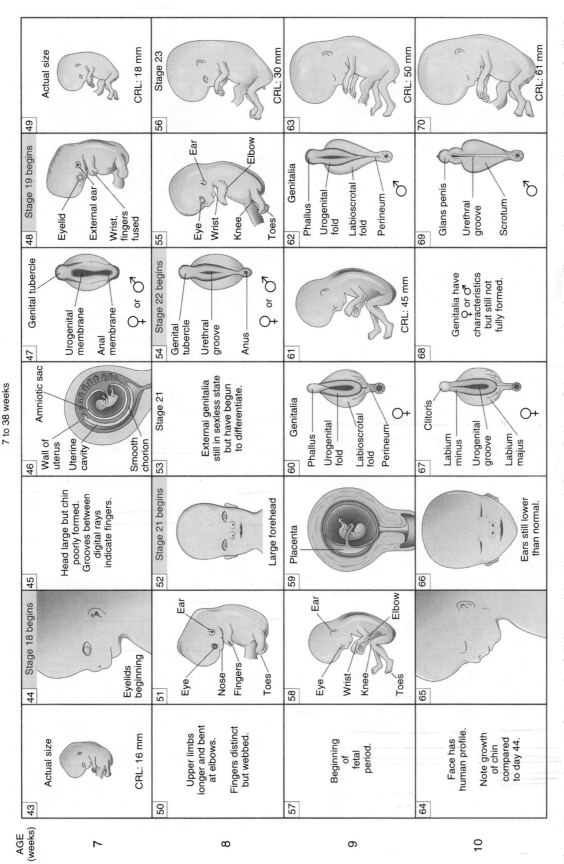

Figure 20-5 Development of an ovarian follicle containing the oocyte, ovulation, and phases of the menstrual cycle are illustrated. Human development begins at fertilization, about 14 days after the onset of the last menstruation. Cleavage of the zygote in the uterine tube, implantation of the blastocyst, and early development of the embryo are shown.

Source: Moore KL, Persaud TVN. *The Developing Human: Clinically Oriented Embryology.* 6th ed. Philadelphia, PA: W. B. Saunders; 1998.

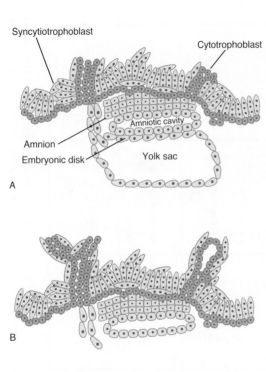

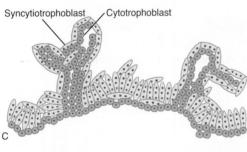

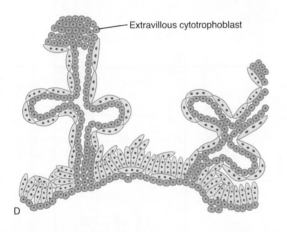

Figure 20-6 (A) Cytotrophoblast columns in early implanted embryo. (B) Extension of columns and differentiation of peripheral cells. (C) Folding of extensions caused by shape of syncytiotrophoblast cells. (C) and (D) Formation of trophoblastic villi.

Source: Cole LA. hCG, the wonder of today's science. *Reprod Biol Endocrinol.* 2012;10:24-28. Published by BioMed Central.

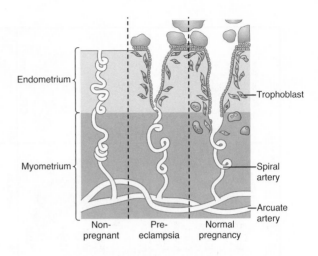

Figure 20-7 Spiral artery invasion in normal and preeclamptic pregnancies.

Source: Jain A. Endothelin-1: a key pathological factor in preeclampsia. *Reprod BioMed Online.* 2012;25:443-449. Copyright 2012 by Reproductive Healthcare Ltd. Reproductive biomedicine online by Reproductive Healthcare Ltd. Reproduced with permission of Reproductive Healthcare Ltd. in the format reuse in a book/textbook via Copyright Clearance Center.

Initially, the vast majority of fluid in the intravillous space is composed of maternal serum and secretions from the endometrial glands, until fetal vessels begin to function at 8 to 9 weeks' gestation (**Figure 20-8**). At term, the placenta weighs approximately 500 grams, is 18 to 22 centimeters in diameter, and is approximately 2 to 2.5 centimeters thick.[24]

The Umbilical Cord

The umbilical cord has two arteries and one vein surrounded by a gelatinous collagen material called Wharton jelly. The vessels within the cord are longer than the cord itself, so they coil in a spiral fashion as the cord lengthens. This coiling may protect the blood flow within the cord if it is subjected to tension or compression. The maximum length of the cord averages 55 to 60 centimeters. The cord epithelium, which is formed by the amnion, typically inserts into the placenta centrally but may insert at any point. The only clinically relevant aspect of cord insertion occurs when the cord inserts marginally at the end of the placenta or when the insertion is velamentous, wherein the cord inserts into the membranes a distance from the placenta. When this occurs, fetal vessels run through the membrane unprotected by Wharton's jelly. If these vessels happen to run through the membranes across the cervix, the presentation is termed vasa previa. Although vasa

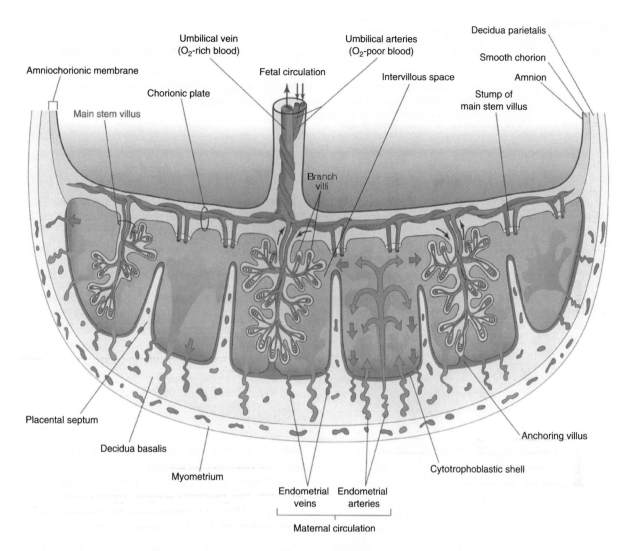

Figure 20-8 Schematic drawing of a transverse section through a full-term placenta, showing (1) the relation of the villous chorion (fetal part of placenta) to the decidua basalis (maternal part of placenta), (2) the fetal placental circulation, and (3) the maternal placental circulation. Maternal blood flows into the intervillous spaces in funnel-shaped spurts from the spiral arteries, and exchanges occur with the fetal blood as the maternal blood flows around the branch villi. It is through the branch villi that the main exchange of material between the mother and embryo/fetus occurs. The inflowing arterial blood pushes venous blood out of the intervillous space into the endometrial veins. Note that the umbilical arteries carry poorly oxygenated fetal blood to the placenta and that the umbilical vein carries oxygenated blood to the fetus. Note that the cotyledons are separated from each other by placental septa projections of the decidua basalis. Each cotyledon consists of two or more main stem villi and their many branches. In this drawing, only one stem villus is shown in each cotyledon, but the stumps of those that have been removed are indicated.

Source: This figure was published in Moore, KL, and Persaud, TVN. *The Developing Human: Clinically Oriented Embryology,* 7th ed., Copyright Saunders 2003. Reprinted by permission of Elsevier.

previa is very rare, fetal mortality is approximately 50% if the vessels rupture.[25]

Placental Transport Mechanisms

Various mechanisms of placenta transport occur within the placenta, including facilitated diffusion, passive diffusion, active transport, pinocytosis, endocytosis, bulk flow, solvent drag, accidental capillary breaks, and independent movement. These mechanisms are described in **Table 20-2**.

Placental Metabolism

Beginning early in pregnancy, the placenta synthesizes glycogen, cholesterol, and fatty acids, all of

Table 20-2	Placental Transport Mechanisms	
Transport Mechanism	Description of Mechanism	Substances Transported via Mechanism
Simple diffusion	Transfer of substances across a membrane down a concentration gradient (from an area of higher concentration of the substance to an area of lower concentration of the substance)	Oxygen, carbon dioxide, electrolytes, water, certain medications including analgesic and anesthetic agents
Facilitated diffusion	Transfer of substances across a membrane down a concentration gradient (like diffusion), but in a manner that allows for more rapid or more specific transfer	Substances such as glucose that are essential for rapid fetal growth but are present in low concentration in maternal blood
Active transport	Transport against a concentration gradient, which requires energy.	Transfer to the fetus of substances that are in higher concentration in the fetus than in the mother, such as iron and ascorbic acid
Pinocytosis	A form of endocytosis that allows small particles to be brought into a cell. The cell membrane folds around the particle and becomes an intracellular membrane.	IgG globulin maternal antibodies, phospholipids used to make cell membranes, lipoproteins are used to transport cholesterol
Breaks between cells	Active capillary breaks allow fetal and maternal cells to mix	Cell trafficking may play a role in fetal immunity and in maintaining maternal tolerance to the fetal allograft
Bulk flow	Movement of water and some solutes in water via aqueous pores	Free movement of water and some solutes maintains equal osmolality in the fetal and maternal compartments

which serve as sources of nutrients and energy for the embryo and growing fetus.

Immunology of the Placenta

The fetus is a semi-allogenic graft, which means it consists of foreign tissue from the same species but has different antigens. The reasons why the woman does not reject the fetus are still being discovered. Most importantly, the trophoblast does not express the cell surface antigens that are the usual targets for maternal antibodies. In addition, the hormones of pregnancy alter the maternal immune response in ways that allow tolerance to contact with the cytotrophoblast and syncytiotrophoblast.

Interestingly, there appears to be more cellular traffic between the fetus and mother than was originally hypothesized.[26] Fetal cells can be found in many maternal tissues and can persist in the mother for decades. Similarly, maternal cells enter the fetal circulation via mechanisms that have not been fully elucidated and may support the development of fetal immunity. The implications of this microchimerism are unknown.[27]

Amniotic Fluid

Amniotic fluid serves multiple functions during pregnancy, including cushioning and protecting the fetus,

providing space for fetal movement and growth, and maintaining consistent temperature and pressure.[28] Substances found in amniotic fluid include electrolytes, urea, creatinine, bile pigments, renin, glucose, hormones, fetal cells, lanugo, and vernix caseosa. The fluid's osmolality and composition change throughout the course of the pregnancy and are similar to the characteristics of dilute fetal urine in a term gestation.

In the latter half of pregnancy, amniotic fluid is produced primarily by the fetus in the form of urine (700–800 mL) and lung fluid. The average amount of amniotic fluid at term is 700–800 mL.[29] Amniotic fluid is removed via fetal swallowing (500–700 mL) and diffusion across the placenta. The fluid secretions from the lungs contain phospholipids, including lecithin and sphingomyelin, which are components of surfactant—a substance that is essential for the function of the neonatal lungs. As pregnancy advances, the absolute and relative amounts of lecithin in amniotic fluid increase. The ratio of lecithin to sphingomyelin is used as means of assessing fetal lung maturity to help guide decisions about delivery prior to term. While the amount of fluid varies in the third trimester and begins to decrease after 40 gestational weeks, the amount of fluid that is turned over (produced and removed) is relatively constant, at approximately 1000 mL per day.

Amniotic fluid is essential for normal growth of the fetus. Oligohydramnios at term is defined as an amniotic fluid index of 5 centimeters or less as noted on ultrasound. Oligohydramnios in the second trimester can inhibit normal fetal lung development. This condition can be caused by fetal renal abnormalities, heart disease, or fetal growth restriction. Maternal conditions that can cause oligohydramnios include severe hypertension, dehydration, and renal disorders.

Polyhydramnios is defined as an amniotic fluid index of more than 24 centimeters and is caused by too much production or too little removal of amniotic fluid. Modest polyhydramnios can be idiopathic, whereas oligohydramnios is most likely to be associated with an abnormal condition in the fetus or mother. Conditions that can cause polyhydramnios include maternal hyperglycemia, obstructed fetal swallowing, fetal cardiac failure, and severe fetal anemia.

Uteroplacental Circulation

The uteroplacental circulation is the lifeline for the fetus and, in turn, this physiology that affects fetal respiration deserves detailed attention. Fetal respiration depends on four factors: (1) adequate maternal blood flow into the intervillous space; (2) sufficient functional placental villi for gas exchange; (3) adequate diffusion, facilitated diffusion, and active transport of gases, nutrients, and fetal waste products; and (4) unimpaired fetal circulation through the placenta and umbilical cord.

The fetus can use either oxygen or glucose for the production of energy that is needed for growth and metabolic processes. Carbon dioxide (CO_2) and water (H_2O) are the end products of using oxygen in what is termed aerobic metabolism. When the fetus does not have sufficient oxygen, glucose is used to create adenosine triphosphate (ATP) for energy. This process is called anaerobic metabolism, and one of its end products is lactic acid ($C_3H_6O_3$), which has important clinical implications.

Lactic acid is acidic and, therefore, needs to be buffered by bicarbonate or hemoglobin so the pH within the circulation and tissue stays within a normal range.[30] Terms that describe fetal acid–base physiology are listed in **Table 20-3**. Carbon dioxide and water cross the placenta via diffusion very rapidly. In contrast, lactic acid transfers slowly;

Table 20-3	Definitions of Terms Related to Hypoxia
Acidemia	Increased concentration of hydrogen ions in the blood.
Acidosis	Increased concentration of hydrogen ions in the tissues of the body.
Aerobic metabolism	Metabolism of glucose using oxygen.
Anaerobic metabolism	Metabolism of glucose without the use of oxygen.
Asphyxia	Comes from the Greek word for "pulseless." A decrease in O_2 and increase in CO_2 secondary to an interference with gas exchange. Asphyxia is a continuum described by degrees of acidosis.
Base	A substance that is capable of accepting hydrogen ions and thereby decreasing acidity.
Base excess (BE)	The amount of base or HCO_3^- that is available for buffering hydrogen ions. As metabolic acidosis increases, the base excess decreases.
Bicarbonate (bicarb)	HCO_3^- is the base or hydrogen acceptor that is part of the primary buffering system within the blood.
Buffer	A chemical substance that is both a weak acid and a salt. Buffers can absorb or give up hydrogen ions, thereby maintaining a constant pH value. The primary buffer involved in fetal oxygenation is HCO_3^-.
Hypercarbia	Excessive carbon dioxide in blood.
Hypoxia	Decreased oxygen in tissue.
Hypoxemia	Decreased oxygen content in blood.
Metabolic acidemia	Low bicarbonate (negative base excess).
pH	The concentration of hydrogen ions in blood. The term pH refers to *puissance hydrogen*, which is French for "strength (or power) of hydrogen." A pH of 7.0 is the same as 0.0000001 mole per liter of hydrogen ions.
Respiratory acidemia	High PCO_2.

consequently, it can become concentrated in the fetal compartment if uterine, placental, or umbilical blood flow is interrupted. If the fetal supply of bicarbonate buffer is used, the pH in the fetal circulation and tissue will drop. As the fetal environment becomes more acidic, normal functions fail. The most common clinical scenario where this might occur is frequent uterine contractions during labor that disallow sufficient time for equilibrium to occur in the intervillous space.

Fetal hypoxia can be either acute or chronic. Acute interruptions in gas exchange can occur at any time in gestation but are most common during labor. Examples include umbilical cord occlusion and maternal supine positioning that results in an interruption in uterine blood flow. Chronic hypoxia is more likely to occur secondary to placental disorders that cause conditions such as preeclampsia. Any maternal condition that might adversely affect the uterine spiral arteries can also cause a chronic decrease in uteroplacental circulation. Examples include diabetes and chronic hypertension.

The Embryo and Fetus

Organogenesis

Returning to the blastocyst, the embryonic period, which is the period of organogenesis, occurs between 2 weeks and 8 weeks following fertilization. The fetal period, which is marked by growth and tissue differentiation, starts at 8 weeks after fertilization and extends to birth. The age of the embryo in "gestational weeks" refers to the number of weeks after fertilization in the embryology and basic science literature. Clinical obstetric texts use the term "gestational weeks" to define the number of weeks

after the woman's last menstrual period. This 2-week discrepancy can be confusing unless the reader understands which terminology the author is using. This chapter follows the convention used by embryologists in this section.

The embryonic disc within the blastocyst gives rise to the three germ layers: (1) endoderm, (2) mesoderm, and (3) ectoderm. The third week of embryo development is marked by rapid growth during which the mesoderm, ectoderm, and endoderm begin to undergo the dramatic transformations that form specific embryonic structures (**Table 20-4**). Most functional organs and organ systems are formed from all three embryonic germ layers. Each germ layer contributes a specific feature but the germ layers do not produce specific structures separately from each other.

Morphogenesis

The genetically controlled process during which cells and cell groups take on a specific form, shape, and function is known as morphogenesis. Initially, the cells in the embryoblast are all the same; that is, they are stem cells, capable of becoming any type of body cell. These unspecialized cells must proceed through two distinct phases: (1) determination, which restricts the cell to a specific type, and (2) differentiation, in which the morphologic and functional characteristics specific to that cell type develop. Cell differentiation often involves a process called induction wherein cells in a local environment signal one another to develop in a specific

Table 20-4	Differentiation of Embryonic Germ Layers	
Ectoderm	**Mesoderm**	**Endoderm**
Central and peripheral nervous system	Connective tissues	Epithelium of the digestive system (except the mouth and anus which are involutions of the ectoderm)
Epidermis including hair, nails and sebaceous glands	Muscle tissue	
	Skeleton (bone)	Liver and pancreas
Epithelium of sensory organs	Cardiovascular	
Nasal and oral cavities	Lymphatics	Respiratory system including alveolar cells of the lung
Salivary glands	Urogenital structures (gonads and kidney)	Thymus, thyroid, parathyroid, pancreas
Adrenal medulla		
Parts of the pituitary gland	Serous lining of body cavities (peritoneum, pleural and pericardium)	

manner. The signaling cell is called the inductor, and the cells that respond to induction are called the inducers. If a disruption occurs during any of the differentiation sequences, the next step in the process will not proceed in the usual fashion and an abnormality will develop. Complete organ agenesis may occur when the process is disturbed at an early stage. Anencephaly is an example of organ agenesis wherein the brain does not form. Some disruptions in differentiation sequences will result in termination of the pregnancy, whereas others may produce a fetal defect that can be undetectable, minor, or clinically significant.

In addition to cell differentiation and induction, several other cellular mechanics are involved in morphogenesis including proliferation, migration, adhesion, and folding. Some of these processes are summarized in **Table 20-5**.

Fetal Growth

All major organs have formed by the beginning of the fetal period. Fetal growth involves both hyperplasia (cellular division that yields a significant increase in cell numbers) and hypertrophy (an increase in cell size). At approximately 32 weeks' gestation, hypertrophy dominates.[31]

The rate and amount of fetal growth are determined by many factors, including genetics, placental metabolism, maternal conditions, maternal behavior, and environmental factors. For example, there is a well-known correlation between maternal smoking and impaired fetal growth.[32]

Adequate fetal growth is also directly associated with optimal functioning of the placenta and the uterine vascular system. Alterations in the trophoblastic invasion of the maternal spiral arterioles, or

Table 20-5	Selected Cellular Mechanisms Involved in Morphogenesis	
Cell Mechanism	**Description**	**Congenital Defects That May Result from Faulty Mechanism**
Cell proliferation (hypertrophy)	A rapid increase in the number of cells by cell division and growth.	Inhibition of cell proliferation can occur when there is a lack of space. A diaphragmatic hernia will allow abdominal contents to be in the thoracic cavity and pulmonary hypoplasia occurs because the lungs are not allowed to continue cell proliferation.
Cell differentiation	Process by which pluripotent cells become more specialized cells.	It is theorized that prenatal exposure to high levels of methylmercury results in failure of cell differentiation in the central nervous system thus, causing neurologic and developmental defects.
Apoptosis	A genetically determined process of cell self-destruction. Cells produce enzymes that lead to their dissolution.	Excessive enzymatic release can lead to excessive cellular destruction and result in defects such as limb shortening. Deficient enzymatic release can lead to defects such as bowel atresia, syndactyly, or imperforate anus.
Migration	A dynamic and cyclical process where layers migrate to a strategic location along the developing embryo. The cell extends protrusions at its front and attaches to the substratum on which the cell is migrating.	Central nervous system abnormalities, such as lissencephaly
Adhesion	The interaction of specific mechanisms on one cell with complementary adhesion molecules on the membrane of another cell.	Cleft palate and neural tube defects occur as a result of alteration in cell recognition and the adhesion process.
Folding	As new cells form, the embryo is forced to conform to the available space. The embryo folds in both the transverse and longitudinal planes. Structures within the embryo also must fold to conform to the space available to them.	Congenital heart defects Diverticula

inadequate development of the chorionic villus, can result in impaired fetal growth.

Fetal Movement and Behavioral States

Limb movement develops at 9 weeks, with reflective leg movements occurring at 14 weeks. Hand-to-face movements become apparent by 12 to 13 weeks, while limb, head, and torso movements develop by 12 to 16 weeks. Fetuses begin to suck on fingers by 15 weeks and continue to develop more complex movement patterns after 24 weeks, when respiratory movements occur.[33]

Discrete fetal behavior states involving sleep–wake patterns and behavioral patterns begin to occur by 32 weeks as the fetus matures. Distinct fetal heart rate patterns, eye movement, gross body movement, and quiet states have been catalogued.[33,34] Although women often report less fetal movement close to term, the underlying fetal physiology is probably maternal perception of the fetus in a quiet state. The average time the fetus spends in this quiet state is 20 to 40 minutes.[32,33]

Fetal Origins of Adult Disease

In the 1990s, David Barker, a physician and researcher, published a theory that was later known by various names, including Barker's hypothesis or fetal origins of adult disease. Today, this widely accepted theory is cited as establishing a link between a number of adult major chronic diseases and the fetal environment, especially in the context of maternal malnutrition. When a pregnant woman experiences poor nutrition, such as during war or related to poverty, her unborn fetus makes metabolic changes in an attempt to prepare for life in a low-resource world. The specific physiologic changes are still being investigated and much remains to be learned. Not surprisingly, though, a child exposed to limited intrauterine nutrition is more likely to be small at birth with a lowered metabolic rate.[35]

Barker's major finding was that fetuses starved in utero had an increased risk for chronic diseases such as obesity, diabetes, coronary heart disease, and hypertension when they grew to adulthood in a developed country with abundant food. His work linked birth records with later health/death records in his home country of the United Kingdom. Approximately a decade after his initial publication, Barker described his basic methodology and acknowledged his debt to the meticulous and complete records of midwives, without whom he would not have had adequate data to discover the associations.[36]

Fetal programming—a newer term derived from recent work on fetal origins of adult disease—has further examined the process whereby a nutritional stress that occurs during a critical phase of development permanently affects fetal physiology and metabolism.[37] The fetal origins of disease theory provides yet more proof of the importance of prenatal care and assurance that a woman is well nourished during pregnancy.

Maternal Anatomic and Physiologic Adaptations to Pregnancy

Pregnant women experience a wide variety of physiologic alterations. While many are normal symptoms of pregnancy, others herald the onset of an abnormal process. One of the most important characteristics of midwifery practice is a broad and deep knowledge of normal variations in combination with accurate and early risk assessment. A thorough knowledge of the maternal anatomic and physiologic adaptations that occur during pregnancy is, therefore, an essential foundation for midwives who care for women during the childbearing cycle.

This section presents an overview of some of the clinically important anatomic and physiologic pregnancy adaptations. Additional information that midwives need for safe practice can be found in the references for this chapter and other texts. Symptoms of pregnancy, the related etiologies, and management are also described in the *Prenatal Care* chapter. Normal laboratory values for common physiologic indices are listed in **Table 20-6**.[38,39]

Anatomic Changes

Anatomic changes are primarily related to weight gain, the growing uterus, the softening effects of progesterone on cartilage in joints, and the laxity of ligaments induced by estrogen and relaxin.[40]

The result of these changes is a gradual increase in lordosis, kyphosis, and altered gait. The changes within the pelvic girdle are the most profound. The sacroiliac joint widens and has more mobility. The symphysis also widens, and the pelvis develops an anterior tilt. Many of the common complaints of pregnancy can be attributed to these anatomic changes, including pelvic pain, sciatica back pain, and carpal tunnel syndrome. A careful history and physical examination is needed to rule out more serious problems that pregnant women are at increased risk for, such as herniated discs and peripheral nerve injury.

Integumentary Changes

Pregnancy is associated with many changes in the integument. Hyperpigmentation occurs as estrogen,

Table 20-6	Normal Laboratory Values in Pregnancy				
Test	**Abbreviation**	**Nonpregnant Adult**	**First Trimester**	**Second Trimester**	**Third Trimester**
Hematology					
Ferritin (ng/mL)[a]		10–150	6–130	2–230	0–116
Folate, serum (ng/mL)		5.4–18.0	2.6–15.0	0.8–24.0	1.4–20.7
Hemoglobin[a] (g/dL)	Hgb	10.4–15.2[b]	11.6–13.9	9.7–14.8	9.5–15
Hematocrit[a] (%)	Hct	32.0–45.0[b]	31–41	30–39	28–40
Iron, total iron-binding capacity[a] (mcg/dL)	TIBC	251–406	278–403	Not reported	359–609
Iron, serum[a] (mcg/dL)		41–141 (mean 135)	72–143 (mean 90)	44–178	30–193
Mean corpuscular hemoglobin (pg/cell)	MCH	23.2–33.3[b]	30–32	30–33	29–32
Mean corpuscular volume	MCV	73.4–98.3[b]	80–100	82–97	81–99
Platelets ($\times 10^9$/L)		172–453[b]	174–400	155–409	146–426
Red blood cell count	RBC	3.70–5.20[b]	3.42–4.55	2.81–4.49	2.71–4.43
Reticulocyte count (%)		0.5–1	1–2	Not reported	Not reported
White blood cell count ($\times 10^3$/mm^3)	WBC	3.9–12.5[b]	5.7–13.6	5.6–14.8	5.9–16.9
Neutrophils ($\times 10^3$/mm^3)		1.4–4.6	3.6–10.1	3.8–12.3	3.9–13.1
Lymphocytes ($\times 10^3$/mm^3)		0.7–4.6	1.1–3.6	0.9–3.9	1.0–3.6
Monocytes ($\times 10^3$/mm^3)		0.1–0.7	0.1–1.1	0.1–1.1	0.1–1.4
Transferrin (mg/dL)		200–400	254–344	220–441	288–530
Basic Coagulation Studies					
International Normalized Ratio	INR	0.9–1.04	0.89–1.05	0.85–0.97	0.80–0.94
Fibrinogen (mg/dL)		233–496	244–510	291–538	373–619
Partial thromboplastin time, activated (sec)	aPTT	26.3–39.4	24.3–38.9	24.2–38.1	24.7–35.0
Prothrombin time (sec)	PT	12.7–15.4	9.7–13.5	9.5–13.4	9.6–12.9
Blood Chemistry					
Alanine transaminase (U/L)	ALT	7–41	3–30	2–33	2–25
Alkaline phosphatase (U/L)	ALP/ALKP	33–96	17–88	25–126	38–229
Amylase (U/L)		20–96	24–83	16–73	15–81
Aspartate transaminase (U/L)	AST	12–38	3–23	3–33	4–32
Bilirubin, total (mg/dL)	T. Bili	0.3–1.3	0.1–0.4	0.1–0.8	0.1–1.1
Bilirubin, conjugated (mg/dL)		0.1–0.4	0–0.1	0–0.1	0–0.1

(continues)

Table 20-6	Normal Laboratory Values in Pregnancy (continued)				
Test	Abbreviation	Nonpregnant Adult	First Trimester	Second Trimester	Third Trimester
Blood Chemistry (continued)					
Bile acids (μmol/L)		0.3–4.8	0–4.9	0–9.1	0–11.3
Calcium, ionized (mg/dL)		4.5–5.3	4.5–5.1	4.4–5.0	4.4–5.3
Creatinine (mg/dL)		0.5–0.9[c]	0.4–0.7	0.4–0.8	0.4–0.9
Lactate dehydrogenase (U/L)	LDH	115–221	78–433	80–447	82–524
Lipase (U/L)		3–43	21–76	26–100	41–112
Potassium (mEq/L)	K	3.5–5.0	3.6–5.0	3.3–5.0	3.3–5.1
Sodium (mEq/L)	Na	136–146	133–148	129–148	130–148
Urea nitrogen (mg/dL)	BUN	7–20	7–12	3–13	3–11
Uric acid (mg/dL)		2.5–5.6[c]	2.0–4.2	2.4–4.9	3.1–6.3
Endocrine/Metabolic					
Hemoglobin A_{1c} (%)	Hgb A_{1c}	4–6	4–6	4–6	4–7
Thyroid-stimulating hormone (μIU/mL)	TSH	0.34–4.25	0.60–3.40	0.37–3.60	0.38–4.04
Thyroxine, free (ng/dL)	fT_4	0.8–1.7	0.8–1.2	0.6–1.0	0.5–0.8
Vitamins/Minerals					
Vitamin B_{12} (pg/mL)		279–966	118–438	130–656	99–526
Vitamin D, 25-hydroxy (ng/mL)		14–80	18–27	10–22	10–18
Hormones					
Estradiol (pg/mL)		< 20–443[c]	188–2497	1278–7192	6137–3460
Progesterone (ng/mL)		< 1–20[c]	8–48		99–342
Blood Gases					
Bicarbonate (mEq/L)	HCO_3^-	22–26	Not reported	Not reported	16–22
PCO_2 (mm Hg)		38–42	Not reported	Not reported	25–33
PO_2 (mm Hg)		90–100	93–100	90–98	92–107
pH		7.38–7.42 (arterial)	7.36–7.52 (venous)	7.40–7.52 (venous)	7.41–7.53 (venous) 7.39–7.45 (arterial)
Renal function					
24-hour protein excretion (mg/24 hr)		< 150	19–141	47–186	46–185

[a]Values are based on populations with and without iron supplementation.

[b]Values for females 19–65 years old.

[c]Values for females only.

Sources: Adapted from Cunningham FG. Appendix B: laboratory values in normal pregnancy. In: Queenan JT, Hobbins JC, Spong CYT, eds. *Protocols for High-Risk Pregnancies: An Evidence-Based Approach,* 5th ed. Oxford, UK: Blackwell; 2010:587-595; Centers for Disease Control and Prevention. Laboratory procedure manual: complete blood count with 5-part differential. NHANES 2005-2006. Available at: http://www.cdc.gov/nchs/data/nhanes/nhanes_05_06/cbc_d_met.pdf. Accessed November 9, 2012.

progesterone, and melanocyte-stimulating hormone induce melanocytes to make and deposit pigment. Hyperpigmentation results in darkening of the areola, the change of the linea alba to the linea nigra, and chloasma (irregular areas of pigmentation on the cheeks), which is also called the "mask of pregnancy."[41]

Thinning of the elastin fibers in connective tissue under the skin predisposes pregnant women to striae gravidarum or stretch marks. As the abdomen and breasts grow in size, the elastin fibers at the dermal–epidermal junction stretch and shift from perpendicular to parallel, which creates the striae.

Vascular nevi called spider angiomas are common as blood vessels dilate and proliferate. These small red lesions have a central puncta and branches that extend from the center. They disappear after birth. More troublesome is the development of varicosities. During pregnancy, connective tissue softens, vascular walls relax, blood volume expands, and pressure in the vessels in lower extremities increases from the uterus compressing the vena cava. The result can be lower limb and vulvar superficial varicosities.

Cardiovascular Changes

Cardiovascular changes begin early in the first trimester.[42] Blood volume increases by 40% to 50% over the course of pregnancy, reaching a maximum by 32 weeks' gestation. Plasma accounts for 75% of this increase. Cardiac output increases 30% to 50%—an increase that begins in the first trimester but peaks at approximately 25 to 30 weeks' gestation, when the total blood volume is approximately 5000 to 6000 mL. Heart rate increases by approximately 10 bpm and blood pressure decreases from prepregnancy values as early as 7 weeks' gestation. This decrease reaches a nadir in the second trimester. A significant decrease in systemic vascular resistance occurs secondary to progesterone-induced vasodilation.

Several common signs and symptoms are related to these changes. The hemodilution that occurs as the volume shifts to favor proportionately more plasma than red cells results in a physiologic anemia, which is evidenced by a drop in hematocrit. Systolic ejection murmurs are a common finding in pregnant women that is attributed to the dramatic increase in cardiac output, though such murmurs are clinically benign. The decrease in systemic vascular resistance in combination with pressure on the vena cava from the growing uterus is responsible for the dependent edema that most pregnant women experience in the third trimester and contributes to the development of varicosities, as previously described.

Careful monitoring of cardiovascular changes can help the midwife detect abnormalities early. For example, when a woman's blood pressure fails to decrease during the second trimester, she may have chronic hypertension or be at increased risk for developing preeclampsia. Cardiovascular changes can also increase the risk for adverse outcomes in women who have preexisting cardiomyopathies; these women should be referred for medical evaluation.[42]

Hematologic Changes

Two aspects of hematologic changes in pregnancy have important clinical implications. First, pregnancy is a hypercoagulable state, as evidenced by the increased clotting factors, decreased fibrinolysis, and decreased anticoagulant activity noted in the pregnant woman. Clotting factors I, II, VII, VIII, IX, and XII are more abundant in such women, whereas protein S levels and activated protein C levels fall. These alterations in the coagulation cascade are probably protective in that they prevent hemorrhage at birth, but they also increase a woman's risk for venous thromboembolism in the prenatal and postnatal periods. In addition, significant placental damage and obstetric hemorrhage are associated with early onset of disseminated intravascular coagulation (DIC), which is not a common component of surgical or traumatic hemorrhage. This occurs because the tissue factor in placental tissue acts as a potent activator of the coagulation cascade, which is already in a hypercoagulable state.[44]

The second clinically important hematologic change in pregnancy relates to iron metabolism and iron-deficiency anemia. The hemodilution of pregnancy causes a decrease in hematocrit of approximately 3% to 5%, with this level reaching its nadir late in the second trimester or early in the third trimester. Hemoglobin (Hgb) decreases by 2% to 10% secondary to fetal uptake that is more than maternal absorption can replace.

Iron is not easily absorbed, so fetal uptake can deplete a woman's iron reserves despite the fact that iron absorption in the second and third trimesters increases more than fivefold.[45] Thus iron stores can be easily depleted in pregnancy.

Respiratory Changes

An increase in thoracic diameter and cephalad rise in the diaphragm (up to 4 cm) change the pregnant woman's lung capacity. Tidal volume increases by 30% to 40%, and vital capacity increases slightly. This hyperventilation probably occurs secondary to the effects of progesterone. It places the woman in a state of respiratory alkalosis, which has the effect of improving carbon dioxide transfer from the fetus to the maternal circulation. It is common for pregnant women to experience dyspnea even when at rest. The actual etiology is unknown, but most sources assume this condition arises secondary to the added respiratory effort and work of breathing.[46] Physiologic dyspnea can be distinguished from pathologic dyspnea by the respiratory rate. Tachypnea is a sign of possible respiratory compromise.

Gastrointestinal Changes

The enlarging gravid uterus shifts gastrointestinal structures. Specifically, the stomach is moved superiorly and the intestines are displaced laterally. Gastric emptying time and gastric motility are decreased secondary to the smooth muscle relaxation effects of progesterone. Thus constipation is common, especially in the first trimester when the growing uterus also places pressure on the descending colon. Heartburn is very common in the second and third trimesters, and gastroesophageal reflux disorder can be aggravated throughout pregnancy.

Renal Changes

Two different aspects of renal changes in pregnancy are responsible for symptoms that must be carefully evaluated to determine normal versus abnormal alterations. First, a marked increase in renal plasma flow is the natural consequence of arterial vasodilation and increased cardiac output. Renal blood flow increases 60% to 80% above prepregnant levels in the first and second trimesters and 50% above prepregnant levels in the third trimester. The glomerular filtration rate (GFR) increases by 50% over prepregnant levels, peaking at 12 gestational weeks.[47] The obvious physiologic consequences of these changes are the commonly reported symptoms of urinary frequency and nocturia.

The increased flow may be great enough that the descending tubule is unable to reabsorb all glucose. This resultant physiologic glycosuria is usually intermittent, but affects as many as 20% of pregnant women. Similarly, protein reabsorption is not as efficient as it is in the nonpregnant state. A small amount of urinary protein in a sample of concentrated urine can cause a dipstick test to be positive, which may be falsely interpreted as a urinary tract infection or preeclampsia. Serum creatinine likewise falls; thus plasma values for creatinine that would be considered normal in a nonpregnant individual may actually reflect renal dysfunction in a pregnant woman.

Conversely, pregnant women are at increased risk for urinary tract infections in pregnancy because the ureters, urethra, and bladder all dilate under the influence of progesterone. The bladder becomes hyperemic and urinary stasis can occur, which occasionally results in stress incontinence. Thus physiologic changes in pregnancy cause symptoms that can be either normal or a sign of urinary tract infection or renal dysfunction, and careful attention to the history, physical examination, and adjunct measures of urinary function are necessary to adequately care for women with urinary symptoms.

Endocrine Changes

Among the many endocrine and metabolic changes of import in pregnancy are changes that occur in the hypothalamus, pituitary, and adrenal glands, often in an interrelated manner. Calcium metabolism and the renin–angiotensin system both exhibit significant alterations in ways that facilitate fetal growth and development.

Thyroid Metabolism

Although all endocrine organs undergo changes in pregnancy, the thyroid is a particularly interesting story. Because both hypothyroid and hyperthyroid states can adversely affect the fetus, it is critical that a euthyroid state be maintained in pregnancy. The thyroid is the first endocrine gland to appear in the fetus, but the fetus does not start secreting thyroid hormone until approximately 18 to 20 weeks. As a consequence, the fetus is dependent on maternal thyroid hormone for the critical metabolic functions fulfilled by this hormone. The thyroid increases in size early in the pregnant woman and may be palpable on an initial prenatal visit as a smooth and regular-shaped mass. The basal metabolic rate also increases by 20% to 25% during pregnancy.

Several changes occur in the production and transport of thyroxine. Higher levels of plasma albumin and thyroxine-binding globulin (TBG) mean that more thyroxine (T_4) is protein bound in serum and, therefore, not available to move into cells. The alpha unit of hCG is able to stimulate the thyroid as would TSH, which causes a decrease in TSH but an increase in total thyroxine levels (i.e., subclinical hyperthyroidism). The TSH level reaches a nadir at approximately 10 gestational weeks; then, as the hCG level declines, the TSH level rises to reach the nonpregnant level by the third trimester and the thyroxine level declines to a normal value. Plasma values for thyroid function are trimester specific and cannot be determined via one measurement. In general, an assessment of TSH and free T_4 or total T_4 is needed to interpret thyroid function (**Table 20-7**).[48]

Overt hypothyroidism is rare, but it is associated with a range of pregnancy complications when

Table 20-7	Tests of Thyroid Function in Pregnancy				
Test	Normal Pregnancy	Hyperthyroidism and Pregnancy[a]	Hypothyroidism (Overt)[b]	Postpartum Thyroiditis with Hyperthyroidism[c]	Hyperemesis Gravidarum
TSH	Normal	Suppressed or undetectable[d]	High	Undetectable	Normal or low
TBG	Increased	Increased	Normal	Normal	Increased
Total T$_4$	Increased	Increased	Low	Increased	Increased
Free T$_4$	Normal	Increased	Low	Increased	Normal or increased
Total T$_3$	Increased	Increased	Low	Increased	Increased
Free T$_3$	Normal	Increased	Low	Increased	Normal or increased

TBG = thyroid-binding globulin; T$_4$ = thyroxine; T$_3$ = triiodothyronine; TSH = thyroid stimulating hormone.

[a]Tests for overt hyperthyroidism are shown; subclinical hyperthyroidism has undetectable serum TSH with normal, total, and free T$_4$ and T$_3$.

[b]Tests for overt hypothyroidism are shown; subclinical hypothyroidism has high TSH with normal, total, and free T$_4$ and T$_3$.

[c]Hypothyroidism may also develop.

[d]TSH may be high in rare cases.

Source: Adapted from Mazzaferro EL. Evaluation and management of common thyroid disorders in women. *Am J Obstet Gynecol.* 1997;176:507-514. Copyright 1997 by Mosby, Inc. *American Journal of Obstetrics and Gynecology* by American Gynecological Society. Reproduced with permission of Mosby, Inc. in the format reuse in a book/textbook via Copyright Clearance Center.

it occurs. Women who enter pregnancy on thyroid replacement medications generally remain euthyroid, but the doses may need to be serially increased over the course of pregnancy.

Overt hyperthyroidism is also uncommon, but it is associated with miscarriage, preterm labor, stillbirth, and other pregnancy complications. Women who are on thyroid-suppressing medication will need medical consultation, as these medications cross the placenta and can adversely affect the fetus.

Glucose Metabolism

Glucose metabolism is significantly altered in pregnancy. Maternal hyperinsulinemia occurs as a compensation for the insulin resistance caused by hPL and other placental hormones. In turn, hPL initiates hyperplasia within the beta cells of the maternal pancreas, so that more production of insulin can occur. Fetal uptake of glucose occurs via facilitated diffusion; thus it is not affected by changes in maternal serum glucose levels. Maternal fasting glucose levels can be lower than usual, for example, yet because of the insulin resistance, postprandial glucose levels can be higher than in the nonpregnant state.

Lower fasting blood glucose levels can worsen nausea and vomiting in early pregnancy but may also play a role in the pregnant woman's enhanced appetite and her need to eat more often. As the placenta increases in size and function, maternal hyperinsulinemia must also increase to keep pace.

Women who are unable to raise insulin production sufficiently will develop diabetes in the latter half of pregnancy.

Immunologic Changes

Immunologic changes in pregnancy are implicated in several important clinical disorders, including recurrent miscarriage, Rh sensitization, and preeclampsia, yet certain autoimmune disorders may improve during pregnancy. Pregnancy is essentially an immunologic paradox: First, how does the mother avoid rejecting the fetus given that fetal cells and maternal cells are in direct contact in the maternal spiral arteries and intervillous space? Second, how do the immunologic changes that take place to accommodate the fetus, a semi-allograft, affect the maternal immune response?

Immune response may be classified as either innate immunity or adaptive immunity; the latter is subdivided into two components called cell-mediated immunity and antibody-mediated immunity. The innate immune response is the first line of defense against "non-self" invaders, which includes inflammation and phagocytosis. Cell-mediated immunity, in contrast, is responsible for elimination of intracellular microbes and involves several immune lymphocytes, including natural killer (NK) cells and T cells. Antibody-mediated immunity involves the production of antibodies by B cells; these antibodies then target extracellular microbes or antigens.

The Fetus as an Allograft

The first part of the immunologic story of pregnancy occurs during implantation and is not yet completely understood. Put simply, the trophoblastic tissue does not express the cell membrane proteins that would stimulate an innate or cellular immune response. In addition, changes in the cell-mediated immune response result in a concentration of NK cells in the decidua; these cells, however, are a variant of NK cells that have minimal cytotoxic abilities but a refined ability to control trophoblast invasion and remodel uterine vasculature. T cells and B cells become scarce in the uterine environment during this period.

Many of the bioactive agents produced by the fetus and placenta effect subtle shifts in maternal immunity. Although there is little overall change in the maternal immune response, subtle changes in each of the three types of immunity have some important clinical implications (**Box 20-1**).

Fetopelvic Relationships

The fetus can lie in any number of positions within the uterus and in relationship to the maternal abdomen pelvis. Some of these positions preclude a vaginal birth; others are associated with a longer labor. For this reason, it is important for the midwife to know all possible fetopelvic relationships and their clinical significance. The terminology used to describe fetopelvic relationships is listed in **Table 20-8**.

The Fetal Skull

The fetal skull is made up of five bones—two frontal bones, two parietal bones, and one occipital bone—that may be palpated during labor to identify the position of the fetus and assess labor progress. In addition, the two temporal bones are located inferior to the parietal bones on each side, but are not involved in the anatomic markers important during labor assessment (**Figure 20-9**). The bones meet at the frontal suture, located between the two frontal bones; at the sagittal suture, located between the two parietal bones; at the two coronal sutures, where the parietal and frontal bones meet on either side of the head; and at the two lambdoid sutures, where the parietal bones and the upper margin of the occipital bone meet on either side of the head. Two fontanels—areas formed by the meeting of sutures—are found on either end of the sagittal suture. The anterior fontanel is the largest, formed as the frontal, sagittal, and two coronal sutures come together in a diamond-like shape. The four sutures can be palpated coming from the four

---

BOX 20-1 Changes in the Immune System During Pregnancy

Primary Host Defense Mechanisms

- Increased number of white blood cells (primarily polymorphonucleic leukocytes), which enhances the pregnant woman's nonspecific immune response.
- Delayed chemotaxis (the movement of phagocytes to the site of foreign invasion), which may delay maternal response to infection.
- Decreased number of natural killer cells, which may delay maternal response to infection.
- Reduced levels of plasma immunoglobulin G (IgG). The hemodilution of pregnancy and passive transfer of Ig antibody to the fetus reduces maternal blood levels of IgG.

Cell-Mediated Immunity

Although the overall number of lymphocytes remains unchanged, there is a decreased number of T-helper cells (CD4 cells) relative to the number of T-suppressor cells (CD8 cells). With fewer CD4 cells, the B-cell function may be slightly impaired.

Antibody-Mediated Immunity

Overall, the antibody-mediated response is unchanged.

Clinical Implications

- Small increase in risk for developing gram-negative organism infections and mycotic or fungal infections.
- Increased morbidity from gram-negative infections, H1N1 flu virus, and varicella if infection occurs.
- Increased infectivity with certain pathogens, including herpes simplex virus, poliovirus, cytomegalovirus, malaria, and hepatitis.
- Changes in autoimmune disease characteristics (rheumatoid arthritis often improves during pregnancy, while systemic lupus erythematosus can flare up).

---

corners of diamond shape, with the frontal suture being more subtle and sometimes difficult to palpate. The sagittal and two lambdoid sutures meet to form the posterior fontanel in a triangle shape; the sagittal and lambdoid sutures can be palpated from the three corners of the triangle. The fetal head also has several diameters of importance in providing maternity care, which are shown in Figure 20-9 **and Figure 20-10**.

Table 20-8	Fetopelvic Relationships
Term	**Definition**
Asynclitism	When the fetal biparietal diameter is not parallel to the planes of the pelvis. The sagittal suture will not be palpable as midway between the front and back of the pelvis.
Attitude	Relation of fetal parts to each other. The basic attitudes are flexion and extension. The fetal head is flexed when the chin is close to the chest; it is extended when the occiput is closer to the cervical spine.
Denominator	An arbitrarily chosen point on the presenting part of the fetus that is used to describe fetal position. The denominator for a vertex presentation is the occiput and for a breech presentation it is the sacrum. The denominator of a face presentation is the mentum or chin.
Engagement	When the widest diameter of the presenting part is at or below the pelvic inlet, engagement has taken place.
Lie	Relationship of the long axis of the fetus to the long axis of the mother. The three possible lies are cephalic, transverse, and breech.
Position	Relationship of the denominator to the front, back, or sides of the maternal pelvis.
Presentation	The part of the fetus that presents first to the maternal pelvis. The three possible presentations are cephalic, shoulder, and breech. Breech presentations are further subdivided based on presentation of the buttocks or feet.
Presenting part	The most dependent part of the fetus that is closest to the maternal cervix.
Station	The number of centimeters above or below the plane between the ischial spines. The ischial spines are designated 0 station; the centimeters above the spines are −1, −2, -3,-4, and -5; and the centimeters below the ischial spines are +1, +2, +3, +4, and +5, which is when the fetal presenting part is visible at the vaginal introitus.

Lie, Presentation, Denominator, Position

Determination of the lie, presentation, and position of the fetus require an understanding of terms and the anatomic landmarks of the fetal skull in relation to the maternal pelvis.

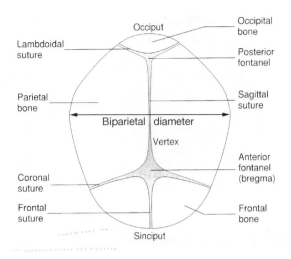

Figure 20-9 Fetal skull: landmarks, bones, fontanelles, sutures, and biparietal diameter.

Lie is the relationship of the long axis of the fetus to the long axis of the mother. Three possible lies are longitudinal, transverse, and oblique (**Figure 20-11**). Transverse and oblique lies in labor are abnormal conditions requiring collaboration with the consulting physician and will likely necessitate cesarean section. Approximately 0.5% of women enter labor with a shoulder presentation.

Presentation is determined by the presenting part, the part of the fetus to first enter the pelvic inlet. The three possible presentations are cephalic, breech, and shoulder. Cephalic and breech presentations are each further subdivided; a cephalic presentation can be vertex, sinciput, brow, or face (**Figure 20-12**), and a breech presentation can be frank (legs extended), full/complete (legs flexed), or footling (single or double). Approximately 3.0% to 3.5% of women enter labor with a breech presentation and 0.5% with a face presentation. The midwife collaborates with a physician

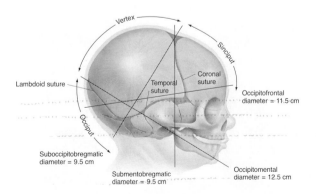

Figure 20-10 Diameters of the term fetal head.

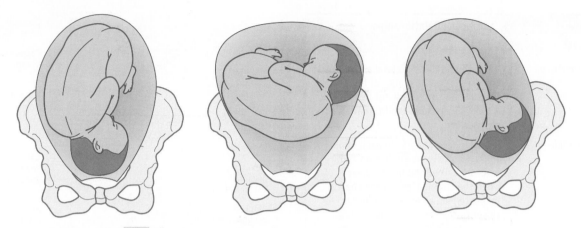

Figure 20-11 Lies: (a) longitudinal; (b) transverse; (c) oblique.

in the management of women with a breech, brow, or face presentation.

The *attitude* of the fetus is its characteristic posture, determined by the relationship of the fetal parts to one another and the effect this has on the fetal vertebral column. The attitude of the fetus varies according to its presentation. For example, a fetus in a vertex presentation has a well-flexed head, flexion of the extremities over the thorax and abdomen, and a convex curved back; the straight upright attitude of a fetus with a sinciput presentation has resulted in the classically defined military attitude; and a fetus with a face presentation has an acutely extended head, flexion of the extremities on the thorax and abdomen, and a vertebral column that is arched to some degree.

Fetal *position* is named using three letters in the following order: the first reference is to the side of the maternal pelvis (Left or Right); the second reference is the denominator (Occiput, Sacrum, or Mentum); and the third reference is where in the maternal pelvis the denominator lies (Anterior, Transverse,

Posterior). These designations serve as a shorthand description for describing the lie, presentation, and position of the denominator within the circle of the pelvis (**Figure 20-13**). For example, the designation LOA indicates that the lie is longitudinal, the presentation is cephalic, and the denominator, which is the occiput, is in the anterior portion of the left side of the pelvis. The possible fetal relationships to the maternal pelvis for each lie and presentation are summarized in **Table 20-9**.

Vertex is the most common presentation associated with a longitudinal lie. With an incidence of approximately 95%, approximately two-thirds of all fetuses will be positioned with the occiput in the left side of the mother's pelvis (LOA, LOT, LOP) and one-third with the occiput in the right side of the mother's pelvis (ROA, ROT, ROP) by the last month of pregnancy. Because the head usually enters the inlet with the occiput directed to the transverse portion of the mother's pelvis, the most common position of the fetus at the onset of labor is left occiput transverse (LOT).

(a)   (b)   (c)   (d)

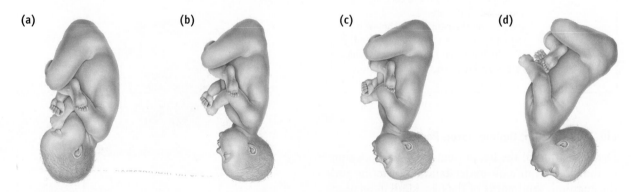

Figure 20-12 Attitude of the fetus in (a) vertex, (b) sinciput (military), (c) brow, and (d) face presentations.

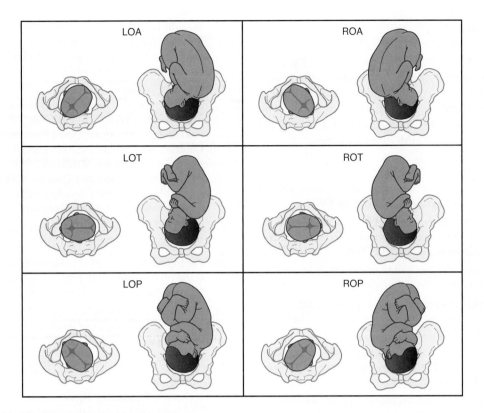

Figure 20-13 Fetal position for occiput presentations.

Table 20-9	Possible Fetal Relationships to the Maternal Pelvis for Each Lie and Presentation		
Lie	**Presentation**	**Denominator**	**Designation for Position**
Longitudinal	Cephalic		
	Vertex	Occiput	ROA LOA
			ROT LOT
			ROP LOP
	Sinciput	Sinciput (bregma, anterior fontanel)	Sinciput and brow presentations usually convert to either a vertex or a face presentation.
	Brow	Brow	
	Face	Mentum (chin)	RMA LMA
			RMT LMT
			RMP LMP
	Breech		
	Frank	Sacrum	RSA LSA
			RST LST
			RSP LSP
	Full/complete	Sacrum	Same as frank presentation
	Footling	Sacrum	Same as frank presentation
Transverse	Shoulder	Acromion	RAA LAA
			RAP LAP
			A transverse variety is not possible.
Oblique	With an oblique lie, the midwife will feel nothing at the inlet. There is no presentation, position, or variety associated with an oblique lie, which is usually a transitory condition.		

Conclusion

Remarkable physiologic changes occur during pregnancy. Physiologic changes underlie every aspect of pregnancy care. A deep understanding of these changes will allow the midwife to interpret signs and symptoms accurately—an essential first step in the provision of quality health care to women.

• • • References

1. Buhimschi CS. Endocrinology of lactation. *Obstet Gynecol Clin North Am.* 2004;31:963-979.

2. Pijneborg R, Vercruysse L, Hanssens M. The uterine spiral arteries in human pregnancy: facts and controversies. *Placenta.* 2006;27:939-958.

3. Damjanov I. Vesalius and Hunter were right: decidua is a membrane [Editorial]. *Lab Invest.* 1985;53:597.

4. Strowitzki T, Germeyer A, Popovici R, Wolff M. The human endometrium as a fertility-determining factor. *Hum Reprod Update.* 2006;12(5):617-630.

5. Murphy CR. Understanding the apical surface markers of uterine receptivity: pinopods or uterodomes: *Hum Reprod.* 2000;15:2451-2454.

6. Gellersen B, Brosens IA, Brosens JJ. Decidualization of the human endometrium: mechanisms, functions and clinical perspectives. *Sem Reprod Med.* 2007; 25(6):445-453.

7. Tingaker BK, Irestedt L. Changes in uterine innervation in pregnancy and during labour. *Curr Opin Anesthesiol.* 2010;23:300-310.

8. Latini C, Frontini A, Morroni M, Marzioni D, Castellucci M, Smith PG. Remodeling of uterine innervation. *Cell Tissue Res.* 2008;334:1-6.

9. Ludmir J, Sehdev H. Anatomy and physiology of the uterine cervix. *Clin Obstet Gynecol.* 2000;43(3): 433-439.

10. Timmons B, Akins M, Mahendroo M. Cervical remodeling during pregnancy and parturition. *Trends Endocrin Metab.* 2010;21(6):353-361.

11. Barnhart KT, Sammel MD, Rinaudo PF, Zhou L, Hummel AC, Guao W. Symptomatic patients with an early viable intrauterine pregnancy: hCG curves redefined. *Obstet Gynecol.* 2004;104:50-55.

12. King TL, Murphy PA. Evidence-based approaches to managing nausea and vomiting in early pregnancy. *J Midwifery Women's Health.* 2009;54:430-444.

13. Verberg MF, Gillott DJ, Al-Fardan N, Grudzinskas JG. Hyperemesis gravidarum, a literature review. *Hum Reprod Update.* 2005;11(5):527-539.

14. Lager S, Powell TL. Regulation of nutrient transport across the placenta. *J Preg.* 2012;2012:179827. doi: 10.1155/2012/179827.

15. Wahabi HA, Fayed AA, Esmaeil SA, Al Zeidan RA. Progestogen for treating threatened miscarriage. *Cochrane Database Sys Rev.* 2011;12:CD005943. doi: 10.1002/14651858.CD005943.pub4.

16. Likis FE, Andrews JC, Woodworth AL, et al. *Progestogens for Prevention of Preterm Birth.* Comparative Effectiveness Review No. 74 (prepared by the Vanderbilt Evidence-based Practice Center under Contract No. 290-2007-10065-I). AHRQ Publication No. 12-EHC105-EF. Rockville, MD: Agency for Healthcare Research and Quality; September 2012. Available at: www.effectivehealthcare.ahrq.gov /reports/final.cfm. Accessed February 17, 2013.

17. Cole LA. hCG, the wonder of today's science. *Reprod Biol Endocrinol.* 2012;10:24-28.

18. Pijnenborg R, Vercruysse L, Hanssens M. The uterine spiral arteries in human pregnancy: facts and controversies. *Placenta.* 2006;27:939-958.

19. Wang A, Rana SA, Karumanchi SA. Preeclampsia: the role of angiogenic factors in its pathogenesis. *Physiology.* 2009;24:147-158.

20. Jain A. Endothelin-1: a key pathological factor in preeclampsia. *Reprod BioMed Online.* 2012;25:443-449.

21. Brosens I, Pijnenborg R, Vercruzysse L, Romero R. The "great obstetrical syndromes" are associated with disorders of deep placentation. *Am J Obstet Gynecol.* 2011;204(3):193-201.

22. Longo LD, Reynolds. Some historical aspects of understanding placental development, structure, and function. *Int J Develop Biol.* 2010;54:237-255.

23. Lillycrop KA, Burdge GC. Epigenetic mechanisms linking early nutrition to long term health. *Best Pract Res Clin Endocrin Metab.* 2012;26:667-676.

24. Schuler-Maloney D. Placental triage of the singleton placenta. *J Midwifery Women's Health.* 2000;45: 104-13.

25. Derbala Y, Grochal F, Jeanty P. Vasa previa. *J Perinat Med.* 2007;1(1):2-13.

26. Dawe GS, Tan XW, Xiao ZC. Cell migration from baby to mother. *Cell Adhes Migration.* 2007;1(1): 19-27

27. Burlingham WJ. A lesson in tolerance: maternal instruction to fetal cells. *N Engl J Med.* 2009;360(13): 1355-1357.

28. Modena AB, Fieni S. Amniotic fluid dynamics. *Acta Biomed.* 2004;75(suppl 1):11-13.

29. Moore TR. Amniotic fluid dynamics reflect fetal and maternal health and disease. *Obstet Gynecol.* 2010;116(3):757-763.

30. Blechner JN. Maternal–fetal acid–base physiology. *Clin Obstet Gynecol.* 1993;36(1):3-12.

31. Murphy VE, Smith R, Giles WB, Clifton VL. Endocrine regulation of human fetal growth: the role of the mother, placenta, and fetus. *Endocrine Rev.* 2006;27:141-169.

32. Lieberman E, Gremy I, Lang JM, Cohen AP. Low birthweight at term and the timing of fetal exposure to maternal smoking. *Am J Public Health.* 1994; 84:1127.

33. de Vries JIP, Fong BF. Normal fetal motility: an overview. *Ultrasound Obstet Gynecol.* 2006;27:701-711. doi: 10.1002/uog.2740.

34. Martin CB. Normal fetal physiology and behavior, and adaptive responses with hypoxemia. *Semin Perinatol.* 2008;32:239-242.

35. Gluckman PD, Hanson MA, Cooper C, Thornburg KL. Effect of in utero and early-life conditions on adult health and disease. *N Engl J Med.* 2008;359: 61-73.

36. Barker D. The midwife, the coincidence, and the hypothesis. *BMJ.* 2003;327(7429):1428-1430.

37. Dyer JS, Rosenfeld CR. Metabolic imprinting by prenatal, perinatal, and postnatal overnutrition: a review. *Sem Reprod Med.* 2011;29(3):266-276.

38. Cunningham FG. Appendix B: laboratory values in normal pregnancy. In: Queenan JT, Hobbins JC, Spong CYT, eds. *Protocols for High-Risk Pregnancies: An Evidence-Based Approach,* 5th ed. Oxford, UK: Blackwell; 2010:587-595.

39. Centers for Disease Control and Prevention. Laboratory procedure manual: complete blood count with

5-part differential. NHANES 2005-2006. Available at: http://www.cdc.gov/nchs/data/nhanes/nhanes_05_06 /cbc_d_met.pdf. Accessed November 9, 2012.

40. Borg-Stein J, Duagn S, Gruber J. Musculoskeletal aspects of pregnancy. *Am J Phys Med Rehabil.* 2005: 84:180-192.

41. Geraghty LN, Pomeranz MK. Physiologic changes and dermatoses of pregnancy. *Int J Dermatol.* 2011; 50:771-782.

42. Ozuounian JG, Elkayam U. Physiologic changes during normal pregnancy and delivery. *Cardiol Clin.* 2012;30:317-329.

43. Vainrib A, Stergiopoulos K. Hypertrophic cardiomyopathy and pregnancy. *Minerva Ginecol.* 2012; 64(5):399-407.

44. James AH, McLintock C, Lockhart E. Postpartum hemorrhage: when uterotonics and sutures fail. *Am J Hematol.* 2012;87:S16-S22.

45. Barrett JF, Whittaker PG, Williams JG, Lind T. Absorption of non-haem iron from food during normal pregnancy. *Brit Med J.* 1994;309:79-82.

46. Wise RA, Polito AJ, Krishnan V. Respiratory physiologic changes in pregnancy. *Immunol Clin North Am.* 2006;26:1-12.

47. Cornelis T, Odutayo A, Keunen J, Hladunewich M. The kidney in normal pregnancy and preeclampsia. *Semin Nephrol.* 2011;31:4-14.

48. Mazzaferro EL. Evaluation and management of common thyroid disorders in women. *Am J Obstet Gynecol.* 1997;176:507-514.

CHAPTER

21

Genetics

GWEN A. LATENDRESSE

Introduction

Essentially all health and disease conditions have a genetic component, and the provision of midwifery care increasingly will include genetics within the context of prevention, screening, diagnosis, and treatment selection. Furthermore, genetic disorders are not rare occurrences. Indeed, approximately 5% of women report a family history of some type of genetic disorder, and at least half of all spontaneous abortions are genetically related.[1] Of all newborns with malformations, 15% of the anomalies are "familial," 10% are chromosomal, 3% to 4% are related to single gene mutations, 23% are multifactorial (i.e., involve multiple genetic and environmental components), and 3% are due to teratogens.[1] It is clear that genetics contributes significantly to newborn/infant mortality, half of which comprises congenital anomalies. These numbers make it clear that genetics knowledge is important in midwifery care.

Genetic science and technology rapidly are evolving, and increasing numbers of genetic tests are becoming available. This dynamic nature of the field can be a challenge for midwives who desire to remain knowledgeable and responsive in provision of healthcare services to women. However, the first-line approach to perinatal genetics includes classic "low-tech" midwifery care activities that are woman/family centered, such as history taking, health education, and informed decision making. Women are increasingly bombarded with genetic information and may

find it difficult to understand this information or apply it to their own lives. It must also be kept in mind that in spite of all available genetics knowledge and testing options, there is no cure for the vast majority of genetic disorders.

Perinatal genetic risk assessment, counseling, screening, and diagnosis have many potential benefits for women, including adequate appraisal of options, well-informed decision making, access to resources, appropriate healthcare planning, psychological preparation, reassurance, and ultimately optimal outcomes for everyone involved. Midwives can play an important role in the provision of genetics-related health care for childbearing women, and for those who are considering childbearing. Furthermore, midwifery care has long facilitated women's access to appropriate technology and the delivery of accurate information to women and families who are engaged in decision making about use of health-related technologies. It is imperative that midwives have a solid understanding of genetics and available technology, as well as essential skills for genetic risk assessment, screening, diagnostic testing, basic counseling, and appropriate referral.

Although midwives indicate that genetics knowledge is important to incorporate into their clinical practice, they often feel a lack of confidence in doing so.[2] This chapter assists the midwife to acquire basic genetics knowledge and to understand contemporary approaches to perinatal genetics within the context of midwifery care.

Foundations in Genetics

The foundations of molecular genetics and heredity provide the basis for understanding perinatal genetics specifically. This section reviews basic principles in molecular genetics, as well as inheritance patterns and the meaning of genetic mutations, gene expression, and chromosomal structure. **Table 21-1** provides a glossary of commonly used genetics-related terms.[3] Readers are also encouraged to access the many excellent genetics resources currently available in print as well as online for more in-depth information. Additional resources are listed at the end of this chapter.

Genes, Genome, DNA, and Chromosomes

Genes, which are the basic unit of inheritance, consist of deoxyribonucleic acid (DNA) that is found within the cell nucleus; genes are contained within the chromosomes found in each and every cell in the body (other than the egg and sperm cells, which contain a set of 23 single chromosomes). Chromosomes consist of long segments of DNA that are tightly wrapped around proteins (**Figure 21-1**).[1] The human cell normally contains 46 chromosomes that are organized in 23 paired sets. In each of these sets, one chromosome is contributed by the individual's biologic mother and the other is contributed by the individual's biologic father. Twenty-two of those pairs are called autosomes and are the same in males and females. The last pair consists of the sex chromosomes: females have two Xs and males have an X and a Y chromosome.

The entire collection of genes in an individual, referred to as the genome, provides a complete set of "instructions" for directing all biologic functions within a living organism. The end product of all gene instruction is the production of a protein, via the processes of "transcription" and "translation" of the DNA that occur as the instructions are translated into actual proteins. Every gene is a sequence of nitrogenous base pairs—molecules of cytosine, thymine, adenine, and guanine—that form the double-stranded DNA molecule, and each genetic sequence encodes for a specific protein with a specific function. The single-stranded ribonucleic acid (RNA) contributes to this process by providing a template for the eventual assembly of amino acids into proteins within the cell's cytoplasm.

Gene expression refers to the eventual production of a gene product, but not all genes are expressed in every cell or in precisely the same way. For example, an epithelial cell (a skin cell) does not look or function the way a myocyte (a muscle cell) does. Although both cell types contain the exact same set of genetic instructions, only those genes that are expressed will contribute to the unique structure and function of the specific cell type.[4] Gene expression is regulated by a very complex set of signals within an organism. This allows undifferentiated cells (i.e., fetal stem cells) to differentiate into a wide variety of cells with differing structures and functions. The term "epigenetic" refers to the regulation of gene expression via modifications of the DNA structure (i.e., histones or chromatin as noted in Figure 21-1), but not the DNA sequence within the genes.[5] Environmental signals (both internal and external to an organism) are now known to make tremendous contributions to the regulation of gene expression.

Genetic Mutations

Mutation refers to any alteration in the DNA sequence within a gene, either by deletion, insertion, repetition, or duplication of a single base pair or larger segments of the DNA strand, entire genes, or piece of chromosome. Mutations occur rather frequently, and are often repaired by the body; a large number of them do not result in a clinical effect or disease.[1] However, a genetic mutation that causes a change in the protein product can subsequently alter the function of the cell. This change results in the disease phenotype (clinically or physically observed or experienced signs or symptoms) that is reflective of the genotype (specific DNA sequence) within the individual. Genetic mutations can either be inherited from a parent or occur spontaneously.

Inheritance Patterns of Genetic and Chromosomal Abnormalities

Genes, as the basic unit of inheritance, contribute significantly to an individual's characteristics, including disposition for health and disease in addition to physical appearance, such as height, eye color, and hair color. Patterns of inheritance are either autosomal, which means the inherited genes are located on the first 22 pairs of chromosomes, or sex linked, which means the inherited genes are located on the X or Y chromosome. In addition, they are either dominant or recessive. Many well-known heritable genetic disorders are caused by a mutation in a single gene. These conditions are referred to as classic "Mendelian" disorders, after the early geneticist Gregor Mendel. Mendel was an Austrian monk who is usually called the "father of genetics" because he was one of the first scientists to clearly establish that physical traits are heritable from one generation to the next.[1] In contrast, most chromosomal abnormalities are not heritable. This is an important clinical

Table 21-1	Genetics Glossary
Term	**Definition/Description**
Allele	One of the two or more versions of a genetic sequence that encodes for the same protein or function at a specific location on a chromosome. In reference to an autosomal recessive disorder, a person must inherit a mutant allele from both parents. In an autosomal dominant disorder, a person requires only one mutant allele from one parent.
Aneuploid	Refers to a chromosomal condition in which there is an abnormal number of chromosomes in the complement of 23 pairs secondary to either a deletion or an addition of a chromosome.
Base pair	Two nitrogenous bases paired together in double-stranded DNA (i.e., adenine paired with thymine, and guanine paired with cytosine). Sequences of various lengths of base pairs make up the various genes.
CFTR	The gene that encodes for chloride channel transmembrane regulation. There are several variations of mutations in this gene that directly cause cystic fibrosis.
Chromosomal abnormality	An alteration in the number or structure of a chromosome. Chromosomal abnormalities can be inherited or occur de novo. Most common chromosomal abnormalities, such as trisomy 21, are not heritable.
DNA	Deoxyribonucleic acid; the double-stranded helix of nitrogenous base pairs within cells that provide instructions for all cell activity, and is passed on from generation to generation. The DNA strand comprises the collection of genes within a chromosome.
Epigenetics	Changes in the regulation of gene expression that occur due to modifications in DNA, rather than changes in DNA sequence. Methylation—the attachment of methyl groups to DNA at cytosine bases—is one example of a DNA modification that alters gene expression.
Exon	The segment of the gene that codes for a specific amino acid. Conversely, introns are generally considered noncoding segments of DNA and are normally spliced out of the sequence prior to formation of amino acids.
Expressivity	Phenotypic variation (i.e., severity) among persons who have a specific genotype.
Gene	The fundamental unit of heredity. An ordered sequence of DNA constitutes a gene; it is found on a specific location on a specific chromosome. Each gene encodes for a specific functional protein.
Genetic disorder	Alterations in genes that code for a particular protein, which results in a heritable disorder.
Genome	The entire DNA sequence and set of genetic instructions found within each cell. This is different for each organism. The Human Genome Project documented the entire DNA sequence of the approximately 25,000 genes held within the 23 pairs of chromosomes in humans.
Genotype	A person's complete collection of specific genes. A person's genotype is largely responsible for determining the phenotype.
Heterozygous	Referring to an individual who has a mutant allele on only one of a pair of specific genes. Autosomal dominant inheritance can occur in a heterozygous individual because only one mutant allele from one parent is required to have a trait, condition, or disease.
Homozygous	Referring to an individual who has a mutant allele on both genes in a specific gene pair (one from each parent). Autosomal recessive inheritance of a trait, condition, or disease occurs only when an individual is homozygous for the specific gene. Cystic fibrosis and sickle cell anemia, for example, occur only in individuals who are homozygous for the specific disease gene.
Karyotype	An individual's full complement of chromosomes. Also used to refer to a photograph of an individual's chromosomes, arranged in the standardized laboratory format (Figure 21-1).
Monosomy	A chromosomal condition in which a single chromosome is found when there should be a chromosome pair. These mutations are almost always lethal when found in autosomal chromosomes.
Multifactorial disease	A condition caused by the interaction between several genes and several environmental factors. Cancer, type 2 diabetes mellitus, and heart disease are commonly encountered multifactorial conditions.
Mutation	A change in DNA sequence that may or may not result in a change in the protein product. Mutations may affect only one base pair or a larger segment in the DNA sequence via deletion, insertion, repetition, or duplication. Genetic mutations cause such disorders as cystic fibrosis, Tay-Sachs disease, and sickle cell anemia.

(continues)

Table 21-1	Genetics Glossary *(continued)*
Term	**Definition/Description**
Nondisjunction	Failure of chromosome pairs to separate properly during meiosis. Meiosis is the type of cell reproduction that results in gametes (eggs and sperm) in which each gamete has only one set of 23 chromosomes rather than a full complement of 46 chromosomes in 23 paired sets.
Penetrance	The proportion of persons with a specific genotype who also express the expected phenotype.
Phenotype	The outward expression or the observable traits of a person, usually resulting from some combination of genotype and environmental influences.
RNA	Ribonucleic acid; single-stranded nitrogenous molecules that mirror the DNA sequence. RNA is essential for moving DNA instructions out of the nucleus (via transcription and translation) into the cell cytoplasm and for subsequent construction of amino acids into final protein products.
Single-nucleotide polymorphism (SNP)	Often called "snip"; any of the common variations found in a single nucleotide of genomic DNA sequence between individuals, as well as between different populations.
Transcription	The synthesis of an RNA strand from a sequence of DNA. It is a first step in gene expression.
Translation	During protein synthesis, the process through which the sequence of bases in a molecule of messenger RNA is read to create a sequence of amino acids.
Trisomy	A chromosomal condition in which three chromosomes occur where there should be only a pair. Trisomy is a form of aneuploidy. The occurrence of trisomy increases in infants born to older mothers. A common trisomy condition is trisomy 21 (Down syndrome).

Source: Adapted from Feero WG, Guttmacher AE, Collins FS. Genomic medicine: an updated primer. *N Engl J Med.* 2010;362:2001-2011.

distinction because tests for chromosomal abnormalities are often referred to as "genetic tests." Use of the word "genetics" when referring to tests for both genetic disorders and chromosomal abnormalities can mistakenly convey the idea that chromosomal abnormalities are inherited. Thus, when a midwife discusses genetic testing with women and their families, inheritance is an important component to include in the discussion.

Alleles and Penetrance

All of the genes on a given maternally inherited chromosome correspond to the same gene in the same location (allele) on the paternal chromosome counterpart. Individuals with a mutant allele on only one of the pair of genes are referred to as "heterozygous," while those with a mutant allele on both genes in the pair are referred to as "homozygous."

Penetrance refers to the percentage of individuals with a specific disease genotype who also express the expected phenotype (the observable characteristics of the genotype). For example, a genetic mutation that is not associated with an expected phenotype 100% of the time has "incomplete penetrance," and a penetrance of 50% indicates that only half of the individuals with a specific disease genotype will also exhibit the phenotype. The variation in phenotype

(i.e., severity) of a particular genetic disorder, which is called expressivity, can be influenced by modifier genes, and perhaps aging or the environment. Expressivity contributes to the wide range of abilities that is observed among individuals with Down syndrome, for example. Knowledge about penetrance and expressivity helps to answer the question of why all individuals with the same genotype do not have the same phenotypic characteristics or severity of the genetic disorder.

Genetic Mutations and Disorders

Autosomal Dominant Inheritance: Definition and Common Disorders

Disease phenotypes expressed only in heterozygous individuals (i.e., those persons with only one mutant allele in a specific gene pair) reflect an autosomal dominant inheritance pattern.[1] Examples of autosomal dominant disorders include achondroplasia (commonly known as dwarfism), neurofibromatosis, Marfan's syndrome, and Huntington disease. The child of a parent affected with an autosomal dominant condition has a 50% probability of inheriting the disease-causing mutation. Males and females are equally likely to transmit and inherit autosomal

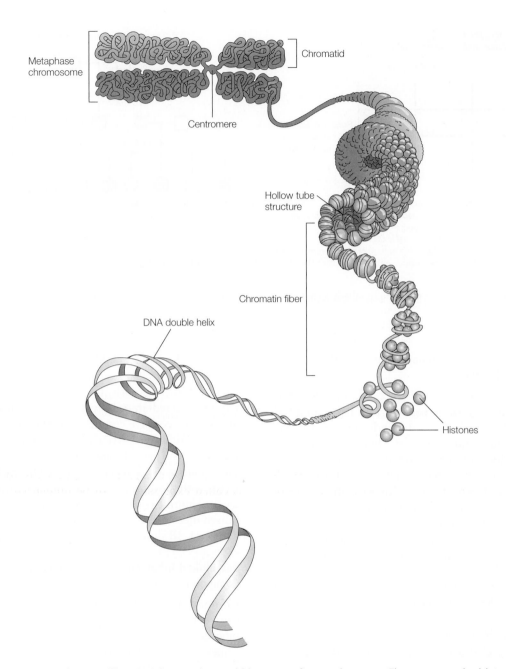

Figure 21-1 Patterns of DNA coiling. DNA is wound around histones to form nucleosomes. These are organized into solenoids, which in turn make up the chromatin loops.
Source: Chiras DD. *Human Biology.* 7th ed. Sudbury, MA: Jones & Bartlett Learning; 2012.

dominant traits. Unlike autosomal recessive disorders, dominant disorders are often observed in most generations of a family tree (pedigree).

Not uncommonly, children with autosomal dominant disorders are born to unaffected parents (i.e., the parents do not have the disease or carry the mutant allele). The most likely explanation for this phenomenon is that a new, spontaneous mutation occurred in either the egg or the sperm that formed the child.[1]

While the parents of these individuals have a low recurrence risk, the affected individuals themselves have a 50% chance of transmitting their new mutation to their children. A diagram, commonly referred to as a Punnett square, is often used to demonstrate the probability of inheritance in offspring of affected and unaffected parents, as shown in **Figure 21-2A**. A typical corresponding pedigree reflective of autosomal dominant inheritance is shown in **Figure 21-2B**.

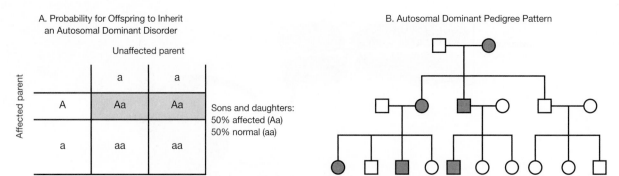

A. Probability for Offspring to Inherit an Autosomal Dominant Disorder

B. Autosomal Dominant Pedigree Pattern

A. This diagram demonstrates the probability of offspring inheriting an autosomal dominant disorder from a heterozygous (affected) parent and an unaffected parent. Shading indicates affected individuals.
  A = chromosome with a dominant disease allele.
  a = chromosome with a normal allele.
B. Pedigree showing inheritance pattern of an autosomal dominant disorder. Both genders are equally affected. Solid shapes represent affected individuals. Open shapes represent unaffected individuals. Circles represent females. Squares represent males.

Figure 21-2 Probability for offspring to inherit an autosomal dominant disorder and dominant pedigree pattern.

Autosomal Recessive Inheritance: Definition and Common Disorders

Disease phenotypes expressed only in homozygous individuals (i.e., those persons with two mutant alleles in the specific gene pair) indicate an autosomal recessive inheritance pattern.[1] Individuals who are heterozygous for an autosomal recessive inheritance pattern are considered "carriers" and are largely unaffected by the disease. However, these carriers can pass the genetic mutation to their offspring. A carrier's single working gene is sufficient for normal function. Cystic fibrosis (CF), Tay-Sachs disease, and sickle cell anemia are examples of autosomal recessive disorders.

When two carriers have children together, each pregnancy has a 25% chance of being affected with the disorder, a 50% chance of being an unaffected carrier of either the maternal or paternal mutation, and a 25% chance of being an unaffected noncarrier.

Couples who have a child with an autosomal recessive disorder often are surprised because they are not aware of anyone with the condition among either parent's immediate relatives, especially because an autosomal recessive condition frequently skips generations. Although carrier status for some autosomal recessive disorders among higher-risk populations is quite common, the incidence of newborns being affected with the disorder actually is much lower (**Table 21-2**). **Figure 21-3A** demonstrates the probability of inheritance in the offspring of carrier parents, and **Figure 21-3B** shows a typical corresponding pedigree.

Sex-Linked Inheritance: Definition and Common Disorders

Compared to autosomal inheritance, disorders caused by mutations on the sex chromosomes are inherited differently, as females have two X chromosomes and males have one X chromosome and one

Table 21-2	Autosomal Recessive Carrier Frequency in Specific High-Risk Populations and Associated Newborn Incidence		
Genetic Disease	**Ethnic Group**	**Carrier Frequency**	**Newborn Incidence**
Tay-Sachs disease	Ashkenazi Jews	1/30	1/3600
Sickle cell disease	African Americans	1/12	1/600
Cystic fibrosis	Northern Europeans	1/25	1/2500
β-Thalassemia	Greeks/Italians	1/30	1/3600
α-Thalassemia	Southeast Asians, Chinese	1/25	1/2500

A. Probability for Offspring to Inherit
an Autosomal Recessive Disorder

B. Autosomal Recessive Pedigree Pattern

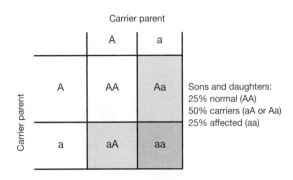

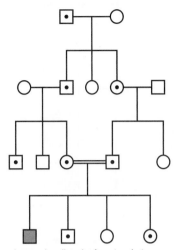

A. Diagram demonstrating the probability of offspring inheriting an autosomal recessive disorder from two heterozygous (carrier) parents. Light shading indicates carrier status. Heavy shading indicates affected individuals.
   A = Chromosome with a normal allele.
   a = Chromosome with the disease allele.
B. Pedigree showing the inheritance pattern of an autosomal recessive disorder. Consanguinity is denoted as a double line in this figure, but should not be interpreted as a requirement for inheritance. Solid shapes represent affected individuals. Open shapes represent unaffected individuals. Circles represent females. Squares represent males. Shapes containing a dot represent carriers of an autosomal recessive mutation.

Figure 21-3 Probability for offspring to inherit an autosomal recessive disorder and autosomal recessive pedigree pattern.

Y chromosome.[1] As very few genes reside on the Y chromosome, Y-linked disorders are unique to men and extremely rare. In contrast, X-linked disorders in which only males are affected and only females are carriers can occur. Female carriers of X-linked recessive disorders (by far the most common inheritance pattern for sex-linked disorders) are usually healthy, as the normal gene on their one X chromosome can compensate for the mutant allele on the other. Males, having only one X chromosome, require only one mutation to have the disease, as they do not have another normal X chromosome to compensate for the mutant allele.

A female who is a carrier for an X-linked recessive mutation has four possible pregnancy outcomes: a 25% chance for a carrier female, a 25% chance for a noncarrier female, a 25% chance for an affected male, and a 25% chance for a healthy male. **Figure 21-4A** illustrates the inheritance probabilities for X-linked disorders among offspring of a carrier mother and an unaffected father. **Figure 21-4B** shows a typical corresponding pedigree.

Hemophilia A and Duchenne muscular dystrophy are among the more common X-linked disorders. One way to distinguish X-linked from autosomal dominant conditions when analyzing a pedigree is to determine whether affected males have affected sons. Male-to-male transmission is observed with autosomal dominant conditions but not with X-linked recessive traits.

X-linked dominant disorders exist, but appear rarely in the population. These conditions also affect heterozygous females. Upon pedigree analysis, none of the sons and all of the daughters of affected males will also be affected.

Multifactorial Inheritance: Definition and Common Disorders

Many common conditions and disorders are described as being due to multifactorial inheritance, meaning that they are caused by the combined effects of several genes (genetic predisposition) and several environmental factors.[1] It is also generally accepted that a "threshold" must be reached for the disease or condition to become manifest. In other words, an additive effect of genetic predisposition and increasing environmental "load" will cause an individual to reach a certain "tipping point" when the disease phenotype will occur. Gender, age, socioeconomic status, lifestyle, nutrition status, geographic area, and ethnic background frequently influence the occurrence of a

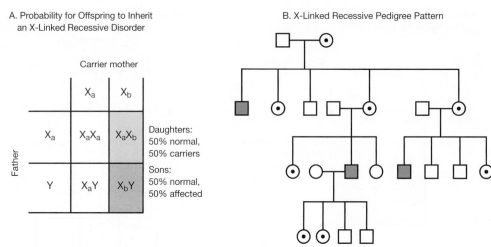

A. Probability for Offspring to Inherit an X-Linked Recessive Disorder

B. X-Linked Recessive Pedigree Pattern

A. Diagram demonstrating the probability of offspring inheriting an X-linked recessive disorder from a heterozygous mother (carrier) and an unaffected, noncarrier father. Light shading indicates carrier status. Heavy shading indicates an affected individual.

Xa = Chromosome with a normal allele.

Xb = Chromosome with the disease allele.

B. Pedigree showing inheritance pattern of an X-linked recessive disorder. Only males are affected. Only females are carriers. For offspring of a carrier mother and a normal father, in each pregnancy there is an independent chance that for males there is a 50% chance the male will be affected and a 50% chance the male will be unaffected. For females there is a 50% the daughter will be a carrier, and a 50% chance the daughter will be unaffected. For offspring of affected males, 100% of daughters are carriers and 100% of sons are normal. Solid shapes represent affected individuals. Open shapes represent unaffected individuals. Circles represent females. Squares represent males. Shapes containing a dot represent carriers of an autosomal recessive mutation.

Figure 21-4 Probability for offspring to inherit an X-linked recessive disorder and linked recessive pedigree pattern.

multifactorial condition or disease. Neural tube defects (spina bifida and anencephaly) and congenital pyloric stenosis are common examples of multifactorial conditions. Cancer, type 2 diabetes mellitus, and heart disease are common multifactorial conditions that usually manifest in adulthood.

Neural Tube Defects

Neural tube defects (NTD) are one example of a multifactorial condition that contributes significantly to adverse birth outcomes. NTDs occur when there is a failure of the neural tube to develop and close properly during very early embryonic life (2–6 weeks' gestational age).[6] Multiple genes—particularly those associated with folate metabolism—contribute to a genetic predisposition for NTDs; environmental factors, such maternal age, diet, geographic area, drug exposure, and socioeconomic status, are associated with such defects as well.[7] Spina bifida (protrusion of the spinal tissue through the vertebral column) and anencephaly (partial or complete absence of the cranial vault and partial or complete absence of the cerebral hemispheres) are the most common NTDs observed.[8] These two conditions are also referred to as open neural tube defects to

differentiate them from the rarer closed neural tube defects in which skin covers the spinal abnormality.

The prevalence of NTDs varies widely among different populations, from 1 to 2 persons per 1000 live births, to as high as 6 persons per 1000 live births in northern Chinese populations. While the pathophysiologic basis for NTDs is complex and not well understood, it is known that folic acid supplementation can reduce the occurrence of NTDs by 60% to 70%. This recognition has led to the widespread recommendation for folic acid supplementation (400–800 mcg per day)[9] prior to conception, as well as during the first 8 weeks of pregnancy.[10] Although women who have had an affected child have a risk of reoccurrence of approximately 2% to 5%, 95% of all NTDs occur in previously unaffected families.[8]

Individuals with spina bifida—the most common NTD—have varying degrees of physical and mental challenges, including hydrocephalus (which is associated with a risk of mental retardation) and physical disability. The severity of disability increases with the severity of the defect. Approximately 35% of infants born with spina bifida do not survive to 10 years of age.[11] Surgical repairs of the defect are the usual approach for improving prognosis.[11]

Anencephaly, understandably, has an extremely high level of mortality. The majority of infants with anencephaly are stillborn, and the remaining newborns do not live longer than a few hours or days after birth.[11]

Chromosomal Disorders

Chromosomal disorders are not the result of single-gene mutations, such as the autosomal dominant and recessive disorders previously discussed, but rather reflect changes in the number or structure of the chromosomes.[1] Chromosomal abnormalities are relatively common, occurring in an estimated 1 in 150 live births and approximately 50% of first-trimester spontaneous abortions.[1,12] Such abnormalities frequently are associated with common phenotypic and physical characteristics, thereby aiding in their early identification (including during fetal ultrasound examination). However, chromosomal evaluation via a karyotype (a visual display of the full complement of an individual's chromosomes) provides the definitive diagnosis.

The most common chromosomal aberrations are caused by aneuploidy—an addition or deletion of an entire chromosome in a normal set of 23 pairs of chromosomes. Aneuploidy most often occurs due to nondisjunction during cell division in the egg or sperm.[13] The resulting absence of a chromosome (monosomy) is almost always lethal, so such a mutation is rarely observed in live-born children. In contrast, the addition of a chromosome (trisomy) leads to one of several disorders depending on which chromosome pair receives the extra genetic material. The most common trisomy is trisomy 21 (Down syndrome), which is caused by an extra chromosome on the 21st pair of chromosomes. **Figure 21-5** shows the chromosomal display (karyotype) for an individual with trisomy 21 below the display for a normal individual. Phenotypic characteristics of individuals with trisomy 21 include easily recognized facial features, such as small upturned eyes, small flat nose, small mouth with large tongue, and small ears (**Figure 21-6**). Mental and physical disabilities of varying severity are also observed. Congenital heart defects, obstructions of the gastrointestinal tract, and frequent respiratory infections are associated with trisomy 21. Trisomy 18 (Edwards syndrome) and trisomy 13 (Patau syndrome) are less frequently encountered conditions, but both result in severe physical and mental disability in offspring, and are usually lethal during gestation or shortly after birth.[1,12]

Other common aneuploid disorders include sex chromosomal aberrations, such as Turner syndrome (XO), Klinefelter syndrome (XXY), trisomy X (XXX), and 47 XYY syndrome. Aneuploidy of sex chromosomes frequently results in less severe consequences than does autosomal aneuploidy, but the conditions also are associated with varying degrees of intellectual disability, sex characteristic effects (including sterility, feminization, or virilization), or frequent minor physical changes specific to the disorder.[1,12] Many individuals who are mildly affected are not identified with a chromosome abnormality for much of their lives unless health care is sought for a seemingly unrelated condition (e.g., infertility) and a karyotype is performed to identify the potential genetic etiology of the condition.[1,14,15]

Rearrangements and small deletions or microdeletions of portions of a chromosome are considered

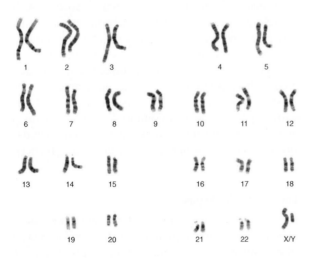

Figure 21-5A Karyotype A: A full complement of 23 pairs of chromosomes in a female individual.

Source: Courtesy of Darryl Leja/National Human Genome Research Institute

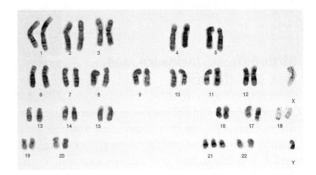

Figure 21-5B Karyotype B: An extra chromosome is observed in this female individual with trisomy 21 (Down syndrome).

Source: © Jens Goepfert/ShutterStock, Inc.

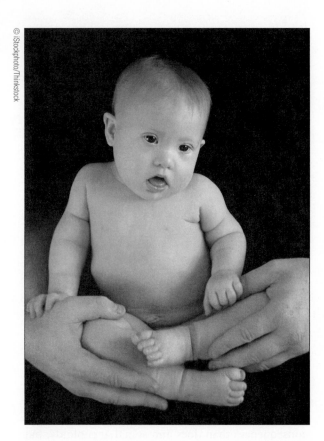

Figure 21-6 Infant with Down syndrome (trisomy 21) chromosomal disorder.

structural abnormalities. They contribute to infrequently occurring genetic conditions, such as cri-du-chat syndrome, which is the result of a deletion of a portion of chromosome 5; Wolf-Hirschhorn syndrome, which is the result of a deletion of a portion of chromosome 4; Prader-Willi syndrome, which is a microdeletion of a portion of chromosome 15; and Williams syndrome, which is a microdeletion of a portion of chromosome 7.[12] Each abnormality has phenotypic characteristics specific to the condition.

Birth Defects, Incidence, and Risk Identification

Genetic disorders and chromosomal disorders are not rare occurrences. An individual's risk for a genetic disorder is based on several factors, including age, gender, and ethnic background. For example, cystic fibrosis has a prevalence of 1 case per 2500 persons among whites of Northern European descent, while sickle cell disease has a prevalence of 1 case per 400 to 600 persons among blacks of African descent.

Another example of a factor affecting the risk for chromosomal disorders is maternal age: women have an increased risk of having a child with trisomy 21 as they get older.[16] **Table 21-3** lists several conditions and diseases with a genetic component, along with their prevalence in specific populations. Understanding particular risks among specific populations and groups can prompt the midwife to probe further when obtaining a medical and family history, provide accurate patient education, recommend specific testing to women and families, or make a referral to a genetic counselor, as appropriate.

Age

Advanced maternal age (AMA), particularly women who are older than 35 years, is a well-documented risk for chromosomal abnormalities, particularly for aneuploidy such as trisomy 21 (Down syndrome).[1,12,16] The graph in **Figure 21-7** demonstrates the escalating risk of a pregnancy being affected by a chromosomal anomaly as maternal age increases. By the maternal age of 45 years, the risk for any chromosomal disorder is approximately 5.3% (the majority being trisomy 21), compared to approximately 0.25% for women who are younger than age 30 years. Presented another way, in **Table 21-4** it is clear that 1 in 30 infants born to women age 45 years will have trisomy 21, compared to 1 in 1250 infants born to women age 25 years.[16] The risk for any chromosomal disorder for women who are 45 years is 1 in 20 newborns.

Although a few studies have shown a very slight increase in the risk of genetic disorders among older men (primarily autosomal dominant disorders such as achondroplasia and neurofibromatosis), most research has not revealed that older fatherhood is associated with an increased risk for chromosomal anomalies.[17,18] Furthermore, unlike the risk associated with advanced maternal age, no clear consensus exists for when a man is considered to be of advanced paternal age. A commonly used criterion is age 40 years, but there are no specific recommendations for couples wherein the father is of advanced paternal age.[17]

Environmental Exposure

Environmental exposure to teratogens may be a genetic risk factor depending on the level and type of exposure (i.e., duration, strength, potency).[19] A teratogen is a drug, virus, chemical, or other substance that can interfere with normal embryonic or fetal development and cause malformations. A list of medications that are known or suspected to be

Table 21-3	Selected Genetic Conditions/Diseases and Approximate Incidence Rates		
Condition/Disease	**Approximate Incidence**	**Condition/Disease**	**Approximate Incidence**
Chromosome Abnormalities		**Multifactorial Disorders: Congenital Malformations**	
Trisomy 21 (Down syndrome)	1/700 to 1/1000	Cleft lip with or without cleft palate	1/500 to 1/1000
Trisomy 18 (Edwards syndrome)	1/6000	Club foot (congenital talipes equinovarus)	1/1000
Trisomy 13 (Patau syndrome)	1/10,000	Congenital heart defects	1/200 to 1/500
Klinefelter syndrome	1/1000 males	Neural tube defects (spina bifida, anencephaly)	1/200 to 1/1000
Turner syndrome	1/5000 females	Pyloric stenosis	1/300
Single-Gene (Mendelian) Disorders		**Multifactorial Disorders: Adult Diseases**	
Cystic fibrosis	1/2500 (Persons of European descent)	Alcoholism	1/10 to 1/20
Sickle cell disease	1/400 to 1/600 African Americans; as many as 1/50 Central Africans	Bipolar affective disorder	1/100 to 1/200
Thalassemias: α-Alpha β-Beta	1/2500 Southeast Asians and Chinese 1/3600 Greeks and Italians	Cancer (all types)	1/3
Tay-Sachs disease	1/3000 to 1/3600 Ashkenazi Jews	Diabetes (types 1 and 2)	1/10
Hemophilia A	1/5000 to 1/10,000 males	Heart disease or stroke	1/3 to 1/5
Duchenne muscular dystrophy	1/3500 males	Schizophrenia	1/100
Achondroplasia (dwarfism)	1/25,000		
Neurofibromatosis	1/3000		
Huntington disease	1/20,000 (persons of European descent)		

Source: Adapted from Jorde L, Carey J, Bamshad M. *Medical Genetics.* 4th ed. Philadelphia, PA: Mosby Elsevier; 2010.

teratogens can be found in the *Pharmacotherapeutics* chapter, and known or highly suspected maternal conditions and environmental toxins are listed in **Table 21-5**.[20,21] A number of environmental exposures have also raised concerns about teratogenicity (e.g., polychlorinated biphenyls [PCBs], some paints, phthalates), but the evidence that would firmly implicate these items as teratogens is lacking at this time.[20,21]

Teratogens may cause genetic mutations, but it is thought that alteration in gene expression during critical embryonic and fetal developmental periods is the more likely mechanism contributing to genetic disorders that occur secondary to teratogen exposure.[4] Epigenetic regulation of gene expression is an increasingly documented and plausible mechanism that may partially explain the link between environmental exposures and birth defects.[4] For example, epigenetic regulation of gene expression may explain the association between chronic hyperglycemia, found among women with poorly managed diabetes (gestational or otherwise), and an increased risk of birth defects, such as heart defects and NTDs.[22] Moreover, epigenetic modifications may endure and confer risk for more than one generation.[23]

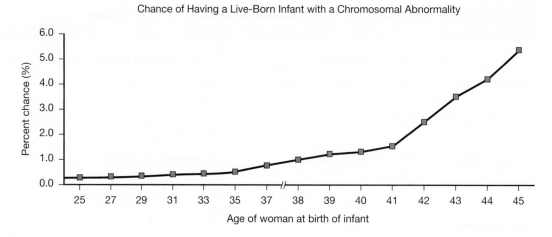

Figure 21-7 Maternal age and risk of chromosomal abnormality.
Source: Data from Hook EB. Rates of chromosomal abnormalities. *Obstet Gynecol.* 1981;58(3):282-285.

The major concern is for exposures to women during pregnancy, particularly during the first trimester. As yet, little to no evidence has been published suggesting that paternal exposure is associated with increased occurrence of birth defects.[19]

Family History and Pedigree Evaluation as Risk Assessment Tools

One of the most effective, low-cost approaches to genetics risk assessment is to conduct a thorough personal health and family history that includes evaluation of a three-generation "pedigree." Obtaining a personal and family history is a "free, well-proven, personalized genomic tool that...can serve as the cornerstone for individualized disease prevention."[24]

Table 21-4	Maternal Age and Risk of Chromosomal Disorders (Live Births)	
Maternal Age (years)	Risk for Trisomy 21	Risk for Any Chromosomal Disorder
20	1 in 1667	1 in 526
25	1 in 1250	1 in 476
30	1 in 952	1 in 384
35	1 in 385	1 in 204
40	1 in 106	1 in 65
45	1 in 30	1 in 20
49	1 in 11	1 in 7

Source: Adapted from Arnold KM, Self ZB. Genetic screening and counseling: family medicine obstetrics. *Prim Care.* 2012;39:55-70.

Many "red flags" that indicate the need for further evaluation, testing, or referral to a genetic counselor can be found by obtaining a thorough family history[25,26] (**Box 21-1**). Furthermore, a number of patient-completed family genetics history tools (see the genetics resources list at the end of this chapter) are available, both in print and online, to facilitate collection of personal and family history. Such patient participation tools can be completed by a woman prior to her prenatal care appointment with the midwife and can be an effective and efficient way for identifying genetic risk. Constructing and evaluating a three-generation pedigree for genetic risk is a basic skill that all healthcare professionals, including midwives, should be comfortable with.[27] Instructions for how to obtain a three-generation pedigree can be found in the appendix to this chapter.

Prenatal Screening and Diagnostic Testing for Genetic Disorders

A major aim of prenatal screening and testing is to provide families (particularly at-risk families) with the information necessary to make well-informed reproductive health decisions. The ultimate goal is to obtain optimal outcomes for an individual woman, her infant, and family. Understanding the differences between screening tests and diagnostic tests can assist midwives in providing the appropriate education for women and can avoid misinterpretation and anxiety about test results, particularly when screening tests are "abnormal."

Table 21-5	Known or Suspected Maternal Conditions and Environmental Toxins as Teratogens (A Short List[a])	
Teratogen	**Associated Defects**	**Percentage of Pregnancies Affected**
Maternal Infections		
Cytomegalovirus	Mental retardation, microcephaly	10–15%
Rubella	Deafness, cataracts, heart defects, mental retardation	Up to 85%
Syphilis (untreated)	Abnormal teeth and bones, mental retardation	Not established
Toxoplasmosis	Hydrocephaly, blindness, mental retardation	5–6%
Varicella	Limb reduction defects, skin scarring, muscle atrophy, chorioretinitis	1%
Maternal Conditions		
Active alcoholism	Miscarriage, fetal alcohol syndrome (minor facial changes, heart defects), IUGR, developmental delay	Up to 50%
Diabetes mellitus HbA1c < 7.9% HbA1c 8.0–9.9% HbA1c > 10%	Heart defects, microcephaly, neural tube defects, skeletal defects, and defects in the urinary, reproductive, and digestive systems	3.2% 8.1% 23.5%
Hyperthermia (fever); early pregnancy only	Neural tube defects, heart and abdominal wall defects, oral cleft	Not established
Seizure disorder (treated)	Cleft lip with or without cleft palate, heart defects	6–8%
Systemic lupus erythematosus (uncontrolled)	Miscarriage, stillbirth, congenital heart block, IUGR, prematurity	Not established
Toxin Exposures		
Mercury poisoning (from contaminated fish)	Small head size, cerebral palsy, developmental delay and/or mental retardation, blindness, muscle weakness, and seizures	Not established

[a]A list of medication teratogens can be found in the *Pharmacotherapeutics* chapter.

HbA1c = hemoglobin A1c, a laboratory measurement that represents the average serum glucose level during the most recent 6 weeks; IUGR = intrauterine growth restriction.

Source: Adapted from the Utah Department of Health Pregnancy Riskline and the Organization of Teratology Information Specialists (OTIS).

Screening Versus Diagnostic Tests

First, screening tests simply separate those who "might" from those who "probably don't" have the specific condition being tested for. Midwives and the women who are receiving care from them should remain cognizant that screening tests are *not* diagnostic. Screening results usually aid in determining the level of risk for a specific disorder, and they identify individuals who might be advised to undergo further, definitive diagnostic testing. In contrast, diagnostic tests, provide a *definitive* answer to whether an individual has a particular disorder. For example, results of a maternal serum screening test for trisomy 21 during the first trimester are not simply "normal" or

"abnormal." Results will indicate the chance (e.g., 1 in 40, 1 in 400, 1 in 4000) of having a fetus with trisomy 21, based on the level of pregnancy-associated plasma protein A (PAPP-A) and human chorionic gonadotropin (hCG) in maternal serum when the fetus has reached a specific gestational age. Screening test results give the midwife and pregnant woman the information necessary to help them decide whether diagnostic testing will be chosen as the next step.

Second, tests are rarely, if ever, 100% accurate. Reliability of tests must be considered. Again using first-trimester maternal serum screening for trisomy 21 as an example, this screening test will not identify

100% of all fetuses with trisomy 21, but it has demonstrated the ability to detect approximately 87% of these fetuses.[28] Thus approximately 13% of fetuses with trisomy 21 will not be detected with this screening test, thus giving false reassurance to the woman, family, and provider that the fetus is normal. Furthermore, screening tests have a false-positive rate, meaning a positive test indicating a high likelihood for trisomy 21, when a perfectly healthy fetus is actually present. The "false alarm" rate for first-trimester screening for trisomy 21 is approximately 5% to 6%,[28] and is a significant contributor to unintended parental anxiety during the prenatal period and potentially unnecessary interventions. **Table 21-6**

provides the sensitivity and specificity of various prenatal tests offered.

Because prevalence of a disorder is often different for different groups of women (e.g., based on ethnicity or geographical location), these differences must be taken into account to accurately interpret test results.[29] Prevalence, predictive value of test results, and ways to interpret these values are illustrated in **Figure 21-8**. Other factors may also affect test results, including gestational age, maternal age, presence of multiple gestation, certain medical conditions such as diabetes, and other coexisting congenital or genetic disorders.[30] A good example of this multifactorial input into test results involves the maternal serum alpha fetoprotein (MSAFP) or alpha fetoprotein (AFP) test. AFP is a protein normally made by the fetal liver and found in the amniotic fluid. It passes through the placenta and circulates in the maternal blood, thereby enabling assessment of AFP via sampling maternal serum. MSAFP is a screening test for NTDs (higher levels are associated with higher risk), but also is used to identify a risk for trisomy 21 (lower levels are associated with higher risk of trisomy 21).[30] In this case, an additional factor influencing the interpretation of results is an accurate estimation of gestational age. The MSAFP test has different normative values at different gestational ages. Thus, if a woman has the test done at 15 weeks' gestation, it will be interpreted based on 15-week norms. However, if the gestational age has not been accurately determined and the pregnancy is actually at 13 gestational weeks, the test results will appear abnormal simply because they have been interpreted incorrectly. This situation also has prompted the use of multiple biochemical markers for screening tests, rather than reliance on a single marker, such as MSAFP.

Currently, the American College of Obstetricians and Gynecologists recommends offering both screening and diagnostic testing to all pregnant women, regardless of age or risk factors present.[31] This recommendation was made in light of the low-risk, reliable, noninvasive methods currently available today, as well as the belief that all women should have a choice in testing, not just "high-risk" women.

There are several time points during pregnancy at which specific screening and diagnostic tests can be performed and will provide the most accurate results. However, the decision whether to engage in testing is always the individual woman's choice. The midwife's role is to provide as much information as needed to facilitate a woman's decision making about what is best for her and her family. **Table 21-7** provides a comprehensive list of both screening and diagnostic tests and the appropriate timing for testing options

Table 21-6	Sensitivity and Specificity for Currently Available Prenatal Tests	
Test	**Sensitivity[a]**	**Specificity[b]**
First-trimester screening (NT and maternal serum)	Trisomy 21: 87% Trisomy 18: 60%	Trisomy 21: 5–6% Trisomy 18: 0.5–1%
Second-trimester screening (anatomic ultrasound and maternal serum)		
Integrated screen (first- and second-trimester screening)	Trisomy 21: 87% Trisomy 18: 60% NTDs: 80%	Trisomy 21: 1–2% Trisomy 18: < 0.5% NTDs: 2–3%
Chorionic villus sampling	Aneuploidy: 98%	
Amniocentesis	Aneuploidy: 99.5% NTDs: 95%	
Noninvasive prenatal testing (trisomy 21, 18, and 13)	Trisomy 21 and 18: 99% Trisomy 13: 92%	0.3–1%
Direct DNA testing: saliva, blood, placental, or skin cell sample for identification of genetic mutation and carrier status	99.9%	< 0.4%

[a] Sensitivity is the "accuracy" or ability of a test to correctly identify those who have a disorder.

[b] Specificity is the ability of a test to correctly identify those who do not have a disorder.

NT = nuchal translucency; NTDs = neural tube defects.

regularly offered in the United States, as well as some that are expected to be adopted soon.

First-Trimester Testing for Aneuploidy

Screening for aneuploidy—particularly trisomies 21, 18, and 13—can be done in the first trimester and is best performed between 10 and 14 weeks of gestation. Risk for aneuploidy can be determined by measuring maternal serum levels of PAPP-A and hCG (expressed as multiples of the median) in relation to maternal weight and age, and gestational age. Generally, an increased risk of trisomy 21 is associated with lower PAPP-A levels and higher hCG levels.[30,32]

Risk can also be calculated during ultrasound measurement of nuchal translucency between 10 and 14 weeks of gestation. Increased thickness (greater than 3 mm) of the nuchal fold (fluid-filled space behind the fetal neck) is associated with an increased risk of trisomy 21, other aneuploidies, and perhaps other defects, such as heart defects, diaphragmatic hernias, skeletal dysplasia, and a variety of genetic syndromes.[28,32] Absence of the fetal nasal bone is also associated with trisomy 21; thus some facilities also include ultrasound assessment of the nasal bone.[30]

Diagnostic tests for aneuploidy and direct DNA genetic testing in the first trimester includes chorionic villus sampling (CVS), which entails collection

of placental tissue between 10 and 14 weeks, transcervically or transabdominally, and completion of karyotyping for detection of aneuploidy using the tissue obtained.[32] One advantage of CVS over amniocentesis is that it can be performed earlier in the pregnancy. This early performance allows more time to consider options and to make decisions (including pregnancy termination), particularly if a woman desires to make difficult decisions earlier in a pregnancy or before the pregnancy becomes known to others. **Figure 21-9A** depicts collection of placental tissue for diagnostic testing, which should be performed by a highly skilled physician (obstetrician or maternal-fetal medicine specialist). If desired, fetal sex can also be identified from a karyotype obtained via CVS. A separate direct DNA testing can be completed, if desired, to identify genetic mutations (e.g., Tay-Sachs disease, cystic fibrosis, hemophilia A, Huntington disease). CVS, however, cannot detect NTDs. The best screening for NTDs consists of MSAFP testing followed by measurement of AFP in amniotic fluid (collected during an amniocentesis). The best diagnostic test for NTDs is anatomic ultrasound examination of the fetus.

CVS is an invasive procedure associated with an additional 1% risk for miscarriage, above the baseline risk of approximately 15% for an average pregnant

Chart A

	Trisomy 21 present	Trisomy 21 absent	Interpretation (predictive value for a 25-year-old woman)
Positive test result	87 will have a true-positive test	6235 will have a false-positive test	A 25-year-old woman with a positive test for trisomy 21 has a 1.4% chance of actually having an infant with trisomy 21 (out of 6322 positive tests, 87 infants had trisomy 21 and 6235 tests were false alarms). This is the PPV.
Negative test result	13 will have a false-negative test	118,665 will have a true-negative test	A woman with a negative test result has a 99.9% chance of *not* having an infant with trisomy 21 (out of 75,918 negative tests, 13 infants actually had trisomy 21). This is the NPV.
	100 infants affected	124,900 not affected	Out of 125,000 infantsborn to 25-year-old women, 100 will have trisomy 21 and 124,900 will not.

Chart A: Sensitivity (87%), specificity (95%), and predictive value of first-trimester screening (NT and maternal serum) for trisomy 21 when the prevalence rate is 1 per 1250 (as it is among 25-year-old women).

Chart B

	Trisomy 21 present	Trisomy 21 absent	Interpretation (predictive value for a 45-year-old woman)
Positive test result	87 will have a true-positive test	145 will have a false-positive test	A 45-year-old woman with a positive test for trisomy 21 has a 37.5% chance of actually having an infant with trisomy 21 (out of 232 positive tests, 87 infants had trisomy 21 and 145 tests were false alarms). This is the PPV.
Negative test result	13 will have a false-negative test	2755 will have a true-negative test	A woman with a negative test result has a 99.3% chance of *not* having a baby with trisomy 21 (out of 2768 negative tests, 13 infants actually had trisomy 21). This is the NPV.
	100 infants affected	2900 infants not affected	Out of 3000 infants born to 45-year-old women, 100 will have trisomy 21 and 2900 will not.

Chart B: Sensitivity (87%), specificity (95%), and predictive value of first trimester screening (NT and maternal serum) for trisomy 21 when the prevalence rate is 1 per 30 (as it is among 45-year-old women).

PPV = positive predictive value, the proportion of all positive tests that truly indicate an infant with trisomy 21.
NPV = negative predictive value, the proportion of all negative tests that truly indicate an infant without trisomy 21.

Note: Test performance (specificity and sensitivity) is the same in both charts. However, the PPV and the NPV are different in the two charts because the prevalence rate for trisomy 21 differs for women who are 25 years old (chart A) and women who are 45 years old (chart B). The interpretation is therefore different for women represented in each of these charts.

Figure 21-8 The impact of prevalence on the predictive value and interpretation of first-trimester screening for trisomy 21 among women of differing age.

woman at a similar gestation.[32] Furthermore, CVS is no longer performed prior to 10 weeks' gestation due to the documented risk of limb reduction birth defects among infants born to women who had CVS testing at an earlier gestational age. Transabdominal CVS is considered safer, technically less difficult, and more accurate than transcervical CVS.[33]

Noninvasive prenatal testing (NIPT) is the newest testing option for identification of trisomies 21, 18, and 13, but is not yet widely available.[34,35] NIPT involves collection of maternal blood, which contains small fragments of circulating cell-free fetal DNA, anytime after 10 weeks' gestation. This newest technology amplifies the fetal DNA and makes it possible to quite accurately identify the extra genetic material that exists when aneuploidy is present in the fetus.[36] Because NIPT has not been extensively used yet, most facilities currently recommend that a positive

Table 21-7 Prenatal Screening and Diagnostic Tests Currently Available

Gestational Age When Test Is Performed	Test	Testing Available for These Conditions			
		Aneuploidy	Neural Tube Defects	Genetic Mutation	Congenital Anomalies
First-Trimester Screening					
10–14 weeks	Ultrasound: nuchal translucency (thickness)	✔			✔
10–14 weeks	Maternal serum: PAPP-A and hCG	✔			
10+ weeks	NIPT (maternal serum)[a]	✔			
Second-Trimester Screening					
15–23 weeks (optimal at 18 weeks)	Ultrasound: anatomic exam	✔	✔		✔
15–18 weeks	Maternal serum: multiple marker (quad): AFP, hCG, uE3, and inhibin-A	✔	✔		
Integrated screening	Combines first- and second-trimester screening as a comprehensive risk assessment	✔	✔		✔
Sequential	First-trimester screening, followed by second-trimester screening, as desired, based on first-trimester results	✔	✔		✔
Anytime	NIPT (maternal serum)[a]	✔			
First-Trimester Diagnostic Tests					
10–14 weeks	Chorionic villus sampling (CVS) For karyotype and/or direct DNA testing	✔		✔	
Second-Trimester Diagnostic Tests					
15–22 weeks	Amniocentesis for karyotype and/or direct DNA testing, and amniotic fluid AFP level	✔	✔	✔	
Anytime: Prepregnancy, Pregnancy, Newborn, Parents					
Direct DNA diagnostic testing	Blood, saliva, and skin cells from parents prior to or during pregnancy, or in the newborn or siblings	✔		✔	

[a]NIPT: Newly developed test for trisomy 21, 18, and 13 that is not yet routinely offered (but expected to rapidly become available). Many predict this test will replace invasive (and more risky) CVS and amniocentesis procedures for diagnosis of aneuploidy. Its performance appears to match that of CVS and amniocentesis at this time.

AFP = alpha fetoprotein; hCG = human chorionic gonadotropin; NIPT = noninvasive prenatal testing; NTD = neural tube defect; PAPP-A = pregnancy-associated plasma protein A; uE3 = unconjugated estriol.

test result be followed with CVS or amniocentesis to confirm the diagnosis. It is predicted that NIPT may replace the more invasive procedures because its test performance (approximately 99% detection rate) nearly matches that of CVS (98% detection rate) and amniocentesis (99.5% detection rate), particularly for the detection of trisomies 21 and 18.[36]

Second-Trimester Testing

Screening for aneuploidy and NTDs during the second trimester currently includes measurement of several markers in maternal serum. Commonly referred to as a maternal serum, multiple marker, or "quad" screen, this test includes the measurement of maternal serum levels (expressed as multiples of the median) of

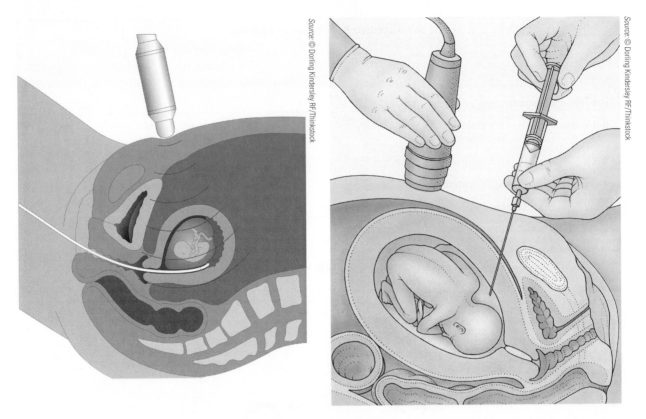

Source: © Dorling Kindersley RF/Thinkstock

Source: © Dorling Kindersley RF/Thinkstock

Figure 21-9 (A) Transcervical chorionic villus sampling. (B) Amniocentesis.

alpha fetoprotein, uE3 (unconjugated estriol), human chorionic gonadotropin, and inhibin-A.[32] The last three of these markers are hormones produced by the placenta and secreted into the maternal circulation. In contrast, AFP is a protein made by the fetus. The AFP test, also known as the maternal serum AFP test, has been in use longer than the other tests included in the quad screen.

Screening options over the past 10 to 20 years have moved rapidly from a single serum marker test (MSAFP) to the addition of other markers as it became established that multiple markers are more effective in screening for abnormalities and decrease the risk of false-positive results compared to a single marker.[37] NIPT can also be conducted anytime during the second trimester.

Ultrasound

Ultrasound examination of the fetus during the second trimester is targeted toward identification of physical characteristics associated with aneuploidy phenotypes, NTDs and other anatomic defects such as heart, kidneys, cranium/brain, and limb defects.[38] For example, ultrasound findings in a fetus that include an absent nasal bone, palmar creases, short femur, and echogenic bowel correspond to characteristics commonly found in the trisomy 21 phenotype.[32] Such findings would arouse suspicion for aneuploidy and prompt recommendations for further testing, such as diagnostic amniocentesis if the woman wants a diagnostic test for this condition. Second-trimester anatomic ultrasounds are usually performed at approximately 18 weeks' gestation for best results.

Diagnostic Testing in the Second Trimester

Diagnostic testing in the second trimester can be accomplished via amniocentesis and entails inserting a fine needle through the woman's abdomen and into the uterus to collect a small sample of amniotic fluid. Fetal cells are found in the fluid, separated, and usually grown in a culture medium until the chromosomes can be examined under a microscope. The final result is a fetal "G-banded" karyotype that is used to identify aneuploidies and other chromosomal derangements. (Figure 21-5 provides an example of a karyotype display.) Other technologies besides the G-banded karyotype that can be used to detect chromosomal abnormalities in fetal cells obtained via CVS or amniocentesis include fluorescent in situ hybridization (FISH), spectral karyotyping, and comparative genomic hybridization (CGH).[4]

Fetal sex can also be determined with an amniocentesis. Amniocentesis is usually performed at 16 to 18 gestational weeks of pregnancy and has an associated risk of pregnancy loss of approximately 1% above the background risk (2.1% versus 1.3% background risk; relative risk [RR]: 1.60; 95% confidence interval [CI]: 1.02–2.52).[32,33] Early amniocentesis (before 15 weeks' gestation) can be performed, but is associated with a higher risk of pregnancy loss (7.6% versus 5.9% background risk; RR: 1.29; 95% CI: 1.03–1.61).[33] Early amniocentesis is also associated with a higher incidence of talipes (club foot) compared to CVS testing (RR: 4.6; 95% CI: 1.82–11.66).[33]

During a CVA or amniocentesis, direct DNA testing can be completed if warranted to identify genetic mutations in the fetus (e.g., Tay-Sachs disease, cystic fibrosis, hemophilia A, Huntington disease). If a woman chooses to have a diagnostic amniocentesis, an amniotic fluid AFP test can be completed at the same time to screen for NTDs.

Integrated, Combined, or Sequential Prenatal Testing for Aneuploidy

First- and second-trimester screening can be combined (ultrasound and maternal serum markers) in an effort to improve the ability to detect trisomy 21.[39] Results can be calculated and returned to the pregnant woman after all testing has been completed (i.e., integrated/combined), or after each trimester's results are known (i.e., sequentially). Calculation of the risk that the fetus has trisomy 21 after all test results are known, however, would preclude the woman's choice to have a CVS, if diagnostic testing is indicated. In contrast, the sequential screen calculates risk based on first-trimester screening tests and returns the results to the woman before proceeding with further screening tests. One advantage of a sequential screen is that a woman and her prenatal care provider can decide whether to continue with the second-trimester screening or to proceed with diagnostic testing (CVS or amniocentesis) if the first-trimester results indicate high risk for chromosomal abnormalities.[30,40]

Future Trends in Genetic Testing

It may come as no surprise that "direct-to-consumer" (DTC) genetic testing is becoming available, given the demand from increasing numbers of well-educated individuals who are used to Internet access and personal autonomy.[41] Nevertheless, there is a heated debate about the harms and benefits of DTC genetic tests. Some countries and locations have banned availability of DTC genetic testing altogether, whereas others have adopted an "over-the-counter" approach in making the tests available. Some argue that provision of such testing options empowers people by increasing their knowledge about their own health and the genetic basis of their health. Others are concerned that most people have low health literacy, particularly regarding genetic information, and are not able to interpret or emotionally process these tests appropriately without the assistance of trained healthcare personnel.[42] A quick Internet search reveals availability of DTC genetic testing for hundreds of genetic mutations. Testing for the entire individual genome is certain to follow.

Individuals can purchase these noninvasive DTC tests from commercial enterprises if they would like to know, for example, the presence of genetic mutations for heritable disorders, including those that indicate carrier status and susceptibility to multifactorial diseases. Some tests are targeted to pregnant women and couples who would like to determine carrier status for specific genetic and chromosomal disorders, paternity, or the sex of the fetus prenatally. Samples (usually saliva/cheek swab or blood spot via finger prick) are collected in the privacy of one's home and returned to the commercial testing facility. This step usually does not require the services of a healthcare intermediary, such as the midwife, obstetrician, or family practice provider, although some tests do. One advantage of DTC testing may be that it enables potential parents to test for carrier status prior to making the decision to attempt pregnancy. This approach raises the prospect of increasing use of preventive options for couples who want to avoid having a child with specific heritable disorders.[42,43]

Factors Influencing Screening, Diagnostic Testing, and Decision Making

Women are faced with many difficult decisions in healthcare settings, and the prenatal genetic screening and testing crossroads is certainly not an exception. Midwives can ease the process by engaging in excellent informed decision making when offering prenatal testing, interpreting test results, and discussing options. Women and their families should have their questions answered adequately and candidly, but with compassion and respect for individual values and wishes. The common questions posed by women should be addressed when offering or recommending any screening or diagnostic test to women and/or their families (**Box 21-2**). The answers to these questions may differ significantly from woman to woman, from setting to setting, and from midwifery practice to midwifery practice. Many factors such as cultural, individual, family, and religious values will play a role in how a woman perceives testing for birth defects. In some settings, the questions in Box **21**-2 will not enter into the conversation at all because the tests are simply not available, are too expensive, or are unacceptable to the woman seeking care.[44-49]

The most important question for a woman is, "What will I do with the information?" This question will need to be answered by the woman for herself with support from her significant others and her midwife. Answering this question can assist her to make the ultimate decision whether she will undergo screening or diagnostic tests or both.[50] A woman can often arrive at an answer by addressing additional, very personal questions: "Would I terminate this pregnancy if I know my baby is affected with (fill in the blank)?" "Do I want to know that my baby is affected before the baby is born?" "Would testing simply make me more anxious rather than less anxious?" "Am I willing to accept the increased risk of miscarriage associated with a diagnostic test such as CVS or amniocentesis?" "Am I strongly opposed to pregnancy termination even if I have a baby affected with (fill in the blank)?" "Why should I have screening or diagnostic tests if I am fine with any outcome the baby might have?" It often helps women to self-identify their stance when the midwife offers statements that begin with "Some women choose to have these tests because…" and "Some women choose not to have these tests because…."

When Genetic Disorders Are Identified

Understandably, when genetic disorders are identified, parents are first shocked and then devastated, they have lots of questions, and are usually in need of resources to help them deal with the situation. Helpful resources will vary depending on the setting and geographic area, and the cultural, societal, personal, and family beliefs. Women may choose to access their families, religious leaders, or mental health counselors for direction and support, and may desire access to medical resources and options, where available. Midwives can be a valuable resource for women who need additional information and discussion of options, and for referrals to appropriate healthcare providers (i.e., geneticists and genetics counselors). If the woman has an established relationship with a midwife, it may also be helpful for her to meet again with the midwife after she has met with and received input from other providers. Making decisions about how to proceed can be emotionally wrenching for women and their families.[50]

Pregnancy termination may be an option, depending on a woman's feelings, the gestational age, and local regulations and laws. Midwives can provide substantial assistance to women by way of nonjudgmental support and appropriate education about options and anticipatory planning. If available, women may need and want additional information obtained from a referral to a maternal–fetal medicine physician or neonatologist.

Many women can appropriately continue with midwifery care during pregnancy and birth, often in consultation or collaboration with other members of the healthcare team. Frequently, affected newborns will need immediate attention after birth, and arrangements for this care will need to be made

---

BOX 21-2 Frequently Asked Questions Regarding Prenatal Testing

- Why is this test offered?
- What will I do with the information?
- How much does the test cost?
- Will insurance cover the test?
- When does the test have to be done?
- Are there any treatments for the conditions being tested for?
- How are the results communicated?
- What if there is a positive result?
- Who will know about the results?
- Should a spouse or others relatives be informed about the test or the test results?
- Will the results affect insurance coverage?
- Can testing be refused?
- What are the options if test results indicate the baby has a serious problem?

Source: Adapted from March of Dimes. *Genetics and Your Practice: Family Health and Social History.* 2012. Available at: http://www.marchofdimes.com/gyponline/index.bm2. Accessed January 19, 2013.

in advance, including the site for the birth. Many proponents of prenatal testing believe that the biggest value in testing lies in the ability for parents to access resources and make arrangements for the care of a special needs child well in advance of the birth.[32] In addition, many support networks exist to help families who have a child with a specific genetic disorder or birth defect, such as the National Down Syndrome Society.[51] Whatever final decision is made by a woman, the midwife can be instrumental in supporting her and directing her and her family to the best resources, and in providing ongoing midwifery care when appropriate.

Genetic Disorder Prevention and Risk Reduction

Midwives and the women to whom they provide services often are left to ponder the fact that in spite of all the testing options available and genetics knowledge developed, there are still no "cures" for the vast number of genetic disorders identified. However, there are some options and preventive approaches that can improve the outcomes for many mothers and babies, of which midwives will want to be aware.

Excellent nutrition (including folic acid supplementation)[8,11] and avoidance of exposures to teratogens[20,21] are two long-standing preventive strategies that are well known in most geographic areas of the world. Furthermore, most developed countries can offer genetic risk assessment and genetic testing to women and couples who are considering childbearing so that options can be considered before a pregnancy occurs. Indeed, some high-risk groups have taken it upon themselves to broadly screen for carrier status of a genetic disorder specific to the group. For example, some Ashkenazi Jewish groups strongly encourage carrier status testing for Tay-Sachs disease prior to conception, to avoid the sorrow that is experienced by families who have a child affected by this devastating disease.[52]

Unfortunately, many couples learn of hereditary disorders only after having a child who is affected. In this situation, the midwife will need to provide the family with accurate information and compassionate care. Preconception and postpartum testing for genetic disorders and carrier status can be obtained by families who have a child with a birth defect. This testing often provides answers to the questions most parents have, such as "What went wrong?" and "How can we prevent this from happening again?" Testing may be able to identify the specific disorder, as well as the risk for reoccurrence in subsequent children.

Moreover, options can be considered once a definitive answer is given. Options include the choice not to bear biological children, addition of future children via adoption, sperm and/or egg donation, and, in some developed countries, pre-implantation genetic testing. Pre-implantation testing involves in vitro fertilization (often with the sperm and/or egg from the prospective parents), genetic testing of a cell collected from the 8-cell blastocyst, followed by selection of only normal embryos for transfer into the uterus of the woman.[53,54] This method assures that only normal embryos without genetic disease mutations will continue forth in a pregnancy. Some couples are delighted with this choice, whereas others are strongly opposed to this approach owing to religious or personal reasons, and others simply find the use of such technology too complex, too expensive, or too reminiscent of eugenics to consider it.[55]

Financial, Ethical, Legal, and Social Issues in Genetics

Along with the rapid increase in genetic knowledge and technology came the need to address a myriad of financial (economic), ethical, legal, and social issues (FELSI). The World Health Organization (WHO) has proposed international guidelines regarding ethics in genetic testing, including in developed countries.[44] These guidelines include respect for the autonomy of individuals, beneficence, nonmalfeasance, and justice in provision of genetics-related services. The WHO guidelines are clear that genetic testing can have a profound impact on women and their families. Thus confidentiality and privacy, the right for persons to receive sufficient information about testing and treatment, and individual autonomy to make decisions about testing and treatment, regardless of geographic area, socioeconomic status, ethnic background, religion, or belief system are emphasized. Midwives have an obligation to understand and act on the principles related to FELSI, including a duty to fully inform women, offer appropriate testing when available, and refer women and families to other resources (i.e., genetic counselor or geneticists) when their own professional or personal limitations have been reached. Some of the more common FELSI concerns and questions are listed in **Box 21-3**.[56]

BOX 21-3 Common Financial, Ethical, Legal, and Social Concerns in Genetic Testing

- Disparities in access to genetic resources due to lack of health insurance coverage, inability to pay, low income economy, other competing priorities in healthcare needs, or geographic location
- Distributive injustice (some populations benefit but not others)
- Religious and cultural beliefs and perceptions about genetic risk, decision making, health and disease, family, privacy, authority, invasive procedures, childbearing, influence over life events, and use of alternatives to Western medicine
- Racial and ethnic discrimination
- Cultural factors that may impact accuracy or interpretation of family history information
- Privacy and confidentiality
- Discrimination or stigmatization by others based on genetic information
- Judgment about family genetic history (is it good or bad?)
- Sensitive issues encountered, such as previously undisclosed adoption, rape, incest, misattributed paternity, substance abuse, mental illness, ethnic origins
- Stigma and legality of consanguinity
- When or if relatives (who may not want to know) should be informed about an individual's genetic testing results
- Implications of family history information and genetic testing results
- The negative impact of false positive test results
- The ethical question of testing for disorders that have no cure or treatment
- Eugenics
- Pregnancy termination
- Cost effectiveness: the high cost of genetic testing versus the possibility of improved health outcomes
- Denial of health insurance or employment based on genetic test results[*]

[*]The Genetic Information Nondiscrimination Act of 2008, also referred to as GINA, is a federal law that prohibits discrimination in health coverage and employment on the basis of genetic information (including genetic test results). More information is available at http://www.genome.gov /Pages/PolicyEthics/GeneticDiscrimination/GINAInfoDoc.pdf.

Source: Adapted from March of Dimes. *Genetics and Your Practice: Family Health and Social History.* 2012. Available at: http://www.marchofdimes.com/gyponline/index.bm2. Accessed January 19, 2013.

Conclusion

In 1990, a collaborative project was begun among several public and private entities in the United States as well as governments and research centers in Europe and Japan with the goal of exploring genetics in more detail. The Human Genome Project focused on sequencing the DNA and mapping the more than 25,000 genes found in the entire genome of *Homo sapiens.* Although the Human Genome Project was completed in the early twenty-first century, applications of its findings and further investigation will continue for the foreseeable future.

In addition to knowledge being gleaned from the Human Genome Project, the information about non-Mendelian inheritance patterns has been growing for several years. For the midwife receiving a report of a CVS, amniocentesis, or direct DNA testing, the results usually are phrased in Mendelian terms (e.g., "autosomal recessive"). However, non-Mendelian inheritance patterns are emerging as potential important etiologies for some human genetic diseases. Among these are mitochondrial inheritance, which is a pattern exclusively from the maternal line; mosaicism, in which cells within the same person have different genetic makeup; and genomic imprinting, which occurs when a child receives only one "working" copy from one parent (instead of both) due to gene "silencing" by epigenetic mechanisms. Research continues into the variety of inheritance patterns because they may be of significant clinical relevance in the future.

This chapter has provided a foundation in genetics for midwives and has included several approaches for the provision of genetics-related healthcare services to women and families. The intention is to increase the confidence that midwives have when addressing prenatal genetic risk assessment, testing options, and decision making. Although genetics is considered a "high-tech" arena, midwives have a particular talent for using the important "low-tech" tools for identifying risk, communicating with women, and assisting families to make decisions. Furthermore, these midwifery care practices are woman/family centered, thereby increasing the satisfaction of women and their families. Although most genetic disorders do not have a cure, prenatal genetic risk assessment, counseling, screening, and diagnosis have many potential benefits to women, including the ability to consider options, make well-informed decisions, access valuable resources, prepare for outcomes in advance, and ultimately optimize the health of mothers and babies. Well-informed midwives can make valuable contributions in this endeavor.

••• References

1. Jorde L, Carey J, Bamshad M. *Medical Genetics*. 4th ed. Philadelphia, PA: Mosby Elsevier; 2010.

2. Crane MJ, Quinn Griffin MT, Andrews CM, Fitzpatrick JJ. The level of importance and level of confidence that midwives in the United States attach to using genetics in practice. *J Midwifery Women's Health*. 2012;57:114-119.

3. Feero WG, Guttmacher AE, Collins FS. Genomic medicine: an updated primer. *N Engl J Med*. 2010; 362:2001-2011.

4. Wilson G, Oligny L. Mechanisms of development and growth: molecular genetics. In: Gilbert-Barness E, ed. *Potter's Pathology of the Fetus, Infant and Child*. 2nd ed. Philadelphia: Mosby Elsevier; 2007:3-64.

5. Meaney MJ. Epigenetics and the biological definition of gene x environment interactions. *Child Dev*. 2010;81:41-79.

6. Ray HJ, Niswander L. Mechanisms of tissue fusion during development. *Development*. 2012;139: 1701-1711.

7. Bassuk AG, Kibar Z. Genetic basis of neural tube defects. *Semin Pediatr Neurol*. 2009;16:101-110.

8. Frey L, Hauser WA. Epidemiology of neural tube defects. *Epilepsia*. 2003;44(suppl 3):4-13.

9. Folic acid for the prevention of neural tube defects: U.S. Preventive Services Task Force recommendation statement. *Ann Intern Med*. 2009;150:626-631.

10. Toriello HV. Policy statement on folic acid and neural tube defects. *Genet Med*. 2011;13:593-596.

11. Neural tube defects (NTDs). 2007. Available at: http://www.nichd.nih.gov/health/topics/neural_tube_defects.cfm. Accessed September 30, 2012.

12. Gilbert-Barness E, Oligny L. Chromosomal abnormalities. In: Gilbert-Barness E, ed. *Potter's Pathology of the Fetus, Infant and Child*. 2nd ed. Philadelphia: Mosby Elsevier; 2007:213.

13. Hassold T, Hall H, Hunt P. The origin of human aneuploidy: where we have been, where we are going. *Hum Mol Genet*. 2007;16(2):R203-R208.

14. Bouchlariotou S, Tsikouras P, Dimitraki M, et al. Turner's syndrome and pregnancy: has the 45,X/47,XXX mosaicism a different prognosis? Own clinical experience and literature review. *J Matern Fetal Neonatal Med*. 2011;24:668-672.

15. Morris JK, Mutton DE, Alberman E. Revised estimates of maternal age specific live birth prevalence of Down syndrome. *J Med Screen*. 2002;9:2-6.

16. Arnold KM, Self ZB. Genetic screening and counseling: family medicine obstetrics. *Prim Care*. 2012;39:55-70.

17. Sartorius GA, Nieschlag E. Paternal age and reproduction. *Hum Reprod Update*. 2010;16:65-79.

18. Wiener-Megnazi Z, Auslender R, Dirnfeld M. Advanced paternal age and reproductive outcome. *Asian J Androl*. 2012;14:69-76.

19. Frias J, Gilbert-Barness E. Teratogenic disruptions. In: Gilbert-Barness E, ed. *Potter's Pathology of Fetal, Infant and Child*. 2nd ed. Philadelphia: Mosby Elsevier; 2007:137.

20. Organization of Teratology Information Specialists. Fact sheets. 2012. Available at: http://www.otispregnancy.org/otis-fact-sheets-s13037. Accessed September 30, 2012.

21. Answers about medications and other exposures during pregnancy and breastfeeding. 2011. Available at: http://www.health.utah.gov/prl/factsheet.htm. Accessed September 30, 2012.

22. Allen VM, Armson BA, Wilson RD, et al. Teratogenicity associated with pre-existing and gestational diabetes. *J Obstet Gynaecol Can*. 2007;29:927-944.

23. Chen M, Zhang L. Epigenetic mechanisms in developmental programming of adult disease. *Drug Discov Today*. 2011;16:1007-1018.

24. Guttmacher AE, Collins FS, Carmona RH. The family history: more important than ever. *N Engl J Med*. 2004;351:2333-2336.

25. National Coalition for Health Professional Education in Genetics. Family history for prenatal providers. 2012. Available at: http://www.nchpeg.org/index.php?option=com_content&view=article&id=53:family-history-for-prenatal-providers&catid=35:todays-highlights. Accessed October 20, 2012.

26. March of Dimes. *Genetics and Your Practice: Family Health and Social History*. 2012. Available at: http://www.marchofdimes.com/gyponline/index.bm2. Accessed January 19, 2013.

27. *Core Competencies in Genetics for Health Professionals*. 3rd ed. Lutherville, MD: National Coalition for Health Professional Education in Genetics; 2007.

28. Driscoll DA, Gross SJ. First trimester diagnosis and screening for fetal aneuploidy. *Genet Med*. 2008; 10:73-75.

29. Fletcher R, Fletcher S. *Clinical Epidemiology: The Essentials*. 4th ed. Baltimore, MD: Lippincott Williams & Wilkins; 2005.

30. Chitayat D, Langlois S, Wilson RD. Prenatal screening for fetal aneuploidy in singleton pregnancies. *J Obstet Gynaecol Can*. 2011;33:736-750.

31. ACOG Practice Bulletin No. 77: screening for fetal chromosomal abnormalities. *Obstet Gynecol*. 2007; 109:217-227.

32. Farrell P, Elias S. Prenatal diagnosis and neonatal screening. In: Gilbert-Barness E, ed. *Potter's Pathology of the Fetus, Infant and Child*. 2nd ed. Philadelphia: Mosby Elsevier; 2007:612.

33. Alfirevic Z, Mujezinovic F, Sundberg K. Amniocentesis and chorionic villus sampling for prenatal diagnosis. *Cochrane Database Syst Rev.* 2003;3:CD003252. doi: 10.1002/14651858.CD003252.

34. National Coalition for Health Professional Education in Genetics and National Society of Genetic Counselors. Non-invasive prenatal testing (NIPT) factsheet. 2012. Available at: http://www.nchpeg.org /index.php?option=com_content&view=article&id= 384&Itemid=255. Accessed January 19, 2013.

35. Canick JA, Palomaki GE. Maternal plasma DNA: a major step forward in prenatal testing. *J Med Screen.* 2012;19:57-59.

36. Palomaki GE, Deciu C, Kloza EM, et al. DNA sequencing of maternal plasma reliably identifies trisomy 18 and trisomy 13 as well as Down syndrome: an international collaborative study. *Genet Med.* 2012;14:296-305.

37. Alldred SK, Deeks JJ, Guo B, Neilson JP, Alfirevic Z. Second trimester serum tests for Down's Syndrome screening. *Cochrane Database Syst Rev.* 2012;6:CD009925. doi: 10.1002/14651858. CD009925.

38. Gagnon A, Wilson RD, Allen VM, et al. Evaluation of prenatally diagnosed structural congenital anomalies. *J Obstet Gynaecol Can.* 2009;31:875-881, 882-889.

39. Cocciolone R, Brameld K, O'Leary P, et al. Combining first and second trimester markers for Down syndrome screening: think twice. *Aust N Z J Obstet Gynaecol.* 2008;48:492-500.

40. Fisher J. Supporting patients after disclosure of abnormal first trimester screening results. *Curr Opin Obstet Gynecol.* 2012;24:109-113.

41. Direct-to-consumer genetic testing. *Lancet.* 2012; 380:76.

42. Howard HC, Borry P. To ban or not to ban? Clinical geneticists' views on the regulation of direct-to-consumer genetic testing. *EMBO Rep.* 2012;13: 791-794.

43. Valles SA. Should direct-to-consumer personalized genomic medicine remain unregulated? A rebuttal of the defenses. *Perspect Biol Med.* 2012;55:250-265.

44. *Medical Genetic Services in Developing Countries: The Ethical, Legal and Social Implications of Genetic Testing and Screening.* Geneva: World Health Organization; 2006.

45. Farrell RM, Nutter B, Agatisa PK. Meeting patients' education and decision-making needs for first trimester prenatal aneuploidy screening. *Prenat Diagn.* 2011;31:1222-1228.

46. Garcia E, Timmermans DR, van Leeuwen E. Women's views on the moral status of nature in the context of prenatal screening decisions. *J Med Ethics.* 2011; 37:461-465.

47. Hodgson J, Weil J. Talking about disability in prenatal genetic counseling: a report of two interactive workshops. *J Genet Couns.* 2012;21:17-23.

48. Usta IM, Nassar AH, Abu-Musa AA, Hannoun A. Effect of religion on the attitude of primiparous women toward genetic testing. *Prenat Diagn.* 2010;30:241-246.

49. Wong AE, Kuppermann M, Creasman JM, et al. Patient and provider attitudes toward screening for Down syndrome in a Latin American country where abortion is illegal. *Int J Gynaecol Obstet.* 2011;115:235-239.

50. Durand MA, Stiel M, Boivin J, Elwyn G. Information and decision support needs of parents considering amniocentesis: interviews with pregnant women and health professionals. *Health Expect.* 2010;13: 125-138.

51. National Down Syndrome Society. 2012. Available at: http://www.ndss.org. Accessed September 30, 2012.

52. Dor Yeshorim. 2012. Available at: http://webexposite .com/preview/dor_yeshorim/about.html. Accessed September 30, 2012.

53. Audibert F, Wilson RD, Allen V, et al. Preimplantation genetic testing. *J Obstet Gynaecol Can.* 2009;31: 761-575.

54. Brezina PR, Brezina DS, Kearns WG. Preimplantation genetic testing. *BMJ.* 2012;345:e5908.

55. Meisenberg G. Designer babies on tap? Medical students' attitudes to pre-implantation genetic screening. *Public Underst Sci.* 2009;18:149-166.

56. Financial, ethical, legal, and social issues. 2012. Available at: http://www.marchofdimes.com/gyp online/index.bm2?uid=gwen.latendresse@nurs.utah .edu&sid=g9XobZ36NS3OpPURwXrF20XF6& cid=00000002&spid=gyp_hp_1&tpid=gyp_felsi_1. Accessed September 30, 2012.

• • • Additional Genetics Resources

Genetics Curriculum Resources

Consensus Panel on Genetic/Genomic Nursing Competencies. *Essentials of Genetic and Genomic Nursing: Competencies, Curricula Guidelines, and Outcome Indicators.* 2nd ed. Silver Spring, MD: American Nurses Association; 2009.

Greco KE, Tinley S, Seibert D. *Essential Genetic and Genomic Competencies for Nurses with Graduate Degrees.* Silver Spring, MD: American Nurses Association and International Society of Nurses in Genetics; 2012.

National Coalition for Health Professional Education in Genetics (NCHPEG). *Core Competencies in Genetics for Health Professionals.* 3rd ed. Lutherville, MD: NCHPEG; 2007. Available at: http://www.nchpeg.org /index.php?option=com_content&view=article&id= 237&Itemid=84. Accessed April 4, 2013.

Genetics Learning Resources

The American Society of Human Genetics Health Provider Genetics Resources:
http://www.ashg.org/press/healthprofessional.shtml

Centers for Disease Control National Office of Public Health Genomics:
http://www.cdc.gov/genomics

Genetic Alliance, a nonprofit health advocacy organization:
www.geneticalliance.org

Genetics/Genomics Competency Center, National Institutes of Health National Human Genome Research Institute:
http://www.g-2-c-2.org

Genetic Science Learning Center:
http://gslc.genetics.utah.edu

March of Dimes for Providers (requires free registration):
http://www.marchofdimes.com/gyponline/index.bm2

National Human Genome Research Institute Educational Resources:
http://www.genome.gov/Education

National Human Genome Research Institute (NHGRI), National Institutes of Health
http://www.genome.gov/glossary/index.cfm

NHGRI online education kit:
http://www.genome.gov/25019879

NHGRI extensive education for both professionals, patients, and the public:
http://www.genome.gov/Health

Public Organizations

American Sickle Cell Anemia Association:
http://www.ascaa.org

Cystic Fibrosis Foundation:
http://www.cff.org

Foundation to Eradicate Duchenne:
http://www.duchennemd.org

Huntington's Disease Society of America:
http://www.hdsa.org

National Down Syndrome Society:
http://www.ndss.org

National Hemophilia Foundation:
http://www.hemophilia.org

National Tay-Sachs & Allied Disease Association of Delaware Valley:
http://www.tay-sachs.org

March of Dimes:
http://www.marchofdimes.com

Thalasaemia International Federation:
http://www.thalassaemia.org.cy

Trisomy 18 Foundation:
http://www.trisomy18.org

Self-Completed Family History Tools

My Family Health Portrait: A tool from the Surgeon General, USDHHS, developed by the American Society of Human Genetics and the Genetic Alliance:
https://familyhistory.hhs.gov/fhh-web/home.action

Family History Tool, NCHPEG:
http://www.nchpeg.org/index.php?option=com _content&view=article&id=61&Itemid=74

Family History for Prenatal Care Providers

ACOG, Family History as a Risk Assessment Tool:
http://www.acog.org/Resources_And_Publications /Committee_Opinions/Committee_on_Genetics /Family_History_as_a_Risk_Assessment_Tool

Family History for Prenatal Providers (in pilot testing); a tablet PD-based tool for personalized risk assessment (an electronic approach to collecting and evaluating genetic risk in the prenatal care setting):
http://www.nchpeg.org/index.php?option=com_ content&view=article&id=53:family-history-for-prenatal-providers&catid=35:todays-highlights

NCHPEG: The Pregnancy and Health Profile: A Risk Assessment & Genetic Screening Tool:
http://www.nchpeg.org/index.php?option=com_ content&view=article&id=53:family-history-forprenatal-providers&catid=35:todays-highlights

Look Up a Gene or Test and What It Does (More Technical)

Genetics and Medicine, National Center for Biotechnology Information:
http://www.ncbi.nlm.nih.gov/guide/genetics-medicine/

Mendelian Inheritance in Man (OMIM), a comprehensive description of single gene disorders:
http://www.ncbi.nlm.nih.gov/Omim/

GeneTests a publicly funded medical genetics information resource. Look up genetic tests, available at no cost to all interested persons:
http://www.genetests.org

APPENDIX

21A

Steps in Constructing a Three-Generation Pedigree

---

1. Use standard symbols and notation for building the pedigree (see **Figure 21A-1**).

2. Computer-generated pedigrees can be constructed, but a simple piece of paper works well.

3. For greater convenience, women can complete a genetic checklist or questionnaire or fill out a computer-generated (i.e., online) pedigree prior to the prenatal visit.

4. Collect information about the individual woman (often called the "proband") and her family members, including grandparents, parents, aunts and uncles, brothers and sisters, and any previous offspring.

5. Collect information about the father of the baby and his family members, including grandparents, parents, aunts and uncles, brothers and sisters, and any previous offspring.

6. Identify any genetic "red flags" and mark affected relatives (i.e., use shading of symbols as appropriate).

7. List any health or medical conditions, or cause of death (if known), for each relative, along with the current age or age at time of death

(if known) next to each corresponding relative on the pedigree.

An example of a three-generation pedigree is shown in **Figure 21A-2**. In this example, the 34-year-old woman is the proband. She has a 2-year-old daughter. Both she and her partner, who is the father of her daughter, are healthy. She has a sister who is healthy, one brother who has type 2 diabetes, and one brother who has a congenital heart defect. Her aunt died of cystic fibrosis at the age of 12.

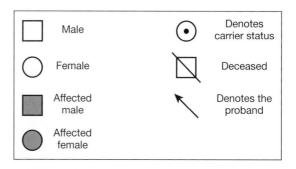

Figure 21A-1 Symbols used in constructing a three-generation pedigree.

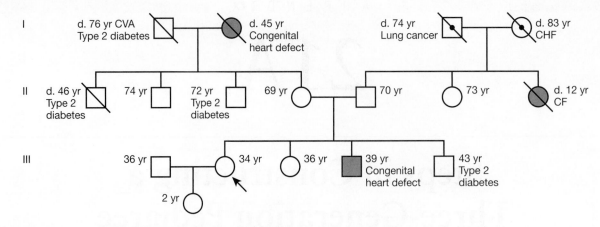

Figure 21A-2 Example of a three-generation pedigree.

CHAPTER

22

Prenatal Care

JENNIFER M. DEMMA

KAREN TRISTER GRACE

Introduction

The delivery of prenatal care, like all other aspects of the childbearing cycle, incorporates basic philosophical beliefs of midwifery. These concepts include promoting natural processes, woman-centered care, continuity of care, and the woman's right to participate knowledgeably in her own childbearing experience. When providing prenatal care, midwives work in partnership with women to help support the normal, physiologic processes of pregnancy.

Prenatal care is one of the most frequently used preventive health services in the United States. Its goal is to optimize the health of the woman and developing fetus. The five basic components of prenatal visits are (1) early and accurate identification of gestational age; (2) identification of the woman at risk for complications and ongoing risk assessment; (3) ongoing assessment of growth and well-being of the embryo/fetus; (4) health promotion in the form of counseling, education, and provision of resources; and (5) interventions and follow-up for existing physical and/or psychosocial illness and/or consultation with specialized providers as needed.[1] Specifically, prenatal care includes diagnosis and management of early pregnancy; assessment and evaluation of the well-being of the woman and embryo/fetus; provision of relief measures for the common discomforts of pregnancy experienced by women; nutritional intervention as needed; anticipatory guidance and instruction addressing health education and planning for birth and parenting; screening for and diagnosis of maternal and fetal complications; and management of maternal and fetal complications via collaboration or referral as indicated.

This chapter reviews the essential components of prenatal care for women who are not at risk for medical or obstetric complications. Detailed information about genetic counseling and screening tests can be found in the *Genetics* chapter. Similarly, detailed information about nutrition and vitamins used in pregnancy is found in the *Nutrition* chapter. Medical and obstetric complications of pregnancy are reviewed in the chapters *Obstetric Complications in Pregnancy* and *Medical Complications in Pregnancy*.

History of Prenatal Care

Throughout history, pregnant women have been accorded a special status and directed to healthy life choices. Organized prenatal care in the United States was introduced in the early twentieth century, initially as home visits conducted by public health nurses. The purpose of these visits, which occurred when the woman was 7 to 8 months pregnant, was to detect and prevent eclampsia using the newly invented sphygmometer.[2]

As medical knowledge and technology advanced, the goals and structure of prenatal care changed and the content of the prenatal care visits expanded. The development of pregnancy tests in 1928 allowed for the concept of "early care," such that women began to access healthcare services earlier in pregnancy. During the same era, a schedule of prenatal visits was recommended for women in the United Kingdom that included elements such as urine testing, assessing fetal heart tones, and assessing uterine growth.[2] By the 1960s, prenatal care had become a ritualized series of 9 to 12 individual visits conducted over the course of the pregnancy. However, the evidence for the individual components of prenatal care had not been established.

Structure of Prenatal Care

In 1989, a U.S. Public Health Service Expert Panel was convened, with its membership being composed of a variety of professionals including midwives. The subsequent publication of *Caring for Our Future: The Content of Prenatal Care*, co-authored by a midwife, provided an analysis of the structure and content of prenatal care.[1] This work was followed by a 2005 update.[3] Recommendations from these reports included a reduction in the number of prenatal visits for women with normal pregnancies and no identified medical problems. It proposed a total of eight visits for nulliparous women and six visits for multiparous women. Another visit at 41 weeks is added for women whose pregnancies continue beyond 40 gestational weeks.

Reaction to these recommendations was varied and included the following objections:

- Concerns that outcomes would be negatively affected—especially with regard to preterm birth and preeclampsia
- Concerns that there would not be enough time and sufficient contact to adequately address the psychosocial concerns of women
- Questions about cost-effectiveness if women instead used the emergency room for pregnancy discomforts (a situation that would theoretically be circumvented with more frequent prenatal visits and related education)[4]

The Expert Panel recommendation was based in part on the smaller number of scheduled visits that are common practice in the United Kingdom. Some concern was expressed about superimposing a prenatal visit schedule predicated on a system of universal health care, like the system in the United Kingdom, onto the United States, where for many women, prenatal care is their first access to regular health care.

A 2010 Cochrane review of seven randomized controlled trials of more than 60,000 women with either standard prenatal care schedules or a reduced number of visits found that clinical outcomes (obstetric and neonatal) were not different for selected low-risk populations, with the exception of a higher rate of perinatal mortality in women with a reduced visit schedule in low-resource countries.[5] In five of the seven trials the relative risk (RR) for perinatal mortality in the reduced number of visit cohorts was 1.14 (95% CI, 1.00-1.31), which the review characterized as borderline statistically significant. In these five studies, the number of maternal deaths among women with reduced visits in developed countries was less than 0.01% (n = 32/5108) and there was no difference between the two groups. Reduced number of visits was also associated with a decrease in reported satisfaction with prenatal care as well as a potential decrease in costs.[5]

Today most models of prenatal care consist of anywhere from 6 to 12 individual or group visits. A woman who is progressing normally through her pregnancy is typically seen every 4 weeks until 28 weeks' gestation, then every 2 weeks until 36 weeks' gestation, and then weekly until she gives birth. Although many clinicians continue with the traditional schedule of visits, some have instituted schedules with a reduced number of visits.[6-9] When considering the level of care recommended for an individual woman, her specific risk factors as well as her needs and concerns must be the first consideration.

Effectiveness of Prenatal Care

Despite significant expansion of the content within prenatal care in the United States, since the mid-1980s, rates of negative birth outcomes such as low birth weight and preterm birth have remained elevated—especially among African American women.[10] Although women who access prenatal care have lower rates of low-birth-weight infants, it is not clear if prenatal care is responsible or if healthier women are better able to access care. This conundrum has haunted the research on effectiveness of prenatal care, and the question remains unresolved.

Much of the existing research on the effectiveness of prenatal care has focused on gestational age at initiation of care or number of visits, finding that more care is associated with better outcomes.[11] However, research to determine the effectiveness of individual components of prenatal care is sorely lacking.[11,12] Additionally, little is known about whether prenatal care affects current or future health behaviors of women and their families.[11] In contrast, ongoing research related to "nontraditional" models of prenatal care such as group prenatal care, home visits, telemedicine, and reduced numbers of visits for low-risk women suggests that these approaches hold promise in this area.[12]

The Role of Midwifery in Provision of Prenatal Care

In the United States, midwifery has a long history and central role in the provision of prenatal care.[13] Some of the initial publications that first documented the effectiveness of midwifery were related to prenatal care. Midwifery in the United States has shown demonstrable benefits in improving many pregnancy outcomes, including lower rates of preterm labor, decreased low birth weight, increased access to care, and lower rates of morbidity and mortality.[13]

The benefits of midwifery care have been demonstrated internationally as well. For instance, in a review of the literature comparing midwife-led care versus physician-led and shared care models of prenatal care from 11 studies in four developed nations, midwife-led care for low-risk women showed benefits in outcomes such as decreased prenatal hospitalization, decreased need for analgesia/anesthesia in labor, decreased number of operative deliveries, fewer episiotomies, and more breastfeeding initiation.[14] Midwifery care in underdeveloped nations has a well-recognized essential role in preventing adverse pregnancy outcomes as discussed in the *International Midwifery and Safe Motherhood* chapter.

When providing prenatal care, midwives work in partnership with the pregnant woman to help support the normal physiologic processes of pregnancy. Skills in culturally competent communication and counseling are integral.

Basic Definitions

The prenatal period covers the time from the first day of the last normal menstrual period to the start of true labor, which marks the beginning of the intrapartum period. **Table 22-1** summarizes the obstetric nomenclature used to signal how many pregnancies (*gravida*, from the Latin word *gravidus*, which means "pregnant") and births (*para*, from the Latin word *parous*, which means "bringing forth or producing") a woman has experienced. Interestingly, there is no clear standard for how these terms are defined, and there is variability in how they are used. Conversely, it is important that the terms are used correctly with an accepted set of definitions.[15,16] The definitions listed in this chapter are those recommended in most obstetric texts. Because parity does not reflect all the possible outcomes of birth, a four-digit system, TPAL is used to better describe a woman's birth history.

Duration of Pregnancy

Gestational Age Versus Embryonic Age

Fertilization takes place at the time of ovulation, which is usually about 14 days after the last menstrual period, assuming a 28-day cycle. Therefore, gestation is approximately 266 days or 38 weeks in length after fertilization. Women are not usually aware of the date of fertilization, but they typically do know the date of their last menstrual period.

Thus, historically, a woman's due date is calculated as 40 weeks (280 days) after her last menstrual period. The terms "gestational age" or "weeks' gestation" are used to refer to the number of weeks subsequent to the last menstrual period. The mean gestational age (i.e., menstrual age) for spontaneous labor in primigravid women is 41 weeks from the last menstrual period (287 days), or 40 weeks 3 days (283 days) for the multiparous woman.[17] Estimates based on pooled data are consistent with this finding and suggest that the mean menstrual age for pregnancy is 283 to 284 days.[17]

The study of embryology prefers language referring to "embryonic age," "postconceptional age," or "ovulation age," reflecting the more precise age of the embryo or fetus. A postconceptional age differs from a gestational age by 2 weeks. When reviewing information about embryonic development or exposure to teratogenic agents, the reader is cautioned to carefully verify which type of calendar weeks is being used—gestational or postconceptional—to avoid confusion.

Trimesters

The prenatal period is divided into three trimesters, which are not evenly divided into 13 weeks or 3 calendar months. In practice, the first trimester is considered to be weeks 1 to 12 (12 weeks) because organogenesis is completed at the end of 12 weeks and the risk for spontaneous abortion is significantly reduced at this time. Historically, the second trimester was considered to be weeks 13 to 28 because prior to the introduction of modern neonatal intensive care techniques 28 weeks was the limit of viability. The third trimester extends from weeks 28 to 40. The term "post dates" or "post term" is typically used to describe a pregnancy beyond 40 weeks.

Estimated Due Date

For many years, the expected date of the end of pregnancy by birth of a full-term newborn was called the estimated date of confinement (EDC). While this term is still used in many settings, a number of healthcare professionals have changed it to estimated date of delivery or estimated due date (EDD). This change was introduced because of a feeling that the word "confinement" connotes illness, limitation, and a passive role based on an archaic practice of isolating women in late pregnancy rather than recognizing pregnancy as a normal event, a healthy process, with active participation. Although there is no national consensus regarding the use of EDC versus EDD, the term used throughout this book is estimated due date or EDD.

Table 22-1	Obstetric Nomenclature
Obstetric Term	**Definitions**
Gravida	The total number of times a woman has been pregnant, regardless of whether the pregnancy resulted in a termination or if multiple infants were born from a pregnancy. A current pregnancy is included in the gravida count.
Nulligravida	A woman who has never been pregnant.
Primigravida	A woman who is pregnant for the first time.
Secundigravida	A woman pregnant for the second time.
Multigravida	A woman who has been pregnant more than twice.
Para	The number of times a woman has given birth to a fetus of at least 20 gestational weeks (viable or not viable), counting multiple births as one birth "event."
Nullipara	A woman who has not remained pregnant beyond 20 weeks' gestation.
Primipara	A woman who has had one pregnancy in which the fetus or fetuses reached 20 weeks' gestation. This woman has given birth once.
Multipara	A woman who has had two or more pregnancies in which the fetus or fetuses reached 20 weeks' gestation. This woman has given birth more than once (counting multiple births as one birth "event").
Gravida/para two-digit nomenclature	Notation of gravida and para status are essential terms used to describe a woman's reproductive history and status. • G2P0: A woman who has been pregnant twice and no births. She may have had abortions or miscarriages. • G2P2: A woman who is currently pregnant, and she had one pregnancy that resulted in an infant born at 38 weeks' gestation.
Gravida/para TPAL four-digit nomenclature	**Term (T):** The number of term births the woman has experienced. Term refers to any gestation of 37 completed weeks or more. **Preterm (P):** The number of preterm births the woman has experienced. Premature in this system refers to any infant born between 20 and 37 completed gestational weeks. **Abortions (A):** The number of pregnancies ending in abortion (either spontaneous or induced). Abortion refers to any fetus delivered before 20 weeks' gestation. **Living (L):** The number of children currently living. Examples: • G3 P2002: A woman who is currently pregnant with her third pregnancy. She gave birth to a full-term baby with each prior pregnancy, both of whom are living. • G2 P0101: A woman who is currently pregnant. She gave birth to one preterm infant and has one live child. • G2 P1103: A woman who is currently pregnant. She gave birth to one full-term infant and preterm twins. All three offspring are alive.

Diagnosis of Pregnancy and Calculation of Gestational Age

Although it is best to conduct the "first" prenatal visit preconceptionally as discussed in the *Preconception Care* chapter, many women are pregnant at the time they seek care. When a woman presents for an initial visit during pregnancy, the first goal for this encounter has three subcomponents: (1) confirm the pregnancy, (2) establish a gestational age, and (3) determine if the pregnancy is viable. Signs and symptoms of pregnancy have historically been categorized into presumptive, probable, and positive signs (**Table 22-2**). While differentiation between these categories is not typically clinically significant today, the importance of these categories remains conceptually important. The distinctions between these categories help the midwife discern those signs or symptoms that (1) grouped together are associated with pregnancy or (2) as single symptoms may potentially be secondary to other causes.

Presumptive symptoms of pregnancy are maternal physiologic changes that the *woman* experiences and that in most cases indicate to her that she is pregnant. Probable signs of pregnancy are maternal physiologic and anatomic changes that are detected upon examination and documented by the *examiner*. Positive signs are those that confirm the pregnancy

Table 22-2	Signs and Symptoms of Pregnancy

Presumptive Signs of Pregnancy (Reported by a Woman on History)

Cessation of menstruation in a woman who previously experienced regular cycles

Nausea and vomiting

Tingling, tenderness, increased nodularity, and/or enlargement of the breasts or nipples

Increased urinary frequency

Fatigue

Sustained elevated basal body temperature (in the absence of infection)

Skin pigmentation changes (e.g., chloasma, linea nigra)

Probable Signs of Pregnancy (Detected by Physical Examination or Laboratory Testing)

Breast changes (e.g., expression of colostrum, enlargement of breasts and nipples)

Skin changes (e.g., chloasma, linea nigra, abdominal striae)

Enlargement of the abdomen

Enlargement of the uterus

Palpable fetal outline

Ballottement

Piskacek's sign

Hegar's sign

Goodell's sign

Chadwick's sign

Palpation of Braxton Hicks contractions

Positive pregnancy test

Palpable fetal movement

Positive Signs of Pregnancy (Confirms Pregnancy)

Sonographic evidence of pregnancy

Audible fetal heart rate

with certainty, although the viability of the fetus may not be assured.

Confirming Pregnancy: Hormonal Pregnancy Tests

The use of a woman's urine to detect pregnancy has a long history. In ancient Egypt, urine was poured over wheat or barley. The growth or nongrowth of the grain was interpreted as a sign of pregnancy or nonpregnancy, respectively.[18] Interpretation of different characteristics of urine was also used in the Middle Ages and up to the twentieth century. Starting in the late 1920s, morning urine was injected into female mice or rabbits, which were then euthanized to detect changes in their ovaries. This test was the

standard pregnancy test for more than 40 years until the 1960s, when immunoassays of human chorionic gonadotropin (hCG) were developed.[18] Current tests consist of immunosorbent assays of monoclonal antibodies to the hCG beta subunit that provide reliable results a few weeks after fertilization.

A qualitative assessment of the presence of the beta subunit of hCG in urine is the basis of the pregnancy tests used in health care facilities and also marketed as home pregnancy tests today. Detection of hCG in plasma can occur as early as 8 to 11 days after fertilization; by the time of the missed menses, hCG is typically detectable in plasma and urine with levels ranging from 50 to 250 mIU/L.[19]

Commercially available urine pregnancy tests can be highly reliable if used correctly. The theoretical effectiveness of home pregnancy tests is superior to typical-use testing, however, and some reports indicate their sensitivity is as low as 75%. False-negative results are more likely if the test is performed prior to the first day of the expected menstrual period.[20] As many as 10% of viable pregnancies do not implant by the first day of the missed menstrual period and, therefore, would register as false-negative pregnancy tests if testing is done at that time.[20]

It is important to note that a positive pregnancy test does not offer any information about the viability of the pregnancy. The percentage of pregnancies that are detected very early and result in a spontaneous abortion has been found to range between 20% and 62%.[21,22]

Serum beta-hCG can be measured as a qualitative "present" or "absent" value or as single values of quantitative serum beta-hCG levels. In early pregnancy, the production of hCG increases exponentially, doubling approximately every 1.5 to 3 days in the first 5 to 6 weeks and then doubling every 3 to 3.5 days in weeks 7 to 8 until it peaks at about 8 to 10 weeks' gestation[17,23–26] (**Table 22-3**). However, there is some variability in the rate that hCG rises in maternal plasma. The embryo may still be viable even if the beta-hCG rises but does not double in 48 hours.[23]

A single quantitative serum beta-hCG value does not provide any information about normal development of the embryo, as individual values at specific gestational ages are highly variable. Therefore, serial quantitative values of serum beta-hCG— at least two values obtained at least 48 to 72 hours apart—are often used to help determine the viability of an early pregnancy, to detect a spontaneous or missed abortion, and to monitor for the presence of an ectopic pregnancy.

Quantitative serum beta-hCG values are often used in conjunction with an early ultrasound and other clinical data to help the midwife determine the

Table 22-3	Discriminatory Levels of Human Chorionic Gonadotropin Levels and Ultrasound Findings by Gestational Age[a]	
Gestational Age in Weeks from LMP	**beta-hCG Level**	**Ultrasound Findings**
3–4 weeks	150–1000 mIU/mL	Decidual thickening
4–5 weeks	> 1000–2000 mIU/mL	Gestational sac visible with TVUS when beta-hCG is approximately 1000 mIU/mL and detectable on abdominal ultrasound when beta-HCG is approximately 1800 mIU/mL
5–6 weeks	1000–7200 mIU/mL	Yolk sac present when gestational sac is larger than 10 mm Embryo present when gestational sac is larger than18 mm Cardiac activity present when crown rump length is greater than 5 mm
6–7 weeks	> 10,800 mIU/mL	Crown-rump length 4–9 mm

TVUS = transvaginal ultrasound.

[a]beta-hCG values are approximate. Each ultrasound department will have institutionally specific values that can be used to guide management.

Source: Adapted from Snell BJ. Assessment and management of bleeding in the first trimester of pregnancy. *J Midwifery Women's Health.* 2009;54:483-491.

presence and viability of an intrauterine pregnancy. For example, when the serum beta-hCG is at least 1500–2000 mIU/L, the value is usually considered to be in the clinical "discriminatory zone," whereby an intrauterine gestational sac should typically be visualized on transvaginal ultrasound.[24–26]

Establishing Gestational Age and Estimated Due Date

Accurate assessment of gestational age is one of the most critical judgments a midwife makes during the course of caring for a pregnant woman. Incorrect estimation of the duration of a pregnancy can lead to inappropriate timing for screening, misinterpretation of data, unnecessary intervention, or a failure to intervene when indicated.[27] Gestational age at the time for birth is the single most valuable predictor of infant health, and timing of an induction of labor is determined by the assessed gestational age. In general, the opportunity for accurate assessment of gestational age decreases with the passage of time. Documenting all available data that will assist in establishing an accurate gestational age as early in pregnancy as possible is an essential part of prenatal care. Several methods can be used to calculate the EDD, all of which have some variability. **Table 22-4** summarizes the range of accuracy of various EDD calculation methods.[28–31]

Estimated Due Date via Last Menstrual Period

The date of the first day of the last menstrual period (LMP) or last normal menstrual period (LNMP) is used as the baseline for an initial determination of gestational age and the EDD. Some women do

not keep a record of their menstrual periods, while other women will have a history of irregular cycles or amenorrhea, which can make determination of a reliable LNMP difficult or not possible. Other confounding variables that may influence the reliability of an LMP date include a woman's use of various medications that affect menses, recent changes in weight, as well as continuing to breastfeed an older child. It is also important to bear in mind that LMP refers to the *first day* of the woman's last normal menstrual period. Some women will mistakenly provide the last day of their last normal menstrual period, unless this point is clarified.

While many women can accurately recall the date of LMP within 1 to 2 days,[32] the reported LMP can also be inaccurate. Women often demonstrate a number preference when reporting LMP with the 15th of the month stated more frequently than other dates. Digit preference extends the EDD by approximately 2.8 days when compared to ultrasound dating.[33]

It is not uncommon for a woman to experience some spotting at the time of implantation of the blastocyst as a result of the invasive activity of the chorionic villi in the endometrial lining. Because implantation in a woman with a 28-day cycle can occur close to the time she would be expecting a menstrual period, a woman can misinterpret this spotting from implantation as a light menstrual period.

Therefore, after determining the date of the LMP, the next step is to inquire whether the LMP was a "normal" period for the woman. To do this, obtain a menstrual history and compare her description of her last menstrual period with her description of her regular menstrual periods. For example, if the woman reports an LMP that was scanty and short when her usual menses were moderately heavy for the first 2 days and had a duration of 5 days, then it is possible that the LMP she reports could have been related to bleeding that was from a source different than the normal monthly cyclic bleed. In this event, questioning the woman about the period before the so-called last one is in order. If this preceding period were normal for her, then it is the one that would be considered her LNMP.

Traditionally the EDD is initially calculated by Naegele's rule (**Box 22-1**), which is based on the assumption of a 28-day menstrual cycle. Franz Karl

Naegele, a German physician, authored a text published in 1812 that contained the advice to estimate that a pregnancy would terminate approximately 40 weeks (280 days) after the first day of the last menstrual period.[32,34] Although this theory is not based on any modern concept of research and its accuracy has been questioned,[32,35] it remains widely used today and is the basis of many pregnancy calculators.

The use of the LMP to calculate an EDD is somewhat reliable (with a 10-day margin of error) if the woman has experienced regular cycles, has recorded her menstrual history, and has not used hormonal contraceptives for at least 3 months prior to conception.[36] However, the length of the menstrual cycle in women who have regular cycles can vary between 23 and 32 days (mean = 27.7; standard deviation = 2.4).[37] The LMP may also be unreliable because there can be considerable variability in the preovulatory interval as well as the timing of implantation. Usually, ovulation occurs approximately 14 days before the next menstrual period and the duration of follicular phase is typically more variable than the luteal phase. Therefore, a woman with a longer follicular phase and, hence, a longer menstrual cycle (more than 28 days) will actually begin her pregnancy later in relation to the LMP and will deliver at a correspondingly later date. Similarly, there can be variation in the timing of implantation, which can occur 5 to 14 days after the ovulatory window.[37] Thus calculation of the EDD using the LMP and Naegele's rule is at best an approximation, as it is the middle of a 10-day time period during which a term infant is most likely to be born and this range is considered physiologically normal.[32,36]

Table 22-4	Criteria and Range of Accuracy for Dating Pregnancy
Clinical or Sonographic Parameters	**Variability Estimates**
Intrauterine insemination or embryo transfer[a]	± 1 day
Ovulation induction[a]	± 3 days
Artificial insemination[a]	± 3 days
Single intercourse record[a]	± 3 days
Basal body temperature chart with coital record, ovulation, and temperature elevation, combined with previous menstrual record	± 2–5 days
Last menstrual period that is normal, regular, and certain	± 10 days
First-trimester ultrasound	± 5 days
Second-trimester ultrasound	± 10 days
Third-trimester ultrasound	± 15 days
First-trimester physical examination of fundal height	± 2 weeks
Second-trimester physical examination of fundal height	± 4 weeks
Third-trimester physical examination of fundal height	± 6 weeks

[a]These are indicators of conception age (menstrual age = conception age + 14 days).

Sources: Adapted from Frank-Herrmann P, Freundl G, Baur S, et al. Effectiveness and acceptability of the symptothermal method of natural family planning in Germany. *Am J Obstet Gynecol.* 1991;165:2008-2011; Chervenak FA, Skupski DW, Romero R, et al. How accurate is fetal biometry in the assessment of fetal age? *Am J Obstet Gynecol.* 1998;178:678-687; Mongelli M, Chew S, Yuxin NG, Biswas A. Third-trimester ultrasound dating algorithms from pregnancies conceived with artificial reproductive techniques. *Ultrasound Obstet Gynecol.* 2005;26:129-131; Hunter L. Issues in pregnancy dating: revisiting the evidence. *J Midwifery Women's Health.* 2009;54:184-190.

BOX 22-1 Naegele's Rule

To use Naegele's rule, 7 days are added to the LMP and then 3 months are subtracted in order to obtain the EDD. For LMPs that occur after the first 3 months of the year, an additional year will be added.

First day of LMP + 7 days – 3 months = EDD

Be careful to use the actual number of days in the month of the LMP if adding 7 days crosses over to the next month. This is illustrated in the following example of calculating the EDD by Naegele's rule: If the LMP is May 28, then 5/28 + 7 days = 6/4 (May has 31 days) – 3 months = EDD is March 4 of the next year. Note that Naegele's rule does not account for the additional day in a leap year.

Information that is supplemental to the LMP, and helpful in validating the EDD, includes coital timing (inclusion or exclusion dates for exposure to conception), use (or not) of contraception (i.e., type, timing, consistency), and date(s), type, and result(s) of any home ovulation timing or pregnancy test that the woman has done prior to seeking prenatal care. When a pregnancy was conceived via an artificial reproductive technique, a woman will know the date of insemination or embryo transfer, and this information can then be used to calculate the EDD.

Estimated Due Date via Pregnancy Wheels

Many drug companies manufacture pregnancy wheels. These instruments have been widely used in obstetrics to calculate EDD and determine gestational age.[32] There can be up to a 5-day difference between different wheels, however, and there has been little investigation of this problem or attempt to standardize the pregnancy wheels. Computer-based software designed for mobile devices or use on the Internet may be more accurate and have less variation between proprietary or free software. For example, the software may reflect calendar variations such as leap years that are unable to be reflected when wheels are used. However, the issue of accuracy of these methods has not been investigated to date.

Estimated Due Date via First-Trimester Ultrasound

Women can become pregnant without having a recent LMP. For example, conception can occur while a woman is breastfeeding and amenorrheic, or it may occur before regular menstruation is established after termination of a pregnancy or discontinuation of hormonal birth control methods. In such instances, the EDD is based on clinical findings and an ultrasound. Ultrasound determination of gestational age is most accurate when it is performed in the first trimester, when fetal biometry is most accurate.[29] Reliability of ultrasound results depends on the gestational age at assessment, the skill of the examiner, the technology available, and the position of the fetus. First-trimester ultrasound estimates based on accurate measurement of crown–rump length are accurate to within 5 days.[30] Second-trimester ultrasound estimates of fetal age are based on combined measurements of the head circumference, biparietal diameter, femur length, and abdominal circumference to give an estimate that is within 7 days of the subsequent date of birth.[29,30]

Last Menstrual Period and Ultrasound Dating Discrepancies

Occasionally, an ultrasound gestational age will change the EDD that was calculated on the basis of the LMP. Because there is some variability in both calculations, the general recommendation is the following: If the ultrasound were performed in the first trimester, the LMP-calculated EDD should be changed to the ultrasound-calculated EDD if there is more than a 7-day discrepancy between the two EDDs. If the ultrasound were performed in the second trimester, the EDD should be changed to the ultrasound-calculated EDD if there is a 10-day discrepancy between the two calculated EDDs.[38] Ultrasound dating has a consistent margin of error of 8%.[32,39] This factor can be used to determine which EDD is the most reliable.

Less Reliable Methods of Dating Pregnancy

Careful review of the literature reveals that although uterine size correlates positively with gestational age, fundal measurement is a much less reliable predictor of EDD than the LMP.[27,40–42] Clinical assessment of uterine size may be affected by distension of the bladder (up to 7 cm), and/or maternal body mass index (BMI),[42] retroversion or retroflexion of the uterus, presence of fibroids, uterine anomaly, position and presentation of the fetus, amniotic fluid volume, and clinician experience.[27] Optimally, symphyseal-fundal heights should be measured by the same professional throughout the pregnancy and in a standard method. There is a common tendency to assess the uterine size as "appropriate for dates" if the menstrual history is known.[39,40] The closest correlation between the fundal height (measured in centimeters) and gestational age (expressed in weeks from the LMP) is most likely between 20 and 32 gestational weeks, when the number of weeks of gestation is close to the number of centimeters measured between the symphysis and fundus.[39] However, the correlation between gestational weeks and fundal heights depends on several factors including maternal habitus and fetal lie. For example, a petite woman who is only 5 feet (1.5 meters) tall may have different fundal measurements than a taller woman of 6 feet (1.8 meters) in height at the same point in pregnancy. Similarly women with different degrees of abdominal fat such as a woman with a BMI of 19 compared to another woman with a BMI of 40 also can have different measurements. The fundus of a uterus containing a fetus in a transverse lie is lower than one for an unengaged fetus in a vertex presentation.

In clinical practice many midwives commonly use a rule of 2 centimeters or 3 centimeters. That is, during 20-32 gestational weeks a woman should have a fundal measurement in centimeters within 2-3 of the number of gestational weeks. No strong evidence supports this approach, most likely because of the maternal and fetal variations noted above. But this deviation from the 2 or 3 rule of thumb alerts the midwife to carefully assess for size dates discordance. Assessment methods range from use of low technology such as verification of an empty maternal bladder and careful Leopold's maneuvers to use of high technology such as ultrasound dating. Fundal heights are continued to be measured until the woman begins labor because steady growth over the last weeks of pregnancy provides reassurance of fetal weight and a wide variation may suggest growth restriction and/or abnormalities of the amniotic fluid. Therefore, if a variation of more than 2 or 3 cm between the fundal height and gestational age is noted, the first step might be to verify that the woman has an empty bladder. If the measurement is still discordant, further investigation of dating should be undertaken—for example, obtaining an ultrasound.

Other indicators such as the onset of quickening along with the clinician's notation of first fetal heart tones by ultrasound or fetoscope or the client's signs and symptoms of pregnancy, are poor predictors of gestational age.[39] However, in low-resource settings, multiple measures of fundal height using a consistent technique can improve estimation of gestational age.[43] **Appendix 22A** reviews reliable methods of determining fundal height.

Maternal Psychological Adjustment

Pregnancy is a time of transition from life circumstances before the addition of a child to the realities of life that include the child. This change can pose psychological challenges. In addition, the emotional experience of pregnancy is different for every woman and every pregnancy. The prenatal period is also a time that family roles and relationships change. The transition to new role expectations can result in varying amounts of turmoil and disruption or, conversely, newfound closeness. Although several sources codify the changes in psychological adaption, each woman and each pregnancy is unique and should not be stereotyped. The following discussion is based on broad groups of women.

First Trimester

Women experience a wide range of emotions upon learning that they are pregnant. Negative reactions to the pregnancy can be part of a normal adaptive response.

The first trimester can also be a time of anxiety as women wait for the pregnancy to be "well established" and then wait for the results of tests for birth defects if these tests have been performed. It is not uncommon for women to feel as if they cannot relax and believe in the pregnancy until after the first trimester, and they may delay telling family or friends about the pregnancy. Other women need the support of their family and friends as they cope with symptoms such as nausea and vomiting and other physical changes in their bodies.

Second Trimester

The second trimester is generally a time of increasingly inward focus and orientation.[44] Quickening or a second-trimester ultrasound may enable the woman to conceptualize her fetus as an individual separate from herself.[45]

Third Trimester

Preparation for childbirth and parenthood occurs in the third trimester as the woman's attention focuses on the forthcoming newborn. A number of fears may surface during the third trimester. Rarely, the woman may fear for her own life and the life of her child; she may worry that she will have a baby with physical or other abnormalities; she may fear labor and birth (pain, loss of control, the unknown). More commonly, she may have concerns that she will not know when she is in labor or that she will not handle the pain of labor well.

It is important that the midwife understand the wide range of normal reactions to pregnancy and to the transition to motherhood, and be able to provide reassurance as well as anticipatory guidance to women who may be concerned about the emotions they are experiencing. Listening to a woman's concerns and normalizing her experience during pregnancy has been identified in the literature as significantly important to her experience of quality prenatal care.[46]

The Initial Prenatal Visit

The initial prenatal visit consists of a complete history, a physical and pelvic examination, and a number of laboratory and adjunctive studies. This visit may require confirmation of pregnancy via one of the methods mentioned earlier in this chapter.

Options Counseling

A woman may come for an initial prenatal visit prior to having made the decision to continue the pregnancy. Therefore reviewing a woman's options about continuing the pregnancy is an essential initial topic for discussion. There are three alternatives depending on the gestational age at which she is first seen: (1) continue the pregnancy and parent the child, (2) continue the pregnancy and place the infant for adoption, and (3) terminate the pregnancy with an abortion if the gestational age is within the allowable time frame. Options counseling is reviewed in detail in the *Family Planning* chapter.

History

When the midwife ascertains that the woman chooses to remain pregnant and pursue prenatal care, a complete history is obtained, including past medical and surgical history, along with family, genetic, social, menstrual, obstetric, gynecologic, sexual, and contraceptive history. The conditions in a woman's medical history that increase her risk for adverse obstetric outcomes are listed in **Table 22-5**. All current medications and allergies are noted. Emphasis is placed on obtaining the date of her last normal menstrual period, calculation of an EDD, determination of the present number of weeks' gestation, and calculation of her gravida and para status.

In planning the sequence in which information is to be obtained during a visit, it may be best to start with the present pregnancy history, although variations can occur based upon the situation. Allowing the visit to be prioritized by the woman's primary concern facilitates obtaining all other information and helps establish a therapeutic relationship.

Physical Examination

A complete physical examination, as presented in the *Introduction to the Care of Women* chapter, is performed during the initial prenatal visit. Additional physical examinations specific for pregnant women include a pelvic examination with clinical pelvimetry and obstetric abdominal examination with auscultation for fetal heart tones if gestational age permits. The techniques for these examinations are detailed in Appendix 22A and **Appendix 22B**.

Some women may be reluctant or decline to have a pelvic examination for personal or cultural reasons. Under no circumstances should a woman be forced or pressured into a pelvic examination. The midwife may explain the benefits of doing the examination and the information that can be obtained from the pelvic examination, but the woman is entitled to decline or to defer the exam to another time.

Laboratory Tests and Adjunctive Studies

Box 22-2 reviews the standard laboratory assessments that are recommended at the initial visit, and **Box 22-3** lists the tests that are recommended for individuals on the basis of their past medical history, race, ethnicity, and other individual factors. The first prenatal visit includes counseling about the benefits and risks of recommended tests, alternatives to them, and documentation if a woman declines a test, including the reasons she provides for declining.

Assessment and Management Plan

At the end of the first prenatal visit, an assessment of the status of the woman's health is made and a plan for follow-up care is developed (**Box 22-4**).

Counseling and Anticipatory Guidance

Anticipatory guidance and instruction at the end of an initial prenatal visit can encompass many health education topics, but should always include instruction about warning or danger signs (**Box 22-5**), an orientation to the plan of care, and information about how to contact the midwife.

Documentation

Thorough and articulate documentation is essential for many reasons. The midwife will need a clear record of personal thought processes, rationales for any interventions, and plan for the visit and follow-up, so that in the future plans that were made can be continued by the same or different provider. Thorough documentation helps codify details that may be forgotten in the interim between visits. Such details also can be used to justify billing and coding for the level of service provided at each visit. Office visits are billed and reimbursed at different rates depending on the level of care, and the level of care is demonstrated by the number of procedures performed, the number of systems assessed, and other measurements of the of care provided. Accurate documentation is critical to support billing and coding and to avoid any appearance of fraud. It is also critical to support the midwife's care if the care given is reviewed at a later date secondary to an unexpected adverse event or review for reimbursement.

Subsequent Prenatal Visits

A template for the basic components for follow-up prenatal visits can be found in **Box 22-6**.

Review of the Prenatal Record

Immediately before seeing a woman for an interval prenatal care visit, the woman's record should be reviewed to determine her EDD, any significant problems that have been noted on a problem list, medications, treatments, and dietary interventions, as well as results of laboratory tests or ultrasound

Table 22-5	Essential Components History at an Initial Prenatal Visit
History Element	**Clinical Significance**
Present pregnancy	Risks for adverse obstetric outcomes: • Signs of pregnancy complications such as cramping, bleeding, or excessive vomiting in the first trimester; signs of preterm labor or preeclampsia in the late second and early third trimesters • Signs of medical complications such as fever, dysuria, rashes • Extreme discomforts of pregnancy • Exposures to teratogens such as drugs or medications, street drugs, alcohol, tobacco, X rays, environmental exposures, occupational exposures
Medical history	Medical conditions that are associated with increased risks for adverse maternal or fetal outcomes, such as diabetes or hypertension, indicate a need for consultation, collaboration, co-management, or referral to a physician.
Surgical history	Uterine surgery such as cesarean section or myomectomy may indicate a need for a repeat cesarean section or physician consultation. If the woman had a prior cesarean section, several additional items need to be discussed: (1) the availability of VBAC, (2) her interest in TOLAC, and (3) whether TOLAC is indicated given her obstetric history will need to be explored. Any significant surgeries on vital organs such as heart, lungs, or kidneys.
Family history	Evidence of genetic disorders such as hemophilia, cystic fibrosis, or mental retardation that may suggest the need for specific genetic counseling or tests.
Social history	Risks that indicate a need for social service or psychology consultation or referral: • Living situation: barriers to care such as transportation, job hours • Stressors: history of sexual abuse, IPV, or emotional abuse
Menstrual history	The menstrual history will determine the reliability of the LMP for use in calculating an EDD: • Regularity of cycles • Cycle length
Obstetric history	A detailed obstetric history is warranted at the initial visit, noting anything that could raise or lower risk or affect care in the current pregnancy: • Gravida, para-TPAL • Dates of previous births, as well as weights of newborns • Pregnancy complications such as gestational diabetes • Birth complications: mode of birth, vaginal lacerations, or episiotomies • Postpartum complications
Gynecologic history	Gynecologic conditions that can adversely affect a current pregnancy: • Past or current STIs, especially herpes simplex virus and HIV • Diagnosed malformations of the reproductive tract • History of female genital cutting or female circumcision • Procedures for treatment of abnormal cervical cytology • Vulvovaginal disorders • Exposure to diethylstilbesterol (DES) in utero
Sexual history	Sexual history can reveal a risk for STIs: • Sexual activity: number of current partners and number of partners in the last year; gender of partners (male, female, or both) • Use of barrier methods for prevention of infections
Contraceptive history	Recent use of hormonal methods may affect accurate dating of the pregnancy: What was the last form of contraception used and when was it discontinued?
Current medications	Medications that can adversely affect a pregnancy need to be identified as soon as possible: • Current medications, dose, and duration of treatment • Vitamins • Regular use of over-the-counter products
Allergies	If the woman reports an allergy, document the allergic response (e.g., anaphylaxis versus rash): • Allergies to medications • Allergies to foods or environmental exposures

EDD = estimated due date; IPV = interpersonal violence; LMP = last menstrual period; STI = sexually transmitted infection; TOLAC = trial of labor after cesarean; VBAC = vaginal birth after cesarean.

BOX 22-2 Common Laboratory Tests for the Initial Visit During Pregnancy

Blood Tests

Blood type

Rhesus (Rh) type and antibody screen

Hemoglobin, hematocrit, and mean corpuscular volume (MCV), or complete blood count (CBC) to include platelet count

Hepatitis B surface antigen (HbsAg)

Human immunodeficiency virus (HIV) screening test

Syphilis screening test (RPR/VDRL)

Rubella titer for immunity

Varicella titer if unknown status

Hemoglobin A1c, random blood glucose, or fasting blood glucose[a]

Urine Tests

Urinalysis or urine dipstick for protein

Urine culture with sensitivities if bacteria are detected

Cultures

Chlamydia screening (often is combined with gonorrhea screening)

Screening Tests

Tuberculin test (PPD)

Pap test if indicated

Additional Tests Based on Gestational Age

18–20 weeks: Ultrasound to confirm gestational age and screen for cardiac anomalies

24–28 weeks: Screen for gestational diabetes

Additional Tests Based on Past Medical History and Demographic Characteristics

History of aneuploidy: CVS or amniocentesis

Intravenous drug use: hepatitis C screening

Tests for diabetes if risk factors present[a]:

- Hemoglobin A1c, fasting blood glucose level
  - Diabetes or history of glucose intolerance
  - History of gestational diabetes mellitus

- BMI > 25
- Older than age 25 years
- History of macrosomia or stillbirth
- First-degree relative with diabetes
- Non-white race

- Test for gonorrhea if risk factors present:
  - Living in an area with high prevalence
  - Report of a new sexual partner
  - Multiple sexual partners
  - History of an STI, or commercial sex worker
  - Age less than 25 years
  - Previous gonorrhea infection

- Lead level if lead exposure risk factors:
  - Recent immigration from an area where the ambient lead contamination is high
  - Residence near a point source of lead
  - Working with lead or living with a person who works with lead
  - Using lead-glazed ceramic pottery
  - Pica
  - Using imported cosmetics or imported food products
  - Using alternative medicines, herbs, or therapies
  - Remodeling a home without lead hazard controls in place
  - Lead-contaminated drinking water
  - Living with someone who has an elevated lead level

- Thyroid function (TSH, T_4) if thyroid disorder risk factors:
  - History of thyroid surgery
  - Hypothyroidism or hyperthyroidism
  - History of multiple miscarriages
  - Goiter or symptoms of thyroid disease

CVS = chorionic villus sampling; STI = sexually transmitted infection; TSH = thyroid-stimulating hormone.

[a]Screening for diabetes is routine in some institutions but not others. It is currently recommended by the International Association of the Diabetes and Pregnancy Study Groups (IADPSG), but not by other professional associations.

BOX 22-3 Genetic Tests Offered at the Initial Prenatal Visit

Genetic Screening Based on Gestational Age at Initial Visit

- Down syndrome screening[a]:
  - 10–14 weeks: first-trimester screening (nuchal translucency ultrasound, PAPP-A, and free beta-hCG blood values)
  - 15–18 weeks: integrated or sequential second-trimester screening
- Down syndrome diagnosis:
  - 10–14 weeks: chorionic villus sampling
  - 12–22 weeks: amniocentesis
  - Anytime if available: direct DNA diagnostic screening

[a]The American College of Obstetricians and Gynecologists recommends that all women be offered invasive testing, regardless of their risk factors.

Genetic Tests Based on Race or Ethnicity

African American	Hemoglobin electrophoresis or sickle cell prep if not already known
Ashkenazi Jewish	Canavan disease, cystic fibrosis, familial dysautonomia, Tay-Sachs disease, Gaucher's disease, Niemann-Pick disease, Bloom syndrome, mucolipidosis IV, Fanconi anemia Group C
African	Sickle cell disease or trait, thalassemia
Asian: Southeast Asian or Chinese	Alpha thalassemia
Asian: Indian	Beta thalassemia
Cajun or French-Canadian	Tay-Sachs disease
Caucasian	Cystic fibrosis

BOX 22-4 Assessment and Management Plan Following an Initial Prenatal Visit

Essential Assessments

1. Diagnosis of pregnancy: Viable, risk for miscarriage, or nonviable?
2. Estimation of gestational age and EDD
3. Any medical or obstetric risk factors
4. Are the woman's reported symptoms normal symptoms of pregnancy or possible complications?
5. Individual learning needs
6. Recommended laboratory tests
7. Is there a need for immediate physician consultation or collaborative management with other healthcare team members?
8. Indicated referrals such as genetic counseling, social services, and nutritionist
9. Are any medications for treatment of minor complications (e.g., vaginitis, asymptomatic bacteriuria, anemia) needed at this time?

Plan of Care

1. Confirm all assessments with the woman
2. Orient to prenatal care, prenatal care providers, and recommended plan of care
3. Arrange for all necessary referrals
4. Arrange for recommended laboratory tests
5. Prescribe any needed medications
6. Schedule return visit
7. Health education topics for initial visit
   - Avoidance of alcohol, drugs, smoking cessation
   - Safe use of medications
   - Common discomforts and relief measures
   - When to call the midwife/warning signs
8. Reconfirm that she understands the recommendations

BOX 22-5 Warning Signs of Pregnancy Complications

First Trimester

- Vaginal bleeding
- Persistent nausea and vomiting
- Fever, chills
- Dysuria, hematuria, or inability to void

Second and Third Trimesters

- Leaking of fluid or abnormal vaginal discharge
- Sudden, sharp, or continuing abdominal cramping or pain
- Vaginal bleeding
- Contractions or cramping

- Pelvic pressure
- Persistent backache
- Persistent severe headache unrelieved by over-the-counter pain relievers
- Facial edema, edema of the hands, or unilateral lower-extremity edema
- Visual changes (e.g., blurring of vision, dizziness, spots before eyes)
- Decreased fetal movement
- Fever, chills
- Dysuria, hematuria
- Protrusion of umbilical cord from the vagina

BOX 22-6 Components of Interval Prenatal Visits

History

- Interval medical history
  - New bodily changes, symptoms, or concerns
  - Status of previous problems and response to treatment
- Interval social history
  - Social support
  - Safety at home
  - Risky maternal behaviors
- Fetal movement
- Vaginal bleeding, leaking fluid, uterine contractions
- Medications

Physical Examination

- Weight and interval weight gain
- Blood pressure
- Urine dipstick for protein at specified intervals
- Obstetric abdominal examination:
  - Fundal height in centimeters
  - Fetal heart tones
  - Fetal presentation after 36 weeks
- Third trimester: assess for inverted nipples

Health Screening

- Intimate-partner violence screening at least once every trimester
- Depression screening[a]
- Alcohol and drug use

Laboratory and Ultrasound Assessments

16–20 weeks	Second-trimester Down syndrome screening test (triple or quad screen)
18–20 weeks	Dating and anatomy ultrasound
24–28 weeks	Diabetes screen[b]
	Repeat hemoglobin and hematocrit
	Antibody screen if Rh negative[c]
Third trimester	Gonorrhea, chlamydia, and syphilis screening for women at increased risk or per state law
35–37 weeks	Group B *Streptococcus* screening culture

[a]Universal depression screening is not formally recommended by all professional associations. Depression screening is encouraged during pregnancy, but there are insufficient data to recommend specific timing of depression screening.

[b]Diabetes screening can be universal or offered to women who do not have risk factors.

[c]A repeat antibody screen at 24–28 weeks if the woman is Rh negative and the initial prenatal visit antibody screen was negative may be deferred in some settings, as it has not been shown to be cost-effective. The incidence of Rh isoimmunization is very low before 28 weeks' gestation.

assessments, including abnormal values and need for any follow-up testing. A purposeful and systematic review of the record is invaluable. It allows the midwife to become reacquainted with the woman, review the care provided to date, and assess the effectiveness of preceding management. Most importantly, this review is essential for prevention of errors that can result from missed information.

Interval History and Physical Examination

The interval history is designed to detect any questions, discomforts, or complications that the woman may have experienced since her last visit. In addition to the standard components of the interval prenatal examination, the physical examination may include a targeted exam to assess specific symptoms. For example, a speculum examination may be performed to assess a vaginal discharge or determine if membranes have ruptured. A bimanual examination may be performed to evaluate cervical ripening or to perform membrane sweeping.

Laboratory Tests and Adjunctive Studies

In many practices, a voided urine specimen is obtained at each prenatal visit to detect proteinuria, glucosuria, or signs of asymptomatic bacteriuria. However, the urine dipstick test—especially in the absence of symptoms or risk factors such as hypertension—is not supported in the literature as a reliable means of detecting asymptomatic bacteriuria[47] or preeclampsia[48,49] and is of questionable benefit in early detection of gestational diabetes.[47] Some authors have advocated for discontinuation of such testing as a part of regular prenatal care.[48,50]

Group Prenatal Care: CenteringPregnancy

In the last decade, alternatives to individual one-on-one prenatal visits have been developed, including group prenatal care. Probably the best studied is the model known as CenteringPregnancy,[51,52] which was started by a midwife and is now being widely adopted. CenteringPregnancy is a group approach to prenatal care that differs from the traditional model by combining the typical elements of a prenatal visit risk assessment with childbirth education and peer support. This model is composed of a standardized approach including 13 Essential Elements that define the group process that makes CenteringPregnancy a self-empowering environment (**Box 22-7**). Groups of 8 to 12 women or couples at approximately the same gestational age are formed between 12 and

16 weeks. The group meets monthly for 4 months, and then biweekly, and once in the early postpartum period for a total of ten 90-minute sessions. Additional individual examination room visits are scheduled if necessary. The largest randomized controlled trial of CenteringPregnancy ($n = 1047$) found that it is associated with high patient satisfaction, cost-effectiveness, and positive pregnancy outcomes, including increased self-esteem, less depression, and higher rates of breastfeeding initiation.[53–56] Studies of adolescents enrolled in CenteringPregnancy have yielded promising evidence that this model may improve birth weight and lower preterm labor rates.

Special Populations

With advances in reproductive technology and the increasing visibility of changing family structures, midwives need to be prepared to effectively engage with a diverse array of individual values and family structures when providing prenatal care. It is important

---

BOX 22-7 Essential Elements of CenteringPregnancy

There are 13 Essential Elements that define the Centering model of care:

1. Health assessment occurs within the group space.
2. Participants are involved in self-care activities.
3. A facilitative leadership style is used.
4. The group is conducted in a circle.
5. Each session has an overall plan.
6. Attention is given to the core content, although emphasis may vary.
7. There is stability of group leadership.
8. Group conduct honors the contribution of each member.
9. The composition of the group is stable, not rigid.
10. Group size is optimal to promote the process. *8–12 women*
11. Involvement of support people is optional.
12. Opportunity for socializing with the group is provided.
13. There is ongoing evaluation of outcomes.

Source: Reprinted courtesy of Centering Healthcare Institute.

for midwives to identify any barriers that may be present in their practice environments and within their personal biases and beliefs. Working to remove barriers and biases will help the midwife develop approaches that honor every woman, show respect for her family, and help her meet her unique needs.

Although a trend toward decreased birth rates among adolescents has been noted recently, the adolescent pregnancy rate in the United States remains higher than in other industrialized nations.[57] Young women often lack education, finances, and sometimes social support. They are at higher risk for living in poverty, having depression, and being exposed to intimate-partner violence (IPV) than their peers who defer childbearing. Pregnant adolescents often need additional support services during pregnancy. Although adolescent pregnancy is associated with an increased risk for preterm birth and low birth weight, it is difficult to ascertain if these outcomes occur secondary to a biologic age effect or to socioeconomic status. Nevertheless, when younger (age 10–14 years) women are compared to older adolescents (15–19 years), adolescents in the younger age group are much more likely to experience preterm birth, low birth weight, late or no prenatal care, and higher infant mortality rates.[58]

Pregnancy-Specific Conditions

Medical and obstetric complications of pregnancy are detailed in the *Medical Complications in Pregnancy* and *Obstetric Complications in Pregnancy* chapters. This section reviews pregnancy-specific conditions that are common variants and, therefore, are part of regular prenatal care.

Anemia in Pregnancy

Approximately 35% to 56% of pregnant women are anemic worldwide.[59] Anemia is the most common nutritional deficiency worldwide. In developing nations, anemia is also frequently a comorbidity of infection (e.g., malaria) or a hemoglobinopathy.

In the United States, approximately 18% of pregnant women are anemic overall, but this rate increases from 6.9% to 14.3% to 29.5% in the first, second, and third trimesters, respectively.[60] Iron deficiency is a continuum that ranges from iron depletion to overt anemia; thus, although fewer than half of all pregnant women are anemic, more women are iron depleted at the end of pregnancy.[61]

Anemia in pregnancy is associated with low birth weight, preterm birth, low iron stores in offspring, and increased susceptibility to infection. Treatment of anemia improves these outcomes.[62]

Although iron-deficiency anemia is by far the most common etiology of anemia in pregnant women, anemia can occur secondary to several different chronic, acute, or genetic conditions. Therefore it is important to know how to evaluate anemia and interpret laboratory tests that depict red blood cell indices and serum constituents involved in iron storage and iron transport. Values for hemoglobin, mean corpuscular volume (MCV), serum iron, and total iron-binding capacity (TIBC) in iron-deficient states are listed in **Table 22-6**.[63,64]

Anemia is categorized as microcytic, macrocytic, or normocytic based on the size of red blood cells. Iron-deficiency anemia is a microcytic anemia. An algorithm for evaluating anemia is presented in **Figure 22-1**.

Pica

Pica is the purposive ingestion of nonfood items. Pica is more common in pregnant women than in women who are not pregnant. The prevalence of pica varies by geographic region and culture, but has been noted to affect as many as 50% of women in some settings.[65] The most common substances eaten are earth, clay, or dirt; raw starches such as cornstarch; and ice and freezer frost. The etiology of pica is unknown, although several theories exist. There is a clear association between ice-ingestion pica and iron-deficiency anemia, but it is not clear if pica causes anemia or if anemia initiates pica. Pica can cause lead poisoning and may be associated with other micronutrient deficiencies. Management consists of diagnosis and treatment of nutritional deficiencies, assessment of hunger or eating disorders, and health education.

Rh Isoimmunization

Today it is possible that a midwife will have a long career caring for pregnant women and never see a woman with Rh (D) isoimmunization. The treatment of this disease is a success story of the twentieth century. The Rhesus factor first was identified in the late 1930s, and an Rh incompatibility was identified shortly thereafter as the etiology for large numbers of fetal deaths and stillbirths for which the reasons previously were unknown. In the late 1960s, an anti-D serum was approved; its introduction changed the landscape entirely.

An individual, including a fetus, who is Rh (D) positive has the Rh antigen on each red blood cell.

Table 22-6	Laboratory Tests Indicative of Iron Deficiency, by Degree of Severity			
	Normal Values	Iron Deficient Without Anemia	Iron Deficient with Mild Anemia	Severely Iron Deficient with Severe Anemia
Hemoglobin (g/dL)	12–13	Normal (> 12)	9–12	6–7
Mean corpuscular volume (MCV) (fl)	80–100	80–100	< 80	< 80
RBC morphology	Normal	Normal	Normal or slight hypochromia	Hypochromic, microcytic
Serum ferritin (ng/mL)	10–150	< 40	< 20	< 10
Serum iron (SI) (mcg/dL)	40–175	60–150	< 60[a]	< 40
Total iron-binding capacity (TIBC) (mcg/dL)	216–400	300–390	350–400	> 410[a]
Transferrin saturation (SI/TIBC) (%)	16–60	30	< 15	< 10
Erythrocyte protoporphyrin (ng/mL RBC)	< 3	30–70	> 100	100–200

Sources: Adapted from American College of Obstetricians and Gynecologists. Anemia in pregnancy. ACOG Practice Bulletin No. 95. *Obstet Gynecol.* 2008;112:201-207; Haider BA, Olofin I, Wang M, Spiegelman D, Ezzati M, Fawzi WW; Nutrition Impact Model Study Group (anaemia). Anaemia, prenatal iron use, and risk of adverse pregnancy outcomes: systematic review and meta-analysis. *BMJ.* 2013 Jun 21;346:f3443.

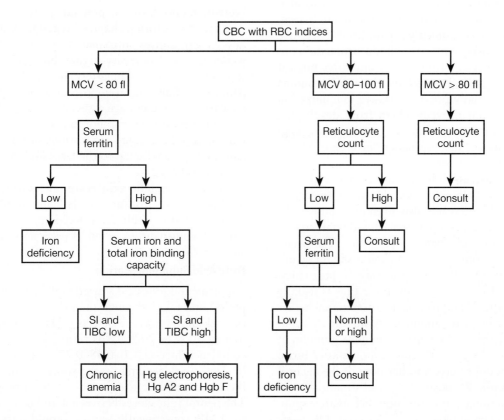

Figure 22-1 Morphologic evaluation of anemia.

Conversely, a person who is Rh (D) negative does not have the Rh (D) antigen on the red blood cell membrane, but is capable of mounting an antibody response when exposed to Rh (D)-positive blood.

In pregnancy and birth, there are several opportunities for fetal blood to mix with maternal blood. During the prenatal period such mixing is not common. During third stage labor, as the placenta separates from the decidua, fetal blood commonly escapes into the maternal circulation. For a woman who is Rh (D) negative with an Rh (D) positive fetus, these physiologic events can cause her to develop immunoglobulin G (IgG) antibodies to the Rh (D) antigen. At birth, it is estimated that approximately 17% of women might potentially become isoimmunized secondary to some fetomaternal blood transfer.[66]

The IgG–type antibodies produced are small. During subsequent pregnancies, they may easily cross the placenta and attach themselves to any antigens found on Rh (D)-positive red blood cells of a fetus, causing catastrophic results such as hemolysis, erythroblastosis fetalis, and stillbirth. Thus, in the 1950s, women who were Rh (D) negative were warned of having a "blue baby" after their first pregnancy. Partners were routinely screened and women whose partners were Rh (D) negative were reassured.

Today Rh isoimmunization in pregnant women and hemolytic disease of the newborn are rarely seen, primarily because women who are Rh (D) negative are given anti-D immune globulin prophylaxis in the third trimester of pregnancy and after birth if the newborn is Rh (D) positive. The anti-D immune globulin essentially provides passive immunization for women that prevents them from developing permanent antibodies. Thus every subsequent pregnancy becomes a "first pregnancy" in terms of Rh (D) antibody development.

Initially Rh (D) globulin was administered in the immediate postpartum period. However, to further minimize risk, today it is also given prenatally in the third trimester when the maternal and fetal circulations are close and when an occult bleed can occur. Therefore, a woman who is pregnant should be initially screened for Rh (D) status early in pregnancy. If she is RH negative, an antibody titer is usually ordered in the second trimester to ascertain whether she has become isoimmunized. Assuming this titer is negative, she is given anti-D immune globulin at 28 gestational weeks. Within 72 hours after birth, she also should receive another dose of the agent if the newborn is Rh positive. Special situations warranting additional administration such as after spontaneous pregnancy loss are discussed in *Obstetric Complications in Pregnancy* chapter.

Health Promotion During Pregnancy

Prenatal care offers protracted access to healthcare services. Given this opportunity, it is incumbent upon all healthcare providers who offer prenatal care to incorporate health promotion and health education into prenatal care visits following the principles of adult learning described in the *Health Promotion and Health Maintenance* chapter.

Each prenatal visit is associated with different evaluations and interventions depending on the woman's gestational age. Many institutions have established road-map templates for what is performed at each visit. A representative template is listed in **Appendix 22C**. The needs of an individual woman can vary substantially, however, so knowledge of the trimester-specific psychological transitions can be used in combination with principles of adult learning to assist the midwife in tailoring health promotion and health education to be congruent with the woman's stage of pregnancy and priorities. The midwife is encouraged to know all of the health promotion and health education activities that are included in prenatal care.

Nutrition and Weight Gain in Pregnancy

Nutritional needs during pregnancy are reviewed in detail in the *Nutrition* chapter. Pregestational weight and weight gain in pregnancy both affect offspring weight gain and adiposity. In turn, birth adiposity affects adult weight and long-term health. Thus weight gain in pregnancy is an important topic in prenatal education.[67] Likewise, an assessment of weight gain, diet, and nutrition is an important component of prenatal care. The average proportions of total weight gain that are attributed to the fetus and mother are listed in **Table 22-7**.[68,69]

Current weight gain recommendations were modified by the Institute of Medicine in 2009 and are presented in **Table 22-8**. Recommended weight gain for women differs based on pregestational BMI.

Folic Acid Supplementation

Supplemental folic acid started in the preconception period and taken through the first trimester lowers the risk of neural tube defects (NTDs) by approximately 30% to 70% (odds ratio [OR], 0.67; 95% confidence interval [CI]: 0.58–0.77), with the amount of decrease depending on the study conducted and the amount of folic acid used by study participants.[70] The neural tube closes between 4 and 6 weeks after the LMP; consequently, women should start supplements in the preconception period if possible, and at

Table 22-7	Disposition of Weight Gain in Pregnancy
Compartment	**Amount of Weight Gain in Pounds (kg)**
Fetus	7–8 (3.2–3.6)
Fat stores	6–8 (2.7–3.6)
Increased blood volume	3–4 (1.4–1.8)
Increased fluid volume	2–3 (0.9–1.4)
Amniotic fluid	2 (0.9)
Breast enlargement	1–3 (0.45–1.4)
Uterine hypertrophy	2 (0.9)
Placenta	1.5 (0.7)
Total	**25–35 (12–15)**

Source: Adapted from Composition and components of gestational weight gain: physiology and metabolism. In Institute of Medicine, National Research Council Committee to Reexamine IOM Pregnancy Weight Guidelines; Rasmussen KM, Yaktine AL, eds. *Weight Gain During Pregnancy: Reexamining the Guidelines.* Washington, DC: National Academies Press; 2009. Available at: http://www.ncbi.nlm.nih.gov/books/NBK32815.

the first prenatal visit if not already taking a prenatal supplement. The recommended dose is 400 mcg per day for women who do not have an a priori risk for neural tube defects. Women who had a previous pregnancy complicated by an NTD should take 4 mg of folic acid per day starting 1 month prior to conception and through the first 4 months of pregnancy. Women who are taking anticonvulsant medications (Valproate [Depakote, Depakene], carbamazepine [Tegretol]) should take 4 mg of folic acid per day starting 1 month prior to conception and continue that regimen throughout the pregnancy, as these medications have an antifolate effect.

Prenatal Vitamins

Prenatal vitamins are specially formulated multivitamins that generally contain higher amounts of iron and folic acid compared to regular multivitamins. The amount of specific vitamins and minerals in commercially marketed prenatal vitamins varies greatly and there is no known advantage for one combination over another. The *Nutrition* chapter details the needs of specific vitamins and minerals during pregnancy.

Many women assume a prenatal multivitamin is required in pregnancy. In reality, it is not recommended that all pregnant women ingest a prenatal multivitamin daily. Folic acid and iron supplementation both are recommended during pregnancy. Prenatal multivitamins usually contain 400 mcg to 800 mcg of folic acid and varying amounts of iron; therefore, they are an easy vehicle for obtaining these two nutrients.

Prenatal multivitamins are recommended for women who are in one of the following categories: does not consume a nutritionally adequate diet, multiple pregnancy, heavy smoker, alcohol abuse, adolescent, vegetarian, substance abuse, history of bariatric surgery, eating disorder, or lactase deficiency.

Prenatal multivitamins can cause increased gastrointestinal distress and constipation in some women. It is presumed that these symptoms arise secondary to the iron content in the vitamin. For women with nausea and vomiting, discontinuing iron-containing pills does appear to improve nausea symptoms.[71] When a prenatal vitamin is discontinued, even if temporarily, it should be replaced with a folic acid supplement.

Iron Supplementation

A woman's need for iron is approximately doubled in pregnancy. Two types of iron exist: heme iron, which is found in meat, and non-heme iron, which is

Table 22-8	Recommended Weight Gain in Pregnancy for Singleton Pregnancy	
Pregestational Weight Category	**BMI (kg/m^2)**	**Recommended Weight Gain in Pounds (kg)**
Underweight	< 18.5	28–40 (12.5–18.0)
Normal weight	18.5–24.9	25–35 (11.5–16.0)
Overweight	25.0–29.9	15–25 (7.0–11.5)
Obese	> 30.0	11–20 (5–9.0)

Source: Adapted from Composition and components of gestational weight gain: physiology and metabolism. In Institute of Medicine, National Research Council Committee to Reexamine IOM Pregnancy Weight Guidelines; Rasmussen KM, Yaktine AL, eds. *Weight Gain During Pregnancy: Reexamining the Guidelines.* Washington, DC: National Academies Press; 2009. Available at: http://www.ncbi.nlm.nih.gov/books/NBK32815.

found in plant and, to a smaller extent, dairy products. Iron is absorbed via the mucosal cells in the jejunum. Approximately 20% to 30% of heme iron is absorbed without being affected by other dietary factors. Non-heme iron is more difficult to absorb; approximately 2% to 10% is absorbed, and absorption requires an acidic environment in the gastrointestinal tract to reduce the ferric iron to ferrous iron for absorption. Tannins found in tea, caffeine, and whole grains can adversely affect non-heme iron absorption. Absorption increases substantially in pregnancy, when more iron is used and iron stores are low.

The absorption of iron in prenatal vitamins can depend on the amount of calcium in the vitamin. For example, more iron may be absorbed from a vitamin with a lower iron content without calcium than from a vitamin containing both calcium and iron. The absorption of iron in supplements depends on the amount of elemental iron in the formulation, whether it is a quick-release or extended-release formulation, and whether the iron is in the ferric, ferrous, or iron polymaltose complex form.[72] The doses and side effects of various iron supplements can be found in the *Nutrition* chapter.

Routine iron supplementation is associated with a decrease in the incidence of low birth weight and maternal anemia. However, it is not clear if routine iron supplements improve birth outcomes in healthy nonanemic women. In turn, routine iron supplementation is somewhat controversial. In addition to gastrointestinal distress and constipation, daily iron supplementation may have adverse effects including reduced absorption of other minerals and increased oxidative stress.[73,74]

Because iron absorption increases in pregnancy, some authors have proposed that intermittent iron supplementation may be preferable to daily iron supplementation. Exposure of the intestinal mucosal cells to iron supplements on an intermittent basis may improve iron absorption because these cells might absorb iron better if not exposed continuously. Randomized controlled trials of intermittent iron supplementation rather than daily iron supplementation demonstrated equally positive pregnancy outcomes when iron supplements were taken one to three times per week rather than daily.[76]

In summary, folic acid supplementation is recommended for all women in the preconception period through the first trimester. Prenatal multivitamins usually contain the recommended daily intake amounts for folic acid and iron, but they may decrease iron absorption secondary to the presence of calcium and other minerals. Intermittent iron supplementation may be as effective as daily supplementation secondary to the physiology of iron absorption. Recommending iron supplements in addition to a prenatal multivitamin may appropriately be a routine component of prenatal care in some practices and not in others. All women should be evaluated for anemia secondary to diet and nutritional status. Iron supplements should be recommended for all women with anemia and considered for others depending on the needs of the individual.

Infection Precautions

Pregnant women, like all individuals, can be exposed to infectious organisms. Some infections can harm a fetus or newborn, and others are more likely to develop into serious or life-threatening illnesses if a pregnant woman becomes infected.

- Infections that can harm the fetus include listeriosis, parvovirus, rubella, syphilis, varicella, and toxoplasmosis.

- Herpes and group B *Streptococcus* can be harmful to the newborn if infected at the time of vaginal birth. Varicella can harm the newborn if contracted near the time of birth.

- Influenza and varicella can become severe illnesses in pregnant women and are associated with an increased risk of death.

Health education related to infection precautions is described in **Table 22-9**.[77] Additional information about management of exposure to these infections in nonimmune individuals is discussed in the *Medical Complications in Pregnancy* chapter.

Immunizations

Maternal immune antibodies of the IgG class cross the placenta and generally provide protection for the fetus. Vaccines that are composed of inactive antigen ingredients or toxoid are safe for use in pregnancy, whereas live-attenuated vaccines have a small risk of causing disease and are not recommended for use by pregnant women. Vaccines that are recommended and those that are contraindicated during pregnancy are listed in **Table 22-10**.[78]

All pregnant women are offered vaccination for tetanus, diphtheria, and pertussis (Tdap) and influenza vaccine during pregnancy. Women who are in the middle of the hepatitis B series, are counseled to finish the series, but women who are in the middle of the human papillomavirus (HPV) vaccine series are counseled to wait until the pregnancy is over before finishing the vaccine series.[79,80] Additional vaccines can be given during pregnancy if the woman is at increased risk for specific infections.

Table 22-9	Health Education for Disease Prevention During Pregnancy
Disease Prevention	**Disease-Causing Agent (Disease)**
Avoid	
Cleaning cat litter boxes. If not avoidable, wear gloves and wash hands after cleaning.	Toxoplasmosis
Working in dirt unless gloves are worn	Toxoplasmosis
Sexual contact with persons who have active herpes lesions	Herpes
Contact with individuals who have chickenpox (unless known immune), whooping cough, or slap-cheek disease	Varicella (chickenpox)
	Parvovirus B19 (fifth disease, slap-cheek disease)
	Pertussis (whooping cough)
Hand Washing	
After handling raw meat	Listeria (listeriosis)
After changing a diaper	Cytomegalovirus
After handling body fluids of a toddler	Cytomegalovirus
Recommended Testing for Diseases	
Rubella, HBsAg, HIV, syphilis, group B *Streptococcus*, chlamydia	
Recommended Vaccines During Pregnancy	
Hepatitis A and hepatitis B vaccine if at increased risk for disease	Hepatitis A
	Hepatitis B
Influenza vaccine	Influenza virus (flu)
Tetanus/diphtheria/pertussis (Tdap)	Pertussis (whooping cough)

Table 22-10	Routine Immunizations That Are Recommended or Contraindicated During Pregnancy	
Vaccine	**Recommended in Pregnancy**	**Type of Vaccine**
Hepatitis A	If at risk[a]	Inactivated
Hepatitis B	If at risk[b]	Inactivated
Human papillomavirus (HPV)	No[c]	Inactivated
Influenza TIV	Recommended for all women during pregnancy	Inactivated
Influenza LAIV	Contraindicated	Live
Measles, mumps, rubella (MMR)	Contraindicated	Live
Meningococcal: polysaccharide or conjugate	If indicated	Inactivated
Pneumococcal polysaccharide	If indicated	Inactivated
Tetanus/diphtheria (Td)	Yes, but Tdap preferred if > 20 weeks	Toxoid
Tetanus/diphtheria/pertussis (Tdap), one dose only	Recommended for all women during each pregnancy irrespective of having received the vaccine previously	Toxoid/inactivated
Varicella	Contraindicated	Live

[a]The hepatitis A vaccine is an inactivated vaccine and should be safe for pregnant women. It is recommended only if the woman has a high risk of exposure.

[b]Risk factors for hepatitis B include having more than one sex partner during the previous 6 months, having been evaluated or treated for an STD, recent or current injection drug use, or having had an HBsAg-positive sex partner

[c]If a woman is in the middle of the HPV vaccine series and becomes pregnant, the rest of the series should be delayed until after the pregnancy.

Source: Adapted from Bridges CB, Woods L, Coyne-Beasley T. Advisory Committee on Immunization Practices (ACIP) recommended immunization schedule for adults aged 19 years and older—United States, 2013. *MMWR Surveill Summ.* 2013;62:9.

The topic of vaccine safety is important to the woman, her fetus, and her newborn. Controversies about purported associations between vaccines and methylmercury poisoning and between vaccines and autism have been reviewed extensively. Although thimerosal was not shown to be harmful in the amounts used in vaccines, it has been removed from all vaccines administered to pregnant women and children so vaccines no longer expose individuals to methylmercury.[81] The hypothesized relationship between vaccines and autism has been found to be spurious.[82]

Substance Abuse Screening

A general health history can be a partial screen for drug, alcohol, and smoking. When seeking an initial or annual history for a woman, use of alcohol, tobacco, caffeine, over-the-counter medications, prescription medications, and illicit drugs should be explored. Because individuals who abuse legal or illegal substances also tend to have a higher incidence of sexually transmitted infections and IPV, it is useful to discuss substance abuse when an STI is diagnosed or IPV is a concern. Signs or symptoms of depression, family dysfunction, sleep disorders, and gastrointestinal problems may all be associated with substance abuse.

Because half of all pregnancies are unplanned, the first prenatal visit represents an important opportunity to identify substance abuse risks. Unfortunately, many women who abuse drugs are reluctant to interact with the healthcare system and may seek care later in pregnancy, if at all. Use of illicit drugs may cause fear of legal actions for the woman and her unborn child and further delay presentation for care.

Screening for alcohol and drug use, depression, and IPV has been shown to improve maternal and fetal outcomes when linked to support services and intervention. Smoking cessation interventions have been shown to lower the incidence of low-birth-weight infants. When a woman is immunized against a disease such as pertussis, her fetus becomes protected from a disease that can have devastating outcomes. These health promotion activities are essential components of prenatal care. Although they are best performed early, the results may be more reliable once a therapeutic relationship has been established.

Alcohol Screening

Fetal alcohol syndrome is one of the most common preventable causes of mental disability in the United States. Surveys conducted by the Centers for Disease Control and Prevention (CDC) have found that 7.6%

of pregnant women report using alcohol and 1.4% report binge drinking.[83]

National guidelines in the United States and many other developed nations recommend that women do not consume alcohol during pregnancy. This recommendation reflects the fact that the dose-response relationship between alcohol intake and fetal effects is unknown. Alcohol freely crosses the placenta, and its elimination from both maternal and fetal systems is dependent upon maternal metabolism. It is thought that genetic regulation of alcohol metabolism may play a role in vulnerability to fetal alcohol syndrome. Fetal damage caused by alcohol ranges from mild to severe; thus, a general category of fetal alcohol spectrum disorder has been described. Alcohol screening followed by education and referral for treatment when indicated improves maternal and newborn outcomes.[84]

Illicit Drug Screening

The complexity of individual motivations, the various physical reactions to drugs and their interactions, and the widespread tendency toward polypharmacy all contribute to the difficulty in assessing for substance abuse. There is no single assessment technique for evaluating substance abuse. The single question validated by Smith et al.[85]—"How many times in the past year have you used an illegal drug or used a prescription medication for nonmedical reasons?"—may be used. The CAGE alcohol screening tool has been adapted for drug use, and other screening tools are available as well.

The care of a woman struggling with substance abuse requires collaboration between her midwife and professionals in multidisciplinary programs who have skills in treating chemical abuse and addictions. These professionals may include social workers, chemical abuse counselors, psychologists, psychiatrists, nutritionists, pharmacologists, and physicians with knowledge and experience in managing withdrawal, detoxification, and long-term treatment. The midwife must coordinate care for the woman with the professionals in substance abuse treatment. It is essential that the woman receive consistent information and that all team members hold the same expectations for her behavior.

A cycle of recovery has been identified that includes a period when the woman does not recognize the need to change behavior, a period of contemplation when the problem is recognized but no action is taken, a period when the woman plans action, a period of action, and a period of maintenance.[86]

The factors that motivate recovery in a woman who has been abusing drugs or alcohol are varied and unpredictable. Sometimes concern about a fetus during pregnancy may be the catalyst to begin the cycle of recovery. Conversely, for some women, any concern for a fetus may be overridden by her concern for acquiring drugs. By providing ongoing care and support while recognizing the recovery/relapse pattern, the midwife can work to minimize maternal and fetal complications, encourage decreased substance use, and support the woman appropriately depending on where she is in the cycle of recovery.[87]

Smoking Cessation

The body of evidence linking smoking to adverse neonatal outcomes is extensive and well accepted.[88,89] Prenatal smoking is associated with fetal growth restriction, low birth weight, sudden infant death syndrome (SIDS), asthma, and other long-term effects in the child. In addition, use of the *Five A's* (referred to in the *Health Promotion and Health Maintenance* chapter) has proven effectiveness. Nevertheless, two surveys of midwives found that although all participants recognized the value of smoking cessation and discussed smoking cessation with their patients, fewer than half provided smoking cessation materials, offered counseling or nicotine replacement therapy, or scheduled follow-up visits for smoking cessation assistance. Insufficient time was cited as one of the more prevalent barriers to providing smoking cessation interventions.[90,91]

Smoking cessation measures that are effective for pregnant women include provision of pregnancy-specific smoking cessation materials, short 2- to 3-minute counseling from a healthcare provider, and follow-up phone calls and letters.[92]

Depression Screening

Depression is common among reproductive-age women. Untreated depression has been associated with adverse perinatal outcomes, impaired maternal–infant attachment, and disordered family relationships.[93] Although universal depression screening is not recommended by all professional organizations[94] others recommend that it be performed as often as every trimester, and some states mandate that all pregnant women be screened for depression.

Intimate-Partner Violence Screening

Screening for IPV deserves a special note. All women can be victims of violence, irrespective of their age, race, ethnicity, socioeconomic status, profession, sexual orientation, or marital status. It is recommended that women be assessed for the risk of intimate-partner violence at least once per trimester[95] because violence may begin during the pregnancy, it may increase in severity, or women may need time to consider whether they want to reveal the violence.[96] Women may be more vulnerable to the effects of violence while pregnant, due to their physical condition or their financial and emotional dependence, and when violence does occur it can have devastating short- and long-term health outcomes for the woman and fetus.[97]

A variety of screening tools for IPV exist.[98] There is no single screening method or tool that has demonstrated consistently high sensitivity and specificity in screening for IPV, especially in outpatient settings with diverse populations.[98] Midwives may choose to screen for IPV in a face-to-face interview, using a patient self-administered questionnaire, or using a computer-assisted self-interview.[99-101] Examples of screening questions and tools are reviewed in the *Health Promotion and Health Maintenance* chapter.

The midwife's primary role in working with a woman who is a victim of IPV is to assess her safety and to help her make a plan for safety if needed, and to accurately document her condition and refer her to appropriate resources. IPV is a very dangerous environment for a woman; when it is revealed, the midwife has an ethical responsibility to provide the woman with needed resources and to follow up as indicated.

Environmental Exposures

The primary environmental exposures of concern in pregnancy are lead, mercury, ionizing and non-ionizing radiation, and endocrine disruptors such as phthalates.

Lead Exposure

Elevated lead levels are associated with miscarriage, gestational hypertension, low birth weight, and impaired neurodevelopment in offspring. Both chronic and acute lead poisoning can be dangerous during pregnancy, because lead is stored in bone and pregnancy is a time of increased bone turnover.[102] Although routine screening for lead exposure is not indicated, women who have important risk factors for lead exposure should be screened. Risk factors for lead exposure are listed in the *Preconception Care* chapter. Maternal venous lead levels of less than 5 mcg/dL do not require any further follow-up. Women whose levels are between 10 mcg/dL and 45 mcg/

dL should have the source of lead identified and be retested within a month, then within 1 month to 3 months, following the schedule recommended by the CDC.[103] Women whose lead level is more than 45 mcg/dL should be referred to a clinician who specializes in caring for lead toxicity.

Mercury

Mercury exists naturally in the environment and is also a pollutant of industrial processes. Mercury poisoning has an interesting history. The term "mad as a hatter" refers to dementia caused by mercury poisoning. In eighteenth- and nineteenth-century England, mercury was used to produce the felt from which hats were made. Persons who worked in the hat factories would develop dementia as a result of mercury poisoning.

Excess mercury can impair neurologic development in a fetus. The primary source of mercury today is the methylmercury that accumulates in large fish. Therefore, pregnant women are counseled to avoid consumption of shark, tilefish, swordfish, and king mackerel. However, fish has several essential nutrients and women should be encouraged to eat fish that have low levels of mercury in up to 2 meals per week (8–12 oz per week). The other possible source of mercury is the thimerosal in vaccines. All vaccines offered to pregnant women and infants are thimerosal free.

Ionizing Radiation

X rays are ionizing radiation. Exposure to X rays between 8 and 25 weeks' gestation can cause miscarriage, fetal growth restriction, mental retardation, and—at very high doses—death or stillbirth. X-ray exposure can also increase the risk for some childhood cancers. Fetal effects are dose dependent and fetal effects of X-ray exposure are not noticeable when the exposure is less than 0.05 Gy (5 rads).[104] Routine X rays expose the fetus to very low doses of ionizing radiation. For example, a chest X ray is approximately 0.00007 rad.[105] Exposure in the first 2 weeks after conception reflects the "all or nothing" phenomenon since it is either fatal or has no adverse effects. Therefore women can be assured that accidental exposure to one diagnostic X ray will not cause fetal harm.[106] If X-ray exposure has occurred, the woman can be referred to a radiologist who will calculate the exact dose and counsel her appropriately.

Non-ionizing Radiation

Ultrasound, microwaves, electric blankets, computers, cell phones, and airport screening devices for metal all emit non-ionizing radiation. Exposure to non-ionizing radiation has not been shown to cause fetal harm.[107]

Endocrine Disrupters

Endocrine disrupters are chemicals that mimic or disrupt the effects of estrogen, androgen, and thyroid stimulation. The primary endocrine disrupters of concern for pregnant women are bisphenol A (BPA) and phthalates. Current evidence suggests that BPA and phthalates might potentially have adverse effects on a fetus based on animal studies and effects on wildlife. Therefore women are counseled to use BPA-free baby bottles, avoid microwaving plastic containers, avoid use of plastic containers with the number 3 or 7 on the container, and limit intake of foods packaged in cans.[108] Phthalates are used to make soft plastics such as cling wrap, some baby toys, many cosmetics, and polyvinyl tubing. The most common phthalate, di(2-ethylhexyl) phthalate (DEHP), is currently voluntarily being removed by some manufacturers from baby toys.

Health Education During Pregnancy

The list of specific health education topics that are recommended over the course of prenatal care is long, and trying to teach too much at one time is a common mistake. It can be helpful to keep a teaching checklist in the woman's prenatal record, so that recommended health education topics can be addressed over the course of prenatal care, providing trimester-appropriate teaching throughout the pregnancy and decreasing the possibility of redundancies. Prenatal health education needs to be tailored to the woman's needs, with a focus on health literacy, health numeracy, and cultural sensitivity. Skills in culturally competent communication and counseling are called upon regularly.

Teaching should be focused first on acute needs, such as "warning signs" of obstetric complications (also referred to as "danger signs"), counseling about genetic tests, and ways to reach the midwife. This section briefly reviews health education topics that are considered essential over the course of prenatal care management. A selected list of health education topics frequently of interest to pregnant women is presented in **Table 22-11**.[108–120]

The details of all health education topics that should be covered during pregnancy are beyond the scope of this text. The reader is encouraged to access resources such as the free *Share with Women*

Table 22-11	Health Education Topics for Pregnant Women
Topic	**Recommendations**
Air travel	No known risks for healthy women. Women with conditions that increase the risk for hypoxia, such as cardiac disease or fetal growth restriction, may need supplemental oxygen or should avoid flying.
	Safe to fly until 36 gestational weeks, when the risk of spontaneous labor increases.
	Flying increases the risk for venous thromboembolism; pregnant women should wear support hose and/or move frequently if traveling a long distance.[115]
Breastfeeding	Breastfeeding is recommended unless contraindicated.
Caffeine	Caffeine crosses the placenta easily and is metabolized more slowly by the fetus than by the pregnant woman.[116]
	Caffeine consumption of less than 300 mg/day (2 cups of coffee) is not associated with miscarriage, congenital anomalies, or fetal growth restriction.[117]
Car seats	Car seats are required by state law in all states, for children up to specific age and weights. State laws vary. Infants should ride in a rear-facing seat until age 2 years.
	State laws for car seats can be found at http://www.iihs.org/laws/safetybeltuse.aspx.
Circumcision	The American Academy of Pediatrics states that the health benefits outweigh the risks of circumcision, but the benefits are not great enough to recommend routine circumcision of all male newborns.[118]
Employment during pregnancy	The Pregnancy Discrimination Act of 1964 protects pregnant women from being fired secondary to being pregnant. It is also illegal to ban a woman from a particular job if she might become pregnant. Complaints about pregnancy discrimination are filed with the U.S. Equal Employment Opportunity Commission at http://www.eeoc.gov/stats/enforcement.html.
Environmental exposures	Information about specific environmental exposures can be obtained from the following sources: • The National Birth Defects Center Pregnancy Exposure Hotline (1-800-322-5014) provides free information on environmental exposures. • REPROTOX (www.reprotox.org) provides commentaries on harmful effects of chemicals and physical agents.
Exercise	Regular exercise is associated with cardiovascular fitness, prevention of low back pain, reduced symptoms of depression, and lower weight gain.
	Avoid activities that increase the risk for falls or abdominal injury. Scuba diving and sky diving are not recommended.
Hair treatments	No data support a relationship between hair dye and teratogenic effects.
Hot tubs and saunas	Maternal fever or increased core temperature is associated with an increased risk of neural tube defects of approximately 50% (OR: 1.62; 95% CI: 1.10–2.17).[120]
	It takes approximately 10 minutes to raise the core temperature to more than 40°C (104°F) in water of 40°C (104°F) and 15 minutes if the water temperature is 39°C (102°F).[119]
	Hot tubs should be avoided in the first trimester.
Lead exposure	Routine screening is not indicated unless 1 of 12 risk factors is present.
Maternity leave benefits	Maternity leave benefits are usually a combination of short-term disability, sick leave, vacation, and unpaid leave.
	Laws and eligibility requirements governing pregnancy-related disability for childbirth vary by state.
	The Family Medical Leave Act (FLMA) mandates 12 weeks of unpaid leave for childrearing in a 12-month period. Parents are eligible if they have worked for an employer 12 months in a facility with at least 50 employees.
	Individual companies have different maternity policies that may be combined with state benefits.
Medication use	Although only a few medications are known teratogens, the safety of most medications for use in pregnancy has not been proven. Women should be counseled to check with a midwife or other healthcare provider before using medications or over-the-counter treatments.
Mercury exposure	The primary sources of mercury are large fish. See Box 22-8.
Seat belts	Three-point seat belts are recommended. The lap belt should be placed across the hips and below the uterus. The shoulder belt should be placed between the breasts and lateral to the uterus.
Sex during pregnancy	Sexual intercourse is not associated with adverse outcomes. Sexual intercourse is contraindicated for women with a placenta previa, preterm labor, or ruptured membranes.
Vaccines in pregnancy	See Table 22-10.

health education series published by the *Journal of Midwifery & Women's Health*, the CDC, the March of Dimes, and the 4women website sponsored by the U.S. Department of Health and Human Services Office of Women's Health.

Food Safety During Pregnancy

Some bacteria that infect foods can have teratogenic or fetotoxic effects. In turn, pregnant women are cautioned to avoid certain foods. Recommendations for food safety are listed in **Box 22-8**.[121]

BOX 22-8 Food Safety During Pregnancy

Foods to Avoid

- Soft cheeses unless they clearly state they are made from pasteurized milk, including brie, feta, camembert, blue-veined cheeses, and Mexican-style cheeses such as queso blanco, queso fresco, and Panela
- Uncooked meats or refrigerated pâtés or meat spreads
- Raw eggs, cookie dough
- Raw fish
- Shark, swordfish, king mackerel, and tilefish[a]
- Deli meat salads or smoked seafood
- Raw sprouts
- Raw unpasteurized fruit juice or unpasteurized dairy products

Food Handling

- Wash cutting boards and equipment used to cut raw meat with hot soap and water
- Wash and peel raw fruits and vegetables before eating
- Wash hands after handling hot dogs, luncheon meats, or deli meats

Food Processing

- Cook all deli meats, hot dogs, and luncheon meats to steaming hot before eating
- Cook meat and eggs to 71.1°C (160°F)
- Cook seafood to 62.8°C (145°F)

[a]One to two fish servings per week are recommended during pregnancy. The fish with the smallest amounts of mercury are shrimp, light canned tuna, catfish, pollock, and salmon. The maximum recommended intake of albacore tuna is 6 oz per week.

Source: Adapted from Food and Drug Administration. Food safety for moms-to-be. Updated February 28, 2013. Available at: http://www.fda.gov/food/resourcesforyou/healtheducators/ucm081785.htm.

Planning for Birth

Planning for birth includes consideration of childbirth education classes, sibling preparation, assessment for postpartum support at home, knowing when to go to the hospital if a hospital birth is planned, and knowing when and how to contact the midwife. If the woman already has children, she also should have arrangements made for childcare based on the birth site she has planned.

Childbirth Preparation Classes

One could argue that childbirth education has existed forever in the form of information shared by women and midwives. Even today, pregnant women get the majority of the information they receive about birth from books or friends and family, rather than healthcare providers or childbirth educators.[122] Nevertheless, childbirth education classes, like prenatal vitamins, are generally recommended without strong evidence for their effectiveness.

In the United States, the first formal childbirth classes in the early 1900s focused on preparation for parenting, nutrition, and health care.[123] Formal childbirth preparation classes that addressed how to cope with labor first started in the United States in 1947, when the Maternity Center Association in New York sponsored Grantly Dick-Read's visit to the United States. Dick-Read is credited with being the founder of childbirth preparation. His book *Childbirth Without Fear*[124] describes how pain in labor can be decreased via knowledge of the fear–tension–pain syndrome wherein fear increases tension, which in turn increases pain. Dick-Read's work served as the foundation for the different models of childbirth preparation taught today.[125] The focus of the childbirth preparation techniques was originally to teach women about the process of labor and to give them techniques for coping with labor pain, with the goal of having an unmedicated birth. Today, most childbirth classes also teach women about medical procedures that can occur during labor and the focus on having an unmedicated birth varies with the particular technique. **Table 22-12** briefly outlines the different types of childbirth education classes that are taught today.

The effectiveness of childbirth education has proved difficult to determine, as the goals of the programs are all somewhat different and there may exist differences between groups of women who seek classes and those who do not. Overall, formal childbirth education appears to improve knowledge, lower anxiety, and increase self-efficacy. The effect of childbirth education on perception of labor pain is modest at best.

Table 22-12	Comparison of Childbirth Education Models/Organizations
Childbirth Education Model	**Teaching Elements**
Lamaze Childbirth Education	Goal is to increase confidence in giving birth by focusing on how to cope with labor pain
	Natural childbirth
	Controlled breathing, used to enhance relaxation and decrease perception of pain
	Communication skills
	Evidence based
	Comfort measures
	Information about obstetrical procedures
	Breastfeeding encouraged
Bradley Method (husband-coached childbirth)	Goal is to facilitate natural birth via breathing techniques and partner support
	Natural childbirth
	Partner's active participation
	Avoidance of medications and medical procedures
	Nutrition and exercise
	Relaxation techniques and guided imagery
	Coping mechanisms
	Immediate contact with newborn and immediate breastfeeding
	Six needs of laboring women: darkness and solitude, quiet, physical comfort during the first stage of labor, physical relaxation, controlled breathing, need to close eyes with the appearance of sleep
International Childbirth Education Association (ICEA)	Family-centered maternity care
	Freedom of choice
	Alternatives in childbirth
	Draws from other models
HypnoBirthing, Mongan Method	Calm, peaceful, natural childbirth
	Relaxation techniques
	Negate the fear–tension–pain cycle
	Education
	Evidence based
Mindfulness Childbirth	Mindfulness techniques used to help couples cope with labor
	Meditation and yoga
	Stress reduction
	Awareness
	Breathing
	Group dialogue
Birthing From Within	Natural childbirth goal
	Based on *primordial knowing* (knowledge of body) and *modern knowing* (knowledge of medical culture and how to give birth within this culture)
	Soulful and holistic approach
	Creative self-expression via artwork and journaling
	Instructor and couples co-create class together
	Coping with challenges
Hospital-based classes	Instructors can be certified in Lamaze, ICEA, or other childbirth education technique
	Philosophy of childbirth educators varies
	Increased focus on institutional policies and procedures with information about medical procedures
	Breathing, relaxation, and massage technique

Source: Adapted from Walker DS, Visger JM, Rossie D. Contemporary childbirth education models. *J Midwifery Women's Health.* 2009;54(6):469-471. Reprinted with permission of Wiley.

Postpartum Contraception

The initial conversation about postpartum contraception should take place prenatally for two reasons. First, postpartum contraceptive choices depend on infant feeding choice, so the options available may be new information for nulliparous women. Second, some women assume that pregnancy cannot occur while they are breastfeeding and not having menses. Although the chance of pregnancy occurring in the first 4 weeks postpartum is unlikely, breastfeeding does not reliably prevent pregnancy even if it prevents return of regular menses unless the requirements of the lactational amenorrheic method are met as outlined in the *Nonhormonal Contraception* chapter. Key items to discuss are the usual timing of ovulation, contraceptive methods that can be used immediately after birth, and the need to avoid hormonal contraception for the first 4 weeks postpartum if breastfeeding exclusively.

Relief Measures for Common Discomforts of Pregnancy

Not all women experience each of the common discomforts listed in this section. However, when they do occur, relief from these discomforts can make a significant difference in how a woman experiences pregnancy. Because uncomfortable symptoms are common in pregnancy, it can be tempting to attribute any symptoms to normal pregnancy effects. However, it is important to make a thorough assessment of every symptom reported to rule out signs of a disorder that needs further evaluation. The common discomforts are presented in the approximate chronologic order of their appearance in pregnancy.

Breast Tenderness

Etiology

The breasts undergo significant changes secondary to the effects of estrogen, progesterone, prolactin, hCG, and human placental lactogen (HPL). The fat layer of the breasts thickens, and there is proliferation and differentiation of the ductal system and glandular tissues of the breasts. Blood flow increases, and it is common for the blood vessels of the breast to appear more prominent when inspecting the breasts. The breasts increase in size and weight, causing many women to experience breast heaviness and/or breast tenderness. Additionally, breast appearance changes, as the areola darkens and increases in size and the Montgomery's tubercles enlarge. Many women will experience tingling or increased sensitivity of the nipples in addition to tenderness of the breast tissue. As the breasts prepare for lactation, it is not uncommon for many women to notice yellow to milky-colored colostrum discharge that can sometimes stain or dry on the woman's bra or sleeping clothes.

Warning Signs and Differential Diagnosis

The expected changes of pregnancy will involve both breasts and typically do not cause acute pain, redness, or warmth—especially in a localized area. Breasts should not demonstrate any of the warning signs of dimpling, puckering, peeling, or retracting skin, and the breasts and axillae should be absent of any dominant or suspicious masses. Consideration of differential diagnoses such as mastitis, fibrocystic breast changes, benign breast mass, and breast cancer should accompany any evaluation of breast complaints.

Relief Measures

The breast size increase that can occur in pregnancy may be either a welcome or an unwelcome change for a woman. Often, wearing a correctly fitted and supportive bra is an effective relief measure. If the tenderness is significant, some women find it helpful to wear a bra while sleeping. Correct fit is important when wearing a bra during pregnancy, and a woman may need to change sizes more than once during the pregnancy. Avoidance of caffeine or other methylxanthines may help prevent additional breast tenderness although effectiveness of this method has not been proven.

Fatigue

Etiology

As many as 95% of pregnant women experience fatigue at some point in pregnancy, making it among the most common pregnancy discomforts.[126] The etiology of pregnancy fatigue is not well known. It is often in evidence during the first trimester and then again in the third trimester. A variety of potential causes have been suggested, such as increased energy requirements, weight gain and musculoskeletal changes that can make regular movement or activity more difficult, and the influence of pregnancy hormones such as progesterone.[127] Fatigue in the third trimester can also be a result of disrupted sleep patterns.[128] Fatigue can also have the effect of increasing the intensity of the psychological responses the woman is having during pregnancy. Sleep deprivation, anxiety, and childbirth fear have been significantly correlated with fatigue in pregnancy.[129]

Warning Signs and Differential Diagnosis

Other causes of fatigue and insomnia should be evaluated, such as thyroid dysfunction, depression, anemia, sleep apnea, cardiac conditions, and viral or other systemic illnesses. Careful consideration of non-pregnancy-related causes is important, especially if fatigue appears to be worsening or is accompanied by other symptoms such as hair loss, temperature intolerance, heart palpitations, shortness of breath, weakness, or dizziness.

Relief Measures

It can be helpful to provide women with reassurance regarding the normality of fatigue and the common experience of gradual, spontaneous remission by the second trimester. Promoting adequate sleep and adequate nutrition may improve fatigue for some women. Making time for frequent rest periods is a common recommendation for relief of fatigue, although not all women experience significant relief of fatigue of pregnancy by increasing rest periods. Increasing exercise may combat fatigue. Pregnant women with insomnia or sleep disruptions may benefit from complementary and alternative therapies that assist with relaxation such as yoga and meditation.[129]

Nausea and Vomiting

Nausea is a common problem in the prenatal period, occurring in as many as 80% of pregnant women.[130] Nausea is so common, in fact, that it is a presumptive sign of pregnancy. The peak prevalence of nausea and vomiting in pregnant women is at 11 weeks' gestation, with the average time of onset between 5 and 6 weeks. For most women, nausea and vomiting in pregnancy (NVP) will resolve by 14 to 16 weeks' gestation, although a small percentage of women will have NVP that persists beyond 20 weeks.[131] Women with a multiple gestation often have longer-lasting and more severe nausea and vomiting.

Etiology

Nausea, with or without vomiting, has erroneously been termed "morning sickness" because, it is not limited to the morning hours but can occur during at any time of day. Nausea is more apt to be present when the stomach is empty, which may be why it can be more noticeable in the morning in some women. The cause of NVP is not fully known, although a number of theories have been advanced. Likely causes include the interplay between hormonal changes of pregnancy (e.g., hCG, estrogen, progesterone, placental prostaglandin E_2), slowed peristalsis, and genetic factors. Other factors such as preexisting gastroesophageal reflux disease (GERD) or *Helicobacter pylori* infection can contribute to the occurrence of NVP in many women.[131]

There is little support for an older theory that NVP, especially severe nausea and vomiting, reflects the transformation of psychological distress into physical symptoms.[131] Rather, it is more likely that biologic, psychologic, and sociocultural factors have an intricate relationship with NVP that is poorly understood. Persistent and severe nausea and vomiting beyond the first trimester may indicate hyperemesis gravidarum or hydatidiform mole.

The severity of NVP and how the symptoms interfere with her ability to maintain daily activities needs to be established for each woman. Standardized measures such as the Pregnancy-Unique Quantification of Emesis/Nausea Index (PUQE) can be a helpful tool to aid the midwife in determining which relief measures to recommend (**Table 22-13**).[132]

Warning Signs and Differential Diagnosis

When NVP is very severe, it is called hyperemesis gravidarum (HG). Hyperemesis is a common reason for hospitalization in pregnancy. Women with persistent nausea and vomiting, inability to retain any liquids or solids, weight loss, ketonuria, or dehydration warrant careful and close evaluation and treatment for hyperemesis gravidarum (see the *Obstetric Complications in Pregnancy* chapter). Differential diagnoses to be considered when evaluating NVP in addition to hyperemesis include thyroid disease and gastrointestinal disorders such as GERD, peptic ulcer disease, cholecystitis, and gastroenteritis.

Relief Measures

There are numerous relief measures for NVP that have not been evaluated for effectiveness. Nonetheless, many dietary strategies are recommended because they are unlikely to cause harm and may be of benefit. **Box 22-9** lists some of the more common recommendations for mitigating the discomfort of pregnancy-induced nausea and vomiting. There is good evidence for use of acupressure, acupuncture, ginger, vitamin B_6, and medication therapies, although their effects may be modest.[131,133]

It is also common for a relief measure or combination of measures to become ineffective after a short time, so that the woman may need to try different strategies. Frequent reassurance and emotional support can help women with NVP, as these symptoms can be distressing, especially when relief measures are not working or stop working.

Table 22-13	Modified PUQE Index

1. On an average day, for how long do you feel nauseated or sick to your stomach?

> 6 hours (5 points)	4–6 hours (4 points)	2–3 hours (3 points)	≤ 1 hour (2 points)	Not at all (1 point)

2. On an average day, how many times do you vomit or throw up?

7 or more (5 points)	5–6 (4 points)	3–4 (3 points)	1–2 (2 points)	None (1 point)

3. On an average day, how many times do you have retching or dry heaves without bringing anything up?

7 or more (5 points)	5–6 (4 points)	3–4 (3 points)	1–2 (2 points)	None (1 point)

Total score is the sum of the points for each of the three questions.

Nausea score: mild NVP = ≤ 6; moderate NVP = 7–12, severe NVP = ≥ 13.

Source: Reprinted from *American Journal of Obstetrics and Gynecology* 198(1), January 2008, Lacasse A et al., "Validity of a modified Pregnancy-Unique Quantification of Emesis and Nausea (PUQE) scoring index to assess severity of nausea and vomiting of pregnancy," Copyright 2008, with permission from Elsevier.

BOX 22-9 Nonpharmacologic Relief Measures for Nausea and Vomiting in Pregnancy[a]

- Eat small, frequent meals, even as often as every 2 hours, as these may be more apt to be retained than three large meals a day.

- Eat dry crackers or toast before getting up in the morning.

- Avoid brushing teeth immediately after eating to avoid stimulating the gag reflex.

- Drink carbonated beverages—ginger ale made with real ginger may be helpful.

- Avoid eating or preparing foods with strong or offensive odors.

- Because fats can decrease gastric emptying time, decreasing fats in the diet may be helpful.

- Avoid consuming liquids and solids at the same time to prevent overfilling of the stomach.

- Suck on a hard candy (tart or sweet) or a mint periodically between meals.

- Acupressure wristbands can be worn daily or the woman can use manual pressure on the P6 acupressure point.

- Promote frequent rest periods and adequate sleep.

- Maintain regular exercise.

- Acupuncture or hypnosis may be beneficial.

- Communicate to the woman's significant others to provide her with considerate, understanding, loving treatment with special attention to the little things that are important to her.

- Discontinue prenatal vitamins (maintain folic acid) until nausea resolves.

- Take ginger, 1 gram in divided doses per day.

[a]Educational counseling is primarily based on expert opinion and common practice. Little strong evidence exists in this area.

Pyridoxine (vitamin B$_6$) and the antihistamine doxylamine (Unisom) are both FDA Category A drugs and have extensive research establishing their safety in pregnancy.[134] The anti-nausea drug known as Bendectin in the United States, which contained pyridoxine (vitamin B$_6$) and doxylamine, was commonly used in pregnancy throughout the 1970s and early 1980s, but it was voluntarily removed from the market because of litigation brought against the manufacturer that claimed congenital malformations resulting from use of the drug.[131] This legal action was taken despite numerous epidemiologic studies and a large meta-analysis that showed no increased risk of congenital malformations in women who used Bendectin.[135] Fortunately, pyridoxine and doxylamine are readily available as over-the-counter remedies. A reformulated delayed-release version of the drug combination is widely used in Canada and now available in the United States under the brand names Diclectin (Canada) and Diclegis (United States). This pharmaceutical has demonstrated effectiveness in research studies.[131] Women with mild NVP who do not experience relief of symptoms with nonpharmacologic relief measures will often experience some relief of symptoms by adding pyridoxine 25 mg, taken orally two to three times per day, with or without doxylamine 12.5 mg, taken two to four times daily. Use of doxylamine can cause drowsiness.

Ptyalism (Excessive Salivation)

Etiology

The etiology of ptyalism is uncertain. Some women may have the sensation of ptyalism related to a reluctance to swallow saliva during periods of nausea and vomiting, but in some cases a woman will have an actual increase in saliva production.

Warning Signs and Differential Diagnosis

Because ptyalism is often associated with nausea and vomiting, the differential diagnoses include hyperemesis gravidarum and GERD.

Relief Measures

Ptyalism usually resolves spontaneously, although resolution may not occur until after the pregnancy is over. Women with severe ptyalism need emotional support, as this condition can be quite distressing. Some women get temporary relief from gum chewing or sucking on hard candies. Many women will need

or want to carry a cup, tissues, handkerchief, or even a small towel with them to be able to have something to spit into when needed.

Urinary Frequency and Nocturia

Etiology

Urinary frequency, defined as urinating more than seven times during the daytime hours, as a non-pathologic discomfort of pregnancy occurs at two different times during the prenatal period. Frequency during the first trimester is due to hormonal changes affecting levels of renal function as well as developing hypervolemia. Urinary frequency during the third trimester occurs most often in primiparous women, after engagement has occurred when the presenting part descends into the pelvis and causes direct pressure against the bladder.

Nocturia also can be caused by increased urine production at night. Venous return from the extremities is facilitated when the woman lies in a recumbent lateral position while sleeping at night, when the uterus is not pressing against the pelvic vessels and inferior vena cava, which results in an increase in urinary output. Additionally, pregnant women have an increase in sodium excretion at night, with an associated increase in fluid excretion, which may also explain nocturia.

Warning Signs and Differential Diagnosis

The differential diagnosis when a woman has urinary frequency or nocturia is urinary tract infection. Symptoms such as dysuria, hematuria, fever, suprapubic pain, or changes in the appearance of the urine deserve further evaluation.

Relief Measures

The only relief measures for urinary frequency are an explanation of why it occurs, reassurance, and decreasing fluid intake before bedtime. Women should be counseled that they should not try to restrict fluids in general.

Constipation

Etiology

Constipation is common early in pregnancy. Many factors contribute to the development of constipation, including decreased peristalsis caused by relaxation of the smooth muscle of the large bowel in the presence of increased amounts of progesterone, as well as changes in fluid reabsorption. The displacement and compression of the bowel by the enlarging uterus or presenting part may also contribute to decreased motility in the gastrointestinal tract and, therefore, to constipation. One of the common side effects of iron medication is constipation; this compounds the problem for a large percentage of pregnant women. Dietary factors as well as a decrease in physical activity and exercise in formerly active women may also contribute to constipation.

Warning Signs and Differential Diagnosis

Constipation associated with severe abdominal pain, fever, or weight loss could indicate a more serious problem and should be evaluated immediately. Other possible causes of constipation include use of opioids or other medications, and other causes of abdominal pain and discomfort, such as preterm labor or gastrointestinal disorders such as irritable bowel syndrome.

Relief Measures

Nonpharmacologic relief measures for constipation are listed in **Box 22-10**. They are most effective when all are used in combination. Medications can be recommended if the nonpharmacologic methods are not sufficient. Mild bulk-forming laxatives, stool softeners, and glycerin suppositories are all safe for use in pregnancy, whereas stimulant laxatives should be avoided.

Flatulence and Gas Pain

Etiology

Flatulence and gas pain are another result of decreased gastrointestinal motility. The slower transit time allows food a longer time for fermentation and gas production in the intestine. The decreased motility results both from the effect of progesterone relaxing smooth muscle and from the displacement of and pressure on the intestines by the enlarging uterus.

Warning Signs and Differential Diagnosis

Other potential causes of flatulence and gas include dietary sensitivities or intolerances, irritable bowel syndrome, celiac disease, and other gastrointestinal disorders. Pain that is not relieved with passage of flatus or pain that is worsening, along with any warning signs such as fever, changes in stool color (i.e., black, tarry stools), diarrhea, or rectal bleeding, warrants further evaluation.

BOX 22-10 Nonpharmacologic Relief Measures for Constipation in Pregnancy[a]

- An adequate fluid intake, defined as a minimum of eight glasses (drinking-glass size) per day.
- Prunes or prune juice; prunes are a natural mild laxative.
- Warm liquids (e.g., water, tea) on rising, to stimulate peristalsis.
- A diet high in nutritious sources of fiber (25–30 grams daily) is helpful in relieving constipation. Foods that contain roughage, bulk, and natural fiber (e.g., greens, celery, bran) can be slowly and gradually added to the diet while assuring adequate water intake as well. Bulk-forming fiber supplements may also be used.
- Exercise, a daily walk, good posture, good body mechanics, and daily exercise of contracting the lower abdominal muscles; all of these measures facilitate venous circulation and promote peristalsis, thereby preventing congestion in the large intestines.

[a]Educational counseling is primarily based on expert opinion and common practice. Little strong evidence exists in this area.

Relief Measures

The only relief measures are maintaining a regular pattern of bowel movements and avoidance of gas-forming foods. Some women may experience flatulence and gas pains if fiber is added to the diet too quickly or without adequate hydration; thus decreasing fiber consumption for a short time and slowly and gradually increasing it along with increasing water intake may be beneficial. Exercise can aid in improving gastrointestinal motility and help with gas expulsion. The knee-chest position may also help with discomfort from unexpelled gas. Some women may benefit from working with a nutritionist for evaluation of the diet to detect possible dietary triggers or food sensitivities.

Dyspnea

Etiology

Pregnant women frequently experience varying degrees of dyspnea, ranging from shortness of breath to hyperventilation. These symptoms, which may begin as early as the first trimester, can provoke significant anxiety, which can in turn exacerbate the experience. The etiology of this condition is largely unknown, but it is thought to relate to an enhanced sensitivity to carbon dioxide levels as well as to hypoxia. Pregnancy is associated with an increase in minute ventilation (i.e., the volume of air inhaled and exhaled in a minute) and in pulmonary blood volume, both of which can contribute to the sensation of dyspnea. Pregnant women often describe the sensation as needing to take an "extra" breath. As the uterus expands into the abdominal cavity in the second and third trimesters, the respiratory effort required by the woman further contributes to dyspnea.

Warning Signs and Differential Diagnosis

The dyspnea of pregnancy is not associated with tachypnea. Any acute or severe episode of dyspnea or any associated symptoms such as fever, upper or lower respiratory infection, or adventitious breath sounds suggest a pathologic disorder such as asthma, pulmonary embolism, pneumonia, bronchitis, or possibly cardiac disorders.

Relief Measures

Relief measures for hyperventilation include encouraging the woman to deliberately regulate the speed and depth of her respirations at normal rates when she is aware of hyperventilating, having the woman periodically stand up and stretch her arms above her head and take a deep breath, teaching the woman to do intercostal breathing as opposed to abdominal breathing, and explaining the physiologic basis for shortness of breath to relieve anxiety.

Bleeding Gums
Etiology

During pregnancy, bleeding gums, especially after brushing teeth, is related to estrogen- and progesterone-mediated inflammation and hyperemia. Elevated levels of estrogen create a favorable environment for the growth of bacteria that can cause gingivitis and gingival inflammation.

Warning Signs and Differential Diagnosis

Bleeding gums may be an indication of thrombocytopenia or periodontal disease, and both of these conditions should be ruled out. An additional complication that may be encountered is the development of epulis, or "pregnancy tumor," which is a benign overgrowth of friable gingival tissue that will typically resolve after birth.

Relief Measures

Reassurance and education about the normalcy of this symptom, in addition to encouraging frequent dental hygiene (regular teeth brushing and flossing) and dental care as regularly scheduled, are usually all that are required.

Heart Palpitations
Etiology

Some pregnant women report feeling changes in cardiac rhythm, which may be described as a skipped beat, an extra beat, a fluttering sensation, or heart palpitations. The majority of these symptoms last for a short time period and are not associated with underlying cardiac disease. They are usually premature ventricular or atrial contractions. The etiology is unclear, but may possibly be related to hormonal changes, fluid and electrolyte imbalance, or an active sympathetic nervous system.

Warning Signs and Differential Diagnosis

Heart palpitations may also be a sign of undiagnosed cardiac disease or structural defect, and should be thoroughly assessed just as they would be in nonpregnant women. Diagnoses such as thyroid disorder and anxiety should be considered as well.

Relief Measures

There are no specific relief measures that stop the sensation. Reassurance and education are usually sufficient.

Leukorrhea
Etiology

Leukorrhea is a profuse, thin or thick vaginal secretion that typically begins during the second trimester. The secretion is acidic because of the conversion of glycogen in the vaginal epithelial cells into lactic acid by lactobacilli, or Döderlein's bacilli. The productivity of the cervical glands in secreting more mucus at this time to form the cervical mucus plug may also contribute to leukorrhea.

Warning Signs and Differential Diagnosis

An increase in vaginal discharge may be a sign of vaginitis, either sexually transmitted or not, ruptured membranes, or premature labor.

Relief Measures

Pregnant women should be encouraged to avoid douching or using feminine hygiene sprays and to clean the perineal and vaginal areas only with water.

Frequent changes of unscented, cotton panty-liners and cotton underwear can increase comfort as well.

Leg Cramps

As many as 25% to 50% of pregnant women experience leg cramps.[136]

Etiology

The physiologic basis for leg cramps during pregnancy is unclear. Potential causes include hormonal and biochemical changes of pregnancy affecting the calcium, magnesium, and phosphorus levels or the ability of calcium to enter the muscles, but these causes have not been proven. Another school of thought suggests that the enlarged uterus exerts pressure either on the pelvic blood vessels, thereby impairing circulation, or on the nerves as they course through the obturator foramen. Additional, non-pregnancy-related causes of leg cramps include electrolyte imbalances, excessive activity, and muscle or neurovascular disorders.[136]

Pregnancy is a known cause of secondary restless leg syndrome, which has the same symptoms as leg cramps but is a distinct disorder.

Warning Signs and Differential Diagnosis

Leg cramps are classified as part of sleep-related movement disorders by the American Academy of Sleep Medicine.[136] Leg cramps should be differentiated from restless leg syndrome through careful history and review of the diagnostic criteria.[136] Other potential causes of leg pain to be considered include radicular pain associated with back injury, musculoskeletal disorders, endocrine or renal disorders that can cause muscle cramps, phlebitis, peripheral neuropathy, deep vein thrombosis, and peripheral vascular disease. Careful muscular, neurologic, circulatory, and skin assessment of the lower extremities is important when evaluating a complaint of leg cramps or pain.

Relief Measures

Common suggestions that may be beneficial include having the woman straighten her affected leg and dorsiflex her ankle. If the woman is in bed, she may need strong, steady pressure against the bottom of her foot—either someone's hand or the footboard of the bed—to push against; if she is standing, the floor serves this function. This measure will frequently alleviate an acute leg cramp. Magnesium supplementation of 350 mg at bedtime has shown to be helpful in some studies, but not all.

Round Ligament Pain

Etiology

The round ligaments attach on either side of the uterus just below and in front of the insertion of the fallopian tubes; they then cross the broad ligament in a fold of peritoneum, pass through the inguinal canal, and insert in the anterior (upper) portion of the labia majora on either side of the perineum. The ligaments are composed largely of smooth muscle that is continuous with the smooth muscle of the uterus. The round ligaments hypertrophy during pregnancy and stretch as the uterus enlarges. It is anatomically mandatory that the round ligaments increase in length as the uterus rises high into the abdomen. Round ligament pain probably results from this stretching and possibly from the pressure of the increasingly heavy uterus on the ligaments.

Warning Signs and Differential Diagnosis

Other potential causes of lower abdominal pain include preterm labor, appendicitis, constipation, gas pain, inguinal hernia, and muscle strain or sprain. One feature that aids in this differentiation is the extension of pain into the inguinal or labial area, which, among the conditions mentioned, is specific to round ligament pain. Round ligament pain also often becomes worse with exercise or turning.

Relief Measures

Relief measures are few and not always effective. Explanations of why the pain is happening may help to alleviate anxieties or fears and may help a woman to cope with the discomfort. Additional measures include pelvic tilt exercises, positions that place less tension on the round ligament (**Figure 22-2**), and wearing a maternity abdominal support or girdle.

Heartburn (Pyrosis)

Heartburn affects as many as 50% of pregnant women.[137] The symptoms can start in the first trimester

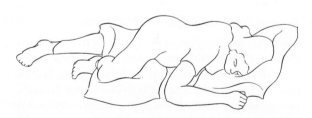

Figure 22-2 Side-lying relaxation position.

and continue throughout pregnancy. As many as 80% of women experience heartburn in the third trimester.[138]

Etiology

Regurgitation, or reflux, of acidic gastric contents into the lower esophagus causes the sensation of heartburn. Several physiologic changes of pregnancy predispose the pregnant woman to heartburn: The lower esophageal sphincter is relaxed, gastrointestinal motility is slower, esophageal function and peristalsis change, and the angle of the gastroesophageal junction is altered as the stomach is displaced by the enlarging uterus.[137]

Heartburn is described as burning sensation in the chest or throat and may lead to development of gastroesophageal reflux disease. Factors such as higher prepregnant BMI; weight gain in pregnancy; smoking; and prepregnant heartburn, GERD, or nausea and vomiting have been associated with increased likelihood of heartburn in pregnancy.

Warning Signs and Differential Diagnosis

Symptoms of heartburn should be distinguished from hiatal hernia, peptic ulcer disease, cholecystitis, and pancreatitis. Although not common in pregnancy, reflux of gastric material may ultimately cause esophagitis. The sensation of heartburn may be described as "chest pain," therefore other causes of chest pain must be ruled out—that is, causes that are cardiac in origin, as well as asthma and pulmonary embolism. Women with epigastric pain should also be evaluated for preeclampsia.

Relief Measures

Relief measures for heartburn are typically the same as those recommended to nonpregnant individuals (**Box 22-11**). Finding the right combination is largely a matter of trial and error.

When medication is needed, a stepwise approach is recommended: starting with antacids, then moving as necessary to medications such as H_2 receptor antagonists (H_2 antihistamines, H_2 blockers), and lastly using proton pump inhibitors for women with intractable symptoms that are unresponsive to other measures.[139] Any recommendation for medication must always involve informed consent so that the woman understands what is and is not known about the safety and effectiveness of these drugs.

Antacids are readily available over-the-counter and work by neutralizing gastric acid secretions. Most magnesium-, calcium-, and aluminum-based

---

> ### BOX 22-11 Nonpharmacologic Relief Measures for Heartburn in Pregnancy[a]
>
> - Consume small, frequent meals, eaten at a slow pace to avoid overfilling the stomach.
> - Avoid foods that trigger symptoms. Foods that commonly make heartburn worse include fried foods, citrus, tea, cola, coffee, chocolate, and spicy foods.
> - Avoid lying down within 3 hours of eating.
> - Elevate the head of the bed by 10 to 30 degrees.
>
> [a]Educational counseling is primarily based on expert opinion and common practice. Little strong evidence exists in this area.

---

antacids are considered safe in pregnancy. They do not have FDA drug categorization and have minimal systemic absorption. Magnesium trisilicate and sodium bicarbonate (Alka-Seltzer, baking soda) should be avoided due to the risk for metabolic alkalosis and fluid overload.[140,141] Women should be counseled not to exceed daily dosage limits, especially with calcium- and aluminum-containing antacids. Antacids have numerous drug–drug interactions; for example, they decrease the absorption of iron. Magnesium-based antacids can cause diarrhea and calcium- and aluminum-based antacids can cause constipation.[141]

H_2 receptor antagonists have been evaluated for their safety in pregnancy. Ranitidine (Zantac) and cimetidine (Tagamet) have the most evidence for their safety.[140] Omeprazole (Prilosec) has been associated with adverse fetal effects in animals, but it has the most research related to its safety of all the proton pump inhibitors and has no known teratogenicity in humans.[141]

Dyspareunia

Etiology

Vulvovaginal pain during sexual activity may stem from a number of causes during pregnancy. Physiologic changes such as pelvic/vaginal congestion may play a role. Vaginal sensitivity may cause dyspareunia, and vascular engorgement may contribute to vulvar varicosities that can also cause pain or discomfort.

Warning Signs and Differential Diagnosis

A woman who reports dyspareunia while pregnant may have a previous experience of sexual dysfunction that she is reporting for the first time during pregnancy. A thorough sexual history can be the most important factor in determining a diagnosis for dyspareunia. Dyspareunia can also be a sign of vaginitis, either sexually transmitted or not, or vulvovaginal disorders. Pain with penetration in early pregnancy may indicate an ovarian cyst or ectopic pregnancy. Dyspareunia is also associated with current or past IPV or a history of sexual assault or abuse.

Relief Measures

Appropriate relief measures depend on the etiology. Treatments for dyspareunia range from simple positional changes to alleviate problems that are caused by an enlarged abdomen or pain from deep penetration to more complex therapies for women who have been sexually abused. Many women will benefit from a frank discussion of sexual positions, changes in sexual technique that might bring greater comfort and pleasure, and contraindications to vaginal penetration and/or orgasm during pregnancy.

Back Pain: Upper and Lower

Approximately 70% of pregnant women experience back pain at some point during pregnancy.

Etiology

Low back pain in the lumbosacral region generally occurs in the last half of pregnancy and increases in intensity as the pregnancy progresses secondary to the increasing weight of the enlarging uterus and relaxation of the sacroiliac ligaments that normally support the uterus and prevent its forward tilt. The normal lordosis of pregnancy strains the back muscles and causes pain. The problem is exaggerated if the woman's abdominal muscles are lax—a condition that is more common in multiparous women. Thus low back pain generally increases in severity with parity.

Backache may also result from excessive bending, walking without rest periods, and lifting. Upper backache develops during the first trimester because of the increase in size and resulting heaviness of the breasts. This enlargement may produce muscular strain if the breasts are not adequately supported.

Warning Signs and Differential Diagnosis

Low back pain can be a symptom of early labor, pyelonephritis, kidney stone, or gastrointestinal disorders such as cholecystitis, pancreatitis, or peptic ulcer disease. Careful musculoskeletal and neurologic assessment is indicated and further investigation is warranted with acute, severe, or worsening pain; pain that radiates down the buttocks or legs; any loss of function or sensation of the lower extremities; or loss of bowel or bladder control.

Relief Measures

Proper body mechanics for lifting may help prevent acute back pain during pregnancy. Women are counseled to stoop, rather than bend, to lift anything (e.g., a toddler, groceries) so that the legs (thighs), rather than the back, bear the weight and strain. They are also advised to spread the feet apart and place one foot slightly in front of the other when stooping so there is a broad base for balance when rising from the stooped position.

Multiple randomized controlled trials have evaluated pregnancy-specific exercises, pelvic tilt exercises, water gymnastics, physical therapy, acupuncture, and use of pillows. Strengthening exercises, sitting pelvic tilt exercises, and water gymnastics can all significantly reduce back pain intensity. Acupuncture may be more effective than physical therapy. The effect of sacroiliac belts is unclear.[142] Nonpharmacologic relief measures are listed in **Box 22-12**.

Sciatica

Etiology

Sciatica refers to pain in the pelvis, buttock, and lower extremity resulting from pressure on the sciatic nerve. In pregnancy, this pressure is produced by the growing fetus and expanding uterus.

Warning Signs and Differential Diagnosis

Any significant worsening in symptoms should be evaluated with a thorough musculoskeletal and neurologic assessment, paying particular attention to diminished strength, diminished reflexes, positive straight-leg raise sign, or other neurologic symptoms in the lower extremities. Additionally, if the woman reports loss of bowel or bladder control, severe symptoms, or loss of sensation or function in the lower extremities, immediate referral is indicated. If the pain is discovered to originate from above the pelvis, a careful evaluation for signs of pyelonephritis is indicated.

Relief Measures

Resting in a side-lying position on the contralateral side from the affected leg may afford some relief. Some women experience relief from use of heat packs, ice, or abdominal support girdles.

BOX 22-12 Nonpharmacologic Relief Measures for Back Pain in Pregnancy[a]

- Proper body mechanics for lifting
- Avoidance of excessive bending, lifting, or walking without rest periods
- Pelvic rock/pelvic tilt exercises
- Supportive low-heeled shoes—high heels are unstable and further exaggerate the problem of the center of gravity and lordosis
- If the problem is severe, external abdominal support (e.g., a maternity girdle or supportive elastic "belly band," or sacroiliac support belt)
- Warmth on the back (e.g., heating pad, warm bath, sitting in a warm shower)
- Ice packs on the back
- Massage therapy or backrub
- Regular exercise as tolerated; yoga or swimming may be helpful
- For resting or sleeping:
  ◆ A supportive mattress
  ◆ Positioning with pillows to straighten the back and alleviate pulling and strain
- For upper back pain, a well-fitting and supportive brassiere
- Evaluation and treatment by a chiropractor experienced in working with pregnant women

[a]Educational counseling is primarily based on expert opinion and common practice. Little strong evidence exists in this area.

Acetaminophen may also mitigate acute pain; the maximum daily dosage is 4000 mg/day when using acetaminophen. Yoga (cat and dog stretches) and muscle stretches that target the hamstrings, gluteal muscles, and hips can decrease symptoms as well. For those women with access to a chiropractor experienced in the care of pregnant women, a chiropractic adjustment may be of benefit. Moderate exercise on a regular basis may also provide relief—specifically, swimming and walking.

Hemorrhoids

Etiology

Progesterone causes relaxation of the vein walls in the rectum, which predisposes the woman to developing hemorrhoids. Then constipation and excessive straining when defecating adds to the risk. In addition, the enlarging uterus causes increasing pressure—specifically in the hemorrhoidal veins; this pressure interferes with venous circulation and causes congestion in the pelvic veins.

Warning Signs and Differential Diagnosis

Causes of constipation need to be considered when evaluating women who are experiencing hemorrhoids in pregnancy. Pain that is severe or getting worse should be carefully evaluated and external examination can help to rule out the presence of thrombosed hemorrhoids, which necessitate referral. Reports of abdominal pain, changes in stool color (i.e., black, tarry stools), diarrhea, or rectal bleeding should also prompt further investigation for other gastrointestinal disorders.

Relief Measures

A number of relief measures for hemorrhoids are available. Some solely give comfort; others both numb and reduce the hemorrhoids. The first step is to avoid constipation and straining during defecation. Sitz baths or ice may give some comfort. Witch hazel compresses or Epsom salt compresses may help reduce the size of the hemorrhoid. Topical anesthetics and topical cortisone creams are safe for use in pregnancy. Hemorrhoids also can be common during the postpartum period and further discussion can be found in the *Postpartum Care* chapter.

Edema

Etiology

Edema is the result of impaired venous circulation and increased venous pressure in the lower extremities. These circulatory disturbances are accentuated by pressure of the enlarging uterus on the pelvic veins when the woman is sitting or standing and on the inferior vena cava when she is supine. Additionally, higher estrogen levels affect the fluid permeability of the vessels as well as sodium retention. Any constrictive clothing that inhibits venous return from the lower extremities can add to the problem. Edema is generally dependent, in the ankles and feet, but may occur in the hands and face.

Warning Signs and Differential Diagnosis

The physiologic edema of pregnancy must be carefully differentiated from edema associated with preeclampsia/eclampsia. If swelling is unilateral, evaluation for signs of deep vein thrombosis is warranted. Potential causes related to musculoskeletal, renal, hepatic, cardiac, or vascular disorders should be considered. Evaluation of the extremities includes the muscular, neurologic, and circulatory systems as well as careful skin assessment.

Relief Measures

Relief measures include elevating the legs periodically throughout the day and positioning on the side when lying down. Graduated compression or support hose can reduce venous pooling in the lower extremities. Knee-high, thigh-high, or full-length hose can be used as tolerated. Women can apply them after rest periods or before getting out of bed when edema is at its lowest point to try to maximize their effectiveness. Regular exercise and avoiding prolonged sitting or standing may help.

Varicosities

Etiology

A number of factors contribute to the development of varicosities during pregnancy. Varicose veins are more apt to occur in women who have a familial tendency or congenital predisposition to this condition. Varicosities result from increased blood volume, impaired venous circulation, and increased venous pressure in the lower extremities. These changes are caused by pressure of the enlarging uterus on the pelvic veins when the woman is sitting or standing, and by pressure on the inferior vena cava when she is supine. Any constrictive clothing inhibiting venous return from the lower extremities or prolonged periods of standing or sitting can add to the problem. Estrogen- and progesterone-induced vasodilation—that is, relaxation of the vein walls and valves—also contributes to the development of varicosities. Increasing maternal age and multiparity can further add to the likelihood of varicosity formation secondary to loss of venous tone and decreased valve patency.[143] Varicosities during pregnancy are most pronounced in the legs and vulva.[144]

Warning Signs and Differential Diagnosis

The majority of women with varicosities do not have significant complications and usually obtain relief or resolution after giving birth. Lower-extremity or vulvar edema may accompany varicosities, and any edema should be carefully evaluated. Assessment of leg pain, pain with activity, skin temperature, skin appearance, nail appearance, and circulation in the lower extremities are elements to assess in the woman with varicosities. Differential diagnoses such as deep vein thrombosis and peripheral arterial or venous disease are important to consider.

Relief Measures

The primary nonpharmacologic treatments for varicosities are rest and use of compression stockings that are put on after elevating the legs before arising in the morning.

Insomnia and Sleep Disorders

Approximately 50% of pregnant women experience poor sleep quality by the third trimester.

Etiology

Insomnia—referring to the inability to fall asleep—and disordered sleep can have many causes in pregnancy, including hormonal changes, physical discomfort, and psychosocial changes, anxiety, or emotional distress. Estrogen, progesterone, cortisol, and prolactin all influence the sleep cycle during pregnancy. The most frequent reasons for altered sleep patterns in pregnancy are nocturia, back pain, heartburn, and hip pain.

Warning Signs and Differential Diagnosis

Women who report poor sleep quality, daytime sleepiness, difficulty sleeping, or insomnia warrant evaluation for other conditions that can affect the sleep cycle, such as anxiety, thyroid disorders, sleep apnea, restless leg syndrome, leg cramps, and cardiac or pulmonary conditions. Screening for substance use, intimate-partner violence, and abuse should also be performed.

Relief Measures

The time-honored relief measures for insomnia listed in **Box 22-13** may or may not be effective during pregnancy. Encourage women to use trial and error to discover which relief measures are helpful. It is important to provide emotional support for the distress that can happen with persistent or prolonged insomnia. Medication therapy is not recommended during pregnancy.

Supine Hypotensive Syndrome

Etiology

Supine hypotensive syndrome causes the woman to feel dizzy and lightheaded. Supine hypotensive syndrome occurs when the woman lies in a supine position (such as for sleep or on an examining table), and the full weight of the enlarged uterus and its contents rests on the inferior vena cava and other vessels of the venous system. Venous return from the lower half of the body is inhibited, which in turn reduces the amount of blood filling the woman's heart and subsequently lowers her cardiac output. Supine hypotensive syndrome is actually arterial hypotension. In addition, the weight of the enlarged uterus compresses the aorta, which also results in deleterious changes in arterial pressure.

BOX 22-13 Nonpharmacologic Relief Measures for Insomnia During Pregnancy[a]

- Warm baths or showers may help promote relaxation.

- Consume a warm noncaffeinated beverage before going to bed.

- Keep a consistent sleep and wake time schedule.

- Reduce stimulation prior to bedtime (i.e., turn off television, computers, or other electronics and keep electronics out of the bedroom).

- Avoid caffeine and simple sugars. Encourage consumption of a healthy, well-balanced diet.

- Regular exercise can be helpful. Vigorous exercise should be avoided near bedtime.

- Promote relaxation with breathing exercises. Meditation or hypnosis tapes may be helpful.

- Create darkness by using sleep shades or eye covers.

- Regulate the temperature in the bedroom to promote sleep.

- Avoid alcohol and smoking.

- Avoid drinking too many fluids prior to bedtime to reduce nocturia.

[a]Educational counseling is primarily based on expert opinion and common practice. Little strong evidence exists in this area.

Warning Signs and Differential Diagnosis

If a pregnant woman does not immediately rouse from a syncopal episode, if she has cognitive changes following the episode, or if the episode is accompanied by abnormal movements consistent with seizure, emergent evaluation is warranted. Other less serious causes include hypoglycemia and sudden change from sitting to standing.

Relief Measures

Supine hypotensive syndrome is alleviated immediately by simply having the woman either turn on her side or sit up. Reassurance and explanation are essential, because the sensation of near syncope or syncope can be frightening.

Tingling and Numbness of Fingers
Etiology

The change in the center of gravity resulting from the enlarged and heavy uterus may cause the woman to assume a posture in which her shoulders, neck, and head are out of their normal alignment. This places pressure or traction on nerves in the arm, which can cause tingling and numbness of the fingers. Physiologic edema can also exert pressure on the nerves supplying the hands, which can cause numbness or tingling or exacerbate preexisting problems such as carpal tunnel syndrome. Hyperventilation may cause finger tingling and numbness as well, but most women do not hyperventilate enough to have this effect.

Warning Signs and Differential Diagnosis

Another possible explanation for finger tingling and numbness is carpal tunnel syndrome. Edema reduces the available space in the carpal tunnel through which the median nerve passes. Compression of the nerve then causes these symptoms, which are usually bilateral, vary in severity, and at times become distressingly painful. Starting in the second or third trimester, the symptoms usually occur at night and resolve spontaneously during the postpartum period. Treatment is designed to alleviate symptoms and consists of wrist splints that keep the wrist in a neutral position and are worn while sleeping or during work or other activities.

Relief Measures

Relief measures include an explanation of the probable cause and encouraging scrupulous attention to good posture. Some women obtain relief simply by lying down. Also, the midwife should review good body mechanics and ergonomics, especially related to lifting and carrying of items, bags, car seats, children, and repetitive motions.

Conclusion

Although protocols and guidelines abound, prenatal care is more than a simple series of visits with scripted interventions. In reality, the complex nature of a pregnant woman's experience requires facile, flexible, and knowledgeable caregivers using a multifaceted approach. For the midwife, prenatal care involves an extensive knowledge of pregnancy, a broad understanding of common primary care topics, and recognition of the continuum of mental health states.

Prenatal care entails more than simply providing prenatal vitamins and scheduling fetal assessment tests, although these actions may be included. This care comprises a holistic approach encompassing important considerations about lifestyle, nutrition, and environmental factors that can affect not only the woman and fetus during this pregnancy, but also the entire family over its lifespan.

The midwife caring for a pregnant woman continually multitasks, holding several different perspectives at the same time, simultaneously offering support and health education, conducting ongoing risk assessment, and monitoring normal fetal development and pregnancy changes. Integrating these perspectives and helping women empower themselves, all in a short series of visits, is a unique and fascinating undertaking—one that can change the caregiver just as it changes the pregnant woman and her family.

● ● ● References

1. U.S. Public Health Service Expert Panel on the Content of Prenatal Care. *Caring for Our Future: The Content of Prenatal Care.* Washington, DC: U.S. Public Health Service, Department of Health and Human Services;1989.

2. Thompson JE, Walsh LV, Merkatz IR. The history of prenatal care: cultural, social, and medical contexts. In: Merkatz IR, Thompson JE, Mullen PD, Goldenbert RL, eds. *New Perspectives on Prenatal Care.* New York: Elsevier Science; 1990:9-30.

3. Gregory KD, Johnson CT, Johnson TRB, Entman SS. The content of prenatal care: update 2005. *Women's Health Issues.* 2006;16(4):198-215.

4. Walker DS, Day S, Diroff C, et al. Reduced frequency prenatal visits in midwifery practice: attitudes and use. *J Midwifery Women's Health.* 2002;47(4):269-277.

5. Dowswell T, Carroli G, Duley L, Gates S, Gülmezoglu AM, Khan-Neelofur D, et al. Alternative versus standard packages of antenatal care for low-risk pregnancy. *Cochrane Database Syst Rev.* 2010;10:CD000934. doi: 10.1002/14651858.CD000934.pub2.

6. Binstock MA, Wolde-Tsadik G. Alternative prenatal care: impact of reduced visit frequency, focused visits and continuity of care. *J Reprod Med.* 1995;40(7):507-512.

7. Walker DS, McCully L, Vest V. Evidence-based prenatal care visits: when less is more. *J Midwifery Women's Health.* 2001;46:148-1451.

8. Villar J, Ba'aqeel H, Piaggio G, et al. WHO antenatal care randomised trial for the evaluation of a new model of routine antenatal care. *Lancet.* 2001;357(9268):1551-1564.

9. McDuffie RS Jr, Beck A, Bischoff K, Cross J, Orleans M. Effect of frequency of prenatal care visits on perinatal outcome among low-risk women: a randomized controlled trial. *JAMA.* 1996;275(11):847-851.

10. Krans EE, Davis MM. Preventing low birthweight: 25 years, prenatal risk, and the failure to reinvent prenatal care. *Am J Obstet Gynecol.* 2012;206(5):398-403.

11. Alexander G, Kotelchuck M. Assessing the role and effectiveness of prenatal care: history, challenges, and directions for future research. *Public Health Rep.* 2001;116:306-316.

12. Hanson L, VandeVusse L, Roberts J, Forristal A. A critical appraisal of guidelines for antenatal care: components of care and priorities in prenatal education. *J Midwifery Women's Health.* 2009;54:458-468.

13. Raisler J, Kennedy H. Midwifery care of poor and vulnerable women, 1925–2003. *J Midwifery Women's Health.* 2005;50(2):113-121.

14. Hatem M, Sandall J, Devane D, Soltani H, Gates S. Midwife-led versus other models of care for childbearing women. *Cochrane Database Syst Rev.* 2008;4:CD004667. doi: 10.1002/14651858.CD004667.pub2.

15. Opara EL, Zaidi J. The interpretation and clinical application of the word "parity": a survey. *BJOG.* 2007;114:1295-1297.

16. Beebe KR. The perplexing parity puzzle. *AWHONN Lifelines.* 2005;9:394-399.

17. Mittendorf R, Williams MA, Berkey CS, Cotter RF. The length of uncomplicated human gestation. *Obstet Gynecol.* 1990;75(6):929-932.

18. Haarburger D, Pillay T. Historical perspectives in diagnostic clinical pathology: development of the pregnancy test. *J Clin Pathol.* 2011;64(6):546-548.

19. Thorstensen K. Midwifery management of first trimester bleeding and early pregnancy loss. *J Midwifery Women's Health.* 2000;45(6):481-497.

20. Wilcox AJ, Baird DD, Dunson D, McChesney R, Weinberg CR. Natural limits of pregnancy testing in relation to the expected menstrual period. *JAMA.* 2001;286(14):1759-1761.

21. Butler SA, Khanlian SA, Cole LA. Detection of early pregnancy forms of human chorionic gonadotropin by home pregnancy test devices. *Clin Chem.* 2001;47(12):2131-2136.

22. Benagiano G. The fate of fertilized human oocytes. *Reprod BioMed Online.* 2010;21:731.

23. Barnhart KT, Sammel MD, Rinaudo PF, Zhou L, Hummel AC, Guo W. Symptomatic patients with an early viable intrauterine pregnancy: hCG curves redefined. *Obstet Gynecol.* 2004;104(1):50-54.

24. Barnhart KT, Simhan H, Kamelle SA. Diagnostic accuracy of ultrasound above and below the beta-hCG discriminatory zone. *Obstet Gynecol.* 1999;94: 583-587.

25. Seeber B. What serial hCG can tell you, and cannot tell you, about an early pregnancy. *Fertil Steril.* 2012; 98:1074-1077.

26. Snell BJ. Assessment and management of bleeding in the first trimester of pregnancy. *J Midwifery Women's Health.* 2009;54:483-491.

27. Nichols C. Dating pregnancy: gathering and using a reliable data base. *J Nurse-Midwifery.* 1987;32(4): 195-204.

28. Frank-Herrmann P, Freundl G, Baur S, et al. Effectiveness and acceptability of the symptothermal method of natural family planning in Germany. *Am J Obstet Gynecol.* 1991;165:2008-2011.

29. Kalish RB, Thaler HT, Chasen ST et al. First- and second-trimester ultrasound assessment of gestational age. *Am J Obstet Gynecol.* 2004;191:975-978.

30. Chervenak FA, Skupski DW, Romero R, et al. How accurate is fetal biometry in the assessment of fetal age? *Am J Obstet Gynecol.* 1998;178:678-687.

31. Mongelli M, Chew S, Yuxin NG, Biswas A. Third-trimester ultrasound dating algorithms from pregnancies conceived with artificial reproductive techniques. *Ultrasound Obstet Gynecol.* 2005;26:129-131.

32. Hunter L. Issues in pregnancy dating: revisiting the evidence. *J Midwifery Women's Health.* 2009;54: 184-190.

33. Wegienka G, Baird DD. A comparison of recalled date of last menstrual period with prospectively recorded dates. *J Women's Health.* 2005;14(3):248-252.

34. Naegele FS. *Erfahrung und Abhandlungen des Weiblichen Geschlechtes.* Mannheim, Germany: Ben Lobias Loeffler; 1812.

35. Alexander GR, Tompkins ME, Petersen DJ, Hulsey TC, Mor J. Discordance between LMP-based and clinically estimated gestational age: implications for research, programs, and policy. *Public Health Rep.* 1995;110(4):395-402.

36. Lynch CD. Research implications of the selection of a gestational age estimation method. *Paediatr Perinat Epidemiol.* 2007;21(suppl 2):86-96.

37. Cole LA, Ladner DG, Byrn FW. The normal variabilities of the menstrual cycle. *Fertil Steril.* 2009;91: 522-527.

38. American College of Obstetricians and Gynecologists. Ultrasonography in pregnancy. ACOG Practice Bulletin No. 101. *Obstet Gynecol.* 2009;113:451-461.

39. Hadlock FP, Deter RL, Harrist RB, Park SK. Estimating fetal age: computer-assisted analysis of multiple fetal growth parameters. *Radiology.* 1984;152:497-501.

40. Neilson JP. Symphysis-fundal height measurement in pregnancy. *Cochrane Database Syst Rev.* 1998; 1:CD000944. doi: 10.1002/14651858.CD000944.

41. Engstrom JL, Sittler CP, Swift KE. Fundal height measurement. Part 5: The effect of clinician bias on fundal height measurements. *J Nurse-Midwifery.* 1994; 39(3):130-114.

42. Jelks A, Cifuentes R, Ross MG. Clinician bias in fundal height measurement. *Obstet Gynecol.* 2007;110(4): 892-899.

43. White LJ, Lee SJ, Stepniewska K, Simpson JA, Dwell SL, Arunjerdja R, et al. Estimation of gestational age from fundal height' a solution for resource-poor settings. *JR Soc Interface.* 2012;9:503-510.

44. Slade A, Cohen LJ, Sadler LS, Miller M. The psychology and psychopathology of pregnancy. In Zeanah CH, ed. *Handbook of Infant Mental Health.* New York: Guilford Press; 2009:22-39.

45. DiPietro JA. Psychological and psychophysiological considerations regarding the maternal–fetal relationship. *Infant Child Dev.* 2010;19(1):27-38.

46. Sword W, Heaman MI, Brooks S, Tough S, Janssen PA, Young D, et al. Women's and care providers' perspectives of quality of prenatal care: a qualitative descriptive study. *BMC Pregnancy Childbirth.* 2012; 12:29-47.

47. Lumbiganon P, Laopaiboon M, Thinkhamrop J. Screening and treating asymptomatic bacteriuria in pregnancy. *Curr Opin Obstet Gynecol.* 2010;22(2): 95-99.

48. Gribble RK, Fee SC, Berg RL. The value of routine urine dipstick screening for protein at each prenatal visit. *Am J Obstet Gynecol.* 1995;173:214-217.

49. Murray N, Homer CSE, Davis GK, Curtis J, Mangos G, Brown MA. The clinical utility of routine urinalysis in pregnancy: a prospective study. *Med J Aust.* 2002;177:477-480.

50. Akkerman D, Cleland L, Croft G, Eskuchen K, Heim C, Levine A, et al. Institute for Clinical Systems Improvement: routine prenatal care. Available at: https://www.icsi.org/_asset/13n9y4/Prenatal-Interactive0712.pdf. Accessed September 11, 2012.

51. Rising SS. CenteringPregnancy: an interdisciplinary model of empowerment. *J Nurse-Midwifery.* 1998; 43(1):46-54.

52. Novick G. CenteringPregnancy and the current state of prenatal care. *J Midwifery Women's Health.* 2004;49(5):405-411.

53. Sheeder J, Weber Y, Kabir-Greher K. A review of prenatal group care literature: the need for a structured theoretical framework and systematic evaluation. *Matern Child Health J.* 2012;16(1):177-187.

54. Ickovics JR, Reed E, Magriples U, Westdahl C, Schindler Rising S, Kershaw TS. Effects of group prenatal

care on psychosocial risk in pregnancy: results from a randomised controlled trial. *Psychol Health.* 2011; 26(2):235-250.

55. Kennedy HP, Farrell T, Paden R, Hill S, Jolivet RR, Cooper BA, et al. A randomized clinical trial of group prenatal care in two military settings. *Milit Med.* 2011;176(10):1169-1177.

56. Picklesimer AH, Billings D, Hale N, Blackhurst D, Covington-Kolb S. The effect of CenteringPregnancy group prenatal care on preterm birth in a low-income population. *Am J Obstet Gynecol.* 2012;206(5): 415-417.

57. Ruedinger E, Cox JE. Adolescent childbearing: consequences and interventions. *Curr Opin Pediatr.* 2012; 24(4):446-452.

58. Menacker F, Martin JA, MacDorman MF, Ventura SJ. Births to 10–14 year-old mothers, 1990–2002: trends and health outcomes. *Natl Vital Stat Rep.* 2004;53(7):1-18.

59. McLean E, Cogswell M, Egli I, Wojdyla D, de Benoist B. Worldwide prevalence of anaemia: WHO Vitamin and Mineral Nutrition Information System, 1993–2005. *Public Health Nutr.* 2009;12:444–454.

60. Mei Z, Cogswell ME, Looker AC, Pfeiffer CM, Cusick SE, Lacher DA, et al. Assessment of iron status in US pregnant women from the National Health and Nutrition Examination Survey (NHANES), 1999–2006. *Am J Clin Nutr.* 2011;93(6):1312-1320.

61. Centers for Disease Control and Prevention. Recommendations to prevent and control iron deficiency in the United States. *MMWR.* 1998;47(RR-3):1-36. Available at: http://www.cdc.gov/mmwr /preview/mmwrhtml/00051880.htm. Accessed March 3, 2013.

62. Allen LH. Anemia and iron deficiency: effects on pregnancy outcome. *Am J Clin Nutr.* 2000;71(suppl): 1280S-1284S.

63. American College of Obstetricians and Gynecologists. Anemia in pregnancy. ACOG Practice Bulletin No. 95. *Obstet Gynecol.* 2008;112:201-207.

64. Haider BA, Olofin I, Wang M, Spiegelman D, Ezzati M, Fawzi WW; Nutrition Impact Model Study Group (anaemia). Anaemia, prenatal iron use, and risk of adverse pregnancy outcomes: systematic review and meta-analysis. *BMJ.* 2013 Jun 21;346:f3443.

65. Young SL. Pica in pregnancy: new ideas about an old condition. *Ann Rev Nutr.* 2010;30:407-422.

66. American College of Obstetricians and Gynecologists. *Prevention of RH Alloimmunization.* Practice Bulletin No. 4. Washington, DC: ACOG; May 1999.

67. Mamun AA, O'Callaghan M, Callaway L, Williams G, Najman J, Lawlor DA. Associations of gestational weight gain with offspring body mass index and blood pressure at 21 years of age: evidence from a birth cohort study. *Circulation.* 2009;119:1720.

68. Composition and components of gestational weight gain: physiology and metabolism. In Institute of Medicine, National Research Council Committee to Reexamine IOM Pregnancy Weight Guidelines; Rasmussen KM, Yaktine AL, eds. *Weight Gain During Pregnancy: Reexamining the Guidelines.* Washington, DC: National Academies Press; 2009. Available at: http://www.ncbi.nlm.nih.gov/books/NBK32815.

69. Pitkin RM. Nutritional support in obstetrics and gynecology. *Clin Obstet Gynecol.* 1976;19(3):489-513.

70. Goh YI, Bollano E, Einarson TR, Koren G. Prenatal multivitamin supplementation and rates of congenital anomalies: a meta-analysis. *J Obstet Gynaecol Can.* 2006;28:680-688.

71. Gill SK, Maltepe C, Koren G. The effectiveness of discontinuing iron-containing prenatal multivitamins on reducing the severity of nausea and vomiting of pregnancy. *J Obstet Gynaecol.* 2009;29(1):13-26.

72. Santiago P. Ferrous versus ferric oral iron formulations for the treatment of iron deficiency: a clinical review. *Sci World J.* 2012;846824.

73. Pena-Rosas JP, De-Regil LM, Dowswell T, Viteri FE. Daily oral iron supplementation during pregnancy. *Cochrane Database Syst Rev.* 2012;12:CD004736.

74. Cao C, Obrien KO. Pregnancy and iron homeostasis: an update. *Nutr Rev.* 2013;71(1):35-57.

75. Barger MK. Maternal nutrition and perinatal outcomes. *J Midwifery Women's Health.* 2010;55(6):502-511.

76. Peña-Rosas JP, De-Regil LM, Dowswell T, Viteri FE. Intermittent oral iron supplementation during pregnancy. *Cochrane Database Syst Rev.* 2012;7:CD009997. doi: 10.1002/14651858.CD009997.

77. Delgado AR. Listeriosis in pregnancy. *J Midwifery Women's Health.* 2008;53(3):255-259.

78. Bridges CB, Woods L, Coyne-Beasley T. Advisory Committee on Immunization Practices (ACIP) recommended immunization schedule for adults aged 19 years and older—United States, 2013. *MMWR Surveill Summ.* 2013;62:9.

79. Pickering LK, Baker CJ, Freed GL, et al. Immunization programs for infants, children, adolescents, and adults: clinical practice guidelines by the Infectious Diseases Society of America. *Clin Infect Dis.* 2009;49:817.

80. ACIP Adult Immunization Work Group, Bridges CB, Woods L, Coyne-Beasley T; Centers for Disease Control and Prevention (CDC). Advisory Committee on Immunization Practices (ACIP) recommended immunization schedule for adults aged 19 years and older—United States, 2013. *MMWR Surveill Summ.* 2013;62:9.

81. Thompson WW, Price C, Goodson B, Shay DK, Benson P, Hinrichsen VL, et al. for the Vaccine Safety Datalink Team. Early thimerosal exposure and neuropsychological outcomes at 7 to 10 years. *N Engl J Med.* 2007;357(13):1281-1292.

82. Price CS, Thompson WW, Goodson B, Weintraub ES, Croen LA, Hinrichsen VL, et al. Prenatal and infant exposure to thimerosal from vaccines and immunoglobulins and risk of autism. *Pediatrics.* 2010; 126:656-664.

83. Alcohol use and binge drinking among women of childbearing age—United States, 2006–2010. *MMWR.* Available at: http://www.cdc.gov/mmwr/preview /mmwrhtml/mm6128a4.htms_cid=mm6128a4_e. Accessed July 19, 2012.

84. Goler NC, Armstrong MA, Taillac CJ, Osejo VM. Substance abuse treatment linked with prenatal visits improves perinatal outcomes: a new standard. *J Perinatol.* 2008;28:597.

85. Smith PC, Schmidt SM, Allensworth-Davies D, Saitz R. A single-question screening test for drug-use in primary care. *Arch Intern Med.* 2010;170(13):1155-1160.

86. Kuczkowski KM. The effects of drug abuse on pregnancy. *Curr Opin Obstet Gynecol.* 2007;19(6):578-585.

87. Greenfield SF, Brooks AJ, Gordon SM, Green CA, Kropp F, McHugh RK, et al. Substance abuse treatment entry, retention, and outcome in women: a review of the literature. *Drug Alcohol Depend.* 2007;86(1): 1-21.

88. Blood-Siegrief J, Rende E. The long-term effects of prenatal nicotine exposure on neurologic development. *J Midwifery Women's Health.* 2010;55:143-152.

89. Castles A, Adams EK, Melvin CL, Kelsch C, Boulton ML. Effects of smoking during pregnancy: five meta-analyses. *Am J Prev Med.* 1999;16:208-215.

90. Price JH, Rodan TR, Dake JA. Perceptions and use of smoking cessation in nurse-midwives practice. *J Midwifery Women's Health.* 2006;51:208-215.

91. Abatemarco DJ, Steinberg MP, Denevo CD. Midwives' knowledge, perceptions, beliefs and practice supports regarding tobacco dependence treatment. *J Midwifery Women's Health.* 2007;52:451-457.

92. U.S. Preventive Services Task Force. Counseling and interventions to prevent tobacco use and tobacco-caused disease in adults and pregnant women: U.S. Preventive Services Task Force reaffirmation recommendation statement. *Ann Intern Med.* 2009;150:551-555.

93. Breedlove G, Frzyelka D. Depression screening during pregnancy. *J Midwifery Women's Health.* 2011; 56(1):18-25.

94. American College of Obstetricians and Gynecologists. Screening for depression during and after pregnancy. Committee Opinion No. 453. *Obstet Gynecol.* 2010; 115:394-395.

95. American College of Obstetricians and Gynecologists. Intimate partner violence. ACOG Committee Opinion No. 518. *Obstet Gynecol.* 2012;119:412-417.

96. Brownridge DA, Taillieu TL, Tyler KA, Tiwari A, Ko Ling Chan, Santos SC. Pregnancy and intimate partner violence: risk factors, severity, and health effects. *Violence Against Women.* 2011;17: 858-881.

97. Chu SY, Goodwin MM, D'Angelo DV. Physical violence against U.S. women around the time of pregnancy, 2004–2007. *Am J Prev Med.* 2010;38(3): 317-322.

98. Rabin RF, Jennings JM, Campbell JC, Bair-Merritt MH. Intimate partner violence screening tools: a systematic review. *Am J Prev Med.* 2009;36(5):439-445.

99. Chen PH, Rovi S, Washington J, Jacobs A, Vega M, Pan KY, et al. Randomized comparison of 3 methods to screen for domestic violence in family practice. *Ann Fam Med.* 2007;5:430-435.

100. Renker PR. Breaking the barriers: the promise of computer-assisted screening for intimate partner violence. *J Midwifery Women's Health.* 2008;53: 496-503.

101. MacMillan HL, Wathen CN, Jamieson E, Boyle M, McNutt LA, Worster A, et al. Approaches to screening for intimate partner violence in health care settings: a randomized trial. *JAMA.* 2006;296:530-536.

102. Alba A, Carlton L, Dinkel L, Ruppe R. Increased lead levels in pregnancy among immigrant women. *J Midwifery Women's Health.* 2012;57:509-514.

103. Ettinger AS, Wengrovitz AG, eds. *Guidelines for the Identification and Management of Lead Exposure in Pregnant and Lactating Women.* Centers for Disease Control and Prevention; 2010. Available at: http ://www.cdc.gov/nceh/lead/publications/leadand pregnancy2010.pdf. Accessed March 3, 2013.

104. International Commission on Radiological Protection, eds. *Annals of the ICRP, Publication 84: Pregnancy and Medical Radiation,* 30(1). Tarrytown, NY: Pergamon/Elsevier Science; 2000.

105. Williams PM, Fletcher S. Health effects of prenatal radiation exposure. *Am Fam Phys.* 2010;82(5): 488-493.

106. American College of Obstetricians and Gynecologists. Guidelines for diagnostic imaging in pregnancy. ACOG Committee Opinion No. 299. *Obstet Gynecol.* 2004;104:647-651.

107. Shaw GM. Adverse human reproductive outcomes and electromagnetic fields: a brief summary of the epidemiologic literature. *Bioelectromagnetics.* 2001;5(suppl):S5.

108. National Institute of Environmental Health Sciences. Since you asked: bisphenol A. Questions and answers about the Draft National Toxicology Program Brief on Bisphenol. Available at: http://www.niehs.nih .gov/news/media/questions/sya-bpa.cfm. Accessed on September 7, 2012.

109. Motozawa Y, Hitosugi M, Abe T, Tokudome S. Effects of seat belts worn by pregnant drivers during low-impact collisions. *Am J Obstet Gynecol.* 2010; 203:62.e1.

110. Read JS, Klebanoff MA. Sexual intercourse during pregnancy and preterm delivery: effects of vaginal microorganisms. The Vaginal Infections and Prematurity Study Group. *Am J Obstet Gynecol.* 1993;168:514.

111. Sayle AE, Savitz DA, Thorp JM Jr, Hertz-Picciotto I, Wilcox AJ. Sexual activity during late pregnancy and risk of preterm delivery. *Obstet Gynecol.* 2001; 97:283.

112. Werler MM, Mitchell AA, Hernandez-Diaz S, Honein MA. Use of over-the-counter medications during pregnancy. *Am J Obstet Gynecol.* 2005;193:771.

113. Wilson DL, Barnes M, Ellett L, Permezel M, Jackson M, Crowe SF. Decreased sleep efficiency, increased wake after sleep onset and increased cortical arousals in late pregnancy. *Aust N Z J Obstet Gynaecol.* 2011;51:38.

114. Freeman M, Ghidini A, Spong CY, Tchabo N, Bannon PZ, Pezzullo JC. Does air travel affect pregnancy outcome? *Arch Gynecol Obstet.* 2004; 269:274.

115. Magann EF, Chauhan SP, Dahlke JD, McKelvey SS, Watson EM, Morrison JC. Air travel and pregnancy outcomes: a review of pregnancy regulations and outcomes for passengers, flight attendants, and aviators. *Obstet Gynecol Surv.* 2010;65:396.

116. Grosso LM, Bracken MB. Caffeine metabolism, genetics, and perinatal outcomes: a review of exposure assessment considerations during pregnancy. *Ann Epidemiol.* 2005;15:460.

117. Brent RL, Christian MS, Diener RM. Evaluation of the reproductive and developmental risks of caffeine. *Birth Defects Res B Dev Reprod Toxicol.* 2011;92:152.

118. Task Force on Circumcision. Circumcision policy statement. *Pediatrics.* 2012;130:585. Available at: http://pediatrics.aappublications.org/content/130/3/585.

119. Harvey MA, McRorie MM, Smith DW. Suggested limits to the use of the hot tub and sauna by pregnant women. *Can Med Assoc J.* 1981;125:50-53.

120. Duong HT, Shahrukh Hashmi S, Ramadhani T, Canfield MA, Scheuerle A, Kim Waller D; National Birth Defects Prevention Study. Maternal use of hot tub and major structural birth defects. *Birth Defects Res.* 2011;91(Pt 1):836-841.

121. Food and Drug Administration. Food safety for moms-to-be. Updated February 28, 2013. Available at: http://www.fda.gov/food/resourcesforyou/healtheducators/ucm081785.htm.

122. Declercq ER, Sakala C, Cory M. *Listening to Mothers II: Report of the Second National US Survey of Women's Childbearing Experiences.* New York: Childbirth Connections; 2006.

123. Zwelling E. Childbirth education in the 1990s and beyond. *JOGNN.* 1996;25(5):425-432.

124. Dick-Reed G. *Childbirth Without Fear.* 1st ed. London: Heinemann Medical Books Ltd; 1942.

125. Walker DS, Visger JM, Rossie D. Contemporary childbirth education models. *J Midwifery Women's Health.* 2009;54(6):469-471.

126. Facco FL, Kramer J, Ho KH, Zee PC, Grobman WA. Sleep disturbances in pregnancy. *Obstet Gynecol.* 2010;115(1):77-83.

127. Hall WA, Hauck YL, Carty EM, Hutton EK, Fenwick J, Stoll K. Childbirth fear, anxiety, fatigue, and sleep deprivation in pregnant women. *JOGNN.* 2009;38:567-776.

128. Lee K, Zaffke M. Longitudinal changes in fatigue and energy during pregnancy and the postpartum period. *JOGNN.* 1999;28:183-191.

129. Beddoe AE, Lee KA, Weiss SJ, Kennedy HP, Yang CP. Effects of mindful yoga on sleep in pregnant women: a pilot study. *Biol Res Nurs.* 2010;11:363-370.

130. Lacroix R, Eason E, Melzack, R. Nausea and vomiting during pregnancy: a prospective study of its frequency, intensity, and patterns of change. *Am J Obstet Gynecol.* 2000;182:931-937.

131. King TL, Murphy PA. Evidence-based approaches to managing nausea and vomiting in early pregnancy. *J Midwifery Women's Health.* 2009;54:430-444.

132. Lacasse A, Rey E, Ferreira E, Morin C, Bérard A. Validity of a modified Pregnancy-Unique Quantification of Emesis and Nausea (PUQE) scoring index to assess severity of nausea and vomiting of pregnancy. *Am J Obstet Gynecol.* 2008;198(1):71e1-71e7.

133. Niebyl JR, Goodwin TM. Overview of nausea and vomiting of pregnancy with an emphasis on vitamins and ginger. *Am J Obstet Gynecol.* 2002;186(5 Pt 2 suppl):S253-S255.

134. Koren G, Clark S, Hankins GD, Caritis SN, Miodovnik M, Umans JG, et al. Effectiveness of delayed-release doxylamine and pyridoxine for nausea and vomiting of pregnancy: a randomized placebo controlled trial. *Am J Obstet Gynecol.* 2010;203:571.e1-571.e7.

135. McKeigue PM, Lamm SH, Linn S, Kutcher JS. Bendectin and birth defects: a meta-analysis of the epidemiologic studies. *Teratology.* 1994;50:881-884.

136. Hensley JG. Leg cramps and restless legs syndrome during pregnancy. *J Midwifery Women's Health.* 2009;54:211-218.

137. Naumann CR, Zelig C, Napolitano PG, Ko CW. Nausea, vomiting, and heartburn in pregnancy: a prospective look at risk, treatment, and outcome. *J Matern Fetal Neonatal Med.* 2012;25(8): 1488-1493.

138. Neilson JP. Interventions for heartburn in pregnancy. *Cochrane Database Syst Rev.* 2008;4:CD007065. doi: 10.1002/14651858.CD007065.pub2.

139. Richter JE. Review article: the management of heartburn in pregnancy. *Aliment Pharmacol Therap.* 2005; 22(9):749-757.

140. Mahadevan U. Gastrointestinal medications in pregnancy. *Best Pract Res Clin Gastroenterol.* 2007;21(5): 849-857.

141. Botehlo N, Emeis CL, Brucker MC. Gastrointestinal conditions. In King T, Brucker MC (eds) *Pharmacology for Women's Health.* Sudbury, MA: Jones and Bartlett; 2011;605-642.

142. Pennick V, Young G. Interventions for preventing and treating pelvic and back pain in pregnancy. *Cochrane Database Syst Rev.* 2007;2:CD001139. doi: 10.1002/14651858.CD001139.pub2.

143. Ponnapula P, Boberg JS. Lower extremity changes experienced during pregnancy. *J Foot Ankle Surg.* 2010;49:452-458.

144. Bamigboye AA, Smyth RMD. Interventions for varicose veins and leg oedema in pregnancy. *Cochrane Database Syst Rev.* 2007;1:CD001066. doi: 10.1002/ 14651858.CD001066.pub2.

APPENDIX

22A

Obstetric Abdominal Examination

JENNIFER M. DEMMA

KAREN TRISTER GRACE

JAN M. KRIEBS

The components of the obstetric abdominal examination include (1) abdominal inspection and palpation; (2) measurement of fundal height; (3) Leopold's maneuvers for determining fetal lie, presentation, position, variety, and engagement; (4) estimation of fetal weight; and (5) detection of fetal heart tones.

While ultrasound can effectively be used to assess fetal growth and position—and should be used when discrepancies arise or assessment is challenging—being able to employ one's hands to gain information about the progress of a pregnancy is an invaluable skill. The standard descriptions in this appendix assume a woman of normal habitus and a singleton pregnancy. Maternal height and weight, uterine abnormalities, fetal growth pattern, and multiple pregnancies are all factors that can challenge the examiner's interpretation of clinical findings, and their effects are discussed here.

Equipment

- Measuring tape with centimeter increments
- Pinard fetoscope or Doppler fetoscope

Abdominal Inspection

1. Surgical scars. The scar of a previous cesarean section is of particular importance. It is useful to know if the woman has undergone an appendectomy so that appendicitis can be ruled out in the event of right-sided abdominal pain during the pregnancy.

2. Bruises or abrasions. Document a description and location of any bruises and discuss their origin with the woman, paying particular attention to the possibility of intimate-partner violence and abuse.

3. Linea nigra. This hyperpigmented vertical line on the lower abdomen may be visible by 20 weeks of pregnancy, or it may be faintly present from a previous pregnancy and begin to darken in the first trimester.

4. Striae gravidarum. Many women develop these pink or red streaks during pregnancy. Silvery white streaks may be present from previous weight changes or previous pregnancy.

5. Inspection to determine the abdominal contours can give some indication of the fetal lie, presentation, position, and variety.

    a. Uterine shape is a longitudinal ovoid: fundal height in the expected range based on the gestational age—suggests a longitudinal lie.

    b. Uterine shape is a transverse ovoid: fundal height lower than expected for gestational age—suggests a transverse lie.

    c. A long smooth curve is prominent on one side of the abdomen—suggests that the back of the fetus is on that side of the abdomen.

    d. A saucer-like depression appears just below the umbilicus and a bulge like a full bladder appears above the symphysis pubis—suggests a posterior position or full bladder.

    e. Movement of fetal small parts can be seen all over the abdomen—suggests a posterior position.

Abdominal Palpation

1. Diastasis recti. The presence and width of a diastasis are palpated by placing one or two fingers parallel to the abdominal midline, just below the epigastric region, and feeling the separation of the rectus abdominis muscle after asking the woman to lift her head while lying supine. This exam is routinely performed at the postpartum visit but may also be useful at the first prenatal visit, especially when a woman has been pregnant in the past, she may have a persistent diastasis recti.

2. Umbilical hernia can be detected on palpation at any point during the pregnancy.

3. Evaluation of uterine irritability, tone, tenderness, consistency, and any contractility is done to assess for signs of preterm labor in the second and third trimesters, and for signs of labor after 37 gestational weeks.

4. Gross evaluation of amniotic fluid volume. When performing an abdominal exam, the midwife can estimate the quantity of amniotic fluid. If a woman has polyhydramnios, it will be difficult to palpate small parts of the fetus and may be difficult to determine fetal position. The opposite will be true if a woman has oligohydramnios.

Measuring Fundal Height

Serial fundal height measurements provide information about the enlargement of the uterus and, therefore, about the growth of the fetus. The height of the fundus from the top of the symphysis pubis to the top of the fundus, as measured in centimeters, is used to monitor fetal growth and can be a screening tool for detection of multiple gestation, fetal growth restriction, polyhydramnios, and other complications of fetal growth. Fundal height is of greatest value when it is measured the same way by the same examiner at successive prenatal visits. **Table 22A-1** lists the approximate expected location of the fundal height at different gestational ages.

Key Points

- Early in pregnancy, the uterus is contained within the pelvic cradle. Only after 10 to 12 gestational weeks can the top of the uterine fundus be palpated above the symphysis pubis. Prior to 18 to 20 gestational weeks,

Table 22A-1	Approximate Expected Fundal Height at Specific Gestational Weeks
Weeks of Gestation	**Approximate Expected Fundal Height**
12	Level of the symphysis pubis
16	Halfway between symphysis pubis and umbilicus
20	Within one fingerbreadth of umbilicus
24	Two to four fingerbreadths above umbilicus
28–30	One-third of the way between umbilicus and xiphoid process (three fingerbreadths above umbilicus)
32	Two-thirds of the way between umbilicus and xiphoid process (three to four fingerbreadths below xiphoid process)
36–38	One fingerbreadth below xiphoid process
40	Two to three fingerbreadths below xiphoid process if lightening has occurred

the uterine size is best described in relation to the level of the uterine fundus between the symphysis pubis and umbilicus, using one's fingerbreadth (fb) as the measuring tool (e.g., 1 fb above symphysis, 4 fb below umbilicus). (See figure in the *Anatomy and Physiology of Pregnancy: Placental, Fetal, and Maternal Adaptations* chapter.)

- Between 20 and 32 weeks of gestation, the measurement should be within 2 or 3 cm of the number of weeks' gestation.

- The pattern of fundal height growth is more important than the absolute number.

- Late in the third trimester, as the fetal presenting part moves into the pelvis, more variation is seen between measurements, and the absolute fundal height may remain stable or decrease slightly.

- Used alone, the fundal height measurement may be specific, but lacks sensitivity. When a measurement is not within the expected value for the woman's gestational age:

  ◆ First assess for confounding factors such as a full bladder or BMI.

  ◆ Refer the woman for ultrasound evaluation if confounding factors do not sufficiently account for the discrepancy.

Procedure for Measuring Fundal Height

Fundal height can be measured in a number of different ways. For an extensive review of fundal height measurement, the interested reader is referred to the series of articles written by Engstrom et al.[1-7]

1. Assessment of the fundal height should take place with the woman in a supine or semi-recumbent position.

2. Some midwives advocate turning the tape measure to hide the centimeter markings and thus, minimize inadvertent bias by the examiner. Alterations in maternal position, a full urinary bladder, multiple examiners, and provider awareness of the weeks of gestation all create bias that leads to inaccurate measurements.

3. Before measuring, both the symphysis pubis and the uterine fundus are identified (**Figure 22A-1**).

   a. The woman may need to partially remove her clothing to allow access to the symphysis and fundus. The abdomen is exposed from the xiphoid process to the top of the pelvis.

   b. Assessment is done with a gentle, firm touch using the palmar surface of the fingers.

   c. Facing the woman's head as she lies semi-reclining, the midwife's hands are placed on each lateral side of the uterus approximately midway between the symphysis and the fundus, with the fingers pointed vertically toward the woman's head.

   d. The uterine fundus is identified by walking one's hands up the sides of the uterus until they meet at the top. Smooth motions avoid the sensation of kneading or poking and will decrease uterine contractility during the examination.

   e. Measuring "over the top" of the fundus is a common error that can be avoided by paying attention to the curve of the uterus, the location of the fetal part highest in the uterus, and any laxity of the maternal abdomen.

4. Two techniques are commonly employed:

   a. Place the zero line of the tape measure on the superior border of the symphysis and measure *upward* in a straight line, following the abdominal midline to the crest of the uterine fundus, and taking care not to cross over the top and begin to measure the posterior aspect of the uterus.

   b. After identifying the fundus, place the tape at that point and measure *downward* to the superior border of the symphysis.

Leopold's Maneuvers

The process of evaluating fetal lie, position, and presentation with Leopold's maneuvers also offers the opportunity to assess the abdomen for muscle tone, uterine tone and contractility, palpable fetal movement, and to estimate fetal weight. The four Leopold's maneuvers and the combined Pawlik's grip are shown in **Figure 22A-2**.

Key Points

1. The woman's bladder should be empty.

2. The woman's abdomen is typically exposed from just below the breasts to the symphysis pubis. Provide privacy and consider cultural variations in comfort with exposure of skin. Ask the woman to move her clothing instead of doing it for her. This allows her to control the extent and amount of skin exposure.

3. Relaxation of the abdominal muscles can be facilitated by:

   a. Placing a pillow under the woman's head and upper shoulders

   b. Asking her to place her arms by her sides or across her chest

   c. Having her bend her knees slightly

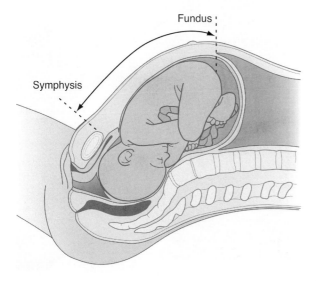

Figure 22A-1 Measurement of fundal height.

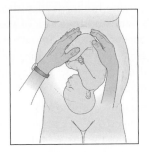

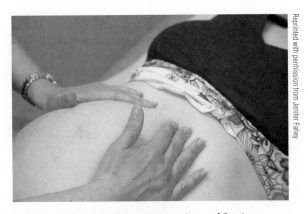

First maneuver. Identify the part of the fetus that resides in the fundus. Curve fingers of both hands around top of fundus.

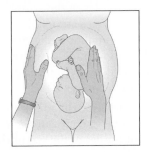

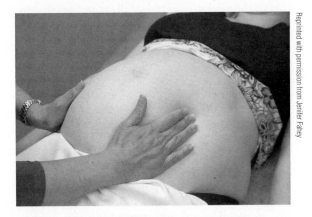

Second maneuver. Identify the location of the small parts and fetal back. Place both hands on side of uterus.

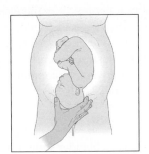

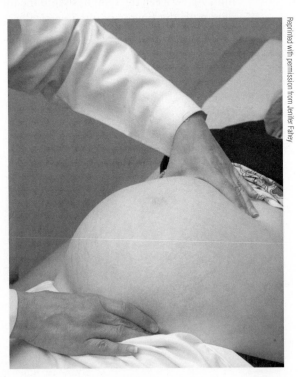

Third maneuver. Identify the presenting part. With thumb and middle finger of one hand, press gently but deeply into the mother's abdomen immediately above the symphysis pubis and grasp the presenting part.

Figure 22A-2 The four Leopold's maneuvers and the combined Pawlik's grip.

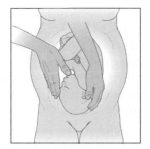

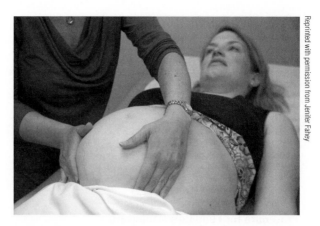

Reprinted with permission from Jenifer Fahey

Fourth maneuver. Check to see if the presenting part is engaged and the location of the cephalic prominence. Place both hands on sides of lower uterus, press deeply, and move fingertips toward pelvic inlet.

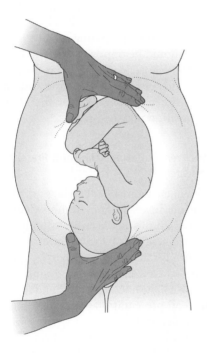

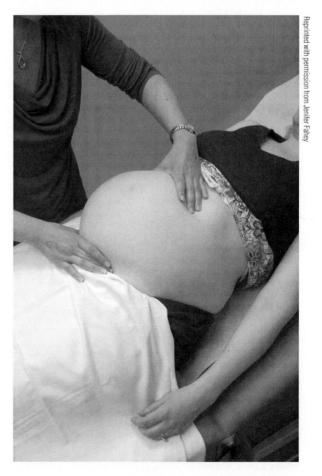

Reprinted with permission from Jenifer Fahey

Combined Pawlik's grip. Combine Leopold's third maneuver with one hand and palpation of the fundus using the other hand. Compare the two poles for final determination of lie and presentation.

Figure 22A-2 The four Leopold's maneuvers and the combined Pawlik's grip. *(continued)*

4. Before palpating, the midwife lightly rests her hand on the woman's abdomen (**Figure 22A-3**). This action gives the woman an opportunity to adjust to the sensation of the midwife's touch and allows any initial muscle-tightening reaction to dissipate.

5. The flat palmar surfaces of the fingers are used for palpating—*not* the fingertips. Smooth, deep pressure is used—as firm as is necessary to obtain accurate findings without causing pain or discomfort.

Procedure for Leopold's Maneuvers

First Maneuver: Determine Fetal Lie and Presentation

Facing the woman's head, palpate the area of the uterine fundus, noting the shape of the fetal part in the fundus. A fetal part that feels round and hard, is readily movable, and can be balloted between the examiner's fingers or hands suggests a fetal head. The mobility arises from the head being able to move independently of the trunk. A fetal part that feels irregular, larger or bulkier, and less firm than a head, and that cannot be well delineated or readily moved or balloted, suggests the fetal breech. The breech cannot move independently of the trunk. In these cases the lie is longitudinal. If neither of the preceding conditions is felt in the fundus, a transverse lie may be present.

Second Maneuver: Determine Location of Fetal Back

1. Continue to face the woman's head. Place the hands on both sides of the uterus about midway between the symphysis pubis and the fundus.

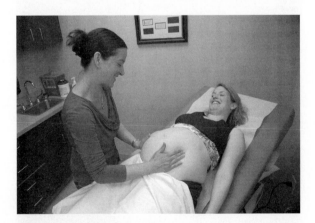

Figure 22A-3 Midwife preparing to do an abdominal palpation.
Source: Reprinted with permission from Jenifer Fahey

2. Apply pressure with one hand against the side of the uterus, thereby pushing the fetus to the other side of the abdomen against the examining hand and stabilizing it there. Maintain this pressure while the examining hand palpates the other side of the uterus to identify fetal parts.

3. Palpate the entire area with the examining hand, from the abdominal midline to the lateral side, and from the fundus to the symphysis. Use firm, smooth pressure and rotary movement.

4. Reverse the procedure to examine the other side of the uterus.

A firm, convex, continuously smooth, and resistant mass extending from the breech to the neck indicates the fetal back. The location of the back in the anterior, lateral, or posterior portion of the abdomen helps to determine the variety (position). Small, knobby, irregular masses that might move when pressed on suggest the fetal small parts—hands, feet, knees, elbows. When palpating the uterus, the fetal small parts should be opposite the fetal back. If the back is difficult to feel and seems to be just out of reach in the posterior portion of the abdomen, and small parts are palpable all over the abdomen, a posterior position may be present.

Third Maneuver: Determine the Fetal Presentation and Engagement

The third maneuver is called Pawlik's grip: Grasp the portion of the lower abdomen immediately above the symphysis pubis between the thumb and middle finger of one hand. It will be necessary to press gently but firmly into the abdomen to feel the presenting part below and between the thumb and finger. Pawlik's grip can be uncomfortable and may be omitted as the fetal presentation can be determined with the fourth maneuver.

If the head is above the pelvic brim, it is readily movable and ballottable, as described for the first maneuver. A procedure that is sometimes added to this maneuver is called the combined Pawlik's grip, in which Pawlik's grip is utilized with one hand and the fundus is grasped in the same way with the other hand at the same time (**Figure 22A-4**). This combination enables the simultaneous comparison of what is in the two poles for final determination of the fetal lie and presentation.

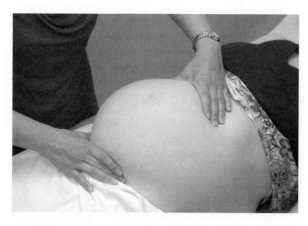

Figure 22A-4 Combined Pawlick's grip.
Source: Reprinted with permission from Jenifer Fahey

Fourth Maneuver: Cephalic Prominence and Fetal Attitude

1. Turn and face the woman's feet.

2. Place both hands on the sides of the uterus with the palms just above the symphysis and iliac crest with the fingers directed toward the symphysis pubis.

3. Press with the fingertips into the lower abdomen slowly but firmly and move them toward the pelvic inlet to determine the cephalic prominence; note if it is on the side of the fetal back or fetal front. If the cephalic prominence is on the same side as the fetal small parts, the fetal attitude is flexed and the fetal head is tucked toward the chin. If the presentation is vertex and the cephalic prominence is on the same side as the fetal back, the fetus is in a face or brow presentation.

At the conclusion of the four maneuvers, share the findings with the woman, and offer to help her feel and identify various parts of her fetus if she would like.

Estimation of Fetal Weight

The estimated fetal weight (EFW) is important in the intrapartum period, when this figure is compared with the clinical evaluation of the pelvis to ascertain the adequacy of a woman's pelvis. During the prenatal period, EFW is used as one clinical measurement in evaluating gestational age and progressive fetal growth starting at 34 to 36 gestational weeks. Neither experienced hands nor a sonogram is necessarily more accurate than the other method when assessing fetal weight in a full-term fetus.[8]

Auscultation of Fetal Heart

The sound of the fetal heart is transmitted best through the convex portion of the fetus closest to the anterior uterine wall, which is usually the fetal back. Thus, if the position of the fetus is known, fetal heart tones can be readily located, allowing for some variation depending on how far the fetus has descended into the pelvis (**Figure 22A-5**). Location of the fetal heart is an additional piece of data that either confirms or calls into question the diagnosis of fetal presentation and position.

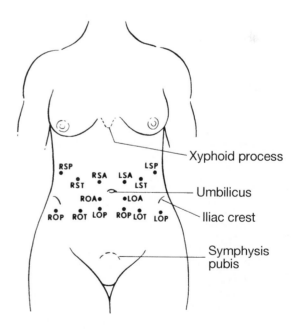

Figure 22A-5 Location of the point of maximum intensity of auscultation of the fetal heart tones for specific fetal presentations and positions.

● ● ● **References**

1. Engstrom JL. Measurement of fundal height. *J Obstet Gynecol Neonatal Nurs.* 1988;17(3):172-178.

2. Engstrom JL, Ostrenga KG, Plass RV, Work BA. The effect of maternal bladder volume on fundal height measurements. *Br J Obstet Gynaecol.* 1989;96(8):987-991.

3. Engstrom JL, Sittler CP. Fundal height measurement. Part 1: techniques for measuring fundal height. *J Nurse- Midwifery.* 1993;38(1):5-16.

4. Engstrom JL, McFarlin BL, Sittler CP. Fundal height measurement. Part 2: intra- and interexaminer reliability of three measurement techniques. *J Nurse-Midwifery.* 1993;38(1):17-22.

5. Engstrom JL, Piscioneri LA, Low LK, McShane H, McFarlin B. Fundal height measurement. Part 3: the effect of maternal position on fundal height measurements. *J Nurse-Midwifery.* 1993;38(1):23-27.

6. Engstrom JL, McFarlin BL, Sampson MB. Fundal height measurement. Part 4: accuracy of clinicians' identification of the uterine fundus during pregnancy. *J Nurse-Midwifery.* 1993;38(6):318-323.

7. Engstrom JL, Sittler CP, Swift KE. Fundal height measurement. Part 5: the effect of clinician bias on fundal height measurements. *J Nurse-Midwifery.* 1994; 39(3):130-141.

8. Chauhan SP, Hendrix NW, Magann EF, Morrison JC, Kenney SP, Devoe LD. Limitations of clinical and sonographic estimates of birth weight: experience with 1034 parturients. *Obstet Gynecol.* 1998;91(1): 72-77.

22B

Clinical Pelvimetry

JENNIFER M. DEMMA

KAREN TRISTER GRACE

TEKOA L. KING

Pelvimetry comes from the Latin word *pelvis* (meaning "basin or bowl") and the Greek word *metron* (meaning "measure").[1] Thus pelvimetry refers to measurement of diameters of the pelvis. It is possible to evaluate the general structure (size and shape) of the pelvis and measure some of the critical diameters of the pelvis during a vaginal examination. This assessment, which is referred to as "clinical pelvimetry," is classically done when an initial vaginal examination is performed during pregnancy and/or during the course of labor.

Pelvic diameters are most accurately measured by X ray or computed tomographic (CT) X ray. However, X-ray pelvimetry is no longer used because of the potential hazards of exposing the fetus to radiation, and CT scans are reserved for prenatal assessment of the pelvis in women who plan a vaginal breech birth.

Historically, clinical pelvimetry was an essential piece of information that was used to guide clinical management. A woman whose pelvis was contracted in one or more dimensions was likely to have cephalopelvic disproportion (CPD) in labor and could be assisted with a cesarean section or use of high or mid-forceps.[2] The shape and size of the pelvis partly determined which method of birth would be safest. Because diseases such as rickets, scurvy, and polio were more common in the past, CPD was a more frequent occurrence and clinical dilemma.[3]

Today the diagnosis of CPD is not made until there is a failure of progress or descent in labor; thus the predictive value of clinical pelvimetry is controversial.[4,5] Nevertheless, it is important that we do not "throw the baby out with the bath water"—the results of clinical pelvimetry can help confirm cephalopelvic disproportion and, therefore, inform and help guide intrapartum management. In addition, clinical pelvimetry continues to have an important role in developing nations wherein a contracted pelvis is more common.[3]

Key Points

1. The examiner should have an understanding of the four classic pelvic shapes and dimensions of the pelvic planes, as described in the *Anatomy and Physiology of the Female Reproductive System* chapter.

2. Before doing clinical pelvimetry, it is important that an examiner measure the lengths of the fingers as well as the width of the fist, as these lengths will used to determine specific measurements.

    a. The length of the reach of the examining fingers is measured from the tip of the longest finger to the juncture of the first finger (palm) and thumb.

    b. The fist is measured from the lateral (ulnar) aspect to the medial (radial) aspect of the tops of the knuckles of the fingers where they attach to the hand. If this does not measure at least 8 cm, then position the thumb in a way that it will be positioned each time and add the joint or knuckle of the thumb into the measurement.

3. Clinical pelvimetry is best performed with the thumb of the examining hand tucked into the palm. If the thumb is extended, it will come in

contact with the clitoris or another part of the external vulva, which disallows use of the full length of the examining fingers in reaching for the sacrum or diagonal conjugate.

4. The procedure for performing clinical pelvimetry can be practiced using a bony pelvis model but must be performed consistently and methodically at the completion of a vaginal examination to truly understand the effects of soft tissue and movements that cause discomfort.

5. Some midwives believe that it is necessary to palpate and evaluate completely both sides of the bony pelvis. Others believe that it is sufficient to palpate only one side of the bony pelvis and assume both sides are equilateral, unless an obvious pelvic deformity is observed or the woman has a history of pelvic trauma. In such cases, both sides of the bony pelvis should be evaluated.

6. Clinical pelvimetry may be performed in several different ways. Some texts advocate assessing the diagonal conjugate first and moving from the back of the pelvis forward; others advocate the reverse order. Some texts do not include assessment of the retropubic arch or sidewalls. The order of maneuvers recommended in this text is designed to cause a woman the least discomfort.

7. Clinical pelvimetry uses measures of the length and shape of pelvic structures to indirectly assess the size of the three pelvic planes as well as the back and forepelvis. The pelvic planes cannot be measured directly. Thus clinical pelvimetry is used to categorize the pelvis as adequate, borderline, or contracted for the birth of an average-size fetus by determining the shape and size of the pelvic inlet, midplane, and outlet.

Procedure for Performing Clinical Pelvimetry

The procedure for performing clinical pelvimetry is presented in **Table 22B-1**. The pelvis is palpated from the forepelvis posteriorly toward the sacrum, and the shape and length of the following structures

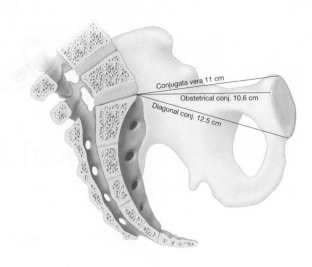

Figure 22B-1 Diameters and planes of the pelvis.

are noted: symphysis pubis, ischial rami, sidewalls, ischial spines, interspinous diameter, sacrospinous ligament, coccyx, sacrum, and diagonal conjugate. The pubic arch is measured as the examiner's hand is removed from the vagina, and the intertuberous diameter is measured externally at the end of the examination. **Figure 22B-1** and **Figure 22B-2** show the pelvic diameters and shape of the sacrum as described in Table 22B-1.

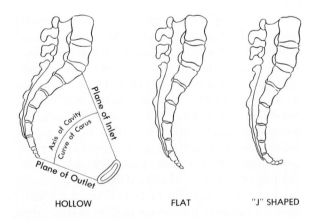

Figure 22B-2 Sacral shapes.

Table 22B-1 Procedure for Performing Clinical Pelvimetry

Step	Obstetric Plane	Area Measured	Technique	Description of Findings	Clinical Implications During Labor
1	Forepelvis and AP diameter of the pelvic inlet	Retropubic arch	Insert two fingers just inside the vagina; rotate so the palmar surface is up. Separate fingers gently to avoid trauma to the urethra, and gently palpate the posterior aspect of the symphysis pubis to determine the inclination.	*Parallel inclination:* The longitudinal axis of the symphysis pubis is parallel to the sacrum. *Anterior inclination:* The superior margin of the symphysis pubis is tilted toward the sacral promontory, and the inferior margin is tilted away from the sacrum. *Posterior inclination:* The inferior margin of the symphysis pubis is tilted toward the sacrum, and the superior margin is tilted away from the sacral promontory.	When the symphysis pubis is not at least approximately parallel to the sacrum, the anteroposterior diameters of the inlet and the outlet can be changed significantly (Figure 22B-1). However, a contracted inlet is uncommon in developed nations today, so this step may be omitted by some practitioners.
2	Transverse diameters of midplane and outlet	Sidewalls (interior surface of the ischium)	Sweep the examining fingers down the pubic rami to the inferior wall of the ischium, and move them back along the ischium toward the ischial spine.	*Convergent:* Sidewalls converge toward the outline. *Divergent:* Sidewalls converge toward the ischial spines and flare toward the outline. *Parallel:* Most common finding in gynecoid pelvis.	Convergent sidewalls are associated with deep transverse arrest.
3	Transverse diameter of midplane	Ischial spines	Proceed along the sidewalls downward and backward to locate the ischial spine. Gentle lateral pressure may be required to locate the spine. If unable to locate the spine in this manner, move the fingers medially to the sacrum and locate the sacrospinous ligament. Follow it laterally to the ischial spine.	*Blunt:* Not easily palpated, more flattened against the pelvic wall; the, the most common finding in gynecoid pelvis. *Prominent:* Easily palpable. *Encroaching:* Easily palpable and long, almost sharp, encroaching toward each other.	The transverse diameter of the midplane is the narrowest diameter that the fetus must traverse. A narrowed midplane can result in deep transverse arrest or failure to descend in the second stage of labor. This dystocia is associated with marked molding and caput.
4	Transverse of midplane	Interspinous diameter	Sweep the finger across the pelvic cavity to the ischial spine on the opposite side of the pelvis to estimate the transverse diameter of the midplane.	Estimate diameter in centimeters (normal is 10 cm or greater).	

(continues)

Table 22B-1	Procedure for Performing Clinical Pelvimetry *(continued)*		
Step	Obstetric Plane	Area Measured	Technique	Description of Findings	Clinical Implications During Labor

Step	Obstetric Plane	Area Measured	Technique	Description of Findings	Clinical Implications During Labor
5	Transverse diameter of midplane and posterior aspect of pelvis	Sacrosciatic ligament	Move the examining finger back to the first ischial spine palpated and follow the sacrosciatic ligament to the sacrum to measure the width of the sacrosciatic notch.	More than 2 FB (3 FB = average). Less than 2 FB (suggests forward inclination of sacrum).	
6	AP diameter of outlet	Coccyx shape and mobility	Press firmly on the coccyx to determine its shape and mobility.	Mobility: Describe as a *mobile* or *fixed*. Shape: *J-shaped* or *flat*.	A coccyx that is J-shaped or immobile may break during childbirth. Labor may or may not be impeded, but postpartum, significant pain in the area of the coccyx can occur when the coccyx does break.
7	AP diameter of midpelvis	Sacrum shape	Palpate the sacrum from sacrococcygeal junction upward; "walk up the sacrum," estimating the degree of curvature and inclination.	Curve is described as *straight* (flat), *angular* (J-shaped), or *hollow*. Inclination is described as *backward, average,* or *forward*.	A hollow sacrum is indicative of an anthropoid pelvis and persistent occiput posterior position.
8	AP diameter of inlet	Diagonal conjugate	Drop both wrists and elbow toward the floor, and extend the fingers posteriorly and cephalad with the inferior margin of the symphysis in contact with the dorsal aspect of the examining hand. Avoid undue pressure on the urethra or clitoris. Most often the sacral promontory cannot be reached.	A diameter of 11.5 cm or greater implies an adequate DC. The obstetric conjugate is approximately 1.5 cm less than the measured DC (Figure 22B-1). Recorded as (1) greater than or equal to the measured distance of the examiner's reach or (2) equal to the measured distance of the examiner's reach.	A narrow diagonal conjugate can result in failure of engagement.
9	Transverse diameter of outlet and forepelvis	Subpubic arch	The examiner's hand is rotated to the side so the fingertips face the side of the pelvis as the hand is removed from the vagina. Just prior to removing the hand, rotate the examining fingers so the palmar surface is up. Evaluate how easily two examining fingers are accommodated under the arch. If two fingers are easily accommodated, the angle is approximately 90°. If the fingers must overlap to fit into the pubic arch, the arch is less than 90°.	Degree of angle relative to 90°. Record as greater than 90° (gynecoid) or equal to 90° or less than 90° (android).	The fetal head must descend lower to traverse a narrow pubic arch, which increases the chance of perineal lacerations.
10	Transverse diameter of outlet	Intertuberous diameter	Measure the transverse diameter of the outlet (intertuberous diameter; biischial diameter) by placing a premeasured fist between the tuberosities.	Record measurement of the intertuberous diameter as greater than, or equal to, or less than the premeasured width of the fist.	

DC = diagonal conjugate; FB = fingerbreadth.

● ● ● **References**

1. Yeomans ER. Clinical pelvimetry. *Clin Obstet Gynecol.* 2006;49(1):140-146.

2. Caldwell WE, Moloy HC. Anatomical variations in the female pelvis: their classification and obstetrical significance. *Proc R Soc Med.* 1938;32(1):1-30.

3. Maharaj D. Assessing cephalopelvic disproportion: back to the basics. *Obstet Gynecol Surv.* 2010;65(6): 387-395.

4. Blackadar CS, Viera AJ. A retrospective review of performance and utility of routine clinical pelvimetry. *Fam Med.* 2004;36(7):505-507.

5. Pattinson RC. Pelvimetry for fetal cephalic presentations at term. *Cochrane Database Syst Rev.* 2000; 2:CD000161.

● ● ● **Additional Resources**

Cunningham F, Leveno K, Bloom S, Hauth J, Rouse D, Spong C. *Williams Obstetrics*, 23rd ed. New York: McGraw-Hill; 2009.

Hamlin RHJ. *Stepping Stones to Labour Ward Diagnosis.* Adelaide, Australia: Rigby; 1959.

Steer CM. *Moloy's Evaluation of the Pelvis in Obstetrics.* 3rd ed. New York: Plenum Medical Book; 1975.

Thoms H. *Pelvimetry.* New York: Hoeber-Harper; 1956.

Ullery JC, Castallo MA. *Obstetric Mechanisms and Their Management.* Philadelphia, PA: F. A. Davis; 1957: Chapter 1.

APPENDIX

22C

Sample Template for Prenatal Care Visits

JENNIFER M. DEMMA

KAREN TRISTER GRACE

Physical Examination	Laboratory or Other Testing	Screenings and Education
Initial Visit		
Height and weight (determine prepregnancy weight and BMI) Vital signs Complete physical examination with pelvic exam and clinical pelvimetry Assessment of uterine size/ gestational age; comparison with LMP	Blood type, Rh and antibody screen Hemoglobin/hematocrit or CBC to include platelet count Hepatitis B surface antigen HIV Chlamydia (with or without gonorrhea screening) Syphilis (RPR/VDRL) Rubella titer Pap test (if indicated) Urinalysis and urine culture Offer cystic fibrosis carrier screening (can be done at any time in pregnancy) Additional testing as indicated (e.g., hemoglobin electrophoresis, monthly urine culture, early diabetes screening, lead level) Consider ultrasound to establish EDD Based on gestational age at first visit: First-trimester screening— nuchal translucency, PAPP-A, and free beta hCG (11w0d–13w6d)	**Screenings:** • Full history (e.g., medical, surgical, obstetric, gynecologic, menstrual, genetic) • Acceptance of pregnancy • Symptoms of pregnancy • Women's concerns • Screening for depression • Intimate-partner violence/domestic abuse screening • Risk assessment and screening • Immunizations **Education:** • Orientation to midwifery care • Schedule of visits • Establishing EDD • Nutrition, weight gain guidelines, food cravings, pica • Exercise/Rest • Anticipatory guidance regarding mood changes • Breast support • Food safety • Travel • Dental care • Perineal and vaginal care • Toxoplasmosis • Avoidance of alcohol and drugs, smoking cessation • Safe use of medications • Sexuality • Myths and superstitions • Fetal growth and development and physiologic changes • Options for genetic/chromosomal anomaly screening • Common discomforts and relief measures • When to call the midwife/signs of complications

Physical Examination	Laboratory or Other Testing	Screenings and Education
Initial Visit to 10 Weeks		
Weight	Review results from initial visit	**Screenings:** • Risk assessment and screening • Woman's symptoms and concerns **Education:** • Fetal growth and development and physiologic changes • Common discomforts and relief measures • Nutrition • Exercise • Food safety • Genetic/anomaly screening options • Address any risk factors present (e.g., preterm labor risk factors, substance abuse, psychosocial stressors, STIs) • When to call the midwife/signs of complications
Blood pressure		
Full physical examination with pelvic exam and clinical pelvimetry (if not done at the initial visit)		
Fetal heart rate with handheld Doppler, after 8 weeks		
Assessment of uterine size and change from previous visit		
10–14 Weeks		
Weight	First trimester screening— nuchal translucency, PAPP-A, and free beta hCG (11w0d–13w6d)	**Screenings:** • Risk assessment and screening • Woman's symptoms and concerns **Education:** • Fetal growth and development and physiologic changes • Common discomforts and relief measures • Nutrition • Exercise • Genetic /anomaly screening options; review prior to testing as needed • Anticipatory guidance (e.g., when to expect quickening) • Address any risk factors present • When to call the midwife/signs of complications
Blood pressure		
Abdominal exam (fundus at symphysis pubis by 12 weeks)	CVS (10–12 weeks)	
Fetal heart rate with handheld Doppler		
14–20 Weeks		
Weight	Follow up on previous screening results	**Screenings:** • Risk assessment and screening • Woman's symptoms and concerns **Education:** • Fetal growth and development and physiologic changes • Common discomforts and relief measures • Nutrition • Exercise • Address any risk factors present • When to call the midwife/signs of complications
Blood pressure	Amniocentesis (after 15 weeks)	
Obstetric abdominal exam (fundus halfway to umbilicus at 16 weeks; 2 fingerbreadths below umbilicus at 18 weeks; immediately below the umbilicus at 20 weeks)	Quad screening or multiple markers (15–20 weeks)	
	Anatomy ultrasound (18–20 weeks)	
Fetal heart rate with handheld Doppler		

Physical Examination	Laboratory or Other Testing	Screenings and Education
20–24 Weeks		
Weight Blood pressure Abdominal exam (measure fundus; measurement in centimeters should equal weeks' gestation ± 2–3 centimeters) Fetal heart rate (fetoscope detects heart rate after 20 weeks)		**Screenings:** • Screening for depression • Intimate-partner violence/domestic abuse screening • Risk assessment and screening • Woman's symptoms and concerns **Education:** • Preterm labor signs and symptoms • Fetal growth and development and physiologic changes • Common discomforts and relief measures • Nutrition • Exercise • Address any risk factors present • When to call the midwife/signs of complications
24–28 Weeks		
Weight Blood pressure Obstetric abdominal exam (measure fundus; measurement in centimeters should equal weeks' gestation ± 2–3 centimeters) Fetal heart rate	Gestational diabetes screening (24–28 weeks) Hemoglobin/hematocrit (28 weeks) Repeat antibody screen if Rh negative at initial visit, in preparation for anti-D serum administration (28 weeks) Follow up on previous screening and ultrasound results	**Screenings:** • Risk assessment and screening • Woman's symptoms and concerns **Education:** • Gestational diabetes • Preterm labor signs and symptoms • Childbirth classes and preparation • Nutrition • Exercise • Sibling preparation • Fetal growth and development and physiologic changes • Common discomforts and relief measures • Address any risk factors present • When to call the midwife/signs of complications
28–34 Weeks		
Weight Blood pressure Obstetric abdominal exam (measure fundus; measurement in centimeters should equal weeks' gestation ± 2–3 centimeters until approximately 32 weeks after which steady growth should continue) Fetal lie and presentation Fetal heart rate	Consider repeat STI testing as indicated by history or state law Follow up on GDM screening and other labs	**Screenings:** • Risk assessment and screening • Fetal kick counts begin now if high risk • Woman's symptoms and concerns **Education:** • Preterm labor signs and symptoms • Nutrition • Exercise • Breastfeeding • Sibling preparation • Sexuality • Fetal growth and development and physiologic changes • Common discomforts and relief measures • Circumcision decision • Issues surrounding employment • Body mechanics • Travel precautions • Address any risk factors present • When to call the midwife/signs of complications

Physical Examination	Laboratory or Other Testing	Screenings and Education
35–40 Weeks		
Weight Blood pressure Obstetric abdominal exam (measure fundus; should demonstrate growth but will be influenced by fetal size and lightening) Abdominal exam and Leopold's maneuvers for fetal lie, presentation, position, variety, and EFW Fetal heart rate	Group B *Streptococcus* (GBS) screening (35–37 weeks, unless unnecessary based on history) Follow up on previous screening results if done	**Screenings:** • Screening for depression • Intimate-partner violence/domestic abuse screening • Risk assessment and screening • Women's symptoms and concerns • Fetal kick counts for all women **Education:** • Preterm labor signs and symptoms • Preeclampsia symptoms • Term labor signs and symptoms • Preparation for labor and birth • Breastfeeding • Contraception plans • Preparation for parenthood • Postpartum preparation • Car seat • Selection of provider for newborn • Sibling preparation • Postpartum depression signs and symptoms • Readiness of home and family for newborn • Anticipatory guidance regarding labor and birth • Circumcision decision • Nutrition • Exercise • Rest • Issues surrounding employment • Body mechanics • Travel precautions • Fetal growth and development and physiologic changes • Common discomforts and relief measures • Address any risk factors present • When to call the midwife/signs of complications

Physical Examination	Laboratory or Other Testing	Screenings and Education
Beyond 40 Weeks		
Weight	Follow up on GBS screening	**Screenings:**
Blood pressure	Educate woman if GBS is positive (also recheck her allergies)	• Risk assessment and screening
Obstetric abdominal exam (measure fundus; should demonstrate growth but will be influenced by fetal size and lightening)		• Woman's symptoms and concerns
		• Fetal kick counts for all women
		Education:
Abdominal exam and Leopold's maneuvers for fetal lie, presentation, position, variety, and EFW		• Post dates education and informed consent regarding any testing protocols
		• Induction education and informed consent
Fetal heart rate		• Preeclampsia symptoms
Cervical exam for Bishop's score		• Nutrition
		• Exercise
Additional antepartum fetal assessment as indicated (e.g., nonstress testing, AFI, biophysical profile)		• Labor signs and symptoms
		• Preparation for labor and birth
		• Anticipatory guidance regarding labor and birth
		• Breastfeeding
		• Contraception plans[b]
		• Address any risk factors present
		• When to call the midwife/signs of complications

[a]Although it is common practice to repeat an antibody screen for women who are Rh negative to document that isoimmunization has not occurred, the change of maternal fetal blood exchange prior to 26–28 weeks' gestation is very small and, therefore, this laboratory test is not required. Anti-D serum may be given without repeating the Rh status or antibody screen.

[b]Contraception counseling may need to be introduced sooner, as women with federal- or state-funded medical assistance must sign the consent for tubal sterilization 30 days or more prior to having the procedure done. The time frames differ by state.

AFI = amniotic fluid index; BMI = body mass index; EDD = estimated due date; EFW = estimated fetal weight; GDM = gestational diabetes mellitus; hCG = human chorionic gonadotropin; LMP = last menstrual period; PAPP-A= pregnancy-associated plasma protein A; STI = sexually transmitted infection.

23

Obstetric Complications in Pregnancy

NANCY JO REEDY

TEKOA L. KING

Introduction

Every woman deserves the personalized care and skill of a midwife during pregnancy and birth. The majority of women experience healthy pregnancies, and midwifery care provides the appropriate support and interventions needed. Women with obstetric complications during pregnancy benefit from midwifery care, but may need physician care as well. For the obstetric conditions and complications addressed in this chapter, the midwife may manage them independently, consult with a physician at intervals, provide care in collaboration with a physician, or refer the woman to a physician for total management. The midwifery role in the woman's care may vary based on assessment at the time of initial diagnosis, after laboratory findings are evaluated, or in the event of increasing severity of a problem. The care provided by a midwife will also depend on the practice setting, the experience and education of the midwife, the availability and collaborative relationship with medical consultants, and the clinical practice agreement in place. This chapter describes the scope of knowledge and care with which all midwives should be comfortable.

Women of all risk categories and complication levels can benefit from the individualized care, education, and support from midwives. Midwives with a strong interest in the care of women with obstetric complications, in turn, may extend their knowledge and skills to provide care for women with specific complications, such as hyperemesis or twins.

Extending midwifery care to women with obstetric complications requires knowledge beyond the core competencies, a system that provides timely consultation and referral, and guidelines established collaboratively with the medical consultants. This chapter is not intended to set limits on midwifery practice, but rather to serve as a starting point from which each midwife may determine the scope of practice and circle of safety appropriate to the population served and the practice setting.

Screening for Complications at the Initial Visit When Pregnancy Is Diagnosed

The process for completing a standard history, physical examination, and laboratory assessment for all pregnant women is discussed in the *Prenatal Care* chapter. At the first visit, risks can be identified and care instituted to minimize adverse effects. **Box 23-1** lists examples of conditions that may require physician consultation.

First Trimester Complications

The most common complications in the first trimester are vaginal bleeding, verification of fetal viability in the case of bleeding, and management of early pregnancy loss. In addition, nausea and vomiting can vary from being mild and perceived as troublesome for the woman, or severe requiring hospitalization and management.

BOX 23-1 Conditions That Indicate a Need for Medical Consultation, Collaboration, or Referral[a]

Medical History

- Uterine anomaly
- Large uterine fibroids
- History of cervical insufficiency
- Previous uterine surgery including prior cesarean section
- Prior unexplained third trimester fetal loss

Obstetric Complications That Develop During Pregnancy

- Abnormal screening results for chromosomal conditions such as aneuploidy or genetic disorders
- Gestational diabetes
- Nausea and vomiting that requires hospitalization
- Cervical length less than 2.0 cm prior to 24 weeks
- Short cervix (less than 3.2 cm) on objective measurement at 24–28 weeks
- Malpresentation of the fetus after 36 weeks
- Multiple gestation
- Post-dates pregnancy (more than 41 0/7 weeks)
- Pyelonephritis
- Labor at less than 35 weeks' gestation
- Ultrasound with abnormal findings such as fetal growth restriction, polyhydramnios, fetal anomalies, or unresolved size/dates discrepancy
- Vaginal bleeding suspected not to be bloody show or related to cervicitis
- Suspected extrauterine pregnancy: ectopic
- Isoimmunization
- Placenta previa with significant bleeding or persisting after 20 weeks
- Pregnancy-induced hypertension

Medical Complications Prior to Pregnancy or That Develop During Pregnancy

- Asthma requiring medication
- Breast mass
- Cholethiasis
- Hypertension
- Deep vein thrombosis or pulmonary embolus: history or current
- Significant gastrointestinal disease such as Crohn's disease, previous bariatric procedure
- Headaches: severe, recurrent, or associated with hypertension
- Hemoglobinopathy
- Mental disorder that requires medication
- Morbid obesity
- Mitral valve prolapse without previous cardiology evaluation
- Varicose veins with pain, swelling, or stasis
- Renal calculi
- Persistent proteinuria
- Severe anemia not responding to oral iron supplementation
- Suspected pneumonia
- Syphilis
- Thyroid disease
- Undiagnosed skin rashes or lesions
- Systemic infections such as tuberculosis, HIV, or bacterial endocarditis
- Cancer
- Diabetes
- Lupus or other autoimmune disorder
- Active seizure disorder
- Cardiac, renal, or hepatic disease

[a]This list is offered for consideration and is not absolute or all inclusive. The list is intended as an adjunct to clinical management based on the individual woman, the midwife, the consulting physician, and institutional guidelines.

First Trimester Bleeding

While normal pregnancy is associated with amenorrhea and a complete lack of vaginal bleeding, many women with a viable pregnancy experience some form of vaginal bleeding in the first trimester. Conversely, women who have a pregnancy loss may not experience bleeding until several weeks after the fetal demise. Vaginal bleeding may be fresh (bright red) or old (dark brown), light and occur just once or twice as vaginal spotting, persist for several days, or present as a sudden onset of heavy menstrual-like bleeding.

Bleeding before 20 weeks' gestation occurs in 20% to 30% of pregnant women.[1,2] Although many of these women ultimately will have uncomplicated pregnancies and the bleeding will not have a clear etiology, the most common abnormal conditions associated with vaginal bleeding in the first trimester include anembryonic pregnancy, incomplete or missed abortion, subchorionic hemorrhage, trophoblastic disease, lesions of the cervix, vaginitis, and rare medical diseases.[2] The most common underlying reasons for miscarriage in the first trimester are chromosomal, with approximately 50% of these losses being associated with chromosomal abnormalities, including trisomies (56%), polyploidy (20%), and monosomy (18%).[2]

The timing of the bleeding is an indicator of potential pregnancy viability. Women who have bleeding toward the end of the first trimester are less likely to have a pregnancy loss than are women who experience bleeding early in the first trimester. Bleeding that occurs after cardiac activity is confirmed (5 to 6 weeks' gestation via ultrasound) lowers the risk of pregnancy loss to less than 6%.[3] Even women with heavy bleeding at 10 to 13 gestational weeks are reported to have a loss rate of less than 11%.[4]

Categories of First Trimester Bleeding

Miscarriage in the first trimester occurs in approximately 30% of all pregnancies. Many of these losses occur prior to missing a menstrual period, so a woman may not know she was pregnant. **Table 23-1**

lists the definitions of conditions associated with first trimester pregnancy loss.

Spontaneous Abortion

Abortion is the natural termination of pregnancy by expulsion of the products of conception prior to the ability of the fetus to survive if born. Spontaneous abortion (SAB)—also known as "miscarriage"—is the term applied when pregnancy loss occurs before 20 weeks' gestation or when the embryo is less than 500 grams in weight. In addition to congenital and genetic etiologies, other conditions associated with miscarriage include abnormal progesterone levels, thyroid abnormalities, uncontrolled diabetes, uterine anomalies, infection, and autoimmune diseases. Within the diagnosis of spontaneous abortion are varied expressions, including threatened abortion, inevitable abortion, missed abortion, and incomplete abortion.

Table 23-1	Definitions of Conditions Associated with Spontaneous Abortion	
Term	**Definition**	**Objective Findings**
Biochemical pregnancy or anembryonic gestation Old term: blighted ovum	Development of gestational sac without development of an embryo	Gestational sac > 18 mm without an embryo Dropping beta-hCG levels after beta-hCG level < 1000 mIU/mL with gestational sac visible on TVUS
Missed abortion	Nonviable products of conception are retained with or without vaginal bleeding	Irregularly shaped/collapsing gestational sac, sac < 5 mm Lack of cardiac motion with fetal pole > 5 mm
Recurrent abortion	Spontaneous abortion has terminated the course of three or more consecutive pregnancies	No diagnostic ultrasound findings
Threatened abortion	Painless vaginal bleeding < 20 weeks' gestation without cervical dilation or effacement	May or may not show sonographic signs of abnormal sac or embryo May show subchorionic bleeding
Inevitable abortion	Less than 20 weeks' gestation with cervical dilation and/or rupture of the membranes in addition to vaginal bleeding and lower abdominal or back pain but no passage of tissue	Embryo > 5 mm in size, without cardiac activity Embryonic bradycardia after 8 weeks' gestation Serum progesterone < 5 ng/mL
Incomplete abortion	Passage of some fetal or placental tissue through the cervix at less than 20 weeks' gestation	Tissue visible in uterus without evidence of viable gestation
Complete abortion	Spontaneous expulsion of fetal and placental tissue from uterine cavity at less than 20 weeks' gestation	Uterus empty on sonogram
Septic abortion	Serious maternal infection that occurs after any abortion	May or may not show retained products of conception on sonogram

In addition to miscarriage, other causes of first trimester bleeding include ectopic pregnancy, cervicitis, cervical lesions, cervical polyp, vaginitis, postcoital bleeding, implantation spotting, subchorionic hemorrhage, or (rarely) hydatidiform mole. Demise of a twin may also cause vaginal bleeding without any expulsion of products of conception. Rectal bleeding, hemorrhagic cystitis, perineal lesions, and vulvar varicosities are uncommon sources of bleeding that may be perceived as coming from the vagina and, therefore, are included in the initial differential diagnosis.[2]

Evaluation of First Trimester Bleeding

Any report of vaginal bleeding during pregnancy must be investigated via a physical examination. The goal of management is first, to recognize and rule out potentially life threatening causes of bleeding such as active hemorrhage or ectopic pregnancy, and second, to determine pregnancy viability. **Box 23-2** reviews the evaluation and management of first trimester bleeding. The first step in assessing vaginal bleeding is to determine the origin of the bleeding, including whether it is from the vagina, cervix, or uterus.

BOX 23-2 Evaluation and Management of First Trimester Bleeding

History

1. Last menstrual period (LMP), regularity of menses, use of contraception prior to pregnancy, confirmation of dates by exam and or sonogram; is there an established estimated date of delivery (EDD)?
2. Pregnancy test results: by urine or blood sample and when positive?
3. Previous pregnancy history: any previous spontaneous abortions (SAB) or ectopic pregnancy?
4. Contraceptive history, specifically for current use of an intrauterine device (IUD).
5. History of bleeding? When did it start? How much bleeding is present? Is it dark or bright red? How frequently do pads need to be changed?
6. Is there pain or cramping? When did it start? Where is the pain (lower front, midline, right or left side, back, rectal, shoulder, painful with breathing)? What is its nature (mild, intense, sharp, dull)?
7. Has she had fever or urinary tract symptoms?
8. Has she had a urinary tract infection or sexually transmitted infection recently or during this pregnancy?
9. Has there been any change in pregnancy symptoms (worsening nausea, suddenly improved nausea, improved breast tenderness)?
10. Has there been recent intercourse? When? Was there any impact on the pain or bleeding either during or after sexual contact?

Physical Examination

1. The first step in assessing vaginal bleeding is to determine whether the bleeding is coming from the vagina, cervix, or uterus.

2. Evaluate the woman's blood pressure, temperature, pulse, and respirations.
3. Confirm a pregnancy test if indicated (this could be delayed menses).
4. Perform an abdominal exam, including the following steps:
   a. Palpation for tenderness/pain
   b. Palpation for fundal height or other masses
   c. Assessment for rebound tenderness
   d. Auscultation for bowel sounds (diminished in appendicitis)
   e. Palpation for costovertebral angle (CVA) tenderness (pyelonephritis can present with referred pelvic pain)
5. Perform a gentle speculum examination of the vagina and cervix.
   a. Screen for vaginitis and cervicitis with cultures and a wet prep if indicated.
   b. Observe the cervical os for dilation, presence of fluid, blood, clots, pus, or fetal parts or membranes.
6. Perform a gentle bimanual examination to assess the following:
   a. Size of uterus
   b. Cervical effacement, dilatation, and status of membranes
   c. Adnexal masses or pain
   d. Cervical motion pain
7. Attempt to auscultate for the fetal heart tones if more than 10 weeks' gestation.
8. Obtain a hemoglobin and hematocrit if indicated.
9. Order an ultrasound if indicated.
10. Serial serum quantitative beta human chorionic gonadotropin (beta-hCG) or progesterone measurement may be indicated.

Bleeding from the Cervix

During early pregnancy, the cervix becomes more vascular. Any situation that would cause inflammation or trauma to the cervix can cause bleeding. If cervical bleeding or cervicitis is noted on a speculum exam, evaluation for infection is indicated. Gonorrhea, chlamydia, and trichomoniasis are all associated with cervical bleeding. A herpetic lesion may be present on the cervix or another site in the vagina. Another possible cause of cervical bleeding is a cervical polyp. In the absence of a specific infectious process, simple increased vascularity of the cervix may be implicated. Irritation or trauma to the cervix or vagina following sexual intercourse may stimulate or worsen the bleeding. Bleeding from the cervix or vagina is rarely associated with pregnancy loss. If all other physical signs are normal, the woman may be reassured that the pregnancy is not in jeopardy. Most clinicians counsel women to refrain from sexual intercourse until a few days or week after the bleeding has ceased.

Bleeding from the Uterus

If the physical examination does not reveal an obvious non-uterine source of bleeding, the primary differential diagnoses are spontaneous abortion and ectopic pregnancy. In addition to history and physical examination, quantification of the beta-hCG and ultrasound can be useful in determining the status of the pregnancy. Although individual settings may have individualized protocols, **Figure 23-1** presents an algorithm for evaluation and management of first trimester bleeding that will help the clinician differentiate between viable pregnancy, spontaneous abortion, and ectopic pregnancy.[5]

Laboratory Evaluation of First Trimester Bleeding
Human Chorionic Gonadotropin Levels

The normal values for beta-hCG in early pregnancy are described in detail in the *Anatomy and Physiology of Pregnancy: Placental, Fetal, and Maternal Adaptations* chapter. Beta-hCG is initially measurable 8 to 9 days after conception. Serial quantitative measurement of beta-hCG can be helpful in determining the viability of a pregnancy. In a healthy pregnancy, the beta-hCG level doubles approximately every 1.6 days through week 5 after the LMP, then every 2 days in week 6, and then every 2.5 days in week 7. Levels rise more slowly after week 7, and they plateau and then fall between 8 to 10 weeks' gestation. By the time the beta-hCG blood level is 1500 mIU/mL, a gestational sac should be visible during a transvaginal ultrasound examination. Transabdominal ultrasound may not be able to visualize a gestational sac until after the beta-hCG reaches 6000 mIU/mL, however. Expected ultrasound findings have been linked to beta-hCG levels, although each institution will have defined specific cut-off values for correlating beta-hCG values with ultrasound findings, as there is significant variability in how beta-hCG is measured.[6]

Ultrasound

First trimester ultrasound examinations can be very useful in evaluating a woman with bleeding early in her pregnancy. The use of beta-hCG levels in combination with ultrasound helps determine the diagnosis and guides management, as shown in Figure 23-1. Ultrasound findings in the first trimester include identification of intrauterine versus extrauterine pregnancy, gestational age (accurate within 5 days), number of fetuses, viability with cardiac activity, adnexal masses (e.g., ectopic pregnancy, ovarian cyst, dermoid cyst), uterine fibroids, and presence of fluid in the cul-de-sac. Ultrasound can also identify subchorionic hemorrhage, incomplete abortion with retention of products of conception, and complete abortion when the uterus is empty of any products of conception. Ultrasound examination also can be diagnostic for hydatidiform mole via the appearance or a cluster of grape like material, a honeycomb effect, or a snow storm on the screen. However, once cardiac activity has been identified at a normal fetal heart rate (FHR), the incidence of spontaneous pregnancy loss drops to approximately 3%[6], providing reassurance to the woman and her provider.

Subchorionic hemorrhage is the term for bleeding that occurs between the chorion and myometrium or between the chorion and placenta. This finding is noted in approximately 18% to 30% of women who present with first trimester bleeding. Although subchorionic hemorrhage is associated with an increased risk for miscarriage, many of these hemorrhages resolve spontaneously without adverse pregnancy outcomes. The etiology is unclear and no consensus exists regarding a specific course of treatment. Larger subchorionic hemorrhages are more likely to result in miscarriage than are smaller ones.

Progesterone

Progesterone is produced by the corpus luteum in the first trimester of pregnancy. If the serum progesterone value is 20 ng/mL or more, it is likely that the pregnancy is a viable pregnancy. Similarly, a value

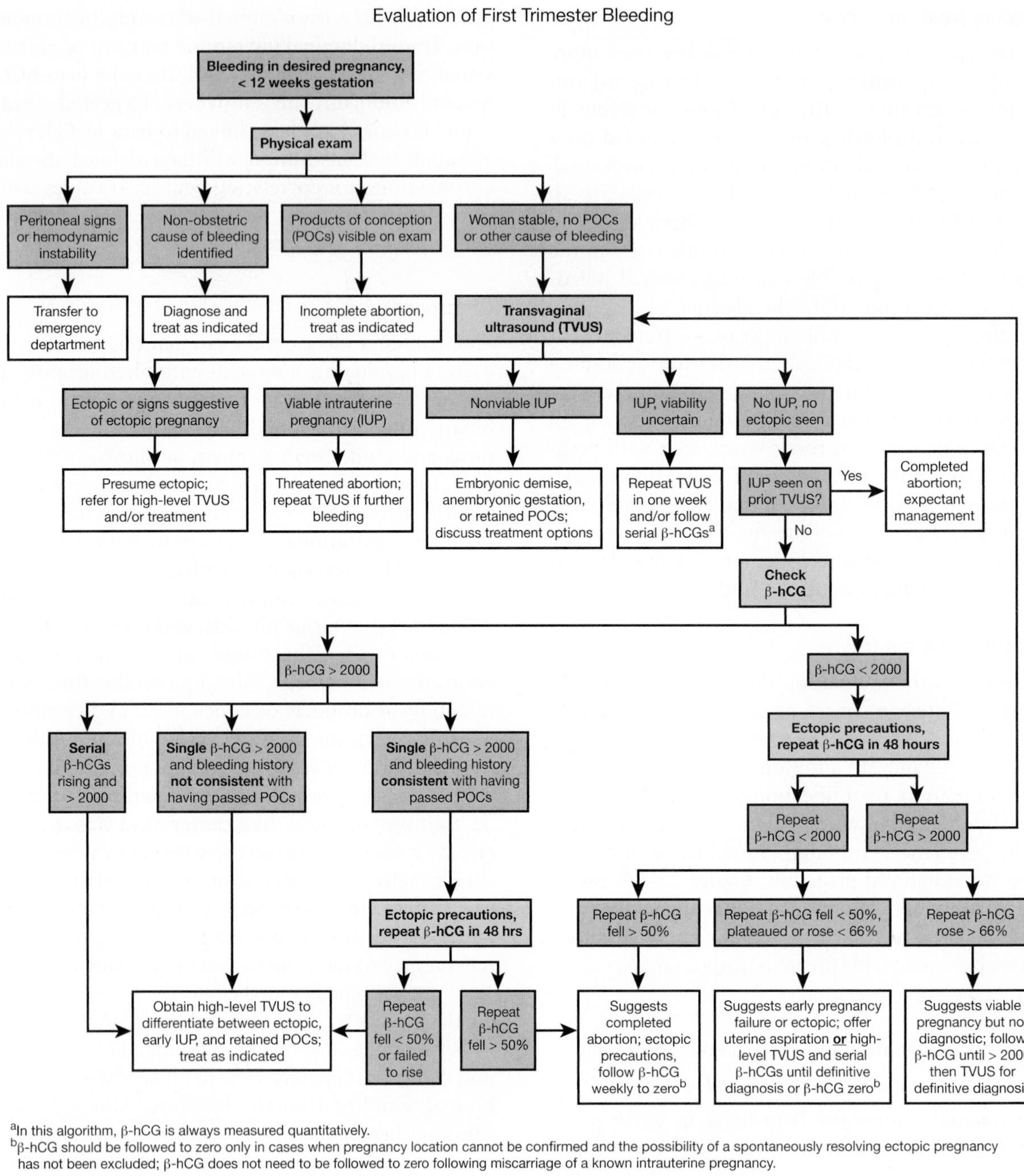

Evaluation of First Trimester Bleeding

Figure 23-1 Evaluation of first trimester bleeding.
Source: Reprinted with permission from the Reproductive Health Access Project. First trimester bleeding algorithm. http://www.reproductiveaccess
.org/m_m/downloads/First_trimester_bleeding_algorithm.pdf.

of 5 ng/mL or less is consistent with an abnormal or failing pregnancy, but the progesterone value alone does not give information about the site of the pregnancy. When the value of serum progesterone is between 5 and 20 ng/mL, further evaluation of the pregnancy is indicated.[7] A potential problem with the use of progesterone is that some laboratories take

several days to return results, which limits the clinical utility of this test as a diagnostic tool.

Management of First Trimester Bleeding

The woman with heavy, bright red bleeding consistent with active hemorrhage needs to be evaluated in a hospital emergency department. A woman with subjective symptoms or physical findings consistent with an ectopic pregnancy or a woman with positive pregnancy test and no intrauterine pregnancy on ultrasound needs immediate medical management to rule out an ectopic pregnancy.

After the two most serious causes of bleeding have been ruled out, management involves determining whether the pregnancy is viable. If the woman is less than 6 weeks' gestation, serial beta-hCG levels can be performed every 48 to 72 hours. After 6 weeks, an ultrasound will provide information about viability quickly and more reliably than serial beta-hCG levels via confirmation of a fetal pole, fetal heart motion, and absence of placental abnormality.

If the woman does not have excessive bleeding or pain, has normal vital signs, is not severely emotionally distressed, and has a previous hematocrit of at least 30%, the rest of the evaluation can occur on an outpatient basis. Any concern that the woman may have an ectopic pregnancy or a lack of intrauterine pregnancy on ultrasound requires immediate physician evaluation.

Management of Missed or Inevitable Abortion

If a woman is hemodynamically stable when an inevitable or missed abortion is diagnosed, she can chose expectant management, medical abortion, or chose to have the pregnancy terminated via a suction dilatation and curettage (D & C). If the woman chooses expectant management, she should be instructed to take her temperature daily (unless she is asleep) or more often if she has chills, and to call if she soaks through a regular sanitary napkin in an hour or less, passes clots larger than 3 centimeters (the size of a 50-cent piece), or has a fever of 38°C (100.4°F) or higher. If she has experienced two or more miscarriages, she may be able to save the products of conception in a container for genetic studies once the miscarriage is completed. The products of conception may also be sent to the laboratory or viewed in the office under a microscope for verification of placental villi to confirm a complete abortion and verify that the pregnancy had been intrauterine.

Approximately 25% to 30% of women with a missed or anembryonic miscarriage will spontaneously expel the products of conception within 7 days and 52% to 60% will expel the products of conception by 14 days. After 14 days the number of women who have a spontaneous miscarriage slowly drops so that only 66% to 76% will have completed the miscarriage by 45 days. Thus, it is common to recommend a waiting period of up to 2 weeks before

offering medical or surgical intervention for women who chose expectant management. That said, there are no clear health risks for the woman who wants to wait longer if it is her desire to do so.

Medical abortion involves vaginal administration of 800 mcg of misoprostol (Cytotec) that is repeated once 24 to 72 hours after initial administration. The success of misoprostol is 80% to 90% within 7 days in women who are up to 10 weeks' gestational age at the time of administration. The success of misoprostol varies somewhat by diagnosis, with slightly lower success rates in anembryonic pregnancies and highest success rates in women who have an incomplete or inevitable abortion. General information about use of misoprostol can be found in the *Family Planning* chapter. When used to help evacuate the uterus in a woman who has a missed or inevitable abortion, counseling about expected symptoms, danger signs, and evaluation that the woman has access to emergency care are essential. Pain medication may be prescribed concomitantly.

Recurrent Abortion

When a woman has experienced three or more miscarriages, genetic counseling and an endocrine evaluation should be considered. The standard evaluation for recurrent abortion includes ultrasound to look for developmental abnormalities of the genital tract (e.g., bicornuate uterus, vaginal septum), genetic testing, and tests for autoimmune disorders and thyroid abnormalities. In some settings, midwives may start the initial steps by ordering initial laboratory tests and assisting the woman schedule follow-up appointments with the appropriate consultants.

Follow-Up

Follow-up for a woman who has experienced a miscarriage includes provision of support through the grieving process, counseling to avoid sexual intercourse until bleeding has ceased, and then counseling about contraception and future pregnancy planning. This is also a good time to perform some preconception counseling and assessment, as outlined in the *Preconception Care* chapter. If she appears to be having significant grief or emotional difficulty, it may be appropriate to offer to continue seeing her or to refer her for counseling.

Regardless of the type of miscarriage or outcome of vaginal bleeding, all women who have had significant bleeding in the first trimester and who are Rh-negative should receive Rh immune globulin (i.e., RhoGAM) within 72 hours of the initial bleeding event.

Ectopic Pregnancy

Ectopic pregnancy occurs whenever the blastocyst implants anywhere except the endometrium. Possible sites for ectopic pregnancy include the cervix, fallopian tubes, ovaries, and abdomen.[8] Risk factors for ectopic pregnancy include pelvic infections, pregnancy with an intrauterine device in situ, previous ectopic pregnancy, and prior tubal surgery. Early symptoms of an ectopic pregnancy usually consist of vaginal bleeding and spotting, and occasionally pelvic pain.

Signs and symptoms of ectopic pregnancy include the triad of pain (particularly on one side of the pelvis), vaginal bleeding, and a palpable adnexal mass; some women with an ectopic pregnancy may be asymptomatic, however. Because the levels of beta-hCG are lower and tend to rise more slowly than normal when an ectopic pregnancy is present, a woman may have fewer presumptive signs of pregnancy. She also may or may not have had a positive pregnancy test.

Uterine changes are not diagnostic for ectopic pregnancy because the uterus can enlarge to the same size and consistency as a pregnant uterus due to the influence of the placental hormones. However, the uterus may be displaced to one side by a tubal pregnancy.

Early diagnosis of ectopic pregnancy in recent years has greatly improved the outcome of tubal patency and diminished the number of catastrophic tubal ruptures. The midwife must always include ectopic pregnancy in the differential diagnosis for a woman who may be pregnant and who has vaginal spotting, bleeding, or lower abdominal pain. There is an old adage, "You have only one chance to miss an ectopic."

Pharmaceutical management of ectopic pregnancy with methotrexate (Trexall) has diminished the need for surgical intervention and improved the potential for preserving tubal function and therefore a woman's fertility.[8] However, appropriate administration of this medication relies on early diagnosis prior to significant distortion of the fallopian tube and rupture of the pregnancy into the abdomen.

Tubal Pregnancy

Tubal pregnancy accounts for more than 95% of all ectopic pregnancies.[8] The evaluation for an ectopic pregnancy is the same as noted in Figure 23-1. Because ectopic pregnancy is a potentially life-threatening condition, the woman with subjective symptoms or slowly rising beta-hCG must be thoroughly evaluated to ensure the pregnancy is in the uterus. Screening with history, physical assessment, and laboratory evaluation, including ultrasound, is within the scope of midwifery care. It is often difficult to palpate the ectopic mass, and the subjective signs of such pregnancy vary widely. Therefore an ultrasound is indicated emergently at any time an ectopic pregnancy is suspected. If this diagnosis cannot be ruled out, the midwife should consult with the physician immediately.

Ruptured ectopic pregnancy is an emergency. Its signs and symptoms vary widely. The classic case of tubal rupture involves a woman who may or may not realize she is pregnant because slight vaginal bleeding or spotting has been interpreted as a menstrual period. Without warning, she suddenly experiences a sharp, stabbing, severe, lower abdominal pain. Hypotension and other signs of shock can develop quickly. Her abdomen is tender, and vaginal examination is quite painful. Movement of the cervix elicits exquisite pain. A tender, boggy mass might be felt to one side of the uterus. The cul-de-sac may be full of blood, thereby causing the posterior vaginal fornix to bulge. Pain in the neck or shoulder, especially on inspiration, may be present as a result of diaphragmatic irritation from blood in the peritoneal cavity. A woman with this profile is experiencing a medical emergency and requires immediate medical assistance.

Ovarian Pregnancy

Ovarian pregnancy is rare. Symptoms besides vaginal bleeding or spotting relate to rupture into the peritoneal cavity and are similar to those of tubal rupture. On examination, an enlarged ovary or ovarian mass might be palpable, which may or may not be painful. The uterus might be slightly enlarged from the endometrial stimulation by progesterone and hCG. Diagnosis is made on the basis of slowly rising beta-hCG levels and ultrasound examination. Referral for medical management is always indicated.

Abdominal Pregnancy

Abdominal pregnancy usually is the result of an early tubal pregnancy rupture or abortion into the peritoneal cavity. In a few exceedingly rare cases, the fertilized ovum makes the abdomen the site of primary implantation. Such pregnancies are so rare that they are reported as case reports and are too few to calculate the incidence of this condition. Signs and symptoms include the inability to outline the uterus and the sensation that the fetal parts are just "under the skin" of the woman. The woman may have severe gastrointestinal symptoms that are not resolving with standard management. Ultrasound examination does not always make the diagnosis, especially later in pregnancy.

Abdominal pregnancy is a life-threatening condition due to the adverse effects of placental implantation on abdominal organs such as the liver. Delivery must be by abdominal route, clearly requiring medical management of multiple subspecialists in maternal–fetal medicine and surgery in a tertiary setting.

Hydatidiform Mole

The term *hydatidiform mole* is derived from the combination of the Greek word *hydatisia*, which means "drop of water," and the Latin word *mola*, which means "false conception." Hydatidiform mole occurs when trophoblastic cells that normally develop into the placenta exhibit atypical growth.[9] An abnormal union of sperm and egg develops with no fetal tissue, but abnormal placental tissue proliferates and fills the uterine space. Placental villi become edematous grape-like structures that can be identified on ultrasound.

Hydatidiform mole occurs in approximately 1 in 15,000 pregnancies.[10] Risk factors for this condition include younger maternal age and older maternal age. The risk is higher for women who have had a previous molar pregnancy.[9]

Hydatidiform mole is classified as either complete or partial. A complete mole occurs when an ovum that has lost its DNA is fertilized by a sperm and the resultant mitosis results in sperm chromosomal DNA only. A partial hydatidiform mole occurs when two sperm fertilize a normal ovum and the result is usually triploid, with both villus changes and nonviable fetal tissue.[11] On rare occasion, a woman may have a twin pregnancy consisting of one normal fetus and placenta and one molar pregnancy.

A hydatidiform mole is usually a benign neoplasm, but it has the potential for becoming malignant. This condition often precedes the extremely malignant—but fortunately rare—trophoblastic neoplasm known as choriocarcinoma. With current chemotherapeutic drugs, the cure rate for choriocarcinoma is nearly 100%.

Rapid growth of the abnormal placental tissue is responsible for many of the symptoms associated with hydatidiform mole, as the beta-hCG values are very high when a complete mole is present. Beta-hCG levels may be normal in a partial mole and diagnosis

---

BOX 23-3 Signs and Symptoms of Molar Pregnancy

- Persistent, often severe, nausea and vomiting
- Uterine bleeding evident by the 12th week of pregnancy
- A large-for-dates uterus
- Shortness of breath
- Often enlarged, tender ovaries (theca lutein cysts)
- No fetal heart tones
- No fetal activity
- Fetal parts not evident with palpation
- Pregnancy-induced hypertension, preeclampsia, or eclampsia before 24 weeks' gestation

---

is made by ultrasound. Signs and symptoms of hydatidiform mole are shown in **Box 23-3**.

Hydatidiform mole has a characteristic ultrasound pattern of an echogenic mass and the classic "snowstorm pattern" of the villi and trophoblastic hyperplasia. A persistently high, or even rising, level of hCG after 100 days from the first day of the last menstrual period is indicative of abnormal trophoblastic growth or a multiple gestation. The woman is referred to the consulting physician for care and follow-up.

A woman presenting with a pregnancy after a previous molar pregnancy needs careful first trimester screening to detect a recurrence. A careful history and review of signs and symptoms associated with mole, a first trimester ultrasound, and a quantitative beta-hCG level should be obtained to rule out a recurrence of hydatidiform mole.

Hyperemesis Gravidarum

Hyperemesis gravidarum is the term used when a woman has excessive nausea and vomiting during pregnancy (NVP). Although there is no standard definition for this condition, most diagnostic criteria include persistent vomiting before 9 gestational weeks, dehydration and/or ketonuria, weight loss greater than 5% of initial body weight, and electrolyte imbalance (hypokalemia).[12] Risk factors for hyperemesis include previous pregnancy complicated by hyperemesis, molar pregnancies, multiple gestation, prepregnancy history of gastrointestinal disorders, clinical hyperthyroid disorders, and prepregnancy psychiatric diagnosis. Interestingly, women 30 years and older and women who smoke have a lower risk of hyperemesis, and women who have hyperemesis are more likely to carry a female fetus.[13,14] In the United States, hyperemesis is the second most common reason for hospitalization during pregnancy (following preterm labor).[15]

Etiology of Hyperemesis Gravidarum

The etiology of hyperemesis is unknown but presumed to be multifactorial. Several hypotheses have been explored, including the role of high levels of hCG, genetic factors, thyroid dysfunction, preexisting gastrointestinal or vestibular disorders, and psychiatric disorders. Although associations between many of these conditions and hyperemesis have been found, none has been determined to be strong enough to be considered the etiologic mechanism for all women.[16]

The relationship between hyperemesis and psychiatric conditions is complicated. Older studies found that women with preexisting psychiatric disorders such as conversion disorder or psychosomatic disorder were more likely to develop hyperemesis during pregnancy. It was incorrectly theorized that these women transfer psychological distress or not wanting a baby into physical symptoms. The methodologies of those studies were not scientifically sound and this misconception needs to be put to rest.[17] More recent work has documented that psychological distress, anxiety, and depression are more often consequences of hyperemesis rather than its antecedents.[13] Thus it appears that the etiology of hyperemesis is multifactorial, which suggests comfort, emotional support, and medications all need to be offered as part of a multipronged approach to care.

Maternal and Fetal Effects of Hyperemesis

Hyperemesis has significant adverse effects on the women who experience this pregnancy complication, including adverse psychosocial effects, concerns about economics and employment, depression, anxiety, and fear about future pregnancies.[18] Among women with severe NVP or hyperemesis, 76% changed plans for future children, 15% terminated their pregnancy secondary to the condition, and 7% reported long-term psychological sequelae.

Women with hyperemesis frequently experience a transient biochemical hyperthyroid state. This occurs because the beta-hCG is structurally quite similar to thyroid-stimulating hormone and is able to stimulate production of thyroid hormone. This hyperthyroid state does not need to be treated and will resolve spontaneously by 18 to 20 weeks' gestation.

Hyperemesis is not associated with adverse pregnancy outcomes if pregnancy weight gain normalizes. Women with hyperemesis who have low-pregnancy weight gains have an increased risk for preterm labor as well as low birth weight when compared to women who have hyperemesis and normal weight gains and women without hyperemesis.[19]

Assessment and Management of Hyperemesis

The PUQE index discussed in detail in the *Prenatal Care* chapter is one diagnostic tool for determining the severity of nausea and vomiting. Women with a PUQE index score of 13 or higher fall into the category of severe NVP or hyperemesis; their treatment usually requires hospitalization to break the cycle of vomiting and establish adequate rehydration.[16] Although management of women with hyperemesis requires medical consultation, collaborative management is common and midwives frequently initiate the assessment and referral for hospitalization, or initial assessment at hospital admission. The evaluation and management of a woman who presents with severe NVP is outlined in **Box 23-4**.

Intravenous fluids are an essential first step for women who are dehydrated. Dextrose-containing fluids should be avoided because Wernicke's encephalopathy can occur in women who are given a large carbohydrate load when they are deficient in thiamine secondary to persistent vomiting. Wernicke's encephalopathy is a neuropsychiatric syndrome that results from thiamine deficiency; it presents with a classic triad of ocular abnormalities, ataxia, and confusion. Persistent vomiting is a risk for thiamine deficiency because vomiting prevents adequate absorption of this essential vitamin.[20] The standard intravenous solution is normal saline, which aids in preventing hyponatremia. Potassium chloride can be added as needed and thiamine (vitamin B_1) or a multivitamin solution that includes thiamine should be added at least once a day to prevent Wernicke's encephalopathy.

Intravenous or intramuscular antiemetics such as metoclopramide (Reglan) or ondansetron (Zofran) are the second pillar of initial treatment for hyperemesis gravidarum. If the woman is not able to tolerate oral fluids or food after an initial course of IV fluids and antiemetics, a physician should again be consulted for further evaluation and management, which may consist of corticosteroids and either parenteral nutrition or nasogastric feeding.

BOX 23-4 Midwifery Management: Evaluation for Severe Nausea and Vomiting of Pregnancy

History

- Frequency of vomiting episodes: PUQE score
- Dietary history (which foods and fluids, amounts, timing, reaction)
- Medication history (medication reactions)
- Elimination (frequency, amount, constipation, diarrhea)
- Blood in vomitus (peptic ulcer or esophagitis from repeated vomiting)
- Fever or chills
- Exposure to viral infection
- Exposure to contaminated food
- Abdominal pain
- History of eating disorders

Physical Examination

- Weight (compare to previous weights)
- Temperature, pulse, respirations
- Skin turgor
- Moistness of mucous membranes
- Condition of tongue (swollen, dry, cracked)
- Abdominal palpation for organomegaly, tenderness, distension
- Bowel sounds
- Assessment of uterine size

Laboratory Tests

- Complete blood count (CBC)
- Urinalysis and urine dipstick for specific gravity and ketones
- BUN and electrolytes

- Liver function tests (rule out hepatitis, pancreatitis, and cholestasis)
- TSH and T_4 (rule out thyroid disease)

Ultrasound

- Confirm pregnancy
- Rule out multiple pregnancy and/or hydatidiform mole

Management

1. Consult with a physician for ongoing management.
2. Administer IV fluids.
3. Place on NPO status or give minimal sips of clear fluid and ice chips for several hours to let the woman's stomach rest.
4. The following antiemetics may be used initially to stop vomiting or dry heaving:
   a. Promethazine (Phenergan) 25 mg intravenous or prochlorperazine (Compazine) 10 mg intramuscular or 2½–10 mg intravenous every 3–4 hours or metoclopramide (Reglan) 10–20 mg intravenous combined with 50 mg of diphenhydramine (Benadryl) to prevent dystonic reactions (do not combine metoclopramide with the other phenothiazines due to possible increased risk of dystonic reactions).
   b. Ondansetron (Zofran) is used on an off-label basis for hyperemesis and appears to be both safe and effective. Initial dose is 4–8 mg over 15 minutes intravenous every 12 hours.

BUN = blood urea nitrogen; NPO = nil per os (no oral food or fluids); T4 = thyroxine; TSH = thyroid stimulating hormone.

Second Trimester Complications

Obstetrical complications are rare in the second trimester of pregnancy. When they do occur, they often are associated with abnormal ultrasound findings. Therefore a brief discussion of use of the ultrasound modality is presented here.

Ultrasound in the Second Trimester

An ultrasound may be requested to provide a general or targeted assessment. The usual application of ultrasound in pregnancy is classified as one of three types of evaluation.

A limited ultrasound, which may be called a level I ultrasound, is performed to address a specific topic such as identification of presentation or position of the placenta. A limited ultrasound maybe done in an office setting. Midwives may acquire advanced skills in performing limited ultrasounds in accordance with American College of Nurse-Midwives (ACNM) guidelines.[21] The standard examination, often called a level II ultrasound, identifies gestational age, fetal number, viability, and placental localization, and completes an assessment of fetal anatomy. Such an ultrasound is offered to all pregnant women between 18 and 20 weeks' gestation, as this examination provides the most accurate information about gestational age and is simultaneously able to detect most major morphologic malformations prior to the time that the fetus would be viable if born.

A specialized or targeted ultrasound is ordered when an anomaly is suspected from the woman's history, laboratory results, or abnormal findings on a standard ultrasound. More complicated visualizing technology can be utilized for specific purposes. For example, fetal echocardiogram can be used to accurately diagnose cardiac malformations. The newer three-dimensional (3D) or four-dimensional (4D) ultrasound is used to detect facial anomalies and some neural tube defects, and is under study for use in detection of congenital heart defects.[22] However, because of the limited clinical evidence supporting the benefit of the 3D mode over two-dimensional ultrasound, the American College of Obstetricians and Gynecologists (ACOG) does not consider 3D ultrasound to be a required modality for routine evaluation of the fetus.[23] The 3D mode is used as a marketing tool in many practices and independent "prenatal baby picture" commercial settings.

Incidental Ultrasound Findings: Echogenic Intracardiac Focus and Choroid Plexus Cysts

Incidental ultrasound findings of anatomic variants in the fetus, often referred to as "soft markers," may or may not be significant—or their significance may not be known. Common second trimester findings include echogenic intracardiac focus (EIF), choroid plexus cyst (CPC), echogenic bowel, renal pelviectasis, and ventriculomegaly.[24]

An EIF or echogenic bowel is noted when ultrasound detects some "floating" particles that are echogenic in the fetal heart or bowel. A CPC is a cyst that forms in the choroid plexus within the ventricles of fetal brain. The choroid plexus is an area within the ventricles that produces cerebrospinal fluid and sometimes small fluid-filled cysts can form as the choroid plexus develops. Both EIF and CPC are more likely in fetuses with trisomy 21, but more typically they are transient findings not associated with any fetal anomaly. If other tests for aneuploidy such as maternal serum alpha-fetoprotein (MSAFP) and nuchal translucency measurements on first trimester ultrasound are normal, CPC and EIF are presumed to be benign.

Echogenic bowel is also a soft marker for cystic fibrosis and fetal growth restriction. Women with normal chromosomal studies whose fetus has findings consistent with echogenic bowel during an 18-week ultrasound may be advised to have either cystic fibrosis testing, serial ultrasounds, or both. Amniocentesis is not warranted on the basis of the soft markers findings alone.[25]

Ventriculomegaly is the term for dilation of the lateral ventricles, a condition that occurs in 1 to 2 of every 1000 pregnancies. It may be associated with brain abnormalities or infection; however, mild ventriculomegaly is also associated with male gender and is considered a normal variant. Marked ventriculomegaly is rare. Pelviectasis is the term for mild enlargement of the renal pelvis, which can be either a result of blockage of the outflow tract of the renal system or a normal variant. Renal pelviectasis is most common in males and is thought to result from posterior urethral valves. Both ventriculomegaly and pelviectasis are usually followed with one or more serial ultrasounds to determine that they are not progressive. If no progression is noted prenatally, they are considered normal anatomic variations. Occasionally a fetal cardiac arrhythmia in a 24 to 28 weeks' gestation is noted. In such a case, a level II ultrasound or fetal echocardiogram is indicated to rule out structural cardiac anomalies.

Although called "soft markers," the impact of these findings on the pregnant woman and her family can be significant. Women can be anxious before any fetal testing is conducted. Normal prenatal test results reduce anxiety, but soft markers may be neither normal nor clearly abnormal. The woman is then left in a situation of ambiguity as more testing or passage of time must occur before the significance of these findings becomes clear. Anxiety and depression associated with the diagnosis of a soft marker in pregnancy may persist throughout pregnancy, postpartum, and into the newborn period.[26] Provision of support and factual information that might need to be repeated several times can help minimize long-term impacts following the detection of a soft marker on ultrasound.

Short Cervix

Identification of a "short cervix" through ultrasound was seen as an incidental finding of unknown importance until a few years ago, when the association between cervical length and preterm labor became clear. A short cervix is defined as a sonographic cervical length of 10 to 20 mm (or less than 25 mm) measured at 18 to 24 weeks' gestation.[27,28] Women with a very short cervix (less than 15 mm) prior to 24 weeks' gestation, regardless of other risk factors, need immediate medical consultation for consideration of cerclage placement. Measurement of cervical length provides an opportunity to institute action that may prevent or delay preterm birth (**Table 23-2**).

The "gold standard" for cervical length measurement is transvaginal ultrasound (TVUS). TVUS measures the distance between the internal and external os. It also determines the shape of the canal, such as "funneling," and the presence of membranes in the canal. Abdominal ultrasound is not reliable for cervical length measurement because of the difficulty

Table 23-2	Predicted Probability (%) of Preterm Birth Before Week 35 by Cervical Length (mm) and Gestational Week at Time of Measurement							
	Cervical Length (mm)							
Week of Gestation	**10**	**15**	**20**	**25**	**30**	**35**	**40**	**45**
16	53.3	45.2	37.3	30.1	23.7	18.3	13.9	10.5
18	50.7	42.6	34.9	27.9	21.8	16.8	12.7	9.6
20	48.1	40.1	32.5	25.8	20.1	15.4	11.6	8.7
22	45.4	37.6	30.3	23.9	18.5	14.1	10.6	7.9
24	42.8	35.1	28.1	22.0	16.9	12.8	9.6	7.5
26	40.5	32.8	26.0	20.3	15.5	11.7	8.7	6.5
28	37.8	30.5	24.0	18.6	14.2	10.6	7.9	5.9

Source: Adapted from Berghella V, Roman A, Daskalakis C, et al. Gestational age at cervical length measurement and incidence of preterm birth. *Obstet Gynecol.* 2007;110:311-317.

in obtaining an appropriate angle. The confounding factors of maternal habitus and the need to fill the bladder may result in a false lengthening of the measurement.

The standard level II ultrasound evaluation between 18 and 24 weeks' gestation may or may not include transvaginal ultrasound (TVUS) to determine cervical length at this time. Accurate TVUS requires a provider, commonly a maternal–fetal medicine specialist with special training, and may not be readily available in all settings. Although cervical length screening at the time of the 18-week ultrasound was recommended by ACOG in 2011, this assessment has not yet been fully implemented in clinical practice. ACNM has also affirmed the recommendation to screen all pregnant women for short cervix and then to implement available strategies to prevent preterm birth.[29]

Cervical length may also be measured with CerviLenz, a disposable device that can be used during a speculum examination (**Figure 23-2**). Measurements of the cervix using the CerviLenz tool are usually shorter than measurements taken by TVUS. A cervical length of less than 30 mm using the CerviLenz tool has been found to be predictive for preterm labor and warrants follow-up with TVUS. This tool may become an excellent, cost-effective method for cervical length screening that could replace serial ultrasound screening once studied sufficiently, but it is not yet used widely in clinical practice.

Women who do not have a prior history of preterm birth but who have a short cervix (less than 25 mm) on screening at 18 to 24 weeks' gestation, will benefit from vaginal progesterone therapy. A large multicenter study (*n* = 458), known as the PREGNANT trial, found that vaginal progesterone

treatment of women with a short cervix resulted in a significant reduction in the incidence of preterm birth at 28 and 35 weeks (8.9% in the progesterone group versus 16.1% in the placebo group).[30] Thus 14 women with a short cervix need to be treated with progesterone to prevent one preterm birth. When the subgroups of women who had a history of preterm birth were evaluated, the results were more nuanced. For the women without a history of preterm birth, treatment with progesterone reduced the preterm birth rate (7.6% versus 15.6%, *P* = .02), but in women who had a previous preterm birth, treatment with progesterone did not significantly reduce the preterm birth rate (15.68% versus 20.6%, *P* = .60).[30]

Cervical Insufficiency

Cervical insufficiency is diagnosed when the cervix effaces and dilates without pain in the second or early third trimester. The typical picture is a woman

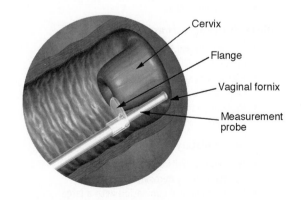

Figure 23-2 Cervilenz.
Source: Reproduced with permission from CerviLenz Inc.

who presents with a report of vaginal bleeding, pelvic pressure, or ruptured membranes and is found on examination to have a cervix with advanced dilation. For women with cervical insufficiency, this sequence of events is repeated in subsequent pregnancies, regardless of the pregnancy interval. Risk factors for cervical insufficiency are listed in **Box 23-5**.

Women with a history of two or more second or third trimester losses need medical consultation and evaluation. Depending on the current and historical circumstances, this woman may be a candidate for weekly or biweekly vaginal ultrasound to measure cervical length and for placement of a cervical cerclage before 24 weeks' gestation. Historically, the management of a woman with two or more midtrimester losses included a placement of a cerclage between 14 and 18 weeks' gestation without consideration of cervical condition. Cerclage, however, has significant risks including infection, rupture of membranes with or without infection, and subsequent pregnancy loss.

As early ultrasound, including TVUS, became more common, cervical length was considered as an indication for cerclage—regardless of past obstetric history. Cerclage was offered to women with a cervical length less than 15 mm in the late first or early second trimester. The ability to monitor cervical length reliably has provided new management options. Currently, the trend in some settings is to monitor cervical length and perform cerclage only if the cervix shortens.

Berghella et al. published a meta-analysis of history-indicated cerclage versus ultrasound cervical length–indicated cerclage.[31] The evidence supports scheduled evaluation of cervical length by ultrasound by 18 weeks' gestation and repeat TVUS every 2 weeks thereafter. Cerclage is reserved for women with a cervical length that has shortened to less than 25 mm before 24 weeks' gestation. It is important to provide detailed education about signs and symptoms of cervical change (e.g., pressure, increased discharge, spotting, cramping) to the woman with this condition so that she can return at the earliest sign of change for reassessment.

If a woman presents with signs or symptoms that suggest possible cervical insufficiency, an initial speculum examination may be performed to check for more common causes of symptoms such as vaginitis. However, cervical dilation or the presence of visible membranes indicates a need for immediate physician consultation. Bimanual and digital exam is best deferred to the physician to avoid potentially rupturing membranes and introducing infection through the actions of multiple examiners. If the membranes are intact and the cervix is amenable, the common treatment is cervical cerclage. Several types of cerclage are used, with the precise technique being selected based on the clinical situation, cervical length and dilation as well as practice experience and preference of the physician.

Preterm Labor: Risk Assessment and Prenatal Management

Preterm birth continues to be the leading cause of neonatal mortality and one of the primary causes of long-term neonatal morbidity in the United States. One in eight infants in the United States is born prematurely.[32] Prematurity is the cause of more than 70% of neonatal deaths and is associated with 50% of long-term neurologic disabilities in infants in the United States.[33] Preterm birth is subcategorized into early preterm, preterm, and late preterm births. Overall, any infant born prior to 37 weeks' gestation is considered preterm. Infants born between 34 0/7 gestational weeks and 36 6/7 gestational weeks are born in the late preterm period, whereas infants born prior to 34 weeks' gestation are categorized as early preterm births.[34]

Overall preterm birth rates in the United States increased 35% between 1981 and 2006, and late preterm rates increased 50% between 1990 and 2006.[35] The rate of early preterm births has remained essentially unchanged at 3.5% since 2006. The late preterm birth rate has declined 7% since 2006, reaching

---

BOX 23-5 Risk Factors for Cervical Insufficiency

Congenital Factors
- Diethylstilbestrol (DES) exposure
- Congenital anomalies
- Uterine anomalies

Obstetric History Factors
- History of fetal loss at 14 weeks' gestation or more
- History of cervical laceration following vaginal or cesarean birth
- Multiple first or second trimester pregnancy terminations

Gynecologic History Factors
- Mechanical dilation from dilation and curettage or hysterosalpingogram
- Previous cervical conization with a large amount of tissue removed

11.99% in 2012.[35] The reduction in late preterm births has resulted in an overall statistical decline in preterm births. It is postulated that the increase in late preterm births seen in the 1990s resulted from an increase in elective induction of labor and scheduled repeat cesarean section prior to 39 weeks' gestation. Following a national effort to eliminate elective delivery prior to well-documented 39 gestational weeks, the drop in the incidence of late preterm births was seen. In addition, progesterone therapy is being used more frequently and may be a factor in reducing the incidence of preterm birth.

The greatest risk factor for infant morbidity and mortality is early preterm birth. In 2008, the mortality rate for newborns born at term (39–41 weeks) was 2.08 per 100 live births. The corresponding rate for infants born early term (37–38 completed weeks) was 3.14 per 100 live births and it was 7.40 per 100 live births for infants born in the late preterm period (35–36 completed weeks).[36] **Box 23-6** summarizes the risks of preterm birth for the infant.[37–40]

Strategies to reduce preterm birth include risk assessment, objective evaluation of threatened preterm labor, evidence-based interventions, and reduction of iatrogenic prematurity. The midwife has an active role in each strategy.

Unfortunately, risk factors are not always predictive of preterm birth; indeed, the majority of preterm births cannot be linked to a specific risk factor or condition.[41,42] However, risk assessment at the first visit and on an ongoing basis over the course of pregnancy does facilitate evidence-based intervention at the earliest point with the potential for best effect. Signs and symptoms of preterm labor are listed in **Box 23-7**.

Pathogenesis of Preterm Labor

The etiology of preterm labor is not well defined. Several theories have been proposed based on histologic studies and epidemiologic associations. There appear to be at least five discrete mechanisms that can initiate premature uterine activity in pregnant women:

- Premature activation of the hypothalamic–pituitary–adrenal (HPA) axis
- Inflammation
- Decidual bleeding
- Overdistension of the uterus
- Genetics[43]

Each of these mechanisms then incites a cascade of pathologic changes that result in uterine contractions.

Risk Factors for Preterm Labor

Risk factors for preterm labor are listed in **Box 23-8**.[42,44,45] It has been known for some time that women who were themselves born preterm have a higher chance of having preterm labors and births during their own childbearing experiences, although

---

BOX 23-6 Morbidity and Mortality of Preterm Birth

Early Consequences

- Mortality
  - Markedly increased risk compared with term infants
- Morbidity
  - Acute respiratory, gastrointestinal, immunologic, and central nervous system complications
- Significant economic and emotional costs

Long-Term Consequences

- Neurodevelopmental disabilities
- Altered pulmonary function
- Metabolic and cardiovascular risk
- Decreased long-term survival

Sources: Adapted from Kramer MS, Demissie K, Yang H, Platt RW, Sauvé R, Liston R, for the Fetal and Infant Health Study Group of the Canadian Perinatal Surveillance System. The contribution of mild and moderate preterm birth to infant mortality. *JAMA.* 2000;284:843-849; Callaghan WM, MacDorman MF, Rasmussen SA, Qin C, Lackritz EM. The contribution of preterm birth to infant mortality rates in the United States. *Pediatrics.* 2006;118:1566-1573; Institute of Medicine of the National Academies. Preterm birth: causes, consequences, and prevention. 2006. Available at: http://www.iom.edu/CMS/3740/25471/35813.aspx; Swarmy GK, Ostbye T, Skaerven R. Association of preterm birth with long-term survival, reproduction, and the next-generation preterm birth. *JAMA.* 2008;299:1429-1436.

BOX 23-7 Signs and Symptoms of Preterm Labor

- Pelvic pressure
- Lower back pain
- Abdominal tightness or "cramps"
- Contractions—more than 6 in an hour
- Fetus dropping low into pelvis before 36 weeks
- Increased vaginal discharge
- Vaginal bleeding
- Diarrhea

BOX 23-8 Risk Factors for Preterm Labor

History Factors

- Previous preterm labor (2× risk). Each recurrent preterm birth increases the risk in subsequent pregnancies. The earlier the preterm birth, the greater the subsequent recurrence risk. A term birth after a preterm birth may reduce, but does not eliminate, the risk of preterm birth in subsequent pregnancies.
- Pregnant woman born preterm
- Short cervical length (cervical length less than 25 mm between 24 and 28 week)
- Prior cervical surgery (cone, dilation and curettage)
- Prior uterine surgery (repair of uterine structural anomalies such as a septum)

Maternal Factors

- Smoking (tobacco and/or marijuana)
- Low maternal body weight (BMI < 19.8)
- Short interpregnancy interval (< 18 months)
- African American ethnicity
- Maternal age < 15 years
- Maternal age > 40 years (women older than age 40 have a 25% greater risk of preterm birth than younger women)
- Stress
- Substance abuse (cocaine, crack, heroin)
- Low socioeconomic status

Current Pregnancy Factors

- Cervical insufficiency/short cervix
- Multiple gestation
- Hydramnios (polyhydramnios)
- Pyelonephritis

- Severe maternal illness (severe pregnancy-induced hypertension/HELLP syndrome, bleeding placenta previa)
- Intrauterine infection
- Imminent fetal jeopardy (isoimmunization with hydrops, fetal growth restriction with evidence of compromise)

Associated Factors with Conflicting Evidence

- Asymptomatic bacteriuria, lower urinary tract infections
- Genital tract infections
- Periodontal disease
- Vaginal bleeding

Preventable Iatrogenic Factors

- Failure to accurately determine gestational age
- Elective induction of labor (provider or woman)
- Ill-timed cesarean birth

Sources: Adapted from Mercer BM, Goldenberg RL, Das A, et al. The preterm prediction study: a clinical risk assessment system. *Am J Obstet Gynecol.* 1996;174:1885-1893; Muglia LJ. The enigma of spontaneous preterm birth. *N Engl J Med.* 2010;362:529-535; McManemy J, Cooke E, Amon E, Leet T. Recurrence risk for preterm delivery. *Am J Obstet Gynecol.* 2007;196:576; Dekker GA, Lee SY, North RA, et al. Risk factors for a preterm birth in an international prospective cohort of nulliparous women. *PLoS One.* 2012;7(7);e39154; Ward K, Argyle VA, Meade M, Nelson L. The heritability of preterm delivery. *Obstet Gynecol.* 2005;106(6):1235-1239; Chen K, Chen SF, Chang H, et al. No increased risk of adverse pregnancy outcomes in women with urinary tract infections: a nationwide population-based study. *Acta Obstet Scan.* 2010;89(7):882-888; Manns-James L. Bacterial vaginosis and preterm birth. *J Midwifery Women's Health.* 2011; 56(6):575-583.

women may not offer this information spontaneously as they do not realize the significance. Ward et al. have recently confirmed these data.[46] A genetic factor, as yet unidentified, may explain the recurrence risk of preterm labor in families and may be a factor in the increased rate of preterm birth in African American women.

Screening for Preterm Labor

Review of maternal history and ongoing assessment with attention to subjective symptoms will alert the midwife to evaluate for preterm labor. Specific screening strategies have varying clinical value. As universal cervical screening is beginning to be considered, concerns about availability of Food and Drug Administration (FDA)–approved progesterone

therapy, and such therapy's cost-effectiveness, are being explored.[47]

The role of screening and treatment of urinary tract and vaginal infections is complex. While most urogenital infections are associated with an increased risk of preterm labor, treatment is not always associated with a lower risk of preterm labor. Nevertheless, diagnosis and treatment of asymptomatic bacteriuria to prevent recurrent urinary tract infection and treatment of chlamydia have been shown to have a role in prevention of preterm birth. The benefit of treating vaginal trichomoniasis is not clear. Treatment of bacterial vaginosis, gonorrhea, and monilia has not been shown to affect the preterm birth rate.[48,49] Periodontal disease is associated with preterm labor, but treatment of the disease does not alter preterm birth rates. This fact suggests that the lifestyle that produces periodontal disease may be the underlying true risk factor.[34] Referral of women for dental care can prevent serious dental infection, such as abscess, that can complicate pregnancy.

Biochemical Markers for Preterm Labor

Fetal fibronectin (fFN) is a glycoprotein that acts as an adhesive between the fetal membranes and the maternal decidua. Normally, fFN is present in cervicovaginal secretions before 20 weeks' gestation and after 37 weeks' gestation. A full discussion of fFN and its use is found in the *Complications During Labor and Birth* chapter.

The classic study of fFN in 1996 demonstrated the value of an fFN assay in preterm labor assessment.[50] A negative test obtained between 24 and 30 weeks' gestation indicated the risk of birth within the next 7 days was 1% or less. With a positive fFN, the risk of birth in the next 7 days was 12%. The risk of birth prior to 37 weeks' gestation was 45%.[51] The fFN test is better at determining who *will not* give birth prematurely rather than who *will* give birth prematurely. It is most effective as an assessment tool in symptomatic women who are between 22 and 36 gestational weeks. It is not recommended for use as a screening tool.[52]

The clinical utility of cervical length measurement versus fFN assays is controversial. Data suggest that when the two modalities are used together, the reliability of the diagnosis is increased.[53] The best information can be obtained when using both cervical length measurement and fFN. If the cervical length is short and/or the fFN is positive, appropriate interventions can be initiated to prevent preterm birth. In the ambulatory setting, the results of fFN testing can help determine the need for hospital evaluation, physician consultation, transfer to hospital or tertiary care, and administration of prenatal steroids in anticipation of preterm birth.

Progesterone Therapy for Women at Risk for Preterm Labor

Evidence supporting the use of progesterone therapy for women at risk for preterm labor is rapidly emerging. The mechanism of action of exogenous progesterone in the prevention of preterm birth is not well understood, however. Progesterone is thought to have an anti-inflammatory effect that curtails the inflammatory process associated with preterm labor. Another theory suggests that exogenous progesterone increases the level of progesterone in maternal tissue and prevents the drop in progesterone associated with the onset of labor.[54,55]

The safety of progesterone for the developing fetus and child has been studied in long-term randomized controlled trials (RCTs).[56] Children who were prenatally exposed to progesterone in the form of 17-alpha-hydroxyprogesterone caproate (17-OHPC) have been followed for an average of 4 years and compared to children who were not exposed to this hormone. No difference in health status, physical examinations, or social, motor, or problem-solving skills have been found between the groups.

The best data available to date indicate that progesterone is safe and has a role in preventing prematurity. Progesterone therapy to prevent preterm labor is initiated in the early second trimester for women with select risk factors.

In multiple RCTs, progesterone administration in the form of 17-OHPC, given to women with a history of preterm birth and a singleton pregnancy, reduced the risk of preterm birth by as much as 26%.[30] The dose of 17-OHPC is 250 mg, administered via weekly injections from 16 to 36 weeks' gestation. The injections are continued until 36 completed weeks; stopping earlier is associated with an increase in preterm birth.[57] Women with a history of spontaneous preterm birth, with or without premature rupture of membranes, can benefit from progesterone therapy.[58] Progesterone is not effective for prevention of preterm birth in multiple-fetus gestations.[59] Likewise, it is not effective for women who have preterm rupture of membranes or as a tocolytic for women in active preterm labor.

Administration of natural progesterone as a vaginal gel provides higher concentrations because this mode of administration avoids the first-pass effect. Although vaginal progesterone gel has not been shown to be effective for women who have a history of preterm birth, it has been shown to prevent preterm birth in women without a history of preterm birth who have a short cervix. Two RCTs have evaluated the use of vaginal progesterone. Fonseca et al. treated women with a TVUS cervical length measurement of less than 15 mm at 20 to 24 weeks' gestation. In this study, 85% of the women had no history of preterm birth. The women were treated with 200 mg of vaginal progesterone nightly beginning at 24 weeks. Preterm birth prior to 34 weeks was reduced by 44%, although a significant decrease in neonatal morbidity was not observed.[60] Hassan et al. treated with women with a TVUS-determined cervical length of 10 to 20 mm at 19 to 23 6/7 weeks' gestation. As in the Fonseca et al. study, 84% of the women in this study had no history of preterm birth.

Women in the Hassan et al. study used 90 mg of progesterone gel daily, beginning as early as 20 weeks and continuing until 36 6/7 weeks. The results of the Hassan et al. study included a 45% reduction in preterm birth prior to 33 weeks and a 43% reduction in neonatal morbidity and mortality.[30] No additive effect was noted when using 17-OHPC and vaginal progesterone gel simultaneously. Similarly, no benefit was found in adding vaginal progesterone to women receiving 17-OHPC.

Iatrogenic Preterm Birth

The decrease in the rate of preterm birth from 2006 to 2011 in the United States has been attributed to a national effort to prevent iatrogenic preterm birth that results from ill-timed cesarean birth or induction of labor. The first step to avoid iatrogenic preterm birth is accurate assessment of gestational age by calculating a due date early in the pregnancy. If a due date is not clear based on the woman's history of her last menstrual period (LMP) that is consistent with an early physical examination, ultrasound for pregnancy dating is indicated. Accurate dating is essential to avoid inducing women who are preterm or initiating unnecessary fetal surveillance for women who are not really post-term.

Pregnancy is best terminated naturally by spontaneous labor, and labor should not be induced prior to term unless there are compelling medical reasons to do so, such as severe preeclampsia or fetal jeopardy.[29,61] When compelling social reasons such as a partner in the military nearing deployment or a serious illness in a child exist, induction should not be offered until at least 39 weeks' gestation. Pressure from a pregnant woman to have an elective induction due to discomfort, exhaustion, or family convenience is best met with education and emotional support.

Pregnant women may not understand the implications of preterm birth. In 2003, Green et al. found that 53% of pregnant women in their study thought an infant at 32 weeks' gestation would be healthy without significant risk for long-term problems. Only 31% of women thought preterm birth was a serious risk, and just 50% thought they knew signs of preterm labor.[62]

Suspected Active Preterm Labor

Women with symptoms of active preterm uterine activity such as backache, contractions, pelvic pressure, or increased vaginal discharge need to be evaluated immediately for preterm labor. If active preterm labor is suspected, obstetric triage/emergency room assessment is warranted to permit full assessment.

Use of tocolytics as outpatient prophylaxis for preterm labor has not been shown to be effective and carries significant maternal risks. Tocolysis is reserved for women with active preterm labor who are remote from term. Triage and management of the woman with active preterm labor is discussed in the *Complications During Labor and Birth* chapter.

Gestational Diabetes

Gestational diabetes (GDM) is the term that has historically been used to define onset or first recognition of abnormal glucose intolerance during pregnancy.[63] Women with type 1 or type 2 diabetes may be first diagnosed during pregnancy if they have not received health care prior to entering prenatal care. Therefore, diabetes diagnosed in pregnancy may actually be previously undetected type 1 or type 2 diabetes. GDM in the general population occurs in 2% to 5% of pregnancies, but its incidence may be as high as 10% in Native American women.[64] Women with GDM have a 45% increased risk of developing GDM in subsequent pregnancies and an increased risk of developing type 2 diabetes later in life that ranges from 17% to 60%, depending on the presence of other risk factors such as obesity.[65] The overall incidence of all types of diabetes is increasing in all U.S. populations concomitant with the rising rate of obesity.

Pathophysiology of Gestational Diabetes

Gestational diabetes is similar to type 2 diabetes in that it is a disease of insulin resistance. Hormonal changes of pregnancy alter cells' receptivity to insulin. In early pregnancy (prior to 20 weeks' gestation), the cells are more responsive to insulin and, therefore, circulating glucose levels may be lower than usual. As the placenta grows, levels of human placental lactogen (hPL) and other diabetogenic hormones rise. These hormones increase cellular resistance to insulin, which results in higher blood glucose levels. In most women, the pancreas is able to increase the supply of insulin to counterbalance the insulin resistance effect of placental hormones. Overt hyperglycemia results when the pancreas is unable to produce adequate insulin. The peak effect of hPL occurs around 26 to 28 weeks of pregnancy, which is the suggested timing for screening for GDM.

Risk Factors for Gestational Diabetes

Risk factors for developing diabetes in pregnancy are the same as the risk factors for developing type 2 diabetes (**Table 23-3**).

Table 23-3	Risk Factors for Gestational Diabetes	
Demographic Characteristics	**Medical and Family History**	**Previous Obstetric History**
Maternal age Member of an ethnic group at increased risk for type 2 diabetes mellitus • Hispanic • African American • Native American • South or East Asian • Pacific Islands for more than 25 years	Prepregnancy weight ≥ 110% of ideal body weight or body mass index > 30 kg/m², significant weight gain in early adulthood or between pregnancies, or excessive gestational weight gain History of abnormal glucose tolerance Current use of glucocorticoids Polycystic ovary syndrome Essential hypertension First-degree relative with diabetes	History of adverse pregnancy outcomes associated with GDM • Infant more than 9 pounds at birth • Unexplained stillbirth • Infant with congenital anomalies History of GDM in prior pregnancy

Complications of Gestational Diabetes

Women with GDM have an increased incidence of hypertension, preeclampsia, and fetal macrosomia. Macrosomia is associated with additional risks for protracted labor, shoulder dystocia, perineal trauma, infection, and operative delivery. Fetal/neonatal risks depend on the timing and degree of maternal hyperglycemia.

Women with poorly controlled or undiagnosed type 1 or type 2 diabetes that predates the pregnancy have a significant risk for congenital anomalies. For the fetus of a woman with GDM whose early pregnancy blood sugars were not elevated, the risk of congenital anomalies is the same as that of the general population. Obstetric risks associated with type 1 and type 2 diabetes are discussed in the *Medical Complications in Pregnancy* chapter.

As maternal blood sugars rise in the second trimester for a woman with GDM, glucose crosses the placenta and enters the fetus. The fetus does not have diabetes, but must increase production of insulin in order to metabolize the higher levels of glucose obtained from the maternal circulation. This response causes a dramatic growth profile in the fetus, which results in macrosomia. Macrosomia is caused by both hyperplasia (an increased number of cells) and hypertrophy (an enlargement of the cells). Thus this is a lifelong change for the fetus that has been shown to increase the likelihood of childhood and adult obesity as well as the risk for diabetes later in life.[66]

Screening and Diagnosis

The best procedure for screening and diagnosis of GDM is a continuing controversy. All strategies involve an oral glucose test. The standard strategy until recently has been a two-step process that involves a screening test and a subsequent diagnostic test. The screening test is a 50-gram 1-hour glucose challenge. With this test, the woman ingests 50 grams of glucose in liquid or jellybean or meal form without previous fasting. A blood glucose level is drawn 1 hour later. If the 1-hour glucose is elevated, usually a level above 130 mg/dL or above 140 mg/dL, a 3-hour glucose tolerance test (GTT) is performed. The two studies that have evaluated glucose loading in the form of a prespecified number of jelly beans found that they have similar sensitivity, specificity, and positive predictive value, as did the 50-gram glucose drink.[67,68] However, because jelly beans are metabolized into circulating glucose at differential rates, "confectionary screening" has not been formally approved by the American Diabetes Association.

The second strategy screens only women with overt risk factors. The problem with this strategy is that the prevalence of risk factors in the general population is 90%, which means that the overwhelming majority of women meet the criteria for screening.[69] However, it is important to remember that women who do not have risk factors for GDM who want to decline screening should be counseled that their choice is a safe one. Characteristics of women who are at low risk for GDM are listed in **Box 23-9**.

Universal screening does have advantages—notably, it will detect women with previously undetected type 1 or type 2 diabetes. In the selective screening strategy, women at the highest risk of GDM (i.e., obesity or history of GDM) or those with risk factors for undetected type 1 or type 2 diabetes are offered initial screening in the first trimester. For the purpose of detecting type 2 diabetes, hemoglobin A1c (HbA1c) may be part of the screening strategy.

The third screening strategy has recently been proposed by the International Association of the Diabetes and Pregnancy Study Groups (IADPSG).[70,71] This group recommends that all women be screened at the first prenatal visit via a fasting blood glucose value, HbA1c, or random plasma glucose. Results are classified as either normal, GDM, or overt diabetes. If results are normal, then a one-step 75-gram GTT diagnostic test for GDM is performed between 24 and 28 weeks' gestation. The diagnostic criteria for both the two-step and one-step strategies are presented in Table 23-4.[71]

The IADPSG criteria diagnose more women with GDM than the other two strategies. Although the lower threshold for diagnosis results in increased prevalence and more treatment, it is not yet clear how treating more women for GDM will affect outcomes of importance.[71]

Management of Gestational Diabetes

Once a diagnosis of diabetes—gestational or otherwise—is made, physician consultation is indicated. Midwives may provide prenatal care to women with GDM or controlled type 2 diabetes in collaboration with a physician, appropriate subspecialists,

Table 23-4	Screening and Diagnostic Criteria for Gestational Diabetes
Organization	**Plasma Glucose Diagnostic Values**
ACOG	1. *50-gram glucose screening test:* GDM diagnosed if > 200 mg/dL If > 130 mg/dL or > 140 mg/dL, move to 3-hour GTT 2. *3-hour GTT at 24–28 weeks:* GDM diagnosed if two values are over the following threshold values: a. Carpenter/Coustan plasma or serum glucose level: fasting > 95 mg/dL; 1-hour > 180 mg/dL; 2-hour > 155 mg/dL; 3-hour > 140 mg/dL b. NDDG plasma level: fasting > 105 mg/dL; 1-hour > 190 mg/dL; 2-hour > 165 mg/dL; 3-hour > 145 mg/dL
IADPSG and ADA	1. *Measure fasting plasma glucose, HbA1c, or random plasma glucose of all women or all high-risk women at initial prenatal visit* a. Overt diabetes diagnosed: fasting ≥ 126 mg/dL; HbA1c ≥ 6.5%; random plasma glucose ≥ 200 mg/dL that is subsequently confirmed via HbA1c or fasting blood glucose value b. GDM diagnosed: fasting ≥ 92 mg/dL but < 126 mg/dL 2. *If initial values do not detect overt diabetes or GDM, do 75-gram 2-hour GTT at 24–28 weeks* a. Overt diabetes diagnosed: fasting ≥ 126 mg/dL b. GDM diagnosed if one value is over the following threshold values: fasting > 92 mg/dL; 1-hour plasma glucose > 180 mg/dL; 2-hour plasma glucose > 153 mg/dL

ACOG = American College of Obstetricians and Gynecologists; ADA = American Diabetes Association; NDDG = National Diabetes Data Group; IADPSG = International Association of the Diabetes and Pregnancy Study Groups.

Sources: Adapted from American College of Obstetricians and Gynecologists. Gestational diabetes. ACOG Practice Bulletin No. 30. *Obstet Gynecol.* 2001;98:525-538; International Association of Diabetes and Pregnancy Study Groups Consensus Panel, Metzger BE, Gabbe SG, et al. International Association of Diabetes and Pregnancy Study Groups recommendations on the diagnosis and classification of hyperglycemia in pregnancy. *Diab Care.* 2010;33:676.

and nutritional support personnel. Management of women with type 1 diabetes or GDM requiring insulin is generally referred for medical management, although the midwife may provide support.

Nonpharmacologic treatment of GDM consists of nutrition and exercise. For women with any form of diabetes, food is medicine and must be planned as carefully as any other medication. Pregnant women at normal weight with GDM need 30–36 kcal/kg per day, whereas women with a body mass index (BMI) higher than 30 need 24 kcal/kg per day. Exercise in the form of walking, swimming, or specialized exercise programs is encouraged but not always possible. Referral to a diabetes educator for extensive nutritional counseling is important to provide education about the appropriate intake and the appropriate timing of meals and snacks.

Women with GDM are asked to monitor and record their fasting and 2-hour postprandial glucose levels every day, and these logbooks are reviewed by their healthcare providers. Fasting levels higher than 105 mg/dL or postprandial levels higher than 120 mg/dL indicate the need for pharmacologic therapy.[71]

Consultation with the physician is needed to determine the medication to be initiated. Metformin (Glucophage) is usually the first-line oral medication, although sometimes glyburide (DiaBeta, Micronase, Glynase) is used. Some physicians prefer to prescribe insulin and do not use oral medications. Women tend to be able to manage oral medications better than insulin, so the standard of care may be moving toward the oral route. If the oral medications do not adequately control the glucose levels, insulin must be used.

Monitoring of the woman and fetus during pregnancy is directed toward minimizing risks. The risk of stillbirth suggests the need for increased surveillance of women with GDM in the third trimester. Women who require insulin or an antiglycemic oral medication to maintain euglycemia (Class A2 GDM) are usually offered antenatal testing twice weekly starting at approximately 32 weeks and asked to perform daily fetal movement counts. Women with GDM who are able to maintain euglycemia via diet and exercise alone (Class A1 GDM) do not appear to be at risk for stillbirth and are not usually referred for antenatal testing.

The risk of macrosomia and its complications for the woman and her infant may tempt providers to seek an ultrasound assessment of fetal weight. Clinical assessment of fetal weight and serially measured fundal height are equivalent to ultrasound in their ability to detect macrosomia, with the caveat that neither clinical assessment nor ultrasound is very accurate. Fetuses of women with diabetes develop respiratory maturity later than do fetuses of women without diabetes, so early delivery poses increased risks for respiratory distress. The temptation to deliver a woman with GDM early to avoid macrosomia or stillbirth has not been supported by research data. Instead, a vaginal birth should be planned unless the ultrasound-determined estimated fetal weight is more than 4500 grams.[71] Because the estimate of fetal weight is not precise, additional factors such as patient obstetric history, clinical pelvimetry, and careful monitoring of labor progress are essential. Timing and mode of delivery are determined with the consulting physician and the woman.

Postpartum care includes follow-up to assess for type 2 diabetes. Women who have GDM should have a glucose tolerance test at 6 to 12 weeks postpartum.[72]

Third Trimester Complications

Third trimester complications include hypertensive disorders, gestational diabetes, fetal growth abnormalities, and placental abnormalities. In the third trimester, management of complications focuses on a balance between the health of the woman and the gestational age of the fetus. Complications that compromise maternal well-being or the fetal environment may require intervention to accomplish an early delivery.

Placental Abnormalities

Placenta abnormalities fall into three categories: abnormal placental structure or size, abnormal placement in the uterus, and abnormal attachment. Although the placenta is considered a "fetal organ," the intrauterine environment affects implantation of the placenta. Placental abnormalities can, in turn, affect fetal growth and fetal oxygenation, cause maternal or fetal bleeding, and potentially require cesarean birth.

Abnormal Placenta Structure

Abnormal placental structures can occur at initial formation or, more rarely, as a result of injury, such as complications following chorionic villus sampling or failed abortion attempt. An abnormally small placenta is associated with intrauterine infection, whereas an abnormally large or edematous placenta is associated with conditions such as maternal diabetes and fetal hydrops.

Velamentous cord insertion is a structural developmental abnormality of the placenta wherein the cord is elevated off the placental disc, leaving a span of vessels not protected with Wharton's jelly. A velamentous cord can occur with a normal placenta or a placenta with succenturiate lobes. The vessels are vulnerable to rupture with vigorous fetal movement and traction on the vessels in labor and at delivery.

Velamentous vessels that precede the fetus or cross the cervix are termed vasa previa. In this situation, the vessels may cross over the cervical os before being fully in the placenta. Women at high risk for vasa previa include those with a velamentous insertion of the cord, low-lying placenta particularly if the cord insertion is not clear, or multilobar placenta. Occasionally a vessel can be palpated on vaginal exam as the cervix dilates in labor. Ultrasound with Doppler flow may be used, although not all vasa previas can be seen with ultrasound.[73] Birth in the presence of a vasa previa creates a risk for life-threatening hemorrhage in the fetus. In a Canadian study, neonatal survival was 97% when early diagnosis permitted administration of prenatal steroids and planned cesarean preterm birth in a center with a neonatal intensive care unit. Neonates delivered following rupture of a vasa previa that was undiagnosed had a 44% survival rate.[73]

Abnormal Placement of the Placenta: Placenta Previa

Placenta previa is the malposition of the placenta in the lower uterine segment, either anteriorly or posteriorly, so that the fully developed placenta extends to or across the cervical os. In a *complete or central* placenta previa, the body of the placenta fills the lower uterine segment, entirely overlying the cervical os. In a *partial* placenta previa, the placental edge covers (totally or partially) the cervical os. A *marginal* previa will have the edge of the placenta near, but not actually over, the internal cervical os. If the edge of the placenta is at least 3 centimeters from the cervical os, it is considered *low-lying* (**Figure 23-3**).

The primary complications associated with placenta previa are hemorrhage and fetal demise when the cervix dilates and the cervical portion of the placenta separates prior to birth of the fetus. The primary risk factor for development of placenta previa is previous uterine scarring secondary to cesarean section or uterine surgery. The incidence of placenta previa is approximately 0.3% to 0.5% of all pregnancies. This risk increases with repeat cesarean sections and is approximately 11% to 25% after one cesarean and 50% to 70% after four cesarean births.[74] Additional risk factors include multiple uterine curettages and

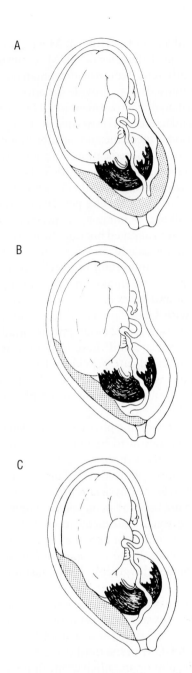

Figure 23-3 Placenta previa: (A) complete; (B) partial; (C) marginal.

uterine surgery that significantly affects uterine structure, such as removal of the uterine septum or myomectomy. Infertility due to endometriosis and tubal factors are also associated with placenta previa.[75] In addition, increasing parity, advanced maternal age, multiple gestation, and smoking have all been associated with placenta previa.

Placenta previa may be diagnosed by ultrasound prior to any symptoms becoming evident. Low-lying placentas and those that touch or cross the cervix are not uncommon findings in first- and second-trimester ultrasounds. Most often, the growing uterus displaces the placenta upward, and the distance between the cervix and the border of the placenta increases as gestational age increases. The more central the placenta implants over the os, the more the placenta needs to grow superiorly and the less likely it is to do so.

A first trimester ultrasound that detects a low-lying or partial placenta previa requires follow-up ultrasound at 24 to 28 weeks' gestation to confirm placental location. A low-lying placenta is considered safe for labor and vaginal birth. If the placenta remains encroaching over the cervix into the third trimester, then vaginal birth is contraindicated. A placenta found to be complete or central at 24 to 28 weeks' gestation indicates the need for continued surveillance via serial ultrasounds to confirm placement prior to determining whether labor and vaginal birth can be safely attempted.

In addition, the abnormally located placenta may not be adequate to support fetal growth. Surveillance includes maternal observation of fetal activity, monitoring of fetal growth clinically with fundal height, and possibly antenatal testing for fetal well-being.

Placenta abnormalities are the major causes of vaginal bleeding in the second and third trimesters. Placenta previa is the cause in 20% of all vaginal bleeding, abruptio placenta is the cause in 30%, and vasa previa is a rare but contributing cause. The remaining 50% of vaginal bleeding is the result of cervical insufficiency or the bloody show of labor.[76]

Sudden, painless vaginal bleeding is the cardinal presentation of a woman with a placenta previa. Eighty percent of women with placenta previa present with this history, while another 20% report contractions.[77] Approximately 10% of women with a placenta previa present in labor without a history of bleeding.[77]

When placenta previa is diagnosed in the first half of pregnancy prior to any symptomatology, no intervention is required. The woman should be informed about the placenta location and told to call immediately with any evidence of vaginal bleeding. If the previa is a complete previa, she may be counseled to avoid intercourse for the duration of the pregnancy.

If a woman has bleeding associated with the placenta previa, management will depend on the gestational age, severity of bleeding, and fetal status. Evaluation will take place in a hospital setting. When the dating criteria are certain, and the fetus is at 37 weeks or more, cesarean section is indicated.

It is common for women with a placenta previa to experience an initial episode of bleeding, which then subsides. If both the woman and her fetus are stable, expectant management may be advised after initial hospitalization (see the *Complications During Labor and Birth* chapter). For some women, hospitalization with or without the use of tocolytics may be required until fetal maturity is achieved, at which point a cesarean section can be performed.[78] These women are counseled to observe pelvic rest, with nothing being inserted into the vagina (i.e., vaginal therapeutics, douches, or penis). In addition, the woman should be counseled to avoid orgasm, because orgasm results in uterine contractions that may exacerbate bleeding.

Gestational Hypertension and Preeclampsia

Hypertensive disorders of pregnancy remain a leading cause of maternal death. Approximately 12% of maternal deaths are attributed to hypertensive disorders in pregnancy.[79] It is estimated that 6% to 10% of women experience hypertensive disease during pregnancy.

Four categories of hypertension in pregnancy are distinguished: (1) chronic hypertension, (2) gestational hypertension, (3) preeclampsia, and (4) preeclampsia superimposed on chronic hypertension. Chronic hypertension is reviewed in the *Medical Complications in Pregnancy* chapter. This chapter reviews gestational hypertension and preeclampsia. The terminology used today was established by the National High Blood Pressure Education Program Working Group,[80] which defined categories for the progressive development of hypertension, proteinuria, and multiple organ system compromise in pregnancy. These definitions are shown in **Table 23-5**.[80]

Risk Factors for Gestational Hypertension

Risk factors for hypertensive disease in pregnancy are shown in **Box 23-10**.

Complications of Gestational Hypertension

Women with hypertension are at risk for multiple complications, including renal failure, liver failure, cerebral hemorrhage, disseminated intravascular coagulopathy, abruptio placenta, emergent operative delivery, and death. The fetus is at risk for fetal growth restriction, oligohydramnios, abruptio placenta, intolerance of labor, and medically indicated preterm delivery.[81]

Table 23-5	Definition and Diagnostic Criteria for Gestational Hypertension and Preeclampsia
Diagnosis	**Definition and Diagnostic Criteria**
Gestational hypertension	Systolic blood pressure ≥ 140 mm Hg and/or diastolic blood pressure ≥ 90 mm Hg in a previously normotensive pregnant woman who is at least 20 weeks' gestation and who does not have proteinuria. Blood pressure readings should be documented on at least two occasions at least 6 hours apart.
Severe gestational hypertension	Blood pressure is sustained for at least 6 hours with a systolic value of at least 160 mm Hg and/or a diastolic value of at least 110 mm Hg.
Preeclampsia	Gestational hypertension with the addition of proteinuria (≥ 300 mg in a 24-hour period or more than 1+ on a dipstick in two random urine samples tested at least 6 hours apart). +1 on a urine dipstick correlates with 30 mg/dL in a random collection.
Severe preeclampsia	Preeclampsia is considered severe if one or more of the following criteria are present:
	Blood pressure of ≥ 160 mm Hg systolic or ≥ 110 mm Hg diastolic on two occasions at least 6 hours apart
	Proteinuria of ≥ 5 grams in 24 hours or ≥ 3+ on two random urine samples collected at least 4 hours apart
	Oliguria of < 500 mL in 24 hours
	Cerebral or visual disturbances
	Pulmonary edema or cyanosis
	Epigastric or right upper-quadrant pain
	Impaired liver function
	Thrombocytopenia
	Fetal growth restriction
HELLP	Hemolysis, elevated liver enzymes, and low platelets. HELLP syndrome may be a severe form of preeclampsia or it may be an independent disorder.
Eclampsia	Grand mal seizures in a woman with preeclampsia.

Source: Adapted from Report of the National High Blood Pressure Education Program Working Group on High Blood Pressure in Pregnancy. *Am J Obstet Gynecol.* 2000;183:S1-S22.

BOX 23-10 Risk Factors for Gestational Hypertension and Preeclampsia

- Nulliparity
- Age > 35 years
- African American race
- Obesity
- Family history of preeclampsia
- Preeclampsia in previous pregnancy
- Chronic hypertension
- Chronic renal disease
- Pre-gestational diabetes
- Multiple gestation
- Vascular and connective tissue disease
- Antiphospholipid antibody syndrome
- Abnormal Doppler studies at 18 and 24 weeks
- Hydatiform mole

Pathophysiology of Gestational Hypertension and Preeclampsia

The etiology of the spectrum of hypertensive disorders in pregnancy is unclear. The "cure" for preeclampsia/eclampsia, except for the rare postpartum initial presentation of preeclampsia, is always delivery of the placenta. The resolution following expulsion of the placenta supports theories related to the placental influence on the disease. One theory suggests that the placental cytotrophoblasts are implanted abnormally where they invade the maternal spiral arteries. Normally, this interface between maternal cells and placental cells leads to spiral artery remodeling so the arteries become large, low-resistance vessels. Preeclampsia is a two-stage event. In the first stage, a series of abnormal processes occur at the interface between cytotrophoblasts and maternal spiral arteries that result in endothelial cell dysfunction within the maternal arteries, poor perfusion, and the release of an unidentified "toxin."[82] The historical term "toxemia of pregnancy" reflects this theory. The key feature in this theory is vasospasm. The second stage occurs later in pregnancy, when symptoms appear.

A genetic component is suspected because of the high incidence of preeclampsia in sisters and daughters of women with eclampsia. A classic study in 1985[83] found that the sisters of women with eclampsia had a 37% risk of preeclampsia and daughters had a 25% risk of preeclampsia. This association may be the result of multifactorial genetic susceptibility, or perhaps a recessive gene. In any event, such a link remains theoretical at this time. Dietary deficiencies in protein, calcium, and vitamin D have also been suggested as etiologic factors, but research has not yielded consistent findings on this front and supplementation has not reliably affected the incidence or severity of hypertensive disorders in pregnancy.[84]

The second stage of preeclampsia is the woman's response to abnormal placentation. The placenta in women with preeclampsia produces inadequate prostacyclin compared to thromboxane. This imbalance increases the sensitivity to angiotensin II, with a concomitant increase in vasoconstriction. As early as 14 weeks' gestation, some women demonstrate a sensitivity to angiotensin II, seen as an occasional isolated elevated blood pressure and/or failure of the blood pressure to exhibit the normal drop in the second trimester.

The vasospasm of preeclampsia has a multisystem effect on the pregnant woman and is responsible for the three classic signs: (1) hypertension, (2) proteinuria, and (3) edema. Renal perfusion and glomerular filtration rate decrease as a result of renal vasospasm. The glomerular damage is clinically evident as proteinuria. Blood urea nitrogen, creatinine, and plasma uric acid levels also rise. Hemoconcentration develops as fluid moves out of the intravascular space and edema becomes evident. Vasospasm in the liver may lead to HELLP syndrome, discussed later in this chapter. Neurologic symptoms resulting from vasospasm include headache, visual disturbances including scotomata, diplopia, and (rarely) transient blindness.

Diagnosis

The diagnosis of gestational hypertension or preeclampsia requires attention to the woman's report of symptoms, accurate measurement of blood pressure, assessment of urinary protein, laboratory assessment of liver and renal indices, and comparison of all parameters over time. Preeclampsia may develop and progress over a period of weeks, or it may develop in a fulminant manner over a few hours. Preeclampsia typically becomes evident after 20 weeks' gestation but rarely occurs prior to 20 weeks if the woman has a hydatidiform mole or hydrops.

Any baseline elevation in blood pressure is a signal for close observation for development of preeclampsia. Historically, edema has been considered a physical sign of preeclampsia. However, edema is common in all pregnancies, so it is not a good marker for the renal compromise associated with preeclampsia. Edema *is* an indication for increased surveillance and laboratory evaluation, particularly 24-hour collection for protein and renal function. Laboratory evaluation for preeclampsia is shown in **Table 23-6**.

HELLP Syndrome

HELLP syndrome—which is an acronym for hypertension, elevated liver enzymes, and low platelets—is either a severe form of preeclampsia or a separate disorder, given that as many as 20% of women with this condition do not have hypertension or proteinuria.[85] Women with HELLP syndrome may report cerebrovascular symptoms of severe headache (predominantly frontal), blurred vision, or scotomata. The persistent epigastric pain of severe preeclampsia and HELLP syndrome is a result of vasospasm in the liver with hepatic compromise. Women with HELLP syndrome are seriously ill and are at risk of subcapsular hematoma or hepatic rupture and disseminated intravascular coagulopathy; they are also at high risk for eclampsia.

Eclampsia

Eclampsia is the occurrence of seizure in a woman with preeclampsia who has no other reason for the seizure, such as epilepsy or drug overdose. Eclampsia is a life-threatening complication of pregnancy that is associated with a high risk of intracranial hemorrhage.

Midwifery Management

The role of the midwife in caring for women who develop hypertension during pregnancy focuses on meticulous screening, early identification, and knowing when to consult, collaborate with, or refer to a physician colleague. Assessment of risk factors early in pregnancy alerts the midwife to those women who will benefit from close surveillance, including, perhaps, more frequent visits in the third trimester. A blood pressure of 140/90 mm Hg or higher indicates the need for laboratory assessment and physician consultation. Baseline laboratory evaluation, including 24-hour urine collection for total protein, hemoglobin, hematocrit, platelets, and liver function tests, will help make the differential diagnosis of gestational hypertension versus preeclampsia.

Table 23-6	Interpretation of Laboratory Findings in Preeclampsia		
Laboratory Test	**Finding**	**Interpretation**	**Pathophysiology**
Hemoglobin and hematocrit	Increased	Hemoconcentration	Fluid moves from intravascular to extracellular spaces, causing edema
Platelet count	Decreased	Reflects severity of preeclampsia	< 100,000 platelets is severe preeclampsia
Serum uric acid	Increased	Decreased renal clearance	Serum uric acid increases as renal excretion of uric acid decreases
Blood urea nitrogen (BUN)	Normal	Mild preeclampsia	
	Increased	Decrease in renal blood flow and glomerular filtration rate indicates increasing severity of preeclampsia	Doubling of BUN represents a 50% reduction in renal blood flow
Serum creatinine	Normal	Mild preeclampsia	
	Increased	Decrease in renal blood flow and glomerular filtration rate indicates increasing severity of preeclampsia	Doubling of serum creatinine represents a 50% reduction in renal blood flow > 1.2 mg/dL in progressive preeclampsia
Creatinine clearance	Decreased	May be normal in mild preeclampsia; is decreased in severe preeclampsia	More useful measure than a single serum creatinine value
Liver function tests:			
• Aspartate transaminase (AST)	Elevated	Liver cell damage	Serious complication of preeclampsia is subcapsular hemorrhage in the liver
• Alanine transaminase (ALT)	Elevated		
Coagulation profile:			
• Fibrinogen	Low	Measures blood clotting ability; abnormal clotting function is indicative of severe disease	
• Fibrin split products	Present		
• Prothrombin time (PT)	Prolonged		
• Partial prothrombin time (PPT)			
Urine protein (dipstick)	Increased	3+ and 4+ in severe disease	2+ indicates need for 24-hour collection
Urine protein (24-hour)	Increased protein	The damaged glomerulus allows proteins to escape into urine	300 mg in 24 hours, or 1 g/L in preeclampsia; 5 g/L in 24 hours in severe disease
Urine volume	Decreased	Hypovolemia, hypoperfusion, renal compromise	Less than 400–500 mL in 24 hours in severe disease

Weight gain assessment can alert the midwife to significant fluid retention. Edema of hands and feet are common in all pregnancies, but edema of the face or trunk is more concerning. A sudden increase in edema or weight gain of more than 2 pounds in a week is an indication of significant fluid retention.

Careful measurement of blood pressure to ensure accurate readings is essential. Appropriate cuff size, measurement of blood pressure when the woman is sitting and has settled comfortably in the examination area, and careful attention to accuracy of the measurement is needed. If automated blood pressure techniques are used, the device needs regular calibrating.

The value of a urine dipstick test for protein at every visit is debatable. Many factors, including urinary tract infection, vaginitis, collection volume, and time of day, may affect the accuracy of this test. Any suspicion of preeclampsia or more than 1+ protein on a dipstick warrants further evaluation with a 24-hour urine collection that will be tested for proteinuria and renal function.

Management of preeclampsia requires a balance between the health of the woman and the health of her fetus. If delivery is not indicated for fetal well-being, then the goal of treatment is to manage the woman's symptoms to allow for the fetus to have more time in utero.

If preeclampsia is mild and appears not to be taking a fulminant course, the woman may remain at home with close observation. This would include modified bedrest, possible home blood pressure measurement by a family member, daily fetal kick counts, biweekly prenatal testing, and frequent office or home visits for assessment of blood pressure and other symptomatology. Women and their families should be educated about the signs and symptoms of worsening preeclampsia. In addition, the woman must be able to access medical care 24 hours a day.

If the woman develops severe preeclampsia or fetal prenatal testing is nonreassuring, hospitalization is required for the duration of the pregnancy. The decision to prolong pregnancy will be revisited daily, based on progression of maternal disease and fetal status.

Fetal Growth Restriction

A fetus whose estimated weight via ultrasound is below the 10th percentile for gestational age is considered small for gestational age (SGA) and may have fetal growth restriction.[86] Although some fetuses who are less than the 10th percentile for their gestational age are constitutionally small without compromise, others have some cause for their growth restriction.

Historically, fetuses who were more than two standard deviations smaller than average were termed "intrauterine growth retarded." This term was changed to "intrauterine growth restriction" (IUGR) or "fetal growth restriction" (FGR), terms that are currently used interchangeably to describe this condition. The term "fetal growth restriction" is used in this text.

Perinatal morbidity and mortality are significantly increased in fetuses with FGR, especially the risk of stillbirth. FGR is associated with 26% of stillbirths.[87] Several etiologies have been proposed for FGR, with the most common being listed in **Table 23-7**.[88]

FGR can be subdivided into three categories. The first category is symmetrical FGR, in which both the fetal body and head are equally small. For example, the head is noted on ultrasound at the 8th percentile and the fetal bone/abdomen/chest are also 8th percentile. The most common cause of symmetrical growth restriction is congenital anomalies. Symmetrical growth restriction that occurs early in gestation and is progressively severe—that is, the delay becomes more pronounced as pregnancy continues—is associated with severe maternal malnutrition, low pre-pregnancy weight/no weight gain, multiple gestation, chromosomal abnormalities, perinatal infections, and exposure to drugs or environmental teratogens. The prognosis for this fetus is poor. The other subcategory of symmetrical FGR includes the fetus who is constitutionally small and can be expected to be normal. If the reduction in growth is symmetrical, occurs prior to 32 weeks' gestation, and is consistent with a 2- to 3-week delay, and growth continues but remains 2 to 3 weeks behind, the growth restriction may be attributed to a constitutionally small but normal fetus.[88]

The second category of FGR is asymmetrical growth restriction. This condition is the result of compromise later in fetal life, typically after 30 weeks' gestation. Asymmetric growth restriction can be caused by any condition that causes decreased placental blood flow or decreased oxygenation of the fetus (described in more detail in the section of this chapter on antenatal testing). In such a case, the fetus's estimated weight is below the 10th percentile but the head circumference is above the 10th percentile. Factors associated with asymmetric FGR include maternal hypertension, renal disease, collagen vascular disease, microvascular disease of diabetes, cyanotic heart disease, and hemoglobinopathies.

Table 23-7	Etiology of Fetal Growth Restriction	
Fetal Factors	**Maternal Factors**	**Placental Factors**
Chromosome abnormalities: primarily trisomy 13, 18, or 21	Maternal conditions: hypertension, autoimmune disease (e.g., systemic lupus erythematosus, antiphospholipid antibody syndrome, or acquired immune-mediated thrombophilia), pregestational diabetes, cardiac, severe renal insufficiency, cyanotic heart disease, and severe anemia	Abnormal placental attachment to the uterus
Genetic gene mutations		Reduced perfusion secondary to maternal vascular disease
Inborn errors of metabolism		
Intrauterine infections: particularly viral		
Multiple gestation	Chronic malnutrition	
	Substance abuse: tobacco, alcohol, drugs (prescribed and illicit)	
	Previous history of fetal growth restriction in a prior pregnancy	
	Stress/depression	
	Exposure to certain medications such as valproic acid (Depakene)	
	Obesity	

Source: Adapted from Nardozza LM, Araujo E, Barbosa MM, Caetano ACR, Lee DJR, Moron AF. Fetal growth restriction: current knowledge to the general Obs/Gyn. *Arch Gynecol Obstet.* 2012;286:1-13.

The third subcategory of FGR is a combination of symmetrical and asymmetrical growth restriction. The etiology of this type is often either maternal infection (e.g., rubella, cytomegalovirus) or exposure to toxins (e.g., medications, illicit drugs).

Detection of Fetal Growth Restriction

The role of the midwife is to identify a woman with FGR and to refer her to a physician for further evaluation. Initial indications of FGR include either no increase or slower than expected increases in fundal height, poor or no maternal weight gain, and development of risk factors such as hypertension. When FGR is suspected, the next step is to obtain an ultrasound evaluation. If the ultrasound finds the fetus is less than the 10th percentile in estimated weight, consultation with the physician is indicated and a plan for surveillance developed. Timing of birth will depend on fetal status.

Use of Fundal Height to Detect Fetal Growth Restriction

The use of fundal heights to accurately detect fetal growth restriction has been evaluated.[89,90] To be useful, fundal height must be measured in a standardized manner within the practice group—that is, all providers must use the same technique. Use of a centimeter tape with a standard procedure such as measuring in the midline from the top of the fundus to the top of the maternal symphysis needs to be established. Ideally, the measurements would be made by the same person; however, given that often is not possible, a common procedure is needed. Several standardized fundal height curves are available that enable plotting of the measurements to provide a visual graph of the fundal height compared to both the low and high limits. The accuracy of prediction of small-for-gestational-age with these two charts ranges from 73% to 84%.[92] A slow growth pattern or even a single measurement that falls below the lower limit of normal curve on the chart warrants further investigation with ultrasound.

Polyhydramnios (Hydramnios)

Polyhydramnios, also called hydramnios, is an excessive amount of amniotic fluid. Polyhydramnios is described as an amniotic fluid index (AFI) of 24 centimeters or more, or the maximum deepest vertical pocket that is 8 centimeters or more.[91] Fifty percent to 60% of polyhydramnios is idiopathic. Several conditions are associated with a higher incidence of polyhydramnios, including multiple gestation, especially monozygotic twins; pre-gestational diabetes and GDM; fetal conditions such as infection, isoimmunization, and fetal–maternal hemorrhage; and fetal chromosomal abnormalities.[92,93] In particular, fetal structural anomalies, such as gastrointestinal tract tracheoesophageal fistula and central nervous system anomalies including anencephaly and meningomyelocele, are associated with polyhydramnios.

Polyhydramnios is initially suspected when uterine enlargement, maternal abdominal girth, and fundal height are larger than expected for the fetus's gestational age. It may be difficult to auscultate fetal heart tones and to palpate the fetal outline and fetal parts. The fetus may have an unstable lie—and a change in lie may be detected during Leopold's maneuvers. In severe cases of polyhydramnios, the woman may experience dyspnea; lower extremity and vulvar edema; pressure pains in the back, abdomen, and thighs; heartburn or nausea; and vomiting. Complications include preterm labor secondary to uterine distension, premature rupture of membranes, malpresentation of the fetus, cord prolapse, abruptio placenta, dysfunctional labor, and postpartum hemorrhage.

If the midwife suspects that a woman has polyhydramnios, consultation with a physician is indicated. An ultrasound is obtained to confirm the diagnosis and identify any coexisting fetal or placental conditions or complications. Additional laboratory evaluation might include rescreening for GDM and an antibody titer to detect if any alloimmunization is present.

Uncomplicated polyhydramnios is not an indication for delivery. The diagnosis warrants increased fetal surveillance and attention to the potential mechanical difficulties of dyspnea and edema for the woman. On rare occasions, the polyhydramnios is so severe that fluid must be removed via controlled amniocentesis to relieve respiratory distress.

Oligohydramnios

Oligohydramnios is an abnormally low volume of amniotic fluid. The amount of amniotic fluid increases throughout pregnancy until it reaches approximately 1000 milliliters by the start of the third trimester, and then it gradually decreases, at approximately 34 weeks' gestation, until it is about 800 milliliters at term.[94]

Measurement of amniotic fluid volume is a standard component of complete ultrasound examinations and is included in the biophysical profile (BPP)

described later in this chapter. An amniotic fluid volume in the third trimester of less than a 5-cm pocket in a singleton pregnancy or less than a 2-cm pocket in a twin pregnancy is considered oligohydramnios.

Oligohydramnios is associated with an increase in perinatal morbidity and mortality. This condition can result from fetal genitourinary abnormalities such as malformed[95] or absent kidneys, premature rupture of membranes, uteroplacental perfusion abnormality, and post-term pregnancy. When oligohydramnios occurs early in the second trimester, the fetus is at risk for developing hypoplastic lungs. Amniotic fluid is required for normal chest expansion and fetal breathing. Oligohydramnios that develops between 24 and 34 gestational weeks is associated with major fetal anomalies, fetal growth restriction, and preterm birth.[96]

Oligohydramnios is also a significant finding suggestive of postmaturity syndrome in a postdate pregnancy. Oligohydramnios at term is associated with an increased incidence of meconium-stained fluid and fetal intolerance of labor. The combination of this condition and fetal growth restriction significantly increases the risk that the fetus will tolerate labor poorly and that operative delivery may be necessary.

A number of conditions have been associated with oligohydramnios, although it is difficult to ascertain which, if any, may be causes and which may be consequences of the condition. These conditions include congenital anomalies (e.g., renal agenesis, Potter's syndrome), viral diseases, FGR, uteroplacental insufficiency, preterm premature rupture of membranes, response to Indocin as a tocolytic, fetal hypoxia, meconium-stained fluid (including meconium aspiration), and postmaturity syndrome.[97]

Oligohydramnios may be suspected on clinical exam but will need to be confirmed via formal ultrasound. Its clinical signs and symptoms include "molding" of the uterus around the fetus, a fetus that is easily outlined, a fetus that is not ballottable, and lagging fundal height.

Oligohydramnios in an indication for physician consultation. An ultrasound will be performed. Conservative management includes bedrest to increase uterine perfusion, good maternal nutrition, and oral hydration. Hydration has been shown to increase amniotic fluid volume. In a Brazilian study, oral hydration with Gatorade and water increased the AFI as much as 20% among women who had normal pregnancies.[98] A subsequent RCT confirmed the benefit of maternal hydration on amniotic fluid volume.[99] Patrelli et al. confirmed that oral hydration of 1500 mL or intravenous hydration with 2500 mL daily resulted in an increase in amniotic fluid volume for women with uncomplicated oligohydramnios. If oligohydramnios is suspected, increasing hydration while undertaking further investigation may be of benefit. Frequent surveillance of fetal well-being that includes fetal movement counts, nonstress tests (NST), a BPP, and possibly color ultrasound to determine the Doppler indices in the umbilical vessels will be initiated.

Oligohydramnios can be associated with variable decelerations in the fetal heart rate.[100] These decelerations are assumed to occur secondary to umbilical cord compression in the absence of fluid that "cushions" the cord. The timing of birth depends on the evidence for fetal well-being during frequent surveillance. Early intervention has not been found to reduce perinatal morbidity or mortality.[101]

Multiple Gestation

Multiple gestation refers to a pregnancy with two or more fetuses. The incidence of multiple gestation in the United States increased 76% between 1980 and 2009, largely because of the increased use of assisted reproductive technologies including ovulation-inducing medications.[102] Since 2004, the prevalence of twin gestations has remained stable at approximately 32 per 1000 live births and the prevalence of higher-order multiple gestations has dropped, presumably because clinicians who perform assisted reproductive technologies now avoid multiple-fetal pregnancies when possible.[103]

The major fetal risks are preterm birth and fetal growth restriction. The preterm birth rate in twins was 50% in 2010.[105] Women with multiple gestations are also at risk for fetal anomalies, early pregnancy loss, stillbirth, FGR, placenta previa, preterm labor and birth, GDM, preeclampsia, malpresentation, and dysfunctional labor. Less common complications include acute fatty liver disease, pruritic urticarial papules and pustules of pregnancy (PUPP), and pulmonary embolus.[105]

Higher-order multiples, defined as triplets or more, are associated with significant risks for perinatal morbidity and mortality. Women with higher-order multiple gestations are referred for physician management. Twins may be collaboratively managed with the physician as determined by the midwife, the physician, and the availability of consultation and tertiary care. Signs and symptoms that are indicative of multiple pregnancy are shown in **Box 23-11**.

It is common for a woman with a multiple gestation who receives prenatal care in the first trimester to have an initial physical exam that is consistent

---

BOX 23-11 Signs and Symptoms Indicative of a Possible Multiple Pregnancy

- Large-for-dates uterine size, fundal height, and abdominal girth, associated with rapid uterine growth during the second trimester
- Severe nausea and vomiting (associated with rapidly increasing hCG levels)
- History of recent use of ovulation-inducing drugs such as clomiphene citrate (Clomid) or menotropins (Pergonal)
- Abdominal palpation of three or more large parts or multiple small parts
- Auscultation of more than one clearly distinct fetal heart tone (differing by more than 10 beats per minute and separate from the maternal pulse)

---

with her dates. The uterus will then be larger than expected in the early second trimester. Diagnosis is confirmed via ultrasound.

Ultrasound will determine fetal number, fetal anatomy, and chorionicity of placentation. Monozygotic twins develop from one egg and one sperm; dizygotic twins develop from two eggs and two sperm. Monozygotic twins may be monochorionic or dichorionic. Dizygotic twins will always be dichorionic and, therefore, diamniotic. Chorionicity is based on when during the early gestational period that the zygote splits and includes the following possibilities:

- Diamniotic/dichorionic, which occurs if cleavage happens by day 3 after fertilization
- Diamniotic/monochorionic, which occurs if the zygote splits between days 4 and 8
- Monoamniotic/monochorionic, which occurs if cleavage happens between days 8 and 13

Monoamniotic/monochorionic chorionicity is rare and increases the risk for perinatal mortality secondary to the high likelihood of cord entanglement and cord strangulation. If the zygote splits after day 13, the embryos have not had time to separate and they develop as conjoined twins. **Figure 23-4** illustrates the possible combinations of chorionicity.

Once the diagnosis of multiple pregnancy is made, prenatal care management changes to include more frequent prenatal visits, increased surveillance for complications, serial ultrasounds to monitor fetal growth, and earlier changes in home and work responsibilities. Ultrasound examinations are generally

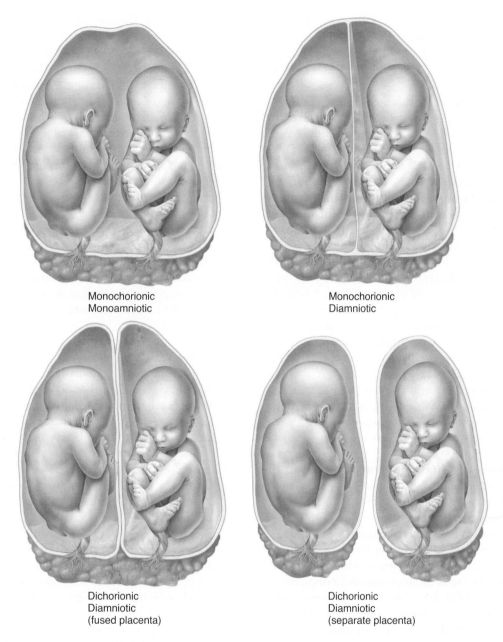

Monochorionic
Monoamniotic

Monochorionic
Diamniotic

Dichorionic
Diamniotic
(fused placenta)

Dichorionic
Diamniotic
(separate placenta)

Figure 23-4 Placentation in twin pregnancies.

performed every 3 to 4 weeks from 20 weeks' gestation until term for assessment of fetal growth and cervical measurements to assess for increased risk for preterm labor. If one of the twins exhibits discordant growth, or if both twins are found to be lagging in growth, there will be heightened concern for FGR or placental abnormalities. Poor fetal growth may occur secondary to the tremendous demands on the woman for nutritional support or because of uteroplacental abnormality. The large size of the placenta can stress the capability of uterine blood flow, especially if there is underlying pathology such as maternal

hypertension, diabetes, or collagen vascular disease. A conjoined placenta increases the possibility of twin-to-twin transfusion.

Women with twin gestations need extra counseling and anticipatory guidance that address several topics. In these areas, midwifery care can complement medical care for women who are pregnant with twins. For example, maternal nutrition is critical for healthy fetal development. Women with twins need more protein and calories. They may have more difficulty getting adequate nutrition as the physical discomforts of pregnancy can be more extreme. Iron supplementation is warranted, as it is very difficult to get enough iron to meet the needs of both fetuses and the woman via diet alone. Family stress can be more pronounced, so planning for help after birth is especially important.

Management also includes limiting activity and increasing rest periods throughout pregnancy. Bedrest has not been found to be an effective means to prevent preterm labor in multiple gestation. Nevertheless, rest periods will become increasingly necessary, and women are advised to avoid exhaustion and long hours spent standing. Instruction regarding sexual activity is based on cervical findings, previous obstetric history, and frequency of Braxton Hicks contractions. Advice may include the use of condoms, because the prostaglandins in semen can cause uterine irritability, or may extend to complete pelvic rest including avoidance of orgasm, based on individual findings.

Plans should be made for a physician to attend the birth, and the mode of birth will depend on the position of both fetuses and physician expertise. The midwife may have a role in the vaginal birth of twins especially when the progress is normal, both fetuses are in a vertex presentation, and a vaginal birth is planned.

Management of Pregnancy with Known Fetal Anomalies

Prior to the advent of prenatal genetic evaluation and routine prenatal ultrasound, many fetal anomalies were not identified until birth. With today's screening and diagnostic technologies, management of known fetal anomalies can become a component of prenatal care. Early identification allows the woman to have a range of options, including pregnancy termination, fetal reduction in the case of high-order multiple gestation, adoption, or possibly fetal surgery. If the woman chooses to remain pregnant, depending on the anticipated condition of the newborn, she will face the additional choices of parenting the child, placing the newborn in foster care, or relinquishing the child for adoption. If the anomaly is a lethal one, the family may access perinatal hospice for assistance.

Planning for care of the infant after birth begins when the woman or couple decide to continue the pregnancy. The complex decision making as well as management of prenatal care and birth alter the role of the midwife, as a team of providers—including genetic counselors, pediatricians, and maternal–fetal medicine experts—will be involved in pregnancy care. The midwife can play an important role in helping women and their families identify important questions they want to ask and in interpreting some of the information they are given. It is most important to provide time for the woman and her support persons to consider options and make decisions based on the values that normally govern their lives. A rule of thumb is that bad news has to be heard at least three times to be truly heard. Tears and anger are signs that the bad news has been understood. Nondirective counseling is difficult and may need to be practiced ahead of time for a midwife to use it competently.[104]

It is not uncommon for a woman with a fetus that has an anomaly to request periodic reconfirmation that the anomaly still exists. A repeat ultrasound should be provided if requested.

Different grieving styles may put the couple at risk for relationship stress. The midwife can prepare the couple for differences in grieving style and help them find a common way of working through their grief and supporting each other. The woman or couple may also need help in planning what to tell family members, other children, and even strangers who see her pregnancy and ask about it. Few tools exist to help with these tasks, although the perinatal hospice staff or the family pediatric provider may be of assistance.

If the anomaly is lethal, the woman may not exhibit the common bonding behaviors because she subconsciously or consciously does not want to fall in love with a child she knows she will lose. If the fetus is expected to survive until birth, a birth/newborn plan can be discussed and documented prior to onset of labor. The hospital may require that the family sign the plan to avoid misunderstanding and ensure they have received adequate discussion of the plan. Specific components of the plan that should be present include whether fetal heart rate monitoring will be used during labor and if a cesarean section for fetal intolerance to labor will be performed. The *Complications During Labor and Birth* chapter reviews labor management for women who have a fetus with a lethal anomaly or intrauterine fetal demise.

Fetal Death and Stillbirth

Classification of Intrauterine Fetal Demise

Pregnancy loss before 20 completed weeks of pregnancy is considered a miscarriage (spontaneous abortion). After 20 weeks, the death is classified as a stillbirth or fetal death. In some states, fetal weight is used to determine the category. The recommendation is that the loss should be classified a stillbirth after 20 weeks if the dates are known or if the fetus weighed more than 350 grams when the dates are uncertain.[105] "Stillbirth" has now replaced the term "fetal death"and the literature has adopted this term in response to women's and families' requests. The rate of early stillbirth (20–27 weeks) is approximately 3.1 per 1000 births, and the rate of late stillbirth (more than 28 weeks) has slowly decreased to 2.97 per 1000 births.[106] The overall stillbirth rate in the United States has remained approximately 6.2 per 1000 births since 2003. Of particular concern is the racial disparity in rates of stillbirth. Hispanic women have a rate that is 14% higher than the corresponding rate for white women, and non-Hispanic black women have a rate that is more than twice the rate of white women. The reasons for the disparity are not clear.[107]

Often the first sign of a stillbirth is the woman's perception of the loss of fetal movement. The loss of fetal movement and inability to detect the fetal heart tones (FHT) are collectively called the "silent uterus." Inability to detect FHT with a Doppler indicates the need for immediate ultrasound to confirm the diagnosis. The midwife should accompany the woman to the ultrasound appointment if at all possible, and notify the ultrasound staff ahead of time that fetal heart tones could not be found. Once the diagnosis is made, immediate physician consultation is recommended. In many states, a physician must make the determination of death, even fetal death. After birth, midwives may be able to complete the required death certificate, but these regulations vary by state.

The decision to induce labor or wait for labor to occur spontaneously will depend on the woman's choice, her cervical status, and any concomitant medical issues that need to be addressed. Although most women chose immediate induction, expectant management is a viable option for a short period of time. The majority of women (80% to 90%) will go into labor spontaneously within 2 weeks following a fetal demise. An unusual chronic form of disseminated intravascular coagulation (DIC) can occur if the fetus is retained in utero for more than 4 to 5 weeks; this DIC occurs secondary to slow release of tissue factor from the fetal tissue.[108] Coagulation studies consisting of prothrombin, partial prothrombin, fibrinogen, and platelets may be performed to screen for DIC prior to induction and at intervals if expectant management continues beyond a week or two.

Most women do not want to wait more than a few days for delivery. However, waiting at least 24 hours can provide a family time to plan, resolve some of the shock, and gather supportive family and friends. Information should be supplied to counteract "old wives' tales" concerning possible causes of the fetal death (e.g., falling down stairs, raising arms over head, lifting heavy objects). The midwife may need to initiate this discussion to elicit specific beliefs held by the woman or family members or significant others.

The determination of the cause of the stillbirth is extremely difficult; indeed, in most cases, no cause can be found. It is best to refrain from discussing any possible cause for the loss until objective facts are clear and the post-delivery studies are completed and results available.

Pregnancy After Stillbirth

When a woman has experienced stillbirth, intensified surveillance is indicated in a subsequent pregnancy. Prior to pregnancy or at the first prenatal visit, a detailed history needs to include a review of all information available about the prior stillbirth. Medical records can be ordered if needed and physician consultation is recommended to determine a management plan. Plans can be made to mitigate any recurrent factors such as smoking, cocaine use, diabetes, or other problems. Genetic counseling, as well as thrombophilia and antiphospholipid antibody assessment, may be considered. Early ultrasound for pregnancy dating and detailed anatomic ultrasound (level II) at 18 to 20 weeks' gestation will identify fetal conditions and provide reassurance to the woman and her family if the ultrasound findings are normal.

The third trimester is likely to be a time of special anxiety for the woman, her family, and the providers. Although there is no evidence that heightened surveillance lowers the risk of a recurrent stillbirth, many providers offer women frequent prenatal visits or serial nonstress tests, and elective delivery at 38 weeks' gestation. Serial ultrasounds for fetal surveillance including fetal growth are recommended every 2 weeks beginning at 28 weeks.

Female Genital Mutilation

Female circumcision or "cutting" is currently more commonly called female genital mutilation (FGM). The procedure is practiced in parts of Africa, Asia, and the Middle East. As women have immigrated to European and American countries, practitioners in areas previously unfamiliar with the practice have found themselves caring for women with FGM who are pregnant.

The World Health Organization classifies the degree of FGM as type I, involving the removal of the prepuce and clitoral tissue; type II, which includes removal of the prepuce, clitoris, and labia minora;

and type III, called infibulation, in which the clitoris, labia minora, and inner surface of the labia majora are excised. The incised sides of the labia majora are then stretched toward each other and stitched together, creating a false hood of skin over the urethra and anterior part of the vaginal orifice, which narrows the vaginal opening and leaves only a small opening at the introitus through which menstrual blood and urine can exit.[109,110] Long-term complications of infibulation include urinary tract infections, menstrual irregularities and retention, dyspareunia, perineal and pelvic pain, recurrent vaginal infections, infertility, pelvic infections, inclusion cysts, and abscess formation.[111]

Although women with type I and type II FGM do not usually experience obstetric complications, type III FGM can cause obstruction from the resulting anatomy and scar tissue, necessitating the need for deinfibulation or "anterior episiotomy" prior to birth. This can be done because the scar tissue that forms during the healing process from infibulation does not fuse with the underlying tissue of the female genitalia.

Discussion of deinfibulation needs to be initiated early in pregnancy. Counseling includes information about the medical and obstetric risks associated with birth and the options for deinfibulation. Deinfibulation can be done in the second trimester under regional anesthesia. Second trimester or early third trimester deinfibulation is preferred to deinfibulation during labor because it enables more accurate assessment of the pelvic organs and pelvic anatomy, facilitates evaluation of the progress of labor, and may decrease the risk of lacerations/incision, sepsis, and postpartum hemorrhage at the time of birth.

Counseling about deinfibulation can take several visits. Fears and apprehensions must be thoroughly explored and usually involve societal and marital concerns. Separate counseling with the partner may be advisable, followed by a counseling session with the couple to arrive at a mutual decision.[112] The decision to undertake repair or reinfibulation at the time of birth needs to be discussed and documented. In the United States, FGM is illegal; however, reinfibulation, at the woman's request, is within the law.

Techniques for Fetal Surveillance

The term "antenatal testing" is used to refer to tests that assess fetal oxygenation in the late second or early third trimester. The goals of antenatal fetal testing include (1) prevention of stillbirth, (2) identification of the fetus whose oxygen status is compromised in order to allow intervention before irreversible metabolic acidosis ensues, and (3) avoidance of unnecessary interventions when other clinical parameters are equivocal. This section reviews the theory, indications, methodology, and normal versus abnormal findings for fetal kick counts, NST, BPP, contraction stress testing (CST), and Doppler indices. Antenatal testing is a classic "screening test" in that if the results are normal, fetal well-being is assured. In contrast, if results are abnormal, further assessment is indicated to determine fetal well-being or fetal compromise.

Tests for fetal well-being are clinically useful primarily because their negative predictive value is 99% or higher.[113,114] The incidence of false-positive tests varies between 50% and 60% depending on the outcome measures utilized. Miller et al. estimated that induction resulting in preterm birth following a false-positive test occurred in approximately 1% of women who were induced for an abnormal prenatal fetal test.[115] This study was conducted in 1996, however, and it is not clear how often false-positive testing results in iatrogenic adverse outcomes today. Additional surveillance technologies such as Doppler ultrasound are better able to accurately detect the fetus at risk, so the incidence of iatrogenic intervention is presumed to be small. Because the positive predictive values are much lower, clinical management of abnormal prenatal test results varies depending on other clinical factors.[116] The interpretation of these testing methods is summarized in **Table 23-8**.

Fetal Physiologic Indices and Factors That Affect Fetal Behavior

Prenatal surveillance of fetal well-being is based on the observation that specific fetal behavior states reflect adequate oxygenation. The fetal heart rate pattern, level of fetal activity, and degree of muscle tone are sensitive to hypoxemia and acidosis. Therefore, fetal oxygenation can be indirectly evaluated by assessing biophysical parameters, just as vital signs are used to assess well-being in an adult or child. Fetal biophysical behavior that is assessed in the various prenatal fetal tests includes fetal heart rate parameters, fetal movement, fetal breathing, and quantification of amniotic fluid (because the amount of amniotic fluid reflects fetal renal function and renal perfusion). Each of these parameters can be affected by a multitude of factors. Therefore a brief review of normal fetal behavior and factors that affect fetal behavior is in order.

Table 23-8	Interpretation of Antenatal Tests	
Name	**Results**	**Criteria**
Contractions stress test (CST) or breast stimulation test (BST)[a]	Negative	Normal FHR without late decelerations
	Equivocal suspicious	Intermittent late decelerations or variable decelerations
	Equivocal hyperstimulation	Decelerations that occur in presence of tachysystole
	Unsatisfactory	Unable to obtain a satisfactory FHR tracing
	Positive	Recurrent late decelerations following ≥ 50% of contractions even if fewer than 3 contractions in 10 minutes
Nonstress test (NST)[b]	Reactive	≥ 2 accelerations with in 20 minutes (some settings extend to 40 minutes)
	Nonreactive	< 2 accelerations in 40 minutes
	Inconclusive	Unable to obtain a satisfactory FHR tracing
		Variable or late decelerations or other Category II FHR tracing
		Reactive NST with FHR decelerations
Biophysical profile (BPP)	Normal	≥ 8/10 or 8/8 if NST excluded
	Equivocal	6/10
	Abnormal	≤ 4/10
Modified NST	Normal	Reactive NST and AFI > 5 cm
	Abnormal	Nonreactive NST and/or AFI ≤ 5 cm

AFI = amniotic fluid index; FHR = fetal heart rate.

[a]This test is interpreted once the woman has at least 3 contractions within 10 minutes.

[b]An acceleration must be 15 beats per minute above the baseline and it must last 15 seconds or more from onset to resolution after 32 weeks' gestation. The acceleration must be 10 beats per minute above baseline and last 10 seconds in a preterm fetus.

Maternal awareness of fetal movement begins in the second trimester; multiparous women usually start feeling the fetus between 16 and 18 weeks, whereas primiparous women usually start feeling the fetus between 18 and 22 weeks. Women who have an anterior placenta may begin detecting fetal movement somewhat later than women whose placenta is posterior. Fetal movement is initially slight and irregular, gradually becoming stronger and more frequent. Fetal movement maximizes around 34 weeks, but then appears to become less frequent. This pattern occurs because, as the central nervous system matures, the fetus begins to exhibit longer and cyclic sleep or quiet alert states wherein movement does not occur. Thus the woman's perception can be one of decreased movement toward the end of the pregnancy. Women usually perceive approximately 50% of isolated limb movements and 80% of movements that involve both the trunk and the limb.[117] A list of maternal factors that affect perception of fetal behavior appears in **Box 23-12.**

Fetal behavior changes as the fetus becomes hypoxic. In general loss of fetal heart rate reactivity, fetal heart rate decelerations, and reduced fetal activity are fetal responses to acute hypoxia whereas oligohydramnios, FGR, and altered umbilical artery blood flow are responses to chronic hypoxia. The progressive fetal response to hypoxia is depicted in **Figure 23-5**. Additional information on the FHR responses to acute hypoxia can be found in the *Fetal Assessment During Labor* chapter.

Indications for Antenatal Testing

Although indications for antenatal testing vary between institutions, those that are common to all settings are listed in **Box 23-13**. Likewise, determining when to start testing will vary depending on the

BOX 23-12 Factors That Influence Maternal Perception of Fetal Movement

Decreased Fetal Movement

- Obesity
- Maternal position (fetal movement perceived best in a recumbent position as compared to sitting or standing)
- Anterior placenta
- Amniotic fluid volume (polyhydramnios and oligohydramnios)
- Drugs:
    - Corticosteroids[a]
    - Sedatives and alcohol prolong quiet sleep states[a]
- Hypoglycemia[a]
- Fetal spine in an anterior position (occiput anterior)
- Short period of time immediately after cigarette smoking[a]

No Difference in Perception of Fetal Movement

- Parity
- Maternal anxiety

Increased Fetal Movement

- Maternal meal or increase in blood glucose levels[a]
- Evening hours: fetal movement is least in the morning[a]

[a]These factors have a direct effect on fetal movement.

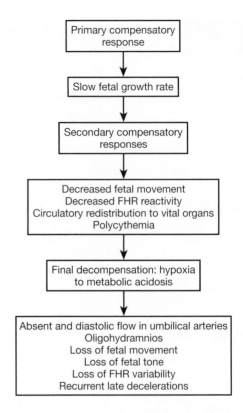

Figure 23-5 Fetal response to chronic hypoxia.

condition. Most antenatal testing is started at 34 to 36 weeks and is conducted either weekly or biweekly.

Fetal Movement Counting (Kick Counts)

The rationale for formal fetal movement counting is that 30% to 50% of stillbirths occur in women with low-risk pregnancies and structurally normal fetuses wherein there were no indications for prenatal testing.[118] Fetal movement starts to decrease several days prior to stillbirth, presumably in an effort to decrease oxygen requirements.[119] This observation became the basis for introducing maternal fetal movement counts for the purpose of preventing stillbirth. Maternal monitoring of fetal movements was first introduced into clinical practice in the 1980s based on a few clinical trials that noted fetal movement counting was associated with fewer stillbirths.[120] Over time, it became clear that formal fetal movement counting

by women who are at low risk for fetal asphyxia was not an effective means of preventing stillbirth.[121,122]

The clinical question has long been, "Should all women perform formal fetal movement counts during the third trimester or just women who are at high risk for stillbirth?" This question has not been definitively answered and the RCTs conducted on routine fetal movement counting have had mixed results.[123,124] Some authors suggest that a general maternal awareness of fetal activity and reduced fetal activity may be a better predictor of fetal risk than formal movement counts. Although most practices use a "count to 10" method for fetal movement counting, the specific fetal movement threshold that is the best "alarm" or trigger for additional evaluation has not been determined.

Currently, some clinicians recommend formal fetal movement counting for all pregnant women, whereas others recommend formal fetal movement counting only for those women who are at increased risk for FGR or stillbirth (i.e., conditions that impose a significant risk for uteroplacental insufficiency and chronic fetal hypoxia). ACOG does not recommend formal fetal movement counting for women who are not at risk for chronic fetal hypoxia.[125]

Decreased Fetal Movement

There is now more than 40 years of literature and research on the relationship between fetal movement and adverse pregnancy outcomes. Formal fetal movement counting does not prevent all stillbirth in unselected populations, but it is clear that women who have a heightened awareness of fetal movement will detect decreased movement and that these women self-select into a higher risk category wherein more intense evaluation is of value. Women who report decreased fetal movement have a higher incidence of fetal growth restriction and stillbirth.[124] Thus these women do need additional evaluation. All pregnant women should be encouraged to pay regular attention to fetal movement and to report decreased or absent movement.

Women's Experiences

A few studies have looked at women's experiences with formal fetal movement counting. Saastad et al., in an RCT of fetal movement counting ($n = 1013$), found that women who performed fetal movement counting reported less concern about their fetuses than did women in the control group, although the frequency of reporting decreased fetal movement was the same in both groups.[126] However, because there is an overall dearth of information on women's experiences and a marked variability in how women perceive risk information, no real conclusions can be drawn about how fetal movement teaching affects the pregnant woman or her response to her fetus or newborn.

Method for Fetal Movement Counts

The method most commonly used is the "Count to 10" method, whereby a woman focuses attention on fetal movement and records how long it takes to document 10 fetal movements. If it takes longer than 2 hours, the woman is to call her midwife; she is then asked to come in for a formal nonstress test (**Figure 23-6**).

Midwifery Management of Decreased Fetal Movement

It is common that women close to term call with a report of decreased fetal movement. If the woman has no risks for uteroplacental insufficiency, it is reasonable to recommend that she eat something, rest in a semirecumbent position, and then count fetal movement. If she notes 10 movements in an hour, she can be reassured and the midwife may recommend that she repeat the formal fetal movement counts for a few days at the same time of day. If she notes fewer than 10 movements, the midwife can either have her count for another hour to see if 10 movements occur or have her be seen for a formal auscultated acceleration test or nonstress test. It is important to remember that women who report decreased fetal movement have an increased risk for adverse outcomes, so the midwife should have a low threshold for having a woman come to the office for additional testing.

Contraction Stress Test

The contraction stress test (CST) was the first antenatal fetal test employed in clinical practice. It is

Name _____

At the same time each day, count the baby's movements. When you have felt 10 movements, record the length of time it took. All movements, even small ones, count toward the total. If you have not felt 10 movements in the usual amount of time, please call your midwife.

Week of_____

Hours taken to feel
10 movements of the baby

Day	Start Time	1	2	3	4	5	6	7	8	9	10
M											
T											
W											
T											
F											
S											
S											

Week of_____

Hours taken to feel
10 movements of the baby

Day	Start Time	1	2	3	4	5	6	7	8	9	10
M											
T											
W											
T											
F											
S											
S											

Week of_____

Hours taken to feel
10 movements of the baby

Day	Start Time	1	2	3	4	5	6	7	8	9	10
M											
T											
W											
T											
F											
S											
S											

Figure 23-6 Fetal movement counting chart.

based on the observation that uterine contractions transiently restrict blood flow to the intervillous space, thereby lowering oxygen availability to the fetus. The compromised fetus will respond with a late deceleration. (For more description of the pathophysiology of the fetal heart rate response to contractions, see the *Fetal Assessment During Labor* chapter.) The CST entails intravenous administration of oxytocin to initiate uterine contractions and continuous electronic fetal monitoring. It can be performed via breast stimulation (BST) to initiate contractions instead of intravenous oxytocin. The procedure for the BST is to have the woman massage one nipple through her clothing for 2 minutes, followed by a rest for 5 minutes and a repeat of the procedure on the other nipple. She should not stimulate the breast during a contraction. The BST and CST are performed in similar fashion, but the BST is associated with more uterine hyperstimulation. Interpretation of results is not different, however.

The test is based on the fetal response to 3 contractions in a 10-minute window (Table 23-8). The CST has the lowest false-negative rate of all antenatal fetal tests (0.04%) but a high false-positive rate of approximately 30% and is expensive to perform. The NST and the BPP have largely replaced the CST except in inpatient settings wherein it is important to establish the fetus's ability to tolerate uterine contractions prior to induction of labor.

Nonstress Test

The NST is the most common method of antenatal testing used in practice today. Its false-negative rate ranges from 0.3% to 0.65%, and the false-positive rate is approximately 55% to 90% depending on the population studied.[127] External fetal monitoring is initiated when the woman is in a side-lying semirecumbent position. The test is concluded when two fetal heart rate accelerations appear within a 20-minute window in a FHR tracing that has moderate variability, no decelerations, and a normal baseline, or when accelerations are unable to be elicited (**Figure 23-7**). If accelerations do not appear in the first 20 to 30 minutes, vibroacoustic stimulation may be applied. Vibroacoustic stimulation lowers the incidence of nonreactive results. The generation of accelerations via vibroacoustic stimulation appears to be as valid as the observation of spontaneous accelerations in predicting fetal well-being. The interpretive criteria for NST results are listed in Table 23-8. Management of inconclusive and nonreactive NSTs varies by practice and by the condition for which the NST was performed.

Because a rise in blood glucose can initiate fetal movement, clinicians have traditionally believed that a sudden infusion of glucose via juice or candy would stimulate fetal accelerations. Studies of the practice have found that glucose does not improve the results of antenatal fetal testing.[128]

Auscultated Nonstress Test

A nonstress test can be performed via auscultation with a fetoscope. During the 1980s, Paine et al. researched the use of auscultation of the FHR as a means of predicting fetal well-being prenatally. From this work, a method of auscultation was devised as a simple alternative to the nonstress test and as a formal method of auscultation for antenatal testing.[129-132]

The auscultated acceleration test (AAT) has been validated as a predictor of both reactive and nonreactive NST results. The procedure and interpretation for an auscultated acceleration test are described in **Appendix 23A**. Anecdotal accounts indicate that use of low-technology techniques such as fetal movement counting and the AAT has led to appropriate management of compromised fetuses that would not otherwise have been identified as high risk by usual prenatal care services in midwifery practice.

Biophysical Profile

The BPP employs both ultrasound and NST. The ultrasound portion is an "intrauterine Apgar score" that includes observation of AFI, fetal breathing, fetal tone, and fetal movement. The NST provides the fifth component of the test. Each examined factor has a possible score of 2, for a maximum total score of 10 (**Table 23-9**). The BPP has a lower false-negative rate (0.08%) and fewer false-positive tests (40% to 50%) when compared to the CST or NST.[113,127]

Individual biophysical activities appear at different stages of fetal development. Fetal tone appears at approximately 8 gestational weeks, fetal movement at 9 gestational weeks, fetal breathing at 21 gestational weeks, and fetal heart rate reactivity by the late second trimester. The biophysical activity that appears first is also the last to disappear when acidemia is present. Thus FHR variability is first to disappear; conversely, the absence of fetal tone predicts fetal acidemia 100% of the time.

The relationship between the BPP score and fetal acidemia has been studied extensively. A fullterm fetus with a score of 8 to 10 has a risk of fetal asphyxia occurring within a week after the test of approximately 1/1000, whereas the risk of fetal asphyxia for a fetus with a score of 1 to 4 is between 91/1000 and 600/1000.[113]

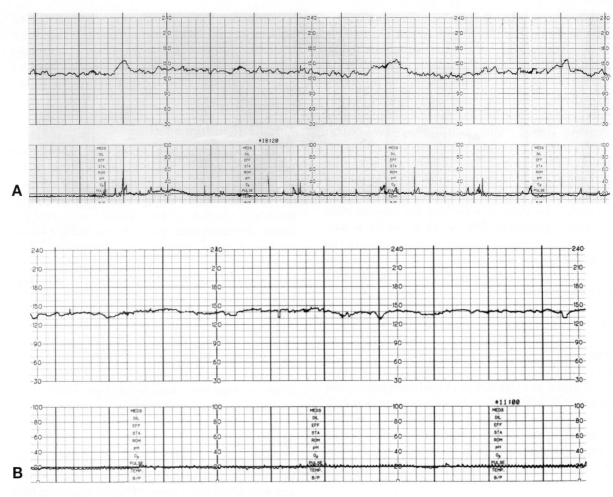

Figure 23-7 (A) Reactive nonstress test. (B) Nonreactive nonstress test.

Table 23-9	Scoring for Biophysical Profile	
Variable	**Adequate Score (Score = 2)**	**Inadequate Score (Score = 0)**
Nonstress test (NST) (reactive FHR)	2 accelerations in 20 minutes, 15 beats above baseline with duration of 15 seconds from onset to return to baseline within a 20-minute observation period	< 2 accelerations in 20 minutes
Fetal breathing movements (FBM)	1 or more episodes of FBM or ≥ 30 seconds duration in 30 minutes of observation	< 30 seconds of sustained fetal breathing movements
Fetal movements (FM)	≥ 3 discrete body/limb movements (simultaneous limb and trunk movements are considered 1 movement)	< 2 episodes of fetal movement
Fetal tone (FT)	1 episode of extension with return to flexion of fetal limb(s), trunk, or hand	Either slow extension with return to partial flexion or movement of limb in full extension or absent fetal movement
Amniotic fluid index (AFI)	< 5.0	Oligohydramnios
	5.1–8	Low normal
	8.1–24	Normal
	> 24	Polyhydramnios

Modified Biophysical Profile

The full BPP can take some time to perform. The modified BPP, composed of an NST and AFI, has similar false-negative and false-positive rates as the full BPP, and has become the most common prenatal testing conducted. Nonstress testing is the reflection of acute hypoxia and decreased amniotic fluid is considered a reflection of chronic hypoxia. The modified BPP has a predictive value similar to that of a full biophysical profile when the NST is reactive and the AFI is higher than 5.0 centimeters. If the NST is nonreactive or if the AFI is less than 5.0 centimeters, a complete BPP should be performed. If all of the ultrasound components of the BPP are reassuring, the NST is not necessary for confirmation of fetal well-being.[125]

Doppler Indices

Doppler ultrasound uses the waveform properties of arteries or veins to analyze the passage of blood through that vessel. Evaluation of the Doppler velocimetry within the umbilical arteries, fetal aorta, and middle cerebral artery are recently introduced antenatal tests used to assess placental function in women who may have a growth-restricted fetus.

Uterine Artery Doppler

The end-diastolic flow in the uterine artery normally increases with advancing gestation secondary to decreased resistance in the placenta. This occurs because more tertiary vessels develop so the pressure within the artery drops slightly. The systolic/diastolic (S/D) ratio of the umbilical artery normally decreases as gestational age increases. This development takes place secondary to the higher diastolic velocity that occurs as the number of placental villi increase. Abnormal umbilical artery Doppler studies have been consistently linked to abnormal fetal outcomes. It is estimated that no diastolic flow reflects a loss of 60% to 70% of placental vascularity. Abnormal elevation of the umbilical artery S/D ratio occurs before fetal heart rate variability decreases, which makes this assessment a useful data point when evaluating a fetus with fetal growth restriction. The rate of perinatal death is decreased when uterine artery Doppler studies are added to standard antepartum testing in the setting of FGR. Assessment of the umbilical artery S/D ratio is a standard component of care for the fetus with fetal growth restriction.[133]

Prediction of fetal risks based on umbilical artery Doppler indices may be improved with the addition of assessments of umbilical vein Doppler indices, the middle fetal cerebral artery and most recently, the ductus venosus. For example, vasodilation and high diastolic flow in the middle fetal cerebral artery reflects the "brain-sparing" response to hypoxia, although tests using this observation are still being evaluated for clinical utility. Flow through the ductus venosus is being used to assess fetal cardiac function.

Conclusion

Although midwives primarily care for women without obstetric complications, an essential component of that care is careful risk screening and early detection of complications. In addition, when a woman does have an obstetric complication, she can be significantly reassured when given accurate information and emotional support. Therefore the midwife who understands the pathophysiology; maternal, fetal, and newborn risks associated with a particular complication; and interventions and risks associated with those interventions will be best positioned to provide continuity of care and the information these women need most.

• • • References

1. Verhaegen J, Gallos ID, van Mello NM, et al. Accuracy of single progesterone test to predict early pregnancy outcome in women with pain or bleeding: meta-analysis of cohort studies. *BMJ.* 2012;345-354.

2. Thorstenson KA. Midwifery management of first trimester bleeding and early pregnancy loss. *J Midwifery Women's Health.* 2000;45:481-497.

3. Tongsong T, Srisomboon J, Wanapirak C, Sirichootiyakul S, Pongsathas S, Polsrisurthikul T. Pregnancy outcome of threatened abortion with demonstrable fetal cardiac activity: a cohort study. *J Obstet Gynecol.* 1995;21:331-335.

4. Pandya PP, Snijders R, Psara N, Hilbert L, Nicolaides K. The prevalence of nonviable pregnancy at 10–13 weeks of gestation. *Ultrasound Obstet Gynecol.* 1996; 7:170-173.

5. Evaluation of first trimester algorithm. Reproductive access.org. Available at: http://www.reproductive access.org/m_m/menu.htm. Accessed January 21, 2013.

6. Simpson JL, Janiaux ERM. Pregnancy loss. In: Gabbe SG, Niebyl JR, Galan HL, et al., eds. *Obstetrics: Normal and Problem Pregnancies,* 6th ed. New York: Churchill Livingstone; 2012:592-608.

7. Lipscomb GH, Stovall TG, Ling FW. Nonsurgical treatment of ectopic pregnancy. *N Engl J Med.* 2000; 343:1325-1329.

8. American College of Obstetricians and Gynecologists. Medical management of ectopic pregnancy.

Practice Bulletin #94. *Obstet Gynecol.* 2008;111(6): 1479-1485.

9. Monchek R, Wiedaseck S. Gestational trophoblastic disease: an overview. *J Midwifery Women's Health.* 2012;57:255-259.

10. American College of Obstetricians and Gynecologists. Diagnosis and treatment of gestational trophoblastic disease. ACOG Practice Bulletin. *Obstet Gynecol.* 2004;103:1365-1377.

11. Hancock BW, Tidy JA. Current management of molar pregnancy. *J Reprod Med.* 2002;47(5):347-354.

12. Lacroix R, Eason E, Melzack R. Nausea and vomiting during pregnancy: a prospective study of its frequency, intensity, and patterns of change. *Am J Obstet Gynecol.* 2000;182(4):931-937.

13. Seng JS, Schrot JA, van De Ven C, Liberzon I. Service use data analysis of pre-pregnancy psychiatric and somatic diagnoses in women with hyperemesis gravidarum. *J Psychosom Obstet Gynaecol.* 2007;28(4):209-217.

14. Attard CL, Kohli MA, Coleman S, et al. The burden of illness of severe nausea and vomiting of pregnancy in the United States. *Am J Obstet Gynecol.* 2002;186(5 suppl):S220-S227.

15. Bacak SJ, Callaghan WM, Dietz PM, Crouse C. Pregnancy-associated hospitalizations in the United States, 1999–2000. *Am J Obstet Gynecol.* 2005; 192(2):592-597.

16. King TL, Murphy PA. Evidence-based approaches to managing nausea and vomiting in early pregnancy. *J Midwifery Women's Health.* 2009;54(6):430-444.

17. Buckwalter JG, Simpson SW. Psychological factors in the etiology and treatment of severe nausea and vomiting in pregnancy. *Am J Obstet Gynecol.* 2002;186:S201-S214.

18. Poursharif B, Korst LM, Fejzo MS, MacGibbon KW, Romero R, Goodwin TM. The psychosocial burden of hyperemesis gravidarum. *J Perinatol.* 2008;28(3): 176-181.

19. Dodds L, Fell DB, Joseph KS, Allen VM, Butler B. Outcomes of pregnancies complicated by hyperemesis gravidarum. *Obstet Gynecol.* 2006;107(2 Pt 1): 2876-2892.

20. Zara G, Codemo V, Palmieri A, et al. Neurological complications in hyperemesis gravidarum. *Neuro Sci.* 2012;33(1):133-135.

21. American College of Nurse-Midwives, Division of Standards and Practice, Task Force for Midwives' Performance of Ultrasound. Midwives' performance of ultrasound in clinical practice. Available at: http://www.midwife.org/ACNM/files/ACNMLibraryData/UPLOADFILENAME/000000000228/Ultrasound%20position%20statement%20June%202012.pdf. Accessed June 25, 2013.

22. Yagel S, Cohen SM, Rosenak D, et al. Added value of three-/four dimensional ultrasound in offline analysis and diagnosis of congenital heart disease. *Ultrasound Obstet Gynecol.* 2011;37:432-437.

23. American College of Obstetricians and Gynecologists. Ultrasonography in pregnancy. ACOG Practice Bulletin, Number 101. *Obstet Gynecol.* 2009;113(2 Pt 1):451-461.

24. Zafar HM, Ankola A, Coleman B. Ultrasound pitfalls and artifacts related to six common fetal findings. *Ultrasound Q.* 2012;28(2):105-125.

25. Dagklis T, Plasencia W, Maiz N, Duarte L, Nicolaides KH. Choroid plexus cyst, intracardiac echogenic focus, hyperechogenic bowel and hydronephrosis in screening for trisomy 21 at 11+0 to 13+6 weeks. *Ultrasound Obstet Gynecol.* 2008;31:132-135.

26. Viaux-Savelon S, Dommergues M, Rosenblum O, et al. Prenatal ultrasound screening: false positive soft markers may alter maternal representations and mother–infant interaction. *PLoS One.* January 23, 2012;7(1).

27. Slager J, Lynne S. Assessment of cervical length and the relationship between short cervix and preterm birth. *J Midwifery Women's Health.* 2012;57:S4-S11.

28. Berghella V, Roman A, Daskalakis C, et al. Gestational age at cervical length measurement and incidence of preterm birth. *Obstet Gynecol.* 2007;110:311-317.

29. American College of Nurse-Midwives. *Position Statement: Prevention of Preterm Labor and Preterm Birth.* Approved by the ACNM Board of Directors, June 2012.

30. Hassan SS, Romero R, Vidyadhari D, et al., for the PREGNANT Trial. Vaginal progesterone reduces the rate of preterm birth in women with a sonographic short cervix: a multicenter, randomized, double-blind, placebo-controlled trial. *Ultrasound Obstet Gynecol.* 2011;38:18-31.

31. Berghalla V, Mackeen AD. Cervical length screening with ultrasound-indicated cerclage compared with history-indicated cerclage for prevention of preterm birth. *Obstet Gynecol.* 2011;118(1):148-155.

32. March of Dimes Birth Defects Foundation. PeriStats. Updated January 2009. Available at: www.marchofdimes.com/peristats. Accessed January 22, 2013.

33. Williamson DM, Abe K, Bean C, Ferré C, Henderson Z, Lackritz E. Report from the CDC: current research in preterm birth. *J Women's Health.* 2008; 17(10):1545-1549.

34. American College of Obstetricians and Gynecologists. Prediction and prevention of preterm birth. Practice Bulletin No. 130. *Obstet Gynecol.* 2012;120: 964-973.

35. Martin JA, Hamilton BE, Ventura SJ, Osterman MHS, Wilson EC, Mathews TJ. Births: final data for 2010. *Nat Vital Stat Rep.* 2012;61(1):13.

36. Mathews, TF, MacDorman MF. *Infant Mortality Statistics from the 2008 Period Linked Birth/Infant Death Data Set. National Vital Statistics Reports,* Vol. 60(5). Hyattsville, MD: National Center for Health Statistics; 2012.

37. Kramer MS, Demissie K, Yang H, Platt RW, Sauvé R, Liston R, for the Fetal and Infant Health Study Group of the Canadian Perinatal Surveillance System. The contribution of mild and moderate preterm birth to infant mortality. *JAMA.* 2000;284:843-849.

38. Callaghan WM, MacDorman MF, Rasmussen SA, Qin C, Lackritz EM. The contribution of preterm birth to infant mortality rates in the United States. *Pediatrics.* 2006;118:1566-1573.

39. Institute of Medicine of the National Academies. Preterm birth: causes, consequences, and prevention. 2006. Available at: http://www.iom.edu/CMS/3740/25471/35813.aspx. Accessed June 13, 2013.

40. Swarmy GK, Ostbye T, Skaerven R. Association of preterm birth with long-term survival, reproduction, and the next-generation preterm birth. *JAMA.* 2008;299:1429-1436.

41. Mercer BM, Goldenberg RL, Das A, et al. The preterm prediction study: a clinical risk assessment system. *Am J Obstet Gynecol.* 1996;174:1885-1893.

42. Iams JD, Goldenberg RL, Mercer BM, et al. The Preterm Prediction Study: can low risk women destined for spontaneous preterm birth be identified? *Am J Obstet Gynecol.* 2001;184:652-655.

43. Muglia LJ. The enigma of spontaneous preterm birth. *N Engl J Med.* 2010;362:529-535.

44. McManemy J, Cooke E, Amon E, Leet T. Recurrence risk for preterm delivery. *Am J Obstet Gynecol.* 2007; 196:576.

45. Dekker GA, Lee SY, North RA, et al. Risk factors for a preterm birth in an international prospective cohort of nulliparous women. *PLoS One.* 2012;7(7);e39154.

46. Ward K, Argyle VA, Meade M, Nelson L. The heritability of preterm delivery. *Obstet Gynecol.* 2005;106(6):1235-1239.

47. Parry S, Himhan H, Elovitz M, Iams J. Universal maternal cervical length screening during the second trimester: pros and cons of a strategy to identify women at risk of spontaneous preterm birth. *Am J Obstet Gynecol.* 2012;207(2):101-106.

48. Chen K, Chen SF, Chang H, et al. No increased risk of adverse pregnancy outcomes in women with urinary tract infections: a nationwide population-based study. *Acta Obstet Scan.* 2010;89(7):882-888.

49. Manns-James L. Bacterial vaginosis and preterm birth. *J Midwifery Women's Health.* 2011;56(6):575-583.

50. Goldenberg RL, Mercer BM, Meis PJ, et al. The Preterm Prediction Study: fetal fibronectin testing and spontaneous preterm birth. *Obstet Gynecol.* 1996; 87:643-648.

51. Peaceman AM, Andrews WW, Thorp JM, et al. Fetal fibronectin as a predictor of preterm birth in patients with symptoms: a multicenter trial. *Am J Obstet Gynecol.* 1997;177:13-18.

52. American College of Obstetricians and Gynecologists. Prediction and prevention of preterm birth. Practice Bulletin No. 130. *Obstet Gynecol.* 2012;120: 964-973.

53. Bolt LA, Chandiramani M, De Greeff A, Seed PT, Durtzman J, Shennan AH. The value of combined cervical length measurement and fetal fibronectin testing to predict spontaneous preterm birth is asymptomatic high-risk women. *J Matern Fetal Neonatal Med.* 2010:24(7);928-932.

54. Sfakianaki AK, Norwitz ER. Mechanisms of progesterone action in inhibiting prematurity. *J Matern Fetal Neonatal Med.* 2005;19:763-772.

55. Zakar T, Hertelendy F. Progesterone withdrawal: key to parturition. *Am J Obstet Gynecol.* 2007;196: 289-290.

56. Northern AT, Norman GS, Anderson K, et al., for the National Institute of Child Health and Human Development (NICHD) Maternal–Fetal Medicine Units (MFMU). Network follow-up of children exposed in utero to 17α-hydroxyprogesterone caproate compared with placebo. *Obstet Gynecol.* 2007; 110:865-872.

57. Rebarber A, Ferrara LA, Hanley ML, et al. Increased recurrence of preterm delivery with early cessation of 17 alpha hydroxyprogesterone caproate. *Am J Obstet Gynecol.* 2007;196:224.e 1-4.

58. Likis FE, Andrews JC, Woodworth AL, et al. *Progestogens for Prevention of Preterm Birth.* Comparative Effectiveness Review No. 74. (Prepared by the Vanderbilt Evidence-based Practice Center under Contract No. 290-2007-10065-I). AHRQ Publication No. 12-EHC105-EF. Rockville, MD: Agency for Healthcare Research and Quality; September 2012. Available at: http://www.effectivehealthcare.ahrq.gov/reports/final.cfm. Accessed June 13, 2013.

59. Lim AD, Schuit E, Bloemenkamp K, et al. 17α-Hydroxyprogesterone caproate for the prevention of adverse neonatal outcome in multiple pregnancies: a randomized controlled trial. *Obstet Gynecol.* 2011;118(3):513-520.

60. Fonseca EB, Celik E, Parra M, Singh M, Nicolaides KH. Progesterone and the risk of preterm birth among women with a short cervix. *N Engl J Med.* 2007;357:462-469.

61. American College of Nurse-Midwives. Induction of labor: position statement. September 2010. Available at: http://www.midwife.org/documents/Induction_of_Labor.pdf. Accessed January 22, 2013.

62. Green N, Ryan C, Shusterman L. Understanding pregnant women's perspectives of preterm birth. *Contemp Obstet Gynecol.* 2003;48(1):70-87.

63. American College of Obstetricians and Gynecologists. Gestational diabetes. ACOG Practice Bulletin No. 30. *Obstet Gynecol.* 2001;98:525-538.

64. Coustan DR. Gestational diabetes. In: National Institutes of Diabetes and Digestive and Kidney Diseases. *Diabetes in America.* 2nd ed. NIG Publication No. 95:1468. Bethesda, MD: National Institutes of Health; 1995:703-717.

65. Kitzmiller J, Dang-Kilduff L, Tasumi MM. Gestational diabetes after delivery. *Diab Care.* 2007;30(suppl 2):S225-S230.

66. Reedy NJ, King TL. Diabetes. In King TL, Brucker MC, eds. *Pharmacology for Women's Health.* Sudbury MA: Jones and Bartlett; 2011:530.

67. Boyd KL, Ross EK, Sherman SJ. Jelly beans as an alternative to a cola beverage containing fifty grams of glucose. *Am J Obstet Gynecol.* 1995;173(6):1889-1892.

68. Lamar ME, Kuehl TJ, Cooney AT, Gayle LJ, Holleman S, Allen SR. Jelly beans as an alternative to a fifty-gram glucose beverage for gestational diabetes screening. *Am J Obstet Gynecol.* 1999;181(5 Pt 1):1154-1157.

69. Danilenko-Dixon DR, Van Winter JT, Nelson RL, Ogburn PL Jr. Universal versus selective gestational diabetes screening: application of 1997 American Diabetes Association recommendations. *Am J Obstet Gynecol.* 1999;181:798-802.

70. Langer O, Umans JG, Miodovnik M. Perspectives on the proposed gestational diabetes mellitus diagnostic criteria. *Obstet Gynecol.* 2013;121(1):117-182.

71. International Association of Diabetes and Pregnancy Study Groups Consensus Panel, Metzger BE, Gabbe SG, et al. International Association of Diabetes and Pregnancy Study Groups recommendations on the diagnosis and classification of hyperglycemia in pregnancy. *Diab Care.* 2010;33:676.

72. American College of Obstetricians and Gynecologists. Postpartum screening for abnormal glucose tolerance in women who had gestational diabetes mellitus. ACOG Committee Opinion No 435. *Obstet Gynecol.* 2009;113:1419-1421.

73. Gagnon R, Morin L, Bly S, Butt K, Cargill YM, Denis N. Guidelines for the management of vasa previa. *J Obstet Gynaecol Can.* 2009;8:748-760.

74. Rosenberg T, Pariente G, Sergienko R, Wiznitzer A, Sheiner E. Critical analysis of risk factors and outcomes of placenta previa. *Arch Gynecol Obstet.* 2011:284(1):47-51.

75. Takemura Y, Osuga Y, Fujimoto A, et al. Increased risk of placenta previa is associated with endometriosis and tubal factor infertility in ART pregnancy. *Gynecol Endocrin.* 2013;29(2):113-115.

76. Clark SL. Placenta previa and abruptio placentae. In: Creasy RK, Reznik R, Iams J, eds. *Maternal Fetal Medicine,* 5th ed. Philadelphia, PA: W. B. Saunders; 2004:715.

77. Silver RM, Landon MB, Rouse DJ, et al. National Institute of Child Health and Human Development Maternal Fetal Medicine Units Network. Maternal morbidity associated with multiple repeat cesarean deliveries. *Obstet Gynecol.* 2006;107:1226-1232.

78. Towers CV, Pircon RA, Heppard M. Is tocolysis safe in the management of third trimester bleeding? *Am J Obstet Gynecol.* 1999;180(6):1572-1578.

79. Berg CJ, Callaghan WM, Syverson C, Henderson A. Pregnancy-related mortality in the United States, 1998 to 2005. *Obstet Gynecol.* 2010;116(6);1302-1309.

80. Report of the National High Blood Pressure Education Program Working Group on High Blood Pressure in Pregnancy. *Am J Obstet Gynecol.* 2000;183:S1-S22.

81. Leeman L, Fontaine P. Hypertensive disorders of pregnancy. *Am Fam Physician.* 2008;78(1):93-100.

82. Sharma S, Noris WE, Kalkunte S. Beyond the threshold: an etiological bridge between hypoxia and immunity in preeclampsia. *J Reprod Immunol.* 2010;85:112-116.

83. Chesley LC. Diagnosis of preeclampsia. *Obstet Gynecol.* 1985;65:423-430.

84. Conde-Agudelo A, Romero R, Kusanovic JP, Hassan SS. Supplementation with vitamins C and E during pregnancy for the prevention of preeclampsia and other adverse maternal and perinatal outcomes: a systematic review and metaanalysis. *Am J Obstet Gynecol.* 2011;204(6):503 e1-12.

85. Sibai BM. Diagnosis, controversies, and management of the syndrome of hemolysis, elevated liver enzymes, and low platelet count. *Obstet Gynecol.* 2004;103:981.

86. American College of Obstetricians and Gynecologists. *Intrauterine Growth Restriction.* Clinical Bulletin No. 12. January 2000.

87. Morrison I, Olsen J. Weight-specific stillbirths and associated causes of death: an analysis of 765 stillbirths. *Am J Obstet Gynecol.* 1985;152:975-980.

88. Nardozza LM, Araujo E, Barbosa MM, Caetano ACR, Lee DJR, Moron AF. Fetal growth restriction: current knowledge to the general Obs/Gyn. *Arch Gynecol Obstet.* 2012;286:1-13.

89. Engstrom JL, Work BA. Prenatal prediction of small and large-for-gestational age neonates. *JOGNN.* 1993;21(6):486-495.

90. Morse K, Williams A, Gardosi J. Fetal growth screening by fundal height measurement. *Best Pract Res Clin Obstet Gynecol.* 2009;23:809-819.

91. Magann EF, Chauhan SP, Doherty DA, et al. A review of idiopathic hydramnios and pregnancy outcomes. *Obstet Gynecol Surv.* 2007;62;795-802.

92. Martinez-Frias ML, Bermejo E, Rodriguez-Pinilla E, Frias JL. Maternal and fetal factors related to abnormal amniotic fluid. *J Perinatol.* 1999;19(7):514-520.

93. American College of Obstetricians and Gynecologists. Ultrasonography in pregnancy. ACOG Practice Bulletin No. 101. *Obstet Gynecol.* 2009;113:451-461. Reaffirmed 2011.

94. Magaan E, Sanderson M, Martin J, Chauhan S. The amniotic fluid index, single deepest pocket and two-diameter pocket in normal human pregnancy. *Am J Obstet Gynecol.* 2000;182:1581-1588.

95. Haws RA, Yakoob MY, Soomro T, Menezes EV, Darmstadt GL, Bhutta ZA. Reducing stillbirths: screening and monitoring during pregnancy and labour. *BMC Pregnancy Childbirth.* 2009;9(suppl 1):S5.

96. Petrozella LN, Dashe JS, McIntire DD, Leveno KL. Clinical significance of borderline amniotic fluid index and oligohydramnios in preterm pregnancy. *Obstet Gynecol.* 2011;117(2):338-342.

97. Larmon JE, Ross BS. Clinical utility of amniotic fluid volume assessment. *Obstet Gynecol Clin North Am.* 1998;25(3):639-661.

98. Borges VT, Rososchansky J, Abbade JF, Dias A, Peraçoli JC, Rudge MV. Effect of maternal hydration on the increase of amniotic fluid index. *Braz J Med Biol Res.* 2011;44(3):263-266.

99. Patrelli TS, Gizzo S, Cosmi E, et al. Maternal hydration therapy improves the quality of amniotic fluid and the pregnancy outcome in third trimester isolated oligohydramnios: a controlled randomized institutional trial. *J Ultrasound Med.* 2012;31(2):239-244.

100. Magann EE, Kinsella MJ, Chauhan SP, McNamara MF. Gehring BW, Morrison, JC. Does an amniotic fluid index of ≤ 5 cm necessitate delivery in high-risk pregnancies? A case-controlled study. *Am J Obstet Gynecol.* 1999;180:1354-1359.

101. Nabhan AF, Abdelmoula YA. Amniotic fluid index versus single deepest vertical pocket as a screening test for preventing adverse pregnancy outcome. *Cochrane Database Syst Rev.* 2008;3:CD006593. doi: 10.1002/14651858.CD006593.pub2.

102. American College of Obstetricians and Gynecologists. *Multiple Gestation: Complicated Twin, Triplet, and High-Order Multifetal Pregnancy.* ACOG Clinical Practice Bulletin No. 56. October 2004.

103. Wright VC, Chang J, Jeng G, Chen M, Macaluso M. Assisted reproductive technology surveillance—United States, 2004. *MMWR Surveill Summ.* 2007;56(6):1-22.

104. Chervanak F, McCullough LB. Responsibly counseling women about the clinical management of pregnancies complicated by severe fetal anomalies. *J Med Ethics.* 2012;38(7):397-398.

105. National Center for Health Statistics. *Model State Vital Statistics Act and Regulations: 1992 Revisions.* Hyattsville, MD: NCHS; 1994. Available at: http://www.cdc.gov/nchs/data/misc/mvsact92h.pdf. Accessed January 22, 2013.

106. MacDorman MF, Kirmeyer SE, Wilson EC. *Fetal and Perinatal Mortality, United States, 2006. National Vital Statistics Reports,* Vol. 60, no. 8. Hyattsville, MD: National Center for Health Statistics; 2012.

107. Stillbirth Collaborative Research Network Writing Group. Causes of death among stillbirths. *JAMA.* 2011;306(22):2459-2468.

108. Maslow AD, Breen TW, Sarna MC, et al. Prevalence of coagulation abnormalities associated with intrauterine fetal death. *Can J Anaesth.* 1996;43:1237.

109. World Health Organization. Management of pregnancy, childbirth and the postpartum period in the presence of female genital mutilation: report of WHO Technical Consultation. Geneva, Switzerland, October 15–17, 1997. Available at: http://www.who.int/reproductivehealth/publications/maternal_perinatal_health/RHR_01_13_/en/index.html. Accessed January 22, 2013.

110. Nour NM. Female genital cutting: clinical and cultural guidelines. *Obstet Gynecol Surv.* 2004;59(4):272-279.

111. Brady CM, Files JA. Female genital mutilation: cultural awareness and clinical considerations. *J Midwifery Women's Health.* 2007;42:154-163, 160.

112. Toubia N. *Caring for Women with Circumcision: A Technical Manual for Health Care Providers.* New York: Research, Action and Information Network for the Bodily Integrity of Women (RAINBO); 1999.

113. Oyelese Y, Vintzileos. The use and limitations of the fetal biophysical profile. *Clin Perinatol.* 2011;38:47-64.

114. Manning FA. Antepartum fetal testing: a critical appraisal. *Curr Opin Obstet Gynecol.* 2009;21:348-352.

115. Miller D, Rabello Y, Paul R. The modified biophysical profile: antepartum testing in the 1990's. *Am J Obstet Gynecol.* 1996;174:812-817.

116. Devoe LD. Antenatal fetal assessment: contraction stress test, nonstress test, vibroacoustic stimulation, amniotic fluid volume, biophysical profile, and modified biophysical profile: an overview. *Semin Perinatol.* 2008;32:247-252.

117. Hijazi ZR, East CE. Factors affecting maternal perception of fetal movement. *Obstet Gynecol Surv.* 2009;64:489-494.

118. Fretts RC, Boyd ME, Usher RH, Usher HA. The changing pattern of fetal death 1961–1988. *Obstet Gynecol.* 1992;79(1):35-39.

119. Richardson BS. Fetal adaptive responses to asphyxia. *Clin Perinatol.* 1989;16:595-611.

120. Neldam S. Fetal movement as an indicator of fetal wellbeing. *Lancet.* 1980;315(8180):1222-1224.

121. Froen JF, Haezell AE, Tveit JV, et al. Fetal movement assessment. *Semin Perinatol.* 2008;32:243-246.

122. Grant A, Elbourne D, Valentin L, Alexander S. Routine formal fetal movement counting and risk of antepartum late death in normally formed singletons. *Lancet.* 1989;2:345-349.

123. Grant A, Elbourne D, Valentin L, Alexander S. Routine formal fetal movement counting and risk of antepartum late death in normally formed singletons. *Lancet.* 1989;2:345–349.

124. Saastad E, Winje BA, Perdersen BS, Froen JF. Fetal movement counting improved identification of fetal growth restriction and perinatal outcomes: a multicentre, randomized, controlled trial. *PLoS One.* 2011;6(12):e28482.

125. ACOG Practice Bulletin. Antepartum fetal surveillance. Number 9, October 1999. *Int J Gynaecol Obstet.* 2000;68(2):175-185.

126. Saastad E, Winje BA, Israel P, Foren JF. Fetal movement counting: maternal concern and experiences: a multicenter, randomized controlled trial. *Birth.* 2012;39(1):10-20.

127. Signore C, Freeman RK, Spong CY. Antenatal testing: a reevaluation. Executive summary of a Eunice Kennedy Shriver National Institute of Child Health and Human Development Workshop. *Obstet Gynecol.* 2009;113(3):687-701.

128. Tan KH, Sabapathy A. Maternal glucose administration for facilitating tests of fetal wellbeing. *Cochrane Database Syst Rev.* 2012;9:CD003397. doi: 10.1002/14651858.CD003397.pub2.

129. Gegor CL, Paine LL, Johnson TRB. Antepartum fetal assessment: a nurse-midwifery perspective. *J Nurse-Midwifery.* 1991;36(3):153-167.

130. Paine LL, Payton RG, Johnson TRB. Auscultated fetal heart rate accelerations: Part I. Accuracy and documentation. *J Nurse-Midwifery.* 1986;31(2):68-72.

131. Paine LL, Johnson TR, Turner MH, et al. Auscultated fetal heart rate accelerations: Part II. An alternative to the nonstress test. *J Nurse-Midwifery.* 1989;31(2):73-77.

132. Paine LL, Benedict MI, Strobino DM, et al. A comparison of the auscultated acceleration test and the nonstress test as predictors of perinatal outcomes. *Nurs Res.* 1992;41(2):87-91.

133. American College of Obstetricians and Gynecologists. *Intrauterine Growth Restriction.* ACOG Practice Bulletin 12. Washington, DC: ACOG; 2000.

APPENDIX

23A

Auscultated Acceleration Test

The auscultated acceleration test (AAT) is used to detect fetal accelerations via a specific counting method via use of an Allen or Doppler fetoscope.[1] The procedure for conducting an AAT should be performed by two clinicians; one auscultates and reports the fetal heart rate (FHR) count, and the other records the findings.[2–6]

Background

FHR accelerations of 15 bpm or more above the baseline that last for 15 seconds or more from onset to return to the baseline are a reliable indicator of fetal oxygenation. When two accelerations are noted in a 20-minute FHR recording, the chance of stillbirth within the next 7 days is less than 1% (the false-negative rate is 0.3%).[7]

Mendenhall et al. evaluated the efficacy of a single acceleration (n =1005 AAT tests, 367 women) and found the single acceleration was associated with no perinatal losses. The nonreactive AAT in this series predicted the 4 stillbirths that occurred in the cohort.[8] Other authors have shown that a clinician listening to a FHR recording will detect 77.7% of all FHR accelerations that are 15 bpm or more above baseline and 94% of the nonreactive FHR recordings.[9]

In settings where electronic fetal monitoring is not available or chosen for use, the AAT is a reliable and valid method of detecting fetal accelerations.

Procedure

- Place the woman in a semirecumbent comfortable position.

- Auscultate the FHR for a maximum of 6 minutes.

- Count every other 5-second interval.

- Record each 5-second count on the AAT graph (**Figure 23A-1** and **Figure 23A-2**).

- If an acceleration of 2 bpm in a 5-second counting interval is noted in conjunction with fetal movement (FM), the test can be stopped.

- If no acceleration is noted after 3 minutes, the maternal abdomen can be gently shaken in an attempt to waken the fetus or elicit a more active state. The clinician grasps the fetal head and buttocks and slowly moves the fetus slightly from side to side in a gentle shaking motion for 5 seconds.

- The FHR auscultation procedure is again repeated for a maximum of 2 to 3 minutes.

- Identify baseline FHR and any accelerations by plotting the numbers obtained on the AAT chart (Figures 23A-1 and 23A-2).

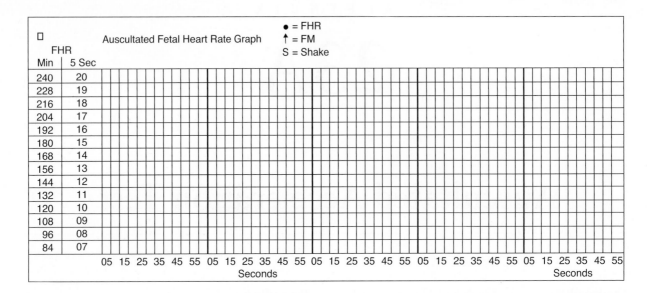

Figure 23A-1 The AAT graph used to document the FHR pattern.

Source: Adapted with permission of Lisa L. Paine from Paine LL, Payton RG, Johnson TR. Auscultated fetal heart rate and accelerations. Part I. *J Nurs Midwifery*. 1986;31(2):68-72.

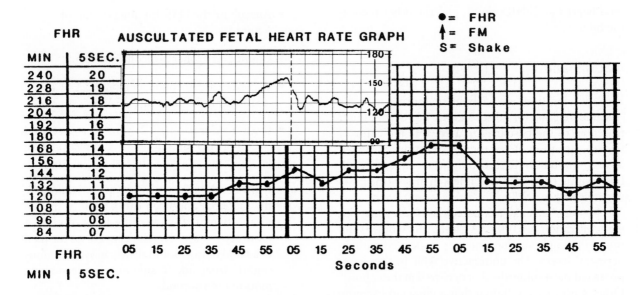

Figure 23A-2 AAT with inset of a nonstress test completed simultaneously.

Source: Reprinted with permission of Lisa L. Paine, who first developed the AAT with colleagues at Malcolm Grow Medical Center, Andrews AFB, Maryland and later studied its validity and refinement at the Johns Hopkins Hospital in Baltimore, Maryland with funding from the NIH National Center for Nursing Research Grant No. R-01-NR-01705-01.

Interpretation

Reactive nonstress test (NST)

- An acceleration is present when the FHR is up by two grid points (2 bpm in a 5-second period).
- A single FHR acceleration indicates reactivity.[8]

Unsatisfactory

- No acceleration and no fetal movement after fetal stimulation are noted.

Nonreactive

- No accelerations are noted.

References

1. Gegor CL, Paine LL, Johnson TRB. Antepartum fetal assessment: a nurse-midwifery perspective. *J Nurse-Midwifery.* 1991;36(3):153-167.

2. Paine LL, Payton RG, Johnson TRB. Auscultated fetal heart rate accelerations: Part I. Accuracy and documentation. *J Nurse-Midwifery.* 1986;31(2):68-72.

3. Paine LL, Johnson TR, Turner MH, et al. Auscultated fetal heart rate accelerations: Part II. An alternative to the nonstress test. *J Nurse-Midwifery.* 1989;31(2):73-77.

4. Paine LL, Benedict MI, Strobino DM, Gegor CL, Larson EL. A comparison of the auscultated acceleration test and the nonstress test as predictors of perinatal outcomes. *Nurs Res.* 1992;41(2):87-91.

5. Daniels SM, Boehm N. Auscultated fetal heart rate accelerations: an alternative to the nonstress test. *J Nurse-Midwifery.* 1991;36(2):88-94.

6. Paine LL, Zanardi RL, Johnson TR, Rorie JA, Barger MK. A comparison of two time intervals for the auscultated acceleration test. *J Midwifery Women's Health.* 2001;46(2):98-102.

7. Signore C, Freeman RK, Spong CY. Antenatal testing: a reevaluation. Executive summary of a Eunice Kennedy Shriver National Institute of Child Health and Human Development Workshop. *Obstet Gynecol.* 2009;113(3):687-701.

8. Mendenhall HW, O'Leary J, Phillips K. The nonstress test: the value of a single acceleration in evaluating the fetus at risk. *Am J Obstet Gynecol.* 1980;136:87:244-246.

9. Baskett TF, Boyce CD, Lohre MA, Manning FA. Simplified antepartum fetal heart assessment. *Br J Obstet Gynaecol.* 1981;88(4):395-397.

C H A P T E R

24

Medical Complications in Pregnancy

JAN M. KRIEBS

The anatomic, physiologic, and hormonal changes of pregnancy affect the course of many preexisting medical conditions. This chapter primarily addresses those complications of pregnancy related to underlying medical disorders. Most have already been discussed in the *Common Conditions in Primary Care* chapter, which can be referred to for basic information. Some dermatologic conditions are included in this chapter that are specific to pregnancy. Health care is not tidy: Women's needs overlap, with one or another taking precedence at any one time. The same is true for the division of material in this book—hence the reader will find reference to some of the conditions reviewed here in several other chapters of this text.

In addition to the needs of women varying, midwives currently practice in a wide variety of settings. Historically midwifery practices were more restricted and women with medical conditions were referred to another healthcare provider, usually an obstetrician or maternal–fetal medicine specialist. This referral often was characterized as transfer to "medical management" and the midwife might never care for that woman again. Today many midwives work in interdisciplinary teams wherein each member has skills and expertise in different aspects of obstetric care. Thus when a woman has a medical condition that would previously have necessitated her transferring from midwifery to physician care, today, she may continue to see her midwife who will provide the midwifery aspects of care and health education that she needs. Woman-centered care should use the best providers for the best care. This caveat should be kept in mind as the reader considers the information in this chapter. Because of the variations in needs of

the woman, the severity of the disease, composition of a team, or accessibility to resources, it would be simplistic to say that all women with a particular condition warrants a consultation, collaboration, or she should be referred to be under "medical management." Midwives need to recognize basics of diagnosis and treatment for the conditions in this chapter so that women-centered care can be promoted and that whenever possible, a woman still can have a midwife for care.

Hematologic Disorders in Pregnancy

Hematologic disorders encompass a broad category of conditions that range from asymptomatic genetic traits to severe illness. Women with hematologic disorders are at increased risk for adverse obstetric outcomes. Although many women with known disorders become pregnant, others may receive the initial diagnosis of a hematologic condition during pregnancy.

Anemia

Anemia is by far the most common hematologic condition seen in pregnant women and is often presumptively treated as iron-deficiency anemia. In reality, anemia may be an outcome of a number of underlying disorders, some of which should not be treated with iron.

Anemia in pregnancy is defined as a hemoglobin level of less than 11 g/dL in the first and third trimesters and less than 10.5 g/dL in the second trimester. This condition is always an indication for further evaluation until the cause has been diagnosed.

Anemia can be caused by (1) decreased production of red blood cells, (2) increased destruction of red blood cells, or (3) blood loss, which can be either acute or chronic. Decreased production of red blood cells most often occurs secondary to a deficiency of iron, folate, or vitamin B_{12}. Physiologic anemia of pregnancy and iron deficiency during pregnancy are reviewed in the *Prenatal Care* chapter. Folate deficiency is rare in the United States, because many foods are fortified with folate. Vitamin B_{12} deficiency can develop among women who follow a vegan diet.

Increased destruction of red blood cells can occur during infection. Although not common in the United States, this cause of anemia is well known in developing nations that have high rates of malaria and other chronic infections. Anemia secondary to heavy bleeding with menses is a more common initiating reason for anemia during pregnancy in women who reside in the United States.

The evaluation of anemia is based on the size of the red blood cells (microcytic, macrocytic, or normocytic). Mild to moderate maternal anemia is not associated with fetal injury. In contrast, severe maternal anemia is associated with abnormal placentation and decreased fetal oxygenation. Regardless of the cause of anemia during pregnancy, maternal blood transfusion is restricted to women with severe anemia (defined as a hemoglobin level less than 6 mg/L).[1]

Hemoglobinopathies: Sickle Cell Disease and the Thalassemias

Individuals who are clinically affected by a hemoglobinopathy or thalassemia will have received medical care for the disorder prior to pregnancy; these individuals will need careful obstetric management during pregnancy. In contrast, women who are asymptomatic carriers for a variant hemoglobin type may not be aware that they have an abnormal hemoglobin prior to pregnancy. The initial diagnosis of hemoglobinopathy or thalassemia trait in pregnancy is important for two reasons. First, these disorders are genetically inherited. If the woman and her partner are both heterozygous asymptomatic carriers, the fetus could be homozygous and have severe disease; thus genetic counseling will be needed. Second, abnormal hemoglobin, even in asymptomatic individuals, can increase the risk for some pregnancy complications.

Recommended screening for hemoglobinopathies and thalassemia is presented in **Figure 24-1**. Standard genetic/inherited risk factor histories taken in pregnancy include questioning about known family history of sickle cell trait or disease and history of thalassemias. Many women will be unaware of the associations of ethnicity and these disorders, or may be unaware of family history details. When in doubt, additional questions or testing should be conducted.

Sickle Cell Disease

All persons of African ancestry should have a hemoglobin electrophoresis to screen for sickle cell disease or trait if such testing has not been performed prior to pregnancy. If the woman has sickle cell disease or sickle cell trait, screening of the partner is recommended, along with genetic counseling, to determine inheritance patterns and the chance that the fetus will have the trait or disease. Sickle cell is an autosomal recessive inheritance pattern. Thus, if the woman has sickle cell trait and her partner does not, there is a 50% chance in each pregnancy that her fetus will have the trait. If she and her partner both have sickle cell trait, there is a 25% chance the fetus will have sickle cell disease and a 50% chance the fetus will have sickle cell trait.

Sickle cell disease is associated with hemolytic anemia and multiorgan dysfunction secondary to microvascular obstruction by red blood cell agglutination. Women with sickle cell disease can accumulate iron and become iron overloaded despite having microcytic anemia. Women with sickle cell disease have an increased risk for sickle cell crisis, spontaneous abortion, preterm labor, preeclampsia, stillbirth, fetal growth restriction, prematurity, and low birth weight.[2,3]

Women with sickle cell trait have an increased risk for urinary tract infections during pregnancy. Additionally, iron does not accumulate, so these women can become iron deficient in pregnancy and need iron supplementation.

Thalassemias

Pregnant women who are of Southeast Asian or Mediterranean descent should be screened for thalassemia if they are have anemia, normal iron indices, and a low mean corpuscular volume (MCV). Partner testing and genetic counseling are indicated if beta or alpha thalassemia trait is identified.

Women with beta thalassemia intermedia or major have an increased risk of diabetes and cardiovascular disease during pregnancy. Homogeneous alpha thalassemia is associated with nonimmune fetal hydrops and intrauterine fetal death. Women with beta thalassemia minor appear to have uncomplicated pregnancies, although increased risks for oligohydramnios and fetal growth restriction have been reported.[4] Fetal evaluation for growth and well-being with serial sonography and fetal testing is recommended although there is no clear consensus on how often.

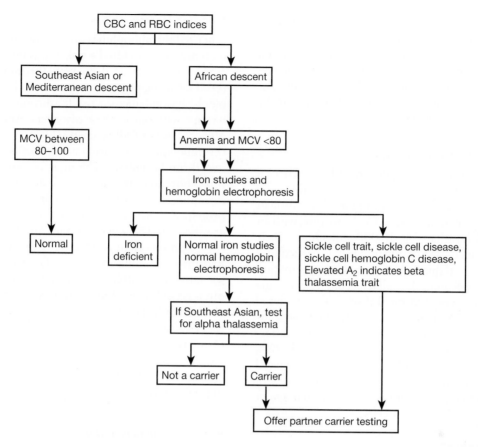

Figure 24-1 Screening for hemoglobinopathies.

G6PD Deficiency

During pregnancy, women who report a personal or family history consistent with G6PD deficiency should be screened. The primary maternal risk associated with G6PD deficiency is the inadvertent use of medications such as nitrofurantoin (Macrobid, Macrodantin) and sulfa derivatives (including Bactrim), which cause hemolysis. Hemolysis as a result of infection or surgery can also occur. Neonatal hemolysis from inherited G6PD deficiency can lead to severe jaundice and kernicterus. Therefore, at the time of birth neonatal providers should be aware of maternal or paternal family history consistent with G6PD deficiency.

Thrombocytopenia

Thrombocytopenia is commonly defined as a platelet count less than 150,000/µL. Causes of low platelet counts during pregnancy include gestational thrombocytopenia, immune thrombocytopenia, thrombotic macroangiopathy, autoimmune disease, drugs, preeclampsia, HELLP syndrome, and other less common conditions. Gestational thrombocytopenia is a form of mild thrombocytopenia that occurs late in pregnancy to a woman who does not have a history of thrombocytopenia. Gestational thrombocytopenia is not associated with fetal thrombocytopenia and is not considered clinically significant as long as the platelet count remains higher than 100,000/µL. Significant bleeding is unlikely with a platelet count higher than 50,000/µL. Regardless of the underlying cause, low platelet levels may affect access to epidural anesthesia as well as other decisions regarding childbirth, such as the use of internal fetal monitoring if there is a concern for fetal thrombocytopenia.[5]

Immune Thrombocytopenia

Immune thrombocytopenia (ITP) is uncommon in pregnancy, occurring in 1 in 1000 to 1 in 10,000 pregnant women. ITP can be a primary diagnosis or may be related to underlying viral infections or autoimmune disorders.[5] Clinical features include bruising, petechiae, and bleeding from mucous membranes.

Because antiplatelet antibodies cross the placenta, fetal thrombocytopenia can occur, although it is rare and not predictable from maternal status.

Corticosteroids are used to treat ITP albeit with caution in pregnancy, because steroids have been associated with oral–facial clefts when used in the first trimester, then glucose abnormalities, and pregnancy-induced hypertension when used later in pregnancy.[6] Neonates of women with primary ITP need to be evaluated for platelet status.

Thrombotic Thrombocytic Purpura

Thrombotic thrombocytic purpura (TTP) and hemolytic uremic syndrome are referred to as thrombotic microangiopathies (TMAs) due to the presentation of hemolysis in the small vessels. TMAs are rare, with an incidence of less than 1 in 10,000 individuals. Their incidence is increased during pregnancy, particularly in the second and third trimesters.[7] The combination of hemolytic anemia, a low platelet count, neurologic dysfunction, fever, and renal disease is considered diagnostic for TMA, although only the first two signs may be present.[5] Plasma exchange is the most effective therapy, achieving success in approximately 80% of cases when the diagnosis is made rapidly. Perinatal loss, including stillbirths, are high for women with TMAs, in large part because the gestational age at birth is often less than 30 weeks.[7]

Clotting Disorders

Antiphospholipid Syndrome

Among the various causes of abnormal blood clotting, antiphospholipid syndrome (APS) is one that is associated with adverse effects during pregnancy. APS is an autoimmune disorder in which antibodies develop to blood proteins that are bound to phospholipids, leading to formation of blood clots and increasing the risk of miscarriage and stillbirth. Women who have APS are at higher risk for miscarriage, severe early-onset preeclampsia, fetal growth abnormalities, and stillbirth. Women who have a history of thrombosis or adverse pregnancy outcomes such as multiple early miscarriages, one or more unexplained stillbirths, or a pregnancy complicated by preeclampsia or placental insufficiency prior to 34 weeks' gestation should be evaluated for APS.[8] Tests for this syndrome include immunoglobulin G (IgG) and immunoglobulin M (IgM) anticardiolipin antibodies and evidence of lupus anticoagulant activity as assessed by Russell viper venom time and activated partial thromboplastin time.

Close fetal surveillance is essential for women with APS. Heparin or low-molecular-weight heparin is prescribed to the woman during pregnancy, along with low-dose aspirin to prevent clotting.[9]

Inherited Thrombophilias

Inherited thrombophilias are genetic conditions that increase an individual's risk for venous thromboembolisms such as deep vein thromboembolism (DVT). During pregnancy, the normal hypercoagulable changes enhance the risk for thromboembolism in women with one of these disorders. Approximately 50% to 60% of all women who develop a venous thromboembolism during pregnancy have an inherited thrombophilia.[10] The most common inherited thrombophilias are factor V Leiden mutation, prothrombin gene mutation, protein S deficiency, and protein C deficiency. The inherited thrombophilias are less clearly associated with specific pregnancy complications than is APS, but women with inherited thrombophilias appear to be at increased risk for late fetal stillbirth. Antepartum fetal testing is often recommended at 36 weeks' gestation. In the absence of homozygous mutations plus family history of venous thromboembolism (VTE), close monitoring is preferred to prophylactic therapy.[9] Women who do have a history of VTE are offered anticoagulation therapy for prevention of recurrent VTE in pregnancy.

Venous Thromboembolism

DVT and pulmonary embolus (PE) are categorized as types of venous thromboembolism. VTE is four times more common in pregnant women than in nonpregnant women. DVT may occur at any time during gestation; by comparison, PE is rarer and most likely to occur in late pregnancy or during the intrapartum period. While pregnancy is always a hypercoagulable state, factors that are associated with an increased risk for VTE include age older than 35 years, African American ethnicity, obesity, smoking, and diabetes, among others.[10] Cesarean section birth also increases the risk for VTE.

The symptoms of common discomforts of advancing pregnancy may mask the symptoms of either DVT or PE, which requires that the midwife be suspicious of sudden changes or onset of severe symptoms. The symptoms of DVT include swelling, pain, and discoloration in the involved extremity. The left leg is more likely to be affected than the right leg. Dyspnea is the first sign of PE, although it also is a common symptom of pregnancy.

Compression ultrasonography followed by d-dimer testing (for thrombus) and chest X ray (for PE) is the recommended initial evaluation.[10] Physician consultation should be obtained, and referral initiated following diagnosis. The treatment for VTE is low-molecular-weight heparin throughout the remainder of the pregnancy. Women are instructed to stop therapy at the onset of labor and notify their care providers.[9] Anticoagulation is reestablished following birth for at least 6 weeks postpartum (or long enough to achieve 3 to 6 months' total therapy).[9,10] Women with lower-extremity DVT will need compression stockings during and after the birth for as long as 2 years as well as during any future pregnancy.[10] After the initial VTE, women should be counseled to inform their care provider of the history of this condition at the start of any future pregnancy so that therapy and clinical monitoring can occur. Factors that increase the risk of recurrence, such as limited mobility and obesity, may require prophylaxis in future pregnancies.

Cardiovascular Conditions: Chronic Hypertension in Pregnancy

The four hypertensive disorders that occur in pregnant women are gestational hypertension, preeclampsia–eclampsia, chronic hypertension, and preexisting hypertension with superimposed preeclampsia.[11] Gestational hypertension and preeclampsia are reviewed in the *Obstetric Complications in Pregnancy* chapter. Chronic hypertension is defined as hypertension that predates pregnancy, is diagnosed prior to 20 weeks' gestation, or first occurs later in pregnancy (gestational hypertension) and persists for more than 12 weeks postpartum. This form of hypertension affects more than 5% of all pregnant women, and its incidence can be expected to increase as the incidence of obesity increases.[11]

The diagnosis of chronic hypertension is made by the presence of a systolic blood pressure higher than 140 mm Hg or a diastolic blood pressure higher than 90 mm Hg, or by documented treatment for hypertension in a woman with normal blood pressure. Among women with underlying renal disease, proteinuria may also be present. Ideally, women with chronic hypertension will have been seen prior to becoming pregnant for a discussion of pregnancy management, including medication changes if needed.

Women with chronic hypertension are at increased risk for preterm birth, fetal growth restriction, and superimposed preeclampsia. Women who have severe hypertension are at higher risk for stroke, left ventricular hypertrophy, pulmonary edema, renal disease, placental abruption, and maternal death.[13] Their fetuses are at higher risk of growth restriction, prematurity, low birth weight, and perinatal death.[13]

Laboratory evaluation is used to obtain a baseline assessment of kidney and liver function early in gestation and to differentiate chronic hypertension that is worsening under the stress of pregnancy from the development of superimposed preeclampsia later in gestation. When a woman with chronic hypertension first presents for prenatal care, initial baseline testing usually includes a serum creatinine level, uric acid, lactic acid dehydrogenase (LDH), serum transaminase levels, and occasionally a 24-hour urine collection for assessment of proteinuria, although there may be minor variations between practices and institutions in which grouping of these tests are recommended. The presence of 1+ proteinuria early in pregnancy requires 24-hour urine testing for protein and creatinine to evaluate for renal dysfunction, assuming common confounders such as vaginitis or UTI have first been ruled out. These tests should be performed even for the woman whose chronic hypertension is currently controlled on medication.[11] Abnormal or rising levels of creatinine, uric acid, transaminases, and LDH suggest preeclampsia, as do alterations in serum albumin, hemoconcentration, and thrombocytopenia.

Many women with mild to moderate hypertension can discontinue medication during pregnancy or delay starting medication, because the normal physiologic pattern of blood pressure changes associated with gestation results in lower blood pressure in the first half of pregnancy. Lowering maternal blood pressure beyond the normal changes associated with pregnancy may decrease placental perfusion and deprive the fetus of oxygen.

Methyldopa (Aldomet) and labetalol (Trandate) are the medications most commonly used during pregnancy for women with chronic hypertension. Some antihypertensive agents taken prior to pregnancy are associated with teratogenic effects and require reevaluation. Angiotensin-converting enzyme (ACE) inhibitors and angiotensin receptor blockers are contraindicated during pregnancy, as are specific drugs from other classes that are associated with increased risk of fetal harm. Nifedipine (Procardia), which is used for preterm labor management, may also be used, but is not a first-line choice. Diuretics are not used during pregnancy primarily because of concerns regarding reduction of plasma volume with possible subsequent diminished placental perfusion. Women should maintain restricted sodium intake.

Whether or not medication is used, careful blood pressure monitoring at home and increased fetal surveillance via ultrasound to assess fetal growth are warranted. Depending on the severity of maternal disease, weekly or biweekly antenatal fetal testing and amniotic fluid assessment may be recommended starting in the early third trimester. Timing of delivery is based on maternal and fetal indications.

After the birth, maternal blood pressure is monitored to determine when and how to change medications or restart prepregnancy medication. Women who did not require therapy prior to pregnancy can monitor blood pressure weekly, have oral medication stopped after 1 month, and be evaluated at 1- to 2-week intervals for a month following cessation, and then at 3- to 6-month intervals for at least a year.[11] Among women with severe disease, there is an increased risk in the immediate postpartum period for pulmonary edema and cardiac failure as well as advancing renal disease. Consideration is given to the effects of breastfeeding on medication choice. In general, beta blockers and calcium-channel blockers are considered to be safe for breastfeeding mothers.

Respiratory Conditions

Respiratory Infections

The physiologic changes of pregnancy predispose women who have upper respiratory infections, including influenza, to develop pneumonia. Symptomatic relief can be provided for women with mild infections, using over-the-counter remedies.

Common Cold

Pregnant women are as susceptible to the common cold as nonpregnant women. The only difference in progression of this disorder is that a cough may take several days longer to resolve. Treatment focuses on mitigating symptoms. Decongestants, both oral and nasal sprays, are the usual treatment for women who have an upper respiratory infection and are not pregnant. Studies have failed to identify strong teratogenic effects associated with these agents; however, many midwives suggest nonpharmaceutical treatments and use of drugs only when the former fail to provide relief. Dextromethorphan, which is available under many brand names either alone or labeled "DM" when with other ingredients, can be used to treat cough.

Influenza

Influenza vaccination, using the injectable trivalent inactivated vaccine, does not cause harm to women or their fetuses.[14] In addition, maternal vaccination reduced infection among one of the highest-risk populations—namely, infants younger than 1 year of age.[15] However, only half of pregnant women receive routine vaccination against influenza.[14] Reasons for this relatively low vaccination rate include both maternal refusal and provider failure to offer and encourage vaccination. Viral upper respiratory infections other than influenza do not require antibiotic therapy. However, when influenza is suspected, at the time of this writing, both oseltamivir (Tamiflu) and zanamivir (Relenza) can be safely used during pregnancy within 2 days of symptom onset to decrease the severity of infection.[14] However, midwives should be aware that these recommendations may change based on development of viral resistance and evolution of new strains of influenza.

The primary concern for pregnant women with influenza or any severe viral respiratory infection is progression to pneumonia. Data from epidemic flu seasons have demonstrated increased rates of hospitalization and increased maternal mortality among pregnant women.[16] Additionally, there are increased risks of preterm birth, low birth weight, and fetal loss among women hospitalized for influenza,[16] while women who were immunized have shown decreased rates of prematurity and low birth weight during influenza season compared to women who were not immunized.

Pneumonia

Community-acquired pneumonia is the most common nonobstetric cause of maternal death in the United States.[17] The symptoms among pregnant women are similar to those experienced by nonpregnant women, and include cough, shortness of breath, sputum production, chest pain, fever, and malaise.[18] On examination, lung consolidation, elevated temperature, tachypnea, and signs of respiratory distress may be present. Women with suspected pneumonia should have a chest X ray, a complete blood count (CBC), metabolic panel (electrolytes, blood urea nitrogen, creatinine, glucose), and blood gases.[18] Because of the likelihood of rapid disease progression and fetal compromise from decreased oxygenation, hospitalization is often necessary during pregnancy, especially during the third trimester.[17] Antimicrobial therapy is chosen based on the microorganism.

In addition to the maternal morbidity directly related to infection, pregnant women with pneumonia have an increased risk of developing preeclampsia. Fetal risks include preterm premature rupture of membranes, fetal growth restriction, prematurity, low birth weight, and small-for-gestational-age infants, as well as morbidity from hypoxemia experienced by their mothers.[17–19]

Asthma

Asthma affects as many as 8% of pregnant women in the United States and is one of the most common medical conditions that affect pregnant women. This disease is often undertreated in adults. The normal physiologic changes of pregnancy may exacerbate asthma symptoms in as many as 30% of women. Asthma severity in pregnancy is usually similar to the severity experienced in the year prior to becoming pregnant. In addition, the more severe or poorly controlled a woman's asthma is in the year prior to pregnancy, the higher the risk she has of worsening disease and hospital admission during pregnancy.[20] Thus, when obtaining a history of asthma, it is important to determine the classification of the woman's asthma and to gather data about the severity, number of episodes, hospitalizations, and medications used in the prior year.

Women with mild intermittent asthma can still experience severe asthma attacks. Thus the management of asthma during pregnancy requires vigilance. In addition to evaluation and medication, midwifery counseling includes avoidance of triggers, the importance of correct medication use, and warning signs of worsening disease. **Table 24-1** describes the recommended evaluation for asthma during pregnancy.

Treatment of Asthma

Although some women will resist using medication out of fear of fetal harm, a fetus needs oxygenation.[21] Long-term management strategies for asthma are not different during pregnancy than for nonpregnant individuals. The criteria for adequate treatment are minimal chronic symptoms or exacerbations, normal pulmonary function, normal daily activity, and minimal use of "rescue" inhalers—all of which are also recommended criteria during pregnancy.[20]

Behavior and lifestyle changes are particularly important for women with asthma who have not had their asthma well controlled prior to becoming pregnant. Indeed, collaborative care of a woman who has asthma is a good example of how a midwife can be an important member of the healthcare team in caring for a woman with a preexisting medical condition. In addition to normal prenatal care that the midwife can provide, these women can need extensive health education and preventative health strategies such as how to avoid triggers, how to take their medication, the importance of influenza vaccine, and how to do fetal movement counts.

Maternal risks associated with asthma include hospitalization for exacerbation, hypoxia, status asthmaticus, increased risk of cesarean section, and preeclampsia. Fetal risks are associated with severe disease and include prematurity and low birth weight.[22] For women with severe asthma or those who require daily medications, fetal assessment during pregnancy will likely include daily fetal movement kick counts and serial fetal ultrasounds to monitor fetal growth.

The National Heart, Lung, and Blood Institute's recommendations for medications during pregnancy include albuterol as a short-acting drug, inhaled corticosteroids (e.g., budesonide [Pulmicort]) for long-term control, and intranasal corticosteroids for relief of comorbid symptoms such as allergic rhinitis.[23] Antihistamines such as loratadine (Claritin) and cetirizine (Zyrtec) may also be used. However, when a woman is well controlled on other medications, she should remain on her current regimen through pregnancy.

Only limited information is available about the fetal effects of asthma medications. An association with isolated omphalocele, esophageal atresia, and anal atresia has been reported but not yet confirmed to be medication related, nor is it clear if the inciting medication is a beta-agonist, steroid, or some combination of the two.[24] Because maternal hypoxia could have an independent adverse effect on the fetus, the

Table 24-1	Office Evaluation of a Woman with Asthma During Pregnancy	
	History/Review of Symptoms	**Physical Examination**
At initial visit	Disease onset, symptoms, frequency of exacerbations, medications, prior hospitalizations, prior intubation	Assessment of physical signs of respiratory difficulty, including nasal flaring, use of accessory muscles Lung auscultation
Monthly (more frequently as needed)	Symptom frequency, nocturnal symptoms, interference with normal activities of daily living, use of rescue inhaler	Lung auscultation Peak flow meter

effects of medications versus the effects of the disease have not been determined or differentiated.

Tuberculosis

Tuberculosis testing during pregnancy may be done with either the intradermal tuberculin screening test (TST; also referred to as a PPD) or the interferon-gamma release assay (IGRA). The IGRA is currently recommended by the Centers for Disease Control and Prevention (CDC).[25] Both tests measure a body's response to tuberculin and both are used in pregnancy. When either test is positive, it usually means the woman has been infected with tuberculosis, but the diagnosis of latent tuberculosis or active tuberculosis is not yet made.

Chest X ray using shielding can be performed during pregnancy and should be done to rule out active disease. If the woman has a positive screening test but does not have active tuberculosis, she is presumed to have latent tuberculosis. At this time, the CDC recommends deferring treatment of latent tuberculosis during pregnancy, unless risk factors are present, such as recent exposure to or the presence of HIV.

If treatment is initiated, isoniazid (INH) is given either daily or twice weekly for 9 months. Vitamin B_6 supplementation of 10 to 25 mg/day is recommended when treating women during pregnancy or while lactating. Pregnant and postpartum women being treated for latent tuberculosis should be monitored for hepatotoxicity.[26]

Gastrointestinal Conditions

Gastroesophageal Reflux Disease

Reflux is a common discomfort of pregnancy, occurring in more than half of all pregnant women.[27] The nutritional counseling normally provided includes avoidance of fatty, spicy, or acidic foods, although many pregnant women may already be doing so. Raising the head of the bed slightly and avoiding eating just before retiring to sleep may help prevent some symptoms as well. Initial treatment with antacids containing calcium and magnesium should be recommended before use of a histamine H_2 receptor antagonist such as ranitidine (Zantac). Because the proton pump inhibitors (PPIs) are more expensive medications, their use should be reserved for resistant cases. If needed, lansoprazole (Prevacid), esomeprazole (Nexium), and pantoprazole (Protonix) are all safe for use in pregnancy. Because information regarding safety during lactation is not available, PPIs are not recommended for use in breastfeeding women.[28]

Cholelithiasis

Gallstones and biliary sludge in pregnancy are associated with increasing parity and obesity. They affect as many as 10% of pregnant women and may persist or occur as a new finding following pregnancy. Most women are asymptomatic.[29] Symptoms of acute epigastric pain, nausea, and vomiting suggest the presence of gallstones; acute upper right quadrant abdominal pain on examination is the primary clinical finding. These findings are not altered in pregnancy. Approximately one-fourth of women fail to respond to conservative management with pain medication and fluids.[30] The risks of conservative treatment include recurrence and poor nutrition due to restriction of oral intake secondary to symptoms. Further, cesarean section birth is more common among women managed conservatively.[31] Laparoscopic surgery is safe in pregnancy, and should be performed during the second trimester when possible.

Pancreatitis

Gallbladder disease is the underlying cause of most acute pancreatitis—a rare complication of pregnancy.[32] Symptoms include nausea and vomiting, abdominal tenderness and guarding, and epigastric pain that radiates to the back. Serum lipase and amylase and white blood count elevations occur. Ultrasound confirms the diagnosis.

Although mild pancreatitis can be treated with pain medication and medical therapy, gallstone pancreatitis is usually treated surgically with cholecystectomy or endoscopic retrograde cholangiopancreatography (ERCP); severe disease will require intensive care unit admission. Surgical therapy improves outcomes and prevents recurrence.[32,33] When treated conservatively, biliary acute pancreatitis will recur in as many as two thirds of women who develop this condition. Pregnancy risks associated with acute pancreatitis include fetal loss and preterm birth.[33]

Viral Gastroenteritis

Nausea, vomiting, and diarrhea are all symptoms that can be common discomforts of pregnancy. However, they may also be the result of viral gastroenteritis or, in the case of diarrhea, be the result of irritable bowel or inflammatory bowel disease. Empiric treatment of new-onset gastrointestinal symptoms includes rehydration and monitoring for electrolyte imbalance. Most viral or bacterial infections are self-limiting and need no additional treatment. Women should be reassured that symptoms that resolve within 24 to 48 hours do not require additional treatment. However, if the woman is unable to hydrate orally at all for 24 hours or more, she may need evaluation and intravenous rehydration. Women who report decreased fetal movement need to be seen and evaluated.

Appendicitis

Appendectomy is the most common nonobstetric indication for surgery during pregnancy.[34] The key to recognizing appendicitis in pregnancy is to remember that the appendix is not where it used to be. The diagnosis of appendicitis in pregnant women is frequently delayed because the location of the appendix has shifted, leukocytosis is common in pregnancy, and the signs and symptoms of pregnancy can mask the significance of maternal reports.

Symptoms in pregnant women that differ from those in nonpregnant women include a superior and lateral shift in the point of greatest pain and decreased reliability of guarding in the lower abdomen. A report of anorexia is an important clue for women presenting with abdominal pain. The diagnosis can be made by ultrasound; however, because ultrasound visualization of the appendix can be obscured in pregnancy, magnetic resonance imaging (MRI) may be necessary to prevent unnecessary surgery.[35] Preterm birth and fetal loss are both more common among women with appendicitis, with their rates being highest among women who have a ruptured appendix.[36] Surgery is the definitive therapy. When appendicitis is misdiagnosed, surgical intervention is also associated with increased risk to the fetus.[36]

Genitourinary System

Asymptomatic Bacteriuria and Lower Urinary Tract Infections

The frequency of bacteriuria is similar among pregnant and nonpregnant women, and affects approximately 2% to 10% of all women.[37] Low socioeconomic status and history of recurrent lower urinary tract infection (LUTI) are associated with increased risk of infection in pregnancy.[38] Urinary infections increase the risk for preterm birth. A Cochrane review[37] determined that antibiotic treatment of asymptomatic bacteriuria (ASB) in pregnancy can reduce the incidence of pyelonephritis and low-birth-weight infants, although the quality of studies reviewed was not excellent.[38]

Both the Infectious Diseases Society of America (IDSA) and the U.S. Preventive Services Task Force support screening for bacteriuria and urinary tract infection in pregnancy.[39] Specifically, the IDSA recommends screening with a urine culture at least once during pregnancy, and treatment consisting of 3 to 7 days of antibiotic therapy if the results are positive. Although it is acceptable to treat empirically based on symptoms, a urine culture should be obtained when a woman is pregnant. Determining sensitivities now is recommended because of the increase in resistant urinary pathogens. A follow-up test-of-cure culture should be performed after treatment. Women who have been treated for ASB or LUTI during pregnancy should be rescreened periodically, although there is no consensus on timing.

When two or more culture-proven infections occur during pregnancy, the woman is placed on suppressive daily therapy for the duration of the pregnancy. Nitrofurantoin (Macrobid, Macrodantin) is preferred if the organisms identified have been susceptible to this agent. Women on suppressive therapy should be followed with urine dipstick that tests for nitrites and leukocyte esterase at each visit or at least one urine culture during the third trimester to ensure that a bacterial breakthrough has not occurred. When the urine dipstick is negative for both nitrites and the leukocyte esterase test is negative, the negative predictive value for bacteriuria is reliable.

Pyelonephritis

Women with bacteriuria have a 20- to 30-fold increase in the risk of developing pyelonephritis when pregnant[39] due to the renal tract structural changes that increase the risk of bacteria accessing the kidney. Multiparity and young maternal age are associated with increased risk, although most pregnant women with pyelonephritis do not have identified risk factors.[40] Pyelonephritis increases the maternal risks of sepsis, adult respiratory distress syndrome, anemia, and renal insufficiency, and the fetal risks of preterm birth and low birth weight.[41] The risks are similar in each trimester; inpatient management even in early gestation can reduce complications of disease.[41] Management is similar to that in nonpregnant women, with one exception: pregnant women should be managed initially in the inpatient setting, regardless of the severity of their disease.

Endocrine Conditions

Pre-gestational Diabetes

Approximately 1% of pregnant women in the United States are affected by preexisting (pre-gestational) diabetes and approximately 60% of those pregnancies are among women with type 1 diabetes. However, the rate of type 2 diabetes among pregnant women is increasing.[42] Care of a woman with pre-gestational diabetes during pregnancy is best started prior to conception.

Maternal risks of poorly controlled diabetes include disease progression and preeclampsia. Poor glycemic control during organogenesis is associated with an increased risk of congenital malformations (heart, central nervous system, and caudal regression), early fetal loss, and stillbirth.[43] The risk of congenital defects among infants of diabetic mothers increases as much as 10-fold among women with poor glycemic control during the period of organogenesis.[44]

The higher risk is found among women who have hemoglobin A_{1c} (HbA1c) levels 1% higher than in normal nondiabetic women and increases with each percent increase in HbA1c. Whether the fetus becomes macrosomic or is growth restricted is an effect of severity of maternal disease and glycemic control. Newborns of women who have diabetes are at increased risk of hypoglycemia, respiratory distress, and hyperbilirubinemia.

Women with pre-gestational diabetes should have an evaluation of HbA1c, thyroid function, and renal function (protein/creatinine ratio) at the initial prenatal visit.[45] Most women will be prescribed insulin during pregnancy, even if they have previously been maintained on oral agents, although the use of oral agents during pregnancy for women with type 2 diabetes is increasing.[46]

Using insulin, glycemic control is established as early during gestation as possible; thus, women are placed on multidose regimens. Daily monitoring of finger stick glucose values while fasting and before and after meals permits adjustments that will be required due to the metabolic demands of pregnancy and the growing fetus.[44] Individualized dietary counseling is essential for the same reasons. Fetal surveillance includes serial ultrasound, fetal echocardiography at 20 to 22 weeks' gestation, weekly antenatal fetal testing beginning at 32 weeks' gestation, and consideration of delivery timing based on maternal and fetal status. Amniocentesis to ascertain lung maturity is required if birth is planned prior to 39 weeks' gestation.

Thyroid Disease

During pregnancy, physiologic changes in thyroid metabolism result in lower levels of thyroid-stimulating hormone (TSH) and alterations in the levels of free T_4 and T_3. Later in pregnancy, TSH values return to the normal nonpregnant range. For this reason, evaluation of thyroid disease during pregnancy should be based on trimester-specific laboratory ranges (**Table 24-2**).[46,47] Laboratory testing of free T_4 and T_3 should be interpreted using a laboratory-specific pregnancy range.

Hyperthyroidism is defined by a low TSH level (lower than the trimester-specific reference range for normal in pregnancy or less than 0.01 mU/L) and elevated free T_4; hypothyroidism is defined by an elevated TSH (higher than the trimester-specific reference range for normal in pregnancy) and low free T_4. Subclinical hypothyroidism is defined as an elevated TSH level with normal T_4 function. The lack of clarity about whether subclinical disease should be treated in pregnancy emphasizes the need for accuracy in interpreting laboratory values.[48]

There is controversy about the role of universal screening for thyroid dysfunction in pregnancy; generally accepted recommendations currently are to screen women based on risk factors.[46,47] **Box 24-1** lists criteria for thyroid screening in pregnancy.

Hypothyroidism in Pregnancy

The prevalence of overt hypothyroidism in the United States, where iodine deficiency is rare, is approximately 0.3%. Most cases are a result of autoimmune thyroiditis, also called Hashimoto's disease rather than iodine deficiency.[49] Maternal risks of untreated hypothyroidism include an increased risk of miscarriage, anemia, preeclampsia, gestational hypertension, placental abruption, and postpartum hemorrhage. Fetal risks include fetal loss, preterm birth, low birth weight, and postnatal cognitive impairment.

Treatment consists of levothyroxine (Synthroid, Levoxyl), which is titrated to maintain the TSH in the normal range by trimester. For women diagnosed prior to pregnancy, an increased dose may be needed early in pregnancy. For women with subclinical hypothyroidism and elevated TSH, therapy can be considered, but there is no universal consensus about whether or not to treat at the time of this writing. For women who are treated for hypothyroidism,

Table 24-2	Normal Thyroid-Stimulating Hormone Values During Pregnancy
Trimester	**TSH**
1	0.1–2.5 mIU/L
2	0.2–3.0 mIU/L
3	0.3–3.0 mIU/L

BOX 24-1 Increased Risk of Thyroid Disease in Pregnancy

Past medical history:
- Thyroid disease or thyroid surgery
- Elevated thyroid peroxidase antibodies
- Irradiation of head or neck or multiple dental X rays
- Infertility
- Multiple miscarriages
- Unexplained preterm birth
- Type 1 diabetes mellitus
- Autoimmune disorder
- Treatment with lithium

Family history of thyroid disease

Symptoms or clinical signs of thyroid disease

Goiter

Age ≥ 30 years

BMI ≥ 40

Environmental or dietary risk of iodine deficiency

laboratory monitoring should be performed every 4 weeks until the second half of pregnancy and then at least once at the beginning of the third trimester.[46,47]

Hyperthyroidism in Pregnancy

Hyperthyroidism occurs in 0.5% of pregnancies; Graves' disease is the predominant cause.[49] When the diagnosis of hyperthyroidism has been made prior to pregnancy, the endocrinologist may offer women surgery or radioactive iodine to destroy thyroid tissue. Following treatment, women should delay pregnancy for at least 6 months to initiate levothyroxine, as they will be hypothyroid following ablation of the thyroid tissue.[46]

Another cause of hyperthyroidism in pregnancy is related to thyroid stimulation by human chorionic gonadotropin; gestational thyrotoxicosis is associated with hyperemesis gravidarum and resolves spontaneously in the early second trimester.[47] Treatment is not necessary for most women in this situation.

Maternal risks of untreated disease include gestational diabetes, preeclampsia, spontaneous abortion, heart failure, and (rarely) thyroid storm. Fetal risks include preterm labor, fetal goiter, fetal

hyperthyroidism, cardiac decompensation, hydrops, stillbirth, and low birth weight.

Treatment with propylthiouracil (PTU) is preferred in early pregnancy, as this medication presents the fewest risks to the fetus during organogenesis. After the first trimester, transition to another drug—methimazole (Tapazole)—may be recommended, as this medication has fewer maternal side effects. Thyroid testing is done at least monthly. Over the course of pregnancy, medication needs may diminish. Women continued on PTU should be screened monthly with liver function testing. Fetal ultrasound for growth and well-being, goiter, and cardiac status should be performed monthly following the anatomy screen.

Following birth, women with well-controlled Graves' disease may experience a relapse. At the time of the postpartum visit, thyroid testing should be repeated.

Neurologic Conditions

The neurologic conditions affected by pregnancy include neuropathies such as carpal tunnel syndrome and Bell's palsy, as well as complex diseases such as migraine, seizure disorders, and multiple sclerosis.

Carpal Tunnel Syndrome

Carpal tunnel syndrome is associated with older age, nulliparity, and gestational edema. The incidence of this condition increases in the third trimester, is more likely to occur bilaterally in pregnant women than in nonpregnant women, and resolves without treatment for most women during the postpartum period. Breastfeeding may delay resolution. The incidence of carpal tunnel syndrome in some studies has been as high as 35%; increased fluid retention and effects of relaxin have been reported to play a role in the increased frequency. If treatment is needed, nighttime use of wrist splints can be employed, as can referral to physical therapy.[50]

Bell's Palsy

Bell's palsy—a peripheral neuropathy affecting the face unilaterally—is more common among women than men and is three times more common among pregnant women than among nonpregnant women.[51] The reasons for this increase are unclear. Onset is most commonly in the third trimester or immediately postpartum. The condition is painful; reports of dry eye (because the eyelid does not completely close), oversensitive hearing, changes in taste, and headache are common.[52] On examination, the face is smooth and the affected side of the mouth droops. One test is to ask the woman to wrinkle her forehead, which she cannot do if Bell's palsy is present.[51] Management in pregnancy is limited to supportive treatment, and occasionally corticosteroids. Recovery in most cases occurs within 3 weeks postpartum. Most other cases will resolve at least partially within 6 months. The more severe the paralysis, the less likely it is that complete healing will occur as it resolves.[52]

Sciatica and Meralgia Paresthetica

Both lumbosacral radiculopathy causing compression of the sciatic nerve and meralgia paresthetica (i.e., compression of the lateral cutaneous femoral nerve) are examples of lower-body neuromuscular problems associated with advancing pregnancy. The sciatic nerve has both motor and sensory function. Symptoms of sciatica include pain and numbness in the buttocks and down the back of the leg, and possible difficulty with walking. The lateral cutaneous femoral nerve is sensory only; no motor defect will develop in association with the numbness or pain in the lateral thigh. Because the underlying causes of both conditions are related to the pregnancy itself, repositioning, exercise therapy, use of a pregnancy support belt, and reassurance can be of value. If symptoms are severe or do not begin to resolve during the postpartum period, lidocaine patch placement for pain can be used.[53] Physical therapy may also be of benefit for women with sciatica.

Migraine Headache

Migraine headaches are the most commonly reported types of headaches during pregnancy. As pregnancy progresses, headache frequency and severity usually decrease; migraine without aura is most likely to improve, and menstrual migraine is least likely to do so. New-onset migraine during pregnancy is rare enough that a woman presenting with headache with migraine-like symptoms should be evaluated for more serious causes such as pseudo-tumor cerebri, preeclampsia, and stroke.[54]

Self-care with avoidance of migraine triggers, adequate fluid and rest, and use of massage or relaxation therapies should be recommended to all women with migraine who are pregnant. Acetaminophen (Tylenol) either alone or with opioids can be used to interrupt migraine pain, if nonpharmacologic methods are not effective. Sumatriptan (Imitrex) can be used during pregnancy by women with severe migraines if other treatment fails.[52] Preventive treatment for migraines is less likely to be needed during pregnancy, as remission frequently occurs; women

with three or more episodes of migraine per month require additional investigation.

Epilepsy

Ninety percent of women with epilepsy will have uncomplicated pregnancies.[54] The likelihood of a normal pregnancy is increased for women who have been seizure free for 9 or more months prior to pregnancy and remain seizure free. However, seizure disorders during pregnancy have been associated with increased risks of preeclampsia, placental abruption, and prematurity, as well as low birth weight, low Apgar scores, and decreased cognitive function in the child.[56] Risks of congenital malformation are increased among women who take valproate (Depakote) or are on polytherapy in the first trimester; the overall risk of a major malformation is 4% to 6%.[57] Cognitive defects are more common among infants of women who are on polytherapy or who take valproate, and possibly among those whose mothers take phenytoin (Dilantin) or phenobarbitol (Luminal).[56] Although it had been thought that epilepsy itself might be responsible for fetal anomalies, current evidence indicates that it is the medications—rather than the disease—that cause the anomalies.[58]

The use of a single drug during pregnancy is preferable, but prevention of maternal seizures is equally important. Treatment of epilepsy is also associated with folic acid deficiency. Folic acid supplementation begun preconceptionally is continued, and vitamin K supplementation of 10 to 20 mg/day is given in the last month of pregnancy. Whether folic acid supplementation above the usual pregnancy recommendation is necessary is unclear.[59] Seizure occurrence may cause a fetal bradycardia, but most fetuses tolerate this condition and recover well.

Multiple Sclerosis

Multiple sclerosis (MS) is a chronic and progressive neurologic disorder that is associated with inflammation and demyelination of the central nervous system. Onset is most common among women of childbearing age, and diagnosis is often delayed by the variability of symptoms. Both genetic and environmental factors have been implicated in the development of MS. Progression is widely variable, demonstrating either progressive or relapsing and remitting patterns.[60] As many as one third of women with MS will have children after their diagnosis.[61]

During pregnancy, MS generally regresses, and women do well. Following delivery, there is an increase in relapses.[62] Overall, pregnancy does not increase disease progression. Prior to becoming pregnant, women with MS should either stop all medications during pregnancy or change pharmacologic therapies if they are known teratogens. If a fetus is inadvertently exposed in the first trimester, consultation regarding potential fetal harm and serial ultrasounds to assess fetal well-being are indicated. Prenatal risks associated with MS include an increase in risk of fetal growth restriction and cesarean birth rates.[61]

Autoimmune Disease in Pregnancy

Systematic Lupus Erythematosus

Other conditions addressed in this chapter—Hashimoto's disease and multiple sclerosis, among others—share aspects of immune disorders with systemic lupus erythematosus (SLE) and illustrate the difficulty of creating distinct categories. SLE is a chronic autoimmune disease (also called a connective tissue disease) that can affect multiple organs. This condition is more common among women than among men, and appears primarily during the reproductive years. African Americans and Asians have a higher prevalence than Caucasians.[63] Common symptoms include fever, fatigue, joint pain, and a red facial rash; because so many organs are at risk, renal disease, cardiac arrhythmias, and other symptoms may occur as well.

The best pregnancy outcomes occur among women who have not had a lupus flare for 6 or more months preceding pregnancy.[64] Maternal risks include exacerbation of disease, new-onset lupus nephritis, thrombocytopenia, thromboembolism, preeclampsia, and pregnancy loss. Fetal risks include fetal heart block, preterm birth, fetal growth restriction, and neonatal lupus.[65,66] Women are followed closely for disease exacerbation, risk of thrombotic events, and hypertensive disorders; the fetus is monitored with a weekly biophysical profile in the third trimester, along with Doppler ultrasound.

Dermatoses of Pregnancy

Pruritic Urticarial Papules and Plaques of Pregnancy

Pruritic urticarial papules and plaques of pregnancy (PUPPP) occurs in 1 in 300 to 1 in 130 pregnant women, but is found more often among nulliparous women and women with a multiple gestation.[66] Typically, PUPPP arises in the late third trimester and persists through the birth. The red, painfully itchy

rash initially presents in the striae, but it may spread to cover the trunk and extremities. The face, palms and soles, and periumbilical area are not involved. Excessive stretching of abdominal skin causing tissue damage and high levels of estrogen and progesterone are theorized to be involved in the development and severity of the outbreaks.

Except for the discomfort, PUPPP is a benign exanthem. Low-potency topical steroids and antihistamines can be used to treat the discomfort. The woman can be reassured that the rash and itching will decrease once her infant is born.

Pemphigoid Gestationis

Pemphigoid gestationis, also called herpes gestationis (HG), is a rare autoimmune disorder that is most common among Caucasians. In contrast to PUPPP, HG does not always occur in the first pregnancy. HG most often presents between 12 and 24 weeks' gestation. A prodrome of malaise, fever, nausea, and headache may precede the skin eruptions.[67] Pruritus and a papular rash begin on the abdomen and rapidly spread, sparing the face, but appearing on the trunk and extremities. Urticaria is followed by vesicular and bullous lesions.[67] Remission is common in the later third trimester. HG frequently flares in the postpartum period before resolving without causing scars. It recurs in most, not all, subsequent pregnancies and tends to worsen with recurrence.[68]

The diagnosis is made with skin biopsy and immunofluorescence. Maternal risks associated with HG include a long-term increase in the incidence of Graves' disease.[66] Unlike PUPPP, HG is associated with adverse effects on the fetus. Low birth weight and prematurity are associated with earlier onset and the formation of blisters.[69] Antenatal fetal testing in the third trimester includes weekly biophysical profiles, along with Doppler studies if placental insufficiency is suspected.[76] Treatment in the early stages of HG includes potent topical steroids, topical or oral antihistamines, and oral prednisolone. If HG progresses to the bullous stage, systemic corticosteroid therapy is required.

Intrahepatic Cholestasis of Pregnancy

Intrahepatic cholestasis of pregnancy (ICP), like PUPPP, is a syndrome of intense itching; unlike in PUPPP, however, there is no rash involved. Slowed emptying of bile from the gallbladder underlies the development of ICP. Older maternal age, family history of hepatic diseases, a personal history of hepatitis C, and multiple pregnancies are all associated with increased risk.[70] Environmental, dietary, genetic, and ethnic influences all contribute to the relative risk of developing this condition. The rate of ICP in the United States is low, affecting less than 0.3% of all pregnant women.[70]

Fetal risks include meconium ileus, preterm birth, and sudden stillbirth. Antenatal fetal testing should be initiated with biophysical profiles and Doppler studies as soon as the diagnosis is made in addition to physician referral. Stillbirth rarely occurs before 36 weeks. However, because stillbirth occurs suddenly among women with ICP, it is unclear how well antenatal fetal testing can be considered reassuring. Delivery is recommended as soon as the fetal lungs are mature, or earlier if fetal testing is no longer reassuring. In one study, there was a 7% stillbirth rate, with 90% of the deaths occurring in term fetuses.[71]

Symptoms develop in the latter half of pregnancy, usually between 25 and 32 weeks' gestation. Intense itching that may be most severe on the palms and soles intensifies at night. Jaundice develops in 10% to 25% of women with ICP.[72] Some women have diarrhea or steatorrhea. Aminotransferase levels rise dramatically, conjugated bilirubin is increased, and bile acids become elevated to more than 10 mmol/L.

Treatment with ursodeoxycholic acid (Ursodiol, Actigall) can be started while bile acid results are pending. The usual dose is 10 to 15 mg/kg body weight daily.[72] The risk of delaying treatment is more significant for the fetus than the risk of misdiagnosis. Maternal risks are limited to the psychological stress of the pruritus, possible vitamin K deficiency that increases the risk of postpartum hemorrhage, and increased risk of future liver disease.

Infectious Diseases

Several infectious diseases can cause congenital anomalies, fetal harm, or fetal death and, therefore, are worthy of review as a group. TORCH is an older acronym for toxoplasmosis, rubella, cytomegalovirus (CMV), and herpes. The O (for "other") in this acronym has variously included varicella zoster, listeria, parvovirus B19, and syphilis. Although the term TORCH is still in use and a single test for TORCH antibodies may be available at laboratories, ordering the specific relevant antibody tests based on risks, exposure, or maternal/fetal signs of infection is more appropriate. Most of these organisms cause mild maternal infection; diagnosis is often made during screening or when fetal abnormalities are seen on ultrasound.

Midwifery management includes knowledge of these disorders, counseling about prevention,

and monitoring for women who are exposed. The *Reproductive Tract and Sexually Transmitted Infections* chapter reviews prenatal considerations for women who have syphilis and herpes. This section reviews other clinically significant infections.

Toxoplasmosis

Toxoplasma gondii is an obligate intracellular protozoan parasite that infects humans and usually remains dormant in neural or muscle tissue for the lifetime of the infected individual. Approximately 10% to 50% of adults have evidence of infection worldwide; in the United States, the prevalence of toxoplasmosis among women of childbearing age is approximately 11%. Typical sources of infection include uncooked or undercooked meat, contaminated soil, and feces of cats that hunt and eat wild birds or rodents. Maternal infection is usually asymptomatic, but the risk of fetal injury increases by trimester. Fetal risks include mild to severe neurologic and ocular lesions, including chorioretinitis, hydrocephalus, and intracranial calcifications. Stillbirth is relatively rare.[73]

Because the rate of *T. gondii* infection is low in the United States and there is no treatment, routine screening is not recommended. Primary prevention counseling is considered part of routine prenatal care, which is in contrast to France where toxoplasmosis is more common and secondary prevention via monthly testing to identify women who seroconvert is part of regular prenatal care. Antibody testing is complex and needs to be performed at a toxoplasmosis reference laboratory if indicated; both IgM and IgG persist for years following infection.[74]

Varicella

Approximately 95% of pregnant women are immune to the varicella zoster virus.[75] If the woman has no history of vaccination or disease, a varicella titer should be obtained at the initial prenatal visit. Maternal risks associated with varicella infection include varicella pneumonia, which is more likely among pregnant women than in nonpregnant adults and has a mortality rate of 28%. Fetal risks when the infection occurs in the first half of pregnancy include miscarriage and congenital anomalies. Approximately 1% to 2% of fetuses whose mothers have varicella infection will develop varicella congenital syndrome. Newborn varicella infection is a life-threatening condition that can occur if the mother contracts varicella 2 days prior to birth or within 5 days after birth. The incubation period for varicella is 10 to 21 days. Nonimmune women who are exposed to varicella during pregnancy should receive varicella zoster immune globulin (VZIG), which can be administered up to 10 days after exposure.[76]

Listeriosis

The bacterium *Listeria monocytogenes* grows in meat, dairy products, and cheese.[77] The source of the infection is usually soil and decaying vegetable matter that contaminates nonpasteurized products or processed food after pasteurization. Although *Listeria* outbreaks are uncommon in the United States, pregnant women are among the groups most at risk for this infection; one in 6 cases of listeriosis occurs during a pregnancy. Infection can cause a mild flu-like malaise, fever, nausea, and vomiting, or it can be asymptomatic. Fetal risks include miscarriage, preterm labor, and stillbirth because the bacterium has a predilection for the placenta and fetal central nervous system.[78] Guidelines for prevention are listed in the section on food safety in the *Prenatal Care* chapter. Listeriosis is often a mild illness in women and may be missed as it is self-limiting. The most common symptoms are a flu-like illness with fever, chills, and possibly backache. The incubation period is 24 hours to 10 days after exposure. If a pregnant woman is diagnosed with acute listeriosis, she will be given antibiotics (usually ampicillin or penicillin) and may be admitted for hospitalization. Intensive follow-up to monitor the fetus will also be initiated.

Parvovirus B19

Parvovirus B19 or erythema infectiosum is a double-stranded DNA virus that is the cause of a common childhood illness called fifth disease, so called because it was the fifth disease identified that presents with a facial exanthem; it is also called "slapped-cheek disease" because of the bright red erythema on both cheeks that is the hallmark of this infection. Seasonal outbreaks occur in early winter. Approximately 50% to 60% of pregnant women are immune to parvovirus

B19. The primary sources of infection are young children who develop fifth disease. Approximately 20% to 30% of susceptible women exposed to parvovirus B19 in a nursery school or school classroom will become infected. Transmission within a household can be as high as 50%.[79] Of the women who do become infected, approximately 30% will transmit the virus to the fetus, 10% of the infected fetuses will die, and the others will recover without sequelae. Parvovirus causes a mild flu-like illness in women, but it may also be asymptomatic. Fetal risks, which are greater during early pregnancy, include miscarriage, fetal anemia, and non-immune hydrops. Women should be counseled to report any exposure to parvovirus B19.

Management of women who are exposed to parvovirus B19 starts with documenting the date of exposure. IgG and IgM titers should be obtained no earlier than 7 days after exposure. Interpretation of laboratory tests are outlined in **Table 24-3**. The fetus will need to be monitored with serial ultrasounds if infection is confirmed.

Rubella

The rubella virus, a member of the togavirus family, is the organism responsible for German measles. Population-level immunization has virtually eliminated maternal rubella infection and congenital rubella syndrome in the United States, but this risk should not be forgotten and outbreaks still can occur. Rubella is transmitted via droplets and has an incubation period of 14 to 21 days. The characteristic rash is a maculopapular eruption with associated fever, malaise, sore throat, and lymphadenopathy. Fetal infection rates vary over the course of pregnancy, being high in the first and third trimesters (80% and 100%, respectively) and somewhat lower in the second trimester (25%).[80] Deafness, cataracts, and cardiac defects are the classic congenital anomalies associated with rubella infection, but the

Table 24-3	Interpretation of Lab Results for Maternal Parvovirus B19 Serology		
IgG[a]	**IgM**[a]	**Interpretation**	**Clinical Management**
Negative	Negative	Nonimmune and no infection	Repeat tests in 14 days[a]
Negative	Positive	Current active infection	Weekly ultrasound to monitor for fetal hydrops
Positive	Negative	Past infection with immunity but cannot rule out recent infection especially if IgG is high	Weekly ultrasound to monitor for fetal hydrops
Positive	Positive	Current active infection	Weekly ultrasound to monitor for fetal hydrops

[a]There is a window of 7 days immediately after infection in which both IgG and IgM are negative.

infection is systemic and can affect virtually all fetal organs; thus miscarriage, preterm birth, fetal growth restriction, and stillbirth are possible. If a woman who is rubella nonimmune is exposed to a child with German measles, successive antibody titers of IgG and IgM should be drawn and physician consultation obtained. Interpretation of maternal rubella serology can be complicated.

Cytomegalovirus

Cytomegalovirus is a virus in the herpes family. Transmission is by droplets and body fluids. Toddlers are the most frequent source of infection. CMV is ubiquitous in the environment, and approximately 50% to 80% of reproductive-aged women in the United States have experienced an asymptomatic infection.[81] Reinfection can occur, however, and the risk of maternal–fetal transmission is as high as 33% for women with a primary infection. Severe fetal central nervous system damage occurs in approximately 20% of cases, especially if the fetus is infected in the first or second trimester.[82]

There are no recommendations for screening women for CMV. Women who work with children are counseled to pay close attention to hand washing. Antibody titers may be of value if confirmed seroconversion can be documented. Serial ultrasounds and possible amniocentesis are necessary to confirm the diagnosis of fetal infection.

Conclusion

When pregnancy is medically complicated, the midwife can often continue to support the woman through her pregnancy. This chapter has not addressed every medical condition that can affect pregnancy. Careful history taking, competent physical examination, and thoughtful listening will provide the midwife with clues to aid diagnosis. The decision to consult, collaborate, or refer to a physician for ongoing care will be based on the woman's condition, practice policies, the midwife's individual scope of practice, and resources available. This collaborative management course of action best serves the woman and her fetus when she experiences complications during her pregnancy.

• • • References

1. Carles G, Tobal N, Raynal P, et al. Doppler assessment of the fetal cerebral hemodynamic response to moderate or severe maternal anemia. *Am J Obstet Gynecol.* 2003;188:794-799.

2. Sun PM, Wilburn W, Raynor BD, Jamieson D. Sickle cell disease in pregnancy: twenty years of experience at Grady Memorial Hospital, Atlanta, Georgia. *Am J Obstet Gynecol.* 2001;184(6):1127-1130.

3. Rogers DT, Molokie R. Sickle cell disease in pregnancy. *Obstet Gynecol Clin North Am.* 2010;37(2):223-237.

4. Sheiner E, Levy A, Yerushalmi R, Katz M. Beta-thalassemia minor during pregnancy. *Obstet Gynecol.* 2004;103:1273-1277.

5. McCrae KR. Thrombocytopenia in pregnancy. *Hematology.* 2010;1:397-402.

6. Provan D, Stasi R, Newland AC, et al. International consensus report on the investigation and management of primary immune thrombocytopenia. *Blood.* 2010;115:168-186.

7. Martin JN Jr, Bailey AP, Rehberg JF, Owens MT, Keiser SD, May WL. Thrombotic thrombocytopenic purpura in 166 pregnancies: 1955–2006. *Am J Obstet Gynecol.* 2008;199:98-104.

8. Del Papa N, Vaso N. Management of antiphospholipid syndrome. *Ther Adv Musculoskelet Dis.* 2010;2(4):221-227.

9. Bates SM, Greer IA, Middeldorp S, Veenstra DL, Prabulos A, VBandvik P. VTE, thrombophilia, antithrombotic therapy, and pregnancy: antithrombotic therapy and prevention of thrombosis, 9th ed.: American College of Chest Physicians evidence-based clinical practice guidelines. *Chest.* 2012;141(2 suppl):e691S -e736S.

10. Marik PE, Plante LA. Venous thromboembolic disease and pregnancy. *N Engl J Med.* 2008;359(19):2025-2033.

11. Report of the National High Blood Pressure Education Program Working Group on High Blood Pressure in Pregnancy. *Am J Obstet Gynecol.* 2000;183:S1-S22.

12. Bateman BT, Shaw KM, Kuklina EV, Callaghan WM, Seely EW, Hernandez-Diaz S. Hypertension in women of reproductive age in the United States: NHANES 1999–2008. *PLoS One.* 2012;7(4):e36171.

13. Bateman BT, Bansil P, Hernandez-Diaz S, Mhyre JM, Callaghan WM, Kuklina EV. Prevalence, trends and outcomes of chronic hypertension: a nationwide sample of delivery admissions. *Am J Obstet Gynecol.* 2012:206:134.e1-134.e8.

14. Fiore AE, Uyeki TM, Broder K, et al. Prevention and control of influenza with vaccines: recommendations of the Advisory Committee on Immunization Practices (ACIP), 2010. *MMWR Recomm Rep.* 2010;59:1.

15. Rasmussen SA, Jamieson DJ, Uyeki TM. Effects of influenza on pregnant women and infants. *Am J Obstet Gynecol.* 2012;207(3 suppl):S17-S20.

16. Omer SB, Goodman D, Steinhoff MC, et al. Maternal influenza immunization and reduced likelihood of prematurity and small for gestational age births: a retrospective cohort study. *PLoS Med.* 2011;8(5):e1000441.

17. Brito V, Niederman MS. Pneumonia complicating pregnancy. *Clin Chest Med*. 2011;32(1):121-132.

18. Sheffield JS, Cunningham FG. Community acquired pneumonia in pregnancy. *Obstet Gynecol*. 2009; 114(4):915-922.

19. Chen Y-H, Keller J, Wang I-T, et al. Pneumonia and pregnancy outcomes: a nationwide population-based study. *Am J Obstet Gynecol*. 2012;207:288.e1-288.e7.

20. Dombrowski MP. Asthma and pregnancy. *Obstet Gynecol*. 2006;108(3 Pt 1):667-681.

21. National Asthma Education and Prevention Program. Working group report on managing asthma during pregnancy: recommendations for pharmacologic treatment updated 2004. Available at: http://www.nhlbi .nih.gov/guidelines/asthma/astpreg.htm. Accessed January 27, 2013.

22. Hardy-Fairbanks AJ, Baker ER. Asthma in pregnancy: pathophysiology, diagnosis and management. *Obstet Gynecol Clin North Am*. 2010;37(2):159-172.

23. National Asthma Education and Prevention Program. Expert panel report: guidelines for the diagnosis and management of asthma (EPR-3). National Heart, Lung, and Blood Institute; 2007. Available at: http://www.nhlbi.nih.gov/guidelines/asthma/asthgdln .htm. Accessed January 27, 2013.

24. Lin S, Munsie JPW, Herdt-Losavio ML, et al. Maternal asthma medication use and the risk of selected birth defects. *Pediatrics*. 2012;129(2):e317-e324.

25. Mazurek GH, Jereb J, Vernon A, LoBue P, Goldberg S, Castro K. Updated guidelines for using interferon gamma release assays to detect *Mycobacterium tuberculosis* infection—United States, 2010. *MMWR Recomm Rep*. 2010;59(RR05):1-25.

26. Centers for Disease Control and Prevention. Latent tuberculosis infection: a guide for primary care providers. Available at: http://www.cdc.gov/tb/publications /LTBI/default.htm. Accessed January 27, 2013.

27. Richter JE. Gastroesophageal reflux disease during pregnancy. *Gastroenterol Clin North Am*. 2003;32: 235-261.

28. Botelho NB, Emets CL, Brucker MC. Gastrointestinal conditions. In King TL, Brucker MC, eds. *Pharmacology for Women's Health*. Sudbury, MA: Jones and Bartlett; 2011:605-640.

29. Ko CW, Beresford SAA, Schulte SJ, Matsumoto AM, Lee SP. Incidence, natural history, and risk factors for biliary sludge and stones during pregnancy. *Hepatology*. 2005;41:359-365.

30. Date RS, Kaushal M, Ramesh A. A review of the management of gallstone disease and its complications in pregnancy. *Am J Surg*. 2008;196:599-608.

31. Othman MO, Stone E, Hashimi M, Parasher G. Conservative management of cholelithiasis and its complications in pregnancy is associated with recurrent symptoms and more emergency department visits. *Gastrointest Endosc*. 2012;76(3):564-569.

32. Hernandez A, Petrov MS, Brooks DC, Blanks PA, Ashley SW, Tavkkolizadeh A. Acute pancreatitis and pregnancy: a 10-year single center experience. *J Gastrointest Surg*. 2007;11(12):1623-1627.

33. Tang S-J, Rodriguez-Frias E, Singh S, et al. Acute pancreatitis during pregnancy. *Clin Gastroentrol Hepatol*. 2010;8(1):85-90.

34. Freeland M, King E, Safcsak K, Durham R. Diagnosis of appendicitis in pregnancy. *Am J Surg*. 2009; 198(6):753-758.

35. Pedrosa I, Lafornara M, Pandharipande PV, Goldsmith JD, Rofsky N. Pregnant patients suspected of having acute appendicitis: effect of MR imaging on negative laparotomy rate and appendiceal perforation rate. *Radiology*. 2009;250(3):749-757.

36. McGory ML, Zingmond DS, Tillou A, Hiatt JR, Ko CY, Crier HM. Negative appendectomy in pregnant women is associated with a substantial risk of fetal loss. *J Am Coll Surg*. 2007;205:534-540.

37. Schnarr J, Smaill F. Asymptomatic bacteriuria and symptomatic urinary tract infections in pregnancy. *Eur J Clin Invest*. 2008;38(S2):50-57.

38. Smaill F, Vazquez JC. Antibiotics for asymptomatic bacteriuria in pregnancy. *Cochrane Database Syst Rev*. 2007;2:CD000490.

39. Nicolle LE, Bradley S, Colgan R, Rice JC, Schaeffer A, Hooton TM. Infectious Diseases Society of America guidelines for the diagnosis and treatment of asymptomatic bacteriuria in adults. *Clin Infect Dis*. 2005;40(5):643.

40. Hill JB, Sheffield JS, McIntire DD, Wendel GD Jr. Acute pyelonephritis in pregnancy. *Obstet Gynecol*. 2005;205(1):18-23.

41. Archibald KL, Friedman A, Raker CA, Anderson BL. Impact of trimester on morbidity of acute pyelonephritis in pregnancy. *Am J Obstet Gynecol*. 2009; 201(4):401.e1-401.e4.

42. Albrecht SS, Kuklina EV, Bansil P, et al. Diabetes trends among delivery hospitalizations in the U.S., 1994–2004. *Diab Care*. 2010;33:768-773.

43. Temple R, Aldridge V, Greenwood R, Heyburn P, Sampson M, Stanley K. Association between outcome of pregnancy and glycaemic control in early pregnancy in type 1 diabetes: population based study. *BMJ*. 2002;325:1275.

44. Kitzmiller JL, Block JM, Brown FM, et al. Managing preexisting diabetes for pregnancy: summary of evidence and consensus recommendations for care. *Diab Care*. 2008;31:1060-1079.

45. American Diabetes Association. Standards of medical care in diabetes—2013. *Diab Care*. 2013;36(suppl 1):S11.

46. Stagnaro-Green A, Abalovich M, Alexander E, et al. Guidelines of the American Thyroid Association for the diagnosis and management of thyroid disease

during pregnancy and postpartum. *Thyroid.* 2011; 21(10):1081-1125.

47. De Groot L, Abalovich M, Alexander EK, et al. Management of thyroid dysfunction during pregnancy and postpartum: an Endocrine Society clinical practice guideline. *J Clin Endocrinol Metab.* 2012;97(8): 2543-2565.

48. Stagnaro-Green A. Overt hyperthyroidism and hypothyroidism during pregnancy. *Clin Obstet Gynecol.* 2011;54(3):478-487.

49. Stagnaro-Green A. Optimal care of the pregnant woman with thyroid disease. *J Clin Endocrinol Metab,* 2012;97(8):2619-2622.

50. Mabie WC. Peripheral neuropathies during pregnancy. *Clin Obstet Gynecol.* 2005;48(1):57-66.

51. Cohen Y, Lavie O, Granovsky-Grisaru S, Aboulafia Y, Diamant YZ. Bell palsy complicating pregnancy: a review. *Obstet Gynecol Surv.* 2000;55(3):184-188.

52. Pearce CF, Hansen WF. Headache and neurological disease in pregnancy. *Clin Obstet Gynecol.* 2012; 55(3):810-828.

53. Sax TW, Rosenbaum RB. Neuromuscular disorders in pregnancy. *Muscle Nerve.* 2006;34(5):559.

54. Martin SR, Foley MR. Approach to the pregnant patient with headache. *Clin Obstet Gynecol.* 2005; 48(1):2-11.

55. Practice parameter: management issues for women with epilepsy (summary statement). Report of the Quality Standards Subcommittee of the American Academy of Neurology. *Neurology.* 1998;51(4):944-948.

56. Harden CL, Meador KJ, Pennell PB, et al. Practice parameter update: management issues for women with epilepsy—focus on pregnancy (an evidence-based review): teratogenesis and perinatal outcomes: report of the Quality Standards Subcommittee and Therapeutics and Technology Assessment Subcommittee of the American Academy of Neurology and American Epilepsy Society. *Neurology.* 2009;73(2):133.

57. Yerby MS. Clinical care of pregnant women with epilepsy: neural tube defects and folic acid supplementation. *Epilepsia.* 2003;44:33-40.

58. Holmes LB, Harvey EA, Coull BA, et al. The teratogenicity of anticonvulsant drugs. *N Engl J Med.* 2001; 344(15):1132.

59. Wlodarczyk BJ, Palacios AM, George TM, Finnell RH. Antiepileptic drugs and pregnancy outcomes. *Am J Med Genet.* 2012;158A:2071-2090.

60. Kantarci O, Wingerchuk D. Epidemiology and natural history of multiple sclerosis: new insights. *Curr Opin Neurol.* 2006;19(3)248-254.

61. Kelly VM, Nelson LM, Chakravarty EF. Obstetric outcomes in women with multiple sclerosis and epilepsy. *Neurology.* 2009;73(22):1831.

62. Confavreux C, Hutchinson M, Hours MM, Cortinovis-Tourniaire P, Moreau T. Rate of pregnancy-related relapse in multiple sclerosis. Pregnancy in Multiple Sclerosis Group. *N Engl J Med.* 1998;339(5):285.

63. McCarty DJ, Manzi S, Medsger TA Jr, Ramsey-Goldman R, LaPorte RE, Kwoh CK. Incidence of systemic lupus erythematosus: race and gender differences. *Arthritis Rheum.* 1995;38(9):1260-1270.

64. Smyth A. A systematic review and meta-analysis of pregnancy outcomes in patients with systemic lupus erythematosus and lupus nephritis. *Clin J Am Soc Nephrol.* 2010;5(11):2060-2068.

65. Kwok L, Tam L, Zhu T, Leung Y, Li E. Predictors of maternal and fetal outcomes in pregnancies of patients with systemic lupus erythematosus. *Lupus* [serial online]. 2011;20(8):829-836.

66. Kroumpouzos G, Cohen LM. Specific dermatoses of pregnancy: an evidence-based systematic review. *Am J Obstet Gynecol.* 2003;188:1083-1092.

67. Ingber A. Herpes (pemphigoid) gestationis. In *Obstetric dermatology.* Berlin: Springer; 2009:111-133.

68. Engineer L, Bhol K, Ahmed AR. Pemphigoid gestationis: a review. *Am J Obstet Gynecol.* 2000;183(2): 483-491.

69. Chi CC, Wang SH, Charles-Holmes R, Ambros-Rudolph C, Powell J, Jenkins R. Pemphigoid gestationis: early onset and blister formation are associated with adverse pregnancy outcomes. *Br J Dermatol.* 2009;160:1222-1228.

70. Pathak B, Sheibani L, Lee RH. Cholestasis of pregnancy. *Obstet Gynecol Clin North Am.* 2010;37(2):269-282.

71. Williamson C, Hems L, Goulis D, et al. Clinical outcome in a series of cases of obstetric cholestasis identified via a patient support group. *BJOG.* 2004; 111(7):676-681.

72. Hay JE. Liver disease in pregnancy. *Hepatology.* 2008;47:1067-1076.

73. Paquet C, Yudin MH. Toxoplasmosis in pregnancy: prevention, screening, and treatment. *J Obstet Gynaecol Can.* 2013;35(1):78-79.

74. U.S. Public Health Service, Department of Health and Human Services, Food and Drug Administration. *FDA Public Health Advisory: Limitations of Toxoplasma IgM Commercial Test Kits.* Rockville, MD: Department of Health and Human Services, Food and Drug Administration; 1997.

75. Watson B, Civen R, Reynolds M, et al. Validity of self-reported varicella disease history in pregnant women attending prenatal clinics. *Public Health Rep.* 2007;122:499.

76. Centers for Disease Control and Prevention. FDA approval of an extended period for administering

VariZIG for postexposure prophylaxis of varicella. *MMWR.* 2012;61(12):212.

77. Delgado AR. Listeriosis in pregnancy. *J Midwifery Women's Health.* 2008;53(3):255-259.

78. Mylonakis E, Paliou M, Hohmann EL, et al. Listeriosis during pregnancy: a case series and review of 222 cases. *Medicine (Balt).* 2002;81:260.

79. Valeur-Jensen AK, Pedersen CB, Westergaard T, et al. Risk factors for parvovirus B19 infection in pregnancy. *JAMA.* 1999;281:1099-1105.

80. Miller E, Cradock-Watson JE, Pollock TM. Consequences of confirmed maternal rubella at successive stages of pregnancy. *Lancet.* 1982;2:781.

81. Carlson A, Norwitz ER, Stiller RJ. Cytomegalovirus infection in pregnancy: should all women be screened? *Rev Obstet Gynecol.* 2010;3(4):172-180.

82. Centers for Disease Control and Prevention. Cytomegalovirus (CMV) and congenital CMV infection. Available at: http://www.cdc.gov/cmv/transmission .html. Accessed March 26, 2013.

V

Intrapartum

Midwifery Care During Labor and Birth

"Not just another day in a woman's life." This conclusion by Penny Simpkin,[1,2] childbirth educator and doula extraordinaire, plays itself over and over in my mind when I am with or think about a woman in labor. They are simple words, yet profound in their description of the importance and permanence of a woman's memory of the day she gives birth. As Simkin's research showed, women remember with exquisite detail and accuracy the words and actions during labor of their providers and partners 15 to 20 years later. What the midwife does and says during labor may affect not only the physiology of the labor process, but also the woman's memory of the important day when she gave birth and welcomed a new child into her life and family. The chapters in this section present all the components of midwifery care of women during the labor process.

The midwife is the guide, consultant, and collaborator for a woman and her family during labor and birth. The midwife helps to ensure a safe physical, psychological, and spiritual place for labor and birth, while functioning in the milieu of the specific birth setting, whether in the home, birth center, or hospital. The midwife serves as the buffer between the laboring woman and whatever system of care surrounds her. It is the midwife's responsibility to ensure that protected space where labor and birth can evolve as the unique process that it is for each woman and each infant she carries. The philosophy of midwifery care includes "watchful waiting and non-intervention into normal processes."[3]

There are few times during the reproductive cycle when inappropriate or ill-timed interventions can have the dire consequences that are possible during labor and birth. The ill-timed amniotomy with a high fetal head can turn an otherwise normal labor into an emergency when a loop of umbilical cord drops into the midwife's hand and the fetal head descends against it. Tachysystole and fetal bradycardia from injudicious exogenous oxytocin administration produce a cascade of additional interventions that create anxiety and further disrupt and may even stop the normalcy of labor. While the availability of medical and surgical interventions during labor can help assure an appropriate safety net for problems that may occur, their injudicious use not only produces more harms than benefits for mother and infant, but also unnecessarily increases the cost of health care.

The midwife is the vigilant protector who ensures safety for a woman and her infant during labor and birth. This vigilance requires an exquisite understanding of the physiology and psychology of human parturition, as well as the scientific basis for midwifery practice during this vulnerable period of transition. The expert midwife is a lifelong student of labor, its many aberrations, and the scientific literature that helps deepen our understanding and expand our expertise.

Although labor is a normal physiologic and developmental process, it is also a period of vulnerability for both mother and infant during which problems can arise requiring the midwife's expert action through timely identification based on comprehensive assessment, treatment, and collaboration with and potential referral to other members of the healthcare team. Regardless of the problem or the treatment regimen required, the laboring woman and respect for her autonomy and self-determination remain the center of the midwife's care.

I am reminded of an adaptation of a writing by Lao Tzu on leadership and being a midwife (Do you think of your role as a midwife as a role of leadership?): "Imagine that you are a midwife; you are assisting at someone else's birth. Do good without show or fuss. Facilitate what is happening rather than what you think ought to be happening. If you must take the lead, lead so that the mother is helped, yet still free and in charge. When the baby is born, the mother will rightly say: 'We did it ourselves!'"[4 p. 33]

Nancy K. Lowe

● ● ● **References**

1. Simkin P. Just another day in a woman's life? Women's long-term perceptions of their first birth experience. Part I. *Birth*. 1991:18(4);203-210.

2. Simkin P. Just another day in a woman's life? Women's long-term perceptions of their first birth experience. Part II. *Birth*. 1992;19(2):64-81.

3. American College of Nurse-Midwives. *Philosophy of the American College of Nurse-Midwives*. Silver Spring, MD: American College of Nurse-Midwives; 2004.

4. Heider J. *The Tao of Leadership: Lao Tzu's Tao Te Ching Adapted for a New Age*. Atlanta, GA: Humanics New Age; 1985.

CHAPTER

25

Anatomy and Physiology During Labor and Birth

CINDY M. ANDERSON

MELISSA D. AVERY

Introduction

Providing care that supports the normal physiologic process requires an understanding of the physiology of labor and birth. The anatomy and physiology of the female reproductive system and changes during pregnancy have been described in the chapters *Anatomy and Physiology of the Female Reproductive System* and *Anatomy and Physiology of Pregnancy: Placental, Fetal, and Maternal Adaptations*. This chapter focuses on the anatomic and physiologic changes that occur during labor and birth in both the woman and the fetus. The uterine changes that proceed from contraction inhibition during pregnancy to uterotropin-associated activation and uterotonin-associated stimulation during latent and active labor are highlighted, followed by a review of the anatomic relationships between the fetus and pelvis during the process of birth.

Physiologic adaptations during labor are required to support the unique demands imposed on both the woman giving birth and her fetus. Traditionally, the processes involved in labor and birth have been conceptualized as those that affect the power (uterus), the passenger (fetus), and the passage (pelvis). A fourth "P" is often included in this rubric—the psyche—and will be addressed in this chapter. However, many more complex adaptations also occur during labor and birth. With this knowledge, midwives are prepared to both appreciate and support the normal physiologic processes of labor and birth, and to recognize situations when labor may not progress as anticipated such that alternative management strategies may be required.

Physiology of Premonitory Signs and Symptoms of Labor

Premonitory signs and symptoms of impending labor may occur in the week or two before labor starts as the uterus slowly shifts from a quiescent state to active ongoing contractions.

Maternal Responses to Fetal Descent

Lightening—that is, the descent of the fetus into the true pelvis—may occur as early as 4 weeks prior to the onset of labor. The movement of the fetus into a lower position into the true pelvis (sometimes referred to as the baby "dropping" or becoming engaged) indicates the initial descent and engagement of the presenting part and is more common among nulliparous women than multiparous women. The anatomic change in fetal position measured objectively by a decrease in fundal height is accompanied by characteristic signs and symptoms in the mother, including partial relief of pressure on maternal structures such as the diaphragm, leading to greater ease of breathing and decreased reflux. In turn, increased pressure on structures adjacent to the pelvis worsens, with symptoms such as urinary frequency, pelvic pressure, leg cramps, and dependent edema in the lower extremities becoming more evident. Partial obstruction by the fetal presenting part on the femoral veins reduces venous return to the heart, particularly when the woman is standing. As blood pools in the lower leg veins, increased intravascular pressure promotes fluid movement out of the vessels and into the surrounding interstitial tissue, resulting in edema. When the woman is supine, venous return is enhanced and intravascular pressure is reduced, resulting in improvement of edema. Tilting a woman to her left side further improves venous return by reducing pressure on the inferior vena cava, which lies slightly to the right of center. The reduced capacity of the maternal bladder due to anatomic pressure of the engaged fetal presenting part, coupled with increased venous return when recumbent, contributes to increased frequency of urination, which can lead to interrupted sleep in the last weeks of pregnancy.

Cervical Anatomic and Physiologic Premonitory Changes

Cervical connective tissue changes are central to the significant remodeling that characterizes cervical changes in labor, including softening, ripening, dilation, and repair.[1] Descent of the fetal presenting part into the true pelvis is due in part to progressive cervical changes that precede labor. Increased distensibility of the cervix, "softening," and effacement are characteristic of the cervical ripening that is initiated approximately 4 weeks prior to labor onset. The rearrangement of collagen is the primary driver of cervical ripening, with realignment of elastin and smooth muscle fibers playing a more minor role in the process.[1,2] The anatomic changes modulated by inflammatory and hormonal influences are accompanied by an increase in water content that causes the softening of the cervix,[3] setting the stage for the full effacement and dilation that precede birth during active labor.

The ripening and softening of the cervix are essential for effacement and dilation, reflecting the enhanced collagen breakdown and elastin remodeling that were previously inhibited by progesterone during uterine quiescence. The tight collagen bundles in the nonpregnant cervix respond to hormonal changes, becoming less dense and more loosely packed at midpregnancy. In later pregnancy and during labor, an increase in water content creates a softer consistency that is also associated with separation of collagen fibrils promoted by the proteoglycan decorin and the reduction in fibronectin.[1] Increases in enzymes that break down connective tissue, including collagenase and elastase, contribute to the process of cervical remodeling. Effacement is the result of the lengthening of the muscle fibers at the internal os, stretching the endocervix upward into the lower uterine segment. Effacement is clinically evaluated in terms of percentage, where no effacement is described as 0% and complete effacement is described as 100% or in terms of actual centimeters of length. As clinicians adopt cervical length screening for all women in pregnancy, the trend is toward documenting the cervix in actual centimeters. However, when a woman is at term and her cervix is being assessed for how likely she is to have a vaginal birth, cervical length may be reported as a percentage of the original length noted before the process of effacement begins. Effacement as a percentage remains one of the parameters in determining the Bishop's score. Use of the Bishop's score is discussed in more detail in the *Complications During Labor and Birth* chapter.

Some cervical dilation may also occur prior to labor, with effacement and dilation continuing over the course of labor. Nulliparous women may have some cervical softening and effacement prior to labor, or they may enter labor with the cervix not yet soft or effaced. In nulliparous women, effacement typically precedes dilation. In contrast, parous women often enter labor with some effacement and dilation having already taken place, and these processes continue to occur simultaneously as labor progresses.

Dilation is the widening of the external os, expanding from an opening of a few millimeters to one that allows the passage of the fetus during birth. The force of contractions, coupled with the hydrostatic action of the amniotic fluid, creates a force for dilation of the low-resistance cervix. In the case of ruptured membranes, the pressure of the presenting fetal part on the cervix also promotes progressive dilation. Dilation is clinically evaluated by measuring the diameter of the cervical opening digitally in centimeters, with 0 centimeters describing a closed external cervical os and 10 centimeters defining complete dilation. The 10-centimeter measure of complete dilation is based on the suboccipito-bregmatic diameter of the fetal head, which is approximately 9.5 centimeters at term; it is the widest anterior-posterior diameter of the flexed head during the normal mechanisms of labor when the fetus is in a cephalic presentation. Fetal head diameters are reviewed in detail later in this chapter.

In addition to placing traction on the cervix to promote ripening, uterine contractions may increase in frequency and lead to discomfort before the onset of labor. Historically referred to as "false labor," these early Braxton Hicks–like contractions do not occur in a regular pattern, nor do they cause the progressive cervical dilation and effacement seen during active labor. However they are not "false" because premonitory uterine contractions probably reflect the changes within the uterine musculature that occur with advancing gestation and preparation for labor.[4] The hormonal milieu that stimulates cervical ripening, combined with anatomic pressure of the presenting part on the cervix and the traction generated by uterine contractions also cause the premonitory sign of the passing of the cervical mucus plug. This blood-tinged mucus is expelled from the cervical canal after cervical change has started. The passage of the mucus plug may occur all at once or, more commonly, over a period of 1 to 2 days. In the absence of trauma or injury to the cervix (e.g., during aggressive vaginal examination), the passing of the mucus plug often indicates impending labor within 48 hours.

Onset of Labor

The onset of labor is classically defined as the occurrence of regular painful contractions that promote dilation of the cervix. Contractions that occur at regular intervals with increasing frequency, duration, and intensity are the hallmark of labor.[5] The primary basis of our understanding of the process of labor onset is based on animal studies extrapolated to explain the human condition. The onset of labor is likely the result of a complex interplay between biochemical and mechanical influences originating both in the maternal and fetal systems. Therefore the wide individual variation in chronology of events associated with labor onset reflects the variability of the human experience.

Factors That Influence Labor Onset

The influence of familial/individual and racial trends in the timing of labor onset provides some evidence for genetic influences of labor onset.[6–8] Gene–environment interactions that occur as a result of maternal, fetal, and intrauterine factors illustrate the complexity of outcomes, including labor onset.[9,10] Genetic polymorphisms in the maternal genome suggest a role for factors associated with stress[11] and inflammation[12–14] in the timing of labor onset.

Endocrinology of Onset of Labor

It is believed that the onset of labor is the result of interplay between the maternal, fetal, and placental units.[15] For example, maternal factors include increased uterine stretch due to the growing fetus and increased amniotic fluid volume, which may promote the start of labor.[16] However, the process is likely a cascade of events that include multiple redundant loops and this may be why no one initiating factor has been found in research on this topic. Two primary mechanisms that are known "players" are a change from progesterone dominance and uterine quiescence to estrogen stimulated uterotropin activation and placental production of corticotropin-releasing hormone.

Contraction onset leading to progressive cervical change is possible following a shift in hormonal dominance from progesterone to estrogen. Under the influence of estrogen, uterine myometrial cells express receptors for prostaglandins and ocytocin and develop gap junctions that allow direct communication between muscle fibers. Gap junctions are transmembrane proteins that create a pore or line of communication between two adjacent myocytes. The action potentials that initiate contraction activity propagate through gap junctions, resulting in synchronous uterine contraction characterized by generation of force along a short distance at low velocity.[19]

Placenta-derived corticotropin-releasing hormone (CRH) levels peak at time of birth, which implicates an important role for the placenta in the timing of labor onset and birth.[16] Placental CRH is transported to the fetus, where it stimulates the fetal hypothalamic–pituitary–adrenal axis, promoting cortisol production by the fetal adrenal gland. Cortisol-induced maturation of fetal lungs promotes increased pro-inflammatory surfactant and phospholipid production, thereby serving as a fetal mechanism for inducing maternal uterine contractions.[15] CRH also stimulates fetal adrenal production of dehydroepiandrosterone sulfate (DHEA-S), which serves as a substrate for estrogen production, enhancing the fetal influence on the onset and progression of labor. Fetal membranes, which represent the maternal–fetal interface, serve as a vehicle for communication of these hormones between the fetal and maternal systems to stimulate labor.[17]

Uterine Myometrial Anatomy and Physiology During Labor

Regardless of whether the fetus, placenta, or maternal hormonal milieu initiates labor, the event takes place within the uterus. The hyperplasia and hypertrophy of the uterine cells that accommodate the 5000-mL uterine capacity at term are accompanied by optimization of the contractile ability of the longitudinal and circular muscles.

Physiologic changes in the uterus specific to pregnancy, labor, and birth are classified into four phases: quiescence, activation, stimulation, and involution (**Figure 25-1**). The transition from long-lasting, irregular contractions of low frequency to high-intensity, high-frequency, regularly spaced contractions is associated with the progressive dilation and effacement of the cervix.[18] Uterine smooth muscle contractions are involuntary, a common characteristic of smooth muscle.

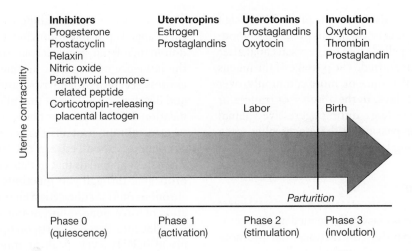

Figure 25-1 Phases of parturition.

Uterine Myometrial Activity in the Activation Phase

The loss of progesterone dominance characterizes the activation phase of labor. The uterus has two forms of progesterone receptor and they have opposing functions. Progesterone's binding preference for the progesterone receptor-B (PR-B) during quiescence switches to preference for the shortened progesterone receptor-A (PR-A) during activation, promoting the dominant pro-inflammatory effects associated with labor.[20] The increased concentration of PR-A in the myometrium opposes the effects of progesterone, leading to a functional progesterone withdrawal without altering circulating progesterone concentrations.[21–24] The removal of the inhibitory effects of hormones, including progesterone, prostacyclin, relaxin, and nitric oxide, during the quiescent period allows for increased uterine activity. Increases in excitability, spontaneous activity, and responsiveness to substances that stimulate uterine contraction are the primary changes that the uterus undergoes in the transition from quiescence to activation.[25]

In the absence of progesterone dominance, several changes combine to promote the frequency, duration, and intensity of uterine contractions, including decreased nitric oxide (NO) synthase activity, increased stimulatory prostaglandin ($PGF_2\alpha$ and PGE_2) production, and more oxytocin receptors and calcium-ion channels in myometrial cells. In labor, PGE_2 favors the prostaglandin EP3 receptor over the EP1 receptor, thereby stimulating uterine contractility through the binding to the EP3 receptor.[26] Prostaglandins facilitate uterine contractions, increase myometrial sensitivity to oxytocin, and stimulate formation of gap junctions.

The declining influence of progesterone and NO also contributes to increased production of CRH from the placenta.[20,27] CRH influences the transition from progesterone to estrogen dominance in labor through stimulation of fetal adrenal activity, which releases DHEA-S. The placenta, in turn, converts DHEA-S to estrogen. Increased uterine perfusion is promoted by CRH-related increased dilation of the blood vessels that supply the uterus, fetus, and placenta. Contractile activity is also modulated by CRH through the promotion of fetal membrane production of the stimulatory prostaglandins $F_2\alpha$ and E_2 and through uterine smooth muscle cell signaling that increases calcium availability.[28]

Role of Inflammation in Labor Initiation

The activation and stimulation stages of labor are characterized by a heightened state of inflammation. At the onset of labor, leukocytes invade the myometrium, cervix, chorio-decidua, and amnion.[29] Pro-inflammatory cytokines released by activated leukocytes promote calcium entry into uterine smooth muscle cells and increased prostaglandin production, enhancing uterine contractions. Neutrophil release of enzymes further degrades extracellular matrix proteins, including fetal fibronectin and collagen, to allow for progressive dilation. Inflammatory cytokines and degrading enzymes are also increased in the fetal membranes, contributing to their weakening and eventual rupture.

Uterine Myometrial Activity in the Stimulation Phase

The onset of regular, progressive uterine contractions characterizes the stimulation phase of the intrapartum period. The influence of oxytocin becomes especially pronounced during the stimulation phase of labor. Produced by the hypothalamus and released via the posterior pituitary, oxytocin is released into the maternal circulation in a pulsatile fashion, reaching peak levels during fetal expulsion.[30] Estrogen dominance also stimulates expression of oxytocin genes in the chorio-decidua, providing a local source of oxytocin. Binding of oxytocin to myometrial oxytocin receptors stimulates the smooth muscle contractions that characterize active labor through a calcium-dependent pathway. Prostaglandin production in the maternal decidua is also stimulated by oxytocin-receptor binding; thus the relationship between prostaglandins and oxytocin is bidirectional.[31,32]

Changes in oxytocin receptor number and sensitivity, rather than the production and release of oxytocin itself, serve as the primary influence on strength and frequency of uterine contractions during active labor.[27] This is an important point with several clinical implications. First, the affinity of oxytocin for its receptor in the uterine fundus increases, maximizing the effect of this hormone even without an increase in oxytocin plasma concentration. Second, the number of oxytocin receptors present on the myometrial cell membranes peak in early labor, reflecting an increase of up to 200-fold from the number of such receptors present on myometrial cells in the nonpregnant state. The plasma level of oxytocin does not change from prelabor levels during the first stage of labor but does increase and peak in the second stage of labor, possibly enhanced by fetal oxytocin release[33] and transport to the maternal side of the placenta. Labor and mechanical stretch also increase oxytocin receptor expression in uterine myocytes, further enhancing the potential for more oxytocin-receptor binding.[32,34]

Similar to the case for other related G-protein–coupled receptors, desensitization of the oxytocin receptor may result from increased concentrations of oxytocin in the maternal circulation, often as the result of increasing concentrations or prolonged exposure to synthetic oxytocin administration during labor.[35] The prolonged or repeated stimulation of the oxytocin receptors may contribute to downregulation, which reduces the number of receptors available for oxytocin binding, Uterine contractions become less forceful and less frequent as a result of attenuation of cell signaling and reduced calcium release, potentially leading to impaired labor progress or uterine atony after birth.

Along with oxytocin, the influence of prostaglandins on the myometrium predominates during the stimulation phase. Produced by the amnion, chorion, and decidua, prostaglandins work in a paracrine fashion to promote uterine contractile activity. Prostaglandin production is also stimulated by inflammatory cytokines. Recent evidence suggests additional effects of these changes may include decreased collagen content and area covered by connective tissue, providing a potential explanation for the higher vaginal delivery rates, tachysystole, and uterine rupture noted with PGE_1 use in labor.[36]

Mechanisms of Uterine Contraction

The uterine myocyte is the excitable smooth muscle cell type that is involved in contractile activity. Triggers for uterine myocyte contraction include mechanical stretch (myogenic) and hormone-receptor binding. Hormones that promote contraction through binding to their receptors include oxytocin, stimulatory prostaglandins, norepinephrine, angiotensin II, and endothelin. Prostaglandins produced by activated myocytes work in a paracrine fashion, stimulating nearby myocytes to depolarize in a wave of contraction,[15] with action potentials being propagated to adjacent myocytes via gap junctions between muscle groups.[5]

Uterine smooth muscle contractions are intermittent, which allows for reperfusion of the uterine muscle, placenta, and fetus between contractions. Each contraction builds in intensity, reaches its peak, and then decreases in intensity until it returns to a state of relaxation, which persists until the next contraction begins. This pattern is often referred to as the increment, acme, and decrement phases of contraction. Contraction of uterine smooth muscle is a phenomenon unique to labor.

The smooth muscle (myometrium) in the uterus is anatomically different from other types of smooth muscle. Located between the decidua and the perimetrium, the myometrium consists of four muscle layers, each of which produces a distinct response to substances that promote or inhibit contractions. The inner circular muscle layer runs perpendicular to the long axis of the uterus in a spiral fashion, while the two outer layers run parallel to this axis. The middle layer has blood vessels running throughout the interlacing fibers. The uterine myocytes are organized in a bundle, contributing to the generation of tension under local stimulation by uterotonic hormones.[19,p.125] Uterine muscle is thickest in the fundus, which generates the area of greatest contractile strength. The fundal portion of the uterus becomes the active segment (**Figure 25-2**). Uterine muscle becomes thinner toward the lower uterine segment in the isthmus; thus this thinner lower uterine segment forms the muscular tube through which the fetus passes.

The propagation of the contraction wave is often called the triple descending gradient of fundal dominance, wherein contractions (1) start in the fundus, (2) last longer in the fundus, and (3) progress from fundus toward the isthmus. Fundal dominance is essential for effective cervical dilation but has not ever been definitely proven to exist. Nonetheless, the

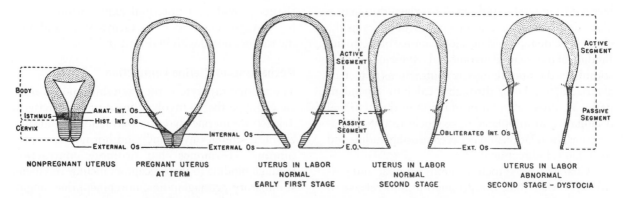

Figure 25-2 Sequence of development of the segments and rings in the uterus in pregnant women at term and in labor. Note comparison between the uterus of a nonpregnant woman, the uterus at term, and the uterus during labor. The passive lower segment of the uterine body is derived from the isthmus; the physiologic retraction ring develops at the junction of the upper and lower uterine segments. The pathologic retraction ring develops from the physiologic ring.

Anat. Int. Os = anatomic internal os; E.O. = external os; Hist. Int. Os = histologic internal os.

Source: Cunningham FG, Cant NF, Leveno KJ, Gilstrap LC III, Hauth JC, Wenstrom KD. *Williams Obstetrics.* 21st ed. New York, NY: McGraw-Hill; 2001. Reproduced by permission of The McGraw-Hill Companies, Inc.

muscle bundles in the uterine fundus progressively shorten with each contraction, causing the upper portion of the uterus to thicken and gradually become a smaller cavity. This reduced fundal capacity, in turn, promotes descent of the fetus toward the more passive lower uterine segment. The lower uterine segment muscle bundles become longer in response to fundal contractions, creating a distensible structure that is able to accommodate the fetus and promote descent. The line of demarcation between the active and passive segments is termed the *physiologic retraction ring.* When labor is obstructed, the active segment becomes so much thicker and shorter that one can sometimes see the line between the two uterine segments when observing the abdomen. This is called a *pathologic retraction ring* or *Bandl's ring.*

At the cellular level, contractile units made of myosin and actin in uterine smooth muscle myocytes promote the generation of tension that leads to synchronous smooth muscle contraction. The interaction between the thin actin and thick myosin filaments is central to the generation of force (**Figure 25-3**). Myosin is arranged in two heavy chains and two light chains, with a globular head attached to a tail that protrudes from the heavy chains at regular intervals. The myosin head also contains a site that binds to actin, generating force that is carried along the myosin tails. Entry of calcium into the myocyte in response to specific stimuli prompts intracellular release of additional calcium from a reservoir in the sarcoplasmic reticulum (SR) through binding of inositol triphosphate (IP$_3$) to SR receptors. Calcium binding to the smooth muscle protein calmodulin causes activation of the myosin light-chain kinase

(MLCK) enzyme. MLCK phosphorylation of the light chain on the myosin head leads to establishment of a structural link between actin and myosin, catalyzed by myosin adenosine triphosphatase (ATPase) enzyme activity on the myosin head. Energy release from myosin ATPase activity causes the structural cross-bridge to shorten the muscle. At this point, the myosin head rotates and pulls on actin, which generates force and shortening. The coordinated effect in myocytes in the uterine smooth muscle bundles leads to coordinated uterine smooth muscle contraction. Decreased intracellular calcium concentrations and the action of myosin light-chain phosphatase enzymatically reverses the actin–myosin linkages through removal of a phosphate from the myosin light chain, prompting smooth muscle relaxation.

Relaxation involves the removal of contractile stimuli or action of factors that inhibit contractions.[37] Factors that may inhibit this process and, therefore, can be used to treat preterm labor contractions include drugs that stimulate the β-adrenergic signaling pathway (e.g., terbutaline [Brethine]), inhibit inflammatory pathways (e.g., indomethacin [Indocin]), calcium-channel blockers (e.g., nifedipine [Procardia]), and agents that inhibit the myosin light chain (e.g., magnesium sulfate). In addition, progesterone is increasingly being used to prevent recurrent preterm labor in women who have experienced a previous preterm birth.

Oxytocin

Oxytocin is a small 9-amino acid peptide that is a potent uterotonic. The word *oxytocin* is derived from the Greek *oxys,* which means "quick," and *tokos,*

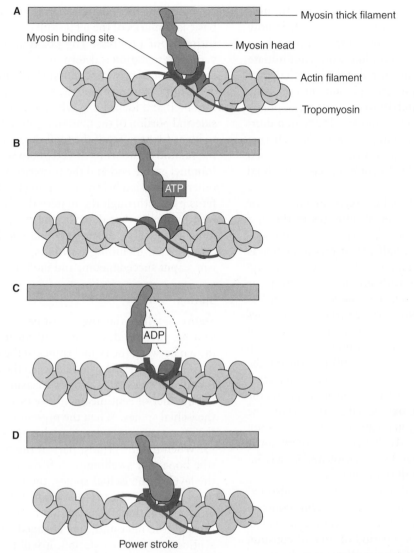

(A) **Attached:** At the start of the cycle, the myosin head is attached to the myosin binding site on the actin filament. (B) **Recharging:** A molecule of ATP binds to a large cleft at the back of the myosin head, which causes a slight change in the conformation of the myosin binding site, which reduces the affinity the myosin head has for the myosin binding site. (C) **Cocked:** The cleft on the myosin head closes around the ATP, which causes a large shape change so that the head is displaced along the actin filament by a distance of approximately 5 nm. (D) **Force-generating:** As ATP is hydrolyzed to ADP, the myosin head once again binds tightly to the next myosin binding site on the actin filament and in this process the myosin head essentially ratchets along the actin filament, creating the muscle contraction.

Figure 25-3 Uterine muscle contraction.

Source: King TL, Brucker MC. *Pharmacology for Women's Health*. Sudbury, MA: Jones and Bartlett; 2011.

which means "birth." Many organs have oxytocin receptors, but especially the uterus, breast, kidney, and central nervous system. Although the primary source of oxytocin is the hypothalamus, oxytocin is synthesized in the uterus, placenta, corpus luteum, and fetus. Along with exerting uterotonic effects, oxytocin stimulates contraction of myoepithelial cells in the lactating breast (i.e., the let-down reflex), increases sexual arousal in women and men, and may have profound effects on initial maternal–infant bonding. In animal studies, oxytocin has been shown to regulate many maternal behaviors.

For many years, oxytocin was thought to initiate the stimulatory phase of parturition. It is now known that this peptide plays an important role in maintaining labor but it most likely does not initiate labor. Oxytocin is manufactured in the hypothalamus and released from the posterior pituitary in a pulsatile fashion. Between 36 and 39 weeks' gestation, pulsations increase in frequency and amplitude in a diurnal rhythm, with maximum plasma levels occurring at night. Oxytocin may play a role in the increased frequency of Braxton Hicks contractions in the final weeks of pregnancy.

During spontaneous labor, oxytocin pulses occur approximately 4 times per 30 minutes in the first stage of labor and 7 times per 30 minutes in the second stage. The biologic half-life of this molecule is approximately 3 to 4 minutes. Plasma levels of oxytocin do not correlate with uterine contractility or cervical dilation. Instead, the number and distribution of oxytocin receptors on the surface membranes of myocytes influence the strength and frequency of uterine contractions in labor. The number of oxytocin receptors in the uterus increases 100-fold during the last weeks of pregnancy, reaching a maximum during labor. This increase in receptor density explains the increased sensitivity to oxytocin displayed by uterine myometrial cells. Early in pregnancy, the uterus is not sensitive to oxytocin. Myometrial receptivity starts at approximately 20 weeks' gestation and slowly increases over the last half of pregnancy.

The pivotal role of oxytocin receptors also explains why oxytocin can cause both uterine contractions and uterine atony. The oxytocin receptors can become saturated after a period of time of constant agonist stimulation and downregulate via endocytosis. Thus, when synthetic oxytocin infusions are used for induction or augmentation of labor, the woman may have an increased risk for uterine atony after birth secondary to downregulation of oxytocin receptors.

Maternal Pelvic Anatomy Related to Labor and Birth

The obstetric pelvic types and fetopelvic relationships are reviewed in the *Anatomy and Physiology of the Female Reproductive System* chapter. Confirmation of the fetal presentation and position is made during a vaginal examination once the cervix is dilated enough to feel the fetal presenting part. Fetal suture lines and fontanels, or portions of the fetal face, breech, external genitalia, or fetal extremities (hands or feet), are palpated. Cephalic vertex presentations are by far the most common, so familiarity with the basic landmarks of the fetal skull is crucial for monitoring labor progress. The position of a fetus in a vertex presentation is determined vaginally by feeling the anterior or posterior fontanel (the fontanel shape and number/direction of the sutures leading off the fontanel) and identifying which fontanel is in which side and portion of the maternal pelvis. When seeking to identify the parts of the fetal skull, remember that the sagittal suture runs directly between the anterior fontanel at one end and the posterior fontanel at the other end and is a helpful beginning landmark. As the fetus passes through the maternal pelvis, additional measurements that describe the relationship of the fetus to the pelvis during labor should be noted and documented including station, synclitism, asynclitism, caput succedaneum, and molding.

Station

Station is where the lowermost part of the fetal presenting part resides relative to an imaginary line drawn between the ischial spines of the woman's pelvis (**Figure 25-4**). The line between the ischial spines is called 0 station. Station is measured in terms of the number of centimeters above or below a level at the ischial spines. When the presenting part is above the spines, station is designated as −1, −2, −3, -4, and -5. When the lowermost part of the presenting part (the bone, not swelling or soft tissue) is lower than the level of the ischial spines, the presenting part is at +1, +2, +3, +4 , or +5 station. When the fetus is at 0 station, the biparietal diameter is most always through the inlet and thus engaged. When the presenting part is at +5 station, it will be visible at the vaginal introitus. It is important to make sure station is determined based on level of the fetal bone (usually the occiput). Soft tissue swelling is variable and if it is used to determine the level of the fetus, one can mistakenly assume the fetal head is engaged when it is not engaged.

Synclitism and Asynclitism

Synclitism and *asynclitism* are terms that describe the relationship of the sagittal suture of the fetal head to the symphysis pubis and the sacrum of the maternal pelvis—a relationship determined when the anteroposterior diameter of the fetal head is in alignment with the transverse diameter of the pelvic inlet. This places the sagittal suture line of the fetal skull in the same line as the transverse diameter of the pelvic inlet and the occiput of the fetal head in the transverse portion of the mother's pelvis. With synclitism, the sagittal suture is midway between the symphysis pubis

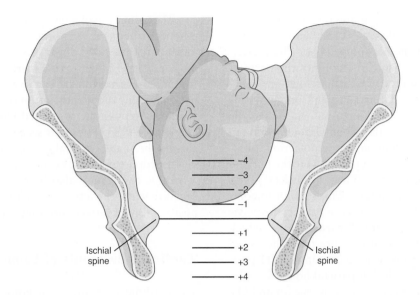

Figure 25-4 Station, or level of descent, of the head of the fetus through the pelvis. The location of the forward leading edge (lowest part of the head) is designated in centimeters above or below the plane of the interspinous line.

and the sacral promontory. With asynclitism, the fetal neck is bent so that the fetal head is tipped laterally toward the fetal shoulder somewhat. Therefore the alignment of the sagital suture and transverse diameter of the maternal pelvis are not exact and the sagital suture tends to be closer to the symphysis pubis or to the sacral promontory (**Figure 25-5**).

Determination of anterior asynclitism or posterior asynclitism is based not on which maternal pelvic structure the sagittal suture is closer to, but rather on which parietal bone is dominant. Therefore, anterior asynclitism occurs when the anterior parietal bone (the one closest to the symphysis pubis) becomes the lowermost part of the presenting part, due to flexion of the head toward the sacral promontory, causing the sagittal suture to lie closer to the sacral promontory. Posterior asynclitism occurs when the posterior parietal bone (the one closest to the sacral promontory) becomes the lowermost part of the presenting part as a result of flexion of the head toward the symphysis pubis, causing the sagittal suture to lie closer to the symphysis pubis. In normal labor, the fetal head usually enters the pelvic inlet with a moderate degree of posterior asynclitism and then changes to anterior asynclitism as it descends farther into the pelvis before the mechanism of internal rotation occurs. This sequential change from posterior to anterior asynclitism facilitates the mechanism of descent; it is an accommodation by the fetus to take advantage of the roomiest portions of the true pelvis.

Molding and Caput Succedaneum

Molding and *caput succedaneum* are both conditions that result from pressure exerted on the fetal head by the maternal structures of the birth canal during labor and birth. Molding is the change in the shape of the head as a result of the soft skull bones' overriding, or overlapping, one another because they are not yet completely fused, so that movement is possible at the location of the sutures. Minor degrees of molding

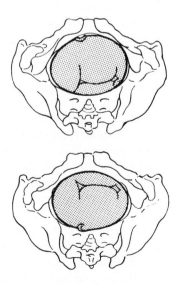

Figure 25-5 Asynclitism: (A) anterior; (B) posterior.

occur as the fetal head negotiates the maternal pelvis and are initially considered a normal finding.

The shape of the head depends on the presentation and attitude, which determines the parts of the skull that present first and, therefore, are being subjected to pressure. Occiput cephalic presentations are most common, so molding usually occurs as the parietal bones override the occipital bone, which in effect obliterates or minimizes the posterior fontanel. A bony ridge may be palpable where the parietal bones override the occiput. When the parietal bones overlap at the sagittal suture, which is not uncommon, the parietal bone that was anterior in the pelvis overlaps with the "posterior" parietal bone, which was depressed because of pressure from the sacral promontory. Therefore, when a fetus in an ROT position rotates to ROA, the left parietal bone overrides the right parietal bone; the reverse is true for an LOT position that rotates to LOA.

In regard to the overriding of the parietal bones, the location of the left and right parietal bones (either anterior or posterior) should not be confused with anterior and posterior asynclitism. Whether the left or right parietal bone is anterior is based solely on whether the occiput is to the left or right of the pelvis, which then determines which one lies closest to the symphysis pubis and which is closest to the sacrum.

Molding involves the entire skull, with overlapping in one area being counterbalanced by movement elsewhere. This creates harmony between the base and the vertex of the skull and prevents destructive tension and possible rupture of the cranial membrane, the dura mater.

Caput succedaneum is the formation of an edematous swelling over the most dependent portion of the presenting fetal head. Pressure around the presenting part by the cervical opening produces congestion and edema of the portion of the fetal head that presents against the cervical opening. If the fetal membranes are ruptured and the fetal head (rather than the membranes) is functioning as the dilating wedge against the cervical opening, a greater amount of caput succedaneum will likely be formed. If the fetal head is unusually molded or there is significant caput, the head may not be engaged in the pelvis at all, thus caput and molding can be clinically quite important. After birth, caput succedaneum can be differentiated from the more serious condition known as cephalohematoma by the fact that caput succedaneum crosses suture lines as a generalized swelling, whereas a cephalohematoma (bleeding beneath the periosteum) may occur over more than one cranial bone but is limited to each individual bone and does not cross any sutures.

The formation of a few millimeters of caput succedaneum is considered normal. A small caput succedaneum may develop during a somewhat prolonged labor resulting from uterine inertia with weak contractions. Formation of extensive caput succedaneum, making the identification of fetal sutures and fontanels impossible, combined with a more severe degree of molding, is usually seen only when the pressure has been great and labor prolonged; cephalopelvic disproportion must be suspected in such a case. A sizable caput may also be seen from positional pressure when the fetus was in an occipitoposterior position for a relatively prolonged period.

Cardinal Movements of Labor

The cardinal movements of labor, also called the mechanisms of labor, describe the movements made by the fetus during labor and immediately before birth to negotiate the diameters of maternal pelvis (**Table 25-1**). Understanding the cardinal movements of labor requires knowing the essential average diameters of the fetal head. Although the majority of fetuses enter labor in a cephalic presentation, knowledge of the cardinal movements of labor for each fetal presentation, position, and denominator is essential. The cardinal movements are engagement, descent, flexion, internal rotation, extension, restitution, and external rotation.

Engagement occurs when the biparietal diameter of the fetal head has passed through the pelvic inlet. *Descent* occurs throughout labor and, therefore, is requisite to and occurs simultaneously with the other cardinal movements. Descent is the result of contractions and maternal pushing efforts during the second stage.

Flexion is essential to further descent. During this third cardinal movement, the smaller suboccipitobregmatic diameter is substituted for the larger fetal head diameters that exist when the fetal head is not completely flexed, is in a military attitude, or is in some degree of extension. Flexion occurs when the fetal head meets resistance; this resistance increases with descent and is first met from the cervix, then from the sidewalls of the pelvis, and finally from the pelvic floor. Some degree of flexion, therefore, may occur prior to engagement.

Internal rotation brings the anteroposterior diameter of the fetal head into alignment with the anteroposterior diameter of the maternal pelvis. Most commonly, the occiput rotates to the anterior portion of the maternal pelvis, beneath the symphysis pubis. If internal rotation has not occurred by

Table 25-1	Cardinal Movements of Labor for Occiput Anterior and Persistent Posterior Positions	
Cardinal Movement	**Occiput Anterior**	**Persistent Posterior**
Engagement	ROT or LOT position	Right or left oblique diameter
Descent	Occurs throughout	Occurs throughout
Flexion	Suboccipitobregmatic diameter presenting	Usually less completely flexed
Internal rotation	45° LOA or ROA, 90° LOT or ROT, 135° LOP or ROP to OA	45° LOP or ROP to OP
Extension	Birth of head by extension	Birth of head by first flexion and then extension
Restitution	45° to LOA or ROA	45° to LOP or ROP
External rotation	45° to LOT or ROT	45° to LOT or ROT
Lateral flexion or expulsion	Birth of shoulders by lateral flexion	Birth of shoulders by lateral flexion

the time the fetal head has reached the pelvic floor, it takes place shortly thereafter. Internal rotation is essential for vaginal birth to occur, except in unusually small fetuses. The pelvic inlet has a larger transverse diameter than anteroposterior diameter; the midplane and the outlet have larger anteroposterior diameters than transverse diameters. Internal rotation is effected by the V-shape of the pelvic floor musculature and the decreased dimensions of the pelvic cavity. The amount of internal rotation is determined by the distance the occiput must travel from its original position on entering the pelvis to the occiput anterior or occiput posterior position that precedes birth. The distance is expressed in degrees, as it is a portion of the arc of a circle that is being traversed.

When the fetus's occiput rotates from an LOP, ROP, LOT, or ROT position, the shoulders also rotate with the head until the LOA or ROA position has been reached. As the occiput rotates the final 45 degrees into the occiput anterior (OA) position, the shoulders do not continue their rotation with the head, but instead enter the pelvic inlet in one of the oblique diameters (the left oblique diameter for an LOA and the right oblique diameter for an ROA). The entire cardinal movement, therefore, has the effect of turning the neck 45 degrees.

Birth of the head occurs by *extension* in occiput anterior births. This cardinal movement of labor is different when the occiput rotates to an occiput posterior (OP) position, as explained later in this chapter. Extension must occur when the occiput is anterior because of the resistant force of the pelvic floor, which has a curve called the curve of Carus that directs the head upward to the vaginal introitus. The curve of Carus is the lower exiting end of the pelvic curve; the

fetus and placenta must follow this curve to be born. The pelvic cavity actually resembles a curved cylinder, such that the direction of either the baby or the placenta coming through it is first downward from the axis of the inlet to just above the tip of the sacrum and then forward, upward, and outward to the vaginal opening. The suboccipital region impinges under the symphysis pubis and acts as a pivot. At this point, the fetal head is positioned so that further pressure from the contracting uterus and maternal pushing serve to further extend the head as the vulvovaginal orifice opens. Thus the head is born by extension as the occiput, sagittal suture, anterior fontanel, brow, orbits, nose, mouth, and chin sequentially sweep over the perineum. The suboccipitofrontal diameter is, therefore, the largest anterior-posterior diameter to pass through the vulvovaginal orifice.

Restitution is the rotation of the head 45 degrees to either the left or the right, depending on the direction from which it rotated into the OA position. In effect, in restitution, the neck turns back so that the head is again at a right angle with the shoulders. The sagittal suture is now in one of the oblique diameters of the pelvis and the bisacromial diameter of the fetus is in the other oblique diameter of the pelvis.

External rotation occurs as the shoulders rotate 45 degrees, bringing the bisacromial diameter into alignment with the anteroposterior diameter of the pelvic outlet. This causes the head to rotate externally another 45 degrees into the LOT or ROT position, depending on the direction of restitution.

Birth of the fetus's shoulders and body is by *lateral flexion* to accommodate the curve of Carus. The anterior shoulder comes into view at the vaginal opening, where it impinges under the symphysis pubis; the posterior shoulder then distends the perineum and is born by lateral flexion. After the shoulders are assisted, the remainder of the body follows the curve of Carus and is readily born.

Cardinal Movements for Occiput Anterior Position

Variations of the eight basic positional movements are determined by the position of the fetus and must be delineated for each. The cardinal movements of labor when a fetus begins labor in the LOA, LOT, LOP, ROA, ROT, or ROP position and delivers in an occiput anterior position are as follows:

1. Engagement takes place for the fetus in the LOT and ROT positions, with the fetal sagittal suture in the transverse diameter of the pelvic inlet and the biparietal diameter of the fetus in the anteroposterior diameter of the pelvic inlet. For LOA, ROA, LOP, and ROP positions, engagement of the fetal head takes place with the sagittal suture in one of the oblique diameters of the pelvis (right oblique diameter for LOA and ROP positions and left oblique diameter for ROA and LOP positions). The biparietal diameter, therefore, is in the oblique diameter of the pelvis opposite from the one the sagittal suture is in. The sagittal suture is used as the fetal landmark that determines in which oblique diameter the fetal head enters the pelvis.

2. Descent occurs throughout labor.

3. Flexion substitutes the suboccipitobregmatic diameter for the diameter that entered the pelvic inlet.

4. Internal rotation takes place: 45 degrees (for LOA and ROA positions), 90 degrees (for LOT and ROT positions), and 135 degrees (for LOP and ROP positions—long arc rotation). The fetal head is now in the OA position in the anteroposterior diameter of the mother's pelvis.

5. Birth of the head occurs by extension.

6. Restitution is 45 degrees to the LOA or ROA position. The fetal head moves left if the fetus started the cardinal movements of labor with the occiput in the left side of the pelvis; it moves right if the fetus started the cardinal movements of labor with the occiput in the right side of the pelvis.

7. External rotation is 45 degrees to the LOT or ROT position. The direction of the rotation of the shoulders is determined by the direction of restitution. External rotation

brings the bisacromial diameter of the shoulders into the anteroposterior diameter of the maternal pelvis.

8. Birth of the shoulders and body occurs by lateral flexion via the curve of Carus.

Cardinal Movements for Persistent OP Position

A persistent posterior position occurs when the fetus in a left or right occiput posterior position (LOP or ROP) undergoes internal rotation through a short arc of 45 degrees to a direct occiput posterior (OP) position in the anteroposterior diameter of the maternal pelvis, instead of the more common long arc rotation of 135 degrees to a direct OA position, as described in the previous subsection. Short arc rotation is much less common, occurring approximately 6% to 10% of the time and most frequently in women with an anthropoid or android type of pelvis.

The cardinal movements of labor for a fetus that begins in the LOP or ROP position and delivers in the OP position are the same as for those fetuses that rotate to an occiput anterior position except as explained here:

1. Engagement takes place in the right oblique diameter for the ROP position and in the left oblique diameter for the LOP position.

2. Descent occurs throughout.

3. Flexion is the same.

4. Internal rotation takes place. The fetal head rotates 45 degrees to an occiput posterior position in the anteroposterior diameter of the mother's pelvis.

5. Birth of the head occurs by the double cardinal movements of flexion and then extension. The sinciput impinges beneath the symphysis pubis and becomes the pivotal point for delivery of the head. The head stays flexed as the occiput distends the perineum and is born to the nape of the neck. The remainder of the head is then born by extension, starting with the anterior fontanel and ending with the chin, as the head falls back toward the rectum, with the face looking upward.

6. In restitution, the fetal head rotates 45 degrees to the LOP or ROP position, depending on whether internal rotation was from the LOP or ROP position.

7. In external rotation, the fetal head rotates 45 degrees to the LOT or ROT position.

8. Birth of the shoulders and body occurs by lateral flexion via the curve of Carus.

Persistent posterior position is considered a variation of normal labor. Its effect on the length of labor may be slightly extended, but this is not always true. A woman with a fetus in a persistent posterior position commonly experiences additional and often severe back pain. Diagnosis of a posterior position is made by abdominal examination and confirmed by vaginal examination or ultrasound. Observation of the contour of the woman's abdomen may give the first clue of a posterior position. A depression in the shape of a saucer is commonly seen at or just below the woman's umbilicus. This depression occurs because the fetus's shoulder is posterior rather than anterior, so there is not a smooth anterior curve but rather what looks like a gap between the cephalic and podalic poles of the fetus. If the head is not engaged, there is a bulge between the symphysis pubis and the saucer-shaped depression.

Maternal Systemic Adaptations in Labor

The adaptations of pregnancy that developed progressively during the quiescent phase of gestation provide the essential preparation for the final stages of pregnancy in the intrapartum period. The significant physiologic demands associated with the activation and stimulation phases of labor require maternal adaptations to meet the transient challenges imposed on the maternal and fetal systems.

Hemodynamic Adaptations

The physiologic demands of the activation, stimulation, and involution phases of labor require hematologic adaptations to promote fetal tolerance. Established during the quiescent phase, the pregnancy adaptations provide the anatomy and physiologic capacity to meet challenges inherent in active labor and through the anticipated blood loss experienced in the third stage of labor. Increased maternal blood volume of approximately 40% reaches its acme in the early third trimester, ensuring hemodynamic capacity of increased cardiac output and left ventricular stroke volume necessary to meet oxygen consumption demands throughout active labor.[38] Oxygen carrying capacity is further supplemented by similar increases in red blood cell (RBC) production, thereby maximizing delivery of oxygen to both the maternal systems and the fetus. Maternal vascular system hypertrophy is promoted by NO-mediated vasodilation and progesterone-mediated reduction in vascular tone and resistance, creating the ability to accommodate the increased blood volume and perfusion requirements of the maternal–placental–fetal unit.[39, p.18] Increased plasma volume and decreased viscosity reduce resistance to flow, further supported by decreased vascular resistance; the result is the development of a physiologic arteriovenous shunt that promotes accommodation of increased blood volume and cardiac output.

Accentuated hemodynamic adaptations occur during active labor to support the additional demands imposed by the labor process.[40] Both systolic and diastolic blood pressure increase during contractions, returning to baseline between contractions. Blood pressure and heart rate may also increase due to pain. Although heart rate often increases, the direction of change is variable, such that both increases and decreases can be observed.[19, pp.259–260] The maternal pulse commonly increases during contractions.

The mother's cardiac output increases by an additional 10% to 15% in first-stage labor and by as much as 50% in second-stage labor, due primarily to increased stroke volume. Cardiac output can also be affected by maternal pain, anxiety, and any anesthetics used.[19, pp.259–260] An inverse relationship exists between myometrial contraction intensity and duration and placental blood flow, with perfusion being reduced during maximal contraction. Restoration of resting tone between contractions provides the opportunity to reestablish perfusion. Approximately 500 mL of blood flows through the placental site each minute. Shifts in blood volume that occur during contractions force 300 mL to 500 mL of blood into the venous system, contributing to increased venous return. Increases in central venous pressure during the second stage of labor can result from pushing efforts, prompting parasympathetic nervous system stimulation during Valsalva maneuvers. Redistribution of blood flow in the maternal system after delivery of the placenta leads to splanchnic circulation vasoconstriction, shunting an additional 500 mL of blood from the uteroplacental circulation to the maternal circulation. This autoinfusion phenomenon serves as a protection against maternal blood loss of approximately 500 mL after vaginal delivery by increasing central venous pressure, ventricular preload, and cardiac output.

Changes in blood factors initiated during quiescence are enhanced during the activation and stimulation stages of labor, promoting rapid hemostasis after placental separation.[19, p.224] Levels of coagulation factors—most notably factor VIII—are markedly increased during active labor. Tissue factor release from the placenta and decidua activates the extrinsic coagulation pathway, promoting clot development. The procoagulant condition reaches its maximal point after placenta separation, with increases in factor V, platelet activation, and fibrin clot formation. Clot development contributes to reduced circulating fibrinogen and platelets as a result of their utilization in the production of fibrin clots. A simultaneous decrease in fibrolytic activity enhances clot development after placental separation, associated with decreased levels of circulating plasminogen.

After birth of the newborn, clot dissolution is associated with increased production of fibrin degradation products and d-dimer may promote an anticoagulant effect, potentially interfering with clot development.[41] Uterine contraction and compression of uterine vessels serve to promote accumulation of clotting factors and hemostasis after placental separation, in turn reducing risk of maternal blood loss.[42] In the event of uterine atony and maternal bleeding, uterine massage and the use of exogenous uterotonics can be used to promote contraction and intrinsic vasoconstriction. As uterine blood flow contributes to cardiac output increases ranging from 1% in the nonpregnant women to 15% at the end of pregnancy, interference with adequate uterine contraction and hemostasis after placental separation can lead to massive maternal hemorrhage.[43]

Respiratory Adaptations

Pregnancy adaptations that lead to reduced total lung capacity, residual volume, and functional residual capacity and increased tidal volume[44] promote the respiratory system changes that support increased oxygen requirements during the activation and stimulation stages of labor. Increased muscular work, metabolic rate, and oxygen consumption represent the major challenges to the respiratory system during labor.[19, pp.302–303]

Oxygen consumption in the woman increases as her muscular activity increases during uterine contractions. Intercontraction periods of relaxation allow reperfusion and restoration of oxygen content to the uterine myometrium. Failure to restore oxygenation to uterine muscle cells over time results in anaerobic metabolism, production of lactic acid, and subsequent ischemic pain that is theorized to contribute to the uterine pain felt during labor.

Pain can also lead to an increased respiratory rate and hyperventilation, promoting respiratory alkalosis. During pushing efforts, voluntary muscle activity further contributes to the increased maternal PCO_2 and base deficit, leading to a decline in maternal arterial pH values. A reduction in respiratory rate in the third stage of labor promotes the return to the usual acid–base balance, which typically normalizes within 24 hours of delivery.

Gastrointestinal Adaptations

The hormonal and anatomic effects on the gastrointestinal system during pregnancy, including delayed motility and reflux, are retained as the quiescent stage transitions into the activation and stimulation stages of labor. The combined effects of decreased gastric motility, relaxation of the gastroesophageal sphincter, and increased intra-abdominal pressure contribute to an increased risk for emesis and aspiration when the laboring woman is sedated or intubated.[44] Delay in gastric emptying time can be further exacerbated by pain, and stress is certainly a consideration during active labor.[45] Transient nausea and vomiting may occur during active labor, particularly during the transition phases.

Nutritional Needs During Labor

There are few objective reports regarding gastrointestinal physiology during labor that can provide evidence to support interventions regarding intake of solid foods and fluids in labor. The restriction of solid food intake during active labor is controversial, often explained by the risk for aspiration should intubation or anesthesia be required. Solid food and fluid restriction must be balanced with the need for energy intake to support the work of labor. Energy demands during the first stage of labor are related to increased cardiac output and work of respiratory and uterine muscles.[46] The additional work required of voluntary muscles in pushing efforts during the second stage further increases the demand for energy.[47,48] Hypoglycemia due to fasting may lead to use of alternative metabolic pathways that lead to accumulation of by-products including lactate[49] and ketones.[50, 51] Strategies that provide energy while limiting risks due to increased volume of gastric contents, including intake of isotonic sports drinks[46,50] and consumption of a light diet,[52] has not produced any adverse outcomes. A recent report[53] indicated that there was no benefit or harm from restriction of food and fluids in laboring women at low risk of needing anesthesia.

Maternal Psychobiological Responses in Labor

The anticipation of pain during labor is a source of concern for many women, which affects the physical, psychological, social, and environmental context of the birth experience. Mechanical pressure on anatomic structures, uterine contractions, and cervical changes are the primary mediators of pain in labor. Pain associated with contractions is conducted from pain receptors (nociceptors) to afferent type A delta and C neurons extending from the uterus to the dorsal spinal cord. The afferent neurons enter the spinal cord via segments of the thoracic spinal nerves (10–12).[54] Fetal descent induces mechanical pressure on the pelvic floor, vagina, and perineum during the second stage of labor, mediating sensory pain impulses via the pudendal nerve to the sacral spinal nerves (2–4). Interpretation of pain is achieved when the pain impulse ascends the spinal cord to higher cortical brain centers.

The influence of anxiety produced in response to anticipated or actual pain in labor can serve as an impediment to labor progress. Fear, previous traumatic birth experience, or other unpleasant memories can exacerbate anxiety, worsening the perception of pain.[55,56] Hormonal influences associated with stress, particularly cortisol, may also be a significant factor influencing women's response to pain during labor.[57] Attenuation of fear, stress, and anxiety has the potential to reduce the perception of pain in labor and extend this response to subsequent births.[58] Strategies to promote an optimal psychobiological response to labor include education and anticipatory guidance, support for decision making, and promotion of emotional well-being[59] as providing the physiologic basis for interventions to reduce fear, stress, and anxiety during the birth experience.

At any point in the transmission of the pain neurologic impulse, modulation can be achieved through interruption of the pain pathway (entry into the spinal cord, spinal neurons, and higher brain centers). This knowledge forms the basis for implementing effective strategies for pain relief.[60] Decreased transmission of the pain sensation can be promoted through stimulation of inhibitory afferent type A beta pain fibers using interventions such as massage. Endogenous substances (e.g., enkephalins) can decrease pain perception via the descending spinal nerves. Cognitive strategies such as distraction can also reduce the pain sensation through the targeting of higher cortical brain centers. Promotion of knowledge, attention to goals, companionship, feelings of reassurance and safety,[61] and implementation of nonpharmacologic strategies (e.g., relaxation, water immersion, acupuncture) have the potential to reduce the sensation of pain intensity, modulate pain, and optimize perceptions of the birth experience.[62,63]

Fetal Response to Labor

Approximately 40% of fetal cardiac output is located in the placental circulation. As a consequence, transient changes in fetal circulation are influenced by maternal uterine activity, which poses a potential risk for impaired fetal perfusion during the first and second stages of labor.[64] Oxygen uptake by the fetus is determined by three factors: (1) placental oxygen diffusing capacity, (2) uterine and umbilical blood flow, and (3) oxygen content in maternal blood available for diffusion from the maternal to fetal circulation across the placental interface. Due to the high metabolic rate of the placenta, the fetus extracts less oxygen than the amount of oxygen delivered to the maternal uterus. Although fetal arterial partial pressure of oxygen is only approximately 25% of the maternal value, the fetus maximizes oxygen delivery via high-affinity fetal hemoglobin, high fetal cardiac output, and the distribution pattern of cardiac output between the placenta and fetus. The low PO_2 creates a "physiologic hypoxia" as compared to the newborn and is considered a normal state of fetal oxygenation.[65] Severe hypoxia beyond that considered "physiologic" redistributes blood flow; in this condition, shunting of blood to the brain, myocardium, and adrenal gland and away from the pulmonary, mesenteric, and renal circulation occurs in conjunction with reductions in the amount of oxygenated blood in the fetal circulation.[64]

Uterine contractions have been demonstrated to reduce fetal oxygenation both when measured physiologically and by assessing uterine activity. In a study of this phenomenon, fetal pulse oximetry readings increased initially, then declined during contractions, returning to baseline after 2 minutes following the end of the contraction without concomitant changes in fetal heart rate.[66] Near-infrared spectrometry has been used to measure changes in fetal brain oxyhemoglobin (HbO_2); deoxyhemoglobin (Hb) showed a negative change in HbO_2 and a positive change in Hb when the interval between contractions was less than 2 minutes, and a positive change in HbO_2 following longer contraction intervals.[67] Contraction intervals less than 2 minutes are uncommon in normal labor, but are seen more frequently with oxytocin use. Shorter uterine relaxation time, longer contractions, and higher contraction amplitude during labor have been associated with acidosis as measured by cord blood pH at birth (umbilical artery pH of 7.11 or less) compared to newborns who experienced less uterine activity during labor.[68]

In another study utilizing fetal pulse oximetry, Simpson et al. assessed the effects of uterine hyperstimulation of 30-minute periods in two defined categories: (1) five or more but less than six contractions in 10 minutes and (2) more than six contractions in 10 minutes. The group with more contractions had greater decreases in fetal oxygen saturation compared to normal contraction patterns.[69] Although the mean fetal heart rate (FHR) was unchanged, the group with more contractions had more periods of reduced or absent FHR variability.[69]

Compensatory responses involving the autonomic nervous system are limited during labor, depending on fetal maturity. Sympathetic responses involving the baroreceptor reflex response, renin–angiotensin system, and blood pressure regulation influence the fetus's ability to respond to decreases in perfusion. Parasympathetic innervation via the vagus nerve is a more mature development in the fetus, with typical responses of reduced heart rate, blood pressure, and increased pulmonary flow becoming evident in the fetus with advancing gestation. Failure or exhaustion of compensatory mechanisms that might otherwise ensure fetal oxygen delivery may result in lactic acidemia, cardiac dysfunction, and acidosis.[70] Provision of supplemental oxygen to the mother increases the partial pressure of oxygen and the overall oxygen delivery to the fetus. Left lateral positioning may help increase uterine perfusion, and reducing or eliminating administration of oxytocin, if in use, may also aid fetal recovery.

Conclusion

The physiology of labor is complex, involving hormonal, mechanical, and biochemical events that lead to birth. Endocrine and anatomic changes involving the maternal and fetal systems contribute to the phases of labor, including the premonitory signs and symptoms that precede labor and the activation and stimulation phases of uterine activity. With a solid foundation in the physiology and maternal and fetal anatomy of the intrapartum period, framed in the context of midwifery philosophy and grounded in the best research evidence, including a healthy respect for individual normal variation, midwives are in an excellent position to support women during this unique period in their lives.

• • • References

1. Leppert PC. Anatomy and physiology of cervical ripening. *Clin Obstet Gynecol.* 1995;38(2):267-279.
2. Banos A, Wolf M, Grawe C, et al. Frequency domain near-infrared spectroscopy of the uterine cervix during cervical ripening. *Laser Surg Med.* 2007;39(8):641-646.
3. Hwang JJ, Macinga D, Rorke EA. Relaxin modulates human cervical stromal cell activity. *J Clin Endocrinol Metab.* 1996;81(9):3379-3384.
4. Norwitz ER, Lye SJ. Biology of parturition. In: Creasy RK, ed. *Creasy and Resnik's Maternal–Fetal Medicine.* 6th ed. Philadelphia, PA: Saunders Elsevier; 2009:69-85.
5. Liao JB, Buhimschi CS, Norwitz ER. Normal labor: mechanism and duration. *Obstet Gynecol Clin North Am.* 2005;32(2):145-164.
6. Centers for Disease Control and Prevention (CDC). Infant mortality and low birth weight among black and white infants—United States, 1980–2000. *MMWR.* 2002;51(27):589-592.
7. Cypher RL. Reducing recurrent preterm births: best evidence for transitioning to predictive and preventative strategies. *J Perinat Neonatal Nurs.* 2012;26(3):220-229.
8. Esplin MS. Preterm birth: a review of genetic factors and future directions for genetic study. *Obstet Gynecol Surv.* 2006;61(12):800-806.
9. Esplin MS, O'Brien E, Fraser A, et al. Estimating recurrence of spontaneous preterm delivery. *Obstet Gynecol.* 2008;112(3):516-523.
10. Roberts CT. IFPA award in placentology lecture: complicated interactions between genes and the environment in placentation, pregnancy outcome and long term health. *Placenta.* 2010;31(suppl):S47-S53.
11. Rodriguez-Dennen F, Martinez-Ocana J, Kawa-Karasik S, et al. Comparison of hemodynamic, biochemical and hematological parameters of healthy pregnant women in the third trimester of pregnancy and the active labor phase. *BMC Pregnancy Childbirth.* 2011;11:33.
12. Warren JE, Nelson LM, Stoddard GJ, Esplin MS, Varner MW, Silver RM. Polymorphisms in the promoter region of the interleukin-10 (IL-10) gene in women with cervical insufficiency. *Am J Obstet Gynecol.* 2009;201(4):372.e1-372.e5.
13. Hsu TY, Lin H, Lan KC, et al. High interleukin-16 concentrations in the early second trimester amniotic fluid: an independent predictive marker for preterm birth. *J Matern Fetal Neonatal Med.* 2013;26(3):285-289.
14. Gervasi MT, Romero R, Bracalente G, et al. Midtrimester amniotic fluid concentrations of interleukin-6 and interferon-gamma-inducible protein-10: evidence for heterogeneity of intra-amniotic inflammation and associations with spontaneous early (32 weeks) preterm delivery. *J Perinat Med.* 2012;40(4):329-343.
15. Mendelson CR. Minireview: fetal–maternal hormonal signaling in pregnancy and labor. *Mol Endocrinol.* 2009;23(7):947-954.
16. Smith R. Parturition. *N Engl J Med.* 2007;356(3):271-283.
17. Golightly E, Jabbour HN, Norman JE. Endocrine immune interactions in human parturition. *Mol Cell Endocrinol.* 2011;335(1):52-59.

18. Norwitz ER, Robinson JN, Challis JR. The control of labor. *N Engl J Med.* 1999;341(9):660-666.

19. Blackburn ST. *Maternal, Fetal, and Neonatal Physiology: A Clinical Perspective*, 4th ed. St. Louis, MO: Elsevier; 2013:115.

20. Tan H, Yi L, Rote NS, Hurd WW, Mesiano S. Progesterone receptor-A and -B have opposite effects on proinflammatory gene expression in human myometrial cells: implications for progesterone actions in human pregnancy and parturition. *J Clin Endocrinol Metab.* 2012;97(5):E719-E730.

21. Kamel RM. The onset of human parturition. *Arch Gynecol Obstet.* 2010;281(6):975-982.

22. Zakar T, Hertelendy F. Progesterone withdrawal: key to parturition. *Am J Obstet Gynecol.* 2007;196(4): 289-296.

23. Vidaeff AC, Ramin SM. Potential biochemical events associated with initiation of labor. *Curr Med Chem.* 2008;15(6):614-619.

24. Chai SY, Smith R, Zakar T, Mitchell C, Madsen G. Term myometrium is characterized by increased activating epigenetic modifications at the progesterone receptor-A promoter. *Mol Hum Reprod.* 2012;18(8):401-409.

25. Shynlova O, Tsui P, Jaffer S, Lye SJ. Integration of endocrine and mechanical signals in the regulation of myometrial functions during pregnancy and labour. *Eur J Obstet Gynecol Reprod Biol.* 2009;144(suppl 1):S2-S10.

26. Arulkumaran S, Kandola MK, Hoffman B, Hanyaloglu AC, Johnson MR, Bennett PR. The roles of prostaglandin EP 1 and 3 receptors in the control of human myometrial contractility. *J Clin Endocrinol Metab.* 2012;97(2):489-498.

27. Weiss G. Endocrinology of parturition. *J Clin Endocrinol Metab.* 2000;85(12):4421-4425.

28. You X, Gao L, Liu J, et al. CRH activation of different signaling pathways results in differential calcium signaling in human pregnant myometrium before and during labor. *J Clin Endocrinol Metab.* 2012;97(10):E1851-E1861.

29. Osman I, Young A, Ledingham MA, et al. Leukocyte density and pro-inflammatory cytokine expression in human fetal membranes, decidua, cervix and myometrium before and during labour at term. *Mol Hum Reprod.* 2003;9(1):41-45.

30. Blanks AM, Thornton S. The role of oxytocin in parturition. *BJOG.* 2003;110(suppl 20):46-51.

31. Blanks AM, Shmygol A, Thornton S. Regulation of oxytocin receptors and oxytocin receptor signaling. *Semin Reprod Med.* 2007;25(1):52-59.

32. Terzidou V, Blanks AM, Kim SH, Thornton S, Bennett PR. Labor and inflammation increase the expression of oxytocin receptor in human amnion. *Biol Reprod.* 2011;84(3):546-552.

33. Dawood MY, Raghavan KS, Pociask C, Fuchs F. Oxytocin in human pregnancy and parturition. *Obstet Gynecol.* 1978;51(2):138-143.

34. Terzidou V, Sooranna SR, Kim LU, Thornton S, Bennett PR, Johnson MR. Mechanical stretch upregulates the human oxytocin receptor in primary human uterine myocytes. *J Clin Endocrinol Metab.* 2005;90(1):237-246.

35. Phaneuf S, Rodriguez Linares B, TambyRaja RL, MacKenzie IZ, Lopez Bernal A. Loss of myometrial oxytocin receptors during oxytocin-induced and oxytocin-augmented labour. *J Reprod Fertil.* 2000;120(1):91-97.

36. Chiossi G, Costantine MM, Bytautiene E, et al. The effects of prostaglandin E_1 and prostaglandin E_2 on in vitro myometrial contractility and uterine structure. *Am J Perinatol.* 2012;29(8):615-622.

37. Webb RC. Smooth muscle contraction and relaxation. *Adv Physiol Educ.* 2003;27(1-4):201-206.

38. Fujitani S, Baldisseri MR. Hemodynamic assessment in a pregnant and peripartum patient. *Crit Care Med.* 2005;33(10 suppl):S354-S361.

39. Anderson C. The physiology of pregnancy, labor and birth. In: *Supporting a Physiologic Approach to Pregnancy and Birth: A Practical Guide.* Ames, IA: Wiley-Blackwell; 2013:13-27.

40. Harris IS. Management of pregnancy in patients with congenital heart disease. *Prog Cardiovasc Dis.* 2011;53(4):305-311.

41. Tripodi A. d-Dimer testing in laboratory practice. *Clin Chem.* 2011;57(9):1256-1262.

42. James AH, McLintock C, Lockhart E. Postpartum hemorrhage: when uterotonics and sutures fail. *Am J Hematol.* 2012;87(suppl 1):S16-S22.

43. McLintock C, James AH. Obstetric hemorrhage. *J Thromb Haemost.* 2011;9(8):1441-1451.

44. Chang J, Streitman D. Physiologic adaptations to pregnancy. *Neurol Clin.* 2012;30(3):781-789.

45. Gordon MC. Maternal physiology. In: Gabbe SG, Niebyl JR, Simpson JL, et al., eds. *Obstetrics: Normal and Problem Pregnancies*, 6th ed. Philadelphia, PA: Elsevier; 2012:49-51.

46. Kardel KR, Henriksen T, Iversen PO. No effect of energy supply during childbirth on delivery outcomes in nulliparous women: a randomised, double-blind, placebo-controlled trial. *J Obstet Gynaecol.* 2010;30(3):248-252.

47. Banerjee B, Khew KS, Saha N, Ratnam SS. Energy cost and blood sugar level during different stages of labour and duration of labour in Asiatic women. *J Obstet Gynaecol Br Commonw.* 1971;78(10):927-929.

48. Hagerdal M, Morgan CW, Sumner AE, Gutsche BB. Minute ventilation and oxygen consumption during labor with epidural analgesia. *Anesthesiology.* 1983;59(5):425-427.

49. Maganha e Melo CR, Peracoli JC. Measuring the energy spent by parturient women in fasting and in ingesting caloric replacement (honey). *Rev Lat Am Enfermagem*. 2007;15(4):612-617.

50. Kubli M, Scrutton MJ, Seed PT, O'Sullivan G. An evaluation of isotonic "sport drinks" during labor. *Anesth Analg*. 2002;94(2):404-408.

51. Scrutton MJ, Metcalfe GA, Lowy C, Seed PT, O'Sullivan G. Eating in labour: a randomised controlled trial assessing the risks and benefits. *Anaesthesia*. 1999;54(4):329-334.

52. O'Sullivan G, Liu B, Hart D, Seed P, Shennan A. Effect of food intake during labour on obstetric outcome: randomised controlled trial. *BMJ*. 2009;338:b784.

53. Singata M, Tranmer J, Gillian ML, Gyte GML. Restricting oral fluid and food intake in labour. *Cochrane Database Syst Rev*. 2010;1:CD003930. doi: 10.1002/14651858.CD003930.pub2.

54. Hawkins JL, Bucklin BA. Obstetrical anesthesia. In: Gabbe SG, Niebyl JR, Simpson JL, et al., eds. *Obstetrics: Normal and Problem Pregnancies*. 6th ed. Philadelphia, PA: Elsevier; 2012:362-365.

55. Alder J, Breitinger G, Granado C, et al. Antenatal psychobiological predictors of psychological response to childbirth. *J Am Psychiatr Nurses Assoc*. 2011;17(6):417-425.

56. Goffaux P, Michaud K, Gaudreau J, Chalaye P, Rainville P, Marchand S. Sex differences in perceived pain are affected by an anxious brain. *Pain*. 2011; 152(9):2065-2073.

57. Giurgescu C. A clinical translation of the research article titled "antenatal psychobiological predictors of psychological response to childbirth." *J Am Psychiatr Nurses Assoc*. 2011;17(6):426-430.

58. Haines HM, Rubertsson C, Pallant JF, Hildingsson I. The influence of women's fear, attitudes and beliefs of childbirth on mode and experience of birth. *BMC Pregnancy Childbirth*. 2012;12(1):55.

59. Meyer S. Control in childbirth: a concept analysis and synthesis. *J Adv Nurs*. 2013;69(1):218-218.

60. Marchand S. The physiology of pain mechanisms: from the periphery to the brain. *Rheum Dis Clin North Am*. 2008;34(2):285-309.

61. Simkin P. Pain, suffering, and trauma in labor and prevention of subsequent posttraumatic stress disorder. *J Perinat Educ*. 2011;20(3):166-176.

62. Jones L, Othman M, Dowswell T, et al. Pain management for women in labour: an overview of systematic reviews. *Cochrane Database Syst Rev*. 2012;3: CD009234. doi: 10.1002/14651858.CD009234.pub2.

63. Smith CA, Levett KM, Collins CT, Crowther CA. Relaxation techniques for pain management in labour. *Cochrane Database Syst Rev*. 2011;12(12):CD009514. doi: 10.1002/14651858.CD009514.

64. Fineman JR, Clyman R. Fetal cardiovascular physiology. In: Creasy RK, Resnik R, eds. *Maternal–Fetal Medicine*. 6th ed. Philadelphia: W. B. Saunders; 2008:159-170.

65. Meschia G. Placental respiratory gas exchange and fetal oxygenation. In: Creasy RK, Resnik R, eds. *Maternal–Fetal Medicine*. 6th ed. Philadelphia: W. B. Saunders; 2008:181-191.

66. McNamara H, Johnson N. The effect of uterine contractions on fetal oxygen saturation. *Br J Obstet Gynaecol*. 1995;102:644-647.

67. Peebles DM, Spencer JAD, Edwards AD, et al. Relation between frequency of uterine contractions and human fetal cerebral oxygen saturation studied during labour by near infrared spectroscopy. *Br J Obstet Gynecol*. 1994;101:44-48.

68. Bakker PCAM, Kuver PHJ, Kuik DJ, Va Geijn HP. Elevated uterine activity increases the risk of fetal acidosis at birth. *Am J Obstet Gynecol*. 2007;196 (313):e1-313e6.

69. Simpson KR, James DC. Effects of oxytocin-induced uterine hyperstimulation during labor on fetal oxygen status and fetal heart rate patterns. *Am J Obstet Gynecol*. 2008;199(1):34.e1-34.e5.

70. Harman CR. Assessment of fetal health. In: Creasy RK, Resnik R, eds. *Maternal–Fetal Medicine*. 6th ed. Philadelphia: W. B. Saunders. 2008;361-395.

C H A P T E R

26

The First Stage of Labor

JEREMY L. NEAL

SHARON L. RYAN

LINDA A. HUNTER

Introduction

A normal physiologic labor and birth is one that is powered by the innate human capacity of the woman and fetus.[1]

Normal labor and birth do not require medical intervention, yet most women in the United States experience childbirth in hospitals, where their labors are closely monitored via electronic fetal monitoring, they frequently have intravenous infusions, and they experience labor while lying in bed. Approximately half of the women who have a hospital birth receive synthetic oxytocin for induction or augmentation. Yet despite recognition that unnecessary intervention is extensive, until recently, there has been little guidance for eliminating commonly used interventions that are not needed and may in fact impede normal labor.

There is now a burgeoning movement to recharacterize normal physiologic labor. In 2012, the American College of Nurse-Midwives (ACNM), Midwives of North America (MANA), and the National Association of Certified Professional Midwives (NACPM) published a consensus document titled *Supporting Healthy and Normal Physiologic Childbirth: A Consensus Statement by ACNM, MANA and NACPM*.[1] This document defined normal physiologic childbirth. It described essential components and factors that disrupt normal physiologic childbirth (**Box 26-1**) and listed factors that affect birth from the perspectives of the woman, clinician, and birth setting (**Box 26-2**). Similar material can be found in the ACNM materials Midwifery Pearls (Box 2-11), the Physiologic Birth Tool Kit which can be found at BirthTOOLS.org, and consensus documents from Canada and the United Kingdom, resources that are listed at the end of this chapter.

This chapter and those that follow in the intrapartum section of this text present the evidence for the recommendations in the *Supporting Health and Normal Physiologic Childbirth* consensus statement.[1] These points are the roadmap to optimal care for women during labor and birth and, as the United States maternity care system begins to step back from the current overuse of unnecessary interventions, the skills and techniques used in midwifery practice are being recognized as a critical component of this roadmap. Only the key points of the statement are presented in Boxes 26-1 and 26-2. The reader is encouraged to read the document in full.

Labor is the process by which childbirth occurs, requiring uterine contractions of sufficient frequency, duration, and intensity to cause demonstrable effacement and dilatation of the cervix.[2] The mechanisms underlying the onset and progress of spontaneous labor remain largely unknown. Indeed, labor is a continuum that does not readily lend itself to measurement. Not only is prospectively defining the onset of labor a significant challenge, but evaluating its progression is limited because cervical examinations are only performed episodically. Attempts to divide the continuum of labor into stages and phases add to the complexity. In spite of measurement difficulties, understanding and supporting normal first-stage labor allows time for the events of physiologic labor to unfold without unnecessary interventions, while simultaneously observing the woman for situations in which interventions may be needed. Only in this way can safe, state-of-the-science midwifery care be provided.

The first stage of labor begins with true labor contractions, as evidenced by progressive cervical

---

BOX 26-1 Normal Physiologic Birth

Normal physiologic childbirth:
- is characterized by spontaneous onset and progression of labor;
- includes biological and psychological conditions that promote effective labor;
- results in the vaginal birth of the infant and placenta;
- results in physiological blood loss;
- facilitates optimal newborn transition through skin-to-skin contact and keeping the mother and infant together during the postpartum period; and
- supports early initiation of breastfeeding.

The following factors disrupt normal physiologic childbirth:
- induction or augmentation of labor;
- an unsupportive environment, i.e., bright lights, cold room, lack of privacy, multiple providers, lack of supportive companions;
- time constraints, including those driven by institutional policy and/or staffing;
- nutritional deprivation, e.g., food and drink;
- opiates, regional analgesia, or general anesthesia;
- episiotomy;
- operative vaginal (vacuum, forceps) or abdominal (cesarean) birth;
- immediate cord clamping;
- separation of mother and infant; and/or
- any situation in which the mother feels threatened or unsupported.

Source: Reprinted with permission from American College of Nurse-Midwives, Midwives Alliance, National Association of Certified Professional Midwives. Supporting healthy and normal physiologic childbirth: a consensus statement by ACNM, MANA, and NACPM. 2012. Available at: http://midwife.org/index.asp?bid=59&cat=3&button=Search. Accessed January 3, 2013.

BOX 26-2 Factors That Influence Normal Physiologic Childbirth

There are multiple factors that influence the ability of a woman to give birth without intervention. These include the following:

For the woman:
- Her individual health status and physical fitness;
- Autonomy and self-determination in childbirth;
- Personal knowledge and confidence about birth, including cultural beliefs, norms, and practices and education about the value of normal physiologic birth;
- Fully informed, shared decision-making; and
- Access to health care systems, settings, and providers supportive of and skilled in normal physiologic birth.

For the clinician:
- Education, knowledge, competence, skill, and confidence in supporting physiologic labor and birth, including helping women cope with pain;
- Commitment to working with women through education to enhance their confidence in birth and diminish their fear of the process;
- Commitment to shared decision making; and
- Working within an infrastructure supportive of normal physiologic birth.

Source: Reprinted with permission from American College of Nurse-Midwives, Midwives Alliance, National Association of Certified Professional Midwives. Supporting healthy and normal physiologic childbirth: a consensus statement by ACNM, MANA, and NACPM. 2012. Available at: http://midwife.org/index.asp?bid=59&cat=3&button=Search. Accessed January 3, 2013.

---

change, and ends when the cervix is completely dilated (approximated at 10 centimeters). It is known as the stage of cervical dilatation. The second stage of labor, known as the expulsive stage, follows.

Signs and Symptoms of Progress Toward True Labor Onset

The onset of spontaneous labor cannot be reliably predicted, although many pregnant women experience premonitory signs or symptoms of impending labor. Common signs and symptoms suggestive of physiologic progress toward labor include descent of the fetus, cervical changes, increase in uncoordinated uterine contractions, rupture of membranes, bloody show or increased mucus discharge from the vagina, maternal perception of increased energy, and gastrointestinal distress. Anticipatory guidance for all women in late pregnancy should include reassurance that these signs and symptoms are normal, promotion of comfort measures, and support for watchful waiting.

Descent of the Fetus

Notable descent of the fetus prior to labor, or "lightening," occurs following the gradual softening of the uterine isthmus (lower uterine segment). The fetal presenting part, most commonly the head, descends to or through the inlet of the maternal pelvis (**Figure 26-1**). Although lightening is not synonymous with engagement of the fetal presenting part (i.e., when the widest diameter of the fetal presenting part is at or below the maternal pelvic inlet), engagement may be the end result of lightening. A small reduction in fundal height is common following this prelabor fetal descent. Leopold's maneuvers will reveal that the presenting part is no longer ballottable above the symphysis pubis. Cervical examination typically discloses the presenting part as "fixed" and not ballottable. Women often subjectively refer to the physical experience of lightening as "the baby has dropped."

Among many but not all nulliparous women, prelabor descent of the fetus may occur two or more weeks in advance of labor and is reassuring for pelvic adequacy at the inlet plane. For women who have previously given birth, notable descent may not occur until labor is advanced.

The fetal descent associated with lightening can result in women having more room in the upper abdomen, allowing for better lung expansion and increased stomach capacity. However, lightening often causes new discomforts because of the pressure imposed by the presenting part on other structures in the area of the true pelvis. Urinary frequency can be caused by compression of the bladder between the fetal presenting part and the maternal pelvis. An increase in generalized pelvic pressure contributes to the straddling walk of late pregnancy, and women may relate a constant feeling of "something needs to come out" or that she needs to defecate. Increased venous stasis and pelvic congestion can cause more dependent edema, development of hemorrhoids, and vulvar or lower extremity varicosities. Feelings of generalized pressure may occur, and spending some time throughout the day in the knee-chest or left side-lying position may temporarily relieve the

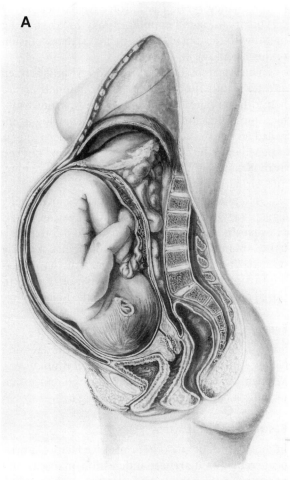
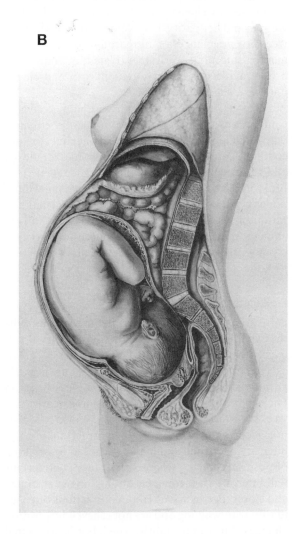

Figure 26-1 Prelightening (A) and postlightening (B).
Source: © Childbirth Connection 2013. Used with permission.

discomforts related to venous stasis. Finally, sciatic nerve pain, characterized by unilateral shooting pain radiating from the buttocks down the back of the leg, can be aggravated or initiated by the fetal descent. This sciatic pain is self-limited to pregnancy and may relieved by massage, application of heat/cold, or gentle stretching exercises. If sciatic nerve pain is debilitating or persists in the postpartum period, referral of the woman for evaluation may reveal vertebral disc herniation.

Cervical Changes

The process of cervical change preparatory to labor is referred to as "ripening." The cervix, which is typically long, closed, and semi-firm throughout pregnancy, becomes soft and malleable during this phase. Effacement, dilation, and anterior rotation of the cervix may be noted. While ripening is a reassuring change suggestive of progress toward true labor, it is not a reliable predictor of actual labor onset. Evaluation of ripeness is relative to the individual woman and her parity. For example, during the final weeks of pregnancy a multiparous woman's cervix may be soft and surprisingly dilated; in contrast, a primigravida's cervix may remain firm and closed until near the onset of labor.

Cervical ripening can occur without perceivable contractions through hormonal influence, collagen matrix changes, and increased extracellular water content. Conversely, the cervix may remain closed and relatively firm even in the presence of regular Braxton Hicks contractions. Unless such an evaluation is being used to inform clinical decision making, routine assessment of cervical ripeness via digital examination in late pregnancy is unnecessary because it is not predictive of labor onset and may be uncomfortable for the woman.

Prelabor or False Labor

False labor is the term historically used to describe the experience of uterine contractions of varying intensity that are not associated with progressive cervical change over time. These contractions are actually an intensification of the usually painless Braxton Hicks contractions, which may begin as early as 6 weeks' gestation and thus the term "false labor" is not accurate. These prelabor contractions do not intensify over time and may be relieved by walking or position changes, whereas true labor contractions will intensify over time, becoming longer, stronger, and closer together. True labor contractions often intensify with walking and are not relieved by position changes. Most importantly, true labor is associated with progressive cervical change. Use of the term "prelabor contractions" in lieu of "false labor" may be more appropriate and also help women understand the discomfort.

Prelabor contractions may occur for days or intermittently for weeks before the onset of true labor. A woman experiencing persistent or recurrent prelabor contractions may fatigue over time and have difficulty coping, as these contractions can be genuinely painful. Anticipatory guidance includes reassurance that the woman will be able to identify a change in the labor pattern and reinforcement of education regarding true labor characteristics and other signs of impending labor can help. Comfort measures for prelabor contractions are the same as those used to support women in latent phase labor.

Bloody Show

A mucus plug, created by cervical secretions from proliferation of the glands of the cervical mucosa early in pregnancy, seals the cervical canal throughout pregnancy, serving as a protective barrier. As the cervix ripens, small capillaries may break, mixing blood with the mucus. Bloody show is the expulsion of this blood-tinged mucus.

The mucus associated with bloody show is thick and tenacious. Both history and examination can help differentiate benign bloody show from frank bleeding. Occasionally the entire mucus plug is expelled en masse. More commonly, the mucus plug is expelled over the course of several days, and noticed by the woman as mild irregular spotting when wiping after urination or defecation.

As a predictive sign of labor, bloody show usually signals the onset of labor within the next few days. However, it is of no value as a sign of labor if a vaginal examination or sexual intercourse has recently occurred, because blood-tinged mucus discharge during this time may be the effect of minor trauma to the ripening cervix or disruption of the mucus plug.

Energy Spurt

Some women perceive an energy spurt in the days preceding labor onset, the cause of which is unknown. Women may benefit by anticipatory guidance that includes a caution against "overdoing it."

Gastrointestinal Distress

In the absence of any other causative factors, a brief occurrence of diarrhea, indigestion, nausea, and vomiting is thought to be indicative of impending labor. These gastrointestinal distress symptoms are likely associated with the increased production of prostaglandins and estrogen and drop in progesterone levels that occurs with the approach of labor.

Prelabor Rupture of Membranes

Rupture of the fetal membranes with associated loss of amniotic fluid prior to the onset of labor is called prelabor rupture of membranes (PROM). PROM occurs in 8% to 10% of women with term pregnancies, the majority of whom begin labor spontaneously within 24 hours, if given this time. Management of PROM varies according to several factors described in more detail in the *Complications During Labor and Birth* chapter. The steps for diagnosing prelabor rupture of membranes are listed in **Appendix 26A**.[3,4]

A special consideration in the woman experiencing PROM is her status related to group B *Streptococcus* (GBS), as it may impact management decisions related to expectant management, antibiotic prophylaxis, and recommendations for induction. The Centers for Disease Control and Prevention (CDC) maintains current guidelines for GBS screening and management, including recommendations for antibiotic prophylaxis in the presence of PROM when GBS status is positive or unknown. The CDC management algorithms are used in almost all institutions in the United States with minor variations. Expectant management of women with PROM varies by the individual's situation and facility or institution. Institutional guidelines and recommendations should be supported by written instructions and included in the anticipatory guidance offered to all women approaching term.

Accurate diagnosis of rupture of membranes can sometimes be difficult. The woman's perceptions of the event, careful physical examination, and possibly laboratory testing may all contribute to confirming the diagnosis. Laboratory tests that may be used to establish the likely status of the fetal membranes include the arborization test (fern test), pH testing (nitrazine test), ultrasound quantification of amniotic fluid volume, and testing for the presence of placental alpha macroglobulin-1 (PAMG-1) or fetal fibronectin in vaginal secretions. Differential diagnoses that need to be excluded include urinary incontinence, vaginal or cervical discharge, semen, and (rarely) rupture of the chorion alone.

The ACNM, in a position statement on PROM at term,[5] affirmed that women with PROM should receive counseling and informed consent about the risks and benefits of various management options. Expectant management at term should be considered a safe alternative to induction of labor under the following conditions: uncomplicated, singleton, vertex pregnancy with clear amniotic fluid; absence of identified infection, including GBS, hepatitis B and C, and HIV; absence of fever; and no evidence of significant risk for fetal acidemia in the fetal heart rate and fetal heart rate pattern. Expectant management requires avoiding all digital cervical examinations, including avoidance of a baseline cervical examination.[5]

Progress in the First Stage of Labor

The rate of cervical dilatation in the first stage of labor, expressed in centimeters per hour (cm/hr), is the backbone of decision making for clinicians providing care to laboring women. Accuracy of determining cervical dilation is dependent on the skill of the examiner and even among experienced professionals the assessment may vary to some degree. There is no objective method to validate the measurements and dilation can change rapidly. However, because cervical dilation rates are highly related to labor duration, measures of labor duration also inform the "normal" boundaries of first-stage labor progression.

The first stage of labor is classically divided into two sequential, albeit rather nebulously defined, phases: latent and active. The *latent phase* begins with the onset of regular uterine labor contractions; the *active phase* begins when the rate of cervical dilation increases. The first stage of labor ends with complete cervical dilatation. The second stage of labor begins with complete cervical dilatation and ends with the birth of the infant. Each phase of labor is characterized by physical and psychological changes. The physical changes are used to evaluate progress in labor; the psychological changes are used to estimate where a woman is within a phase of labor without resorting to a cervical examination and to guide the midwife in devising appropriate support and comfort measures.

Latent Phase

The latent phase encompasses the period of time from the beginning of regular contractions to the point when dilation begins to progress rapidly. Application of this definition is difficult at both ends of the spectrum. First, the onset of the latent phase is difficult to determine objectively, as women typically do not seek labor care until after the onset of labor. Thus identification of latent-phase onset often depends on maternal memory and discernment between uterine activity causing discomfort and true labor contractions. Second, the end of the latent phase is difficult to determine due to the wide variability in the onset of active dilation. In multiparous women, the rate of cervical dilation commonly accelerates after 6 cm dilatation; however the average labor curve for nulliparous women does not show a clear inflection point of dilation acceleration that marks the end of the latent phase.[6]

Contractions become established during the latent phase as they increase in frequency, duration, and intensity. It is common for contractions during latent labor to initially be of mild intensity, occurring every 10 to 20 minutes and lasting 15 to 20 seconds. As latent labor advances, contractions typically increase to moderate intensity, occurring approximately every 5 to 7 minutes and lasting 30 to 40 seconds. These parameters alone do not define latent labor, however, as the experience of contractions may vary greatly between women at similar points of the labor process. Only demonstrable effacement and dilation of the cervix truly define labor. Little to no descent of the presenting part occurs during the latent phase.

A woman in latent labor typically experiences a mixture of emotions: she may be excited, happy, and relieved that the end of pregnancy has come and the long period of waiting has ended, but simultaneously feel a sense of anticipation and apprehension about what is yet to come. Many women cope well with this situation. For some women, however, the latent phase of labor may be a time of fear and increased sensitivity to pain and external stimuli. This is the ideal time for the midwife to assess coping skills, establish rapport, and develop an initial management plan.

Active Phase

The active phase of labor encompasses the period of time from an increase in the rate of cervical dilation (the end of the latent phase of labor) until complete dilatation (the beginning of the second stage of labor). Progressive descent of the fetal presenting part also typically occurs during the latter part of the active phase and during the second stage of labor. Accurately diagnosing active labor is of utmost importance because a woman's rate of cervical dilation (cm/hr) in this phase serves as the basis against which her labor progress is assessed, admission decisions are made, and the need for intervention is determined. It is critical that expectations of cervical dilation during active labor be appropriately defined, based on the most current research.

Onset and Duration of the Active Phase of Labor

Unfortunately, true active labor can never be diagnosed prospectively, which is limiting to clinicians; rather, it can be determined only retrospectively based on an assessment of adequate cervical dilation over time.[7,8] However, both the time intervals for cervical dilation rates and cervical dilatation at the onset of the active phase—factors used for the last several decades by clinicians in practice to guide management—have been recently reevaluated for their validity in assessing progression of labor.

Friedman Studies

Clinical expectations of cervical dilation and fetal descent during labor continue to be heavily influenced by the research of Emanuel Friedman, a physician whose work began in the 1950s.[7–12] Friedman depicted the progress of labor as a sigmoid (S-shaped) curve, varying in duration and slope between parities. Active labor, most often beginning between 2 and 3 cm, was divided into three sequential subphases: an acceleration phase, a phase of maximum slope, and a deceleration phase. Friedman reported that the active phase averaged 4.4 to 4.9 hours for nulliparous women[7,8,11,12] and had an upper "normal" limit of 11.7 hours (mean + 2 standard deviations [SD]).[1,8,12] For multiparous women, the active phase averaged 2.2 to 2.4 hours,[9–12] with a statistical limit of 5.2 hours.[9,12] Regardless of parity, approximately half of the total active phase time for aggregate groups was spent in the acceleration phase, when little progress in dilation is made. Cervical dilation rates in Friedman's phase of maximum slope for nulliparous and multiparous women at the mean were 3.0 cm/hr and 5.7 cm/hr, respectively; the slowest acceptable rates (i.e., mean − 2 SD) were reported to be 1.2 cm/hr and 1.5 cm/hr, for nulliparous and multiparous women respectively.[7,8,11,12] Unfortunately, these aggregate active phase dilation rate estimates are of limited prospective use for individual women because the cervical dilatation at which active labor begins varies widely among women.[6]

Partograph Studies

Partographs are tools that allow labor progress to be graphically recorded and visually assessed. They aid in the early detection of abnormal labor progress and are credited by some for decreasing rates of prolonged labor, oxytocin use, cesarean sections, and intrapartum morbidity/mortality as compared to usual care, although a 2012 Cochrane systematic review did not find that use of a partograph was associated with improved outcomes.[13] Common partograph designs display time (in hours) on the x-axis and cervical dilatation (in centimeters) on the y-axis. Use of the partograph is initiated during presumed active labor. Many incorporate a graphically straight "alert" line, first introduced by Philpott and Castle,[14,15] that represents a dilation rate of 1 cm/hr based on findings from Emanuel Friedman in the mid-1950s (**Figure 26-2**). Alert line incorporation was meant to represent the cervical dilation rate of the slowest 10% of nulliparous women in active labor, so that timely transfer from lower- to higher-resource settings could be accomplished.[14] An "action" line is conventionally placed a number of hours to the right of the "alert" line, most commonly 4 hours. A 4-hour action line can be crossed only when dilation averages less than 0.64 cm/hr for partographs initiated at 3 cm, less than 0.60 cm/hr for partographs initiated at 4 cm, and less than 0.56 cm/hr for partographs initiated at 5 cm. Only when the "action" line is reached are more aggressive management interventions, such as oxytocin augmentation, typically initiated in an attempt to accelerate labor progress.

Although the "alert" line is purported to discriminate only the slowest 10% of nulliparous labors,[14] studies spanning the past four decades have consistently reported that approximately 18% to 56% of nulliparous women cross the "alert" line following partograph initiation.[14–24] Among exclusively multiparous or mixed-parity cohorts, 10% to 42% of cross the "alert" line.[16,17,22–25] With these findings, it became evident that a linear active labor cervical dilation rate expectation of 1 cm/hr is overly stringent for a large percentage of women diagnosed as being in active labor. Indeed, *it is the "action" line rather than the "alert" line that better segregates the slowest 10% of women*, although even the 4-hour "action" line is crossed by 10% to 45% of women.[15–19,21–24,26]

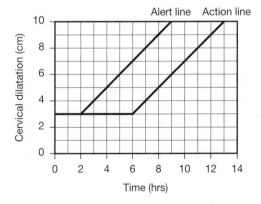

Figure 26-2 Central component of common partographs.
Source: "Cervicographs in the management of labour in primigravidae. I. The alert line for detecting abnormal labour." by Philpott RH, Castle WM. *Journal of Obstetrics and Gynaecology British Commonwealth* 79(7), pp. 592-598. Copyright © 1972 by John Wiley & Sons Ltd. Reproduced with permission of John Wiley & Sons Ltd.

Contemporary findings regarding the hyperbolic progression of labor indicate that most existing partographs are not physiologically based. Even so, the potential for physiologically based partographs to provide an evidence-based framework for homogeneous labor assessment is great.[28] Such instruments may go a long way toward improving birth outcomes in both low- and high-resource settings.

Contemporary Studies

In 1996, Friedman wrote, "the majority of patients are in active-phase labor by the time the cervix reaches 4 cm, but many are not."[29] Data from the National Collaboration Perinatal Project (CPP), a large, multicenter study conducted from 1959 to 1966 including 54,390 births experienced by 48,197 women, was recently evaluated by Zhang et al. using modern statistical interval measure techniques as opposed to simple mathematical means modeling.[30,31] The CPP data-set detailed the labors of women giving birth during the time when Friedman's labor curves were introduced. Zhang et al. found important differences from Friedman's work, including that the active phase of labor may not start until 5 cm of cervical dilation in multiparous women and even later in nulliparous women.[31] Moreover, the labor curve was hyperbolic in shape, with dilation becoming more rapid as labor advanced and without the deceleration phase reported by Friedman. The median time to dilate from 4 to 10 cm was 3.7 hours (16.7 hours at the 95th percentile) and 2.2 hours (14.2 hours at the 95th percentile) for nulliparous and multiparous women, respectively.[31]

When labor progress in the CPP (1959–1966) was compared to labor progress from the Consortium on Safe Labor (CSL; 2002–2008) database that contains records of contemporary women giving birth, it became evident that the first stage of labor in the CSL cohort was longer by a median of 2.6 hours in nulliparas and 2.0 hours in multiparas, after adjusting for differences in maternal and pregnancy characteristics (e.g., older age, higher body mass index [BMI], and higher birth weight in the CSL) when compared to the CPP cohort.[30] There are multiple differences in practice patterns between the 1950s and practice today. In Friedman's era, all women received an episiotomy and the second stage of labor was terminated at 2 hours via a forceps delivery if the woman did not give birth spontaneously within 2 hours of complete cervical dilation. Today women frequently use epidural analgesia to manage labor pain and in the 1950s women used sedatives and morphine to manage labor pain. Differences in labor duration may be partially attributed to these significant changes in practice patterns, but it is also clear that Friedman's analysis was simple by today's more sophisticated standards and did not generate accurate values for the normal time intervals between successive centimeters of cervical dilation.

Thus it is worthwhile to review labor duration studies that have included contemporary labor practices and current populations of women who reside in the United States. In 1989, Kilpatrick and Laros[32] reported that nulliparous ($n = 2302$) and multiparous women ($n = 3767$) who gave birth spontaneously without the use of oxytocin or anesthesia required a mean of 8.1 ± 4.3 hours and 5.7 ± 3.4 hours, respectively, to progress from the onset of regular, painful contractions occurring every 3 to 5 minutes and leading to cervical change, to 10 centimeters or complete dilatation.

Many midwives use criteria commonly associated with active-phase onset in their admission decision process, which is suggested by some to begin between 3 cm and 5 cm, in the presence of regular uterine contractions.[33,34] However, these starting points do not validly describe true active labor onset for many women with spontaneous labor onset. Peisner and Rosen[35] found that 75%, 50%, and 24% of low-risk women with regular contractions admitted for spontaneous labor ($n = 1699$) at 3, 4, and 5 cm, respectively, did not dilate at rates indicative of active labor, as traditionally defined by Friedman. In 2010, investigators reported that dilation rates indicative of active labor do not begin for many women until 6 cm or more.[6] Such findings highlight two important realities of contemporary clinical practice: (1) many women are presumed to be in active-phase labor and managed as such, before actually being in active labor; and (2) expected rates of cervical

dilation during traditionally defined active-phase labor are overly stringent. In addition, in situations where there are multiple professionals performing cervical examinations, the inter-rater reliability may cause doubt in accuracy.

Careful consideration must be given to how these shortcomings contribute to overdiagnosis of dystocia and overuse of interventions aimed at accelerating labor progress. Allowing sufficient time for the events of physiologic labor to progress without unnecessary interventions, balanced with an understanding of when particular interventions may be justified, optimizes the safety and health outcomes of labor and birth for both the woman and her fetus.

Spontaneous Labor Onset

Zhang et al. provided compelling evidence about the duration of first-stage labor and the pattern of labor progression among women with spontaneous labor onset.[6,30,36] This research team most recently used data from the CSL, a multicenter, retrospective, observational study detailing the labor and delivery records of 228,668 women delivering in different areas of the United States; 87% of births occurred in 2005–2007.[6,30] Women included in this data set may have received care including interventions such as amniotomy, oxytocin augmentation, and epidural analgesia. Most importantly, these researchers measured the time interval between one cervical dilation and the next (i.e., how long it took to progress from 4 cm to 5 cm and the time interval between 5 cm and 6 cm). This is in contrast to previous studies that usually determined the mean time interval for a particular phase of labor (i.e., the active phase). Durations of the first stage of labor for women of different parity are shown in **Table 26-1**. Importantly, the average labor curve for nulliparous women did

Table 26-1	Duration of First-Stage Labor with Spontaneous Onset in Hours, by Parity, Beginning with Cervical Dilations Commonly Associated with Active Labor Onset		
	Parity 0 **($n = 43,576$)**[a] **Median (95%)**	**Parity 1** **($n = 27,471$)**[a] **Median (95%)**	**Parity 2+** **($n = 27,312$)**[a] **Median (95%)**
4 cm to complete dilatation, hours	6.5 (24.0)	—	—
5 cm to complete dilatation, hours	3.6 (15.1)	3.0 (15.0)	2.8 (15.5)
6 cm to complete dilatation, hours	2.2 (10.0)	1.6 (8.9)	1.3 (8.9)

[a]Data from the Consortium on Safe Labor.

Note: Parous women tended to be admitted at more advanced dilations than nulliparous women; thus, measures of labor duration started at 5 cm for these women.

Source: Adapted from Laughon SK, Branch DW, Beaver J, Zhang J. Changes in labor patterns over 50 years. *Am J Obstet Gynecol.* 2012;206:419. e1-419.e9.

not show a clear inflection point of dilation acceleration, whereas labor appeared to accelerate after 6 cm in multiparous women and again there is no deceleration phase.[6]

A critical finding in the study by Zhang et al. is that the slope of cervical dilation is not linear; instead, dilation rates progressively accelerate with each passing centimeter, thereby forming a hyperbolic curve for the aggregate (**Figure 26-3**).[6,30,36] In their 2002 study with a focus on nulliparous women (*n* = 1162), median dilation rates for each centimeter of progression between 3 and 10 cm were 0.4, 0.6, 1.2, 1.7, 2.2, 2.4, and 2.4 cm/hr, respectively.[36] At the 5th percentile, these dilation rates were 0.1, 0.2, 0.3, 0.5, 0.7, 0.8, and 0.7 cm/hr, respectively, never exceeding 1 cm/hr. Accordingly, the time needed to dilate from one centimeter to the next is commonly shorter with each passing centimeter after the spontaneous onset of labor for both nulliparous and multiparous women (**Table 26-2**). Moreover, as rates of cervical dilation accelerate with advancing labor, the time necessary to dilate from one centimeter to the next is typically less variable.[6,36] While no appreciable change in dilation for 4 hours may be normal in between 6 and 7 cm, waiting 4 hours before intervening may be too long if a woman is more than 7 cm dilated.[6]

Today, assessments of active labor progression are best based on appropriate hyperbolic labor curves; linear conceptualizations of cervical dilatation, although common in contemporary practice,

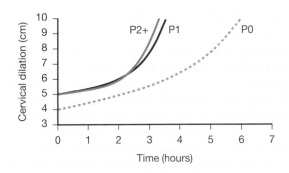

Figure 26-3 Average labor curves by parity in singleton term pregnancies with spontaneous onset of labor, vaginal delivery, and normal neonatal outcomes (95th percentile curves are not shown). P0, nulliparous women; P1, women of parity 1; P2+, women of parity 2 or higher.

Source: Zhang J, Landy HJ, Branch DW, et al. Contemporary patterns of spontaneous labor with normal neonatal outcomes. *Obstet Gynecol.* 2010;116:1281-1287. Copyright 2010 by Lippincott Williams & Wilkins. *Obstetrics and Gynecology* by American College of Obstetricians and Gynecologists; American Academy of Obstetrics and Gynecology. Reproduced with permission of Lippincott Williams & Wilkins in the format reprint in a book/textbook via Copyright Clearance Center.

are fundamentally flawed and should be abandoned. It must be borne in mind that many patterns of labor progression culminate in hyperbolic curves for aggregate populations; thus individual women without a consistent pattern in progression of active labor often still achieve vaginal birth with normal neonatal outcomes.

Table 26-2	Duration of Labor from One Centimeter to the Next Centimeter, by Parity, in Women with Spontaneous Onset of Labor		
Cervical Dilatation (cm)	**Parity 0** (*n* = 25,624)[a] **(hr)** Median (95%)	**Parity 1** (*n* = 16,755)[a] **(hr)** Median (95%)	**Parity 2** (*n* = 16,219)[a] **(hr)** Median (95%)
3–4	1.8 (8.1)	—	—
4–5	1.3 (6.4)	1.4 (7.3)	1.4 (7.0)
5–6	0.8 (3.2)	0.8 (3.4)	0.8 (3.4)
6–7	0.6 (2.2)	0.5 (1.9)	0.5 (1.8)
7–8	0.5 (1.6)	0.4 (1.3)	0.4 (1.2)
8–9	0.5 (1.4)	0.3 (1.0)	0.3 (0.9)
9–10	0.5 (1.8)	0.3 (0.9)	0.3 (0.8)

[a]Data from the Consortium on Safe Labor.

Source: Zhang J, Landy HJ, Branch DW, et al. Contemporary patterns of spontaneous labor with normal neonatal outcomes. *Obstet Gynecol.* 2010;116:1281-1287. Copyright 2010 by Lippincott Williams & Wilkins. *Obstetrics and Gynecology* by American College of Obstetricians and Gynecologists; American Academy of Obstetrics and Gynecology. reproduced with permission of Lippincott Williams & Wilkins in the format reprint in a book/textbook via Copyright Clearance Center.

Spontaneous Active-Phase Labor

Labor and birth is a normal physiologic process. Thus the sparseness of studies reporting on the duration and progress of *spontaneous* active phase labor indicates an important knowledge gap that is difficult to study especially today due to the frequency of various interventions in contemporary practice. Albers[37,38] and Jones and Larson[39] specifically aimed to identify the duration of spontaneous active labor (i.e., no oxytocin, no epidurals, no operative deliveries) among low-risk women who gave birth vaginally in a primarily Hispanic population. In these studies, active labor was defined as the time necessary for the cervix to dilate from 4 to 10 cm (**Table 26-3**). Viewed linearly, active labor dilation rates in these studies averaged 0.8 to 1.0 cm/hr for nulliparous women and 1.1 to 1.4 cm/hr for multiparous women; at the mean – 2 SD, rates were 0.3 to 0.5 cm/hr and 0.4 to 0.5 cm/hr, respectively.

In their recent systematic review limited to nulliparous women (*n* = 7009), Neal et al.[40] conclude that the weighted mean duration of active labor for nulliparous women at term who spontaneously start labor is 6.0 hours (13.4 hours at mean + 2 SD) and the weighted mean rate of cervical dilatation, based on linear calculations, is 1.2 cm/hr, when beginning with criteria commonly associated with the onset of active labor (i.e., dilatation of 3 to 5 cm and regular contractions). The weighted cervical dilation rate at the mean – 2 SD is 0.6 cm/hr. Studies included in this review reflect the diverse care patterns in contemporary practice—for example, epidural analgesia, amniotomy, and oxytocin augmentation. These findings confirm those of Perl and Hunter,[41] who suggest that nulliparous labors progressing at 0.5 cm/hr or faster, in the absence of other problems or symptoms, be considered within normal limits. In their study, 89.7% of term, nulliparous women with a spontaneous labor onset (*n* = 453 of 505) progressed at a rate of 0.5 cm/hr or faster. Only 8.6% of this cohort required a cesarean section (*n* = 37 of 453) and 0.8% required oxytocin (*n* = 4 of 453).

In sum, many contemporary studies indicate that a dilation rate approximating 0.5 cm/hr is achievable for approximately 90% of nulliparous laboring women with spontaneous labor onset. However, this *linear* rate must be evaluated judiciously in light of the physiologic acceleration of dilation that occurs during typical labor. The variability of normal first-stage labor is sufficiently broad that management must be individualized to provide every woman with complete and accurate information so she can make informed health decisions. Current research suggests there may be racial and ethnic differences in normal labor progress that have not been fully elucidated. Women who have a high BMI also progress in labor differently than do women with lower BMIs, and induced labor is different than spontaneous labor. However the development of population-specific labor curves that can be used to guide clinical management of labor are not yet available.

Clinical Correlates of Duration of Labor Studies
Dystocia

The expectation of cervical dilation during active labor is intimately linked to diagnoses of labor

Table 26-3	Duration and Dilation of Spontaneous Active Phase Labor					
		Dilatation Used as Evidence of Active Phase Onset (cm)[a]	Nulliparous Women			
			Active Phase Duration (hrs)		Rate of Dilation (cm/hr)[b]	
Trial	*n*		Mean (SD)	Mean + 2 SD	Mean	Limit
Albers et al., 1996[10]	949	4	7.7 (5.9)	19.4	0.8	0.3
Albers, 1999[11]	2511	4	7.7 (4.9)	17.5	0.8	0.3
Jones et al., 2003[12]	240	4	6.2 (3.6)	13.4	1.0	0.5
			Multiparous Women			
Albers et al., 1996[10]	949	4	5.7 (4.0)	13.7	1.1	
Albers, 1999[11]	2511	4	5.6 (4.1)	13.8	1.1	
Jones et al., 2003[12]	240	4	4.4 (3.4)	11.6	1.4	

[a]Absolute value taken as evidence of active phase onset (cm).

[b]Calculated based on assumption that the cervical dilation phase ends at 10 cm, which approximates complete cervical dilatation.

Source: Adapted from Laughon SK, Branch DW, Beaver J, Zhang J. Changes in labor patterns over 50 years. *Am J Obstet Gynecol.* 2012;206:419.e1-419.e9.

dystocia, which is broadly characterized as slow, abnormal progression of active labor. In practice, diagnoses of dystocia are most often based on ambiguously defined delays in cervical dilation beyond which labor augmentation is deemed justified. When clinicians have expectations for cervical dilation rates that are faster than physiologic reality, women with normal labor progression are at risk of being misdiagnosed with dystocia and receiving subsequent interventions aimed at expediting birth. Indeed, dystocia is known to be "overdiagnosed,"[33] indicating that existing definitions lack clinical relevance because they neither differentiate normal from abnormal labor progression nor discriminate labors that are more prone to adverse outcomes. This tendency is of concern because dystocia is the leading indication for primary cesarean deliveries,[1,33] accounting directly for approximately 50% of all cesarean sections performed in nulliparous women.[42,43] At present, cesarean deliveries account for one-third of all births in the United States.[44] It is believed that best birth outcomes for women and their newborns reportedly occur with cesarean rates of 5% to 10%, while rates higher than 15% are associated with more harm than good.[45,46] Specific definitions of dystocia based on contemporary population-based criteria are needed.

Pre-active Labor Admissions

The timing of when a woman is admitted for labor care significantly influences the labor process and outcomes; indeed, the admission decision is one of the most important decisions that is made. As noted earlier, true active labor can be determined only retrospectively based on an assessment of adequate cervical dilation over time. As a result, many women are inadvertently admitted prior to being in active labor, yet they are held to dilation expectations of active labor. Women who are admitted early (e.g., less than 4 cm dilation) are approximately twice as likely to be augmented with oxytocin when compared to women admitted in active labor.[47–49] Indeed, the rate of oxytocin use is inversely related to cervical dilatation at admission ($r = -0.79$, $P < 0.05$).[50] Moreover, the cesarean rate following early labor admission is reported to be more than twice as high as the reference group rate in most studies.[47,48,51–53] Cesarean sections for dystocia are more frequent in early-admission groups in studies reporting specific surgical indications ($P < 0.001$ in each study).[47,52] These findings corroborate those from a study reporting that before 4 cm dilatation, the earlier a woman is admitted for labor is linearly related to her cesarean delivery risk.[53] Half of all cesarean sections performed in nulliparous women for dystocia occur at 5

cm or less dilatation.[43] This raises concern that many cesarean sections may be performed prior to active-phase labor onset.

Zhang et al.'s[6] findings can be used to illustrate the shortcomings of viewing cervical dilation linearly and how it pertains to dystocia. From 3 cm forward, calculations based on their data demonstrate that dilation rates conceptualized as linear are faster than actual rates until some point after 5 cm dilatation, when the linear rates become slower than actual rates, as described previously (**Figure 26-4**).[54] As a consequence, diagnoses of dystocia and interventions aimed at correcting "slow" labor are much more likely in earlier active labor when linear dilation expectations are less likely to be met. For this reason, it is important that clinicians base cervical dilation expectations on an evidence-based, hyperbolic labor curve.

Augmentation of Labor

Once a woman in spontaneous labor enters the active phase, attempts to accelerate labor may be justified if the dilation rate becomes slower than the accepted minimum rate for the population. Accelerative interventions are primarily used to decrease the number of dystocia-related cesarean sections that are performed. However, the main interventions used by clinicians in an attempt to accelerate labor—that is, amniotomy and oxytocin augmentation—are used at surprisingly high rates in contemporary practice.

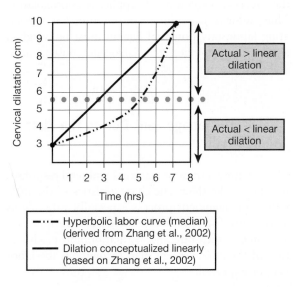

Figure 26-4 Hyperbolic, median nulliparous labor curve with linear conceptualization.

Source: Neal JL, Lowe NK, Patrick TE, Cabbage LA, Corwin EJ. What is the slowest-yet-normal cervical dilation rate among nulliparous women with spontaneous labor onset? *J Obstet Gynecol Neonatal Nurs.* 2010;39(4):361-369.

For example, when Zhang et al. limited their analyses of the CPL database to only women with spontaneous labor onset, vertex presentation, vaginal delivery, and normal neonatal outcome (*n* = 62,415), approximately 45% were found to have received oxytocin augmentation during labor.[6] Oxytocin is a "high-alert medication"[55] and the drug most commonly associated with preventable adverse perinatal outcomes.[56] Misuse of this agent is involved in half of all paid obstetric litigation claims.[57]

While studies comparing oxytocin use to no treatment are sparse, a recent Cochrane Collaboration review found that early versus delayed oxytocin use results in a higher risk of uterine tachysystole associated with fetal heart rate changes requiring intervention (relative risk [RR] = 2.51; 95% confidence interval [CI] = 1.04–6.05).[58] Early oxytocin use reduces the mean duration of labor by approximately 2 hours, but this medication has not proved to be effective in reducing the cesarean section rate, the role for which it is primarily used (RR = 0.88; 95% CI = 0.66–1.19).[58]

With regard to amniotomy, there are no statistically significant differences between outcomes of women in amniotomy and control groups in terms of first-stage labor duration or cesarean section rates.[59] Clinicians should bear in mind that the extent to which the relationship between prolonged labor and labor morbidity is causal is by no means certain; that is, it remains unclear if the risks associated with longer labors are more related to time in labor or to the interventions commonly applied to shorten labor. Thus, prior to using interventions aimed at accelerating labor, any potential benefit must be weighed against disadvantages, risks, iatrogenic consequences, and their attendant costs.

Midwifery Management During the First Stage of Labor

The dynamic nature of maternal and fetal responses to labor make the cyclic characteristics of the midwifery management process especially valuable as a structure for planning labor care. Continual reassessment with ongoing evaluation and modification of the management plan throughout the labor is to be expected.

Initial Evaluation of the Woman and Fetus

Initial evaluation of a woman presenting with signs and symptoms of labor includes review of history, physical assessment, and, often, laboratory investigations. The initial assessment of a woman who presents in labor not only ascertains the current physical well-being of the woman and fetus, but also assesses the encounter within the context of her medical and obstetric history, her social situation, and her expectations. A comprehensive approach is necessary to identify actual and potential problems and to create a mutually agreeable and appropriate plan of care.

History

If the woman's prenatal record is available, it can be used as the source of information for much of the history. Specifically, personal information, past obstetric history, past medical and primary healthcare history, and family history should be reviewed. Present pregnancy history should be reviewed to confirm gestational age and estimated date of delivery, significant prenatal events, and presence of a personalized plan for birth. This spares the woman from having to reiterate history she has given before and from being disturbed at a time when she may be coping with the demands and stresses of labor. Critical items of the history should be double-checked with the woman to verify the existence of drug allergies, blood transfusions and reactions, and major obstetric or medical complications during her pregnancy. Documentation that the prenatal record was reviewed should be included in her intrapartum medical record. An interim history that includes any change in health status from the time of the last documented visit to the present encounter, chief complaint, and history of present illness, coupled with a brief review of pertinent systems, will complete the history database and give direction to the physical examination.

A woman presenting for labor evaluation without an available prenatal record presents a special challenge for caregivers. The woman may have been receiving regular prenatal care but simply not have records available for a variety of reasons, such as miscommunication about expected birth location or travel. However, women who have received less than adequate prenatal care are at increased risk of unexpected adverse obstetric complications including preterm birth and stillbirth, giving birth to infants who are large or small for gestational age, and early neonatal death.[60] In the absence of a prenatal record, the midwife must skillfully elicit essential information beginning with those data most relevant to the acuity of the clinical scenario. **Table 26-4** outlines the essential components of the health history when evaluating a woman presenting for labor evaluation and identifies their significance.

Physical Examination

Essential components of the physical and pelvic examination performed at the initial labor evaluation are presented in **Table 26-5**. A physical examination that was performed prenatally can be reviewed as a baseline for the current physical examination when a prenatal record is available. An abbreviated examination can then be performed that focuses on any problem areas identified. Documentation that

the previous examination was reviewed should be included in the woman's healthcare record. A comprehensive physical examination is indicated when a woman has no prenatal records available or has received inadequate prenatal care.

Physical examination findings or vital signs indicative of a potential or actual complication require further evaluation. For example, an elevated blood pressure is an indication for eliciting and evaluating reflexes and for assessing for the presence of clonus.

Controversy exists about the role of digital cervical examinations in the initial and ongoing evaluation

Table 26-4	Essential Components of Health History When Evaluating a Woman Presenting with Signs and Symptoms of Labor
History Element	**Significance**
Age	Birth at the extremes of the reproductive lifespan is associated with an increased risk for adverse perinatal outcomes
Parity	Parity influences labor progress and labor duration (e.g., progress is typically slower in nulliparous women compared to multiparous women)
Estimated date of delivery and estimated weeks of gestational age	Identifies potential for newborn complications related to prematurity or postmaturity and establishes a baseline for evaluating fetal size as related to gestational age
Complications of current pregnancy including group B streptococcus status	Identifies existing or potential problems that may influence management of the current labor and birth
Major complications of previous pregnancies, including prenatal, intrapartum, and postpartum periods	Identifies potential recurring problems that may affect the current labor and birth
Previous labor experience, including duration	Previous labor experience influences expectations for labor progress and makes known previously used labor coping strategies
Mode of previous births/deliveries	Identifies previous operative vaginal deliveries or cesarean sections, which may influence management of current labor and birth
Size of previous babies	Suggests an estimate of pelvic adequacy
Fetal movement pattern	Reflects fetal well-being
Vaginal bleeding	Differentiated from bloody show, vaginal bleeding is abnormal and will typically contraindicate performance of a digital cervical examination and indicate necessity for further evaluation and physician consultation, collaboration, or referral
Status of membranes	Duration of ruptured membranes and characteristics of amniotic fluid will influence management decisions
Time of onset of contractions, and character of contractions from onset to the present, including frequency, duration, intensity, and aggravating and relieving factors	Establishes the probable start of labor and helps discriminate false labor from true labor
Last oral intake	Provides a baseline from which to assess energy reserves and fluid status; also useful in anesthesia management in the event of surgery

Table 26-5	Essential Components of the Physical Examination When Evaluating a Woman Presenting with Labor Signs and Symptoms	
Physical Examination Element	**Significance**	
Vital signs: blood pressure, temperature, pulse, respirations	Elevated blood pressure may indicate a hypertensive disorder, while lowered blood pressure may indicate shock. In the presence of a normal diastolic measurement, elevation in systolic blood pressure usually indicates anxiety or pain	
	Elevated temperature indicates an infectious process or dehydration	
	Elevated pulse and/or respirations may indicate infection, shock, dehydration, or anxiety	
Auscultation of heart and lungs	Screens for and identifies acute or previously unrecognized conditions that could potentially adversely affect the current labor and birth	
Abdominal palpation to determine contraction pattern and fetal lie, presentation, position, and engagement	Contraction pattern helps determine labor status	
	Fetal lie, presentation, and position influence the course of labor and guide care decisions regarding mode of delivery and necessity for consultation, collaboration, or referral	
	Engagement of the fetal presenting part is reassuring for pelvic adequacy	
Abdominal palpation to determine estimated fetal weight and fundal height	In relation to gestational age, identifies the possibility of inaccurate dating, smaller or larger than expected fetus or multiples, oligohydramnios or polyhydramnios, or other abnormalities and their associated complicating factors	
Visual inspection for abdominal scars	Confirms surgical history or identifies previously unidentified surgical procedures, including previous cesarean sections	
Assessment for presence of peripheral or facial edema	Facial edema alone or in association with peripheral edema is a classic sign of preeclampsia	
Cervical Examination to Evaluate:		
Cervical effacement and dilatation	Progressive cervical effacement and dilatation is the mark of true labor	
Position of the cervix	Location of the cervix in an anterior or middle position is associated with greater readiness for labor	
Station of fetal presenting part	Progressive fetal descent is indicative of pelvic adequacy and labor progression	
Presence of molding or caput succedaneum	The presence or absence of molding and/or caput indicates fetal adaptation to the maternal pelvis and indirectly signifies pelvic adequacy	
Fetal lie, presentation, and position	Digital examination findings confirm and enhance abdominal examination findings relative to fetal lie, presentation, and position	
Tone and elasticity of vagina and perineum	Potential for lacerations or need for episiotomy may be suggested by assessment of the tone and elasticity of the vagina and perineal body	
Confirmation of membrane status	Palpation of intact fetal membranes or amniotic fluid expulsion with cervical examination is suggestive of membrane status	
Visual inspection of perineum	Identification of lesions, vulvar varicosities, and vaginal discharge including frank bleeding will impact the management plan	
Assessment of fetal heart rate	Indicates fetal well-being	
Optional and Supplemental Physical Examination Elements	**Significance**	
Measurement of maternal weight	Relevant when compared to prepregnancy weight to ascertain total weight gain during pregnancy or to previous prenatal visit measurements to assess interval weight gain	
Clinical pelvimetry	Supports clinical judgment when estimating pelvic adequacy	
Evaluation of reflexes and determining the presence of clonus	Hyperreflexia and clonus are signs of severe preeclampsia/eclampsia	
Speculum examination	Provides visualization of the cervix and vaginal vault to confirm rupture of membranes, collect laboratory specimens, and estimate cervical dilatation and effacement.	

of a woman with labor signs and symptoms. The unique clinical situation of the laboring woman and her desires along with the clinical judgment and expertise of the midwife are taken into consideration when considering the necessity of performing a digital cervical examination.

It is common practice in institutions that have continuous electronic fetal monitoring capability to obtain an initial baseline fetal heart rate (FHR) recording (e.g., 20 minutes) as the means of initial evaluation of fetal well-being for most, if not all, women presenting for evaluation of labor. This practice, when applied to women who are at at low obstetric and medical risk for fetal acidemia, does not improve maternal or neonatal outcomes and, when compared to initial assessment by intermittent monitoring, may be associated with an increase in intrapartum interventions including continuous electronic fetal monitoring and cesarean delivery.[61] National guidelines are silent on the preferred method of evaluation of fetal heart rate for women presenting for evaluation with labor signs and symptoms, but are clear regarding the appropriateness of intermittent auscultation for ongoing evaluation of low-risk women in labor.[62,63]

Laboratory Investigation

Available prenatal records can be reviewed to identify the woman's blood type and Rh status, anemias, glucose tolerance testing, and specific perinatal infections including GBS, hepatitis B, and HIV. In the case of a woman presenting with no prenatal record, all routine prenatal lab work will need to be collected to provide a baseline for development of a management plan.

Clinical judgment and institutional policy will influence the decision to order further laboratory studies. If the woman will be having an intravenous infusion, blood specimens can be obtained concurrently with intravenous line placement. Common laboratory studies for evaluation of a woman with labor signs and symptoms are presented in **Table 26-6**.

Confirmation of Labor Status

A diagnosis of labor warrants admission to the birth center/hospital or continuous attendance when a home birth is planned. Because dilation rates indicative of active labor do not begin for many women until 6 cm or more,[6] labor status determinations must be based on at least two adequately spaced cervical examinations—for example, 2 to 4 hours apart. In the presence of regular, painful contractions and complete or near-complete effacement, it is reasonable to consider a woman to be in active labor at 4 cm or 5 cm dilatation *if immediately preceded by cervical change over time* (i.e., 1 cm or more in a 2-hour or shorter window) or at 6 cm or more regardless

Table 26-6	Common Laboratory Investigations for a Woman Presenting with Labor Signs and Symptoms
Laboratory Test	**Significance**
Complete blood count (CBC)	Provides baseline measures of hemoglobin and hematocrit, thereby evaluating for anemia, a risk factor for postpartum hemorrhage
	Provides a baseline for the white blood cell count, which can indicate infection—although transiently high values are common with labor
	Provides a baseline platelet count
Blood type, Rh status, and antibody screen[a]	To confirm prenatal blood group and Rh status
	Provides a comparative value to prenatal results to assess development of maternal antibodies
	Provides basic information for a blood bank in the event of blood transfusion
Urinalysis	Identifies the presence of protein, a marker for preeclampsia
	Identifies the presence of glucose, a marker for poorly controlled diabetes
	Identifies the presence of ketones, a reflection of fat metabolism and current nutrition status
	Provides indication of hydration status through specific gravity measure
	Identifies abnormal components in the urine that may direct differential diagnosis toward urinary tract infection

[a]Test can also be ordered as a "type and hold," which identifies the blood type and Rh status but holds further evaluation of a coagulated sample until the need for a blood transfusion is identified.

of the rate of previous cervical change. Unless labor is clearly advanced, a single-point cervical dilation measurement does not reliably differentiate labor phases. When a diagnosis of labor cannot be made with relative certainty, observation before admission to the birthing unit is prudent assuming the woman is opting to give birth in the hospital.

It may take several hours of ongoing assessment to differentiate between pre labor, latent labor, and active labor. Between assessments and after fetal well-being is confirmed, the woman may be encouraged to walk, rock, sit on a birthing ball, or simply rest. In hospital and birth center settings, when no change in dilation is noted at the next examination, the woman may safely go home if she lives nearby, has no transportation problems, and wants to go home.

In making a diagnosis of labor, clinicians must carefully differentiate not only between true and pre labor, but also between labor and any obstetric or nonobstetric discomforts or complications that masquerade or can be misinterpreted as labor, such as urinary tract infections or placental abruption.

Components of Midwifery Care for Laboring Women

Labor Support and Pain Management

Labor support and pain management are intertwined. Labor support consists of techniques and interventions that support the physical and emotional experience of the woman in labor and includes recognizing the therapeutic value of human presence, a hallmark of the art and science of midwifery. Covered in detail in the *Support for Women in Labor* chapter, the inclusion of labor support and pain management as a basic component of midwifery care reflects the importance of intentionally and continually evaluating and modifying the midwifery care provided throughout labor. Women who receive continuous labor support are more likely to have a spontaneous vaginal birth, use less pain medication, have slightly shorter labors, and are more satisfied with their birth experiences than women who do not receive such support.[64]

While some practice environments essentially preclude the midwife from personally acting as the exclusive continuous labor support provider, midwives remain in the unique position of advocating for this essential care. Midwives can engage with and support local doulas and/or other labor support caregivers so that they are engaged in the labor support process.

Maternal Position and Level of Activity

The level of physical activity and positions used during labor are ideally those of the laboring woman. It is rare that a woman would have a contraindication to assuming any position that she prefers. When given a choice, many women prefer an upright position or ambulation throughout much of their labor. However, the birth environment may impact the level of comfort a woman has to assert her desires, and many hospital labor settings have a culture of lying in bed during the first stage of labor. While laboring in bed is considered to be convenient to some providers, it may not be optimal for the progress of physiologic labor or for the comfort of the laboring woman. Upright positions are associated with a 1-hour shorter labor duration and fewer epidurals as compared to recumbent positions.[65] Creative use can be made of furniture, pillows, birthing balls, or an adjustable bed to support a laboring woman in a variety of upright positions, including hands and knees, sitting, standing, and squatting.

The midwife can support unlimited activity and freedom of choice of positions for low-risk women in labor by routine utilization of intermittent fetal auscultation and becoming comfortable with the process of assessing fetal heart rate and contractions with the woman in a variety of positions.

When resting in bed is necessary or desired, lateral recumbent positions are preferred to supine positions because they reduce the potential for aortic/vena caval compression with resulting maternal hypotension and potential fetal compromise. Lateral positions also facilitate kidney function and do not interfere with coordination and efficiency of uterine contractions.

Rupture of the fetal membranes is not usually a contraindication to ambulatory and upright activity. Once fetal well-being is assured, if there is a cephalic presentation and the fetal presenting part is engaged in the pelvis or well applied to the cervix, there is no reason to restrict ambulation or assumption of upright positions. These activities may be desirable to the woman as the intensity of the contractions often increases after rupture of membranes and upright positioning facilitates maternal comfort. Ambulation or upright positioning may be contraindicated upon rupture of membranes if the fetal head is unengaged or in a malpresentation because of the heightened risk of umbilical cord prolapse.

Women with medical or obstetric conditions such as severe preeclampsia, placental abruption, or acute infections will necessarily have their activity restricted due to their physiologic instability, the effect of medications, or increased fetal risk.

Hydration and Nutrition

Hydration and nutrition are potentially important variables for optimal uterine perfusion and myometrial function and, therefore, may be related to uterine efficiency during labor. However, contemporary management of labor in the United States typically involves limited oral nutritive intake and noncaloric intravenous fluid administration. Decreasing the risk of gastric content aspiration during general anesthetic induction—an extremely rare but serious syndrome first described by Mendelson in 1946[66]—remains the primary rationale for withholding food and fluid during labor. Obstetric anesthesia has changed considerably since the 1940s, with greater use of regional anesthesia and better general anesthetic technique. Moreover, fasting does not guarantee an empty stomach or less acidity. Overall, modern evidence shows no benefits or harms associated with oral intake during labor, so there is no justification for the restriction of fluids and food in labor for women at low risk for complications.

Adequate hydration during labor would seemingly assist in the delivery of oxygen and nutrients as well as facilitate the elimination of waste from the contracting uterus, akin to how proper hydration benefits the skeletal muscle of athletes.

Five randomized studies investigated maternal hydration as a potential variable in labor progress, all focusing on nulliparous women.[67–71] In the earlier studies, Garite et al.[67] and Eslamian et al.[68] randomized low-risk, nulliparous women in spontaneous labor to receive 125 or 250 mL/hr of intravenous isotonic fluids while receiving little or nothing by mouth. In the 250 mL/hr groups, Eslamian et al. report a shorter first stage of labor duration (3.9 ± 1.4 versus 6.1 ± 1.8 hours, respectively; $p < 0.0001$), while Garite et al. demonstrated a strong trend toward a shorter first-stage labor. Both research teams found fewer prolonged labors in the 250 mL/hr group, and Eslamian et al. reported that oxytocin augmentation was significantly less likely in this group (8.1% versus 20.4%, respectively; $p < 0.001$).

Coco et al.[69] studied whether giving low-risk, nulliparous women more intravenous fluid reduced labor duration when oral intake was unrestricted (e.g., water, juice, or even carbonated soft drinks). This team found that increased intravenous hydration does not decrease labor duration when women are permitted to drink freely, nor does it decrease rates of oxytocin augmentation or cesarean sections.

Likewise, Kavitha et al.[70] found no significant differences in labor duration, oxytocin augmentation, or mode of delivery between women receiving oral fluids only or intravenous fluids at either 125 or 250 mL/hr, although those women who received intravenous hydration were less likely to vomit during labor. In 2012, an Iranian team reported that women offered only oral fluids (no intravenous fluids administered), compared to women receiving intravenous fluids at 240 mL/hr and oral fluids, had significantly longer first stage labors (4.2 ± 0.7 versus 3.5 ± 0.6 hours, respectively; $p < 0.001$), had longer second-stage labors (1.1 ± 0.2 versus 0.8 ± 0.2 hours, respectively; $p = 0.01$), and received oxytocin augmentation more often (53.3% versus 20.0%, respectively; $p = 0.02$).[71]

A significant shortcoming in all five of these randomized hydration studies is that none measured maternal hydration by scientific means (e.g., urine specific gravity). Thus the women's actual hydration status remained unknown.

Nutrition needs during labor are not well understood, although it has been reported that women in the third trimester of pregnancy exhibit a state of "accelerated starvation" with rapid rises in plasma beta-hydroxybutyric acid (the principal labor ketone) and a concomitant fall in plasma glucose. This process of accelerated lipolysis conserves glucose for the fetus. Ketones are produced in the liver as a byproduct of fat catabolism when glycogen stores are unavailable (e.g., in starvation states or during exercise) and are normally oxidized to carbon dioxide, water, and alternate energy that is usable by tissues such as a contracting uterus.[72,73] Production of ketones in quantities above the level of need results in ketosis, which may have deleterious effects on uterine function.[72] A Cochrane review published in 2010 found no significant differences in duration of labor, augmentation of labor, cesarean sections, or Apgar scores between women with and without oral fluid and food restriction during labor.[74]

Intravenous Access

Routine prophylactic insertion of intravenous access is a practice that may be eliminated in the provision of normal labor and birth care for women who have no significant obstetric or medical risks. Instead, the decision to initiate and maintain intravenous access during labor should be based on actual or potential risk factors for each individual. Women who cannot tolerate oral fluid intake may require intravenous fluids. Intravenous access is necessary for administration of some medications such as antibiotic prophylaxis for women who are carriers of GBS, pain medications, or oxytocin augmentation. Prior to epidural anesthesia, intravenous access allows for administration of isotonic fluid blood volume expansion to mitigate epidural-related hypotension; continuing access after epidural placement allows for ongoing fluid administration and medication administration should complications develop. Institutional policies that require intravenous access exist in many hospital birth settings, and eliminating these policies is one example of changes needed so that policies are in line with existing evidence to support normal physiologic labor and birth.

Membrane Management

Historically, being born "in the caul" or with intact membranes was considered a sign of good fortune and occasionally magic gifts. Yet artificial rupture of membranes (AROM) during labor has commonly been believed to accelerate the progress of labor and is used frequently in contemporary practice. AROM can be employed to induce labor either alone or with other agents, used routinely during labor to speed progress, or used selectively as a treatment for dystocia. Because AROM is associated with adverse outcomes, however, the efficacy of each of these uses must be examined. Risks associated with AROM include umbilical cord compression with resultant fetal heart rate decelerations, umbilical cord prolapse, discomfort from the procedure, increased risk of infection, and rarely, rupture of fetal vessels (vasa previa).[75]

AROM was compared to prostaglandins for induction of labor in one randomized trial that included 260 nulliparous and primiparous women.[76] Application of prostaglandin gel resulted in a significant reduction in the need for oxytocin augmentation (odds ratio [OR] = 0.27; 95% CI = 0.12–0.61) and induction to delivery intervals was shorter in the women who were treated with prostaglandins. Although no differences in the cesarean section or chorioamnionitis rates were noted, all women were induced with oxytocin within 6 hours after the induction intervention if labor was not active.

Two trials have evaluated the effectiveness of early amniotomy (during latent labor) as an adjunct during induction. Macones et al.[77] evaluated outcomes of nulliparous women who were induced at term who had an amniotomy before 4 cm dilatation compared to women who had an amniotomy after they were at 4 cm dilatation. More women in the early amniotomy group delivered within 24 hours (68% versus 56%, $P = 0.002$) and there was a mean 2-hour shorter labor in the early amniotomy group.

The use of AROM to treat dystocia has also been investigated. Rouse et al. randomized women with active-phase arrest to amniotomy with oxytocin or oxytocin alone ($n = 108$). There were no significant differences in mode of birth or duration of labor between the groups. The women in the amniotomy group had a trend toward more chorioamnionitis and endometritis. Because they had internal uterine pressure catheters and fetal scalp electrodes placed at the time of amniotomy, it is not clear if AROM or the other interventions increased this risk for infection; however, there is known relationship between intrauterine pressure catheters and an increased risk for infection.[78] Wei et al. evaluated early versus late use of amniotomy and oxytocin augmentation for both prevention and treatment of dystocia in a Cochrane meta-analysis ($n = 7792$).[79] In the prevention of dystocia trials, women in the early amniotomy/oxytocin groups had a modest reduction in cesarean section rates (RR = 0.88; 95% CI = 0.77–0.99) and shorter labor (mean difference: –1.11 hour). In the treatment of dystocia trials, there was no reduction in cesarean section rates (RR = 1.54; 95% CI = 0.75–3.15), nor was there a reduction in the duration of labor between women who had early versus late amniotomy and oxytocin augmentation. There were no differences in the rate of infection or neonatal outcomes.

Current evidence suggests that when amniotomy is used in conjunction with oxytocin for induction or as a method of preventing dystocia in women who have mild labor delays, the diminution in labor duration associated with amniotomy may be statistically significant but may not be clinically relevant. The reduced risk of cesarean section is significant but modest. In contrast, amniotomy alone does not appear to be a beneficial treatment for women with active phase arrest.

The use of AROM as a routine measure to speed the progress of labor in women without dystocia has been evaluated in several randomized trials and a Cochrane meta-analysis. Unlike in the dystocia trials, AROM was associated with a trend toward an increased risk for cesarean section (RR = 1.26; 95% CI = 0.98–1.62; $n = 4893$; 14 trials)[75] without a concomitant shortening of the first stage of labor. There was a similar trend toward more fetal heart rate abnormalities (RR = 1.09; 95% CI = 0.97–1.23) but no differences in the risk of infection.

If an amniotomy is to be performed, a cephalic presentation and engagement in the pelvis should be confirmed first. Before performing the procedure, the midwife carefully reassesses the fetal station and ensures the fetal head is well applied to the cervix.

Keeping the fingers in the cervix, the membranes can be gently disrupted with the amnihook, ideally during a contraction. Care should be taken to avoid scratching the fetal head and the fingers should be left in place during the initial gush of fluid to ensure a prolapsed cord does not occur. The fetal heart rate should be monitored during the procedure and for a short time afterwards.

In summary, routine amniotomy for women in spontaneous term labor may do more harm than good. This procedure should be reserved for treatment of dystocia and as an adjunct intervention for women who have a clear indication for induction of labor. In addition to performing an AROM only with appropriate indication, it is prudent to avoid commonly used language such as "break the bag," because for many women this phrase connotes a painful activity. The woman should be reassured that aside from the potential discomfort associated with any vaginal examination, there is no pain associated with AROM. Finally, the woman should give consent for this procedure and a formal informed consent that reviews the benefits, risks, and alternatives should be conducted.

Fetal Monitoring

Fetal monitoring does not necessarily imply "continuous electronic fetal monitoring," but rather reflects an attitude of heightened sensitivity on the part of the midwife to fetal well-being, via ongoing evaluation of the fetal heart rate through the method most appropriate to the individual woman and fetus. The *Fetal Assessment During Labor* chapter details the methods and indications for intermittent auscultation of the fetal heart rate as well as continuous external and continuous internal fetal heart rate assessment.

Uterine Contraction Monitoring

Uterine activity can be evaluated by correlating the woman's perceptions of contractions with observation and abdominal palpation and/or one of two electronic monitoring methods: an external tocodynamometer or an intrauterine pressure catheter.

Labor progress is the best indicator of adequate contractions. Nevertheless, it is generally accepted that three contractions within 10 minutes is the minimum frequency necessary to achieve progressive cervical change in active labor. "Adequate" labor contractions typically do not allow indentation of the uterine fundus when palpated abdominally at their acme. The maternal response to contractions provides insights into the frequency, duration, and intensity of contractions, but it is important to keep in mind that women's responses to labor vary widely. The intensity of a woman's external response to a contraction is influenced by environment, culture, and individual coping ability.

When considering application of electronic uterine monitors, the need for uterine activity data must be weighed against the need of the woman for mobility and freedom of movement. The rise of the uterus within the abdomen during a contraction can be easily visualized on a woman of average or low BMI. It is this change in abdominal shape that is the mechanism by which an external electronic tocodynamometer functions, capturing the graphic image of a contraction as the abdomen lifts against the pressure transducer, which is held in place by the resistance of an abdominal band. External tocodynamometry can present graphically the frequency and duration of uterine contractions, but it relies on correct placement and calibration and may not work well for women who are overweight or obese. In addition, the tocodynamometer is unable to provide accurate information regarding the intensity of contractions. It is highly sensitive to maternal movement, predisposing the graphic data to artifacts and errors.

To counter limitations of the traditional tocodynamometer, researchers are presently investigating the use of electrical uterine myography. This emerging method of electronic uterine monitoring uses noninvasive electrodes placed on the maternal abdomen to report electrical activity of the uterine muscle, similar to how an electrocardiogram records the electrical conduction of the heart. This promising technology is able to graphically represent the same information as a tocodynamometer while having the advantage of being less sensitive to maternal body type and movement.

Women generally sense contractions when they reach approximately 15 mm Hg of pressure; this is also the minimum level of contraction that can be detected by an observer's hand. In contrast, internal uterine monitoring detects the increase in tonus slightly sooner than the woman or her attendants[80] (**Figure 26-5**). Internal uterine monitoring is the most accurate but most invasive method of evaluating uterine activity (**Figure 26-6**). The intrauterine pressure catheter requires membranes to be ruptured and carries with it a low—albeit real—risk of uterine or placental perforation and infection. When placed correctly (i.e., within the amniotic fluid compartment), the intrauterine pressure catheter provides information regarding frequency, duration, and intensity of contractions. The intrauterine pressure

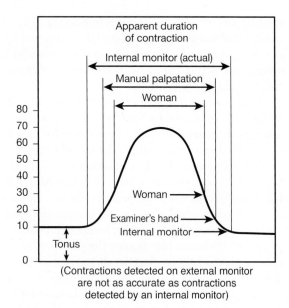

Figure 26-5 Relative sensitivity of various methods available for detection of uterine contractions.

Source: Freeman, RK, Garite, TJ, Nageotte, MP, *Fetal Heart Rate Monitoring* 3rd edition, p. 57. Copyright © 2003. Reprinted by permission of Lippincott Williams & Wilkins and the author.

catheter has the added feature of enabling the instillation of fluid into the uterus (amnioinfusion) to treat certain fetal heart pattern aberrations or to thin meconium, if present.

Montevideo units (MVUs) are used to assess the effectiveness of uterine contractions measured via intrauterine pressure catheter. MVU levels are

determined by taking the numeric amplitude of all contractions that occur in a 10-minute window in millimeters of mercury (mm Hg) minus the baseline uterine tonus amplitude and summing the total rise in amplitude over that 10-minute time period. Historically, 200 to 250 MVUs has been used to define "adequate" contractions based on Calderyo-Barcia's studies from the 1960s that determined which minimum MVU values reliably predict vaginal birth.[81]

Introduction of an intrauterine pressure catheter may be indicated during labor augmentation when labor dystocia is suspected. However, this device has no place in the management plan for labor in the absence of fetal or obstetric complications.

Continuing Evaluation of Maternal Well-Being, Fetal Well-Being, and Labor Progress

Continuing evaluation during labor has three primary focuses: (1) maternal well-being, (2) fetal well-being, and (3) labor progress. Assessing maternal status includes monitoring maternal vital signs, urinary output, coping status, and general well-being. Continuing evaluation of the fetus includes the monitoring of fetal heart rate. In addition to monitoring cervical dilation over time, evaluation of fetal presentation and position, and adaptation to the maternal pelvis, is an essential component of evaluating of labor progress.

Maternal Well-Being

Vital Signs

The frequency with which vital signs are checked in the absence of complications may vary between settings, typically being detailed in an institutional policy to ensure adherence to a minimum standard. Unfortunately, the standards for the frequency of vital signs for low-risk women in labor may be based in nursing and institutional tradition rather than on evidence of clinical relevance in laboring women. The following schedule for checking vital signs is frequently encountered as policy for a woman (without epidural anesthesia) during the first stage of labor who does not have a specific condition that would require more frequent monitoring:

- Blood pressure, pulse, and respirations: every hour
- Temperature: every 2 to 4 hours when the temperature is normal and the membranes are

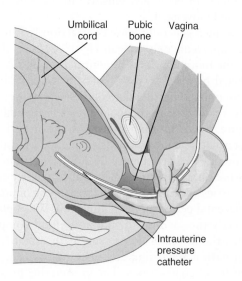

Figure 26-6 Insertion of intrauterine pressure catheter.

intact, and every 1 to 2 hours if the temperature is abnormal and/or after the membranes have ruptured

As a woman's status may change over the course of her labor, the frequency of assessing vital signs should be adjusted to match the individual's situation.

Urinary Output

The bladder is a pelvic organ. A distended bladder can impede the progress of labor by preventing fetal descent as well as increasing the discomfort and pain in the lower abdomen that women frequently experience during labor. A woman in labor should be encouraged to empty her bladder at least every 2 hours during the active phase of the first stage of labor. This provides an opportunity for the clinician to evaluate maternal hydration status. Presence of ketones or protein in the urine may be helpful in developing the management plan and can be assessed as indicated.

With deepening descent of the fetal presenting part into the true pelvis during labor, the bladder may be compressed to the point at which even small urine volumes cause distension. In the third stage of labor, a distended bladder can inhibit the ability of the uterus to contract effectively, increasing the risk of postpartum hemorrhage secondary to uterine atony. Bladder hypotonicity, urine stasis, and infection during the postpartum period can result from traumatic pressure exerted on a distended bladder during labor.

A distended bladder may appear as a bulge above the symphysis pubis and, in severe cases, may extend as high as the umbilicus. When the fetus is in a posterior position, the contour of the woman's abdomen may look as though she has a full bladder; bladder distension must then be ruled out.

In the event of bladder distension, the first step is to facilitate spontaneous voiding. The best method is for her to walk to the toilet if she has no contraindications to ambulating. If she is unable to be out of bed and if the common methods (having her listen to the sound of running water; running warm water over her perineum; applying light suprapubic pressure; and having her practice perineal relaxation) do not initiate urination, then catheterization may be considered. Bladder distension can occur in any laboring woman but is especially likely in women with epidural anesthesia who receive a bolus of fluid prior to initiating the epidural. Once the epidural is active, the woman cannot feel the urge to urinate and may not have the muscle control to void. Intermittent insertion of a urinary catheter to drain the bladder should be considered to minimize the risk of urinary retention or infection for these women, especially if they are remote from delivery.

General Condition

Continuing evaluation of maternal status includes evaluation of several areas that interrelate and overlap: the woman's level of fatigue and physical depletion, her behavior and responses to labor, her perception of pain, and her ability to cope with labor.

A woman's level of fatigue and physical depletion is affected by her state at the start of labor, maintenance of hydration during labor, length of labor, and her ability to cope with the demands placed upon her by labor. This can be a vicious cycle. A woman's lack of ability to cope may increase fatigue, and fatigue can decrease her ability to cope. Occasionally a woman enters labor truly exhausted and dehydrated from days of the general aches and symptoms characteristic of the end of pregnancy or from a prolonged latent phase. A mutually agreed-upon hospital-based management plan for such a woman might include considering an early epidural and intravenous fluids.

A woman's behavior normally changes throughout labor, and these changes can be used in evaluating her response to labor. Her behavior is also affected by her degree of self-efficacy, anxiety or fear, and the amount of pain she is experiencing. In another cycle of interplay, these factors affect her coping ability, and her ability to cope in turn affects her self-efficacy, anxieties, and fears. Evaluation of behavior during labor will aid in determining the support and comfort measures needed, including consideration for medication.

Fetal Well-Being

Ongoing and standardized fetal heart rate assessment is essential to evaluating fetal well-being throughout labor regardless of the method chosen. The *Fetal Assessment During Labor* chapter provides details on fetal assessment in labor.

Labor Progress
Digital Cervical Examinations

Internal cervical examinations are intrusive and often uncomfortable for women; however, appropriately timed digital cervical dilatation examinations are critical in informing labor progress. Use of contemporary guidelines that account for normal duration of labor and rate of cervical dilation is important. As noted earlier, use of the Friedman curve is likely to result in overdiagnosis of dystocia. Therefore, while it is appropriate to wait several hours prior to doing a cervical examination as the cervix changes in early active labor (e.g., from 4 cm to 5 cm), it may be inappropriate to wait as long later in labor (e.g., between 8 cm and 9 cm).[82]

Supplemental indicators of labor progress in addition to cervical dilatation can and should be obtained from each digital cervical examination that is performed during labor, including (1) cervical effacement; (2) position (posterior, mid-position, anterior); and (3) consistency (firm or soft), station and position. The frequency with which cervical examinations are performed depends on the woman's condition and on the midwife's ability to use other parameters for evaluating progress in labor. It is not always necessary to perform an internal examination to gain insights into the progress of labor. The traditional practice of conducting cervical examinations every 1 to 2 hours simply subjects the woman to unnecessary discomfort, intrusion, and increased risk of infection. Astute observation of the woman—her behavior, contraction pattern, signs and symptoms of transition into second-stage labor, change of location of back pain, change in location of maximum intensity of fetal heart tones, and change in position of fetal heart tones—can give insights into labor progression. This information does not negate performance of a cervical examination if there is a question of progress, however.

During normal first-stage labor, a cervical examination may be indicated in the following situations:

1. To establish an informational baseline
2. Before deciding on the kind, amount, and route of any medication
3. To verify complete dilatation to either encourage or discourage maternal pushing effort
4. After spontaneous rupture of the membranes if a prolapsed cord is a suspected risk (e.g. ballotable presenting part).
5. To check for a prolapsed cord when fetal heart rate decelerations do not resolve with the usual maneuvers

Unfortunately, digital cervical examinations rely on the clinical experience and proprioceptive skill of the examiner. Labor care providers accurately determine actual cervical dilatation in only half of all cases,[83–86] but are accurate to ± 1 cm from actual cervical dilatation in approximately 90% of cases.[83–85] This is a significant shortcoming for accurately evaluating labor progress, considering that a laboring woman who is truly dilated to 4 cm may be determined to be 3 cm to 5 cm by a labor care clinician, and so on for subsequent examinations. Thus true cervical change over time is only *estimated* by cervical examinations. Because of this shortcoming in labor progress evaluation, it is recommended that cervical examinations be performed by the same professional whenever possible, and be interpreted conservatively so that unnecessary interventions aimed at accelerating labor are not imposed on women who are adequately progressing in labor.

Fetal Presentation, Position, and Station

Descent and internal rotation of the fetal presenting part is as equally important as is progressive cervical dilation to monitor labor progress. It is not uncommon to find no cervical dilation between one digital examination and the next, but to find instead, progressive changes in fetal descent. Conversely, arrest of descent is an important finding that may indicate true cephalopelvic disproportion. Because cephalic presentations are by far the most common, it is vital that a midwife be proficient in identifying the essential landmarks of the fetal skull as described in the *Anatomy and Physiology During Labor and Birth* chapter. Cervical examination provides information regarding (1) fetal presentation; (2) position; (3) station; (4) the adaptation of the fetus to the pelvis—specifically, synclitism, or asynclitism of the fetal head; (5) the presence or absence of molding; and (6) the presence or absence of caput succedaneum. Each one of the items should be determined at every cervical examination conducted during active labor.

The formation of a few millimeters of caput succedaneum is not unusual or abnormal. A small caput succedaneum may be indicative of a somewhat prolonged labor resulting from uterine inertia with weak contractions. Formation of extensive caput succedaneum, which makes the identification of fetal sutures and fontanels difficult, combined with severe amounts of molding, is usually seen only when the pressure has been great and labor prolonged. Cephalopelvic disproportion must be suspected when significant molding or overriding sutures are noted. A sizable caput may also be seen from positional pressure when the fetal position was occipitoposterior.

Conclusion

Normal physiologic labor is an intricate interplay of physiologic and psychological forces within the woman. Caring for women during labor involves attention to three different but equally important variables: the well-being of the woman, the well-being of the fetus, and labor progress. Historical measures for evaluating labor progress have been found to be unreliable, but new indices are not yet available for all populations. With the evident labor pattern differences existing between Friedman's traditional findings and contemporary research, it is inappropriate to base clinical expectations of cervical dilation during labor on Friedman's work. Instead, contemporary patterns of labor should be used as this body of research continues to grow.

● ● ● **References**

1. American College of Nurse-Midwives, Midwives Alliance, National Association of Certified Professional Midwives. Supporting healthy and normal physiologic childbirth: a consensus statement by ACNM, MANA, and NACPM. 2012. Available at: http://midwife.org/index.asp?bid=59&cat=3&button=Search. Accessed January 3, 2013.

2. ACOG Practice Bulletin Number 49, December 2003: dystocia and augmentation of labor. *Obstet Gynecol.* 2003;102:1445-1454.

3. de Haan HH, Offermans PM, Smits F, et al. Value of the fern test to confirm or reject the diagnosis of ruptured membranes is modest in nonlaboring women presenting with nonspecific vaginal fluid loss. *Am J Perinatol.* 1994;11:46-50.

4. Abdelazim IA, Makhlouf HH. Placental alpha microglobulin-1 (AmniSure(®) test) for detection of premature rupture of fetal membranes. *Arch Gynecol Obstet.* 2012;285:985-989.

5. American College of Nurse-Midwives. Position statement: premature rupture of membranes at term. 2012. Available at: http://midwife.org/ACNM/files/ACNMLibraryData/UPLOADFILENAME/000000000233/PROM%20Mar%202012.pdf. Accessed January 5, 2013.

6. Zhang J, Landy HJ, Branch DW, et al. Contemporary patterns of spontaneous labor with normal neonatal outcomes. *Obstet Gynecol.* 2010;116:1281-1287.

7. Friedman E. The graphic analysis of labor. *Am J Obstet Gynecol.* 1954;68:1568-1575.

8. Friedman EA. Primigravid labor: a graphicostatistical analysis. *Obstet Gynecol.* 1955;6:567-589.

9. Friedman EA. Labor in multiparas: a graphicostatistical analysis. *Obstet Gynecol.* 1956;8:691-703.

10. Friedman EA, Kroll BH. Computer analysis of labour progression. *J Obstet Gynaecol Br Commonw.* 1969;76:1075-1079.

11. Friedman EA, Kroll BH. Computer analysis of labor progression. III. Pattern variations by parity. *J Reprod Med.* 1971;6:179-183.

12. Friedman EA, ed. *Labor: Clinical Evaluation and Management.* 2nd ed. New York: Appleton-Century-Crofts; 1978.

13. Lavender T, Hart A, Smyth RMD. Effect of partogram use on outcomes for women in spontaneous labour at term. *Cochrane Database Syst Rev.* 2012; 8:CD005461.

14. Philpott RH, Castle WM. Cervicographs in the management of labour in primigravidae. I. The alert line for detecting abnormal labour. *J Obstet Gynaecol Br Commonw.* 1972;79:592-598.

15. Philpott RH, Castle WM. Cervicographs in the management of labour in primigravidae. II. The action line and treatment of abnormal labour. *J Obstet Gynaecol Br Commonw.* 1972;79:599-602.

16. Drouin P, Nasah BT, Nkounawa F. The value of the partogramme in the management of labor. *Obstet Gynecol.* 1979;53:741-745.

17. World Health Organization, Division of Family Health, Maternal Health and Safe Motherhood Programme. *The Partograph: The Application of the WHO Partograph in the Management of Labour. Report of a WHO Multicentre Study 1990–1991.* 1994;WHO/FHE/MSM/94.4.

18. Lavender T, Alfirevic Z, Walkinshaw S. Partogram action line study: a randomised trial. *Br J Obstet Gynaecol.* 1998;105:976-980.

19. Lavender T, Wallymahmed AH, Walkinshaw SA. Managing labor using partograms with different action lines: a prospective study of women's views. *Birth.* 1999;26:89-96.

20. Pattinson RC, Howarth GR, Mdluli W, Macdonald AP, Makin JD, Funk M. Aggressive or expectant management of labour: a randomised clinical trial. *BJOG.* 2003;110:457-461.

21. Lavender T, Alfirevic Z, Walkinshaw S. Effect of different partogram action lines on birth outcomes: a randomized controlled trial. *Obstet Gynecol.* 2006;108:295-302.

22. Mathews JE, Rajaratnam A, George A, Mathai M. Comparison of two World Health Organization partographs. *Int J Gynaecol Obstet.* 2007;96:147-150.

23. Orji E. Evaluating progress of labor in nulliparas and multiparas using the modified WHO partograph. *Int J Gynaecol Obstet.* 2008;102:249-252.

24. van Bogaert L. Revising the primigravid partogram: does it make any difference? *Arch Gynecol Obstet.* 2009;279:643-647.

25. Dujardin B, De Schampheleire I, Sene H, Ndiaye F. Value of the alert and action lines on the partogram. *Lancet.* 1992;339:1336-1338.

26. World Health Organization partograph in management of labour. World Health Organization Maternal Health and Safe Motherhood Programme. *Lancet.* 1994;343:1399-1404.

27. Fahdhy M, Chongsuvivatwong V. Evaluation of World Health Organization partograph implementation by midwives for maternity home birth in Medan, Indonesia. *Midwifery.* 2005;21:301-310.

28. Neal JL, Lowe NK. Physiologic partograph to improve birth safety and outcomes among low-risk, nulliparous women with spontaneous labor onset. *Med Hypotheses.* 2012;78:319-326.

29. Friedman EA. The length of active labor in normal pregnancies. *Obstet Gynecol.* 1996;88:319-320.

30. Laughon SK, Branch DW, Beaver J, Zhang J. Changes in labor patterns over 50 years. *Am J Obstet Gynecol.* 2012;206:419.e1-419.e9.

31. Zhang J, Troendle J, Mikolajczyk R, Sundaram R, Beaver J, Fraser W. The natural history of the normal first stage of labor. *Obstet Gynecol.* 2010;115:705-710.

32. Kilpatrick SJ, Laros RKJ. Characteristics of normal labor. *Obstet Gynecol.* 1989;74:85-87.

33. Cunningham FG, Leveno KJ, Bloom SL, Hauth JC, Rouse DJ, Spong CY, eds. *Williams Obstetrics.* 23rd ed. New York: McGraw-Hill; 2010.

34. Battista LR, Wing DA. Abnormal labor and induction of labor. In: Gabbe SG, Niebyl JR, Simpson JL, eds. *Obstetrics: Normal and Problem Pregnancies.* 5th ed. Philadelphia: Churchill Livingstone; 2007.

35. Peisner DB, Rosen MG. Transition from latent to active labor. *Obstet Gynecol.* 1986;68:448-451.

36. Zhang J, Troendle JF, Yancey MK. Reassessing the labor curve in nulliparous women. *Am J Obstet Gynecol.* 2002;187:824-828.

37. Albers LL, Schiff M, Gorwoda JG. The length of active labor in normal pregnancies. *Obstet Gynecol.* 1996;87:355-359.

38. Albers LL. The duration of labor in healthy women. *J Perinatol.* 1999;19:114-119.

39. Jones M, Larson E. Length of normal labor in women of Hispanic origin. *J Midwifery Women's Health.* 2003;48:2-9.

40. Neal JL, Lowe NK, Ahijevych KL, Patrick TE, Cabbage LA, Corwin EJ. "Active labor" duration and dilation rates among low-risk, nulliparous women with spontaneous labor onset: a systematic review. *J Midwifery Women's Health.* 2010;55:308-318.

41. Perl FM, Hunter DJ. What cervical dilatation rate during active labour should be considered abnormal? *Eur J Obstet Gynecol Reprod Biol.* 1992;45:89-92.

42. *Evaluation of Cesarean Delivery* [Developed under the direction of the Task Force on Cesarean Delivery Rates, Roger K. Freeman et al.]. Washington, DC: American College of Obstetricians and Gynecologists; 2000.

43. Gifford DS, Morton SC, Fiske M, Keesey J, Keeler E, Kahn KL. Lack of progress in labor as a reason for cesarean. *Obstet Gynecol.* 2000;95:589-595.

44. Hamilton BE, Martin JA, Ventura SJ. Births: preliminary data for 2011. *Natl Vital Stat Rep.* 2012;61:1-29.

45. Althabe F, Belizan JM. Caesarean section: the paradox. *Lancet.* 2006;368:1472-1473.

46. World Health Organization. Joint Interregional Conference on Appropriate Technology for Birth, Fortaleza, Brazil, April 22-26, 1985.

47. Bailit JL, Dierker L, Blanchard MH, Mercer BM. Outcomes of women presenting in active versus latent phase of spontaneous labor. *Obstet Gynecol.* 2005;105:77-79.

48. Holmes P, Oppenheimer LW, Wen SW. The relationship between cervical dilatation at initial presentation in labour and subsequent intervention. *BJOG.* 2001;108:1120-1124.

49. McNiven PS, Williams JI, Hodnett E, Kaufman K, Hannah ME. An early labor assessment program: a randomized, controlled trial. *Birth.* 1998;25:5-10.

50. Incerti M, Locatelli A, Ghidini A, Ciriello E, Consonni S, Pezzullo JC. Variability in rate of cervical dilation in nulliparous women at term. *Birth.* 2011;38:30-35.

51. Impey L, Hobson J, O'Herlihy C. Graphic analysis of actively managed labor: prospective computation of labor progress in 500 consecutive nulliparous women in spontaneous labor at term. *Am J Obstet Gynecol.* 2000;183:438-443.

52. Rahnama P, Ziaei S, Faghihzadeh S. Impact of early admission in labor on method of delivery. *Int J Gynaecol Obstet.* 2006;92:217-220.

53. Mikolajczyk R, Zhang J, Chan L, Grewal J. Early versus late admission to labor/delivery, labor progress and risk of caesarean section in nulliparous women. *Am J Obstet Gynecol.* 2008;199:S49.

54. Neal JL, Lowe NK, Patrick TE, Cabbage LA, Corwin EJ. What is the slowest-yet-normal cervical dilation rate among nulliparous women with spontaneous labor onset? *J Obstet Gynecol Neonatal Nurs.* 2010;39:361-369.

55. Institute for Safe Medication Practices. ISMP's list of high-alert medications. 2008. Available at: http://www.ismp.org/tools/highalertmedications.pdf. Accessed November 10, 2012.

56. Clark SL, Simpson KR, Knox GE, Garite TJ. Oxytocin: new perspectives on an old drug. *Am J Obstet Gynecol.* 2009;200:35.e1-35.e6.

57. Clark SL, Belfort MA, Dildy GA, Meyers JA. Reducing obstetric litigation through alterations in practice patterns. *Obstet Gynecol.* 2008;112:1279-1283.

58. Bugg GJ, Siddiqui F, Thornton JG. Oxytocin versus no treatment or delayed treatment for slow progress in the first stage of spontaneous labour. *Cochrane Database Syst Rev.* 2011:CD007123.

59. Smyth RMD, Alldred SK, Markham C. Amniotomy for shortening spontaneous labour. *Cochrane Database Syst Rev*. 2007:CD006167.

60. Balayla PS. Inadequate prenatal care utilization and risks of infant mortality and poor birth outcome: a retrospective analysis of 28,729,765 U.S. deliveries over 8 years. *Am J Perinatol*. 2012;29:787-794.

61. Devane D, Lalor JG, Daly S, McGuire W, Smith V. Cardiotocography versus intermittent auscultation of fetal heart on admission to labour ward for assessment of fetal wellbeing. *Cochrane Database Syst Rev*. 2012;2:CD005122.

62. Intermittent auscultation for intrapartum fetal heart rate surveillance (replaces ACNM Clinical Bulletin #9, March 2007). *J Midwifery Women's Health*. 2010;55:397-403.

63. ACOG Practice Bulletin No. 106: intrapartum fetal heart rate monitoring: nomenclature, interpretation, and general management principles. *Obstet Gynecol*. 2009;114:192-202.

64. Hodnett ED, Gates S, Hofmeyr GJ, Sakala C. Continuous support for women during childbirth. *Cochrane Database Syst Rev*. 2012;10:CD003766.

65. Lawrence A, Lewis L, Hofmeyr GJ, Dowswell T, Styles C. Maternal positions and mobility during first stage labour. *Cochrane Database Syst Rev*. 2009:CD003934.

66. Mendelson CL. The aspiration of stomach contents into the lungs during obstetric anesthesia. *Am J Obstet Gynecol*. 1946;52:191.

67. Garite TJ, Weeks J, Peters-Phair K, Pattillo C, Brewster WR. A randomized controlled trial of the effect of increased intravenous hydration on the course of labor in nulliparous women. *Am J Obstet Gynecol*. 2000;183:1544-1548.

68. Eslamian L, Marsoosi V, Pakneeyat Y. Increased intravenous fluid intake and the course of labor in nulliparous women. *Int J Gynaecol Obstet*. 2006;93:102-105.

69. Coco A, Derksen-Schrock A, Coco K, Raff T, Horst M, Hussar E. A randomized trial of increased intravenous hydration in labor when oral fluid is unrestricted. *Fam Med*. 2010;42:52-56.

70. Kavitha A, Chacko KP, Thomas E, et al. A randomized controlled trial to study the effect of IV hydration on the duration of labor in nulliparous women. *Arch Gynecol Obstet*. 2012;285:343-346.

71. Direkvand-Moghadam A, Rezaeian M. Increased intravenous hydration of nulliparas in labor. *Int J Gynaecol Obstet*. 2012;118:213-215.

72. Foulkes J, Dumoulin JG. The effects of ketonuria in labour. *Br J Clin Pract*. 1985;39:59-62.

73. Watanabe T, Minakami H, Sakata Y, et al. Effect of labor on maternal dehydration, starvation, coagulation, and fibrinolysis. *J Perinat Med*. 2001;29:528-534.

74. Singata M, Tranmer J, Gyte GM. Restricting oral fluid and food intake during labour. *Cochrane Database Syst Rev*. 2010:CD003930.

75. Smyth RMD, Alldred SK, Markham C. Amniotomy for shortening spontaneous labour. *Cochrane Database Syst Rev*. 2007;4:CD006167. doi: 10.1002/14651858. CD006167.pub2.

76. Mahmood TA, Rahyner A, Mith NC, Beat I. A randomized prospective trial comparing single dose prostaglandin E$_2$ vaginal gel with forewarte amniotomy for induction of labor. *Eur J Obstet Gynecol Reprod Biol*. 1995;58(2):11107.

77. Macones GA, Cahill A, Stamilio DM, et al. The efficacy of early amniotomy in nulliparous labor induction: a randomized controlled trial. *Am J Obstet Gynecol*. 2012;207:403.e1-e5.

78. Rouse DJ, McCullough C, Wern A, Woen J, Hauth JC. Active-phase labor arrest: a randomized trial of chorioamnion management. *Obstet Gynecol*. 1994;83:937-940.

79. Wei S, Wo BL, Xu H, Luo ZC, Roy C, Fraser WD. Early amniotomy and early oxytocin for prevention of, or therapy for, delay in first stage spontaneous labour compared with routine care. *Cochrane Database Syst Rev*. 2009;2:CD006794. doi: 10.1002/14651858. CD006794.pub2.

80. Freeman RK, Garite TJ, Nageotte MP. *Fetal Heart Rate Monitoring*. 3rd ed. Philadelphia, PA: Lippincott Williams and Wilkins; 2003:57.

81. Krapohi A, Myers GG, Caleryo-Barcia R. Uterine contractions in spontaneous labor: a quantitative study. *Am J Obstet Gynecol*. 1970;106(3):378-387.

82. Suzuki R, Horiuchi S, Ohtsu H. Evaluation of the labor curve in nulliparous Japanese women. *Am J Obstet Gynecol*. 2010;203:226.e1-226.e6.

83. Buchmann EJ, Libhaber E. Accuracy of cervical assessment in the active phase of labour. *BJOG*. 2007;114:833-837.

84. Huhn KA, Brost BC. Accuracy of simulated cervical dilation and effacement measurements among practitioners. *Am J Obstet Gynecol*. 2004;191:1797-1799.

85. Phelps JY, Higby K, Smyth MH, Ward JA, Arredondo F, Mayer AR. Accuracy and intraobserver variability of simulated cervical dilatation measurements. *Am J Obstet Gynecol*. 1995;173:942-945.

86. Tuffnell DJ, Bryce F, Johnson N, Lilford RJ. Simulation of cervical changes in labour: reproducibility of expert assessment. *Lancet*. 1989;2:1089-1090.

● ● ● **Additional Resources for Normal Birth**

1. World Health Organization, Department of Reproductive Health and Research. Care in normal birth: a practical guide. Geneva, Switzerland: World Health Organization, 1997. Available at: www.who.int/reproductivehealth/publications/maternal_perinatal_health/MSM_96_24_/en. Accessed June 16, 2013.

2. Making normal birth a reality: Consensus statement from the Maternity Care Working Party, our shared views about the need to recognize, facilitate and audit normal birth. Royal College of Obstetricians and Gynaecologists. Available at: http://www.pbh.gov.br/smsa/bhpelopartonormal/estudos_cientificos/arquivos/normal_birth_consensus.pdf. Accessed June 14, 2013.

3. The Society of Obstetricians and Gynaecologists of Canada. Joint policy statement on normal childbirth. Available at: http://sogc.org/guidelines/joint-policy-statement-on-normal-childbirth-policy-statement. Accessed June 16, 2013.

4. American College of Nurse-Midwives, Midwives Alliance, National Association of Certified Professional Midwives. Supporting healthy and normal physiologic childbirth: a consensus statement by ACNM, MANA, and NACPM. 2012. Available at: http://midwife.org/index.asp?bid=59&cat=3&button=Search. Accessed January 3, 2013.

5. Sakala C, Corry MP. *Evidence-Based Maternity Care: What It Is and What It Can Achieve.* New York, NY: Milbank Memorial Fund; 2008.

6. Romano AM, Lothian JA. Promoting, protecting, and supporting normal birth: A look at the evidence. *J Obstet Gynecol Neonatal Nurs.* 2008; 37(1): 94-105.

7. Goer H, Romano A. *Optimal Care in Childbirth; The Case for a Physiologic Approach.* Classic Day Publishing: Seattle, WA; 2012.

8. Childbirth Connection. Blueprint for action: steps toward a high-quality, high-value maternity care system. Available at: http://transform.childbirthconnection.org/blueprint. Accessed May 4, 2012.

9. www.BirthTOOLS.org. This website is a joint venture among ACNM, AWHONN, NCAP, and Lamaze. The website has tools for clinicians to help them optimize the outcomes of labor safely. Content includes tools for coping in labor, promoting spontaneous onset of labor, nutrition and hydration, and physiologic second stage, to name just a few.

26A

Evaluation and Diagnosis of Ruptured Membranes

JEREMY NEAL

SHARON RYAN

LINDA HUNTER

When evaluating a woman whose history suggests rupture of membranes, the differential diagnoses include urinary incontinence, vaginal or cervical discharge, semen, and (rarely) rupture of the chorion alone.

Several laboratory tests can confirm or support a diagnosis of rupture of membranes (ROM), including the arborization test (fern test), pH testing (nitrazine test), ultrasound assessment of amniotic fluid volume, and testing for the presence of placental alpha macroglobulin-1 (PAMG-1) or fetal fibronectin in vaginal secretions. Several of these tests can be directly performed on samples of fluid obtained during the physical examination.

for a fern-like pattern (arborization) caused by crystallization due to the high sodium chloride and protein concentrations in amniotic fluid.

The sensitivity and specificity of the fern test among nonlaboring women are 51.4% and 70.8%, respectively; for women in labor, these results improve to 98% and 88.2%, respectively.[1] Cervical mucus and semen can also show fern-like patterns, which may cause a false-positive result. The results of a fern test must be viewed within the context of the history and physical examination and may best be viewed as a supportive test rather than a

Tests for Rupture of Membranes

1. Observation of fluid coming from the cervical os is diagnostic for ROM.

2. The *fern test* is a classic method of assessing for ROM and is considered diagnostic in many settings when the classic pattern of ferning is clearly seen (**Figure 26A-1**). During a sterile speculum examination, a sterile cotton swab is used to obtain a specimen of the fluid from the posterior vaginal fornix. Care must be taken not to touch the cervical os to avoid collecting cervical mucus. The specimen is spread thinly onto a microscope slide and allowed to dry thoroughly. The slide is then inspected using a microscope at 10× power

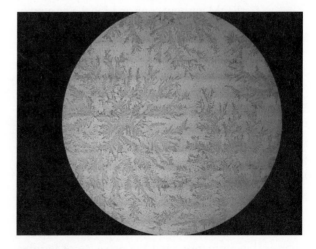

Figure 26A-1 Fern pattern of amniotic fluid under 10x power.
Source: Courtesy of Paul_12

conclusive one if active leaking from the cervical os is not visible.

3. The *nitrazine test* uses limited-range pH paper or a commercially prepared swab to detect the rise in pH in vaginal discharge associated with the presence of amniotic fluid. The normal pH of the vagina of most women is acidic (approximately 4.5), whereas amniotic fluid is neutral to slightly alkaline (7.0–7.5). The mustard-gold nitrazine will turn dark blue in the presence of alkaline material. Collecting a sample of fluid from the posterior fornix with a sterile cotton swab and then touching the nitrazine paper with the saturated swab is the procedure for using nitrazine paper. A well-saturated cotton swab can be used to prepare a slide for the fern test, then touched to the nitrazine paper. Alternatively, the paper can be touched in the fluid collected at the tip of the sterile speculum when it is withdrawn from the vagina. Commercially prepared nitrazine swabs are available and are accompanied by manufacturer instructions that must be carefully followed.

The sensitivity and specificity of the nitrazine method in confirming ROM are approximately 87% and 81%, respectively.[2] False-positive results can occur in the presence of vaginal infections, blood, semen, or other alkaline substances, while false-negative results can be caused by a "high" or minimal leak of amniotic fluid.

4. Pooling of fluid in the posterior fornix of the vagina is a helpful sign, but it is not diagnostic for ROM without confirmation via ferning or nitrazine testing.

5. Ultrasound quantification may also be used, although a woman can have ruptured membranes and still have a normal amount of amniotic fluid, especially if the membranes are only leaking. Ultrasound documentation of oligohydramnios does not confirm ROM but may be helpful in making a management plan.

Diagnosis of ROM

Most of the time, the diagnosis of ruptured membranes is made via the constellation of history, physical examination, and the presence of ferning. When two or more of these tests are positive, the accuracy of the diagnosis is approximately 93%.[3] This method is generally considered acceptable for women at term. For women who are preterm, accurate diagnosis is more critical. Physician consultation is needed if the diagnosis is inconclusive for a woman who is at a preterm gestation.

Evaluation for Ruptured Membranes

1. History

   a. Inquire about the time, amount, color, consistency, odor, and pattern of leaking (e.g., large gush, continued trickling).

      i. These data are especially important for development of a management plan because the length of time from rupture of membranes to delivery is directly correlated with risk of maternal–fetal infection. The characteristic of the fluid can reveal clues to fetal well-being.

      ii. ROM typically will cause a large gush of fluid, followed by a continuous watery discharge necessitating use of sanitary pads or even washcloths or towels.

      iii. In some instances of ruptured membranes, the only symptom the woman may notice is a feeling of moistness on her undergarments from a small, continuous discharge. Assessing the woman's ability to control the leakage with contraction of the pelvic floor muscles (Kegel) helps to differentiate PROM from urinary incontinence.

   b. Inquire about any recent fever, abdominal pain, vaginal bleeding, abnormal discharge, urine symptoms, and last intercourse.

      i. Semen expelled from the vagina can sometimes be mistaken for amniotic fluid.

   c. Inquire about signs of labor: contractions, bloody show, fetal movement, recent cervical assessments or intercourse.

   d. Confirm pregnancy dating (this is especially important if less than 37 weeks' gestation).

   e. Review the prenatal record for past obstetric history, prenatal issues, or current medical problems.

2. **Physical Examination**

The earlier an examination is performed after the rupture of membranes occurs, the easier it is to diagnose ruptured membranes. When more than 6 to 12 hours passes, many of the diagnostic observations become unreliable because of lack of fluid.

a. Measure temperature, pulse, respirations, and blood pressure.

b. Perform heart and lung auscultation.

c. Palpate abdomen for fundal tenderness.

d. Perform Leopold's maneuvers to assess fetal position, estimated fetal weight, and presenting part.

   i. Ultrasound confirmation of the presenting part may be required.

e. Perform fetal assessment with Doppler or electronic fetal monitoring (EFM) per institutional or practice guidelines. Continuous EFM is required for women who are gestational ages 24 to 37 weeks.

f. Perform a sterile speculum examination.

   i. Note the color, consistency, and amount of any fluid leaking from the vaginal introitus.

   ii. As the speculum is carefully inserted, be alert for any evidence of prolapsed cord, bulging forebag, or protruding fetal parts.

   iii. Visualize the cervical os and note any pooling of fluid in the vaginal vault or fluid leaking directly from the os.

     1. Normal amniotic fluid can be clear, straw colored, or cloudy. Flecks of white or creamy vernix may be noted in the amniotic fluid of preterm or near-term infants. Dark yellow or green fluid indicates the presence of meconium in the amniotic fluid. Meconium-stained fluid increases the risk for chorioamnionitis and can be an indication of fetal compromise.

     2. Amniotic fluid has a distinct musty odor, which differentiates it from urine, while foul-smelling fluid can be an indicator of infection.

     3. If there is no visible fluid leaking from the os:

       a. Have the woman perform a Valsalva maneuver or cough.

       b. Alternatively, one can consider having an assistant apply gentle fundal pressure or gently elevate the presenting part abdominally to allow fluid to pass by the presenting part and flow through the cervical os.

       c. The other option is to have the woman remain semi-reclining for 30 to 60 minutes and then repeat the sterile speculum examination.

   iv. Obtain sterile swab specimens of any fluid or discharge seen, avoiding the cervical mucus.

     1. Using a sterile swab, collect a sample of fluid for 10–15 seconds from the vaginal pool at the posterior fornix or along the vaginal wall. Avoid the cervix.

     2. If a nitrazine swab is being used, the color change can be read directly from the swab.

     3. If nitrazine paper is being used, apply the swab to pH paper before proceeding. A pH of 6.5 or higher is suggestive of amniotic fluid rupture.

     4. Immediately roll the swab across a dry, clean slide to create a thin film. Thick specimens may obscure ferning. Set aside for 10 minutes.

       a. Ferning is based on crystallization of the sodium chloride in amniotic fluid. This occurs as the liquid evaporates, so false-negative results are possible if the slide is examined before it is completely dry.

     5. Obtain a wet mount of any discharge.

   v. If 32 to 34 weeks' gestation, obtain a sample of fluid for fetal lung maturity using a 5- to 10-cc syringe and intravenous catheter with the needle removed.

vi. Obtain a specimen for gonorrhea chlamydia culture per protocols as required.

vii. Obtain GBS culture if the woman's status is unknown or if it has been more than 5 weeks since the last GBS result.

viii. Visualize the cervix for dilatation and length/effacement.

ix. *Do not* perform a digital vaginal/cervical examination unless signs of active labor are present.

3. **Microscopy Evaluation**

i. Examine the dry slide under low power (10×) for the presence of ferning (see Figure 26A-1).

ii. Examine the wet mount slide for the presence of yeast, bacterial vaginosis, or trichomoniasis.

● ● ● **References**

1. de Haan HH, Offermans PM, Smits F, Schouten HJ, Peeters LL. Value of the fern test to confirm or reject the diagnosis of ruptured membranes is modest in nonlaboring women presenting with nonspecific vaginal fluid loss. *Am J Perinatol.* 1994;11:46-50.

2. Abdelazim IA, Makhlouf HH. Placental alpha microglobulin-1 (AmniSure test) for detection of premature rupture of fetal membranes. *Arch Gynecol Obstet.* 2012;285:985-989.

3. Canavan TP, Simhan HN, Caritis S. An evidence-based approach to the evaluation and treatment of premature rupture of membranes: Part 1. *Obstet Gynecol Surv.* 2004;59(9):669-677.

C H A P T E R

27

Fetal Assessment During Labor

TEKOA L. KING

Introduction

Assessment of fetal well-being is a critical component of intrapartum management. The goal of all fetal assessment techniques used during labor is to identify the fetus with impaired gas exchange. None of the current fetal heart rate assessment methods directly measures fetal oxygenation or acid–base balance in fetal tissue. To date, there is no single indicator that has a high positive predictive value for detecting clinically significant fetal acidemia. It may be that the threshold for permanent damage differs among individual fetuses; perhaps today's instruments are not individually or collectively sensitive enough; or both of these theories can play a role.[1,2] Therefore it is important to know the value of the fetal assessment technologies that are in use and the extent of their capabilities. This chapter reviews fetal acid–base physiology, continuous electronic fetal heart rate monitoring (EFM), intermittent auscultation techniques, umbilical cord gas assessments that reflect fetal acid–base balance immediately prior to birth, and midwifery management of fetal heart rate patterns.

History of Fetal Heart Rate Monitoring

The safe passage of the fetus is of paramount concern to everyone involved in the birth process. Historically, the presence of fetal movement was the method used to determine that a fetus was viable. Jean Alexandre Lejumeau, the Vicomte de Kergaradec, who used a stethoscope hoping to hear the noise of the water in the uterus, first heard fetal heart sounds in 1821.[3] Although he probably was not the first person to identify fetal heart sounds, he

was the first to publish on the topic of possible clinical uses for fetal heart rate auscultation. In 1833, British obstetrician William Kennedy published the first descriptions of "fetal distress" by describing a late fetal heart rate (FHR) deceleration and associating it with poor prognosis.[4] Other discoveries from early research using intermittent auscultation that remain clinically relevant today include the relationship between maternal fever and fetal tachycardia, fetal heart rate effects of uterine hyperstimulation, and acceleration of the FHR in association with fetal movement.[3]

In the 1960s, animal studies elucidated the mechanisms of variable decelerations and hypoxia secondary to umbilical cord occlusion.[5] This body of research supported the beliefs of the time that cerebral palsy was a consequence of intrapartum asphyxia and that umbilical cord occlusion was the most common cause of oxygen deprivation in the fetus.

The electronic fetal monitor was introduced as an instrument for monitoring women with high-risk pregnancies in the 1960s. Clinicians originally anticipated that electronic fetal heart rate monitoring would become a screening test that would identify early fetal asphyxia in time to intervene before fetal damage occurred. Unfortunately, continuous EFM was rapidly adopted in clinical practice before adequate research studies could determine the sensitivity, specificity, positive predictive value, and negative predictive value of FHR interpretation. The first observational studies of FHR monitoring documented a significant decrease in the intrapartum stillbirth rate in women who were continuously monitored during labor.[6] The decrease in intrapartum stillbirths still is one of the acknowledged benefits of EFM. However, other results from use of EFM are less clear.

No randomized controlled trials (RCTs) have compared continuous EFM to no monitoring. RCTs comparing continuous EFM to FHR monitoring with a Pinard stethoscope or a handheld Doppler device were conducted in the 1990s. Most of these trials included one-to-one nursing and several included women at high risk for adverse outcomes only. Neither the RCTs nor the meta-analyses that followed found one method of fetal heart rate assessment led to improved outcomes when compared to the others in terms of Apgar scores, cerebral palsy, or perinatal mortality.[7,8] However, continuous EFM was associated with an approximately 50% increase in rates of cesarean section (relative risk [RR], 1.66; 95% confidence interval [CI], 1.30–2.13) and a slight increase in operative vaginal birth (RR, 1.16; 95% CI, 1.01–1.32).[9] The largest RCT performed in Dublin, Ireland, found EFM resulted in a decrease in neonatal seizures, but no long-term adverse effects were observed when the newborns who had seizures were followed into childhood.[10,11]

The findings of the meta-analysis based on all the RCTs conducted included more than 37,000 women resulted in many clinicians thinking that EFM has no clinical value. However, the advantages of hindsight are many. When looking back through the lens of FHR research conducted after the RCTs were done, it became clear that the RCTs failed for many reasons. These studies did not find a lower rate of cerebral palsy in children of women monitored with EFM because the largest proportion of children with cerebral palsy acquired the brain lesion prenatally or after birth. Thus it is not surprising that intrapartum management did not affect the incidence of cerebral palsy.[12,13] The marked increase in cesarean sections noted in the EFM-recipient groups may be at least partially attributed to the criteria used to define fetal distress in the trials. Because the importance of FHR variability was not yet known, cesarean sections were performed for indications such as clinician judgment, fetal scalp sampling results of a pH less than 7.2, late decelerations, FHR baseline rate less than 120 bpm, FHR baseline rate more than 160 bpm, and severe variable decelerations for more than 30 minutes. In short, the RCTs did not answer the question of whether EFM improves neonatal outcomes because they had the wrong outcome measures, they did not have a standardized interpretation of FHR characteristics that indicate fetal compromise, and few of them incorporated assessment of FHR baseline variability into the management protocols.

Over the years it became apparent that some of the variability in practice and difficulty in comparing findings across different studies was due to lack of a consensus of definitions in the field. In 1997, the National Institutes of Child Health and Human Development (NICHD) convened an expert panel charged with developing a standard terminology for interpreting FHR patterns. The panel created mutually exclusive definitions for each FHR characteristic that are used in clinical practice today; the same definitions have been used in FHR research over the last decade (**Table 27-1**).[14]

An NICHD expert panel met again in 2008 to reevaluate the prior decade of research. The results of this meeting were a reaffirmation of the 1997 terminology, formulation of new definitions for uterine tachysystole, and recommendation of a three-tier system for interpreting FHR patterns as normal (Category I), indeterminate (Category II), or abnormal (Category III) (**Table 27-2**).[15] Research on the validity and effectiveness of these categories is currently being conducted.[16,17]

The recommended terminology and interpretation guidelines from the two NICHD expert panels apply to intrapartum FHR tracings for term fetuses. Although the terminology is used for preterm fetuses, there is a paucity of research on the relationship between fetal heart rate patterns and neonatal outcomes in preterm births.

Despite use of a standard terminology and the three-category system for interpretation, even Category III FHR patterns are not good predictors of fetal acidemia. For example, although absent variability and bradycardia are more frequent antecedents in infants who develop neonatal encephalopathy when compared to infants who do not have neonatal encephalopathy, many infants born after a period of bradycardia with absent variability are vigorous and do well. When the positive predictive value is calculated, absent variability with bradycardia correctly predicts newborn acidemia 50% of the time.[18] The false-positive rate of other FHR patterns is higher. The poor sensitivity and high rate of false-positive FHR patterns from EFM represent a clinical conundrum that has not yet been solved.

The controversy about the value of continuous EFM continues today, yet use of EFM in hospital birthing units is almost universal. There are many possible reasons for this enigma. It has been suggested that continuous EFM monitoring reassures women and caregivers alike, whereas the risks associated with cesarean section births are not considered as significant in comparison. In addition, FHR monitoring allows for remote surveillance without the need for a continuous bedside provider.

Based on the extensive use of EFM, midwives and some obstetric nurses may be the only healthcare

Table 27-1	Terminology for Fetal Heart Rate Characteristics
Term	**Definition**
Baseline rate	Mean FHR rounded to increments of 5 bpm during a 10-minute segment excluding periodic or episodic changes, periods of marked variability, and segments of baseline that differ by > 25 bpm. Duration must be ≥ 2 minutes.
Bradycardia	Baseline rate of < 110 bpm
Tachycardia	Baseline rate of > 160 bpm
Variability	Fluctuations in the baseline FHR ≥ 2 cycles/minute.
Absent variability	Amplitude from peak to trough undetectable.
Minimal variability	Amplitude from peak to trough > undetectable and ≤ 5 bpm.
Moderate variability	Amplitude from peak to trough 6–25 bpm.
Marked variability	Amplitude from peak to trough > 25 bpm.
Acceleration	Visually apparent abrupt increase (onset to peak is < 30 seconds) of FHR above baseline. Peak is ≥ 15 bpm. Duration is ≥ 15 bpm and < 2 minutes. In gestations less than 32 weeks, peak of ≥ 10 bpm above baseline and duration of ≥ 10 seconds is an acceleration.
Prolonged acceleration	Acceleration ≥ 2 minutes and < 10 minutes' duration. An acceleration ≥ 10 minutes is a baseline change.
Early deceleration	Visually apparent *gradual* decrease (onset of deceleration to nadir is ≥ 30 seconds) of FHR below baseline. Return to baseline associated with a uterine contraction. The nadir of the deceleration occurs *at the same time* as the peak of the contraction. Generally, the onset, nadir, and recovery of the deceleration occur at the same time as the onset, peak, and recovery of the contraction, respectively.
Late deceleration	Visually apparent *gradual* decrease (onset of deceleration to nadir is ≥ 30 seconds) of FHR below baseline. Return to baseline associated with a uterine contraction. The nadir of the deceleration occurs *after* the peak of the contraction. Generally, the onset, nadir, and recovery of the deceleration occur after the onset, peak, and recovery of the contraction, respectively.
Variable deceleration	Visually apparent *abrupt* decrease (onset of deceleration to nadir is < 30 seconds) in FHR below baseline. Decrease is ≥ 15 bpm below baseline. Duration is ≥ 15 seconds and < 2 minutes from onset to return to baseline.
Prolonged deceleration	Visually apparent decrease in FHR below baseline. Decrease is ≥ 15 bpm below baseline. Duration is ≥ 2 minutes but < 10 minutes from onset to return to baseline.

Source: Adapted from National Institute of Child Health and Human Development Research Planning Workshop. Electronic fetal heart rate monitoring: research guidelines for interpretation. *Am J Obstet Gynecol.* 1997;17:1385-1390; *JOGNN.* 1997;26:635-640.

professionals with the knowledge and skill to safely use intermittent auscultation for fetal assessment during labor. As the incidence of cesarean section rises and risks of procedure become more apparent, it is possible that more frequent use of intermittent auscultation in low-risk women will help lower the cesarean section rate. Thus it is important that the skill not be lost. Before reviewing techniques for fetal assessment, a brief review of fetal oxygenation and acid–base physiology is in order.

Fetal Physiology

Uteroplacental Circulation and Gas Exchange

Optimal transfer of oxygen, carbon dioxide, and nutrients from the maternal circulation into the fetal circulation can occur only when the following five components function well: (1) adequate maternal blood flow into the intervillous space, (2) a large enough placental area to facilitate gas and nutrient exchange, (3) efficient diffusion of gases and nutrients

Table 27-2	Fetal Heart Rate Interpretive Categories
Category	**FHR Patterns Assigned to This Category**
Category I (normal) Baseline rate 110–160 bpm, moderate variability and absence of late or variable decelerations must *all* be present.	Baseline rate: 110–160 bpm Baseline FHR variability: moderate Late or variable decelerations: absent Early decelerations: present or absent Accelerations: present or absent
Category II (indeterminate) All FHR tracings not categorized as Category I or Category III. Includes *any* of these patterns.	Baseline rate: • Bradycardia not accompanied by absent baseline variability • Tachycardia Baseline FHR variability: • Minimal baseline variability • Absent baseline variability • Marked baseline variability Accelerations: • Absence of induced accelerations after fetal stimulations Periodic or episodic decelerations: • Recurrent variable decelerations accompanied by minimal or moderate baseline variability • Prolonged deceleration greater than 2 minutes but less than 10 minutes • Recurrent late decelerations with moderate baseline variability • Variable decelerations with other characteristics, such as slow return to baseline, "overshoots," or "shoulders"
Category III (abnormal) Includes *either* pattern.	Absent baseline FHR variability and any of the following: • Recurrent late decelerations • Recurrent variable decelerations • Bradycardia Sinusoidal pattern

Source: Adapted from Macones GA, Hankins GD, Spong CY, Hauth J, Moore T. The 2008 National Institute of Child Health and Human Development Research Workshop report on electronic fetal heart rate monitoring. *Obstet Gynecol.* 2008;112:661-666; *JOGNN.* 2008;37:510-515.

across the three membranes that separate the maternal and fetal circulations, (4) unimpaired umbilical vein circulation into the fetus, and (5) adequate oxygen transport capacity in the fetus.

In women without preexisting medical disorders, placental growth is usually adequate, gas and nutrient exchange is efficient, and an adequate amount of amniotic fluid cushions the umbilical cord well. In addition, the fetus has extra oxygen-carrying capacity relative to the adult secondary to several physiologic differences: Fetal hemoglobin binds to oxygen more easily than does adult hemoglobin, which favors transfer of oxygen from the maternal circulation to the fetal circulation; the fetus has more

hemoglobin in circulation than do adults (the average fetal hematocrit ranges from 43% to 63%); the fetus has a higher cardiac output and heart rate for an overall faster circulation; and organs that need oxygen such as the heart and brain are over-perfused. These mechanisms allow the fetus to survive well at a PO_2 of approximately 35 mm Hg, which is approximately the same as the maternal venous system; these same mechanisms also provide a buffer during the intermittent decreases in oxygenation that occur during uterine contractions. Thus the components of uteroplacental function most likely to adversely affect fetal gas exchange are decreased placental perfusion (e.g., uterine tachysystole, maternal supine positioning) and decreased umbilical vessel perfusion (e.g., cord compression).

Approximately 500 to 600 mL of maternal blood flows to the uterus each minute at term. The majority of this blood (70% to 90%) enters the maternal spiral arteries that run perpendicular through uterine muscle. Uterine contractions constrict these arteries, which temporarily interrupts blood flow in and out of the intervillous space.

The spiral arteries become deinnervated during pregnancy when their endothelial linings are replaced with trophoblastic tissue. This process of deinnervation causes the arteries to lose their ability to constrict if pressure in the vessel drops. As a consequence, the arteries become maximally dilated, in order to facilitate blood flow into the intervillous space.

The clinical significance of this placental structure is that maternal hypotension, hypertension, and uterine contractions can all decrease blood flow into the intervillous space. Very little can be done physiologically to increase uterine blood flow if it is needed (**Figure 27-1**). Maximal arterial flow to the spiral arteries can be supported via use of side-lying positions to prevent compression of the inferior vena cava and administration of tocolytics that stop uterine contractions for a short time.

Factors That Control the Fetal Heart Rate

The fetal heart rate is controlled by sympathetic, parasympathetic, chemoreceptor, baroreceptor, and central nervous system (CNS) inputs.

Sympathetic and Parasympathetic Input

The average baseline heart rate in the normal term fetus before labor is 140 bpm (range: 120–160 bpm). Early in pregnancy, the FHR is even higher, although not significantly higher. The FHR of a preterm fetus is likely to be on the higher end of this range.

The sympathetic fibers that innervate the myocardium are responsive to catecholamine stimulation and cause an increase in FHR. As the parasympathetic nervous system matures during the second trimester, parasympathetic input—which is mediated via the vagus nerve—becomes dominant over sympathetic stimulation and the baseline heart rate gradually slows.

The fetal heart is similar to the adult heart in that it has intrinsic pacemaker activity. The sinoatrial node, in the right atrium, has the highest intrinsic rate and, therefore, the sinoatrial node sets the pace.[19, p54] The vagus nerve originates in the medulla oblongata and terminates in the sinoatrial node of the fetal heart, where vagal stimulation changes the

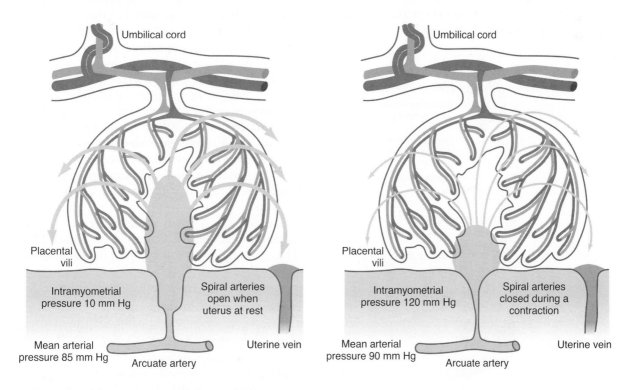

Figure 27-1 Effect of uterine contraction on blood flow into the intervillous space in the placenta.

FHR by causing the interval between successive beats to vary.[20]

Chemoreceptors and Baroreceptors

Chemoreceptors found in the aortic arch and central nervous system are sensitive to changes in oxygen and carbon dioxide content within the blood. Increased carbon dioxide causes the chemoreceptors to signal the medulla oblongata, which stimulates the vagus nerve and slows the FHR. In the adult, central chemoreceptor detection of hypercarbia produces tachycardia, whereas peripheral chemoreceptor detection of hypercarbia produces bradycardia. In the fetus, the parasympathetic system is dominant and the mechanisms of chemoreceptor trigger are not totally understood, but the result of transient hypercarbia is clearly a slowing of the FHR.

Baroreceptors are found in the aortic and carotic arches, where they rapidly detect changes in pressure. When blood pressure rises, a quick reflex occurs (via the vagal nerve) to slow the heart rate (**Figure 27-2**).

Fetal Response to Hypoxia

Basic definitions related to hypoxia are listed in the *Anatomy and Physiology of Pregnancy: Placental, Fetal, and Maternal Adaptations* chapter.[21] The fetus responds to hypoxia with (1) a transient bradycardia that decreases oxygen consumption by as much as 60%, (2) redistribution of blood to vital organs, and (3) use of anaerobic metabolism.[19,p.64]

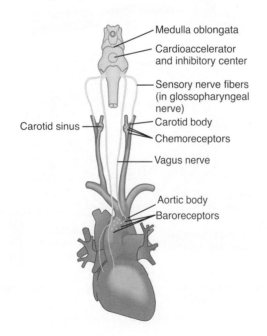

Medulla oblongata

Cardioaccelerator and inhibitory center

Sensory nerve fibers (in glossopharyngeal nerve)

Carotid body

Chemoreceptors

Carotid sinus

Vagus nerve

Aortic body

Baroreceptors

Figure 27-2 Chemoreceptors and baroreceptors.

During normal aerobic metabolism, the fetus produces carbonic acid (H_2CO_3), which dissociates into water and carbon dioxide (CO_2). Both CO_2 and water diffuse across the placenta very quickly. When oxygen is not available for aerobic metabolism, anaerobic metabolism occurs. Anaerobic metabolism utilizes glucose and glycogen to produce energy, with the final dissociation product being lactic acid ($C_3H_6O_3$). Unlike water and CO_2, lactic acid does not cross the placenta quickly. When anaerobic metabolism persists, the accumulating lactic acid will overcome the buffering capacity within the fetal circulation and lower the pH so that a state of metabolic acidosis exists.

Mechanism of Asphyxia

Asphyxia is a state of extreme deficiency of oxygen and excess in the concentration of carbon dioxide. Severe asphyxia results in metabolic acidosis and ultimately organ failure.[21] The term "perinatal asphyxia" refers to asphyxia that is the result of compromised fetal gas exchange. Because asphyxia is a continuum that cannot be directly measured, and because the individual response to asphyxia varies, there is no clear threshold at which one can say metabolic acidosis will have long-term adverse effects in the fetus/newborn. Thus the term asphyxia should not be used clinically or during written documentation when describing newborn behavior.

When metabolic and respiratory acidosis become severe, normal metabolic processes begin to fail. Neurons have a high metabolic rate and the brain does not store glucose, so the fetal brain is particularly vulnerable to asphyxial damage. In addition, oxygen deficiency in brain tissue results in both acidemia and ischemia because the cardiovascular adaptive mechanisms that preserve cerebral perfusion become overwhelmed when the arterial O_2 falls below a critical threshold. Autoregulation of cerebral blood flow fails, such that cerebral perfusion becomes pressure dependent and then, in the presence of hypotension, the brain becomes ischemic.[22] Cellular metabolism is quickly compromised (**Figure 27-3**). Thus the final pathway to brain injury is termed "hypoxic-ischemic."

Hypoxic Ischemic Encephalopathy

Hypoxic ischemic encephalopathy (HIE) is the diagnostic term that describes the type of lesion seen in the brains of newborns who survive a severe asphyxial insult. Hypoxic ischemic encephalopathy occurs in approximately 1.5 per 1000 term births.[23] Approximately 66% of newborns with severe HIE

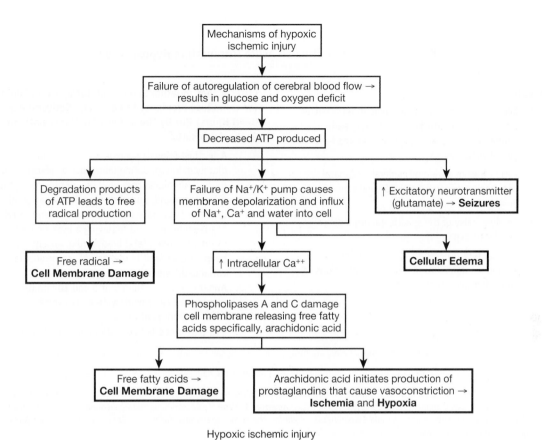

Hypoxic ischemic injury

Figure 27-3 Mechanism of hypoxic-ischemic encephalopathy.
Source: King TL, Parer JT. Physiology of fetal heart rate and asphyxia. *J Perinat Neonat Nurs.* 2000;14:19-40. Used with permission.

will die or have long-term sequelae. Conversely, most infants with mild HIE have no adverse effects.[24]

The region of the brain that is damaged depends on the gestational age of the fetus, as hypoxic-ischemic injury typically occurs in border zones between the ends of major cerebral vessels. Spastic quadriplegia cerebral palsy may result from hypoxic ischemic injury in term infants because the regions of the brain that are most likely to suffer insult at that point of gestation are those involved in motor cordination.[25,26]

The relationship between hypoxic-ischemic injury secondary to oxygen deprivation during labor and subsequent development of cerebral palsy is complex. There are multiple etiologies of cerebral palsy, yet many of the symptoms exhibited in the newborn are part of a common pathway that was originally started by any one of several different pathologic events. For example, placental lesions, intrauterine infection, and intrauterine stroke are all potential inciting events that result in fetal brain damage and subsequent cerebral palsy.

Neonatal Encephalopathy

Neonatal encephalopathy is the term for the clinically defined syndrome of disturbed neurologic function in the earliest days of life in an infant born at more than 35 weeks' gestation. Neonatal encephalopathy manifests as subnormal level of consciousness or seizures, often associated with difficulty initiating and maintaining respiration and depression of tone and reflexes. Hypoxic-ischemic injury is a subset of neonatal encephalopathy, but because these symptoms can be secondary to many different pathologic events, it is recommended that the term(s) *hypoxic-ischemic injury* or *hypoxic-ischemic encephalopathy* not be used unless very specific criteria are met. The criteria necessary to assign the etiology of cerebral palsy to intrapartum asphyxia are listed in **Box 27-1**. These criteria are currently being modified by the American

---

BOX 27-1 Criteria to Define an Acute Intrapartum Hypoxic Event

Essential Criteria[a]

1. Evidence of a metabolic acidosis in intrapartum fetal, umbilical arterial cord, or very early neonatal blood samples. pH < 7.00 and base deficit ≥ 12 mMol/L.

2. Early onset of severe or moderate neonatal encephalopathy in infants 35 weeks or more gestational age.

3. Cerebral palsy of the spastic quadriplegic or dyskinetic type.

4. Exclusion of other identifiable etiologies such as trauma, coagulation disorders, infectious conditions, or genetic disorders.

Criteria That Together Suggest an Intrapartum Timing (Within Close Proximity to Labor and Delivery; e.g., 0–48 Hours) But by Themselves Are Nonspecific to Asphyxial Insults[b]

1. A sentinel (signal) hypoxic event occurring immediately before or during labor such as placental abruption, umbilical cord prolapse, or uterine rupture.

2. A sudden, rapid, and sustained deterioration of the fetal heart rate pattern usually when the FHR has been normal and following a hypoxic sentinel event: sustained fetal bradycardia, absent fetal heart rate variability, persistent (recurrent) late or variable decelerations.

3. Apgar scores less than 5 at 5 and 10 minutes.

4. Early evidence of multisystem involvement, within 72 hours of birth.

5. MRI performed between 24 hours and 96 hours.

[a]All three of the essential criteria are necessary before an intrapartum hypoxia can be considered the etiology of the cerebral palsy.

[b]If evidence for some of the criteria is missing or contradictory, the timing of the neuropathology becomes increasingly in doubt.

Sources: Adapted from MacLennan A. A template for defining a causal relation between acute intrapartum events and cerebral palsy: international consensus statement. *BMJ.* 1999;319:1054-1059; American College of Obstetricians and Gynecologists, American Academy of Pediatrics. *Neonatal Encephalopathy and Cerebral Palsy: Defining the Pathogenesis and Pathophysiology.* Washington, DC: American College of Obstetricians and Gynecologists; January 2003.

College of Obstetricans and Gynecologists based on recent research regarding the etiology and outcomes of neonatal encephalopathy.[26,27]

Fetal Assessment During Labor

Fetal well-being can be assessed during labor via intermittent auscultation of the FHR as well as continuous or intermittent EFM. Fetal scalp stimulation can be used as an adjunctive test to determine if the fetal pH is in the normal range.

Intermittent Auscultation

Auscultation of the fetal heart rate may be performed with a fetoscope, a Doppler device, or even the external ultrasound transducer of the electronic fetal monitor. The DeLee-Hillis and the Allen fetoscopes utilize bone conduction in the listener's cranium to amplify the sounds of the FHR. Because fetoscopes that do not use Doppler all require use of bone conduction and close proximity of the examiner's head to the pregnant abdomen, maternal position and activity can limit assessment of the FHR with a fetoscope.

Doppler ultrasound technology projects an ultrasound wave into the uterus. This wave is reflected off the moving fetal ventricle, and the waveform changes as it is reflected back to the Doppler transducer. The transducer translates the heart movement of each heartbeat and creates an electronically created sound that can be counted or displayed digitally. The Doppler can detect the fetal heart movement when the woman is in most positions and some models can be safely used underwater, allowing for their use during hydrotherapy in labor and birth. Auditory counting of the fetal heart rate by Doppler technology and by fetoscope has been demonstrated to be equivalent in nonlaboring women.[28,29]

Use of the EFM Doppler transducer for intermittent documentation is somewhat controversial. Advocates find use of the EFM ultrasound transducer to be convenient, and a hard copy can be made of the tracing. Caution is warranted, however: When a FHR tracing is obtained, data including the FHR variability and possible accelerations or decelerations are evident and must be interpreted according to continuous EFM guidelines. There is no standard in this regard; each institution and individual clinician must consider the pros and cons. The technique for performing intermittent auscultation is presented in **Appendix 27A**. Benefits and limitations of intermittent auscultation are presented in **Table 27-3**.

Electronic Fetal Heart Rate Monitoring

The electronic fetal monitor displays the fetal heart rate pattern and the uterine contraction pattern. It can be used with either external or internal devices. The fetal monitor record has both upper and lower display areas. The upper portion displays the fetal heart rate pattern with increments of 10 bpm graphed on the vertical axis. The lower portion displays the uterine contractions with gradations for 0 to 100 Montevideo units on the vertical axis. The horizontal is divided into 10-second and 1-minute segments. Therefore, the FHR pattern, the contraction pattern, and the timing and relationship between the two are displayed on the device.

External Monitoring

For external fetal heart rate monitoring, a Doppler transducer is secured to the maternal abdomen, over the area of the fetal heart, by an elastic strap. The monitor counts the interval between fetal heartbeats and calculates a per-minute rate. It then plots this rate on the graph paper that scrolls continuously so that the individual plot points merge into a jagged line. The line is jagged because the time interval between each beat typically varies between 6 and 25 bpm. The recorded jagged line is termed fetal heart rate variability. Because the vagus nerve is responsive to input from the central nervous system and the frequent change in timing between beats occurs secondary to vagus input, the variability seen on EFM is the primary reflection of central nervous system function and well-being.

More specifically, the Doppler technology records a number of points on the changed wavelength that occurs during each fetal heartbeat and constructs a replica from these points. This technique, which is called autocorrelation, has improved over the last decade such that the FHR recorded using an external Doppler transducer now closely approximates the exact FHR recorded on an EKG. Early fetal monitors did not have the autocorrelation function and often displayed too much interference to allow accurate interpretation of baseline variability. Today external fetal monitoring can be used with the same reliability as internal monitoring for assessment of all FHR characteristics.

External fetal monitoring is appropriate for the majority of women who choose to have continuous EFM during labor. In most situations, with careful placement of the abdominal transducer and tocodynamometer (toco), the FHR and contractions will be visually displayed adequately for interpretation. The equipment and its electrical cords limit the distance a woman can move about unless a telemetry unit is available. The telemetry units currently in use allow women to walk long distances, shower, or be in a tub. However, maternal movement can cause interference in the signal, occasionally obscuring or making the data being collected unreadable.

Internal Fetal Heart Rate Monitoring

Internal monitoring is used when the fetal heart rate or the contractions need to be monitored continuously and an adequate tracing is not available via external monitoring. This can occur for example when a woman with a high BMI is in labor. Internal

Table 27-3	Benefits and Limitations of Intermittent Auscultation	
Benefits	**Limitations**
Neonatal outcomes are comparable to those with EFM.	The use of a fetoscope may limit the ability to hear the FHR (e.g., in cases of maternal obesity or increased amniotic fluid).
Cesarean section rates are lower.	
The technique is noninvasive.	FHR variability cannot be detected.
The woman's freedom of movement is not impaired.	The type of FHR decelerations cannot be determined with accuracy (e.g., late vs variable deceleration)
The FHR can be assessed if the woman is immersed in water.	There is no permanent visual record of the data.
The equipment is less costly than EFM equipment and is more durable.	There is a potential need to increase or to realign staff to meet the 1:1 nurse-to-woman ratio that is recommended based on RCTs that compare auscultation and EFM.
Hands-on, individualized care must be provided.	Some women may feel auscultation is more intrusive.

monitoring requires ruptured membranes. A fetal scalp electrode (FSE) is placed a few millimeters into the fetal scalp. The wires extending from the electrode are entrapped in an electronic transmission device that is secured to the woman's thigh with an elastic or Velcro belt. The fetal scalp electrode transmits the fetal electrocardiogram to the monitor, which displays a digital signal of the FHR as well as a continuous graph of the heart rate. The procedure for placing an FSE is described in **Appendix 27B**.

Uterine Activity Monitoring

Uterine contractions can be monitored via maternal perception, manual palpation, external tocodynamometer attached to an electronic fetal monitor, or internal placement of an intrauterine pressure catheter (IUPC).

Although there is significant variability between individuals, maternal perception of a painful contraction usually occurs when the intrauterine pressure reaches a minimum of 15 mm Hg.[30] This pressure is the amount required to distend the lower uterine segment and create pressure on the cervix. A uterine contraction is first detectable via manual palpation when the intrauterine pressure exceeds 10 mm Hg.[30]

A uterine pressure tocodynamometer (toco) is placed on the maternal fundus and secured with a belt that goes around the woman's abdomen. The toco records changes in pressure that occur when the fundus tightens during a contraction. Although this device records contraction duration and frequency, it does not record intensity accurately. In fact, tightening the monitor straps or changing the position of the toco can show very different apparent intensity of contractions.

Internal uterine monitoring is accomplished by placing an intrauterine pressure catheter through the cervix and into the uterine cavity. The IUPC has the advantage of providing specific information about the resting tone of the uterus, the actual pressure generated by the contractions, and accurate timing of the onset, peak, and completion of the contraction. If amnioinfusion is needed, it will be done through the same catheter as the IUPC. However, IUPCs increase the risk of infection if left in place an extended period of time and internal monitoring requires that the woman is tethered to a bed.

If the progress of labor is slower than expected, an IUPC may be used to determine a quantitative measure of uterine contraction intensity in Montevideo units, a concept first introduced by Caldeyro-Barcia in 1957.[30,31] The Montevideo unit is calculated by adding together the peak pressures of all contractions that occur in a 10-minute window. Montevideo units of approximately 200 when subtracting the baseline tone, or 240 when the baseline tone is included, are considered adequate for labor that progresses normally.

Benefits and limitations of EFM are presented in **Table 27-4**.

Table 27-4	Benefits and Limitations of EFM	
Benefits	**Limitations**
Recorded data are provided for collaborative decision making and education.	The rate of cesarean sections is increased.
Continuous recording is perceived by nursing administrators to decrease the need for 1:1 bedside nursing care.	Interrater reliability is poor.
	EFM prevents normal movement and ambulation during labor unless telemetry units are available.
EFM is an excellent predictor of fetal well-being.	EFM may create a false sense of security that EFM will detect all fetal health problems.
The recorded strip demonstrates FHR and contractions simultaneously.	
	There is no consensus on guidelines for interpretation of Category II FHR patterns.
Some women are reassured with the use of high-technological devices.	There is no agreement regarding need for or timing of interventions.
EFM may offer assistance with coaching by being able to identify the onset of contractions before the woman perceives them.	There are increased rates of operative vaginal delivery (forceps and vacuum assist).
	EFM uses equipment that is expensive to purchase and maintain.
	There is a high false-positive rate for suspected fetal compromise.

Source: Adapted from Schmidt JV. History and development of fetal heart rate assessment: a composite. *JOGNN*. 2000;29(3):295-305.

Fetal Heart Rate Patterns

The characteristics of the fetal heart rate are classified as baseline, periodic, or episodic.[14] The baseline features, which include the heart rate, variability, and accelerations, are assessed between uterine contractions. Periodic changes occur in association with uterine contractions. Episodic changes are not clearly associated with uterine contractions.

Baseline Fetal Heart Rate

Fetal tachycardia alone is not usually associated with poor outcomes in the term fetus. Tachycardia is common in the fetus of less than 28 weeks' gestation because parasympathetic (vagal) tone does not predominate until the third trimester. Thus heart rates of 140 to 160 bpm often comprise normal baseline rates in a preterm fetus.

The most common cause of sustained tachycardia in a term fetus is maternal and/or fetal infection. Other causes include administration of beta-mimetic drugs or ephedrine given to correct maternal hypotension. More rarely, fetal tachycardia occurs secondary to fetal anemia (Rh isoimmunization), acute fetal blood loss (placental abruption), an abnormal fetal conduction system (fetal arrhythmia), or poorly controlled maternal hyperthyroidism.

Short periods of tachycardia are a normal compensatory response to transient hypoxemia. Sustained tachycardia, especially if accompanied by minimal variability and recurrent decelerations, may indicate that the fetal ability to compensate for repeated hypoxia is limited.[32] This pattern can appear after recurrent decelerations are present for some period of time but before a terminal bradycardia becomes evident and may be part of a pattern evolution when increasing acidemia is developing.

Both asphyxial and non-asphyxial causes of fetal bradycardia are possible. Non-asphyxial causes include fetal heart block and maternal hypothermia. A mild bradycardia in the 100 bpm to 120 bpm range can be idiopathic and is most likely to be seen in postmature gestations. More commonly, bradycardia occurs during rapid descent or at the end of the second stage of labor when fetal head compression causes increased intracranial pressure, which then initiates a vagal response and bradycardia. In such a case, the fetus will maintain cerebral oxygenation at a FHR higher than 80 bpm and variability will be retained.

Fetal bradycardia also can occur after administration of intrathecal opioids or local anesthetics for epidural analgesia. This etiology is usually attributed to maternal hypotension that occurs secondary to the sympathetic block, which causes a subsequent decrease in uteroplacental blood flow. These transient bradycardias or prolonged decelerations usually maintain normal FHR variability and are rarely associated with adverse outcomes.

Asphyxial causes of bradycardia include acute emergency events such as prolapsed cord, placental abruption, uterine rupture, or vasa previa. A FHR of less than 60 bpm is an obstetric emergency. At this heart rate, the fetus is unable to increase stroke volume to sustain adequate circulation through the heart and supply the coronary arteries.

Fetal bradycardia that is accompanied by moderate variability is not associated with fetal acidemia. The presence of moderate variability during an end-stage bradycardia can reassure the midwife that no intervention is required.[33]

When an acute bradycardia occurs, its depth, its duration, and the presence or absence of variability are the key factors associated with subsequent neonatal morbidity. An acute drop in FHR to less than 60 bpm usually results in rapid fetal asphyxial decompensation and is managed as an obstetric emergency. The goal is to deliver the newborn before a hypoxic-ischemic injury occurs.

Fetal Heart Rate Variability

The presence of moderate FHR variability signifies an intact cerebral cortex, midbrain, vagus nerve, and cardiac conduction system. Moderate variability is the single best indication that the fetus does not have cerebral tissue hypoxia or ischemia.[33,34] Approximately 98% of all fetuses with moderate variability will not have clinically significant acidemia at the time the variability is observed, even if recurrent fetal heart rate decelerations are present (**Figure 27-4**).[35,15]

Minimal variability should be interpreted based on the presence or absence of accelerations and/or recurrent decelerations. When variability is minimal, without the presence of decelerations, it is rarely caused by asphyxia.[12] Fetal sleep cycles are associated with uncomplicated minimal variability. These periods of minimal variability typically last 20 to 40 minutes but can persist for as long as 75 to 80 minutes.[35] Administration of opiates (e.g., morphine, butorphanol, fentanyl), promethazine (Phenergan), or beta-adrenergic agents such as terbutaline (Brethine) will also decrease the FHR variability.

Absent variability without decelerations can be idiopathic and not consistently associated with acidemia. Minimal or absent variability in the presence of recurrent late or variable decelerations is one of the FHR patterns most consistently associated with fetal acidemia and requires urgent assessment and intervention.[15,33,36] The evolution of moderate to

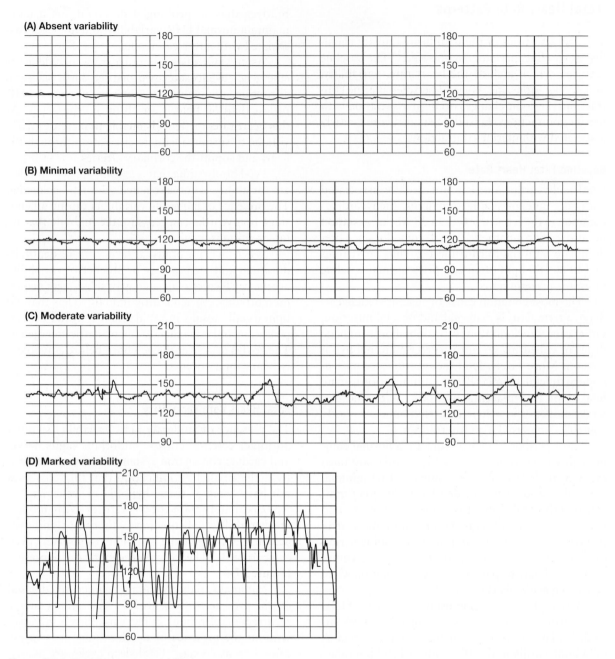

Figure 27-4 Fetal heart rate variability.

minimal to absent variability in the presence of recurrent decelerations is one classic pattern evolution that reflects developing fetal acidemia.[16,37]

Marked variability is relatively rare. It is thought to be a fetal response to a short period of hypoxia. Marked variability is not associated with adverse newborn outcomes.

Accelerations

Accelerations are transient increases of the fetal heart rate above the baseline (**Figure 27-5**). They are a reassuring indicator of fetal well-being in that they are associated with a normal pH at the time the acceleration occurs. Accelerations are often associated with fetal movement. Fetal scalp stimulation and acoustic stimulation can be used to induce an acceleration.

Fetal Heart Rate Decelerations

Early Decelerations

The mechanism underlying early decelerations has not been conclusively determined. These

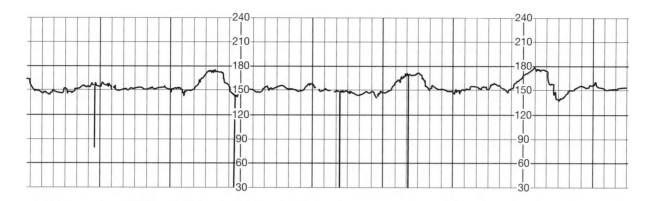

Figure 27-5 Accelerations of the fetal heart rate.

decelerations appear in active labor and are associated with moderate variability. One theory suggests that early decelerations are caused by head compression. Early decelerations are benign and do not require intervention, although it is important to carefully differentiate between early and late decelerations (**Figure 27-6**).

Late Decelerations

Late decelerations are a fetal response to transient decreases in oxygen tension. This mechanism starts with a uterine contraction that causes a decrease in uteroplacental perfusion, which is followed by lower oxygen levels in the fetal circulation. The hypoxemia is detected by chemoreceptors in the fetal carotid artery, carotid sinus, and aortic arch. Chemoreceptor

activation signals a vagally mediated drop in fetal heart rate. The nadir of the fetal bradycardia is "late" relative to the peak of the uterine contraction because the physiologic pathway that results in chemoreceptor stimulation takes time. The relatively deoxygenated blood must first traverse the umbilical vein before reaching the chemoreceptors (**Figure 27-7**).

Uteroplacental insufficiency is often the precursor of late decelerations in labor. Causes of chronic uteroplacental insufficiency include fetal growth restriction, maternal hypertensive disorders, diabetes, hyperthyroidism, autoimmune disorders such as lupus, and abnormal placentation. All of these disorders are associated with narrowed spiral arteries, small placentas, and/or placental infarcts that decrease the placental area available for transfer of oxygen and nutrients. Postmaturity is also associated with uteroplacental insufficiency, as the placenta no longer grows and therefore loses the ability to meet the needs of the postmature still growing fetus. Acute uteroplacental insufficiency can arise secondary to tachysystole or maternal hypotension caused by supine positioning, induction of conduction anesthesia, or (rarely) septic shock. Finally, fetal anemia secondary to fetal–maternal hemorrhage, Rh sensitization, or nonimmune hydrops will effectively lower the oxygen-carrying capacity of the fetus so that the transient decreases in oxygen present in the intervillous spaces associated with uterine contractions result in significant drops in fetal oxygen tension.

Late decelerations in the presence of moderate variability can be viewed as a physiologic response to transient hypoxemia. These decelerations do not indicate the presence of acidemia. Conversely, recurrent late decelerations in the presence of absent variability is classified as Category III, one of the FHR patterns most commonly associated with fetal acidemia.[15,33] Although recurrent late decelerations with minimal variability are classified as Category

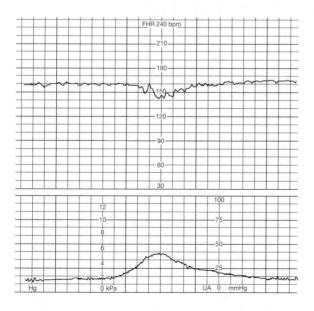

Figure 27-6 Early decelerations.

II, the ability to discriminate between minimal and absent variability can be difficult. In addition, the early studies that noted an association between decreased variability with late decelerations and subsequent newborn acidemia did not distinguish between minimal and absent variability. Therefore, in clinical practice, recurrent late decelerations with minimal variability are often part of a pattern evolution that suggests the fetus may be acidemic or at significant risk for acidemia.

Late decelerations can be classified as mild (equal to or less than a 15-bpm drop from baseline

(A) Late deceleration with moderate variability

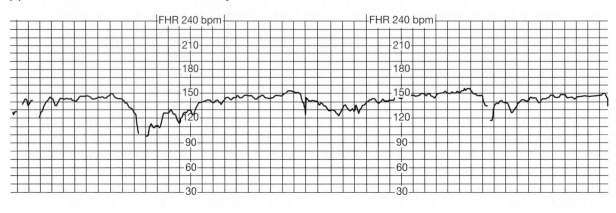

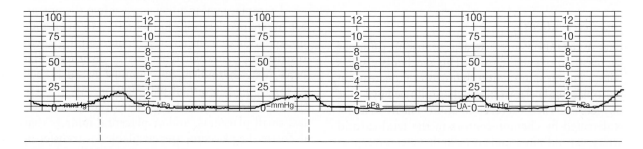

(B) Late deceleration with absent variability

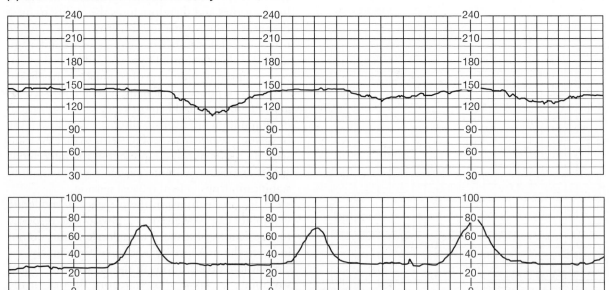

Figure 27-7 Late decelerations.

to nadir), moderate (more than a 15-bpm drop but less than a 45-bpm drop from baseline to nadir), or severe (equal to or more than a 45-bpm drop from baseline to nadir). Although these classifications are not part of the NICHD terminology, there is good evidence that late decelerations become progressively deeper as fetal acidemia worsens.[15]

Variable Decelerations

Variable decelerations occur secondary to an interruption in umbilical blood flow. A variety of causes of umbilical cord compression have been postulated. In vertex presentations, these include cord occlusion secondary to the cord around the neck or body, true knots in the cord, frank and occult prolapse of the cord, and compression due to decreased amniotic fluid that cushions the cord. Variable decelerations are common in the second stage of labor. These variable decelerations are presumed to be secondary to head compression and the increased intracranial pressure then has a direct effect on the vagus nerve. Variable decelerations can be either episodic and occur at random times or periodic, occurring with each uterine contraction.

Variable decelerations are the most common variant FHR pattern, seen in approximately 45% to 75% of all labors.[38,39] The association between variable decelerations and fetal acidemia depends on the frequency, depth, duration and associated baseline fetal heart rate variability. Variable decelerations that return to baseline in less than 60 seconds with concomitant normal baseline and moderate variability are not associated with fetal acidemia. Recurrent variable decelerations with minimal or absent variability, similar to recurrent late decelerations with minimal or absent variability, are associated with fetal acidemia and require urgent evaluation (**Figure 27-8**).

Categorizing variable decelerations as mild, moderate, or severe has not proved to be clinically useful. Variables have been categorized as typical or atypical based on different shapes. For example, variable decelerations often have a short increase in FHR above the baseline that precedes or is part of the final variable complex. These short increases are called shoulders and overshoot. Several authors have tried to determine which characteristics of variable decelerations are most likely to be associated with acidemia, aside from the companion baseline variability.[34,40,41] Variable deceleration characteristics that increase the risk for acidemia include the following:

1. Although there is no clear time frame, variable decelerations that occur more frequently than every 5 minutes appear to increase the risk for acidemia, whereas a deceleration interval of more than 5 minutes is sufficient for normalization of acid–base balance.[32]

2. The nadir is more than 60 bpm below the baseline rate.

3. The nadir reaches 60 bpm.

4. Deceleration lasts longer than 60 seconds.

5. Two or more of the "sixties rule" characteristics detailed above appear to be more prognostic than just one.

A slow return to baseline and loss of variability within the deceleration may increase the risk of acidemia, although these characteristics have not been studied in sufficient detail to draw definitive conclusions. The presence of shoulders or overshoot and the shape of the deceleration do not appear to have a correlation with acidemia per se.[41]

Prolonged Decelerations

Prolonged decelerations have multiple causes. Known precipitating factors include umbilical cord compression; maternal hypotension related to supine positioning, epidural, or spinal anesthesia; paracervical anesthesia (which can cause decelerations by direct fetal uptake of local anesthetic, maternal hypotension, or uterine hypertonus); uterine tachysystole; maternal hypoxia associated with seizures or acute respiratory depression; and rapid descent of the fetal head (**Figure 27-9**).

Management of prolonged decelerations depends on the putative etiology, length of deceleration, baseline at nadir, and baseline variability. It is common for the fetus to recover with a period of tachycardia, decreased variability, or occasional late decelerations for a short time following a prolonged deceleration. If the precipitating cause is alleviated, the FHR generally returns to the previous baseline. Intermittent prolonged decelerations are not associated with an increased risk for fetal acidemia in the presence of moderate variability.

Sinusoidal Pattern

A sinusoidal pattern is characterized by an undulating, recurrent uniform fetal heart rate equally distributed 5 to 15 bpm above and below the baseline (**Figure 27-10**). The undulation occurs at a rate of 2 to 6 cycles per minute and is identified by an absence of short-term variability. True sinusoidal patterns are extremely rare.

The sinusoidal fetal heart rate pattern is seen when the fetus is experiencing clinically significant

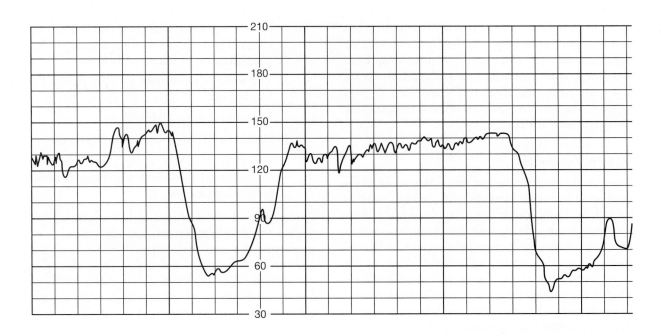

12/07   3 cm/min

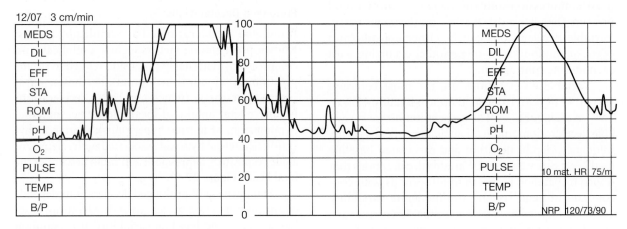

Figure 27-8 Variable decelerations.

anemia, such as Rh isoimmunization, vasa previa, uterine rupture, or placental abruption. It may also appear shortly before death in the severely asphyxiated fetus. A sinusoidal heart rate pattern is always an ominous fetal heart rate pattern, and immediate intervention is indicated. The midwife should notify the consulting physician immediately and prepare the woman for emergency cesarean section. The neonatal team should be notified to prepare for a potentially anemic and hypovolemic newborn.

Pseudo-sinusoidal Fetal Heart Rate Pattern

A pseudo-sinusoidal FHR pattern is somewhat similar to the real sinusoidal pattern with three important exceptions: Variability is retained, there are more than 2 to 6 cycles per minute, and this pattern

is not associated with fetal acidemia. The pseudo-sinusoidal pattern is not an NICHD recognized FHR pattern because it is most often the result of opioid administration rather than being an intrinsic FHR characteristic. This clinically insignificant pattern is intermittent and bracketed by periods of moderate variability.

Wandering Baseline

The wandering baseline is not an official NICHD FHR term, but it continues to be used in clinical practice and, therefore, deserves mention. The wandering baseline is a very late development in the progression of fetal deterioration. It is often within the normal baseline parameters of 120 to 160 bpm and is identifiable by absent variability. This pattern is

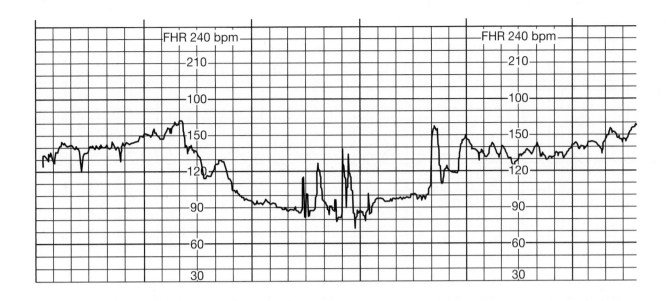

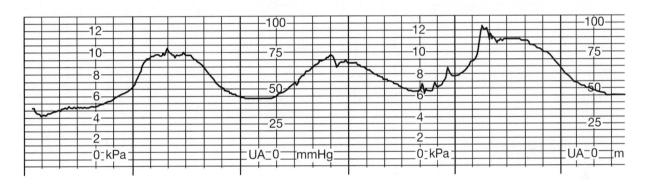

Figure 27-9 Prolonged decelerations.

an ominous indicator of fetal acidemia and requires immediate notification of a consulting physician and preparation for emergency operative birth if vaginal birth is not imminent. Pediatric providers should be present at the birth. The key characteristic is the absence of variability more than the fact that the baseline changes over the course of several minutes.

Fetal Arrhythmias

Fetal arrhythmias occur among approximately 1% to 3% of fetuses at term.[42] Approximately 90% of fetal arrhythmias are transient and benign in nature. A consulting physician should evaluate any fetus with an arrhythmia, and a plan should be made for ongoing collaboration as long as the arrhythmia is present. Arrhythmias can be heard on audible Doppler devices and can be seen on FHR tracings, but cannot be accurately diagnosed via EFM (**Figure 27-11**). Thus pediatric attendance at birth may be

recommended depending on the rate and persistence of the arrhythmia.

Pattern Evolution

Clinically significant metabolic acidosis can be the result of either frequent, unremitting hypoxic insults or an acute bradycardia. In a term healthy fetus, it takes approximately 1 hour to develop significant acidemia once a pattern of recurrent late or variable decelerations and diminishing variability begins.[33] Midwives, nurses, and physicians interpreting EFM should recognize the typical pattern evolution that occurs as acidemia is accumulating as well as the specific Category III FHR patterns that herald a significant risk for fetal acidemia (**Figure 27-12**).

Fetal Heart Rate Patterns and Uterine Activity

The 2008 NICHD expert panel on FHR monitoring defined tachysystole as more than 5 contractions

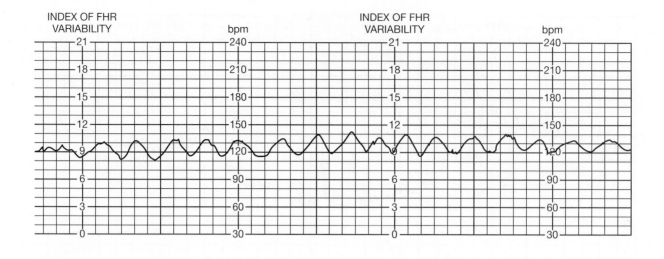

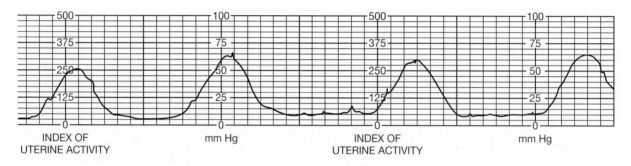

Figure 27-10 Sinusoidal pattern.

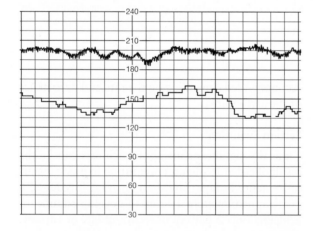

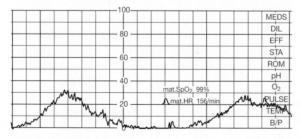

Figure 27-11 Fetal arrhythmia.

within a 10-minute window.[15] Tachysystole is more likely among women whose labors are induced or augmented with oxytocin. Because 23% of women in the United States have their labors induced, and the incidence of tachysystole in induced labors is approximately 40%, the FHR response to tachysystole is an important clinical consideration.[43,44] The most common FHR response to brief episodes of tachysystole is a prolonged deceleration.

Studies of fetal oxygenation have found that an interval of approximately 60 seconds between contractions is associated with stable fetal cerebral oxygenation, whereas intervals between contractions that are less than 60 seconds are associated with lower umbilical artery pH levels.[30,45,46] Simpson et al. measured fetal oxygenation ($FSpO_2$) via pulse oximetry among women who were being induced at term.[45] These researchers found that when fewer than 5 contractions occurred in a 10-minute window, fetal saturation was unaffected; when 5 or more contractions occurred in a 10-minute window, fetal $FSpO_2$ dropped 20% in 30 minutes; and when more than 6 contractions occurred in 10 minutes, fetal $FSpO_2$ dropped 29% in 30 minutes. A suggested

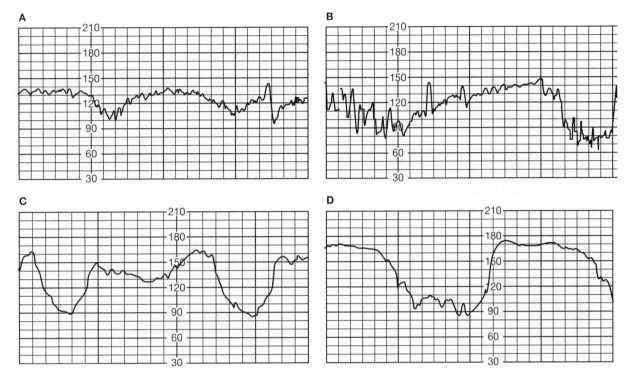

Figure 27-12 Fetal heart rate pattern evolution from normal to fetal acidemia.

management plan for tachysystole is presented in Box 27-2.[46,47]

Relationship Between Fetal Heart Rate Patterns and Newborn Outcomes

Several different dependent variables have been used in studies linking fetal heart rate patterns to neonatal outcomes, including Apgar scores, newborn seizures, umbilical cord blood gases, and—more recently—magnetic resonance imaging (MRI) findings in newborns with signs of neonatal encephalopathy.

Apgar Scores

The Apgar score has been used for many years as a surrogate for the diagnosis of perinatal asphyxia and predication of neurologic outcome. However, Apgar scores were created to assess the adaptation of the infant to extrauterine life and not as a measure of pre-birth acidemia. This may seem like a trivial distinction but, in fact, it is an important one. While a 5-minute score of 7 or higher virtually negates the possibility of fetal acidemia prior to birth, the converse is not true. Apgar scores can be markedly affected by drugs given prior to birth, infant resuscitation techniques, gestational age, and infection—all of which will result in a lower score.[48] Likewise, Apgar scores do not reliably predict newborn outcomes except in the extreme range of or less than 5 at 5 minutes. Therefore another index is needed that accurately reflects fetal status prior to birth and predicts newborn outcomes. Umbilical cord blood gases meet both requirements.

Umbilical Cord Blood Gases

The biochemical indicator of acidemia is pH. Umbilical artery cord blood gases reveal the presence or absence of respiratory acidosis, metabolic acidosis, or a mixed acidosis. pH is an indication of the degree of acidemia. The PCO_2 value is a reflection of the respiratory component, and the base deficit (or base excess if negative numbers are used) indicates the severity of metabolic acidosis. The base deficit is a calculation of how much buffer has been lost as lactic acid accumulates in the fetal circulation and tissue (**Table 27-5**).[49] Umbilical artery cord pH values in the normal range exclude intrapartum development of acidemia as the etiology of neonatal encephalopathy in a depressed or compromised newborn.[50]

Umbilical cord blood gases are obtained by collecting a sample of umbilical arterial blood and then a sample of umbilical venous blood in a heparinized syringe, from a section of umbilical cord that has been clamped at both ends. The fetal vessels on the surface of the placenta may be used if a length of

BOX 27-2 Suggested Clinical Protocol for Oxytocin-Induced Uterine Tachysystole

Category I FHR Tracing (Normal)

1. Reposition the woman to her left or right side.
2. Give an intravenous fluid bolus of lactated Ringer's solution.
3. Decrease the oxytocin rate by at least half.
4. If tachysystole has not resolved after 10 minutes, discontinue the oxytocin until contractions slow to fewer than five in 10 minutes.

Category II FHR Tracing (Indeterminate)

1. Reposition the woman to her left or right side.
2. Give an intravenous fluid bolus of lactated Ringer's solution.
3. Turn the oxytocin infusion down by at least half or discontinue the oxytocin.
4. If the initial interventions do not resolve the abnormal FHR tracing, administer oxygen at 10 L/min via nonrebreather face mask until the FHR improves.
5. If no response, consider one dose of terbutaline (Brethine) 0.25 mg subcutaneously.
6. Notify the consulting physician.

Category III FHR Tracing (Abnormal)

1. Discontinue oxytocin.
2. Administer terbutaline (Brethine) 0.25 mg subcutaneously.
3. Perform intrauterine resuscitation measures and prepare for delivery if the FHR pattern does not quickly revert to a Category II or Category I pattern.

Resuming Oxytocin After an Episode of Tachysystole

1. Ensure FHR is normal (Category I).
2. Ensure contraction frequency and duration are normal.
3. If less than 30 minutes: restart oxytocin at half the rate that caused the tachysystole.
4. If more than 30 minutes: restart oxytocin at 1 mU/min.
5. Titrate the infusion per the institution's guidelines.
6. Monitor contraction frequency and FHR closely.

Source: Adapted from Simpson KR. *Cervical Ripening, Induction and Augmentation of Labor* (AWHONN Practice Monograph; 3rd ed.). Washington, DC: Association of Women's Health, Obstetric, and Neonatal Nurses; 2009. Used by permission.

umbilical cord is not available. The umbilical artery (UA) reflects the status of the fetus, whereas the umbilical vein (UV) reflects the status of the intervillous space. Thus the values of import are those obtained from the umbilical artery. However both UA and UV samples are needed so the results can be correctly interpreted. When only one sample is obtained or when the samples have the same results, one cannot be certain if the values are from the UA or the UV.

Umbilical cord blood gases should be obtained if a concern arises that the fetus might have experienced clinically significant acidemia. Recommended

Table 27-5	Guidelines for Interpretation of Umbilical Arterial Cord Gases in Term Newborns			
Diagnosis	**pH**	**PCO$_2$ (mm Hg)**	**Bicarbonate (HCO$_3$)**	**Base Deficit[a] (mEq/L)**
Normal[b]	7.26 (± 0.07)	53 (± 10)	22.0 (± 3.6)	4 (± 3)
Respiratory acidemia	< 7.20	> 65	Normal	Normal
Metabolic acidemia[c]	< 7.20	Normal	≤ 17	≥ 15.9 ± 2.8
Mixed (metabolic–respiratory) acidemia[c]	Low	> 65	≤ 17	≥ 9.6 ± 2.5

[a]May be reported as base excess (negative values) or base deficit (positive value); however, the numeric value is the same.

[b]Data from term infants with an Apgar score ≥ 7 at 5 minutes.

[c]There is a clinical association with adverse neonatal outcomes when pH < 7 and base deficit > 12 meq/L.

Sources: Adapted from Helwig JT, Parer JT, Kilpatrick SJ, Laros RK Jr. Umbilical cord blood acid–base state: what is normal? *Am J Obstet Gynecol.* 1996:1807-1814; Gilstrap LC, Cunningham G. Umbilical cord blood acid–base analysis. In *Supplement #4: Williams' Obstetrics* (19th ed.). Raritan, NJ: Ortho Pharmaceutical; 1994:1-24.

indications for umbilical cord blood gas analysis are listed in **Box 27-3**.[51]

If the infant is vigorous, there is no need for cord blood sampling. Current evidence suggests that all newborns will benefit from delayed cord-clamping, but especially those who may need resuscitation. The effect of delayed cord-clamping on umbilical cord blood gases is a current area of study. It appears that delayed cord-clamping may result in a higher number of cords with an inadequate amount of blood for analysis. It is not yet clear how delayed cord-clamping affects the blood gas parameters. The few studies that have compared cord blood samples in healthy newborns following immediate versus delayed sampling have yielded conflicting results.[52,53] In those studies that have found delayed cord blood sampling results in lower values for the umbilical artery pH and base excess, the clinical implications of these changes has not been determined.

Interpretation of Umbilical Cord Blood Gases

The risk of neonatal morbidity is inversely related to pH, although the precise level of acidemia that is pathologic remains unknown. The result of fetal acidemia is an interaction between the magnitude of the stress and the responsiveness of the individual wherein there is a great deal of variability. In addition, the concept of a "continuum of causality" may not be correct in the fetal response to hypoxia. One might expect a small amount of asphyxia to cause a small amount of damage and larger amounts to have more adverse consequences. In reality, the fetal response to hypoxia is probably a threshold effect wherein damage becomes evident after a certain threshold has been exceeded.

Despite these caveats, pathologic acidemia is generally defined as a UA pH value of less than 7.0 and a base deficit of greater than 12 mEq/L.[54] The risk of complications increases in newborns with umbilical cord gas values that reflect a metabolic acidosis rather than a respiratory acidosis, so the base deficit is more important than the pH.[54]

Approximately 25% of infants with a pH less than 7.0 will experience neonatal morbidity or mortality. The majority will be vigorous and have normal Apgar scores.[23] Many infants with a low pH have a respiratory acidosis that is quickly corrected following an initial few breaths. Newborns with a base deficit higher than 12 mEq/L are more likely to have significant neonatal morbidity or mortality.[55]

Infants with a UA pH between 7.0 and 7.1 have an increased risk for short-term neonatal problems such as transient tachypnea, need for supplemental oxygen, or hypothermia. Newborns with pH values in this range rarely experience long-term complications. A clinically significant metabolic acidemia is highly unlikely in newborns with a UA pH higher than 7.1.

Umbilical cord blood gases have an important limitation. Measurements of the UA pH and base deficit provide information about the severity of the asphyxial insult but do not provide any information about the duration, whether the insult was continuous or intermittent, or the ability of the individual fetus to compensate for the insult.

Fetal Heart Rate Patterns and Risk for Newborn Acidemia

Clinically significant acidemia is a rare event, yet variant FHR patterns are quite common. Although Category III FHR patterns are the best predictors of fetal acidemia, their positive predictive value is low because many newborns who are vigorous at birth had one of these FHR patterns in the hour just prior to birth.

Nonetheless, FHR patterns correlate well with UA cord blood gases,[56] and UA cord blood gases are the best indicator of fetal acid–base balance that are currently available. In addition, the relationship between UA pH and base deficit and subsequent neonatal morbidity is known at the low and high ends of pH and base deficit values.

BOX 27-3 Suggested Indications for Umbilical Cord Blood Gas Analysis

- Cesarean section birth for fetal compromise
- Operative vaginal birth
- Preterm birth
- Fetal growth restriction
- Breech presentation
- Hypertension/preeclampsia
- Low 5-minute Apgar score
- Category III FHR pattern in last hour prior to birth
- Maternal thyroid disease
- Intrapartum fever
- Multiple gestations
- Diabetes
- Maternal thyroid disease
- Breech
- Meconium
- True knot in cord
- Substance abuse or no prenatal care

Interpretation and Management of Fetal Heart Rate Patterns

By now it should be clear that FHR variability is the key reflection of intact cerebral and cardiovascular function. However, FHR decelerations play a critical role in the development of acidemia. Decelerations must be present for an oxygen debt to start to accrue. Parer et al. reviewed the FHR research published between the 1960s and 2005 that evaluated the relationship between FHR patterns and newborn outcomes in term gestations. Four consistent themes were identified that explain the relationship between FHR patterns and neonatal outcomes:

1. Moderate variability is strongly predictive of neonatal vigor independent of the presence of variant patterns. Moderate FHR variability has a negative predictive value of 98% to 99% in a term fetus.

2. Minimal and absent variability in the presence of late or severe variable decelerations are the FHR patterns most likely to be associated with fetal acidemia, although the positive predictive value is only in the range of 10% to 30%.

3. There is a positive relationship between the depth and severity of decelerations or bradycardia and the degree of acidemia.

4. Newborn acidemia with decreasing FHR variability in combination with decelerations develops over a period of time approximating 1 hour in a previously healthy term fetus.

Three Categories for FHR Interpretation

The three-category system for FHR interpretation has some benefits and some challenges. Category I FHR tracings signify fetal well-being and, if no other risk factors are present, women with a Category I FHR pattern can be monitored with intermittent auscultation during labor. Category III is similarly clear-cut, as these FHR patterns are the ones most likely reflect significant fetal acidemia. A Category III FHR pattern requires urgent evaluation and preparations for emergent delivery.

Category II FHR patterns constitute a heterogenous group with differing risks for fetal acidemia and are an area of current research.[37,57,58] Management of these patterns should be based first on the FHR variability (and accelerations, if present) and

second on the presence or absence of recurrent decelerations. Management of specific patterns also needs to be based on institutional resources and guidelines. It is unlikely that one management paradigm for Category II FHR patterns will be applicable to all settings.

Finally, when a Category II FHR pattern is present, it must be considered in reference to other factors in the clinical scenario that can affect the fetal ability to tolerate repeated hypoxic events (**Box 27-4**).[59]

Fetal Scalp Stimulation, Vibroacoustic Stimulation, and Fetal Blood Sampling

Fetal scalp stimulation or vibroacoustic stimulation that elicits an acceleration provides reassurance that the fetal pH is higher than 7.2 at that time.[60] Vibroacoustic stimulation is performed using a handheld vibroacoustic stimulator (artificial larynx), which is applied to the maternal abdomen over the

---

BOX 27-4 Selected Clinical Considerations That Affect Management of FHR Patterns in Labor

1. Maternal complications that increase the risk for uteroplacental insufficiency (e.g., preeclampsia, hypertension, diabetes, lupus erythematosus)
2. Fetal factors that increase the risk for uteroplacental insufficiency (e.g., post dates, fetal growth retardation, decreased amniotic fluid index)
3. Presence or absence of tachycardia and/or decreased variability (Chorioamnionitis may increase vulnerability to brain damage that causes cerebral palsy.[59])
4. Whether or not attempts to correct the underlying problem are successful
5. Acid–base status of the fetus determined either through scalp or acoustic stimulation or via direct fetal scalp blood sampling
6. Presence or absence of meconium
7. Gestational age (with the preterm fetus having a lower tolerance for hypoxia than the term infant)
8. Anticipated time until birth
9. Availability of consultant physician, emergency operative staff, and facility

region of the fetal head, where it delivers a sound stimulus for 3 to 5 seconds. Approximately 50% of fetuses who do not respond with an acceleration will have a normal pH. Thus this test is useful only if the scalp stimulation, which is performed between contractions, results in a FHR acceleration. If the acceleration occurs, one can be assured that the fetus is not acidemic. Conversely, when an acceleration does not occur, the presence or absence of fetal acidemia has not been determined and management must be based on other clinical factors.

Although fetal blood sampling is rarely performed in the United States, it remains a core aspect of FHR management in other developed nations. Fetal blood sampling involves collection of blood from the fetal scalp in a capillary tube and laboratory assessment of the blood gases. Fetal blood sampling is technically challenging and requires a laboratory available to analyze the blood sample as soon as it is collected. Fetal blood sampling also has the problem that fetal scalp stimulation has—namely, a reassuring fetal pH does not predict how long the pH will stay reassuring. Therefore, management must be based on clinical factors and the FHR pattern.

Fetal oxygen saturation monitoring ($FSpO_2$), also known as fetal pulse oximetry, was introduced in the early 1990s. It was hoped that fetal pulse oximetry would be an adjunct to EFM and accurately identify the fetus at risk for developing acidemia when the FHR pattern could not be interpreted easily. It was intended to determine the actual level of fetal oxygenation so the clinician could make decisions regarding the continuation of labor versus the need to expedite the birth. Randomized trials of fetal pulse oximetry did not show that use of this technique lowered cesarean section rates for fetal compromise; thus, at this time, it is used for research purposes only.

In summary, fetal scalp stimulation or vibroacoustic stimulation is most useful in the setting of minimal variability and decelerations or minimal variability without decelerations. For example, if a woman has been given opioids, the FHR variability will be iatrogenically decreased. If this woman has a FHR pattern that includes late or variable decelerations, it may be of value to perform a scalp stimulation test.

Corrective Measures for Category II FHR Patterns

Some Category II FHR patterns will resolve with corrective measures. These corrective measures, which are also referred to as intrauterine resuscitation techniques, are summarized in **Table 27-6**.[61-64]

Labor Admission Test with Fetal Heart Rate Monitoring

An initial EFM assessment of the fetus is commonly used in hospital birth settings to assess fetal status at the time of admission. The underlying concept assumes that if the FHR pattern shows a reactive nonstress test (NST) or a negative oxytocin challenge test (OCT), no decelerations, and moderate variability, this can be interpreted as a reassuring sign of fetal well-being for the duration of the labor. However, the EFM assessment upon labor admission has not been shown to have adequate predictive value to warrant its use as an admission screening tool in women who are either high-risk or low-risk for developing fetal acidemia during labor.[65] An admission EFM tracing does appear to increase the risk of having continuous monitoring throughout labor (RR, 1.30; 95% CI, 1.14–1.48) and a trend toward a higher risk for cesarean section (RR, 1.20; 95% CI, 1.00–1.44). The admission test did not affect rates of fetal or neonatal deaths.

Preterm Fetus

The preterm fetus has different FHR characteristics when compared to a term fetus. The baseline heart rate is higher, averaging 155 bpm at 20 gestational weeks. FHR accelerations in association with fetal movement are a developmental process. By 28 gestational weeks, approximately 80% of fetuses will have accelerations adequate to meet the standard NST criteria. Prior to 32 weeks' gestation, the amplitude of an acceleration may be only 10 bpm with a duration of 10 seconds, which satisfies the requirement for NST reactivity in a preterm fetus. Baseline variability may be decreased in the very preterm fetus, but no standards have been established in this regard. Indications for prolonged FHR monitoring for a preterm fetus are often related to complications of pregnancy, such as preterm labor, preterm premature rupture of membranes (PPROM), or maternal hypertension. Therefore, fetal tachycardia (still defined as FHR greater than 160 bpm) may be related to use of tocolytics or maternal fever.

Most importantly, the preterm fetus is more vulnerable to cerebral injury from a hypoxic event. Pattern evolution that includes diminishing variability and deeper decelerations occurs more rapidly among such fetuses.

Table 27-6	Corrective Measures for Category II FHR Patterns
Corrective Measure	**Underlying Mechanism**
Variable Decelerations	
Position change	Alters relationship between umbilical cord and fetus to relieve cord compression.
Amnioinfusion	Increases the amount of amniotic fluid available in the uterus to protect the cord from compression.
Intravenous fluid bolus	Increases the amount of amniotic fluid available in the uterus to protect the cord from compression.
Open glottis pushing	Reduces the frequency and severity of variable decelerations.
Late Decelerations	
Lateral position	Increases uterine blood flow so intervillous space is adequately perfused.
Reduce uterine activity via discontinuing oxytocin, tocolysis	Decreases frequency of uterine contractions so that the fetus has more time to equilibrate acid–base balance between contractions.
Intravenous fluid bolus	Increases uterine blood flow and dilutes plasma oxytocin levels.
Oxygen administration	Oxygen administration to a laboring woman increases fetal oxygenation. The effect lasts approximately 30 minutes after supplemental oxygen is stopped. It relieves late decelerations. There is a theoretical risk that supplemental oxygen may produce free oxygen radicals that could be harmful to the fetus. Therefore supplemental oxygen should be removed once the FHR pattern improves.
Prolonged Decelerations	
Intravenous fluid bolus	Increases uterine blood flow and dilutes plasma oxytocin levels.
Reduce uterine activity via discontinuing oxytocin, tocolysis	Decreases frequency of uterine contractions so that the fetus has more time to equilibrate acid–base balance between contractions.
Correct maternal hypotension via intravenous fluids, lateral positioning	If prolonged deceleration occurs secondary to maternal hypotension from supine positioning or following placement of regional analgesia, maternal hypotension will result in a prolonged deceleration from decreased uteroplacental perfusion. If lateral positioning and intravenous fluids do not resolve the deceleration, intravenous ephedrine can be administered.

Sources: Adapted from Simpson KR. Intrauterine resuscitation during labor: should maternal oxygen administration be a first-line measure? *Semin Fetal Neonatal Med.* 2008;13(6):362-367; Briozzo L, Martinez A, Nozar M, et al. Tocolysis and delayed delivery versus emergency delivery in cases of non-reassuring fetal status during labor. *J Obstet Gynaecol Res.* 2007;33(3):266-273; Simpson KR, James DC. Efficacy of intrauterine resuscitation techniques in improving fetal oxygen status during labor. *Obstet Gynecol.* 2005;105(6):1362-1368; Simpson KR. Intrauterine resuscitation during labor: review of the current methods and supportive evidence. *J Midwifery Women's Health.* 2007;52:229-237.

Conclusion

The assessment of fetal well-being is a critical component of midwifery management of the maternal–fetal dyad during labor. Regardless of the use of intermittent auscultation, electronic fetal monitoring, or a combination of the two, the focus must be on the care of both the woman and her fetus, not just documentation of electronically generated data.[66] Like many other areas of practice, assessment of the fetus in labor is complex, and research information is being gathered continuously.

All midwives can use the methodologies that promote normal labor and birth while screening for and managing deviations from normal. The midwife may be the primary supporter of intermittent auscultation and the educator of other professionals in the birthing environment. Use of intermittent auscultation is a clear opportunity to blend the art and science of midwifery in a way that can make substantive positive change in clinical practice.

● ● ● References

1. Gilstrap LC, Leveno KJ, Burris J, Williams ML, Little B. Diagnosis of birth asphyxia on the basis of fetal pH, Apgar score, and newborn cerebral dysfunction. *Am J Obstet Gynecol.* 1989;161:835-840.

2. Nelson KB, Dambrosia JM, Ting TY, Grether JK. Uncertain value of electronic fetal monitoring in predicting cerebral palsy. *N Engl J Med.* 1996;334: 613-618.

3. Surreau C. Historical perspectives: forgotten past, unpredictable future. *Bailliere's Clin Obstet Gynecol.* 1996;10;162-184.

4. Kennedy E. *Observations of Obstetrical Auscultation.* Dublin: Hodges and Smith; 1833:311.

5. Myers RE. Two patterns of perinatal brain damage and their conditions of occurrence. *Am J Obstet Gynecol.* 1972;112:246-276.

6. Yeh SY, Diaz F, Paul RH. Ten year experience of intrapartum fetal monitoring in Lost Angeles County/University of Southern California Medical Center. *Am J Obstet Gynecol.* 1982;143:496-500.

7. Thacker SB, Stroup DF, Peterson HB. Efficacy and safety of intrapartum electronic fetal monitoring: an update. *Obstet Gynecol.* 1995;86(4):613-620.

8. Vintzileos AM, Nochimson DJ, Guzman ER, et al. Intrapartum electronic fetal heart rate monitoring versus intermittent auscultation: a meta-analysis. *Obstet Gynecol.* 1995;85(1):149-155.

9. Alfirevic Z, Devane D, Gyte GML. Continuous cardiotocography (CTG) as a form of electronic fetal monitoring (EFM) for fetal assessment during labour. *Cochrane Database Syst Rev.* 2006;3:CD006066. doi: 10.1002/14651858.CD006066.

10. MacDonald D, Grant A, Sheridan-Periera M, Chalmers I. The Dublin randomized controlled trial of intrapartum fetal heart rate monitoring. *Am J Obstet Gynecol.* 1985;152:524-539.

11. Grant S, O'Brien N, Joy MT, Hennessy E, MacDonald D . Cerebral palsy among children born during the Dublin randomized trial of intrapartum monitoring. *Lancet.* 1989;2:1233-1235.

12. Parer JT, King T. Fetal heart rate monitoring: is it salvageable? *Am J Obstet Gynecol.* 2000;182(4): 982-987.

13. Freeman RK. Problems with intrapartum fetal heart rate monitoring interpretation and patient management. *Obstet Gynecol.* 2002;100:813-826.

14. National Institute of Child Health and Human Development Research Planning Workshop. Electronic fetal heart rate monitoring: research guidelines for interpretation. *Am J Obstet Gynecol.* 1997;17: 1385-1390; *JOGNN.* 1997;26:635-640.

15. Macones GA, Hankins GD, Spong CY, Hauth J, Moore T. The 2008 National Institute of Child Health and Human Development Research Workshop report on electronic fetal heart rate monitoring. *Obstet Gynecol.* 2008;112:661-666; *JOGNN.* 2008;37: 510-515.

16. Di Tommaso M, Seravalli V, Cordisco A, Consorti G, Mecacci F, Rizzello F. Comparison of five classification systems for interpreting electronic fetal monitoring in predicting neonatal status at birth. *J Matern Fetal Neonatal Med.* 2013;26(5):487-490.

17. Bannerman CG, Grobman WA, Antoniewicz L, Hutchinson M, Blackwell S. Assessment of the concordance among 2-tier, 3-tier, and 5-tier fetal heart rate classification systems. *Am J Obstet Gynecol.* 2011;205(3):288.e1-288.e4.

18. Larma JD, Silva AM, Holcroft CJ, Thompson RE, Donohue PK, Graham EM. Intrapartum electronic fetal heart rate monitoring and the identification of metabolic acidosis and hypoxic–ischemic encephalopathy. *Am J Obstet Gynecol.* 2007;197(3): 301.e1-301.e8.

19. Parer JT. *Handbook of Fetal Heart Rate Monitoring.* 2nd ed. Philadelphia: W. B. Saunders; 1997.

20. Parer JT. Physiological regulation of the fetal heart rate. *JOGNN.* 1976;5:265-295.

21. Fahey J, King TL. Intrauterine asphyxia: clinical implications for providers of intrapartum care. *J Midwifery Women's Health.* 2005;50:498-506.

22. King, TL, Parer JT. Physiology of fetal heart rate and asphyxia. *J Perinat Neonat Nurs.* 2000;14:19-40.

23. Graham EM, Ruis KA, Hartman AL, Northington FJ, Fox HE. A systematic review of the role of intrapartum hypoxia–ischemia in the causation of neonatal encephalopathy. *Am J Obstet Gynecol.* 2008; 199(6):587-595.

24. Shah PS, Beyene J, To T, et al. Postasphyxial hypoxic–ischemic encephalopathy in neonates: outcome prediction rule within 4 hours of birth. *Arch Pediatr Adolesc Med.* 2006;160:729.

25. Rennie JM, Hagmann CF, Robertson NJ. Outcome after intrapartum hypoxic ischaemia at term. *Semin Fetal Neonatal Med.* 2007;12:398-407.

26. American College of Obstetricians and Gynecologists, American Academy of Pediatrics. *Neonatal Encephalopathy and Cerebral Palsy: Defining the Pathogenesis and Pathophysiology.* Washington, DC: American College of Obstetricians and Gynecologists; January 2003.

27. MacLennan A. A template for defining a causal relation between acute intrapartum events and cerebral palsy: international consensus statement. *BMJ.* 1999;319:1054-1059.

28. Paine LL, Payton RG, Johnson TRB. Auscultated fetal heart rate accelerations. Part I: accuracy and documentation. *J Nurse-Midwifery.* 1986;31(2):68-72.

29. Paine LL, Johnson, TRB, Turner, MH, Payton RG. Auscultated fetal heart rate accelerations. Part II: an alternative to the nonstress test. *J Nurse-Midwifery.* 1985;31(2):73-77.

30. Bakker PCAM. Uterine activity monitoring during labor. *J Perinat Med.* 2007;35:468-477.

31. Caldeyro-Barcia R, Sica-Blanco Y, Poseiro JJ, et al. A quantitative study of the action of synthetic oxytocin on the pregnant human uterus. *J Pharmacol Exp Ther.* 1957;121:18-31.

32. Westgate JA, Wibbens B, Bennet L, Wassink G, Parer JT, Gunn AJ. The intrapartum deceleration in center stage: a physiologic approach to the interpretation of fetal heart rate changes in labor. *Am J Obstet Gynecol.* 2007;197:236.e1-236.e11.

33. Parer JT, King TL, Flanders S, Fox M, Kilpatrick SJ. Fetal acidemia and electronic fetal heart rate patterns: is there evidence of an association? *J Matern Fetal Neonat Med.* 2006;19:289-294.

34. Krebs HB, Petres RE, Dunn LJ, Jordan HVF, Segreti A. Intrapartum FHR monitoring. I. Classification and prognosis of fetal heart rate patterns. *Am J Obstet Gynecol.* 1979;135(7):762-772.

35. Patrick J, Campbell K, Carmichael L, Natale R, Richardson B . Patterns of gross fetal body movements over 24-hour observation intervals during the last 10 weeks of pregnancy. *Am J Obstet Gynecol.* 1982;142:363-371.

36. Williams KP, Galerneau F. Intrapartum fetal heart rate patterns in the prediction of neonatal acidemia. *Am J Obstet Gynecol.* 2003;188:820-823.

37. Coletta J, Murphy E, Rubeo Z, et al. The 5-tier system of assessing fetal heart rate tracings is superior to the 3-tier system in identifying fetal acidemia. *Am J Obstet Gynecol.* 2010;206:226.e1-226.e5.

38. Sameshima H, Ikenoue T, Ikeda T, Kamitomo M, Ibara S. Unselected low-risk pregnancies and the effect of continuous intrapartum fetal heart rate monitoring on umbilical blood gases and cerebral palsy. *Am J Obstet Gynecol.* 2004;190:118-123.

39. Hader A, Sheiner E, Hallak M, et al. Abnormal fetal heart rate tracing patterns during the first stage of labor: effect on perinatal outcome. *Am J Obstet Gynecol.* 2001;185:863-868.

40. Hamilton E, Warrick P, O'Keefe D. Variable decelerations: do shape and size matter? *J Matern Fetal Neonat Med.* 2012;25(6):648-653.

41. Spong CY, Collea JV, Engliton GS, Ghidini A. Characteristics and prognostic significance of variable decelerations in the second stage of labor. *Am J Perinatol.* 1998;15(6):369-374.

42. Larma HJ, Strasbruger JF. Differential diagnosis and management of the fetus and newborn with an irregular or abnormal heart rate. *Pediatr Clin North Am.* 2004;51:1033-1050.

43. Martin JA, Hamilton BE, Ventura SJ, et al. Births: final data for 2009. *Natl Vital Stat Rep.* 2011;60(1):1-70.

44. Kunz MK, Loftus RJ, Nichols AA. Incidence of uterine tachysystole in women induced with oxytocin. *Obstet Gynecol Neonatal Nurs.* 2013;42(1):12-18.

45. Simpson KR. Effects of oxytocin-induced uterine hyperstimulation during labor on fetal oxygen status and fetal heart rate patterns. *Am J Obstet Gynecol.* 2008;199:34.e1-34.e5.

46. Simpson KR. Clinician's guide to the use of oxytocin for labor induction and augmentation. *J Midwifery Women's Health.* 2011;56:214-221.

47. Simpson KR. *Cervical Ripening, Induction and Augmentation of Labor* (AWHONN Practice Monograph; 3rd ed.). Washington, DC: Association of Women's Health, Obstetric, and Neonatal Nurses; 2009.

48. *The Apgar Score.* ACOG Committee Opinion no. 333. Washington, DC: American College of Obstetricians and Gynecologists; May 2006.

49. Helwig JT, Parer JT, Kilpatrick SJ, Laros RK Jr. Umbilical cord blood acid base state: what is normal? *Am J Obstet Gynecol.* 1996:1807-1814.

50. Gilstrap LC, Cunningham G. Umbilical cord blood acid–base analysis. In *Supplement #4: Williams' Obstetrics* (19th ed.). Raritan, NJ: Ortho Pharmaceutical; 1994:1-24.

51. ACOG Committee on Obstetric Practice. ACOG Committee Opinion No. 348, November 2006: umbilical cord blood gas and acid–base analysis. *Obstet Gynecol.* 2006;108:1319-1322.

52. Andersson O, Hellstrom-Westas L, Andersson D, Clausen J, Domellof M. Effects of delayed compared with early umbilical cord clamping on maternal postpartum hemorrhage and cord blood gas sampling: a randomized trial. *Acta Obstet Gynecol Scand.* August 22, 2012. doi: 10.1111/j.1600-0412.2012.01530.x.

53. Valero J, Desantes D, Perales-Puchalt A, Rubio J, Diago Almela VJ, Perales A. Effect of delayed umbilical cord clamping on blood gas analysis. *Eur J Obstet Gynecol Reprod Biol.* 2012;162(1):21-23.

54. Ross MG, Gala R. Use of umbilical artery base excess: algorithm for the timing of hypoxic injury. *Am J Obstet Gynecol.* 2002;187:1-9.

55. Low JA, Lindsay BG, Derrick EJ. Threshold of metabolic acidosis associated with newborn complications. *Am J Obstet Gynecol.* 1997;177:1391-1394.

56. Sameshima H, Ikenoue T. Predictive value of late decelerations for fetal acidemia in unselective low-risk pregnancies. *Am J Perinatol.* 2005;22:19-23.

57. Jackson M, Holmgren CM, Esplin MS, Henry E, Varner MW. Frequency of fetal heart rate categories and short-term neonatal outcome. *Obstet Gynecol.* 2011;118:803-808.

58. Miller DA. Intrapartum fetal heart rate definitions and interpretation: evolving consensus. *Clin Obstet Gynecol.* 2011;54(1):16-21.

59. Girard S, Kadhim H, Roy M, et al. Role of perinatal infection in cerebral palsy. *Pediatr Neurol.* 2009;40(3): 168-174.

60. Clark SL, Gimovsky ML, Miller FC. The scalp stimulation test: a clinical alternative to fetal scalp blood sampling. *Am J Obstet Gynecol.* 1984;148:274-277.

61. Simpson KR. Intrauterine resuscitation during labor: should maternal oxygen administration be a first-line measure? *Semin Fetal Neonatal Med.* 2008;13(6): 362-367.

62. Briozzo L, Martinez A, Nozar M, Fiol V, Pons J, Alonso J. Tocolysis and delayed delivery versus emergency delivery in cases of non-reassuring fetal status during labor. *J Obstet Gynaecol Res.* 2007;33(3): 266-273.

63. Simpson KR, James DC. Efficacy of intrauterine resuscitation techniques in improving fetal oxygen status during labor. *Obstet Gynecol.* 2005;105(6): 1362-1368.

64. Simpson KR. Intrauterine resuscitation during labor: review of the current methods and supportive evidence. *J Midwifery Women's Health.* 2007;52: 229-237.

65. Devane D, Lalor JG, Daly S, Fiol V, Pons J, Alonso J. Cardiotocography versus intermittent auscultation of fetal heart on admission to labour ward for assessment of fetal wellbeing. *Cochrane Database Syst Rev.* 2012;2:CD005122.

66. Albers LL. Monitoring the fetus in labor: evidence to support the methods. *J Midwifery Women's Health.* 2001;46(6):366-373.

APPENDIX

27A

Intermittent Auscultation During Labor

TEKOA L. KING

The purpose of intrapartum assessment of the fetal heart rate (FHR) is to monitor fetal well-being over the course of labor and to identify the fetus at risk for clinically significant acidemia. Effective methods of evaluation and accurate interpretation of the FHR during labor have long been the subjects of clinical debate. Continuous electronic fetal monitoring (EFM) is the most commonly used method of intrapartum fetal surveillance use, but has not been shown to be more efficacious than intermittent auscultation (IA).[1]

Professional organizations' recommendations for fetal heart rate assessment during labor are primarily based on protocols used in randomized clinical trials conducted during the 1990s that compared IA to EFM.[2-4] Handheld Doppler or Pinard-type fetoscopes were used for the IA groups and those women had continuous one-to-one nursing during labor. Since those studies were performed, the understanding of the relationship between specific FHR patterns and adverse neonatal outcomes has vastly improved.[5,6] Intermittent auscultation is typically conducted using a handheld Doppler fetoscope; although Pinard-type fetoscopes are used on a prenatal basis, they have limitations for intrapartum use. A handheld Doppler device can effectively monitor the fetus if the technique is done appropriately.[2-4,7] Conversely, intermittent auscultation can miss significant fetal heart rate decelerations if it is not done appropriately. This appendix presents the technique for intermittent auscultation, interpretation of findings from IA,

and management recommendations based on current knowledge of fetal heart rate characteristics.

Intermittent Auscultation Versus Electronic Fetal Monitoring

Both EFM and IA have benefits and limitations that will assist the midwife to choose the most appropriate monitoring modality for specific situations. Auscultation allows the woman freedom of movement and permits fetal assessment if the woman is in water. Auscultation also requires one-to-one continuous care, but may not be technically feasible for women who are overweight or obese. EFM will monitor the fetus continuously during labor and provides a record that can be examined by others as needed, often from a central monitoring site. However, EFM limits the woman to a bed or sitting near a bed unless telemetry units are available for her use. Moreover, if a supportive person is not present, she may miss the additional advantages of having someone with her continuously throughout her labor.

The RCTs that evaluated EFM versus IA did not find that either modality was a better option for improving Apgar scores, lowering the incidence of cerebral palsy, or improving perinatal mortality rates.[1] EFM was associated with a significant increase in the rate of cesarean section compared to IA. The value of these findings and limitations of the RCTs have been reviewed extensively elsewhere.[8-11] Until another RCT comparing EFM to IA that uses modern definitions of FHR characteristics is published, it is unlikely that the question of which modality is superior will be answered. Therefore the focus of this appendix is on safe use of IA based on current knowledge.

FHR Characteristics Detectable on Intermittent Auscultation

Table 27A-1 lists the FHR characteristics that can be detected via IA and EFM. Auscultation has been shown to be able to identify baseline FHR and changes in the rhythm of the heart rate and to appreciate accelerations of the heart rate.[12-14] The *Auscultated Acceleration Test* appendix of the *Obstetric Complications in Pregnancy* chapter describes the methods used to identify and document FHR accelerations in nonlaboring women. Although these methods have not been assessed in a laboring population, it is reasonable to assume that they are valid. Studies assessing reliability have not been conducted. IA cannot identify FHR variability.[15] Decelerations can be identified as a decrease of the heart rate, but specific timing of the decelerations in relationship to uterine contractions cannot be determined with assurance, nor can the degree of decline of the heart rate, such as "sudden with a variable deceleration" or "gradual

with an early or late deceleration." Thus decelerations cannot be categorized as early, variable, or late in character. Instead, auscultation of decreases in the FHR can be described as brief or prolonged by the auscultated duration and by the slowest rate counted or registered on the Doppler device.

Moderate FHR variability is the most reliable indicator that a fetus is not experiencing clinically significant acidemia.[16] As a consequence, the inability of IA to detect FHR variability or to discriminate between types of FHR decelerations must be addressed.

There are several reasons why IA is a viable option for low-risk women at term despite the fact that it cannot detect FHR variability:

- IA is recommended only for women who do not have an a priori risk for developing fetal acidemia during labor, because it is the metabolic acids produced during anaerobic metabolism that are most closely correlated with adverse neurologic outcomes. The incidence of clinically significant metabolic acidemia in newborns in a healthy population of women is approximately 3 per 1000 births.[17,18] Of these infants, only a small proportion will have adverse outcomes.

- When significant fetal acidemia does occur in the intrapartum period in a previously healthy fetus, recurrent FHR decelerations that are detectable on IA[19] will appear. In addition,

Table 27A-1	FHR Characteristics Determined via Auscultation Versus Electronic Fetal Heart Rate Monitoring		
FHR Characteristic[a]	**Fetoscope**	**Doppler Without Paper Printout**	**Electronic Fetal Heart Rate Monitor**
Variability	No	No	Yes
Baseline rate	Yes	Yes	Yes
Accelerations	Detects increases[b]	Detects increases[b]	Yes
Decelerations	Detects decreases	Detects decreases	Differentiates types of decelerations
Rhythm[c]	Yes	Yes	Yes
Double-counting or half-counting EFM	Can clarify	May double-count or half-count	May double-count or half-count
Differentiation of maternal and fetal FHR	Yes	May detect maternal heart rate instead of fetal heart rate	May detect and record maternal heart rate instead of fetal heart rate

[a]Definitions of each FHR characteristic per the NICHD 2008 criteria.[6]

[b]Per method described by Paine et al.[12,13]

[c]Determined as regular or irregular. None of these devices can diagnose the type of fetal arrhythmia.

Source: Reprinted with permission from American College of Nurse-Midwives. Intermittent Auscultation for Intrapartum Fetal Heart Rate Surveillance no. 11 (replaces ACNM Clinical Bulletin #(March 2007). *J Midwifery Women's Health.* 2010;55:397-403.

labor abnormalities that signal the need for additional surveillance or intervention are also those that are likely to be associated with diminishing FHR variability and recurrent decelerations (e.g., maternal fever, labor dystocia and need for oxytocin augmentation, or acute sentinel event).[20]

- Most FHR patterns that are associated with adverse neonatal outcomes develop over a period of time, approximating 1 hour.[5] Thus, when recurrent fetal heart rate decelerations are detected, there is usually ample time to initiate and obtain EFM tracings and transfer the woman to a setting where operative birth is available if needed.

Professional Guidelines for Intermittent Auscultation

The American College of Nurse-Midwives (ACNM) published a Clinical Bulletin that summarizes the technique and interpretation of IA.[3] The method described in this appendix is concordant with the ACNM guidelines. Individual institutions or practices may have protocols specific for their setting and population. Protocols for IA should define the method of conducting IA, frequency and duration of IA, indications for IA, and indications for transfer to EFM.

Frequency, Timing, and Technique for Intermittent Auscultation for Women in Labor

The frequency and timing of IA in current professional association guidelines[2-4] are based on the frequency and timing used in the RCTs comparing EFM with IA. ACNM recommends auscultating the FHR every 15 to 30 minutes in the active phase of labor and every 5 minutes in the second stage of labor.[4] However, using protocols designed for RCTs in daily clinical practice has some limitations.

Frequency

With regard to frequency, strict adherence to a 15- or 30-minute interval fails to account for changes in labor status that could potentially affect the FHR. The frequency of auscultation should be individualized based on labor characteristics such as the frequency of contractions, clinical signs of fetal descent (e.g., spontaneous rupture of membranes, bloody show, urge to push, nonrecurrent decelerations), and institution of hydrotherapy or other interventions that may affect the FHR.

Duration

With regard to duration, current guidelines recommend auscultating between contractions. Listening between contractions can result in missing significant variable decelerations that occur during a contraction. As a consequence, midwives who use IA extensively periodically listen throughout a contraction and for 30 to 60 seconds after the contraction is over. If no abnormal FHR decreases are noted, they may begin to listen at the peak of a contraction and continue listening for 30 to 60 seconds after the contraction is over for subsequent assessments. Listening between contractions is not an appropriate technique.

Multicount Strategy

A multicount technique has been shown to be more reliable than counting once throughout the period of assessment.[21] In a study conducted by Shiffrin et al., the multicount strategy identified approximately 93% of FHR decelerations; by comparison, a single-count strategy identified 74% of the FHR decelerations.[21] When using a multicount strategy, the listener counts the FHR for a period of 6, 10, or 15 seconds several times over the course of the listening period. A defined rest period of 5 or 10 seconds occurs between each count. Each count is then multiplied by the appropriate number to obtain a FHR-per-minute rate. The counts can be plotted to diagram the FHR changes over the course of the auscultation period, as shown in **Figure 27A-1**. There is some anecdotal evidence that this technique will reveal FHR variability but this has not been evaluated scientifically.

Interpretation of IA FHR Characteristics

FHR changes identifiable on IA have been evaluated in concert with the 2008 NICHD FHR interpretative categories for EFM that have been adopted by all relevant professional associations.[4,6,22] FHR changes detected on IA are classified as either Category I or Category II, as outlined in **Table 27A-2**. There is no Category III using IA because Category III FHR patterns have absent variability that cannot be detected via IA.

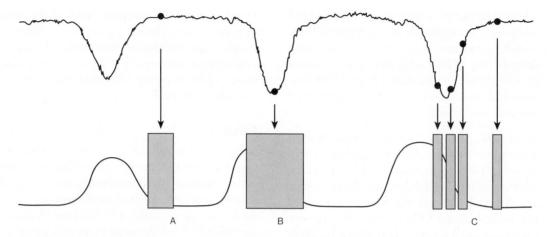

A. Single count strategy for less than 1 minute between contractions may miss a deceleration.
B. Single count strategy for 30–60 seconds that starts after the peak of the contraction will detect presence of a deceleration qualitatively.
C. Multi-count strategy for 10 seconds with a 5–10 second break between counts allows the clinician to graphically sketch the deceleration.

Figure 27A-1 Multicount strategy for assessing the fetal heart rate via intermittent auscultation.

Management of Category II FHR Changes on Intermittent Auscultation

Category II FHR changes require increased surveillance. A longer listening period may be initiated, the frequency of auscultation increased, or transfer to EFM may be indicated. If recurrent decelerations are noted or the FHR is bradycardic, the woman should be turned to her side and the FHR reevaluated. Oxygen therapy and intravenous fluids may be initiated or increased depending on the clinical situation. If concern for the fetus is such that birth should occur as soon as possible, frequent auscultation and documentation of results should continue while transferring the woman to a setting where EFM and operative delivery are available.

Documentation of Intermittent Auscultation

The type of Doppler technology used and the multicount procedure employed should be documented. Documentation of IA is critical in management of the course of labor as well as for retrospective review of the chart to evaluate care of the fetus in labor. As

Table 27A-2	Interpretation of Auscultation Findings	
Category 1	**Category II**
Category 1 FHR characteristics by auscultation include the following:	Category II FHR characteristics by auscultation include any of the following:
• Normal FHR baseline between 110 and 160 bpm • Regular rhythm • Absence of FHR decreases or decelerations from the baseline	• Irregular rhythm • Presence of FHR decreases or decelerations from the baseline • Tachycardia (baseline > 160 bpm) • Bradycardia (baseline < 110 bpm)
FHR increases or accelerations from the baseline may or may not be present but should be assessed for and documented if present. If present, FHR accelerations signify fetal well-being at the time they are noted.	

Source: Fetal Heart Monitoring: Principles and Practices, 4th edition, p. 129. Adapted with permission from Association of Women's Health, Obstetric and Neonatal Nurses (AWHONN).

with other vital signs, IA must be documented after each episode of auscultation, as no printed version is recorded (as there is with a fetal monitor strip).[23] The graph for documentation of IA should be simple and straightforward, allowing for little extra time to be wasted with excess documentation.

Key Points

- Intermittent auscultation is recommended for women at term gestations who do not have an a priori risk for fetal acidemia at the onset of labor.[2–4]
- Randomized controlled trials of IA included one-to-one nursing care, which may have an independent positive effect on labor outcomes. Thus use of IA presumes continuous labor support is also in effect.
- Current professional guidelines for conducting IA are based on the protocols used in previously conducted RCTs. These guidelines specify the time intervals for IA that were needed for an RCT. The time intervals between IA assessments in clinical practice should also be based on labor characteristics and the frequency of uterine contractions.

- Multicount strategies are more accurate than single-count strategies.

Equipment

Fetoscope

- Several Pinard-type stethoscopes are available. All rely on bone conduction from the listener's cranium to amplify the sound. The most commonly used version is the Allen fetoscope, which can be obtained with short or long tubing. The midwife can use these devices without pressing her/his forehead to the headpiece, although this practice decreases the accuracy in detecting the FHR. The DeLee-Hillis fetoscope has a headpiece that fits over the listener's head, which facilitates the bone conduction. The Pinard-type fetoscopes identify the sounds associated with the opening and closing of ventricular valves and must be placed on the maternal abdomen where the fetal heart is closest, over the fetal scapula or chest. With the Allen fetoscopes, the short tubing is more likely to detect the FHR but requires the provider to bend close to the woman's abdomen (**Figure 27A-2**).

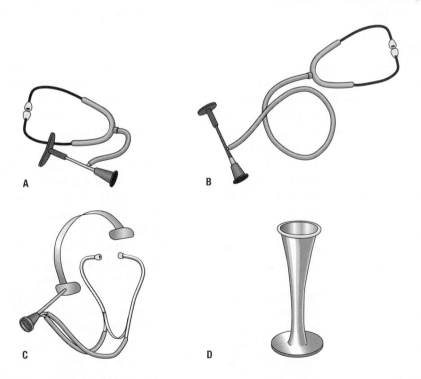

Figure 27A-2 Pinard-type fetoscopes: (A) Allen fetoscope with short tubing. (B) Allen fetoscope with long tubing. (C) DeLee-Hillis fetoscope. (D) Pinard fetoscope.

- The fetoscope can detect the baseline fetal heart rate, changes from the baseline rate, and irregular rhythms.[12-14] The midwife must count the heart rate that is heard. Because the actual heart sounds are detected, the fetoscope will not detect a maternal heart rate—unlike with EFM, wherein either the Doppler or a fetal scalp electrode can misinterpret the maternal heart rate as a fetal heart rate.

- If using a DeLee-Hillis or Allen fetoscope, the bell must be placed tightly against the maternal abdomen to achieve a good air seal, and the headpiece must be against the listener's forehead to utilize bone conduction. Similarly, the bell of a Pinard fetoscope is placed firmly on the woman's skin, ensuring contact with the entire rim of the bell; the listener then places an ear firmly against the earpiece for best transmission of sound.

- Although some of the RCTs of EFM versus IA used a Pinard-type fetoscope during labor, these devices are not good choices for detecting the FHR during a contraction. Given current knowledge about the role of FHR decelerations as a reflection of developing fetal acidemia,[5] most midwives do not use these devices for monitoring the FHR during labor today, and they are not recommended by the authors of this text.

Doppler Fetoscopes

- The Doppler device uses ultrasound to detect the movement—that is, opening and closing—of the ventricular valves by noting the change in ultrasound wave length that is caused by heart movement. The machine converts the wavelength change into a visual digital recording and audible sound. Some handheld devices will generate a printout record. Most Doppler fetoscopes are water-proof and can be used to record the FHR when a woman is in water.

- The Doppler fetoscope detects baseline rate and changes in baseline rate. An irregular rhythm may be audible, but the Doppler device does not reliably detect irregular rhythms. Methods have been devised and validated for accurately detecting FHR variability in non-laboring women, but have not been tested scientifically in laboring women. In addition, a maternal heart rate can be detected by the Doppler device in the presence of fetal demise;

thus the midwife must make sure the heart rate that is detected is fetal.

- Doppler devices require use of a gel between the face of the transducer and the maternal skin to ensure transmission of sound without air interference.

Technique for Performing Intermittent Auscultation

1. Determine the fetal lie to optimize the quality of the heart sounds. Listening through the fetal back provides the clearest sound.

2. Determine the duration and frequency of uterine contractions.

3. Determine baseline FHR:

    a. If using a Doppler device, check the maternal radial pulse at the same time to be certain the Doppler fetoscope is detecting the FHR. The maternal heart rate may be documented in the medical record.

    b. Initial auscultation should be for a minimum of 60 seconds, between contractions, to determine the baseline FHR and to listen for regularity of the rate.

    c. Listen between contractions for several intervals within a 10-minute period to confirm consistency of the FHR and to identify the baseline.

    d. Count for 6 to 10 seconds several times with a 5- or 10-second pause between counts then multiply each count by 10 or 6, respectively, to obtain the FHR-per-minute numeric value.

4. Listen for the presence of FHR accelerations. Noting the presence of FHR accelerations can be done qualitatively or quantitatively. Accelerations do not need to be present to identify the FHR as Category I if the FHR rate has a normal baseline and no decelerations are present. However, FHR accelerations are a sign of fetal well-being when present and should be assessed for and documented if auscultated. The *Auscultated Acceleration Test* appendix in the *Obstetric Complications in Pregnancy* chapter describes the procedure for detecting FHR accelerations quantitatively.

5. Determine the presence of FHR decelerations. Begin listening at the peak of the contraction and

continue for at least 30 to 60 seconds after the contraction is over.

   a. If a deceleration is heard, listen through successive contractions or several contractions in a 10-minute window to determine if they are recurrent or nonrecurrent.

   b. Use a multicount method to document the drop in FHR baseline and depth of the decrease.

6. Document the FHR-per-minute rate for each assessment and inform the laboring woman of the findings.

● ● ● References

1. Alvrevic Z, Devane D, Gyte GML. Continuous cardiotocography (CTG) as a form of electronic fetal monitoring (EFM) for fetal assessment during labour. *Cochrane Database Syst Rev.* 2006;3:CD006066. doi: 10.1002/14651858.CD006066.

2. Lyndon A, Ali LU, eds. *Fetal Heart Monitoring Principles and Practices.* 4th ed. Dubuque, IA: Kendall-Hunt; 2009.

3. American College of Nurse-Midwives. Intermittent auscultation for intrapartum fetal heart rate: Surveillance no. 11 (replaces ACNM Clinical Bulletin #9 March 2007). *J Midwifery Women's Health.* 2010; 55:397-403.

4. American College of Obstetricians and Gynecologists. Management of intrapartum fetal heart rate tracings: Practice Bulletin number 116 November 2010. *Obstet Gynecol.* 2010;116:1232-1240.

5. Parer JT, King TL, Flanders S, Fox M, Kilpatrick SJ. Fetal acidemia and electronic fetal heart rate patterns: is there evidence of an association? *J Matern Fetal Neonatal Med.* 2006:19:289-294.

6. Macones GA, Hankins GD, Spong CY, Hauth J, Moore T. The 2008 National Institute of Child Health and Human Development Research Workshop report on electronic fetal heart rate monitoring. *Obstet Gynecol.* 2008;112:661-666. *JOGNN.* 2008;37: 510-515.

7. Feinstein NF. Fetal heart rate auscultation: current and future practice. *JOGNN.* 2000;29:306-315.

8. Parer JT, King T. Fetal heart rate monitoring: is it salvageable? *Am J Obstet Gynecol.* 2000;182(4): 982-987.

9. Parer JT, King TL. Fetal heart rate monitoring: the next step. *Am J Obstet Gynecol.* 2010;203:520-521.

10. Freeman RK. Problems with intrapartum fetal heart rate monitoring interpretation and patient management. *Obstet Gynecol.* 2002;100(4):813-826.

11. Resnik R. Electronic fetal monitoring: the debate goes on...and on...and on. *Obstet Gynecol.* 2013;121(5):917-918.

12. Paine LL, Payton RG, Johnson TRB. Auscultated fetal heart rate accelerations: Part I. Accuracy and documentation. *J Nurse-Midwifery.* 1986;31(2):68-72.

13. Paine LL, Johnson TR, Turner MH, et al. Auscultated fetal heart rate accelerations: Part II. An alternative to the nonstress test. *J Nurse-Midwifery.* 1989;31(2): 73-77.

14. Paine LL, Benedict MI, Strobino DM, Gegor CL, Larson EL. A comparison of the auscultated acceleration test and the nonstress test as predictors of perinatal outcomes. *Nurs Res.* 1992;41(2):87-91.

15. Feinstein NF. Fetal heart rate auscultation: current and future practice. *JOGNN.* 2000;29(3):306-315.

16. Low JA. Determining the contribution of asphyxia to brain damage in the neonate. *J Obstet Gynaecol Res.* 2004;30(4):276-286.

17. Graham EM, Petersen SM, Christo DK, Fox HE. Intrapartum electronic fetal heart rate monitoring and the prevention of perinatal brain injury. *Obstet Gynecol.* 2006;108(3 Pt 1):656-666.

18. Kurinczuk JJ, White-Koning M, Badawi N. Epidemiology of neonatal encephalopathy and hypoxic-ischaemic encephalopathy. *Early Hum Dev.* 2010; 86(6):329-338.

19. Low JA, Pickersgill H, Killen H, Derrick EJ. The prediction and prevention of intrapartum fetal asphyxia in term pregnancies. *Am J Obstet Gynecol.* 2001;184(4):724-730.

20. Badawi N, Kurinczuk JJ, Keogh JM, et al. Intrapartum risk factors for newborn encephalopathy: the Western Australian case-control study. *BMJ.* 1998;317(7172):1554-1558.

21. Shiffrin BS. The accuracy of auscultatory detection of fetal cardiac decelerations: a computer simulation. *Am J Obstet Gynecol.* 1992;166(2):566-576.

22. American College of Nurse-Midwives. Standardized nomenclature for electronic fetal monitoring: position statement. Division of Standards and Practice approved: ACNM Board of Directors, March 2010 reviewed; August 2011.

23. Feinstein NE, Sprague A, Trepanier M. Fetal heart rate auscultation: comparing auscultation to electronic fetal monitoring. *AWHONN Lifelines.* 2000;4(3):35-44.

APPENDIX

27B

Attaching a Fetal Scalp Electrode

A fetal scalp electrode (FSE) is a very small, thin, spiral electrode that, when attached to the fetal scalp, detects the fetal EKG. The FSE is attached to a cord that connects to an electronic fetal monitor, which turns the EKG into an audible and written continuous recording. An FSE requires that membranes are ruptured and the cervix is at least 1 to 2 centimeters dilated.

This device is not recommended for routine use. An FSE is used *only* when a continuous legible recording is considered necessary as a basis of clinical management and an external Doppler fetoscope is *not* able to supply such a record. Although there are no specific indications for use of an FSE in the United States, it is commonly used when an external Doppler device is unable to continuously detect the FHR and the fetus is at risk for metabolic acidemia or perinatal death. Examples of such situations include severe preeclampsia or prior cesarean section birth wherein an increased risk for uterine rupture is present.

First-generation electronic monitors exaggerated FHR variability when the abdominal Doppler device was used, thus an FSE would be applied to provide a more accurate rendition of FHR variability. However, the electronic fetal monitors in use today have an auto-correlation feature that allows portrayal of FHR variability with an accuracy almost equal to that shown if an FSE is used.[1] Thus the need to better assess variability is not an indication for use of an FSE if a legible tracing is present. Nevertheless, it is important to note that the external Doppler device can erroneously detect a maternal heart rate or double or halve the signal, which can, in rare situations, confound interpretation of its output.[1,2] In turn, doubt about the Doppler signal accurately portraying a fetal heart rate is another indication for FSE.

The FSE penetrates into the fetal scalp approximately 2 mm.[3] It is contraindicated for use among women who have infections that might potentially be vertically transmitted to the fetus, such as active herpes, hepatitis, or HIV. An FSE is also contraindicated if the fetus has a known or possible coagulation disorder. Some clinicians consider chorioamnionitis to be a relative contraindication to the use of an FSE. This type of electrode should not be attached if the fetus is in a face presentation, or if the presentation is unknown. Likewise, it should not be placed on genitalia in breech presentations, or over the fontanelle in a vertex presentation.[1]

Complications following FSE use include scalp laceration, localized infection, and (rarely) abscess. Some case reports describe facial injury, or insertion in the eye or ear when the FSE is placed without accurate diagnosis of fetal position. An FSE provides a potential pathway for ascending infection. Early studies found a correlation between prolonged use of an FSE (more than 12 hours) and neonatal sepsis.[4] Subsequent retrospective analyses have found that FSE alone has not been associated with an increased risk for neonatal sepsis.[5,6] To date, none of the studies conducted has been sufficiently powered to definitely answer this question. When attachment of an FSE is done in a known vertex presentation and the procedure is performed under aseptic conditions, complications are very rare.

Mechanism of Action

The FSE spiral electrode contains two electrodes in close proximity. One penetrates the fetal scalp to the depth of approximately 2 mm, with vaginal secretions providing electrical conduction between the two wires; the difference in voltage between the two electrodes is then measured and recorded. A third reference electrode that helps eliminate electrical interference is placed on the maternal thigh.

Contraindications

- Active infection such as HIV or herpes, hepatitis B or C
- Placenta previa
- Unknown fetal presentation or position
- Face presentation
- Do not place on genitalia or a fontanelle

Equipment

- Sterile fetal spiral electrode
- Sterile gloves
- Electronic fetal monitor
- Leg plate with Velcro strap or adhesive patches and cable to fetal monitor
- Water-based lubricant

Procedure for Attaching a Fetal Scalp Electrode

1. Explain to the woman the indication for use of an FSE, and review the procedure, along with its benefits and risks. Answer any questions the woman or her support personnel have. Obtain an informed consent prior to placement and perform hand hygiene.
2. Attach the leg plate to the woman's thigh.
3. Open the FSE packaging.
4. Put on sterile gloves.
5. Remove the wires from between the drive tube and the guide tube.
6. Perform a vaginal examination; confirm lie, presentation, and position. Keep examining hand on the area of the presenting part where the FSE will be applied.
7. Select the FSE with the nonexamining hand. Verify that the spiral end of the electrode is withdrawn so it is completely within the guide tube. This assures that the device will not inadvertently injure any tissue of the woman or the examiner (**Figure 27B-1**).

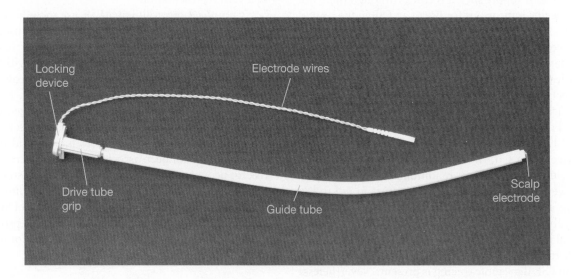

Figure 27B-1 Fetal monitoring spiral electrode assembly.

8. Advance the guide tube between the examining fingers and position it firmly against the fetal presenting part, avoiding sutures, fontanelles, or genitalia. If uncertain about the exact presentation, do not attach the FSE.

9. Advance the drive tube until it touches the fetal presenting part.

10. Maintain pressure on the guide tube so it remains touching the fetal presenting part and rotate the drive tube clockwise approximately 1.5 rotations until mild resistance is felt and the drive tube recoils. Rotating causes the tip of the spiral electrode to penetrate the fetal scalp and be attached.[1]

11. Release the end of the electrode wires from the locking device at the end of the drive tube grip.

12. Carefully retract the guide tube a few inches and check the placement of the scalp electrode with examining hand.

13. Remove the guide tube from the woman's vagina and dispose of per institutional policy.

14. Remove gloves.

15. Attach the electrode wires to the leg plate and the cable from the leg plate to the fetal monitor.

16. Evaluate the FSE recording of FHR for at least 5 to 10 minutes before leaving the room.

17. Explain the findings to the woman and her support team.

Procedure for Removing a Fetal Scalp Electrode

1. To detach the electrode, put on sterile gloves.

2. With the examining hand on the electrode, rotate it counterclockwise until it is free of the fetal presenting part.

3. Do not pull the electrode directly, as this could cause a scalp laceration.

● ● ● ● **References**

1. Freeman RK, Garite TJ, Nageotte MP, Miller LA. *Fetal Monitoring*. 4th ed. Philadelphia PA: Wolters Kluwer Health; 2012:49-50.

2. Bernardes J, Ayres-de-Campos D. The persistent challenge of foetal heart rate monitoring. *Curr Opin Obstet Gynecol.* 2010;22(2):104-109.

3. Tucker SM, Miller LA, Miller DA. *Fetal Monitoring: A Multidisciplinary Approach*. 6th ed. St, Louis, MO: Mosby Year Book; 2009:45-51

4. Yancey MK, Duff P, Kubilis P, Clark P, Frentzen BH. Risk factors for neonatal sepsis. *Obstet Gynecol.* 1996;87(2):188-194.

5. Nakatsuka N, Jain V, Aziz K, Verity R, Kumar M. Is there an association between fetal scalp electrode application and early-onset neonatal sepsis in term and late preterm pregnancies? A case-control study. *J Obstet Gynaecol Can.* 2012;34(1):29-33.

6. Harper LM, Shanks AL, Tuuli MG, Roehl KA, Cahill AG. The risks and benefits of internal monitors in laboring patients. *Am J Obstet Gynecol.* April 2, 2013. doi: pii:S0002-9378(13)00350-5.10.1016/j.ajog.2013.04.001. [Epub ahead of print.]

C H A P T E R

28

Support for Women in Labor

KIMBERLY K. TROUT

LADAN ESHKEVARI

Introduction

Every labor and birth is unique. While most women experience pain in labor, interpretation of labor pain is highly individual. The actions of the midwife can make a significant difference in how a woman copes with labor pain and views her experience of labor. If a woman feels that she is being neglected emotionally, labor pain can become suffering.[1] Conversely, if she is feeling emotionally supported and coping reasonably well, even though still experiencing pain, she may feel a sense of accomplishment. Her perception of how she is treated by those who care for her during labor and the memory of her child's labor and birth persists for many years, likely for her lifetime.[2] This chapter reviews the physiology of labor pain and considers how the experience of pain may differ among women. Nonpharmacologic and pharmacologic techniques that can be used to assist women during labor are presented.

Nature and Experience of Pain

The formal definition of pain used in health care today comes from the International Association for the Study of Pain:

> Pain is an unpleasant sensory and emotional experience…Pain is always subjective. Each individual learns the application of the word through experience related to injury early in life.[3]

The neuromatrix theory of pain based on Melzack's pioneering work regarding the nature of pain recognizes that all pain, including the pain of labor, is the result of a complex interplay between physical, biological, psychological, and cultural factors, each of which contributes to the overall perception of the experience.[4,5]

Pain Physiology: Receptors and Pathways

Pain is generally characterized as either acute or chronic. Acute pain serves the purpose of alerting the individual to a stimulus; chronic pain, in contrast, can be a maladaptive response with no physiologic purpose. Pain is caused by stimulation of sensory neurons known as nociceptors and is further characterized as somatic (deep or superficial) or visceral. Deep somatic pain is dull and aching but poorly localized, whereas superficial somatic pain is sharp and well localized. Visceral pain is caused by ischemia or inflammation in visceral structures (internal organs). Over the course of labor, visceral, deep somatic, and superficial somatic pain can all be experienced. What is curious about labor pain is that labor is a normal physiologic phenomenon; thus it may be the only physiologic event that usually is described as severely painful.

Pain is transmitted from nociceptors in the periphery and viscera via fast, lightly myelinated A-delta fibers and slower, unmyelinated C fibers (**Figure 28-1**). Pain traveling along the A-delta fibers is felt within 0.1 second, whereas pain transmitted along the C fibers takes about 1 second or more, and sometimes up to several minutes, to be felt by the individual. Numerous types of stimuli, such as mechanical, thermal (temperature related), and chemical agents, can cause pain. For example, uterine stretching during labor causes mechanical pain, whereas chemical substances generated when there is a lack of oxygen in uterine muscle secondary

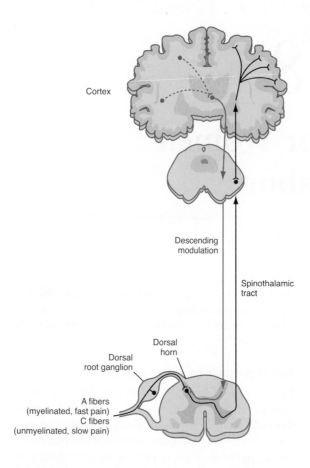

Cortex

Descending
modulation

Spinothalamic
tract

Dorsal
horn

Dorsal
root ganglion

A fibers
(myelinated, fast pain)
C fibers
(unmyelinated, slow pain)

Figure 28-1 Transmission of pain periphery to the central
nervous system.

to recurrent frequent uterine contractions are also
responsible for pain felt during labor. Some examples
of these chemical mediators of pain include substance
P, glutamate, bradykinin, acetylcholine, serotonin,
and histamine. Pain management of the parturient is
aimed at minimizing or allaying the effects of both
mechanical and chemical mediators.[6]

Once pain is transmitted from the nociceptors at
the anatomic source of the pain, the impulse is transmitted via A-delta and C fibers to the dorsal column
of the spinal cord, where these fibers synapse with
other neurons in the cord. During the first stage of
labor, the pain from the contracting uterus enters the
spinal cord at T10 to L1 levels, whereas during the
second stage the fibers enter the cord at S2–S4 levels.[7]

Nerves within the spinal cord transfer the impulse to the contralateral spinothalamic tract, where
nerves ascend to the cerebral cortex. The pain impulse can be modulated via several different mechanisms as it crosses from one side of the spinal cord
to the other prior to ascending to the central nervous system (CNS). The gate-control theory of pain

modulation is based on the hypothesis that stimulation of A-delta fibers via massage, sterile water injections, or transcutaneous electric nerve stimulation
(TENS) gets impulses to the dorsal horn quickly,
where they effectively close a "gate" that blocks impulses from the slower C fibers.[4]

The pain impulse travels to the brain via two
pathways: the neospinothalamic tract and the
paleospinothalamic tract. Most of the fibers of the
neospinothalamic tract terminate in brain areas such
as the brain stem and the thalamus, where the pain
signal is transmitted to basal areas of the brain as well
as the somatosensory cortex, where the parturient
"feels" pain. The paleospinothalamic tract fibers terminate in the brain stem, in the areas of the medulla,
pons, mesencephalon, and the periaqueductal gray
region. These lower regions of the brain also play a
role in the perception of pain. The perception of pain
is the result of the brain integrating pain information
from the thalamus, lower brain areas, and the cortex.

Just as the brain perceives pain, so it also has
the capability of modifying the perception of that
pain. The pathways of pain perception are not "one
way only." That is, inhibitory neurons in the CNS
can dampen pain sensation via an endogenous opiate
system. In fact, the brain has a fairly elegant analgesic system that varies from person to person, which
partially explains some of the individual differences
in pain perception across the population.

The periaqueductal gray and the periventricu-
lar areas (areas around the third and fourth ventricles of the brain) possess neurons that transmit
anti-nociceptive impulses to the dorsal horns of the
spinal cord. The impulses from these fibers block
pain before it is relayed to the brain, via release of
neurotransmitters such as enkephalin and serotonin
at their terminus in the dorsal horn of the spinal cord.
Serotonin promotes release of enkephalin, which is
known to inhibit both presynaptic and postsynaptic
type C and A-delta pain fibers at the dorsal horns.
Several other naturally occurring physiologic opiates
also play a similar role to enkephalin, such as beta-
endorphin and dynorphin. Most of the opioids we
now use exogenously to treat pain are derived from
opium, a naturally occurring opiate with a similar
structure to that of the endogenous opiates found in
the brain and dorsal horn of the spinal cord.

Physiologic Response to Pain

Pain during the first stage of labor is generally believed to be caused by mechanical distension of the
lower uterine segment, cervical dilatation, and perhaps acidemia in uterine muscle after several hours
of contraction activity.

A number of physiologic systems are affected by pain. One of the first responses elicited is that of the neuroendocrine system, leading to release of stress-related hormones such as cortisol, catecholamines, and cytokines. There is a concomitant rise in angiotensin II, antidiuretic hormone, growth hormone, and glucagon. The effect of these hormones is heightened alertness, increased cardiac output, increased heart rate, elevated blood pressure, higher serum glucose levels, and more extracellular fluid in the periphery and lungs. The catecholamines contribute greatly to the increase in heart rate, blood pressure, and activation of the renin–angiotensin system, which causes systemic vasoconstriction and further elevations in blood pressure. Pain-induced release of catecholamines can also slow gastrointestinal and genitourinary motility, leading to vomiting and urinary retention, respectively. Coagulation and immune responses may also be negatively affected by pain-induced stress.

The relationship between catecholamine release (norepinephrine and epinephrine) and uterine contractility during labor is poorly understood. It has been theorized and noted in observational studies with small numbers of laboring women that the uterus does not contract well if the catecholamine levels are very high.[8] In general, the well-being of the woman and her fetus are affected by release of the hormones and cytokines related to pain and stress. Poorly controlled pain can lead to anxiety, fear, and a loss of confidence by the woman, and can promote the release of even more catecholamines and cytokines which may result in a positive feedback process.

Women's Experiences of Labor Pain

The neuromatrix theory of pain helps to elucidate why such great variability is noted in regard to individual perception and response to labor pain.[5,9,10] The perception of pain by any individual, including the laboring woman, is a dynamic process with physical, psychological, and behavioral components.

The interplay of psychological preparation, expectations, past experience, and emotional support all affect the degree of pain perceived by the woman in labor. Notably, psychological preparation and expectations appear to play a large role in a woman's perception and ability to cope with the pain of labor.[11] Multiple studies have looked at the relationship between women's expectations and their labor experiences. In a review of this body of work, Lally et al. found that, in general, there is a significant gap between expectations and experience, with most women reporting more pain than expected and expectations that were not met.[11] There is a great deal

of work to be done in learning how to help women prepare for labor and in learning how the healthcare system can better meet women's expectations.

Research on the effects of age, gender, and culture on pain perception has yielded conflicting results. Consequently, it is best to discuss the woman's personal past experiences with pain and her general pain tolerance when reviewing pain management options as part of her birthing preferences.[12]

Numerous studies have also demonstrated that genetic variability can affect both pain sensation, by altering peripheral nociceptive pathways, and its modulation by the descending pathways.[13-15] Additionally, genetic differences in the microsomal enzymes involved in metabolizing drugs play a role in a woman's ability to metabolize the opioids often used in pain management. For example, the microsomal enzyme superfamily in the cytochrome CYP2D6 has several polymorphisms that render some individuals unable to metabolize codeine and, therefore these individuals do not obtain adequate pain relief from medication that contains codeine because the biologically active effect of codeine is caused by its metabolite, which is morphine.[16]

Women's Reports of Labor Pain

Labor pain is felt in three general locations. Virtually all women in labor experience lower abdominal pain, approximately 74% experience contraction-related back pain, and approximately 33% experience continuous low back pain.[17] In Melzack's classic study of 42 nulliparous women and 37 multiparous women who completed hourly pain assessments throughout labor, there was a good deal of variability in the spatial distribution of where pain was felt.[18]

In addition to spatial variation, variation in intensity of labor pain is apparent. Generally, nulliparous women report higher average intensity levels of pain than multiparous women on the McGill Pain Questionnaire, especially nulliparous women who have had no preparation for childbirth.[18] However, there is significant variability in the pain reported at hourly intervals by individuals, just as there is a great deal of variability among different women. Although the average intensity of pain increases as labor progresses for most women, nulliparous women often report more pain in early labor whereas multiparous women tend to report more pain in active labor. A few women report consistently low levels of pain throughout labor and birth.[9] In addition, many women report periods during active labor where pain does not increase or when it actually decreases for a short time. In summary, labor pain can be independent of cervical dilatation for both nulliparous and multiparous women and there is a great deal of interindividual variability in the location, intensity, and progression of pain during labor.[6,9]

Predictors of Labor Pain

Several physiologic and demographic characteristics of women are associated with more labor pain. Specifically, women who have severe dysmenorrhea are more likely to have severe labor pain. This outcome may be related to increased prostaglandin synthesis, which results in intense uterine contractions.[6] Pain tends to be worse at night than in the daytime, and unfamiliar settings increase self-reports of pain intensity. Fear of labor and lack of self-efficacy are also associated with severe labor pain. A woman's ability to use mental strategies to cope with labor pain is directly related to her self-confidence in being able to use those strategies.[6]

Women's Experience of Labor and Birth

The goal when caring for women in labor is to facilitate a safe and satisfying birth experience. It is logical to assume that dissatisfaction with labor and birth must solely be derived from complications, such as unrelieved pain or an operative delivery. In actuality, birth satisfaction is a much more complex phenomenon.[12,19]

Birth Satisfaction

In 2002, Hodnett performed a systematic review that analyzed results from 137 studies (both qualitative and quantitative) involving more than 14,000 women to determine the major factors that influence birth satisfaction.[12] This author identified four major components of birth satisfaction: (1) prenatal expectations, (2) support from caregivers, (3) quality of the caregiver–woman relationship, and (4) involvement in decision making. These results have been validated and replicated in multiple studies since the publication of this seminal analysis.

Surprisingly, adequate pain relief is not one of the four factors that affect birth satisfaction. In conclusion, Hodnett stated: "The influences of pain, pain relief and intrapartum medical interventions on subsequent satisfaction are neither as obvious, as direct, nor as powerful as the influence of the attitude and behaviors of the caregivers"[12 p.S160]

Childbirth Connection (formerly Maternity Center Association) administered the Listening to Mothers II national survey in 2006 to women who gave birth in United States hospitals in 2005.[19] The goal of the survey was to obtain a broad understanding of the experience of childbirth in the United States and to identify gaps in care. The Listening to Mothers II survey also corroborated many of Hodnett's findings.[12,19] Specifically, the survey found that women too often feel uninformed and without any degree of self-determination or decision-making power during their labor and birth.

It is clear from the consistent findings of women's reports of their labor experiences that keeping a laboring woman informed not only about labor process, but also about the risks, benefits, and alternatives for any interventions, medications, or procedures is an essential component of care.[20] Cultural humility and respect in all discussions, with consistent mindfulness of the identified four key components of the labor experience that are related to birth satisfaction when discussing comfort/pain relief measures for labor and birth, is essential.

Coping During Labor

One important concept is that pain and coping are not the same thing. Research suggests that for the laboring woman, the ability to cope is more important to birth satisfaction than relief of pain.[21] The typical numerical rating scale (NRS) that is used for pain assessment for most pathological conditions is, therefore, not particularly suitable for use by laboring women or by the professionals who care for them.[20] The NRS is the 0 to 10 scale that is used for most pain conditions for adults in hospital settings in the United States (where 0 is no pain and 10 is the worst possible pain).[22]

Women in labor may be annoyed at being asked how they would rate their pain on a scale of 0 to 10, especially if they have a goal of avoiding pharmacologic methods of pain relief. Yet, adequate pain relief is considered an important patient right by The Joint Commission (formally Joint Commission on Accreditation of Hospitals).[23] Fortunately, alternative algorithms have been developed to assess the more important variable of "coping" for the laboring woman. Gulliver et al. developed a Coping with Labor Algorithm that was pioneered at the University of Utah and better captures the variable of coping for the laboring woman, while at the same time meeting compliance with The Joint Commission standards.[24] This algorithm is presented in **Figure 28-2**. Simply asking "How well are you coping on a scale of 1 to 10?" instead of "How bad is your pain on a scale of 1 to 10?" can generate information the midwife needs most to help a woman during labor.

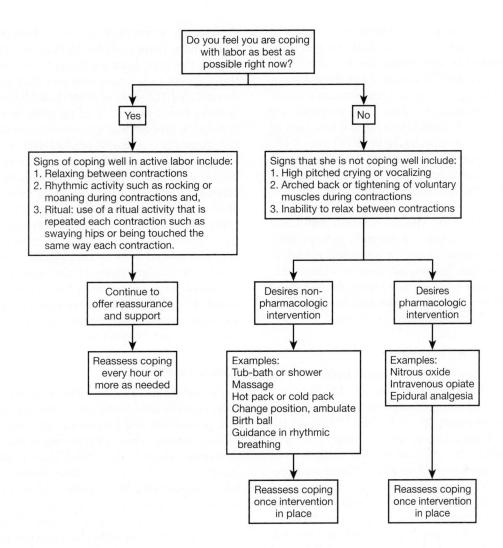

Figure 28-2 Coping with labor algorithm.
Source: Adapted from Roberts L, Gulliver B, Fisher J, Cloyes K. The coping with labor algorithm: an alternate pain assessment tool for the laboring woman. *J Midwifery Womens Health.* 2010;55(2):107-116.

Simkin analyzed the behaviors of women who were coping well in labor and found three consistent behaviors that serve as cues in addition to what the woman tells her caregivers: (1) relaxation during or between contractions, (2) use of a ritual (repeated use of a meaningful rhythmic activity), and (3) rhythmic activity (breathing, rocking, swaying).[25] If a woman is coping well with the pain of labor, then one can reliably presume she is not suffering or experiencing acute emotional distress. The authors noted that "Although pain and suffering often occur together, one may suffer without pain or have pain without suffering...one can have pain coexisting with satisfaction, enjoyment and empowerment. Loneliness, ignorance, unkind or insensitive treatment during labor, along with unresolved past psychological or physical distress, increase the chance that the woman will suffer."[1 p.489]

Signs of not coping well or signs of suffering include crying, thrashing in bed, and inability to focus. Performing a secondary analysis of data from the National Institutes of Health–funded Second Stage Labor Project, Bergstrom et al. reviewed videotapes of 23 women in the second stage of labor who eventually gave birth vaginally. The researchers observed four broad categories of behavior during the second stage: (1) no pain or distress, (2) low-level pain, (3) focused working, and (4) severe pain.[26] In all but the last category, women were able to maintain their sense of self-control.

When pain was severe and women were not able to maintain a sense of self-control, an effective technique identified by the researchers was the "talking down" method. This method has three distinct steps: (1) calling out (getting the woman's attention), (2) positioning very close to the woman's face (en face position), and (3) talking in a low tone of voice so that the woman has to be quiet to hear. The researchers found that when the "talking down" method was used, women went back to a lower level of pain intensity that allowed them to maintain their sense of control.

Women who have effectively coped with labor pain often report a sense of triumph, perhaps analogous to the satisfaction of a marathon runner at the end of a race. In contrast, there is a reasonable assumption that when women report dissatisfaction with their birth experiences, this may be related to a feeling of inability to cope, or "suffering."

Traumatic Birth Experiences

A critical review of the literature from 1977 to 2003 determined that approximately 1% to 6% of women have symptoms consistent with the diagnosis of post-traumatic stress disorder (PTSD) in the immediate postpartum period following birth and approximately 2% continue to have symptoms of PTSD at 6 months postpartum.[27] Consistent predictors of PTSD after birth are preexisting anxiety disorders, obstetric procedures, negative staff interaction, and feelings of loss of control over the birth. More recently, a review of data from the Listening to Mothers II survey found the rate of PTSD after childbirth in women who gave birth in the United States to be approximately 9%.[21,28] More information about postpartum depression is found in the *Mental Health Conditions* chapter.

Prenatal Factors That Influence Labor Pain

Knowledge of the physiology of labor pain and the ability to assess how a woman is coping with labor pain are important but not enough to ensure a midwife has the ability to support women sufficiently in labor. There are multiple antecedents that affect labor pain and many tools to help alleviate it, which are reviewed next.

Women with Childbirth Fear or Anxiety

Fear of childbirth can range from mild anxiety to avoidance of childbearing because the fear is so great; the latter extreme is defined as *tokophobia*. Most of the research on fear of childbirth has been conducted in Northern Europe. Although there is a paucity of data on this topic from the United States, significant fear appears to be more common than previously thought. A 2012 study of more than 2200 women in Norway found that 7.5% of pregnant women who enrolled to give birth at a university hospital identified themselves as fearful of childbirth when given a self-administered, validated questionnaire at 32 weeks' gestation.[29] Subsequently, women who expressed fear of childbirth had a longer mean duration of labor (47 minutes) than those women who did not express fear ($p < 0.001$).[29] The authors suggested that fear-induced elevation of maternal catecholamines may have inhibited uterine contractility, although this conclusion was speculative. Other studies have also examined pregnant women's fear of childbirth and found increased fear is often associated with nulliparity, young maternal age, preexisting psychological conditions, and a history of abuse.[30,31]

Cultural Expectations

Each woman comes into labor with her own cultural expectations, fears, preparation, pain threshold, personality and behavioral makeup, and way of experiencing what is happening to her. The predominant culture in the United States promotes the use of technology as the means to a better birth, even when unsupported by scientific evidence. However, within the United States, there are many different subcultures that vary by race, class, ethnicity, and level of acculturation within the predominant society. Cultural expectations and birth rituals are a part of every community. It is not expected that midwives will be knowledgeable about every possible cultural practice related to the relief of pain in labor; thus asking the woman about her cultural practices can be an important part of the assessment process. An attitude of interest and humility is the most important factor in adapting labor and birth care to a woman's individual cultural practices.

Childbirth Education and Labor Experiences

Throughout much of human history, information about childbirth was handed down from woman to woman, from one generation to the next. Women lived in communities where they supported one another for labor and birth, and passed along their cultural rituals of birth in the United States, an abrupt change to this pattern occurred when childbirth moved to the hospital setting.[32,33]

Accompanying birth in a hospital setting was the advent of "twilight sleep" to relieve labor pain.

Starting around 1914, suffragist groups demanded that twilight sleep be made available to women, citing the relief of pain in childbirth as a women's rights issue.[32] This method of analgesia involved use of the amnesic drug scopolamine, a medication that did not erase the pain of childbirth very well, but rather erased the *memory* of the pain and sometimes even the memory of the birth itself. In the subsequent aftermath of the widespread use of "twilight sleep," some women began to perceive that something was missing from their childbirth experience. Different methods of childbirth preparation were developed as women demanded to become more active and aware participants in their births.

Starting with the first edition of Dick-Read's classic *Childbirth Without Fear* published in the 1930s, various childbirth preparation programs evolved, and by the 1970s childbirth education classes became the *de rigueur* means of obtaining childbirth preparation information.[34] The initial focus of these classes was to reduce the fear–pain–tension cycle with knowledge about the labor process so pain medications could be avoided during labor. Grantly Dick-Read postulated that fear generates physical tension, which in turn increases pain; he also suggested that fear could be alleviated with knowledge and skills. Subsequent natural psychoprophylactic methods of childbearing vary in the emphasis they place on preparatory muscular and breathing exercises, but all educate the woman about the processes of labor and various means of coping with pain, thereby reducing fear.

Despite some differences in methods of teaching and the underlying philosophy of various childbirth preparation programs, common goals exist in educating women and their families:

- To increase knowledge about the physiologic changes of pregnancy and birth
- To increase knowledge about options in preparation for childbirth (e.g., use of nonpharmacologic and pharmacologic means for coping with the pain of labor)
- To increase confidence in one's own level of preparation for birth and parenting
- To provide an opportunity for socialization with other women and their partners[34,35]

How effective is childbirth education? According to a rigorous Cochrane review, "the effects of antenatal education for childbirth or parenthood remain largely unknown," with the researchers citing multiple methodological flaws in the trials that made up their systematic review of this topic, including no information about details of randomization procedures in many studies, and small to moderate sample sizes.[36] However, since publication of the Cochrane review, a large randomized trial that involved intention-to-treat analysis has found some significant benefits of childbirth education. In this study, women were randomly assigned to a group that received 9 hours of formal childbirth education versus a group that received usual care. The researchers found that women in the usual-care group were more likely to be admitted in the active phase of labor and less likely to request epidural analgesia for labor.[37]

Childbirth preparation courses have continued to evolve, as practice styles change. For example, women who participate in group prenatal care such as CenteringPregnancy often receive much of the educational content and socialization that would have typically occurred in conventional childbirth education classes during the course of their care. Modern communication technology is having an impact on childbirth education as well, with programs such as *text4baby* demonstrating effectiveness in helping low-income women feel more confident in their preparation for childbirth. In a randomized, controlled pilot study that involved 123 initial participants who received prenatal care in the setting of an urban county health department, the intervention of receiving regular text messages throughout pregnancy had a significant effect on increased agreement with the statement, "I am prepared to be a new mother" (odds ratio [OR], 2.73; 95% confidence interval [CI], 1.04–7.18).[38]

In conclusion, the knowledge imparted to a woman (or couple) in formal childbirth education classes may empower her with information that will assist her in achieving satisfaction with her care, but to date the overall effect of childbirth education on pain and coping during labor appears to be modest.

General Principles for Comfort Care and Labor Support

In addition to nonpharmacologic techniques and pharmacologic medications, several general principles form the foundation of supporting a woman during labor, including support techniques and basic care activities (**Box 28-1**).

The Environment

The midwife caring for a woman in labor is responsible for creating and maintaining the general environment within the room. An environment that is soothing to the laboring woman is usually one that is quiet, clean and not cluttered, family centered, and

---

BOX 28-1 General Support and Comfort Measures to Mitigate Pain During Labor

Basic Principles
- Ensure privacy and prevent exposure
- Help support persons work effectively
- Use calm, quiet, purposeful communication

Physical Care Activities
- Support relaxation to prevent fatigue
- Help the woman maintain an empty bladder
- Alleviate leg cramps
- Perineal care: keep clean and dry
- Mouth care (sips of fluids, lip moistening)
- Fanning (can use glove package or washcloth)
- Support position changes (e.g., propping pillows as needed)

Support During Vaginal Examinations During Labor

The following steps may help to make vaginal examinations during labor less uncomfortable:
- An empty bladder
- Explanation of why the examination is being performed
- Position of the woman's arms beside her body if comfortable for her
- Help with relaxation breathing and encouragement throughout the examination
- Use of a calm, gentle verbal and physical approach
- Warning and explanation if pain is anticipated before performing the maneuver
- Explanation of findings as the examination is being performed

---

home-like. To promote generalized relaxation, a side-lying position or whatever position the woman finds comfortable may help, as well as bolstering with pillows and blankets, as needed.

Assurance of Privacy and Prevention of Exposure

Assurance of privacy and prevention of exposure are of particular importance in a hospital. Privacy refers to respecting the woman's choice regarding who will be with her. For women who give birth in a hospital, any hospital-based staff should be introduced to the woman personally, so that their first contact, if she grants permission, is person-to-person rather than eyes-to-body. If the woman is assured that her sense of privacy and space will be honored, she will feel

more relaxed. Ideas of modesty vary widely, often according to the woman's culture. Some women may not feel the need to be carefully draped to prevent exposure of external genitals, whereas other women will be uncomfortable exposing their body to anyone other than their partner and need as much draping as possible.

Knowledge: Explanation of the Process and Progress of Labor

Two of the four most important determinants of satisfaction with labor are support from caregivers and the quality of the midwife–woman relationship. The latent phase of labor is an ideal time to assess a woman's understanding about the labor progress, understand her expectations, and learn her goals. Instructional support about what to expect and what she will experience can be shared. This conversation needs to be geared toward her desire for knowledge and presented at her level of health literacy.

If a woman is in active labor at first contact, explanations about labor progress will be necessarily brief. Careful individually tailored explanations can reduce anxiety or fear, which may decrease the pain resulting from tension caused by fear. Explanations are a form of instructional support and, when provided in a culturally sensitive manner, they improve the quality of support between the midwife and the laboring woman by establishing a rapport. Finally, instructional support can help a woman to feel more in control, thereby increasing her sense of satisfaction.[12]

Ideally, the midwife should explore the woman's preferences for labor pain management prenatally. It is important to explore with each woman which comfort measures have worked for her in the past, which measures have not worked, and even which measures could potentially be damaging. For example, touch therapies may not be experienced as comforting for a woman who has a history of sexual abuse, but may be quite comforting for a woman who has previously used massage to decrease discomfort. Prenatal preparation will allow the woman to identify her own personal repertoire of coping resources for stress, anxiety, and pain. How does she deal best with stress and anxiety in her life? If she is unable to identify anything specific, introducing her to the evidence-based options described in this chapter can allow her to "try out" suggestions before the actual event of labor.

Role of Support Persons/Significant Others

In most cultures, women have sought the support of other women while giving birth, whether in the form of other female relatives, midwives, nurses, or doulas. Today women may have no support persons or many support persons with them during their labor. It is the midwife's job to incorporate these individual(s) and facilitate their roles and support activities.

The significant others, partners, and support persons a woman brings with her into the labor setting also experience the highly emotionally charged event. Thus, just as there are known determinants that affect the woman's experience, so too are there specific caretaker activities that affect the experience of the support person (**Figure 28-3**). In a literature review of studies from developed nations, Genrdoni and Tallandini found that fathers frequently feel helpless, anxious, and in need of psychological support during a woman's labor and birth.[39] Although there has been little research on how partners of women in the United States feel about the labor experience, recent data from Sweden found that the factors associated most strongly with a positive birth experience were support from the midwife, the midwife's continuous presence in the delivery room, and information about the progress of labor.[40] The promotion of family-centered care and the facilitation of healthy family relationships are both, in fact, identified as important hallmarks of midwifery practice.[40]

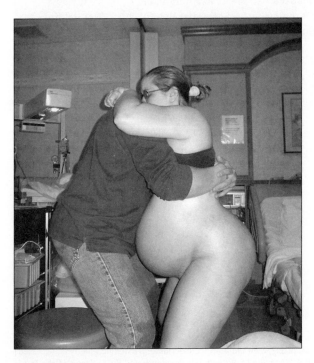

Figure 28-3 Partner supporting woman.
Source: Reprinted with permission from Amy Maschio

Prevention of Exhaustion and Provision for Rest

Prevention of exhaustion and provision for rest between contractions are also important general support and comfort measures. Unnecessary exhaustion can be prevented by the following means:

- Have the woman use the most relaxed form of breathing possible. For example, panting is a physically taxing type of breathing, and should be used only when the goal is to help a woman not bear down. Controlled types of breathing, whether Lamaze or abdominal, can also be tiring if used in early, latent-phase labor before they are needed.

- Organize or plan procedures so that as many as possible are done sequentially in the shortest possible time (or number of intervals between contractions).

- Control the environment in accord with what is most restful to the individual woman. This includes controlling lighting, air, external noises, restriction of loud noises, and room arrangement.

Physical Care to Mitigate Pain

Empty Bladder

A full bladder can impede fetal descent into the birth canal. In addition, a prolonged period of time without normal voiding increases the risk for bladder hypotonicity, urinary stasis, and bladder infection. A full bladder can also accentuate lower abdominal pain—a factor that is often forgotten. Frequent assessment and helping the woman keep her bladder empty are part of the package of basic care activities needed by women in labor and are specifically part of helping them manage pain.

Support During Vaginal Examinations

Box 28-1 describes specific steps that help mitigate the discomfort of a vaginal examination during labor.

Alleviation of Leg Cramps

Cramps in the calf muscles or gluteal muscles during labor are common and can be so acute that they capture the woman's total attention and require immediate relief. A pregnant woman's legs should never be deeply or aggressively massaged secondary to her increased risk for thromboembolism. Instead, straighten her leg and dorsiflex her foot. Alternating relaxation with dorsiflexion of her foot increases the speed of the relief for cramps in calf muscles. The dorsiflexion should be gentle but forcibly exaggerated to effect relief.

Labor Pain Relief Methods Used in the United States

Laboring women can choose many methods of mitigating labor pain. **Table 28-1** presents findings from the second and third national Listening to Mothers surveys (LTM II and LTM III) conducted in 2006 and 2012.[41] This survey interviews women who have given birth in the previous year and provides a wealth of information about birth practices in the United States today. Interestingly, the rate of epidural use appears to be dropping as techniques such as birth balls and nitrous oxide are being adopted. Although epidurals are consistently rated as very helpful by women who use them, other pharmacologic methods such as opioids are not rated as highly as some nonpharmacologic methods such as immersion in water.[19]

Nonpharmacologic Methods of Mitigating Pain

Some nonpharmacologic techniques for addressing labor pain are quite simple, whereas others require specialized training to perform. These techniques are reviewed here in the general order of the evidence for their use, although in some cases comparisons are difficult due to different outcome measures, populations, and experimental designs used for the various studies.

Table 28-2 reviews purported mechanisms of action of each of the following nonpharmacologic methods of labor pain relief.[1]

Continuous Labor Support/Doula Care

Multiple randomized controlled trials (RCTs) have shown that continuous labor support improves labor outcomes and has a positive influence on a woman's childbirth experience.[1,42] The word *doula* is derived from the Greek word *doulē*, meaning "female slave," or "one who serves." Doulas do not have any requisite medical training, but rather are companions for women during labor. Doulas assist women in coping with childbirth. The primary role of the doula is to provide continuous nonmedical care during the woman's' labor, including physical comfort, emotional support (reassurance and encouragement), information (nonmedical advice, anticipatory guidance), and facilitation of communication with health care providers.

Doulas can provide many of the comfort measures during labor that are detailed in this chapter.

Table 28-1	Methods of Pain Relief Used by Women in the United States			
Technique	**Who Used This Technique 2012 (%)**	**Who Used This Technique 2006 (%)**	**It Was Helpful or Somewhat Helpful 2006 (%)**	**It Was Not Helpful 2006 (%)**
Epidural or spinal analgesia	67	76	91	9
Breathing techniques	48	49	77	22
Position changes	40	42	77	24
Mental strategies	21	25	77	23
Opioids	16	22	75	25
Touch or massage	22	20	91	9
Birthing ball	10	7	64	33
Immersion in water	8	6	91	8
Application of hot or cold	12	6	81	17
Changes to environment such as music	2	4	78	22
Shower	10	4	78	19
Nitrous oxide	8	Not assessed		

Source: Adapted from Declercq ER, Sakala C, Corry MP, Applebaum S. *Listening to Mothers II: Results of the Second National U.S. Survey of Women's Childbearing Experiences.* New York: Childbirth Connection; 2006. Available at: http://www.Childbirthconnection.org/listeningtomothers. Accessed January 22, 2013; Declercq ER, Sakala C, Corry MP, Applebaum S, Herrlich A. *Listening to Mothers III: Pregnancy and Birth: Report of the Third National U.S. Survey of Women's Childbearing Experiences.* New York: Childbirth Connection; 2013. Available at: http://transform.childbirth connection.org/wp-content/uploads/2013/06/LTM-III_Pregnancy-and-Birth.pdf. Accessed August 10, 2013.

Table 28-2   Mechanism of Action for Reducing Pain in Selected Nonpharmacologic Methods

Mechanism	Acupuncture/ Acupressure	Aromatherapy	Breathing/ Focus	Childbirth Education	Cold	Emotional Support	Heat	Hydrotherapy	Hypnosis	Intradermal Water Block	Massage/ Touch	Movement & Positioning	Music/ Audioanalgesia	Relaxation	TENS
Counter-irritation analgesia					✓					✓					✓
Increases endorphins	✓									✓			✓		✓
Provides stimuli from peripheral sensory receptors to inhibit pain awareness		✓			✓		✓	✓			✓		✓		✓
Increases joint mobility								✓				✓			
Alters pressures within pelvis and on soft tissue							✓	✓			✓	✓			
Improves energy flow along meridians crucial to labor progress and comfort	✓				✓*										
Decreases muscle tension	✓						✓	✓	✓		✓			✓	
Alters nerve conduction velocity (slows pain transmission to central nervous system)					✓										
Decreases anxiety/fear, provides reassurance		✓	✓	✓		✓			✓		✓	✓	✓	✓	
Increases woman's sense of control, reducing pain perception			✓	✓		✓			✓		✓	✓	✓	✓	✓
Distraction of attention from pain		✓	✓		✓	✓	✓	✓	✓		✓	✓	✓	✓	✓
Enhances or changes mood, reducing pain perception		✓				✓					✓		✓	✓	
Cues rhythmic activity and rituals			✓			✓					✓	✓	✓	✓	

Source: From Simkin P, Bolding A. Update on non-pharmacologic approaches to relieve labor pain and prevent suffering. *J Midwifery Womens Health.* 2004;49:489–505. Reprinted with permission of Wiley.

They sometimes will also provide postpartum support and assistance with breastfeeding and infant care. Doulas have become increasingly important in the provision of continuous labor support, especially for women who give birth in the hospital setting.

The effects of a doula have been evaluated in more than 20 RCTs that have included more than 15,000 women.[42] In addition several meta-analyses have assessed the role of doula care for young, low-income nulliparous women, intermittent versus continuous doula care, and use of nurses as doulas. The overall benefits of doula care include the following:

- Shorter duration of labor (mean duration: −0.58 hour; 95% CI, −0.85 to −0.31)

- Reduced need for pharmacologic pain relief (relative risk [RR], 0.90; 95% CI, 0.84–0.96)

- Lowered risk of operative vaginal births (RR, 0.90; 95% CI, 0.85 to 0.96)

- Lowered risk of cesarean births (RR, 0.78; 95% CI, 0.67 to 0.91)

- Increased likelihood of spontaneous vaginal birth (RR, 1.08; 95% CI, 1.04–1.12)

Findings also include less maternal negative perceptions of childbirth experiences (RR, 0.69; 95% CI, 0.59–0.79). Newborn effects include a reduced risk for low 5-minute Apgar scores (RR, 0.69; 95% CI, 0.50–0.95). There were no significant differences found in the use of synthetic oxytocin, newborn admission to a special care nursery, or breastfeeding at 1 to 2 months postpartum. It is speculated that the emotional support provided by doulas decreases anxiety and fear, mentally distracts women from pain perception, and may increase some mood-elevating neurotransmitters.[1]

Surprisingly, there was no increase in the spontaneous vaginal birth rate when hospital-employed nurses in North America offered doula care as part of an RCT of doula care, although laboring women reported that they did favor continuous labor support from a nurse as opposed to usual care (where the nurse would be assigned to more than one laboring woman).[43] Although it is not known why nurses were unable to replicate the positive effects of nontrained personnel, it is postulated that general rates of intervention in North American hospital settings are stronger variables with regard to vaginal versus operative delivery rates than is the effect of continuous support. The positive effects of continuous support are more robust in settings where other forms of pain relief and support are not available.

Water Immersion/Tub Baths

Midwives in many countries promote the use of water immersion for labor.[44] The Cochrane Collaboration completed a systematic review of the effects of water immersion on labor and birth by examining 12 clinical trials involving more than 3400 women.[45] Water immersion during the first stage of labor was associated with a reduction in the use of epidural/spinal analgesia (RR, 0.90; 95% CI, 0.82–0.99) and a shorter first stage of labor (MD: −32.4 minutes; 95% CI, −58.67 minutes to −6.13 minutes) and no difference in the risk for chorioamnionitis (RR, 0.99; 95% CI, 0.50–1.96). There were no differences in the use of oxytocin, operative vaginal delivery, or adverse neonatal outcomes.

However, in one RCT, women who used water immersion in latent labor had longer labors and were more likely to require pain medication and oxytocin use for labor.[46] It appears that hydrotherapy results in a diminution of uterine activity if used during the latent phase of labor. Thus it may be that this technique is of most benefit for women who are in active labor.

Hydrotherapy has been used as a form of medical treatment for various conditions for many years. The primary mechanism of action comprises an increase in hydrostatic pressure; shift of extracellular fluid into the circulation, which provides a central blood volume bolus; increased cardiac output; and subsequent decrease in circulating catecholamine levels. The tub needs to be deep enough for the water to cover the woman's abdomen. It is postulated that improved blood flow results in improved uteroplacental perfusion and increased uterine efficiency.[47,48]

Acupressure/Acupuncture

Traditional Chinese medicine recognizes acupuncture as a means to correct imbalances in vital energy, also known as "qi," Acupuncture involves the needling of specific points along meridian pathways, thereby stimulating the flow of "qi" for pain reduction. Specific acupuncture points successfully used for labor pain are the large intestine 4 point (also known as the Hoku point) and the bladder 67 point (4 fingerbreadths above the inner malleolus). Explaining the efficacy of acupuncture through the conceptual framework of Western medicine, acupuncture is thought to stimulate the body to produce endogenous opioids (endorphins). Diminution of the stress response may be another mechanism of action underlying acupuncture efficacy.[49,50]

In a Cochrane Collaboration meta-analysis of acupressure and acupuncture for pain relief in labor,[51] both acupressure and acupuncture were associated with significant decreases in pain and a lower risk for operative vaginal delivery (RR, 0.67; 95% CI, 0.46–0.98) and cesarean section (RR, 0.24; 95% CI, 0.11–0.54).[52]

Midwives who are knowledgeable about acupressure points can easily incorporate this knowledge into care for a laboring woman by stimulating the acupressure LI4 point (**Figure 28-4**) with thumb and forefinger pressure during contractions (or helping the woman to stimulate the point herself) with the use of an ice or cold pack wrapped in a washcloth.[53] The services of a licensed acupuncturist must be obtained to perform actual needling of points. In some areas, licensed acupuncturists may be difficult to find, and some institutions may not grant privileges for acupuncture practice.

A theoretical risk of acupuncture would be possible infection if sterile needles are not used, although any licensed practitioner would be expected to use sterile needles. Contraindications to the use of the Hoku or bladder 67 acupressure/acupuncture points would be preterm gestation or any other clinical condition that would make uterine contractions contraindicated (such as placenta previa).

Sterile Water Injections

Sterile water injections, or sterile water papules, involve intradermal injections of sterile water administered in four places in the lower lumbosacral area of the back to form papules. The goal is to specifically relieve back pain in labor. It is speculated that sterile water injections work by providing noxious

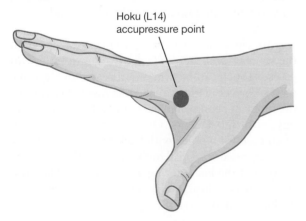

Hoku (LI4)
accupressure point

Figure 28-4 Correct positioning of small ice bag for massage stimulation of LI4.
Source: Reprinted with permission from Waters B JMWH 2004.

stimulation of nociceptors that results in a subsequent release of endorphins and stimulation of A-delta fibers, which overwhelm the visceral sensations transmitted to the brain by the slower C fibers. This hypothesis is based on the gate-control theory. A 25-gauge needle with 0.6 to 1.0 mL of sterile water is used to inject 0.1 to 0.15 mL of sterile water at each of the four sites described in **Appendix 28A**. Women experience an intense stinging sensation for approximately 30 to 90 seconds during (and immediately following) the injection and then relief from their back pain for approximately 2 to 3 hours.

Sterile water injections have been found to significantly reduce severe back pain. Nevertheless, the overall need for additional pain medication is not reduced, presumably because the effect dissipates before the labor is concluded. Derry et al. performed a meta-analysis of seven RCTs and concluded that the evidence is insufficient to recommend this practice, due to perceived limitations of the studies involved.[54] In contrast, the meta-analysis of eight RCTs performed by Hutton et al. found sterile water papules associated with a significant reduction in Visual Analog Scores (VAS) for pain in women and a decreased rate of cesarean births in the sterile water group (4.6%) versus the comparison groups (9.9%) (RR, 0.51; 95% CI, 0.30–0.87).[55]

Position Changes/Ambulation

During labor, a woman should assume whatever position is the most comfortable for her. When women are not confined to bed or acculturated to believe they should be in bed, they frequently change positions throughout the course of labor. Pelvic dimensions change with various postures, and maternal movement (such as walking, dancing, or swaying) is thought to facilitate optimal fetal positioning (**Figure 28-5**). Contraindications to ambulation and movement would include ruptured membranes with high fetal station and presenting part not well applied to cervix, or any other condition for which bedrest is necessary.

The many studies that have compared upright to recumbent positions during labor have found that in early labor, upright positions are associated with the least pain and supine positions are the most painful. In active labor, women tend to prefer side-lying positions. Women who use upright positions are less likely to use epidural analgesia, and upright positions appear to shorten labor by approximately a mean of 1 hour, which is statistically significant but only modestly clinically significant.[56]

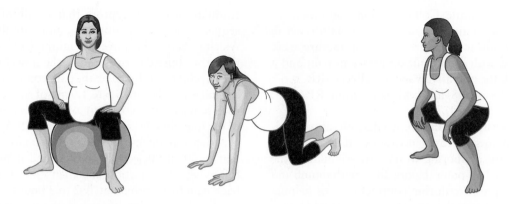

Figure 28-5 Positions for laboring women.

The effect of upright positions during the second stage of labor is interesting. A meta-analysis of women who did not have epidural analgesia and who assumed upright positions in the second stage of labor ($n = 7280$; 22 RCTs) revealed that they did not have shorter second stages but did have fewer operative vaginal deliveries, fewer abnormal fetal heart rate patterns, fewer episiotomies but more second-degree lacerations, and an increased risk of an estimated blood loss of more than 500 mL.[57] Clinically, these findings suggest that upright positions have benefits but that preserving the perineum at birth may be technically more difficult.

Birthing Ball

A physiotherapy or "birth ball" is a recent addition to the pantheon of nonpharmacologic methods of mitigating labor pain. A physiotherapy ball of the right size and sturdiness can withstand the woman's weight and use for labor. Generally a 65-centimeter ball is the right size for women more than 5 feet 5 inches tall and a 55-centimeter ball is the right size for women less than 5 feet 5 inches tall. The ball is then adjusted for an individual "fit" by adding or letting out air so that it is firm but gives to the touch, and rolls easily, with the woman's legs being bent at a 90-degree angle when sitting on the ball. Women sit on the ball with their feet about 2 feet apart and flat on the floor. Good posture is necessary to maintain balance on the ball. This puts the woman in an upright position from which she can rotate her hips in a circular or figure of eight pattern that both relieves back pain and encourages fetal descent. A woman can also sit on the ball and lean forward or use a birthing ball to lean against either in a kneeling (ball on floor) or standing (ball on a bed or table) position. This supports the woman's body and provides a position in which the mother can rest. It also aligns the long axis of the uterus and the fetus with the mother's pelvis and facilitates occiput anterior positions.

Research on the effect of the birth ball on pain is limited to a few RCTs with a small number of subjects, yet results have been consistent in that women who use the birth ball report lower pain scores when compared to women who do not use the birth ball during labor. More research is needed about this method.

Touch and Massage

Massage and touch significantly reduce pain intensity during the first stage of labor (standardized mean difference: -0.82; 95% CI: -1.17 to -0.47; $n = 225$).[58] However, studies that have evaluated the use of massage or touch have used many different methods, so it is not clear exactly which massage or touch techniques are the most helpful. In addition, touching is effective only if the woman is comfortable being touched. Even women who do not like to be touched, however, may find holding the hand of a midwife or doula reassuring.

Touching can be extremely effective when both the toucher and the touched are comfortable with its use. Touch can be firm and repeated in a specific pattern or very light (called effleurage). Massage of the foot can be informal or part of a formal reflexology set of movements. One specific form of touch often used for women with back pain is firm, steady counterpressure applied to the center of the sacroiliac portion of the back during a contraction. The pressure increases during the contraction and decreases as the contraction wanes.

Hypnosis

Hypnosis employs specific mind–body techniques that are used to induce profound relaxation. The goal of using hypnosis during labor is to induce a state of deep relaxation within a state of focused attention, thereby reducing perception of external stimuli and increasing receptivity to specific suggestions by the hypnotist. An example of a hypnotic pain relief technique would be imagining "glove anesthesia"; in other words, the laboring woman can imagine that her hand is numb and that by placing her hand on other areas of her body, she can also make those areas numb.[59]

Studies that have evaluated the use of hypnosis to mitigate labor pain have yielded conflicting findings to date.[60] It appears that women who practice self-hypnotic techniques during the prenatal period may reduce the use of analgesia during labor and have shorter labors when compared to women who use other childbirth preparation techniques. The beneficial effects of introducing hypnosis for the first time to women in labor, however, have not been confirmed.[61]

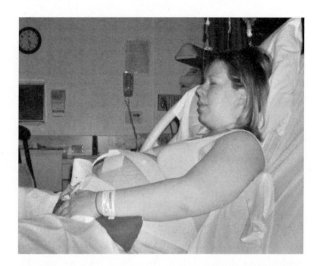

Figure 28-6 Woman with warm pack to abdomen.
Source: Courtesy of Kimberly Trout and Sarah Martyn

Transcutaneous Electrical Nerve Stimulation

TENS uses a low-voltage electric current to stimulate nerves. The device is applied to the skin and battery operated to provide electric stimulation that is lower than what is needed to generate a motor response. The mechanism of action of TENS is based on the gate-control theory of pain, in that transcutaneous stimulation of A-delta nerve fibers purportedly increases endorphins and prevents transmission of pain from the periphery to the brain by closing the synapse in the dorsal horn that transmits pain signals from C fibers.

TENS has been used to treat chronic pain conditions, but its efficacy is unclear. Women who use TENS in labor have not reported lower pain scores overall, nor have they used less analgesia; nevertheless, women who use TENS are less likely to report severe pain and may request analgesia later in labor.[62] It is theorized that the TENS treatment may work for labor pain temporarily, and may produce best effects if started early in labor, when a buildup of endorphins can be most helpful. TENS has also been used to treat postoperative incision pain and may be of some value for women who have cesarean sections.

Application of Heat/Cold

Heat applied to the lower abdomen or the woman's lower back in the area where the fetal head presses against the spine may decrease pain (**Figure 28-6**). Topical application of heat increases circulation to the area, thereby combating tissue anoxia. Caution is warranted, however: Burns can be caused by using too high a temperature or by putting heat on an area

to which creams or ointments have already been applied. It is recommended that at least one layer of cloth be placed between the woman's skin and hot or cold pack, and that the pack be tested on an arm or other portion of skin by someone other than the laboring woman before being placed against her skin. Using a microwave to heat hot packs can be particularly dangerous, as microwaves heat elements at different temperatures; thus the hot pack can be differentially heated in different places within the pack.

Some women have found that the application of cold decreases the pain when heat does not. Supposedly, the relief secondary to topical application of cold results from a numbing effect, probably due to superficial vasoconstriction. Some women find alternating heat and cold comforting. To date, no RCTs have evaluated the use of heat and cold, so further study is needed to determine if either approach is truly efficacious. Contraindications to use of cold include sickle cell anemia, cold hypersensitivities, cryoglobulinemia, Raynaud's phenomenon, and cultural proscriptions.[1] Fever is a contraindication to using heat. Use of heat or cold should also be avoided in the dermatomes anesthetized by an epidural due to concern that women may not be able to perceive if the temperature is too hot or cold.

Breathing and Relaxation Exercises

Breathing and relaxation exercises can help a woman in labor by decreasing her anxiety and fear, and increasing her sense of control or self-efficacy.[1] Thus use of these techniques is directly related to childbirth satisfaction, and they are essential components of most childbirth education programs.[1] Approximately 48% of women in the United States use breathing and relaxation methods during labor, and 77% of those women report that these techniques were either somewhat helpful or very helpful.[19] Practice may play a large role in how well these techniques work. Specific breathing techniques work best in early labor but do not help women cope with labor well if introduced for the first time during active labor.

Breathing techniques that focus on progressive relaxation may be more effective than specific types of breathing patterns. Progressive relaxation can be practiced prenatally, so that the woman can quickly relax between contractions during labor. A knowledgeable caregiver can also teach some relaxation techniques during labor. **Box 28-2** reviews specific breathing techniques that midwives can use to help women relax between contractions.

Audioanalgesia and Aromatherapy

Audioanalgesia may positively affect pain perception via elevation of mood and an increase in pain tolerance.[63] Audioanalgesia can also cue women to breathe rhythmically. Like favored scents, music is extremely personal. The extreme variation in personal choices may account for the lack of sufficient evidence to make recommendations for the use of music for labor support. Studies that have found music is effective for managing labor pain have been hampered by small sample sizes. Clearly, further study is needed before recommendations can be made, although no evidence of harm has been shown with the use of music in labor.

Aromatherapy uses concentrated essential oils from plants for therapeutic properties. It is used to decrease fear, pain, anxiety, and nausea and vomiting. Rose oil has been rated as more helpful than lavender or frankincense by laboring women, and approximately 50% of the women who used it liked it.[64] However, aromatherapy has not been shown to lower pain scores or affect any aspect of labor progress. In addition, volatile oils can cause nausea or headache, so their use should be tried by the woman prior to labor.[64]

BOX 28-2 Breathing Techniques

Breathing/relaxation exercises may help a woman in labor by also decreasing anxiety and fear and increasing her sense of control.[1] It is best if breathing techniques are practiced during the prenatal period so that they are more familiar during labor, but they can also be taught in early labor for the woman who has had no prior preparation.

Progressive Relaxation

This type of relaxation can be practiced so that a woman can quickly will herself to relax her muscles between contractions. The exercise involves deliberately tightening a single muscle group (e.g., hand, arm, leg, face) as tight as possible and then letting it go as limp as possible. Muscles are tightened sequentially and progressively from one end of the body to the other.

Deep Breath and Sigh After Each Contraction

This relaxation can be taught when a woman is in active labor. It consists simply of the woman taking a deep breath and letting it all out in "a big heavy sigh" after the contraction is over. This serves a double function: It promotes relaxation and it acts as a cleansing breath to counteract any possible hyperventilation during the contraction or to break a pattern of rapid breathing at this time. Relaxation is further promoted if the woman has a mental image of how she should look and feel after her sigh. For example: "Let yourself sink into the bed and be loose like a rag doll."

Abdominal Breathing

Abdominal breathing involves taking a deep breath in which the woman imagines filling her *belly* with air, and then releasing that air.

Panting

During transition, the woman may no longer be able to do abdominal breathing, and she can be taught to pant–pant–blow or a superficial chest breathing for use during the contraction. This type of breathing has one caution: If she breathes rapidly and deeply from her chest (which is what often happens as part of the sympathetic nervous system's "fight or flight" response to pain), she can easily hyperventilate.

Panting is also used when a woman has an urge to push and the midwife wants her to avoid pushing, for example:

1. To deliver the head of the fetus between contractions. The woman may be instructed to pant through her contraction and then push without a contraction.
2. If the cord is wrapped tightly around the infant's neck after the head is born the midwife may not want the mother to push until the nuchal cord has been reduced.

Pharmacologic Methods of Mitigating Pain

Midwives do not exclusively care for women who want unmedicated births. The term *unmedicated* as used in this chapter refers specifically to not using pain medications during labor. Medications such as antibiotics or any other necessary medications should always be used as recommended. Women can be knowledgeable and prepared; want active participation in the natural, normal process of childbearing; and yet still desire to use medication to mitigate labor pain. The goal of midwifery care is a safe, satisfying birth experience for each woman, based on her individual goals. As Varney Burst stated in an editorial on "real" midwifery:

> If we believe that every woman has the right to receive care from a midwife, then the practice of midwifery must encompass all women regardless of their normalcy or risk status, the setting in which they receive their care, or the practices within that setting.... Real midwifery is "with woman," wherever she may be, in whatever circumstances she may be in, in whatever condition her pregnancy, in whatever health care system.[65]

Medication may be used during labor to relieve pain, decrease anxiety and apprehension, provide sedation, or control nausea and vomiting. All medications used by laboring women must be evaluated for (1) effectiveness, (2) safety for the laboring woman, (3) safety for the fetus and newborn, and (4) effects on labor progress. Prior to administering any medication during labor, a careful assessment of the woman's vital signs, fetal heart rate pattern, other medications being used, and stage of labor should be made and documented. The choice of medication will be tailored to the degree of pain relief the woman wants to attain and what is safe for the stage of labor she is in. Medications used to treat labor pain can be systemic, inhaled, or neuraxial.

Systemic Medications

Systemic medications were the mainstay of drugs used to assist laboring women for most of the first half of the twentieth century. The primary limitation to these drugs is that they adversely affect the fetus to varying degrees.

Sedatives and Hypnotics

As reviewed in the *Complications During Labor and Birth* chapter, helping women who have a prolonged prelabor or latent phase of labor remain comfortable can be difficult. Sedatives and hypnotics are most often used to facilitate sleep and augment the pain relief provided by morphine when it is used to treat prolonged latent-phase labor. These medications also lessen nausea and vomiting, a side effect of morphine. The most common combination for treating prolonged latent-phase labor is 10 mg morphine sulfate and 50 mg of promethazine (Phenergan) given intramuscularly.

There is some controversy about the effect of sedatives on labor pain. Two randomized trials compared meperidine (Demerol) with promethazine (Phenergan) to meperidine alone and found the combination of meperidine with promethazine did not improve pain relief over meperidine alone.[66] Promethazine does, however, produce significant sedation, which results in women appearing as though they are in less pain but may actually just prevent them from communicating their level of pain. Thus, although anecdotally the combination of an opiate with a sedative results in pain relief potentiation, this potentiation effect has not been unambiguously proven. Sedatives and hypnotics should be used with caution.

Opiates

The opiates most commonly used to treat labor pain are listed in **Table 28-3**. These drugs are readily available and fast acting. There is no apparent effect on labor progress if they are administered during the active phase of labor. Some women feel an unwelcome loss of control after being given an opiate, although this is not common. More common side effects include euphoria and sedation. Potential side effects include nausea and vomiting and urinary retention. Opiates can cause respiratory depression, but this outcome is rare with the doses and methods of administration typically used to treat labor pain.

All opiates are lipid soluble, so they cross the placenta easily and concentrate in the fetus. Fetal effects include decreased fetal heart rate variability and neonatal respiratory depression; in addition, there is controversy about whether opiates adversely affect early neurobehavioral scores in the newborn.

Until recently, meperidine (Demerol) was the most frequently used opiate for treating labor pain worldwide; now, however, it has largely fallen out of favor. Meperidine does not provide strong pain relief and when women who have used it are queried, more than half report that it was ineffective.[66] In addition, meperidine has a long half-life and active metabolites, so its use is associated with a high risk of neonatal respiratory depression. Infants exposed to

Table 28-3	Opioid Doses for Management of Pain During Active Labor				
Opioid Generic (Brand)	IM Dose (Dose/Peak/ Duration)	IV Dose (Dose/Peak/ Duration)	Agonist Effect	Maternal Side Effects	Fetal/ Neonatal Effects
Fentanyl (Sublimaze)	50–100 mcg/ 1–2 hours/ 1–2 hours Maximum dose usually 500–600 mcg	50–100 mcg/ 3–5 minutes/ 1–2 hours Maximum dose usually 500–600 mcg	Pure agonist at mu receptor,[a] kappa receptor,[b] sigma receptor,[c] and delta receptor[d]	Short-acting; less effective than morphine or Demerol, but very few side effects noted	None reported
Meperidine (Demerol)	75 mg/ 40–50 minutes/ 2–4 hours	75–80 mg/ 5 minutes/ 2–4 hours	Pure agonist at mu and kappa receptors	Nausea and vomiting, urinary retention, respiratory depression, sedation	Respiratory depression 1–4 hours after dose; effect is independent of dose Neonatal developmental depression 20–60 hours after last dose
Morphine	10 mg/ 1–2 hours/ 2–4 hours	2.5–5 mg/ 20 minutes/ 2–4 hours	Pure agonist at mu and kappa receptors	Pruritus, nausea and vomiting, urinary retention, respiratory depression[e]	Decreased fetal heart rate variability Cumulative effect respiratory depression
Butorphanol (Stadol)	2 mg/ 30–60 minutes/ 3–4 hours	1–2 mg/ 30 minutes/ 2–4 hours	Kappa agonist and sigma agonist	Ceiling effect	Transient pseudo-sinusoidal fetal heart rate pattern
Nalbuphine (Nubain)	10–20 mg/ 30–60 minutes/ 2–4 hours	10–20 mg/ 30–60 minutes/ 2–4 hours	Mu antagonist and kappa partial agonist	Ceiling effect	Transient pseudo-sinusoidal fetal heart rate pattern

[a]Mu-receptor stimulation causes slowed gastrointestinal motility, nausea and vomiting, respiratory depression, spinal and supraspinal analgesia, sedation, urinary retention, pruritus, and euphoria.

[b]Kappa-receptor stimulation causes sedation, spinal analgesia, and miosis.

[c]Sigma-receptor stimulation causes dysphoria, hallucination, and mydriasis.

[d]Delta-receptor stimulation causes spinal and supraspinal analgesia.

[e]Morphine causes more pruritus and urinary retention when administered via epidural or intrathecally. Maternal respiratory depression can be a late effect in epidurally administered morphine sulfate secondary to slow uptake into the CNS.

meperidine have lower Apgar scores, more difficulty establishing breastfeeding, and less alert behavior.

Morphine and fentanyl (Sublimaze) are the two mu-opioid receptor agonists commonly used in the United States. Morphine is used to treat prolonged latent labor, as it decreases uterine activity prior to active labor but does not inhibit active labor contractions. Fentanyl can be used to decrease the pain of active labor because it has a very short half-life and, therefore, has not been associated with neonatal respiratory depression.

Butorphanol (Stadol) and nalbuphine (Nubain) are kappa-receptor agonists and mu-receptor antagonists. Anecdotally, these drugs provide better pain relief than fentanyl, and they have a longer period of duration. Both are contraindicated for use by women who have a history of drug abuse or addiction because the mu-receptor antagonist effect can elicit withdrawal symptoms.

Naloxone (Narcan) is the opioid antagonist given to the newborn to reverse the respiratory depression effect of opiates given during labor. All midwives who use opiate medications should have naloxone available and know the dose and expected response. The dose is 0.01 mg/kg of body weight, and the effect becomes evident 2 to 5 minutes after an intramuscular injection and 1 to 2 minutes after an intravenous injection. The peak effect occurs in 5 to 15 minutes.[67]

Inhaled Analgesics: 50:50 Nitrous Oxide/Oxygen

The combination of 50% nitrous oxide and 50% oxygen (N_2O/O_2) as an inhalation analgesic has only recently been reintroduced in the United States; in contrast, it is in widespread use in Northern Europe and Canada. This agent is widely considered both safe and effective.[68,69] Nitrous oxide is a weak anesthetic when used in high doses and has an analgesic and anxiolytic effect at low doses.[68] For labor anagesia, it is administered as a 50:50 N_2O/O_2 mixture. The mixture is blended in a machine attached to nitrous oxide and oxygen tanks or attached to piped nitrous oxide and oxygen if the hospital has these gases available in labor rooms (**Figure 28-7**). N_2O/O_2 can be used as the sole analgesic or can be administered in combination with opioids or opioid agonist-antagonists.

Women have generally reported satisfaction with the use of N_2O/O_2 for pain relief in labor. The analgesic effect of N_2O/O_2 is relatively mild with the doses used for labor, but in combination with the anxiolytic effect, it effectively reduces the perception of pain.[69] An additional factor that may contribute to the decreased perception of pain is, at least in part, secondary to maternal control, as N_2O/O_2 is self-administered.

Self-administration is not only empowering for the woman, but also acts as a safety mechanism (**Figure 28-8**) because it is almost impossible to overdose with N_2O/O_2 when it is self-administered. Guidelines for use of this agent are listed in **Table 28-4**.

Potential side effects of N_2O/O_2 include nausea and vomiting, dizziness, and dysphoria, although the occurrence of these side effects is rare. Administration of N_2O/O_2 must occur in settings where scavenging of the exhaled gases is possible to avoid contamination of the environment. No fetal heart rate abnormalities have been attributed to its use.[70] Adverse effects on the fetus or newborn have not been seen in the extensive history of this agent as a labor analgesic but there are some theoretical risks associated with higher doses than those used for labor analagesia that have not been well studied. Likewise there are

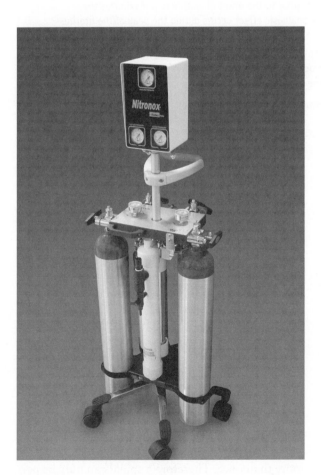

Figure 28-7 A nitrous oxide machine.
Source: Courtesy of Porter Instrument Division, Parker Hannifin Corp.

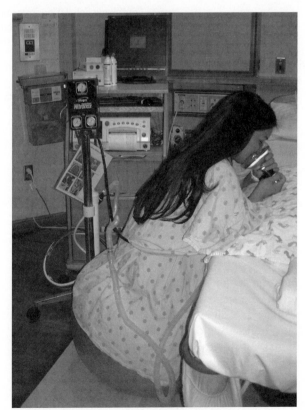

Figure 28-8 Woman using 50:50 nitrous oxide/oxygen for pain relief during labor.
Source: Courtesy of Judith Bishop, CNM, MPH, MSNg

Table 28-4	Clinical Application: Use of 50% N₂O/O₂ for Labor Analgesia
Steps	**Description**
Precautions	1. Determine that there are no contraindications such as inability to hold face mask, impaired oxygenation, or hemodynamic instability.
	2. Use with caution if other sedating drugs are administered concomitantly.
Preparation	1. Inform the woman of the potential side effects of nausea, vomiting, and/or dizziness.
	2. Instruct her on how to hold the mask so it creates a seal; instruct her on timing of inhalation.
	3. Review with the woman and any labor support persons that only the woman can hold the mask.
	a. Sedation from N₂O/O₂ is possible only if the woman continues to inhale the gas after she can no longer hold the mask tightly to her face. N₂O/O₂ dissipates rapidly with exhalation and the effects resolve very quickly.
	b. Self-administration gives the woman personal control of management of pain, and this control may potentiate the analgesic effect.
Procedure	1. The woman holds mask over her mouth and nose, creating a seal that allows activation of a second-stage regulator.
	2. She begins breathing the gas 30 seconds before a contraction starts because the onset of action is approximately 30 seconds and the full analgesic effect occurs in 50 seconds. It often takes three to four contractions to learn the correct technique.
	3. She should exhale into the mask to facilitate scavenging.
Intermittent versus continuous inhalation	1. Intermittent inhalation 30 seconds prior to the onset of contraction maximizes the peak effect of N₂O/O₂ so the peak analgesic effect occurs during the peak of the uterine contraction.
	2. Continuous inhalation is easier to initiate, but in this scenario the woman is exposed to the effects of the gas between contractions when the central nervous system effects of dizziness or dysphoria could be bothersome.

Source: Rooks JP. Safety and risks of nitrous oxide labor analgesia: a review. *J Midwifery Women's Health.* 2011;56:557-565. Reprinted with permission of Wiley.

no risks to healthcare personnel who are in a room where N₂O/O₂ is being used.[69]

Neuraxial Analgesia

Neuraxial analgesia encompasses both epidural and spinal analgesic techniques. These pain relief methods are performed by anesthesia specialists (nurse anesthetists and anesthesiologists), and the specific technique depends on the needs of the laboring woman as well as the availability and choice of the anesthetist. Regional analgesic techniques include spinal (intrathecal injection), epidural, or combined spinal/epidural injections. The effect depends on where the medication is placed, which medications are used, and what dose is administered.

Spinal Analgesia

With spinal anesthesia, a medication is placed in the intrathecal (subarachnoid) space that contains cerebrospinal fluid, spinal nerves, and blood vessels, all of which are enclosed by the membrane of the dura mater. Small doses of opioids are placed into the intrathecal space for relief of labor pain. Spinal analgesia provides excellent relief within a few moments and the effect lasts approximately 90 minutes.

Spinal analgesia has no effect on motor ability, so women can ambulate or assume any position they want. It is often called "the walking epidural" despite the fact that this technique does not deliver analgesia into the epidural space. Spinal analgesia is associated with transient fetal heart rate abnormalities such as prolonged decelerations and a transient increase in uterine contractions and uterine tone.[71] Thus close observation of the fetal heart rate is necessary for a period of time after the injection. The major drawback to spinal analgesia is that it requires a dural puncture, which is not safe to do more than once. Therefore a spinal can only be performed once and because it is not easy to predict when during labor a woman will need analgesia the most, spinal analgesia is not used as often as is epidural analgesia.

Side effects of intrathecal analgesia include pruritus or nausea and vomiting, which occur secondary to the effect of the opioid rather than the technique itself. Pruritus (skin itching) is the most common side effect, occurring in varying degrees of severity in 50% to 90% of women. Diphenhydramine (Benadryl; 25 mg given intravenously) can be of value in this situation, or in severe cases naloxone (Narcan) can be administered with caution. If naloxone is needed, the anesthetic effect of the spinal analgesia will also be reversed. Urinary retention and respiratory depression are less common side effects.

Spinal analgesia is more often today used as part of a combination spinal/epidural, wherein the spinal technique is used to inject a small dose of opioid and, as the needle is withdrawn, a catheter is placed in the epidural space. When the spinal analgesia wears off, medication is injected to initiate epidural analgesia.

Epidural Analgesia

Over the past three decades, the use of epidural analgesia/anesthesia for managing labor pain has dramatically increased due to improvement in the techniques, greater access to the procedure, and consumer demand.

Overall, epidurals provide the most effective relief of labor pain compared to opiates and inhalation anesthetics. Women using epidurals have lower pain scores and are more satisfied with their analgesia than women using parenteral opioids when the experience of pain is evaluated.[72]

Mechanism of Action

The epidural space is exterior to the dura mater, bounded posteriorly by the ligamentum flavum. It contains nerve roots, fat, lymphatics, and blood vessels. Some of the individual differences noted in the quality of neuraxial blocks, despite use of consistent technique, may reflect individual anatomic variations that occur in the epidural space, such as nerve root size or the presence of membranes that disallow equal spread of the medication to all nerves passing through the epidural space (**Figure 28-9**).

The effect of epidural analgesia depends greatly on the drug and dose that are placed in the epidural space. Bupivicaine is an amide local anesthetic with a long duration of action. Bupivacaine provides an excellent sensory block, while preserving some motor function when used at low doses. A concentration of 0.25% or 0.5% is often used for labor analgesia. Fentanyl and remifentanil are synthetic opioids with

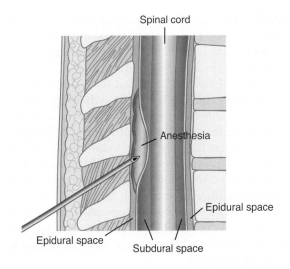

Figure 28-9 Epidural space.

a potency 100 times greater than that of morphine; one of these opioids is frequently added to the anesthetic to augment the analgesic effect. The anesthetic and opioids are extremely lipid soluble and can cross into the fetal circulation in small amounts depending upon what gets into the maternal circulation. Although the doses of opiates used for spinal and epidural analgesia are fairly low, respiratory depression, nausea, vomiting, and pruritus in the woman, as well as fetal depression, can potentially occur.

Indications and Contraindications

Indications for the use of epidural analgesia/anesthesia include relief of pain in active labor, operative vaginal birth, cesarean section, and need to diminish maternal expulsive efforts (e.g., maternal cardiac or ophthalmologic disease). Epidural analgesia also allows the woman to rest during a protracted, exhaustive labor.

If a woman's medical or obstetric condition places her at increased risk for needing an emergent cesarean section, an epidural may be recommended to avoid any loss of time if the emergency does, in fact, occur. This "double setup" is often done, for example, if membranes must be ruptured when the fetal presenting part is not in the pelvis, for a vaginal breech birth, or for a woman with a multiple gestation. If a woman requires an operative vaginal delivery and does not have an epidural, it may be initiated prior to application of the vacuum or forceps.

Effective analgesia can also be helpful for women who have a history of sexual abuse. For some of these women, labor brings great anxiety about painful stimuli in the vaginal/rectal area, and/or flashbacks of abusive events. Thus the "numbing" effect of an epidural can mitigate some aspects of the post-traumatic stress caused by labor and birth.

Absolute contraindications to epidural or spinal anesthesia include refusal or inability to cooperate, skin or soft-tissue infection at the site of needle placement, frank coagulopathy, untreated sepsis, and maternal hemodynamic instability. Relative contraindications include heparin therapy or a low platelet count, and neurologic disease of the spinal cord. In addition, women with the conditions listed in **Box 28-3** should be offered consultation with an anesthesia provider prior to labor. Contrary to popular belief, a tattoo is not a contraindication to epidural analgesia.

Informed Decision Making

Some authors have suggested that informed consent or refusal is difficult to obtain when a woman is in acute pain or under the influence of intravenous opioids.[73] However, a woman is able to give informed consent if she understands the nature and purpose of the procedure, the consequences of declining, and the alternative interventions. Women in active labor are able to give consent for neuraxial analgesia.

BOX 28-3 Risk Factors Indicating the Need for an Anesthesia Consult Prior to Labor

- Scoliosis, spina bifida, or other spinal column abnormalities
- Previous back surgery
- Arthritides
- Preexisting tracheostomy
- Neurologic or neuromuscular disease (e.g., multiple sclerosis or muscular dystrophy)
- Cardiac disease
- Pulmonary disease other than mild asthma
- Low platelet counts (≤ 100,000) or use of anticoagulants in pregnancy
- Coagulopathies
- Any history of complications with an epidural or other anesthetic
- Family history of major anesthesia complications
- Allergy to anesthetics
- Morbid obesity (BMI > 40)

The anesthetic provider will review the risks, benefits, side effects, adverse effects, and alternative therapies prior to initiating the procedure. However, midwives who care for women with epidurals should know the effects of this procedure and be prepared to manage complications. Often the anesthesia provider focuses on maternal risks associated with the procedure or the block, while the obstetric provider addresses the effect of neuraxial analgesia on labor progress and the fetus or newborn.

Preparation of the Woman for Epidural Analgesia

All women requiring epidural analgesia/anesthesia will receive a bolus of intravenous fluids prior to administration of the anesthetic drug to prevent maternal hypotension, which is an expected side effect of the vasodilation caused by the regional block. Continuous electronic fetal monitoring is required. The epidural catheter can be placed with the woman in either a side-lying position or sitting at the side of the bed. After identifying the L2–L3, L3–L4, or L4–L5 interspace, the area is cleansed using sterile technique. A small amount of local anesthetic is injected to numb the skin, followed by insertion of a 17-gauge Tuohy needle, until a loss of resistance is felt and the epidural space is reached. Local anesthetic alone is instilled as a test dose, to ensure that the needle is not inadvertently placed intrathecally or intravenously. Once correct placement is confirmed, a catheter is threaded through the needle to the epidural space and secured to the woman's back.

Intrathecal or Intravenous Injection

Inadvertent intrathecal (subarachnoid) or intravascular placement can result in toxicity as described in **Table 28-5**.[74] Total spinal anesthesia occurs in 0.03% of cases when the level of the anesthesia rises dangerously high, resulting in paralysis of the respiratory muscles including the diaphragm. When this occurs, the woman will suffer anxiety, numbness of the hands and fingers, and dyspnea. Treatment is accomplished with assisted respiration until the anesthesia resolves.

Intermittent Versus Continuous Versus Patient-Controlled Epidural Analgesia

Additional medication can be given through the epidural catheter in intermittent boluses, in a continuous small dose by pump, or by patient-controlled epidural analgesia (PCEA). Evidence supports the use of PCEA, which appears to result in greater maternal satisfaction (along with greater maternal sense of control) and lower overall medication requirements.[75] The combination of a local anesthetic and

Table 28-5	Signs of Toxicity Following Epidural Injection
Placement of Anesthetic	**Signs and Symptoms of Toxicity**
Intrathecal	Rapid cephalad spread of anesthesia
	Profound hypotension
	Respiratory depression
	Loss of consciousness
Intravascular	Tinnitus
	Dizziness
	Metallic taste in the mouth
	Disorientation
	Seizures
	Cardiac dysrhythmias
	Cardiac arrest

opioid injected into the epidural space has been found to offer excellent pain relief with less of a motor block than when anesthetic is used alone. In addition, a smaller overall dose of anesthetic can be used.[76]

Maternal Side Effects and Adverse Effects of Neuraxial Analgesia

Side effects related to local anesthetics include hypotension, urinary retention, and leg numbness and weakness, all of which are attributable to relaxation of muscle tone. Side effects related to performance of the procedure include postdural puncture headaches, back pain, and, very rarely, epidural abscess or spinal cord injury.

Local anesthetics cause a sympathetic blockade that leads to decreased vascular tone, peripheral vasodilation, and subsequent drop in blood pressure. Hypotension (systolic blood pressure less than 100 mm Hg) is noted in as many as 50% of women following administration of epidural analgesia.[77–79] Significant complications are uncommon, but blood flow to the uterus diminishes with hypotension, and fetal heart rate decelerations frequently occur for a short time 10 to 20 minutes after the epidural is emplaced. These fetal heart rate patterns are associated with moderate fetal heart rate variability, usually resolve spontaneously or with a bolus of intravenous fluids, and are not associated with adverse newborn outcomes. In rare cases, ephedrine is required to elevate maternal blood pressure and restore blood flow to the uterus. This is most commonly accomplished with incremental doses (5–10 mg administered

intravenously) of ephedrine, a mixed catecholamine agonist that increases blood pressure and heart rate without constricting uterine blood vessels.

Bladder distension can occur when there is loss of the sensation to void, relaxation of overall bladder tone, and loss of control of the urinary sphincter. Intermittent catheterization during labor and/or at the time of birth is common. If many hours will elapse between initiation of an epidural and birth, and the woman is unable to void on her own, an indwelling catheter may be considered. The catheter should be discontinued during the second stage of labor.

An increase in the incidence of maternal fever, defined as equal to or higher than 38°C (100.4°F), has been demonstrated in women who have epidural analgesia during labor.[80,81] Women who develop temperature elevations tend to have increases that start immediately after the epidural is initiated and average 0.18°C (0.33°F) per hour. The occurrence of fever equal to or higher than 38°C (100.4°F) is apparent after approximately 4 hours.[82]

The fever related to a labor epidural has not been associated with an increased incidence of infections. Most likely, epidural-related fever is attributable to thermoregulatory alterations such as a decrease in heat dissipation secondary to sympathetic block of sweating. Some women who develop a fever after epidural initiation may have subclinical chorioamnionitis.[80–82] Unfortunately, it is not possible to distinguish fever of benign versus infectious origin; therefore all women who develop a fever in labor are treated for chorioamnionitis. Infants of women who develop a fever during labor are more likely to be subjected to evaluations for sepsis in the first few days of life.[83]

Postdural puncture headaches occur in 1% to 4% of women who receive an epidural or combined spinal/epidural (CSE).[84] If the epidural needle inadvertently pierces the dura and cerebrospinal fluid leaks into the epidural space, the drop in intrathecal pressure can cause a positional headache, which increases in severity when the woman is in the sitting or standing position. Resolution of the headache occurs spontaneously within 4 to 5 days. If not severe, this headache may be treated with oral hydration, caffeine, and simple analgesics such as acetaminophen (Tylenol) or ibuprofen (Motrin, Advil). If the headache is severe or prolonged, it can be treated with a blood patch, which is an epidural injection of the woman's blood that seals the leaking membrane.[85]

Back pain is a common side effect of labor and birth, with or without an epidural. When lower back pain occurs following regional analgesia, the epidural is often thought to be the causative factor. General tenderness at the site of the epidural injection may be present for several days; however, long-term back pain following pregnancy and birth is present in similar numbers of women regardless of the anesthesia method employed.[80] Permanent injury to the spinal cord is extraordinarily rare, occurring in 0.06% of women who receive spinal anesthetics and in 0.02% of all women post epidural.[86] These rare cases are related to either epidural hemorrhage or development of a spinal abscess.

Effect of Neuraxial Analgesia on Labor Progress

Throughout the years that epidurals have been in use, there has been a great deal of controversy regarding the potential effects of epidurals on the course and outcomes of labor.[78,80,87] Length of labor and the effects of epidural analgesia are very difficult to determine due to many confounding variables. The meta-analyses of RCTs that compared labor outcomes in women with and without epidurals have not found epidurals to be associated with a prolongation of the first stage of labor in the aggregate (mean difference: 18.51 minutes; 95% CI: −12.91 to 49.92; 11 trials; 2981 women).[77] However, aggregate mean values for duration of labor do not tell the full story.

In general, it is felt that epidurals may slow the rate of cervical dilatation in the first stage of labor, especially if such analgesia is initiated during the latent phase of labor. Women who need an epidural in the latent phase of labor for pain relief, however, may have an underlying uterine dysfunction that results in a longer labor. Thus it is not clear if epidurals slow the first stage of labor or if women who need epidural analgesia have inherent differences that result in slower labors.

Conversely, some women have an accelerated course of labor after epidural analgesia is initiated. This may be due to improved uterine contractility after previous inhibition from markedly elevated catecholamine levels in women who had severe pain. Conversely, the higher level of pain that initiated the request for an epidural could also have been a reflection of rapid dilation that occured spontaneously. Thus the combination of some women whose labors are slowed by the epidural with some women whose labors are faster after epidural use results in an aggregate mean duration of the first stage that is no different than the duration of the first stage in women who do not use epidural analgesia and it is difficult to draw clinically meaningful conclusions from these data.

In contrast, epidural analgesia is associated with a prolongation of the second stage of labor (mean difference: 13.66 minutes; 95% CI: 6.67–20.66; 13 trials; 4233 women).[77] This outcome is presumed to occur secondary to the lack of sensation for bearing down and perhaps the relaxation of the levator ani muscles that make up the pelvic floor. Pelvic relaxation is also the presumed etiology of the increase in persistent occiput posterior malpositions that are associated with epidural analgesia.[89]

Epidural analgesia is not associated with an increase in cesarean sections, but women who have epidurals are more likely to have an operative vaginal delivery (RR: 1.42; 95% CI: 1.28–1.57).[77] The incidence of instrumental deliveries can be reduced with the use of a more dilute solution of local anesthetic.[88] Delayed pushing or "laboring down" techniques also appear to reduce the incidence of operative vaginal births in women who have epidural analgesia.[89] Some practitioners have advocated cessation of epidural analgesia during second-stage labor to enable the woman to experience the urge to push and to be able to actively participate in expulsive efforts. For a few women, this is a successful approach; for many others, the reoccurrence of severe pain and anxiety can interfere with the woman's ability to push. Discontinuing the epidural infusion is not recommended.

Fetal and Neonatal Side Effects and Adverse Effects of Neuraxial Analgesia

Neonatal outcomes such as poor 5-minute Apgar scores and low umbilical artery pH have not been shown to be significantly different between women using epidurals and those using intravenous opioids or no medications.[80,87] Neurologic studies of epidural-exposed infants, opioid-exposed infants, and nonmedicated infants have not identified significant differences in performance between any of these groups.

The effect of epidural analgesia on breastfeeding outcomes has been controversial. Women cannot be randomized prospectively to epidural or no-epidural groups and because women who have epidurals tend to have longer second stages, more fevers, and a higher rate of operative delivery, it is not clear if lower rates of breastfeeding initiation is secondary to the epidural or the labor course. Overall, rates of breastfeeding initiation and continuation through 6 weeks postpartum appear to be unchanged regardless of the method of analgesia.[80]

Midwifery Management

When midwives care for women who have epidural analgesia, they must consider a variety of logistical issues. Clinical practice guidelines that are agreed upon by the midwife and the consulting physician should address use of epidurals, indications for their use, and any special circumstances that might require additional assistance. Too often, technology is allowed to take center stage. The midwife's role in de-emphasizing the technology and centering the focus of the birth environment on the laboring woman cannot be understated.

General Anesthesia

General anesthesia refers to the use of an inhaled anesthetic agent to induce sleep for obstetric applications, primarily for emergency cesarean birth. Induction of anesthesia is accomplished with short-acting agents that render the woman unconscious, such as thiopental or propofol. After the induction agent is administered, a muscle relaxant such as succinylcholine is typically given to facilitate intubation. Intubation generally proceeds without complications; however, in pregnant women, intubation is approximately seven times more complicated than in the nongravid patient. For this reason, general anesthesia is avoided when possible, due to maternal and fetal side effects that are undesirable and possibly life-threatening. General anesthesia complications due to inability to intubate and maternal aspiration remain leading causes of anesthesia-related maternal mortality. Even so, true emergencies such as cord prolapse and acute placental abruption may necessitate the use of general anesthesia if neuraxial anesthesia is not already in place. For many clinical situations where a surgical birth becomes necessary, there is adequate time for placement of spinal anesthesia, which has less potential for maternal–fetal complications.

Conclusion

Unmedicated or medicated, easy labor and birth or complicated labor and birth, the midwife sets the tone for all involved in the care of the laboring woman. Speaking in a low voice, dimming bright lights, and making all involved as comfortable as possible help women feel cared for and supported. The midwife always has a special opportunity to make each birth experience one that shows respect for birth, even if the birth takes place in the midst of a high-technology environment. Thus providing support to the woman in labor and facilitating her choices for coping with the pain of labor are key responsibilities for the midwife, regardless of birth setting.

● ● ● **References**

1. Simkin P, Bolding A. Update on nonpharmacologic approaches to relieve labor pain and prevent suffering. *J Midwifery Women's Health*. 2004;49(6):489-505.

2. Simkin P. Just another day in a woman's life? Part II. Nature and consistency of women's long-term memories of their first birth experiences. *Birth*. 1992; 19(2):64-81.

3. Merskey H, Bogduk N, eds. Part III: pain terms, a current list with definitions and notes on usage. In: IASP Task Force on Taxonomy. *Classification of Chronic Pain*. 2nd ed. Seattle WA: IASP Press; 1994:209-214.

4. Melzack R. From the gate to the neuromatrix. *Pain*. 1999;S121-S126.

5. Trout, KK. The neuromatrix theory of pain: implications for selected nonpharmacologic methods of pain relief for labor. *J Midwifery Women's Health*. 2004;49(6):482-488.

6. Lowe NK. The nature of labor pain. *Am J Obstet Gynecol*. 2002;186:S16-S24.

7. Eltzchig HK, Lieberman ES, Camann WR. Regional anesthesia and analgesia for labor and delivery. *N Engl J Med*. 2003;348:419-432.

8. Lowe NK, Corwin EJ. Proposed biological linkages between obesity, stress, and inefficient uterine contractility in humans. *Med Hypotheses*. 2011;76:755-760.

9. Melzack R. The myth of painless childbirth: the John J. Bonica lecture. *Pain*. 1984;(19):321-327.

10. Melzack R. Evolution of the neuromatrix theory of pain: the Prithvi Raj lecture: presented at the third World Congress of World Institute of Pain, Barcelona 2004. *Pain Pract*. 2005;5(2):85-94.

11. Lally JE, Murtagh MJ, Macphail S, Thomson R. More in hope than expectation: a systematic review of women's expectations and experiences with pain relief in labour. *BMC Med*. 2008;6:7.

12. Hodnett ED. Pain and women's satisfaction with the experience of childbirth: a systematic review. *Am J Obstet Gynecol*. 2002;186:S160-S173.

13. Mogil S. Pain genetics: past, present and future *Trends Genet*. 2012;28(6):258-266.

14. Muralidharan A, Smith MT. Pain, analgesia and genetics. *J Pharm Pharmacol*. 2011;63(11):1387-1400.

15. Stamer UM, Stüber F. The pharmacogenetics of analgesia. *Expert Opin Pharmacother*. 2007;8(14): 2235-2245.

16. Ingelman-Sundberg M. Genetic polymorphisms of cytochrome P4502D6 (CYP2D6): clinical consequences, evolutionary aspects and functional diversity. *Pharmacogenom J*. 2005;5(1):6-13.

17. Melzack R. Low-back pain during labor. *Am J Obstet Gynecol*. 1987;156:901-905.

18. Melzack R, Kinch R, Dobkin P, Lebrun M, Taenzer P. Severity of labor pain: influence of physical as well

as psychological variables. *Can Med Assn J.* 1984; 30(5):579-584.

19. Declercq ER, Sakala C, Corry MP, Applebaum S. *Listening to Mothers II: Results of the Second National U.S. Survey of Women's Childbearing Experiences.* New York: Childbirth Connection; 2006. Available at: http://www.childbirthconnection.org/listening tomothers. Accessed January 22, 2013.

20. Lowe NK. Context and process of informed consent for pharmacologic strategies in labor pain care. *J Midwifery Women's Health.* 2004;49:250-260.

21. Spilby H, Slade P, Escott D, et al. Selected coping strategies in labor: an investigation of women's experiences. *Birth.* 2003;30(3):189-194.

22. McCaffery M, Pasero C. *Pain Clinical Manual,* 2nd ed. Philadelphia, PA: Mosby; 1999.

23. *Joint Commission Resources: 2004 Comprehensive Accreditation Manual for Hospitals.* Oak Brook Terrace, IL: Joint Commission for Accreditation of Healthcare Organizations; 2003.

24. Gulliver BG, Fisher J, Roberts L. A new way to assess pain in laboring women: replacing the rating scale with a "coping" algorithm. *Nurs Women's Health.* 2008;12(5):405-408.

25. Simkin P. The three R's in childbirth preparation: relaxation, rhythm and ritual. Available at: http://www .pennysimkin.com/articles/Three_r's.pdf. Accessed November 28, 2011.

26. Bergstrom L, Richards L, Morse JM, Roberts J. How caregivers manage pain and distress in second stage labor. *J Midwifery Women's Health.* 2010;55(1);38-40.

27. Olde E, van der Hart O, Kleber R, van Son M. Posttraumatic stress following childbirth. *Clin Psychol Rev.* 2006;26:1-6.

28. Beck CT, Gable RK, Sakala C, Declercq ER. Posttraumatic stress disorder in new mothers: results from a two-stage U.S. national survey. *Birth.* 2011;38(3): 216-227.

29. Adams SS, Eberhard-Gran M, Eskild M. Fear of childbirth and duration of labor: a study of 2206 women with intended vaginal delivery. *BJOG.* 2012; 119(10):1238-1246.

30. Laursen M, Johansen C, Hedegaard M. Fear of childbirth and risk for birth complications in nulliparous women in the Danish National Birth Cohort. *BJOG.* 2009;116(10):1350-1355.

31. Rouhe H, Salmelo-Aro K, Halmesaki G, Saisto T. Fear of childbirth according to parity, gestational age, and obstetric history *BJOG.* 2009;116(1):67-73.

32. Wertz RW, Wertz DC. *Lying-in: A History of Childbirth in America.* New Haven, CT: Yale University Press; 1979:178.

33. Zwelling E. Childbirth education in the 1990s and beyond. *J Obstet Neonatal Nurs.* 1996;25:425.

34. Dick-Read, G. *Childbirth Without Fear,* 2nd ed. New York: Harper and Row; 1959.

35. Walker DS, Visger JM, Rossie D. Contemporary childbirth education models. *J Midwifery Women's Health.* 2009;54:469-476.

36. Gagnon AJ, Sandall J. Individual or group antenatal education for childbirth or parenthood, or both. *Cochrane Database Syst Rev.* 2007;3:CD002869. doi: 10.1002/14651858.CD002869.pub2.

37. Maimburg RD, Vaeth M, Durr J, et al. Randomised trial of antenatal training sessions to improve the birth process. *BJOG.* 2010; 117:921.

38. Evans WD, Wallace JL, Snider J. Pilot evaluation of the text4baby mobile health program. *BMC Pub Health.* 2012;12:1031.

39. Genesoni L, Talladini MA. Men's psychological transition to fatherhood: an analysis of the literature 1989–2008. *Birth.* 2009;36(4):305-310.

40. Hildingsson I, Cederlof L, Widen S. Fathers' birth experience in relation to midwifery care. *Women Birth.* 2011;24:129-136.

41. Declercq ER, Sakala C, Corry MP, Applebaum S, Herrlich A. Listening to Mothers III: Pregnancy and Birth: *Report of the Third National U.S. Survey of Women's Childbearing Experiences.* New York: Childbirth Connection; 2013. Available at: http ://transform.childbirthconnection.org/wp-content /uploads/2013/06/LTM-III_Pregnancy-and-Birth.pdf. Accessed August 10, 2013.

42. Hodnett ED, Gates S, Hofmeyr GJ, Sakala C. Continuous support for women during childbirth. *Cochrane Database Syst Rev.* 2012;10:CD003766. doi: 10.1002/14651858.CD003766.pub.4.

43. Hodnett ED, Lowe NK, Hannah ME, et al. Effectiveness of nurses as providers of birth in North American hospitals: a randomized controlled trial. *JAMA.* 2002;288:1373.

44. Royal College of Midwives. Immersion in water during labor and birth. Available at: http://www.rcm.org .uk/college/policy-practice/guidelines/joint-guidelines /joint-statements/. Accessed January 22, 2013.

45. Cluett ER, Burns E. Immersion in water in labour and birth. *Cochrane Database Syst Rev.* 2009;2:CD000111. doi: 10.1002/14651858.CD000111.pub3.

46. Eriksson M, Mattson LA, Ladfors L. Early or late bath during the first stage of labor: a randomized study of 200 women. *Midwifery.* 1997;13(3):146-148.

47. Benfield RD, Hortobagyi T, Tanner CJ, Swanson J, Heltkemper MM, Newton ER. The effects of hydrotherapy on anxiety, pain, neuroendocrine response, and contraction dynamics during labor. *Bio Res Nurs.* 2010;12(1):28-36.

48. Benfield RD. Hydrotherapy in labor. *J Nurs Schol.* 2002;34(4):347-352.

49. Wang SM, Kain ZN, White P. Acupuncture analgesia: I. The scientific basis. *Anesth Analg.* 2008;106(2):602-610.

50. Eshkevari L, Egan R, Phillip D, et al. Acupuncture at ST36 prevents chronic stress-induced increases in neuropeptide Y in rat. *Experi Biol Med.* 2012;237(1):18-23.

51. Smith CA, Collins CT, Crowther CA, Levett KM. Acupuncture or acupressure for pain management in labour. *Cochrane Database Syst Rev.* 2011;7:CD009232. doi: 10.1002/14651858.CD009232.

52. Jones L, Othman M, Dowswell T, et al. Pain management for women in labour: an overview of systematic reviews. *Cochrane Database Syst Rev.* 2012;3:CD009234. doi: 10.1002/14651858.CD009234.pub2.

53. Waters BL, Raisler J. Ice massage for the reduction of labor pain. *J Midwifery Women's Health.* 2003;48:317-321.

54. Derry S, Straube S, Moore RA, Hancock H, Collins SL. Intracutaneous or subcutaneous sterile water injection compared with blinded controls for pain management in labour. *Cochrane Database Syst Rev.* 2012;1:CD009107. doi: 10.1002/14651858.CD009107.pub2.

55. Hutton EK, Kasperink M, Rutten M, Reitsman A, Wainman B. Sterile water injection for labor pain: a systematic review and meta-analysis of randomized controlled trials. *BJOG.* 2009;116(9):1158-1166.

56. Lawrence A, Lewis L, Hofmeyr GJ, Dowswell T, Styles C. Maternal positions and mobility during first stage labour. *Cochrane Database Syst Rev.* 2009;2:CD003934. doi: 10.1002/14651858.CD003934.pub2.

57. Gupta JK, Hofmeyr GJ, Shehmar M. Position in the second stage of labour for women without epidural anaesthesia. *Cochrane Database Syst Rev.* 2012;5:CD002006. doi: 10.1002/14651858.CD002006.pub3.

58. Smith CA, Levett KM, Collins CT, Jones L. Massage, reflexology and other manual methods for pain management in labour. *Cochrane Database Syst Rev.* 2012;2:CD009290. doi: 10.1002/14651858.CD009290.pub2.

59. Ketterhagen D, VandeVusse L, Berner M. Self-hypnosis: alternative anesthesia for childbirth. *Am J Matern/Child Nurs.* 2002;27:335-340.

60. Madden K, Middleton P, Cyna AM, Matthewson M, Jones L. Hypnosis for pain management during labour and childbirth. *Cochrane Database Syst Rev.* 2012;11:CD009356. doi: 10.1002/14651858.CD009356.pub2.

61. Landold AD, Millin LS. The efficacy of hypnosis as an intervention for labor and delivery pain: a comprehensive methodological review. *Clin Psychol Rev.* 2011;31:1022-1031.

62. Bedwell C, Dowswell T, Neilson JP, Lavender T. The use of transcutaneous electrical nerve stimulation (TENS) for pain relief in labour: a review of the evidence. *Midwifery.* 2011; 27(4):e141-e148.

63. Phumdoung S, Good M. Music reduces sensation and distress of labor pain. *Pain Manage Nurs.* 2003;4:54.

64. Burns EE, Blamey C, Ersser SJ, et al. An investigation into the use of aromatherapy in intrapartum midwifery practice. *J Altern Complement Med.* 2000;6:141.

65. Burst HV. "Real" midwifery. *J Nurse-Midwifery.* 1990;35(4):189-191.

66. Bricker L, Lavender T. Parenteral opioids for labor pain: a systematic review. *Am J Obstet Gynecol.* 2002;186:S94-S109.

67. Guinsburg R, Wyckoff MH. Naloxone during neonatal resuscitation: acknowledging the unknown. *Clin Perinatol.* 2006;22:121-132.

68. Rooks JP. Safety and risks of nitrous oxide labor analgesia: a review. *J Midwifery Women's Health.* 2011;56:557-565.

69. Rosen MA. Nitrous oxide for relief of labor pain: a systematic review. *Am J Obstet Gynecol.* 2002;186:S110-S126.

70. Stewart LS, Collins M. Nitrous oxide as labor analgesia. *Nurs Women's Health* 2012;16(5):398-409.

71. Mardirosoff C, Dumont L, Boulvain M, Tramèr MR. Fetal bradycardia due to intrathecal opioids for labour analgesia: a systematic review. *BJOG.* 2002;109:274.

72. Schrock SD, Harraway-Smith C. Labor analgesia. *Am Fam Physician.* 2012;85(5):447-454.

73. Gerancer JC, Grice CS, Dewan DW, Eisenach J. Evaluation of informed consent prior to epidural analgesia for labor and delivery. *Int J Obstet Anesth.* 2009;9:168-173.

74. Weinberg GL. Current concepts in resuscitation of patients with local anesthetic cardiac toxicity. *Reg Anesth Pain Med.* 2002;27:568.

75. Saito M, Okutomi T, Kanai Y, et al. Patient-controlled epidural analgesia during labor using ropivacaine and fentanyl provides better maternal satisfaction with less local anesthetic requirement. *J Anesth.* 2005;19:208.

76. Soetens FM, Soetens MA, Vercauteren MP. Levobupivicaine-sufentanil with or without epinephrine during epidural labor analgesia. *Anesth Analg.* 2006;103:182.

77. Anim-Somuah M, Smyth R, Jones L. Epidural vs nonepidural or no analgesia in labor. *Cochrane Database Syst Rev.* 2011;CD000331.

78. Mayberry LJ, Clemmens D, De A. Epidural analgesia side effects, co-interventions, and care of women during childbirth: a systematic review. *Am J Obstet Gynecol.* 2002;86(5, pt. 2):S81-S93.

79. Pham LH, Camann WR, Smith MP, Datta S, Bader AM. Hemodynamic effects of intrathecal sufentanil compared with epidural bupivacaine in laboring parturients. *J Clin Anesth.* 1996;8:497.

80. Leighton BL, Halpern SH. The effects of epidural analgesia on labor, maternal, and neonatal outcomes: a systematic review. *Am J Obstet Gynecol.* 2002;186:S69-S77.

81. Goetzl L, Cohen A, Frigoletto F, Ringe SA, Lang JM, Lieberman E. Maternal epidural use and neonatal sepsis evaluation in afebrile mothers. *Pediatrics.* 2001;108(5):1099-1102.

82. Goetzl L. Epidural analgesia and maternal fever: a clinical and research update. *Curr Opin Anaesthesiol.* 2012;25(3):292-299.

83. Shatken S, Greenough K, McPherson C. Epidural fever and its implications for mothers and neonates: taking the heat. *J Midwifery Women's Health.* 2012;57(1): 82-85.

84. Vallejo MC, Mandell GL, Sabo DP, Ramanathan S. Postdural puncture headache: a randomized comparison of five spinal needles in obstetric patients. *Anesth Analg.* 2000;91:916.

85. Thew M, Paech MJ. Management of postdural puncture headache in the obstetric patient. *Curr Opin Anesthesiol.* 2008;21:288.

86. Wong CA. Neurologic deficits and labor analgesia. *Reg Anesth Pain Med.* 2004;29:341.

87. Lieberman E, O'Donoghue C. Unintended effects of epidural analgesia during labor: a systematic review. *Am J Obstet Gynecol.* 2002;186(5, pt. 2):S31-S68.

88. Comparative Obstetric Mobile Epidural Trial (COMET) Study Group UK. Effect of low-dose mobile versus traditional epidural techniques on mode of delivery: a randomized controlled trial. *Lancet.* 2001;358:19.

89. Fraser WD, Marcoux S, Krauss I, Douglas J, Goulet C, Boulvain M. Multicenter, randomized, controlled trial of delayed pushing for nulliparous women in the second stage of labor with continuous epidural analgesia. The PEOPLE (Pushing Early or Pushing Late with Epidural) Study Group. *Am J Obstet Gynecol.* 2000;182(5):1165-1172.

APPENDIX

28A

Injection of Intradermal Sterile Water Papules for Relief of Low Back Pain in Labor

Approximately 30% of women experience severe continuous low back pain in labor.[1] Back pain in labor, especially when caused by an occiput posterior position, is one of the most challenging conditions for the midwife to treat effectively. The tension caused by this pain has been associated with prolonged labor, increased need for pain medication, and prevention of the spontaneous rotation of the vertex to an anterior position. Several techniques have been reported to be helpful, including massage, counterpressure, applied heat or ice, transcutaneous electrical nerve stimulation (TENS), and hydrotherapy. However, most of these measures offer only partial relief with constant application by another person.

Several randomized controlled trials (RCTs)[1–6] and two meta-analyses[7,8] have shown that intradermal sterile water papule injections have greater analgesic effects than massage, TENS, or counterpressure. The pain relief has been shown to last approximately 1 to 3 hours in 85% to 90% of women,[2–6] and intradermal injections appear to reduce pain by approximately 60%.[7,8] This technique offers the advantages of needing minimal, readily available equipment; moreover, it is adaptable to any birth setting and simple to administer. There are no systemic maternal or fetal side effects. Laboring women are able to ambulate and move freely. There is no need for additional fetal heart rate monitoring or other supplemental interventions. The main disadvantage is the sensation of intense burning or stinging at time of application—an effect that lasts 30 to 90 seconds. Uneven or inadequate relief of pain is also an undesirable side effect.[7–9]

The mechanism of action seems to be primarily counter-irritation, which is thought to inhibit multireceptive neurons to the brain.[10] The gate control mechanism of pain control may also be involved in the effectiveness of this procedure.[7,11]

The onset of relief occurs within 2 minutes of injection and usually lasts 2 to 3 hours. The technique may be repeated up to three times, but some women will decline reapplication because of the initial burning. Some women will experience no relief or only partial relief. The exact location of the injected papules can influence the effectiveness of this technique. Hence, prior to injection, the midwife should assess both fetal position and the woman's preferred focal points for pressure.

Method to Inject Sterile Water Papules

1. Prior to beginning the procedure:
   - Prepare a 1-cc syringe with 0.6 mL of sterile water (do not use normal saline) and a 25-guage needle. Use two syringes if two midwives will do the injections simultaneously.
   - Gather alcohol swabs, pen(s) for marking the skin, and sterile gloves to avoid introduction of pathogens and to protect the provider from exposure to the woman's blood.

2. Explain the procedure to the woman and her support persons.
   - Benefits include relief of back pain, lack of systemic maternal or fetal side effects, and continued ability to ambulate or move as desired.

- Risks include intense burning pain at the injection sites for 30 to 90 seconds and less effective pain relief than desired.
- Relief occurs by 2 minutes of completion of injections. Prepare the woman and her support persons with methods of maintaining a stable position and coping with discomfort during the procedure.

3. Place the woman in a sitting, kneeling, or standing position, stabilizing herself with her arms and hands as she leans forward slightly. The injection sites in the sacral area will be more visible when the woman leans forward and flattens her back.

4. Expose her lower back enough to visualize the sacral dimples, which correspond to the dorsal sacral foramina. Place and press the pads of the thumbs on the superior iliac spines. Mark these landmarks with a pen. Place the index finger at these marks and move the thumbs about 3 to 4 cm down and 1 to 2 cm inward into the sacral dimples so that the fingertips touch the corners of a trapezoid (**Figure 28A-1**); mark these points as well.[12] Put pressure on these four points, moving them very slightly laterally and vertically until the woman indicates the points of greatest relief.[8]

5. To mark the points of greatest relief most accurately, ask an assistant to place an X or draw a half-circle around the provider's fingertips while they remain in place.

6. Clean the sites with an alcohol swab, taking care not to erase the circular marks around the area to be injected. Put on sterile gloves. Remind the woman that she will feel temporary burning and stinging as the papules are placed.

7. Plan to do the injections quickly during a contraction unless the woman prefers having the injections done between contractions.[7]
   - Inject 0.1 to 0.15 mL intradermally in each of the four points that have been delineated (within the half-circle mark) until the distended skin forms a blanched 1-cm bleb or papule.
   - If possible, have another clinician inject two papules simultaneously to reduce the burning episodes. Do not touch or rub the injection sites when complete.[7]

8. The onset of relief should occur within 2 minutes.

9. If the relief is uneven, the area of less analgesia is often consistent with a bleb that is noted to absorb too quickly, is misplaced, or was injected too deeply. Replacing the papule slightly laterally or vertically often achieves the desired effect.

10. Reevaluate the areas with finger pressure as initially applied, and then repeat the injection.

11. Once the effects have worn off (in 1 to 3 hours depending on the woman and the fetal position and station), the papules may be replaced with the woman's consent. More than three applications may not be advisable.

12. Document the woman's consent for the procedure. Also document the time of injections and patient pain scores both before and after the procedure.

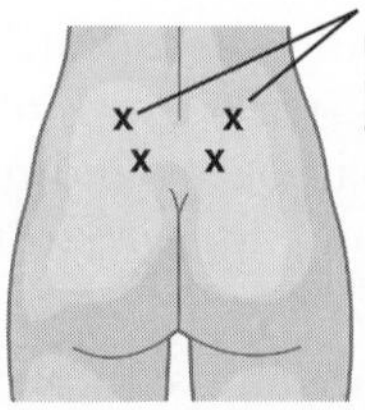

Figure 28A-1 Injection sites for sterile water papules.

Source: From Simkin P, Bolding A. Update on non-pharmacologic approaches to relieve labor pain and prevent suffering. *J Midwifery Womens Health*. 2004;49:489-505. Reprinted with permission of Wiley.

● ● ● References

1. Bahasadri S, Ahmadi-Abhari S, Dehghani-Nik M, Habibi GR. Subcutaneous sterile water injection for labour pain: a randomised controlled trial. *Aust N Z J Obstet Gynaecol*. 2006;46 (2):102-106.

2. Trolle B, Moller M, Kronborg H, Thomsen S. The effect of sterile water block on low back labor pain. *Am J Obstet Gynecol*. 1991 5(1):1277-1281.

3. Ader L, Hansson B, Wallin G. Parturition pain treated by intracutaneous injections of sterile water. *Pain*. 1990;41(2):133-138.

4. Kushtagi P, Bhanu BT. Effectiveness of subcutaneous injection of sterile water to the lower back for pain relief in labor. *Acta Obstet Gynecol Scand*. 2009;88,(2):231-233.

5. Reynolds JL. Intracutaneous sterile water for back pain in labour. *Can Fam Physician*. 1994;40:1785-1788, 1791-1792.

6. Martenson L, Wallin G. Sterile water: labor pain treated with cutaneous injections of sterile water: a randomized controlled trial. *Br J Obstet Gynaecol.* 1999;106:633-637.

7. Fogarty V. Intradermal sterile water injections for the relief of low back pain in labour: a systematic review of the literature. *Women Birth.* 2008;21;157-163.

8. Mårtensson L, McSwiggin M, Mercer JS. US midwives' knowledge and use of sterile water injections for labor pain. *J Midwifery Women's Health.* 2008; 53:115-122.

9. Jaynes AC, Scott KE. Intrapartum care the midwifery way: a review. *Prim Care.* 2012;39(1):189-206.

10. Martensson L, Wallin G. Sterile water injections as treatment for low-back pain during labour: a review. *Aust N Z J Obstet Gynecol.* 2008;48(4):369-374.

11. Huntley AL, Coon JT, Ernst E. Complementary and alternative medicine for labor pain: a systematic review. *Am J Obstet Gynecol.* 2004;191(1):36-44.

12. Simkin P, Bolding A. Update on nonpharmacologic approaches to relieve labor pain and prevent suffering. *J Midwifery Women's Health.* 2004;49(6):489-505.

C H A P T E R

29

The Second Stage of Labor and Birth

LISA KANE LOW

TEKOA L. KING

SARASWATHI M. VEDEM

Introduction

Midwives provide women-centered care by creating a circle of support and safety that encourages rather than disrupts the normal processes that facilitate the labor and birth process. In this capacity, the role of the midwife has best been described as "the art of doing nothing well."[1] The midwife anticipates a woman's needs and provides vigilance in the assessment of the woman and fetus. Simultaneously the midwife remains cognizant of the wide range of what constitutes normal and where boundaries of abnormal begin. The interactions between the midwife and the laboring woman unfold in the form of a dialectic, a give-and-take interaction, with the midwife being responsive, not reactive; supportive, not directive; but all within the boundaries of evidence-based care and safety. This chapter reviews midwifery management during the second stage of labor and through the event of birth.

Definition of Second Stage Labor

Anatomically, second stage labor is defined as beginning with complete dilation of the cervix (10 cm) and ending with expulsion of the fetus. However, the clinical and physiologic demarcation between the final dynamics of first-stage labor and the beginning of second stage labor is less distinct. Subtle changes indicative of the second stage may appear in the final phases of active labor, or there may be a lull in the frequency and intensity of contractions at the end of first-stage labor prior to active second stage events.[2] Although the anatomic definition is primarily still in use in clinical practice, physiologically, second stage labor may be defined as the onset of the urge to bear down until birth of the infant. Using this definition, second stage labor is initiated when the vertex or presenting part of the fetus has descended to a station wherein an involuntary maternal urge to bear down occurs. The urge to push typically occurs when the fetal presenting part reaches +1 station.

Normal Course of the Second Stage of Labor

Observations of women who have no anesthesia and are not coached to push regardless of lack or urge have found that the second stage sometimes has subphases depending on the fetal station and urge to push when complete dilation occurs (Box 29-1).[2,3] If the fetus is above zero station when the cervix becomes completely dilated, the first phase can be a short lull or pause during which uterine contractions may be less frequent and the woman may have no urge to push. This is followed by an expulsive phase or period of linear descent during which the urge to push and pushing efforts become progressively stronger. The final perineal phase occurs when the fetal head is visible at the introitus. During this last phase, women often push even without contractions.

Signs and Symptoms of Second Stage Labor

The most common symptom that heralds the onset of the second stage is an urge to push. Women who do not have epidural analgesia usually have an irresistible need to push or bear down, but this is not universally true. Many women interpret this feeling as needing to have a bowel movement.

Signs of second stage labor include finding the fetal heart rate (FHR) in progressively lower locations

BOX 29-1 Three Subphases of Physiologic Second Stage of Labor

1. Latent period:
   a. Lull in contractions
   b. No desire to push; woman may sleep or doze
   c. Fetus at −1 to +1 station
2. Phase of linear descent:
   a. Regular contractions
   b. Spontaneous maternal efforts
   c. Fetus internally rotates and descends to +2 to +4
3. Expulsive phase:
   a. Vertex distends vaginal walls; pressure on pelvic floor
   b. Regular contractions; more frequent contractions
   c. Increased maternal discomfort; may desire to push between contractions
   d. Vertex visible with contractions; crowning and delivery

Source: Adapted from Roberts JE. A new understanding of the second stage of labor: implications for nursing care. *J Obstet Gynecol Neonatal Nurs.* 2003;39:794-801.

BOX 29-2 Factors That Influence the Duration of the Second Stage of Labor

- Parity
- Fetal station at complete cervical dilatation
- First-stage dystocia
- Uterine contraction activity: strength and frequency of contractions
- Presence or absence of infection
- Fetal position
- Effectiveness of maternal pushing efforts
- Pelvic architecture
- Birth weight
- Maternal weight
- Epidural analgesia
- Induction of labor
- Maternal fear or anxiety
- Maternal pain or discomfort

in the maternal abdomen, rectal bulging, perineal bulging, and progressive visibility of the fetal head at the vaginal introitus. In addition, there may be an increase in bloody show, and the FHR pattern may demonstrate variable decelerations. Interestingly, an almost infallible signal of imminent birth is the woman saying, "The baby's coming!" a verbal expression that occurs in most cultures and languages.

Fetal Descent During Second Stage Labor

During the second stage of labor, the fetus descends, internally rotates, and is born via extension of the fetal neck and external rotation. (See the *Anatomy and Physiology During Labor and Birth* chapter to review the cardinal movements of fetal descent.) This process can occur very quickly, as is often the case in multiparous women, or it can occur over a period of time, which is more common in nulliparous women.

Duration of Second Stage Labor

The factors that influence the duration of the second stage of labor are listed in **Box 29-2**. For women who have no medical or obstetric complications at the onset of labor, the three factors that have the strongest effect on the duration of the second stage are parity, fetal position, and the presence or absense of regional analgesia.

The traditional norms used for duration of second stage labor were based on investigations conducted in the 1950s and early 1960s by a physician, Emanuel A. Friedman.[4] However, labor management strategies varied greatly from contemporary practice today. Approximately 55% of the women in Friedman's observations had their labors terminated by low or mid-forceps. Thus Friedman's analysis of second-stage duration was more an observation of practice patterns at the time than the natural course of the second stage. According to Freidman, the average length of the second stage was 46 minutes for women having a first vaginal birth and 14 minutes for women having subsequent births.[4]

Recent evidence argues for a more nuanced evaluation of second stage labor duration, taking into consideration if the woman has an epidural in place, fetal position, and duration of active pushing time combined with a period of passive descent. The duration of the second stage of labor from contemporary reviews of women with and without epidural analgesia who had a spontaneous vaginal birth is shown in **Table 29-1**.[5–7]

Abnormalities of the Second Stage of Labor

Second stage abnormalities have traditionally been categorized as either prolonged in duration or descent abnormalities, which can be further subdivided into protracted descent, failure of descent, or arrest of descent.

Table 29-1	The Duration of the Second Stage of Labor in Hours			
	Mean	Median	95% Limit	
	Kilpatrick et al. 1975–1987	Zhang et al. 2002–2008	Kilpatrick et al. 1975–1987	Zhang et al. 2002–2008
Nulliparous without epidural, hours	1.0 ± 0.65	0.6	2.2	2.8[a]
Nulliparous with epidural, hours	1.3 ± 0.8	1.1	3.0	3.6
Multiparous without epidural, hours	0.3 ± 0.3	0.2	1.0	1.3
Multiparous with epidural, hours	0.75 ± 0.75	0.4	2.2	2.0

[a] Data from Kilpatrick et al. was conducted before laboring down or a period of passive descent was included in practice guidelines. It is theorized that one factor in the difference between Kilpatrick's findings and the findings of Zhang et al. may reflect the incorporation of "laboring down" that occurred in the time interval between when these two studies were performed.

Source: Adapted from Kilpatrick SJ, Laros RK. Characteristics of normal labor. *Obstet Gynecol.* 1989;74(1):85-87; Zhang J, Landy HJ, Brancy DW, et al. Contemporary patterns of spontaneous labor with normal neonatal outcomes. *Obstet Gynecol.* 2010;116:1281-1287.

Prolonged Second Stage Labor

Abnormal duration of the second stage has been historically defined as longer than 2 hours for a primigravida and longer than 1 hour for a multigravida, according to Freidman criteria.[4] In 1989, Kilpatrick and Laros[5] published an analysis of the durations of labor (*n* = 6991) in women who had a spontaneous vaginal birth at term without use of oxytocin. These researchers determined the means and 95% confidence intervals for women with and without epidural analgesia and stratified by parity. The natural limit (95% confidence interval [CI]) of the second stage of labor was 3 hours for nulliparous women who had epidural analgesia, 2 hours for multiparous women who had regional analgesia, 2 hours for nulliparous women who did not have epidural analgesia, and 1 hour for multiparous women who did not have epidural analgesia. This 1-2-3 rule became the standard values used for the definition of prolonged second stage, until the more recent recognition of the value of an initial period of passive descent was introduced into clinical practice.

Duration of the Second Stage

Today labor management has changed. Specifically, women who enter the second stage of labor without an urge to push are often allowed to rest for a period of time. Women who have an epidural often are in this category so that this period of "passive descent" or "laboring down" allows the fetus to descend to the pelvic floor before the woman begins voluntary pushing efforts. Passive descent of the fetus among laboring women who have epidural analgesia increases the spontaneous birth rate and decreases the risk of operative vaginal delivery and active pushing time. In addition, passive descent results in less maternal exhaustion.[8–11]

The use of passive descent extends the duration of the second stage, however, and the determination of "how long is too long" has not been fully elucidated. In a secondary analysis of a randomized controlled trial wherein 94% of the participants had an epidural, Rouse et al. found that 85% of women who pushed less than 1 hour had a spontaneous vaginal birth. For women who pushed between 1 and 2 hours, 78.7% had a spontaneous vaginal birth; for women who pushed between 2 and 3 hours, the rate was 59.1%; and for women who pushed between 3 and 4 hours, the rate was 24.7%. When women pushed 5 hours or more, the vaginal birth rate was 8.7%.[12] Thus, it appears there is a duration at which the chance of vaginal birth diminishes significantly. However, the authors did not record how many of the participants underwent a period of passive descent, so it is still unclear if complications of second stage duration are secondary to time alone or secondary to time of maternal pushing. Studies of passive descent, reviewed later in this chapter, have found no adverse maternal or neonatal effects.

There was no increased neonatal or other maternal morbidity associated with a longer second stage in this particular investigation, but others have noted an increased risk of postpartum hemorrhage and infection associated with longer second stages.[12,13] Other investigations have found vaginal birth rates higher than 10% for women who have a 3- to 4-hour second stage, though rates did not exceed 25%.[12–15]

To date, no prospective randomized trial has been conducted to address the question of "how long is too long" for the duration of second stage labor.[16] Differences between second stage labor in the presence of an epidural compared to physiologic second stage labor further challenge investigators regarding how best to answer this question. **Box 29-3** provides evidence-based recommendations to consider when assessing the duration of second-stage labor for an individual woman based on current research.

In summary, the criteria for a diagnosis of prolonged second stage labor have evolved from the strict limitations of Freidman to the latest recommendations outlined in **Box 29-4**,[17] which offer greater latitude in evaluation of an arrest in second stage. In brief, in the absence of maternal exhaustion, other maternal complications, or fetal intolerance, there are no clear reasons for a rigid adherence to any preset time limit for duration of second stage labor.

Descent Abnormalities in the Second Stage

Descent abnormalities can occur secondary to malpositions such as persistent occiput posterior or asynclitism, uterine hypocontractility, or cephalopelvic disproportion. Failure of descent is present if the fetal presenting part makes no descent after 1 to 2 hours of adequate contractions and maternal pushing efforts. At that point, one can assume that some degree of cephalopelvic disproportion is present and consultation with a physician is necessary. Relative cephalopelvic disproportion may also manifest as protracted descent and prolonged second stage. Protracted descent is more common than failure of descent or arrest of descent, and malpositions are a common cause of protracted descent. From a clinical standpoint, it is important not to confuse molding or caput with true descent.

Maternal Complications from Prolonged Second Stage Labor

Increasing duration of the second stage is associated with some maternal complications. Actively pushing for more than 3 hours in one study[12] and for more than 2 hours in another study[13] was associated with an increased risk for postpartum hemorrhage and chorioamnionitis in the short term. Prolonged pushing may also contribute to long-term adverse outcomes in the pelvic floor such as levator ani muscle tears, which can lead to uterine prolapse.[18]

Fetal Complications from Prolonged Second Stage Labor

Research on second stage labor has shown that there is no significant relationship between second-stage

---

BOX 29-3 Clinical Implications Associated with Duration of Second-Stage Labor

- Negative neonatal outcomes previously associated with longer duration of second-stage labor have been significantly reduced with improved fetal surveillance.
- Use of a combination of passive descent followed by active pushing may contribute to improved neonatal outcomes.[10,30]
- Close observation of continuing progress, descent, fetal well-being, and maternal fatigue are essential elements of evaluation during the second stage of labor.
- Three to four hours of active pushing for a woman with an epidural having her first child appears to be a more realistic timeline for the limit of duration of second-stage labor.[17]
- After active pushing for 3 hours, women are at higher risk for postpartum hemorrhage and chorioamnonitis.[12,13,15]
- After 3.5 hours of active pushing in second-stage labor, fewer than 20% of women will have a spontaneous birth.[15] The effect of passive descent on long-term maternal outcomes such as pelvic organ prolapse are unknown.[18,36]

Sources: Adapted from Fraser WD, Marcoux S, Krauss I, et al. Multicenter randomized, controlled trial of delayed pushing for nulliparous women in the second stage of labor with continuous epidural analgesia. *Am J Obstet Gynecol.* 2000;182:1165-1172; Rouse DJ, Weiner SJ, Bloom SL, et al. Second-stage labor duration in nulliparous women: relationship to maternal and perinatal outcomes. *Am J Obstet Gynecol.* 2009;201(4):357.e1-e7; LeRay C, Audibert F, Goffinet F, Fraser W. When to stop pushing: effects of duration of second-stage expulsion efforts on maternal and neonatal outcomes in nulliparous women with epidural analgesia. *Am J Obstet Gynecol.* 2009;201(4):361.e1-e7; Allen VM, Baskett TF, O'Connell CM, McKeen D, Allen AC. Maternal and perinatal outcomes with increasing duration of the second stage of labor. *Obstet Gynecol.* 2009;113:1248-1258; Spong CY, Berghella V, Wenstrom KD, Mercer BM, Saade GR. Preventing the first cesarean delivery: summary of a joint Eunice Kennedy Shriver National Institute of Child Health and Human Development, Society for Maternal–Fetal Medicine, and American College of Obstetricians and Gynecologists Workshop. *Obstet Gynecol.* 2012;120(5):1181-1193; Kearney R, Miller JM, Ashton-Miller J, DeLancey JOL. Obstetric factors associated with levator ani muscle injury after vaginal birth. *Obstet Gynecol.* 2006;107(1):144-149; Simpson KR, James DC. Effects of immediate versus delayed pushing during 2nd-stage labor on fetal well-being: a randomized clinical trial. *Nurs Res.* 2005;54(3):149-157.

duration and perinatal mortality, 5-minute Apgar scores of less than 7, neonatal seizures, or admission to the newborn intensive care unit as long as the FHR pattern does not indicate an increasing risk for fetal acidemia.[13,19]

Protracted Descent and Occiput Posterior Position

One of the most common reasons for protracted fetal descent is persistent occiput posterior position. Approximately 15% of fetuses are in an occiput posterior (OP) position prior to labor, yet only 5% of fetuses are born in this position.[20] Persistent occiput posterior is associated with several adverse labor events, including prolonged first-stage labor, arrest disorders in second stage labor, a twofold increase in the risk for operative delivery, and an increased incidence of perineal tears. Anecdotally, it has been reported that women experience more intense back pain when the fetus is in an OP position, although the veracity of this supposition has been neither proven nor disproven.[19]

The cardinal movements of labor when the fetus is in an OP position are slightly different. Flexion can be incomplete, which makes the diameters of the presenting part larger. When the fetus is in an occiput anterior (OA) position, the occiput descends down the 5-cm anterior-posterior diameter of the posterior symphysis pubis, and then the fetal head is born by extension of the neck. In contrast, when the fetus is in an OP position, the occiput descends the 10-cm distance between the top of the sacrum to the bottom of the coccyx and the final few centimeters along the floor of the birth canal before being born via flexion, with the occiput presenting in the lower portion of the introitus, then extension as the occiput fully exits the vagina.

Diagnosis of an OP position can be obtained via a digital examination or ultrasound. There is a high degree of discordance between digital and ultrasound determinations, however. Although ultrasound is more likely to be accurate than is a digital examination, approximately 10% of ultrasounds are not able to determine the fetal position.[20]

Practices purported to assist internal rotation of an OP fetus to the OA position include having the woman labor on her hands and knees for a period of time, digital rotation with the examiner's fingers, and manual rotation with the examiner's hands. Although only one randomized controlled trial (RCT) has evaluated the effect of hands-and-knees positioning during labor, 16% of the OP fetuses rotated to anterior in the hands-and-knees group versus 7% in the control group.[21] In addition, the women who assumed a hands-and-knees position reported less back pain and high satisfaction with laboring in this position. Other maternal maneuvers—such as lunging, asymmetric kneeling, walking, or side-lying (if the fetus is in a right occiput posterior position, have the woman lie on her right side so the fetal back is toward the bed and gravity pulls the fetus into an occiput transverse position)—have not been rigorously studied but do have theoretical positive effects on pelvic diameters and may aid the fetus in finding the "best fit." Frequent changes of position may be more useful than any specific position.

Either digital or manual rotation reduces the incidence of OP birth.[23] The techniques for digital and manual rotation are described in **Box 29-5**. Although there is a theoretical risk of umbilical cord prolapse or trauma to the fetal neck, these complications appear to be rare and the procedures are considered safe.

Assessment of Maternal and Fetal Well-Being in Second Stage Labor

Assessment during the second stage of labor includes evaluation of maternal well-being, fetal well-being, and progress of labor (**Box 29-6**).

BOX 29-5 Technique for Digital and Manual Rotation of Occiput Posterior Position

Digital Rotation

1. Review the risks and benefits of the procedure and obtain informed consent.

2. Make certain the woman's bladder is empty.

3. Place the tips of the gloved index and middle fingers in the anterior portion of the lambdoidal suture near the posterior fontanelle.

4. Place the thumb of the same hand over the parietal bone.

5. Move the fetal head up toward the pelvic brim slightly and flex it with upward pressure from the two fingers.

6. Rotate the fetal head to the occiput anterior position via the shortest arc during a contraction and when the woman is pushing (i.e., if the fetus was right OP, then rotate to right OA).

Manual Rotation

1. Review the risks and benefits of the procedure and obtain informed consent.

2. Make certain the woman's bladder is empty.

3. Place four gloved fingers behind the posterior parietal bones with the palm and fingers resting on the occipital bone.

4. Place the thumb of the same hand over the anterior parietal bone.

5. Flex and rotate the fetal head anteriorly during a contraction and when the woman is pushing. Mild upward pressure of the fetal head toward the pelvic brim may facilitate rotation.

BOX 29-6 Midwifery Assessment During Second Stage Labor

1. Maternal vital signs and well-being:

   a. Blood pressure taken between contractions every 15 minutes unless more frequent evaluation is indicated.

   b. Temperature, pulse, and respirations every hour unless more frequent evaluation is indicated. Maternal pulse normally increases during contractions.

   c. Bladder: Assess for distension periodically during the second stage.

      i. Intermittent catheterization may be needed if the woman is unable to void spontaneously.

      ii. If an indwelling catheter is in place at the onset of the second stage, it should be removed when the woman is pushing to minimize trauma to the urethra when the fetal head compresses it.

   d. Hydration and nutrition: Dehydration can contribute to ineffectual uterine activity. Frequent intake of small amounts of oral fluids is recommended.

   e. Pain and coping:

      i. Fear or anxiety about giving birth.

      ii. Maternal fatigue.

      iii. Coping versus suffering behaviors.

   f. Fatigue: Maternal pushing efforts will become less effective if the woman becomes too fatigued after pushing for a prolonged period of time.

2. Fetal heart rate:

   a. Every 15 to 5 minutes, with increasing frequency as the fetal presenting part descends unless more frequent evaluation is indicated.

3. Labor progress

   a. Contraction pattern.

   b. A sterile digital cervical examination is performed intermittently when the results will inform a change in management. Assessments are made of each of the following during each examination:

      i. Fetal position.

      ii. Fetal station.

      iii. Fetal movement in response to maternal pushing effort.

      iv. Fetal adaptation to the pelvis including:

         (a) Synclitism or asynclitism

         (b) Molding or caput succedaneum

Evaluation of Maternal Well-Being in the Second Stage of Labor

Vital Signs

Maternal blood pressure between contractions (which is when it should be taken) is normally increased by an average of 10 mm Hg if the woman has been pushing compared to values obtained in the first stage of labor. Similarly, the maternal pulse increases during contractions.

Bladder

The use of an epidural in labor results in reduced ability to void and leads to increased risk for postpartum urinary retention and distension. In addition, the bladder often has residual urine in larger volumes compared to women who have not had an epidural, which may occur partially secondary to the intravenous fluids used to maintain systemic blood pressure following the sympathetic block induced by the epidural.[24,25] If a woman enters the second stage with an indwelling Foley catheter in place, the catheter should be removed when a woman is actively pushing to avoid undue stress on the urethra.

If the woman has a distended bladder and is unable to void, intermittent catheterization can be performed. If catheterization must be performed during second stage labor and the fetal head is in the true pelvis, the direction of the catheter is different from usual. The urethra is displaced by the fetal head and conforms to its contour. Therefore, immediately after inserting the catheter into the urethra, it is necessary to direct it upward and over the fetal head while concomitantly directing the catheter into the bladder. Sometimes it is helpful to splint the urethra by placing a finger into the vagina, below the urethra, as the catheter is being inserted.

Hydration

The second stage of labor is active physical work; in turn, the risk for dehydration increases. Prolonged fasting in labor is associated with an increased production of ketones, which may result in ketosis for the laboring woman.[26] Consequences of limited fluid intake or dehydration can include a rising pulse rate or fetal heart rate and limited energy or fatigue. Theoretically, ketosis could cause dysfunctional uterine contractions, although this has not been definitively shown. An added consequence of limiting oral intake is women's perception of this restriction adding to the stress of coping with labor.[27] The midwife can encourage oral hydration by offering a drink or ice chips after each pushing effort.[28] The presence of an epidural should not alter the recommendation to maintain oral hydration during labor if the woman desires.[28] If the woman is unable to maintain oral hydration, intravenous fluids may be indicated.

Assessment of Pain and Coping

During the second stage of labor, new physical sensations occur as the woman progresses toward birth. Anticipatory guidance as the second stage progresses can help the woman cope with pushing sensations, perineal stretching, and the uncontrollable urge to bear down.

If a woman is crying out rather than grunting and bearing down, or is unable to sustain any position of comfort, she may be suffering acute distress instead of actively coping.[29] Occasionally a woman will experience significant fear and anxiety with the sensations of vaginal stretching, and pain relief that ameliorates this perineal sensation may be necessary so she can push. A pudendal block can be used if an epidural is not available or desired. Women who have experienced past sexual abuse or assault may be at particular risk for fear or anxiety that escalates when the fetal presenting part causes sensation in the pelvic floor or perineum.[30]

Maternal Fatigue

The amount of added energy a woman requires for the process of pushing varies greatly, as does the average duration of second stage labor. Some women begin the active process of pushing with renewed energy and excitement. The entire energy level in the labor and birth room may increase as the activity and excitement of impending birth grow. Family members present may become engaged as well and can add to the level of encouragement provided to the woman to aid her in overcoming fatigue.

Evaluation of Fetal Well-Being

The assessment of the FHR or fetal heart tones during the second stage of labor is reviewed in more detail in the *Fetal Assessment During Labor* chapter. Variant FHR patterns are more common in the second stage than in the first stage, especially variable decelerations, prolonged decelerations, and bradycardias. Thus the FHR is evaluated more frequently in second stage labor. Current standards recommend assessment every 15 minutes for women without a risk for fetal acidemia and every 5 minutes for women who have a risk for acidemia.[31] In practice, the FHR is evaluated more frequently as the second stage progresses and is often checked every two to three contractions in the final phases of the second stage.

Midwifery Management of the Second Stage of Labor

The support and encouragement of everyone present in the birthing room can be highly effective in helping a woman maintain focus and call on reserve energy when she starts pushing. The role of the midwife is to assess the manner in which the woman is responding to the support being offered by those around her. Are the comments and words helpful or distracting? The midwife can model how to offer the woman encouragement and facilitate the efforts of everyone in ways that best help the individual parturient.

The Family-Centered Birth Environment

The decision of who to include in the birth room is an important one. Home settings and freestanding birth centers generally have few to no restrictions on the number of persons present. Most hospitals allow any number of support persons in the labor room, but restrictions on the number of persons able to be in the operating room are common. Hospitals today also often allow siblings to be present during labor and birth; if children will be present, however, the institution usually requires the presence of an adult whose primary responsibility will be care of the child. Children may want or need to leave the birthing environment, so an adult present who is assigned the job of caring for the child should be available. Children should be prepared for the sights and sounds of birth and be involved in preparations for the birth.

Maternal Pushing Efforts

There are several management options for helping women push during the second stage of labor.[32] A key consideration is to determine whether a period of passive descent would be beneficial for the woman who has an epidural or who does not have an urge to push. Once active pushing begins, coaching can be directive versus supportive, and pushing efforts can be open glottis versus closed glottis (Valsalva). Each of these methods is reviewed.

Delayed Pushing: Passive Descent Versus Immediate Maternal Pushing Efforts

The use of passive descent as a management strategy was initially introduced for the purpose of reducing the incidence of instrumental delivery for women using epidural anesthesia. During the process of passive descent, the fetus descends owing to force generated from contractions alone and begins to internally rotate once the presenting part reaches the pelvic floor. This initial period of maternal rest prior

to engaging in active pushing efforts allows for conservation of the woman's energy until there is a stimulus to actively push. Once the woman does engage in active pushing, her efforts tend to be more effective and efficient in the presence of physical cues from pressure of the presenting part on the pelvic floor.[33]

Several RCTs and two meta-analyses have compared maternal and fetal outcomes in women who rested for a period of approximately 1 hour prior to pushing versus women who started pushing as soon as the cervix was found to be fully dilated.[8–11,34–37] The majority of RCTs defined the process of passive descent as not encouraging active pushing for 1 to 2 hours unless an uncontrollable urge to push developed or the fetal head was visible at the perineum. Vause et al. allowed a delay of up to 3 hours before active pushing began.[37] The meta-analysis by Brancato et al. found delayed pushing was associated with an increased chance of spontaneous deliveries (relative risk [RR]: 1.08; 95% CI: 1.01–1.15; $P = .025$), fewer operative deliveries (RR: 0.77; 95% CI: 0.77–0.85; $P < .001$), less maternal exhaustion, and no increase in adverse maternal or newborn outcomes.[9] In contrast, the meta-analysis by Tuuli et al. did not find a statistically significant difference in the operative delivery rate when they assessed only those RCTs that they deemed of appropriate quality.[8]

Contraindications to delayed pushing include any variant fetal heart rate pattern that indicates an increased risk for fetal acidemia, chorioamnionitis, or another maternal condition wherein a delay would increase the risk for adverse outcomes.

Despite evidence that suggests passive descent has advantages, identification of how long to wait and when to transition to active pushing efforts requires careful consideration. Longer duration of the second stage is associated with an increased risk for chorioamnionitis and postpartum hemorrhage. As yet, no consistent data have emerged regarding how longer second stages may affect long-term outcomes such as maternal urinary incontinence or uterine prolapse.[38–40] Although there are no specific guidelines at this time, it is common practice to offer a period of 1 to 2 hours for passive descent, as these are the time periods used in most of the investigations. It may be prudent to encourage active pushing whenever the vertex reaches +1 station. The midwife should assess the effectiveness of pushing efforts soon after they start. If the woman is able to push effectively, then she can continue to do so until she gives birth. If her initial efforts do not result in any fetal movement and the fetal station is above 0 station, the midwife can consider allowing a time of passive descent.

Some authors have suggested reducing the concentration of anesthetic in the epidural infusion so the sensory block is less strong and the woman can better feel the urge to push. This strategy can be effective if the woman wants to have more sensation, the epidural is able to be titrated, and the woman gives her consent, but totally discontinuing the epidural is not recommended because it results in more pain and no increase in the spontaneous vaginal birth rate.[41,42] Completely removing pain relief from a woman who has used an epidural during labor can result in the sudden onset of intense pain, and this can be more detrimental to her pushing efforts than having the epidural in place.

Open-Glottis Versus Closed-Glottis (Valsalva) Pushing

Traditionally, women have been counseled to take a deep breath, hold their breath, and push forcefully throughout the duration of a uterine contraction. The use of breath holding combined with prolonged bearing down results in a Valsalva maneuver that can decrease cardiac output and subsequent blood flow to the uterus. Conversely, open-glottis pushing is similar to the semi-voluntary grunting pushing associated with defecation. Because the glottis is not closed, there is no increase in intrathoracic pressure and, therefore, no drop in cardiac output.

Studies that have compared Valsalva-type closed-glottis pushing to open-glottis pushing have found that Valsalva-type pushing is associated with more fetal heart rate decelerations;[3] a higher incidence of perineal trauma (lacerations, episiotomy);[43] maternal exhaustion; and an increased risk for cystocele and urinary stress incontinence.[3,44,45] This evidence is compelling and closed-glottis pushing is not recommended in practice today.

Spontaneous Versus Directed Pushing

Spontaneous pushing occurs when the parturient responds with bearing-down efforts and open-glottis pushing based on her bodily sensations. This compares to directed or coached pushing wherein the healthcare provider instructs the woman to push in a specific manner, including the traditional teaching to hold her breath for a sustained period while performing Valsalva or closed-glottis pushing efforts. Directed pushing can include pushing before the woman feels an urge and may ask her to hold the push beyond what she would do spontaneously. Table 29-2 summarizes the effects of spontaneous pushing versus directed pushing. While there are gaps in the literature regarding the benefits of the spontaneous pushing strategy, its use has not been shown to cause harm to either the woman or her newborn.[30,46]

Table 29-2	Comparison of Physiologic Self-Directed Pushing to Valsalva Directed Pushing	
Effects of Different Pushing Techniques	**Physiologic**	**Directed**
Directions given to the woman	Spontaneous based on natural urges. Usually results in 5–6 bearing down efforts of 3–10 seconds each per contraction	Provider directed, repeated counts to 10 with sustained breath holding. Usually results in 2–3 bearing down efforts per contraction
Breathing	Exhale, mouth open with occasional Valsalva maneuver	Valsalva, breath holding
Noise	Grunting, exhaling, low groaning	Silence encouraged
Legs	No leg holding	Held up and back toward abdomen
Fatigue	Less fatigue when compared to directed pushing	Can be pronounced depending on duration of pushing
Fetus	Variable decelerations not as frequent compared to directed pushing	Variable decelerations more likely
Perineum	Gradual distension	Rapid distention during forceful pushing
Duration	Longer second stage but shorter period of active pushing	Shorter second stage but longer period of active pushing
Long-term effects	Preliminary evidence that physiologic pushing is associated with better urodynamic measures in the first 3 months postpartum	Unclear

The effect of pushing techniques on long-term urogenital outcomes is undetermined. A small RCT (*n* = 128) found that postpartum urodynamic measures were poorer in women who were coached during the second stage of labor versus those not coached.[45]

In its purest form, the use of spontaneous pushing would not result in any direction being offered by the midwife. Instead, the role of the midwife would be to offer encouragement and to observe for evidence of progress.[47] However, occasionally a woman will experience significant distress and need some directive counseling. Roberts[48] identified a category of care during second stage labor called supportive direction that is used in conjunction with maternal pushing efforts. In this capacity, the midwife tailors instructions to what the woman is asking about or may need to facilitate progress.

Maternal Position During the Second Stage of Labor

A woman can push in any position—on her side, on her hands and knees, kneeling, standing, or squatting. Her position depends on her preference, her status, and the status of the fetus. Many RCTs have examined upright versus supine positions during the second stage of labor. A meta-analysis of maternal position in second stage labor of women without epidural analgesia published in 2012 failed to find any one position to be better than another with regard to the duration of the second stage.[49] However, upright positions are associated with a decreased incidence of episiotomy, abnormal fetal heart rate patterns, more operative deliveries, and a modest increase in second-degree perineal tears and estimated blood loss.

Despite modest findings in randomized trials, older knowledge about the effects of position on maternal pelvic diameters suggests that upright positions in the latter stages of the second stage may have marked advantages.[50,51] Upright positions increase both the anterior–posterior and transverse diameters of the pelvic outlet, which results in approximately 20% more area in the outlet.[50,51] Optimal positions to promote labor progress are listed in **Box 29-7**.

Preparing for the Birth

The midwife has the responsibility to ensure that all the necessary preparations are made including preparing for the birth itself and ensuring that everyone who is involved is prepared and aware of the plans going forward. Management decisions involve ongoing risk assessment to inform the decision about

---

BOX 29-7 Principles to Consider When Recommending Positions to Promote Progress in Second Stage Labor

1. Avoid the supine or lithotomy positions, as they are associated with uterine pressure on the vena cava, maternal hypotension, decreased uterine perfusion, and variant fetal heart rate patterns.
2. Upright positions are associated with less pain and stronger contractions.
3. Encourage spinal flexion: When a woman rounds her back rather than arching it, the uterus and fetal presenting part are better aligned with the pelvis.
4. Upright positions leaning forward: This increases the angle between the uterus and the spine, thereby directing the fetal presenting part toward the larger posterior segment of the pelvis.
5. Changing positions frequently promotes changes in pelvic diameters, which could aid the fetus finding the "best fit" during the cardinal movements.
6. Squatting increases the area within the pelvic outlet by approximately 20% and can be most beneficial in the final phase of second stage labor.
7. Regardless of the position a woman is in, her legs should not be abducted laterally in an exaggerated manner (lithotomy position) because these positions put increased stress and tension on the perineum.

---

the best location for this birth and timing of transfer if moving from one room to another is indicated. Additionally, it is important to consider the need for other personnel such as a pediatric provider, additional nursing support, or an anesthesia provider.

Maintaining a Circle of Safety in the Birth Environment

The goal of midwifery care during birth is to create a circle of safety and support about the woman, which is accomplished by orchestrating the activities of the room so that everyone present is prepared and appropriately participating in the process. The midwife must be aware of everything happening in the room and redirect any activity that is potentially disruptive to the process. The process of preparation for birth can be reviewed through the use of drills or role-playing using manikins or through the use of virtual simulations of the birthing environment.

Location of the Birth

If the birth is taking place in a hospital, birth locations may include the labor room, a single maternity care room (often called a labor–delivery–recovery room), an in-hospital birthing room, a delivery room, or an operating room. Each of these sites requires different preparation for the woman and her support persons. The midwife should be aware of any institutional policies that dictate criteria for use of a specific location. For example, in some settings the presence of meconium-stained fluid may require added personnel to be in attendance and the location of the birth to change from an in-hospital birth center room to a single-room maternity care room.

When to Prepare for Birth

Experience is required to achieve the best timing for when to prepare for the actual birth. However, a few guidelines exist. In general, if labor is progressing normally, it is best to begin preparations for birth before complete dilatation if the parturient is multiparous and at the beginning of second stage labor if the parturient is nulliparous.

Preparation of the Woman and Her Family for Birth

As the event of birth is approaching, the midwife should ensure that everyone in the room is prepared for what to expect. In particular, the midwife should verify that the woman, her support persons, and any staff who will be in the room know the roles and responsibilities of all involved so that they can complement one another as much as possible.

Confirm with the woman that she is comfortable having the newborn placed on her abdomen immediately following birth if the infant is stable. While most women desire this interaction, some women may choose to have the infant dried and wrapped in a blanket before they hold their newborn. This conversation also gives the midwife the opportunity to explain the advantages of skin-to-skin contact.

When the birth is imminent, the midwife and the woman may need to communicate directly without others giving the woman guidance. At the very final perineal phase of second stage labor, the midwife may want the woman to breathe or pant instead of bearing down so that the infant can be born between contractions; this is easier to accomplish if the midwife is the only person coaching the woman during that time.

It is also good to review the roles of support persons in the birth process. This also allows individuals to voice any concerns or fears or to indicate that they have changed their minds since the original plans were made. For example, if the woman's partner wants to participate in the process of "catching" the baby, the midwife can explain which aspects of hands-on care are possible and which aspects the midwife may need to perform (e.g., if there is a nuchal cord or perineal tearing).

Preparation of the Room, Resources, and Personnel

Care during and immediately following birth is unique, in that both the mother and the newborn may need care simultaneously. Thus two healthcare providers should be present. In the hospital setting, this usually means that a nurse will be present. In the home birth setting, the second provider may be a birth assistant or another midwife who comes to the location when the woman is in active labor. The presence of additional personnel will also be based on risk factors present. Most hospital settings have guidelines for when pediatric or anesthesia staff need to be present at the birth. It is the responsibility of the midwife to consider the unique risk factors of the mother and newborn, to request the necessary resources in anticipation of the birth, and to know how to activate the call for emergency support should an unexpected complication occur. In the out-of-hospital situation, everyone should know what to do in case an emergency transport is required.

The instruments provided in a prepared "delivery kit" vary from setting to setting. At a minimum, a midwife uses sterile gloves, two clamps, a pair of scissors, two surgical clamps (e.g., Kelly clamp) for clamping the cord, an umbilical cord clamp, something in which to place the placenta when it is delivered, clean disposable pads to place beneath the woman's buttocks, sterile 4 × 4 gauze, a receiving blanket, and a head covering for the newborn.

While most newborns will not require any additional support other than drying and stimulation, the equipment to provide a higher level of care should be available and ready for use. A warm blanket and space to manage and assess the newborn should be available. In addition, the following items should be available: oxygen, including the Ambu-bag and appropriately sized mask to deliver it; a method of suctioning to clear secretions; and equipment for intubation, including a laryngoscope and endotracheal tube should neonatal resuscitation become necessary. Regardless of where birth takes place, essential instruments, supplies, and personnel are needed.

General preparations for the site of the birth are outlined in **Box 29-8**.

Midwife Preparation for Attending the Birth

As the birth approaches, the midwife should follow basic principles of sterile technique and scrubbing that are outlined in the chapter *An Introduction to the Care of Women*. The midwife will need to decide when to don protective wear, including a waterproof gown or clothing and eye protection. Consistent with the principles of universal precautions, the midwife should be protected against the risk of splash. If a water birth is planned, the midwife will also need to ensure the use of longer gloves or a gown that is fully waterproof to maintain universal precautions.

Continuing Family-Centered Care

The final moments when the newborn's head is crowning is an exciting time for all involved in the birth. Family, doulas, and other maternity care staff may all become a chorus of encouragement for the woman giving birth. The midwife may need to request that support persons not coach the woman at

this time so that the midwife and the woman can jointly work to facilitate the birth and minimize genital tract trauma.

The birth of a newborn involves both a list of memorized sequences and steps and a need for constant situational awareness. Birth is a fluid and changing situation that can shift from totally normal to an emergency within minutes. Thus, the midwife attending a birth needs to be able to move from quietly facilitating and supporting the bonding of a new family to assertively managing a critical emergency such as postpartum hemorrhage. This ability to adjust management on a moment's notice is an essential midwifery skill.

Management of the Birth

Management of the birth includes using the proper hand maneuvers to assist with the birth, immediate assessment of the newborn, and immediate assessment of maternal status after the birth. In managing the birth, the midwife must make sequential decisions about the following management techniques:

BOX 29-8 Preparation for Birth

1. A decision has been made about where the birth should take place. If there is a need to better visualize the perineum or a risk for complications that require more assistance, the woman is informed, additional help is requested, and the woman is moved to the appropriate setting.
2. The woman is supported as comfortably as possible in the birth location.
3. The woman's partner, family, and others know that birth is imminent and know their roles and what to expect.
4. If in a hospital setting, the nursing staff has been notified that the woman is nearing birth. If in an out-of-hospital setting, an assistant is present.
5. Newborn resuscitation equipment and supplies are present and in working condition.
6. Blankets are warmed for the newborn.
7. Necessary instruments and materials are in a place of ready access. It is helpful to have additional sterile gloves, or for them to be very accessible, should they be needed.
8. Protective eyewear/facewear should be donned and then scrub hands in preparation for the birth.

9. Dry hands and arms, using surgical technique.
10. Put on protective clothing, which may be a gown or other waterproof garment, and then glove using sterile technique.
11. The sterile equipment is arranged in a manner that makes it readily accessible. Maintain the instruments in a sterile field. It is helpful to separate what is needed for the birth of the infant (i.e., two surgical clamps and a pair of scissors for clamping and cutting the umbilical cord; a cord clamp). The instruments can be reorganized as events progress and different items are needed.
12. Drape the woman in accord with the drapes provided and institutional procedure. In the context of a birth anywhere other than the delivery room, this generally involves covering the bed or area the woman is positioned in to maintain a dry, clean area for the newborn.
13. Continue to keep the woman and her significant others informed and involved in the ongoing progress and activities.

(1) how to coach the woman through the final perineal phase of the second stage of labor; (2) whether to use warm compresses, perineal massage, or a "hands-off" or "hands-on" approach; (3) whether to use a Ritgen maneuver; (4) whether to cut an episiotomy; (5) where to place the newborn immediately after birth—that is, whether to facilitate skin-to-skin contact on the mother; and (6) when to clamp and cut the umbilical cord. Hand maneuvers for the clinician attending the birth of a newborn are reviewed in **Appendix 29A**.

Perineal Integrity

As the actual birth begins, the first focus is on promoting perineal integrity and preventing lacerations. Birth positions known to decrease the incidence of genital tract trauma include lateral and semi-upright positions. Squatting is associated with more second-degree lacerations, but this may be because it is a position wherein the provider has difficulty in controlling extension of the fetal head. The position associated with the most genital tract trauma is lithotomy. This is most likely because marked abduction of the thighs stretches the perineum so it is a tight band without significant ability to flex around the emerging head.

Most women who have a vaginal birth sustain some perineal trauma.[52] A systematic technique for inspecting the vagina and perineum for lacerations immediately after the birth is presented in **Appendix 29B**. The types of perineal lacerations are described in **Table 29-3**. Perineal lacerations can cause both short-term and long-term morbidity and pain. Perineal support techniques that are purported to decrease the incidence of genital tract trauma include warm compresses, perineal massage, and "hands-off" versus "hands-on" perineal support. Strategies that reduce the risk of perineal tearing are described in **Box 29-9**.[53]

A meta-analysis of perineal support techniques has been conducted.[54] Researchers have found that warm wet compresses placed on the perineum and held there continuously during the perineal phase of second stage labor and perineal massage with lubricant (two gloved fingers just inside the vagina and outside on the perineum, moving side to side with some downward pressure during the perineal phase) do not improve the rate of intact perineum but do appear to decrease the incidence of third- and fourth-degree lacerations.[54–56]

"Hands off" means not touching the perineum until the fetal head is crowning (i.e., the biparietal

Table 29-3	Types of Perineal Lacerations
Perineal Laceration	**Description**
First degree	Involves the skin, vaginal mucosa, and posterior fourchette
Second degree	Involves the skin, vaginal mucosa, and posterior fourchette, extending into the perineal body fascia and musculature but not the anal sphincter. Includes the superficial and deep transverse perineal muscle and fibers of the pubococcygeus and bulbocavernosus muscles.
Third degree	Involves the skin, vaginal mucosa, posterior fourchette, perineal muscles, and external anal sphincter
	3a. < 50% of the external anal sphincter
	3b. > 50% of the external anal sphincter
	3c. Complete rupture of the external anal sphincter and internal anal sphincter is torn
Fourth degree	Involves the skin, vaginal mucosa, posterior fourchette, and perineal muscles, extending through the anal sphincter and anterior rectal mucosa
Sulcus tears	Vaginal mucosa and underlying tissue lacerate along one or both sides of the posterior column of the vagina instead of the middle inferior part of the vagina
Labial	A laceration that extends from the fourchette anteriorly in one or both of the labia majora bodies
Periurethral	Longitudinal or transverse tear in the labia minora very near the urethra
Clitoral	A periurethral tear that extends into or near the clitoral body
Cervical	Laceration on any part of the cervix, usually on one or both of the lateral sides at approximately 3 o'clock and 9 o'clock where the anterior and posterior aspects join

BOX 29-9 Promoting an Intact Perineum and Reducing the Incidence of Lacerations

- Making certain the thighs and legs are not abducted laterally reduces the risk of perineal tearing.
- Warm compresses, perineal massage, and "hands-off" or "hands-on" techniques used during the perineal phase may decrease the incidence of third- and fourth-degree lacerations. Vigorous or sustained perineal massage during the second stage can cause perineal edema and tearing.
- When the fetus is delivered slowly between contractions, there is less chance of a laceration. If blanching of the perineum is observed, encourage the woman to breathe instead of push, to support slower birth of the fetal head.

Sources: Adapted from Low LK. Promoting physiological labor and birth in supporting a physiologic approach to pregnancy and birth. In: Avery M, ed. *Supporting a Physiologic Approach to Pregnancy and Birth.* Ames, IA: Wiley; 2013; Aasheim V, Nilsen ABV, Lukasse M, Reinar LM. Perineal techniques during the second stage of labour for reducing perineal trauma. *Cochrane Database Syst Rev.* 2011;12:CD006672. doi: 10.1002/14651858.CD006672.pub2; Albers LL. Midwifery care measures in the second stage of labor and reduction of genital tract trauma at birth: a randomized trial. *J Midwifery Women's Health.* 2005;50:365-372.

hospital in California. The chairman of obstetrics at this hospital noted that women cared for by midwives rarely had third- or fourth-degree perineal lacerations compared to the women who were cared for by resident and attending physicians. The only practice difference between the two professional groups that shared one population was that the midwives did not cut episiotomies routinely. This observation prompted a 2-year retrospective review of births and publication of a seminal study that showed that episiotomies are more likely to result in third- or fourth-degree lacerations than are spontaneous perineal tears.[57] Many subsequent studies have validated these findings, and today routine episiotomy is not recommended.[56–60] The incidence of episiotomy in the United States fell from 60.9% in 1979 to 24.5% in 2004.[59]

Today the primary indication for an episiotomy is an abnormal fetal heart rate pattern suggesting the need to expedite birth. An additional argument can be made that an episiotomy is beneficial in anticipation of using forceps or vacuum, or if there are risk factors present for shoulder dystocia. Nevertheless, there is no evidence that an episiotomy is necessary in these situations, and this procedure clearly increases the risk for an extension to or through the anal sphincter. An episiotomy is not recommended for a woman who has a risk for shoulder dystocia because shoulder dystocia risks are not predictive.

Type of Episiotomy to Perform

The two types of episiotomy are reviewed in **Table 29-4**. A mediolateral episiotomy is less likely to result in a third- or fourth-degree laceration than is a midline episiotomy. Interestingly, in the United States there is a greater tendency to perform midline episiotomies, whereas in other Western and European countries the primary approach is to use a mediolateral episiotomy. If the distance between the posterior fourchette and the rectal sphincter is unusually short, a mediolateral episiotomy may be preferable to prevent laceration through the rectal sphincter, especially if the woman has any condition that impairs healing ability, which would increase the chance of breakdown. A midline episiotomy is less painful than a mediolateral episiotomy during the healing process because there are fewer nerve branches in the locale of a midline episiotomy and its repair, but the risk of a fourth-degree laceration is higher when a midline episiotomy is used.

Need for Analgesia or Anesthesia–Analgesia

If there is a need to perform an episiotomy, there is also the need for anesthesia. The midwife can

diameter of the fetal head is through the vulva). "Hands on" entails using one hand to maintain flexion of the fetal occiput and the other hand to guard the perineal body by placing fingers on both sides of the perineum. Studies of these two techniques have not found one method to be superior to the other. However, a multivariate analysis of the elements of delivery technique associated with reduced genital tract trauma in one of the RCTs performed found that controlled delivery of the fetal head between uterine contractions is associated with the lowest rate of genital tract trauma (RR: 0.82; 95% CI: 0.67–0.99).[56]

Indications for Episiotomy

Routine episiotomy was part of standard obstetric management until the 1990s, as it was believed to decrease the incidence of perineal lacerations. The change from routine episiotomy to rare episiotomy occurred over the course of a decade in the 1990s. The seminal study that initiated this change in practice is credited to a midwifery practice in a large city

Table 29-4	Types of Episiotomy
Episiotomy	**Description**
Midline	A midline incision that starts at the posterior fourchette and extends inferiorly through the central tendon of the perineal body including the transverse perineal muscle. Involves the skin, vaginal mucosa, and posterior fourchette and perineal muscles but not the anal sphincter. Equivalent to a second-degree laceration.
Mediolateral	Incision that begins at the midline in the posterior fourchette and extends laterally and inferiorly away from the rectum. May be right or left mediolateral incision.

select either a pudendal block or local infiltration. The different techniques used for performing a local infiltration both prior to birth (for cutting an episiotomy) and after birth (for repair of a laceration or episiotomy) are reviewed in **Appendix 29C**. The technique and necessary equipment and materials for performing a pudendal block are presented in **Appendix 29D**, and **Appendix 29E** reviews the technique for cutting an episiotomy and for repairing a laceration or episiotomy.

Birth of the Fetal Head

An ideal time for birth of the head is between contractions. The combination of the uterine contraction and the maternal pushing effort exerts a double force at the moment of birth, which makes birth of the head more rapid and the release of restraining pressure more abrupt. In contrast, between contractions, the woman is usually better able to focus on what the midwife may be counseling. As a result, the midwife can work with the woman to control the pace of her pushing, asking her to provide less forceful pushes so that the midwife can slowly guide the perineum over the head and face of the fetus. This process of observation of the perineum looking for blanching or beginning tears and feedback between the midwife and the woman is a team approach to help the woman gently give birth while making every effort to protect perineal integrity.

Ritgen Maneuver

Rarely there is a need to speed the delivery of the head, either to encourage birth when there is concern

for fetal well-being or to slowly control the final extension to theoretically reduce risk of lacerations. The Ritgen maneuver, or modified Ritgen maneuver, is a technique by which the clinician applies pressure behind woman's rectum to support extension of the fetal head (**Figure 29-1**). The steps involved in performance of this maneuver are detailed in **Box 29-10**.

Routine use of the Ritgen maneuver is not recommended. Instead, it should be reserved for those limited circumstances when there is a need to actively direct extension of the fetal vertex to enact a rapid birth. A combination of an episiotomy and a Ritgen maneuver will shorten the final perineal phase of the fetal head being born over the perineum.

Hand Maneuvers

The hand maneuvers for birth when the fetus is vertex (OA) and the mother is in various positions are outlined in detail in Appendix 29A. The hand maneuvers for a persistent OP position are the same as for an OA position, except for control of the fetus's head. The direction of pressure to help maintain the head in flexion and then to allow gradual extension when the head is occiput posterior is exactly opposite from the direction of the pressure exerted for the same purpose when the head is occiput anterior. The use of birth simulators or review of virtual birth simulations may aid in the process of skill development for the new midwife as well.

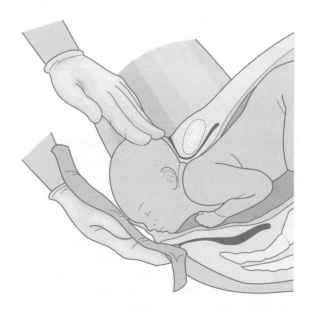

Figure 29-1 Ritgen maneuver.

BOX 29-10 Steps for Ritgen Maneuver

The Ritgen maneuver was first described by Ferdinand von Ritgen in 1828 as a method of protecting the perineum from laceration. The initial technique was to use one hand to press against the perineum, thereby pushing the fetal head into more of a flexed position until after the vertex has crowned. He later modified the technique so that both hands are used, one to maintain flexion by pushing down on the occiput under the symphysis and then the other hand to find the underside of the fetal chin between the coccyx and the rectum and to extend the chin by pulling forward on it. The goal was to control the birth of the head by controlling both flexion and extension. Today the maneuver is often used to speed the birth by speeding the process of extension via forward pressure on the fetal chin.

1. One hand remains on the occiput as the fetus is crowning to maintain flexion until after the biparietal diameters are visible.
2. The other hand uses a gauze or sterile towel to protect against rectal contamination and feels for the fetal chin under the skin in the area between the coccyx and rectum. Some authors have advocated putting a finger in the rectum to find the fetal chin but this increases the risk of perineal tearing and possible buttonhole tear in the rectum.
3. Forward and outward pressure is then exerted on the underneath side of the chin, and the head is controlled between this hand and the hand exerting pressure on the occiput to direct the process of extension to support and control the pace of the birth of the infant's head.

Immediately Following the Birth

Placing the Newborn in Skin-to-Skin Contact

The ideal placement for the newborn is on the mother's abdomen, in skin-to-skin contact, promoting a positive transition from intrauterine to extrauterine life. Skin-to-skin contact promotes thermoregulation of the newborn, reduces physiologic stress, enhances successful breastfeeding both initially and at 3 months postpartum, and results in improved scores on maternal–infant bonding.[61,62] Evaluation of the infant, the assignment of Apgar scores, and initial vital signs can be completed while the newborn remains skin-to-skin with the mother.[61]

Healthy newborns who have uninterrupted contact with their mother begin to make crawling movements toward her breast after approximately 20 minutes, and by an average of 50 minutes most are correctly sucking and breastfeeding.[63] Newborn procedures should be delayed until at least an hour after the birth so skin-to-skin placement can occur while the newborn adapts to post-gestational life.

Clamping and Cutting the Umbilical Cord: Delayed Cord Clamping

Delaying cord clamping is an evidence-based practice that promotes the transition from intrauterine to extrauterine life and offers other additional health benefits.[64–66] Delayed cord clamping involves waiting at least 30 seconds and as long as 4 to 5 minutes after the birth before the cord is clamped and cut. In practice, once the cord has stopped pulsating, there is no more transitional blood flow that could benefit the newborn; thus clamping and cutting the cord can be performed.

If the infant is preterm, good evidence indicates that delayed cord clamping can offer significant benefit to the newborn. Deliberately holding the preterm infant at or below the level of the vaginal introitus, which is itself at or below the level of the placenta, can result in additional blood volume for the newborn. Lowering the infant, combined with delayed cord clamping, will result in a transfusion of approximately 80 mL of blood from the placenta into the newborn. This transfusion is thought to facilitate physiologic processes involved in the transition from fetal life to life after birth that may be critical for the very-low-birth-weight preterm newborn.[64]

Delayed cord clamping action must incorporate the newborn's need for warmth and possible resuscitation. One workable compromise suggested by Mercer et al. is to receive the newborn into a warm blanket. The newborn is then lowered the length of the umbilical cord, without tension on the cord, to obtain maximum placental infusion for 30 to 45 seconds before clamping and cutting the cord.[64,65] Delayed cord clamping is not indicated if there is a known blood incompatibility between the mother and the infant.

The umbilical cord is clamped by placing two surgical clamps on the cord with just enough room between them to allow for easy cutting of the cord. After applying the first clamp, the midwife can milk the cord for the distance to the planned location of the second clamp. This prevents blood from spurting from a distended umbilical vessel that is between the two clamps at the time of cutting. Once one clamp has been applied, it should be supported so the weight of the clamp is not allowed to exert pull or tension on the newborn's abdomen. Once both clamps are placed, the midwife or a support person can cut the cord as a way of participating in this significant moment.

Inspection of the Perineum and Laceration Repair

The third stage of labor begins as soon as the infant is born, and this is the time during which the risk for postpartum hemorrhage is the greatest. As soon as the infant is safely being observed/cared for by an assistant, the midwife observes vaginal bleeding while inspecting the vagina and perineum for lacerations and arterial bleeding. The systematic inspection process and laceration repair techniques are summarized in Appendix 29B and Appendix 29E.

The Apgar Score

Parents today often refer to the Apgar score as their baby's first report card. This scoring system was devised during the mid-twentieth century by Virginia Apgar, an anesthesiologist who worked at a time when heavy maternal sedation and anesthesia was common during labor. Thus it was not unusual for newborns to have respiratory depression and low tone at birth secondary to the large doses of morphine administered late in labor. It is reported that Apgar personally was upset that small apneic newborns were not resuscitated so she developed the Apgar score as a way of assessing the effects of maternal anesthesia on the newborn.[66] Although the actual reason Dr. Apgar developed the score is not known for certain, she instituted a mandate that the newborn

be assessed at 1 and 5 minutes of age. The simplicity of the system as well as the need for attention to the neonate caused it to be adopted quickly. Today the Apgar score is universally used in the United States.

Apgar scoring uses five components to assess the newborn's successful adaptation of extrauterine life.[67] Occasionally it is misinterpreted as a surrogate for assessing the presence of perinatal asphyxia. The Apgar score was designed to assess adaptation to extrauterine life, which is different than an assessment of intrauterine status prior to birth. Although some components of the Apgar score are related to prebirth acid–base balance, the Apgar score alone is not a reliable measure of perinatal asphyxia. Apgar scores are an indicator of resuscitation success, however, and are continued every 5 minutes if resuscitation efforts are ongoing. Moreover, resuscitation efforts should not depend upon the first Apgar score for initiation since the first minute of life can be a critical one.

The five components of the Apgar score include key reflections of cardiovascular and circulatory status, lung function, and neuromuscular integrity. A score of 7–10 denotes a vigorous neonate, a newborn with a score of 4–6 requires some focused resuscitation efforts, and a newborn with a score of 3 or less requires intensive resuscitation procedures. Several years after the scoring system was publicized, an acronym was devised using Virginia Apgar's surname. Therefore, some professionals know the scoring system as Appearance, Pulse, Grimace, Activity, and Respirations, as noted in **Table 29-5**.

In order to decrease bias, optimally, the Apgar score is awarded by a birth attendant or nurse who is not the individual responsible for conducting the birth. The 1-minute Apgar score is not associated

Table 29-5	The Apgar Score			
Classic Component	**Acronym**	**Score of 0**	**Score of 1**	**Score of 2**
Color	**A**ppearance	Blue/pale over entire body	Acrocyanosis Body pink	Body and extremities pink
Heart rate	**P**ulse	Absent	< 100	≥ 100
Reflex irritability	**G**rimace	No response to stimulation	Grimace/weak cry when stimulated	Cry or attempt to pull away when stimulated
Muscle tone	**A**ctivity	None	Some flexion	Flexed extremities that resist extension
Respiratory efforts	**R**espirations	Absent	Week, irregular, gasping	Strong cry

Source: Apgar V. A proposal for a new method of evaluation of the newborn infant. *Curr Res Anesth Analg*. 1953 Jul-Aug;32(4):260-267. Reprinted by permission of Lippincott Williams & Wilkins.

with long-term outcomes. Neonatal mortality is associated with the 5-minute Apgar score and studies in this century continue to demonstrate that relationship, even after the advent of umbilical cord blood sampling and other assessment methods.[68,69]

Conclusion

In summary, the responsibility of the midwife is to maintain safety and security for the woman, fetus, and newborn during the birth process. To do so, the midwife must have full awareness of the desires and expectations of the woman and persons who share her labor and birth. This will allow the midwife to orchestrate an optimal birth experience within the boundaries of the individual circumstances, birth environment, and clinical factors that affect that mother and newborn.

• • • References

1. Kennedy HP, Rousseau AL, Low LK. An exploratory metasynthesis of midwifery practice in the United States. *Midwifery*. 2003;19(3):203-214.

2. Roberts JE. A new understanding of the second stage of labor: implications for nursing care. *J Obstet Gynecol Neonatal Nurs*. 2003;39:794-801.

3. Roberts JE. The "push" for evidence: management of the 2nd stage. *J Midwifery Women's Health*. 2011;47(1):2-15.

4. Friedman EA. *Labor: Clinical Evaluation and Management*. 2nd ed. New York, NY: Appleton-Century-Crofts; 1978.

5. Kilpatrick SJ, Laros RK. Characteristics of normal labor. *Obstet Gynecol*. 1989;74(1):85-87.

6. Zhang J, Landy HJ, Brancy DW, et al. Contemporary patterns of spontaneous labor with normal neonatal outcomes. *Obstet Gynecol*. 2010;116:1281-1287.

7. Laughon SK, Branch W, Beaver J, Zhang J. Changes in labor patterns over 50 years. *Am J Obstet Gynecol*. 2012;206:419.e1-e9.

8. Tuuli M, Frey HA, Odibo AO, Macones, GA, Cahill AG. Immediate compared with delayed pushing in the second stage of labor: a systematic review and meta-analysis. *Obstet Gynecol*. 2012;20:660–668.

9. Brancato R, Church S, Stone P. A meta-analysis of passive descent versus immediate pushing in nulliparous women with epidural analgesia in the second stage of labor. *J Obstet Gynecol Neonatal Nurs*. 2008;37:4-12.

10. Fraser WD, Marcoux S, Krauss I, et al. Multicenter randomized, controlled trial of delayed pushing for nulliparous women in the second stage of labor with continuous epidural analgesia. *Am J Obstet Gynecol*. 2000;182:1165-1172.

11. Fitzpatrick M, Harkin R, McQuillan K, et al. A randomised clinical trial comparing the effects of delayed versus immediate pushing with epidural analgesia on mode of delivery and faecal continence. *Br J Obstet Gynaecol*. 2002;109(12):1359-1365.

12. Rouse DJ, Weiner SJ, Bloom SL, et al. Second-stage labor duration in nulliparous women: relationship to maternal and perinatal outcomes. *Am J Obstet Gynecol*. 2009;201(4):357.e1-e7.

13. LeRay C, Audibert F, Goffinet F, Fraser W. When to stop pushing: effects of duration of second-stage expulsion efforts on maternal and neonatal outcomes in nulliparous women with epidural analgesia. *Am J Obstet Gynecol*. 2009;201(4):361.e1-e7.

14. Myles TD, Santolaya J. Maternal and neonatal outcomes in patients with a prolonged second stage of labor. *Obstet Gynecol*. 2003;102:52-58.

15. Allen VM, Baskett TF, O'Connell CM, McKeen D, Allen AC. Maternal and perinatal outcomes with increasing duration of the second stage of labor. *Obstet Gynecol*. 2009;113:1248-1258.

16. Caughey AB. Is there an upper time limit for the management of the second stage of labor? *Am J Obstet Gynecol*. 2009;201:337-338.

17. Spong CY, Berghella V, Wenstrom KD, Mercer BM, Saade GR. Preventing the first cesarean delivery: summary of a joint Eunice Kennedy Shriver National Institute of Child Health and Human Development, Society for Maternal–Fetal Medicine, and American College of Obstetricians and Gynecologists Workshop. *Obstet Gynecol*. 2012;120(5):1181-1193.

18. Kearney R, Miller JM, Ashton-Miller J, DeLancey JOL. Obstetric factors associated with levator ani muscle injury after vaginal birth. *Obstet Gynecol*. 2006;107(1):144-149.

19. Menticoglou SM, Manning F, Harman C, Morrison I. Obstetrics: perinatal outcome in relation to second-stage duration. *Am J Obstet Gynecol*. 1995;173(3):906-912.

20. Peregrine E, O'Brien P, Jauniaux E. Impact on delivery outcome of ultrasonographic fetal head position prior to induction of labor. *Obstet Gynecol*. 2007;109:618.

21. Simkin P. The fetal occiput position; state of the science and a new perspective. *Birth*. 2010;37(1):61-71.

22. Stremler R, Hodnett E, Petryshen P, et al. Randomized controlled trial of hands and knees positioning for occiput posterior position in labor. *Birth*. 2005;32(4):243-251.

23. Shaffer BL, Cheng YW, Vargas JE, et al. Manual rotation of the fetal occiput: predictors of success and delivery. *Am J Obstet Gynecol*. 2006;194:e7.

24. Liang CC, Wong SY, Tsay PT, et al. The effect of epidural analgesia on postpartum urinary retention in women who deliver vaginally. *Int J Obstet Anesth*. 2002;11(3):164-169.

25. Weiniger CF, Wand S, Nadjari M, et al. Post-void residual volume in labor: a prospective study comparing parturients with and without epidural analgesia. *Acta Anaesthesiol Scand*. 2006;50(10):1297-1303.

26. Scrutton MJ, Metcalfe GA, Lowy C, Seed PT, O'Sullivan G. Eating in labour: a randomised controlled trial assessing the risks and benefits. *Anaesthesia*. 1999;54:329-334.

27. Sharts-Hopko NC. Oral intake during labor: a review of the evidence. *Matern Child Nurs*. 2010;35:197-203.

28. American College of Nurse Midwives. Providing oral nutrition to women in labor. Clinical Bulletin Number 10. *J Midwifery Women's Health*. 2008;53:276-283.

29. Bergstrom L, Richards L, Morse J, Roberts J. How care givers manage distress in second stage labor. *J Midwifery Women's Health*. 2010;55(1):38-44.

30. Sperlich M, Seng JS. *Survivor Moms: Women's Stories of Birthing, Mothering and Healing After Sexual Abuse*. Eugene, OR: Motherbaby Press; 2008.

31. American College of Nurse-Midwives. Intermittent auscultation for intrapartum fetal heart rate surveillance. Clinical Bulletin Number 11. *J Midwifery Women's Health*. 2010;55(4):397-403.

32. Yildirim G, Kizilkaya N. Effects of pushing techniques in birth on the mother and fetus: a randomized study. *Birth*. 2008;35(1):25-30.

33. Roberts J, Hanson L. Best practices in second stage labor care: maternal bearing down and positioning. *J Midwifery Women's Health*. 2007;52(3):238-245.

34. Simpson KR, James DC. Effects of immediate versus delayed pushing during 2nd-stage labor on fetal well-being: a randomized clinical trial. *Nurs Res*. 2005;54(3):149-157.

35. Plunkett BA, Lin A, Wong CA, Grobman WA, Peaceman AM. Management of the second stage of labor in nulliparas with continuous epidural analgesia. *Obstet Gynecol*. 2003;102(1):109-114.

36. Gillesby E, Burns S, Dempsey A, et al. Comparison of delayed versus immediate pushing during second stage of labor for nulliparous women with epidural anesthesia. *J Obstet Gynecol Neonatal Nurs*. 2010;39(6):635-644.

37. Vause S, Congdon HM, Thornton JG. Immediate and delayed pushing in the second stage of labour for nulliparous women with epidural analgesia: a randomised controlled trial. *Br J Obstet Gynaecol*. 1998;105(2):186-188.

38. Dietz HP, Lanzarone V. Levator trauma after vaginal delivery. *Obstet Gynecol*. 2005;106(4):707-711.

39. Shek KL, Dietz HP. Intrapartum risk factors for levator trauma. *Br J Obstet Gynaecol*. 2010;117:1485-1492.

40. Chan SS, Cheung RY, Yiu AK, et al. Prevalence of levator ani muscle injury in Chinese primiparous women after first delivery. *Ultrasound Obstet Gynecol*. 2012;39:704-709.

41. Torvaldsen S, Roberts CL, Bell JC, Raynes-Greenow CH. Discontinuation of epidural analgesia late in labour for reducing the adverse delivery outcomes associated with epidural analgesia. *Cochrane Database Syst Rev*. 2004;CD004457.

42. Mhyre JM. What's new in obstetric anesthesia? *Int J Obstet Anesth*. 2011;20(2):149-159.

43. Sampselle CM, Hines S. Spontaneous pushing during birth: relationship to perineal outcomes. *J Nurse Midwifery*. 1999;44(1):36-39.

44. Bloom SL, Casey BM, Schaffer JI, McIntire DD, Leveno KJ. A randomized trial of coached versus uncoached maternal pushing during the second stage of labor. *Am J Obstet Gynecol*. 2005;194:10-13.

45. Schaffer JI, Bloom SL, Casey BM, et al. A randomized trial of the effects of coached vs uncoached maternal pushing during the second stage of labor on postpartum pelvic floor structure and function. *Am J Obstet Gynecol*. 2005;192(5):1692-1696.

46. Cheng YW, Hopkins LM, Caughey AB. How long is too long: does a prolonged second stage of labor in nulliparous women affect maternal and neonatal outcomes? *Am J Obstet Gynecol*. 2004;191(3):933-938.

47. Sampselle CM, Miller JM, Luecha Y, et al. Provider support of spontaneous pushing during the 2nd stage labor. *J Obstet Gynecol Neonatal Nurs*. 2005;34(6):695-702.

48. Roberts JE, Gonzalez C, Sampselle C. Why do supportive birth attendants become directive of maternal bearing down efforts in second stage? *J Midwifery Women's Health*. 2007;52:134-141.

49. Gupta JK, Hofmeyr GJ, Shehmar M. Position in the second stage of labour for women without epidural anaesthesia. *Cochrane Database Syst Rev*. 2012;5:CD002006. doi: 10.1002/14651858.CD002006.pub3.

50. Fenwick L, Simkin P. Maternal positioning to prevent or alleviate dystocia in labor. *Clin Obstet Gynecol*. 1987;30:83-89.

51. Russell JGB. Moulding of the pelvic outlet. *J Obstet Gynaecol Br Commonw*. 1969;76:817-820.

52. Albers LL. Reducing genital tract trauma at birth: launching a clinical trial in midwifery. *J Midwifery Women's Health*. 2003;48:109.

53. Low LK. Promoting physiological labor and birth in supporting a physiologic approach to pregnancy and birth. In: Avery M, ed. *Supporting a Physiologic Approach to Pregnancy and Birth*. Ames, IA: Wiley; 2013.

54. Aasheim V, Nilsen ABV, Lukasse M, Reinar LM. Perineal techniques during the second stage of labour for reducing perineal trauma. *Cochrane Database Syst*

Rev. 2011;12:CD006672. doi: 10.1002/14651858. CD006672.pub2.

55. Moore ER, Anderson GC, Bergman N, Dowswell T. Early skin-to-skin contact for mothers and their healthy newborn infants. *Cochrane Database Syst Rev.* 2012;5:CD003519.

56. Albers LL. Midwifery care measures in the second stage of labor and reduction of genital tract trauma at birth: a randomized trial. *J Midwifery Women's Health.* 2005;50:365-372.

57. Green JR, Soohoo SL. Factors associated with rectal injury in spontaneous deliveries. *Obstet Gynecol.* 1989;73(5 Pt 1):732-738.

58. Carroli G, Mignini L. Episiotomy for vaginal birth. *Cochrane Database Syst Rev.* 2009;1:CD000081. doi: 10.1002/14651858.CD000081.pub2.

59. Frankman EA, Wang L, Bunker CH, Lowder JL. Episiotomy in the United States: has anything changed? *Am J Obstet Gynecol.* 2009;200(5):573.e1-e7.

60. Albers LL, Borders N. Minimizing genital tract trauma and related pain following spontaneous vaginal birth. *J Midwifery Women's Health.* 2007;52:246-253.

61. Haxton D, Doering J, Gingras L, Kelly L. Implementing skin-to-skin contact at birth using the Iowa model: applying evidence to practice. *Nurs Women's Health.* 2012;16(3):220-229.

62. Anderson GC, Moore E, Hepworth J, Bergman N. Early skin-to-skin contact for mothers and their healthy newborn infants. *Cochrane Database Syst Rev.* 2003;2:CD003519. doi: 10.1002/14651858. CD003519.

63. Righard L, Alade MO. Effect of delivery room routines on success of first breastfeed. *Lancet.* 1990;336: 1105-1107.

64. Mercer J, Erickson-Owens D. Delayed cord clamping increases infants' iron stores. *Lancet.* 2006;367(9527): 1956-1958.

65. Mercer JS. Current best evidence: a review of the literature on umbilical cord clamping. *J Midwifery Women's Health* 2001;46(6):402-414.

66. Finster M, Wood M. The Apgar score has survived the test of time. *Anesthesiology.* 2005 Apr;102(4): 855-857.

67. Apgar V. A proposal for a new method of evaluation of the newborn infant. *Curr Res Anesth Analg.* 1953 Jul-Aug;32(4):260-267.

68. Casey BM, McIntire DD, Leveno KJ: The continuing value of the Apgar score for the assessment of newborn infants. *N Engl J Med.* 2001; 344:467-471

69. Vahabi S, Haidari M, Akbari Torkamani S, Gorbani Vaghei A. New assessment of relationship between Apgar score and early neonatal mortality. *Minerva Pediatr.* 2010 Jun;62(3):249-252.

29A

Hand Maneuvers for Birth

LISA KANE LOW

SARASWATHI VEDAM

MAVIS SCHORN

MARY C. BRUCKER

TEKOA L. KING

The hand maneuvers used to facilitate birth are designed to ensure a safe birth of the infant and minimize perineal trauma. The basic hand maneuvers can be adapted for a woman in any position or a fetus in any position.

Hand Maneuvers for Birth When the Fetus Is in the Occiput Anterior Position and the Woman Is in a Semi-Sitting, Lateral, or Dorsal Position

1. Ensure both access to the perineum and visibility of the vulvar-perineal area.

   a. The midwife stands or sits in a position that allows for a clear visual field and comfortable access to the woman's perineum.

   b. A sterile drape is placed on a surface within easy reach, on which instruments and a bowl for the placenta are placed

2. Control extension of fetal vertex. During extension of the head, the transverse diameter of the fetal vertex gradually changes from the suboccipitobregmatic diameter (9.5 cm) to the occipitofrontal diameter (11.5 cm) and then to the occipitomental diameter (12.5 cm). Gradual extension prevents perineal trauma as these increasing diameters stretch the perineum during the birth. The primary goal is to prevent sudden extension of the fetal head, which increases the likelihood of perineal tearing.

   a. To control extension of the fetal head during crowning, the midwife places the pads of the fingertips on the occiput of the portion of the vertex showing at the vaginal introitus. The position of the woman may dictate the easiest hand to use, but the use of the nondominant hand leaves the dominant hand free to handle any equipment or supplies that may be suddenly and quickly needed (e.g., a right-handed person would use the left hand on the head, leaving the right hand free for other actions). Some midwives advocate an exact placement of the hand. Given that midwifery hands vary in size and women deliver in many different positions, the actual placement may be less important than identifying a manner in which the individual midwife can provide the needed control and simultaneously be able to visualize the entire perineum.

   b. Keeping the fingers flat or parallel to the palm of the hand, the midwife guides extension by exerting a controlling, but not prohibitive, pressure. If the fingers and palm are not in a flat plane, they can easily slip and the vertex can extend suddenly into the midwife's cupped hand.

3. Technique for providing perineal support. Although the studies comparing "hands off" and "hands on" techniques for supporting the perineum prior to birth have been inconclusive with regard to their effect on perineal lacerations, many midwives use some method of perineal support.[1-3] Therefore, although not conclusively evidence-based, a technique for such is presented here as an option for use during the birth. The

goal of perineal support is to reduce tension in the midline plane of the perineum.

a. Using the hand that is not controlling the pace of extension of the occiput, the midwife places a thumb and one finger on the perineum below the fourchette so that the midline area that is likely to tear is between the thumb and finger.

b. Applying pressure with the thumb and fingers inward toward each other and the middle of the perineum (perineal body) reduces tension on the midpoint (**Figure 29A-1**).

c. As the vertex is born via extension, the midwife observes the tension placed on the perineum. The appearance of thin white lines or blanching during this final period of tension indicates increased risk of perineum tearing. If this is present, it would be an indication to increase perineal support.

4. Check for a nuchal cord. As soon as the head is born, the midwife places the fingertips of one hand on the occiput and slides them along the curve of the infant's head toward the neck, sweeping them along the neck in both directions, to determine if the umbilical cord is coiled around the neck (**Figure 29A-2**). If a nuchal cord is present, it is important to assess how tight the cord is by placing the fingertips over the cord and attempting to pull it toward the occiput. There are four options for proceeding with the birth if a nuchal cord is present:

a. *Cord reduction:* If the cord is loose, slip it forward over the head before delivery of the

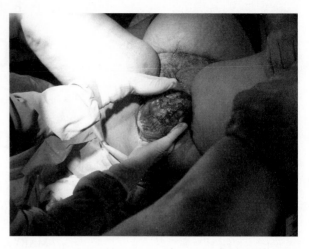

Figure 29A-2 Check for nuchal cord after birth of head.

shoulders (referred to as reducing the cord over the head).

b. *Birth through the cord:* If the cord is too tight to reduce but still has some mobility, slip it back over the shoulders as the infant is born, allowing the infant to be born through the cord.

c. *Somersault maneuver:* If the cord is too tight to slip over the shoulders but loose enough to permit some movement, use one hand to keep the head close to the maternal thigh throughout the delivery of the body and the other hand to "somersault" the body through the tight cord.[4,5] The somersault maneuver is depicted in **Figure 29A-3**.

d. *Clamp and cut:* If the cord is too tight to accomplish the other preferred steps, double-clamp and cut the cord between the clamps

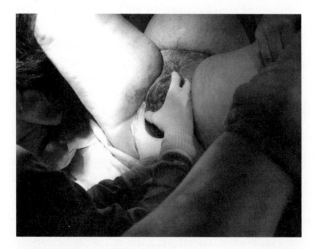

Figure 29A-1 The right hand is controlling extension of the head and the left hand is at the perineum ready to provide support as needed.

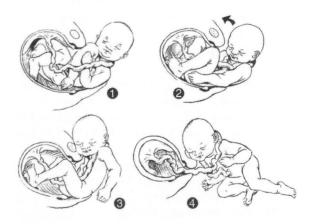

Figure 29A-3 Somersault maneuver for tight nuchal cord.
Source: Copyright © by Judith Mercer. Reprinted with permission of Judith Mercer.

at the neck before the infant's body is born. The midwife informs the woman that she will need to refrain from pushing until the cord has been clamped, cut, and unwound from the infant's neck.

5. While waiting for external rotation and the next contraction, the midwife or assistant can wipe fluid from the neonate's face, nose, and mouth with a soft, absorbent cloth. Suctioning with a bulb syringe of the fetal nasal and oral passages is not necessary.[6]

   a. It is important to wait for a contraction and for restitution and external rotation to occur, as indicated when the occiput rotates 90°. Unless the cord has been cut, there is no need to hurry or interfere by rotating the head manually. If the cord has been cut, and external rotation is not yet completed, assist rotation of the shoulders, as described in the management of shoulder dystocia in the *Complications During Labor and Birth* chapter, into the anteroposterior diameter of the pelvis.

   b. When restitution is complete, the midwife shifts her own position a little to the right or left to align with the infant's back. If the head rotates to the LOT position, then shift toward the woman's left. If the head rotates to the ROT position, then shift toward the woman's right. Wait for the onset of the next contraction.

6. Deliver the shoulders.

   a. Place one hand, straightened so it is flat, on each side of the infant's head over the cheek bones so that the fingers point toward the fetal face and nose and the little fingers are closest to the woman's perineum. This means that for a fetus in the LOT position, the fetus will be facing the woman's right leg, the midwife's left hand will be the bottom hand underneath the fetal head, and the midwife's right hand will be the hand on top of the fetal head; for a fetus in the ROT position, the fetus will be facing the woman's left leg, the midwife's right hand will be the bottom hand underneath the head, and the midwife's left hand will be the hand on top of the head. Colloquially, some midwives term this "sandwiching" the newborn's head between the midwife's hands (**Figure 29A-4**).

   b. Assist the woman to deliver the anterior shoulder. Avoid gripping the infant's neck

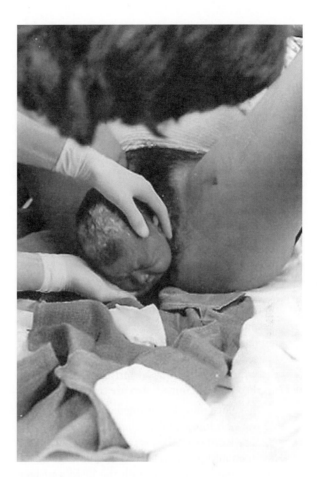

Figure 29A-4 Placement of hands for birth of shoulders.

by keeping the fingers straight so the hands are flat on the sides of the head. During the next contraction, while the woman pushes, exert gentle, downward pressure on the side of the head with the top hand until the top of the anterior shoulder and axilla can be seen beneath the symphysis pubis.

   c. Apply gentle upward pressure on the side of the fetal head with both hands lifting the infant's head following the natural arc of the curve of Carus toward the woman's abdomen. Some midwives suggest that the perineum can be protected during the birth of the posterior shoulder by sliding the bottom hand over the shoulder and keeping the infant's arms and hands close to the body during the birth.

   d. As the posterior shoulder is being born, pivot the bottom hand under the fetal head so that the palmar side of the hand is facing the woman's perineum and cup the neck between the thumb and fingers to support the head. The midwife's thumb will be wrapped around the neck near the back and the fingers will be on the neck near the infant's thorax. The head is resting near the midwife's forearm. This is the first secure grip that will be maintained.

e. Slide the hand that was on the top of the fetal head down the infant's back and grasp the infant between the legs, holding both legs in this hand. This is the second secure grip that will be maintained.

7. Complete the final phase of birth. As the body of the infant emerges, she or he can (1) be placed immediately onto the woman's abdomen or (2) remain being held by the midwife, with the infant supported by the hand that was originally on the bottom side of the head while an initial assessment is completed or in anticipation of handing the infant to another clinician. Which option is used depends on the status of the infant and the woman at the time of birth and if there is a need to initiate immediate care or resuscitation.

a. To place the infant immediately on the woman's abdomen, move the infant in a smooth arc from over the perineum onto her abdomen and position the infant laterally on the woman's abdomen with the head and face slightly lower than the body to facilitate drainage of oral and nasal fluids.

i. While moving the infant onto the abdomen, confirm that there is no tension on the umbilical cord.

ii. Hold one hand on the infant until the woman is holding her newborn.

b. To prepare to hand the infant to another clinician:

i. Pivot the hand cupping the infant's neck so that the head is now supported by the palmar surface of the outstretched index and middle fingers, the suboccipital region and back of the neck are in the palm of the hand, and the thumb and remaining fingers are *resting*—not pressing—against the sides of the neck. The top hand continues its grasp around legs during this maneuver.

ii. The infant's legs are tucked between the midwife's arm (the arm holding the infant's head) and body at waist level. The infant's back is supported on the lower arm. This maneuver allows the midwife to have one hand free to clamp and cut

the umbilical cord as indicated. An initial assessment can be conducted very quickly at this time.

Hand Skills for Birth of a Fetus in the Occiput Posterior Position

The same hand maneuvers described for the woman whose fetus is OA are applicable for the fetus in OP with one exception. The direction of pressure exerted to maintain flexion of the head is maintained by upward pressure instead of downward pressure because the occiput is closer to the rectum than it is to the symphysis. Once the biparietal diameters are visible, releasing the upward pressure on the occiput, in a controlled manner, controls extension. This hand skill also is used for the fetus in a face presentation; in a face presentation, the mentum (chin) will be under the symphysis and, as it is born, the rest of the head will be born by flexion of the neck. A face presentation that rotates so the mentum is posterior will not deliver vaginally because the neck is too short. Once the head is out, the remaining hand maneuvers are the same as described previously.

Hand Skills for Birth When the Woman Is in a Hands-And-Knees Position

While the mechanisms of labor are not changed by this maternal position, the manner in which the infant emerges appears reversed and requires variations in the direction of support and positioning of hands as a result. Visibility and access to effect maneuvers are enhanced in this position, but while the woman can hear the midwife, she is not able to see the midwife when in this position. As a result, anticipatory guidance to the woman about what to expect, and where she will need to position herself to receive the newborn, should all be communicated prior to birth if possible. In addition, there may be increased stress on the anterior labia and on the periurethral area when the woman assumes a hands-and-knees position for birth. **Figures 29A-5 through 29A-8** show a birth when the woman is in a hands-and-knees position and the fetus is in an occiput anterior position.

1. As the head emerges, the midwife places fingertips, palm up, on the occiput, with the fingertips pointing toward to the woman's abdomen. As the head begins to emerge, exert a slight pressure with the length of the fingers on the occiput to

maintain flexion of the fetal head. Be careful to avoid touching the clitoris.

2. Allow the head to extend gradually, maintaining a steady but gentle counterpressure until the biparietal diameter is out and the ears can be visualized. Maintaining flexion until the occiput passes under the symphysis pubis and extension begins will reduce the possibility of perineal trauma.

3. It is possible to support the perineum with the other hand alone or with a warm moist towel. Many women appreciate moist heat on the rectal area as the head crowns and extends.

4. The hand maneuvers involved in checking for a nuchal cord, wiping the infant's head, and watching for restitution and external rotation are the same as the maneuvers for birth described previously. In the hands-and-knees maternal position, the hand checking for the presence of a nuchal cord will be palm up and sliding back under the infant's head. Wiping the infant's face will be easier to effect as the face is up.

5. To effect birth of the shoulders, the hand positions are the same as described previously. Some practitioners deliver the shoulder under the symphysis first just as though the woman were in a dorsal position, and others reverse the order and deliver the shoulder nearest the woman's rectum first.

6. As the upper half of the infant is born and the elbows and hands have cleared the perineum, the same steps are completed as outlined previously.

7. The newborn can be passed to the woman through her legs, keeping a secure hold on the infant until she has a firm grasp on her newborn. The midwife then moves to face the woman and helps her to sit down. It is important to observe for tension on the umbilical cord if this maneuver is selected.

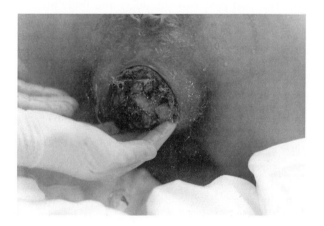

Figure 29A-5

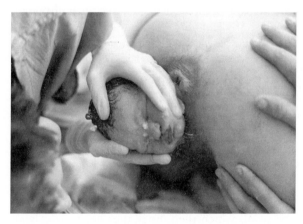

Figure 29A-6

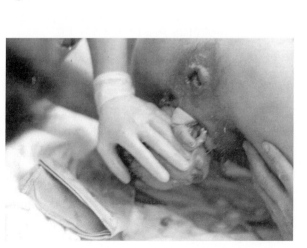

Figure 29A-7

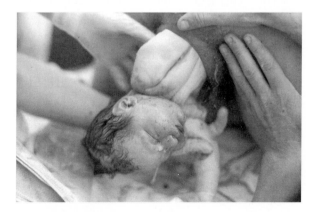

Figure 29A-8

8. Alternatively, the woman can carefully lift one leg and the newborn and cord is passed under her leg as she completes the turn to sit down facing the midwife. The newborn can then be placed on her abdomen.

9. Immediately after birth, many women will naturally lower their haunches to sit back. If the woman sits before passage of the newborn to her arms, she may sit on the cord or newborn. To prevent this problem, the midwife instructs the woman and others assisting with the birth on what to expect both prior to and during the birth process.

Hand Maneuvers for Birth of the Infant When the Woman Is in a Squat or Supported Squat Position

To facilitate visibility, access, and control when the woman is in a squat position, the midwife must also be positioned differently, sitting on a low stool or the floor in front of the woman. In a true squat, the woman's legs are bent and abducted with weight bearing distributed between her legs and feet. This position brings the perineum close to the surface she is squatting on, so the infant emerges just inches above the surface. Moreover, the curve of Carus is such that the natural arc of the infant's path is into the woman's arms as an extension of the arc.[7]

In the supported squat, the woman's buttocks are partially supported by the edge of a broken birthing bed, a birthing chair, or a stool, or the woman is supported in a semi-squat position by another person. The woman may use a squatting bar or handles on the stool, which then distributes her weight bearing between her hands, buttocks, legs, and feet. The perineum is usually suspended above the surface of the bed or floor.

For a fetus in OA position, the following adaptations to the hand maneuvers are made to support the woman giving birth in a squatting position.

1. As the vertex appears at the vaginal introitus, the midwife places the pads of the fingertips of one hand on the crown of the head, with the fingertips pointing toward the woman's abdomen and her elbow pointing to the floor.

2. When the head begins to emerge, the midwife exerts a slight downward pressure with the fingers on the occiput, being careful to avoid touching the clitoris. As the woman pushes, the head gradually extends into the hand, which is maintaining a steady but gentle counterpressure until the biparietal diameter and ears are visible.

3. Perineal support can be provided in the same manner described previously for other positions, but is done by feel—not by sight—in this position.

4. It is important to watch the introitus while the head extends and is born, paying attention to the labial borders. When the vertex emerges with the woman in a true squat position, the pressure exerted on the introitus is distributed between the labia and the perineum. Lacerations along the labial borders are more common but tend to be shallow if the birth is controlled.

The hand maneuvers involved in checking for a nuchal cord, wiping the infant's head, watching for restitution and external rotation, and delivering the anterior and posterior shoulders and body are the same as described previously.

• • • References

1. Aasheim V, Nilsen ABV, Lukasse M, Reinar LM. Perineal techniques during the second stage of labour for reducing perineal trauma. *Cochrane Database Syst Rev.* 2011;2:CD006672. doi: 10.1002/14651858. CD006672.pub.

2. Albers LL. Midwifery care measures in the second stage of labor and reduction of genital tract trauma at birth: a randomized trial. *J Midwifery Women's Health.* 2005;50:365-372.

3. Albers LL, Borders N. Minimizing genital tract trauma and related pain following spontaneous vaginal birth. *J Midwifery Women's Health.* 2007;52:246-253.

4. Schorn MN, Blanco JD. Management of the nuchal cord. *J Nurse Midwifery.* 1991;36:131-132.

5. Mercer JS, Skovgaard RL, Peareara-Eaves J, Bowman TA. Nuchal cord management and nurse-midwifery practice. *J Midwifery Women's Health.* 2005;50: 373-379.

6. Velaphi S, Vidyasagar D. The pros and cons of suctioning at the perineum (intrapartum) and post-delivery with and without meconium. *Semin Fetal Neonatal Med.* 2008;13:375-382; epub May 13, 2008.

7. Golay J, Vedam S. The squatting position for second stage labor: effects on the evaluation and progress of labor and on maternal and fetal well-being. *Birth.* 1993;20(2):73-78.

29B

Genital Tract Injury: Immediate Postpartum Inspection of the Vulva, Perineum, Vagina, and Cervix

Inspection of the vulva, perineum, vagina, and cervix for the presence of lacerations or hematomas takes place immediately after the birth. During this inspection, the midwife identifies:

- The location and type of lacerations
- Whether the lacerations require repair[1,2]
- The presence of any arterial bleeding that needs immediate repair.
- Presence or absence of a hematoma

Key Points

1. Pain relief: Inspection of the vagina and cervix can be uncomfortable or painful. Unless a woman is bleeding heavily and a laceration is suspected as the source of the bleeding, there is no need to proceed with inspection or repair before a woman has adequate pain control. Therefore, the first step is to determine if the woman needs an analgesic for the inspection; this will depend both on how extensive the inspection is likely to be and what the woman's pain threshold is. If an extensive inspection or repair is likely, a woman may need an intravenous dose of an opiate such as fentanyl or morphine. If she has an epidural, the anesthesiologist should be made aware that an inspection is needed so that the epidural can be used to provide the necessary pain relief.

2. Adequate lighting: Ensure that an adequate lighting source is available. The midwife will need to insert three or four fingers into the vagina to provide space to allow visualization of the cervix and possibly the apex of a vaginal tear. Inadequate lighting can cause the midwife to miss identification of a laceration or unnecessarily prolong the process of inspection and repair. It may be necessary to move the woman to a different place or different room to ensure adequate visualization.

3. Positions for the woman and the provider: Position the woman in a manner that will maximize her comfort and also allow the midwife to conduct an adequate examination. For most inspections, having the woman assume a modified lithotomy position by reclining and flexing her knees and placing her feet on the bed or other surface is sufficient. However, if an upper vaginal vault or cervical laceration is suspected, positioning the woman in foot rests or stirrups may be preferable if available.

4. When a laceration is visualized:
   - Assess whether the laceration is hemostatic or bleeding.
   - Identify the exact location of the laceration so that it can be described in the woman's chart and to other providers who may be involved in the postpartum care of the woman.
   - Determine which type of laceration is present (Table 29-3) and whether the laceration requires repair.

Equipment

- Sterile gauze
- Two ring forceps

Procedure for Examination of the Vulva and Perineum

1. Inspection of the vulva and the perineum is achieved by using sterile, gloved fingers to gently separate the labia. A sterile cloth or gauze may be used to gently clean away blood or clots that obscure a laceration.

2. Areas that are completely visualized include the following: periurethral, periclitoral, labia, fourchette, perineum, rectum.

3. If a third- or fourth-degree laceration is suspected, don an additional glove and insert a finger into the rectum to assess the integrity of the rectal sphincter. It may help to ask the woman to squeeze her rectal sphincter if possible. Remove this glove and discard it after the rectal examination.

Procedure for Examination of the Vaginal Vault

For the purpose of this procedure, the vaginal vault is divided into four sections: posterior, anterior, and two lateral walls. Each section is visualized to identify lacerations in the vaginal mucosa. A systematic approach to this examination ensures that all areas are quickly, yet thoroughly inspected.

1. A 4 × 4 gauze folded in fourths and clamped with a long-length ring forceps can be used to clean away blood. The forceps can also be used to gently retract the cervix to inspect the lateral, posterior, and anterior fornices of the vaginal vault.

2. To examine each section of vaginal wall, insert the full length of several fingers of one sterile, gloved hand palmar side down and exert pressure away from the area being examined. Once one area has been inspected, pressure is released and the vaginal hand is repositioned in the new area to be inspected before force is applied again.

3. Insert the ring forceps with the gauze on it by sliding it down the top of the vaginal fingers. This maneuver assists in avoiding the tender anterior structures and minimizes the amount of gauze touching the vaginal walls, as the gauze is abrasive to these tissues. The gauze serves as a sponge to blot the area being exposed of blood and other fluids to facilitate visualization. If the gauze becomes saturated, remove the ring forceps, dispose of the saturated gauze, clamp on another gauze, and reinsert the ring forceps. During this procedure, the midwife should be careful to monitor use of gauze so gauze is not inadvertently left behind in the vagina.

4. Both the fingertips and the end of the ring forceps are to be located visually and should be in the posterior fornix. Press against the cervix with the ring forceps, and press against the vaginal wall with fingers. Inspect the area between the fingers and gauze for lacerations.

5. Repeat the procedure after sequentially locating fingertips and the tip of the ring forceps in each of the lateral fornices, the posterior fornix, and the anterior fornix.

Procedure for Postpartum Inspection of the Cervix

An assistant, if one is available, will make this procedure easier and more efficient.

1. Insert three or four sterile, gloved fingers of the nondominant hand palmar side down along the posterior vaginal wall to the area just in front of the cervix. This hand is used to exert pressure to retract the posterior vaginal wall posteriorly and facilitate visualization of the cervix.

2. Once the cervix is in view, with the dominant hand, grasp the anterior lip of the cervix with one of the ring forceps. The first forceps is used to help bring the anterior part of the cervix into view. The second ring forceps is used to grasp the posterior part of the cervix (**Figure 29B-1**).

3. Hold the handles of both ring forceps in the dominant hand. Pull on the forceps gently, if necessary, to bring the cervix more into view. Move the handles of the forceps toward one side of the perineum, thereby slightly pulling the cervix so the lateral apex of the cervix can be visualized.

4. Visually inspect the area of the cervix between the two ring forceps on one side.

5. If necessary, confirm the visual inspection by using the index finger of the vaginal hand to feel the edge of the cervix.

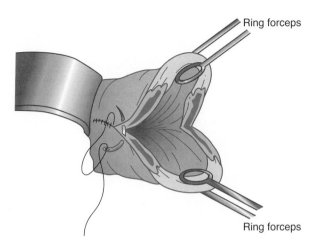

Figure 29B-1 Visualization of the cervix.

6. Repeat the procedure, moving the handles of the forceps toward the other side of the perineum to visualize and inspect the other lateral side of the cervix.

7. If the cervix is very patulous, all of the cervix may be difficult to visualize adequately between the ring forceps placed on the anterior and posterior lips of the cervix. In such a case, the entire circumference of the cervix can be visualized by placing one ring forceps on the anterior lip of the cervix and the second forceps next to it. Release the first forceps and place it on the other side of the second. Continue to leap-frog or "walk" the ring forceps around the cervix. This technique can also be used when the posterior lip of the cervix cannot be located easily.

8. If there are no cervical lacerations, remove the ring forceps and the vaginal hand.

9. If the cervix is bleeding from a cervical laceration, the forceps can be used to exert direct pressure on the laceration to decrease or stop the bleeding. This method can help to significantly reduce the amount of blood lost.

Hematomas

During pregnancy the vagina and vulva have rich and full vascular beds that are at risk for trauma during childbirth. When one of these vessels is torn or damaged, a hematoma can occur and enlarge very quickly. Most hematomas develop from vessels torn during a vaginal or perineal laceration (or episiotomy), but vessels can also be injured without obvious laceration. Hematomas develop rapidly and are extremely painful for women who do not have regional anesthesia. A classic presentation is pain that is unrelieved or getting worse despite administration of pain medication. The most common symptom in women who have epidural anesthesia is rectal pressure or rectal pain. Hematomas are reviewed in more detail in the *Third and Fourth Stages of Labor* and *Postpartum Complications* chapters.

Because hematomas often occur secondary to a tear in an artery, significant blood can be lost and the woman can develop signs of shock. The most common locations for hematoma are the vulva, the vagina, and the retroperitoneum.[3]

1. Vulvar hematomas develop secondary to damage to one of the branches of the pudendal artery. Because the Colles' fascia and urogenital diaphragm or anal fascia prevent their expansion, these hematomas grow superficially toward the skin and loose subcutaneous tissue. They present as swellings in the labia majora.

2. Vaginal hematomas are the result of injury to the uterine artery. These vessels are not surrounded by fascia, and bleeding into the paravaginal area can be extensive.

3. Retroperitoneal hematomas that extend between the folds of the broad ligament are more rare than the other two types. These hematomas are caused by injury to the branches of the internal iliac artery and are more common following uterine rupture or as an extension of a paravaginal hematoma. Hemorrhage can be significant and hemodynamic instability can develop quite quickly. Bleeding can be either arterial or venous. Women who are hemodynamically stable usually have a venous bleed; conversely, women who become hemodynamically unstable are more likely to have an arterial bleed.

• • • References

1. Cioffi JM, Swain J, Arundell F. The decision to suture after childbirth: cues, related factors, knowledge and experience used by midwives. *Midwifery*. 2010;26(2):246-255.

2. Cioffi JM, Arundell F, Swain J. Clinical decision-making for repair of spontaneous childbirth trauma: validation of cues and related factors. *J Midwifery Women's Health*. 2009;54(1):65-72.

3. Mirza FG, Gaddipati S. Obstetric emergencies. *Semin Perinatol*. 2009;33:97-103.

29C

Local Infiltration for Laceration Repair

LISA KANE LOW

TEKOA L. KING

Local infiltration of an anesthetic solution can be placed in the perineum just prior to birth before cutting an episiotomy or administered specifically in the areas or structures involved that need to be sutured after a spontaneous laceration occurs.

Anesthetic Agent for Local Injection

The medication recommended for local infiltration of tissue that requires sutures is 1% lidocaine hydrochloride (Xylocaine) 10 mg/mL. Lidocaine *without* added epinephrine should be used for local infiltration performed before the birth. Pharmacokinetic studies have found that lidocaine is detected in maternal plasma within a minute of injection and that placental transfer is quite rapid.[1] It is theorized that potential adverse effects of epinephrine on the uterine blood flow and fetus could be significant. Because of this risk, lidocaine with added epinephrine should not be used prior to birth. In contrast, lidocaine *with* added epinephrine is used for local infiltration after birth because less overall drug is needed and the anesthetic effects last longer.[2]

Lidocaine Dose and Pharmacokinetics

The recommended dose of lidocaine 1% *without* added epinephrine is typically 5 to 10 mL (50–100 mg). The maximum dose is 30 mL.[2] Peak plasma concentrations occur in 3 to 15 minutes, and the onset of action may take up to 3 minutes. It is important to wait until the anesthetic has taken effect. The duration of action is approximately 30 to 60 minutes.

The total maximum dose of lidocaine *with* added epinephrine is 20 mL (200 mg). The pharmacokinetics when epinephrine is added are unchanged.

Lidocaine Toxicity

Toxicity is usually the result of intravenous injection, rapid absorption from a very vascular area such as mucous membranes, or overdose. Toxic levels of lidocaine can be administered if accidental intravascular injection occurs or if the total volume of medication injected is not monitored. Toxic levels are based on the weight of the woman, the concentration of the medication, and an identified safe range for administration.

Signs of lidocaine toxicity include light-headedness, dizziness, tinnitus, abnormal taste, and confusion. Severe toxicity results in loss of consciousness and respiratory arrest. If lidocaine without epinephrine is injected intravascularly, the first signs may be hypotension and bradycardia. If lidocaine with epinephrine is injected intravascularly, the first signs may be hypertension and tachycardia.

Case reports of toxic levels of lidocaine in the fetus have been described secondary to direct injection into the fetal scalp. The risk of this unanticipated event is more likely if the fetus is in an OP position or if the large amounts are injected more than 4 minutes prior to the birth.

Equipment for Local Infiltration

Equipment used to perform local infiltration is listed in **Box 29C-1**.

Local Infiltration Prior to Cutting an Episiotomy

Local infiltration prior to cutting an episiotomy is done when the perineal body has been thinned and flattened considerably by the crowning of the fetal head or pressure from the presenting fetal part. At this point, there is typically little anteroposterior tissue and only one plane that requires anesthesia. While the thin and flatted perineal body allows for easier administration of anesthetic and identification of the area where infiltration has occurred, it also presents the challenge of potentially piercing the posterior perineal wall and inserting local anesthetic uselessly into the vagina or dangerously into the fetus. To void this risk, the following procedure is recommended.

General Principles

1. Always inject slowly.
2. Aspirate regularly during injection to check for blood return and to avoid intravascular injection.

Procedure

1. Place two fingers of the nondominant hand 3–4 cm into the vagina between the fetal presenting part and the flattened perineal body. Bring a small amount of pressure onto the posterior perineal surface to create a space between the area where the local infiltration is going to occur and the presenting fetal part.

2. Either of two techniques for local infiltration of the perineal body may be used.

   a. Insert the needle at the center of the fourchette and direct the needle straight down the midplane toward the rectum. After aspirating, up to a maximum of 10 mL (100 mg) of lidocaine is injected as the needle is slowly withdrawn. The desired effect is to create a large, visible, and palpable perpendicular wheal approximately 2–2.5 centimeters wide and extending from top to bottom in the center of the perineal body (**Figure 29C-1**).

   b. Insert the needle point at the center of the fourchette and aspirate. The needle is then introduced in a manner that creates an upside-down fan shape centrally in the perineum body while the medication is being injected. This technique provides more anesthesia in a wider section of the perineum, but takes more time to perform and involves pulling the needle back up and repositioning it. The goal is to avoid multiple sticks by drawing the needle up but not removing it before re-angling and moving the needle down the perineum in the next direction (**Figure 29C-2**).

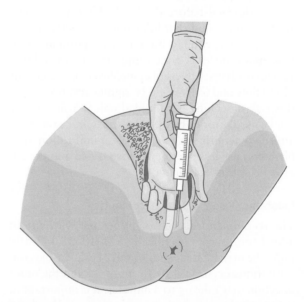

Figure 29C-1 Technique 1 for local infiltration for midline episiotomy.

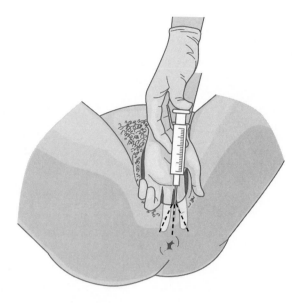

Figure 29C-2 Technique 2 for local infiltration for midline episiotomy.

3. If the plan is to cut a mediolateral episiotomy, the direction of the needle and resultant wheal should not be placed centrally but instead directed to the side, following the intended path of the mediolateral cut that will be made.

Local Infiltration for Repair After Birth

Local infiltration for repair of a laceration may be needed if predelivery anesthesia has dissipated, a postdelivery pudendal block has failed, or local infiltration is the mode of choice. The primary disadvantage of local infiltration for repair is that it distorts the tissue, thereby making tissue approximation potentially more challenging.

Procedure

1. Identify all tissue that requires anesthesia and repair.

2. Place the needle tip at the end or corner of the laceration nearest the posterior fourchette and insert it the length of the wound, reaching the areas where the suture needle will be either entering or exiting the tissue.

3. Aspirate to confirm that the needle is not in a vessel.

4. Inject the anesthetic as the needle is withdrawn along the line of the wound edge.

5. Discontinue injecting medication when the needle point is at the point where it entered the wound, without withdrawing the needle.

6. Redirect the needle along the open wound in any tissue just under the wound that will require suturing.

7. Inject anesthetic as the needle is withdrawn back to the point of entrance.

8. Repeat this process until the area that needs suturing has been anesthetized.

9. Once the area requiring anesthesia is fully infiltrated, the needle is withdrawn and another, noncontiguous area can be anesthetized following the same process.

● ● ● References

1. Phillipson EH, Kuhnert BR, Syracuse CD. Maternal, fetal, and neonatal lidocaine levels following local perineal infiltration. *Am J Obstet Gynecol.* 1984; 149(4):403-407.

2. Colacioppo PM, Riesco MLG. Effectiveness of local anaesthetics with and without vasoconstrictors for perineal repair during spontaneous delivery: double blinded randomised controlled trial. *Midwifery.* 2009;25:88-95.

APPENDIX

29D

Pudendal Block

LISA KANE LOW

TEKOA L. KING

Pudendal block is a regional anesthesia technique that anesthetizes the pudendal nerve, resulting in a reduction or elimination of pain perception in the muscles and tissue innervated by the pudendal nerve. Pudendal nerve block offers the following advantages:

- It provides anesthesia to the perineum and vulva, including the clitoris, labia majora, labia minora, perineal body, and rectal area, thereby offering broader anesthesia coverage than is accomplished with local infiltration.

- There is no alteration of the strength or conduct of uterine contractions.

- There is minimal risk to the woman, fetus, or newborn when a pudendal block is properly administered using the appropriate medication within the safe dosage range.

- Unlike local infiltration, a pudendal block does not cause disruption of the tissues that requires repair.

- A pudendal block can be used prior to birth to provide anesthesia for perineal discomfort at the end of second stage labor, for use of vacuum or forceps, or immediately following birth to provide anesthesia for laceration repair.

Anesthetic Agent for Pudendal Block

The anesthetic agent typically used in pudendal block is 1% (10 mg/mL) lidocaine hydrochloride (Xylocaine) *without* added epinephrine.[1] The duration of anesthesia depends on the success of the pudendal block and on the medication used. An effective block with 1% lidocaine will last approximately 1.5 hours. Lidocaine, as compared to other ester or amide anesthetic agents, has the advantage of being fast acting. The amount used is 10 mL (100 mg) per side. The maximum safe total dosage of 1% lidocaine is 300 mg or 30 mL. Thus, when 200 mg (20 mL) is used for the pudendal block, another 100 mg (10 mL) is available for a local infiltration of the perineal body if needed.

Equipment for Pudendal Block

The equipment needed to perform a pudendal block is listed in **Box 29D-1**.

BOX 29D-1 Equipment for Pudendal Block

- Sterile gloves
- Prepackaged kit for pudendal block or an Iowa trumpet (needle guide) and a 12- to 15-cm (5- to 6-inch) 20- or 22-gauge spinal needle
- 10-mL syringe with a Luer-Lok attachment and 18- to 20-gauge needle for drawing up the anesthetic
- Local anesthetic: usually lidocaine (Xylocaine) without epinephrine

---

Pudendal Block for Perineal Anesthesia

The pudendal nerve is a major branch of the sacral plexus (**Figure 29D-1**). This nerve travels through the gluteus muscle and exits the pelvis through the sacrosciatic foramen. It then travels anteriorly to the sacrospinous ligament, then posteriorly around the ischial spine, before entering the pudendal canal and terminating in three branches:[2]

- Dorsal nerve of the clitoris, which innervates the clitoris
- Perineal branch, which innervates the muscles of the perineum, labia majora and labia minora, and vestibule
- Inferior hemorrhoidal nerve, which innervates the external anal sphincter and mucous membranes of the lower half of the anal canal and perianal skin

A pudendal nerve block places anesthetic solution at the nerve trunk where it enters the sciatic foramen, approximately 1 cm inferior and medial to the ischial spine. The pudendal nerve lies between the posterior surface of the sacrospinous ligament and the internal pudendal artery and vein. Thus taking care not to inject the anesthesia intravascularly is an important consideration during this procedure.

A pudendal block can be performed via a transvaginal or transperineal technique. This appendix reviews the transvaginal technique, because it is the one most commonly employed.

General Principles

1. Accurate knowledge of anatomic landmarks used to identify placement location for the anesthetic is essential.

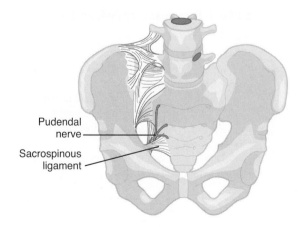

Figure 29D-1 Anatomy of the pudendal nerve.

Pudendal nerve

Sacrospinous ligament

2. Using palpation, the ischial spine and the sacrospinous ligament must be accurately identified.
3. The anesthetic agent must be correctly placed in relation to the ischial spine.

Procedure for Administration of a Transvaginal Pudendal Block

1. Insert the right hand and palpate the right ischial spine and sacrospinous ligament. The sacrospinous ligament runs posteriorly from the ischial spine toward the sacrum.
2. Insert the needle guide and, using the left hand, position the end of it 1 cm medial and posterior to the inferior, medial border of the ischial spine. A small amount of pressure is needed to maintain the exact position (**Figure 29D-2**).
3. The needle, which is attached to the syringe, is then inserted into the needle guide and the protrusion of the needle is inserted posterior to the ischial spine, through the sacrospinous ligament to the space occupied by the pudendal nerve and vessels. There will be a slight give as the needle exits from the sacrospinous ligament and enters this space. This is a distance of approximately 1 to 1.5 cm from the end of the needle guide. Do not extend the needle more than 1–1.5 cm beyond the end of the needle guide.
4. Aspirate once to ensure the needle is not in a blood vessel, and then rotate the needle 180° and aspirate again to ensure the needle is not in a blood vessel and that the lack of blood return on the first aspiration was not caused by the bevel of the needle being snug against the inner wall of the vessel.
5. Inject 3 mL of 1% lidocaine *without* epinephrine (30 mg).
6. Advance the needle slightly until the sensation of resistance from the sacrospinous ligament is lost. This is the area where the perineal nerve lies.
7. Aspirate again to make sure the needle is not in a blood vessel, and inject the next 7 mL of 1% lidocaine without epinephrine (70 mL).
8. Repeat the procedure on the other side.
9. After injecting both sides, wait 2 to 4 minutes and then test the effectiveness of the block by using a sharp object, such as a needle or Allis clamp, to pinch each side of the perineal

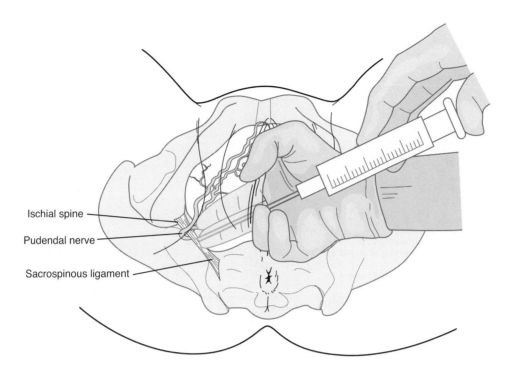

Ischial spine

Pudendal nerve

Sacrospinous ligament

Figure 29D-2 Pudendal block procedure.

area near the rectum (both sides need to be evaluated). Confirmation will come from two sources: (1) the woman will report no pain or no feeling, and (2) there will be no reflex anal sphincter or vaginal orifice contraction. Some midwives gently but firmly stroke the sides of the area near the rectum to ascertain if an anal "wink" or response is apparent.

10. Maximum anesthesia occurs at approximately 10 minutes, so waiting to begin suturing may be necessary.

Outcomes Associated with Pudendal Block

Approximately 10% to 50% of pudendal blocks will be ineffective on one side. However, it may be suggested that, like many procedures, the more it is performed, the likely it is to result in effective anesthesia.

Nevertheless, a pudendal block provides excellent analgesia when it is effective.[3] This relatively simple procedure has few adverse effects. Potential complications, which are all very rare, include hematoma, infection at the site of injection, systemic toxicity from intravascular injection, and temporary ischial paresthesia or sacral neuropathy.

• • • References

1. Schrock SD. Labor analgesia. *Am Fam Physician.* 2012;85(5):447-454.

2. Mahakkanukrauh P, Patcharin S, Vaidhayakarn P. Anatomical study of the pudendal nerve adjacent to the sacrospinous ligament. *Clin Anatomy.* 2005;18: 200-205.

3. Novikova N, Cluver C. Local anaesthetic nerve block for pain management in labour. *Cochrane Database Syst Rev.* 2012;4:CD009200. doi: 10.1002/14651858. CD009200.pub2.

29E

Repair of Lacerations and Episiotomy

LISA KANE LOW

MARY C. BRUCKER

SARASWATHI VEDEM

TEKOA L. KING

Introduction

Approximately 85% of women have a genital tract laceration following birth.[1] These lacerations can be either minor or extensive, and many will need some repair. In addition, an episiotomy—which is a surgical incision of the perineal body—can be performed to expedite birth when necessary. Thus repair of genital tract lacerations is an essential midwifery skill.

This appendix reviews general principles for suturing, different stitches used in repairing genital tract lacerations, and techniques for repairing common genital tract lacerations sustained at birth. A brief review of current controversies regarding different repair techniques is included, and the last section reviews the technique for cutting an episiotomy.

Genital Tract Lacerations

Genital tract lacerations are categorized according to tissue and muscle involvement, as noted in Table 29-3. Lacerations are spontaneous events; in contrast, an episiotomy is intentional. This appendix first addresses how to repair both lacerations and episiotomies, as the principles for repair are the same regardless of how the perineal disruption occurred. The final section addresses the procedure for cutting an episiotomy should one be needed.

Figure 29E-1 illustrates the general anatomy of a common perineal laceration. The anatomy that is disrupted includes the vaginal mucosa, hymenal ring, fourchette, bulbocavernosis muscle, transverse perineal muscle, and—if the laceration extends into the rectum—the external rectal sphincter, internal rectal sphincter, and rectal mucosa.

Episiotomy

Only a generation ago, most women giving birth in the United States routinely experienced an episiotomy, or surgical incision of the perineal body at the time of birth. It was believed that an episiotomy had multiple benefits, including a decrease in the incidence of rectal lacerations, ease of repair, and protection of the fetal head, especially that of the premature infant. Like a host of other traditional interventions that have been reevaluated scientifically, routine episiotomies have been found to provide fewer advantages than originally believed. A 2009 systematic review of eight randomized trials found that women who gave birth in sites with restrictive

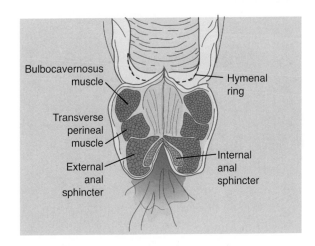

Figure 29E-1 Anatomy of a perineal laceration or midline episiotomy.

episiotomy policies compared to women who gave birth in sites with routine episiotomy policies less frequently had severe perineal trauma (RR: 0.67; 95% CI: 0.49–0.91), less requirement for suturing (RR: 0.71; 95% CI: 0.61–0.81), fewer healing complications (RR: 0.69; 95% CI: 0.56–0.89), and no difference in pain, urinary incontinence, or dyspareunia, although they had a higher risk of anterior perineal damage (RR: 1.84; 95% CI: 1.61–2.10).[2]

The incidence of this procedure, which is also termed a perineotomy, varies throughout the world. Today, however, the use of episiotomies is declining in the United States.[3] Yet, because every birth is unique, cutting and repair of an episiotomy is a skill to be included in the repertoire of a midwife so that, when needed, it can be performed competently. An understanding of perineal anatomy is critical to the discussion of episiotomies/lacerations and can be found in the *Anatomy and Physiology of the Female Reproductive System* chapter.

Episiotomies should be discussed with women prior to labor so they are aware of the indications and procedure should it be necessary. The one accepted indication for an episiotomy is a need to expedite birth secondary to a fetal bradycardia or other fetal heart rate pattern that suggests there is a significant risk of newborn acidemia. Other suggested but controversial indications include operative birth, suspected shoulder dystocia, and short perineum (with a mediolateral episiotomy to avoid a spontaneous fourth-degree laceration).

Equipment for Repair of Genital Tract Trauma

- Sharp scissors
- Sterile gauze sponges (4×4)
- Needle holder (also termed a needle driver)
- Tissue forceps without teeth for "pickups"
- Suture

Optional as needed:

- 1% lidocaine *without* epinephrine
- Syringe and 18-gauge needle for lidocaine
- 22-gauge needle for local infiltration
- Iowa trumpet and needle for pudendal block

Third- or fourth-degree laceration:

- Gelpi retractors
- Allis clamps

General Principles and Suture Technique

Repair of an episiotomy or laceration accomplishes three goals: (1) hemostasis, (2) return to functional integrity, and (3) cosmetic repair. Multiple sources exist electronically on the Internet that demonstrate various aspects of perineal laceration repair for learners who need a visual demonstration. Active practice using models and under direct supervision of an experienced midwife or physician cannot be underestimated.

In addition to differing opinions regarding which type of episiotomy to perform and when it should be performed, different suturing techniques have been evaluated as means to suture a perineal disruption.

Achieving Hemostasis

Hemostasis is obtained first before a wound is closed. Blood clots increase the inflammatory reaction and serve as a culture media for bacteria. Large clots can cause tissue necrosis as they create pressure on adjoining tissue.

Hemostasis is accomplished by tying off bleeding vessels, by eliminating dead space, and by using techniques that minimize trauma to the tissue. The following techniques also aid in promoting hemostasis:

1. Gently probe the depth of the wound before suturing to identify the true depth that needs repair beneath the mucosal layer.
2. Start any line of suture at least 1 cm beyond the apex of the wound to include any retracted blood vessels.
3. Use sutures that facilitate hemostasis in the most vascular areas, such as the continuous locked or blanket suture.
4. Use an atraumatic (tapered) needle instead of a cutting needle.

Promoting Wound Healing

Wound healing involves three phases: inflammation, proliferation, and maturation.[4] Although healthy women tend to heal well, it is critical that aseptic technique is maintained to avoid the risk of infection. This may include changing gloves following the birth and redraping the area if necessary to create a sterile field; using an extra sterile glove over the sterile glove(s) already on an examining hand when checking the rectum and discarding the extra glove immediately after use; and careful placement of suture on the sterile field as the process of the repair is conducted. **Table 29E-1** lists interventions to promote wound healing through the perinatal year.

Table 29E-1	Promotion of Wound Healing
Time Frame	**Examples of Interventions**
Prenatal	Prevention of nutritional deficiencies, including anemia
Intrapartum	Prevention of maternal exhaustion and dehydration
	Strict adherence to aseptic technique
	Avoidance of unnecessary further trauma to the incisional tissues:
	• Use of suture with suture gauge and needle size larger than needed
	• Inappropriate use of a traumatic cutting needle rather than an atraumatic round needle
	• Misplacement of sutures, requiring removal and replacement
	• Placement of sutures too close together
	• Tissue strangulation resulting from too-tight sutures
	• Repeated unnecessary sponging, prodding, and probing of the wound
	• Use of instruments that crush tissue
	Removal of blood clots and debris before closure
	Establishing visible hemostasis before closure to avoid formation of hematomas
	Precise approximation of tissues
	Closure that obliterates all dead space
Postpartum	Adequate nutrition
	Perineal cleanliness

Selection of Suture Material

Types of suture include standard synthetic sutures, rapidly absorbing synthetic sutures, glycerol-impregnated catgut sutures, standard synthetic sutures with rapidly absorbing synthetic monofilament sutures, and catgut.[5] Synthetic sutures are preferred, as they were associated with less pain during the postpartum period when compared to catgut in a systematic review.[6] Catgut has the additional disadvantage of causing a marked tissue inflammatory reaction that produces edema, which places tension on the sutures and may cause tissue necrosis. Ultimately scarring can result, which results in a weaker functional repair. The two most common absorbable synthetic suture types are polyglycolic acid (Dexon, Davis & Geck Ltd., United Kingdom) and polyglactin 910 (Vicryl, Ethicon Ltd., Edinburgh, United Kingdom).

Selection of Suture Gauge and Needle Type

Muscle heals by deposition of scar tissue and requires a stronger suture than does other tissue, which regenerates itself. The larger the gauge number, the finer the suture (e.g., 4-0, 6-0, 8-0); the smaller the gauge number, the heavier the suture and the stronger the tensile strength of the suture (e.g., 2-0, 1-0). The suture gauges used for various conditions are listed in **Table 29E-2**.

Table 29E-2	Gauge and Use of Suture Material		
	Gauge	**Common Repair Sites**	**Usual Types of Stitches**
Thinner	4-0	Clitoral lacerations	Continuous, interrupted
		Shallow periurethral lacerations	Continuous, interrupted
		Anterior wall of rectum (repair of fourth-degree laceration)	Continuous, locked
	3-0	Vaginal mucosa	Continuous, locked
		Deep periurethral lacerations	Subcutaneous, continuous
		Pelvic muscles that are not extensive	Deep interrupted
Thicker	2-0	External anal sphincter	Continuous, deep interrupted
		Cervical lacerations	Continuous, deep interrupted
		Lateral wall lacerations	Continuous, deep interrupted
		Deep pelvic muscles	Deep interrupted

The use of an atraumatic or tapered round needle is recommended instead of a cutting needle to reduce tissue trauma and the risk of increased hemostasis (**Figure 29E-2**). A cutting needle is triangular in shape, and each edge has a sharp surface; in contrast, the atraumatic needle is a round needle with a tapered point. The latter moves through soft tissues more easily than a cutting needle and is less likely to lacerate a blood vessel. The anatomy of a needle is identified in **Figure 29E-3**.

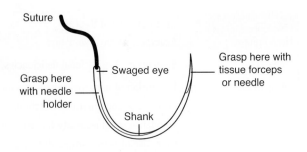

Figure 29E-3 Anatomy of a needle.

Suturing

Key Points

1. General suturing techniques and appropriate sutures for different tissue types should be reviewed before beginning the repair. The tissue should be carefully visualized and landmarks identified.

2. Excess suture can be gathered up in the palm of the hand holding the needle holder to prevent the length of suture from dangling over or dragging across areas of contamination.

3. The needle is clamped by the tip of the needle holder so that the plane of the curve of the needle is perpendicular to the plane of the needle holder. Clamp the needle just proximal to the junction of the needle and the suture.

4. Do not place a clamp on the needle holder at the junction of the needle with the suture, or on the suture, to avoid weakening the suture.

5. The needle holder is controlled by wrist action. It should be held so that the thumb holes are in the palm of the hand and secured by the ring and little fingers. With this positioning, the thumb and middle fingers are on either

lateral side of the shaft, with the index finger on one side (usually the upper) of the broad side of the shaft. This is opposed to placing fingers through the holes. Some midwives refer to this placement as "shaking hands" with the needle holder (**Figure 29E-4**).

6. Because of the need for universal precautions, the midwife always should use forceps to grasp or "pick up" the point and guide the needle through the tissue.

7. The needle should be guided through tissue along the angle of its curve. Follow the circle of the needle rather than pulling it straight up. Turning the wrist to have the same angle as the needle promotes smooth movement.

8. Suturing is begun by holding the needle with its curved midportion turned so the tissue can be entered with the point of the needle perpendicular to the tissue. Therefore, the hand holding the shaft of the needle holder will be positioned so that the back of the hand is up and then further pronated as the needle point is positioned for entry. As the needle enters the tissue, the wrist is rotated approximately 180° so that the needle follows the necessary directional path for exit, completing the stitch.

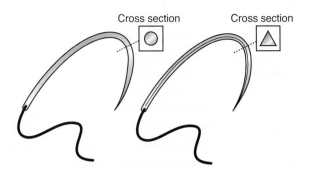

Figure 29E-2 Types of curved needles usually attached to suture material.

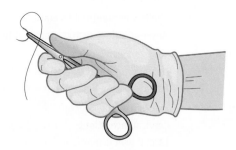

Figure 29E-4 How to hold a needle holder.

9. As the point of the needle emerges, it should be grasped either by tissue forceps or by releasing the needle holder from its original position and repositioning it to grasp the emerging point (**Figure 29E-5**). Tissue forceps always should be used when possible, as the amount of tissue is often large enough that it is impossible to release the needle holder and realign it for this purpose without losing the tip of the needle in the tissue. Do not grasp the point of the needle with fingers—doing so may cause a needle puncture.

10. Avoid an excessive number of needle punctures, an unnecessary number of stitches, placement of stitches in very close proximity, and misplacement of stitches that have to be removed. Excessive suture in the wound slows the healing process by causing an inflammatory reaction to foreign material.

Knots

A square knot is the basic knot used for repairing an episiotomy or a laceration (**Figure 29E-6**). A square knot results after a left-handed overhand knot is created, followed by a right-handed knot. Most experts advocate completing not only the square knot, but also one more action to ensure that the stitch does not come undone. This knot, which may be colloquially termed a "knot and a half," is made in case either the first or third action becomes loose or the suture dissolves more rapidly than anticipated. In either case, the complete square knot would remain.

A square knot can be tied by hand, instrument, or both, as all of these options can ensure that the knot is appropriately tied and placed flat against the tissue. Instrument ties are recommended, as they are safest for the provider. Another advantage of an instrument

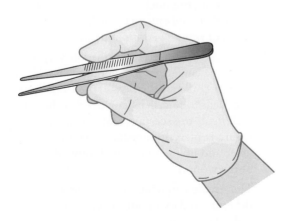

Figure 29E-5 Tissue (pickup) forceps without teeth.

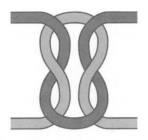

Figure 29E-6 Square knot.

tie is that the knot can be tied with a short suture length, whereas a hand tie requires longer suture to complete tying the knot. Skill in tying knots requires practice. Multiple resources on this topic exist on the Internet, including a variety of digital recordings illustrating how to tie a knot by hand or instrument in real time (a topic beyond the scope of this chapter). Knot-tying boards are available, although not essential for practice.

Key Points for Tying Knots

1. The knot should be as small as possible to minimize the use of excessive suture material. Therefore, the ends should be as short as possible. Extra ties do not necessarily provide extra security, but they do provide additional and unwarranted suture material that can irritate healing tissue.

2. Friction between the strands, also called sawing, should be avoided as much as possible because it can weaken the integrity of the suture.

3. Crimping of the suture should be avoided except when grasping the free end of the suture during an instrument tie.

4. Sutures used simply to approximate tissue should not be tied with excessive tension, because this condition may contribute to tissue strangulation.

5. As the knot is tied, tension should be as equal as possible on each step and the final tension should be made as nearly horizontal as possible. The midwife may need to change personal position to tie the most effective knot.

Types of Stitches

Challenges in any discussion of the types of stitches used in repairing genital tract lacerations include the existence of many, often minor, variations to a basic technique and multiple names for both the same stitch and those variations. The most commonly used stitches—continuous, continuous locked, interrupted, subcuticular, figure of eight, and crown—are illustrated in **Figure 29E-7**. A description of each of these techniques follows for a right-handed practitioner. The direction should be reversed if suturing in a left-handed manner.

Continuous Locked (Blanket) and Continuous (Running) Stitches

A continuous stitch is often called running or "whip" stitch. However, each stitch can also be locked to provide additional security. This locking is the differentiating factor between the two most common types of continuous stitches.

1. The needle is inserted into the right side of the wound and brought through the incision to emerge on the left side of the wound. The amount of tissue on each side should be approximately the same. Based on the amount of the tissue, it may be advisable to bring the point of the needle out into the midline of the wound to verify positioning before continuing to the left side.

2. An anchoring knot is tied on the left side of the stitch and one end is cut short.
   a. For a continuous locked (blanket) stitch, the point emerges in front of the previous stitch but under a loop or section of the suture. As the needle exits the tissue, the section of suture remains behind it. This maneuver locks the stitch.
   b. For a continuous (running) stitch, the needle point should emerge in front of the previous stitch—*not* under a loop or section of the suture.

3. The needle and suture should be guided through the tissue, following the curve of the needle.

4. a. A continuous locked (blanket) stitch is secured or locked along the left side of the wound line.
   b. A continuous (running) stitch lies across the line of the closed wound at an angle. In the tissue, the suture crosses the wound perpendicular to the line of the laceration so the wound approximates accurately, but an angle is visible externally that reflects the distance needed to move forward between each stitch.

These steps should be repeated until the wound is closed.

Interrupted Suture

An interrupted stitch consists of a single stitch and knot (both ends cut short).

1. The suture is placed on the right side of the wound, but the end is neither cut nor tied.

2. The needle should be inserted into the right side of the wound and brought through the wound to emerge on the left side of the wound directly across from the origination on the right side. The amount of tissue on each side should be approximately the same. Based on the amount of the tissue, it may be advisable to bring the needle out in the midline of the wound and then take another stitch into the left side of the wound to verify positioning and ensure that the needle does not try to grasp too much tissue.

3. A square knot should be tied by instrument, and both ends tied. If the interrupted stitch is used for deep muscle, the needle and suture should include the apex of the wound to avoid leaving any unsutured dead space behind the closed wound.

Separate interrupted stitches should be inserted as needed by following these steps.

Subcuticular (Mattress) Stitch

This technique is a buried horizontal stitch used for closing the subcuticular perineal skin during a laceration or episiotomy repair so that the suture is not visible on the skin.

1. An anchoring stitch is placed in the appropriate site going through the skin if necessary, a knot is tied, and one end is cut short. When subcuticular sutures are used to close the perineum during repair of a second-degree laceration, this anchoring stitch is not needed because the subcuticular stitches will follow a series of running continuous stitches.

2. The needle is inserted on the left side of the incision. Unlike with other stitches, this insertion could be shallow. Traditionally this is called "one cell layer" deep, although it is difficult to ascertain that benchmark. The suture is placed immediately below the skin layer and in a parallel line following the line of the wound.

3. The needle can penetrate the tissue between the entry and exit points deeper than the one cell layer to provide for greater security of sutures.

Suture	Alternative nomenclature	Illustration
Continuous locked	Blanket	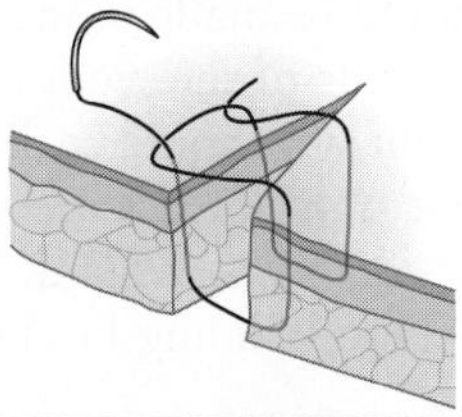
Continuous	Running	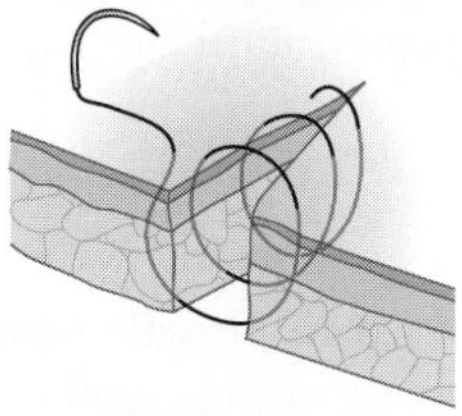
Interrupted		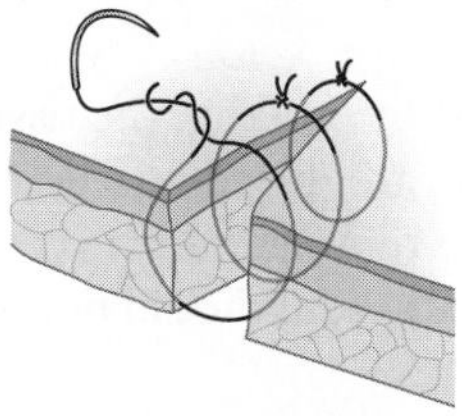
Double interrupted for third-degree laceration		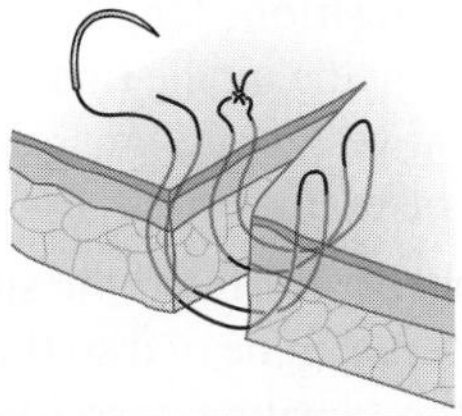
Subcuticular	Mattress	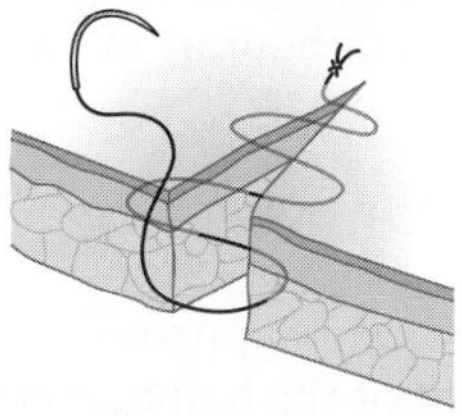
Crown		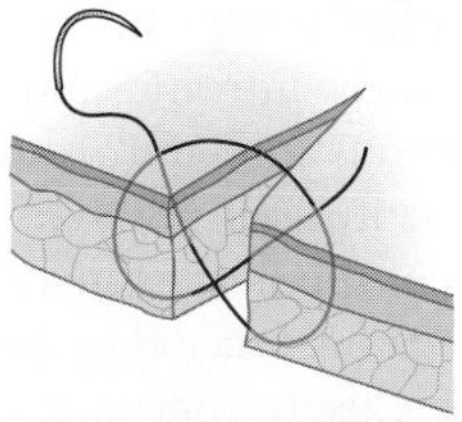
Figure of eight		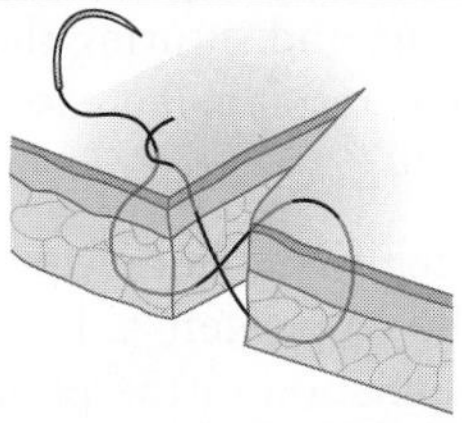

Figure 29E-7 Sutures.

4. The suture should be gently guided through the tissue for approximately 0.5 cm in length.

5. The next suture should be made in the same manner on the right side of the wound. The entry point on the right side should be directly across from the exit point of the preceding stitch on the other side of the wound. Some individuals liken this to building bricks in a vertical manner.

6. These steps are repeated until the wound is closed.

Figure of Eight Stitch

A figure of eight stitch is used to provide hemostasis and tie off actively bleeding vessels (colloquially called pumpers).

1. The stitch is started by entering the tissue on the left side behind the bleeding vessel and emerges out on the right side in front of the bleeding vessel. This suture should not be tied or cut.

2. The needle is then repositioned, and a second stitch is performed starting on the right side in front of the bleeding vessel and emerging on the left behind the bleeding vessel.

3. After cutting the needle off from the suture, the two ends of suture can be tied so that the suture constricts the bleeding vessel within the figure of eight configuration that has been created.

Crown Stitch

The crown stitch is used to reapproximate the perineum at the attachment of the bulbocavernosus muscle (also called the bulbospongiosus muscle). This restores the anatomy of the introitus and labial junction at the mucocutaneous junction. Although similar to a figure of eight suture, it involves a different technique. The ends of the sutures in a crown stitch are proximate to each other when they are tied. Care must be taken to only closely approximate the muscle in repairing it; pulling and suturing the two sides together too tightly may result in increased scar tissue and dysparunia.

1. Begin by entering the tissue in an upper diagonal slant at the upper-left side of the wound line at the junction of the perineum and vagina. Adequate space should be allowed away from the edge of the incision to enable subcutaneous continuous stitches and potentially a subcuticular closure over the completed crown stitch. The suture should not be tied or cut.

2. The needle then should be directed so that it follows a sequence of moving upward, then laterally, downward, and medially so that it exits in the same plane, but posterior to the original entry site. Experience is essential to perform this technique well, because the amount of lateral thrust must be adequate only to reach the retracted cut end of the bulbocavernosus muscle if possible. The more lateral tissue obtained, the more vascular the area and the higher the risk of a potential hematoma. Whether the bulbocavernosus muscle has been included in the suture can be verified by grasping the two ends of the suture a short distance from the tissue and gently pulling them. If the bulbocavernosus muscle has been sutured, the entire left side labia will be pulled.

3. The needle then should enter the tissue at the right side of the wound directly across from the exit point on the left side. The needle should be directed in a manner that mirrors the action in Step 2. The correct placement through the bulbocavernosus muscle can be ascertained using the same technique as described in Step 2.

4. After cutting the needle, the two ends of suture should be next to each other and are knotted, with the ends cut short. The cut ends of the bulbocavernosus muscle should be closely joined, but not too tightly. The placement of the two halves of the stitch ensures the approximation of the muscle.

Repair of a Second-Degree Laceration or an Episiotomy

Following are the steps that are used to repair a second-degree laceration or episiotomy. As with several other midwifery skills, this is only one of several possible methods. This method includes both continuous and interrupted stitches. It has been found that closures dependent only on interrupted suturing techniques are associated with more pain.[7]

Repair of midline and mediolateral episiotomies is essentially the same. However, the midwife should be aware that with a mediolateral episiotomy, the medial aspect of the incision tends to retract more than the lateral aspect, indicating the need for special care to avoid the rectum when suturing. In addition, the stitches for this repair follow the incisional line and are performed at a slant, rather than straight across as done for repair of a midline episiotomy or laceration, with slightly more tissue on the lateral side than on the medial side. When completed, the stitches may be closer than for a midline closure. Sometimes a laceration may occur at an angle, and the same comments may apply.

Key Points Prior to Repair

1. Good visualization of the area of repair is critical. Lighting and positioning may need to be adapted. Rarely, if a woman must be positioned using stirrups, the time should be limited to less than 90 minutes to decrease the risk of impaired circulation or thrombophlebitis.

2. Visualize the vulva, labia, vestibule, vaginal walls, cervix, and perineum to identify all sites of bleeding and tissue disruption prior to beginning the repair.

3. Identify and tie off any active bleeding vessels with a figure of eight stitch prior to repairing the main laceration.

4. An aseptic field must be established and meticulously maintained.

5. Appropriate anesthesia is required. Local infiltration or a pudendal block can be performed when needed.

6. Maintenance of good communication between the woman, the midwife, and other support personnel as appropriate is essential.

Technique for Repair of Second-Degree Laceration or Episiotomy

1. A sponge or other absorbent material that has a tail, which remains outside the vagina, may be inserted as a tampon if necessary to maintain a dry field.

    a. Insert two fingers along the posterior vaginal wall, apply downward pressure, and slide the rolled tampon against the posterior aspect of the fingers toward the posterior fornix of the vagina.

    b. Secure the tail with a clamp to a drape where it can be seen and will not be forgotten or left in the vagina when the repair is complete.

2. Check the integrity of the anal sphincter. Feel the depth of the defect and ascertain that the anal sphincter is intact. Place a second glove over the examining hand if necessary to insert an examining finger into the anus to determine the integrity of the sphincter and rectal mucosa; discard this glove immediately after examining the rectum. The provider should be careful to probe the tissue gently and not cause additional trauma. In rare occasions, the midwife actually can slip a finger through a very thin rectal mucosa, causing a "button-hole fourth degree" where a disruption had not previously occurred.

3. Before starting to sew, gently support the tissue so that it falls together naturally and identify key landmarks that will be anatomically approximated, including the hymenal ring, apex of vaginal mucosa, mucocutaneous junction, and perineal apex.

4. *Vaginal mucosa:* The vaginal mucosa is repaired with a 3-0 synthetic absorbable suture using an atraumatic, tapered needle with locked continuous suturing (**Figure 29E-8**).

    a. Visualize the vaginal apex by placing both fingers along the wound edges and apply gentle downward pressure. The anchoring stitch is placed approximately 1 cm beyond

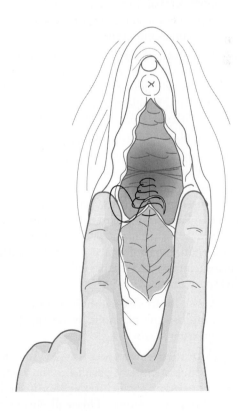

Figure 29E-8 Repair of vaginal mucosa using continuous locked (blanket) stitches.

the vaginal apex of the incision to provide hemostasis for any retracted blood vessels. This stitch is tied and one side cut close to the knot, leaving an approximately 0.5-cm tail.

b. The vaginal mucosa is closed to the junction of the vaginal mucosa and the posterior aspect of the hymenal ring with the long, untied end of the suture using the locked continuous (blanket) suture. The stitches should be approximately 1–1.5 cm apart.

c. The first one or two stitches should include adequate tissue on each side of the incision to close the incision completely. Thereafter, the stitches include only the vaginal mucosa and not the underlying muscle.

d. If the incision is deep, the vaginal mucosa is closed only to the back of the hymenal ring so that placement of deep interrupted stitches can be well visualized.

e. Avoid placing suture through the hymenal ring. It is theorized that suture in the hymenal tissue may cause subsequent dyspareunia, although no clear evidence to support this theory has been published. The needle is repositioned from a horizontal placement to a more vertical (forward toward the introitus) approach and guided under the hymenal ring so it comes out in the defect.

f. The needle is clamped with an instrument so that the point is contained in the clamp. This needle and remaining suture will be used later for closing the subcutaneous and subcuticular spaces. The needle/clamp is then placed onto a sterile drape.

5. Muscle layer under the vaginal mucosa: A layer of interrupted stitches usually is needed to close dead space that is below the vaginal mucosal layer. Insert a finger below the vaginal mucosal area that has been repaired to determine whether more than 1 cm of space is present. If there is more than 1 cm of space below the sutured mucosa, interrupted stitches will be used to close this space (**Figure 29E-9**).

a. A 2-0 absorbable synthetic suture with an atraumatic needle should be obtained for the interrupted stitches.

b. Place these interrupted stitches in a horizontal plane that is parallel to the woman's buttocks, or parallel to the floor if she is in lithotomy position. This will ensure that the stitch does not accidently go into the rectal mucosa. The needle holder will be

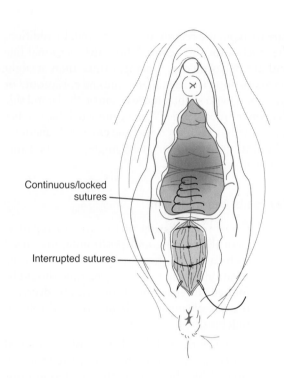

Figure 29E-9 Repair of muscles using interrupted stitches.

perpendicular to the floor and introitus. The amount of tissue to be taken up is often too much for one bite, so the first action directs the needle to come out into the back of the defect, the needle is replaced correctly in the needle holder, and a second stitch is taken to incorporate the other side.

c. The goal of the deep interrupted stitches is to obliterate dead space. Second-degree lacerations can require anywhere from 2 to 6 interrupted sutures.

d. After the interrupted stitches are placed, a rectal examination is performed to determine whether any of the stitches can be palpated within the rectal mucosa. To maintain sterility, either a new glove is placed over the hand used for the examination and then discarded, or the single glove must be replaced. If a suture is palpated in the rectum, the repair must be dismantled until the suture is removed to prevent infection or creation of a sinus tract. The risk of a rectal suture is diminished if all interrupted stitches are placed carefully in the horizontal plane.

e. Crown stitch (**Figure 29E-10**): Historically, a crown stitch has been performed to ensure approximation of the bulbocavernosus

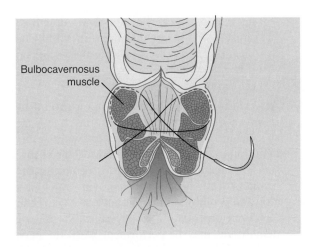

Figure 29E-10 Crown suture.

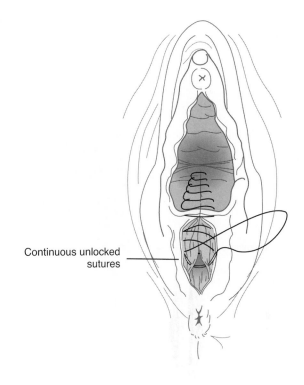

Figure 29E-11 Repair of perineal subcutaneous fascia using continuous stitches.

muscle. Today, however, it is not performed routinely as there is some controversy about whether the crown stitch increases the risk for dyspareunia without added benefit for an anatomic repair. For some incisions or lacerations, the repair of the bulbocavernosus will have already been incorporated into the standard repair process when interrupted stitches are placed and a crown stitch is unnecessary. Thus paying close attention to the anatomy with a clear mental picture of where the two bulbocavernosus muscles come together in the perineum is necessary so the decision to place a crown stitch or not can be made appropriately.

6. *Subcutaneous tissue*: At this point, the suture that had been set aside is used to repair the subcutaneous tissue under the fourchette and down the length of the laceration toward the anus. The goal is to obliterate space that would be created by closing the skin edges over a subcutaneous defect.

   a. The perineal subcutaneous fascia is closed using continuous (unlocked, running) stitches, as illustrated in **Figure 29E-11**.

   b. Resume using the original suture used to close the vaginal mucosa, and take a stitch through the vaginal mucosa (being careful to keep the last vaginal mucosal stitch locked) so that the suture emerges in the subcutaneous tissue just under the hymenal ring.

   c. Close the subcutaneous tissue with a running stich moving down the defect toward the inferior perineal apex close to the anus.

   Do not bring the needle out too close to the skin, as the layer of tissue immediately under the skin will be closed with a final layer of subcuticular stitches.

   d. Stitches are placed approximately 1 cm apart.

   e. Bring the needle out in the perineal apex of the laceration.

   f. Change the direction of the needle on the needle holder for the subcuticular stitches.

7. Subcuticular stitches: Sufficient and equilateral room is to be left on both sides for the final layer of continuous stitches, and the last stitch exits at the central point of the perineal apex. This stitch should be shallow and immediately inside but not through the skin.

   a. A subcuticular, or mattress, stitch is performed using the same suture that was used for the subcutaneous stiches.

   b. Stitches are taken alternatively from side to side moving superiorly toward the fourchette. Each stitch is started exactly parallel to the point on the opposite side where the last suture emerged (**Figure 29E-12**).

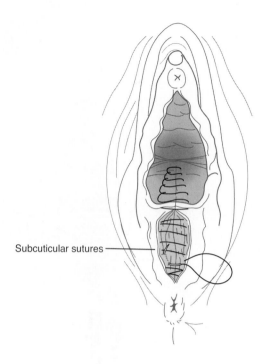

Subcuticular sutures

Figure 29E-12 Reapproximation of skin using subcuticular (mattress) stitches.

i. Bring the suture across to see where to place the needle for the next stitch.

ii. Shorter stitches are usually placed at the perineal apex near the anus, whereas longer stitches can be made closer to the mucocutaneous junction.

iii. Do not pull too tightly—edges should not overlap.

c. Approximate the mucocutaneous junction exactly, and then continue a few subcutaneous stitches back toward the hymenal ring. The depth of the fourchette or space between the mucocutaneous junction and hymenal ring varies among women. Some will require one or two stitches, and some may require as many as three or four stitches.

d. *Final knot*: Bring the suture up into the fourchette just anterior to the hymenal ring and tie it off with a square knot. The entry point should be on the same side as, and close to the exit point of, the preceding stitch; the exit point should be straight across on the opposite side of the repaired laceration. The suture is not guided through the tissue entirely, but instead a loop is left and becomes one side of the tied knot. The knot should be made securely, but not tight enough to cause tissue strangulation, and should be positioned far enough inside the vagina so that the ends do not cause discomfort for the woman.

8. After suturing, any type of tampon should be removed if one was used. The suture line is inspected and verified to be intact and without any hematoma or active bleeding along the suture lines. Other actions include ascertaining the firmness of the fundus and removing any blood clots. Depending on the circumstances, a rectal examination to rule out any rectal sutures or hematomas may be performed. Wash the perineal area, thighs, and buttocks as needed. Assist in helping the woman assume a comfortable position. Apply ice to the repaired laceration.

9. During and after the procedure, the midwife should continually communicate with the woman and family and provide anticipatory guidance and health education.

Repair of First-Degree Lacerations

The majority of first-degree lacerations are small skin disruptions that barely lacerate the vaginal mucosa and will heal spontaneously without suturing. More extensive first-degree lacerations can be repaired using continuous running stitches. In some situations, a single interrupted stitch or two may accomplish closure. The midwife should assess the area to be repaired, approximate the laceration prior to suturing, and visualize all appropriate landmarks; the midwife should then plan the number of stitches that may be required in advance with the principle of placing the fewest possible to accomplish hemostasis and tissue edge reapproximation.

Repair of Sulcus Tears

Sulcus tears are a type of second-degree laceration in which the vaginal mucosa and underlying tissue are lacerated along one (unilateral) or both (bilateral) sides of the posterior column of the vagina instead of up the middle. The posterior column of the vagina is a longitudinal ridge of the inner surface of the lining extending the length of the vagina. The lateral edges of the column as they meld into the lateral vaginal walls create a slight groove (sulcus) from which this type of laceration derives its name.

Repair of sulcus tears differs only from the repair of the vaginal mucosa if a bilateral sulcus tear is involved. In this event, two apices and two separate lines of continuous locked stitches are needed to close the separate tears in the vaginal mucosa. At their common base, one line of sutures is tied with a final stitch and a square knot, while the other continues to draw the larger base opening together. Sulcus tears usually are deep lacerations and may require two layers of deep interrupted stitches when the deep muscle layer is repaired. To provide better access for placing the deep interrupted stitches, the vaginal mucosa may be repaired with a few sutures in the common base of the bilateral tear for approximation of the tissues, followed by interrupted stitches, followed by the return to the repair of the vaginal mucosa. Because of the depth and potential difficulty with visualization, a second person may also be requested to assist with the repair process to aid in visualizing the wound.

Repair of Periurethral, Clitoral, and Labial Lacerations

Periurethral and labial lacerations usually are longitudinal lacerations that follow the general contour of the vestibule of the perineum. They vary in depth as well as in length, with the longest extending into the clitoris. At other times, they may be transverse lacerations extending into the labia minora and occasionally across the labia majora so that it is torn into two sections.

Repair of periurethral lacerations depends on their depth, bleeding, and the need for a cosmetic repair. Repair of any periurethral laceration close to the urethra should be preceded by insertion of a urinary catheter to prevent accidental closure of the urethra. Small superficial periurethral lacerations that are not bleeding will often heal spontaneously without stitches.

When hemostasis is needed, most periurethral lacerations should be repaired with 4-0 or occasionally 3-0 gauge suture using an interrupted technique. Prior to beginning the repair, an assessment should be made of the best approach, using the least number of stitches while accomplishing reapproximation and hemostasis. There is no precise pattern or sequence of stitches to use, as each laceration is unique.

Repair of labial lacerations is also done with 4-0 gauge suture using an interrupted stitch technique. The stitches can be approximately 0.5 to 1 cm apart and should not be tied too tightly, as this tissue can become edematous very easily.

Repair of Third- and Fourth-Degree Lacerations

The experienced midwife may be credentialed to perform repairs of third- or fourth-degree lacerations. Appropriate education, experience, and institutional privileges are needed in such a case.

Key Points

1. Good visualization and adequate anesthesia are essential to accurately repair a third- or fourth-degree laceration. Assistance may be needed to secure the visualization needed.

2. Fourth- and third-degree lacerations are always repaired before repairing the rest of the perineal laceration, if present.

3. The goal is to reconstruct the muscular cylinder of the rectal sphincter, which is approximately 2 cm thick and 3 cm long.

4. The area may be irrigated with saline prior to being repaired; however, in contrast to practice years ago, antiseptic solutions generally are no longer employed, as they may irritate this tissue.

Repair of Fourth-Degree Lacerations

Fourth-degree lacerations involve the external anal sphincter, internal sphincter, and anterior rectal mucosa. The rectal mucosa and the internal anal sphincter are always repaired before the external rectal sphincter is repaired. After identifying the tear in the anterior rectal wall and the torn ends of the anal sphincter, the repair begins by rejoining the anterior rectal mucosa. This area is repaired in two layers with 4-0 polyglactin suture on an atraumatic needle.

1. The first layer starts at the internal apex and consists of a row of interrupted stitches placed in the rectal submucosa to approximate the rectal mucosa without placing stitches in the lumen of the bowel. The use of a smaller, atraumatic curved needle is essential to take smaller amounts of tissue, thereby decreasing the risk of extending into the lumen of the bowel.

2. The second layer is the internal anal sphincter; it appears as a shiny pink, thick tissue that lies just above the rectal mucosa. It often retracts laterally and superiorly. Repair is made with a continuous technique using 3-0 polyglactin suture. This repair also starts at

the internal apex and is brought out to the cutaneous junction, where it is tied off.

3. After verification that no sutures are in the rectal lumen, repair of the external anal sphincter as described in the next section, followed by standard repair of the laceration or episiotomy, is completed. Special care must be taken in rebuilding the muscle layers of the perineal body, which have been totally lacerated.

Repair of Third-Degree Lacerations

A third-degree laceration differs from a fourth-degree laceration in that it does not include the rectal mucosa. Otherwise, repair of the anal sphincter is the same for both types of lacerations.

1. The torn external anal sphincter is identified. As the torn ends retract, they are found flush with, or as dimples in, the lateral walls at the bottom of the perineal aspect of the wound near the surface. The muscle fibers of the sphincter are visually different from the surrounding fascia. Often one side is dimpled, and the muscle can be visualized emerging from the other side.

2. Both torn ends are grasped with an Allis clamp and pulled toward each other, causing them to meet. The suture of choice is 2-0 synthetic, absorbable suture. Some midwives prefer to first anchor a 3-0 absorbable suture within the inferior apex of the skin extension of the laceration and take a few subcuticular stitches in the posterior anal capsule, then lay this suture aside until the end. This approach is intended to avoid later difficulty in repairing the subcuticular area over the rectal sphincter, as it is sometimes difficult to visualize this apex after repair of the sphincter.

3. A lacerated external anal sphincter is repaired with either doubled interrupted stitches or a figure of eight stitch after approximating the torn ends grasped by the Allis clamps.

a. Inclusion of the anterior and posterior fascial layers surrounding the sphincter muscle strengthens the repair.

b. The sphincter can be repaired by placing the torn section "end-to-end" or by overlapping the torn section as shown in **Figure 29E-13**. Some preliminary research suggests that the overlapping technique is superior and associated with less fecal incontinence and pain, but there is no clear consensus at this time.[8,9]

c. Technique for a doubled interrupted stitch:

i. Put the needle into the right side of the muscle and bring it out in the left side of the muscle.

ii. Put the needle in the left side of the muscle near where it came out and bring it out in the right side.

iii. The suture now has two strands and will be tied off on the side where it was started.

d. *End-to-end repair:* Four doubled interrupted sutures are placed, starting at the posterior aspect as illustrated in Figure 29E-13A, with one in each quadrant at the 6 o'clock, then 9 o'clock, then 12 o'clock, then 3 o'clock positions.

e. *Overlapping technique:* Using the Allis clamp, overlap the ends of the sphincter and place three doubled interrupted sutures in both parts of the muscle where they overlap (Figure 29E-13B).

4. After repairing the sphincter and before continuing with the remainder of the repair, a rectal examination is needed to make sure that sutures

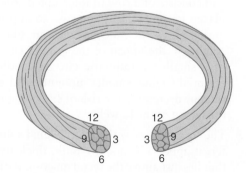
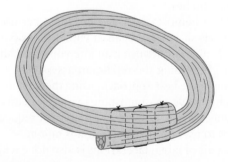

Figure 29E-13 Repair of anal sphincter: (A) End-to-end technique. (B) Overlapping technique.

have not been placed in the rectal mucosa as previously described. Repair of the laceration or episiotomy then continues in standard fashion.

5. When a woman has a third- or fourth-degree perineal laceration, it is common practice to order stool softeners, oral analgesics, and sitz baths for her initial postpartum recovery.

Repair of Cervical Lacerations

Key Points

1. Good visualization is necessary as noted earlier, including effective use of the ring forceps on the cervix to bring the cervix and its laceration into full view, and a well-contracted uterus so any potentially obscuring bleeding is minimal (**Figure 29E-14**).

2. An assistant may be invaluable in this situation to hold the retractors that will enable good visualization. If an assistant is not available, use of an instrument such as a Gelpi retractor can provide better visualization.

3. Anesthesia will not only benefit the woman, but also provide relaxation that will promote better visualization so that the midwife can perform a good repair.

4. Cervical lacerations more than approximately 1 cm in length or a laceration of any length that is bleeding should be repaired.

5. Cervical lacerations are repaired with 2-0 absorbable synthetic suture.

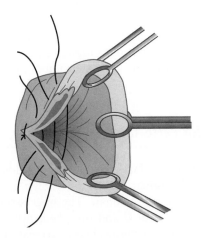

Figure 29E-14 Repair of cervical laceration using interrupted stitches.

Steps to Repair Cervical Lacerations

1. Approximation of the two sides of the tear is facilitated by the placement of a ring forceps on each side of the laceration. The forceps should be placed close enough to the edges to be of use, but far enough away from the edges that the stitches can be taken without sewing through the ring of the forceps.

2. Cervical lacerations are repaired with either interrupted stitches, a continuous stitch, or a continuous locked stitch if additional hemostasis is required.

3. The first stitch should be placed approximately 1 cm above or beyond the apex of the laceration to include any retracted blood vessels.

4. Care should be taken in the placement of each stitch approximating the two sides of the tear so that only the sides of the wound are included in the stitch, thereby maintaining the patency of the cervical canal.

Controversies Regarding Laceration and Episiotomy Repair

To Repair or Not to Repair

Controversy has emerged about when to repair genital lacerations versus when to allow them to heal spontaneously. Because every laceration is unique, meaningful evidence has been difficult to find regarding this question. In general, if the edges of the laceration appear to be well approximated when the tissue is not being handled or when the woman's legs are relaxed in a natural position, then the use of suture for repair may be avoided. Today, some professionals question whether even a second-degree laceration might heal in that manner, but available evidence on this topic is scant and inconsistent.[10]

To Repair Skin Edges or Not to Repair Skin Edges

Some authors have suggested that leaving the skin edges unsutured may result in less pain or dyspareunia, as the sutures themselves can cause irritation. A randomized trial of two-layer versus three-layer repair found that leaving the skin edges unrepaired does result in less pain and dyspareunia at three months postpartum, without disadvantages such as infection or repair breakdown.[11]

Cutting an Episiotomy

Key Points: Preparation

1. During labor, when it becomes apparent that an episiotomy may be indicated, the midwife should discuss the indication and recommendation with the woman and her support personnel. Continuous communication as the procedure is performed informs the woman of events, especially if she has regional anesthesia and impaired sensation.

2. Appropriate equipment should be available.

3. Anesthesia is a prerequisite before an episiotomy is performed, and the level of anesthesia should be appropriate for the extent of surgical repair. Although nitrous oxide or parenteral opioids may be of some value as analgesia, an epidural or a pudendal nerve block will be more effective. Under some circumstances, local infiltration may be performed prior to cutting an episiotomy, although this intervention may distort tissue and cause edema. A description of the techniques for local infiltration and pudendal block can be found in the *Local Infiltration for Laceration Repair* and *Pudendal Block* appendices. A woman's allergies may preclude use of some anesthesia methods.

Determining the Type of Episiotomy to Cut

Two types of episiotomy are performed: midline incision and mediolateral incision. The midline episiotomy is more commonly used in the United States.

Midline Episiotomy

The midline episiotomy has a vaginal apex at the central tendinous point of the perineum and separates the bulbocavernosus and superficial transverse perineal muscles. Depending on the depth of the cut, the deep transverse perineal muscle may also cut into two sides. The perineal apex is above the anal sphincter.

The primary advantage of a midline episiotomy is ease of repair and better cosmetic result. Although retrospective studies of postpartum pain have found that midline episiotomies are associated with less pain than mediolateral episiotomies, prospective studies have not found a significant difference. Because the inferior apex of the midline episiotomy is directly above the rectal sphincter, extension into a third- or fourth-degree laceration is possible.[12]

Mediolateral Episiotomy

A mediolateral episiotomy also has a vaginal apex at the central tendinous point of the perineum. This incision incises through the bulbocavernosus and the superficial and deep transverse perineal muscles, and into the pubococcygeus (levator ani) muscle. Whereas a midline incision is directly anterior/posterior, the mediolateral is cut on the diagonal (right or left) starting at the midline of the posterior fourchette, with the points of the scissors directed right or left toward the ischial tuberosity on the same side as the incision (**Figure 29E-15**).

The primary advantage of a mediolateral episiotomy is that fewer extensions into a third- or fourth-degree laceration occur as compared to the outcomes of median episiotomies. Some studies have found mediolateral episiotomies to be associated with more blood loss; others have not. Compared to median episiotomies, mediolateral episiotomies can be more challenging to repair.

Determining When to Cut an Episiotomy

There is little evidence to guide a midwife regarding when to cut an episiotomy. Performing this procedure too early may result in extra blood loss. Waiting until the perineum is paper thin and the tissue bulging, however, may result in a rapid and perhaps uncontrolled birth of the fetal head, with resulting extension of the episiotomy. Many midwives advocate incision when the head is crowning and not retracting between contractions, such that birth is expected within a few contractions. When the head is well applied to the perineum, it also provides a type of tamponade to decrease bleeding.

After the episiotomy is performed, the midwife should continue to apply gentle pressure to the fetal head to control and direct a slow extension of the head. This will help avoid a rapid birth, sudden pressure on the perineum, and extension of the incision.

Steps for Performing an Episiotomy

1. The midwife places the index and middle fingers into the vagina, palmar side down and facing away from the woman. The fingers should be slightly separated and provide gentle outward pressure on the perineal body to create adequate space between the perineum and the head, and to allow the scissors to slip between the fingers using them as a guide. Thus the fetal head is

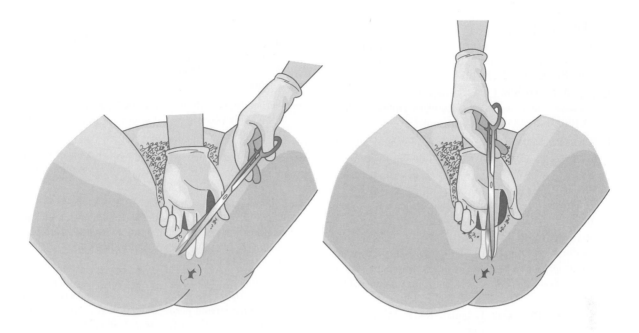

Figure 29E-15 Types of episiotomies.

not touched, yet protected. The pressure also slightly flattens the perineal area, providing an easier incision.

2. The blades of the scissors are placed in the appropriate direction—either straight anterior/ posterior or diagonally, depending upon the type of episiotomy to be cut. One blade of the scissors should be against the posterior vaginal wall, while the other blade should be against the skin of the perineal body, with the point where the blades cross at the midline of the posterior fourchette.

3. The external anal sphincter can be located by palpation using fingers in the vagina and the thumb of the same hand placed externally to the perineal body. Knowing the location of the external anal sphincter minimizes hesitation in cutting an adequate episiotomy due to fear of accidentally cutting through the sphincter.

    a. When cutting a midline episiotomy, the length of the blades of the scissors on the perineal body should be adjusted to the projected length of the incision and terminate above the anal sphincter.

    b. When cutting a mediolateral episiotomy, the blades should be positioned so that there is approximately 1 cm of levator ani muscle between the incision and the sphincter. This directs the incision far enough laterally to avoid the sphincter during the process of

cutting the episiotomy and when performing the repair. Care should be taken not to start the incision on the lateral aspect of the fourchette or to direct the incision too far laterally to avoid incising the Bartholin gland on that side.

4. The perineum should be incised with a single cut that is sufficient to open the perineal body and extend into the vaginal vault. Incising in this manner opens the vagina and the perineum. Performing a single incision through both the vagina and the perineum with one cut avoids the need for multiple incisions and increased trauma to the tissue.

5. After the initial incision, the area should be observed and evaluated to identify any active bleeding. Adequate visualization usually requires use of sponges to blot away blood, although excessive and aggressive blotting or using the sponges to wipe can further harm the tissue.

6. If a second incision is necessary, it can be performed at this time. Extension of an incision is best made by using fingers in the vagina to guide the incision and protect the fetal head.

7. By palpating for a band of tight, restricting vaginal tissue just inside the introitus, the midwife can further evaluate the adequacy of the incision. If such a band is present, it can be determined whether the band must be cut to be released.

● ● ● **References**

1. Albers L, Garcia J, Renfrew M, et al. Distribution of genital tract trauma in childbirth and related postnatal pain. *Birth.* 1999;26:11-17.

2. Carroli G, Mignini L. Episiotomy for vaginal birth. *Cochrane Database Syst Rev.* 2009;1:CD000081. doi: 10.1002/14651858.CD000081.pub2.

3. Albers LL, Sedler KD, Bedrick EJ, et al. Factors related to genital tract trauma in normal spontaneous vaginal births. *Birth.* 2006;33(2):94-100.

4. Leffell DJ, Brown MD. *Manual of Skin Surgery: A Practical Guide to Dermatologic Procedures.* New York: Wiley; 1997.

5. Bharathi A, Reddy DB, Kote GS. A prospective randomized comparative study of Vicryl Rapide versus chromic catgut for episiotomy repair. *J Clin Diagn Res.* 2013;7(2):326-330. doi: 10.7860/JCDR /2013/5185.2758.

6. Kettle C, Dowswell T, Ismail KMK. Absorbable suture materials for primary repair of episiotomy and second degree tears. *Cochrane Database Syst Rev.* 2010;6:CD000006. doi: 10.1002/14651858. CD000006.pub2.

7. Kettle C, Dowswell T, Ismail KMK. Continuous and interrupted suturing techniques for repair of episiotomy or second-degree tears. *Cochrane Database Syst Rev.* 2012;11:CD000947. doi: 10.1002/14651858. CD000947.pub3.

8. Fernando RJ, Sultan AH, Kettle C, et al. Repair techniques for obstetric anal sphincter injuries. *Obstet Gynecol.* 2006;107(6):1261-1268.

9. Leeman L, Spearman M, Rogers R. Repair of obstetric perineal lacerations. *Am Fam Physician.* 2003; 68(8):1585-1590.

10. Elharmeel SMA, Chaudhary Y, Tan S, et al. Surgical repair of spontaneous perineal tears that occur during childbirth versus no intervention. *Cochrane Database Syst Rev.* 2011;8:CD008534. doi: 10.1002/14651858. CD008534.pub2.

11. Gordon B, Mackrodt C, Fern E, et al. The Ipswich childbirth study: 1. A randomized evaluation of two stage postpartum perineal repair leaving the skin unsutured. *Br J Obstet Gynecol.* 1998;105:435-440.

12. Sooklim R, Thinkhamrop J, Lumbiganon P, et al. The outcomes of midline versus medio-lateral episiotomy. *Reprod Health.* 2007;4:10-16.

CHAPTER

30

Complications During Labor and Birth

LINDA A. HUNTER

Introduction

Even under the most normal of circumstances, intrapartum complications can occur. While many of these situations develop gradually or are associated with an already known high-risk condition, some will arise suddenly and without warning. This chapter provides a basic overview of selected complications and conditions that can occur during the intrapartum period. Familiarity with intrapartum complications and emergencies is essential to midwifery practice and requires frequent review of current management guidelines. Additional resources and study may be necessary for a more thorough exploration of the underlying pathophysiology associated with certain preexisting high-risk conditions.

When intrapartum complications are encountered, initiation of interventions is often progressive as the situation evolves and requires the midwife to be vigilant for worsening signs or symptoms. In addition, the need for intervention may disrupt the normal process of labor and will necessitate a careful evaluation of the risk–benefit ratio of intervention versus nonintervention. Shared decision making with the woman and her support persons regarding changes in the plan of care is an important component of midwifery management when a deviation from normal is encountered. In less urgent circumstances, there may be time to thoroughly explore these pros and cons; an obstetric emergency, however, will require prompt recognition and action to avoid serious adverse maternal or fetal outcomes.

In many cases, a collaborative management plan with the consulting physician will already be in place prior to the onset of labor. The development of a new intrapartum complication or deviation from normal labor progress will also require the midwife to seek physician consultation or to establish a collaborative relationship for the continued plan of care. Within this shared model of care, the midwife provides continuity of care and advocacy for the woman, and protects normal labor progress as the clinical situation allows. Additionally, the midwife contributes to medical decision making while promoting family-centered care and keeps the consulting physician informed of any changes in the woman's condition. The medical rationale for consultation, collaboration, and referral as well as the resultant personnel involved in a woman's care are always clearly documented in her obstetric record. The midwife must also be ready and able to manage acute emergent situations within the appropriate institutional and legal boundaries of midwifery practice until the complication is resolved or the consulting physician can take over.

In cases where referral of care is needed, the midwife can maintain an active role in the supportive care of the woman and her family, seeking the most appropriate balance of medicine and midwifery in collaboration with the physician. This supportive role is ongoing throughout the woman's intrapartum clinical course and continues into the postpartum period as needed. Women who experience an unanticipated obstetric complication or emergency greatly benefit from the continuity and emotional support provided by their midwife.

Preterm Labor/Birth

Background

Infants born prior to 37 weeks' gestation face the prospect of many lifelong disabilities, such as cerebral palsy, intellectual impairment, vision defects, and hearing loss.[1] As outlined in the *Obstetric Complications in Pregnancy* chapter, many prevention strategies have been developed to reduce these risk factors and the preterm birth rate in the United States has finally begun a slow but steady decline (from 12.8% in 2006 to 11.99% in 2010).[2]

Preterm births can be subdivided into early preterm (less than 34 weeks) and late preterm (34 to 37 weeks). The threshold of viability is considered to be approximately 22 to 25 weeks' gestation, and many factors affect the decision to resuscitate an infant born within these gestational parameters.[3] Medical indications for delivery (i.e., severe preeclampsia or fetal compromise) account for approximately 30% to 35% of all preterm births and 70% of the late preterm births in the United States.[4] The remaining preterm deliveries occur as a result of either preterm premature rupture of membranes (PPROM) or spontaneous preterm labor (PTL).

Despite years of investigation, the absolute cause of spontaneous preterm labor has yet to be identified. Some researchers believe that, unlike the normal labor physiologic pathway that occurs in full-term gestations, preterm labor results from one or several complex pathologic "triggers."[5] Intrauterine infection or inflammation, hormonal disorders, cervical insufficiency, uterine overdistension, and hemorrhage have all been implicated as potential precursors to preterm labor. Racial disparities have also been identified and here, too, it is thought that the underlying mechanism is probably a complex multifactorial interaction of biologic responses to inflammation, epigenetic responses to environmental stresses, and perhaps other factors that have not yet been elucidated.

Fortunately, the majority of women who have preterm contractions will go on to give birth at term gestations. In cases of true preterm labor, however, even a brief delay in treatment could adversely affect both maternal and fetal outcomes.

Fetal Fibronectin

One biochemical marker that has been shown to aid triaging women with symptoms of preterm labor is fetal fibronectin (fFN). Fetal fibronectin is an extracellular glycoprotein found in the amniochorionic membrane that serves as an adhesive binder between the membranes and the decidua. It is normally present in cervicovaginal secretions prior to 20 weeks' gestation and again after 37 weeks' gestation as cervical remodeling takes place in preparation for normal full-term labor. Between 24 and 34 weeks, the presence of fFN is atypical and could indicate

inflammation or uterine activity—both of which are precursors to preterm birth.[6]

Unfortunately, studies have found fFN has a limited positive predictability of only 25.9% among women who present with preterm labor symptoms.[7] Conversely, fFN has a high negative predictability of 97.6% that birth will not occur within 7 days.[7] These findings are consistent with earlier studies that also demonstrated similar negative predictive values.[8,9] From a clinical practice standpoint, women with symptoms of preterm labor between 24 and 34 weeks' gestation with a negative fFN culture (or assay) have only a 1% to 2% chance of giving birth within the next 7 to 14 days.[7–9]

It is important to remember that fFN predictability exists only in symptomatic women; this biomarker is not recommended for use as a screening test to identify preterm labor risk. In addition, fFN is collected in a sample of vaginal secretions and must be collected prior to any other vaginal examinations. fFN sampling is contraindicated if there is evidence of ruptured membranes. The accuracy of fFN is decreased in the presence of lubricants, blood, recent intercourse, or cervical manipulation within the previous 24 hours. A sample of vaginal secretions should not be collected for fFN testing in these situations or if the cervix is more than 3 cm dilated or 80% effaced.

Typically, fFN is collected at the outset of the examination of a woman presenting with preterm labor symptoms and set aside until the results of a digital cervical examination are available. The culture can then be sent or discarded depending on the clinical situation. The fFN collection technique is outlined in **Figure 30-1**.

Cervical Length Measurement

As discussed in the *Obstetric Complications in Pregnancy* chapter, a transvaginal ultrasound cervical length measurement of 25 mm or less at 18 to 24 weeks' gestation is associated with an increased risk of preterm birth. For women at more than 24 weeks' gestation who have symptoms of preterm labor, cervical length assessment can also be used as a helpful adjunct to fFN testing. Some researchers now advocate combining fFN and cervical length in standardized preterm labor algorithms.[6,10] In these suggested protocols, women presenting with preterm labor symptoms between 24 and 34 weeks' gestation would have an fFN collected (if not contraindicated) during their initial speculum examination, followed by a cervical length measurement. The results of the cervical length measurement would determine whether the fFN test was needed.

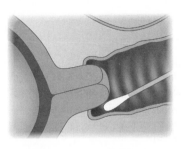

Step 1
During speculum examination,
    lightly rotate swab across posterior
    fornix of vagina for 10 seconds to
    absorb cervicovaginal secretions

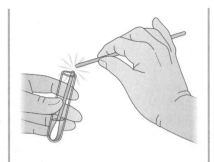

Step 2
Remove swab and immerse
    polyester tip in buffer; break shaft
    at score even with top of tube

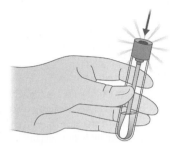

Step 3
Align the shaft with hole inside the
    tube cap and push down tightly
    over shaft, sealing tube; ensure
    shaft is aligned to avoid leakage

Figure 30-1 Fetal fibronectin specimen collection procedure.
Source: Courtesy of HOLOGIC, Inc. and affiliates.

For example, a cervical length of 30 mm or more is considered normal, with preterm birth being unlikely to occur. The fFN culture could then be discarded and the woman discharged home pending any other clinical problems that need to be addressed. If the cervical length is between 16 and 29 mm, the fFN is sent for analysis. A negative fFN would again be reassuring and indicates preterm birth is unlikely. In contrast, a positive fFN in this situation or a cervical length of less than 15 mm would warrant admission and initiation of preterm labor treatment. While these algorithms may reduce false-positive diagnoses and decrease unnecessary hospital admissions, the availability of cervical length ultrasound is limited in many areas and its performance requires specialized training and credentialing.

Midwifery Management of Preterm Labor

Pregnant women who are experiencing painful uterine contractions or more than six contractions per hour, vaginal bleeding, or any loss of fluid prior to 37 weeks' gestation should be evaluated promptly for possible preterm labor. Other less specific symptoms, such as cramping, pelvic pressure, abdominal pain, back pain, and watery vaginal discharge, could also indicate preterm labor, especially if persistent or unrelieved with rest or oral hydration. The differential diagnoses for spontaneous PTL includes physiologic causes such as Braxton Hicks contractions, dehydration, lax vaginal tone, and round ligament pain. Other, more serious etiologies such as infection (intrauterine, renal, genital tract), abruption, trauma, or appendicitis must also be considered and assessed for when obtaining a history and conducting a physical examination. The evaluation procedure for preterm labor is outlined in **Box 30-1**.

For women in preterm labor between 34 and 37 weeks' gestation, the midwife should consult with a physician regarding a collaborative management plan depending on individual practice guidelines and institutional resources. If the woman is less than 34 weeks' gestation and her initial cervical examination is more than 3 cm dilated or 80% effaced, preterm labor treatment should be initiated and the woman referred for immediate medical management. Many smaller institutions will transfer women in preterm labor at less than 36 weeks' gestation to a tertiary center, especially because of availability of specialized neonatal care. Midwives in all practice settings should be aware of the current preterm labor treatment recommendations and initiate these interventions as the clinical situation requires. Any other abnormalities encountered by the midwife during the initial data collection should be managed and treated according to individual practice guidelines.

The more challenging situation for the midwife is formulating a management plan for women with vague preterm labor symptoms and women having painful regular contractions with minimal or no cervical dilatation. In these cases, serial digital cervical examinations (ideally by the same examiner) over an hour or two after rest and hydration may provide a helpful reassurance to both the midwife and the woman that preterm labor is not the cause of these

BOX 30-1 Evaluation for Preterm Labor

1. History and Chart Review
   a. Confirm the gestational age using the most credible data available.
   b. Review the woman's history for any preterm birth risk factors, especially for prior preterm deliveries or unexplained second-trimester loss.
   c. If there is a history of prior preterm birth:
      i. Has the woman been receiving 17-hydroxy-progesterone injections?
      ii. Are serial cervical lengths documented on prenatal record by ultrasound or other cervical measurement instrument (e.g., CerviLenz)?
   d. Inquire about recent intercourse, strenuous physical activity, abdominal trauma, vaginal bleeding, loss of fluid, fever, nausea, vomiting, urinary tract infection symptoms, or abnormal vaginal discharge.
2. Physical Examination
   a. Note the woman's demeanor, distress, and/or coping.
   b. Assess temperature, pulse, respirations, and blood pressure.
   c. Palpate the lower back and assess for CVAT tenderness to rule out independent or concomitant UTI.
   d. Palpate the abdomen for rebound tenderness; note any guarding.
   e. Palpate the uterus for fundal tenderness, contraction strength, and fetal position (Leopold's maneuvers).
   f. Place the woman on continuous electronic fetal monitoring to assess fetal well-being and uterine activity.
   g. Perform a sterile speculum examination:
      i. If there is pooling fluid, check nitrazine, ferning, or other assessment method to rule out PPROM.
      ii. If there is no history of bleeding, vaginal examinations, or intercourse in the past 24 hours, obtain a fetal fibronectin (fFN) culture (see Figure 30-1 for collection technique).
      iii. Obtain cultures for gonorrhea and chlamydia.
      iv. Obtain a specimen for wet mount to assess for bacterial vaginosis or trichomoniasis infection.
      v. Obtain a sample from the proximal third of the vagina and through the rectal sphincter for group B *Streptococcus* (GBS) culture.
   h. If there is no evidence of PPROM, perform a digital cervical examination to assess dilatation, effacement, station, and presenting part.
   i. Laboratory tests:
      i. Clean catch urinalysis (with micro) and urine culture
      ii. Complete blood count
      iii. Other labs as clinically indicated
   j. Ultrasonography
      i. Confirm the presenting part.
      ii. Perform transvaginal assessment of cervical length (depending on institutional protocols and availability).

CVAT = costovertebral angle tenderness; LMP = last menstrual period; PPROM = premature rupture of membranes.

symptoms. Sending the fFN culture or performing a cervical length measurement (if available) can also be considered and may prevent unnecessary hospitalization or interventions.

Treatment of Preterm Labor

In the past, strategies such as bedrest, home contraction monitoring, maintenance tocolysis, hydration, periodontal care, and abstinence from intercourse were used to prevent preterm labor and birth. More evidence has not found these methods to be effective in reducing the preterm birth rate; thus they are no longer used as specific preventive or treatment therapies.[11] There is also extensive evidence regarding the use of tocolytic medications to prolong pregnancy. Several different agents have been studied over the past 50 years, but none has effectively reduced the preterm birth rate or decreased neonatal mortality and morbidity (**Table 30-1**).[12]

Tocolytics

All tocolytic agents slow uterine contractions to some degree, but at best will delay birth for only 2 to 7 days.[12–14] In the past, magnesium sulfate and beta-mimetics (terbutaline [Brethine]) were the most commonly used tocolytic medications. Evidence has found calcium-channel blockers (nifedipine [Procardia]) and prostaglandin synthetase inhibitors

Table 30-1	Summary of Tocolytic Medications Used in Preterm Labor			
Drug (Brand Name)	**Standard Dose**	**Common Maternal Side Effects**	**Fetal Effects**	**Contraindications/ Cautions**
Nifedipine (Procardia)	Loading dose: 10–40 mg orally given in divided doses Then 10–20 mg orally every 4–6 hours (numerous dosing protocols exist)	Transient nausea, flushing, headache, palpitations, hypotension, dizziness	Secondary to maternal hypotension	Cardiovascular disease or hemodynamic instability Do not use concurrently with terbutaline Do not use concurrently with magnesium sulfate
Indomethacin (Indocin)	Loading dose: 50–100 mg orally or 50 mg rectally Then 25–50 mg orally every 6 hours, for 48 hours	Gastrointestinal: nausea, vomiting, reflux, gastritis Platelet dysfunction	Premature closure of ductus arteriosus Oligohydramnios	Not recommended for more than 48 hours of continuous use Not recommended for gestations of 32 weeks or greater Allergy to aspirin or other nonsteroidal anti-inflammatory drugs
Magnesium sulfate	Loading dose: 4–6 g intravenously (IV) over 20–30 min Then 2 g/hour by continuous IV infusion (pump required)	Flushing, nausea, blurred vision, headache, lethargy, muscle weakness, hypotension Rare effects: pulmonary edema, respiratory or cardiac arrest	Decreased fetal heart rate variability Decreased neonatal tone	Impaired renal function Myasthenia gravis Do not use concurrently with nifedipine Toxicity: loss of patellar reflexes, decreased urine output < 30 mL/hr, respiratory rate < 12/min Toxicity risks increase with serum creatinine > 1.0 mg/dL

Sources: Adapted from Abramovici A, Cantu J, Jenkins SM. Tocolytic therapy for acute preterm labor. *Obstet Gynecol Clin North Am.* 2012;39: 77-87; Lowe NK, King TK. Labor. In: King TL, Brucker MC, eds. *Pharmacology for Women's Health.* Sudbury, MA: Jones and Bartlett; 2011:1086-1116.

(indomethacin [Indocin]) have the best clinical efficacy and a lower incidence of toxicity and maternal side effects when compared to magnesium sulfate and terbutaline.[12] As a result, terbutaline is no longer recommended for acute tocolysis, and magnesium sulfate should be reserved for clinical situations in which nifedipine and indomethacin are contraindicated or fetal/newborn neuroprotection is sought.[12]

Regardless of the agent chosen for tocolysis, the primary goal is to delay birth long enough to administer a full course of corticosteroids and arrange for transfer to a tertiary center if needed. These two interventions have demonstrated dramatic improvements in neonatal outcomes and are the mainstay of preterm labor management. The administration of corticosteroids to women in preterm labor between 24 and 34 weeks' gestation has been conclusively shown to improve fetal lung maturity and decrease other morbidities associated with prematurity.[15] Either betamethasone (Celestone) 12 mg intramuscularly (IM) given in two doses 24 hours apart or dexamethasone (Decadron) 6 mg IM given in four doses 12 hours apart can be used.[15] Once the woman has received a complete course of steroids, tocolysis is discontinued. If she does not give birth, the full steroid course can be repeated once as a "rescue dose" if more than 2 weeks have passed, the gestational age is less than 33 weeks, and the woman has a risk of birth within 7 days.[15]

Group B Streptococcus Prophylaxis

Another important intervention in the treatment of preterm labor is the administration of antibiotics to prevent group B *Streptococcus* (GBS) disease.

Preterm infants are especially susceptible to GBS sepsis, and the woman will likely have unknown colonization status because the standard screening culture is not performed until 35 to 36 weeks' gestation. All women in preterm labor prior to 37 weeks with unknown GBS status should receive antibiotic prophylaxis.[16] The Centers for Disease Control and Prevention (CDC) website maintains updated GBS treatment guidelines and algorithms for GBS prevention strategies.[16]

Magnesium Sulfate for Neuroprotection

Lastly, the administration of magnesium sulfate to women in preterm labor may reduce the risk of cerebral palsy in infants born prior to 32 weeks' gestation. This promising therapy is slowly gaining popularity across the United States, and many institutions now include it as part of preterm labor management. Although the exact mechanisms of fetal neuroprotection are unknown, it is hypothesized that the administration of magnesium sulfate improves fetal cerebral blood flow and provides safeguards against hypoxic stress. Given that prematurity and low birth weight are the most significant risk factors for cerebral palsy, fetal neuroprotection has the potential to greatly improve the neurodevelopmental future of children born prior to 32 weeks' gestation.

Institutions that use magnesium sulfate for fetal neuroprotection should have written guidelines and dosing protocols for this therapy in place.[17] These guidelines should also include an informed consent and discussion with the woman and her family regarding the risks and potential benefits of magnesium sulfate in preventing cerebral palsy for informed decision making. It is important for the midwife to be aware of these guidelines and the distinction of using magnesium sulfate for this indication *separately* from tocolysis. More importantly, the full dosing protocol for neuroprophylaxis differs from the magnesium sulfate doses used in the past for tocolysis and the dosing regimen currently in place for the treatment of preeclampsia/eclampsia.

Follow-Up

Women admitted for threatened preterm labor will typically remain in the hospital for at least 24 hours. Once the full course of steroids is completed, tocolysis is usually discontinued and expectant management is resumed if the woman has not given birth. Women with advanced cervical dilatation may need prolonged inpatient care and monitoring, especially if they are at a very early preterm gestation. The midwife should maintain an active supportive role in the woman's care during hospitalization and discuss the continued management plan with the physician as the clinical scenario changes. Prior to the woman's discharge from the hospital, the midwife should reassess her for preterm birth risk factors and initiate any necessary treatments or interventions.

Outpatient monitoring will include weekly prenatal visits for the remainder for the pregnancy with either the midwife or the physician, or both, according to the plan of care. The woman should also be counseled about any signs of preterm labor and advised to call with any if any symptoms are noted. If symptoms do occur, the woman should be reassessed promptly in the hospital and the appropriate treatments repeated if needed.

Post-Term Pregnancy

Background

A post-term or prolonged pregnancy is one that continues beyond 42 0/7 weeks (294 days) of gestation.[18] The term "postdates" is no longer used and should be avoided when discussing prolonged or post-term pregnancy management.[18] The reported frequency of prolonged pregnancy in the United States has remained approximately 5.5% for the past several years.[2] Despite the fact that differences exist in how the absolute endpoint of pregnancy should be defined, the most common cause of post-term pregnancy is an error in calculation of a woman's estimated due date (EDD). Menstrual dating has been used reliably for more than 100 years, but has many potential sources of inaccuracy, such as irregular cycles and poor recall. Ultrasound dating, by comparison, provides a more precise estimate of the due date, typically within 7 days when performed in the first trimester.[19] Studies on ultrasound dating also show a decrease in both prolonged pregnancy and post-term inductions when compared with menstrual dating.[19] Methods of estimating and calculating the EDD are an important component of the initial pregnancy database and are thoroughly reviewed in the *Prenatal Care* chapter.

Beyond an error in the dating, the causes of a truly prolonged pregnancy are unknown. The incidence is higher among nulliparous women and women with a history of a prior post-term birth.[20] Caucasian women are more likely to have a post-term pregnancy than are women of other racial/ethnic groups. Rare causes of prolonged pregnancy include placental sulfatase deficiency, fetal adrenal insufficiency, and fetal anencephaly.[20]

Increased fetal and maternal risks are associated with pregnancies that last beyond 42 weeks' gestation. The perinatal mortality rate (which includes both stillbirths and early neonatal deaths) more than doubles among infants whose pregnancies continue beyond 42 weeks compared with infants born at 40 weeks.[21] Factors such as placental insufficiency, meconium aspiration, and intrauterine infection have been identified as possible etiologies for this difference. Birth weight also increases with prolonged gestation, but there is no evidence that early induction of labor reduces the incidence of fetal macrosomia. Other fetal risks include post-maturity syndrome, oligohydramnios, and fetal intolerance of labor.

Maternal risks of post-term pregnancy include an increased incidence of labor dystocia, along with consequences associated with larger newborns such as perineal injury, shoulder dystocia, and postpartum hemorrhage. There is also a twofold increased risk of cesarean birth, especially for a nulliparous woman with an unfavorable cervix.[22,23]

Expectant Management Versus Induction of Labor

One of the main problems for women who are between 40 and 42 weeks' gestation who do not have medical indications for delivery is determining when labor induction would improve maternal and/or fetal outcomes. In the absence of obstetric complications, there are no reliable means of predicting when the risks of continuing the pregnancy outweigh the risks associated with induction of labor. Many studies have conclusively shown the incidence of stillbirth increases with prolonged gestation.[21,24] In a large retrospective study involving more than 3 million women, the risk of stillbirth was 4.2 per 10,000 women at 40–41 weeks, 6.1 per 10,000 at 41–42 weeks, and 10.8 per 10,000 at 42–43 weeks.[21] These data support the commonly held belief that beyond 42 weeks' gestation, the risk of stillbirth far outweighs the benefits of expectant management and the woman's labor should be induced.

For many years, cesarean section has been considered the primary adverse outcome associated with induction of labor. This relationship has been based on observational studies that compared outcomes of women who were induced versus those who presented in spontaneous labor. Some authors have suggested that it is more appropriate to compare induction of labor to expectant management because this is the actual choice women must make.[25] Expectant management could potentially result in spontaneous labor or a medically indicated induction. In addition, it can result in a vaginal birth or a cesarean section. Thus a cohort of women who are expectantly managed is the proper control group when comparing perinatal outcomes to planned induction of labor. Systematic reviews of randomized trials comparing elective induction to expectant management have found a slightly lower risk of cesarean birth among the women who were induced.[25,26] A Cochrane meta-analysis also found a lower risk for cesarean section in women who were induced after 41 weeks' gestation when compared to expectant management after 41 weeks, as well as a lower incidence of stillbirth and meconium aspiration.[24]

In contrast to these findings, a week-by-week retrospective analysis of more than 40,000 births in the United States found that induction of labor was associated with a higher risk of cesarean birth.[27] Rather than using expectant management of all women who continue being pregnant as the control group, this study examined the outcomes of all women who entered labor at or after the gestational age at which the inductions took place. As a result, the unadjusted cesarean birth rate was higher with induction of labor than with spontaneous labor, regardless of how the comparison group was defined.[27] These differing results have not established a clear evidence-based advantage for recommending induction of labor over expectant management for women between 41 and 42 weeks' gestation; nor have they established whether induction of labor leads to an increased risk of cesarean birth, despite the fact that many authors recommend induction at 41 weeks' gestation.[20,28]

Studies on the benefits of antepartum testing (nonstress test or biophysical profile) in women who are post-term have not included an unmonitored control group for ethical reasons. Unfortunately, antepartum testing has not been shown to decrease perinatal mortality.[29] Regardless, starting antepartum testing at 41 weeks' gestation has provided some reassurance to continue the pregnancy and is a commonly accepted practice.

Prevention of Post-term Pregnancy

Membrane sweeping, acupuncture, and unprotected intercourse have been recommended as techniques that can facilitate the onset of labor and decrease the risk of post-term pregnancy. Membrane sweeping is reviewed later in the section on induction of labor. It is a common procedure that has both risks and benefits, all of which should be discussed with the woman prior to obtaining consent and performing the procedure.

The prostaglandins in semen that is placed near the cervix during unprotected intercourse may stimulate uterine contractions. In fact, the prostate gland was named "prostate" after the discovery of prostaglandins in seminal fluid. Based on the results of one randomized trial, it appears that unprotected intercourse may reduce the post-term pregnancy rate by a modest amount, but more data are needed before this practice can be definitively recommended. Similarly, there are currently insufficient data about the effects of acupuncture to recommend it as a means to prevent post-term pregnancy.

Midwifery Management of Post-term Pregnancy

The ongoing prenatal management of every pregnant woman includes discussion regarding her goals for her labor and birth. Given that midwives promote and support normal physiologic labor, as the woman reaches her due date, this discussion will focus on expectant management between 39 and 41 gestational weeks. Some women will be anxious to end their pregnancies at the soonest possible time and will request induction of labor at 41 weeks. The risks and benefits of induction and expectant management should be thoroughly reviewed with the woman and if her cervix is favorable, a post-term induction can be scheduled at 41 weeks. If the cervix is unfavorable, the woman can be encouraged to wait and antepartum testing begun at 41 weeks. A plan to initiate membrane stripping or incorporate the use of hormonal cervical ripening agents may also be indicated; these methods are discussed later in this chapter.

For women who decline induction at 42 weeks' gestation, consultation with a physician should occur for a continued plan of care that may include more frequent antepartum testing (e.g., every other day). Women whose pregnancies continue beyond 42 weeks' gestation have a higher risk of stillbirth, and careful monitoring and ongoing discussion with the woman are mandatory to explore her reasons for refusal of induction and her goals for birth. This discussion and the results of antepartum testing should be documented in the woman's health record.

Premature Rupture of Membranes

Background

Premature rupture of membranes (PROM) is technically defined as rupture of the membranes prior to the onset of labor. When this event occurs in women who are less than 37 weeks' gestation, it is referred to as preterm premature rupture of membranes (PPROM). Premature rupture of the membranes at term gestations, which is also referred to as prelabor rupture of membranes, is a normal process associated with physiologic weakening of the amniotic membrane as labor nears. Preterm PROM, in contrast, is thought to result from some type of underlying pathology, such as infection. The recommended management

differs considerably for term and preterm PROM; thus these conditions are considered separately here.

The Term PROM Controversy

As discussed in the chapter *The First Stage of Labor*, the primary risks associated with PROM include umbilical cord compression and intrauterine infection (chorioamnionitis). Infection risk increases with the length of the latency period and may be more prevalent among women colonized with group B *Streptococcus*. Research on expectant management of the latency period in term pregnancies was conducted in the 1990s, but has not been replicated specifically with this subgroup of women. Even though 95% of the women in one large clinical trial of PROM at term delivered spontaneously within 28 hours, conflicting opinions remain regarding the safest management options for women with PROM.[30]

This controversy revolves around weighing the risks of expectant management versus the risks associated with induction of labor.[31] Midwifery management of PROM has historically (and philosophically) favored expectant management for women at low risk for infection. This approach does result in a longer latency period, but in the 1996 TermPROM Study the rates of neonatal infection were similar in both the expectant management and induction groups.[31] The rate of maternal infection was slightly higher in the expectant management group, but the study protocol used a lower temperature threshold (37.5°C) for diagnosis of chorioamnionitis than the threshold used in clinical practice (temperature higher than 38°C). Women in the expectant management group also received more digital cervical examinations, which may have further increased their risks for chorioamnionitis.

Citing the data from the TermPROM Study, the American College of Obstetricians and Gynecologists (ACOG) published guidelines in 2007 recommending prompt induction of labor for women diagnosed with PROM at term.[32] This opinion was based on the premise that a shorter latency period would reduce the incidence of chorioamnionitis. As a result of this publication, midwifery protocols for expectant management came into question and many women were no longer given the option of expectant management for PROM. The American College of Nurse-Midwives (ACNM)'s Position Statement on Premature Rupture of Membranes at Term reaffirms the woman's rights to self-determination and supports the option of expected management for low-risk women.[33] **Box 30-2** summarizes these recommendations. Midwives should familiarize themselves with this document as well as the findings of the original TermPROM Study

BOX 30-2 Criteria for Expectant Management of Prelabor Rupture of Membranes

- Full term (more than 37 gestational weeks)
- Singleton pregnancy
- Vertex presentation
- Clear amniotic fluid
- No fever
- No infection including HIV; hepatitis B and C negative
- Not a group B *Streptococcus* carrier (GBS negative)
- No evidence of risk for fetal acidemia in fetal heart rate pattern
- No health or obstetric condition that requires immediate induction of labor

Source: Adapted from American College of Nurse-Midwives position statement: premature rupture of membranes at term. ACNM Division of Standards and Practice, Clinical Practice Section 2008 (reviewed 2012). Available at: http://www.midwife.org.

when counseling women on the risks and benefits of expectant management versus induction of labor when PROM is encountered.

Preterm PROM

Unlike women with term PROM, women who present with ruptured membranes prior to 37 weeks' gestation are likely experiencing an underlying infectious or inflammatory process that weakened the membranes. Preterm PROM occurs in only 3% of all pregnant women, but is associated with 20% to 30% of all preterm births in the United States.[32,34] The management of PPROM is based on weighing the risks of prematurity against the risks of infection with prolonged latency and delayed delivery. In general, the latency period with PPROM lasts an average of approximately 1 week with expectant management, but in some cases it may last several weeks. Similar to preterm birth, neonatal outcomes following PPROM are directly related to the gestational age and the presence of overt infection or other signs of fetal compromise at the time of birth. In addition, fetal malpresentation is more common in earlier gestations, increasing the risks for umbilical cord prolapse when the membranes rupture. Pregnant women with confirmed PPROM at less than 34 weeks' gestation

should be referred to a consulting physician for the continued plan of care.

PPROM at 32–34 Weeks

For women who present at 32 to 34 weeks' gestation, there is a possibility that the fetal lungs could be mature. A sample of the amniotic fluid pooling in the vagina can be collected during an initial sterile speculum examination and sent for fetal lung maturity testing (see the *Evaluation and Diagnosis of Ruptured Membranes* appendix of *The First Stage of Labor* chapter). An attempt should be made to obtain as much fluid as possible, avoiding cervical mucus and vaginal discharge debris. If the fetal lung maturity is confirmed, or if the gestational age is more than 34 weeks, induction of labor is usually recommended.[32] A collaborative management plan can be considered between the midwife and the physician in these situations, and will also depend on institutional and individual practice guidelines for midwifery management of women in preterm labor.

PPROM at 24–32 Weeks

In gestations between 24 and 32 weeks, expectant management is preferred if there are no clinical signs of infection, fetal compromise, or labor. Transfer to a tertiary center should be arranged if necessary. In addition, a full course of corticosteroids is administered to improve fetal lung maturity, as well as latency antibiotics administered to the woman to prevent intra-amniotic infection. The regimen for latency antibiotics varies among institutions but always includes an antibiotic that is appropriate for GBS prophylaxis.[16] The CDC guidelines for GBS prophylaxis, which can be found on the CDC website, detail evaluation and management of women with PPROM with regard to culturing for GBS, how long to administer antibiotics, and management if the woman does or does not go into labor. Maintenance tocolysis is not recommended, but magnesium sulfate for fetal neuroprotection can be administered if birth seems imminent within the next 12 to 24 hours. Digital cervical examinations are contraindicated, in order to reduce the risk of chorioamnionitis. A baseline cervical examination should not be performed.

In situations where PPROM occurs prior to 24 weeks' gestation (a previable state), an individualized collaborative approach that includes the neonatal team is necessary to best determine the course of treatment. Extensive counseling and shared decision making with the woman and her family should occur. Midwives can provide a valuable role in listening and helping the woman understand all the complex information she will be given in this situation.

Evaluation for Ruptured Membranes

The evaluation of women who present with a history of leaking fluid is the same regardless of gestational age. The midwife should pay particular attention to the woman's history, as these details may improve diagnostic accuracy. For example, in situations where the history suggests ruptured membranes but the physical examination is inconclusive, the woman can be placed in a semi-reclining position and the speculum examination repeated in 30 to 60 minutes. A final option for women with preterm gestations wherein the diagnosis of suspected PPROM is essential to dictate management is installation of indigo carmine dye into the uterus via amniocentesis. A tampon is then inserted into the woman's vagina and inspected in 15 to 30 minutes for any blue discharge leaking from the cervix.[32]

Midwifery Management of Women with Ruptured Membranes at Term

Initially, the plan of care will depend on whether the woman is in labor or if there are any signs of maternal infection or fetal compromise. Spontaneous labor is likely to occur; if this is the case, the woman is treated the same as any other laboring woman. Fetal heart rate abnormalities such as variable decelerations are common when there is less amniotic fluid present around the fetus. In addition, fetal tachycardia may be a sign of chorioamnionitis and may be accompanied by maternal tachycardia, fundal tenderness, and fever. Any of these signs or symptoms requires admission, physician consultation, and prompt initiation of the appropriate treatment interventions.

Women who are not in labor and who meet the criteria for expectant management should be given this option in accordance with the midwife's practice (Box 30-2). Risks and benefits of both labor induction and expectant management should be discussed with the woman, and her choice should be supported. Women who require (or opt) for induction of labor are admitted, and the plan of care proceeds per institutional guidelines for cervical ripening and/or oxytocin infusion.

If expectant management is chosen, the woman may be allowed to return home for a predetermined time to await the onset of labor. The evidence and effectiveness of the use of other induction agents such as castor oil or nipple stimulation to initiate cervical ripening or labor are reviewed later in this chapter. Women who return home for expectant management should be advised to monitor their temperature (with a thermometer) every 2 to 4 hours as well as contraction frequency and fetal movement. It is important to also counsel the woman to avoid inserting anything into her vagina. Lastly, home management always includes a plan for follow-up evaluation. The woman should be advised to call immediately if she has a temperature of 38°C (100.4°F) or higher, decreased fetal movement, signs of active labor, and either meconium-stained or foul-smelling amniotic fluid.

Intra-amniotic Infection (Chorioamnionitis)

Chorioamnionitis is acute inflammation or infection of the amniotic sac, the amnion, and the chorion. This serious intrauterine infection can lead to neonatal sepsis, meningitis, pneumonia, and ultimately cerebral palsy as the result of fetal infection.[35] The most common cause of chorioamnionitis is ascending bacteria from the woman's lower genital tract. Organisms such as group B *Streptococcus*, *Escherichia coli*, *Ureaplasma urealyticum*, *Fusobacterium* species, and *Mycoplasma hominis* have all been implicated as causative pathogens.[34] Because the amniotic membrane provides some protection against fetal infection, prolonged rupture of membranes and long labor are risk factors for chorioamnionitis. Manipulative vaginal or intrauterine procedures and frequent digital cervical examinations also increase the likelihood of infection and should be avoided unless absolutely necessary once the membranes have ruptured.[30]

The definitive diagnosis of chorioamnionitis can be made only after the birth through histological examination of the placenta and membranes.[35] When clinical signs such as maternal fever of 38°C (100.4°F) or higher, maternal tachycardia, fetal tachycardia, uterine tenderness, and foul-smelling amniotic fluid are present, the condition is referred to as clinical chorioamnionitis. Technically the diagnosis is not made until the fever is persistent for more than an hour and is higher than 38°C. In practice antibiotic therapy is usually initiated as soon as the fever is recognized.

Maternal fever during labor is the primary clinical marker of chorioamnionitis and associated with 95% of cases of chorioamnionitis. However, fever can also be caused by maternal dehydration, overheated room temperature, and possibly prolonged time in the shower or tub. Maternal fever is also frequently seen in women who have epidural analgesia. Although the exact mechanism for this phenomenon is not known, the fetal risks associated with chorioamnionitis can be severe and some authors have postulated that fever without concomitant bacterial infection may increase the fetal risk for cerebral palsy. Therefore, all women who have a fever are treated with antibiotics.

Midwifery management includes preventive measures such as promoting hydration during labor and remaining vigilant for early trends such as a gradual rise in maternal temperature or pulse or a rising fetal heart rate baseline. Vaginal examinations should be limited once the membranes have ruptured. If the maternal temperature begins to rise, an intravenous fluid bolus can be given initially and the temperature rechecked in an hour. Any maternal temperature of 38°C (100.4°F) or higher, however, is an indication of an intra-amniotic infection; in such a case, the woman should be assessed for other signs and symptoms and a physician consulted for a continued plan of care.

Even in cases where the suspicion for intrauterine infection is low, intravenous antibiotic prophylaxis is always initiated in the presence of maternal fever. Although no randomized trials have compared the various antibiotic regimens, broad-spectrum antibiotics such as ampicillin or penicillin, used in combination with gentamicin (Garamycin), are the most commonly recommended treatment for suspected infection.[36,37] Given intravenously until the woman delivers, these antibiotics have consistently demonstrated the highest efficacy against the two leading causes of neonatal sepsis—namely, group B *Streptococcus* and *E. coli.*[37] **Figure 30-2** shows the recommended dosing regimens, including alternatives for women with penicillin or ampicillin allergy.

One important reminder is that women who are being given penicillin or ampicillin for GBS

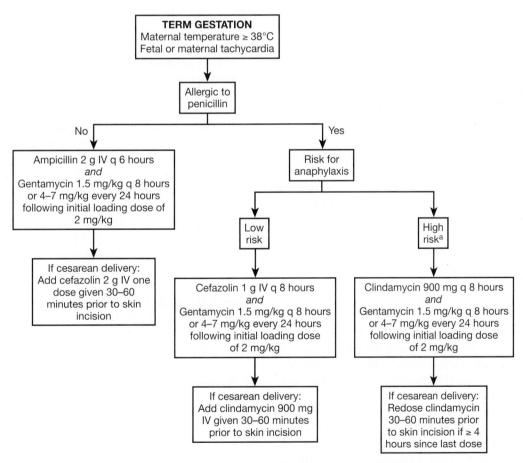

ªHigh risk for anaphylaxis is anyone who has a history of angioedema, respiratory distress, urticaria (hives), or anaphylaxis after exposure to penicillin.

Figure 30-2 Treatments for suspected chorioamnionitis.
Source: Adapted from Fahey JO. Clinical management of intra-amniotic infection and chorioamnionitis: a review of the literature. *J Midwifery Women's Health.* 2008;53:227-235; Fishman SG, Gelber SE. Evidence for the clinical management of chorioamnionitis. *Semin Fetal Neonatal Med.* 2012;17:46-50.

prophylaxis are not sufficiently treated for chorio-amnionitis. If a woman who is receiving penicillin for GBS prophylaxis develops a fever during labor, a broad-spectrum antibiotic that is effective against anaerobic bacteria must be initiated.

Oral acetaminophen (Tylenol) 975 mg should also be given to the woman, especially if her temperature continues to rise. If labor is not progressing normally, active management should be initiated to expedite birth when chorioamnionitis is suspected. The woman's condition and labor progress should also be monitored closely. If a cesarean birth is performed, the woman may need additional anaerobic antibiotic coverage with either cefazolin (Ancef) or clindamycin to prevent postpartum endometritis. Once birth occurs, the placenta is sent to the pathology laboratory for histologic evaluation and the infant closely monitored for any signs of sepsis or infection. Intravenous antibiotics are typically continued for at least one additional dose after the delivery, although many institutions will extend postpartum dosing until the woman has remained afebrile for at least 24 hours.[36,37]

Induction of Labor

Background

Induction of labor refers to stimulation of contractions through artificial means. Methods for inducing labor include both hormonal and nonhormonal approaches. The decision to induce labor involves assessing the risks associated with continuing the pregnancy versus the risks associated with labor induction for both the woman and the fetus. Induction of labor can be elective or medically indicated. Examples of evidence-based medical indications for an induction of labor include gestational hypertension, preeclampsia/eclampsia, fetal growth restriction, cholestasis of pregnancy, diabetes mellitus, fetal demise, chorioamnionitis, oligohydramnios, and nonreassuring fetal status.[22] Other medical indications include prelabor rupture of membranes and post-term pregnancy.

Elective induction is controversial. Factors such as maternal or provider convenience, history of fast labors, maternal distance from the hospital, relief of physiologic pregnancy discomforts, avoidance of certain calendar dates or holidays, institutional staffing concerns, and patient satisfaction have all been cited as reasons for elective induction.[38] Disadvantages include neonatal morbidity from iatrogenic prematurity if the estimated gestational age is incorrect as well as increased costs and possible risks of cesarean section.

The practice of elective induction (i.e., no medical indication for induction), especially prior to 39 weeks' gestation, has come under close scrutiny as the risks associated with late preterm birth have become more evident. Strict criteria for gestational age dating are now in place, and elective induction prior to 39 weeks' gestation is contraindicated.[22] Some institutions have adopted stringent guidelines for elective induction at term that also require a favorable Bishop's score, a signed consent form, and a preinduction checklist for providers.[39–41] The Bishop's score is a numeric assessment of four different characteristics of the cervix and fetal station. The Bishop's score is used to predict the success of induction. The currently used modified version of the Bishop's score is shown in **Table 30-2**. The American College of Nurse-Midwives (ACNM) Position Statement on Induction of Labor (2010) remains clearly against the practice of elective inductions of labor. Midwives in clinical practice will find valuable information in this document.[42]

The risks related to labor induction are the same regardless of the indications for which it is performed. These risks include excessive uterine activity (tachysystole), fetal intolerance to labor, postpartum uterine atony, and an increased risk of cesarean birth.[22] The relationship between cesarean section and induction of labor may be more nuanced than previously thought (see the "Post-term Pregnancy" section). Although the risk of cesarean section secondary to induction for women at term has not been fully elucidated, it is clear that the risk of cesarean birth is approximately twofold greater for nulliparous women who have an unfavorable cervix.[22,23]

Table 30-2	The Modified Bishop Scoring System			
Point Value	**0**	**1**	**2**	**3**
Dilatation (cm)	0	1–2	3–4	> 5
Effacement (%)	0–30	40–50	60–70	> 80
Station	−3	−2	−1/0	+1/+2
Consistency	Firm	Medium	Soft	
Position	Posterior	Midposition	Anterior	

Source: Adapted from Bishop EH. Pelvic scoring for elective induction. *Obstetrics and Gynecology* 24, pp. 266-268. Copyright © 1964 by Lippincott Williams & Wilkins. Reprinted by permission of Wolters Kluwer.

Induction of labor should occur only in a hospital and is contraindicated in any situation that precludes vaginal birth such as placenta previa, vasa previa, transverse lie, umbilical cord prolapse, previous myomectomy entering the endometrial cavity, previous classical uterine incision, active genital herpes infection, or presence of a category III fetal heart rate tracing. Prior to the initiation of any cervical ripening or induction methods, the woman should be counseled about the medical indication for induction as well as the risks and benefits to her and her fetus that are associated with induction and expectant management. Lastly, a collaborative management plan between the midwife and the consulting physician regarding the plan of care for cervical ripening and induction of labor is required. **Box 30-3** summarizes key midwifery considerations when caring for women who require an induction of labor and/or cervical ripening.

Cervical Ripening Techniques

As pregnancy approaches full term, the cervix gradually begins to soften, efface, and move anteriorly in the vaginal vault. This process, which is commonly referred to as "ripening," occurs as a result of normal remodeling of the collagen fibers and other glycoprotein connective tissues within the cervix. Cervical ripening occurs more readily in multiparous women, and the process may begin in the days to weeks before the onset of labor.

The degree of ripening can be quantified using the modified Bishop's score, which takes into consideration all of the factors associated with cervical remodeling (Table 30-2).[43] This scoring system indicates whether the woman's cervix is "favorable" or "unfavorable" with regard to predicting the success of labor induction and is the best predictor of induction success known to date.

For example, women who have a modified Bishop's score higher than 8 are considered to have a favorable cervix and a high probability for vaginal birth with induction of labor.[22] By comparison, women with a Bishop's score of 6 or lower have an unfavorable cervix, such that cervical ripening may improve their labor induction success rates. Cervical ripening agents can advance the Bishop's score by acting directly on the glycoproteins within the cervix (hormonal) or through mechanical dilation of the cervix. Because cervical dilation is considered to be the component of the Bishop's score that is most predictive of induction success, mechanical methods are often used concurrently either with hormonal

---

BOX 30-3 Clinical Considerations Prior to Induction of Labor and/or Cervical Ripening

1. Physician consultation should occur prior to the initiation of cervical ripening or oxytocin induction. In some cases, a collaborative management plan is required.

2. The medical indications for induction should be discussed with the woman and her support person(s). The risks and benefits of each proposed agent (or technique) should be thoroughly reviewed. The woman's preferences should be taken into consideration. This discussion should be documented in her health record.

3. The pre-induction (or cervical ripening) database should include the following information:

   a. Documentation of the gestational age and criteria used to establish the final estimated due date.

   b. Bishop's score.

   c. Indications for induction or cervical ripening.

   d. No contraindications for induction.

   e. Clinical pelvimetry.

   f. Confirmation of a vertex presentation.

   g. Confirmation of Category I fetal heart rate pattern. Induction may proceed with oxytocin if a Category II fetal heart rate pattern is present, following consultation with a physician.

4. The physician should be notified if the woman refuses a medically indicated induction of labor.

5. Caution should be exercised when prescribing or recommending alternative methods of cervical ripening or induction of labor not supported in the scientific literature.

6. During an induction, practices that encourage the normal process of labor (e.g., ambulation with telemetry, oral hydration) should be encouraged.

7. Water immersion in the shower or tub (with waterproof fetal telemetry monitoring) may be considered during induction of labor with oxytocin.

ripening or during oxytocin induction. No cervical ripening method should be employed before 40 weeks' gestation unless there is a medical indication for induction.

Foley Balloon Catheter

The most common method of mechanical dilation is use of a Foley balloon catheter, although hydroscopic vaginal dilators (laminaria) are still used in some locations. Using aseptic technique, a Foley catheter with a 30-cc balloon is inserted directly into the cervix and advanced beyond the internal os. The balloon is then inflated to the full 30 cc with sterile water or saline and the end of the catheter taped to the woman's leg, applying mild tension. Insertion can be done with direct visualization of the cervix using a speculum or during a digital examination. The balloon falls out on its own when the cervix dilates to 3 cm, which typically occurs within 6 to 12 hours. The insertion procedure may cause some discomfort for the woman and continued lower abdominal cramping may be experienced. Accidental rupture of the membranes or cervical bleeding can also occur. The risks, benefits, and expected side effects should be explained to the woman prior to the insertion of a

balloon catheter and documented with a procedure note in the woman's medical record.

Prostaglandin Agents for Cervical Ripening

The two hormonal agents currently in use for cervical ripening are prostaglandin E_2 (dinoprostone [Prepidil, Cervidil]) and the synthetic prostaglandin E_1 analogue (misoprostol [Cytotec]). The current preparations, dosing regimens, and clinical considerations for these agents are outlined in **Table 30-3**. There is considerable research comparing hormonal agents alone or in combination with mechanical dilation.[44] This body of evidence has conclusively demonstrated that cervical ripening prior to initiation of oxytocin shortens the time of induction onset to birth and may increase the vaginal birth rate. To date, no one preferred strategy has emerged; instead, many variables—such as provider preference, availability, and institutional guidelines—will determine which agents or methods are used. All hormonal agents can cause excessive uterine activity (tachysystole) or induce labor. Therefore, assessment of fetal well-being is an important prerequisite before hormonal ripening is started. The midwife should monitor the woman's response to cervical ripening and remain

Table 30-3	Hormonal Cervical Ripening Agents[a]		
Agent	**Brand Name**	**Dose/Route**	**Clinical Considerations**
Prostaglandin E_2 (Dinoprostone)	Prepidil Gel	0.5 mg intracervical (endocervix) *or* 2.5 mg vaginally (posterior fornix)	May be repeated every 6 hours × 3 doses Can be used for outpatient ripening in selected women Monitor fetal heart rate for 1–2 hours after each dose Oxytocin may be started 6–12 hours after last dose
	Cervidil Vaginal Insert	Vaginal 10 mg slow release at 0.3 mg/hour	Inpatient only with continuous fetal heart rate monitoring Left in place for up to 12 hours Remove insert if more than 5 contractions/10 minutes (tachysystole) Oxytocin may be started 30–60 minutes after removal
Prostaglandin E_1 (Misoprostol)	Cytotec	Vaginal: 25 mcg every 3–6 hours × 5 doses (inserted in posterior fornix) *or* Oral: 50–100 mcg every 3–6 hours × 5 doses	Contraindicated in women with a scarred uterus Inpatient only with continuous fetal heart rate monitoring Vaginal doses of 50 mcg are associated with higher incidence of uterine tachysystole and are not recommended Oxytocin may be started 4 hours after last dose

[a]Cervical ripening agents are contraindicated if there is an abnormal FHR tracing or more than 3 contractions in a 10-minute window.

Source: Adapted from American College of Obstetricians and Gynecologists. ACOG Practice Bulletin no. 107: induction of labor. *Obstet Gynecol.* 2009;114:386-397.

vigilant for signs of tachysystole or fetal intolerance to uterine activity.

Misoprostol (Cytotec)

Misoprostol is available as a 100- or 200-microgram (mcg) tablet. Misoprostol is marketed and FDA approved for managing the symptoms of peptic ulcer disease. These tablets are not formulated for vaginal use, and misoprostol is not FDA approved for cervical ripening. Nevertheless, it is effective for cervical ripening and is commonly used on an off-label basis for this indication. Misoprostol is contraindicated for women who have had a prior cesarean section or uterine surgery.

Misoprostol may be administered either orally or vaginally. The recommended vaginal dose of misoprostol is 25 mcg, with the broken tablet portion simply being inserted into the posterior fornix of the vagina during a digital examination. The oral dose is slightly higher, at 50 to 100 mcg. These doses are repeated every 3 to 6 hours depending on institutional guidelines. Due to the potential dosing inaccuracies from splitting up the tablets, the uterine response can be somewhat unpredictable and unreliable, especially with vaginal dosing. Although a variable response can also occur with other prostaglandin ripening agents, the repeated dosing of misoprostol can lead to delayed uterotonic effects that are not easily reversed.[44] As a precaution, the dose should not be administered if the woman experiences more than three contractions in a 10-minute period or any signs of fetal compromise become apparent. Terbutaline should always be readily available to treat tachysystole that is associated with abnormal or indeterminate fetal heart rate patterns. Interestingly although caution is warranted, episodes of fetal heart rate decelerations that occur in response to misoprostol tachysystole in all the misoprostol studies have not been associated with adverse neonatal outcomes.

Induction of Labor Techniques

Membrane Sweeping

Membrane sweeping, historically called strippping of the membranes, is a common practice among both midwives and physicians to aid women at term who desire intervention to speed the onset of labor. Numerous studies have demonstrated that membrane sweeping increases the likelihood of spontaneous labor with oxytocin.[45] Evidence has also found membrane sweeping to be safe with no increased risks of fetal or maternal infection.[45] There may be discomfort during the examination, and the woman may experience slight vaginal bleeding and irregular contractions after membrane sweeping. Accidental rupture of the membranes could also occur but is rare. Membrane sweeping is an elective procedure done only after the woman is informed of the risks and benefits and gives her consent for the procedure. Membrane sweeping should not be offered or performed prior to 40 weeks' gestation.

Amniotomy

Planned artificial rupture of the membranes (AROM) may be used as a method of labor induction either alone or concurrently with oxytocin. Studies have shown amniotomy to be more effective when the cervix is favorable, but individual response to amniotomy can be unpredictable and result in long intervals before the onset of regular uterine contractions.[22] There is a potential risk of infection from a prolonged labor if amniotomy is performed when the cervix is unfavorable. When amniotomy is combined with oxytocin, the induction-to-birth interval is decreased; however, the best timing for AROM has not been clearly established. In addition, once the membranes have been ruptured, the woman is committed to giving birth and no longer has the possibility of further cervical ripening or reverting to a period of expectant management if a trial of oxytocin fails to initiate labor. On the other hand, for women with cervical dilation of 4 cm or more, early amniotomy is not associated with adverse maternal or neonatal outcomes and may shorten labor by 2 hours or more.[46]

The primary risk associated with amniotomy is umbilical cord compression—or, more emergently, a prolapsed umbilical cord. Variable decelerations are commonly seen when the umbilical cord is compressed; the management of this fetal heart rate abnormality is discussed in the *Fetal Assessment During Labor* chapter. Umbilical cord prolapse is an obstetric emergency regardless of whether the membranes ruptured spontaneously or following amniotomy and is the primary reason why amniotomy should not be performed if the fetal head is not engaged in the pelvis. See the "Obstetric Emergencies" section of this chapter for detailed management guidelines for a prolapsed umbilical cord.

Induction of Labor with Oxytocin (Pitocin)

Oxytocin is a small, nine-amino-acid peptide hormone made in the hypothalamus and secreted from the posterior pituitary gland. This hormone is similar to vasopressin and has a direct antidiuretic effect on the kidney. Most importantly, oxytocin is a potent uterotonic agent that causes uterine contractions. Although pituitary secretion appears to be the primary source of oxytocin, this hormone is also synthesized and secreted by the placenta and fetus. Synthetic oxytocin, which is chemically identical to endogenous oxytocin, is one of the most commonly prescribed medications in midwifery practice today.

When this medication is used appropriately, the clinical benefits are undeniable, especially for treating postpartum hemorrhage. However, oxytocin is associated with adverse fetal and maternal outcomes and frequently implicated in obstetric litigation cases.[47] As a result, oxytocin is now considered a "high alert" medication, which mandates the inclusion of safety measures to reduce the increased risks of error that result in maternal or neonatal morbidities.[48] Some of the safeguards currently in place include standardized intravenous concentrations, mandatory use of an infusion pump, continuous fetal heart rate monitoring, and lower-dosing protocols.[47,49]

Ocytocin exerts its effect via agonist action on oxytocin receptors that are present in the uterine myometrium. These receptors become active or "upregulate" more than 100-fold during early labor. The uterotonic effect mediated by receptor function is theorized to be the reason there is marked interindividual variability in response to this drug. The oxytocin receptors also downregulate or become desensitized following prolonged exposure to oxytocin, which may partially explain why women who are exposed to long periods of oxytocin for labor induction are at increased risk for postpartum hemorrhage.[50]

The onset of action of synthetic oxytocin is 3 to 4 minutes, and the half-life is approximately 15 minutes. Uterine response reaches a steady state after 30 to 40 minutes.[51] The individual response to a particular dose is quite variable. Response is also dose dependent: As the infusion is increased, the frequency and intensity of contractions follow. The dose can be titrated until the desired contraction response is met. Nevertheless, it is important to wait at least 30 to 40 minutes before increasing the dose to evaluate the full effects of the prior dose. This time frame allows the oxytocin to reach a steady-state plasma concentration and reduces the chance of dysfunctional uterine activity or tachysystole. There appears to be a ceiling effect wherein further increases in dose do not result in uterine contractions that are stronger or more frequent. Moreover, during the first stage of labor, there may be a small baseline concentration of endogenous oxytocin in the woman's circulation, which may combine with the intravenous oxytocin infusion to produce a cumulative effect on uterine contractions. In light of these physiologic considerations, many individuals recommend a low-dose, cautious oxytocin dosing regimen of 1–2 mU/min at intervals of at least every 30 to 40 minutes.[47,49,52]

Side Effects and Adverse Effects of Oxytocin

Ocytocin has an antidiuretic effect, so it must be used with caution in women who need fluid restriction or who are at increased risk for pulmonary edema. This agent can cause hypotension, tachycardia, and transient myocardial ischemia that results in EKG changes if given as a bolus dose.

The most commonly encountered side effect of oxytocin is excess uterine activity or tachysystole. Tachysystole is defined as more than five contractions in 10 minutes averaged over a 30-minute window.[53] Due to the short half-life of oxytocin, decreasing or stopping an oxytocin infusion will rapidly slow the frequency of contractions. In many cases, tachysystole does not result in obvious fetal compromise but still requires an oxytocin dose adjustment to allow for adequate fetal oxygenation in between contractions. Titration of the infusion is highly individualized and often requires some finesse in finding a balance between the desired effect and avoidance of tachysystole. Women receiving oxytocin also require an assessment of maternal and fetal status every 15 minutes during the active phase of labor and every 5 minutes during second-stage labor.[49,52] This important safeguard ensures prompt recognition and treatment of tachysystole and/or abnormal fetal heart rate patterns.

Regardless of the contraction pattern, any sign of fetal compromise requires immediate discontinuation of the oxytocin infusion. Additional interventions include lateral repositioning of the woman, a 500-mL intravenous fluid bolus of lactated Ringer's solution, and administration of oxygen. A single dose of terbutaline 0.25 mg should be administered subcutaneously if these initial interventions fail to ameliorate the uterine contraction pattern. The midwife should notify the consulting physician and remain at the bedside with the woman until fetal well-being is ensured, in which case after 15 to 30 minutes the oxytocin infusion can be resumed. Refer to the *Fetal Assessment During Labor* chapter for suggested tachysystole management guidelines.

In some cases, induction with oxytocin takes longer than anticipated, especially if cervical ripening was clinically contraindicated or was ineffective in improving the Bishop's score. Desensitization ("downregulation") of the oxytocin receptor sites on the uterus from continuous exposure to oxytocin over a prolonged period of time may occur.[49] When this happens, oxytocin becomes less effective and further increases in the dose merely add to the risk of tachysystole and inefficient uterine contraction activity without necessarily dilating the cervix. As previously mentioned, prolonged use of oxytocin can also increase the risk of postpartum hemorrhage from uterine atony for the same reasons. Midwives should be alert for this possibility and consider active management of third-stage labor to minimize the risk for postpartum hemorrhage in women who have been exposed to exogenous oxytocin for several hours (see the chapter *The Third and Fourth Stages of Labor*).

In addition to postpartum hemorrhage, the use of oxytocin for augmentation or induction of labor is associated with an increased risk of uterine rupture. Uterine rupture in an unscarred uterus is a rare event in the United States (fewer than 1 incident per 10,000 pregnant women).[54] By comparison, in resource-poor areas with limited access to cesarean birth, the incidence of uterine rupture is more common, especially among women with higher parity experiencing an obstructed labor. In developed countries, however, uterine rupture is almost exclusively associated with women attempting a trial of labor after cesarean (TOLAC). Although oxytocin for induction or labor augmentation is not contraindicated for women who are attempting TOLAC, higher doses significantly increase the risks of uterine rupture and should be avoided.[55] A more thorough discussion of uterine rupture and TOLAC can be found later in this chapter.

If the woman's condition is stable and she is not yet in active labor, it is reasonable to discontinue the oxytocin infusion after 10 to 12 hours. This conservative approach will correct any receptor downregulation and enable the woman to rest. It will also reduce the risk of postpartum uterine atony from a prolonged infusion. In addition, this approach allows time for additional cervical ripening overnight if needed. The oxytocin can then be restarted the next day and the induction plan will proceed accordingly. For some women, achieving a vaginal birth from a labor induction requires considerable patience on the part of the caregivers. The criteria for a diagnosis of "failed induction" are not clearly defined in the literature, and this possibility should be considered only after the woman reaches the active phase of labor.[22]

High-Dose Versus Low-Dose Protocols

Currently both high- and low-dose oxytocin protocols can be used.[22] The high-dose protocol initiates oxytocin at 6 mU/min with increases of 4–6 mU/min every 15 minutes to a maximum of 40 mU/min. In contrast, low-dose protocols start at 1–2 mU/min and increase by 1–2 mU/min every 30 to 40 minutes. As noted above, some authors advocate for the conservative approach, in part due to the wide variation in individual response to oxytocin and the increased risks of tachysystole seen with higher doses.[47,49] Moreover, low-dose protocols improve the overall safety of labor induction and augmentation by minimizing the adverse side effects associated with more aggressive dose increases.

The high-dose oxytocin regimens originated as part of the active management of labor (AML) protocol developed by O'Driscoll et al. in the 1970s.[56] In addition to high-dose oxytocin, AML included admission only in active labor, one-to-one labor support (with midwives), routine early amniotomy, and strict criteria for monitoring labor progress. As a package of care, AML resulted in slightly lower cesarean section rates and shorter labors with no differences in maternal or fetal complications.[57] These findings led to the commonly held belief that high-dose oxytocin protocols alone would shorten the induction to birth time. Research has supported the small decrease in cesarean section with high-dose protocols, albeit at the expense of substantially increased risks of tachysystole.[58] While some high-risk clinical scenarios warrant expedited labor, the potential for fetal compromise from excessive uterine activity may not justify aggressive oxytocin dosing as a routine practice and it is being used less often in the United States today.[47]

One last issue with oxytocin is the conflicting goals and miscommunication that sometimes occur between the nurses at the bedside managing the infusion and the ordering providers.[47] Often this conflict revolves around the dosing intervals of the oxytocin infusion. One possible solution is to implement mutually agreed-upon checklist-based protocols for oxytocin administration.[39,52] These checklists focus on the fetal and uterine response to oxytocin instead of specifying a specific dosing regimen, allowing time for normal labor progress rather than more oxytocin. Also included are other safety measures such as appropriate staffing ratios and standard order sets for treating tachysystole. Prompt initiation of interventions without additional orders from the provider is an essential component of best practice recommendations for oxytocin use.[52]

Other Methods of Induction

Midwives have long relied upon nonintervention and alternative approaches when caring for pregnant women. The use of more natural techniques to stimulate labor or facilitate cervical ripening is no exception to this tradition. In many cases, these methods have been endorsed in an attempt to help women avoid an induction of labor with oxytocin.

Nipple Stimulation

Researchers have evaluated the safety and effectiveness of nipple or breast stimulation as a method to stimulate or induce labor.[59] Stimulation of the nipples is known to induce the release of endogenous oxytocin from the pituitary gland, which in turn causes uterine contractions similarly to synthetic oxytocin. In fact, nipple stimulation protocols have been used as an alternative to oxytocin for performing a contraction stress test (see the *Fetal Assessment During Labor* chapter). Various techniques have been employed, such as rolling one or both nipples between the fingers or using a manual or electric breast pump.

A systematic review of the available studies on nipple stimulation reported that low-risk women with a favorable cervix who used this technique were likely to be in labor within 72 hours.[59] Other significant findings were a decreased incidence of postpartum hemorrhage and no episodes of uterine tachysystole or abnormal fetal heart rate changes. One remaining concern is the effect of nipple stimulation and endogenous oxytocin on placental perfusion. Because the existing evidence has not specifically examined nipple stimulation for women who are at risk for fetal acidemia, its use is discouraged with this population.[59]

Herbal Preparations

Several herbal preparations, such as castor oil, evening primrose oil, raspberry leaf, and blue or black cohosh, have been used for the purposes of stimulating labor. Midwives who use herbal preparations believe these methods are safe, are inexpensive, and help women avoid medical induction and prolonged pregnancy.[60] They can also be self-administered by the woman at home or used in a birth center where oxytocin and prostaglandin use is contraindicated. Information regarding herbal methods of labor induction is often shared informally among colleagues and likely based on anecdotal experiences, folklore, and traditional practices. There is also wide variation among midwives in how and when these preparations are prescribed.

A review of the literature regarding herbal methods of labor induction reported an overall lack of scientific evidence regarding these treatments' efficacy or clinical benefit to women.[61] Blue cohosh has been associated in case reports with perinatal stroke and acute myocardial infarction; it should not be used.[62] Currently, there is no scientific literature that documents the safety or efficacy of black cohosh. Until scientific studies can be conducted to refute these concerns, blue and black cohosh either together or in combination with other substances should not be used in clinical practice.[61,62] Evening primrose oil and raspberry leaf, in contrast, have demonstrated no evidence of harm over many years of use. Whether they actually cause contractions or promote cervical ripening is not conclusively seen in the evidence, but their use during pregnancy is considered to be safe.[61]

The use of castor oil can be traced back to Egyptian times, and this product is still commonly used today to induce or stimulate labor. Although the exact mechanism of action is not completely understood, ingestion of castor oil produces a powerful cathartic effect that in turn induces uterine contractions. Some women have reported rapid tumultuous labors after ingesting castor oil, and use of this preparation may be associated with an increased risk of meconium-stained amniotic fluid. The evidence from several studies remains inconclusive regarding the efficacy of castor oil, but many still believe women who receive castor oil are likely to be in labor.[61] Although castor oil ingestion is safe for women during pregnancy, midwives who elect to use it for labor induction should be aware of the inconsistent evidence as well as a lack of standard dosing protocols.

In summary, caution should be exercised when prescribing or recommending alternative methods of cervical ripening or induction of labor not supported in the scientific literature. The midwife should also inform the woman of the known risks, benefits, and safety concerns prior to prescribing or endorsing the use of any herbal preparations.

Labor Abnormalities

Background

As discussed in the chapter *The First Stage of Labor*, normal labor is characterized by regular uterine contractions that cause progressive dilation and effacement of the cervix, ultimately resulting in a spontaneous vaginal birth. Vaginal birth also requires the coordinated interplay of physiologic and psychologic forces within the woman that are commonly referred to as the powers, passage (pelvis), passenger, and psyche.

A variety of factors can affect these components and interfere with the expected course of labor and birth. Specifically, dysfunctional uterine contractions, abnormal fetal position, and disproportion between the size or shape of the maternal bony pelvis and the size of the fetus (cephalopelvic disproportion) are the most common causes of labor abnormalities. These abnormalities are collectively referred to as *dystocia*, which literally means "difficult labor" that is characterized by abnormally slow progress in the first stage of labor.

In the United States, dystocia is the most commonly cited indication for primary cesarean births.[63,64] Many experts believe dystocia is overdiagnosed—which has led to the rising cesarean rates among nulliparous women. Terms such as "failed induction of labor," "active-phase arrest," and "failure to progress" have been used interchangeably to describe dystocia. Other classic phrases commonly used to describe abnormal labor progress include "prolonged latent phase," "protracted (or prolonged) active phase," and "prolonged second stage"; these terms are related more to the timing of the labor abnormality than to the cause, and there is no consensus on their diagnostic criteria.[63]

One of the main problems has been defining the parameters of normal labor progress, especially in regard to the endpoint of the latent phase.[65,66] The original labor curve data published more than 50 years ago by Friedman described the upper limits of latent labor as 20 hours for a nulliparous woman, with the rate of cervical dilation in active phase as 1.2 cm per hour.[67] When a woman's labor progress fell outside these long-accepted time frames, an "arrest" or a "protraction" disorder was diagnosed and interventions such as oxytocin augmentation and insertion of intrauterine pressure catheters were initiated. Ultimately, a cesarean birth was recommended if labor did not progress for 2 hours.

More evidence has challenged Friedman's criteria, now suggesting that labor progress for women today is actually much slower for both nulliparous and multiparous women.[66,68] One key finding is that many nulliparous women are not in the active phase of labor until their cervices are 6 cm dilated. Contemporary research on the normal progress of labor has found that extending the 2-hour rule to a 4-hour minimum in active-phase labor before considering intervention, especially if the woman has received an epidural, results in more vaginal births.[69] In addition, it is strongly recommended that the diagnosis of an arrest of labor not be made until the woman is clearly in the active phase.[64]

Causes of Labor Dystocia

The most common cause of dystocia is dysfunctional uterine activity. This can be further subdivided into hypertonic or hypotonic uterine dysfunction. A second less common cause is failure of descent, which can be secondary to fetal malposition or true cephalopelvic disproportion.

In *hypertonic* uterine dysfunction, the contraction gradient within the uterine muscle is distorted, causing uncoordinated forceful contractions. Typically seen in the latent phase of labor and more common among nulliparous women, this disorder often leads to maternal exhaustion and prolonged labor from ineffective painful contractions.

In contrast, *hypotonic* uterine dysfunction is characterized by infrequent, low-amplitude contractions that do not generate enough pressure to dilate the cervix. This disorder occurs after the woman has progressed normally into the active phase of labor and her contraction intensity and frequency decrease. Although not associated with worsening pain, hypotonic contractions will slow or stop cervical dilation, which can also prolong labor.

In addition to dysfunctional uterine activity, malposition of the fetal head can cause slow progress or failure of descent if the presenting fetal diameter is larger than the corresponding diameter within the maternal pelvis. During the normal cardinal movements of labor, descent is facilitated by flexion of the vertex and rotation to either left or right occiput anterior position. Prolonged labor and arrest of descent can occur when the fetus enters the maternal pelvis in an occiput posterior (OP) position, an asynclitic misalignment, or a face or brow presentation. These types of cephalic malpositions are more commonly seen in nulliparous women and have also been associated with administration of epidural anesthesia.[63]

Labor with a Fetus in Occiput Posterior Position

The most common fetal malposition associated during labor is occiput posterior. Labor abnormalities associated with persistent OP include prolonged duration of both first and second stages. Other complications include a twofold increase in the incidence of operative vaginal births, and threefold increase in the incidence of cesarean birth.[70] Additional complications include an increased incidence of perineal tears, 4th-degree lacerations, birth trauma, 5-minute Apgar scores less than 7, and umbilical artery acidemia.[70]

Cephalopelvic Disproportion

Cephalopelvic disproportion (CPD) refers to a disproportion between the size of the fetal head and the size of the maternal bony pelvis. When this diagnosis is used, it implies that either the fetus was too big or the maternal pelvis was too small. In reality, there are no established criteria for this diagnosis, even though it is commonly listed as a reason for primary cesarean section. The incidence for CPD is increased with large fetal size or contracted maternal pelvis (i.e., android or platypelloid), but the actual cause of this type of labor dystocia is more likely related to fetal malposition.[69] When cesarean birth is performed for dystocia, a more accurate diagnosis of the labor abnormality—that is, arrest of dilation or arrest of descent—is preferred."[63]

Midwifery Management of Labor Dystocia

When dystocia is suspected, other assessments—listed in **Box 30-4**—should be added to the ongoing database for normal labor management. There is considerable overlap for many of these parameters, as fear and anxiety can be factors in both hypertonic and hypotonic labor. Strategies that promote hydration, relaxation, and rest are an important component of management regardless of the underlying cause. There are many situations in which normal labor will fall outside of the commonly accepted parameters for duration of labor. Midwives are experts in the variations of normal physiologic birth and have historically had considerable patience

in managing labor progress. Within each midwife's practice guidelines, however, there should be an upper limit time frame delineating when a physician should be consulted. These parameters will vary according to practice and institutional settings.

The diagnosis of labor dystocia increases the woman's risk for prolonged labor, which can lead to maternal or fetal stress, an increased risk for chorioamnionitis, and uterine atony after birth. The woman should be informed of these risks and her options for continued management. As long as there continues to be a reassuring fetal assessment and no other signs of maternal compromise, many techniques and strategies can be initially used to reduce maternal fear, facilitate rest and coping, stimulate labor, and correct cephalic malposition. These interventions are also discussed in the chapters *The First Stage of Labor* and *The Second Stage of Labor and Birth*. Induction or augmentation of labor, however, is always indicated in situations where the birth should be expedited. The final plan of care should be discussed with a consulting physician, especially if the woman needs to receive oxytocin.

Hypertonic Labor: Prolonged Latent Phase

The formal definition of prolonged latent phase has traditionally been regular painful uterine contractions for more than 20 hours in a nulliparous woman or more than 14 hours in a multiparous woman. However, the distinction between prelabor contractions and labor contractions is subjective, which makes a definition based on time somewhat problematic. Clinically, when a woman has regular painful contractions without progressive cervical dilation, she may need support and intervention whenever she is no longer able to tolerate the process.

Management of prolonged latent labor can be particularly challenging for both the midwife and the woman. A first-line strategy for women who do not desire a home birth is to avoid admission to the birth setting until the active phase of labor is clearly established.[65] Providing the woman with home management guidelines that promote rest allows time for labor to progress naturally. Among these strategies are a warm bath or shower, hydration and food, comfort measures (e.g., massage), ambulation and rhythmic movement, music, and aromatherapy.[65,70] Medications such as diphenhydramine (Benadryl), doxylamine (Unisom), or zolpidem (Ambien) can also be prescribed to promote rest at home if non-pharmacologic strategies prove ineffective.[65]

If the woman becomes dehydrated or too sleep deprived secondary to prolonged latent-phase labor, she may need admission to a hospital. The two

---

BOX 30-4 Assessment for Labor Dystocia

1. Observe the woman for signs of exhaustion, decreased coping, or dehydration.
2. Explore the possibility of an underlying maternal fear or anxiety related to labor or the pending birth to determine ways to improve the woman's coping ability.
3. Check maternal vital signs for fever or tachycardia.
4. Palpate the contractions for frequency and intensity, and note any trends or changes.
5. Reassess fetal size and estimated fetal weight with Leopold's maneuvers.
6. Assess fetal well-being with intermittent auscultation or continuous electronic fetal monitoring.
7. Review the labor progress up until this point.
8. If the membranes are not ruptured, perform a cervical examination and carefully assess dilatation, effacement, station, and position of the fetal head. Note any asynclitism, molding, or caput.
9. During the cervical examination, perform clinical pelvimetry; note any obvious narrowing of the pelvic diameters.
10. If the membranes are ruptured, perform this examination only if clinically indicated.

treatment options are either therapeutic rest to stop contractions and allow a period of rest or uterotonic drugs to encourage organized effective contractions.

Therapeutic rest typically involves a single dose of morphine sulfate administered intramuscularly (or intravenously) in combination with either promethazine (Phenergan) or hydroxyzine (Vistaril).[65] A variety of dosing strategies are used, all of which have a primary goal of inducing heavy sedation or sleep. Commonly encountered maternal side effects include respiratory depression, euphoria, sedation, dizziness, and nausea and vomiting. Neonatal respiratory depression is also a potential concern especially if morphine is administered close to the time of birth. In the majority of cases, however, women managed with therapeutic rest will sleep for several hours and awaken in active labor.

Hypotonic Labor: Protracted Active Phase

A delay in dilation may be a normal variation of a particular woman's labor. Analyses of labor progress in contemporary women conducted by Zhang et al., for example, found significant individual variability in the time interval in dilating from 1 centimeter to the next during the active phase of labor.[68] Continued expectant management is reasonable if there are no clinical indications to expedite birth. Strategies to stimulate or augment labor should be presented to the woman and the risks and benefits of each option reviewed. Depending on the woman's preferences, the least invasive strategies should be attempted first. For example, if the woman is rested, and coping well, ambulation or position changes should be encouraged initially. Although evidence does not support ambulation as a method to shorten the time spent in labor, there is some evidence that upright positions increase contraction strength and women cope better or report less pain when in upright positions.

Theoretically labor progress may slow or stall secondary to acute stress, and it is believed by many that fear or anxiety can interfere with labor progress. The catecholamines, norepinephrine and epinephrine, that are released during the stress response normally have an inhibitory or tocolytic effect on uterine contractility. If labor, fatigue, and/or pain cause an acute stress response, a diminution of uterine contractility may occur. A few small studies have correlated plasma epinephrine levels and uterine contractility in which the results supported this hypothesis.[71] However it is not known if beta-adrenergic receptors for endogenous catecholamines are significantly upregulated in the uterus during term labor, and the research that supports this theory is not robust. Thus the relationship between significant fear or anxiety

and slow labor progress remains somewhat theoretical. However, strategies that promote a sense of emotional well-being and safety are worth considering if labor progress slows without an obvious reason. Decreasing unnecessary stimulation from caregivers, dimming the lights, and allowing alone time with her support persons may help decrease the physiologic stress response.

Relief of pain is another important component of managing prolonged labor. Unrelieved pain is also associated with increased circulating catecholamines. Inability to cope well may indicate the need for medication and, for some women, epidural anesthesia. While this strategy may increase the likelihood of other interventions being used to stimulate labor, ensuring adequate relief of pain is always a priority.

Amniotomy can also stimulate or augment labor when slowed progress or hypotonic contractions are encountered. Large clinical trials have found that when amniotomy is performed after the woman's cervix is 5 cm dilated, labor is accelerated by 1 to 2 hours.[46] In addition, amniotomy performed during the active phase of labor was not associated with an increased need for oxytocin or a higher cesarean section birth rate. Obtaining clear, adequate fluid at the time of amniotomy also is a reassuring aspect of normalcy. For women desiring a natural approach to labor management, labor augmentation with amniotomy may be a more attractive option than use of an oxytocin infusion. Amniotomy does not require intravenous fluids or continuous electronic fetal monitoring unless complications such as variable decelerations from cord compression are encountered. Amniotomy is also discussed in the "Induction of Labor" section of this chapter.

A final strategy for managing hypertonic labor is to start intravenous oxytocin. The same cautions and clinical considerations exist regardless of whether oxytocin is used for augmentation or induction of labor. Additionally, in cases of prolonged labor, starting oxytocin in effect "starts the clock" for a possible "arrest of labor" diagnosis. Insertion of an intrauterine pressure catheter is not mandatory unless external monitoring is unable to detect contraction frequency. The consulting physician should be informed of the ongoing plan of care during labor augmentation with oxytocin and the woman's labor progress and fetal response monitored closely. The woman should also be kept informed of her progress, especially if active-phase arrest and cesarean birth become a possibility.

Failure of Descent

Finally, it is important to remember that fetal position and station are as important as cervical dilation during labor. It is all too easy to focus on cervical dilation and the easy set of integers between 1 and 10 that are used to monitor cervical dilation, as the sole measure of progress in labor. Fetal malpositions and/or asynclitism are also frequent causes of dystocia. Interventions that may help a woman who has dystocia secondary to a fetal malposition (besides an oxytocin infusion) include watchful waiting and/or position changes that increase pelvic diameters.

Trial of Labor After Cesarean

Background

For the past several decades, women presenting with a history of one or more previous cesarean sections have faced a series of changing opinions regarding the best mode of birth for subsequent pregnancies. Prior to the early 1980s, the predominant philosophy was "once a cesarean, always a cesarean." Early reports of successful vaginal births after cesarean (VBAC), however, began to challenge this longstanding practice. As a result, the National Institutes of Health (NIH) published a landmark statement in 1980 endorsing a trial of labor for women who had one previous lower transverse cesarean section.[72] Over the next 10 years, VBAC continued to grow in popularity, with several large studies reporting a 60% to 80% success rate for women who underwent a trial of labor after cesarean (TOLAC).[73] These studies also demonstrated that elective repeat cesarean delivery (ERCD) was associated with more maternal morbidity than a TOLAC and subsequent VBAC.

The NIH had hoped promoting a trial of labor would reduce rising cesarean section rates. This strategy appeared to decrease the rising cesarean section birth rates, with their associated costs in terms of morbidity and economic expense. By 1996, the rate of cesarean section in the United States reached an all-time contemporary low of 20.7%.[74] As the cesarean section birth rate fell and more women underwent TOLAC, safety concerns regarding uterine rupture during a trial of labor began to emerge. Until the mid 1990s, rates of uterine rupture during attempted VBAC were approximately 1%. In 1996, a large clinical trial was published that found major complications (uterine rupture, hysterectomy, and operative injury) were nearly doubled among women who opted for TOLAC when compared with women who had an ERCD.[75]

Almost immediately, enthusiasm for TOLAC began to decrease and VBAC rates steadily fell. Concern about the risk of uterine rupture and its associated liability led ACOG to amend its VBAC practice guidelines in 1999 to mandate the immediate in-house availability of an obstetrician and an anesthesiologist to perform an emergent cesarean section birth if needed.[76] Many hospitals and providers subsequently stopped offering TOLAC services, radically altering women's childbirth choices. By 2007, cesarean section rates had risen to an alarming 32.8% and VBAC rates plummeted to 8.9%.[74] While many factors have been cited for the cesarean section epidemic, decreased access to available TOLAC services has remained a frequently cited cause of this unfortunate trend.[77,78]

Concerns about the rising primary cesarean section rates and the morbidities associated with cesarean section led the NIH to revisit the comparative safety of having a VBAC versus ERCD.[77] The NIH Consensus Development Conference Statement was published in 2010 and concluded that women with a previous low transverse cesarean section can be safely offered a trial of labor when no other contraindications to vaginal birth exist.[77] The NIH statement also encouraged obstetric providers to improve access to TOLAC services and support women's preferences when possible. ACNM has subsequently published a position statement and an updated clinical practice bulletin fully supporting the NIH's consensus report.[79,80]

Risks of TOLAC

Table 30-4 lists the comparative risks of TOLAC versus ERCD. The most serious and catastrophic risk for a woman who elects a TOLAC is that of uterine rupture. Generally speaking, the term "uterine rupture" describes an anatomic separation of the uterine muscle.[77] This outcome can be further differentiated between uterine scar dehiscence and full separation of all uterine layers. Occult scar dehiscence does not include the serosa layer and is an incidental, asymptomatic finding with no adverse maternal or fetal consequences. A complete uterine rupture, in contrast, is a symptomatic life-threatening emergency. Currently, the risk of uterine rupture is cited as 0.5% to 0.7% for women attempting TOLAC compared to 0.03% in women who opt for ERCD.[77]

A history of previous classical or "T" uterine incision, previous uterine rupture, or any type of fundal uterine surgery (i.e., myomectomy) significantly increases the risk for uterine rupture.[81] Women presenting for prenatal care with any of these risk factors are not candidates for TOLAC; instead, it is recommended that they undergo a ERCD. Under these circumstances, ERCD may be scheduled at 36 to 37 weeks' gestation after documentation of fetal

Table 30-4	Comparative Risks of Elective Repeat Cesarean Delivery and Trial of Labor After Cesarean	
Outcomes	**ERCD**	**TOLAC**
Uterine rupture	2.6 per 10,000 women	3.8 per 1000 women
Maternal mortality	9.6 per 10,000 women at term	1.9 per 100,000 women
Hysterectomy	2.8 per 1000 women	1.57 per 1000 women
Blood transfusion	4.6 per 1000 women at term	6.6 per 1000 women
Operative injury	2.5–4.4 per 1000 women	4.0–5.1 per 1000 women
Infection	32 per 1000 women	46 per 1000 women
Hospital stay	3.92 days	2.5 days

ERCD = elective repeat cesarean section; TOLAC = trial of labor after cesarean section.

Source: Adapted from King TL. Can a vaginal birth after cesarean delivery be a normal labor and birth? Lessons from midwifery applied to trial of labor after a previous cesarean delivery. *Clin Perinatol.* 2011;38:247-263.

lung maturity to avoid the likelihood of spontaneous labor.[82] In addition, these women require prompt evaluation in the hospital with continuous fetal monitoring and physician consultation should regular contractions occur before the scheduled date of surgery.

Factors such as a history of two or more previous (low transverse) cesarean section, previous preterm cesarean section, short interpregnancy interval, and single-layer uterine closure all increase the risks of uterine rupture to varying degrees. A review of the existing evidence found weak associations for these factors and concluded that most of the previously identified factors that increased the risk for uterine rupture were minimal to nonexistent.[81] Consequently, women with these obstetric histories can now safely be offered a TOLAC.

Induction or Augmentation of Labor During TOLAC

Abnormal labor progress is associated with an increased risk of uterine rupture,[81] and some studies have shown a slight increased risk of uterine rupture when oxytocin is used for either augmentation of labor in women who attempt TOLAC.[83,84] The increased risk of uterine rupture associated with oxytocin augmentation is minimal and does not prohibit its use when medically indicated.[85] Because the upper limits for oxytocin dosing with TOLAC have not been established, a conservative approach is preferred, accompanied by close monitoring of fetal well-being, uterine activity, and labor progress.

Similarly, the risk of uterine rupture is not significantly increased when labor is induced with oxytocin. However, induced labor is less likely to result in a successful VBAC, especially if the woman has an unfavorable cervix.[85] Therefore induction of labor should be considered only when medically indicated and only in hospital settings with available physician consultation for a cesarean birth.

The use of cervical ripening agents for women who desire TOLAC is more controversial. Prostaglandins and misoprostol (Cytotec) are medications commonly used to facilitate cervical remodeling and have been shown to improve labor induction success rates. A large retrospective review of discharge data from Washington state that was published in 2001 by a midwife and colleagues, Lydon-Rochelle et al., found significantly increased risks of uterine rupture associated with use of prostaglandins and misoprostol.[86] This study had several limitations including use of discharge coding data and birth certificate codes, which have been found to have high inaccurate rates, and although several subsequent studies failed to replicate these findings, cervical ripening with misoprostol is now contraindicated in women attempting VBAC based on findings of the Lydon-Rochelle study. The use of prostaglandin agents for cervical ripening is also discouraged.[85] Mechanical methods (i.e., cervical Foley balloon), however, have not been associated with increased risks of uterine rupture and can be used for cervical ripening.[81,85]

Predictors for Successful TOLAC

Approximately 60% to 80% of the time, women who attempt TOLAC will have a successful vaginal birth.[74] Factors associated with higher success rates include prior vaginal birth or successful VBAC; prior cesarean birth for fetal distress, breech presentation, or other malpresentations; and presenting in spontaneous labor with a cervix at more than 4 cm dilated on admission.[80] Lower success rates have been seen in women who require induction or augmentation of labor, those in whom the indication for the prior cesarean section was dystocia, cephalopelvic disproportion, or failure to progress; birth weight heavier than 4000 grams; and maternal body mass index (BMI) greater than 30 kg/m².[80] These factors are summarized in **Table 30-5**.

Informed Decision Making

Pregnant woman with a history of a prior low transverse cesarean section birth and no contraindications to vaginal birth should receive formal counseling regarding the risks and benefits of both TOLAC and ERCD (Table 30-4).[87] A checklist may be used and the discussion and management plan clearly documented in the woman's health record. Depending on institutional or practice guidelines, the consulting physician may be required to provide this counseling and obtain the informed consent for the chart. Midwives, however, are qualified to provide prenatal and intrapartum care to women who elect TOLAC as well as to perform ongoing risk assessment, counseling, and education.

The choice (and availability) of birth setting should also be thoroughly reviewed with women who desire TOLAC. Women at low risk for uterine rupture can consider out-of-hospital birth centers (within policies of the site) but should be informed that the best outcomes for mothers and newborns occur when a cesarean section birth can be performed within 15 minutes.[80,87]

Despite the relative safety of TOLAC, some women will request an ERCD. To avoid iatrogenic prematurity, pregnancy dating criteria should be carefully reviewed to ensure elective surgery is not performed prior to 39 weeks' gestation.[85] The woman's choice should be supported and the risks and comorbidities of both TOLAC and ERCD presented in an unbiased manner. A consulting physician should be informed of the woman's desired plan of care. Women should also be reassured that they can change their mind regarding the final choice about mode of birth and encouraged to explore their fears and ambivalence regarding both TOLAC and ERCD throughout their pregnancy. This is a discussion that may be best communicated over several prenatal visits.

Intrapartum Management for Women During TOLAC

Box 30-5 outlines intrapartum management guidelines for women attempting TOLAC. When the woman with a history of previous cesarean section birth presents for a labor evaluation, the prenatal record should be reviewed along with any previously discussed labor management options. The woman's continued desire for TOLAC should be reaffirmed and the informed consent documentation reviewed. The intrapartum database should also include a thorough review of her obstetric history, paying particular attention to the indications for and circumstances surrounding the previous cesarean section birth. Equally important is confirming the type of uterine incision (if known) and ascertaining whether the woman has undergone any other uterine surgeries since her last birth. Lastly, a consulting physician should be notified if there is any contraindication to a VBAC or if the woman is opting for an ERCD.

Midwifery management for women in labor who desire TOLAC is similar to the care of any laboring woman (see the chapter *The First Stage of Labor*) with a few exceptions, including the recommendation for continuous fetal heart rate and uterine contraction monitoring and possibly a requirement for

Table 30-5	Factors Associated with Probability of Successful VBAC	
Factor	**Probability of Successful VBAC (%)**
Prior Vaginal Birth	
VBAC	90
Any vaginal birth	87
Indication for Previous Cesarean	
Malpresentation	84
Fetal distress	73
Dystocia	64
Obstetric Factors	
Spontaneous labor	81
Oxytocin augmentation	74
Labor induction	67
Admission cervical examination ≥ 4 cm	84
Admission cervical examination < 4 cm	67
Medical complication	70
Birth weight < 4000 g	75
Birth weight ≥ 4000 g	62
Epidural anesthesia	73

Source: Used with permission from American College of Nurse-Midwives. ACNM Clinical Bulletin no. 12: caring for women desiring vaginal birth after cesarean. *J Midwifery Women's Health.* 2011; 56:517-525.

BOX 30-5 Intrapartum Management Guidelines for Women Attempting TOLAC

---

1. A consulting physician should be notified when a woman desiring TOLAC is admitted in labor.[80]

2. Intravenous access (i.e., heparin or saline lock) may be required according to institutional policies.

3. Clear liquid intake is not contraindicated; however, some institutional policies may restrict this intake to ice chips or sips of water.

4. More frequent fetal heart rate monitoring is required—either continuous electronic monitoring or intermittent monitoring per high-risk guidelines (i.e., every 15 minutes in active labor and every 5 minutes in second-stage labor).[80] A telemetry monitor can be used to encourage freedom of movement.

5. The woman should be monitored closely for indications of uterine rupture. The most common initial sign is either recurrent fetal heart rate decelerations that become progressively deeper or an abrupt fetal heart rate bradycardia. Other signs include changes or cessation of uterine contractions, vaginal bleeding, or a sudden loss of fetal station.[80]

6. Epidural anesthesia is not contraindicated and will not mask the most common signs and symptoms of uterine rupture.[81]

7. Labor progress should be closely monitored for signs of dystocia. Oxytocin should be used with caution and only after other nonpharmacologic methods to promote labor progress have been attempted. Physician consultation should be obtained prior to initiating labor augmentation with oxytocin.

8. High-dose oxytocin protocols are contra-indicated.[85]

9. Intrauterine pressure catheters have not been shown to accurately depict an impending uterine rupture and should not be used solely for that purpose.

10. Water immersion (i.e., tub or shower) is not contraindicated as long as waterproof fetal monitoring is available, although it is frequently restricted according to individual policies.

11. There are no contraindications to alternative positions for birth as long as fetal assessment guidelines are followed.

12. Management of third-stage labor is the same following a VBAC birth as it is following a normal vaginal birth. The midwife and woman can opt for either expectant or active management of the third stage. There is no need to explore the uterine scar for signs of asymptomatic dehiscence after the delivery of the placenta.

13. Women with a previous uterine scar have an increased risk of abnormal placentation (e.g., placenta accreta). A physician should be consulted for a retained placenta prior to any attempts for manual removal.

---

intravenous access. Some of these interventions are not evidence based and will vary according to individual practice settings and institutional policies.

In addition, women who have experienced a previous unplanned cesarean section often present with intense feelings regarding their past birth. They may have psychological milestones to overcome at the point in labor in which the events leading to the cesarean section birth occurred. The midwifery model of care supports practices that promote normal labor and birth and are beneficial for women who desire TOLAC. All interventions, therefore, should be evaluated for safety and interference with normal labor progress and mechanisms.

Intrapartum Management for Women with Coexisting Medical Conditions

The two most common medical conditions that can have adverse effects for a pregnant woman and her fetus are diabetes and hypertension. When caring for a woman with diabetes or hypertension, it is understood that a collaborative plan of care between the midwife and a consulting obstetrician is already in place. As these women enter labor, the balance of management authority will greatly depend on individual policies, the evolving clinical situation, and the experience of the midwife. It is important for midwives to have knowledge of what to expect for these women and to recognize that the intrapartum clinical course could suddenly change, necessitating immediate referral of care to the obstetrician. Ongoing and clear communication between the physician and the midwife is paramount throughout labor to ensure the best outcome for the mother and her infant.

There are many other medical conditions that can adversely affect pregnancy including epilepsy, autoimmune disorders, and heart conditions to name a few. Although this text cannot address every possible condition, management is contingent on knowledge of the physiology of the disorder, diagnosis, and the effects on pregnancy. The midwife also needs to know when to obtain a consultation, and/or transfer of care. In the following text, diabetes and hypertension are used as examples of the midwifery management process when caring for a woman who had a co-existing medical condition.

Women with Diabetes

Regardless of whether the woman has type 1, type 2, or gestational diabetes, these women account for as high as 6–7% of pregnancies in the United States, 90% of which are associated with gestational diabetes.[88] Women with diabetes receive antepartum fetal testing and are typically induced between 39 and 40 weeks' gestation.[88] Women with diabetes also have an increased risk of shoulder dystocia due to macrosomia and should be offered an elective cesarean birth if the estimated fetal weight (by ultrasound) is more than 4500 grams.[89] (See **Appendix 30A** for management of shoulder dystocia.) Fetal lung maturity may be delayed in women with diabetes, and these seemingly full-term infants can exhibit respiratory distress and other related complications immediately following birth.

During labor, monitoring of the woman's blood glucose and maintaining glycemic control have been shown to reduce the incidence of neonatal hypoglycemia.[88] For women who have controlled their diabetes solely with diet, it may not be necessary to monitor glucose levels during labor. Women who are on insulin or oral glycemic agents, however, will require finger-stick glucometer testing of their blood glucose approximately every 2 hours. Any evidence of intrapartum hyperglycemia should be treated promptly with intravenous insulin, balanced with dextrose 5% in lactated Ringer's solution. The goal is to maintain the woman's blood glucose between 80 and 110 mg/dL.[88] There will be institutional variations on these guidelines, and the midwife should develop the most appropriate plan of care with a consulting physician. When a woman in labor has an insulin infusion, she is best cared for collaboratively by a physician who manages the diabetes and a midwife who manages her labor progress.

Careful assessment of fetal size by Leopold's maneuvers is performed when the woman is admitted, and labor progress is monitored closely. Continuous fetal monitoring is required if an insulin infusion is administered. The midwife should be prepared for the possibility of shoulder dystocia at the time of birth and have a low threshold for requesting the presence of the consulting obstetrician during the second stage of labor. The pediatric team should also be notified, especially if there was poor glycemic control or there is any chance of fetal lung immaturity.

Women with a Hypertensive Disorder

The diagnostic criteria for hypertensive disorders in pregnancy are described in the *Medical Complications in Pregnancy* chapter. In all cases, these diagnoses may become medical indications for delivery, but the timing will vary according to the severity of the woman's condition and the gestational age of her fetus. Although some fetal risks are associated with these disorders, maternal mortality and morbidity are the primary concern and treatment is focused on preventing end-organ damage. It is most important for clinicians to recognize that hypertension and preeclampsia exist on a continuum that is often unpredictable. For this reason, women admitted with either of these diagnoses require vigilant monitoring during labor for subtle changes or a sudden acceleration of worsening symptoms. The midwife should work closely with the collaborating physician to develop the most appropriate plan of care, especially if the woman is diagnosed with preeclampsia.

The most serious consequence of preeclampsia is the development of an eclamptic seizure. Magnesium sulfate remains the standard of care for the prevention and treatment of this obstetric emergency. Women diagnosed with severe preeclampsia will have a magnesium sulfate infusion during labor that is continued for 24 hours post birth. Differences of opinion exist as to whether women with gestational hypertension or nonsevere (mild) preeclampsia require seizure prophylaxis with magnesium sulfate. Some feel the risk of seizure is low in these circumstances and that treatment is not needed.[90] Others argue that 20% to 30% of women who present with an eclamptic seizure have no prior symptoms.[91] Regardless of the side taken by the individual midwife on this debate, a physician should be notified and magnesium sulfate started immediately if there is any evidence the woman's condition is progressing to severe preeclampsia.

Other intrapartum considerations include an ongoing assessment of the woman for the presence of headache, visual changes, or epigastric pain. Any headache should be taken seriously and reported to the consulting physician, especially if unrelieved with oral acetaminophen. Visual changes such as scotomata (loss of visual field) or scintillating spots and epigastric or right upper quadrant pain are also worrisome symptoms that require prompt evaluation and consultation with the physician. Careful monitoring of fluid balance is also essential. Although women with preeclampsia are intravascularly fluid restricted, they are at risk for pulmonary edema secondary to the need for intravenous fluids in the presence of impaired kidney function. **Box 30-6** outlines specific assessments that should be included in the plan of

---

BOX 30-6 Labor Assessment for Women with Preeclampsia

1. Hourly blood pressure monitoring[a]
   a. Any result higher than or equal to 160 mm Hg systolic or 110 mm Hg diastolic requires immediate physician consultation and administration of an intravenous antihypertensive medication.
2. Lung auscultation and/or pulse oximetry:
   a. Any shortness of breath, abnormal breath sounds (crackles, wheezes), or other signs of pulmonary edema require the immediate presence of a physician.
   b. Obtain pulse oximetry if the woman has any shortness of breath
3. Deep tendon reflexes:
   a. Hyper-reflexes or the presence of clonus requires physician consultation. (See Box 30-7 for assessment of clonus.)
4. Serum creatinine, AST, complete blood count (hemoglobin, hematocrit, and platelets):
   a. Obtain on admission and every 8 hours per practice/institutional guidelines. Abnormalities are reported to a consulting physician.
5. Strict intake/output:
   a. Urine output at least every 2 to 4 hours. If the urine output is averaging 30mL/hour or less, the physician should be notified. Intravenous and oral fluids are also carefully monitored.
6. If magnesium sulfate is infusing:
   a. Perform hourly assessments of respiratory rate, deep tendon reflexes, and urine output. The infusion should be discontinued and a physician should be notified immediately for any signs of magnesium toxicity (respiratory rate less than 12, absent or diminished deep tendon reflexes, or urine output less than 30 mL/hour).
   b. The antidote for magnesium toxicity is calcium gluconate 10 mL of a 10% solution administered intravenously over 3 minutes.

AST = aspartate aminotransferase.

[a]Manual blood pressure measurements are preferred as they are the most accurate.

BOX 30-7 Assessing for Clonus

What Is Clonus?

Clonus is involuntary, rapid, repetitive, rhythmical contractions and relaxations of a muscle when it is sharply stretched and the stretch is maintained in either flexion or extension. Clonus can be elicited at a number of sites; in obstetrics, most commonly the ankle is used.

What Causes Clonus?

The presence of clonus is associated with a hyper-reflexive state and could indicate abnormal CNS excitability. It is always associated with abnormal (+4) deep tendon reflexes and may be a precursor to an eclamptic seizure.

Assessment for Clonus

1. Position the woman so her knee is partially flexed. Support this position with one hand underneath the bend in her knee.
2. With the other hand grasping her foot, sharply dorsiflex the foot and maintain pressure to keep it in dorsiflexion.
3. Beats of clonus will be seen and felt as the muscle contractions and relaxations cause rhythmical alternation between dorsiflexion and plantar flexion. The muscles being stretched are the same as for the ankle jerk reflex—the gastrocnemius and soleus muscles.

---

is one indication that a seizure is imminent and thus, hyperreflexia is an important piece of information to obtain when a woman presents with hypertension. Conversely, a sign of magnesium toxicity is absent or depressed DTRs. Therefore when a magnesium sulfate is infusing, DTRs are assessed hourly.

Lethal Anomalies and Stillbirth

Every midwife in clinical practice will inevitably encounter a woman who has an unanticipated intrauterine fetal demise (IUFD) or provide care for a woman whose fetus has been diagnosed with a lethal anomaly. The term stillbirth refers to death of a fetus in utero after 20 weeks of gestation. As discussed in the *Obstetric Complications in Pregnancy* chapter, the birth plan will vary according to the woman's choices, her cervical status, and any other medical

care during labor, and **Box 30-7** describes how to determine the presence or absence of clonus.

Deep tendon reflexes (DTRs) are part of both the initial evaluation and ongoing assessments. Normally DTRs are 1+ or 2+. Hyperreflexia (i.e., 3+ or more)

conditions. The woman may arrive in spontaneous labor or she may present for a scheduled induction. In either case, hospital staff should be informed of the diagnosis before the woman's arrival and have a labor room arranged for her that will ensure privacy and liberal visitation from family members. Many labor and birth units have mechanisms in place that discreetly communicate a fetal demise (or lethal anomaly) to the entire staff (e.g., a special door magnet). It is especially important that the woman is not accidently approached by a staff member who is unaware of her diagnosis and assumes she is a "normal" labor patient expecting a healthy newborn.

The midwife's role in the care of a woman with a stillbirth or lethal anomaly will vary according to individual practice guidelines and the specific clinical circumstances. A physician should be consulted to establish the most appropriate plan of care, which may in some cases require referral for medical management. The midwife's continued presence and availability, however, can provide emotional support and comfort for the woman and her family, especially in the immediate postpartum period. Midwives caring for women in these situations will have their own emotions and sadness to deal with, especially during the birth. While this is a normal reaction, the midwife should try to maintain an emotional demeanor that best supports the woman. The priority is always to focus on the woman's immediate needs during labor and birth.

Once the woman is admitted, the midwife should thoroughly review the prenatal chart and all documentation of previous discussions regarding the proposed plan of care. A complete blood count and coagulation studies (especially platelets and fibrinogen) should be obtained on admission due to the potential risk of disseminated intravascular coagulation (usually seen with prolonged fetal retention of more than 2 weeks).[92] If an induction of labor is planned, a physician should be consulted to determine the most appropriate method of induction and cervical ripening. The specific agents and protocols used will depend on the woman's diagnosis, fetal gestational age, past obstetric history, and current Bishop's score.[92] This plan should be reviewed again with the woman and her family, with clear explanations of what to expect as labor and birth progresses. The midwife must be prepared for a wide variety of reactions and emotions that will range from shock and confusion to profound grief, anger, and disbelief. The woman may also need information repeated and should be given opportunities to express her feelings and ask questions. Every effort must be made to honor the woman's choices and requests.

Intrapartum Care of a Woman with a Stillbirth

The majority of women experiencing birth of a known stillbirth will opt for an in-hospital birth. The following discussion addresses that situation. Most labor and birth units have specific protocols and checklists in place for bereaved parents that include referrals to social services, the availability of a chaplain, assistance with burial plans, and collection of photographs, footprints, and other keepsakes from the baby after the birth has occurred. These services should be offered to the woman at the appropriate times and her choices respected. Many families will have already contacted their own community pastor or religious support person. These individuals should be allowed to visit or remain with the woman as long as she needs. Religious and cultural choices should be supported and respected (e.g., desire to baptize the infant).

The woman and her partner must also be informed about the availability of detailed fetal evaluation after the birth. This includes a standard autopsy (with or without facial disfigurement), collection of blood or tissue samples, and a pathology evaluation of the placenta and umbilical cord.[92] Less invasive options may also be available such as photographs, X-ray imaging, and ultrasonography.[92] In this time of emotional crisis, the woman may not want to hear about these options, and sensitivity must be used when discussing these procedures. It should be gently emphasized that this information may be useful to her and her family in planning future pregnancies. Tissue or amniotic fluid samples for fetal karyotype, in particular, may diagnose a syndrome or chromosomal abnormality without the results from a full autopsy.[92] If the woman and her partner decline autopsy or tissue sample collection, the placenta and umbilical cord should still be sent to pathology after the birth.

One of the most difficult aspects of managing labor for a woman with a stillbirth is the absence of the fetal heartbeat on the fetal monitor. Everyone in the room will be painfully aware of the lack of this reassuring sound. Tocodynamometer contraction monitoring may still be required, but this can often be performed intermittently to assess contraction frequency. The necessity and frequency of monitoring should be discussed with the woman beforehand. The woman should be offered all standard labor pain relief options without hesitation regardless of the stage of labor. Some women will want to labor as normally as possible, whereas others will want all pain and discomfort relieved immediately. These choices should be respected and honored throughout labor.

Grief-stricken parents often have difficulty making firm decisions, especially in regard to seeing or holding the infant after birth. As the birth nears, there may be a normal surge of grief emotions from the woman and her partner. The birth itself represents facing their worst fears as they prepare to see their newborn. The midwife should remain present during second-stage labor and allow the woman to push in whatever way she is physically and emotionally able. If the woman has previously stated that she does not want to see the infant after the birth, the nursing staff should be prepared to take the infant to another location after the birth occurs. Women often change their minds about this point, however, and the midwife should remain open to all possibilities.

The birth itself is managed the same as with any other vaginal birth, except that there may be softening or overriding of the fetal skull bones or anomalies not previously identified. In addition, there may be an increased risk of shoulder dystocia. Caution should be used when applying even gentle traction to any part of the fetus during the birth; instead, it is best to rely mostly on the woman's expulsive efforts. The umbilical cord should be clamped and cut as close to the abdomen as possible and the newborn gently dried and wrapped in a towel. Depending on the woman's wishes, the infant will either be handed to her, to a support person, or to the awaiting staff. The placenta should be delivered in the usual fashion and any lacerations repaired.

After the birth, the infant, umbilical cord, and placenta should be carefully examined for any recognizable abnormalities. Any deviations from normal (e.g., a true knot in the umbilical cord) should be shown to the woman and her partner. Sometimes seeing an obvious cause of death is reassuring for grieving families who are searching for answers. Unfortunately, the majority of intrauterine deaths cannot be attributed to a known cause, so it is important not to offer a potential diagnosis without clear evidence.

The woman and her family should be encouraged to view, touch, and hold the infant and allowed as much time as needed for this important component of perinatal bereavement. Often photographs are taken and keepsakes (e.g., a lock of hair and footprints) are obtained and given to the parents. Once they are ready to say goodbye, the infant can be brought to the morgue per hospital policy. The woman should be given the option of where she receives her postpartum care. Some women feel comforted to hear other newborns around them, but in most cases bereaved women will prefer a nonobstetric unit for the remainder of their hospital stay.

Intrapartum Care: Lethal Anomalies

Due to improvements in diagnostic technology, more parents have advanced knowledge of a fetal diagnosis that is life-threatening. While in some cases this early diagnosis may enable prenatal transfer to a tertiary center and neonatal specialists capable of interventions that will improve the infant's survival, in other cases the woman and her partner have the overwhelming task of deciding whether to continue the pregnancy to term. Depending on the gestational age at the time of diagnosis and individual state laws, elective termination of the pregnancy beyond the second trimester or a preterm induction of labor may not be an option. This section focuses on pregnant women with a known lethal fetal anomaly who present at full-term gestations either in spontaneous labor or for a planned induction.

In the majority of cases, the woman and her family will have had time to prepare emotionally for the birth and will likely be receiving care from a multidisciplinary team that includes neonatology, maternal fetal medicine, genetics specialists, and social services. Often a perinatal palliative care plan has been established and many of the decisions facing grieving parents during labor and birth have already been discussed with the woman and her partner. Perinatal palliative care is an emerging field that moves beyond traditional bereavement support and is initiated at the time of diagnosis rather than during labor and birth.[93] This holistic approach incorporates the principles of bereavement care by integrating the woman's choices and understanding with realistic goals for care of the baby after birth, including perinatal hospice care. Ensuring quality of life, reducing pain and suffering, and honoring the baby's life and death are at the core of this framework.[93]

Once the woman is admitted to the labor unit, a collaborative plan of care will be required with a consulting physician. Other care team providers (e.g., neonatology, pediatrics, chaplaincy) should be notified of the impending birth. Depending on the type of anomaly, the gestational age, the expected perinatal outcome, and maternal medical conditions, physician management may be necessary. As a member of the woman's multidisciplinary care team, the midwife's continued presence and support will greatly benefit the woman and her family during this difficult time.

The intrapartum management in this situation is similar to the care of a woman with a stillbirth. Regardless of the amount of prenatal counseling and support, the woman may exhibit a wide range of emotional responses during labor. All pain relief options should be available if requested, but the woman may be hesitant to use any sedative or narcotic medications for fear of the medication's effect on the infant. In addition, as second-stage labor nears, she may experience more difficulty coping and become quite conflicted about pushing. The birth represents facing the confirmation that the infant is going to die, and "holding on" subconsciously prevents this outcome from happening. Providing gentle encouragement, support, and patience will allow the woman to work through any emotional tethering and facilitate her sense of control over the situation.

If the neonatal team is planning to examine the newborn after birth, it may be less distracting for the woman to have them wait outside the room until after the birth occurs. The woman may also be anxious for this examination to occur, as there may still be hope that the prenatal diagnosis was wrong and the infant is healthy and normal. Having a perinatal palliative care plan in place will facilitate the seamless transition from birth to end-of-life care.[93] Normal birth practices such as skin-to-skin contact and immediate breastfeeding should be encouraged if the infant's condition allows. The most important priority is maximizing the woman's time with her infant.

Obstetric Emergencies

Every midwife in clinical practice will inevitably encounter an obstetric emergency. Fortunately, most of obstetric emergencies are rare occurrences, and in some cases they can be anticipated. Regardless, midwives are responsible for the care of women during the intrapartum period, which requires a thorough understanding of how to manage emergent events during labor and birth. Prompt recognition and immediate action are imperative until the situation is resolved or the consulting physician can assume management. The following sections review the clinical management for several intrapartum emergencies, including intrapartum hemorrhage, shoulder dystocia, prolapsed umbilical cord, twin gestation, and breech birth. Also included are intrapartum guidelines for performing a deinfibulation procedure for a Type III female genital mutilation. These are not the only obstetric emergencies midwives will encounter. They do, however, represent clinical circumstances that often require a sequence of management steps to resolve the problem and, therefore, are deserving of a separate discussion.

Intrapartum Hemorrhage

Evaluation of a woman with vaginal bleeding in the second or third trimester includes the differential diagnosis of placenta previa, placental abruption, uterine rupture, and vasa previa.

Initial Midwifery Management

The midwife's role in the care of a woman bleeding is to initiate stabilization measures until the collaborating physician can take over the primary management. Birth will be expedited, regardless of gestational age, if the mother is hemodynamically unstable or the fetus is in jeopardy.

Initial evaluation of hemodynamic status includes assessment of vital signs, mental status, skin color (pallor), and a visual evaluation of blood loss. If there is evidence of significant blood loss on the woman's clothes or body with any signs of hemodynamic compromise, two large-bore IVs should be started and the consulting physician notified immediately. The woman should be given oxygen and placed on continuous electronic fetal monitoring. Laboratory evaluation should include a complete blood count, coagulation studies, blood type, antibody screen, and cross-match for a minimum of 4 units of blood if the woman is actively bleeding. In addition, a Kleihauer-Betke test should be obtained on all women who are Rh negative to quantify the degree of fetomaternal transfusion to guide the dosing of Rh-immune globulin (RhoGAM).

Anesthesia, the operating room team, and the neonatal/pediatric team should also be mobilized and on standby for an emergent cesarean birth and possible neonatal resuscitation. No digital examinations should be performed when a woman presents with vaginal bleeding. Prenatal ultrasound records should be obtained and reviewed as quickly as possible. If previous ultrasound studies confirm a normal placental location, placenta previa can be ruled out but other possibilities such as placental abruption or vasa previa will be considered.

Placenta Previa

When the placenta implants over the inner cervical os, it is referred to as a placenta previa. Placenta previa occurs in approximately 0.4% of all pregnancies and often is diagnosed during routine ultrasonography in the second trimester.[94] The degree of placenta previa is characterized by how close the placental edge is to the internal cervical os (**Figure 30-3**). Terms used to describe a placenta previa include *complete previa* (the entire inner os is covered), *partial previa*

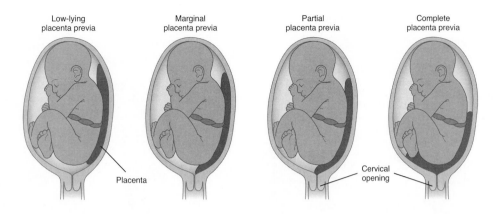

Figure 30-3 Placenta previa: low-lying, marginal, partial, complete.

(the inner os is partially covered), *marginal previa* (the edge of the placenta is at the margin of the os), and *low-lying* (the placental edge is in close proximity to the os). If the placental vessels are at the internal os, this is referred to as a *vasa previa*.

Once a placenta previa is diagnosed, the woman will have repeat ultrasounds to monitor the placental location, as the placenta may migrate away from the internal os as the pregnancy progresses. Vaginal birth is possible only if there is transvaginal sonographic evidence prior to the onset of labor that the placental edge is more than 2 cm from the internal cervical os.[95] In all other cases, a cesarean birth will be required. Risk factors for placenta previa include previous cesarean section, advanced maternal age, multiparity, and cigarette smoking.[94]

Midwifery Management

In the majority of cases, women with a placenta previa will present with an initial episode of painless vaginal bleeding prior to 36 weeks' gestation. If the bleeding has stopped and the woman and fetus are stable, expectant management in the hospital is appropriate. For earlier preterm gestations, administration of steroids to enhance lung maturity and/or magnesium sulfate for neuroprotection may be considered. While in the hospital, the woman's care should be managed by a consulting physician. The midwife may continue in a collaborative role to provide emotional support and anticipatory guidance. Preparation for breastfeeding and parenting as well as family adjustments to hospitalization are an important midwifery component of the woman's plan of care.

Placental Abruption (Abruptio Placentae)

One of the leading causes of obstetric hemorrhage in the second and third trimesters is a placental abruption, defined as a premature separation of a normally implanted placenta.

Placental abruption occurs in approximately 1% of all pregnancies and is associated with significant perinatal mortality and morbidity.[96] In most cases of abruption, bleeding occurs between the membranes and the decidua and passes through the cervix into the vagina. Less commonly, the abruption is concealed and the blood accumulates behind the placenta with no obvious vaginal bleeding. In such a case, the blood may penetrate through the uterine decidua and escape into the peritoneum. This phenomenon is also termed a Couvelaire uterus. An abruption can be either total (involving the entire placenta) or partial (involving only a portion of the placenta) (**Figure 30-4**). A total abruption is a catastrophic obstetric event often leading to fetal death and significant maternal morbidity.

Although the specific etiology of abruption is unknown, several associated factors have been identified (**Box 30-8**). The most common of these risk factors is hypertensive disorders, especially chronic hypertension with superimposed preeclampsia.[96] A history of previous abruption, maternal smoking, and cocaine use also significantly increase the risks of placental abruption. In addition, any maternal trauma (falls, abdominal injury, intimate partner violence, or motor vehicle accidents) warrants an evaluation in the hospital to rule out an abruption. Women who are more than 24 weeks' gestation should have continuous fetal monitoring for a minimum of 4 hours

Concealed bleeding

Bleeding

Placenta

Placenta

Concealed
hemorrhage

Hemorrhage

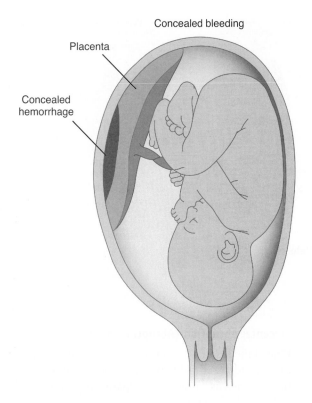

Figure 30-4 Placental abruption.

BOX 30-8 Risk Factors for
Placental Abruption

Maternal Risks

- Advanced maternal age
- Smoking during pregnancy

Obstetric Risk Factors

- Chorioamnionitis
- Hypertensive disorders (chronic, gestational, preeclampsia)
- Premature rupture of membranes
- Fetal growth restriction
- History of placental abruption
- Polyhydramnios

Acute Etiology

- Trauma (falls, abdominal injury, motor vehicle accidents)
- Cocaine or other illicit drug use
- External cephalic version for breech presentation

Source: Adapted from Oyelese Y, Ananth CV. Placental abruption. *Obstet Gynecol.* 2006:108:1005-1016.

---

following trauma to the abdomen. If more than six contractions occur in any given hour, the monitoring should be continued for 24 hours.[97]

Clinical Signs and Symptoms

The clinical presentation of an abruption will depend on the degree of separation and blood loss. Maternal symptoms can vary widely, from mild generalized back discomfort or abdominal cramping to the classic symptoms of vaginal bleeding and severe abdominal pain. Early signs of an abruption can mimic those of labor, and the woman may report periodic mild contractions with what may be perceived as bloody show or bloody amniotic fluid. Low backache may be the only symptom if the placenta is posterior and there is a concealed abruption. The woman may report decreased fetal movement or even a recent surge in fetal activity.

On examination, the woman's demeanor or distress may be out of proportion to the objective clinical signs. The maternal vital signs may be normal with no obvious signs of hemodynamic compromise. The abdomen may be mildly tender with palpable contractions or may feel firm, rigid, and diffusely painful. A pelvic examination may reveal minimal to no bleeding, but this will not correlate with the amount of blood loss from a concealed hemorrhage. In most cases, frequent, low-amplitude contractions are seen on the external fetal monitor. Fetal status will also greatly depend on the degree of separation and blood loss. Thus a variety of fetal heart rate patterns have been associated with a placental abruption, including recurrent late or variable decelerations, loss of fetal heart rate variability, bradycardia, or sinusoidal pattern.[96] Fetal demise is associated with more than a 50% placental separation; rarely does this degree of abruption occur without other overt symptoms.[96]

Ultrasonography is not typically helpful in confirming the diagnosis of placental abruption or in determining the degree of separation. Research has found that the sonographic appearance of placental separation varies considerably depending on how much time has passed from the acute bleeding event.[96] Ultrasound evaluation of a pregnant woman who presents with vaginal bleeding, however, will identify the placental location and the presence of a placenta previa. Although some degree of separation may be seen with a placenta previa, it is considered a distinctly separate diagnosis and would in effect rule out placental abruption as the cause of bleeding.

Midwifery Management

When a woman presents with symptoms of abruption, she should immediately be assessed for signs of hemodynamic compromise and the fetus assessed for signs that suggest an increased risk for fetal acidemia. The continued management will depend in part on the gestational age and in part on the condition of the woman and fetus. The consulting physician should be notified immediately of the midwife's clinical assessment and evaluation to determine the most appropriate plan of care. The midwife should also initiate the maternal/fetal stabilization measures and laboratory assessments discussed in the previous section.

Although management may vary depending on the degree of maternal/fetal compromise, a diagnosis of placental abruption near term will warrant an expedited birth. In many cases, the placental abruption will stimulate vigorous contractions and labor will rapidly progress on its own. The midwife can collaboratively manage this situation with a consulting physician and conduct the birth as planned. During labor, the fetus should be monitored continuously and any signs of fetal compromise promptly reported to the physician. Even with a mild abruption, the situation could deteriorate rapidly, and the woman is at significant risk for coagulopathy and hypovolemic shock. In addition to blood transfusions, the woman may need aggressive replacement of coagulation factors. After the birth, the placenta should be sent to pathology and the woman closely monitored collaboratively with a physician until her condition stabilizes.

Shoulder Dystocia

Shoulder dystocia is impossible to predict with any reliable accuracy and can result in significant maternal and fetal morbidity. Its true incidence is likely underreported due to variations in research design, definition of shoulder dystocia, and differences in the population studied.[98] For example, retrospective studies have reported an incidence of 0.6% to 1.4%,[89] while prospective studies have shown a higher frequency of 3% to 7%.[98] The incidence is thought to rise with increasing fetal size, especially among infants born to women with diabetes. Diabetes is associated with a sixfold increased risk for shoulder dystocia.[99]

Although there is no standard definition for shoulder dystocia, accepted definitions include (1) impaction of the anterior or (less commonly) the posterior shoulder, (2) failure to deliver the fetal shoulders by the usual methods, (3) prolonged head-to-body delivery time (more than 60 seconds), and (4) need for ancillary maneuvers.

Even when managed appropriately, a shoulder dystocia can result in neonatal injuries, such as a fractured humerus or clavicle and either temporary or permanent damage to the infant's brachial plexus (Erb's palsy). Prolonged fetal asphyxia during a difficult shoulder dystocia can also result in neonatal encephalopathy, seizures, and infant death. Maternal complications include excessive blood loss (e.g., from postpartum hemorrhage) and perineal, vaginal, or rectal lacerations. Last-resort maneuvers such as cephalic replacement or abdominal rescue via cesarean section significantly increase the risks for both maternal morbidity and perinatal mortality.

The neonatal consequences of shoulder dystocia are at the root of many lawsuits. For this reason, brachial plexus injury in particular has received considerable attention in the obstetric literature. This injury is thought to occur from forceful stretching or hyperextension of one side of the neck causing avulsion or rupture of one or all of the brachial plexus nerves. Lateral traction applied to the infant's neck while attempting to deliver the anterior shoulder is the likely cause. While research has attempted to quantify the degree of force needed to cause a brachial plexus injury, this injury can also occur prior to birth and may be unavoidable in certain circumstances.[98]

Current evidence has now shifted toward shoulder dystocia management techniques that avoid placing any traction on the infant's neck. Passive maneuvers such as prompt delivery of the posterior arm or immediate rotation of the anterior shoulder to an oblique diameter (Rubin's maneuver) decrease the incidence of brachial plexus injury.[100,101] The risk factors, key points, and maneuvers for managing a shoulder dystocia are included in Appendix 30A.

Risk Factors for Shoulder Dystocia

Antepartum risk factors for shoulder dystocia include fetal macrosomia, maternal diabetes, and a history of shoulder dystocia in prior pregnancy. Other associated factors known to increase the risks of macrosomia, such as maternal obesity, excessive weight gain, and post-term gestation, have also been identified. When these factors are seen in combination, the risks for shoulder dystocia are increased. For example, women with diabetes who have poor glycemic control during pregnancy are more likely to have a fetus with accelerated growth. In addition, women who have experienced a shoulder dystocia in a previous pregnancy have a recurrence rate of 6% to 20%, especially if the estimated weight of the current fetus is higher than the birth weight of the previous infant.[98] Although many shoulder dystocias involve newborns who weigh less than 4000 grams at birth, the incidence steadily increases with each 500-gram increment in birth weight. Accordingly, there is a 23.9% (a 10-fold increase) risk of shoulder dystocia in infants weighing more than 4500 grams at birth.[98]

The principal intrapartum risk factors for shoulder dystocia are a precipitous second stage and operative vaginal birth. Rapid descent of the fetus during second stage labor may not allow enough time for normal internal rotational maneuvers and compression of the shoulders toward the thorax, which results in impaction of the anterior shoulder behind the pubic bone. The unpredictability of this seemingly normal intrapartum event, which precedes as many as 30% of shoulder dystocias, is a key reason why all obstetric providers should be able to recognize and immediately respond to a shoulder dystocia. Likewise, the use of forceps and vacuum extraction has been associated with as many as 35% of shoulder dystocias, especially if other risk factors, such as suspected macrosomia or maternal diabetes, exist. Midwives managing the second stage of labor in women with any of these risk factors should have a low threshold for requesting the immediate availability of their consulting obstetrician.

Prevention Strategies

Because cesarean birth is the only absolute way to prevent a shoulder dystocia, it would seem logical to offer this option to women with risk factors or suspected macrosomia. Unfortunately, ultrasound determination of fetal weight is inaccurate at term. When using ultrasound to estimate fetal macrosomia (more than 4000 grams), one study reported that it would take 2345 elective cesarean births to prevent one permanent brachial plexus injury.[102] Elective induction of labor prior to 41 weeks' gestation performed solely for suspected macrosomia has not been found to reduce the incidence of shoulder dystocia and is also not recommended.[89] Currently, ACOG recommends elective cesarean section be offered after 39 weeks' gestation *only* to women with sonographic evidence of a fetus weighing more than 5000 grams, or more than 4500 grams if the woman has diabetes.[89] Nevertheless, it may be reasonable to discuss the risks and benefits of a planned cesarean section with women who have experienced a previous shoulder dystocia, especially if any permanent neonatal injury was incurred or the estimated fetal weight of the current fetus is higher. A woman with this history will benefit from a physician consultation and prenatal development of a birth plan.[89]

In addition to these recommendations, midwives should assess each pregnant woman for the presence of shoulder dystocia risk factors and closely monitor weight gain for those women with a BMI of more than 29. Referral to a nutritionist may encourage compliance with weight gain goals, and early diabetic screening should be performed.

Shoulder Dystocia Simulation

Unfortunately, half of the shoulder dystocia cases occur in women with no appreciable risk factors and average-weight newborns (less than 4000 grams).[98] Given that the incidence of shoulder dystocia is relatively low, obtaining competency in management of this complication is challenging. While popular mnemonics are helpful memorization tools, evidence suggests simulation and team training are more likely to improve skills and confidence in managing a shoulder dystocia.[101,103–105] Research on simulation specifically related to shoulder dystocia has also shown that the use of high-fidelity manikins is preferred, especially when trying to learn and practice rotational maneuvers.[101,103–105] "High fidelity" also refers to the ability of the equipment, the environment, and the learners to simulate and act as if the learning scenario is a real-life situation.[106]

Another advantage of simulation is to train groups of learners together as a multidisciplinary team working on a specific clinical emergency, such as a shoulder dystocia. At the end of the scenario, participants have an opportunity to debrief on the experience under the guidance of a skilled simulation coordinator. Teaching points are highlighted and the team is given constructive feedback related to the original learning objectives for the session. Studies have shown both improvements in confidence[103] and skills[101,104] when simulation is used for shoulder dystocia training. Even though high-fidelity simulation centers may not be immediately available to all students and providers, the benefits of this type of learning experience in improving critical thinking and skills with shoulder dystocia management cannot be overstated.

Management of Shoulder Dystocia

The detailed management of shoulder dystocia can be found in Appendix 30A. For many years, the management of shoulder dystocia followed a specific protocol that began with external manipulation, which was often repeated several times before internal rotational maneuvers were attempted. Current evidence on brachial plexus injuries suggests shoulder dystocia management should focus first on assisting internal rotation. Touching the infant's head should be avoided and lateral traction should not be applied to the neck. This shift in practice, referred to as a "hands-off" protocol, has resulted in a decrease in brachial plexus injury and improved communication between team members.[101] In addition, the majority of maneuvers and manipulations are done without the woman pushing to facilitate rotation of the shoulders and/or to properly direct assistants.

Clear, calm communication with the woman and the healthcare team is essential. All maneuvers should be performed with a deliberate, systematic approach, avoiding jerky movements or any manipulation of the infant's head. Lastly, there should be no hesitation to insert the entire hand into the posterior vaginal area along the sacral hollow. Simply inserting two fingers will not enable access to the posterior arm or exert enough pressure for rotation.

Prolapsed Umbilical Cord

There are three types of umbilical cord prolapse: occult, funic, and overt. An *occult* cord prolapse occurs when the umbilical cord is compressed alongside the presenting part in the lower uterine segment or inner cervix. The cord may not be palpable during a cervical examination but will often cause variable decelerations or fetal heart rate bradycardia similarly seen with umbilical cord compression (see the *Fetal Assessment During Labor* chapter). In a *funic* umbilical cord prolapse, the cord is palpable in front of the presenting part. In an *overt* umbilical cord prolapse, the cord slips completely out of the uterus through the cervix and may be protruding at the vaginal introitus. Variant fetal heart rate patterns may be present depending on the degree of cord compression from the presenting part.

When a frank or complete umbilical cord prolapse is encountered, the woman will need an emergent cesarean birth and immediate interventions to improve fetal oxygenation. Risk factors and emergency management of a prolapsed umbilical cord are outlined in **Appendix 30B**.

Twin Gestation

In recent years, the incidence of twins and higher-order multiple gestations has increased primarily due to the availability of assisted reproductive technologies. Currently, twin gestations occur in approximately 3% of all pregnancies in the United States and account for 17% of preterm births.[2] Twins are associated with a sevenfold increased perinatal mortality rate compared to singleton gestations.[107,108] In addition, higher rates of congenital anomalies, fetal growth restriction, and maternal complications such as gestational hypertension, preeclampsia, and diabetes are all found among women with multiple gestations.[107] Lastly, intrapartum complications such as malpresentation, prolapsed umbilical cord, placental separation, and postpartum hemorrhage all occur more frequently in twin gestations.[109]

When referring to twin gestations, it is critical to know the chronicity (one or two placentas) and the amnionicity (one or two amniotic sacs)—that is, the twins will be, dichorionic–diamniotic (di-di), monochorionic–diamniotic (mono-di), or monochorionic–monoamniotic (mono-mono). Chorionicity is explained further in the *Obstetric Complications in Pregnancy* chapter.

In some practice settings, the diagnosis of twins will mandate physician referral, especially if an intervening amniotic membrane has not been identified (mono-mono). For either mono-di or di-di twins, a collaborative management plan with the consulting physician can be considered (per practice guidelines) with strict criteria for referral of care. The woman will need ongoing surveillance for both maternal and fetal complications throughout the remainder of her pregnancy. An individualized plan of care regarding the optimal timing and mode of birth with the appropriate informed consent discussion will also be needed.

Mode of Birth

The mode of birth depends on the fetal presentation. Therefore, as the pregnancy progresses, the presentation and lie of each fetus will be carefully assessed and documented in the woman's prenatal record. Regardless of the gestational age or estimated fetal weight, when the presenting fetus is breech, cesarean birth is recommended.[107] Approximately 40% of twins, however, will be in a vertex–vertex presentation at the time of birth; these women are ideal candidates for a trial of labor and vaginal birth.[109] This option should be discussed with the woman well before the onset of labor and the risks and benefits of vaginal birth versus elective cesarean section thoroughly reviewed. Current evidence has not found cesarean birth improves perinatal outcomes in vertex–vertex presentations, and vaginal birth should be encouraged for all vertex–vertex presenting twins.[107,110]

The more controversial situation is a vertex presentation of the first twin and a breech or transverse presentation of the second twin. In some cases, a vertex presenting second twin can convert to a noncephalic presentation after the vaginal birth of the first newborn. For this reason, some sources recommend that twin births occur under the direction of an obstetrician experienced in breech extraction with the immediate availability of an emergency cesarean section. In most settings, twin births occur in the operating room with a full operating room team on standby to perform an emergency cesarean birth if needed.

Upon admission in labor, the presentation and lie of each fetus should be reassessed with ultrasound. The midwife should notify a consulting physician and a collaborative management plan should be established if the woman desires a trial of labor. The intrapartum management guidelines for twin gestation can be found in **Appendix 30C**.

Breech Birth

By 35 to 36 weeks' gestation, the majority of fetuses will spontaneously settle into a vertex presentation. In approximately 3% to 4% of cases, however, at term,

the fetus will be in a breech presentation with the buttocks or feet presenting.[111] There are three types of breech presentation: frank, complete, or footling (see Appendix 30D). In a *frank* breech presentation, the hips are flexed and the knees extended, with the infant's feet near the head. The buttocks (breech) are presenting at the pelvic inlet. A *complete* breech is similar, with the buttocks as the presenting part in the pelvis. The lower knees are flexed, however, and the infant is in a crossed-legged position. If one or both feet are extended down below the buttocks, this is referred to as a single or double *footling* breech. When assessing position in a breech presentation, the fetal sacrum is used as the point of reference—for example, *left sacrum anterior (LSA)* (**Figure 30-5**).

Prematurity, multiple gestation, multiparity with lax uterine tone, polyhydramnios or oligohydramnios, previous breech presentation, and placenta previa have all been associated with an increased risk of breech presentation.[111] In addition, uterine anomalies such as a bicornate uterus or the presence of large fibroids in the lower uterine segment may impede a normal vertex presentation.[111] Breech presentation is also associated with an increased incidence of fetal anomalies such as hydrocephaly or anencephaly.[111]

Diagnosis of Breech Presentation

A breech presentation is often identified during a prenatal visit using Leopold's maneuvers when the firm ballottable vertex is palpated in the upper fundal region. The woman may report feeling increased movement in the lower pelvic area and the fetal heart rate may be found in the upper abdomen. Prior to 35 weeks' gestation, this finding is normal but should be noted in the prenatal chart, especially if the woman has any of the known predisposing risk factors. Only approximately 10% of breech fetuses will spontaneously revert to vertex presentation after 36 weeks' gestation.[111] The midwife should, therefore, have a low threshold for ordering an ultrasound at 35 to 36 weeks' gestation if breech presentation is suspected.

Even with careful assessment techniques, some women will present in labor with an undiagnosed breech presentation, thus a breech presentation may be first diagnosed during a vaginal examination. Palpation of fetal small parts, usually the feet, or the buttocks may be encountered, although sometimes it is very difficult to distinguish the fleshy part of the breech from soft-tissue caput on the fetal vertex. In some cases, the breech presentation is not discovered until the woman is well into active labor when fresh meconium stool is seen coming from the vagina. Once a breech presentation is confirmed, the woman should be informed and a consulting

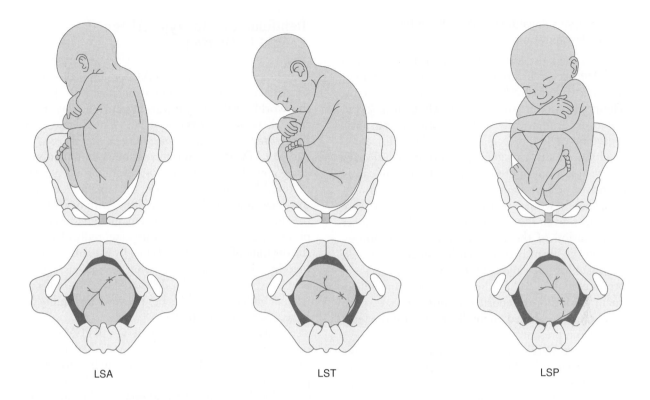

LSA   LST   LSP

Figure 30-5 Breech positions.

physician notified immediately. If the birth is imminent or a cesarean section is not immediately available, the midwife should be prepared to perform a vaginal breech birth. **Appendix 30D** reviews the management steps for a vaginal breech birth, and all midwives caring for laboring women should be thoroughly familiar with these techniques.

External Cephalic Version

If a breech presentation is diagnosed after 35 weeks' gestation but before the onset of labor, the midwife should consult with a physician to determine if the woman is a candidate for an external cephalic version. During this procedure, external pressure is manually exerted on the woman's abdomen to physically rotate the fetus to a vertex presentation. External cephalic version is successful in approximately 50% of cases.[111,112] Factors that decrease the chance of external cephalic version success include oligohydramnios, anterior placenta, breech engaged in the pelvis, fetal back located posteriorly ("back down"), and maternal obesity.[112] External cephalic version should not be performed if the woman has any contraindication to vaginal birth (e.g., placenta previa) or if any of the following conditions are present: ruptured membranes, fetal or uterine anomalies, nonreassuring

fetal heart rate patterns, hyperextended fetal head, placental abruption, or multiple gestation.[112]

External cephalic version is performed only in a hospital setting, ideally between 36 and 37 weeks' gestation. In addition to a prerequisite reassuring fetal heart rate assessment, the woman is given a dose of subcutaneous terbutaline (0.25 mg) to induce uterine relaxation before the procedure is attempted. External cephalic version is done under direct ultrasound guidance with continuous monitoring of the fetal heart rate (by an assistant). Often, women experience considerable discomfort during the procedure, so external cephalic version is sometimes attempted under epidural or spinal anesthesia. The most common fetal side effect of external cephalic version is a transient nonreassuring fetal heart rate pattern such as a prolonged deceleration.[114] In rare circumstances, external cephalic version has been reported to cause vaginal bleeding, placental abruption, fetal compromise, fracture of fetal limbs, emergency cesarean birth, and fetal death.[112] Midwives often assist during external cephalic version by providing ultrasound guidance during the procedure and/or emotional support and comfort to the woman. After the procedure, fetal heart rate and contraction monitoring should continue for at least 1 hour depending on institutional policies.

Controversies Regarding Mode of Birth for Breech Presentation

Prior to the late 1990s, vaginal breech birth was a common occurrence and an important component of obstetric training for both midwives and physicians. The publication of the Term Breech Trial in 2000, however, dramatically changed practice patterns regarding vaginal breech births.[113] This multicenter, randomized study originally reported that elective cesarean section for breech presentation significantly decreased perinatal morbidity and mortality. Almost immediately, women with a breech presentation were no longer given the option for vaginal birth. Closer examination of the definitions and methodology used in the Term Breech Trial has since challenged the reliability and validity of these findings.[114] Several protocol violations have been identified, and subsequent studies have reported no differences in perinatal outcomes based on mode of birth for the fetus in a breech presentation.[114]

Unfortunately, these updated findings have failed to completely reverse the clinical changes brought about by the Term Breech Trial. The current medico-legal environment has continued to influence practice, with the result that women with a breech presentation today are still often advised to have an elective cesarean birth. More importantly, since the Term Breech Trial was published, expertise in vaginal breech birth and clinical learning opportunities have diminished. As a result, vaginal breech birth is now included in simulation training curricula along with other high-risk obstetric skills such as shoulder dystocia management. Midwives are encouraged to participate in these training experiences whenever possible.

Some women with a breech presentation will decline surgery or seek out a provider who will perform a planned vaginal breech birth. Current guidelines for these circumstances have been established and institutions that can safely offer this service are encouraged to develop protocols for intrapartum management.[115] The option for planned vaginal breech birth is always predicated on the availability (and willingness) of an obstetrician experienced in this mode of birth. A thorough informed consent discussion with the woman is also mandatory. Some sources have outlined specific selection criteria shown to improve success rates such as sonographically determined estimated fetal weight between 2500 and 4000 grams, frank or complete breech, no fetal anomalies, adequate maternal pelvis, adequate amniotic fluid, and flexion of the fetal head (documented by ultrasound).[115–117]

Deinfibulation for Type III Female Genital Mutilation

Female genital mutilation (FGM) for nonmedical reasons affects millions of young women worldwide. Per the World Health Organization's current classification, there are four types of FGM, as reviewed in the *Obstetric Complications in Pregnancy* chapter.[118] A type III FGM is also referred to as "infibulation" and is considered to be the most severe form of genital cutting.[118] During infibulation, the labia minora and the inner tissue of the labia majora (with or without the clitoris) are removed. The remaining tissue is purposefully fused or sewn together, essentially blocking the opening of the vagina. Typically a small opening (neo-introitus) remains, allowing for the passage of urine and menstrual blood. This obstruction of the vaginal outlet greatly impedes the woman's ability to have a normal vaginal birth.

Consequently, women with a type III FGM should be offered a deinfibulation procedure to separate this fused scar tissue.[119] Deinfibulation can be performed prior to pregnancy, prenatally, or during labor under either local or regional anesthesia.[119,120] Ideally, it is performed by a physician or midwife who has been previously trained in this procedure.[119] There may be clinical circumstances, however, in which a recently immigrated woman presents in labor with no prenatal care and a deinfibulation procedure is needed to facilitate a normal vaginal birth. Deinfibulation is a simple procedure that is performed similarly to episiotomy. Research has demonstrated minimal complications and no differences in perinatal outcomes after a deinfibulation procedure has been performed.[119,120]

Deinfibulation Procedure

When midwives encounter a woman in labor with any type of FGM, the vulvar area must be carefully assessed to determine (1) the type of FGM, (2) the extent of the infibulation and vulvar adhesions, and (3) the diameter of the vaginal opening. The consulting physician may also need to collaboratively examine the vulvar area to determine if a deinfibulation procedure is needed. It does not matter when the deinfibulation is performed, although releasing the scar tissue earlier in labor will enable vaginal examinations and the ability to perform obstetric procedures if needed.[120] The woman's informed consent is necessary and the procedure should be performed using sterile aseptic technique with adequate anesthesia.

Prior to the procedure, the woman should be placed in lithotomy position and the vulvar area cleaned with an antiseptic solution (i.e., Betadine). The index and middle fingers of the nondominant hand are then gently inserted into the vaginal opening and extended upward alongside the inner aspect of the fused "hood." If the woman does not have an epidural, the central area between the fingers can be infiltrated with 1% lidocaine solution, similarly to the method used when infiltrating the perineum prior to episiotomy. Once the tissue is anesthetized, the scar between the two fingers is very carefully cut apart with sterile blunt Mayo scissors. Care must be taken as the scissors advance toward the urethral area, as the clitoris may still be intact underneath the fused tissue. Although there is usually minimal bleeding from the avascular scar tissue, suturing of the raw edges can be done if needed. During the birth, an episiotomy may still be necessary to further enlarge the vaginal opening or prevent damage from any remaining scar tissue near the urethral/clitoral area.

After the birth, the vulva and perineum is carefully inspected for any extension of the deinfibulation incision or other lacerations. One source recommends placing subcuticular or interrupted polyglactin (Vicryl) sutures along the raw edges of the infibulation scar to prevent fusion during the healing process.[119] Insertion of a Foley catheter post birth for 24 hours may also facilitate healing.[120] Otherwise, routine postpartum care and recovery can be anticipated.

Conclusion

Complications during labor and birth can occur at any time and knowledge of these conditions is essential for midwifery practice. Understanding the condition, its natural course, effects on the woman and her fetus, and what degree of consultation, collaboration, or referral are the basic competencies needed for all obstetric complications. In addition, because emergencies are unpredictable, management of those that are most common will enable midwives to care for women safely. All women who experience a complication intrapartally will greatly benefit from the continuity, education, and support that a midwife provides.

• • • References

1. Cypher RL. Reducing recurrent preterm births. *J Perinat Neonat Nurs.* 2012;26(3):220-229.

2. Martin JA, Hamilton BE, Ventura SJ, Osterman MJK, Wilson EC, Mathews TJ. Births: final data for 2010. *Natl Vital Stat Rep.* 2010;61(1). Available at: http ://www.cdc.gov/nchs/data/nvsr/nvsr61/nvsr61_01.pdf. Accessed January 31, 2013.

3. American College of Obstetricians and Gynecologists. ACOG Practice Bulletin no. 38: perinatal care at the threshold of viability. *Obstet Gynecol.* 2002;100: 617-624.

4. Goldenberg RL, Culhane JF, Iams JD, Romero R. Preterm birth 1: epidemiology and causes of preterm birth. *Lancet.* 2008;371:75-84.

5. Romero R, Espinoza J, Kusanovic JP, et al. The preterm parturition syndrome. *BJOG.* 2006;113(suppl 3):17-42.

6. Wax JR, Cartin A, Pinette MG. Biophysical and biochemical screening for the risk of preterm labor. *Clin Lab Med.* 2010;30:693-707.

7. Sanchez-Ramos L, Delke I, Zamora J, Kaunitz AM. Fetal fibronectin as a short-term predictor of preterm birth in symptomatic patients. *Obstet Gynecol.* 2009;114(3):631-640.

8. Leitich H, Egarter C, Kaider A, Hohlagschwandtner P, Berghammer P, Husslein P. Cervicovaginal fetal fibronectin as a marker for preterm delivery: a meta-analysis. *Am J Obstet Gynecol.* 1999;180:1169-1176.

9. Peaceman AM, Andrews WW, Thorp JM, et al. Fetal fibronectin as predictor of preterm birth in patients with symptoms: a multicenter trial. *Am J Obstet Gynecol.* 1997;177:13-18.

10. Rose CH, McWeeney DT, Brost BC, Davies NP, Watson WJ. Cost-effective standardization of preterm labor evaluation. *Am J Obstet Gynecol.* 2010;203: e1-e5.

11. American College of Obstetricians and Gynecologists. ACOG Practice Bulletin no. 127: management of preterm labor. *Obstet Gynecol.* 2012;119:1308-1317.

12. Haas DM, Imperiale TF, Kirkpatrick PR, et al. Tocolytic therapy: a meta-analysis and decision analysis. *Obstet Gynecol.* 2009;113(3):585-594.

13. Abramovici A, Cantu J, Jenkins SM. Tocolytic therapy for acute preterm labor. *Obstet Gynecol Clin North Am.* 2012;39:77-87.

14. Lowe NK, King TK. Labor. In: King TL, Brucker MC, eds. *Pharmacology for Women's Health.* Sudbury, MA: Jones and Bartlett; 2011:1086-1116.

15. American College of Obstetricians and Gynecologists. ACOG Committee Opinion No. 475: antenatal corticosteroid therapy for fetal maturation. *Obstet Gynecol.* 2011;117:422-424.

16. Centers for Disease Control and Prevention. Prevention of perinatal group B streptococcal disease: revised guidelines from CDC 2010. *MMWR.* 2010; 59(RR-10). Available at: www.cdc.gov/mmwr/pdf/rr /rr5910.pdf.

17. American College of Obstetricians and Gynecologists. ACOG Committee Opinion No. 455: magnesium sulfate before anticipated preterm birth. *Obstet Gynecol.* 2010;115:669-671.

18. American College of Obstetricians and Gynecologists. ACOG Practice Bulletin no. 55: management of postterm pregnancy. *Obstet Gynecol.* 2004;104:639-646.

19. Hoffman CS, Messer LC, Mendola P, Savitz DA, Herring AH, Hartman KE. Comparison of gestational age at birth based on last menstrual period and ultrasound during the first trimester. *Paediatr Perinat Epidemiol.* 2008;22(6):587-596.

20. Norwitz ER, Snegovskikh VV, Caughey AB. Prolonged pregnancy: when should we intervene? *Clin Obstet Gynecol.* 2007;50:547-557.

21. Rosenstein MG, Cheng YW, Snowden JM, Nicholson JM, Caughey AB. Risk of stillbirth and infant death stratified by gestational age. *Obstet Gynecol.* 2012; 120(1):76-82.

22. American College of Obstetricians and Gynecologists. ACOG Practice Bulletin no. 107: induction of labor. *Obstet Gynecol.* 2009;114:386-397.

23. Clark SL, Miller DD, Belfort MA, Dildy GA, Frye DK, Myers JA. Neonatal and maternal outcomes associated with elective term delivery. *Am J Obstet Gynecol.* 2009;200:156.e1-156.e4.

24. Gulmezoglu AM, Crowther CA, Middleton P, Heatley E. Induction of labor for improving birth outcomes for women at or beyond term. *Cochrane Database Syst Rev.* 2012;6:CD004945. doi: 10.1002/14651858 .CD004945.pub3.

25. Caughey AB, Sundaram V, Kaimal AJ, et al. Systematic review: elective induction of labor versus expectant management of pregnancy. *Ann Intern Med.* 2009; 151:252-263.

26. Sanchez-Ramos L, Oliver F, Delke I, Kaunitz AM. Labor induction versus expectant management for postterm pregnancies: a systematic review with meta-analysis. *Obstet Gynecol.* 2003;101:1312-1318.

27. Glantz JC. Term labor induction compared with expectant management. *Obstet Gynecol.* 2010;115: 70-76.

28. Clark SL, Fleischman AR. Term pregnancy: time for a redefinition. *Clin Perinatol.* 2011;38:557-564.

29. American College of Obstetricians and Gynecologists. ACOG Practice Bulletin no. 55: management of postterm pregnancy. *Obstet Gynecol.* 2004;104:639-646.

30. Hannah ME, Ohlsson A, Farine D, et al. Induction of labor compared with expectant management for prelabor rupture of membranes at term. *N Engl J Med.* 1996;334:1005-1010.

31. Marowitz A. Management of prelabor rupture of membranes at term: using the evidence. In: Anderson B, Stone S, eds. *Best Practices in Midwifery.* New York: Springer; 2012:139-151.

32. American College of Obstetricians and Gynecologists. ACOG Practice Bulletin no. 80: premature rupture of membranes. *Obstet Gynecol.* 2007;109:1007-1019.

33. American College of Nurse-Midwives position statement: premature rupture of membranes at term. ACNM Division of Standards and Practice, Clinical Practice Section 2008 (reviewed 2012). Available at: http://www.midwife.org.

34. Goldenberg RL, Hauth JC, Andrews WW. Mechanisms of disease: intrauterine infection and preterm delivery. *N Engl J Med.* 2000;342:1500-1507.

35. Evers AC, Nijhuis L, Koster MP, Bont LJ, Visser GH. Intrapartum fever at term: diagnostic markers to individualize the risk of fetal infection: a review. *Obstet Gynecol Surv.* 2012;67:187- 200.

36. Fahey JO. Clinical management of intra-amniotic infection and chorioamnionitis: a review of the literature. *J Midwifery Women's Health.* 2008;53:227-235.

37. Fishman SG, Gelber SE. Evidence for the clinical management of chorioamnionitis. *Semin Fetal Neonatal Med.* 2012;17:46-50.

38. Simpson KR. Reconsideration of the costs of convenience: quality. operational, and fiscal strategies to minimize elective labor induction. *J Perinat Neonat Nurs.* 2010;24:43-52.

39. Clark S, Belfort M, Saade G, et al. Implementation of a conservative checklist-based protocol for oxytocin administration: maternal and newborn outcomes. *Am J Obstet Gynecol.* 2007;197:480.e1-480.e5.

40. Fisch JM, English D, Pedaline S, Brooks K, Simhan HN. Labor induction process improvement: a patient quality-of-care initiative. *Obstet Gynecol.* 2009:113: 797-803.

41. Reisner DP, Wallin TK, Zingheim RW, Luthy DA. Reduction of elective inductions in a large community hospital. *Am J Obstet Gynecol.* 2009:200:674.e1-e7.

42. American College of Nurse-Midwives position statement: induction of labor. ACNM Division of Standards and Practice; 2010. Available at: www.midwife.org.

43. Bishop EH. Pelvic scoring for elective induction. *Obstet Gynecol.* 1964;24:266-268.

44. Swamy GK. Current methods of labor induction. *Semin Perinatol.* 2012;36:348-352.

45. Boulvain M, Stan C, Irion O. Membrane sweeping for induction of labour. *Cochrane Database Syst Rev.* 2001;2:CD000451. doi: 10.1002/14651858. CD000451.

46. Macones GA, Cahill A, Stamilio DM, Odibo AO. The efficacy of early amniotomy in nulliparous labor induction: a randomized controlled trial. *Am J Obstet Gynecol.* 2012;207:403.e1-e5.

47. Clark SL, Simpson KR, Knox GE, Garite TJ. Oxytocin: new perspectives on an old drug. *Am J Obstet Gynecol.* 2009;200:35.e1-35.e6.

48. Institute for Safe Medication Practices. *High alert medications*. Huntingdon Valley, PA: Institute for Safe Medication Practices; 2007. Available at: www.Ismp .org.

49. Simpson KR. Clinicians guide to the use of oxytocin for labor induction and augmentation. *J Midwifery Women's Health*. 2011;56:214-221.

50. Gimpl G, Fahrenholz F. Oxytocin receptor system: structure, function, and regulation. *Physiol Rev*. 2001; 81(2):629-683.

51. Gosner M. Labor induction and augmentation with oxytocin: pharmacokinetic considerations. *Arch Gynecol Obstet*. 1995:256:63-66.

52. Simpson KR, Miller L. Assessment and optimization of uterine activity during labor. *Clin Obstet Gynecol*. 2011;54:40-49.

53. Macones GA, Hankins GD, Spong CY, Hauth J, Moore T. The 2008 National Institute of Child Health and Human Development workshop report on electronic fetal monitoring: update on definitions, interpretations, and research guideline. *Obstet Gynecol*. 2008;112:661-666.

54. Hofmeyr GJ, Say L, Gulmezoglu AM. World Health Organization systematic review of maternal mortality and morbidity: the prevalence of uterine rupture. *BJOG*. 2005;112:1221-1228.

55. Cahill AG, Waterman BM, Stamilo DM, et al. Higher maximum doses of oxytocin are associated with an unacceptably high risk for uterine rupture in patients attempting vaginal birth after cesarean delivery. *Am J Obstet Gynecol*. 2008;199:32.e1-32.e5.

56. O'Driscoll K, Stronge JM, Minogue M. Active management of labour. *Br Med J*. 1973;3:135-137.

57. Brown HC, Paranjothy S, Dowswell T, Thomas J. Package of care for active management in labour for reducing cesarean section rates in low-risk women. *Cochrane Database Syst Rev*. 2008;4:CD004907. doi: 10.1002/14651858.CD004907.pub2.

58. Wei S, Luo Z, Qi H, Xu H, Fraser WD. High-dose vs low-dose oxytocin for labor augmentation: a systematic review. *Am J Obstet Gynecol*. 2010;203:296-304.

59. Kavanagh J, Kelly AJ, Thomas J. Breast stimulation for cervical ripening and induction of labour. *Cochrane Database Syst Rev*. 2005;3:CD003392. doi: 10.1002/14651858.CD003392.pub2.

60. McFarlin BL, Gibson MH, O'Rear J, Harman P. A national survey of herbal preparation use by nurse-midwives for labor stimulation. *J Midwifery Women's Health*. 1999;44:205-216.

61. Hall HG, Mckenna LG, Griffiths DL. Complementary and alternative medicine for inductions of labor. *Women Birth*. 2012;25:142-148.

62. Dugoua JJ, Perri D, Seely D, Mills E, Koren G. Safety and efficacy of blue cohosh (*Caulophyllum thalictroides*) during pregnancy and lactation. *Can J Clin Pharmocol*. 2008;15:e66-e73.

63. Peaceman A. Abnormal labor. In: Queenan JT, Hobbins JC, Spong CY, eds. *Protocols for High Risk Pregnancies*. West Sussex, UK: Wiley-Blackwell; 2010:505-508.

64. American College of Obstetricians and Gynecologists. ACOG Practice Bulletin no. 49: dystocia and augmentation of labor. *Obstet Gynecol*. 2003;102:1445-1454.

65. Greulich B, Tarrant B. The latent phase of labor: diagnosis and management. *J Midwifery Women's Health*. 2007;52:190-198.

66. Neal JL, Lowe NK, Ahijevych KL, Patrick TE, Cabbage LA, Corwin EJ. "Active labor" duration and dilation rates among low-risk, nulliparous women with spontaneous labor onset: a systematic review. *J Midwifery Women's Health*. 2010;55:308-318.

67. Friedman EA. Primigravid labor: a graphicostatistical analysis. *Obstet Gynecol*. 1955;6:567-589.

68. Zhang J, Landy HJ, Branch DW, et al. Contemporary patterns of spontaneous labor with normal neonatal outcomes. *Obstet Gynecol*. 2010;116:1281-1287.

69. Rouse D, Owen J, Savage K, et al. Active phase labor arrest: revisiting the 2-hour minimum. *Obstet Gynecol*. 2001;98:550-554.

70. Sizer AR, Nirmal DM. Associated factors and obstetric outcomes in nulliparous patients. *Obstet Gyencol*. 2000;96:749-752.

71. Lowe N, Corwin E. Proposed biological linkages between stress, obesity, and inefficient uterine contractility during labor in humans. *Medical Hypothesis*. 2011;76:755-760

72. National Institutes of Health. *Consensus Development Conference on Cesarean Childbirth*. Publication No. 82:2067. Bethesda, MD: National Institutes of Health, Department of Health and Human Services; 1981.

73. Flamm BL, Newman LA, Thomas SJ, Fallon D, Yoshida MM. Vaginal birth after cesarean delivery: results of a 5-year multicenter collaborative study. *Obstet Gynecol*. 1990;76(5 suppl 1):750-754.

74. Guise JM, Denman MA, Emeis C, et al. Vaginal birth after cesarean: new insights on maternal and neonatal outcomes. *Obstet Gynecol*. 2010;115(6):1267-1278.

75. McMahon MJ, Luther ER, Bowes WA, Olshan AF. Comparison of a trail of labor with an elective second cesarean section. *N Engl J Med*. 1996;335(10): 689-695.

76. American College of Obstetricians and Gynecologists. *ACOG Practice Bulletin no. 5: vaginal birth after previous cesarean delivery*. Washington, DC: American College of Obstetricians and Gynecologists; July 1999.

77. National Institutes of Health consensus development conference statement on vaginal birth after cesarean: new insights March 8–10, 2010. *Obstet Gynecol*. 2010; 115(6):1279-1295.

78. Leeman LM, King VJ. Increasing patient access to VBAC: new NIH and ACOG recommendations. *Am Fam Physician.* 2011;83(2):121-122, 127.

79. American College of Nurse-Midwives position statement: vaginal birth after cesarean delivery. ACNM Board of Directors; revised and reapproved 2011. Available at: www.midwife.org.

80. American College of Nurse-Midwives. ACNM Clinical Bulletin no. 12: caring for women desiring vaginal birth after cesarean. *J Midwifery Women's Health.* 2011;56:517-525.

81. Landon MB. Predicting uterine rupture in women undergoing trial of labor after prior cesarean delivery. *Semin Perinatol.* 2010;34:267-271.

82. Spong CY, Mercer BM, D'Alton M, Kilpatrick S, Blackwell S, Saade G. Timing of indicated late-preterm and early-preterm birth. *Obstet Gynecol.* 2010;118(2 Pt 1):323-333.

83. Landon MB, Hauth JC, Levino KJ, et al. Maternal and perinatal outcomes associated with a trial of labor after prior cesarean delivery. National Institute of Child Health and Human Development Maternal–Fetal Medicine Units Network. *N Engl J Med.* 2004; 351(25):2581-2589.

84. Macones GA, Peipert J, Nelson DB, et al. Maternal complications with vaginal birth after cesarean delivery: a multicenter study. *Am J Obstet Gynecol.* 2005;193(5):1656-1662.

85. American College of Obstetricians and Gynecologists. ACOG Practice Bulletin no. 115: vaginal birth after previous cesarean delivery. *Obstet Gynecol.* 2010; 116(2 Pt 1):450-463.

86. Lydon-Rochelle M, Holt VL, Easterling TR, Martin DP. Risk of uterine rupture during labor among women with a prior cesarean delivery. *N Engl J Med.* 2001;345:3-8.

87. King TL. Can a vaginal birth after cesarean delivery be a normal labor and birth? Lessons from midwifery applied to trial of labor after a previous cesarean delivery. *Clin Perinatol.* 2011;38:247-263.

88. American College of Obstetricians and Gynecologists. ACOG Practice Bulletin no. 115: gestational diabetes mellitus. *Obstet Gynecol.* 2013;122(2 Pt 1):406-416.

89. American College of Obstetricians and Gynecologists. ACOG Practice Bulletin no. 40: shoulder dystocia. *Obstet Gynecol.* 2002;100:1045-1050.

90. Cahill AG, Macones GA, Odibo AO, Stamilio DM. Magnesium seizure prophylaxis in patients with mild preeclampsia. *Obstet Gynecol.* 2007;110:601-607.

91. Sibai BM. Diagnosis, prevention, and management of eclampsia. *Obstet Gynecol.* 2005;105:401-410.

92. American College of Obstetricians and Gynecologists. ACOG Practice Bulletin no. 102: management of stillbirth. *Obstet Gynecol.* 2009;113:748-761.

93. Kobler K, Limbo R. Making a case: creating a perinatal palliative care service using a perinatal bereavement model. *J Perinat Neonat Nurs.* 2011;25:32-41.

94. Faiz AS, Anath CV. Etiology and risk factors for placenta previa: an overview and meta-analysis of observational studies. *J Matern Fetal Neonatal Med.* 2003;13:175-190.

95. Society of Obstetricians and Gynaecologists of Canada. SOGC Clinical Practice Guideline no. 189: diagnosis and management of placenta previa. *J Obstet Gynaecol Can.* 2007:29:261-266.

96. Oyelese Y, Ananth CV. Placental abruption. *Obstet Gynecol.* 2006:108:1005-1016.

97. Brown HL. Trauma in pregnancy. *Obstet Gynecol.* 2009:114:147-160.

98. Gurewitsch ED, Allen RH. Reducing the risk of shoulder dystocia and associated brachial plexus injury. *Obstet Gynecol Clin North Am.* 2011;38:247-269.

99. Politi S, D'Emidio L, Cignini P, Giorlandino M, Giorlandino C. Shoulder dystocia: an evidence-based approach. *J Perinat Med.* 2010;4:35-42.

100. Hoffman MK, Bailit JL, Branch W, et al. A comparison of obstetric maneuvers for the acute management of shoulder dystocia. *Obstet Gynecol.* 2011; 117:1272-1278.

101. Inglis SR, Feier N, Chetiyaar JB, et al. Effects of shoulder dystocia training on the incidence of brachial plexus injury. *Am J Obstet Gynecol.* 2011;204:322. e1-e6.

102. Rouse DJ, Owen J, Goldenberg RL, et al. The effectiveness and costs of elective cesarean delivery for fetal macrosomia diagnosed by ultrasound. *JAMA.* 1996;276:1480-1486.

103. Andrighetti TP, Knestrick JM, Marowitz A, Martin C, Enstrom JL. Shoulder dystocia and postpartum hemorrhage simulations: student confidence in managing these complications. *J Midwifery Women's Health.* 2012;57:55-60.

104. Crofts JF, Fox R, Ellis D, Winter C, Hinshaw K, Drawycott TJ. Observations from 450 shoulder dystocia simulations: lessons for skills training. *Obstet Gynecol.* 2008;112:906-912.

105. Fahey JO, Mighty HE. Shoulder dystocia: using simulation to train providers and teams. *J Perinat Neonat Nurs.* 2008;22:114-122.

106. Maran NT, Glavin RT. Low- to high-fidelity simulation: a continuum of medical education? *Med Educ.* 2003;37(suppl 1):22-28.

107. American College of Obstetricians and Gynecologists. ACOG Practice Bulletin no. 56: multiple gestation: complicated twin, triplet, and higher order multifetal pregnancy. *Obstet Gynecol.* 2004;104: 869-883.

108. Cruikshank DP. Intrapartum management of twin gestations. *Obstet Gynecol.* 2007;109:1167-1176.

109. Lee YM. Delivery of twins. *Semin Perinatol.* 2012; 36:195-200.

110. Peaceman AM, Kuo L, Feinglass J. Infant morbidity and mortality associated with vaginal delivery in twin gestations. *Am J Obstet Gynecol.* 2009;200: 462-466.

111. Glezerman M. Planned vaginal breech delivery: current status and the need to reconsider. *Expert Rev Obstet Gynecol.* 2012;7:159-166.

112. Hofmeyr GJ, Kulier R. External cephalic version for breech presentation at term. *Cochrane Database Syst Rev.* 2012;10:CD000083. doi: 10.1002/14651858. CD000083.pub2.

113. Hannah ME, Hannah WJ, Hewson SA, Hodnett ED, Saigal S, Willan AR. Planned cesarean section versus planned vaginal birth for breech presentation at term: a ramdomised multicentre trial. Term Breech Trial Collaborative Group. *Lancet.* 2000;356: 1375-1383.

114. Lawson GW. The Term Breech Trial ten years on: primun non nocere? *Birth.* 2012;39:3-9.

115. American College of Obstetricians and Gynecologists. ACOG Committee Opinion no. 306: mode of term singleton breech delivery. *Obstet Gynecol.* 2006;108:235-237.

116. Alarab M, Regan C, O'Connell MP, Keane DP, O'Herlihy C, Foley ME. Singleton vaginal breech delivery at term: still a safe option. *Obstet Gynecol.* 2004;103:407-412.

117. Yeomans ER, Gilstrap LC. Breech delivery. In: Queenan JT, Spong CY, Lockwood CJ, eds. *Queenan's Management of High-Risk Pregnancy: An Evidence-Based Approach.* 6th ed. Malden, MA: Wiley-Blackwell; 2012:424-428.

118. World Health Organization. Classification of female genital mutilation. 2008. Available at: http://www .who.int/reproductivehealth/topics/fgm/overview /en/#.

119. Nour NM, Michels KB, Bryant AE. Defibulation to treat female genital cutting. *Obstet Gynecol.* 2006: 108:55-60.

120. Rouzi AA, Al-Sibiani SA, Al-Mansourri NM, Al-Sinani NS, Al-Jahdali EA, Darhouse K. Defibulation during vaginal delivery for women with Type III female genital mutilation. *Obstet Gynecol.* 2012:120;98-103.

30A

Shoulder Dystocia

Shoulder dystocia is an obstetric emergency that most midwives will inevitably encounter in clinical practice. Management is focused on systematic steps that are designed to minimize adverse outcomes, especially injury to the infant's brachial plexus. This appendix reviews the key points and management steps required for safe intrapartum practice in the event of a shoulder dystocia.

Clinically, signs of an impending shoulder dystocia occur while the woman is pushing as the infant's head slowly extends and emerges over the perineum. Instead of fully extending, the vertex partially retracts back into the vagina, commonly referred to as the "turtle sign" (**Figure 30A-1**). Restitution and external rotation do not occur as the infant's shoulders have not followed the normal cardinal movements through the pelvis and are impacted in an anterior–posterior position. In cases of maternal

obesity, it may appear as if the "turtle sign" is occurring when there is simply excess maternal soft tissue that impedes the extension and rotation of the infant's head. Abducting the hips, called McRoberts' maneuver, causes the symphysis to shift up over the anterior shoulder of the newborn, which usually allows enough room for normal delivery mechanisms to occur (**Figure 30A-2**).

While accurate diagnosis of a shoulder dystocia is critical, it is equally important to remain calm and fully assess the situation. After the head is delivered, waiting for the next contraction to allow for normal restitution and allowing the woman to push the infant out of the vagina unassisted may reduce the incidence of shoulder dystocia. If restitution does not occur, it is equally important to first assess the location of the

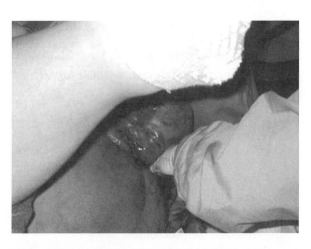

Figure 30A-1 Turtle sign. Note that the infant's chin cannot be seen because the head has retracted into the vagina.

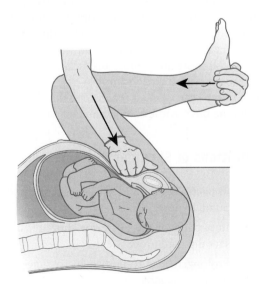

Figure 30A-2 McRoberts' maneuver and suprapubic pressure.

1015

shoulders prior to initiating any maneuvers (other than repositioning the mother). Midwives who are attending births at home or in a birth center may need to enlist the assistance of the woman's partner and/or family if a shoulder dystocia is encountered. Even if the dystocia is resolved quickly, resuscitation assistance and ambulance transfer to the nearest hospital may still be needed for both the woman and her newborn.

After a shoulder dystocia occurs, a carefully written delivery note documenting the details of the birth and the sequence of events/maneuvers should be completed. Some institutions have specific delivery note templates or forms that are used following a shoulder dystocia. At a minimum, this note should include the position of the head at birth, which shoulder was anterior, time of the delivery of the head, who was present or called, maneuvers that were done and in which order, time of the delivery of the body, newborn weight and Apgar scores, cord blood gas results if obtained, disposition of the newborn, and any motor deficit in the upper extremities noted on initial newborn examination; any maternal injuries should also be identified. In addition, using the term "traction" or trying to quantify the amount of force should be avoided. From a medico-legal standpoint, it should also be noted that fundal pressure was *not* used. The events should be explained clearly and simply with no attempts to editorialize or speculate.

A shoulder dystocia is a traumatizing event for all involved. It may be helpful for the midwife to organize a debriefing with the other staff and providers who were present as soon as possible to discuss what happened in a nonthreatening, supportive way. The midwife should also stay in close contact with the woman and her support persons. In the event of a serious shoulder dystocia, they may be facing devastating neonatal consequences and need ongoing support and follow-up. It is also essential that the midwife provides honest and accurate information to the woman regarding what happened during the birth without any blame or judgment.

Definitions of Shoulder Dystocia

1. Impaction of the anterior shoulder behind the pubic bone
2. Impaction of the posterior shoulder on the sacral promontory
3. Prolonged head-to-body delivery time greater than 60 seconds
4. Need for ancillary maneuvers to deliver the shoulders

Incidence[1,2]

1. Retrospective studies: 0.6% to 1.4%
2. Prospective studies: 3% to 7%
3. Likely underreported due to variations in study design, definition, and population
4. Incidence rises with increasing fetal weight (23.9% at 4500 grams)
5. Incidence is highest in women who have diabetes and a macrosomic fetus (likely 50%)

Risk Factors[2,3]

1. Prenatal risk factors
   a. Fetal macrosomia (more than 4000 grams)
      i. 23.9% risk in infants weighing more than 4500 grams at birth
   b. Maternal diabetes (sixfold increased risk)
   c. History of shoulder dystocia in a previous pregnancy
      i. 6% to 20% recurrence rate
2. Intrapartum risk factors
   a. Precipitous second stage
      i. Rapid descent that does not allow enough time for normal rotational maneuvers
   b. Operative vaginal delivery (forceps or vacuum extraction)
   c. Prolonged second stage (increases the risk for operative delivery)
3. Associated risks (all increase incidence of macrosomia)
   a. Obesity
   b. Excessive weight gain
   c. Post-term gestation (more than 41 weeks)

Key Points

1. Stay calm and clearly communicate to the woman and the team.
2. Do not panic and do not rush.
3. Be systematic and deliberate in moving through the procedures.
4. Keep hands off the infant's head as much as possible and avoid excessive traction on the head.

5. Most of these maneuvers are done when the woman is *not* pushing.

6. Do *not* let anyone perform suprapubic pressure until asked for by the person attending the birth.

7. Under *no* circumstances should anyone *ever* perform fundal pressure.

8. Try a maneuver once and then move on to another one; spend no more than 30 seconds on each maneuver.

9. Keep the team informed as each maneuver is performed.

10. Cut an episiotomy *only* if unable to get an entire hand into the vagina.

11. Start an intravenous line and obtain blood for a type and screen if this has not been done.

12. Continuously monitor the fetal heart rate and administer oxygen to the woman if needed.

13. Do not clamp or cut a nuchal cord during a shoulder dystocia; plan to deliver the infant with the somersault maneuver once the dystocia is resolved (see the *Hand Maneuvers for Birth* appendix in *The Second Stage of Labor and Birth* chapter).

14. Be prepared for a postpartum hemorrhage after the infant is born.

15. Be prepared for a full neonatal resuscitation. Cord blood gases should be sent if the shoulder dystocia was prolonged or if there is any sign of neonatal distress after the birth.

16. Neonatal asphyxia becomes a significant risk by 5 minutes. Rescue maneuvers (cephalic replacement or abdominal rescue) should be considered by 4 minutes. These will require transfer to the operating room and the availability of an obstetrician.

Management Steps

There is no clear superiority of one maneuver versus another, and many of these steps occur simultaneously. Delivering the posterior arm may have the highest rate of success because it reduces the shoulder diameter by 2 to 3 cm. In general, McRoberts' maneuver and suprapubic pressure are recommended as the first step, followed by delivery of the posterior arm.

1. The moment shoulder dystocia is suspected, have the woman *stop* pushing and immediately assess the position of the fetal shoulders with a vaginal exam.

2. If the anterior shoulder is impacted, calmly and clearly state, "I have a shoulder dystocia."

3. Request help—additional nurses, the consulting physician, the neonatal team, and anesthesia should be called immediately.

4. Have the woman brought to the edge of the bed and then placed in *McRoberts' position* (head down and knees/hips hyperflexed toward abdomen; **Figure 30A-3**). Hyperflexing the legs does not increase pelvic diameters but it causes cephalic rotation of the symphysis so the symphysis slides up and over the anterior shoulder. Do not let the woman push.

5. Direct another person to perform *suprapubic pressure* at a slight angle in the direction you are trying to rotate the shoulder toward the fetal chest. Do this in between contractions first.

6. *The combination of McRoberts' maneuver and suprapubic pressure* will likely relieve the majority of shoulder dystocias. If it is not working, the fetus may be too large to fit in this alignment and will need rotational maneuvers.

7. *Rubin's maneuver.* Insert a hand (or as many fingers as possible) behind the anterior shoulder on the fetal back and try to rotate the shoulder forward into an oblique position in the pelvis. This is also referred to as "collapsing the shoulders" and may help reduce the bisacromial shoulder diameter. The woman can attempt to push in coordination with your hand rotating the shoulder and the directed suprapubic pressure by an assistant. Use minimal and very gentle lateral traction (on the shoulder—not the head or the neck). If this does not easily relieve the dystocia, repeated attempts increase the force and the risk of brachial plexus injury and should not be continued.

8. *Delivery of posterior arm.* Insert an entire hand in the posterior aspect of the vagina and follow the posterior arm to the infant's elbow. If the arm is extended, try to reach the forearm and bend the arm at the elbow until you can feel the infant's hand. Either grasp the hand or put gentle forward pressure on the elbow to sweep the arm across the chest and out of the vagina. There is an increased risk of humerus or clavicle fracture, but in the majority of cases, delivery of the posterior arm will relieve the dystocia. This maneuver is also associated with the lowest risk of

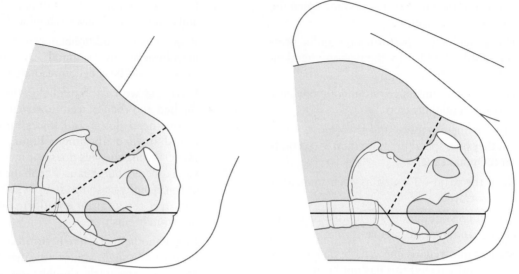

Adduction of the legs toward the woman's abdomen moves the symphysis up so it slides over the fetal anterior shoulder.

Figure 30A-3 Effect of McRoberts' maneuver on the symphysis.

brachial plexus injury some providers choose to try this before trying Rubin's maneuver.

9. Move gently, deliberately, and with purpose. Imagine you are inserting your hand into a circular can of potato chips or through a tight bangle bracelet. Continue to let the team know what you are doing (i.e., "I am going to try to deliver the posterior arm").

10. Cut an episiotomy *only* if more room is needed to insert your hand.

11. Continue to coach the woman not to push and keep her informed—her continued cooperation is critical.

12. *Gaskin maneuver.* Have the woman move onto her hands and knees. If the dystocia is not immediately resolved with repositioning, resume a supine McRoberts' position. (This maneuver can be repeated and/or attempted prior to other maneuvers, even if the woman has an epidural. Rotational maneuvers can also be done in this position.)

13. *Wood screw maneuver.* With a hand firmly against either the posterior or anterior shoulder, push the shoulder clockwise or counterclockwise in an attempt to rotate it in a 180-degree arc. Continue to rotate the shoulders back and forth in whichever direction

they will move until the impaction is dislodged and the infant is born. This maneuver may require both hands (one anterior and one posterior) pushing in opposite directions (**Figure 30A-4**).

14. When the consulting physician or another provider enters the room, step aside and let that person try to facilitate the birth.

15. Intentional fracture of the clavicle may decrease the bisacromial diameter but may be difficult to perform in an emergent situation.

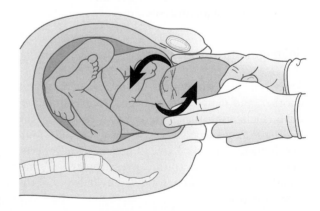

Figure 30A-4 Wood screw maneuver.

16. By 5 minutes, the risk of neonatal asphyxia starts to rise and rescue maneuvers must be considered. This will necessitate transfer to the physician and the availability of anesthesia and a full operating room team.

17. *Rescue maneuvers* include cephalic replacement (Zavanelli maneuver) or abdominal rescue, which both require a full operating room team and a physician capable of performing a cesarean delivery.

● ● ● **References**

1. Gurewitsch ED, Allen RH. Reducing the risk of shoulder dystocia and associated brachial plexus injury. *Obstet Gynecol Clin North Am*. 2011;38:247-269.

2. American College of Obstetricians and Gynecologists. ACOG Practice Bulletin no. 40: shoulder dystocia. *Obstet Gynecol*. 2002;100:1045-1050.

3. Politi S, D'Emidio L, Cignini P, Giorlandino M, Giorlandino C. Shoulder dystocia: an evidence-based approach. *J Perinat Med*. 2010;4:35-42.

APPENDIX

30B

Emergency Interventions for Umbilical Cord Prolapse

An overt umbilical cord prolapse is an obstetric emergency that will require the woman to undergo an immediate cesarean section. Often the first sign of a cord prolapse is a sudden fetal bradycardia or recurrent variable decelerations that rapidly get more severe. Management of this acute situation requires prompt action on the part of the midwife in recognizing the prolapse, performing the appropriate lifesaving interventions while an operating room team and the consulting physician are mobilized. **Figure 30B-1** depicts the types of umbilical cord prolapse.

Definitions

1. *Overt:* The cord slips completely out of the cervix and is protruding in the vagina.

2. *Occult:* The cord is compressed alongside the presenting part in lower uterine segment or inner cervix.

   a. Maternal repositioning or gentle upward pressure on the fetal head during a cervical exam can relieve an occult cord prolapse.

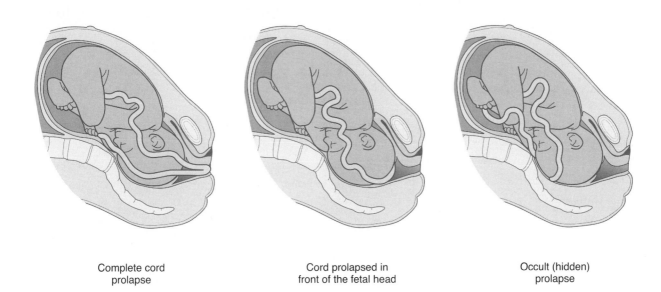

Complete cord prolapse

Cord prolapsed in front of the fetal head

Occult (hidden) prolapse

Figure 30B-1 Umbilical cord prolapse.

b. If fetal heart rate (FHR) decelerations are present, intrauterine resuscitation measures should be initiated (see the *Fetal Assessment During Labor* chapter).

3. *Funic:* The cord is palpable in front of the presenting part.

   a. A funic presentation requires consultation with the collaborating physician to develop the most appropriate management plan.

Risk Factors

1. Prematurity
2. Multiple gestation
3. Multiparity
4. Polyhydramnios
5. Fetal malpresentation
6. Rupture of membranes: intentional or spontaneous with an unengaged head

Management Steps

1. Call for help immediately and do not leave the woman.
2. Clearly state, "I have a prolapsed umbilical cord."
3. Direct others to page a physician and notify the operating room team.
4. Inform the woman of what is happening and tell her she will need an emergency cesarean section.
5. Reposition the woman in the bed, tipped on her side (lateral Sims), or place her in knee–chest position.
6. Do *not* attempt to replace the cord in the uterus.
7. Put a sterile glove on and get into or on the bed, insert a hand into the vagina and firmly push up on the presenting part to relieve any compression on the cord. *Do not remove your hand or let up on the presenting part.*
8. Monitor the fetal heart rate continuously.
9. Administer oxygen and an intravenous fluid bolus.
10. Be prepared to accompany the woman into the operating room in this position riding on the bed.
11. The operating room staff will place the sterile drapes over you, and the physician will let you know when the newborn is safely out of harm's way and you can remove your hand.

APPENDIX

30C

Intrapartum Management of Twin Gestation

Midwifery management of a planned twin birth should always occur in a hospital in close collaboration with a physician capable of performing a cesarean section. Many institutions require vaginal delivery of twins to occur in the operating room with anesthesia and an operating room team on standby. The neonatal (or pediatric) team should also be notified as soon as possible of a twin labor admission to ensure there are adequate nursing staff and personnel capable of full neonatal resuscitation of both newborns. Regardless of how the fetuses were identified during pregnancy, the first twin to deliver is referred to as "Baby A" and the second twin is "Baby B."

Incidence

1. 3% of all births
2. 40% will be vertex–vertex at onset of labor[2]

Types of Twins[2]

1. Monochorionic–monoamniotic (mono-mono)
   a. Requires referral for medical management
   b. Delivery by cesarean section typically at 32 weeks[2]
2. Monochorionic–diamniotic (mono-di)
3. Dichorionic–diamnionic (di-di)

Risks Associated with Twin Deliveries[2]

1. Preterm birth
2. Malpresentation
3. Prolapsed umbilical cord
4. Placental separation (especially with Twin B)
5. Postpartum hemorrhage
6. Preeclampsia
7. Placenta previa

Intrapartum Management Guidelines for Twin Gestations

1. Upon arrival in labor, the presentation and lie of each fetus should be reassessed with ultrasound.
2. These findings should be reviewed with the consulting physician to determine if the planned vaginal delivery is still an option. This plan should be shared with the woman and her informed consent obtained.
3. The woman should have an intravenous line inserted with blood drawn for a blood type, antibody screen, and cross-match.
4. Management of labor pain is no different for twins, including use of epidural anesthesia if the woman desires. Epidural analgesia is

recommended in many institutions as it can provide anesthesia for an emergency cesarean section if needed.

5. Continuous fetal monitoring of both fetuses is required throughout labor with an electronic fetal monitor that can record both heart rates simultaneously. A fetal scalp electrode should be inserted on Baby A only if medically indicated.

6. The consulting physician should be in the hospital and present in the room during the births. It is generally recommended that the births occur in an operating room as the risk of needing an emergency cesarean section for Baby B is approximately 2% to 30%.

7. The management of Baby A's birth is no different than a singleton gestation. An episiotomy should be done only if medically indicated.

8. The umbilical cord from Baby A should be clamped and marked so that it is clear that this cord is from Baby A. For example, use one extra clamp for Baby A and two extra clamps for Baby B.

9. After the birth of Baby A, Baby B's position and presentation should be immediately assessed with ultrasound and the woman's cervix checked for dilation and station of the presenting part.

10. Baby B's fetal heart rate should be monitored continuously as this is the period of risk for umbilical cord prolapse.

11. If Baby B is presenting vertex, care should be taken when rupturing the membranes to avoid a prolapsed umbilical cord. Do not rupture the membranes if Baby B is unengaged.

12. If Baby B is not vertex, the physician should take over the management, especially if a breech extraction is anticipated.

13. A postpartum hemorrhage should be anticipated and the appropriate uterotonic medications and/or blood products should be immediately available.

14. The umbilical cords should be carefully marked to differentiate Baby A from Baby B and the placenta(s) sent to pathology.

● ● ● **References**

1. Martin JA, Hamilton BE, Ventura SJ, Osterman MJK, Wilson EC, Mathews TJ. Births: final data for 2010. *Natl Vital Stat Rep*. 2010;61(1). Available at: http://www.cdc.gov/nchs/data/nvsr/nvsr61/nvsr61_01.pdf.

2. Lee YM. Delivery of twins. *Semin Perinatol*. 2012; 36:195-200.

APPENDIX

30D

Breech Birth

As discussed in the chapter, there may be circumstances when a woman with a known breech presentation is planning a vaginal delivery. Planned vaginal breech births should always take place within a hospital setting under the primary management of an obstetrician. Midwives in clinical practice are more likely to encounter a woman in advanced labor with a previously unknown breech presentation. While every attempt should be made to mobilize a team to perform a cesarean section, if the birth is imminent, it will occur vaginally. This appendix reviews the management techniques for a breech birth, and midwives are encouraged to periodically review these steps. As with other obstetric emergencies, participation in vaginal breech simulation drills has been shown to improve provider confidence and team communication. If available in their practice settings, midwives are encouraged to participate in these types of training experiences.

Incidence of Breech Presentation

3% to 4% of all pregnancies at term[1]

Types of Breech Presentations[1]

See **Figure 30D-1**.

1. *Frank breech (50%–70%)*. The lower extremities are flexed at the hips with the legs extended and the feet near the infant's head ("pike" position). The presenting part is the infant's buttocks.

2. *Complete breech (5%–10%)*. Both the hips and knees are flexed, with both feet above the infant's buttocks ("cannonball" position). The presenting part is the infant's buttocks.

3. *Footling breech (10%–30%)*. One or both feet extend below the infant's buttocks and present in the vagina. This can be either a single or double footling presentation. A single footling is sometimes referred to as an "incomplete breech."

Predisposing Factors[2]

1. Preterm gestation

2. Multiple gestation

3. Multiparity with lax uterine tone

4. Polyhydramnios

5. Oligohydramnios

6. Uterine anomalies (bicornate uterus)

7. Uterine fibroids (especially in the lower uterine segment)

8. Placenta previa

9. Fetal anomalies (hydrocephaly, aneuploidy, nuchal masses)

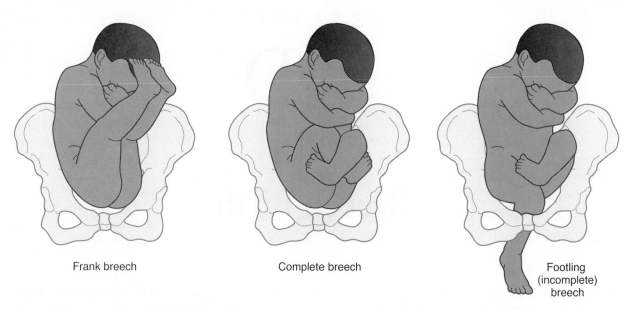

Frank breech   Complete breech   Footling (incomplete) breech

Figure 30D-1 Types of breech presentation.

Factors That May Improve the Success of Vaginal Breech Birth[3,4]

1. Average-size fetus (2500–3800 g) with no known anomalies
2. Proven adequate pelvis
3. Frank or complete breech
4. Documentation of fetal head flexion (by ultrasound)
5. Spontaneous labor with normal progress
6. Easy spontaneous delivery of the buttocks and thighs

Key Points

1. Leopold's maneuvers are an important assessment tool but may be unreliable in determining presentation during active labor.
2. When performing a cervical exam on a woman in labor, palpation of the fetal skull sutures confirms a vertex presentation.
3. *Any* suspicion for breech presentation should always be confirmed with ultrasound.
4. In out-of-hospital sites, the midwife must rely on Leopold's maneuvers and a careful vaginal exam to palpate the fetal skull sutures. There should be no hesitation to transfer the woman to a hospital if a breech presentation is suspected. The midwife should also call 911 for additional help and notify the consulting physician, especially if the woman refuses transfer or the birth is imminent.
5. The infant's sacrum is the denominator (anatomic landmark for determitning the position in the pelvis; Figure 30-5).
6. When a breech birth is imminent, the midwife should request the assistance of any available obstetrician (or a more experienced midwife if a physician is not available). The neonatal or pediatric team should also be called and staff prepared for full infant resuscitation. Anesthesia and an operating room team should be on standby in the event that surgical intervention is needed.
7. During the birth, the infant may pass thick meconium stool from compression of the breech in the vagina. This is often the first indication during labor of a "missed breech" presentation.
8. The fetal heart rate should be monitored continuously. The woman should also have an intravenous line inserted if possible and should be given oxygen if there are any signs of fetal acidemia.
9. The key management steps in a breech birth require a "hands-off" approach until the breech is delivered to the level of the umbilicus and considerable patience to allow for spontaneous progression of the normal

cardinal movements. The woman should be allowed to push and her progress monitored closely.

10. If the woman has any contraindications to a vaginal breech birth, transfer to a hospital or operating room and preparation for a cesarean section is indicated. If contraindications are present, the midwife should assist with a vaginal birth only if the birth occurs before a cesarean section can be facilitated.

Cardinal Movements and Management Techniques for a Breech Birth

1. Descent occurs throughout and is facilitated by maternal pushing efforts.

2. Engagement of the hips usually takes place when the infant's bitrochanteric diameter (the distance between the outer points of the hips) enters the oblique diameter of the maternal pelvis. The position will then be either right sacrum anterior (RSA) or left sacrum anterior (LSA).

3. The anterior hip usually descends more rapidly than the posterior hip.

4. As resistance from the pelvic floor is encountered, internal rotation of 45 degrees will occur and the anterior hip will pass under the pubic bone. The bitrochanteric diameter of the hips is now in the anterior–posterior diameter of the woman's pelvis in either a right sacrum transverse (RST) or left sacrum transverse (LST) position.

5. As descent continues, the anterior hip provides a pivot for the posterior hip, which usually crosses the perineum first. Delivery of the anterior hip will follow through lateral flexion of the spine.

6. Until this point in time, the woman should be allowed to push as needed and descent of the breech observed closely. Resist the temptation to pull the buttocks out and allow the maternal pushing efforts to continue as in any normally progressing second stage. If the infant is born too quickly, the head may not have time to flex, which is necessary for birth of the head.

7. Once the buttocks are born and the umbilicus is visible at the perineum, the legs should be gently released one at a time through the vaginal opening.

8. This should be done in between pushing efforts by following the thigh to the knee and sweeping the flexed leg across the infant's abdomen.

9. If the infant is in a frank breech presentation and the full extension of the legs has hindered descent, *Pinard's maneuver* can be used to "break up the breech" (**Figure 30D-2**). Insert either the right or left hand (depending on the sacrum's position) and follow the thigh to the popliteal fossa behind the knee. The thumb should be on the anterior side of the thigh. Gently press on the popliteal fossa and move the leg laterally away from the midline. This will cause the leg to flex at the knee, thereby bringing the foot down to where it can be grasped. Bring the leg down and out of the vagina by drawing it across the infant's abdomen in its natural range of motion. Repeat the maneuver for the other leg if needed.

10. After the trunk, legs, and feet are delivered, external rotation will occur, aligning the infant's back into a sacrum anterior position. This will cause the shoulders to rotate internally into the oblique diameter of the maternal pelvis and pass under the pubic bone.

11. The remainder of the birth should occur within the next 3 to 5 minutes to avoid hypoxia from compression of the umbilical cord. A generous loop of the umbilical cord can be pulled down to prevent stress at the umbilical insertion site.

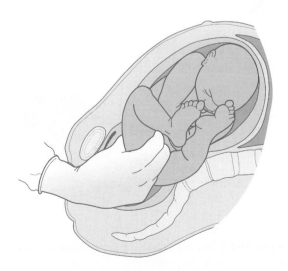

Figure 30D-2 Pinard's maneuver.

12. Wrap a warm towel around the infant's lower body just below the umbilicus. This will keep the infant warm and provide a nonslippery hold on the hips (**Figure 30D-3**).

13. To facilitate birth of the shoulders, grasp the hips by placing the thumbs on the sacrum and the fingers on the corresponding iliac crests. Avoid any pressure on the soft-tissue areas of the abdomen or flank.

14. Provide downward and outward traction on the body with coordinated pushing from the mother, and gently rotate the infant to either an RST or LST position (**Figure 30D-4**).

15. Continue downward traction with maternal pushing efforts until both the scapula and the axilla of the anterior shoulder are visible.

16. *Delivery of shoulders and arms.* There are different techniques for delivery of the shoulders and arms, and it does not matter which shoulder is delivered first. Typically, the anterior shoulder will appear as a result of the downward traction placed on the body. Once the axilla is visible, the arm can then be delivered by reaching in to the elbow and sweeping the arm up across the chest. Once the anterior arm is out, the infant should be rotated 180 degrees, keeping the back up. This will bring the posterior scapula and axilla into view anteriorly, and this arm can be delivered in the same manner.

17. *Delivery of the posterior arm.* If the anterior shoulder does not appear with downward traction, the posterior arm can be delivered first. Grasp the feet securely in one hand and lift the body up and over toward the abdominal side until the scapula and axilla are visible posteriorly at the perineum. Insert the other hand along the upper arm to the elbow and sweep the arm across the chest. Now the infant can be either repositioned with downward traction again or rotated until the anterior shoulder and axilla are in view (**Figure 30D-5**).

18. Engagement of the head usually occurs in one of the oblique pelvic diameters. Internal rotation is facilitated by delivery of the shoulders; once the arms are released, the head is generally in an occiput anterior position, with the back of the neck visible at the vaginal introitus.

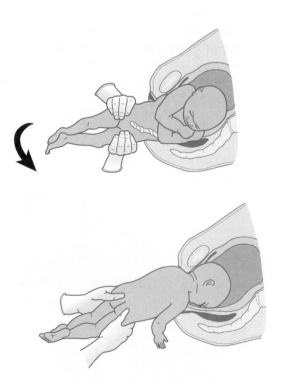

Figure 30D-3 Midwife's hands placed on lower body with thumbs over sacral iliac joint.

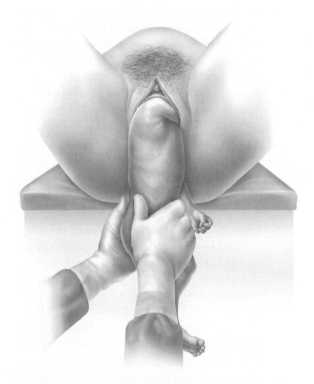

Figure 30D-4 Birth of the anterior shoulder by downward traction. Note placement of the hands on the infant's hips.

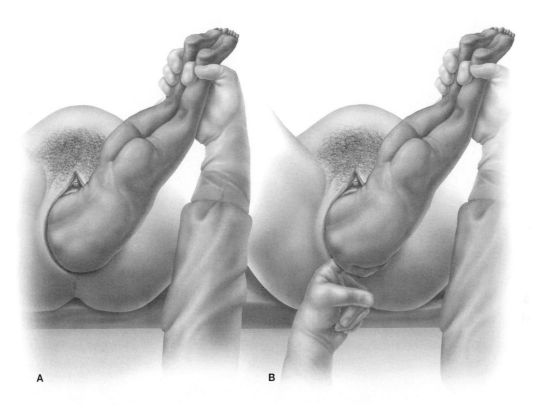

Figure 30D-5 Delivery of the posterior arm: (A) birth of the posterior shoulder by upward traction; (B) freeing the posterior arm.

19. It is very important *not* to let the head rotate to the occiput posterior position, as any traction on the body will cause extension of the head and increase the chances of entrapment.

20. Delivery of the head is best accomplished using the *Mauriceau-Smellie-Veit maneuver* (**Figure 30D-6**). There are several variations of this maneuver, in which the hand is inserted posteriorly into the vagina and the fingers are positioned carefully in and/or around the baby's mouth to facilitate flexion of the head. Most commonly, the index and middle fingers are placed on either side of the nose on the maxilla and downward pressure is applied to maintain flexion of the head. Extreme care must be taken to avoid any pressure on the lower jaw or accidently inserting the fingers into the orbit of the eyes. Although insertion of a finger into the infant's mouth is sometimes described as part of this maneuver, this modification could cause serious damage to the tongue and surrounding tissues.

21. Once the fingers of the posterior hand are in place on the maxilla, rest the infant's body astride the length of the arm. Place the other hand on top of the infant and hook the index and middle fingers of this hand onto the shoulders on each side of the infant's neck. The fingers can also be placed along the occiput to splint the infant's head between the hands to prevent any extension of the neck and head.

22. An assistant should be directed to perform suprapubic pressure to maintain flexion of the head during this part of the birth.

23. Continue to apply downward traction with the infant sandwiched between the arms/hands until the hairline is visible under the symphysis pubis. Care must be taken to avoid pressure on the brachial plexus.

24. Once the hairline is visible, upward traction is applied while elevating the body of the baby. Following the curve of Carus, the chin, face, brow, anterior fontanelle, and the remainder of the head are delivered in sequence across the perineum.

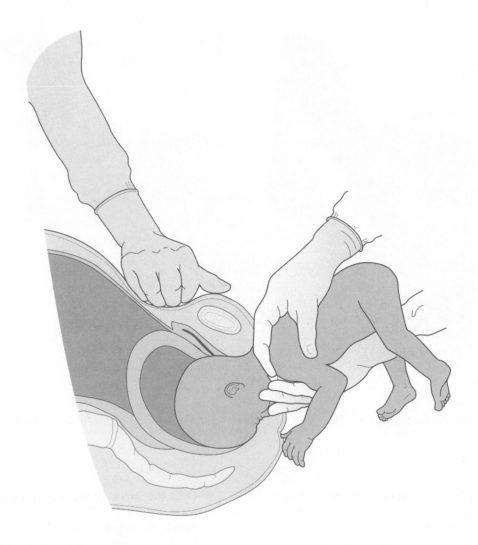

Figure 30D-6 Mauriceau-Smellie-Veit maneuver with suprapubic pressure.

● ● ● References

1. Yeomans ER, Gilstrap LC. Breech delivery. In Queenan JT, Spong CY, Lockwood CJ, eds. *Queenan's Management of High-Risk Pregnancy: An Evidence-Based Approach*. 6th ed. Malden, MA: Wiley-Blackwell; 2012:424-428.

2. Glezerman M. Planned vaginal breech delivery: current status and the need to reconsider. *Expert Rev Obstet Gynecol*. 2012;7:159-166.

3. Alarab M, Regan C, O'Connell MP, Keane DP, O'Herlihy C, Foley ME. Singleton vaginal breech delivery at term: still a safe option. *Obstet Gynecol*. 2004; 103:407-412.

4. American College of Obstetricians and Gynecologists. ACOG Committee Opinion no. 306: mode of term singleton breech delivery. *Obstet Gynecol*. 2006; 108:235-237.

C H A P T E R

31

The Third and Fourth Stages of Labor

MAVIS N. SCHORN

TEKOA L. KING

Introduction

The birth of a child is exciting and the zenith of an intense and emotional period for the birthing woman and her family. However, the time immediately following the birth is also a critical one for both the woman and her newborn. The expulsion of the placenta and physiologic stabilization immediately following this event represent a period of great vulnerability. Postpartum hemorrhage (PPH) is one of the leading causes of childbirth-related maternal morbidity and mortality, both worldwide and in the United States; when it occurs, it most often does so during the third or fourth stage of labor.[1] Moreover, the first hour after birth is a "sensitive period" psychologically and physiologically, wherein continuous contact potentially has significant benefits for both the woman and her infant.[2] This chapter reviews the third and fourth stages of labor, methods for facilitating normal physiologic adaptation, complications that can occur during these time periods, and management strategies for these complications.

Physiology of the Third Stage of Labor

The third stage of labor is defined as the period following the birth of the newborn through the expulsion of the placenta. The length of time for this stage is usually within 10 minutes.[3] Based on a review of more than 12,000 births, only 3% of third stages take longer than 30 minutes to complete.[4] Thus more than 30 minutes without placental expulsion is commonly considered a retained placenta.

Placental Separation

Contraction frequency and intensity in the third stage of labor are similar to their counterparts during the second stage of labor,[5,6] although the intensity of the contractions often is felt minimally if at all by the woman, especially in comparison to contractions immediately before the birth of the neonate. These post-birth contractions constrict the blood vessels that supply the placenta, thereby causing hemostasis. Placental separation is the result of an abrupt decrease in size of the uterine cavity during and following the birth of the neonate. As the uterus contracts, the placental implantation surface area decreases without a corresponding change in the placental size. This sudden disproportion between the area of implantation and placental size causes the placenta to buckle and separate from the decidua.[7]

After the placenta separates, it descends through the lower uterine segment and into the upper vaginal vault, causing clinical signs of placental separation. Table 31-1 lists the common signs of placental separation. During placental separation, women who do not have analgesia may experience a slight increase in the perception of contraction intensity and pelvic floor discomfort.

Placental Expulsion

After placental separation, the placenta passes through the cervix into the vaginal vault and is expelled. Expulsion of the placenta occurs by one of two mechanisms: Shultz or Duncan.[7] The majority of the time the Schultz mechanism occurs, although both mechanisms are considered normal.

Table 31-1	Signs of Placental Separation
Signs of Placental Separation	**Explanation**
A small gush of blood	With separation, some blood escapes from between the placenta and the decidua.
Lengthening of the umbilical cord	As the placenta descends into the vagina, the cord lengthens at the vaginal introitus.
Rise of the uterus into the abdomen	As the placenta descends into the vagina, the uterus is displaced cephalad.
The uterus becomes firm and rounded	Once the placenta is expelled from the uterus, the uterine smooth muscles contract more firmly, altering the shape of the uterus.

The Schultz mechanism results when the placenta separates centrally; the fetal side of the placenta—the side with a smooth, shining membrane continuous with the sheath of the chorion (which also covers the umbilical cord)—drops to the lower portion of the uterus, and then exits through the cervix into the vagina and on to the woman's pelvic floor. At that point, the placenta is expelled, fetal side first. The membranes are expelled last, with the maternal side of the placenta inside the amniotic sac. This mechanism, in effect, inverts the placenta and amniotic sac and causes the membranes to peel off the remainder of the decidua and trail behind the placenta. The majority of bleeding that occurs during this mechanism may remain hidden until the placenta and membranes are expelled, as the blood is captured behind the placenta and inside the amniotic sac (**Figure 31-1**).

Schultz

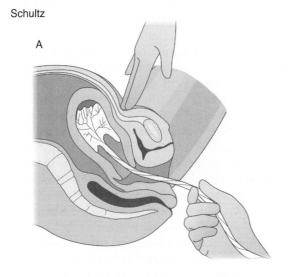

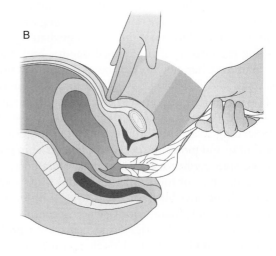

Duncan

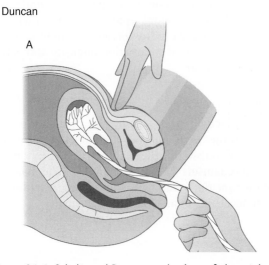

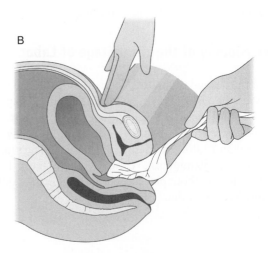

Figure 31-1 Schultz and Duncan mechanisms of placental expulsion.

In contrast, the placenta that separates marginally is known as the Duncan mechanism. This mechanism allows the placenta to slide to the cervical opening without inverting, so that the maternal side of the placenta, with dark red cotyledons, is expelled at the same time as the fetal side. Blood escapes between the membranes and uterine wall and is more likely to be visible externally earlier in the separation process. The amniotic sac is not inverted but trails behind the placenta.

The memory aid for correctly identifying the mechanisms of placental expulsion is based on the appearance of the two different sides of the placenta first seen at the vaginal introitus. The fetal side is shiny and glistening from the fetal membranes covering the placenta, whereas the maternal side is dark and beefy—hence the sayings "Shiny Schultz" and "Dirty Duncan." In past years, some sources have suggested that there is a higher risk of postpartum bleeding when trailing membranes are apparent (as in the Duncan mechanism), but no evidence has been found to substantiate this belief.

Length of the Third Stage

The third stage of labor can occur rapidly, within a few minutes after the birth of the neonate, or it can take several minutes longer. The outer limit of normalcy has not been determined. Because the risk of complications increases with longer duration of the third stage, an understanding of normal third-stage timing is important. A study of more than 45,000 births found that 90% of term placentas will be expelled spontaneously within 15 minutes and 97.8% will be expelled within 30 minutes.[8] When third-stage labor is longer than 30 minutes, the odds of having a postpartum hemorrhage are 6 times higher than if the third stage is less than 30 minutes.[8]

Techniques Used in the Management of Third-Stage Labor

Although research in the area of third-stage management has been increasing, little is known about how the first or second stages of labor affect the third stage. Evidence-based management of the third stage is controversial and practices vary. Best practice is rapidly evolving as ongoing research reveals more information about how to provide safe care while also promoting holistic, physiologic management.

Physiologic Versus Active Management

The two recommended approaches of third-stage management are commonly described as physiologic (expectant) management and active management.[9,10] Table 31-2 compares these two approaches. The physiologic approach is a noninterventionist approach[10,11] and the strategy that is more commonly followed by midwives in many parts of the world.[9,10,12] In contrast, active management is an approach recommended by the International Confederation of Midwives (ICM), the International Federation of Gynecologists and Obstetricians (FIGO), and the World Health Organization (WHO).[13–15] Studies have shown that birth attendants and birth facilities often use a mixed approach that incorporates portions of each approach rather than strictly following one or the other.[12,16]

Active management of the third stage has been shown to decrease the risk of postpartum hemorrhage in a general obstetric population.[10] Thus, this strategy is of particular import in low-resource settings where treatment of postpartum hemorrhage is not readily available. The active management approach initially evaluated in randomized controlled trials (RCTs) included three facets: (1) controlled cord traction to facilitate placental expulsion, (2) early cord clamping and cutting, and (3) the routine administration of a prophylactic uterotonic.[17] However, the single components of active management were not well studied, and each has possible adverse consequences when examined individually. Thus the recommended components of active management of the third stage have evolved over time as new information has emerged.[10,18] The most recent evidence suggests that the administration of a uterotonic agent during the third stage of labor is the most effective treatment for prevention of postpartum hemorrhage and perhaps the only component within the active management triad that has consistent clinical utility.[19]

The current joint ICM/FIGO statement recommends three steps: (1) controlled cord traction (once pulsation stops in a healthy newborn); (2) use of a uterotonic agent; and (3) fundal massage after delivery of the placenta.[14] Early cord-clamping was not included secondary to reflect evidence that delayed cord-clamping has significant benefits for the newborn.[20] WHO recommends use of a uterotonic agent in all settings, but controlled cord traction only in settings wherein a skilled obstetric attendant is present; in support of this recommendation, WHO cites evidence that both controlled cord traction and early cord-clamping can be harmful to the mother and the infant, respectively.[15] Sustained fundal massage is not recommended.[15]

A variety of uterotonic drugs are available, and debate continues about the best route and dose. Current guidelines from ICM/FIGO and WHO

Table 31-2	A Comparison of Physiologic and Active Management Approaches to Management of the Third Stage of Labor	
Interventions	**Physiologic Management**	**Active Management**
Maternal positioning	Upright positioning of the mother to promote gravity assistance	Not addressed
Delayed cord-clamping	Yes	WHO recommends delayed cord-clamping ICM/FIGO has a footnote attached to the recommendation for controlled cord-clamping stating that delaying cord-clamping by 1 to 3 minutes reduces anemia in the newborn
Cord traction	No—generally a "hands-off" approach with spontaneous expulsion by the mother	Yes—continuous gentle cord traction following signs of placenta separation
Maternal efforts to expel the placenta	Yes	Not addressed
External uterine massage following placental expulsion	No—generally a "hands-off" approach to the uterus	Yes (ICM/FIGO only)
Routine administration of a uterotonic agent	No	Yes
Early infant suckling	Yes	Not addressed
Draining the umbilical cord	Not addressed	Not addressed
FIGO = International Federation of Gynecology and Obstetrics; ICM = International Confederation of Midwives; WHO = World Health Organization		

recommend oxytocin (Pitocin) 10 IU administered intramuscularly or intravenously in solution as the first choice.[13–15] Although the guidelines refer to administration of oxytocin after the birth of the infant, this medication can be given as the anterior shoulder is released under the symphysis pubis, during the birth of the neonate, after the birth of the infant, or after placental expulsion. The timing does not influence the amount of bleeding or the rate of postpartum hemorrhage.[21] Administration of a uterotonic agent with the birth of the neonate is effective and safe unless the woman has a multiple gestation and another fetus present in the uterus. Some midwives have expressed concern that administering the uterotonic before the placenta is delivered will increase the risk of an entrapped placenta; however, this has not occurred in any of the studies of uterotonics and is therefore a theoretical concern without supporting clinical evidence.

Physiologic Management

Physiologic management of the third stage includes no routine uterotonic administration, delayed cord-clamping, and gentle—if any—cord traction. Maternal efforts to expel the placenta are encouraged. Begley et al. conducted a meta-analysis of RCTs that compared active management of labor to physiologic management for the Cochrane Collaboration.[10] Although there was heterogeneity in how the components of physiologic management were implemented in the studies, the analysis found that there was no significant differences in the risk for severe PPH (relative risk [RR], 0.31; 95% confidence interval [CI], 0.05–2.17; $n = 2941$) in women who did not have an a priori risk for postpartum hemorrhage. However, the women in the active management arm did have a significant reduction in estimated blood loss more than 500 mL (RR, 0.33; 95% CI, 0.20–0.56; $n = 2941$), blood transfusion (RR, 0.30; 95% CI, 0.10–0.88; $n = 3134$), and need for therapeutic uterotonic administration (RR, 0.15; 95% CI, 0.11–0.21; $n = 3134$).[10] Therefore women who are at low risk for postpartum hemorrhage may be offered physiologic management in settings that have ready access to treatments for PPH, whereas active management may be more efficacious in low-resource settings.

Mixed Management

Mixed management consists of some components of both active and physiologic management of the third stage. The primary change in practice that has resulted in a mixed management strategy is the introduction of delayed cord-clamping, which has proven benefits for the newborn. In this scenario, a midwife may routinely administer a uterotonic agent after the birth but delay clamping the cord either for an arbitrary period of time or until it stops pulsating, then apply gentle controlled cord traction.[22]

Uterotonic Medications

The uterotonic most frequently used to prevent postpartum hemorrhage is oxytocin (Pitocin). This inexpensive agent has the fewest side effects compared to other uterotonic medications. Oxytocin may be administered as an intramuscular injection or intravenously in solution, although never as an undiluted intravenous bolus. However, oxytocin may not be as effective for women who received large doses of this medication during labor for induction or augmentation. In this case, an additional uterotonic agent may be indicated. **Table 31-3** summarizes the dose,

contraindications, and side effects of the uterotonics used in clinical practice.[23] Complementary treatments such as homeopathy, herbs, and Chinese medicine may be considered if the midwife is proficient in these techniques, although research documenting these interventions' effectiveness has not been published.

Cord Traction

Continuous cord traction initially was recommended as part of the active management package, along with early cord-clamping, because of the concern that with early administration of a uterotonic agent, the placenta should be expelled quickly to avoid entrapment.[1] Now that delayed cord-clamping has been shown to improve newborn outcomes and entrapment of the placenta has not been found to occur,[24] the rationale for controlled cord traction is less convincing.

To perform cord traction, following signs of placental separation, the midwife applies gentle counter-traction to the lower uterine segment abdominally

Table 31-3	Uterotonics for the Third and Fourth Stages of Labor		
Generic Drug (Brand)	**Dose and Route**	**Contraindications**	**Side Effects**
First-Line Therapy			
Oxytocin (Pitocin)	20–40 U in 1000 mL of normal saline or lactated Ringer's solution run continuously *or* 10 U intramuscular injection	Never give undiluted as a bolus injection	Cramping Water intoxication (hyponatremia)
Second-Line Therapy			
Misoprostol (Cytotec)	800 mcg per rectum, one dose (Range: 400–1000 mcg)		Shivering and fever are most common side effects Diarrhea and abdominal pain possible
Methylergonovine maleate (Methergine)	0.2 mg intramuscular injection May repeat in 5 minutes Thereafter every 2–4 hours	Hypertension	Cramping Nausea and vomiting Hypertension, seizure, and/or headache
15-methyl-$F_{2\alpha}$-prostaglandin (Hemabate)	0.25 mg intramuscular injection May repeat every 15–90 minutes up to 8 doses	Asthma or active cardiac, pulmonary, renal, or hepatic disease	Vomiting and diarrhea, nausea, temperature elevation
Dinoprostone (Prostin E_2)	20 mg vaginal or rectal suppository May repeat every 2 hours	Hypotension	Vomiting and diarrhea, nausea, temperature elevation

Source: Adapted from Lowe N, King TL. Labor. In: King TL, Brucker MC, eds. *Pharmacology for Women's Health.* Sudbury, MA: Jones and Bartlett; 2011:1102.

with one hand, while the other hand applies continuous gentle downward traction on the cord. An instrument such as a hemostat is used to clamp the umbilical cord close to where it exits the introitus; alternatively, a piece of gauze can be wrapped around the cord to allow tension to be easily applied. The traction should follow the curve of Carus. For example, if the woman is in a semi-recumbent position, the cord is guided inferiorly as the placenta descends to the pelvic floor, and as the placenta becomes visible at the introitus, the cord is guided superiorly.

If the woman is in a squatting or other upright position, cord traction is likely not necessary and may even be dangerous. Excessive cord traction increases the risk for uterine inversion—a risk that theoretically might be further increased if the woman is in an upright position. A woman in an upright position will likely feel the pressure of the placenta as it descends to the pelvic floor and spontaneously expel it.

Umbilical Cord Drainage

Umbilical cord drainage in the third stage of labor involves the removal of the clamp from the previously clamped and cut umbilical cord (after necessary cord blood samples have been obtained) and allowing the blood from the cord and placenta to drain. In a meta-analysis of three RCTs ($n = 1257$), Soltani et al. found that cord drainage may reduce the length of the third stage of labor by approximately 3 minutes and total blood loss by less than 80 mL when compared to no cord drainage.[25] It is questionable whether this is a clinically important finding. No decrease in third-stage complications was found when the umbilical cord was drained as compared to when the umbilical cord was not drained.[25] If umbilical cord drainage is incorporated into third-stage management, the blood should not be counted in the maternal blood loss, as this is fetal blood.

External Uterine Massage Following Placental Expulsion

Uterine massage following the expulsion of the placenta is a component of active management of the third stage of labor that is recommended by both ICM and FIGO.[13,14] However, the precise benefit, if there is one, of routine external uterine massage is still undetermined. One RCT has been published that compared uterine massage to no uterine massage in three groups of women who received uterine massage, uterotonics, or both, respectively.[26] The incidence of blood loss of more than 300 mL and need for more uterotonics was statistically higher in the women who received uterine massage only.[27] Nevertheless, when oxytocin was used, there appeared to be no

additional benefit from uterine massage. If a uterotonic agent is administered, external massage may not further increase the protection against an early postpartum hemorrhage; moreover, it can cause significant maternal discomfort.[27] Uterine massage before expulsion of the placenta is not recommended because if the uterus is massaged before the placenta separates from the uterine wall, the massage may cause incomplete separation of the placenta, resulting in iatrogenic hemorrhage.

Blood Loss Measurement

Measurement of blood loss at birth provides objective data about the woman's health status following birth. Visual estimation of blood loss has been routine practice for many years, although repeated studies have demonstrated the inaccuracy of this simple method.[28] If there is a large blood loss, the amount is usually underestimated visually. If visual estimation is the usual method of evaluating blood loss, it is beneficial to have experience through regular laboratory simulation to improve estimation accuracy.

Although training improves the accuracy of blood loss estimation, alternative quantitative methods of assessing blood loss can be used. Two methods that are relatively easy to implement are measuring and weighing. A calibrated under-buttocks drape can be used to measure blood loss. If a calibrated drape is not available or the woman gives birth in a position that does not allow for an under-buttocks drape (e.g., supported squat), weighing blood-saturated items can be implemented. Because *1 gram is equivalent to 1 milliliter in volume*, weighing blood-saturated items and subtracting the weight of the item when dry provides a relatively accurate quantitative measurement of blood loss. Either the pads or calibrated drapes should be used immediately after birth to limit additional content such as amniotic fluid or urine from being mixed with postpartum blood.

Some birth sites routinely obtain a quantitative measure of blood loss; however, this step can also be instituted if blood loss is estimated to be higher than normal to improve accuracy and guide management. **Figure 31-2** presents a sample worksheet with the weight of commonly used items that can be used to expedite the process of calculating a quantitative measure of blood loss.[29]

Midwifery Management of the Third Stage of Labor

The sequential steps for midwifery management of the third stage of labor are presented in **Appendix 31A**.

Item	Approximate dry weight (grams)	Number of items weighed	Wet weight (grams)	Wet weight minus dry weight equals milliliters (mL) of fluid/blood	Total per category
Blue Chux	35				
Kendall Curity Maternity Pads	14				
Maxithins	11				
Cloth soaker pad	465				
Dry lap sponge (large)	22				
Dry lap sponge (small)	14				
Graduated container volume	Estimated amniotic fluid volume = 100	Number of containers			
	Total estimated blood loss (mL)				

EXAMPLE

Item	Approximate dry weight (grams)	Number of items weighed	Wet weight (grams)	Wet weight minus dry weight equals milliliters (mL) of fluid/blood	Total per category
Blue Chux	35	1	135	135 – 35 = 100 mL	100 mL
Kendall Curity Maternity Pads	14	2	124	124 – 28 = 96 mL	96 mL
Maxithins	11				
Cloth soaker pad	465				
Dry lap sponge (large)	22	10	600	600 – 220 = 380 mL	380 mL
Dry lap sponge (small)	14				
Graduated container volume	Estimated amniotic fluid volume = 100	1 container	250	250 – 100 = 150 mL	150 mL
	Total estimated blood loss (mL)				726 mL

Figure 31-2 Sample measurement of blood loss report.
Source: Reprinted with permission from California Maternal Quality Care Collaborative/California Department of Public Health MCAH Division.

Supporting Women's Choices

Maternal requests for not intervening in the natural progress of the third stage are important to address prior to labor. It is important to discuss how to support normalcy during the third stage while also recommending interventions known to minimize the risk for postpartum hemorrhage. Prenatal preventive measures such as a healthy diet that prevents anemia will lessen adverse effects of blood loss at birth. Avoiding procedures during labor and birth that increase blood loss, such as induction, augmentation, and episiotomy, also decreases the risk of hemorrhage. Conversely, delaying the use of uterotonics until bleeding is excessive may increase a woman's risk of hemorrhage.

The placenta, cord, and membranes have special cultural or spiritual significance in many cultures.

Additional maternal requests for third-stage management may be quite varied. Rituals related to the placenta exist in many cultures today. Thus the woman or family may want to save the placenta for a variety of purposes. The ritual of burying the placenta may be undertaken for the purpose of protecting the child, protecting the woman, or establishing a spiritual or sacred link between the land and the child.[30] Parents may also be interested in leaving the placenta attached to the newborn until the cord falls off spontaneously, often referred to as a lotus birth.[31,32] Some women consume the placenta, raw or cooked, or encapsulated in pill form with the hope of preventing postpartum depression.[33,34]

Rituals also may involve the umbilical cord and even the membranes. The cord may be kept as a charm or used for medicinal purposes. Traditionally, when a newborn is born in a caul (i.e., with membranes over the head), it means that the child will never drown; thus these membranes have been sold to sailors for protection. When a woman has a special request, the focus should be on safety while also attempting to honor her request. Honoring the variety of beliefs surrounding this amazing organ is important whenever possible.

The Placenta

After the uterus is evaluated and massaged, and the uterine bleeding has slowed, a methodical inspection of the placenta should be performed. Routine inspection of the placenta assists in recognition of abnormal findings and reduces the likelihood of overlooking a significant finding. The steps for inspection of the cord, placenta, and membranes are reviewed in **Appendix 31B**.

Table 31-4 lists common variations noted with the cord, placenta, and membranes. Some variations, such as a true knot in the cord, may be simple incidental findings yet also associated with an increased risk for newborn morbidity. When observed, their presence should be noted in the health records of both the woman and the newborn.

Routine placental evaluation by a pathologist usually is not indicated for all placentas. **Table 31-5** lists some of the findings that are commonly used as indications for a pathology examination.[35,36]

The Fourth Stage of Labor

The term *fourth stage of labor* refers to the first postpartum hour following placental expulsion. Immediately following the expulsion of the placenta, a number of maternal changes occur as the physical and emotional stresses of labor and birth resolve and postpartum recovery and bonding begin. Close observation and frequent assessment are needed during the fourth stage of labor, as this is a time of both physical vulnerability to emergent complications and heightened sensitivity as the woman is introduced to her newborn. **Box 31-1** reviews basic management of the fourth stage of labor.

Bonding and Attachment: Birth of a New Family

Emotional attachment between a woman and her newborn has lifelong implications. The term *bonding* refers to the emotional tie the parent has to the infant; the term *attachment* generally refers to the infant's tie to a caregiver.

The theory that there is a biologically determined critical period immediately after birth during which maternal–newborn bonding takes place was first proposed by Klaus and Kennell in the 1970s.[37] They found that skin-to-skin contact between the woman and her newborn in the first hour after birth resulted in more attachment behavior by a woman toward her infant up to a month after birth. Subsequent animal and human studies of bonding in the first postpartum hour have found that healthy newborn infants do undergo a predictable series of behaviors immediately after birth, including crawling toward the mother's breast, rooting and suckling, and looking at the mother's face.[38] It is theorized that this behavior is stimulated by maternal odor and voice recognition.[39]

There is an important caveat to the bonding theory, however: Much of this work is based on animal studies, wherein immediate imprinting of the infant to the caregiver is biologically species specific. Superimposing the results of animal studies on human behavior may result in beliefs that have no scientific basis. Thus it is important that midwives know what human studies have shown with regard to maternal–infant bonding

Early Continuous Contact and Skin-to-Skin Contact

Early skin-to-skin contact involves placing a naked newborn prone on the woman's abdomen or chest immediately or soon after birth. The infant is dried and the area of the infant's body that is not touching the mother's skin is covered with a blanket to assist in maintaining warmth. A cap may be applied to the dried head of the newborn to assist with temperature maintenance. The vital signs of the newborn and woman are monitored with the infant on the maternal chest. Other procedures are delayed for at least 1 hour or until after the first successful breastfeeding.

Continuous maternal–neonatal contact and skin-to-skin touching have been found to improve maternal affectionate behavior, regulate the newborn's behavior, and increase the duration of breastfeeding.[38] Early contact also has been found to increase maternal sensitivity and the infant's self-regulation and irritability at 1 year after birth.[40] Moore et al. conducted a meta-analysis of 30 RCTs of early skin-to-skin contact ($n = 1925$) and found that skin-to-skin contact improved breastfeeding and breastfeeding duration at 1 to 4 months. Positive trends in improved summary scores for maternal affectionate love/touch, maternal attachment behavior, and shorter duration of infant crying were also noted in

Table 31-4	Umbilical Cord, Placenta, and Membrane Variations
Variation	**Significance**
Variations in Appearance of the Umbilical Cord	
Two-vessel cord	A two-vessel cord occurs in 0.5% to 1% of neonates. Two-vessel cords are associated with gastrointestinal, genitourinary, and cardiovascular abnormalities.
Long cord	A long cord, more than 75 cm, is associated with knots and fetal entanglement, as well as increased amniotic fluid and fetal activity.
Short cord	Short cords, less than 32 cm, are associated with disorders that limit fetal movement, such as Down syndrome, neuromuscular disorders, and fetal limb dysfunction. Short cords are associated with fetal heart rate abnormalities in labor as a result of traction on the cord with fetal descent.
Thin cord	Associated with oligohydramnios and poor fetal growth.
Thick cord	Associated with polyhydramnios and macrosomia.
Marginal (Battledore) insertion	The cord is inserted at or within 1.5 cm of the margin of the placenta. May be an insignificant finding but is associated with preterm labor, abnormal fetal heart rate patterns in labor (compression), and bleeding in labor (vessel rupture).
Velamentous insertion	The umbilical cord vessels run through the amnion and chorion before entering the placenta, leaving the vessels unprotected. This type of insertion may lead to rupture and fetal hemorrhage, particularly if associated with vasa previa (transcervical position). This finding is more common in twin placenta.
Knots, loops, torsion, or strictures	These variations are associated with increased fetal mortality and morbidity.
Variations in Appearance of the Placenta	
Pale placenta	A pale placenta is associated with immature neonates and anemia. Edematous, pale, and bulky placentas are seen with immune and nonimmune hydrops fetalis, twin-to-twin transfusion syndrome, fetal congestive heart failure, and infection.
Green-stained placenta	With extended exposure to meconium, a placenta may be stained green.
Calcifications	The maternal surface is usually smooth but may have gritty white areas of calcification. Generally, the quantity of calcifications has no clinical importance.
Missing cotyledon	Incomplete expulsion of the placenta. It is associated with uterine atony and postpartum infection.
Small, light placenta	A small placenta is less than the 10% percentile for gestational age and may be associated with intrauterine infections, genetic mutations, or hypertension.
Large, heavy placenta	A large placenta, more than the 90% percentile for gestational age, is often due to various maternal or fetal conditions such as maternal diabetes, fetal erythroblastosis and fetal hydrops, fetal congestive heart failure, and maternal–fetal syphilis.
Infarctions	A localized area of ischemic tissue necrosis that occurs when there is an obstruction of the villus blood supply. Placental infarctions are most common at the periphery of the placenta. Small infarctions are normal variants. Larger infarctions are associated with hypertension, stillbirth, placental abruption, and fetal growth restriction. Any condition that interferes with uteroplacental circulation can lead to placental infarcts.
Nodules or plaques on the fetal surface	Associated with oligohydramnios and renal agenesis, squamous metaplasia (benign), and infection.
Foul odor	Associated with infection.

Table 31-4	**Umbilical Cord, Placenta, and Membrane Variations** *(continued)*
Variation	**Significance**
Variations in Appearance of the Placenta *(continued)*	
Circumvallate placenta	The membranes appear to arise not from the edge of the placenta but a short distance inward toward the umbilical cord. The area of the chorionic plate is thus reduced. Fetal membranes fold back upon themselves, creating a dense, gray/white ring around the outer margin of the placenta. The fetal vessels stop at this ring. The risk of placental abruption is increased with this variation. Possible causes include a variety of developmental abnormalities. Usually this finding is insignificant, but it has been associated with threatened abortion, preterm labor, painless vaginal bleeding after 20 weeks' gestation, placental insufficiency, fetal growth restriction, and intrapartum and postpartum hemorrhage.
Marginate or circummarginate placenta	A form of circumvallate placenta wherein the fetal membranes do not fold back, creating the white ring. In this variation, it appears as placental tissue extending beyond the marginate ring where the membranes arise. Usually this finding is insignificant.
Succenturiate placenta	One or more smaller accessory lobes of placenta are developed in the membranes and are attached to the main placenta by fetal vessels. This finding is more common in multiple gestations. The accessory lobes may be retained, leading to postpartum hemorrhage or infection. These placentas can be associated with velamentous insertion of the cord.
Bilobate placenta	Also referred to as bipartite or duplex. A placenta with three or more lobes is referred to as multilobate.
Variations in Appearance of the Membranes	
Cloudy membranes	Associated with infection.
Incomplete membranes	Remnants of membranes are usually spontaneously expelled after the birth; however, they can cause subinvolution of the uterus, uterine atony, or infection if retained.

Table 31-5	**Clinical Conditions That Are Indications for Pathology Examination of the Placenta**	
Maternal Indications	**Fetal or Neonatal Indications**	**Placental Indications**
Maternal fever or chorioamnionitis	Gestational age < 34 weeks or > 42 weeks	Cord abnormalities
Abruption, unexplained third-trimester bleeding, or excessive bleeding	Stillbirth/early neonatal death	Gross placental abnormalities
Systemic disorder with clinical concerns for mother or neonate (e.g., diabetes, hypertension, collagen disease, seizures, severe anemia, autoimmune disease)	Newborn with abnormal umbilical cord blood gas values or low Apgar scores	
	Multiple gestation	
Infection during this pregnancy (e.g., HIV, syphilis, cytomegalovirus, primary herpes, toxoplasmosis, rubella)	Fetal growth restriction	
	Thick meconium	
Severe oligohydramnios or polyhydramnios	Very-low-birth-weight infant	
Substance abuse	Neonatal neurologic problems	

Sources: Adapted from Curtin WM, Krauss S, Metlay LA, Katzman PJ. Pathologic examination of the placenta and observed practice. *Obstet Gynecol.* 2007;109:35-41; Gibbs RS, Rosenberg AR, Warren CJ, Galan HL, Rumack CM. Suggestions for practice to accompany neonatal encephalopathy and cerebral palsy. *Obstet Gynecol.* 2004;103:778-779.

BOX 31-1 Management of the Fourth Stage of Labor Following Normal Spontaneous Vaginal Birth

Physical Examination and Management

Vital Signs

Check vital signs regularly every 5 to 15 minutes depending on the amount of bleeding present.

Bleeding

Evaluate vaginal bleeding every 5 to 15 minutes immediately after the birth of the infant. The majority of postpartum hemorrhages occur during the fourth stage of labor. Continue to assess maternal bleeding frequently.

Uterus

Evaluate the uterus every 5 to 15 minutes.

- *Position*. Assess the uterus by abdominal palpation; it is usually midline in the middle of the abdomen, approximately two-thirds to three-fourths of the way up between the symphysis pubis and the umbilicus. If the uterus is above the umbilicus or significantly deviated to one side of the umbilicus, it may be due to the presence of blood and clots in the uterus or displacement from a full bladder. Evacuation of the uterus or emptying of the bladder should be considered.

- *Tone*. Assess the tone of the uterus; it should be firm to the touch. A soft, boggy uterus is not well contracted. External uterine massage and assessment of bleeding are indicated in such a case. Assess for postpartum hemorrhage and presence of blood or clots in the uterus if the uterus does not become firm following abdominal massage.

Bladder

Evaluate the bladder immediately after the third stage and at least 30 minutes after birth. A distended bladder can cause increased uterine bleeding, as the uterus is unable to contract when the bladder is full and displacing it.

A woman without regional anesthesia usually can void spontaneously. If she has regional anesthesia, she may need a catheterization to empty the bladder.

Perineum

Evaluate the perineum immediately after the birth or after the third stage of labor. Inspect the vagina and perineum for lacerations, bruising, or early hematoma formation. Inspect the cervix if indicated. Edema or bruising at the introitus or throughout the perineal area should be noted and documented.

Additional Assessments and Care Practices

- Count needles and gauzes used in the birth to ensure that no gauze is inadvertently left in the vagina and all sharps are disposed of safely. Remove any sharps from the sterile field.

- Clean the mother and bed as needed.

- A perineal pad or ice pack may be placed against the perineum to reduce edema and provide pain relief. Ice may be placed next to the perineum intermittently for the first 24 hours post delivery.

- Position the mother to promote infant latch. Skin-to-skin placement of the neonate following birth allows mothers to notice when their neonates are beginning to root.

- Assess for maternal comfort. Tremor not associated with infection can be common in the fourth stage of labor and can be relieved with warm blankets, reassurance, and relaxation techniques.

- Assess maternal intake and encourage intake of oral fluids.

- Assess family dynamics.

---

the group that experienced early skin-to-skin contact. In addition, premature infants have better cardiorespiratory stability when exposed to skin-to-skin contact with their mothers.[41] Some hospitals in the United States now institute skin-to-skin contact in the operating room and recovery room when a woman has a cesarean section (**Figure 31-3**).

Newborn Self-Latching

When healthy term infants are placed in skin-to-skin contact during the first hours following birth, they frequently crawl and find the areola by themselves, and most will initiate suckling spontaneously.[38]

Supporting newborn interaction with the parents may enhance the newborn's ability to self-regulate his or her behavior over the long term (i.e., improved sleep, social-interactive behavior, and language development).[38] The wide-ranging positive effects of unrestricted maternal–newborn contact reinforce the importance of protecting the family in the first hours after birth from unnecessary intervention.

Inclusion of the Father, Partner, and/or Significant Others

Involvement of the woman's partner, newborn's father, or other support persons during the third and

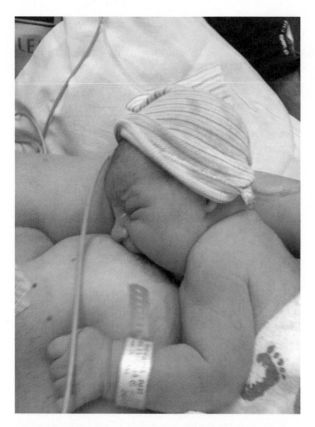

Figure 31-3 Skin-to-skin contact and breastfeeding immediately after cesarean section.

fourth stages of labor has been found to help the woman during the postpartum period,[42] increase the partner's emotional involvement with the neonate,[43] and increase the sense of security experienced by the partner.[44] Men and lesbian partners have expressed feeling helpless, useless, anxious, out of place, and vulnerable during birth; thus, including family members in the experience is an important component of family-centered midwifery care.[45,46]

For all these reasons, it is important to assess and address the partner's needs during the third and fourth stages of labor to facilitate the transition to parenthood. Strategies include anticipatory guidance and explanations to the woman and her significant others. Support via midwifery presence and information has been found to enhance the birth experience of the partner.[47] Engaging partners in activities such as cutting the cord and skin-to-skin contact has been found to enhance their emotional involvement with the neonate.[43] Additional activities may include encouraging continued support for the woman during required genital tract repair, engaging in observation of neonatal transition, and assistance with initial breastfeeding.

Early Breastfeeding

Evidence that breastfeeding improves health outcomes for women and their infants is overwhelming and reviewed in detail in the *Breastfeeding and the Mother–Newborn Dyad* chapter. Initiation of breastfeeding in the first few hours after birth is recommended, as the infant is alert and awake during this time period. Activities during the fourth stage of labor that have been found to promote early breastfeeding include skin-to-skin contact between the newborn and mother following birth and maintaining this contact for the first few hours of life.[48] If the woman and her neonate must be separated for medical indications, skin-to-skin contact in the intensive care nursery, early effective breast milk expression, and support from peers and staff can be implemented and are very important to the promotion of breastfeeding in neonatal units.[49]

Complications of the Third and Fourth Stages of Labor

Although most births end with an uneventful third stage of labor, some of the most severe childbirth complications occur during the third stage, including retained placenta, placenta accreta, and uterine inversion. Postpartum hemorrhage can occur in the third stage of labor or in the first hours postpartum.

Retained Placenta

A third stage of labor that lasts 30 minutes or longer is generally considered prolonged and is termed a retained placenta.[10] Nevertheless, there is no universal definition for when the diagnosis of retained placenta should be made. With the use of active management, the length of the third stage should be less than 20 minutes, and 98% of women will have delivered the placenta by 30 minutes after birth of the newborn.[50] Following physiologic management of third-stage labor, 98% of women will have delivered the placenta by 60 minutes after birth of the newborn.[51] While most settings in the United States recommend intervention after 30 minutes, WHO recommends that intervention not be initiated until 60 minutes in the absence of bleeding.[52]

Risk factors for a retained placenta include previous retained placenta, previous uterine curettage, preterm birth, preeclampsia, augmented labors, birth in a dorsal position, nulliparity, and use of ergotamine (Methergine).[50,53] It is theorized that ergotamine may trap the placenta when this medication is used routinely prior to delivery of the placenta, as it causes a clonic or tetanic contraction. The mechanism of action of ergotamine is in contrast to oxytocin (Pitocin), which is not associated with an increased risk for a retained placenta.

The primary risk associated with retained placenta is hemorrhage. The risk of hemorrhage begins to increase at approximately 20 minutes after birth with the placenta undelivered and continues to increase until it plateaus at approximately 75 minutes after birth.[53] A consultation should be obtained once a prolonged third stage has been diagnosed. The midwife may initiate several interventions when the third stage is increasing in length, including encouraging an upright position for the woman, nipple stimulation via encouraging the newborn to breastfeed or manual nipple stimulation, and ensuring an empty bladder, by means of catheterization if indicated.

If the placenta still has not separated following conservative measures and the time interval has passed 30 minutes, the next step is manual removal of the placenta. Nonemergency manual removal of the placenta should occur in a hospital setting, both for reasons of safety and to enable the woman to receive anesthesia or deep analgesia for this usually painful procedure. **Appendix 31C** reviews the procedure for manual removal of the placenta. In the nonemergency situation, the midwife can manually remove the placenta in consultation with a physician or wait for a physician to conduct the procedure. If the woman is hemorrhaging, the midwife may need to manually remove the placenta emergently.

Evulsed Cord

Excessive cord traction before complete placental separation can cause the umbilical cord to detach or evulse from the placenta, necessitating manual removal of the placenta—an intervention that exposes the woman to unnecessary pain and an increased risk of infection. A sensation of tearing will be felt as the cord is detaching. If this is noticed, cord traction should be stopped and signs of placental separation should be apparent before resuming. Repositioning the woman in an upright position may facilitate placental expulsion.

Uterine Inversion

Uterine inversion occurs when the fundus collapses into the endometrial cavity, which turns the uterus partially or completely inside out. Uterine inversion is a rare event, occurring in approximately 1 in 20,000 births; however, it has been found to occur primarily in women who have low-risk pregnancies.[54] Strong umbilical cord traction and fundal placental implantation are associated with this condition, although it may also occur spontaneously. The uterine inversion can be incomplete (fundus within endometrial cavity), complete (fundus protrudes through the cervical os), prolapsed (fundus protrudes to or beyond vaginal introitus), or total (both the uterus and the vagina are inverted). Incomplete or complete inversions feel like a soft tumor that can be felt in the cervical or vaginal orifice, while abdominally a funnel-like depression may be felt instead of a rounded fundus.

Uterine inversion causes maternal shock and disseminated intravascular coagulation (DIC). Thus, this complications can be a life-threatening emergency. Uterine inversion should be suspected and a vaginal examination performed if the woman develops symptoms of shock after giving birth without obvious reason. Excessive bleeding and severe uterine pain may or may not be present. **Appendix 31D** presents the management of uterine inversion and describes the position of the midwife's hands during this maneuver.

Placenta Accreta

Placenta accreta is the term for a placenta that is abnormally adherent to the uterine wall. Placenta accreta is further subcategorized as *placenta increta*, when the placenta invades the myometrium, and *placenta percreta*, when it has extended through the myometrium and uterine serosa and into adjacent tissue, often the bladder. Placenta accreta most often occurs when the placenta implants over an area wherein there is a deficiency of decidual formation, such as over a uterine scar or in the lower uterine segment.[55] Women who have a cesarean birth are at increased risk for placenta accreta in subsequent pregnancies. Women who have had one or more previous cesarean births and who have a placenta previa in the current pregnancy are especially at risk for placenta accreta. The risk of occurrence increases with increasing number of cesarean births.

The overall rate of placenta accreta has been reported to range from 1 in 2500 pregnancies to (more recently) 1 in 500 pregnancies.[55] It has been proposed that the increasing rate of placenta accreta is occurring secondary to the rising rate of cesarean births.

If the placenta is completely adherent; there usually is minimal bleeding. If it is partially separated or partially adherent, there will likely be bleeding that may or may not be visible. If placenta accreta is suspected due to a retained and adherent placenta, physician consultation and in-hospital care are necessary. Hysterectomy while leaving the placenta intact is generally the recommended treatment for placenta accreta.

Postpartum Hemorrhage

Approximately 800 mL to 1000 mL of blood flows to the gravid uterus each minute. Thus significant blood loss can occur quite quickly. Postpartum hemorrhage has been defined in several ways. The generally accepted definition is a blood loss of more than 500 mL after a vaginal birth or more than 1000 mL blood loss following a cesarean birth.[56] However, most healthy women can tolerate a blood loss of 1000 mL without adverse consequences. Moreover, estimated blood loss is very often underestimated in clinical settings.[28,57] In fact, when blood loss is measured, it appears that 500 mL is the average blood loss following a normal spontaneous vaginal delivery. Thus the "greater than 500 mL" definition is somewhat arbitrary and not evidence based.

Other authors have suggested that a postpartum hemorrhage occurs when the postpartum hematocrit represents more than a 10-point drop from the prenatal value. This retrospective definition is not clinically helpful during the third or fourth stage of labor.

Finally, signs and symptoms of hypovolemia can be used to define a postpartum hemorrhage. However, symptoms such as hypotension and tachycardia appear after 15% of blood volume is lost. Therefore symptoms are not a sensitive indicator that the midwife can use to identify a postpartum hemorrhage in the early stages when the excessive bleeding needs to be recognized. In clinical practice, postpartum hemorrhage is a subjective assessment of an estimated blood loss that threatens hemodynamic stability. It is important to not wait until any of these thresholds are met before implementing steps to control postpartum bleeding. Early action in the presence of excessive bleeding may prevent actual hemorrhage.

Postpartum hemorrhage is termed *early* or *primary* when it occurs within the first 24 hours postpartum and *late* or *secondary* when it occurs after 24 hours and up to 6 weeks postpartum.[56] In the United States, postpartum hemorrhage occurs in 2% to 3% of all births; thus all providers must be prepared to identify and manage this complication.[58] More than half of all maternal deaths occur within 24 hours of birth, most commonly from excessive bleeding or early postpartum hemorrhage.[56] Most importantly, more than half of all obstetric deaths attributed to hemorrhage are preventable. In developed nations where adequate resources are present, these deaths are mostly attributed to failure to coordinate the management of this emergency.[59] Identification of

risk factors, preventive measures, and early detection and management can help mitigate the adverse consequences of this complication.

Etiology of Immediate Postpartum Hemorrhage

Table 31-6 lists the most common causes of postpartum hemorrhage, along with a mnemonic (tone, tissue, trauma, thrombin) to help providers remember them.[46,58–63] Uterine atony or retained placental fragments are the cause of approximately 80% of early postpartum hemorrhages.[56] Late postpartum hemorrhage is often caused by retained placental fragments, infection, coagulopathies, or subinvolution at the placental site.

Many strategies have been used to identify women who are at risk for excessive blood loss. Stratifying women into low-, medium-, and high-risk groups is valuable as a guide for anticipatory preparation. Even so, most postpartum hemorrhages occur in women who have no risk factors.[63]

Stages of Postpartum Hemorrhage

As shown in **Table 31-7**, symptoms of hypovolemia are usually parallel the amount of blood lost. Thus postpartum hemorrhage can be categorized as compensated, mild, moderate, or severe depending on symptoms and the amount of blood loss. Women who are already volume depleted, such as those with preeclampsia, may decompensate more rapidly.

The first physiologic compensation that occurs when blood loss is excessive is systemic vasoconstriction, which is clinically evident as a narrowed pulse pressure. Systolic blood pressure begins to fall and pulse rises after 15% to 25% of blood volume is lost. Hypotension and tachycardia are relatively late signs of hemorrhage. Narrowing trends in pulse pressure are a better vital sign to initially monitor when bleeding becomes excessive.

Complications of Postpartum Hemorrhage

Postpartum hemorrhage can result in anemia, hypotension, and, in severe cases, hypovolemic shock that can lead to DIC, adult respiratory distress syndrome (ARDS), and/or Sheehan's syndrome.

DIC is a consumptive coagulopathy that results in depletion of platelets and coagulation factors. Its etiology is widespread activation of the clotting and fibrolytic systems. This cascade of events is stimulated by circulatory exposure to large amounts of tissue factor, which is present in the placenta. The result is uncontrolled bleeding. Recent studies of postpartum hemorrhage have found that DIC occurs earlier than previously thought.[64] Early treatment of

Table 31-6	The "Four Ts" Mnemonic for Causes of Immediate Postpartum Hemorrhage		
	Cause	**Etiology (%)**	**Clinical Presentation**
Tone	Overdistended uterus—large fetus, multiple gestation, polyhydramnios	70	Bright red bleeding, clots, boggy or soft uterus
	Prolonged labor (all stages)		
	Rapid labor		
	Oxytocin-induced or augmented labor		
	High parity		
	Postpartum hemorrhage with previous birth		
	Chorioamnionitis		
	Poorly perfused myometrium—hypotension		
	Medications such as magnesium sulfate, nifedipine, and some general anesthetics		
	Uterine abnormalities such as fibroids		
Tissue, retained	Avulsed cotyledon, succenturiate lobe	20	Bright red bleeding, clots, boggy or soft uterus
	Abnormal placentation—accreta, increta, percreta		
	Retained blood clots		
Trauma	Episiotomy, especially mediolateral	10	Lacerations: bright red bleeding, clots, firm uterine fundus
	Hematoma		
	Lacerations of perineum, vagina, or cervix		Hematomas: intense pain at site of bleeding
	Ruptured uterus		
	Uterine inversion		Uterine inversion: shock out of proportion to what is expected
Thrombin	Coagulopathies	1	
	Acquired coagulopathies such as placental abruption, amniotic fluid embolism, disseminated intravascular coagulation, HELLP syndrome, stillbirth, or sepsis		
	Congenital coagulation defects such as von Willebrand's disease		
	Therapeutic anticoagulation		

Table 31-7	Clinical Findings in Postpartum Hemorrhage			
	Compensated PPH	**Mild PPH**	**Moderate PPH**	**Severe PPH**
Blood volume loss (mL)	< 1000	1000–1500	1500–2000	> 2000
Percentage of blood volume lost (%)	10–15	15–25	25–35	35–45
Heart rate (bpm)	< 100	> 100	> 120	> 140
Systolic blood pressure (mm Hg)	Normal	Orthostatic	70–80	50–70
Respiratory rate	Normal	Mild	Tachypnea	Tachypnea
Urine output (mL/hr)	> 30	20–30	5–20	Anuria
Mental status	Normal	Weakness, sweating, agitation	Restless, pallor, confusion	Air hunger, collapse, lethargy

DIC can significantly improve maternal outcomes. Evaluation of coagulation studies is part of the initial response to postpartum hemorrhage, and transfusion protocols for postpartum hemorrhage recommend treating DIC as soon as it is determined to be a significant risk.

ARDS and Sheehan's syndrome are rare complications of postpartum hemorrhage. ARDS is the result of damage to the endothelial cells in the pulmonary vasculature. Fluid then leaks into the alveoli, producing respiratory distress. Sheehan's syndrome is the result of pituitary necrosis.[65] The pituitary is perfused via venous pressure, which makes it vulnerable to ischemia and damage in the presence of hypotension. The most common initial symptom of Sheehan's syndrome is failure of lactogenesis II. Amenorrhea, adrenal insufficiency, hyponatremia, and hypoglycemia are possible complications of pituitary hypofunction.

Preventive Measures

Strategies to minimize the adverse effects of postpartum hemorrhage include correction of anemia preconceptionally or in the prenatal period, elimination of routine episiotomies, and avoidance of genital tract lacerations.[60] The best prevention strategy is active management of the third stage of labor, starting with administration of a uterotonic agent during or immediately following the birth of the infant.[10] **Box 31-2** lists recommended preparations to implement for women at a moderate or high risk of early hemorrhage.

Management Steps for Postpartum Hemorrhage

Vital signs such as narrowing pulse pressure or quantified blood loss can be used as a trigger or alert to initiate treatment guidelines and team assistance. **Appendix 31E** lists the steps recommended for managing a postpartum hemorrhage, and **Appendix 31F** reviews the steps taken to explore the intrauterine cavity if needed.[60–63] Standard procedures that are practiced in simulations or as simple dry runs can improve the response time when a real postpartum hemorrhage occurs.

Many sources delineate the sequential steps the midwife should proceed through when managing a postpartum hemorrhage. In addition, the midwife can find some excellent flowcharts that institutions use to guide management of a postpartum hemorrhage. One example obstetric hemorrhage flowchart is shown in **Figure 31-4**.[64]

A combination of bimanual compression and uterotonic drugs controls bleeding in the vast majority of postpartum hemorrhages. If management

---

> ### BOX 31-2 Management Plan for a Woman at Moderate or High Risk of a Postpartum Hemorrhage
>
> 1. Provide anticipatory guidance to the woman and her significant other/family (with the woman's permission).
> 2. Choose the birth site based on risk assessment.
> 3. Prepare a plan of care and communicate to all healthcare team members, including nursing and anesthesia staff, when a woman is in labor. A physician may be alerted when the woman enters labor based on her level of risk.
> 4. Based on her risk, the plan of care for the woman in labor may include the following:
>   a. Order a blood type and screen or type and cross-match for blood if needed.
>   b. Initiate a large-bore intravenous line during labor (at least 18 gauge) for rapid access.
>   c. Catheterize the woman's bladder if it is full and she is unable to void, as a full bladder may impede postpartum uterine contractions.
>   d. Consider pain management methods that will support the steps undertaken to manage a postpartum hemorrhage, and make a plan with the woman early in her labor.
>   e. Administer an uterotonic agent with the release of the neonate's anterior shoulder, assuming there is assurance that a second twin does not exist.
>   f. Promptly initiate and maintain uterine massage after placental expulsion and continue close observation for bleeding.
>
> If hemorrhage occurs, proceed to the steps outlined in Appendix 31E.

---

steps are initiated rapidly, excessive blood loss can be avoided. Calling an interprofessional team to address the emergency should be initiated if the hemorrhage continues despite bimanual compression and use of uterotonic drugs, or if the woman has signs of hypovolemia. The use of agreed-upon vital sign "triggers" that signal the need for more aggressive treatment can help standardize management of postpartum hemorrhage and minimize morbidity. For example, triggers that could signal the need to initiate a hemorrhage protocol could be if a maternal pulse is more than 110 bpm, estimated blood loss is more than 500 mL, or systolic blood pressure is less than 85 mm Hg. The

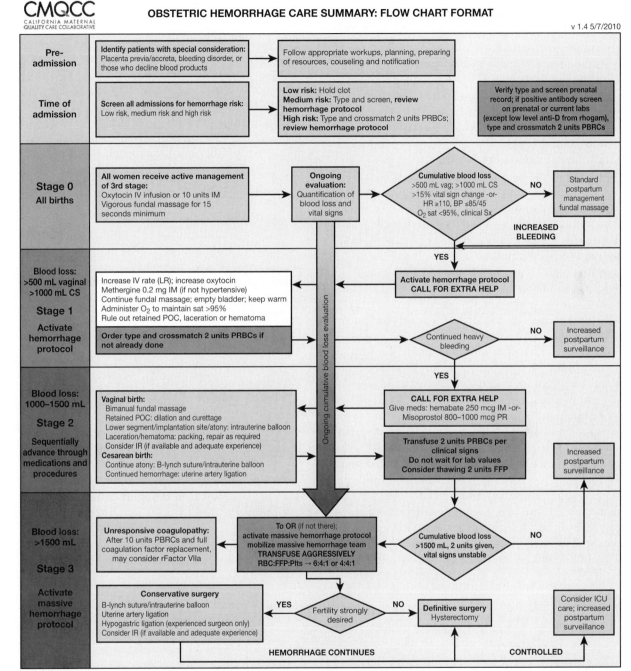

CMQCC
CALIFORNIA MATERNAL
QUALITY CARE COLLABORATIVE

OBSTETRIC HEMORRHAGE CARE SUMMARY: FLOW CHART FORMAT

v 1.4 5/7/2010

California Maternal Quality Care Collaborative (CMQCC), Hemorrhage Taskforce (2009) visit: www.CMQCC.org for details
This project was supported by Title V funds received from the State of California Department of Public Health, Center for Family Health; Maternal, Child and Adolescent Health Division

Figure 31-4 Sample postpartum hemorrhage flow chart.
Source: Reprinted with permission from California Maternal Quality Care Collaborative/California Department of Public Health MCAH Division.

team that responds to such emergencies commonly includes an anesthesia provider, an obstetric physician, and additional nursing staff. Once the hemorrhage is controlled, close postpartum surveillance is maintained until bleeding is minimal and the woman is stable.

Hematoma

Hematomas are the result of damage to blood vessels, and when they occur, they are most likely apparent during the intrapartum or postpartum periods. The most common locations for hematomas are (1) the vulva, (2) the vagina, and (3) the retroperitoneum.[66] The types of hematomas and their initial presentation are described in more detail in Appendix B of *The Second Stage of Labor and Birth* chapter.

Hematomas are very painful in women who do not have epidural analgesia such that pain is the cardinal sign of a developing hematoma.[53] Women who have a functioning epidural may report sudden rectal pressure. The other clinical indicators of hematoma besides pain are signs and symptoms of blood loss such as hypotension or tachycardia.

Because a hematoma may not be visible externally, a gentle internal digital exam is necessary to establish the diagnosis. If there is a firm, rounded swelling into the vaginal canal or on the vulva that is small and not expanding quickly, it can probably be managed expectantly with frequent observation to make sure it is not expanding, placement of cold packs, and establishing intravenous access in case volume resuscitation is needed (**Table 31-8**). A Foley catheter may be needed to aid urination and a complete blood count to establish a baseline may be indicated. The midwife should communicate to the woman and caregivers (nurses in the hospital or family members if out of the hospital) the importance of reporting increasing pain or swelling.

If the pain is severe, the hematoma is increasing rapidly, or signs of hypovolemia develop, emergency measures are needed. If the woman is in an out-of-hospital setting, emergency transport is begun. The midwife's consulting physician and anesthesia staff should be notified and immediate assistance requested. The midwife should not incise the hematoma without additional medical help because of the potential for hemorrhage. Measures to initiate intravenous fluid volume replacement and possible blood transfusion should be initiated while waiting for the medical team.

Rare Emergency Complications

If a newly postpartum woman experiences respiratory impairment, cardiovascular collapse, altered mental status, or loss of consciousness, emergency measures are indicated. The differential diagnoses include pulmonary embolus, anaphylactoid syndrome of pregnancy (i.e., amniotic fluid embolus), septic shock, peripartum cardiomyopathy, and atypical eclampsia, among others. Sudden and rapid deterioration of the woman necessitates a quick response. Initial management steps for any obstetric emergency are listed in **Appendix 31G**.[57-59]

Life support measures focusing on adequate oxygenation are important regardless of the cause of the emergency. Once the emergency team is in place, the midwife plays an important role in communicating the past history including the labor and birth, reviewing how the emergency presented, and identifying which management steps were implemented. Finally, maintaining communication with the family members to keep them informed is a critical component of the management of any obstetric emergency that a midwife can perform.

Conclusion

The third and fourth stages of labor are critical for a healthy start for the new family. Attention to prevention and early identification and treatment of complications can mitigate potential long-term effects. Witnessing the welcome of a newborn into a family is a sweet reward for the midwife. No matter

Table 31-8	Genital Tract Hematoma: Expectant Management
Management	**Rationale**
Frequent assessment	The frequency will depend on when the hematoma is diagnosed, whether it is changing, and how much maternal discomfort is present. Assessments may be spaced out once the hematoma is determined to be stable.
Encourage ice packs to the affected area for 24–48 hours	Ice packs assist with vasoconstriction, thereby decreasing bleeding and edema.
Offer pharmacologic pain management	Even minor hematomas may be uncomfortable. Nonsteroidal anti-inflammatory drugs (NSAIDs) should be adequate for minor hematoma pain, but opioids may be required for larger hematomas.
Encourage side-lying positioning	A side-lying position may relieve pressure and decrease pain. This is often an effective position for assessment and diagnosis of a hematoma. Positioning does not alter the hematoma progression.

how hard the midwife may have worked to assist the woman and her significant others through the labor and birth, complimenting her and stressing her accomplishment is a gift the midwife can offer in return.

● ● ● References

1. Haeri S, Dildy GA. Maternal mortality from hemorrhage. *Semin Perinatol.* 2012;36:48-55.

2. Atzil S, Hendler T, Feldman R. Specifying the neurobiological basis of human attachment: brain, hormones, and behavior in synchronous and intrusive mothers. *Neuropsychopharmacology.* 2011;36:2603-2615.

3. Soltani H, Hutchon DR, Poulose TA. Timing of prophylactic uterotonics for the third stage of labour after vaginal birth. *Cochrane Database Syst Rev.* 2010;8:CD006173. doi: 10.1002/14651858. CD006173.pub2.

4. Combs CA, Laros RK. Prolonged third stage of labor: morbidity and risk factors. *Obstet Gynecol.* 1991;77:863-867.

5. Schorn MN. Uterine activity during the third stage of labor. *J Midwifery Women's Health.* 2012;57: 151-155.

6. Dombrowski MP, Bottoms SF, Saleh AA, Hurd WW, Romero R. Third stage of labor: analysis of duration and clinical practice. *Am J Obstet Gynecol.* 1995;172:1279-1284.

7. Blackburn ST. *Maternal, Fetal, and Neonatal Physiology.* 4th ed. Maryland Heights, MO: Elsevier; 2013:142.

8. Magann EF, Evans S, Chauhan SP, Lanneau G, Fisk AD, Morrison JC. The length of the third stage of labor and the risk of postpartum hemorrhage. *Obstet Gynecol.* 2005;105:290-293.

9. McDonald S. Management of the third stage of labor. *J Midwifery Women's Health.* 2007;52:254-261.

10. Begley CM, Gyte GML, Devane D, McGuire W, Weeks A. Active versus expectant management for women in the third stage of labour. *Cochrane Database Syst Rev.* 2011;11:CD007412. doi: 10.1002/14651858. CD007412.pub3.

11. Fahy K, Hastie C, Bisits A, Marsh C, Smith L, Saxton A. Holistic physiological care compared with active management of the third stage of labour for women at low risk of postpartum haemorrhage: a cohort study. *Women Birth.* 2010;23:146-152.

12. Tan WM, Klein MC, Saxell L, Shirkoohy SE, Asrat G. How do physicians and midwives manage the third stage of labor? *Birth.* 2008;35:220-229.

13. International Confederation of Midwives, International Federation of Gynecology and Obstetrics. Joint statement: prevention and treatment of postpartum hemorrhage: new advances for low-resource settings. Available at: http://www.pphprevention.org /files/FIGO-ICM_Statement_November2006_Final .pdf. Accessed December 16, 2012.

14. International Confederation of Midwives, International Federation of Gynecology and Obstetrics. Joint statement: management of the third stage of labour to prevent post-partum hemorrhage. Available at: http ://www.pphprevention.org/files/ICM_FIGO_Joint_ Statement.pdf. Accessed December 16, 2012.

15. WHO recommendations for the prevention and treatment of postpartum hemorrhage. 2012. Available at: http://apps.who.int/iris/bitstream/10665 /75411/1/9789241548502_eng.pdf. Accessed December 12, 2012.

16. Winter C, Macfarlane A, Deneux-Tharaux C, et al. Variations in policies for management of the third stage of labour and the immediate management of postpartum haemorrhage in Europe. *BJOG.* 2007; 114:845-854.

17. Prendiville WJP, Elbourne D, McDonald SJ. *Active versus expectant management in the third stage of labour* [Cochrane review]. Chichester, UK: Cochrane Library; 2000.

18. Gülmezoglu AM, Lumbiganon P, Landulsi S, et al. Active management of the third stage of labour with and without controlled cord traction: a randomized, controlled, non-inferiority trial. *Lancet.* 2012;379:1721-1727.

19. Afaifel N, Weeks AD. Active management of the third stage of labor: oxytocin is all you need. *BMJ.* 2012;345:e4546.

20. Andersson O, Hellström-Westas L, Andersson D, Domellöf M. Effect of delayed versus early umbilical cord clamping on neonatal outcomes and iron status at 4 months: a randomised controlled trial. *BMJ.* 2011;343:d7156.

21. Soltani H, Hutchon DR, Poulose TA. Timing of prophylactic uterotonics for the third stage of labour after vaginal birth. *Cochrane Database Syst Rev.* 2010;8:CD006173. doi: 10.1002/14651858. CD006173.pub2.

22. Mercer JS, Nelson CC, Skovgaard RL. Umbilical cord clamping: benefits and practices of American nurse-midwives. *J Midwifery Women's Health.* 2000;45: 58-66.

23. Lowe N, King TL. Labor. In: King TL, Brucker MC, eds. *Pharmacology for Women's Health.* Sudbury, MA: Jones and Bartlett; 2011:1102.

24. Jackson KW, Albert JR, Schemmer GK, et al. A randomized controlled trial comparing oxytocin administration before and after placental delivery in the prevention of postpartum hemorrhage. *Am J Obstet Gynecol.* 2001;185(4):873-877.

25. Soltani H, Poulose TA, Hutchon DR. Placental cord drainage after vaginal delivery as part of the management of the third stage of labour. *Cochrane Database*

Syst Rev. 2011;9:CD004665. doi: 10.1002/14651858. CD004665.pub3.

26. Abdel-Aleem H, Singata M, Abdel-Aleem M, Mshweshwe N, Williams X, Hofmeyr GJ. Uterine massage to reduce postpartum hemorrhage after vaginal delivery. *Int J Gynaecol Obstet.* 2010;111:32-36.

27. Hofmeyr GJ, Abdel-Aleem H, Abdel-Aleem MA. Uterine massage for preventing postpartum haemorrhage. *Cochrane Database Syst Rev.* 2008;3:CD006431. doi: 10.1002/14651858.CD006431.pub2.

28. Schorn MN. Measurement of blood loss: review of the literature. *J Midwifery Women's Health.* 2010;55: 20-27.

29. Gabel KT, Weeber, TA. Measuring and communicating blood loss during obstetric hemorrhage. *JOGNN.* 2012;41:551-558.

30. Buckley SJ. Placenta rituals and folklore from around the world. *Midwifery Today Int Midwife.* 2006;80: 58-59.

31. Crowther S. Lotus birth: leaving the cord alone. *Practicing Midwife.* 2006;9(6):12-14.

32. Graff K. The bridge of life: options for placentas. *Midwifery Today.* Winter 2007; 67-68.

33. Higham B. Waste product or tasty treat? *Practicing Midwife.* 2009;12(10):33-35.

34. Ainsworth S. Striking a cord. *Practicing Midwife.* 2009; 12(2):42.

35. Curtin WM, Krauss S, Metlay LA, Katzman PJ. Pathologic examination of the placenta and observed practice. *Obstet Gynecol.* 2007;109:35-41.

36. Gibbs RS, Rosenberg AR, Warren CJ, Galan HL, Rumack CM. Suggestions for practice to accompany neonatal encephalopathy and cerebral palsy. *Obstet Gynecol.* 2004;103:778-779.

37. Klaus MK, Jerauld R, Kreger NC, McAlpine W, Steffa M, Kennel JH. Maternal attachment: importance of the first post-partum days. *N Engl J Med.* 1972;286:460-463.

38. Widström A-M, Lilja G, Aaltomaa-Michalias P, Dahllof A, Lintula M, Nissen E. Newborn behavior to locate the breast when skin-to-skin: a possible method for enabling early self-regulation. *Acta Pædiatr.* 2011;100:79-85.

39. Sullivan R, Perry R, Sloan A, Kleinhous K, Burtchen N. Infant bonding and attachment to the caregiver: insights from basic and clinical science. *Clin Perinatol.* 2011;38:643-655.

40. Bystrova K, Ivanova V, Edhborg M, et al. Early contact versus separation: effects on mother–infant interaction one year later. *Birth.* 2009;36:97-109.

41. Moore ER, Anderson GC, Bergman N, Dowswell T. Early skin-to-skin contact for mothers and their healthy newborn infants. *Cochrane Database Syst*

Rev. 2012;5:CD003519. doi: 10.1002/14651858. CD003519.pub3.

42. Kainz G, Eliasson M, von Post E. The child's father, an important person for the mother's well-being during the childbirth: a hermeneutic study. *Health Care Women Int.* 2010;31:621-635.

43. Brandão S, Figueiredo B. Fathers' emotional involvement with the neonate: impact of the umbilical cord cutting experience. *J Adv Nurs.* 2012;68(12): 2730-2739.

44. Persson EK, Fridlund B, Kvist LJ, Kykes A. Fathers' sense of security during the first postnatal week: a qualitative interview study in Sweden. *Midwifery.* 2011;28(5):e697-e704.

45. Genesoni L, Tallandini MA. Men's psychological transition to fatherhood: an analysis of the literature, 1989–2008. *Birth.* 2009;36:305-317.

46. Spidsberg BD, Sørlie V. An expression of love: midwives' experiences in the encounter with lesbian women and their partners. *J Adv Nurs.* 2012;68:796-805.

47. Hildingsson I, Cederlöf L, Widén S. Fathers' birth experience in relation to midwifery care. *Women Birth.* 2011;24:129-136.

48. Chung M, Raman G, Trikalinos T, Lau J, Ip S. Interventions in primary care to promote breastfeeding: an evidence review for the U.S. Preventive Services Task Force. *Ann Intern Med.* 2008;149;565-582.

49. Renfrew MJ, Dyson L, McCormick F, et al. Breastfeeding promotion for infants in neonatal units: a systematic review. *Child: Care, Health and Development.* 2009;36:165-178.

50. Magann EF, Doherty DA, Briery CM, Niederhauser A, Chauhan SP, Morrison JC. Obstetric characteristics for a prolonged third stage of labor and risk for postpartum hemorrhage. *Gynecol Obstet Invest.* 2008;65:201-205.

51. Weeks AD. The retained placenta. *Best Pract Res Clin Obstet Gynaecol.* 2008;22:1103.

52. World Health Organization (WHO). *WHO Guidelines for the Management of Postpartum Haemorrhage and Retained Placenta.* Geneva, Switzerland: WHO; 2009.

53. Combs CA, Laros RK Jr. Prolonged third stage of labor: morbidity and risk factors. *Obstet Gynecol.* 1991;77:863.

54. Witteveen T, van Stralen G, Zwart J, van Roosmalen J. Puerperal uterine inversion in the Netherlands: a nationwide cohort study. *Acta Obstet Gynecol Scand.* 2012;92(3):334-337.

55. Oyelese Y, Smulian JC. Placenta previa, placenta accreta, and vasa previa. *Obstet Gynecol.* 2006;107: 927-941.

56. ACOG Practice Bulletin: postpartum hemorrhage. *Obstet Gynecol.* 2006;108:1039-1047.

57. Maslovitz S, Barkal G, Lessing JB, Viz A, Many A. Improved accuracy of postpartum blood loss estimation as assessed by simulation. *Acta Obstet Gynecol Scand.* 2008;87(9):929-934.

58. Bateman BT, Berman MF, Riley LE, Leffert LR. The epidemiology of postpartum hemorrhage in a large, nationwide sample of deliveries. *Anesth Analg.* 2010; 110:1368-1373.

59. Bingham D, Jones R. Maternal death from obstetric hemorrhage. *JOGNN.* 2012;41:531.9.

60. Anderson JM, Etches D. Prevention and management of postpartum hemorrhage. *Am Fam Physician.* 2007;75:875-882.

61. Maughan KL, Heim SW, Galazka SS. Preventing postpartum hemorrhage: managing the third stage of labor. *Am Fam Physician.* 2006;73:1025-1028.

62. Rajan PV, Wing DA. Postpartum hemorrhage: evidence-based medical interventions for prevention and treatment. *Clin Obstet Gynecol.* 2010;53:165-181.

63. Lyndon A, Lagrew D, Shields L, Melsop K, Bingham B, Main E, eds. *Improving Health Care Response to Obstetric Hemorrhage: California Maternal Quality Care Collaborative Toolkit to Transform Maternity Care.* Developed under contract #08-85012 with California Department of Public Health, Maternal, Child and Adolescent Health Division. Published by California Maternal Quality Care Collaborative; July 2010. Available at: http://www.cmqcc.org /resources/ob_hemorrhage/ob_hemorrhage_care_ guidelines_checklist_flowchart_tablechart_v1_4. Accessed October 7, 2012.

64. Mcclintock C, James AH. Obstetric hemorrhage. *J Thrombos Haemost.* 2011;9:1441-1451.

65. Schrager S, Sabo L. Sheehan syndrome: a rare complication of postpartum hemorrhage. *J Am Board Fam Prac.* 2001;14(5):389-392.

66. Mirza FG, Gaddipati S. Obstetric emergencies. *Semin Perinatol.* 2009;33:97-103.

APPENDIX

31A

Management of the Third Stage of Labor

History

- Previous birth complications during the third stage, including postpartum hemorrhage
- Risk factors for postpartum hemorrhage
- Course of this labor and birth
- Maternal requests for specific management in the third stage of labor

Physical Examination

- Maternal response to birth
- Vital signs stable
- Continuing evaluation of any previous significant findings
- Evaluation of new findings—for example, nausea is unusual in the third stage
- Evaluation of progress of the third stage, including signs of placental separation
- Continual assessment of bleeding

Management Steps[a]

1. Maintain or reinstate a calm environment to reduce anxiety and facilitate management of normal progress and treatment of complications if they occur.

2. Communicate the next steps and reassurance to the woman.

3. Check the newborn heart rate by palpating at the base of the umbilical cord and abdomen. If the heart rate is faster than 100 bpm, the newborn is breathing, and there are no obvious abnormalities, place the newborn in skin-to-skin contact on the woman's abdomen or arrange to have the newborn placed skin to skin with a person whom the woman designates for this initial period with the infant.

4. Continue to observe the neonatal transition to extrauterine life while the newborn is in skin-to-skin contact when possible. Note that the midwife conducting the birth has a primary responsibility to the woman during the third stage of labor, not management of the newborn.

5. Administer or request administration of a uterotonic agent, if not already given during birth of the anterior shoulder (optional depending on the woman's risk for postpartum hemorrhage, policies, and amount of bleeding present).

6. Consider upright positioning, which uses gravity to assist with placental expulsion if feasible.

7. If cord blood gases are not indicated, two clamps are needed:

   a. Clamp the cord with two clamps placed close together near the newborn's umbilicus after at least 1–3 minutes or when the cord stops pulsating

   b. Cut the cord between the two clamps or guide the father, partner, other support person, or birthing woman to do this.

---

[a] These steps include components of both physiologic management and active management of the third stage of labor. Individual situations may require some alterations in the order of individual steps.

8. If cord blood gases are indicated, four clamps are needed:

   a. Place an initial clamp on the cord near the woman's introitus.

   b. Place two clamps in close approximation to each other on the cord distal (toward the newborn's umbilicus) to the first clamp.

   c. Cut the cord (or have another person cut it) between the last two clamps, and place the newborn on the maternal abdomen or hand off the newborn to another provider as indicated.

   d. Place a fourth clamp close to the first clamp that was placed near the woman's introitus, and cut the cord between these two last clamps. There is now a sealed double-clamped section of cord that can be used to obtain cord blood gases (**Figure 31A-1**).

   e. Obtain a sample of blood from the umbilical artery first, and then a sample from one of the umbilical veins, in a heparinized syringe, marking each syringe correctly as from the artery or vein. Once the syringe is capped, the blood is stable for up to 30 minutes before the blood gas measurement has to be obtained.

9. Inspect the cut end of the umbilical cord and count the number of umbilical vessels.

10. Open the clamp nearest the woman's introitus and allow blood from the placenta to fill a non-heparinized blood collection tube. Approximately 5–10 mL are needed. This blood will be used to determine the type and Rh status of the newborn. Do not milk the cord as tissue thromboplastin can interfere with the analysis.

11. Observe for signs of placental separation (Table 31-1) and do not massage the uterus before placental separation. Massaging the uterus prior to complete separation may increase uterine bleeding or lead to incomplete expulsion of the placenta.

12. Guard the uterus. Place a hand suprapubically, anterior to the uterine fundus, to assess for uterine position in the abdomen and prevent uterine inversion as the placenta is expulsed.

13. Determine whether the placenta has separated:

   a. Use the Brandt-Andrews maneuver (**Figure 31A-2**). Apply slight downward pressure just above the pelvic brim with the hand that is guarding the uterus while holding the cord taut with the other hand. If the placenta is still in the uterus, the cord will become taut as the uterus is displaced upward into the abdomen by pressure from the abdominal hand. If the placenta has separated and is in the vagina, upward displacement of the uterus will not cause the cord to retract, and additional cord traction can be safely provided while maintaining abdominal counter-traction.

   b. Another method of checking for placental location is to slide one finger (using sterile gloves) beside the umbilical cord into the

Figure 31A-1 Double-clamped cord.
Source: Courtesy of Tekoa L. King

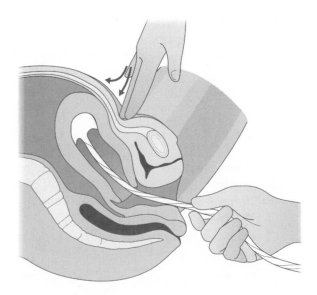

Figure 31A-2 Brandt-Andrews maneuver.

vagina. If the placenta is in the vagina, it will be felt by the tip of the finger. The cord insertion into the placenta feels somewhat like an inverted umbrella. If the cord goes past the cervix, the placenta has not been expelled from the uterus. If the placenta is palpated in the vagina, additional traction can be safely performed.

14. Once the placenta has separated, the woman may spontaneously expel it by pushing. The midwife can also use a combination of the Brandt-Andrews maneuver and controlled cord traction.

15. Cord traction should *not* be performed without guarding the uterus, as this maneuver may result in an evulsed cord or inverted uterus.

16. Grasp the placenta with both hands as it is being expelled to gently tease out the membranes. Slowly guide the placenta out, perhaps following the curve of Carus to allow membranes to follow and not tear. If there appear to be more membranes than immediately are expelled, continue to hold the placenta and either twist it slowly or grasp the membranes with ring forceps to gently extract the membranes—a process commonly known as "teasing" out the membranes.

17. Palpate the fundus abdominally to assess if the fundus is firm. Routine vigorous massage to stimulate uterine contraction has not been shown to decrease the incidence of hemorrhage. Such massage may be indicated to express clots through the cervix if excessive bleeding is present, but it is not indicated if the estimated blood loss is normal.

18. Inspect the cord, placenta, and membranes as described in Appendix 31B (Table 31-4).

19. Show the placenta to the woman and family if interested.

20. Measure or weigh blood loss.

21. Weigh the placenta.

22. Send the placenta for pathology evaluation if indicated.

APPENDIX

31B

Inspection of the Umbilical Cord, Placenta, and Membranes

Inspection of the umbilical cord, placenta, and membranes is performed as soon as the woman and her newborn are stable and comfortable. Any abnormal findings are documented in the maternal and neonatal records. In some situations, a photograph may be of value for documentation.

Inspection of the Umbilical Cord

Count the Number of Vessels

Wipe off the cut end with a gauze or towel if needed. Apply pressure; the apertures of the vessels will be visible. If vessels have collapsed, reclamp and recut the cord then look for the vessels at the site of the new cut (**Figure 31B-1**).

There should be three vessels: two small arteries and one large vein. A two-vessel cord occurs in 0.5% to 1% of neonates. Two-vessel cords are associated with gastrointestinal, genitourinary, and cardiovascular abnormalities. Any two-vessel cord should be submitted for pathology examination, and neonatal providers should be informed.

Measure the Length of the Cord

If the cord appears abnormally long or short, it should be measured. Remember to include the length of cord cut off the newborn's end when the cord was clamped and cut.

The normal length of a term umbilical cord is approximately 55 to 60 cm (range: 30–90 cm). A long cord, more than 75 cm, is associated with knots and fetal entanglement. Short cords, less than 32 cm, may be associated with limited fetal movement.

Inspect the Cord for Abnormalities

Look for knots, hematomas, tumors, cysts, edema, and the amount of Wharton's jelly (**Figure 31B-2**). The normal width of an umbilical cord is 1 to 2 cm.

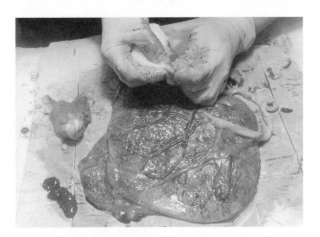

Figure 31B-1 Counting the number of cord vessels.
Source: Photography courtesy of Carrie Klima, CNM, MSN

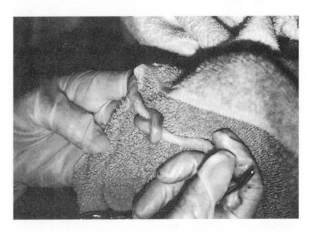

Figure 31B-2 True knot in the umbilical cord.
Source: Photography courtesy of Carrie Klima, CNM, MSN

The width is affected by the amount of Wharton's jelly.

Inspect the Cord Insertion

Observe the insertion site for where the cord inserts in relation to the body of the placenta—central, eccentric, or marginal (Battledore placenta). Determine whether the cord is inserted directly into the placenta or is attached by exposed vessels (velamentous cord insertion) (**Figure 31B-3**). Centric and eccentric (off-center) insertions are variations of normal; however, velamentous and marginal insertions are unusual and associated with a risk of vasa previa should one of these vessels tear when the membranes rupture.

Inspection of the Placenta

Inspect the Placenta for Color, Shape, Size, and Consistency

Lay the placenta flat on a surface. Look at the fetal and maternal sides. If necessary, invert the membranes to see both surfaces.

The placental shape is usually round to slightly oval and approximately 2 to 3 cm in thickness. The fetal surface is smooth. The maternal surface is usually smooth with indentations at the edges of cotyledons, but may have gritty white areas of calcification. Generally, the quantity of calcifications has no clinical importance. A pale placenta is associated with immature neonates and anemia. With extended exposure to meconium, a placenta may be stained green.

Inspect the Smooth, Shiny Fetal Side of the Placenta

Inspect for distribution of vessels from the umbilical cord over the surface of the placenta. The fetal blood vessels traverse the surface of the fetal surface from the cord insertion toward the placental margin before turning into the parenchyma, toward the maternal surface. Inspect for cysts and to determine whether this is an extrachorial placenta (either a placenta circumvallata or a placenta marginata). If necessary, invert the membranes to visualize the entire fetal surface. The fetal surface should also be examined closely for torn or intact blood vessels leading into the membranes in order to identify a missing or intact succenturiate (accessory lobe).

Inspect the Maternal Side

Examine the placental margin for torn blood vessels leading into the membranes to look for evidence of succenturiate lobe. A cotyledon missing from the main placental mass is identified by a defect in the placental mass with a rough surface where it tore away or a torn vessel at the edge of the placenta. This must be differentiated from a simple tear in the placenta without loss of tissue, which also leaves a rough surface. Differentiation is made by holding the placenta, maternal surface up, so that the cotyledons fall into place against each other (**Figure 31B-4**). A missing cotyledon is then evident because, as in a jigsaw puzzle, the surrounding pieces will not fit together smoothly. Observe for infarcts, cysts, tumors, and edema.

Figure 31B-3 Velamentous insertion of the umbilical cord.
Source: Courtesy of Tekoa L. King

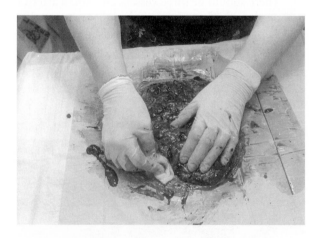

Figure 31B-4 Midwife examining the maternal side of the placenta. The placenta is intact.
Source: Photography courtesy of Carrie Klima, CNM, MSN

Measure and Weigh the Placenta

Measuring and weighing the placenta are usually dictated by policy and are not always routinely performed. A term placenta usually weighs between 400 and 4600 grams. Regardless of the policy in place, if the placenta appears to be of abnormal size, weighing and referring for pathology examination are indicated. This information is then recorded on the both the woman's and newborn's medical record.

Inspection of the Membranes

Place the placenta maternal side down, and then place a hand inside the membranes on the fetal surface of the placenta and hold the membranes up to simulate the sac they once were (**Figure 31B-5**). If the membranes are ragged and do not form a sac, they may be incomplete. If a portion of the membranes is missing, membranes may still be within the uterus although this is not a sensitive indicator of retained membranes.

When inspection and documentation are complete, the placenta should be disposed of appropriately. In some cases, families may wish to keep the organ for culturally appropriate disposal, such as planting in their gardens. Others may desire to make impressions of it for a type of placental art. However, midwives should be aware that the placenta has bodily fluids and should be treated with universal precautions.

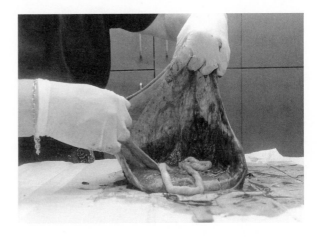

Figure 31B-5 Midwife examining the fetal side of the placenta. The membranes are incomplete.
Source: Photography courtesy of Carrie Klima, CNM, MSN

APPENDIX

31C

Manual Removal of the Placenta

A retained placenta occurs in approximately 0.01% to 6.3% of women who have a vaginal birth.[1,2] Although there is no clear consensus on the length of time a placenta is undelivered that warrants the diagnosis of retained placenta, the World Health Organization considers the placenta retained if it remains undelivered longer than 30 minutes but recommends waiting another 30 minutes before manually removing the placenta unless the woman is actively bleeding.[3] In the United States, the placenta is generally considered retained if not expelled at 30 minutes after the birth, and manual removal is recommended between 30 and 60 minutes if the woman is not actively bleeding.[2]

History

Retained placenta as ascertained by prolonged time

Physical Examination

- Evaluation of progress of the third stage of labor, including signs of placental separation.
- Continual assessment of bleeding: Active bleeding may be apparent in the presence of an undelivered placenta even if time since birth is not prolonged. Active bleeding requires prompt intervention.

Management Steps

1. Explain to the woman and others/family in attendance (with the woman's permission) the problem and the steps needed to resolve the problem.

2. Discuss options of pain management such as opioids, redosing of epidural, and/or nitrous oxide.

3. Alert the birth team (e.g., birth assistant, nurses) regarding the problem and plan for manual removal. Based on the birth site, another provider (e.g., physician, other midwife) with more experience may be immediately available and consulted as appropriate.

4. If an intravenous line is not already in place, insert one using a large-bore, at least 18-gauge needle, in case there is a hemorrhage and intravenous fluids are needed.

5. Verify that the newborn is being cared for appropriately. If the woman is holding the neonate, ask another responsible individual to hold the infant or place the newborn in a safe site.

6. Catheterize the woman's bladder as needed, as a full bladder may impede uterine contractions needed after placental removal.

7. Change gloves or put on second pair so that the procedure is as sterile as possible. Gloves of a regular length can be used, but a longer length that overlaps a sterile gown provides more protection from infection.

8. Reduce the diameter of the hand by squeezing the extended fingers close together, and gently insert one hand slowly and steadily through the vagina and past the cervix. The entire hand is inserted to facilitate the ability to perform the procedure. Once inserted, the hand should not be removed until the procedure is complete. Repeated insertion and removal of the hand increases pain and risk of infection for the woman.

9. Using the internal hand, sweep the margin of the placenta to find any area of separation. Once a point of separation is found, rotate the hand so the back of the hand is next to the uterine wall. This placement results in the hand being in a cup-like position and minimizes the risk of inadvertent uterine rupture.

10. Insinuate fingers between the placenta and the uterus to establish a line of cleavage and separate the placenta by sweeping back and forth from side to side, cutting through the decidua with the outer edge of the hand, fingertips, and first finger (**Figure 31C-1**).

11. Separate the entire placenta before attempting to extract it. If uncertain whether the placenta is totally separated, sweep the uterine wall again, feeling for and separating any remaining areas of attachment. Extraction while a section remains adherent increases the woman's risk of uterine inversion.

12. *Stop* the attempt to remove the placenta if it or its components are adherent. This finding is suggestive of a placental abnormality such as a placenta accreta. Immediate consultation/referral with a physician is required at this point.

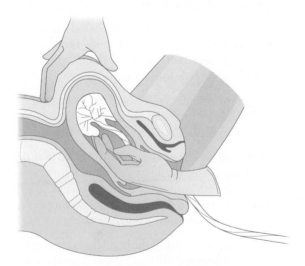

Figure 31C-1 Manual removal of the placenta.

13. Extract the placenta slowly after ascertaining that the placenta is not adherent; simultaneously continue to use the external hand to maintain fundal contraction.

14. Membranes may need to be slowly teased out, as described in Appendix 31A.

15. The placenta should be carefully inspected as described in Appendix 31B. If the placenta does not appear complete, consider performing a uterine exploration to remove any retained tissue (Appendix 31F).

16. Maintain uterine contractility through uterine massage (as needed) and administration of a uterotonic agent. Continue close observation to rule out uterine atony.

17. After the placenta is removed:

    a. If the woman experienced excessive blood loss, assess her response by repeated laboratory evaluations, including hemoglobin or hematocrit values, and the woman's symptoms during the first 24 to 72 hours postpartum. Because tolerance of blood loss is contingent upon many factors, some women will be symptomatic (e.g., syncope) at higher levels than others. Management including blood transfusions will need to be individualized.

    b. Antibiotic therapy is controversial, and lacks strong evidence to either support or refute its use. Individualization is indicated, and consultation may be a reasonable action.

    c. Document all procedures and the woman's response. Include consultations/referrals if appropriate.

● ● ● **References**

1. Cheung WM, Hawkes A, Ibish S, Weeks AD. The retained placenta: historical and geographical rate variations. *J Obstet Gynaecol.* 2011; 31:37.

2. Weeks AD. The retained placenta. *Best Pract Res Clin Obstet Gynaecol.* 2008;22:1103.

3. World Health Organization (WHO). WHO guidelines for the management of postpartum haemorrhage and retained placenta. Geneva: WHO; 2009.

31D

Initial Management of Uterine Inversion

A uterine inversion is an obstetric emergency. When a uterine inversion occurs, the risk for postpartum hemorrhage and disseminated intravascular coagulation (DIC) is quite high. The uterus may need to be repositioned when the woman is under general anesthesia. The most common symptom of uterine inversion is maternal shock that occurs very quickly. Treatment for shock should be instituted immediately even before symptoms are evident.

1. Inform the nurse or other birth assistant of the diagnosis. Request emergency obstetrician and anesthesiology consultation and additional nursing support. Initiate emergency transfer steps if in an out-of-hospital setting.

2. Have a family member or someone else hold the newborn.

3. Explain to the woman and others in attendance that the uterus is inverted, and briefly describe the steps needed to reposition the uterus.

4. Attempt to reposition the uterus immediately. Repositioning will be more successful if attempted as soon as the inversion is recognized, and before the lower uterine segment and cervix contract and form a constriction ring.

    a. Do *not* remove the placenta if still attached. Removing the placenta while the uterus is inverted will increase the blood loss and increase the risk of complications.

    b. Manual repositioning is accomplished by placing one entire hand in the vagina.

        i. Initially place the fingertips on the sides of where the uterus has turned on itself so that the inverted fundus is in the palm of the hand (**Figure 31D-1**).

        ii. Pressure is then applied with the palm of the hand on the fundus and the fingertips on the uterine walls. The fingertips gently walk up or slide up the uterine walls so the fundus is folded back into its original position. Care must be taken not to puncture or rupture the soft uterine wall.

    c. The fundus is held in place by forming the hand into a fist while waiting for the uterus to contract around the examiner's fisted hand. This puts tension on the uterine ligaments, which keeps the uterus in place, and the fist forms a ball that does not allow the fundus to fold in on itself.

    d. Keep the hand in the vagina/uterus until a consulting physician is present and can take over the maneuver, even if it appears that the inversion has been corrected.

    e. Use the abdominal hand to guard the uterus so it is lifted out of the pelvis, above the level of the symphysis, and held there for several minutes.

5. Simultaneously:

    a. Have the woman placed in Trendelenburg position.

    b. Ask that an intravenous line be placed with a large-bore needle.

c. Discontinue uterotonics.

d. Evaluate for signs of shock.

e. Request operating room and team preparation.

f. Request blood type and cross-match for 2 units of packed red blood cells, or initiate the postpartum hemorrhage protocol if one is in place.

g. Initiate quantitative evaluation of blood loss.

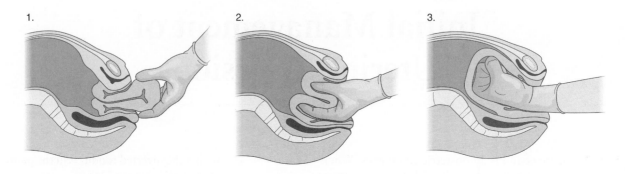

Figure 31D-1 Repositioning uterine inversion.

31E

Management of Immediate Postpartum Hemorrhage

Introduction

The management of a woman who is bleeding excessively during or immediately after the third stage of labor depends on the severity of bleeding, whether or not the placenta is delivered, and the available resources at hand. The steps listed in this appendix take the reader through the process of assessing and managing a woman who has just delivered the placenta and whose bleeding is brisk but not life threatening. In practice, management will be modified by the individual situation. For example, if the woman is hemorrhaging and the uterus is not firm, bimanual compression may be the indicated first response. Conversely, if the bleeding is less severe, the clinician may check for lacerations before other steps are taken. Similarly, if the placenta is not delivered, the first step will be manual removal of the placenta. There are multiple algorithms available that outline recommended components of care of a woman who is hemorrhaging after birth. The reader is encouraged to know all possible management responses so that they may be individualized as appropriate.

Management Steps

1. Maintain or reinstate a calm environment to reduce anxiety and facilitate management.

2. Palpate the woman's uterus, as approximately 80% of immediate postpartum hemorrhages occur secondary to uterine atony. External uterine massage may be the only intervention necessary.

3. If bleeding continues, proceed to the next steps.

4. Explain to the woman and others/family in attendance (with the woman's permission) that vaginal bleeding is excessive and explain the steps needed to resolve the problem.

5. Have a family member or other responsible adult hold the newborn. Alternatively, place the newborn in a safe site under observation.

6. Consult with other members of the healthcare team involved in the birth, including a physician if bleeding continues unabated. At this point, depending on the amount and rate of bleeding, asking for another practitioner to come to the bedside, or if in an out-of-hospital setting, emergency transport may be initiated.

7. Rule out bleeding from a laceration by efficiently performing an examination of the perineum, vulva, vagina, and cervix. Suture any active bleeding vessels appropriately.

8. If bleeding is not secondary to a laceration or the uterus is atonic, proceed to the next steps.

9. Catheterize the woman's bladder so a full bladder will not interfere with uterine contraction.

10. Order a uterotonic agent, assuming one was not administered with release of the anterior shoulder of the newborn. Oxytocin (Pitocin) is the most commonly used agent, either 10–40 units in 1000 mL solution administered intravenously at a rapid rate (500 mL/hr), titrated to uterine tone, or 10 units given intramuscularly while intravenous access with a large-bore needle (usually 18-gauge) is initiated. If a uterotonic agent has been administered with the

birth of the neonate, consider a second agent (e.g., misoprostol [Cytotec], 15-methyl PG-F2a [Hemabate]). See Table 31-3 for dose, route of administration, and side effects of uterotonic drugs used to treat postpartum hemorrhage.

11. If bleeding continues after the previous steps have been taken and the woman is in an out-of-hospital site, initiate emergency transfer to a hospital. If the excessive bleeding is controlled quickly, the transfer can be cancelled.

12. Verify that a physician has been called; while waiting for emergency medical services arrival, proceed to the following steps.

13. Initiate *bimanual compression* (**Figure 31E-1**) of the woman's uterus to treat uterine atony.

    a. Extend the fingers of one hand and squeeze the extended fingers close together, gently insert this hand into the vagina, and close the fingers into a fist as the hand enters the vagina.

    b. Position the fist palmar side up into the anterior fornix.

    c. Direct pressure to the lower uterine segment/uterine corpus by applying pressure inward and upward against the anterior wall of the uterus.

    d. Simultaneously, place the other hand externally on the abdomen and grasp the uterus between the two hands.

    e. Apply pressure to the uterus trapped between the two hands by massaging it using pressure directed against the posterior wall of the uterus, primarily in the area of the fundus and corpus of the uterus with the abdominal hand. This compression places direct pressure on the bleeding uterine vessels while stimulating the uterus to contract, an action that will also provide continuing compression.

    f. Continue bimanual compression until bleeding is controlled and uterine atony is resolved. The effectiveness of this intervention can be ascertained by momentarily releasing the pressure on the uterus and then evaluating uterine consistency and bleeding.

    g. Be aware that atony may seem to be resolved before it actually is, so bimanual compression should not be discontinued until the uterus is firm for several minutes. Removal of the hand and reinsertion increases pain/discomfort and risk of infection.

    h. If bimanual compression provides a response but uterine atony does not resolve, continue compression until a physician is present.

14. If retained products of conception are suspected to be the cause of the bleeding, proceed to performing an *intrauterine exploration*. Additional anesthesia or pain management methods may be needed at this point.

15. After bleeding has been controlled, discuss and explain situation to the woman and her family as she desires.

16. Initiate quantitative evaluation of blood loss.

17. Assess the woman's response to postpartum hemorrhage by repeat laboratory evaluations, including hemoglobin or hematocrit values, and the woman's symptoms during the first 24 to 72 hours postpartum. Because tolerance of blood loss is contingent upon many factors, some women will be symptomatic (e.g., syncope) at higher hemoglobin levels than others. Management, including blood transfusions, will need to be individualized.

18. Antibiotic therapy following uterine exploration is controversial, lacking strong evidence to either support or refute its use. Individualization is indicated, and consultation may be a reasonable action.

19. Document all procedures and the woman's responses. Include any consultations/referrals if appropriate.

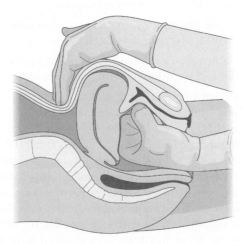

Figure 31E-1 Bimanual compression.

31F

Intrauterine Exploration

To perform an intrauterine exploration:

1. Change gloves or put on second pair so that the procedure is as sterile as possible. Gloves of a regular length can be used, but a longer length that overlaps a sterile gown provides more protection from infection.

2. Wrap one gauze sponge (e.g., 4 × 4) around two or four fingers, with the thumb stabilizing the gauze against the side of the first finger. The rougher surface of the gauze tends to be an effective modality to pick up placental fragments, ragged membranes, or blood clots. Use only one gauze so that it can easily be accounted for and to minimize the risk of leaving a gauze pad in the uterus or vagina.

3. Place the external hand on the woman's abdomen and grasp her uterus in a similar manner to that performed during bimanual compression, thereby stabilizing the organ.

4. Reduce the diameter of the internal hand by squeezing the extended fingers close together, and gently insert this hand slowly and steadily through the vagina and past the cervix. The entire hand is inserted to facilitate the ability to perform the procedure. Multiple insertions and removals of the hand increase pain and infection risk for the woman, so it is advisable to proceed carefully and intentionally.

5. Using the internal hand, sweep the inside of the uterus with the back of the hand while maintaining contact with the uterine wall so that the entire cavity is explored.

6. Remove the hand slowly from the uterus/vagina and unwrap, assess, and discard the gauze. If uncertain whether all the tissue was removed, repeat the procedure once for any remaining tissue or clots.

7. Maintain uterine contractility through uterine massage and administration of a uterotonic agent. Continue close observation to rule out uterine atony. An extended recovery period may be indicated.

8. Count the number of gauzes used and confirm that none has been left in the vagina or uterus.

9. *Stop* the procedure at any time if portions of the placenta are felt to be adherent. This finding is suggestive of a placental abnormality such as a placenta accreta. Immediate consultation/referral with a physician is required at this point, and preparation of the operating room team is indicated.

31G

Sudden Postpartum Cardiovascular or Neurologic Emergencies

Physical Examination

- Maternal consciousness
- Vital signs, including temperature
- Oxygenation (O_2 saturation)
- Skin color
- Evaluation of new findings (i.e., bleeding from unexpected sites)
- Continue monitoring uterine tone and vaginal bleeding

Management

- Initiate measures to obtain emergency medical assistance. If out of the hospital, implement the emergency transport protocol. If in the hospital, call for an emergency response team.
- Initiate a large-bore intravenous line if not already in place (18 gauge or larger). If already in place, ensure patency.
- Provide calm explanations to the woman and other friends or family who are present at her birth.
- Assign someone to provide care to the neonate.
- Administer crystalloid, 0.9% sodium chloride, or lactated Ringer's solution rapidly if the woman is hypotensive.
- Apply oxygen at a 10–12 L/min flow rate via a nonrebreather face mask.
- Obtain blood pressure, pulse, temperature, and oxygen saturation levels frequently. If blood pressure is maintained, do not overload the woman with intravenous fluids because fluid overload can contribute to pulmonary edema.
- Be prepared to initiate cardiopulmonary resuscitation. Prepare for and assist with intubation and ventilation if needed.
- Position the woman in semi-Fowler's position.
- Order arterial blood gases, complete blood count, platelet count, fibrinogen, partial thromboplastin time, blood type and crossmatch for 2 units of red blood cells, and chest X ray.
- Catheterize the bladder with an indwelling Foley catheter to drain to a urometer so output is monitored accurately.

CHAPTER

32

Birth in the Home and Birth Center

ALICE J. BAILES

MARSHA E. JACKSON

Introduction

Birth is profoundly affected by the environment in which it takes place. Ideally, every laboring woman and the team that supports and facilitates her efforts to birth will work together in an environment that is most comfortable and safe for the birthing woman. For many women, families, and providers, that safe, comfortable place to birth is in the home or birth center.

The midwife who works in the home or birth center has an opportunity to develop the hands-on, low-tech skills that are quintessential midwifery. Expertise in and fascination with normal birth make midwives keenly aware of how much they depend on the woman's natural abilities to complete the birth process herself. Midwives finely tune their perception and interaction skills that amplify the woman's abilities. The women who give birth in these birth settings are active in creating a network of support that enables them to optimize their health, and to birth safely, effectively, and with great satisfaction. These women are true partners with their midwives and their supporters as together they create the process of care. As described by Varney in an earlier edition of this text:

> If one were to place the control and responsibility assumed by the woman on a continuum, the continuum would stretch from the hospital delivery room at one end to home birth at the other. There are two important breaks in this continuum where power is transferred to the woman. The first break is when birth moves out of the hospital. The second break is when it moves from a freestanding out-of-hospital childbirth center to the home. In each instance the woman moves further away from external regulations and policies that are imposed on her childbirth experience.[1]

In the United States and beyond, data are obtained and are continuing to emerge about the safety of home birth. Data about home birth comes from small individual practices, larger networks of practices, analyses of birth certificates, and large-scale government-sponsored epidemiologic studies.[2–19] The majority of these studies have demonstrated that planned home and birth center births for healthy women experiencing normal pregnancy at term are at least as safe as—and in some cases safer than—birth in the hospital.[2–5,7–9,12,16,18,20–26] Research has documented that rates of obstetrical interventions are lower for women who begin their labors planning to give birth out of the hospital.

Perinatal mortality rates for women who give birth in home or birth center settings range from 0.35 to 3.0 deaths per 1000 live births.[4,5,15,27,28] In-labor transfer rates for women planning to birth at home or in a birth center range from 7.4% to 16.5%.[6,7,9,13–15] Cesarean birth rates for women transferred after starting labor at home or in a birth center are between 1.4% and 7.2%.[5,9,13,14,16,27] For infants born at home or in a birth center, only 0.7% of 5-minute Apgar scores are less than 7.[27] Women who give birth in a freestanding birth center or home have a lower incidence of meconium staining, fetal distress, shoulder dystocia, birth injury, neonatal respiratory distress, and postpartum hemorrhage.[5,27] In the United States in 2010, 47,028 births occurred in out-of-hospital settings, so that 1 in 85 infants born in the United

States was born at home or in a freestanding birth center.[29] Home births in the United States increased by 29% over a 6-year period from 2004 (23,150 home births) to 2010 (31,500 home births), representing the highest increase since these data were first reported in 1989.[29,30]

Hospitals often advertise their labor and delivery suite as a birth center or an alternative birthing center (ABC). These labels can be very confusing, as they also have been used to refer to both in-hospital and out-of-hospital centers. The birth centers under discussion in this chapter are either freestanding or, if within the hospital, physically separate from the main hospital labor and delivery area. In most cases, they are administratively autonomous units and have specific policies and procedures for operating both the facility and the program for the childbearing families they serve.

In recent years, interest in out-of-hospital birth has increased even as hospitals continue to change labor and birth units to make them more home-like and appealing to birthing families. A number of factors have contributed to this heightened interest. Widespread childbirth education and new published evidence supporting the safety of home birth have led many consumers to seek out-of-hospital care. Popular media, the Internet as a platform for sharing birth experiences and information, and the release of a documentary, *The Business of Being Born*, have also heightened public awareness of out-of-hospital birthing options. In addition, vocal consumers organizing to support out-of-hospital midwives and women fearing the increased rate of unnecessary technologic interventions—especially cesarean birth—have led many families to seriously explore their birth options.[31,32]

The American College of Nurse-Midwives (ACNM) and the American Association of Birth Centers (AABC) support women having a choice in birth setting attended by skilled midwives.[33–35] Unfortunately, the renewed consumer interest in out-of-hospital birth has been accompanied by controversy. In 2011, the American College of Obstetricians and Gynecologists (ACOG) reissued its committee opinion on home birth, strongly amplifying its opposition to this option.[36] In response, ACNM, the Midwives' Alliance of North America (MANA), and other professional and consumer organizations issued their own statements supporting evidence-based maternity care and the importance and availability of safe, satisfying out-of-hospital birth options for women.[37,38]

There will always be women who prefer to give birth outside of the institutional walls of a hospital—either in the home or in the birth center. Midwifery education programs of the twenty-first century are adopting strategies to enable all students to have clinical experiences in these settings. This chapter describes how the midwife works with the woman who chooses home or birth center as her preferred birth site, and presents evidence-based guidelines for safe practice in these settings.

Normal Birth

The home and birth center environments have distinctive care process characteristics that support healthy women experiencing normal birth. According to the World Health Organization:

> [A] low-risk pregnant woman should give birth in a place where she feels safe...that place may be at home, at a small maternity clinic, or birth center in town, or perhaps at the maternity unit of a larger hospital. It must be a place where all the attention and care are focused on her needs and safety, as close to home and her own culture as possible.[21]

Normal birth has been defined as spontaneous in onset, low risk at the start of and throughout labor and birth, and spontaneous birth in vertex position between 37 and 42 + 0 completed gestational weeks.[39] Normal birth has become a maternity care research focus, with seven international "Normal Labour and Birth Research Conference[s]" being convened between 2002 and 2013. In an effort to reform maternity care, English and Canadian maternity care providers and consumers produced joint statements defining normal birth.[39–41] The British Royal College of Midwives initiated a "Campaign for Normal Birth" encouraging midwives to be patient in considering whether interventions are necessary, instill security and confidence in the woman, get the woman "off the bed," listen to the woman's nonverbal signals, act as a role model for both the woman and her birth partner, give her reassurance, and immediately place the newborn in skin-to-skin contact with the mother after the birth.[42] These normal birth practices are commonly implemented in both home and birth center settings.

In the United States, maternity care providers and consumers have also turned their attention to normal birth.[43,44] In 2012, a consensus statement supporting healthy and normal physiologic childbirth was released by ACNM, MANA, and National Association of Certified Professional Midwives (NACPM). This document states that "a normal physiologic labor and birth is one that is powered by the innate human capacity of the woman and fetus. This birth is more likely to be safe and healthy because there is no unnecessary intervention that disrupts normal physiologic processes."[45]

A Home Birth Consensus Summit convened in 2011 brought together a multidisciplinary group of health professionals and consumers in an effort to increase dialogue and explore home birth in the context of maternity care in the United States. Consensus was reached at the Summit as evidenced by nine statements regarding issues related to safety, access to care, and client choice; these statements can be found at the Home Birth Consensus Summit website.[46]

Complex technologies are intentionally kept at a distance during home and birth center births. Minimizing technology may prevent some complications and increase the likelihood of normal birth. The cascade of interventions that are often utilized in the hospital setting is well known.[32] Simply putting the woman to bed may have the effect of slowing down labor progress or increasing the possibility of posterior fetal position. Hampering mobility with an intravenous infusion (IV) or discouraging an upright position by attaching a fetal monitor may reduce the woman's comfort and cause her to become anxious. Maternal anxiety increases blood levels of catecholamines, which may then inhibit uterine contractions and interfere with the action of endogenous oxytocin. Adding an exogenous oxytocin infusion may increase maternal discomfort from augmented or induced contractions, and pharmacologic pain relief may be needed to enable the woman to cope. These more complex technologies are not benign—some of them cause problems that can be remedied only with still more technologies.[25]

Characteristics of Birth Center and Home Birth

The essential characteristics of birth center and home birth are outlined in **Box 32-1**. Attributes of these settings broaden labor and birth management choices for nonpharmacologic childbirth.

Care Process Characteristics

The centrality of the birthing woman is easy to recognize in the small and intimate environments provided in a home or birth center. Distracting events are minimized, allowing the laboring woman and

---

BOX 32-1 Essential Characteristics of Birth Center and Home Birth

- Centrality of the birthing woman is clearly recognized as essential
- Consumers in these settings are:
  - Healthy women experiencing normal pregnancy
  - Actively working to promote their own health
  - Taking a partnership role in decision making
- Midwife and birthing family have increased authority
- Privacy is more accessible to the laboring woman
- Safety is preserved by adherence to essential principles
- Varying levels of family participation are encouraged
- Environments are optimal for normal birth
- Complex technologies are deliberately kept at a distance
- Practices are often owned by midwives
- Independence in midwifery practice is fostered
- Bureaucracy is minimized

---

practitioners to focus on her all-important task of giving birth. Anticipating birth in a low-tech environment, the woman and the midwives who work with her make a commitment to health promotion. They acknowledge that it is the pregnant woman herself who potentiates an excellent outcome, by engaging in activities that will enhance her health.

A number of factors make these environments optimal for normal birth. First, the woman's natural efforts are respected, and all who work with her are dedicated to the concept that birth is normal. Within these environments, it is expected that the woman has the ability to give birth. She can do so with physical, social, and psychological support and without the use of complex technology. She surrounds herself with only the people she chooses, meeting her needs for privacy or companionship. Her team may be as small as four (the woman and her birth partner, the midwife, and the birth assistant) or as large as the home or birth center can accommodate. Able to focus only on the woman as she labors, the team offers their skills, presence, and support. They work to enhance her comfort, helping her to use her energy efficiently. They provide an environment of safety and instill confidence, communicating their belief that she is doing well and has the capacity to get the job done.

The environment itself communicates this expectation of normalcy. It is familiar, without elements foreign to the woman. There is no physical evidence of machinery designed to do the job for her. She is not attached to equipment. She is free to move around and to be in any position she chooses. She can easily alter her environment or make changes within it. She can go outdoors for walks that can invigorate her, occupy her attention, and promote labor progress. She can get in and out of a shower or tub to promote relaxation. Her privacy is protected. She can make sounds without fear of being overheard by strangers close by. She has her own clothes to wear or not wear as she sees fit. Familiar food and drink that she and her family have provided are available to nourish her. At home or the birth center, women are also less likely to encounter pathogenic bacteria and invasive procedures in their birth environment, which in turn reduces the risk of nosocomial infection or adverse outcomes. In the home especially, maternal immunities to familiar bacteria protect the newborn, lessening the likelihood of infection for the mother–infant pair.

In home and birth center practice, emphasis is placed on labor as a dynamic entity wherein progress may be rapid at some times and slow at others. These ebbs and flows are viewed as essentially normal. An important task for the midwife is to watch the woman's available energy and work with her to maximize its efficient use. When the woman is tired and contractions are flagging, quieting the environment is a simple task, minimizing interruptions to promote rest. Encouraging food and fluid intake to assure adequate fuel helps prevent dehydration and fatigue. When rest and nourishment have helped her regain strength, the woman can change her activity to increase the effectiveness of the contractions. In the hospital environment, there is pressure from a variety of sources to alter these normal ebbs and flows of progress. These pressures may be physical, as in the need to make space available to accommodate other laboring women. In addition, there may be active management policies and protocols mandating progress. In contrast, away from the hospital, attention can be focused on addressing the woman's needs, enabling her to progress or rest, expecting and accommodating plateaus of progress.

All births are owned by the woman and the others she selects to share in her maternity experience. At home and in the birth center, this ownership is easier for the woman and her providers to recognize. As a result, the woman has authority to exert control over the birth's environment, management, and outcome.

In this personalized milieu, the woman is able to communicate her birth plans directly with the practice administration prior to labor. She feels assured that her preferences will be honored and looks forward to her birth, confident that the providers have a management philosophy congruent with her own. She feels that the only surprises she will encounter are the ones labor brings, and that she has a right not to be distracted from her work while she is in labor.

Safety Characteristics

To preserve safety at home and in the birth center, it is necessary to adhere to the following essential principles[4–8,10,11,14,16,22,47,48]:

1. **The woman must be committed to actively engage in health promotion.**

   Without good health, it is unsafe to plan birth at home or in a birth center.

   Women need to work to build or maintain excellent health during pregnancy.

2. **The place of birth must be planned before the onset of labor.**

   Adequate planning for the place of birth includes determination that the woman's health and the pregnancy are within normal limits when labor begins and that preparations for appropriate support are in place.

3. **The attendant must be skilled, able to screen appropriately, provide vigilant care, and manage emergency complications should they occur.**

   In addition to assisting with health promotion in the prenatal period, a skilled home or birth center midwife is vigilant in observation, communication, data collection, and care. This vigilance identifies reassuring signs of normalcy, as well as deviations from normal that may preclude a home or birth center option. If problems occur or persist at any time in the maternity cycle, the midwife acts to correct the problem or, if necessary, works to stabilize the woman's condition and transfer the woman to hospital-based care.

4. **There is a system in place for access to medical consultation, hospitalization, and emergency transport.**

   Clinical practice guidelines outline indications for consultation and a mechanism for transport. The midwife has established relationships with hospital-based practitioners to assure a smooth transition into the hospital should a transfer be indicated.

Administrative Characteristics

Home and birth center services primarily are owned by the midwives who practice in that service. The midwives render care within a structure that they create and maintain themselves, fostering independent midwifery practice and leadership skills. These practices tend to be small, minimizing bureaucracy and simplifying communication and policy. The organization is client friendly and can, therefore, be more responsive to the needs of the woman, her family, and the midwife when compared to larger institutions.

Characteristics That Differ Between Home and Birth Center Settings

Although both home and birth center practices share philosophical and administrative characteristics, the primary difference between home and birth center births is that a birth center is still the professional's territory to which the woman comes, whereas a home birth takes place in the woman's territory to which the midwife goes.[1] The balance of power in each setting is different.

A woman who decides to remain in her own home to give birth is in her own territory and has more authority. The midwife and the birth assistant are the guests, and the woman is the host. Familiarity and privacy are present, reducing the psychological stresses that may accompany labor and birth. Because the midwife is the one who travels to the woman, her labor, birth, and postpartum care are not disturbed by travel that can slow or stop early labor, cause intense discomfort in active labor, or incur the risk of giving birth en route. When families have their babies at home, there is little interruption in family routines for adults as well as for children, and there is uninterrupted bonding. When the woman and the newborn are stable and settled postpartum, the midwife and the birth assistant tuck the woman and her newborn into bed and quietly leave the home.

The birth center concept is a replicable model that has become a well-recognized birth option for families. According to the AABC:

> The birth center is a homelike facility, existing within a healthcare system with a program of care designed in the wellness model of pregnancy and birth. Birth centers are guided by principles of prevention, sensitivity, safety, appropriate medical intervention, and cost effectiveness. Birth centers provide

family-centered care for healthy women before, during and after normal pregnancy, labor and birth.[49]

Because our society has become accustomed to conducting birth in an institution, birth centers provide a compromise for families who wish to avoid the hospital, but feel that home birth is not their birthplace of choice or perhaps not appropriate. Some families choose the birth center alternative to gain more privacy than they could achieve in their own busy household. Birth centers can provide out-of-hospital options to families who live outside of a home birth midwife's service territory. Because birth centers are more accepted by the general population than birth at home, families may feel that if an unexpected poor outcome occurs at the birth center, other family members and friends will be somewhat less accusatory than if the birth had occurred at home.

Accreditation is another factor that enhances family and practitioner confidence in the birth center choice. The Commission for the Accreditation of Birth Centers (CABC) provides a mechanism for external review, giving guidance to professionals planning birth centers and practicing in them.[50] There is no comparable agency for home birth.

Midwife–Client Relationships

In every setting, the relationship between the midwife and the woman is vital. In the home and birth center, it is particularly important to specify the roles each participant assumes as they share responsibility and work together in a partnership based on mutual trust. Goals and criteria for normal are clearly delineated. Together, along with the woman's support system, all share responsibility for both the process of care and the outcome. Working in this way requires clear and ongoing communication throughout the maternity cycle.

Women who choose to birth in their homes and in birth centers often are seeking control over management of their maternity care from preconception through early parenting and seek a birth attendant who will use a labor management philosophy matching their own. They choose an attendant very intentionally, searching for a good fit, and seeking a collaborative nonhierarchic relationship. They want to find a midwife who will share power and decision making.

Midwives who choose home and birth center practice need a clear sense of their own strengths and limitations. They must be comfortable with sharing power and occupying a role that is not central. This requirement challenges midwives to sharpen their communication skills, to be open to discovering how to expand flexibility, and to know how to set and explain evidence-based limits and boundaries. Home and birth center midwives must be able to determine where philosophical gaps lie and strategize to resolve them. They must be comfortable in situations where management does not revolve around the midwife but rather around the woman.

While home and birth center midwives welcome and expect the woman's active participation in decision making and management, these midwives must also feel comfortable taking a leadership role in the midwife–client partnership. Using scientific knowledge, evidence, clinical skills, past experience, and sensitive communication, the midwife guides the woman through the preparation process that will enable her to reach her goal of birthing in her preferred site. It is critical to convey the importance of the health promotion model, of a commitment to natural birth, and of the necessity to prepare both physically and psychologically. The midwife must also be assertive as she describes the limits of her practice in the home or birth center environments.

During the prenatal visits, the midwife works to enhance the woman's self-confidence and self-reliance. By giving reassurance regarding the normalcy of pregnancy's changes, and by communicating faith in her ability to give birth, the midwife assists the woman in amplifying her strengths and helps her to compensate for any limitations. The midwife gives positive feedback as the woman takes on the necessary preparation responsibilities by creating her framework of maternity resources, such as a partner for labor support and a social network for her care postpartum. The midwife strengthens the woman's confidence further by describing and assuring access to the healthcare system's safety net should it be needed.

During the intrapartum period, the midwife's role is to be the guardian of the birth environment. The woman and her support team depend on the midwife to provide a reassuring presence. This presence provides physical and psychological labor support, as well as attention to comfort and progress using simple interventions when necessary. The woman depends on the midwife's ability to assess for continued normalcy. Should any complication occur, the midwife must have the skills needed to manage, stabilize, and in many cases resolve the situation, consulting other resources if indicated. If complications cannot be resolved in the home or birth center setting, the midwife implements a transfer to the hospital.

Health status is a dynamic entity throughout life. This is especially true for the woman and her fetus/newborn during pregnancy, labor, and birth. It is important to assist the woman to recognize and understand the significance of this fluidity. Changes in health may require changes in care. The woman, midwife, and medical system recognize that the woman's changing health status may mandate movement back and forth among providers within the healthcare system, sometimes requiring a change in the planned site of services. Transfer from home to hospital may be difficult for both the midwife and woman. The woman may be very emotionally attached to the idea of birthing at home or in the birth center, and grieves leaving her dreams behind. The midwife without hospital privileges may be reluctant to make the referral because in doing so she may lose or limit her opportunity to work with the woman. Neither reason, however, should prevent or delay a prompt transfer from occurring when necessary

The woman plays the central role in her childbearing experience. The midwife is an advocate and a coordinator. The woman knows she can depend on the midwife, and vice versa. Together they maintain the safety of the maternity process within a circle of trust and respect.

Initial Visit During Pregnancy

At the first prenatal visit between the midwife and woman, the midwife introduces the family to the services and philosophy of the practice. The midwife takes the opportunity to explain that when birth occurs in the home or birth center, both midwife and woman need to have a strong commitment to health promotion, to keeping birth normal, and to nonpharmacologic comfort measures for childbirth. The midwife, the woman, and her family discuss their needs and explore how the woman envisions getting her needs met. This visit also provides an opportunity for both woman and midwife to assess their abilities to work together. It is important that adequate time be allotted to cover all of these tasks.

The components of an initial visit include the following:

1. Selection of the birth site and analysis of the client's choice

2. Informed decision making

3. Review of midwife responsibilities

4. Review of family responsibilities

5. Outline of safety criteria and outcome statistics

6. Discussion about possibility of transfer of care

7. Complete history and physical examination

8. Calculation of accurate due date

Selection of Birth Site

At their initial visit, the midwife and the woman consider the advantages and disadvantages of all available birth options. They work together in considering the best birth setting, delineating what can and cannot be done in each site. When discussing birth site options, both positive and negative aspects of each site should be explored. The comparison of the three birth sites in **Table 32-1** lists factors that women may consider when selecting a birth site. Influences on choice of birthplace may include the philosophy of the woman and the caregivers, preferences regarding technology, the woman's health state, her feelings about previous birth experiences, societal and family considerations, and financial concerns. Fewer than 2% of women in the United States choose to give birth at home or in a birth center.[29] Thus an understanding of the woman's motivation for her birth choice will enable the midwife and woman to work together more effectively. The attitudes of the woman's support partner should also be included in this discussion.

Some women seek home and birth center services because they lack financial resources. Although the usual profile of the home or birth center client is an educated middle-class person,[2,29] many women who do not fit this picture desire to educate themselves and work to keep themselves and their babies well. The economically disadvantaged woman may benefit from the personalized, nonbureaucratic, respectful, one-on-one care associated with midwifery, which she may not often encounter elsewhere in the healthcare system. As long as the woman can accomplish the needed preparation for the birth and the pregnancy remains normal, she is a good candidate for out-of-hospital birth. Although a home or birth center birth may be less expensive if everything is normal, it may be more expensive than a hospital birth if complications arise. To that end, women should be discouraged from seeking services purely for financial reasons.

Informed Decision Making

The midwife and the woman should review and sign an informed decision document detailing essential considerations regarding home or birth center birth. This document should enumerate the points listed in **Box 32-2**. Information exchange empowers the woman to make decision about her own health.[51,52] The informed decision form should not be approached as a substitute for a trusting, nurturing relationship among the midwife, the client, and her family, however:

> The woman's signature means only that she has heard the information, understands it, and agrees to the care offered. Therefore, a good form should prompt good discussion, which is also documented in the record.... The challenge is how to inform without creating a climate of doubt about birth, and how to address fear and uncertainty without undermining the birth process.[53]

There should be ongoing communication and exploration of concerns throughout the maternity cycle. In this way, self-care is fostered, good decision making takes place, and the woman and her family are empowered.

Midwife Responsibilities

The midwife's responsibilities are outlined during the initial visit to clarify the woman's expectations regarding the midwife's role. The midwife explains the concept of working in a midwife–client partnership, each with their own set of responsibilities. Throughout the maternity cycle, the midwife provides education, guidance, and health care, with particular emphasis on signs of normalcy and signs of deviation from normal. The role of the primary support partner is discussed, and the midwife makes 24-hour midwifery on-call services available to the woman. Finally, the midwife describes the referral and transport services available; resources to cover remuneration to both midwife and consultant in case of transfer are also important factors to discuss.

Client Responsibilities

When a woman plans to give birth in the home or the birth center, it is easier for her to see the connections between her actions and the outcomes. Her responsibilities for care are clear, including recognition that her actions can make a difference. At the initial visit, enumerating these responsibilities gives the woman an overview of the tasks that she will need to undertake to promote optimal health and to maximize the likelihood of having a normal pregnancy with labor and birth occurring in the birth site that the she has chosen.

Table 32-1	Factors Influencing Birth Site Selection		
Factor	**Hospital**	**Birth Center**	**Home Birth**
Normal birth promoted	Possible, not assured	✔	✔
Personalized relationship with provider	Possible, not assured	✔	✔
Extended time for prenatal visits		✔	✔
Education is core component	Possible, not assured	✔	✔
Shared decision making promoted	Possible, not assured	✔	✔
Culturally sensitive environment	Possible, not assured	✔	✔
Sensitivity to family preferences	Possible, not assured	✔	✔
Children may be included	Possible, not assured	✔	✔
Insurance company limitations	✔	✔	✔
Cost-effective	Possible, not assured	✔	✔
Small, intimate environment		✔	✔
Minimal bureaucracy		✔	✔
Familiar environment	Possible, not assured	✔	✔
Increased control regarding choice and timing of most procedures	Possible, not assured	✔	✔
Society's expected birth site	✔		
Considered safer by general population	✔	✔	
Minimum interruption in activities of daily living			✔
Low-tech, high-touch birth environment	Possible, not assured	✔	✔
Birth takes place outside the hospital		✔	✔
Nonpharmacologic labor comfort measures maximized	Possible, not assured	✔	✔
No separation from baby	Possible, not assured	✔	✔
No limitations on persons attending birth	Possible, not assured	✔	✔
Medication for pain relief available	✔	Possible, not assured	
Complex technology on site	✔		
Birth treated as a medical event	✔		
Manages complicated pregnancy and birth	✔		
Transport necessary for high-tech interventions		✔	✔
Feeling that home environment is unsatisfactory	✔	✔	
Out-of-hospital alternative for families geographically too far for home birth		✔	
No trip to or from birthplace			✔
Decreased chance of infection		✔	✔
Family not responsible for cleanup	✔	✔	

BOX 32-2 Components of the Informed Decision Process for Home Birth and Birth Center Birth

- Information regarding advantages and disadvantages of the decision to give birth on an out-of-hospital basis while attended by a midwife
- Woman's active participation in decision making
- Qualifications of the midwife
- Woman's consent to examination, treatment, and institution of emergency procedures should they be necessary
- Responsibilities of the woman and the midwife
- Possible complications associated with childbirth
- Definitions of common terms used during the maternity cycle
- Emergency equipment present at the home or birth center
- Agreement to hospital transfer if indicated per the midwife's professional judgment

---

Basic health promotion includes good nutrition, adequate rest and exercise, stress reduction, keeping scheduled appointments, and avoiding drugs, alcohol, and smoking. The woman's responsibilities also include assuring the participation of a support partner who will take primary responsibility to be available during pregnancy, labor and birth, and the postpartum period. When small children are to be present at the birth, an adult other than the primary support partner must provide their care.

Other responsibilities introduced during the initial visit will be addressed again later in the pregnancy, including breastfeeding preparation, attending childbirth education classes, touring the hospital, gathering birth supplies, and arranging for the services of a pediatric healthcare provider. Women may also be required to meet with the consultant service during the pregnancy.

In most birth center and home birth practices, birth assistants work alongside the midwives. The client needs to understand the importance of this assistant's role in increasing safety at the birth. Some practices have birth assistants on-call for laboring clients, whereas others may have the client hire a birth assistant. A birth assistant is a person with supportive and technical labor, birth, and postpartum skills. These skills include not only evaluation of the woman's physical and emotional needs and status during labor, but also the ability to monitor maternal, fetal, and newborn vital signs, certification in adult cardiopulmonary resuscitation (CPR), and familiarity with the Neonatal Resuscitation Program (NRP). These are all essential birth assistant skills. The birth assistant should also be able to provide assistance with breastfeeding and postpartum care. Some birth assistants are registered nurses, emergency medical technicians, or even individuals preparing to ultimately attend midwifery programs, but it is not necessary for the birth assistant to be a medical professional. Childbirth educators, La Leche League leaders, and doulas can obtain the additional skills needed to become good birth assistants.

Finally, financial arrangements must be clear for both self-pay and insured clients. A written payment plan should be arranged, including insurance information and a schedule for payments. Financial concerns should be discussed openly by all responsible parties.

Safety Criteria and Transfer

The issue of transfer of care, should a complication arise, should be addressed at the initial visit. Problems that can occur during pregnancy, labor, or birth, or in the immediate postpartum period, and their frequency of occurrence should be reviewed with the woman and her family. The importance of self-care and early intervention to promote health should be reemphasized. The midwife reviews the woman's health needs to assure the choice of an appropriate birth site, making the woman aware that some health conditions are best addressed in the hospital (**Box 32-3**).

It is important to note that problems can occur that can be remedied through self-care, that need the midwife to resolve, or that need a physician to treat. Some problems may require referral or discharge out of the service. The midwife has ultimate responsibility for establishing the link to the hospital system, even though some women arrange or lay the groundwork for consultation/hospital services. Although urgent emergencies are rare in the home or in the birth center,[13,15] women need to explore their feelings regarding the worst possible birth outcome for them. This is a very sensitive issue that they may not be ready to discuss at the initial visit; given this possibility, introducing this subject during the first visit and revisiting it during subsequent prenatal visits is the best way to make sure this topic is fully explored.

BOX 32-3 Common Indications for a Change in Birth Site from Home or Birth Center to Hospital

- Severe chronic hypertension and/or preeclampsia requiring management with medication
- Current mental illness that the midwife deems would have a harmful effect on the perinatal course
- Thromboembolic event requiring heparin
- Current substance abuse including alcohol, cigarettes, and other drugs
- Insulin-dependent diabetes
- Clinically significant blood antibodies during current pregnancy
- Two or more cesarean sections
- No or undocumented prenatal care
- Medical indication for induction of labor
- Placenta previa at term

- Active preterm labor that cannot be stopped
- Post dates more than 42 weeks' gestation
- Nonreassuring fetal surveillance results
- Active herpes lesions of cervix, vagina, introitus, labia, or anus during labor
- Multiple gestation diagnosed before or during labor
- Persistent noncephalic presentation during labor
- Febrile condition in labor with or without spontaneous rupture of membranes that does not resolve with hydration
- Evidence of chorioamnionitis
- Evidence of fetal intolerance of labor
- Thick meconium-stained amniotic fluid
- Irresponsible attitude or action of parents
- Unsafe home or location for birth

This list is not all-inclusive, and the midwife's clinical judgment may determine that additional conditions indicate a hospital birth. It must also be noted that some recognized religious communities, such as Amish or Plain people, claim religious exemptions, choosing to give birth in the home or birth center setting even though they have conditions such as breech presentation or multiple gestation. The midwives caring for these women are responsible for acquiring the clinical skills necessary to manage these conditions, for obtaining an informed decision document from the woman, and for having a consultation agreement in place.

Complete History and Physical Examination

During the initial visit, the midwife will assess the client for predictors of normalcy and predictors of deviation from norm in the woman's history and physical examination. A woman and her partner need to provide accurate family, medical, menstrual, and conception histories. Records from other healthcare providers should be requested if needed. With the information obtained through the history and physical examination, the woman and the midwife can identify factors that have the potential to develop into problems. Instituting prevention strategies early increases the likelihood that the woman will birth in her chosen birth site.

Calculation of an Accurate Due Date

Particular attention must be paid to calculation of an accurate due date, because for most out-of-hospital practices there is a 5-week window of safety for planned home or birth center birth. A pregnancy is full term from 37 weeks' gestation until 42 weeks' gestation. Births occurring at less than 37 weeks' gestation or more than 42 weeks' gestation are more safely accomplished in the hospital, but occasionally the window of safety can be expanded a few days with careful fetal surveillance and appropriate consultation. When labor occurs before 37 weeks'

gestation, fetal lung maturity may not be present.[54] The woman whose preterm labor cannot be stopped is referred to the hospital, where appropriate staff and technology can give long-term support to the newborn if needed. Likewise, women who labor after 42 completed weeks of pregnancy are at increased risk for meconium staining and variant fetal heart rate patterns during labor, both of which have been implicated as causes of morbidity and mortality.[13]

Return Visits

During each return visit, the woman and the midwife identify reassuring signs of normalcy or identify problems, through an interim history, physical examination, and laboratory and adjunctive studies. In the role of educator, the home and birth center midwife teaches the woman about symptoms that could indicate deviation from norm. In this way, the woman is enabled to continue to take a principal role in early identification of problems, allowing for early intervention. To remain a candidate for an out-of-hospital to birth, it is especially vital to intervene early, before problems occur that are not correctable. Women know that if they encounter specific complications, they will lose their opportunity to have the birth they had planned—this knowledge is a powerful motivator for women to engage in health promotion.

The Family's Preparation for Birth and the Postpartum Period

Planning for birth involves readying the participants and requires considerable time, thought, and energy. More preparation on the part of the family is required when birth occurs in an out-of-hospital setting. A list of family responsibilities appears in **Box 32-4**.

As the due date nears, childbirth classes help the woman and her primary support partner focus on the upcoming birth. The classes that are most useful emphasize the woman's inner strengths and are presented by an instructor who is knowledgeable about home and/or birth center births, teaching with confidence that unmedicated birth is possible, given that few pharmaceutical options are available outside the hospital. Women will rely on techniques learned in class to enhance comfort and relaxation, to relieve pain, and to augment labor. Childbirth classes located in hospitals are often intended as an orientation to the hospital system and prepare the woman for labor and birth in that setting.

Writing a birth plan gives women and their partners an opportunity to discuss what is important to them for their birth. These plans detail preferences about the environment, social interaction, and comfort measures. Women and their partners identify the persons who will be present at the birth, the specific duties they may have, the role of siblings, religious or spiritual observance, and planned events with family and friends. Birth plans also describe coping measures learned from previous births, desired positions for labor and birth, and preferences for privacy and company at various points in labor. Plans for music, photography, and audio and/or video recording may be outlined. To promote realistic thinking about possible transfers, families should be encouraged to write a hospital birth plan in addition to a home or birth center birth plan. This plan would focus on preferences regarding interventions and contact with the newborn. Families must realize that when a transfer to the hospital is indicated, medical interventions are needed and should be expected.

Most home and birth center practices anticipate that women will breastfeed their babies unless there are extenuating circumstances. Breastfeeding is an essential safety factor for women giving birth in an out-of-hospital setting. When the woman is home without professional assistance, breastfeeding helps to keep the uterus contracted, thereby helping to

> ### BOX 32-4 The Family's Preparation for Birth and Postpartum
>
> - Continuing commitment to a jointly created plan of care
> - Keeping the midwife informed of any life changes
> - Doing specified reading
> - Attending childbirth education classes
> - Writing a birth plan
> - Confronting and resolving fears
> - Preparing prenatally for breastfeeding
> - Preparing invited participants for their responsibilities
> - Preparing siblings for their participation
> - Paying fees for care and/or conveying insurance information
> - Collecting and organizing specified supplies for home birth
> - Obtaining and packing supplies to take to the birth center
> - Arranging birth assistant availability
> - Having a clean house
> - Arranging for pet safety and care at the time of labor and birth
> - Obtaining an infant car seat and assuring proper installation
> - Making an accurate, detailed map to the home or checking Global Positioning System (GPS) accessibility
> - Visiting an obstetric consultant, if needed
> - Making emergency plans and posting them by each telephone and in the chart
> - Having a vehicle available with a full tank of gasoline
> - Knowing how to get to the hospital
> - Arranging pediatric care

control bleeding postpartum. La Leche League, other breastfeeding support groups, and lactation consultants are invaluable resources for prenatal breastfeeding preparation and support on a postpartum basis.

Participants who will be present for the birth also require preparation. If children are to be present, they need to be prepared for birth events, including sights and sounds. They also need the services of an adult whose primary responsibility is child care. This adult needs preparation for the labor and birth and for his or her role. Children must be cared for to allow the woman and her partner to focus their complete attention on managing labor. Also, if transport occurs, someone must be available to be with the children continuously until the woman and/or her partner return from the hospital.

The people attending the birth should be selected carefully. It should be made clear that people invited to attend the birth may be asked to leave if the woman seems to be distracted by their presence. Some participants may have fears about out-of-hospital births. Addressing their fears before the birth may change attitudes, and their attendance at the birth can be a transformative experience.

Bags should be packed and supplies ready by 36 weeks' gestation for families planning to labor and give birth in a birth center (**Box 32-5**). Supplies needed for home birth should be organized by 36 weeks' gestation and located in or close to the room in which the woman intends to birth (**Box 32-6**). An up-to-date electronic or paper copy of the woman's health record should also be available. Siblings can take an active role in preparing supplies. Last-minute details to be accomplished when labor starts can be posted on a "to do" list.

Prenatal Home Visit

A home visit by the midwife or the birth assistant around 36 weeks' gestation assures that the family is ready for the home or birth center birth. The family prepares a detailed map or ensures global positioning system (GPS) accessibility that can be tested for accuracy when this home visit is made. An emergency plan and important telephone numbers should be posted by each telephone in the home and in the woman's chart. The family should make a "practice run" to the back-up hospital to ensure that they know the fastest route, the traffic patterns, the location to park, and the point at which to enter the building should a transfer become necessary. The car that will be used for emergency transportation needs adequate fuel to get to the hospital. Having hospital admission forms completed online or a completed paper copy in the chart before labor begins decreases stress if a transfer to the hospital becomes necessary.

For home birth, a relatively clean house and pet control are obvious responsibilities of the family. Most pets can be present at births without causing any difficulties.

The Intrapartum Period at Home or in the Birth Center

When labor begins, the family contacts the midwife, the birth assistant, and the other people who are invited to the birth. In some practices, the midwife

---

> **BOX 32-5 Family Supplies for a Birth Center Birth**
>
> **Items to Be Packed for Easy Transport to the Birth Center by 36 Weeks' Gestation**
>
> - Nutritious, easy-to-prepare meals and snacks for you and your birth team
> - At least 3 quarts of juice, energy drink, tea, and broths
> - Honey
> - Comfortable clothing to wear during labor and extra clothing to wear home
> - Extra pillows
> - Music (CDs or electronic device)
> - Camera and/or video camera
> - Swim trunks/suit and extra towels for partner
> - Entertainment for older children (e.g., books, games, videos)
> - Nutritious postpartum meal for the new parents
> - Hydrogen peroxide and ammonia for spot removal and laundry
> - For the infant:
>   - Clean thermometer
>   - Four receiving blankets
>   - Petroleum jelly
>   - Five disposable newborn-size diapers
>   - Baby clothes suitable for the weather
>   - Car seat, in place, adjusted to fit the newborn
>
> *Source:* © BirthCare & Women's Health, Ltd. Reprinted by permission.

---

directly contacts the birth assistant. The midwife is the primary attendant and is responsible for coordinating care. During the initial labor call, the midwife gathers data about how the woman is experiencing her labor, her needs, and her support systems. The midwife, the woman, and her support network review choices and make appropriate management plans, taking into account the woman's perceptions and prenatal history. Plans may include further telephone contact or a decision for the midwife to meet the woman for additional assessment.

If the woman is comfortable at home and has the support she needs, and there are no concerns that require immediate follow-up, continued telephone contact with her midwife may be all that is necessary during the early phases of labor. The woman may want to continue her activities of daily living while

---

BOX 32-6 Family Supplies for a Home Birth

Most midwives request that the family assemble and organize supplies by 36 weeks' gestation. Some of the supplies are common household items; others can be purchased through a company that customizes birth kits to the specifications of the midwife or the family.

- Mattress cover (e.g., plastic dropcloth, shower curtain liner)
- Extra pillows covered with plastic
- Food and fluids for labor
- Flexible straws
- Clean towels
- Antiseptic solution (e.g., povidone-iodine, benzalkonium chloride)
- Wash cloths or 4 × 4 gauze pads
- Flashlight with batteries and extra batteries
- Mirror
- Two quart-size bowls (for placenta)
- Bulb syringe
- Heating pad
- Baby hats
- Baby receiving blankets/soft towels
- Thermometer
- Measuring tape
- Peri pads and underpants
- Squeeze bottle for perineal rinse
- Disposable waterproof underpads
- Baby supplies, including clothes, diapers, and car seat
- Large plastic garbage bags
- Plastic freezer bags
- Two lightweight plastic containers for emesis
- Paper towels
- Tissues
- Hydrogen peroxide for removal of blood stains
- Check photography supplies and charge batteries
- Organize audio/music devices

Source: © BirthCare & Women's Health, Ltd. Reprinted by permission.

---

emphasizing hydration, nutrition, and increased rest. A variety of food choices for the laboring woman should be provided, and food should be available for the entire birth team. Friends and family may come to help with final preparation and management of other household activities, freeing the woman and her primary support partner to focus on the labor.

A woman planning a home birth may "double-make" her bed to protect the mattress. The bed can be made with a full set of linen and then completely covered with plastic such as a plastic mattress cover, a drop cloth, or a shower curtain. A clean old sheet is placed on top of the plastic so that the bed may be used as desired for labor or birth. When the birth is completed, it is a simple matter to remove the top sheet and the plastic. Clean linen is then readily available for the woman's comfort postpartum.

The midwife may do the first physical assessment of labor in the woman's home, the birth center, or the midwife's office, regardless of where the birth is planned. The midwife may also choose to delegate this assessment to the birth assistant. The initial assessment should include a review of the prenatal record, a physical examination to assess presentation, vital signs of the woman and fetus, uterine contractions, and maternal response to labor. A pelvic examination may be part of the initial physical assessment to confirm labor progress, verify the presenting part, or provide information that the woman requests.

As labor intensifies, the midwife or birth assistant's presence is required to assess maternal well-being and fetal heart tones per clinical practice guidelines or according to ACNM's clinical bulletin on intermittent auscultation.[55] Families very often have birth plans that outline the families' preferences for birth. Care provided is individualized for the woman, her family, and the unique labor. The time frame varies during labor in which the midwife should be in close or continuous attendance in labor. The midwife or birth assistant also may augment the birth partner's support measures, give reassurance, and guide the woman to conserve her energy. The woman is free to move around and assume any position she chooses. The midwife may suggest positions that promote comfort, encourage progress, and maintain fetal well-being. In the birth center or home, women very frequently birth out of bed.

During the second stage of labor, it is not unusual for the woman to continue to change positions, moving from the bed to other locations within the home or birth center. The midwife must be alert, flexible, and able to anticipate the woman's movements. Sterile instruments should be placed on a portable sterile surface, allowing the midwife to move while following the woman's lead. Good communication among the midwife, the woman, and her birth team helps everyone work together effectively. When the woman describes where and how she feels the fetus's descent, the midwife can give feedback confirming or correcting her perceptions. If the woman is reluctant to change position, the midwife may need to use persuasive communication to suggest positions that will facilitate the birth.

As the fetal head emerges, the woman and/or her partner often reach down to complete the birth (**Figure 32-1**). Within the first few seconds, the midwife can feel and see the newborn's muscle tone, enabling quick evaluation of infant well-being. She and the birth assistant continue observation of the newborn's heart rate and respiratory effort. Parents place the infant in skin-to-skin contact with assistance as needed, thereby supporting newborn thermal regulation. The midwife is responsible for directing the birth assistant's care and continuing to observe for successful transition from intrauterine to extrauterine life.

It is normal for some newborns to latch on immediately, whereas others are more interested in exploring this change in their environment—looking, listening, nuzzling, and licking, and taking their time to find the nipple and latch on. Most of the time, the woman is eager to get her newborn on the breast. Some women prefer to take a moment to regroup from the intensity of giving birth, and are then ready to welcome their newborn. While the midwife is attentive to the progress of the third stage of labor,

the birth assistant checks the newborn's vital signs without disturbing family–infant bonding. The newborn can remain skin to skin in the birthing woman's arms while the birth assistant checks the vital signs every 30 minutes, or more frequently if indicated. The focus of the family is directed toward welcoming the newborn. Siblings are often present at the birth or they can be invited in when the woman wishes.

Birth of the placenta is usually unhurried. If the woman needs or chooses to do so, she may squat or sit on the toilet to facilitate the completion of the third stage. Both attendants remain alert and in good communication regarding any normal postpartum signs and symptoms or maternal or infant deviations from normal. The midwife may dispose of the placenta through a hazardous waste company. Some families desire to keep their placenta to bury under a plant or tree. Placental encapsulation has become a recent interest, whereby the family requests that the placenta be dried and encapsulated to be used for purported medicinal purposes.

Birth is simple. In the home and birth center settings, where interruptions are limited to those

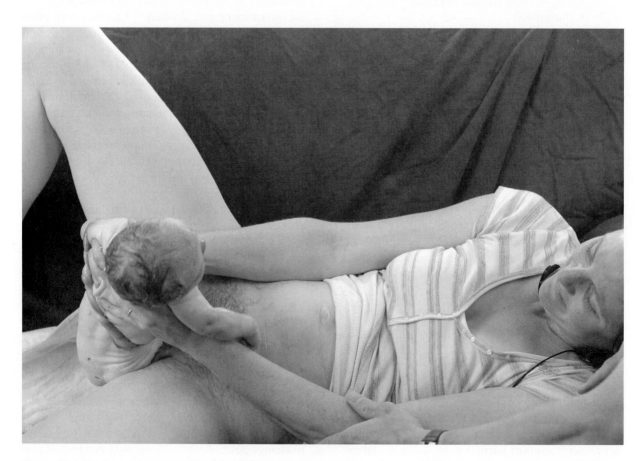

Figure 32-1 Mother reaches to complete the birth.
Source: Photo Credit: Sue Baelen for Wisewoman Childbirth Traditions

necessary to ensure safety, birth can more easily unfold. Welcoming the newborn can take place as the family has planned. An out-of-hospital birth can have long-lasting, positive effects on parental and sibling bonding and attachment, confidence for parenting, and memories of the birth as a peak emotional experience for the family.

The Early Postpartum Period and Follow-Up

The first 2 to 4 hours postpartum is a special time for the new mother, her family, and friends to welcome and bond with the newborn.[56] The midwife and the birth assistant in the home and birth center setting are participants during this time of welcome. The tasks that must be accomplished are both similar to and different from tasks in the hospital environment. It is not unusual for the midwife to spend this period actively working at jobs typically accomplished in the hospital by nursing, secretarial, housekeeping, and dietary staff.

The woman and her newborn are more likely to remain stable after breastfeeding is established. Once it is assured that vital signs, lochia, uterine position, and uterine consistency, as well as infant status, are within normal limits, the midwife can leave the birthing room, facilitating a period of privacy and continued bonding time for the family. Most often, eye prophylaxis and vitamin K administration are delayed until after this time of family bonding. Some families make an informed choice to waive these newborn procedures. While bonding continues, the midwife can accomplish the usual postpartum responsibility of documenting the birth.

The midwife, along with the birth assistant, assure proper nourishment for the woman, help with breastfeeding, assist the woman to shower and void, wash the instruments, and put the birth site in order. Quite often, family and friends who have attended the birth as guests become helpers during this postpartum family time.

The midwife does a complete newborn physical examination, often using a heating pad for a warm surface. As long as the newborn is transitioning appropriately, the physical examination is usually done after a period of bonding according to the family's preference. This examination provides an opportunity for teaching, usually taking place in the woman's bed in the presence of excited children greeting the new sibling. Family members often participate in weighing, measuring, and dressing the newborn in the midst of friends taking photographs and a great deal of socializing and celebration.

The very positive side of this time is the intimacy, emotion, and social closeness involved in spending this time with a family. For many midwives, the tenderness, bonding, and beauty of these postpartum hours fuel their love for midwifery and out-of-hospital birth on a fundamental level.

After the midwife departs the home or the family leaves the birth center, it is recommended that the newborn and mother stay close together. To aid in temperature stabilization, a bath may be delayed for the first 24 to 48 hours. The woman and newborn are assessed in the first 2 days either at a home or office visit or via a telephone assessment. Breastfeeding, the developing family relationships, adequacy of help in the home, infant caretaking abilities, and follow-up appointments with the newborn's healthcare provider are also assessed at this visit.[1] During the 6-week postpartum recovery period, the family may be seen in the midwife's office to evaluate maternal involution and other maternal, infant, or family needs.

Maintaining Safety

Maintaining safety is the primary priority in all settings where midwifery is practiced. The personnel and equipment needed in the home or birth center during the intrapartum period to assist with normal birth and to intervene if problems occur are elegantly simple: a midwife, a birth assistant, and the equipment listed in **Table 32-2**. Access to medical consultation is crucial in all midwifery practices, regardless of birth site. When women plan to birth at home or in a birth center, not only do they need access to consultation, but they also need access to hospitalization should the need for it arise. Wherever birth takes place—at home, at a birth center, or at a hospital—the mechanism for handling problems must be clearly outlined by providers and institutions. When in the hands of a skilled practitioner in the home and birth center environments, the equipment listed in Table 32-2 meets the basic needs of the woman during normal birth.

Appropriate birth site selection, familiarity with the research, and sound clinical knowledge enable the midwife to plan appropriately for prevention, correction, or stabilization of problems and—if necessary—for transport of the woman and/or the newborn to the hospital. When intrapartum transfer is needed, it is usually accomplished by car. The incidence of urgent emergency (when an ambulance may be needed) is rare, ranging from 1% to 2.4%.[6,15]

In a hospital practice, the infrastructure and personnel provide layers of support. Away from the

Table 32-2	Midwife Equipment for Birth at Home or in the Birth Center
Essentials	**Extras to Consider**
Up-to-date electronic or paper copy of chart available	Otoscope/ophthalmoscope
Paper or electronic forms for intrapartum, postpartum, and newborn charting	Hot-water bottle or heating pad
	Flexible straws
Birth certificate forms	Electrolyte replacement drink (e.g., Pedialyte, Gatorade)
Blood pressure cuff, stethoscope	Massage roller
Fetoscope/Doppler stethoscope	Instruments:
Gloves (sterile and nonsterile)	• Tissue forceps
Lubricant (sterile and nonsterile)	• Allis clamps
Sterile instruments	• Hemostats
Scissors (2 pairs)	Combs for acupressure points
Large clamps (Kelly or Rochester-Ochsner)	Antibiotics and 150-cc normal saline bags for administration of antibiotics IV
Needle holder	
Ring forceps	Lidocaine jelly for topical use
Amnihook	Slow-cooker pot for hot perineal compresses
Cord clamp or cord tape	Laryngeal mask airway
Sterile 4 × 4 gauze pads	Adult positive-pressure resuscitation bag and mask
Heating pad for baby blankets	Cotton baby hats
Bulb syringe	Culturettes
Baby scale	Camera
Measuring tape	Apron or gown
Vitamin K	Protective eyewear
Erythromycin ophthalmic ointment	Change of clothes
Sharps box and mechanism for hazardous waste disposal	Toilet articles
	Mirror
Light source (e.g., flashlight)	Speculum
DeLee suction trap or suction machine	Blood glucose monitoring sticks and/or glucometer
Infant positive-pressure resuscitation bag and mask	
Laryngoscope with infant blade (size 1)	
Endotracheal tubes, size 3.5 mm and 4 mm, with stylets	
Oral airways (infant, adult)	
Small oxygen tank, oxygen tubing, mask (neonatal and adult)	
Postpartum hemorrhage control: injectable oxytocin, injectable and oral methylergonovine maleate, and misoprostol tablets	
Urinary catheters	
Suture with needles	
Local anesthetic, syringes, and needles	
Urine dipsticks	
pH indicator paper	
Intravenous fluids: lactated Ringer's and 5% dextrose in Ringer's lactate	
Angiocatheters, long intravenous tubing, tape, antiseptic ointment, gauze pads	
Blood collecting supplies: tourniquet, tubes, syringes, needles and vacutainer	

hospital, clinical judgment takes into account the known delay between some decisions and the implementation of necessary interventions. Management of problems depends on written clinical practice guidelines, characteristics of the woman and her support system, the network of medical support, and the midwife's ability to perform clinically.[51] Other factors that influence decision making may include the following:

- The CNM's/CM's level of experience
- Distance from the hospital
- Quality of the consultant relationship
- Road conditions
- The woman's previous birth experiences and commitment to out-of-hospital birth
- Quality of communication between the CNM/CM and the parents

Management strategies for selected clinical situations may be divided into three categories for home and birth center management: preventive, non-urgent, and emergency.

Personnel and Equipment

Most home and birth center practices utilize two intrapartum providers: the primary midwife and a birth assistant.[51] Inclusion of both as caregivers assures adequate staff are available to meet the laboring family's needs for support and safety maintenance without compromising privacy. Labor is often long, and to meet the woman's needs, the midwife may need periodic rest. Limiting attendants to a midwife and a birth assistant reduces distracting staff changes while providing adequate help.

Each time the midwife and the birth assistant set up for a birth, they organize and check the equipment. A review of the woman's chart and her birth plan will focus attention on her individual needs. The pair ready equipment and review skills needed to address potential problems. The midwife and birth assistant will work together more smoothly if time for practice drills is regularly scheduled. For complications such as shoulder dystocia, postpartum hemorrhage, and neonatal resuscitation, the midwife values a skilled birth assistant's help. The assistant should also be able to perform emergency measures as needed, including suprapubic pressure, fundal massage, and assistance with the administration of medication.

Preventive Management

Prevention is the first line of defense to maintain safety. Safety is most effectively maintained when strategies to reduce risk are actively implemented. Most women who choose home or birth center birth understand that to achieve their goal of birthing in their preferred site, they must build an optimal maternity experience by bolstering excellent health and promoting a pregnancy free of complications. Appropriate birth site planning also reduces the incidence of problems during labor and birth. For example, when the woman is sensitive to the location of fetal movement prenatally, and the midwife uses Leopold's maneuvers to assess fetal position, a breech presentation can be identified early. In turn, appropriate interventions may be implemented prenatally to encourage vertex presentation, thereby decreasing the need for a transfer of care for a hospital birth.

Management of Non-urgent Clinical Situations

Prolonged Labor

Multiple studies have identified prolonged labor in nulliparous women as the most common reason for transfer from home or a birth center into the hospital.[4,6,9,12] Patience and attention to supporting the woman's efficient use of energy during labor are the most important interventions that the midwife can use to avoid prolonged labor secondary to uterine inertia or maternal exhaustion. Adequate hydration and nutritional sources of energy are essential. The midwife may encourage periods of rest when labor ebbs. The variety of environments found within the birth center and home, such as a kitchen, living room or lounge area, and easy access to the outdoors can help the woman pass the time and maintain progress.

With experience, the midwife develops hand skills that can be used to assess the relationship of the fetal head to the maternal pelvis. These hands-on skills also enable the midwife to guide the fetus into more favorable positions, thereby promoting rotation, descent, and birth.

When slow progress becomes a concern, it must be clearly understood that oxytocin cannot be administered to augment or induce labor in the home or birth center. Exogenous oxytocin may cause tachysystole, which reduces placental blood flow and can result in fetal hypoxia. If labor stimulation cannot be accomplished by means such as walking, nutritional support, castor oil, making love, or nipple stimulation, then a hospital transfer may be indicated.

Sometimes when labor continues without progress, the woman may lose her ability to cope with labor pain and may find that strategies for nonpharmacologic pain relief are no longer effective. If the woman's need for pain relief cannot be met by the limited choices available in the out-of-hospital setting, a transfer to the hospital is indicated. A nonurgent transfer may take place in the family car as long as maternal and fetal vital signs are within normal limits. Women transferred for prolonged labor with their first birth can usually complete subsequent births in out-of-hospital settings.

Prolonged Ruptured Membranes

In cases of prolonged rupture of the membranes at home or in the birth center, concern about infection is reduced, but not eliminated. Pathogenic bacteria are not in abundance as long as the woman is not a carrier of group B *Streptococcus* (GBS), and avoiding vaginal examinations decreases the risk of infection. Nevertheless, monitoring for signs of infection remains of critical importance. Setting a time limit before transfer to the hospital, if necessary, will depend on the midwife's preferences, the woman's preferences, and negotiations with the healthcare system, including consideration of obstetric and neonatal community standards.

Group B Streptococcus Colonization

Women who are colonized with GBS may give birth safely at home or in a birth center. When intravenous antibiotic prophylaxis is indicated, it may be administered in the home or birth center. Women who are colonized with GBS should discuss neonatal follow-up plans with their pediatric care provider during the prenatal period. Families may be taught to monitor and record the newborn's vital signs, enabling them to convey information about the newborn's health to the pediatric care provider within 12 to 48 hours after birth.

Vaginal Birth After Cesarean Birth

A vaginal birth after cesarean birth (VBAC) may be undertaken in the out-of-hospital setting provided the proper systems are in place for informed decision making, appropriate prenatal screening and care, and ready access to hospital-based services should they be needed. Studies show that 60% to 80% of women with a previous cesarean birth who elect to labor successfully give birth vaginally. The chances of giving birth vaginally after a prior cesarean section may be increased depending on the woman's specific history. Careful prenatal screening is necessary before attempting VBAC, including documentation of a low transverse uterine incision, sonographic documentation of placental location, and consideration of the indication for previous cesarean birth.

Informed decision making specific to VBAC should be obtained from the outset with careful review of the practice's successful VBAC rate, repeat cesarean rate, possible complications, arrangement for transport to the hospital, and discussion of realistic expectations. Establishing a clear, jointly agreed-upon management plan with the obstetrical consultant is necessary. The laboring woman's birthplace should be close to a hospital that has available staff, including anesthesia services, and access to immediate cesarean birth.

Midwifery-led care processes such as balancing activity and rest, nutritional support, continuity of care, shared decision making, and respect for the woman's own preferences may facilitate VBAC. In addition, intermittent auscultation reduces restrictions on maternal movement imposed by continuous electronic fetal monitoring. All of these practices are available in the home and birth center settings.

The woman who experienced a previous cesarean section needs support to empower herself to labor and to protect herself from disappointment, particularly if she feels that the initial cesarean procedure was unnecessary. It may be liberating for her not to go back to the hospital. Feelings of profound hurt may not be totally resolved until after the current pregnancy is completed and the woman births either vaginally or via repeat cesarean section.[57–62]

Meconium Staining

If meconium appears at any time after rupture of the membranes, consistency of the meconium should be evaluated. Notification of the consultant depends on the consultation agreement and the type of meconium present. Meconium-stained amniotic fluid combined with a fetal assessment that evidences fetal well-being does not always indicate a need to transfer the woman to the hospital. However, a discussion with the woman and her support partner regarding the midwife's assessment, possible consequences of meconium aspiration, and treatment options both in and out of the hospital should always be initiated and documented. The decision to transport or not should occur with the midwife's guidance and with consideration of the family's preferences. If the decision is made to remain out of hospital for the birth, a DeLee suction trap and other resuscitation equipment should be readied. Amniotic fluid with thick meconium indicates that the woman should be transferred to the hospital before the birth, if there is adequate time.

Management of Urgent Emergency Clinical Situations
Abnormal Fetal Heart Rate Patterns

Abnormal fetal heart rate patterns may require emergency transport to the hospital. Similarly, if at any point during the labor the midwife feels a need to monitor the fetus more closely than intermittent use of the fetoscope or Doppler imaging allows, then the woman should be moved to the hospital rather than a fetal monitor moved to the woman. Variant fetal heart rate patterns that do not resolve with increased hydration, a change in maternal position, and a brief period of oxygen by mask indicate that the fetus is at increased risk for clinically significant acidemia at birth. A transfer to the hospital is indicated to allow access to the needed personnel and technology to manage the problem.

Breech Presentation

Women diagnosed prenatally with a fetus in breech presentation should have an informed decision discussion about (1) external version, (2) planned hospitalization for vaginal breech birth, or (3) cesarean section for breech. If by the onset of labor the breech presentation persists, a plan for hospitalization is recommended. Rarely, a woman in labor at home or in the birth center may present with a previously undetected breech. If time permits, the midwife may call 911 for extra personnel and equipment. In this situation, the midwife facilitates the mechanisms of labor for breech presentation with appropriate hand maneuvers to accomplish the breech birth. The midwife notifies the consultant, and transports the woman to the hospital if indicated.

Newborn Complications

"What if the baby doesn't breathe?" is the number one fear that the general population has regarding home and birth center birth. The reality is that resuscitation is very rare when a healthy pregnant woman experiences a normal pregnancy, has an unmedicated and uncomplicated intrapartum course, and gives birth at home or in a birth center.[17,63] However, dealing with fear is essential. Neonatal Resuscitation Program certification or an equivalent is a critical skill for both the midwife and the birth assistant who attend home and birth center births. Having two trained people present for all births is advisable. When a need for resuscitation occurs in these settings, help is remote and the midwife is truly on her own. The resuscitation equipment and skills provided by home and birth center midwives are usually successful in stimulating the newborn's respiratory effort, and the newborn is very likely to recover immediately. If this does not occur, the goal is to stabilize the newborn, oxygenating the infant adequately until transport to a neonatal intensive care unit is completed.

Postpartum Hemorrhage

Another common fear regarding home or birth center birth is "What if the woman bleeds too much?"

The reality is that postpartum hemorrhage requiring transport is *extremely* rare, with incidence reported as ranging from 0.2% to 1%.[6,13,15] In research that examined out-of-hospital births with a comparison low-risk group birthing in the hospital, a greater incidence of hemorrhage was found in the hospital group.[27]

In out-of-hospital settings when postpartum bleeding is excessive, intravenous volume expanders with added oxytocin (Pitocin) can be started, methylergonovine maleate (Methergine) can be administered intramuscularly or orally, and/or misoprostol (Cytotec) administration may be effective. Management of postpartum hemorrhage can take place safely and successfully in the home or birth center, with the exception of the administration of blood or blood products, which are not available in these settings. However, when a woman has a hematocrit of less than 30% or a hemoglobin of less than 10 g/dL, she may be unable to sustain even a normal postpartum blood loss; in this circumstance, prenatal transfer to hospital-based care may be considered.

If an immediate or delayed postpartum blood loss causes symptoms of hypovolemia, making ambulation difficult, reducing self-care abilities, delaying lactogenesis II, or reducing the woman's ability to compensate, the woman may need postpartum professional assistance beyond the capabilities of family and friends. She may require hospitalization for evaluation and treatment. It is important to remember that women birthing at home or in a birth center will not have continuous professional postpartum support beyond 3 to 12 hours postpartum.

Coping with Unexpected Outcomes

If transfer to the hospital due to complications becomes necessary, women who had planned a home or birth center birth must cope with two concerns: worrying about their health and/or their newborn's health, and experiencing the feelings associated with the loss of their planned home or birth center birth. Anticipatory guidance prenatally can reduce the family's distress if transport becomes a reality. Reminding families late in pregnancy of the possibility that transfer could be necessary, reviewing practice statistics, and describing actual transport experiences may be helpful. Discussion may include a review of the decision-making process, consultation, the trip to the hospital, and admission. Women need help to understand that if they are going to the hospital, they will receive the technical interventions they may have hoped to avoid, but now need.

During the process of informed decision making at the first visit, and again around 36 weeks' gestation, women should be made aware of the possibility that their fetus/newborn could be injured or die during the birth process regardless of their chosen birth setting.[51] Although most people hesitate to focus on this frightening issue, women need to ask themselves what they would do and how they would cope. They also need to explore how they would respond to family or friends who may not have been supportive of their decision to give birth outside the hospital.

Facilitating Access to Hospital Care

Even when the midwife and the woman have worked together to select the birth site that matches the woman's needs, challenges and problems may occur during the pregnancy, labor, birth, or early postpartum period. When the midwife determines that more personnel and complex technologies are needed, previously arranged plans are implemented for transfer of care.[4–6,10,13,17,48,64,65]

Some CNMs/CMs attend births out of hospital and also maintain hospital privileges, thereby enabling them to transfer and provide care for the woman who needs interventions that are more safely implemented within the hospital. Other out-of-hospital midwives elect to maintain consultation relationships and transfer care of their clients to hospital-based CNMs/CMs, family physicians, or obstetricians. The midwife may consult with a solo practitioner, a group practice, several different practices, or the house staff employed by the hospital. Each option has both benefits and drawbacks.

The main benefit of working with a single solo practitioner is consistency and predictability in joint clinical management. The main difficulty is that there may be no other provision for coverage if the consultant is away or unavailable. In addition, the solo consultant may feel overwhelmed if called upon to manage several complicated referrals in quick succession. Having an agreement with a hospital staff provides 24-hour coverage, but the practitioner who receives the woman in a transfer situation may be completely unfamiliar with home or birth center birth, and have a clinical philosophy extremely different from the referring midwife's practice. Because this limits the midwife's ability to know what to expect, anticipatory guidance in various clinical situations becomes extremely difficult. Having a small number of familiar, reliable consultants who cross-cover for one another works well. Sometimes, several midwifery practices may hire a physician to provide consultation services if legally appropriate in their locale. The midwives benefit by sharing the cost. However, in covering more than one midwifery service, the physician may become over-extended.

While some home and birth center midwives maintain hospital privileges, others, for several reasons, elect not to seek them or are unable to get them. Out-of-hospital midwives may feel that their first commitment is to serve women who are planning to birth out of the hospital. They may believe that if they also tried to serve women planning hospital births, there would not be enough space in their practices to meet the needs of their out-of-hospital census. Others may worry that they would not be able to keep up with the bureaucratic and political administrative tasks associated with hospital privileges at the various hospitals that may be close to their clients' homes. In most of these scenarios, continuity of care can be accomplished by accompanying the women requiring transfer into the hospital. Making a consultation agreement with hospital-based midwifery practices affords a means of access to the hospital, fostering a collegial relationship among midwives. Women appreciate this arrangement because even if they transfer to the hospital, they still may have their birth attended by a midwife.

When developing a consultation relationship, the midwife writes the clinical practice guidelines on which the practice is based and identifies those situations for which consultation, collaboration, or referral would be needed. Negotiations with the consulting practice for the desired services may then take place. The final document is a contract spelling out consultant services only; in no way is it a supervisory agreement. Some consultants may be hesitant to put an agreement in writing due to concerns about professional liability insurance, loss of hospital privileges, or putting themselves at professional risk with their colleagues. In recent years, several states have passed legislation repealing the requirement that midwives have written collaborative practice agreements with physicians or hospitals.[66] This legislation helps to remove a barrier to midwifery practice and, therefore, gives women more choices and increased access to midwifery care. Because a written collaborative practice agreement may not be required by law, it is even more important that the midwife establishes a relationship with the consultant or the hospital that is built upon mutual trust, open communication, and respect.[67,68]

As the midwife and the hospital-based consulting service become more comfortable working together, required prenatal consult visits may become few to none. Women may still want to meet with the consultant and should be encouraged to do so if they desire. Because access to the hospital is essential for safety, the consultant arrangement must be nurtured.

Intrapartum transfer to medical management is often a time of stress for providers and families alike. On arrival at the hospital, the credibility of the midwife will be increased if a professional image is maintained. In most situations, the problem necessitating transfer is identified as it is emerging. Decision making, clinical skills, and good communication among midwife, woman, family, and consulting practice take the midwife's full concentration and attention. Unfortunately, transfers often occur when labor has been long, and both the woman and the midwife are tired. The client and her family may be disappointed, and sometimes may blame the midwife for letting them down. Although under such circumstances it may be difficult to find time and mental ability to document the care given completely and accurately, it is even more critical in these circumstances to do so.

The transfer summary (**Figure 32-2**) is a simple, easy-to-read form that elicits pertinent data, relieving the midwife and birth assistant of the worry that some important documentation is being omitted. Communication by phone with the clinicians who will receive the woman is also important. If using a paper chart, it is convenient to have no-carbon-required (NCR) forms or to make a copy of the chart before arriving at the hospital. The midwife transferring the woman to the hospital must retain the original copy of all records.

When interaction with the hospital system, including transfer, is needed, a concise, complete chart is an effective ambassador for the woman and the referring midwifery service. This consideration is especially important in home and birth center practice, because the hospital staff who receive the woman may not be familiar with home or birth center birth. These staff may not be aware of the statistics that have demonstrated the safety of this birth option, and may believe that the woman's original plans were unwise. The chart can sway the attitudes of the clinicians who render care and may determine which care the woman receives. In addition, hospital providers actually see only the women for whom transfers are needed. Their experience has not been shaped by the reassurance and satisfaction of seeing the other 85% to 90% of labors and births that proceed safely and superbly at home or in the birth center.[2,5,6,10]

Home and birth center midwives need to remember that in an urgent emergency, the midwife has ultimate responsibility for decision making. If time permits, the birthing woman and her family may provide input. Consultation with a colleague or a physician may be possible only by telephone, but time constraints and birth setting may mandate decision making and clinical action by the midwife alone, usually with the help of a birth assistant.

When working with consultants, management dilemmas may occur that have political implications. If the woman's desires conflict with accepted medical community standards, it may be difficult to convince a consultant to implement a plan that may be safe, but unpopular in the medical community. The resulting situation can become very uncomfortable. The out-of-hospital midwife now has a dilemma that pits the medical community on one side against the woman's desires on the other side. The out-of-hospital midwife and the consultants are caught in the middle. This conundrum has the potential to jeopardize the relationship with the consultants and, therefore, access to the hospital for the entire home or birth center practice. Compromise will be necessary on all sides when working through this type of conflict.

Many times the midwife will be tempted to be led by her heart instead of her head. Families who wish that their midwife would attend them in labor in spite of complications may also pressure the midwife to embrace this course of action. Wish management does not work. Learning to say "no" is not just important—it is critical. Midwives must be brutally honest with themselves in describing their own skills, their own comfort level, and their own experience.

Business Aspects of Out-of-Hospital Birth Settings

Although most birth centers and home birth services are small, regulatory and business issues still must be addressed when opening any midwifery practice. The same legal and professional documents that are necessary when starting a hospital practice are necessary for a home or birth center practice. A reliable financial management system must also be in place. Combining the on-call lifestyle with practice management may cause the midwife to overlook either clinical or administrative issues. These are not easy tasks to accomplish, particularly when a night of sleep is missed. A midwife needs administrative help to run a service.

Birth Center Practice Models

Two childbirth center models have been developed: the closed model and the open model. The closed

Name _____

Date	Time	
		Reason for transfer:
		Review with client and family:
		Name of consultant:
		Name of hospital:
		Consultation and plan:
		Transport called (if applicable):
		Arrival of transport vehicle (if applicable):
		Mode of transport:
		Mother: T ____ P _____ R _____ BP_____ Condition _____
		Baby: FHT _____ T _____ P_____ R _____ Condition _____
		Departure from home/birth center (circle one)
		Arrival at hospital/accompanied by:
		Receiving provider:
		Type of intervention:
		Initiation of treatment:
		Birth information: SVD Inst. Asst. C/S Apgar ___/___
		Outcome summary:
		CNM departure from hospital:
		Breastfeeding status:
		Release for hospital records sent:
		Hospital records received:

© BirthCare & Women's Health, Ltd. 2004

Signature _____

Figure 32-2 Transfer summary.
Source: © BirthCare & Women's Health, Ltd. Reprinted by permission.

model is a birth center that is used by a single practice of midwives and/or physicians. Only women who seek care from that practice may give birth at the center; privileges are not extended to any other providers in the community. In contrast, the open model birth center is a facility usually owned by a separate corporation that extends birth privileges to practices in the community that submit applications to use the facility. These practices may include midwifery, family practice, and obstetrical practices. Although most birth center models offer full-scope midwifery care, some centers provide only intrapartum and immediate postpartum care. Some practitioners prefer to provide regular scheduled visits in the client's home or maintain space at other sites for these routine visits.[1]

The majority of birth centers in the United States are owned and run by midwives. Some centers may be hospital or physician owned, employing the midwifery staff. Other centers may be Federally Qualified Health Centers (FQHC), assuring that low-income women have the birth center option available. FQHCs also have the advantage of avoiding the high cost of professional liability insurance. In some communities, the birth center may be run by a board of directors, and created by either consumers or business-minded individuals who want to expand birth options. Many birth centers become a community meeting place for events or classes. Some birth centers offer other services, such as childbirth and breastfeeding classes and parenting groups. Some sell cloth diapers, infant carriers, clothing for pregnant and breastfeeding women, breast pumps, and other products of interest to birthing families.[69]

Home Birth Practice Models

Home birth practices are usually midwife owned, and may be either solo or group practices. Solo home birth practice can be very rewarding, but is also quite challenging. The relationship between the solo midwife and the client gives each great satisfaction.[70,71] However, the intensely personalized relationship can make each party reluctant to get assistance, if needed, from another midwife. It may be difficult for the midwife to manage more than one labor at a time due to the distance between the clients' homes, and the small number of CNMs/CMs in home birth practice may make cross-coverage hard to find.

Group home birth practices allow the midwife more collegial support, and help decrease the occurrence of practitioner burnout. When women meet more than one midwife from the outset, they often accept having any of the group attend their births. However, relinquishing the unique one-to-one relationship created within the solo practice may decrease satisfaction for both midwife and client.

For midwives who may not be interested in owning their own practice, a collaborative practice model is an option. Such a practice, which may be owned by either a physician or a corporation, hires a solo midwife or a group of midwives to provide home birth services for interested families. This model encourages independent practice for the midwife, while the owner of the practice provides for administration. The financial arrangements used in such a case may vary. The midwife may have a set salary, or there may be other incentives such as profit sharing, bonuses, or payment according to the number of office visits and births attended.

Combination Practice Models

Many birth center and home birth practices offer a combination of services: home/hospital, home/birth center, birth center/hospital, and home/birth center/ hospital. Offering more than one birth option may not only increase the number of families interested in midwifery care, but also allows women to easily change the planned birth site while maintaining continuity of care. In a combination practice, the midwife also has an opportunity to explore birthplace options with women who never would have considered a home or birth center birth. Moreover, the practice's reception area provides a convenient place for families to connect with one another and share experiences while waiting for their appointments.

Social networking sites, books, childbirth organizations, and classes also provide families an opportunity to share resources. The woman, armed with information, develops the self-assurance needed to take an active role in selecting her birthplace.

Other Business Issues

A self-employed independent midwife has more control over decision making and administration. There is less vulnerability to losing the practice due to a change in priority on the part of a physician, a health insurance plan, or a hospital administration. Knowing the cost of every item used, the midwife is able to determine the economic advantages and disadvantages of specific business strategies. By the same token, there is much more responsibility, time involved, and financial risk in self-employment. The midwife understands when to go "that extra mile" to keep the practice alive.

Financial management can make or break a practice, and administrative structure may need to be adjusted often. There may not be much of a budget to work with in the beginning, so it is important to make realistic predictions. If the overhead of the practice can be kept low, salaries may be adjusted higher. Even in established practices, it is not uncommon for home birth or birth center midwives to have lower salaries than their hospital-based colleagues.

Salaries for clinical staff should amount to approximately 50% of the income generated. However, when the practice first opens, overhead may encompass all of the income from services, leaving little for the owner(s). In most practices, the person in charge of billing and collections is key to financial survival. Interpersonal skills and a commitment to the practice help keep the service afloat financially.

The major changes that have occurred in the insurance industry in recent years have affected all providers. Many home birth and birth center midwives are providers on managed care panels, and are reimbursed by Medicaid and indemnity plans. Some insurance companies require accreditation through the Commission for Accreditation of Birth Centers for birth center–based midwives to become participating providers. Negotiations with insurance companies require patience, persistence, and expertise. ACNM has developed materials to help midwives become skillful negotiators, thereby keeping services viable and available to women.[51,72–75] Unfortunately, insurance coverage may limit provider choices for women plan members unless they have the resources to pay out of pocket. Facing such a limit can be especially sad for returning clients whose insurance has changed, precluding birth with their previous midwifery service.

Financial arrangements with consulting practices should be clear. The consultant may elect not to charge a consultation fee to the midwife for providing services, but will charge the woman for services actually rendered. This arrangement works out well financially for the midwife, as long as the families pay the consultant. If women have past-due balances with the consulting practice, it is wise for the midwife to pay the consultant directly, adding the woman's unpaid balance to her bill from the referring midwife's office. By assuring prompt payment of fees, the midwife fosters a good relationship with the consultant.

A mechanism for statistical collection should be in place before a practice opens. Accurate statistics facilitate evaluation, quality management, validation of effective practice, peer review, and research. These practice statistics should be collected regularly and analyzed at least annually. Both AABC and MANA have web-based statistical programs that are comprehensive and user friendly. When arrayed clearly, statistics also serve as a public relations tool conveying important information to families about outcomes and transfers.

Although the home and birth center environments are less bureaucratic, they are not less political. Emotions run high about out-of-hospital-birth. People in the medical community are often unfamiliar with and hesitant to show support for birth center and home births, harboring misconceptions that are not based on fact. Their attitudes can pose a significant barrier to practice. Sometimes when physicians serve as consultants for home and birth center practices, they may benefit from referrals not only from the midwife practice, but also from client networks and sympathetic childbirth educators. Such support can, however, have its costs within the larger medical community. As the consultant's practice grows, competition among physicians may also grow. Some physician colleagues may refuse to cross-cover for a midwife's consultant physician.

Midwives practicing in the home and birth center settings need to be astutely aware of who wields power, both in their local medical community and in the legislative and regulatory arenas. ACNM has legislative liaisons and lobbyists both nationally and at the affiliate level to keep members aware of political and practice issues. To break down barriers, safeguard the profession, and protect the healthcare rights of women and their families, midwives have to be alert and proactive.

Conclusion

Working in the home and birth center environments, midwives have increased access to the important resources of time, place, and social interaction. In the hospital, the staff may become inured to and unconscious of interruptions:

> [S]tudies found that a woman with a low risk delivery giving birth to her first child in a teaching hospital could be attended by as many as 16 people during 6 hours of labor and still be left alone for most of the time. Routine, though unfamiliar, procedures, the presence of strangers and being left alone during labor and/or delivery caused stress, and stress can interfere with the course of birth by prolonging it...[21]

In birth centers and homes, midwives are able to provide more time and privacy to the birthing woman and her birth partner, observing unobtrusively and vigilantly for continued normalcy and for early signs and symptoms of problems. As long as birth remains normal, midwives limit their role to helping the woman be as comfortable as possible, validating the efforts the woman makes to give birth, and, at times, augmenting and redirecting the partner's supportive efforts.

All laboring women seek ways in which they can be most comfortable and most productive.[76] In the home and birth center, women and their partners feel that they have more permission to be creative in finding ways to help themselves birth their babies. The woman can help herself and do her best when she is not limited to laboring within a labor room. Home and birth center environments offer a variety of spaces that may promote the woman's coping ability. The woman also conserves labor energy simply by knowing where things are and not having to ask for permission to enter a space or touch things within the space.[48] It is she who makes choices about who to invite and when she wishes them to come and go as labor proceeds.

Within the home and birth center environment, continuity of care takes on a new meaning for the midwife. She has more freedom to offer a continuous presence during labor. This continuity enables the midwife to observe the way the woman and her partner work with labor and to watch how labor energy is being used. Because home and birth center birth depends on the woman's natural abilities, continuity provides the midwife with an opportunity to watch the dynamic process of labor as it ebbs and flows, enabling the midwife to know when it is beneficial to wait and when to push labor along through natural means.

The midwife carefully selects interventions and utilizes them only when the woman needs them and without interrupting the flow of labor. Being aware of and encouraging changes in place, time, and social interaction are special tasks of the midwife in the home and birth center settings. In these small and personalized environments, midwives maximize opportunities to practice "the art of doing nothing well."[77]

● ● ● References

1. Varney H. *Varney's Midwifery*. 4th ed. Sudbury, MA: Jones and Bartlett; 2004.

2. Fullerton JT, Navarro AM, Young SH. Outcomes of planned home birth: an integrative review. *J Midwifery Women's Health*. 2007;52:323-333.

3. Fullerton J, Jackson D, Snell BJ, Besser M, Dickinson C, Garite T. Transfer rates from freestanding birth centers: a comparison with the National Birth Center Study. *J Nurse Midwifery*. 1997;42:9-16.

4. de Jonge A, van der Goes, BY, Ravelli ACJ, et al. Perinatal mortality and morbidity in a nationwide cohort of 529,688 low-risk planned home and hospital births. *BJOG*. 2009;116(9):1177-1184.

5. Janssen PA, Saxell L, Page LA, et al. Outcomes of planned home birth with registered midwife versus planned hospital birth with midwife or physician. *CMAJ*. 2009;181:377-383.

6. Anderson RE, Murphy PA. Outcomes of 11,788 planned home births attended by certified nurse-midwives: a retrospective descriptive study. *J Nurse Midwifery* 1995;40:483-492.

7. Johnson K, Daviss B. Outcomes of planned home births with certified professional midwives: large prospective study in North America. *Br Med J*. 2005;330(7505):1416.

8. Burnett CA, Jones JA, Rooks J, Chen CH, Tyler CW Jr., Miller CA. Home delivery and neonatal mortality in North Carolina. *JAMA*. 1980;244:2741-2745.

9. Durand AM. The safety of home birth: the farm study. *Am J Public Health*. 1992;82:450-453.

10. Cheng YW, Snowden JM, King TL, Caughey AB. Selected perinatal outcomes associated with planned home births in the United States. *Am J Obstet Gynecol*. 2013;Jun 18. pii: S0002-9378(13)00630-3. doi: 10.1016/j.ajog.2013.06.022. [Epub ahead of print]

11. Hinds MW, Bergeisen GH, Allen DT. Neonatal outcome in planned v unplanned out of hospital births in Kentucky. *JAMA*. 1985;253:1578-1582.

12. Stapleton SR, Osborne C, Illuzzi J. Outcomes of care in birth centers: demonstration of a durable model. *J Midwifery Women's Health*. 2013;58(1):1-12.

13. Murphy PA, Fullerton J. Outcomes of intended home births in nurse-midwifery practice: a prospective descriptive study. *Obstet Gynecol*. 1998;92:461-470.

14. Tyson H. Outcomes of 1001 midwife-attended home births in Toronto, 1983-1988. *Birth*. 1991;18:14-19.

15. Rooks JP, Weatherby NL, Ernst EK, et al. Outcomes of care in birth centers: the national birth center study. *N Engl J Med*. 1989;321:1804-1811.

16. Olsen O, Clausen JA. Planned hospital birth versus planned home birth. *Cochrane Database Syst Rev*. 2012 Sep 12;9:CD000352. doi:10.1002/14651858. CD000352.pub2

17. Springer NP, Van Weel C. Homebirth: safe in selected women, and with adequate infrastructure and support. *BMJ*. 1996;313:1276-1277.

18. Wax JR, Lucas FL, Lamont M, Pinette MG, Cartin A, Blackstone J. Maternal and newborn outcomes in planned home birth vs planned hospital births: a meta-analysis. *Am J Obstet Gynecol*. 2010 Sep;203(3):243.

19. Tew M. *A Safer Childbirth: A Critical History of Maternity Care*. 2nd ed. London/New York: Chapman and Hall; 1995.

20. Lubic RW, Ernst EKM. The childbearing center: an alternative to conventional care. *Nurs Outlook*. 1978;26:754-760.

21. World Health Organization, Maternal and Newborn Health/Safe Motherhood Unit. *Care in Normal Birth: A Practical Guide*. Geneva: World Health Organization; 1996.

22. Royal College of Obstetricians and Gynaecologists and Royal College of Midwives joint statement No. 2. Home births. January 4, 2007. Available at: http://www.rcog.org.uk/print/womens-health/clinical-guidance/home-births. Accessed July 4, 2010.

23. Campbell R, MacFarlane A. *Where to Be Born? The Debate and the Evidence*. 2nd ed. Oxford, UK: National Perinatal Epidemiology Unit, Radcliffe Infirmary; 1994.

24. Fullerton JT, Severino R. In-hospital care for low-risk childbirth: comparison with results from the national birth center study. *J Nurse-Midwifery*. 1992;37: 331-340.

25. Goer H, Romano A. *Optimal Care in Childbirth: The Case for a Physiologic Approach*. Seattle, WA: Classic Day Publishing; 2012.

26. Rooks JP, Weatherby NL, Ernst EKM. The national birth center study: part III—intrapartum and immediate postpartum and neonatal complications and

transfers, postpartum and neonatal care, outcomes, and client satisfaction. *J Nurse-Midwifery.* 1992;37: 361-397.

27. Hutton EK, Reitsma AH, Kaufman K. Outcomes associated with planned home and planned hospital births in low-risk women attended by midwives in Ontario, Canada, 2003-2006: a retrospective cohort study. *Birth.* 2009;36:180-189.

28. Van der Kooy J, Poeran J, de Graaf JP, et al. Planned home compared with planned hospital births in the Netherlands. *Obstet Gynecol.* 2011;118:1037-1046.

29. MacDorman MF, Declercq E, Mathews MS. Recent trends in out-of-hospital births in the United States. *J Midwifery Women's Health.* 2013;58(4). [In press]

30. MacDorman MF, Matthews TJ, Declercq E. *Home Births in the United States, 1990-2009.* NCHS Data Brief, No. 84. Hyattsville, MD: National Center for Health Statistics; 2012.

31. Lake R, Epstein A. *The Business of Being Born: A Documentary Film.* 2007. Available at: info@the businessofbeingborn.com. Accessed July 10, 2010.

32. *Childbirth Connection: Information for Women on Pregnancy & Childbirth.* Available at: http://www .childbirthconnection.org. Accessed January 21, 2013.

33. American College of Nurse-Midwives. *Midwifery: Evidence-Based Practice.* Silver Spring, MD: American College Nurse-Midwives; April 2012.

34. American College of Nurse-Midwives. *Position Statement: Home Birth.* Silver Spring, MD: American College of Nurse-Midwives; 2011.

35. American Association of Birth Centers. *Letter to Douglas Laube, MD.* Perkiomenville, PA: American Association of Birth Centers; November 2006. Available at: http://www.bellytales.com/2006/12/03 /the-out-of-hospital-debate-continues. Accessed August 3, 2013.

36. American College of Obstetricians and Gynecologists. *Committee Opinion on Planned Home Births.* Washington, DC: American College of Obstetricians and Gynecologists; February 2011.

37. American College of Nurse-Midwives. *Issue Brief: ACOG Committee Opinion on Planned Home Birth: Opening the Door to Collaborative Care.* Silver Spring, MD: American College of Nurse-Midwives; 2011.

38. Midwives Alliance of North America. *It Is Time to Reframe the Homebirth Conversation: Focus on Optimal Maternity Care and the Practitioners Who Can Provide It.* Washington, DC: Midwives Alliance of North America; January 2011.

39. Executive and Council of the Society of Obstetricians and Gynecologists of Canada, et al. Joint policy statement on normal childbirth. *J Obstet Gynaecol Can.* 2008;30:1163-1165.

40. Royal College of Midwives. *Position Statement on Normal Childbirth.* London: Royal College of Midwives; 2006.

41. Maternity Care Working Party. *Making Normal Birth a Reality. Consensus Statement from the Maternity Care Working Party: Our Shared Views About the Need to Recognise, Facilitate and Audit Normal Birth.* National Childbirth Trust; Royal College of Midwives, Royal College of Obstetricians and Gynaecologists; 2007.

42. Campaign for Normal Birth. [Internet] Royal College of Midwives. Available at: http://www.rcmnormal birth.org.uk/practice/ten-top-tips/. Accessed October 30, 2012.

43. Kennedy HP. The problem of normal birth. Editorial for continuing education issue on normal birth. *J Midwifery Women's Health.* 2010;55(3):199-292.

44. Kennedy HP, Shannon MT. Keeping birth normal: research findings on midwifery care during childbirth. *JOGNN.* 2004;33:554-560.

45. American College of Nurse-Midwives, Midwives Alliance of North America, National Association of Certified Professional Midwives. *Supporting Healthy and Normal Physiologic Childbirth: A Consensus Statement by ACNM, MANA, and NACPM.* Silver Spring, MD: ACNM, MANA, and NACPM; April 2012.

46. Home Birth Consensus Summit [Internet]. Available at: http://www.homebirthsummit.org. Accessed October 30, 2012.

47. Sakala C, Corry M. *Evidence-Based Maternity Care: What It Is and What It Can Achieve.* New York, NY: Milbank Memorial Fund; October 2008.

48. Jackson ME, Bailes A. Home birth with certified nurse-midwife attendants in the United States: an overview. *J Nurse-Midwifery.* 1995;40:493-506.

49. American Association of Birth Centers. The birth center experience. Available at: http://www.birthcenters .org/open-a-birth-center/birth-center-experience. Accessed October 30, 2012.

50. *Manual for the Accreditation of Birth Centers.* Perkiomenville, PA: Commission for the Accreditation of Birth Centers; 2009.

51. American College of Nurse-Midwives. *ACNM Handbook: Home Birth Practice.* Washington, DC: American College of Nurse-Midwives; 2004.

52. Goldberg H. Informed decision making in maternity care. *J Perinatal Educ.* 2009;18:32-40.

53. Spindel PG, Suarez SH. Informed consent and home birth. *J Nurse-Midwifery.* 1995;40:541-554.

54. Toepke ML, Albers LL. Neonatal considerations when birth occurs at home. *J Nurse-Midwifery.* 1995; 40:529-533.

55. American College of Nurse-Midwives. Clinical bulletin: intermittent auscultation for intrapartum fetal heart rate surveillance. *J Midwifery Women's Health.* 2010;55:397-403.

56. Anderson GC, Moore E, Hepworth J, Bergman N. Early skin-to-skin contact for mothers and their healthy newborn infants. *Cochrane Database Syst Rev.* 2003;(2):CD003519.

57. Cohen NW, Estner JL. *Silent Knife.* South Hadley, MA: Bergin & Garvey Publishers; 1983.

58. King T. Can a vaginal birth after cesarean delivery be a normal labor and birth? Lessons from midwifery applied to trial of labor after a previous cesarean delivery. *Clin Perinatol.* 2011;38:247-263.

59. American College of Nurse-Midwives. *Care for Women Desiring Vaginal Birth After Cesarean.* Clinical Bulletin No. 12. Silver Spring, MD: American College of Nurse-Midwives; May 2011.

60. National Institutes of Health. *Consensus Development Conference Statement: Vaginal Birth After Cesarean: New Insights.* Washington, DC: National Institutes of Health; March 8-10, 2010.

61. Lieberman E. Risk factors for uterine rupture during a trial of labor after cesarean. *Clin Obstet Gynecol.* 2001;44:609-621.

62. Caughey AB, Shipp TD, Repke JT, Zelop CM, Cohen A, Lieberman E. Rate of uterine rupture during a trial of labor in women with one or two previous cesarean deliveries. *Am J Obstet Gynecol.* 1999;181:872-876.

63. American Academy of Pediatrics and American Heart Association. *Neonatal Resuscitation.* 6th ed. Elk Grove, IL: American Academy of Pediatrics; 2011.

64. Rooks JP, Weatherby NL, Ernst EKM. The national birth center study: part I—methodology and prenatal care and referrals. *J Nurse-Midwifery.* 1992;37:222-253.

65. Rooks JP, Weatherby NL, Ernst EKM. The national birth center study: part II—intrapartum and immediate postpartum and neonatal care. *J Nurse-Midwifery.* 1992;37:301-330.

66. American College of Nurse-Midwives. State legislative and regulatory developments. Available at: http://www.midwife.org/index.asp?sid=14&BUTTON=Search&TextSearchWordList=state+legislative+and+regulatory+. Accessed October 30, 2012.

67. American College of Nurse-Midwives. *Collaborative Agreement Between Physicians and Certified Nurse-Midwives (CNMs) and Certified Midwives (CMs): Position Statement.* Silver Spring, MD: American College of Nurse-Midwives; 2009.

68. Darlington A, McBroom K, Warwick S. A northwest collaborative practice model. *Obstet Gynecol.* 2011;118:673-677.

69. Commission for the Accreditation of Birth Centers. President: Susan Stapleton, CNM, DNP. Personal correspondence, August 18, 2010.

70. Frye A. *Holistic Midwifery: A Comprehensive Textbook for Midwives in Homebirth Practice: Volume I.* Portland, OR: Labrys Press; 1995.

71. Bailes A, Jackson ME. Shared responsibility in home birth practice: collaborating with clients. *J Midwifery Women's Health.* 2000;45:537-543.

72. American College of Nurse-Midwives. *ACNM Handbook: Getting Paid: Billing, Coding and Payment for Nurse-Midwifery Services.* Silver Spring, MD: American College of Nurse-Midwives; 2001.

73. Vedam S, Kolodji Y. Guidelines for client selection in the home birth midwifery practice. *J Nurse-Midwifery.* 1995;40:508-521.

74. American College of Nurse-Midwives. *ACNM Handbook: Marketing and Public Relations: A Complete Resource Guide.* Silver Spring, MD: American College of Nurse-Midwives; 2000.

75. American College of Nurse-Midwives. *ACNM Handbook: Minding Your Own Business: Business Plans for Midwifery Practice.* Silver Spring, MD: American College of Nurse-Midwives; 2000.

76. Simkin P. *The Birth Partner: Everything You Need to Know to Help a Woman Through Childbirth.* Boston: Harvard Common Press; 2001.

77. Kennedy HP. The essence of nurse-midwifery care: the woman's story. *J Nurse-Midwifery.* 1995;40:493-507.

VI

Postpartum

Postpartum: Care as a New Family Is Born

The postpartum woman is not "post" anything. She is actively in transition from being pregnant to being a mother—a critical time period when a midwife provides integral care and support that can affect her and her child for a lifetime.

As soon as the newborn is born and the placenta is delivered, the woman's body begins an exquisitely complicated, wondrous set of processes that return her body to its nonpregnant condition, albeit with some permanent changes—and her soul turns to her child. The brain of a woman who is "post" a normal physiologic birth is saturated with endogenous oxytocin, released directly into her brain undeterred by the blood–brain barrier that prevents exogenous oxytocin, which may have been used to augment labor, from affecting her emotions. Endogenous oxytocin is the real thing, the physiologic underpinning of the trust-and-love cement of the mother–baby dyad. Most women who do not have a normal, uncomplicated physiologic birth bond with their newborns anyway; humans are a resilient species—and we need to be, because nearly one-third of all infants born in the United States in 2011 were delivered by cesarean section.[1] Many of those women were having their first babies. It is a loss when the woman who is besotted with oxytocin and physiologically primed to share the experience with her newborn does not get the intense joy of meeting her newborn immediately after birth. In the slightly longer run, a midwife can help the woman achieve similar joy without the chemical assist.

The *Anatomy and Physiology of Postpartum* chapter describes the truly fascinating physiology of puerperal involution. Like everything in nature, it is complex and tuned by evolution; what needs to happen to minimize risk usually occurs. The *Postpartum Complications* chapter describes the complications that occur when that process fails. The midwife's first responsibility is vigilance to ensure early suspicion and recognition of complications and thoroughly learned and practiced rapid responses in the face of the most serious postpartum complications, such as massive maternal hemorrhage, preeclampsia, thromboembolism, and thyroid storm. But, as Kantrowitz-Gordon explains in the *Postpartum Care* chapter, the midwife must go beyond that focus on complications to provide optimal care to a woman during this period of multiple transitions.

Women can gain strength from their experience of being pregnant and giving birth. During her first pregnancy and birth, a woman changes from being only a daughter to being a mother as well. By understanding the social and cultural context in which the woman experiences this transition, a midwife can help her move through the postpartum period with well-being and good health, no matter how her labor and birth occurred.

The *Postpartum Care* chapter uses the work of Goulet et al.[2] to describe the development of a two-way attachment between the parent and infant, requiring *proximity* (to use all the senses—hearing, touch, sight, and smell, and an awareness of the infant's individuality with needs that are different from the parents' needs), *reciprocity* (parents and newborn responding to and adapting to one another, with the parents becoming sensitive to the infant's cues and body language and the infant reinforcing the parents' behaviors), and *commitment* (the parents feeling and acting responsibly for the safety, growth, and development of their infant, placing the child in the central position in the family, and incorporating parenting as an important part of their adult identity).

The *Breastfeeding and The Mother–Newborn Dyad* chapter details the physiology of breastfeeding and picks up from the *Postpartum Care* chapter in describing clues parents can use to know when an infant wants to feed; the importance of the woman feeling confident that she can read her infant and meet both nourishment and suckling needs; following the infant's cues regarding when, how often, and how long to breastfeed; and the importance of skin-to-skin contact (with the father, if the mother is recovering from a cesarean section) and interacting (eye-to-eye contact, talking, and stroking) while the infant feeds.

A successful pregnancy results in a healthy baby and a happy, competent, and confident mother. These chapters are rich in information to help midwives be with women in a way that results in success.

Judith P. Rooks

● ● ● References

1. Hamilton BE, Martin JA, Ventura SJ. *Births: preliminary data for 2011. National Vital Statistics Reports,* Vol. 61, No 5. Hyattsville, MD: National Center for Health Statistics; 2012.
2. Goulet C, Bell L, Tribble DS, Paul D, Lang A. A concept analysis of parent–infant attachment. *J Adv Nurs.* 1998;28(5):1071-1081.

CHAPTER

33

Anatomy and Physiology of Postpartum

JENIFER O. FAHEY

Introduction

Physiologically, the postpartum period begins with birth of the placenta and continues through to the involution of the uterus and return of other reproductive organs to a nonpregnant state. This is not the same prepregnant state the woman experienced prior to pregnancy because pregnancy can have some lasting effects on a woman's body.

Classically, the postpartum period is considered to last between 6 to 8 weeks. However, this time period is not precise and varies among women. Among breastfeeding women, the anatomy and physiology of the mammary glands will continue to be different than in the nonpregnant, nonlactating woman for the duration of lactation and beyond.

A woman's ability to complete the important tasks of bonding and caring for her new infant(s) or, in the case of a stillbirth or other loss, the task of grieving and healing, will be affected to a significant degree by her physical well-being. Her physical well-being can also influence the probability of her developing postpartum depression. It is crucial, therefore, that the midwife possess an accurate understanding of normal postpartum anatomy and physiology and be vigilant for any signs of complications.

Postpartum Hemostasis

Following placental separation and expulsion from the uterus, a series of events must immediately occur in order to ensure maternal hemostasis at the placental attachment site. This series of events begins prior to placental separation with oxytocin-induced contractions of the myometrium that cause a permanent and progressively increasingly shortening of the muscle fibers. In addition to promoting the separation of the placenta from the uterine wall, this shortening and retraction of muscle fibers compresses the maternal arteries that served as the vascular supply to the placenta.[1] As the myometrium contracts, the uterine walls press against each other and may also promote hemostasis.

Therefore, the mechanical compression caused by myometrial contractions remains the primary mechanism of hemostasis in the immediate postpartum period. However, a clotting response is initiated at the time of placental expulsion that will further contribute to hemostasis at the placental attachment site. Uterine atony during the first hour following delivery can lead to massive maternal hemorrhage especially if the contractions are inadequate.

During normal pregnancy, a series of changes in coagulation and fibrolytic systems promote adequate utero-placental circulation. During the postpartum period these same physiologic changes permit adequate coagulation at the placental attachment site following placental detachment. These changes help protect the woman from hemorrhage following birth. In brief, during pregnancy (and particularly in the third trimester) the woman experiences an increase in a number of clotting factors (I, II, VII, VIII, IX, and XII), a decrease in protein S levels, and a progressive fall in the activity of activated protein C as gestation advances.[2] Postpartally, these clotting factors promote coagulation of the sheared maternal vessels at the placental attachment site after the birth. However, while the clotting factors protect a woman from hemorrhage, they also predispose her to thromboembolic events.[3,4] The relative proportions of coagulation factors appear to return to their non-pregnant state by 3 weeks postpartum, but certain clotting cofactor levels, such as protein S levels, may not return to normal levels until 8 weeks postpartum or later.[3,5]

Reproductive Organ Involution

Uterine Involution

Uterine involution is the process of uterine contraction, myometrial cell shrinkage, reestablishment of the endometrium through necrosis and removal through shedding of decidual tissue (lochia), and regeneration of the endometrium. This process starts immediately after birth of the infant and takes approximately 6 weeks to complete.

The uterus weighs approximately 1000 grams after the birth and the fundus can be palpated as a firm mass in the abdominal midline several centimeters below the umbilicus. In the first few days postpartum, the uterus lies in a slightly retroverted position that "drapes" over the sacral promontory, and is easily palpable in the abdomen.[6] As the uterus contracts further, it undergoes a rotation of 100–180° along the axis of the internal os and assumes an upright position by postpartum day 7.[6] By the end of the first week, the uterus weighs approximately 500 grams and is still palpable above the symphysis pubis. By 2 weeks postpartum, the uterus weighs approximately 300 grams; at this point, it has typically taken on its nonpregnant anatomic position in the pelvis, which in most women is in an anteverted inclination, and is no longer able to be palpated abdominally.[7,8]

Uterine contractions are not the only factor involved in involution of the uterus. The organ also loses mass because of decrease in placental hormones that trigger myometrial cell autolysis. The result is a marked decrease in the size—rather than the number—of myometrial cells. Approximately 90% of the excess cellular protein is broken down by proteolytic enzymes that are released by myometrial cells, endothelial cells of uterine blood vessels, and macrophages.[8,9]

In early pregnancy, the uterine endometrium undergoes significant remodeling during implantation. This process, known as the decidual reaction, promotes the normal development and growth of the placenta and the embryo. The remodeled endometrium, or decidua, is divided into multiple layers or strata. Postpartally, the placenta separates at the spongy portion of the layer known as the decidua basalis, most of which is sloughed off with the placenta or in

the early postpartum period. In the second and third postpartum days, the remaining decidua becomes differentiated into two layers, identified as the superficial and basal layers. The superficial layer is formed through leukocyte invasion and protects the desquamated endometrium from infection.[8] Ultimately, this layer becomes necrotic and is sloughed off. In contrast, the basal layer remains intact and gives rise to the new endometrium through proliferation of the remaining glandular and stromal tissue. By 1 week postpartum, the endometrial surface has become epithelized; by 2 to 3 weeks postpartum, the endometrium has regenerated and resembles a nonpregnant endometrium excluding the placental implantation site. The remaining thrombosed vessels at the placental implantation site takes approximately 6 weeks to heal through an "exfoliation" process of sloughing infarcted and necrotic tissue, followed by a process of endometrial remodeling.[8,10]

Lochia

The postpartum vaginal discharge that begins immediately at birth and continues for approximately 4 to 8 weeks is termed lochia. The median total duration of lochia is 33 days.[11] Lochia further is described as lochia rubra, lochia serosa, and lochia alba based on its changing color.[12] This color results from the changing composition of the tissue that is sloughed and expelled in the postpartum endometrial restoration process.

Initially, the lochia consists primarily of blood; as a result, *lochia rubra* is red or brownish red in color. As the uterine bleeding decreases at approximately 3 to 5 days postpartum, leukocyte infiltration occurs and the placental implantation site undergoes exfoliation; at this point, the discharge contains some blood but primarily wound exudate and leukocytes and, therefore, *lochia serosa* is a pinkish brown color. The median duration of lochia serosa is 22 days.[11] Some women will experience a transient increase in bleeding 7 to 14 days postpartum secondary to sloughing of the placental eschar, or scab at the placental site. Toward the end of the process of uterine involution, the endometrium has been primarily restored. *Lochia alba* is composed predominantly of leukocytes and some decidual cells and is white or yellowish white in color.

Cervical and Vaginal Involution

During labor, the maternal cervix becomes soft, dilated, and edematous. It may also be bruised and lacerated during this time. In the first few postpartum days, the cervix reconstitutes and, by the end of the first week, the endocervical canal has reappeared and the os usually is only approximately 1 centimeter dilated.[8] The external cervical os usually does not return to its previous nonpregnant form with its dimple shape characteristic of most cervices of a nulliparous women, but rather takes the form of a slit (**Figure 33-1**). The cervical endothelium also undergoes remodeling during the postpartum period, which has been associated with regression of high-grade cervical intraepithelial lesions.[13]

The vagina is initially edematous and bruised after a vaginal birth and has lost its prepregnant tone and rugae. The vaginal rugae return at approximately 3 to 4 weeks postpartum, but the prepregnant vaginal tone may never be completely restored.[10] The vaginal epithelium is usually healed by 6 to 10 weeks postpartum.

Mammary Involution

During pregnancy, and particularly during the first pregnancy, the breasts undergo significant changes in preparation for breastfeeding. The changes of lactogenesis I and breastfeeding physiology are described in the *Breastfeeding and the Mother–Newborn Dyad* chapter. The timing and process of mammary involution depend on breastfeeding status. In women who do not breastfeed, prolactin decreases within the first postpartum week since there is no stimulation by a suckling infant. The change in this hormone, accompanied by any milk stasis, leads to mammary epithelial cell apoptosis (cell self-destruction) and mammary involution.[14] Women who do not breastfeed, as well as those who abruptly wean an infant, may have an increased risk of mastitis. A gradual weaning by a woman who has been breastfeeding invokes a different process of inhibition of lactation and mammary involution without acute milk stasis, wherein a progressive autocrine inhibition of milk production occurs in response to gradual decreased intake by the infant.[14] Mammary involution following lactation takes place over the course of months.

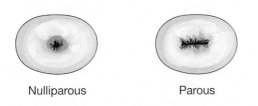

Nulliparous   Parous

Figure 33-1 Postpartum anatomic changes in the cervix.

Source: Schuiling KD, Likis FE. *Women's Gynecologic Health.* 2nd ed. Burlington, MA: Jones & Bartlett Learning; 2013.

Regardless of whether a woman breastfeeds her child, some of the mammary epithelium that was produced during pregnancy is retained. The breasts, therefore, never return to their prepregnant state.

Wound Healing

Some women will experience perineal lacerations during the process of vaginal birth, or from the use of forceps, vacuum, or cutting of an episiotomy. Identification, categorization, and repair of perineal and vaginal lacerations are described in the appendices of *The Second Stage of Labor* chapter. The wound healing process is divided into three phases: hemostasis and inflammation, granulation and proliferation, and remodeling.[9,15,16]

Hemostasis and Inflammation

The hemostatic process begins immediately at the time of injury and continues for a few days. First, platelets adhere to damaged tissue and combine together to form a platelet plug. Fibrinogen is attracted to this platelet plug, where it is subsequently cleaved into fibrin via the action of thrombin. Fibrin is an elastic, insoluble protein that forms an interlacing fibrous network that stabilizes the area of blood vessel injury. Platelets also release growth factors that call fibroblasts to migrate to the area, and cytokines that mediate the initial inflammatory response.

The inflammatory response begins within the first 6 to 8 hours following the perineal injury.[15] Poly-morphonuclear leukocytes (PMNs) from blood vessels in and surrounding the injured area migrate to the area of injury. These white blood cells work to rid the area of bacteria, damaged cells, and cell debris. The PMNs also assist in the recruitment of monocytes to the area, which differentiate into macrophages and also cleanse the area of foreign cells as well as damaged and dead cells via the process of phagocytosis. Unlike the PMNs, which are part of the initial inflammatory response and are short-lived, the macrophages can live for months. After approximately 3 or 4 days, in addition to their work in ridding the area of debris and foreign and dead cells, the macrophages begin to release key growth factors that trigger the growth of new tissue in the area.

During this phase, the woman may experience swelling, burning, or pruritus in the localized area. If the area has been sutured, these sensations may be intensified. She may notice exudate, although this can be indistinguishable to her from lochia. The woman should be aware that neither lochia nor the exudate should have a foul odor. She should also know that it is not normal to have a fever and should one occur, she should contact her midwife immediately.

Granulation and Proliferation

Approximately 5 to 7 days after injury, the fibroblasts that were recruited in the initial inflammatory response migrate to the area of the wound and begin to lay down the extracellular matrix and collagenous tissue in the area that serve as the "framework" for the rebuilding of the new tissue. Revascularization (angiogenesis) is essential to feed the new (granulation) tissue with nutrients and oxygen. New vessels arise as branches from intact vessels in the area. Regrowth of the epithelial layer occurs with migration of epithelial cells from the edges of the injured area or from adjacent tissues. This process can take up to 4 to 5 weeks.

As the granulation tissue grows to fill the wound, the area will take on a red or pebbled pink appearance, particularly if the tissue is healing via secondary intention (not approximated by sutures). This new tissue is highly vascular and friable. It is important that the woman keep the area clean and that she be advised to blot the area dry after urinating/defecating or after washing. Blotting is preferred instead of wiping, to avoid damaging this new tissue. Women who have sutures in place should be made aware that, depending on the suturing material, it may take 6 weeks or longer for the sutures to be fully absorbed.

Remodeling

During the last phase of wound healing, the collagen tissue undergoes remodeling to become similar to the prebirth tissue. This process includes regression of many of the new blood vessels created during the proliferative stage of wound healing. Wound contracture occurs secondary to the action of specialized contractile fibroblasts known as myofibroblasts. This phase can last for years. The collagen scar tissue, and particularly the initial scar tissue that has not undergone remodeling, will feel thicker and less distensible. This change may contribute to postpartum dyspareunia. As the healing process continues, some women describe the scar tissue as transitioning from feeling painful to feeling numb. The woman should be advised that with time, the tissue will regain most of its elasticity and sensation. She should also be aware that the scar tissue is not as strong or elastic as normal tissue and that there is an increased risk of lacerations along the scar tissue with subsequent births.

Postpartum Physiology in Nonreproductive Organs

Pregnancy results in anatomic and/or physiologic changes in every organ system of the body, all of which are altered again during the puerperium (**Table 33-1**). These physiologic changes may disappear over time depending on the organ involved and the underlying health of the individual woman. Because of their importance and profound changes, the postpartum changes that affect the cardiovascular and endocrine systems are described in detail here.

Cardiovascular and Hematologic Changes

A series of significant and rapid cardiovascular changes occur immediately postpartally that include loss of blood, auto-transfusion of 10% to 15% of blood volume secondary to removal of the low-pressure fetal–placental unit,[17] and mobilization of extracellular fluid back into circulation. These dramatic fluid shifts make the postpartum period a period of maternal cardiovascular instability and a time of increased risk for adverse outcomes, including pulmonary edema, cardiac failure, and death, in women with preexisting cardiac disease, hypertension, or preeclampsia.

In the first 10 to 15 minutes after the birth, maternal stroke volume and cardiac output are increased approximately 80% above pregnancy levels.[18] Theoretically, this effect is hypothesized to be due to increased cardiac preload that results from auto-transfusion of utero-placental blood back into maternal systemic circulation and improved venous return with decompression of the vena cava secondary to removal of mechanical pressure from the gravid uterus. In the first postpartum hour, stroke volume and cardiac output remain elevated and heart rate decreases, but mean arterial blood pressure is unchanged.[18]

Mobilization of extracellular fluid back into circulation in the first few postpartum days also contributes to increased blood volume. This acute increase in blood volume helps compensate for the normal blood loss of parturition. Following the sudden increase in cardiac output immediately after birth, blood volume declines to prepregnant levels over a period of approximately 2 weeks. Normal return of cardiovascular function depends in part on a physiologic diuresis in the first week postpartum. Without normal excretion of the extracellular fluid into the intravascular system, there is an increased risk of pulmonary edema, particularly among women with cardiac disease or preeclampsia.

Table 33-1	Postpartum Maternal Physiologic Adaptations		
System or Organ	**Postpartum Change**	**Timing of Return to Nonpregnant Status**	**Clinical Notes**
Cardiovascular changes	Auto-transfusion of 10% to 15% of blood volume secondary to removal of placenta and shift of extracellular fluid into intravascular system. Stroke volume and cardiac output increase by 80%.	Immediate	Women with hypertension, preeclampsia, or cardiac disease have an increased risk for pulmonary edema or cardiac failure in the first 24–48 hours postpartum.
	Blood volume slowly returns to nonpregnant value.	2 weeks postpartum	Women have a natural diuresis and diaphoresis in the initial postpartum period.
Hematologic changes	See Table 33-2		
Respiratory	Removal of the weight of the gravid uterus at birth relieves intra-abdominal pressure and allows elevation of the diaphragm that normal excursion of the diaphragm is reestablished.	Immediate	The dyspnea related to pregnancy usually resolves rapidly after birth. Therefore, complaints of shortness of breath or chest pain in the post-partum period should be evaluated immediately, especially because of the increased risk of thromboembolic events in the postpartum period.
	Decrease in tidal volume back to normal.	Immediate	
	Loss of placental progesterone production, a mediator of many respiratory changes of pregnancy, indicates rapid return of normal nonpregnant respiratory parameters		
	Return of normal RV and ERV that were decreased during pregnancy.	RV returns immediately ERV takes several months to return to nonpregnant values	
Renal and urinary	Gradual return to nonpregnant values of GFR, renal plasma flow, plasma creatinine, BUN, and creatinine clearance that were all altered during pregnancy.	2–3 months postpartum	Alterations may reflect changes of pregnancy that have not returned to nonpregnant levels.
	Mild proteinuria may develop in the first few postpartum days.	3–5 days	New-onset proteinuria may be related to normal postpartum changes. However, evaluation for preeclampsia should occur if new-onset proteinuria is noted in the first 2–3 weeks postpartum.
	Natriuresis (sodium excretion) and diuresis (increased urine production) lead to a decrease in blood volume back in order to return to nonpregnant levels.	3 weeks or less	Oxytocin promotes reabsorption of water. The decrease in oxytocin contributes to postpartum diuresis. Urine production in postpartum days 2–5 can reach 3000 mL. In addition to increased urine production, many women will experience episodes of diaphoresis in the first postpartum week.

(continues)

Table 33-1	**Postpartum Maternal Physiologic Adaptations** *(continued)*		
System or Organ	**Postpartum Change**	**Timing of Return to Nonpregnant Status**	**Clinical Notes**
Renal and urinary *(continued)*	Gradual return of bladder tone and normal size and function of bladder, ureters, and renal pelvis, all of which were dilated during pregnancy.	6–8 weeks, although it may take longer	Changes of pregnancy and trauma, including interventions, during birth of an infant can lead to increased risk of urinary tract infections and urinary retention during the postpartum period.
Hepatic	Increases in liver function indices (AST, ALT, LDH) from labor return to normal.	3 weeks or less	Interpretation of lab tests drawn in the postpartum period must reflect the knowledge that alterations from pregnancy and/or labor may not have returned to nonpregnant levels.
	Increase in alkaline phosphate from pregnancy also returns to normal.	6 weeks	
Gastrointestinal	Gastric tone and motility remain decreased for 2–3 days postpartum.	Bowel movements resume 2–3 days postpartum, normal GI function and bowel patterns return in 1–2 weeks postpartum	Decreased GI motility in the postpartum period can lead to abdominal distension, constipation, and, in severe cases, ileus.
Perineal and abdominal musculature	Ligaments and muscles are lax, so the abdominal wall remains soft and flaccid in the immediate postpartum. Separation of the rectus muscle (diastasis recti abdominis) may be present.	Variable	The recovery of abdominal muscular tone and resolution of diastasis recti abdominis are somewhat related to activity/exercise.
	Muscles and associated tissues that were stretched during childbirth gradually regain tone.	Variable, but can take months to years	Stretching and injury of the pelvic and perineal musculature and associated structures increase the risk of urinary and anal incontinence as well as pelvic organ prolapse. Prevention of these complications includes avoidance of episiotomy and performance of postpartum pelvic exercises.
Integumentary (skin and hair)	Hyperpigmentation (including linea nigra and melasma), striae gravidarum (stretch marks), varicosities, and other skin changes of pregnancy will fade or regress.	6 months or less	Many skin changes do not disappear completely. Striae commonly progress from red to silvery-white in approximately 3 months.
	With return of estrogen levels to nonpregnant levels, hair growth slows and follicles enter into a hair-shedding phase, which results in a period of alopecia or postpartum telogen effluvium.	Normal hair growth is reestablished by 4–6 months postpartum for most women	Reports by women of hair loss in the postpartum period are common, and the provider can offer reassurance. Women with excessive hair loss leading to bald patches or with hair loss lasting longer than 6 months should be evaluated for thyroid dysfunction or nutritional deviations.

Table 33-1	Postpartum Maternal Physiologic Adaptations *(continued)*		
System or Organ	**Postpartum Change**	**Timing of Return to Nonpregnant Status**	**Clinical Notes**
Metabolism of nutrients (carbohydrates, fats, and protein)	Demand for nutrients and hormone levels drop abruptly. Maternal metabolism of nutrients begins to return to normal. Maternal insulin resistance seen during pregnancy begins to resolve shortly after removal of the placenta.	Fasting glucose plasma levels and plasma free fatty acid levels return to prepregnant levels in first 3–5 days for women with normal glucose metabolism in pregnancy; triglyceride levels normalize within 2–3 weeks	Insulin resistance resolves nearly immediately following birth, which may require medication adjustment for women with Class A2, GDM. Maternal glucose values should be back to normal by the 6-week postpartum visit. Women with GDM should be screened for continued glucose intolerance at 6–12 weeks postpartum.
Calcium metabolism	The increase in intestinal calcium absorption seen during pregnancy resolves to nonpregnant levels of calcium absorption.	6 weeks in nonlactating women	Among women who are lactating, increased calcium needs for breast milk are supported by increased resaborption of calcium from the skeleton. This is associated with a reversible decrease in maternal bone density.
Endocrine	Thyroid-binding globulin decreases, which leads to a drop in T_3 and T_4.	First 3–4 days	After giving birth, women are at increased risk for Graves' disease, postpartum thyroiditis, and thyroid storm. Diagnosis can be complicated.
Pituitary	FSH and LH levels are low	2 weeks Nonpregnant values return by 4–6 weeks in nonlactating women	Ovulation is highly unlikely in the first 2 weeks postpartum. Return of FSH and LH levels is related to lactation status and ovulation occurs earlier among nonbreastfeeding women than those who lactate.
	Prolactin and oxytocin	Fall to normal nonpregnant values in 7–14 days if not lactating	See the *Breastfeeding and the Mother–Newborn Dyad* chapter for a review of lactogenesis II. Pituitary disorders can cause an alteration in prolactin levels that interfere with lactogenesis.

ALT = alanine aminotransferase; AST = aspartate aminotransferase; BUN = blood urea nitrogen; ERV = expiratory reserve volume; FSH = follicle stimulating hormone; GDM = gestational diabetes; GFR = glomerular filtration rate; LDH = lactic dehydrogenase; LH = leutinizing hormone; RV = residual volume.

Sources: Adapted from Chiarello CM, Falzone LA, McCaslin KE, et al. The effects of an exercise program on diastasis recti abdominis in pregnant women. *J Women's Health Phys Ther.* 2005;29(1):11-16; Sminakis KV, Chasan-Tabe L, Wolf M, Markenson G, Ecker JL, Thadhani R. Postpartum diabetes screening in women with a history of gestational diabetes. *Obstet Gynecol.* 2005;106:1297-1303.

The increase in stroke volume first during pregnancy and then during the postpartum period leads to a temporary increase in the size of the left atrium of the heart.[19] This physiologic ventricular hypertrophy resolves more slowly than the increase in stroke volume and cardiac output. Left ventricular size does not return to normal until approximately 6 months postpartum.[19]

The blood loss that occurs during birth causes a marked decrease in the red blood cell volume. In addition, a period of hemodilution arises in the first postpartum week due to the increase in plasma volume that occurs as interstitial fluid is mobilized. The loss of red blood cells (RBCs) combined with this hemodilution leads to a decrease in hemoglobin and hematocrit in the first postpartum week. A woman's hemoglobin and hematocrit gradually return over a 4–6 week period to a prepregnant value as plasma volumes and RBC production also return to normal. Postpartum changes in key components of the complete blood count (CBC) are summarized in **Table 33-2**.

Endocrine Changes

An abrupt drop in the blood levels of multiple hormones, including human placental lactogen (hPL), human chorionic gonadotropin (hCG), estrogen, and progesterone, occurs when the placenta is expelled. The abrupt drop in plasma levels of these hormones, in turn, set in motion a series of endocrine alterations, including changes in glucose and lipid metabolism and the initiation of lactogenesis II.

With decreasing levels of circulating estrogen, the thyroid-binding globulin level (which was elevated in pregnancy) also drops. This change, in turn, leads to less production of triiodothyronine (T_3) and thyroxine (T_4) and a gradual return to nonpregnant thyroid function. However, the incidence of thyroid dysfunction is more common in the postpartum period than in other times during a woman's life (7–10% in the postpartum period versus 3–4% in times other than the postpartum period).[18] Postpartum thyroid dysfunction, including postpartum thyroiditis, is often transient. Postpartum thyroiditis—a thyroid disorder that manifests during the first postpartum year—is thought to be an autoimmune disorder that is unmasked in the postpartum period due to the rebound in immunologic function that follows pregnancy.[19] In approximately 23% of women, thyroid dysfunction will become permanent.[20]

It is often postulated that the marked changes in the maternal hormonal milieu in the postpartum period may be the cause of postpartum mood disorders, including postpartum depression. Studies that have evaluated the link between hormonal changes and the development of depression have yielded contradictory results and, in general, have not found a consistent link between hormone levels and postpartum depression.[22] Significant methodological difficulties arise when trying to identify a causal link between any given biologic factor and the development of mood disorders, particularly at a time of significant change in all physiologic and psychosocial systems. However, lack of evidence does not necessarily mean that no such link exists. Currently, hormone levels cannot be used to effectively predict the development of postpartum mood disorders or to determine need for treatment.

Table 33-2	Normal Hematologic Values During the Postpartum Period		
Blood Factor	**Normal Nonpregnant Values (Female 19–65 Years)**	**Alterations During Pregnancy**	**Time to Reestablish Nonpregnant Values**
Red blood cell count (RBC) ($\times 10^6/mm^3$)	3.7–5.2	Increased (approximately 50% of increase lost at time of birth with normal blood loss)	4–6 weeks
Hemoglobin (g/dL)	10.4–15.2	Decreased	4–6 weeks
Hematocrit (%)	32.0–45.0	Decreased	4–6 weeks
White blood cell count (WBC) ($\times 10^3/mm^3$)	3.9–12.5	Increased (further increased to $25–30 \times 10^3/mm^3$ in the intrapartum and immediate postpartum periods)	4–7 days
Platelets ($\times 10^3/mm^3$)	174–452	Remain stable during pregnancy and postpartum	N/A

Source: Centers for Disease Control and Prevention. Laboratory procedure manual: complete blood count with 5-part differential. NHANES 2005–2006. Available at: http://www.cdc.gov/nchs/data/nhanes/nhanes_05_06/cbc_d_met.pdf. Accessed November 9, 2012.

Resumption of Pituitary Function and of Menstruation and Ovulation

Throughout pregnancy, the hypothalamic–pituitary–ovarian (HPO) axis is suppressed and, as a result, production of the follicle-stimulating hormone (FSH) and luteinizing hormone (LH) is also suppressed. Following birth, FSH and LH levels remain low for the first 2 postpartum weeks, but then rise gradually thereafter. Ovarian production of estrogen and progesterone is, therefore, also low during the first few postpartum weeks.

Pituitary function returns to nonpregnant levels by 4 to 6 weeks postpartum.[8] However, return of nonpregnant levels and patterns of gonadotropin-releasing hormone (GnRH), FSH, and LH secretion are related directly to lactation status. For a breast-feeding woman, the return of ovulation and menstruation is variable and related to both duration and frequency of breastfeeding. Elevated levels of prolactin, and other endocrine alterations related to frequent and regular infant suckling, disrupt the pulsatile release of GnRH, which in turn leads to suppression of the LH surge. This cascade of events culminates in the suppression of ovulation. Even once ovulation is resumed, women who are breast-feeding are more likely to experience nonfertile ovulation.[23] This breastfeeding-related suppression of ovulation and menstruation is referred to as "lactational amenorrhea."

In nonlactating women, the return of ovulation occurs sometime between the 45th and 94th postpartum days.[24] As many as 70% of these ovulations may be fertile, and in 20% to 70% of women, ovulation precedes the first menses.[24] Therefore, appropriate contraceptive counseling is essential for the postpartum women since many, particularly those not breastfeeding, may ovulate and be fertile prior to their first postpartum visit. For women who desire to defer another pregnancy for a period of time, timely initiation of the woman's chosen method of contraception is an important management intervention.

Weight Loss in the Postpartum Period

Weight loss following pregnancy is a common concern for women. Aside from the immediate weight loss that occurs directly related to the birth of the baby, expulsion of the placenta, and loss of fluid in the first postpartum week, the physiology of weight loss, which is outside the scope of this chapter, does not appear to differ in the postpartum period from the physiology of weight loss at other times in a woman's life. The rate and amount of weight loss in the postpartum period seem to be determined by the same factors that determine weight loss at any point in a woman's life, including existing weight/BMI, diet, age, and activity level.[25] Furthermore, studies indicate that pregnancy weight retention is not a significant determinant of excessive weight. A study of 7000 women who were followed from the beginning of one pregnancy to the beginning of the next pregnancy found that the average increase in weight between the first pregnancy and the next was 3.4 kg.[26]

In recognition that humans tend to gain weight as they get older, additional studies that controlled for age found an increase of only 0.3 to 0.5 kg between pregnancies.[26] These finding suggest that interventions to reduce rates of maternal obesity should focus not only on the loss of weight gained in pregnancy, but also on primary prevention of obesity and weight management at a preconceptional visit.

Conclusion

The postpartum period is a time of remarkable and rapid physiologic adjustment. Knowledge of postpartum physiology is necessary to determine the difference between normal and abnormal progression during this period. Moreover, although the vast majority of women in the postpartum period have a normal course, it is important to teach all women about signs of danger and worrisome symptoms in the postpartum period. Finally, despite a relatively rapid change from the physiology of pregnancy to a nonpregnant physiologic state, it is important to remember and remind the woman that it is quite normal for her not to feel completely back to "herself" during the weeks and even months following the birth of a newborn. The postpartum period is a profound role transition and life-changing event that cannot be described via a review of anatomic and physiologic changes.

• • • References

1. Khan RU, Refaey HE. Pathophysiology of postpartum hemorrhage. In: Lynch CB, Keith LG, Lalonde AB, Karoshi M, eds. *A Textbook of Postpartum Hemorrhage: A Comprehensive Guide to Evaluation, Management and Surgical Intervention.* Lancashire, UK: Sapiens Publishing; 2006:171-182.

2. O'Riordan MN, Higgins JR. Haemostasis in normal and abnormal pregnancy. *Best Pract Res Clin Obstet Gynaecol.* 2003;17(3):385-396.

3. Bremme KA. Haemostatic changes in pregnancy. *Best Pract Res Clin Haematol.* 2003;16(2):153-168.

4. Brenner B. Haemostatic changes in pregnancy. *Thromb Res.* 2004;114(5-6):409-414.

5. Dahlman T, Hellgren M, Blomback M. Changes in blood coagulation and fibrinolysis in the normal puerperium. *Gynecol Obstet Invest.* 1985;20:37-44.

6. Mulic-Lutvica A, Bekuretsion M, Bakos O, Axelsson O. Ultrasonic evaluation of the uterus and uterine cavity after normal, vaginal delivery. *Ultrasound Obstet Gynecol.* 2001;18:491-498.

7. Clueet ER, Alexander J, Pickering RM. What is the normal pattern of uterine involution? An investigation of postpartum uterine involution measured by the distance between the symphysis pubis and the uterine fundus using a paper tape measure. *Midwifery.* 1997;13(1):9-16.

8. Williams AB, Brown ED, Kettritz UI, et al. Anatomic changes in the pelvis after uncomplicated vaginal delivery: evaluation with serial MR imaging. *Radiology.* 1995;195:91-94.

9. Coad J, Dunstall M. *Anatomy and Physiology for Midwives.* 3rd ed. New York: Elsevier; 2011:363-378.

10. Cunningham F, Leveno K, Bloom S, et al. *Williams Obstetrics.* 23rd ed. New York: McGraw-Hill Medical; 2010:646-659.

11. Oppenheimer LW, Sherriff EA, Goodman JDS, et al. The duration of lochia. *BJOG.* 1986;93:754-757.

12. Sherman D, Lurie S, Frenkel E, et al. Characteristics of normal lochia. *Am J Perinatol.* 1999;16(8):399.

13. Yost NP, Santoso JT, Mcintire DD, Iliya FA. Postpartum regression rates of antepartum cervical intraepithelial neoplasia II and III lesions. *Obstet Gynecol.* 1999;93:359-362.

14. Quarrie LH, Addey CYP, Wilde CJ. Programmed cell death during mammary tissue involution induced by weaning, litter removal, and milk stasis. *J Cell Phys.* 1996;168:559-569.

15. Guo S, DiPietro LA. Factors affecting wound healing. *J Dent Res.* 2010;89(3):219-229.

16. Salamonsen LA. Tissue injury and repair in the female human reproductive tract. *Reproduction.* 2003;125:301-311.

17. Duvekot JJ, Peeters LL. Maternal cardiovascular hemodynamic adaptation to pregnancy. *Obstet Gyne-col Surv.* 1994;49(12):S1-S14.

18. Creasey RK, Resnik R, Iams JD, et al. *Maternal Fetal Medicine.* 6th ed. Philadelphia: Saunders-Elsevier; 2009.

19. Mone SM, Sanders SP, Colan SD. Control mechanisms for physiological hypertrophy of pregnancy. *Circulation.* 1996;94:667-672.

20. Stagnaro-Green A. Postpartum thyroiditis. *J Clin Endoc Metab.* 2002;87(9):4042-4047.

21. Premawardhana LDKE, Parkes AB, Ammari F, et al. Postpartum thyroiditis and long-term thyroid status: prognostic influence of thyroid peroxidase antibodies and ultrasound echogenicity. *J Clin Endoc Metab.* 2000;85(1):71-75.

22. Hendrick V, Altshuler V, Suri R. Hormonal changes in the postpartum and implications for postpartum depression. *Psychosomatics.* 1998;39(2):93-100.

23. Kennedy KI, Visness CM. Contraceptive efficacy of lactational amenorrhoea. *Lancet.* 1993;339(8787):227-230.

24. Glasier JE. A return of ovulation and menses in postpartum nonlactating women: a systematic review. *Obstet Gynecol.* 2011;117:657-662.

25. Schauberger CW, Rooney BL, Brimer LM. Factors that influence weight loss in the puerperium. *Obstet Gynecol.* 1992;79(3):424-429.

26. Gore SA, Brown DM, Smith West D. The role of postpartum weight retention in obesity among women: a review of the evidence. *Ann Behav Med.* 2003;26(2):149-159.

27. Chiarello CM, Falzone LA, McCaslin KE, et al. The effects of an exercise program on diastasis recti abdominis in pregnant women. *J Women's Health Phys Ther.* 2005;29(1):11-16.

28. Sminakis KV, Chasan-Tabe L, Wolf M, Markenson G, Ecker JL, Thadhani R. Postpartum diabetes screening in women with a history of gestational diabetes. *Obstet Gynecol.* 2005;106:1297-1303.

29. Centers for Disease Control and Prevention. Laboratory procedure manual: complete blood count with 5-part differential. NHANES 2005-2006. Available at: http://www.cdc.gov/nchs/data/nhanes/nhanes_05_06/cbc_d_met.pdf. Accessed November 9, 2012.

C H A P T E R

34

Postpartum Care

IRA KANTROWITZ-GORDON

Introduction

The postpartum period is a time of transition for women. The end of pregnancy initiates physiologic changes as many body systems return to their nonpregnant states. The uterus involutes, cardiac output and blood volume decrease, and estrogen and progesterone levels drop. In women who choose to breastfeed, lactogenesis II begins and lactation may continue for months or years. Yet the postpartum period is so much more than just these physical changes—it transforms the social and emotional context for the woman and her family. The midwife can have a profound impact on the woman's experience during the postpartum period by guiding her through this transition. This chapter addresses the various facets of postpartum midwifery care, including the psychological response to childbirth, evaluation and management of the normal transition and common deviations, and the provision of health education and guidance. A key to providing effective postpartum care is understanding the woman in her social and cultural context so that the care provided is culturally sensitive and competent. Only then can health and well-being continue beyond the postpartum period.

Definition of the Postpartum Period

Pregnancy comes to a definitive end when the delivery of the placenta and membranes occurs. At this time, the woman begins the physiologic transition to the nonpregnant state. Traditionally the postpartum period, or puerperium, has been defined as lasting 6 weeks, because by 6 weeks most women have completed the last of the physiologic transitions: Uterine involution is complete, lochia has ceased, and lactation is well established. This is a somewhat arbitrary—and an arguably short—time frame for the transition to parenting. An alternative label for the postpartum period is the "fourth trimester," which suggests a transition that lasts approximately 3 months.

While "recovery" implies healing from illness or trauma, the postpartum transition, as a normative life experience, is more than that. With the arrival of the newborn, family members assume new roles both within the family and in the community. Parents become grandparents, children become siblings, and partners become parents. For many families, employment status may change for either parent. As definitions of family have expanded in recent decades, it has been recognized that there is wide variation in a family's adjustment after childbirth. Despite the significance of these changes, women and families may receive less attention and support during the postpartum period than they did during the third trimester of pregnancy and during the intrapartum period. As a consequence, the postpartum period is a time of both opportunity and challenges to health.

Cross-cultural Perspective

Across the world, the importance of the postpartum period has been marked with cultural practices and rituals. For example, Mexican American immigrant families may practice the *cuarentena*, or 40 days of postpartum recovery.[1] In an ethnographic study of Mexican American immigrants in Colorado, 23 women and their family members provided valuable information about the *cuarentena*. During this time, the woman's body is considered open and vulnerable to illness. Practices to protect the woman include sexual abstinence, wrapping the abdomen in tight garments (*fajas*), avoiding strong foods and cold substances, and remaining at home as much as possible.

Similarly, Chinese women may follow the practice of *zuoyuezi*, or sitting the month. During the month postpartum, they are cared for by their mothers, mothers-in-law, or grandmothers; avoid cold foods; and keep themselves warm by wearing long clothing and staying indoors. In addition to its protective qualities, sitting the month was seen as a way to show respect to elders' beliefs and traditions that have been held for millennia.[2]

Postpartum beliefs and practices in Vietnam were explored through questionnaires and interviews of 115 Vietnamese women in a postpartum clinic in Ho Chi Minh City. Vietnamese women viewed the postpartum state as a cold state (*duong*) and, therefore, protected themselves through warmth (*am*). Cultural practices include warm water for bathing and stimulating lactation, staying indoors, and consuming foods that have warm qualities, such as meat, eggs, ginger, and wine. Rest during the months postpartum was facilitated by women family members helping with housework.[3]

In Southeast Turkey, women engaged in surprisingly similar practices to both the Asian and Latin cultures described. These practices included tightly wrapping the abdomen and other interventions to keep the woman warm, avoiding cold foods, and remaining at home on reduced activity for 40 days. As evident in the other cultural practices described, Turkish women were seen as vulnerable and needing protection during the 40 days postpartum. Protective activities included never being left home alone and placing the Koran, bread, or garlic under the woman's pillow.[4]

A common characteristic of all these cultural practices is the provision of additional social support to the woman after childbirth. When circumstances such as immigration, socioeconomic limitations, and other factors put distance between the woman and her extended family, her ability to follow these practices may be challenged. Part of the work of these new families, then, is learning how to incorporate cultural practices, balance these practices with the beliefs in their new country, and overcome the barriers of distance from family.[2]

In developed countries, there is a wide variation in the amount of financial support provided to women after childbirth. In the United States, unpaid parental leave is guaranteed for 12 weeks under certain conditions. For many families, however, taking time off to care for the woman or infant in the postpartum period places the family at significant financial risk. This economic challenge in the United States stands in contrast to policies in most other developed countries, where paid maternal leave extends from 14 weeks in Singapore and Switzerland to longer than a year in Japan and Finland. In those countries, there is a similar range of paid paternal leave.[5]

For the midwife, it is important not only to have knowledge about other cultures and practices, but also to incorporate this knowledge into clinical practice with curiosity and humility, so that women and families are treated as *they* wish to be treated. To accomplish this requires an ongoing process of clinical inquiry and negotiation with women to provide care that is culturally congruent—that is, care that fits with the family's values and meanings.[6] Questions that can help the midwife conduct a cultural assessment are listed in **Box 34-1**. Resources for providing culturally congruent midwifery care can be found at the end of this chapter.[7]

BOX 34-1 Postpartum Cultural Assessment

Consider the following questions when caring for women and families postpartum:

- Is the postpartum period viewed as a normal physiologic process, a wellness experience, a time of vulnerability and risk, or a state of illness? What does the postpartum experience mean to the woman?
- Is the postpartum period a time for privacy or socialization?
- What support is given during the postpartum period, and who appropriately gives that support?
- Are there culturally expected practices in regarding diet, nutrition, treatments (including pharmacologic), and activity?
- Which maternal precautions or restrictions are necessary during the postpartum period?
- How is postpartum pain managed?
- How is the newborn viewed, and what are the patterns regarding care of the infant and relationships within the nuclear and extended families? Are there supports and patterns to breastfeeding?

Source: Adapted from Callister LC, Eads MN, Diehl J. Perceptions of giving birth and adherence to cultural practices in Chinese women. *Am J Matern Child Nurs.* 2011;36(6):387-394.

History of Postpartum Care in the United States

During the first half of the twentieth century, the location of birth in the United States shifted from the home to the hospital. From 1935 to 1949, the percentage of hospital births in the country more than doubled, from 37% to 87%.[8] This increase represented a change from giving birth in the home under the care of midwives and the family to delivering in the hospital under the care of physicians and nurses. In the hospital, childbirth often was treated as an illness requiring obstetric interventions.[8] Routine obstetric interventions such as anesthesia, forceps delivery, and episiotomies became entrenched in clinical practice. Because puerperal sepsis was a leading cause of maternal morbidity and mortality, hospital nursing care focused on the dangers of infection, which generated care practices that restricted contact among mothers, fathers, and newborns.[8] Newborns were segregated into aseptic-looking central nurseries, placed on strict feeding schedules, and almost exclusively formula fed. While postpartum lengths of stay were 9 to 11 days in the 1930s, nursing shortages during World War II in the 1940s resulted in average stays of 6 days.[9] Early ambulation was introduced in some areas as one strategy to alleviate overcrowding of maternity wards.[8]

As infant psychologists proposed new theories of infant development in the 1940s, the first program of rooming-in was established at Yale–New Haven Hospital. Newborns remained with their mothers in the postpartum ward under the care of postpartum and newborn nurses.[8] During the postwar baby boom, the absolute number of births, as well as percentage of births taking place in the hospital, continued to rise. It was not until decades later, however, that rooming-in became more common in U.S. hospitals.

The 1960s and 1970s saw the rise of the natural childbirth movement as a reaction to unnecessary interventions in childbirth and a desire for more family-centered care. The exclusion of fathers from the delivery room and long postpartum hospital stays were no longer acceptable to consumers who wanted to stay together as a family. Work by Klaus and Kennel[10] regarding maternal–newborn attachment provided a scientific basis for keeping women and their newborns together during the immediate postpartum period. Thus there was a renewed interest in rooming-in, in which infants were moved from the central nursery back to their mother's room for care to promote maternal–newborn attachment and parenting competence before hospital discharge. Rooming-in also developed as a response to nursing shortages,

because it allowed women and their newborns to be cared for more efficiently by the same nurse. Furthermore, rooming-in addressed an increasing prevalence of nosocomial infections found in central newborn nurseries.[11]

Early postpartum discharge was initially developed in the 1970s and 1980s to meet consumer demand. As part of the natural childbirth movement, families that avoided obstetric interventions did not see the need to recover during prolonged hospital stays and risk hospital-based infections. These early discharge programs were implemented initially for low-risk mothers, although increasingly they became the norm for all families. Average lengths of stay decreased from 4 days in the 1970s to 2 days by the 1990s. Concern arose, however, that owing to early discharge, newborn complications such as excessive weight loss and hyperbilirubinemia were being missed. Various strategies to fill the care gap were utilized, including home visits, support groups, telephone calls, and postpartum clinics.[12,13] A public backlash against limits to hospital stays by third-party payers led to the passage of the Newborns' and Mothers' Postpartum Protection Act in 1996, which mandated a 48-hour stay for childbirth.[8] This legislation protected discharge as a decision to be made by providers and families, although it did not mandate insurance payment for longer postpartum stays or for early postpartum follow-up after discharge, nor did it reflect the practices at birth sites that already had a supportive family focus.

Women who give birth at home or at a freestanding birth center have a different context in which postpartum care is delivered. The question of postpartum discharge is moot, because the needs for support, education, and follow-up care are met through home visits by the midwife, as needed. These different models of support are limited in the United States by the low numbers of women choosing to give birth outside the hospital.

Regardless of the site of birth, additional support for women may include hiring a postpartum doula who may help with household tasks, breastfeeding support, and self-care. These support services are available for families that can pay for the care as third-party payment for postpartum care services is not usually available.

Standard postpartum care in the United States today follows the traditional model of an office visit with the prenatal care provider at 4 to 6 weeks postpartum, although women who were followed prenatally in a group setting such as the CenteringPregnancy model usually have a group reunion at 1 to 2 months. Thus, after hospital discharge, many women do not have contact with their healthcare provider until the traditional 6-week postpartum office visit. It is unclear why this specific time frame was selected, and in some centers it has been replaced by an earlier examination at 2 to 3 weeks. An additional office visit at 1 to 2 weeks postpartum has been proposed to bridge the gap in care from discharge until 6 weeks, and to support breastfeeding, contraception, and the psychosocial transition postpartum.[14] The financial pressures of clinical practice deter many providers from providing this extra visit, however, as there often is no additional reimbursement for it. In the twenty-first century, the controversy about lengths of stay continues, and a health system that provides a consistently high standard of care at reasonable cost remains elusive.

Psychological Adaption During the Postpartum Period

Attachment: Formation of the Parent–Infant Relationship

Birth is a transformative moment in the lives of women and their families. The response of parents to their infant and to their experience in childbearing is individual; therefore the response of one parent may differ from the other. Midwives can help families process and integrate the events of the birth into their family story and help the parents who live together transform their relationship with the fetus into a strong and lasting relationship with the child. This action is crucial for the physical, cognitive, and social development of the child. Medical, psychosocial, and environmental conditions during the postpartum period may either facilitate or interfere with that relationship.

Definition of Parent Attachment

Definitions of parent–infant attachment have included concepts such as bonding, love, or an instinctual connection. These definitions may focus on one direction in the relationship: either the parent bonding to the newborn or the newborn bonding to the parent. Goulet et al.[15] used concept analysis methodology to examine the vast literature on attachment to develop a clearer understanding and definition. Based on this analysis, they identified three key attributes in the mutual relationship between parents and newborns (**Figure 34-1**):

- *Proximity.* Physical closeness allows interaction across multiples senses (hearing, touch,

sight, and smell), facilitates a strong emotional connection, and creates an awareness of the infant's individuality and needs that are different from the parent's needs.

- *Reciprocity.* Parents and newborns interact in a responsive and adaptive manner. Parents become sensitive to the infant's cues and body language in their caregiving. The infant contributes to the interaction by reinforcing the parents' behaviors.

- *Commitment.* Feeling and acting responsibly for the safety, growth, and development of the infant place the infant in a central position in the family and identify the parenting role as an important part of the adult's identity.[15]

Relationships develop over time and depend on the participation of parents and infant. Goulet et al. characterized four events or conditions that may enable successful parent–infant attachment: (1) acceptance of the pregnancy and the infant; (2) becoming acquainted with the fetus prenatally and (3) becoming acquainted with the newborn after the birth; and (4) a favorable environment, including the family, social supports, and resources.[15] The quality of parent–infant attachment is mediated by culture and the context of the individual family. For example, in a longitudinal study of 217 pregnant Hispanic

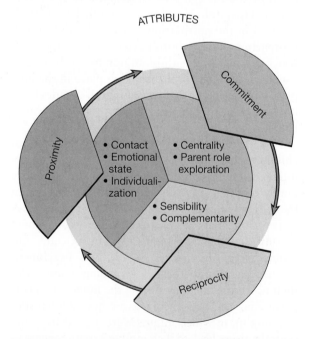

Figure 34-1 Key attributes of parent–infant attachment.
Source: Goulet C, Bell L, Tribble DS, Paul D, Lang A. A concept analysis of parent-infant attachment. *J Adv Nurs.* 1998;28(5):1071-1081. Reprinted by permission of John Wiley.

women, negative feelings about the pregnancy and depressive symptoms in late pregnancy were inversely associated with maternal–infant attachment at 2 months, whereas no association was found between maternal–infant attachment and pregnancy intention or strength of the partner relationship.[16] In a sample of 195 first-time fathers in Taiwan, social support, partner support, and marital intimacy measurements in the third trimester were moderately correlated with paternal–infant attachment at 1 week after birth.[17]

The first hour after birth has been described as an important sensitive period among humans, in which the newborn is alert and receptive to exploring the environment and forming attachment with the parents.[10] The idea of the sensitive period was an extension of research on animals, where interference during the sensitive period was found to sometimes lead to rejection of the newborn by the parents or the newborn animal bonding to alternatives such as other animals or objects. Recognition of the sensitive period has led to changes in maternity practices in which newborns are lifted to the woman's abdomen for skin-to-skin care immediately after birth, an action that has benefits such as conservation of the heat of the newborn as well as promotion of attachment.[18]

The underlying premise that this sensitive time is necessary for the maternal–newborn relationship has been criticized. Because attachment in people is formed over time, overemphasis on the first hour may be harmful in situations where it is missed, such as when the medical condition of the woman or the newborn must be attended to or the second parent is absent due to deployment in the military. Fortunately, there are countless opportunities to develop attachment, as demonstrated by parents who adopt children at a variety of ages. Continuing reciprocal responses, strengthening of the relationship, and changing roles occur throughout life, including during the postpartum period.

Early Parenting Behaviors: The Effect of Skin-to-Skin Contact

In many settings, women are encouraged to practice skin-to-skin care (kangaroo care) immediately after the birth if the newborn's condition allows it. Skin-to-skin care has been evaluated in randomized controlled trials (RCTs) and one meta-analysis.[19] Moore et al. found that skin-to-skin care shared by women and their healthy term neonates ($n = 703$; 13 RCTs) resulted in significant positive effects on breastfeeding at 1 to 4 months (relative risk [RR]: 1.27; 95% confidence interval [CI]: 1.06–1.53). Breastfeeding duration appeared to be extended, although the finding did not reach statistical significance and improved trend scores for maternal attachment behavior were noted.[19]

Immediate skin-to-skin care also facilitates physiologic regulation in the newborn. Newborns who experience skin-to-skin care may attain heart rate stability and have lower salivary cortisol levels when compared to infants who do not share skin-to-skin contact with their mothers immediately after birth.[20]

The benefits of skin-to-skin care have also been demonstrated for fathers when the mother is unavailable to hold the infant (**Figure 34-2**). In the first 2 hours after cesarean birth, neonates who were held in skin-to-skin contact with the father demonstrated less crying, became calmer, and were more drowsy than newborns left in a crib.[21]

Another early behavior demonstrated by parents while doing skin-to-skin care is vocalization. In a controlled trial immediately after cesarean birth, newborns in skin-to-skin care with either the mother or the father demonstrated more soliciting calls than did newborns placed in a crib. Parents reciprocated with more vocalizations directed at the newborn and fathers also communicated more with the mother.[22] Thus the proximity of skin-to-skin care promoted increased vocalization interaction between parents and the newborn.

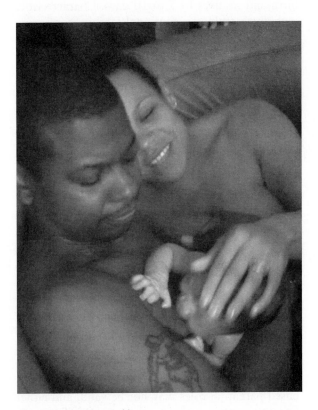

Figure 34-2 Skin-to-skin care.
Source: Reprinted with permission from Melisa Scott

Psychological Response to Childbearing

Childbirth may leave a woman feeling both exhilarated and exhausted. She has experienced dramatic physical and physiologic changes in her body after the exertion of labor. Once the infant is born, she then undergoes the stimulation and excitement of holding her newborn for the first time and incorporating the infant into the family. Over the next few days, she must get to know and care for her newborn and meet the demands of this 24-hour responsibility, under conditions of interrupted sleep. It is not surprising, then, that many new mothers feel overwhelmed and exhibit signs of the "postpartum blues."

Postpartum Blues

The phenomenon of early "postpartum blues" or "baby blues" is a common sequela of childbirth, occurring in as many as 70% to 80% of all women. Various causes have been proposed, including an unsupportive birth environment, rapid hormonal changes, or insecurity in a new role. None of these suggested etiologies has been demonstrated to be a consistent underlying cause. However, all of these factors, in addition to the inevitable sleep deprivation experienced by new mothers, are certainly involved.

Postpartum blues typically begins a few days after birth and resolves by 7 to 10 days. Characteristics include tearfulness, emotional lability, confusion, low mood, anxiety, and agitation.[23] The key to helping a woman through this period is consistent support from family and caregivers, reassurance that she is not mentally impaired, and provision of opportunities for increased rest. Additionally, positive reinforcement of her successes in parenting the newborn can help restore the woman's confidence in her abilities. Postpartum depression is a true depression that usually occurs later in the postpartum period. Postpartum depression is reviewed in the *Mental Health Conditions* chapter.

Beyond Gender

Parenting is a gendered, socially constructed experience. Couples who include lesbian or transgender parents may have different psychosocial reactions to childbirth, but little is known about their postpartum experiences. These families may experience difficulty interacting with the healthcare system due to heterocentric practices in language use and history forms, discriminatory practices, and lack of support from the extended family.[24] Assumptions about gender-based parenting roles may not be valid, and either female parent may choose to breastfeed. Transmen (female-to-male transgender individuals) may give birth yet identify as the father, be unable or unwilling to breastfeed, and react to the physical aspects of childbirth differently from other parents.[25] Due to the additional stress facing these families, a supportive environment, healthcare team, and social network are important for birth and postpartum care.

Reactions to the Birth Experience

The events of childbirth are difficult to predict and often do not match the couple's birth plan. Differences between the planned labor and birth and the reality may include use of analgesia or anesthesia, mode of delivery, gender of the newborn, and the quality of support provided in labor. In the Listening to Mothers II national survey of childbirth, 9% of women met diagnostic criteria for post-traumatic stress disorder (PTSD) and 18% of women experienced significant levels of post-traumatic stress symptoms 7 to 18 months after childbirth.[26] For some families, the experience goes beyond disappointment, as the parents must grieve after a loss. Examples of losses include stillbirth or early neonatal death, loss of fertility after an emergency hysterectomy, the discovery of congenital birth defects, voluntary or involuntary relinquishment of the newborn to adoptive parents or the legal system, and admission to the neonatal intensive care unit. The couple's grief reactions to these outcomes will be unique to their specific circumstances, coping strategies, and social support.

Early Postpartum Period

During the first 72 hours after birth, or the early puerperium period, the frequency with which the midwife evaluates the woman and newborn may depend on the birth setting and other circumstances of the birth. In most settings, the midwife assesses the woman at least once daily. Each visit includes a chart review; interval history, including physical, psychological, and emotional changes since the birth; physical examination, including observation of family interactions; and management plans that focus on treatments for symptoms and conditions of the puerperium, follow-up visit plans, and health education.

Chart Review

Before the midwife begins a visit, the woman's prenatal and birth care should be reviewed, so that the professional can speak knowledgeably with the woman. Even if the midwife is not responsible for the newborn's health management, the midwife should be aware of any complications in the newborn's health status. The newborn's health status may directly influence the management plan for the woman, including timing of the discharge from the facility and follow-up plans. Reviewing the chart entries since the birth also familiarizes the midwife with the record of the woman's vital signs, laboratory results, medication use, and any comments from other caregivers. Previous orders and progress notes are reviewed as well. Medications that were temporarily stopped during the pregnancy or labor should be evaluated and a decision about restarting them made.

Time elapsed since birth, in hours or days, is ascertained to identify expected physical findings. When documenting postpartum notes in the health record, it is important to indicate precise time information. For example, postpartum day 1 may denote that the woman is within 24 hours postpartum or between 24 and 48 hours postpartum. Since indicating postpartum days may generate confusion based on time of birth and calendar days, it may be preferred to specify how many *hours* have elapsed since the birth.

History

Listening to the Birth Story

At some time during the early puerperium it is helpful for the midwife to inquire about the woman's experience of the birth. Asking "How was your labor and birth for you?" provides an opening for the woman and family to talk about the events of the birth. This open-ended question can elicit valuable information about the woman's perspective on her experience— a feeling that can differ markedly from that of the midwife or other healthcare providers involved in her care. The midwife should be especially attentive to symptoms that suggest symptoms of PTSD. While it is not possible to make a formal diagnosis of PTSD so soon after the birth, an awareness of these symptoms may alert the midwife to provide additional resources or referrals (**Table 34-1**). In most situations involving fearful events, the act of listening is by itself therapeutic.

Emotional Assessment

Early postpartum visits should always include an assessment of maternal mood. If the woman contacts her midwife with concerns about depression and/or if a depressed mood is identified during a routine contact, a more detailed assessment to distinguish postpartum blues from postpartum depression is necessary. Persistent depressed mood past the first few weeks postpartum or symptoms of real

Table 34-1	Symptoms Suggestive of Post-traumatic Stress Disorder
Reexperiencing the trauma	Intrusive memories
	Upsetting dreams
	Flashbacks
Avoidance of stimuli associated with the trauma	Avoiding thoughts, feelings, or conversations
	Avoiding activities, situations, or people
	Avoiding once enjoyable activities
	Detachment and emotional numbing
	Amnesia, loss of concentration
	Loss of hope for future
Changes in arousal and reactivity	Sleep disturbances (e.g., insomnia)
	Hypervigilance
	Exaggerated startle response
	Irritability or anger

Source: Adapted from American Psychiatric Association. *Diagnostic and Statistical Manual of Mental Disorders.* 5th ed. Arlington, VA: American Psychiatric Association; 2013.

depression early in the postpartum period may indicate postpartum depression. Methods of evaluation and the differential diagnosis for these two conditions are presented in detail in the *Mental Health Conditions* chapter.

Physical Adaptation to the Postpartum State

Physical assessments for each postpartum visit include a variety of factors: maternal nutrition, bladder and bowel function, amount of lochia, activity level, breastfeeding, and level of pain or discomfort, if applicable. Whether or not the midwife is the primary healthcare provider for the infant, information about the infant feeding method, infant behavior, and sleep–wake cycles should be collected. When a home visit is conducted, the midwife should arrange the visit to coincide with those times when the infant is likely to be awake if possible. This enables an evaluation of the parent–newborn interaction and the parents' skill and comfort in handling the newborn, which may indicate areas of learning needs. Examples of criteria for assessment of parent–newborn interactions are listed in **Box 34-2**.[28] These behaviors may be noted as evidence for the development of parent–newborn attachment. Midwives should be careful to consider cultural factors when evaluating the parent–newborn interactions.[29]

Physical Examination

The examination during the early postpartum period is focused on the physiologic changes that occur after birth. It is important to ensure privacy is maintained according to the woman's wishes. A comfortable location for the exam should be used, and pillows for support may be helpful. Because the woman may have an expected level of discomfort during the exam, a gentle touch should be used and permission requested before examining any part of her body. Physical assessments during the early puerperium include the heart, lungs, breasts, abdomen, perineum and anus, and lower extremities. The midwife may provide teaching about the physiologic changes of the puerperium during the examination. The postpartum examination procedure is outlined in **Appendix 34A.** Expected physical examination findings in the early puerperium are detailed in **Table 34-2.**

The examination of the heart and lungs during the early puerperium is performed in the same manner as when the woman is not pregnant or postpartum. During the phases of lactogenesis, the breast consistency may be soft, filling (i.e., tense, increasing firmness, slightly enlarged), or engorged (i.e., enlarged, hard, reddened, shiny; skin temperature elevated; painful, dilated veins). Soft swelling in the axilla may be evidence of accessory mammary tissue that can cause discomfort, but is otherwise benign. In some situations during the postpartum period, it is of value to express colostrum or milk

from the woman's nipples, as demonstrating this provides an opportunity to educate and assist her with breastfeeding. The woman can be guided to perform manual expression herself by compressing the areola below the nipple between her thumb and fingers. Expression of a drop or two of colostrum or milk helps the newborn learn where to suckle through immediate gratification. When the breasts, and especially the areola, are engorged, it will be easier for the newborn to latch on properly if some milk is first expressed, which diminishes the rigid hardness of the area so that it is soft enough that the newborn can compress the lactiferous sinuses. Additional information about breastfeeding is found in the *Breastfeeding and the Mother–Newborn Dyad* chapter.

Examination of the abdomen during the puerperium begins with the uterus, which will be the largest palpable organ. The fundal height decreases gradually until the uterus is again a pelvic organ by 4 to 6 weeks postpartum, as illustrated in **Figure 34-3.**

The REEDA scale provides a mnemonic for documentation of healing lacerations or incisions. This midwife-developed instrument was created to provide a standard description of perineal healing, but today it is used widely for documentation of any healing incision. REEDA refers to Redness, Ecchymosis, Edema, Discharge/Drainage, and Approximation. Although a scoring system has been used with this scale in the past, today most midwives use descriptors for each component.[30]

Part of the postpartum perineal examination is educating the woman about what to expect when she sees or touches her perineal and vaginal area, including the normal changes such as general edema, as well as the appearance of repaired lacerations or episiotomy. Gentle palpation will help distinguish

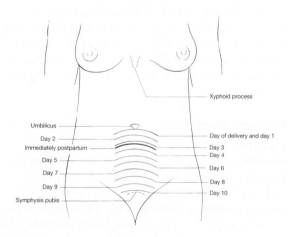

Figure 34-3 Fundal height.

Table 34-2	Subjective and Objective Data in Early Puerperium	
	Expected Findings	**Deviations from Normal**
Subjective Data		
General	Tired, ambulatory without assistance, repeating birth events, usually happy	Inability to ambulate without assistance; sad or teary
Neurologic	Oriented to person, place, and time; bilateral and frontal headaches are normal the first week; normal reflexes	Disoriented Headache—sudden onset or severe Hyperreflexia
Cardiovascular	No chest pain. May feel heartbeat increasing with minimal activity.	Chest pain, palpitations
Pulmonary	No shortness of breath or difficulty breathing	Shortness of breath
Breasts	Neonate is nursing frequently with a good latch Nipples sore, but not painful Colostrum for 3–5 days with breast fullness before milk is seen	Neonate is not latching well or frequently Painful nipples No breast filling by days 4–5
Genitourinary	Urinary: voiding spontaneously, diuresis, and natriuresis normal, especially between days 2 and 5 Mild external burning, some retention and/or incontinence, and lack of sensation or urge to void are common in the first 2 days postpartum if the woman had epidural analgesia, an operative vaginal birth, or extensive perineal trauma, but should resolve rapidly Tender or sore at area of repair	Pelvic pressure or pain increasing Persistent retention or incontinence
Gastrointestinal	Eating and drinking without difficulty. Bowel movements usually return after 2–3 days with normal bowel patterns by 2 weeks. Abdomen: uterine contractions/cramping particularly with nursing	Nausea or vomiting, abdominal pain, constipation or diarrhea
Lower extremities	No pain Generalized muscle soreness	Pain, aching, or swelling, particularly in one leg
Objective Data		
Laboratory tests: routine assessment is unnecessary.	Hemoglobin: decreases slightly in the first 24 hours after birth, then plateaus for 4 days, followed by a slow rise to day 14 WBC count: falls to 6000–10,000/mm^3, then returns to normal values by 6 days	A 500-mL blood loss will usually result in approximately a 1-g reduction in hemoglobin or 3% reduction in hematocrit. These values return to normal by 4–6 weeks postpartum.
Vital signs	Temperature: normal or low-grade elevation Blood pressure: returns to normal by 24 hours Pulse: 65–80 bpm at rest Respirations: 12–16/min at rest	Temperature: higher than 38°C (100.4°F) Blood pressure: higher than 140/90 mm Hg or lower than 85/60 mm Hg Pulse: higher than 100 bpm
General	Comfortable, appears happy	Manner suggesting pain, discomfort, dissatisfaction, unhappiness
Neurologic	Alert and oriented Not in apparent pain	Excessively sedated or somnolent, unable to easily awaken Excessive or unexplained pain or restlessness
Cardiovascular	Regular rate and rhythm	Tachycardia

(continues)

Table 34-2	Subjective and Objective Data in Early Puerperium *(continued)*	
	Expected Findings	**Deviations from Normal**
Objective Data *(continued)*		
Pulmonary	Clear to auscultation	Adventitious sounds
Breasts	Soft for 1–2 days; some fullness beginning days 3–5 Nipples intact and erect when stimulated	Nipples: flat, inverted, cracked, bruised, blistered, or bleeding Breasts: erythema, engorged
Gastrointestinal	Abdomen: nontender, nondistended; bowel sounds present; muscle tone is decreased; distension in the first 2–3 days is common Uterus: fundus firm, nontender, midline, height normal for postpartum day (Figure 34-3)	Abdomen: distended, tender, or no bowel sounds Uterus: increasing fundal height, deviation from midline, or tender
Urinary	Bladder: nondistended—not palpable	Bladder: distended
Perinum	Perineum: mild erythema, edema, or bruising may be present Repair: approximated without drainage Lochia: amount decreasing, color, odor	Costovertebral angle tenderness Perineum: increasing tenderness, erythema, edema, bruising Laceration repair: separation of repair, suppuration, or excessive edema, signs of hematoma Lochia: malodor, clots, soaked or overflowing pads
Anus	Normal in appearance Hemorrhoids: pink	Hemorrhoids: deep blue/purple
Lower extremities	Edema is common Reflexes normal	Positive Homan's sign, deep calf tenderness, one calf larger in the transverse diameter than the other, heat, varicosities that are erythematous and/or painful on palpation
Integument	Normal color No immediate changes. Hyperpigmentation may be retained although will fade with time. Striae, spider nevi, capillary hemangiomas, varicosities, and skin tags regress but may not completely disappear.	

normal edema from hematomas. Examination of the posterior end of a repair and the anal area for external hemorrhoids is best performed when the woman lies on her side with the top leg bent and slightly in front of her bottom leg. Gentle elevation of the upper buttocks provides good exposure for visualization of the area. Evaluation of the lochia on the sanitary pad should include color, extent of saturation on the pad, and the length of time since the pad was last changed.

Evaluation of the extremities has traditionally included Homan's sign to assess for deep vein thrombosis. This test is not diagnostic and could theoretically loosen a thrombus that might be present. Therefore, Homan's sign is not recommended today. DVT is increased 60-fold in the first 3 months postpartum compared with women who are not pregnant or postpartum.[31] Other signs that are more predictive of DVT than a positive Homan's sign include unilateral calf tenderness, erythema, and swelling.

Management in the Early Puerperium

Care during the early puerperium may be very different based on the woman's parity, length and difficulty of labor, site of birth, and postpartum comfort. In many institutional settings, routine or standing orders for the first postpartum days may exist. It is imperative to consider whether these orders are appropriate for the specific woman. The orders may need to be individualized—for example, by modifying pain management routines, deleting intravenous fluids, or ordering a referral to a lactation consultation. The midwife should be certain the issues outlined in **Table 34-3** are addressed if written orders are prepared, or

Table 34-3	Postpartum Orders and Plans
Topic	**Details/Options**
Hydration	Oral hydration preferred; should specify when to discontinue any intravenous hydration
Nutrition	Consider food allergies, cultural preferences, and diabetes
Activity level	Generally unrestricted; first time out of bed with assistance after epidural anesthesia, cesarean section, or postpartum hemorrhage
General postpartum medications	Rh immune globulin (RhoGAM) if needed, vitamins and iron, stool softeners or laxatives, analgesics, sleep medications as needed
Other medications	Continue or reinstate medications such as thyroid replacement, antidepressants per plan that was made prenatally. Consult with a physician colleague as indicated
Perineal care	Ice packs, topical medications, peri-bottle
Management for inability to void	Peppermint oil, catheterization
Breast care	Purified lanolin cream or hydrogel for nipple soreness, breast pump for engorgement, binder/supportive bra for not breastfeeding
Laboratory tests	Hemoglobin and hematocrit if symptoms of anemia; Rh screen of newborn if woman is Rh negative
Vaccinations	Rubella, varicella, for nonimmune women; influenza if needed; HPV series can be resumed if discontinued during pregnancy; Tdap if not received during pregnancy
Contraception	Prescription for self-administered contraceptives; DMPA before discharge in selected clients
Discharge	Depends on family readiness, status of newborn
Follow-up	Postpartum clinics, home visits, 2 or 6 weeks in office
DMPA = depot medroxyprogesterone; Tdap = tetanus, diphtheria, and acellular pertussis.	

that they are considered in the care of women delivering in out-of-hospital settings. Medications that are commonly prescribed during the early puerperium are listed in **Table 34-4**.[32,33]

Postpartum Teaching

Fatigue, excitement, and feeling overwhelmed may limit the ability of parents to take in new information. Therefore, teaching in the early puerperium should be prioritized and targeted to the needs of each woman and her family. Assessing the parents' learning needs is the first step in teaching. Assumptions may be misleading, such as expecting that a woman with previous children already has a wealth of knowledge and that a woman having her first baby is unfamiliar with personal or neonatal care. For example, nulliparous women may have experience with newborns through caring for a sibling or other infant relatives, and a woman who gave birth at a young age may have had that child cared for by a mother or older relative. Women who have given birth previously may appreciate a review as well. Health professionals who have become parents often prefer to receive the same

teaching as other couples. It may be helpful to focus on essential topics, supplement teaching with written materials or electronic sources, and provide contact information for further help in the community. Including available family members in postpartum teaching will maximize the benefits. Topics that may be covered are listed in **Table 34-5**. Important signs of compliations are listed in **Table 34-6**. Discomforts specific to breastfeeding (nipple tenderness and cracked nipples) are discussed in the *Breastfeeding and the Mother–Newborn Dyad* chapter.

Management of Common Discomforts

Afterbirth and Perineal Pain

Afterbirth pains are caused by the continuing sequential contraction and relaxation of the uterus. This phenomenon is more common in multiparous women and in women who breastfeed. Women with increasing parity may have decreased uterine tone as compared to women who have given birth for the first time and can note the pains more intensely. In breastfeeding women, the suckling of the infant stimulates the production of oxytocin by the

Table 34-4	Medications Commonly Prescribed for Women in the Early Puerperium				
Class	**Drug (Brand)**	**Formulations**	**Indications and Dose**	**Clinical Considerations**	**Lactation**
Analgesics	Acetaminophen (Tylenol)	325, 500 mg	*Mild to moderate pain* 500, 650, 1000 mg every 6 hours	Maximum 4 g/day acetaminophen from all sources	Safe
	Ibuprofen (Motrin, Advil)	200, 400, 600 mg	*Mild to moderate pain* 600 mg every 6 hours	Take with food. Maximum 2400 mg/day	Safe
	Ketorolac (Toradol)	15, 30, 60 mg IM 10 mg PO	*Short-term treatment for postoperative pain* 60 mg IM × 1 dose	Reduces postoperative opiate use	Safe
	Acetaminophen (Tylenol)/ codeine No. 3	300/30 mg	*Moderate pain* Tylenol No. 3 every 4–6 hours	Take with food May cause excessive sedation in women and newborns who are rapid metabolizers	Moderately safe but observe for sedation, excessive sleepiness, and poor feeding
	Hydrocodone/ acetaminophen (Vicodin)	5/300 mg	*Moderate pain* 1–2 tables every 4–6 hours	Maximum 4 g/day acetaminophen from all sources	Moderately safe but observe for sedation or constipation
	Oxycodone/ acetaminophen (Percocet)	2.5/325, 5/325, 7.5/325 mg	*Moderate pain* 1–2 tablets every 4–6 hours	Maximum 4 g/day acetaminophen from all sources	Moderately safe but observe for sedation
	Fentanyl (Sublimaze)	50 mcg/mL	*Severe pain* 50–100 mcg IM or IV every 1–2 hours	Short-term use for procedures and painful examinations	Safe
	Morphine sulfate	Varies	*Severe pain* 5–10 mg IM or IV every 3–6 hours		Moderately safe but observe for sedation
	Meperidine (Demerol)	50, 100 mg/mL	*Severe pain* 50–100 mg IM every 3–4 hours		Moderately safe but observe for sedation
Stool softeners	Docusate sodium (Colace)	50, 100 mg	100 mg once or twice daily	Discontinue with diarrhea	Safe
Immuno-biologics	Rho(D) immune globulin (RhoGAM)	Immune globulin	*Rh-negative women with Rh-positive newborn* 300 mcg IM within 72 hours postpartum	Each 300 mcg dose will protect against 15 mL fetal–maternal transfusion	Safe
	Measles/ mumps/rubella (MMR)	Live attenuated virus	*Women nonimmune to rubella* 0.5 mL SQ		Safe
	Varicella (Varivax)	Live attenuated virus	*Women nonimmune to varicella* 0.5 mL SQ, repeat in 4–8 weeks		Safe
	Tetanus/ diphtheria/ acellular pertussis (Tdap) (Adacel)	Combination toxoid and vaccine	*Postpartum women who have not previously received Tdap* 0.5 mL IM		Safe

Sources: Adapted from Rhode MA. Postpartum. In: King TL, Brucker MC, eds. *Pharmacology for Women's Health*. Sudbury, MA: Jones and Bartlett; 2011:1117-1145; Hale TW. *Medications and Mothers' Milk*. Amarillo, TX: Pharmasoft Medical; 2012.

Table 34-5	Early Postpartum Teaching
Physical Care	**Relational Care**
Perineal care	Sibling rivalry
Breast care during breastfeeding and engorgement	Partner's needs and fears
	Transitional family relationships
Abdominal exercises	Need for time together with partner and separate from the baby
Pelvic floor exercises (Kegel)	
Activity, exercise, and rest	Family planning
Nutrition	Postpartum sexuality
Hygiene, including tub bath or shower as preferred	Emotional self-care (postpartum blues)

Table 34-6	Postpartum Signs of Complications
Mother	**Newborn**
Heavy bleeding	Feeding difficulties
Increased abdominal pain or vulvar pain	Yellowing skin (jaundice)
Fever or chills	Fever
Redness, heat, firmness, or pain in one breast	Inability to console
	Insufficient wet/dirty diapers
Calf pain, heat, or swelling	Diarrhea
Significant mood changes	Listless behavior, not alert when awake
Sudden-onset headache, visual changes, or epigastric pain	Respiratory difficulties, turning blue

posterior pituitary. The release of oxytocin not only triggers the let-down reflex in the breasts, but also causes the uterus to contract. Women may reduce afterbirth pains if they urinate frequently to prevent the bladder from displacing the uterus upward, which is associated with more painful contractions. Use of heating pads or lying prone with a pillow or blanket roll under the lower abdomen also may relieve the discomfort of afterbirth pains. Use of analgesics as described later in this section will provide relief for most women.

A number of comfort measures can alleviate perineal discomfort or pain resulting from a laceration or episiotomy and subsequent repair or, more uncommonly, from a hematoma. After assessment, several suggestions can be offered to the woman. A helpful toileting technique includes hand washing, rinsing with warm water from a peri-bottle during urination, wiping front to back, and patting any incision area dry instead of rubbing it. Other comfort measures for the perineum are listed in **Table 34-7**. If perineal discomfort does not progressively improve with time, reexamination should be performed to rule out pathology, including infection.

Multiple choices of analgesics are available to help women with afterbirth pains and perineal pain after vaginal birth. Individual medications for specific women usually are chosen based on past experience of the woman, her allergies, and woman/provider preferences. Most midwives have a preferred pain relief regimen that is based more on clinical experience than on scientific study. Ibuprofen and acetaminophen may be prescribed or purchased over the counter. All

Table 34-7	Comfort Measures for Woman with Perineal Pain
Ice packs	Ice packs are most useful for reducing swelling and numbing the perineum in the first 24 hours. All ice packs should be wrapped in a soft covering, absorbent side out, for protection against freezing injury. Optimal benefit is achieved with 30-minute applications as needed.
Topical anesthetics	Anesthetic sprays (Dermoplast, Americaine) deliver 20% benzocaine. These may be used for pain from vulvar lacerations or hemorrhoids.
Sitz baths	Washing the perineum three times daily may be accomplished using a disposable, fit-in-the-toilet sitz bath. Alternatively, women may soak in a warm bath or pour warm water over the perineum. Water temperature should be tested first on an area such as the inside of the wrist. Some women will prefer the use of cold water or ice baths.
Witch hazel	Witch hazel compresses may be applied to the perineum or anal area and held in place by the sanitary pad. 4 × 4 gauze soaked in witch hazel or ready-to-use Tucks pads may be used.

analgesics should be decreased in dose and frequency as the postpartum discomfort improves. Women who have experienced an uncomplicated vaginal birth should not require anything stronger than ibuprofen by the second or third postpartum day. Significant pain that persists warrants an examination to identify its cause. Women should be instructed that the maximum dosage from all medications containing acetaminophen should not exceed 4000 mg in 24 hours, and women prescribed opioid–acetaminophen combination analgesics such as Vicodin should be cautioned about self-administering additional doses because they can accidentally exceed the maximum dosage of acetaminophen. Women also should be advised that ibuprofen should be taken with food to avoid gastrointestinal discomfort.

Teaching women to perform pelvic floor exercises (also known as Kegel exercises) is another strategy for promoting long-term perineal comfort and strength. Performing pelvic floor exercises has been shown to reduce the prevalence of stress urinary incontinence in women during pregnancy and postpartum[34] and to improve sexual function postpartum.[35] Kegel exercises may also increase circulation to the area, promote healing, restore tone to the pelvic musculature, and facilitate ease of movement. The woman may tighten her perineum, drawing it up and in and maintaining this contracted state while moving in bed or lowering herself onto a chair. For strengthening muscle tone, the exercises can be done in sets of 10, repeatedly tightening and relaxing the muscles for 5 to 10 seconds. It is helpful to repeat these sets two to three times daily—a regimen that will avoid direct pressure to the sensitive areas. If the woman has undergone a mediolateral episiotomy, tightening the muscles when performing Kegel exercises pulls on the posterior end of the suture line because the incision interrupts muscles diagonally and may be too uncomfortable to perform until the perineum is healed.

Breast Engorgement

It is theorized that engorgement of the breasts is due to a combination of milk accumulation and stasis as well as increased vascularity and congestion. This combination results in further congestion by virtue of lymphatic and venous stasis. Engorgement occurs as the milk supply increases, usually beginning on approximately the third postpartum day in both breastfeeding and nonbreastfeeding women, and lasts approximately 24 to 48 hours. The breasts become distended, tense, and tender to the touch. The skin is warm to the touch, with visible veins, and is taut across the breasts. The nipples are firmer and may become difficult for the infant to grasp. For some women, breast tenderness becomes painful, particularly if the infant is having difficulty with nursing or if the woman does not have adequate breast support. Although engorgement is not an inflammatory process, the increased metabolism associated with milk production may cause a mildly elevated temperature. However, a fever of 38.0°C (100.4°F) or higher suggests the presence of mastitis or another infection, as discussed in more detail in the *Postpartum Complications* chapter.

When a woman is not lactating, comfort measures are targeted toward relief of discomfort and cessation of milk production. There are no medications approved for lactation suppression in the United States. Several strategies may be implemented to help with the discomfort and inhibit milk production: the use of good breast support by a supportive bra or breast binder, application of ice packs, and the use of analgesics. These women should use a bra or breast binder to firmly support the breasts, and may be more comfortable if the bra is also worn at night while sleeping. No attempt should be made to express milk from the breasts, either manually or by using heat, as this will simply promote milk let-down and further milk production. For example, the woman should avoid standing in a warm shower and letting the water run over the breasts. When using ice for comfort, caution should be used to not apply the ice directly to the skin. Engorgement will improve within 24 to 48 hours, although the milk supply may take several weeks to resolve completely.

Alternatively, women who are breastfeeding may use the application of heat, frequent feeding, and use of mild analgesics to relieve the discomfort of engorgement. Women who begin breastfeeding immediately after the birth, nurse frequently on both breasts, and avoid the use of supplements or pumping to express milk for bottle feeding, are less likely to experience painful engorgement.

Hemorrhoids and Painful Bowel Movements

In the first 24 to 48 hours postpartum, preexisting hemorrhoids are often painful. Hemorrhoids can be traumatized and edematous during the pushing of the second stage of labor. Relief measures, which are listed in **Box 34-3**, may be used in combination, except cold and warm should not be used during the same time span. External hemorrhoids may be replaced inside the rectum. A lubricated finger cot is used and the hemorrhoids are gently pushed into the rectum. After the hemorrhoids are inserted, the woman tightens her rectal sphincter both to give them support and to contain them within her rectum.

Women with deep lacerations, particularly those that penetrate the rectal sphincter, may have fear of pain or disruption of the repair with defecation. A mild stool softener can prevent painful bowel movements that occur when the stool is hard. Increased fluid intake and a high-fiber diet also will promote normal function. Stool softeners or laxatives should be discontinued if the stools become too soft or liquid. Suppositories should be avoided when lacerations penetrate the anal sphincter or rectum.

Excessive Perspiration

Women experience excessive perspiration during the first week postpartum as a mechanism to eliminate the excess extracellular fluid that is normally accumulated during pregnancy. Women may be reassured that this phenomenon is normal and instructed to keep clean and dry and not to decrease fluids in a misguided attempt to decrease perspiration.

Management of Common Complications

Traumatic Birth

After listening to women tell their experiences of birth during the early postpartum period, midwives may identify those who could benefit from formal counseling after traumatic birth. There are mixed results from randomized trials of debriefing after traumatic birth in reducing symptoms of PTSD or postpartum depression. Women most likely to benefit are those who request counseling or already meet some of the criteria for PTSD.[36] Conversely debriefing can cause a reexperience of the trauma and be more harmful than helpful.

Gamble developed a counseling model for midwives to use with women after traumatic birth who demonstrated risk for developing PTSD. In an RCT including 103 women with trauma symptoms, brief counseling 72 hours after traumatic birth and again at 4 to 6 weeks postpartum was found to be associated with reduced symptoms of traumatic stress (RR: 0.45; 95% CI, 0.20–0.98) and depression (RR: 0.25; 95% CI, 0.09–0.69) at 3 months postpartum.[37] This counseling model is presented in **Table 34-8**. Midwives should be aware of how to refer women to therapists with expertise in perinatal populations in the community.

Postoperative Care

Midwives in collaboration with physicians often participate in the postpartum care of women after surgery. While the goals of postpartum care are similar after cesarean birth, there are unique circumstances to consider. The increased risk of deep vein thrombosis in the puerperium is magnified by the immobility after surgery. Strategies to mitigate this risk include pneumatic compression devices until the woman is fully ambulating and early ambulation. Removal of the urinary catheter by the next morning after surgery will further encourage ambulation to the bathroom and restores independent function. While institutional guidelines may vary, there is no evidence for benefit from withholding food or liquids after cesarean birth.[37] Unrestricted oral intake after cesarean accelerates the return of gastrointestinal function, and bowel sounds should be audible within 12 to 24 hours after surgery.

Postoperatively, there is an increased risk of uterine infection or endometritis, as well as wound infection, in women who have a cesarean section compared to women who have a vaginal birth. Antibiotic therapy is unnecessary after cesarean birth if a single antibiotic dose was administered before the incision is made or after umbilical cord clamping. Women who were receiving group B *Streptococcus* (GBS) prophylaxis will similarly have this treatment discontinued immediately after surgery. However, if the woman develops chorioamnionitis during labor, antibiotics typically are continued until the she is afebrile for 24 hours. The midwife should monitor the woman for signs of postpartum infection, including careful consideration of uterine pain, vital signs, and appearance of the incision. A routine complete blood count may not be helpful in detecting infection because the total white blood cell count is normally elevated as high as 16,000 cells/microliter in the absence of infection.

Postpartum anemia is more likely after a cesarean section, because the typical average blood loss at cesarean birth is 1000 mL. Strategies for pain control after surgery may vary, but the goal is to transition to oral pain medications by time of discharge. When

Table 34-8	A Counseling Model for Postpartum Women
Strategy	**Key Elements of Counseling Intervention**
Therapeutic connection between midwife and woman	Show kindness; affirm competence of the woman, simple nonthreatening and open questions about the birth, attentive listening, and acceptance of woman's perspective.
Accept and work with women's perceptions	Prompt the woman to tell her own story, listen with encouragement and without interruption.
Support expression of feelings	Encourage expressions of feelings with open questions, actively listening, and reflecting back the woman's concerns.
Filling in missing pieces	Clarify misunderstandings, offer information, answer questions realistically and factually, and ask questions about key aspects to check understanding. Do not defend or justify care provided.
Connect event with emotions and behaviors	Ask questions to determine if the woman is connecting current emotions and behaviors with the traumatic event(s). Acknowledge and validate grief and loss. Gently challenge and counter distorted thinking such as self-blame and a sense of inadequacy. Encourage the woman to see that inappropriate or hasty decisions may be a reaction to the birth.
Review the labor management	Ask if the woman thought that anything should have been done differently during the labor. Offer new or more generous or accurate perceptions of the event. Realistically postulate how certain courses of action may have resulted in a more positive outcome. Acknowledge uncertainty.
Enhance social support	Initiate a discussion of the woman's existing support networks. Talk about ways to receive additional emotional support. Help the woman understand that the persons who usually support her may be struggling with their own emotional distress.
Reinforce positive approaches to coping	Reinforce comments by women that reflect a clearer understanding of the situation, plan for the way forward, or outline positive action to overcome distress. Counter oblique defeatist statements.
Explore solutions	Support women to explore and decide on potential solutions, such as support group(s), further one-to-one counseling, seeking specific information, and accessing the complaint system.

Source: Gamble J, Creedy D, Moyle W, Webster J, McAllister M, Dickson P. Effectiveness of a counseling intervention after a traumatic childbirth: a randomized controlled trial. *Birth.* 2005;32(1):11-19. Reprinted by permission of John Wiley and Sons.

staples have been used to close the abdominal incision, the staples may be removed before discharge from the hospital or at a return visit to an ambulatory site within the first week. Timing of the removal depends on the surgeon's preference and individual risks for wound dehiscence. A woman usually is discharged from a hospital, assuming no major complication, approximately 48 to 72 hours after the cesarean birth. Postpartum instructions should include warning signs for surgical-site infections and appropriate instructions regarding physical activity after major abdominal surgery. These recommendations often include advising the woman to lift nothing heavier than the infant and to avoid other activities that may put excessive strain on the surgical site.

Another common surgery during the postpartum period is postpartum tubal sterilization after vaginal birth. Deviations from the routine postpartum care may include nothing by mouth (NPO) status for 6

to 8 hours prior to the sterilization procedure. If an epidural was used during labor or birth, the epidural catheter should be retained in place and used during the sterilization procedure. Typically the surgical incisions for tubal sterilization are small, dressed with simple adhesive bandages, and require no special postoperative care. No additional restrictions or instructions are needed for the postpartum tubal sterilization. Additional information regarding types of sterilization and health education can be found in the *Nonhormonal Contraception* chapter.

Urinary Retention

The inability to urinate is an urgent complication during the early puerperium. Potential causes of urinary retention include slow recovery of sensation after epidural anesthesia, excessive vulvar edema that compresses the urethra, trauma and edema of the bladder neck, and injured bladder innervation.

Postpartum urinary retention should be suspected when the woman has not urinated in 6 to 8 hours, there is palpable bladder distension above the symphysis pubis, the uterine fundus becomes displaced upward and to the side of the midline, or ultrasound is used to estimate bladder volume. Initially, noninvasive care should be implemented to help the woman successfully urinate. Such measures included maintaining privacy, adequate analgesia, warm water immersion, placement of a few drops of peppermint oil in the toilet water or bedpan, and the sound of running water, although there is little research evidence of effectiveness for any of these strategies. If these measures are unsuccessful, then urinary catheterization should be used to effectively empty the bladder.

Urinary catheterization has been the subject of increased discussion, especially given that the Centers for Medicare and Medicaid Services now requires hospitals to report the incidence of catheter-associated urinary tract infections (CAUTIs). General guidelines suggest that intermittent catheterization has less risk of a CAUTI than an indwelling catheter for individuals with bladder-emptying dysfunction. The guidelines do caution that when intermittent catheterization is used, it should be delayed until the bladder is distended. If an indwelling catheter is used, it should be used for the shortest period possible.[39] In practice, it is not uncommon to order an indwelling catheter following a traumatic vaginal birth or dense epidural block. In that situation, a common approach is to leave the indwelling catheter in place overnight, to be removed in the morning. If the woman is unable to urinate the next day, it may be necessary to leave the catheter in place for several days. It is important to clean the catheter and area around the insertion twice a day, as catheter use increases the risk for urinary tract infection.

Figure 34-4 provides a sample algorithm for management of a woman who has postpartum urinary retention. Note that if a woman is able to successfully void after catheterization, she should be assessed for adequate urinary output for the next two or three occasions to evaluate whether she is still experiencing retention to some degree.

Postpartum Fever

The definition of puerperal fever has been standardized as an oral temperature greater than 38°C (100.4°F) on more than two occasions within the first 10 days postpartum. This definition excludes the first 24 hours after birth, as it is normal to have a mild and transient temperature elevation as a physiologic reaction to childbirth. It is also common for a low-grade temperature elevation to be associated with engorgement as milk production increases 3 to 5 days after birth. The differential diagnoses for pathologic postpartum fever include endometritis, mastitis, wound infections, and urinary tract infections. Less commonly, fever may be caused by septic pelvic thrombophlebitis, transfusion reactions, and drug reactions. The presence of a fever warrants a physical examination to determine the source of the fever and to guide prompt treatment of the infection. Laboratory evaluation can include a complete blood count, blood culture, or urine culture. Note that protein found in the urine is likely to be of no clinical significance in an otherwise healthy woman. Consultation with a physician may be warranted depending on the etiology and severity of the infection.

Uterine Subinvolution

Uterine subinvolution is the most common cause of secondary postpartum hemorrhage, or excessive bleeding that occurs after 24 hours postpartum. Symptoms of subinvolution include uterine tenderness, cramping, and increased bleeding or clots. Upon examination, the fundal height is higher than expected and the uterus will feel soft or boggy. There may be signs of infection, as an inflammatory response can be responsible for the lack of uterine contractility.

The initial treatment of subinvolution is use of uterotonic agents to slow bleeding (Table 34-4). If there is suspicion of endometritis, such as fever or malodorous lochia, then it will be necessary to also treat the woman with antibiotics. If treatment is ineffective in reducing the bleeding, then ultrasound examination of the uterus will be helpful in determining whether retained placental fragments are responsible for the bleeding. Ultrasound has a high negative predictive value and will effectively rule out a retained placenta. It may be difficult to interpret positive findings on ultrasound, however, because it is normal within the first 2 weeks after birth for blood clots and fluid to be present in the endometrial canal. Doppler flow may help distinguish clots from retained placenta. Consultation or referral is indicated when there is clinical concern for retained products that are not expelled by the uterus with medical therapy.

Anemia

It is not necessary to routinely screen for postpartum anemia. Instead, such screening should be reserved for women with risk factors such as prenatal anemia, postpartum hemorrhage, and cesarean birth. It can take several hours for the hemoglobin and hematocrit

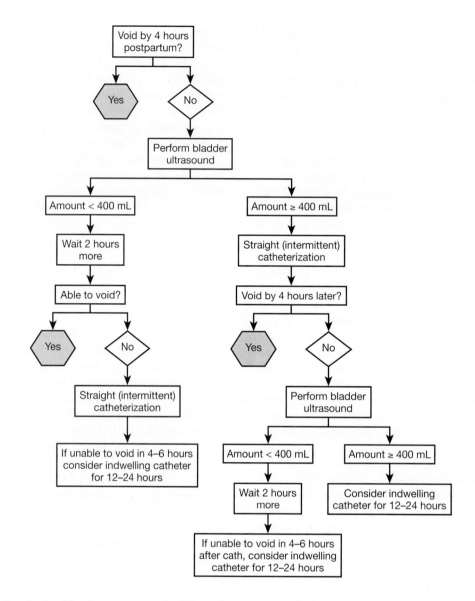

Figure 34-4 Sample algorithm for assessment of voiding and management of urinary retention after vaginal birth.

to equilibrate after acute blood loss; thus it is prudent to wait at least 4 hours after birth and preferably 24 hours after birth before screening for anemia. Treatment of anemia includes increased intake of iron-rich foods, oral iron therapy, and measures to address potential gastrointestinal side effects such as stomach upset and constipation.

Special Considerations

Smoking

While many women are successful in quitting smoking during pregnancy, relapse is common during the postpartum period. In a multistate study using the population-based Pregnancy Risk Assessment Monitoring System (PRAMS), 48% of women resumed smoking within 6 months postpartum, and those women who received smoking cessation interventions in pregnancy were no more successful than the majority of women who had not received prenatal intervention.[40] In a qualitative study of 24 women who quit smoking during pregnancy, the participants' intention regarding remaining abstinent was explored before hospital discharge postpartum. Different themes that the women expressed included feeling uncertain about their ability to remain abstinent, having confidence that they could protect the infant from their smoking, and being in control and not needing help to remain abstinent.[41]

Some interventions to help postpartum women remain abstinent from smoking have shown promise, although there is no single intervention that is effective for all women. One telephone support program based on motivational interviewing and relapse prevention principles provided phone calls at 3, 6, 9, and 12 weeks; it was tested in an RCT. Of the women receiving the intervention, 74% remained abstinent at 12 weeks, compared to 37% in the control group.[42] In a different study, mailing self-help booklets proved helpful in maintaining higher abstinence rates, particularly for low-income women.[43] Midwives should offer women information about available community programs for maintaining abstinence and educate them on the important health benefits for themselves and their children.

Adolescents

Becoming a parent at a young age may have negative consequences for both the adolescent mother and her infant. Social and economic factors, rather than a biology, are likely responsible for these consequences. Adolescent women in the postpartum period are more likely than peers who delay pregnancy to have postpartum depression, lower self-esteem, substance abuse, and poverty. Further, women who are adolescent parents are less likely to attain higher levels of education and are more likely to experience intimate-partner violence than their peers.[44]

A variety of programs exist for providing care to adolescent mothers postpartum. The goals of these programs usually include improving the teenager's parenting skills, provision of social support, supporting educational attainment, and prevention of repeat pregnancy through use of contraception. Programs may be provided in the home, in the community or school, or in clinics.[45] A home mentoring program that was based on adolescent development and negotiation skills was tested in an RCT among African American adolescent women who gave birth in the Baltimore area. By 24 months, women who participated in the program were less likely to have had a second infant compared to those in the intervention group (odds ratio [OR]: 3.3; 95% CI, 3.0–5.1).[46]

Providing effective contraception to adolescent mothers can be a challenge. In a qualitative study of 21 adolescents' postpartum use of contraception, barriers to contraceptive use included insufficient parental involvement, loss of health insurance, lack of information, and discontinuity of care. The participants in this study had a high level of contraceptive method switching.[47] Many researchers have investigated the ideal method of contraception for adolescents during the postpartum period and have focused on long-term reversible contraceptive (LARC) methods such as intrauterine devices, implants, and injectable progestins. Three-year etonogestrel implants

(Nexplanon) inserted prior to postpartum discharge if in a hospital or birth center had longer continuation rates and longer delays to next pregnancy as compared to intrauterine devices (IUDs), depot medroxyprogesterone acetate (DMPA), and oral contraceptives.[48] In a study that specifically examined IUD use in adolescents postpartum, researchers found that the 1-year postpartum continuation rate of IUDs in adolescents was only 55%, with expulsion and the pain being the most common reasons for discontinuation.[49]

Infant in the NICU

The admission of the newborn to the neonatal intensive care unit (NICU) after birth presents a major challenge for new parents. Prematurity is the most likely reason for a newborn to need intensive care, with approximately 12% of all newborns being born prematurely in the United States. Other reasons for NICU admission include hyperbilirubinemia, hypoglycemia, infection, meconium aspiration, birth asphyxia, congenital anomalies, and respiratory distress. Having an infant in the NICU can interfere with the developing maternal–newborn attachment through restricted access to the newborn, difficulty in reading the infant's cues, and inability to commit one's time exclusively to the newborn owing to competing demands both at home and at the hospital.[50] The hospitalization of a newborn is associated with high rates of post-traumatic stress and symptoms of depression.[51] Breastfeeding the hospitalized infant is particularly a challenge when the infant is premature and lacks the neuromuscular development to successfully suckle.

Midwives can do much to support these families when the focus of the healthcare team turns toward the fragile infant.[52] Support for the establishment and continuation of breastfeeding includes initiating pumping within 6 hours of the birth, and continuing to pump milk at least 6 times a day. Milk supplies may be increased by using techniques such as "hands-on pumping."[53] Midwives may advocate for parents to be able to hold their ill infants in skin-to-skin contact even with monitors and ventilation equipment in place.[54] Parents should be monitored for psychological consequences of the infant hospitalization, with attention being paid to their emotional health. When the birth was traumatic, midwives may debrief women about the experience. A prolonged hospitalization is itself a traumatic event for many families, and parents should be screened for postpartum depression and PTSD. The American College of Nurse-Midwives endorses universal screening for depression in women as a regular component of primary care.[55] When parents return for the 6-week postpartum office visit, this is a further opportunity to review the events of the birth and to explore strategies to optimize future childbearing in light of the recent experience.

Relinquishment/Adoption of an Infant

Women may relinquish the care of their infant voluntarily through adoption or surrogacy, or involuntarily through the legal system. Under these circumstances, midwives might be involved in the care of the birth parents, the adoptive or receiving parents, and/or the newborn. The circumstances around the adoption or removal of the infant and emotional reactions are complex and unique to each family. In a survey of 97 nurses across the United States, Foli identified a range of family needs and nursing interventions in the context of adoption.[56] Support for the woman who gave birth included providing psychosocial support, therapeutic communication, follow-up services, and advocacy. Midwives should talk with the woman about her emotions in a nonjudgmental way, validating her feelings and acknowledging that feelings may be conflicted. As the woman's advocate, the midwife should ensure that the decision to relinquish an infant for adoption was not coercive except under the condition of legal removal by child protective services. Referrals to social workers and counselors may be offered to address ongoing issues of grief and visitation.

As primary care providers for women, midwives may also be in the position of caring for women who adopt an infant. The decision to adopt often follows failed attempts at getting pregnant and possibly multiple miscarriages. Thus the emotional reaction to adoption can be complex, as these parents struggle with a sense of legitimacy as parents and fear that the infant will be returned to the biological parents. Postpartum depression is possible for women who become mothers by adoption as they experience stressors similar to women who have given birth.[57] Women who adopt will likely have educational needs about infant care. Referral to resources and support groups for adoptive families may be helpful.[56] Laws regarding adoption vary according to jurisdiction, so midwives should be aware of credible agencies and attorneys in this field.

Women in Prison

Incarceration presents another circumstance in which the infant will be separated from the woman during the postpartum period. The number of incarcerated women and adolescents in the United States is estimated to be 250,000, with approximately 10,000 of them being pregnant.[56] This group of women presents special challenges for the provision of postpartum care due to the likelihood of separation of the infant from the woman when she returns to the correctional facility. In a qualitative study of 12 incarcerated women during the early postpartum period, the women described the strong connection that they developed during the pregnancy, but after the birth they felt empty and experienced a deep sense of loss when their infants were separated from them.[59]

Prison nurseries, in which infants are housed with their incarcerated mothers, represent an alternative to the forced separation of infants from their mothers. According to the Women's Prison Association, only nine such programs existed in the United States in 2009. Such programs promote better attachment, lead to reduced recidivism, and keep women with their babies.[60] When prison nurseries are unavailable, community-based residential parenting programs or placement of the infant with relatives are options for continuing the care of the infant within the family.[58]

Midwives are in a position to advocate for these families and to coordinate with prison health providers to provide comprehensive perinatal and postpartum care. While providing care to women who are prisoners, it is important to maintain privacy while in the presence of guards and to avoid the use of restraints for reasons of safety and respect.[61]

Separation at Discharge

The timing of newborn discharge from hospital or birth centers depends on local institutional criteria and practice patterns. For example, when a woman tests positive for GBS during pregnancy or otherwise has indications for GBS prophylaxis during labor, closer observation of the newborn for signs of infection can delay discharge from hospital settings for as long as 48 hours after the birth. This delay will depend on newborn symptoms of sepsis and whether adequate antibiotic prophylaxis was given during labor. In out-of-hospital birth settings, observation of the newborn for the infection may be accomplished cooperatively by parents and midwives through home visits and by parents monitoring for signs of infection. GBS management plans of the newborn are discussed in more detail in the *Neonatal Care* chapter.

Postpartum sexuality and contraception should both be discussed before discharge, because many women will initiate sexual activity prior to follow-up at 6 weeks postpartum. Prior to discharge from the hospital, or in the first few days after out-of-hospital birth, it is also important to provide vaccinations to the woman to protect her and the infant.

Vaccinations

Vaccinating the woman during the puerperium provides an opportunity to protect her and her newborn against several infections. All women should be offered seasonal influenza vaccine regardless of their pregnancy status and should be offered this vaccine postpartum if the woman did not receive it during her pregnancy. In addition, live-virus vaccines against rubella and varicella should be offered to nonimmune women during the postpartum period. The woman is not likely to be contagious from these live-virus vaccines, and no increased risk of congenital anomalies from conception within 1 to 3 months of vaccine administration has been demonstrated. Nevertheless, it is recommended to delay conception at least 1 month after live-virus vaccine administration. Booster vaccination with tetanus–diphtheria–acellular pertussis (Tdap) is ideally provided in the second half of pregnancy, but may be provided in the postpartum period as well. Vaccination of all family members will also protect the infant from acquiring pertussis.[62]

Rhesus Non-immune

Women with an Rh-negative blood type are at risk of becoming sensitized to Rh-positive blood after giving birth. Most women experience a small transfer of fetal blood into the maternal circulation during childbirth, primarily at the time of placental separation. If the fetal blood type is Rh positive, the fetal blood can engender an immune response in the maternal immune system that could endanger future pregnancies. The newborn's blood type usually is tested on a small sample from the umbilical cord, and Rh immune globulin is given to the woman if the newborn has Rh-positive blood and the woman has not been previously sensitized. Ideally Rh immune globulin, also known as $Rh_o(D)$ immune globulin or the brand name RhoGAM, should be given within 72 hours of birth, as studies have found this timing will prevent the woman's immune system from reacting to any fetal red blood cells that enter her circulation. If blood typing of the newborn's cord blood is not available, the benefits of Rh immune globulin administration outweigh the theoretical risks of unnecessary administration. Administration after 72 hours may be protective, and Rh immune globulin should be given even up to 14 days after the birth, as no studies have been conducted that address the latest period for which the agent is effective. Rh immune globulin is a blood product with only theoretical risks of infection, and midwives should discuss its benefits and risks carefully with women, especially with women who object to the use of blood products.

The standard 300 mcg dose of Rh immune globulin is sufficient to treat a fetal–maternal bleed containing 15 mL of red blood cells or 30 mL of whole blood. While rare, it is important to know when the fetal–maternal hemorrhage exceeds this amount because additional Rh immune globulin will be needed in this situation. In some institutions, when there is a suspicion of a larger bleed, a Rosette test is performed to ascertain whether Rh-positive blood is detectable in the maternal blood.[63] If the Rosette test is positive, a Kleihauer-Betke test is performed. In other facilities, a Kleihauer-Betke test is the only test ordered because it entails the quantitative measurement of fetal red blood cells in maternal blood; the test results are used to determine if and how much additional Rh immune globulin should be administered.

Sexuality and Contraception Postpartum

It is important to be realistic when discussing sexual function postpartum. There is wide variation in the time after childbirth that women resume sexual activity with their partners, as well as cultural variations in prescribed waiting times. Factors that are correlated with less sexual activity and dyspareunia include operative vaginal delivery, episiotomy, third- and fourth-degree lacerations, and urinary incontinence.[64] Other circumstances that may interfere with postpartum sexuality are reduced privacy, increased interruptions, and fatigue. There is no scientific basis for the traditional recommendation to delay sexual activity until the 6-week postpartum examination. Instead, a more nuanced approach is that the woman should wait until she feels comfortable and ready to resume sexual activity. Additional recommendations include using vaginal lubrication, particularly if the woman is lactating; trying alternative positions for comfort during penetrative vaginal intercourse; and engaging in other sexual and nonsexual forms of intimacy.

The early postpartum period is an opportune time to explore contraceptive plans with the woman. While sexual activity may be far from the mind of the woman who has recently given birth, as many as 50% of women will have initiated sexual activity by the time they return to an office for the traditional postpartum examination at 6 weeks.[65] It is best to open the discussion with an inquiry regarding the woman's desire for future pregnancy and perceived need for contraception. If the midwife has concerns that the woman may not return for postpartum follow-up or will initiate sexual activity before the postpartum visit, consideration should be given to early initiation of contraception. DMPA (Depo-Provera) may be offered at the time of postpartum discharge. IUD insertion may be performed safely after delivery of the placenta, although expulsion rates are higher than if insertion is performed earlier than 4 weeks postpartum.[66] However, because a woman in the postpartum period is still in a state of hypercoagulation, estrogen-containing methods should not be used until at least 3 weeks postpartum according to the U.S. Medical Eligibility Criteria for Contraceptive Use, although other sources suggest a longer waiting period.[67]

The impact of the woman's lactation status on contraceptive options and timing is controversial. According to the U.S. Medical Eligibility Criteria,[67] lactation is not a contraindication to the use of any contraceptive options. Other authorities warn against the use combined hormonal contraceptives such as oral contraceptive pills, patches, and vaginal rings because of concerns these contraceptive methods reduce milk supply.[33] For similar reasons, they may recommend delaying use of high-dose progestins such as DMPA for several weeks. Another concern is the postpartum use of the progestin-only pill (POP) by Hispanic women who had gestational diabetes. In a study of 904 Latina women, POP use was associated with an almost three times greater risk of developing type 2 diabetes within 2 years relative to use of nonhormonal or combined hormonal contraceptives (adjusted RR: 2.87; 95% CI: 1.57–5.27). This risk increased with duration of uninterrupted use.[68] Additional studies of DMPA among women in this population found an increased risk of developing diabetes, especially for breastfeeding women, but one that was not statistically significant.[69]

Late Postpartum Period

Postpartum Follow-Up in the First Two Weeks

A midwife can use a variety of methods to stay in contact with the woman and her newborn between the early postpartum period and a 4- to 6-week examination. Some midwives make telephone calls, some do home visits, and others see the woman and/or infant for a 2-week office visit. In addition, some midwives may work with nurses or train birth assistants to initiate the telephone calls or perform the home visits. Many midwives combine these activities depending on the needs of the woman, infant, and family. These activities have a number of purposes, as noted in **Box 34-4**.

There is a lack of clear evidence and consensus on the best approach to maternal and newborn

> ### BOX 34-4 Purposes of Early Postpartum Contacts
>
> - To evaluate the postpartum course and well-being of the mother
> - To evaluate the well-being of the baby
> - To evaluate progress and comfort in caretaking ability and assumption of the parental role
> - To review with the mother her labor and birth experience
> - To be accessible for questions and concerns and to establish a contact for the mother to feel comfortable calling when she has questions or concerns
> - To provide needed teaching and counseling

follow-up postpartum. One large RCT of home visits by nurses at 3 to 5 days after uncomplicated birth compared to standard office-based care found no difference in the number of unplanned office visits, postpartum depression rates, or rehospitalization rates. Women and newborns with specific health problems such as infection or hyperbilirubinemia were excluded from the study. Families with home visits had modest, albeit nonsignificant, improvements in breastfeeding rates by 2 weeks postpartum (92.3% versus 88.6%; $p = .04$) and increased parenting self-confidence scores at 2 weeks and at 2 months.[70]

Phone Calls

Telephone calls are usually made the day after the birth or the day after the woman returns home from the birth center or hospital, and again a few days later. Calls often are combined with a 2-week visit in the ambulatory site. During the telephone call, the midwife screens for problems by asking about both maternal and infant well-being. Limitations of phone calls include the decreased ability to directly screen for neonatal hyperbilirubinemia and excessive infant weight loss and the requirement of reliable telephone service for the woman. A comprehensive assessment of the woman's condition by telephone may include obtaining her self-report of physical and emotional well-being, breastfeeding success, and coping with the significant family changes associated with childbirth. The midwife should ask about the presence of signs or symptoms for postpartum complications. Content for the phone call is listed in **Table 34-9**.

Table 34-9	Postpartum Telephone Call: Maternal Assessment
System	**Assessment**
General	Food and fluid intake
	Sleep quality and quantity
	Fever or chills
	Headaches
Breasts	Breast engorgement, nipple condition, pain, masses
	Progression from colostrum to milk
	Feeding frequency and success
Abdomen	Abdominal pain, cramping, epigastric pain
	Bowel function, constipation, incontinence
	Urinary pain or incontinence, urgency
Pelvis	Lochia amount, color, and odor
	Perineal pain, swelling, or redness
	Hemorrhoids
Lower extremities	Edema, pain, redness, varicosities
Adjustment	Emotional changes (postpartum blues or depression)
	Coping with life changes and response to newborn
	Social support and help with household chores
	Physical activity level
	Abdominal and perineal exercises
	Family adjustment to newborn
	Confidence in infant care

Table 34-10	Postpartum Telephone Call: Newborn Assessment
System	**Assessment**
General	Temperature
	Sleep patterns
	Consolability
	Alert and interacting with parents
Feeding	Frequency and amounts of formula feeding
	Breastfeeding latch, milk supply, frequency
	Infant satisfaction with feeding
Diaper patterns	Frequency of voids and stools
	Appearance of stools
Skin color	Jaundice
	Cyanosis
Umbilicus	Presence of erythema or exudate at umbilical site
	Cord stump fallen off
Circumcision	Appearance of glans if circumcised male

Home Visits

A home visit involves the same set of questions as does a telephone call but also allows the midwife to observe the following: the woman's responses to the infant's needs and cues, the parent–newborn interaction, the place of the newborn in the home's social environment, and resources in the home (e.g., plumbing, water supply, refrigeration, air conditioning/heat, window screens, supplies for baby care). A home visit may also include a brief physical examination of the woman and newborn.

Two-Week Office Visits

The 2-week visit involves the same set of questions as the telephone call, adjusted for expected physical, physiologic, and psychological changes by 2 weeks postpartum. Particular attention should be paid to how well the woman is coping with these changes and her new parental responsibilities. The midwife may or may not conduct an abbreviated physical examination of the woman or newborn during this visit.

If the woman brings her infant to the 2-week visit, the midwife can observe the woman's interaction with her infant and her responsiveness to the infant's needs and cues. Every contact with a new mother is an opportunity to share with her the developmental capabilities of her infant and to discuss

The telephone call also provides an opportunity to check on the newborn's condition, regardless of whether the midwife is the primary healthcare provider for the newborn. The call can be an important opportunity to triage for adequacy of infant feeding and signs of hyperbilirubinemia, infection, or heart disease. Assessment of the newborn by telephone is outlined in **Table 34-10**.

Using a telephone call to assess the mother–infant pair's well-being, particularly if the birth occurred in a setting where the family will be alone with their infant shortly after birth, allows the midwife to triage for emergent problems that might require a trip to the office, the pediatric provider's office, or even the emergency room.

safety, infant stimulation, and parenting skills. This is also a good time to verify that the infant either has already seen or has an appointment to see a pediatric healthcare provider and to discuss the need for these visits and for immunizations. For breastfeeding women, the 2-week visit also can be used as a time to encourage effective breastfeeding and to target any nursing problems.

Finally, if the woman needs to select a contraceptive method, the 2-week visit is an excellent opportunity to review available options. Many couples will choose to begin sexual intercourse shortly after the woman's lochia resolves, if not before, and women who are formula feeding may ovulate before a routine postpartum physical is performed at 4 to 6 weeks.

Four- to Six-Week Postpartum Visit

The defined endpoint of the puerperium is 6 weeks, a benchmark likely chosen because by that time the woman's uterus has completed its involution to the nonpregnant state. The exact timing of the postpartum examination is flexible and may be done as early as 4 weeks postpartum. The significance of this office-based midwife visit goes beyond the confirmation of the woman's return to the nonpregnant state. As the final visit related to maternity care, it marks the end of the heightened attention the woman received from the healthcare system during the childbearing year. For many women who received Medicaid insurance during their pregnancy, their health insurance may abruptly end at 2 months postpartum.

The idea that the woman's health needs are now met takes a very narrow view of women's health. In a prospective longitudinal survey of more than 1500 Australian women giving birth for the first time, symptoms were measured through 18 months postpartum. The results showed a very different view of the postpartum "recovery." At 3 months postpartum, 36% of these women reported breast problems, 29% painful perineum, and 11% pelvic pain. While the prevalence of these three conditions gradually declined by 18 months, other symptoms persisted. At 18 months postpartum, 61.7% of the women reported extreme fatigue, 39.3% frequent coughs or colds, 25% severe headaches, 42% lower back pain, 27% urinary incontinence, and 5% fecal incontinence.[71] Thus 6 weeks postpartum was not a meaningful mark of postpartum recovery for the majority of the women in this study. Ideally the postpartum visit will be the beginning of a new phase of supportive health care, rather than merely the end of a maternity package of services.

The 4- to 6-week postpartum visit often consists of a complete history, physical examination, and pelvic examination, as outlined in the chapter *An Introduction to the Care of Women*. Available records of the prenatal, intrapartum, and postpartum care during this pregnancy should be reviewed. An interval history since the last encounter includes questions from Table 34-9 and **Table 34-11**. If not already done, the midwife should address contraception. Two additional topics that deserve special attention during this visit are sleep and postpartum depression.

Sleep Postpartum

It is well accepted that women have difficulty getting enough sleep during the postpartum period. Montgomery-Downs et al. studied the sleep of 72 women without depression from 2 to 16 weeks postpartum.[72] These researchers found that women slept an average of 7.2 hours per night during the first 4 months postpartum. The fragmentation of their sleep resulted in spending an additional 2 hours awake in the middle of the night during the early postpartum period. By the end of the 4 months, the awakenings had decreased, although the total sleep time remained the same. Thus the time that these women spent in bed became more efficient, with more time asleep. After the second week postpartum, fewer than half of the women studied took any daytime naps,

Table 34-11	Additional Postpartum History for 6-Week Postpartum Visit
Healthcare encounters	Calls to the midwife or the physician
	Visits to the hospital emergency room
	Hospital admissions
Sexual activity	Resumption of sexual activity and number of times
	Woman's/partner's enjoyment and satisfaction
	Dyspareunia
Contraception	Contraceptive used or desired
	Past contraceptive experience
Exercise	Exercise and activities since childbirth
	Pelvic floor exercises
Vaginal bleeding	Resolution of lochia
	Episodes of excessive bleeding
	Resumption of menses
Infant	Attendance at well-child visits
	Growth and well-being of the infant

and among those who did, only two naps per week were reported. The percentage of time in bed spent asleep—that is, the sleep efficiency—increased from a mean of 80% to 90% by the 16th week postpartum. The authors concluded that the nature of sleep disturbance postpartum is sleep fragmentation rather than sleep deprivation.

Women whose sleep patterns are outside the expected patterns for the postpartum period might benefit from evaluation and treatment by a sleep specialist. Excessive sleep disturbance might contribute to postpartum depression, retention of prenatal weight gain, and impaired maternal–newborn attachment.[73] A systematic assessment of sleep postpartum should include the points described in **Box 34-5**.[74]

Warning signs of disordered sleep include frequent use of sleep medications, taking 30 minutes or more to fall asleep most nights, total sleep time of less than 6 hours per night, three or more nighttime awakenings, and sleepiness that significantly interferes with daily activities or results in unintentional falling asleep.[75] The midwife should not assume that sleep changes are always a normal part of the postpartum state, but should also consider conditions that have been correlated with disordered sleep, such as postpartum depression, thyroid disease, anemia, restless leg syndrome, and sleep apnea.[73] Evidence-based recommendations for helping women obtain improved sleep postpartum are listed in **Box 34-6**.[75,76]

Depression Screening

Universal screening for postpartum depression is an important component of postpartum care.[55] Multiple depression screening tools have been used in pregnancy and postpartum, including the 10-question Edinburgh Postnatal Depression Scale (EPDS) and the 20-question Center for Epidemiological Studies Depression Scale (CES-D).[77] These questionnaires have been validated in multiple languages, and may be self-administered. Caution should be exercised when an elevated score is identified, because even a high risk of depression is not equivalent to a diagnosis of depression. Because these questionnaires address symptoms noted by the woman within the past week, repeated testing in 1 to 2 weeks may demonstrate spontaneous improvement. Furthermore, most of the depression screening tests do not distinguish between

---

BOX 34-5 Assessment of Postpartum Sleep

- Employment status and work hours
- Use of medications, herbal remedies, or alcohol to facilitate sleep
- Perception of sleep quality; how often the woman wakes up feeling refreshed
- Time in bed: the time between turning off the lights at bedtime and the final awakening in the morning
- Time asleep: the total time in bed minus the awakenings for infant care activities
- Difficulty in falling asleep (usually should be less than 15 minutes)
- Number of nighttime awakenings, for infant care or other reasons
- Daytime sleepiness

Source: Adapted from Lee KA, Ward TM. Critical components of a sleep assessment for clinical practice settings. *Issues Ment Health Nurs.* 2005;26(7):739-750.

BOX 34-6 Postpartum Sleep Recommendations

- Minimize the disruption of nighttime awakenings.
- Obtain assistance with nighttime awakenings.
- Keep the newborn in close proximity when asleep at night, but not in the same bed.
- Continue to breastfeed at night. Breastfeeding at night results in more sleep than formula feeding.
- Sleep in an area away from noise and disruptions and turn off baby monitors.
- Minimize interactions during nighttime infant care activities.
- Keep lighting as low as possible during nighttime infant care.
- Do not stay up late after the infant goes to bed at night.
- Avoid short daytime naps.
- Naps less than 90 minutes do not allow a full cycle through the stages of sleep and are not restorative.
- The early afternoon is the best time to nap, as such napping is more likely to include deep sleep stages.
- Try to lengthen the infant's wake times during the day to promote more sleep at night.

Sources: Adapted from Lee KA. Sleep dysfunction in women and its management. *Curr Treat Options Neurol.* 2006;8(5):376-386; Hunter LP, Rychnovsky JD, Yount SM. A selective review of maternal sleep characteristics in the postpartum period. *J Obstet Gynecol Neonatal Nurs.* 2009;38(1):60-68.

epression and other illnesses such as anxiety and bipolar disorder.

If a risk is identified, it is important to inquire whether the woman has thoughts of self-harm or suicide and then to determine the next steps for further evaluation and treatment. Midwives should identify resources for postpartum depression that are available in their community to help direct women to the most appropriate care. Even if the midwife is not responsible for the management of a woman's postpartum depression, screening scores can be used to monitor progress in treatment. Depression is discussed in more detail in the *Mental Health Conditions* chapter.

Limited Postpartum Physical Examination

The physical examination for a woman in the remote postpartum period can be a complete physical evaluation, or it can be a limited examination. If a limited examination is performed, it should include the thyroid gland, breasts, abdominal examination for diastasis recti, pelvic examination, and lower extremities. The thyroid gland may be enlarged, indicating postpartum thyroiditis. The heart and lungs should have returned to the nonpregnant state, with no detectable murmurs or adventitious lung sounds. The abdomen should be assessed for the separation

of the rectus abdominus muscles and the appearance of any surgical scars. By 4 weeks postpartum, a well-healed surgical incision will appear as a thin pink line and adjacent areas will have minimal tenderness. Some numbness around the scar is found in many women and will slowly resolve over several months.

The pelvic examination should begin with a visual inspection of the perineum for healing. The bimanual examination will include assessment for vaginal tone by having the woman do a Kegel exercise with one of the examiner's fingers inserted in the vagina. Vaginal walls will be inspected for decreased rugae and atrophy. On palpation, the uterus may be noted to be slightly larger than the nonpregnant size, but it should be a firm pelvic organ. A speculum examination is not necessary unless the woman is due for a Pap test. Due to the discomfort of the speculum examination, the midwife should wait for complete healing of birth lacerations or episiotomies before inserting a speculum. While minor lacerations may be completely healed, more extensive repairs can take months to fully heal and for pain to resolve. Finally, the anus and rectum will be assessed if there is a history of hemorrhoids or a fourth-degree laceration. The lower extremities should be examined for varicosities, edema, and signs of thrombophlebitis. Laboratory assessment may be required based on history, as indicated in **Table 34-12**. Under current

Table 34-12	Postpartum Laboratory Tests		
Laboratory Tests	**Indications**	**Timing**	**Normal Range**
Hemoglobin (Hgb) or hematocrit (Hct)	Prenatal anemia, postpartum hemorrhage, cesarean birth	At least 4 weeks postpartum unless symptomatic of acute anemia	Hgb ≥ 12 g/dL Hct ≥ 36%
Thyroid-stimulating hormone (TSH)	Current or recent thyroid disease, history of postpartum thyroiditis, enlarged thyroid, symptoms of postpartum depression	6-week postpartum visit, 3 months and 6 months postpartum	TSH: 0.4–5.0 mU/L
Cervical cytology	Age 21 or older and history of unresolved abnormal cytology or HPV tests, or 3 years since last test	After perineal and vulvar healing is complete	Negative for intraepithelial lesion or malignancy
Sexually transmitted infection screening (gonorrhea, chlamydia, syphilis, HIV)	History of sexually transmitted infections, unprotected sexual intercourse, multiple sexual partners in past 12 months	Annually and within 3 months of past infection	Negative
2-hour 75-g glucose challenge	Gestational diabetes	6 to 12 weeks postpartum and annually thereafter	Fasting glucose < 100 mg/dL 2-hour glucose < 140 mg/dL

cervical cytology screening guidelines, women who are at least 21 years old who do not have a history of abnormal Pap tests need a Pap test every 3 years.[78]

Management Plans

Based on the history and physical examination, the midwife may be asked to complete an authorization for maternity leave or return to employment. Proper evaluation should include an understanding of the type of work that the woman performs. Midwives are in a position to advocate for women who desire to continue breastfeeding after returning to work and to offer guidance on strategies to continue lactation. Women who need contraception should receive necessary prescriptions, appointments, and education. It is not necessary to wait for menses to resume before starting oral contraceptives or inserting an IUD. If the woman has engaged in unprotected penile–vaginal intercourse, use of emergency contraception and/or urine pregnancy testing after 2 weeks of abstinence or condoms can reasonably ensure that the woman is not pregnant. The postpartum visit is also an opportune time to discuss future plans for pregnancy and provide preconception counseling.

A review of the prenatal record will identify conditions from the pregnancy that have not resolved. For example, a woman may need follow-up care for an ovarian or renal cyst identified by ultrasound during the pregnancy. Based on the scope of the midwife's practice, follow-up care should be arranged within the service or by referral to another primary care provider.

Nutrition and exercise are topics of great importance to many women. By 6 weeks postpartum, most women should be physically ready to resume regular exercise routines, in addition to abdominal and pelvic floor exercises to restore tone to those muscle groups most impacted by pregnancy and childbirth. According to the Physical Activity Guidelines for Americans, women should get at least 150 minutes of moderate exercise per week.[79] It may be advisable to gradually increase to this level of exercise when reinitiating activity postpartum. Based on limited evidence, there is no concern that exercise or calorie restriction will adversely impact lactation or infant growth.[80,81] Many women desire weight loss to achieve prepregnancy weight or another weight goal. The best way to achieve these goals is through a combination of healthy nutrition and exercise and by identifying what constitutes a healthful weight goal based on body mass index and other factors. Women should be cautioned against rapid weight loss postpartum; a useful reminder is that it took 9 months to gain the weight, so it may take at least the same time to lose it.

Conclusion

The puerperium is a time of great physical and psychological change. Midwives can provide effective care by attending to the woman in the context of her environment, family, and culture. It is important to remember that the postpartum period is not just the end of the childbearing year, but also the beginning of the nonpregnant phase of the woman's life. There is a need to address the high rates of problems such as incontinence, dyspareunia, and depression that can be unintended consequences of otherwise normal pregnancy and childbirth. By moving beyond the care of individual women, midwives can also address the health of women in general through advocacy at the system level. In the context of rising healthcare costs and the desire to increase healthcare access to the underserved, there will be new challenges and opportunities for promoting the health of women.

• • • References

1. Waugh LJ. Beliefs associated with Mexican immigrant families' practice of la cuarentena during postpartum recovery. *J Obstet Gynecol Neonatal Nurs.* 2011;40(6):732-741.

2. Callister LC, Eads MN, Diehl J. Perceptions of giving birth and adherence to cultural practices in Chinese women. *Am J Matern Child Nurs.* 2011;36(6):387-394.

3. Lundberg PC, Trieu TNT. Vietnamese women's cultural beliefs and practices related to the postpartum period. *Midwifery.* 2011;27(5):731-736.

4. Geçkil E, Sahin T, Ege E. Traditional postpartum practices of women and infants and the factors influencing such practices in south eastern Turkey. *Midwifery.* 2009;25(1):62-71.

5. Earle A, Mokomane Z, Heymann J. International perspectives on work-family policies: lessons from the world's most competitive economies. *Future Child.* 2011;21(2):191-210.

6. Schim SM, Doorenbos A, Benkert R, Miller J. Culturally congruent care: putting the puzzle together. *J Transcult Nurs.* 2007;18(2):103-110.

7. Callister LC. Cultural meanings of childbirth. *J Obstet Gynecol Neonatal Nurs.* 1995;24(4):327-331.

8. Martell LK. The hospital and the postpartum experience: a historical analysis. *J Obstet Gynecol Neonatal Nurs.* 2000;29(1):65-72.

9. Temkin E. Driving through: postpartum care during World War II. *Am J Public Health.* 1999;89(4):587-595.

10. Klaus MH, Kennell JH. *Maternal–Infant Bonding: The Impact of Early Separation or Loss on Family Development.* Saint Louis, MO: Mosby; 1976.

11. Temkin E. Rooming-in: redesigning hospitals and motherhood in Cold War America. *Bull Hist Med.* 2002;76(2):271-298.

12. Keppler AB, Roudebush JL. Postpartum follow-up care in a hospital-based clinic: an update on an expanded program. *J Perinat Neonat Nurs.* 1999;13(1):1-14.

13. Kronborg H, Vaeth M, Kristensen I. The effect of early postpartum home visits by health visitors: a natural experiment. *Public Health Nurs.* 2012;29(4):289-301.

14. Wheeler LA. *Nurse-Midwifery Handbook : A Practical Guide to Prenatal and Postpartum Care.* 2nd ed. Philadelphia, PA: Lippincott Williams & Wilkins; 2002.

15. Goulet C, Bell L, Tribble DS, Paul D, Lang A. A concept analysis of parent–infant attachment. *J Adv Nurs.* 1998;28(5):1071-1081.

16. Perry DF, Ettinger AK, Mendelson T, Le HN. Prenatal depression predicts postpartum maternal attachment in low-income Latina mothers with infants. *Infant Behav Dev.* 2011;34(2):339-350.

17. Yu CY, Hung CH, Chan TF, Yeh CH, Lai CY. Prenatal predictors for father–infant attachment after childbirth. *J Clin Nurs.* 2012;21(11-12):1577-1583.

18. Bystrova K, Widström AM, Matthiesen AS, et al. Skin-to-skin contact may reduce negative consequences of "the stress of being born": a study on temperature in newborn infants, subjected to different ward routines in St. Petersburg. *Acta Paediatr.* 2003;92(3):320-326.

19. Moore ER, Anderson GC, Bergman N, Dowswell T. Early skin-to-skin contact for mothers and their healthy newborn infants. *Cochrane Database Syst Rev.* 2012;5:CD003519. doi: 10.1002/14651858.CD003519.pub3.

20. Trakahashi Y, Tamakoshi K, Matsushima M, Kawabe T. Comparison of salivary cortisol, heart rate and oxygen saturation between early skin-to-skin contact with different initiation and uration times in healthy full-term infants. *Early Hum Dev.* 2001;87(3):151-157.

21. Erlandsson K, Dsilna A, Fagerberg I, Christensson K. Skin-to-skin care with the father after cesarean birth and its effect on newborn crying and prefeeding behavior. *Birth.* 2007;34(2):105-114.

22. Velandia M, Matthisen AS, Uvnäs-Moberg K, Nissen E. Onset of vocal interaction between parents and newborns in skin-to-skin contact immediately after elective cesarean section. *Birth.* 2010;37(3):192-201.

23. Edhborg M. Comparisons of different instruments to measure blues and to predict depressive symptoms 2 months postpartum: a study of new mothers and fathers. *Scand J Caring Sci.* 2008;22(2):186-195.

24. Renaud MT. We are mothers too: childbearing experiences of lesbian families. *J Obstet Gynecol Neonatal Nurs.* 2007;36(2):190-199.

25. Adams ED. If transmen can have babies, how will perinatal nursing adapt? *J Matern Child Nurs.* 2010;35(1):26-32.

26. Beck CT, Gable RK, Sakala C, Declercq ER. Posttraumatic stress disorder in new mothers: results from a two-stage U.S. national survey. *Birth.* 2011;38(3):216-227.

27. American Psychiatric Association. *Diagnostic and Statistical Manual of Mental Disorders.* 5th ed. Arlington, VA: American Psychiatric Association; 2013.

28. Fowles ER, Horowitz JA. Clinical assessment of mothering during infancy. *J Obstet Gynecol Neonatal Nurs.* 2006;35(5):662-670.

29. McCollum JA, Ree Y, Chen YJ. Interpreting parent–infant interactions: cross-cultural lessons. *Infants Young Child.* 2000;12(4):22-33.

30. Davidson N. REEDA: evaluating postpartum healing. *J Nurse Midwifery.* 1974;19(2):6-8.

31. Pomp ER, Lenselink AM, Rosendaal FR, Doggen CJ. Pregnancy, the postpartum period and prothrombotic defects: risk of venous thrombosis in the MEGA study. *J Thromb Haemost.* 2008;6(4):632-637.

32. Rhode MA. Postpartum. In: King TL, Brucker MC, eds. *Pharmacology for Women's Health.* Sudbury, MA: Jones and Bartlett; 2011:1117-1145.

33. Hale TW. *Medications and Mothers' Milk.* Amarillo, TX: Pharmasoft Medical; 2012.

34. Kocaöz S, Eroğlu K, Sivaslıoğlu AA. Role of pelvic floor muscle exercises in the prevention of stress urinary incontinence during pregnancy and the postpartum period. *Gynecol Obstet Invest.* 2012;75:34-40

35. Citak N, Cam C, Arslan H, et al. Postpartum sexual function of women and the effects of early pelvic floor muscle exercises. *Acta Obstet Gynecol Scand.* 2010;89(6):817-822.

36. Meades R, Pond C, Ayers S, Warren F. Postnatal debriefing: have we thrown the baby out with the bath water? *Behav Res Ther.* 2011;49(5):367-372.

37. Gamble J, Creedy D, Moyle W, Webster J, McAllister M, Dickson P. Effectiveness of a counseling intervention after a traumatic childbirth: a randomized controlled trial. *Birth.* 2005;32(1):11-19.

38. Mangesi L, Hofmeyr GJ. Early compared with delayed oral fluids and food after caesarean section. *Cochrane Database Syst Rev.* 2002;3:CD003516.

39. Gould CV, Umscheid CA, Agarwal RK, Kuntz G, Pegues DA; Healthcare Infection Control Practices Advisory Committee. Guideline for prevention of

catheter-associated urinary tract infections 2009. *Infect Control Hosp Epidemiol.* 2010;31(4):319-326.

40. Tran T, Reeder A, Funke L, Richmond N. Association between smoking cessation interventions during prenatal care and postpartum relapse: results from 2004 to 2008 multi-state PRAMS data [published online ahead of print August 2012]. *Matern Child Health J.* doi: 10.1007/s10995-012-1122-8.

41. Von Kohorn I, Nguyen SN, Schulman-Green D, Colson ER. A qualitative study of postpartum mothers' intention to smoke. *Birth.* 2012;39(1):65-69.

42. Jiménez-Muro A, Nerín I, Samper P, et al. A proactive smoking cessation intervention in postpartum women. *Midwifery.* 2012;29(3):240-245

43. Brandon TH, Simmons VN, Meade CD, et al. Self-help booklets for preventing postpartum smoking relapse: a randomized trial. *Am J Public Health.* 2012;102(11):2109-2115.

44. Ruedinger E, Cox JE. Adolescent childbearing: consequences and interventions. *Curr Opin Pediatr.* 2012;24(4):446-452.

45. Quinlivan JA, Box H, Evans SF. Postnatal home visits in teenage mothers: a randomised controlled trial. *Lancet.* 2003;361(9361):893-900.

46. Black MM, Bentley ME, Papas MA, et al. Delaying second births among adolescent mothers: a randomized, controlled trial of a home-based mentoring program. *Pediatrics.* 2006;118(4):e1087-e1099.

47. Wilson EK, Samandari G, Koo HP, Tucker C. Adolescent mothers' postpartum contraceptive use: a qualitative study. *Perspect Sex Reprod Health.* 2011;43(4):230-237.

48. Lewis LN, Doherty DA, Hickey M, Skinner SR. Implanon as a contraceptive choice for teenage mothers: a comparison of contraceptive choices, acceptability and repeat pregnancy. *Contraception.* 2010;81(5):421-426.

49. Teal SB, Sheeder J. IUD use in adolescent mothers: retention, failure and reasons for discontinuation. *Contraception.* 2012;85(3):270-274.

50. Fenwick J, Barclay L, Schmied V. Craving closeness: a grounded theory analysis of women's experiences of mothering in the Special Care Nursery. *Women Birth.* 2008;21(2):71-85.

51. Lefkowitz DS, Baxt C, Evans JR. Prevalence and correlates of posttraumatic stress and postpartum depression in parents of infants in the neonatal intensive care unit (NICU). *J Clin Psychol Med Settings.* 2010;17(3):230-237.

52. Kantrowitz-Gordon I. Expanded care for women and families after preterm birth. *J Midwifery Women's Health.* 2013 (in press).

53. Morton J, Hall JY, Wong RJ, Thairu L, Benitz WE, Rhine WD. Combining hand techniques with electric pumping increases milk production in mothers of preterm infants. *J Perinatol.* 2009;29(11):757-764.

54. Nyqvist K, Anderson G, Bergman N, et al. Towards universal kangaroo mother care: recommendations and report from the First European conference and Seventh International Workshop on Kangaroo Mother Care. *Acta Paediatr.* 2010;99(6):820-826.

55. American College of Nurse-Midwives. *Depression in Women: Position Statement.* 2003.

56. Foli KJ. Nursing care of the adoption triad. *Perspect Psychiatr Care.* 2012;48(4):208-217.

57. Mott SL, Schiller CE, Richards JG, O'Hara MW, Stuart S. Depression and anxiety among postpartum and adoptive mothers. *Arch Women's Ment Health.* 2011;14(4):335-343.

58. Clarke JG, Adashi EY. Perinatal care for incarcerated patients: a 25-year-old woman pregnant in jail. *JAMA.* 2011;305(9):923-929.

59. Chambers AN. Impact of forced separation policy on incarcerated postpartum mothers. *Policy Polit Nurs Pract.* 2009;10(3):204-211.

60. Villanueva CK. *Mothers, Infants and Imprisonment.* New York, NY: Women's Prison Association; 2009.

61. Committee on Health Care for Underserved Women. ACOG Committee Opinion health care for pregnant and postpartum incarcerated women and adolescent females. *Obstet Gynecol.* 2011;118(5):1198-1202.

62. Centers for Disease Control and Prevention. Updated recommendations for use of tetanus toxoid, reduced diphtheria toxoid and acellular pertussis vaccine (Tdap) in pregnant women and persons who have or anticipate having close contact with an infant aged <12 months: Advisory Committee on Immunization Practices (ACIP), 2011. *MMWR.* 2011;60(41):1424-1426.

63. Kolialexi A, Tounta G, Mavrou A. Noninvasive fetal RhD genotyping from maternal blood. *Expert Rev Mol Diagn.* 2010;10(3):285-296.

64. Leeman LM, Rogers RG. Sex after childbirth: postpartum sexual function. *Obstet Gynecol.* 2012; 119(3):647-655.

65. Rowland M, Foxcroft L, Hopman WM, Patel R. Breastfeeding and sexuality immediately post partum. *Can Fam Physician.* 2005;51:1366-1367.

66. Chen BA, Reeves MF, Hayes JL, Hohmann HL, Perriera LK, Creinin MD. Postplacental or delayed insertion of the levonorgestrel intrauterine device after vaginal delivery: a randomized controlled trial. *Obstet Gynecol.* 2010;116(5):1079-1087.

67. Centers for Disease Control and Prevention. U S. medical eligibility criteria for contraceptive use, 2010. *MMWR Recomm Rep.* 2010;59(RR-4):1-86.

68. Kjos SL, Peters RK, Xiang A, Thomas D, Schaefer U, Buchanan TA. Contraception and the risk of type 2

diabetes mellitus in Latina women with prior gestational diabetes mellitus. *JAMA*. 1998;280(6):533-538.

69. Xiang AH, Kawakubo M, Kjos SL, Buchanan TA. Long-acting injectable progestin contraception and risk of type 2 diabetes in Latino women with prior gestational diabetes mellitus. *Diab Care*. 2006;29(3): 613-617.

70. Paul IM, Beiler JS, Schaefer EW, et al. A randomized trial of single home nursing visits vs office-based care after nursery/maternity discharge: the Nurses for Infants Through Teaching and Assessment After the Nursery (NITTANY) study. *Arch Pediatr Adolesc Med*. 2012;166(3):263-270.

71. Woolhouse H, Perlen S, Gartland D, Brown SJ. Physical health and recovery in the first 18 months postpartum: does cesarean section reduce long-term morbidity? *Birth Issues Perinat Care*. 2012;39(3): 221-229.

72. Montgomery-Downs HE, Insana SP, Clegg-Kraynok MM, Mancini LM. Normative longitudinal maternal sleep: the first 4 postpartum months. *Am J Obstet Gynecol*. 2010;203(5):465.e1-e7.

73. Wolfson A, Lee KA. Pregnancy and the postpartum period. In: Kryger MH, Roth T, Dement WC, eds. *Principles and Practice of Sleep Medicine*. 5th ed. St. Louis, MO: Elsevier; 2011:1278-1286

74. Lee KA, Ward TM. Critical components of a sleep assessment for clinical practice settings. *Issues Ment Health Nurs*. 2005;26(7):739-750.

75. Lee KA. Sleep dysfunction in women and its management. *Curr Treat Options Neurol*. 2006;8(5):376-386.

76. Hunter LP, Rychnovsky JD, Yount SM. A selective review of maternal sleep characteristics in the postpartum period. *J Obstet Gynecol Neonatal Nurs*. 2009;38(1):60-68.

77. Breedlove G, Fryzelka D. Depression screening during pregnancy. *J Midwifery Women's Health*. 2011;56(1):18-25.

78. Moyer VA, U.S. Preventive Services Task Force. Screening for cervical cancer: U.S. Preventive Services Task Force recommendation statement. *Ann Intern Med*. 2012;156(12):880-891, W312.

79. U.S. Department of Health and Human Services. 2008 physical activity guidelines for Americans. *Be Active, Happy and Healthy*. 2008 Available at: http://www.health.gov/paguidelines/pdf/paguide.pdf. Accessed June 25, 2013.

80. Daley AJ, Thomas A, Cooper H, et al. Maternal exercise and growth in breastfed infants: a meta-analysis of randomized controlled trials. *Pediatrics*. 2012;130(1):108-114.

81. Weaver K. Review: dietary restriction, with or without aerobic exercise, promotes weight loss in postpartum women. *Evid Based Nurs*. 2008;11(1):14.

● ● ● Additional Resources

Transcultural Resources

CulturedMed
http://culturedmed.binghamton.edu/index.php/home
Refugee and immigrant health resources.

Ethnomed
www.ethnomed.org
Information on health care and cultures organized by clinical topic, culture, and language. Includes information for practitioners and patients.

Office of Minority Health, Cultural Competency Section
http://www.minorityhealth.hhs.gov/templates/browse.aspx?lvl=1&lvlID=3
A guide to provision of culturally competent care from the U.S. Department of Health and Human Services.

Transcultural Aspects of Perinatal Care: A Resource Guide
Focusing on perinatal care, this volume raises awareness of cultural, ethnic, and religious issues and helps providers become "culturally competent," incorporating awareness and knowledge of cultural values and beliefs in their practice. Chapters cover health and illness, pregnancy and prenatal care, labor and delivery, postpartum, and newborn care.

34A

Physical Examination During the Early Postpartum Period

Examination of the woman during the immediate postpartum period, like any examination, begins with the midwife performing a personal greeting, ascertaining if the moment is an appropriate time for the examination, and adapting the environment to provide comfort and privacy. Throughout the examination, the midwife can clarify questions, integrate teaching, and provide anticipatory guidance.

- Perform hand hygiene, preferably in the woman's sight, and don nonsterile/clean gloves
- Assist the woman in assuming a comfortable supine or dorsal position.

General

- Vital signs: temperature, blood pressure, pulse, respiratory rate
- Observe general affect, mobility, signs of pain or splinting

Breasts

- Observe breasts for symmetry.
- Palpate to assess engorgement if present.
- Palpate axilla to assess for accessory mammary tissue. Inspect the nipple epithelium for erythema, bruising, petechial, and cracks or bleeding.
- Observe the integrity of the areola and inspect for blisters or cracks.

- Roll or gently squeeze the nipple to assess erectility; express colostrum.
- If the woman is not breastfeeding, verify she has a bra that provides comfortable support.
- If the woman is breastfeeding, verify adequate bra support.

Note: The immediate postpartum period is not a time for a reliable clinical breast exam for cancer screening.

Heart

Auscultate the heart (rate, rhythm, cardiac sounds).

- Systolic ejection murmur persists past the first week of puerperium in 20% of women.
- Heart rate decreases to the nonpregnant level within 10 days postpartum.

Lungs

Auscultate the lungs, and percuss as appropriate (the midwife may assist the woman to a sitting position for evaluation of the inferior lobes).

- Respiratory volume increases to the nonpregnant rate within the first postpartum week.
- Diminished breath sounds or crackles in lung base suggest pulmonary edema or pneumonia.

Abdomen

- Position the woman in supine position.
- Palpate the fundus abdominally and verify its location.
  - Immediately after birth, the fundus is several centimeters below the umbilicus.
  - On the first day postpartum, the fundus slightly relaxes and rises to the level of the umbilicus.
  - From 4 to 6 weeks postpartum, there is a gradual decrease in the height of the fundus until it is not palpable abdominally (Figure 34-3).
  - Deviations may exist if the woman is at extremes of height or weight.
- Palpate the suprapubic area to rule out distended bladder.
  - There is a high index of suspicion that the bladder is full if the uterus is displaced upward and to one side (generally the right side).
- If post cesarean section, inspect the incision using REEDA for later documentation.
- Assess the costovertebral angle for tenderness (CVAT).
- Request the woman to lift her head onto her chest while the midwife simultaneously palpates the center of the abdomen to assess the degree of separation of the rectus abdominis, or the rectus diastasis, and determine the size of the separation in centimeters or fingerbreadths for later documentation.

Extremities

- Observe for unilateral calf tenderness, erythema, or swelling that may suggest deep vein thrombosis.

Perineum

Because it is likely that the midwife will come in contact with bodily fluids, most clinicians defer examination of the perineum until after assessment of the woman's extremities.

- Obtain adequate visualization (a flashlight, penlight, or flashlight app works well) with good lighting.
- Ask the woman to lie on her side:
  - Choose the side based on the woman's comfort and the layout of the room.
  - Lateral view and gentle elevation of the upper buttocks allows visualization of the posterior aspect of the repair and the anus.
- Observe the woman for discomfort throughout the examination.
- Consider use of a large mirror to show the woman her perineum if she desires.
- Change to a new pair of nonsterile gloves.
- If laceration or episiotomy is present, inspect the full length of the suture line using the REEDA scale for later documentation.
  - Mild edema is normal in the first 2–3 days postpartum.
  - If signs of a hematoma are present, use a gloved hand to palpate gently with thumb and forefinger to distinguish between normal edema and hematoma. Signs of hematoma include unilateral labial swelling, black/blueish area of erythema, report of vaginal or rectal pressure, or sudden onset of severe pain.
- Evaluate lochia on a sanitary pad, observing the color and extent of saturation and noting the length of time since the pad was changed.
  - If needed, discard the soiled pad and provide a new one to the woman.
- Discard used gloves, and perform hand hygiene.

CHAPTER

35

Postpartum Complications

DEBORAH BRANDT KARSNITZ

Introduction

Most women experience an uneventful postpartum (puerperium) rich in the attainment of new or familiar roles of motherhood. Occasionally, however, complications arise that must be recognized and managed appropriately. Knowledge of normal physiologic and anatomic changes of the puerperium is essential to differentiate between the discomforts associated with healing after childbirth and abnormal conditions. Early recognition of complications of the puerperium facilitates prompt treatment and expedites physician consultation, collaboration, or referral as needed.

Complications of the puerperium discussed in this chapter include infection, subinvolution, late postpartum hemorrhage, hematoma, superficial and deep venous thrombosis, postpartum thyroiditis, and postpartum preeclampsia. Postpartum mood and anxiety disorders and breastfeeding complications are discussed elsewhere in this text.

Puerperal Morbidity

Puerperal morbidity, or illness in the first 10 days postpartum, has long been defined by the Joint Committee on Maternal Welfare as a temperature greater than 38°C (100.4°F) occurring on any 2 of the first 10 days postpartum, exclusive of the first 24 hours after giving birth.[1] Puerperal morbidity and infection are sometimes thought of as synonymous, although that is incorrect. Puerperal morbidity may be caused by conditions other than uterine infection, such as dehydration, urinary tract infection (UTI),

upper respiratory infection, and mastitis. Other causes, such as late preeclampsia, venous thrombosis, and mood and anxiety disorders, as well as other medical conditions, are all causes of illness and sometimes death during or after childbirth.

Historically, infection, hemorrhage, and blood pressure were the three main causes of maternal mortality and morbidity.[2] Today, although the three complications in this "lethal triad" continue to occur, other medical conditions, such as cardiovascular complications associated with childbirth (or not), occur at a high rate.[3-5p661] Puerperal morbidity and mortality remain a concern in the United States despite a decline in incidence with the advent of frequent hand washing and antimicrobial therapy.

Maternal mortality is defined as maternal death during pregnancy or within 42 days of birth or termination of a pregnancy, regardless of cause.[6] In a recent report by the World Health Organization, United Nations Children's Fund, United Nations Population Fund, and the World Bank, global trends from 1990 to 2010 showed that the maternal mortality ratio is decreasing in most countries.[6] Despite this optimistic report, the U.S. maternal mortality ratio did not decrease. In fact, the maternal mortality ratio in the United States has steadily increased over the past two decades.[6] The U.S. maternal mortality ratio (MMR) was 12 maternal deaths per 100,000 live births in 1990, rising steadily to 18 per 100,000 live births in 2005 and then to 21 per 100,000 live births in 2010.[3,4,6] The United States MMR ranks behind most other developed countries.

Speculation about the causes of the increasing trend in MMR in the United States has focused on the escalation of body mass index; high cesarean section rates; medical conditions such as diabetes, hypertension, and heart disease; and increased maternal age.[6] **Figure 35-1** presents the causes of maternal mortality in the United States today.[7]

In addition, disparities in maternal mortality exist for different races and ethnicities. Barriers to services and incongruent treatments continue to be significant factors for inequality in health care. African American women are four times more likely to die from childbirth complications than white women, even though the incidence of postpartum complications for the two groups is similar.[8]

To accurately identify postpartum complications, a midwife needs to comprehensively assess the entire scenario, gather pertinent data to guide diagnostic evaluation, and consider all possible differential diagnoses. Making a differential diagnosis entails determining (1) whether evidence of puerperal morbidity reflects puerperal infection or one of the other causes; (2) if the morbidity is a result of puerperal infection, where the source of that infection resides; and (3) if the morbidity is a result of infection, which offending organism is responsible and which antibiotics are useful in treating infections caused by that organism. For example, a urinary tract infection may be difficult to diagnose during the immediate postpartum period. Initial symptoms of a UTI are similar to those of other puerperal infections and also may vary depending on whether the woman has a simple cystitis or pyelonephritis.

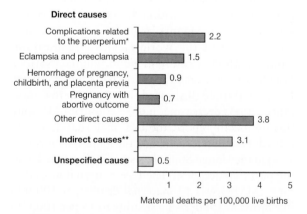

Direct causes

Complications related to the puerperium* — 2.2
Eclampsia and preeclampsia — 1.5
Hemorrhage of pregnancy, childbirth, and placenta previa — 0.9
Pregnancy with abortive outcome — 0.7
Other direct causes — 3.8
Indirect causes** — 3.1
Unspecified cause — 0.5

Maternal deaths per 100,000 live births

*Deaths occurring in the period immediately after delivery.
**Deaths from preexisting conditions complicated by pregnancy.

Figure 35-1 Leading causes of maternal mortality, 2007.
Source: Xu J, Kochanek K, Murphy S, Tejada-Vera B. Deaths: *Final Data for 2007.* National Vital Statistics Reports No. 58:19, Hyattsville, MD: National Center for Health Statistics; 2010.

Puerperal Fever and Puerperal Infection

Puerperal Fever

Puerperal infection is a leading cause of hospital readmission following childbirth.[9] Puerperal fever often occurs secondary to infection (genital tract or other), but it can also be related to dehydration, breast engorgement, pyelonephritis, respiratory illness, or thrombophlebitis.[10] Puerperal pyrexia or fever is defined as a temperature greater than 38.0°C (100.4°F), occurring after the initial 24 hours and on any 2 of the first 10 days postpartum. Fever lasting 24 hours or less is usually not related to infection. However, a fever spiking to 39.0°C (102.2°F) or higher within 24 hours after a cesarean section could indicate a group B *Streptococcus* infection.[5] All fevers occurring during the postpartum period require evaluation.

Puerperal Infection

Puerperal infection is defined as any infection of the genital tract following childbirth, miscarriage, or pregnancy termination. Historically, and well into the twentieth century, puerperal infection was a significant factor causing maternal morbidity and mortality. Currently, according to the Pregnancy Mortality Surveillance System (PMSS), puerperal infections are no longer a leading cause of maternal mortality (they are responsible for approximately 10.7% of all maternal mortality).[4] Since the advent of asepsis and antimicrobial therapies, the incidence of puerperal infection has decreased significantly. Nevertheless, postpartum morbidity from infection remains a significant problem from wound or tissue trauma, and most notably secondary to cesarean section.[4,11] Despite the fact that most puerperal infections occur within the first few weeks postpartum, the 2-week postpartum visit has been discontinued in many practices in favor of a single visit occurring at 6 weeks postpartum.[10] Without earlier postpartum follow-up, many infections could go unreported.

A study of 1871 postpartum women in Denmark (2007–2008) revealed that 24% of women self-reported an infection within 4 weeks postpartum. Breast infections (12%) occurred most frequently, followed by wound, vaginal, urinary, and respiratory infections (3% each) and endometritis and other infections (2% each). Only 66% of women reported symptoms to their healthcare provider and 9% to a hospital facility. Breastfeeding was discontinued by 21% of women with infections.[12]

Pathogenesis

Infections following a vaginal birth primarily occur at the site of a laceration, an episiotomy, or the placental implantation site. However, access to an abdominal incision can occur once the amniotic membrane ruptures; at that point, colonized bacteria can ascend into the uterus, causing infection within the uterus and fallopian tubes as well.

Infectious Organisms

Organisms in puerperal infections come from two sources: (1) those that normally exist in the lower genital tract or in the bowel, and (2) bacteria that are found in the nasopharynx, on the hands of attending personnel, or in the air and dust of the environment. Bacteria from the first source are considered endogenous and become pathogenic secondary to obstetrical manipulation or tissue trauma. Women should be routinely screened and treated prenatally for infections of the lower genital tract. Infection from the second source is best prevented with scrupulous attention to hand washing and asepsis.

Organisms commonly associated with puerperal infection include gram-positive aerobes, such as *Streptococcus* species (A, B, and D), *Enterococcus*, and *Staphylococcus aureus* and *epidermis*; gram-negative aerobes, such as *Escherichia coli*, *Klebsiella*, *Enterobacter*, and *Proteus* species; and gram-variable organisms, such as *Gardnerella vaginalis*. Anaerobes include *Peptostreptococcus*, *Peptococcus*, *Bacteroides* species, *Clostridium*, and *Fusobacterium*. Other organisms implicated in puerperal infection include *Mycoplasma*, *Chlamydia*, and *Neisseria gonorrhoeae*.[5]

Signs and Symptoms of Puerperal Infection

Signs and symptoms of puerperal infection include elevated temperature, general malaise, pain, and malodorous lochia. Degree of temperature elevation and chills, along with increased pulse rate, may be indicative of the severity of infection. Because symptoms for uterine infection may be generalized, the differential diagnosis includes appendicitis, pyelonephritis, and pneumonia.[5,13]

It is important to note the possibility of extended infections. These infections originate from a localized infection and extend via the path of venous circulation or the lymphatics to produce bacterial infection in more distant sites. Extended sites of puerperal infection include pelvic cellulitis, salpingitis, oophoritis, peritonitis, pelvic and femoral thrombophlebitis, and bacteremia.

Endometritis

Uterine infection, most often referred to as endometritis or endomyometritis, may occur anywhere within the uterus (i.e., myometrium, endometrium). Endometritis usually occurs within 2 to 4 days postpartum or as late as 2 to 6 weeks postpartum, and can be either a mild or a very severe infection. Although endometritis may occur in 1% to 2% of vaginal births, cesarean section significantly increases the risk (up to 27%).[13] The American College of Obstetrics and Gynecologists (ACOG) recommends use of one dose of prophylactic antimicrobial therapy administered within 60 minutes before a cesarean section and this has become standard practice in the United States.[14,15]

Risk Factors for Endometritis

The risk factors for, and signs and symptoms of, endometritis are listed in **Table 35-1**. Risk factors for this type of infection are often correlated. A long labor can increase the number of vaginal exams performed, which increases the risk for infection; prolonged labor itself, however, is a risk factor for infection. Improper management could lead to retained placental fragments. Awareness of risk factors can increase attention to preventive practices such as decreasing the number of vaginal exams performed.

Signs and Symptoms of Endometritis

Signs and symptoms of endometritis can be quite generalized, including malaise, chills, and general flu-like symptoms. The classic triad is fever, foul-smelling lochia, and uterine tenderness. The onset of these signs and symptoms varies depending on the organism. Other women may develop minor symptoms that are not fulminant and do not cause them to contact a healthcare provider until a few weeks after giving birth.

Management of Endometritis

Evaluation for postpartum endometritis includes physical exam, interpretation of laboratory cultures and sensitivities (urine and blood), complete blood count, and chest X ray to rule out pneumonia if indicated. The diagnosis is based on ruling out other

Table 35-1	Risk Factors and Signs and Symptoms of Postpartum Endometritis	
Risk Factors	**Signs and Symptoms**
Operative birth/cesarean section	Persistently elevated fever 38°C–39°C (100.4°F–102.2°F) up to 40°C (104°F), depending on the severity of the infection
Prolonged rupture of membranes	
Prolonged labor	Malaise, anorexia
Frequent vaginal exams	Chills often associated with a temperature that spikes or rises quickly
Internal fetal or uterine monitoring	Tachycardia
Uterine manipulation or exploration	Uterine tenderness extending laterally
Retained placental fragments	Pelvic pain with bimanual examination
Medical conditions such as diabetes or immunoinsufficiency	Scanty, odorless lochia, or malodorous, seropurulent lochia
Untreated infection prior to birth	White blood cell count may be elevated beyond the physiologic leukocytosis of the puerperium($> 20,000$ mm^3)
Obesity	Subinvolution of uterus is common in endometritis that presents after the first week postpartum
Postpartum hemorrhage	
Tissue trauma	
Low socioeconomic status	

sources of infection. Consultation is required for women who have a mild case, and collaboration or referral with a consulting physician is required for moderate to severe infections. The differential diagnosis includes appendicitis, pyelonephritis, and pneumonia.

The broad-spectrum antibiotics listed in **Box 35-1** are the treatment of choice for endometritis. Most infections are polymicrobial in nature, and frequently include a combination of aerobes and anaerobes from the genital tract, which increases the risk of virulence.[5] Women with a mild case of endometritis can be treated with oral antibiotics if they have had a vaginal birth. Mild endometritis can be treated with oral ampicillin (Principen) and gentamycin (Garamycin). Women with moderate to severe endometritis will be referred for broad-spectrum intravenous antimicrobials and hospital admission. The "gold standard" intravenous treatment for endometritis comprises a combination of clindamycin (Cleocin) and gentamicin. Most women (90%) respond to intravenous treatment within 24 to 48 hours and do not require follow-up with oral antibiotics.[16]

The spread of endometritis, if left untreated, can lead to salpingitis, septic thrombophlebitis, peritonitis, or necrotizing fasciitis. Suspicion of worsening infection, unexplained symptoms, or acute pain warrants physician consultation and referral.

BOX 35-1 Recommended Antibiotics for Postpartum Endometritis

Generic (Brand)

Clindamycin (Cleocin) 900 mg

+

gentamicin (Garamycin) 1.5 mg/kg, every 8 hours intravenous

OR

Clindamycin (Cleocin) 900 mg every 8 hours
+
ampicillin-sulbactam (Unasyn) 1.5 g every 6 hours[a]

OR

Ampicillin (Amoxil) 2 g every 6 hours

+

Gentamicin (Garamycin) 1.5 mg/kg every 8 hours

[a] For individuals with renal dysfunction in whom gentamycin is contraindicated.

Prevention of Endometritis

Reducing cesarean section rates will significantly lower the rate of postpartum endometritis. Likewise, judicious obstetrical practice—that is, prenatal treatment of infections, limited vaginal exams during labor, avoidance of unnecessary inductions of labor-delayed rupture of membranes, and minimal uterine manipulation during birth—will diminish the risk for developing infection postpartum.

Wound Infection

Etiology and Pathogenesis of Wound Infections

Wound infections may develop in an abdominal incision following a cesarean birth or in a repaired perineal laceration or episiotomy following a vaginal birth. Scrupulous hand washing and administration of prophylactic antibiotics within 60 minutes of the commencement of a cesarean birth has reduced the incidence of infection within an abdominal incision dramatically.[14,15] Common pathogens associated with wound infections include *S. aureus*, *Streptococcus*, and both aerobic and anaerobic bacilli.

Signs and Symptoms of Wound Infections

The signs and symptoms of infection are similar for both abdominal and perineal wounds. Women usually experience a low-grade temperature, seldom greater than 38.3°C (101°F). Localized pain and edema are accompanied by red and inflamed repair edges. Exudate and wound separation or dehiscence may occur as well. Dysuria is often associated with perineal wound infection.[17]

Management of Wound Infections

Management of an infected laceration or episiotomy repair includes removal of sutures; opening, debriding, and cleansing the wound; and administering a broad-spectrum antimicrobial drug. Most wound infections do not need to be repaired again unless a third- or fourth-degree perineal extension is present; a physician referral is indicated for this procedure. A reduction in wound infections has been reported with the administration of prophylactic antimicrobials when a third- or fourth-degree laceration occurs.[16]

Abdominal wound infections often require antibiotics with occasional drainage. Culture of exudates is not usually required. Reclosure of an abdominal wound may be indicated if dehiscence occurs. Depending on the degree of infection and dehiscence, management includes daily debridement, wound packing, antibiotic treatment, and drainage if necessary. Physician consultation or referral is indicated. Persistent fever (lasting for 3 or more days) should be evaluated for complications such as sepsis, septic pelvic thrombophlebitis, abscess, and, rarely, septic shock.

Urinary Tract Infection and Pyelonephritis

Urinary tract infection is the most common cause of puerperal fever.[10] The organisms responsible for UTIs during the puerperium are similar to those observed in nonpregnant women. The organisms most commonly responsible for postpartum UTI include *Escherichia coli* (accounting for 80% to 90% of such UTIs), *Proteus mirabilis*, and *Klebsiella pneumoniae*.

Pregnant and postpartum women are predisposed to urinary stasis resulting from decreased bladder tone and increased bladder volume. Along with decreased sensitivity resulting from various factors such as epidural or local anesthesia, incomplete bladder emptying adds to the increased risk of UTI. Furthermore, women catheterized during labor or those who sustain anterior vaginal trauma are likely to be at greater risk for this complication.

Urinary tract infections may cause urinary frequency, urgency, dysuria, and, occasionally, lower abdominal pain.[5] In contrast, the onset of pyelonephritis is characterized by low-grade fever with spikes, flank pain, costovertebral angle (CVA) tenderness, nausea, and vomiting. Definitive diagnosis of UTI is made by culture of a clean-catch urine specimen demonstrating a significant number of a single type of bacteria.

Uterine Subinvolution

Etiology and Pathogenesis of Uterine Subinvolution

Subinvolution occurs when the uterus does not return to its prepregnant size and position within a standard time frame during the postpartum period. The uterus should not be palpable abdominally by 2 weeks postpartum. Typically, subinvolution occurs when the myometrial fibers do not contract effectively. The process of involution may be hampered for various reasons, most commonly by retained placental fragments, myomata, or infection. Interruption of involution may also occur when maternal activity is excessive; although the direct etiology is not clear, it is postulated that excessive activity might slow the healing process.

Subinvolution of the placental site—an under-recognized condition—occurs when the uteroplacental arteries (modified spiral arteries during pregnancy) have inadequate physiologic closure. Without proper closure, the arteries become filled with thrombi, have inadequate sloughing, and do not regenerate an endothelial lining.[18] Placental site subinvolution has been identified as a cause of delayed postpartum hemorrhage, which can occur between 7 and 40 days following birth, but most often occurs during the second postpartum week.[19]

Signs and Symptoms of Uterine Subinvolution

The usual history of uterine subinvolution includes a longer-than-normal period of lochia, followed by leukorrhea and irregular, heavy bleeding. Pelvic examination will reveal a soft uterus that is larger than expected for the postpartum week during which the woman is being examined. Subinvolution may present with signs and symptoms of uterine infection such as malodorous lochia, tenderness or pain in the adnexa on movement of the uterus, or cervical motion tenderness elicited during a vaginal examination. In this scenario, a lochial culture should be obtained to rule out infection.

Management of Uterine Subinvolution

Management depends on the individual's symptoms. Subinvolution may be diagnosed during a routine 2-week postpartum examination or when a woman calls with a concern about increased or persistent bleeding. If infection is suspected, broad-spectrum antimicrobial therapy is initiated. If retained placental fragments are suspected secondary to the presence of persistent or heavier lochia, ultrasound is indicated. If placental fragments are not identified on ultrasound, uterine exploration may be indicated. Ultrasound is not always definitive, however, and if the diagnosis is equivocal, the ultrasound may not differentiate between placental fragments and blood clots.[20]

If the bleeding is heavier than usual but not markedly so, and there is no indication of infection or retained placental fragments, outpatient treatment may begin with ergonovine (Ergotrate) or methylergonovine (Methergine), 0.2 mg by mouth, every 4 hours for 24 to 48 hours. Women taking either of these uterotonics should be informed that bleeding and cramping may increase during the course of therapy. Reevaluation occurs in 2 weeks.

If pathology is ruled out and increased or excessive maternal activity is suspected as the cause of the subinvolution, attention to daily activities is pertinent. In a society that demands progress, many women return to their usual activity level sooner than the recommended recovery period for complete involution. Encourage women to slow down, increase rest periods, accept help or ask for help, and maintain proper nutrition. Methylergonovine can aid in relieving involution, but its efficacy for treating mild suspected subinvolution based on maternal symptoms of increased bleeding is uncertain.

Delayed (Secondary) Postpartum Hemorrhage

The two most common bleeding complications after initial postpartum hemorrhage are delayed postpartum hemorrhage and postpartum hematoma. As yet, no well-designed randomized control studies have looked at effective treatment for secondary postpartum hemorrhage.[21]

Secondary Postpartum Hemorrhage

Secondary (delayed) postpartum hemorrhage is described as increased bleeding that occurs any time after the first 24 hours postpartum and until 12 weeks postpartum.[22] Although this complication is uncommon, 1% of women experience a secondary postpartum hemorrhage.[22] Most cases of secondary postpartum hemorrhage occur within the first 2 weeks postpartum and are often related to subinvolution (80%).[22]

Risk Factors for Delayed Postpartum Hemorrhage

Risk factors for delayed postpartum hemorrhage include uterine atony, retained placental fragments or membranes, a previously undiagnosed reproductive tract laceration, genital hematoma, uterine infection, placental site subinvolution, and von Willebrand disease (VWD) or other coagulopathies.

The presence of a hemorrhage occurring between 2 to 5 days postpartum could indicate von Willebrand disease. Six different subtypes of VWD are distinguished, although 80% of VWD cases identified during the postpartum period are due to decreased levels of factor VIII. Management depends on the specific subtype. Factor VIII level increases during pregnancy, which usually provides protection from bleeding and consequently is not a concern until approximately 2 days postpartum, when factor VIII levels decrease.[23,24] Postpartum hemorrhage risk secondary to VWD persists for as long as 4 months postpartum. Approximately 50% of women with a diagnosis of VWD are likely to experience a postpartum hemorrhage.[24]

History of menorrhagia or previous postpartum hemorrhage may indicate VWD, and laboratory assessment is suggested in such circumstances. The initial work-up is not directed at diagnosing VWD, but rather at ruling out other causes of bleeding. Preliminary laboratory evaluation includes a complete blood count, platelet count, activated thromboplastin time (aPTT), prothrombin time, and fibrinogen levels. If laboratory results are normal, further testing and physician management are indicated.[24]

Signs and Symptoms of Delayed Postpartum Hemorrhage

Signs and symptoms of secondary postpartum hemorrhage include obvious external vaginal bleeding and, potentially, signs and symptoms of shock or anemia. Persistent or heavier-than-usual lochia rubra or diminished lochia with return to heavy bleeding (not loss of eschar, which typically is short-lived) is indicative of secondary postpartum hemorrhage.

Management of Delayed Postpartum Hemorrhage

Women who experience a sudden, severe delayed postpartum hemorrhage will often present to the emergency department for care. The initial diagnosis of the condition's origin (e.g., uterine atony, reproductive tract laceration, retained placental fragment, infection) will direct management. Treatment may include administration of uterotonics such as methylergonovine (Methergine), laceration repair, or uterine curettage. Ultrasound may be used to assess for retained placental fragments. Curettage is not often the treatment of choice, as the uterus is soft and perforation is a concern.[22] Collaboration with or referral to a consulting physician is advised for diagnosis of the cause and recommendation of appropriate treatment.

Genital Tract Hematomas

A hematoma is a localized collection of extravasated blood that is usually clotted. The dangers of hematoma development are hemorrhage, anemia, and infection. The incidence of postpartum hematoma varies from 1/300 to 1/1500 births; this condition is most often the result of trauma from instrumental birth or episiotomy.[5,26] A hematoma arises following spontaneous or traumatic rupture of a blood vessel. Development occurs most often during birth or within a few hours after the birth. The most common sites for hematoma formation include the vulva, the vagina, and the broad ligament (**Figure 35-2**). Because postpartum hematomas vary in size from small to large, some may be overlooked, which could account for the disparity in incidence estimates.

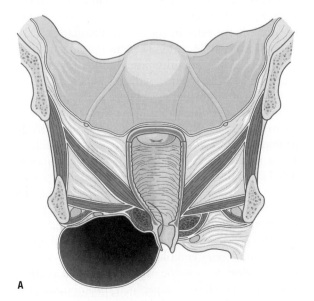

A

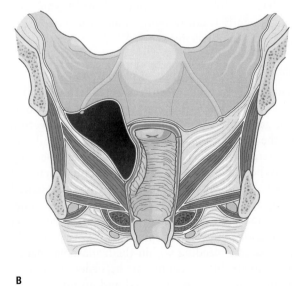

B

Figure 35-2 (A) Vulvar hematoma. (B) Broad ligament hematoma.

Risk Factors for Hematoma

Risk factors for postpartum hematoma formation include operative birth and unrepaired laceration of a torn blood vessel, which can occur during injection of local anesthesia or during repair of an episiotomy or laceration. Failure to achieve hemostasis or ligate torn vessels above the vaginal apex prior to repair of an episiotomy or laceration also increases the risk of hematoma formation. Other risk factors include primiparity, multiple gestation, preeclampsia, coagulopathies, vulvovaginal varicosities, and prolonged second-stage labor.[26]

Signs and Symptoms of Genital Tract Hematoma

Presenting signs and symptoms of a vulvar or vaginal hematoma include: (1) perineal, vaginal, urethral, bladder, or rectal pressure and severe pain; (2) a tense, fluctuant swelling; and (3) bluish or blue-black discoloration of tissue. The characteristic sign of a hematoma is extreme pain out of proportion to the expected amount of discomfort and pain at that time period and pain that develops quite rapidly in the first 2 to 6 hours after birth. Women who have epidural analgesia may report sudden onset of rectal pressure as the only symptom.

Presenting signs and symptoms of a broad ligament hematoma include lateral uterine pain sensitive to palpation, extension of pain into the flank, a painful swelling identified on high rectal examination, a ridge of tissue just above the pelvic brim extending laterally (this is the edge of the swollen broad ligament), and possibly abdominal distention. Subperitoneal hematoma formation (rarely occurs with vaginal birth) leads to unrestricted bleeding and subsequently is not recognized until the woman experiences hypovolemic shock.[26]

Management of Genital Tract Hematoma

Vulvar hematomas are the most obvious of this class of complications, while vaginal hematomas are generally identifiable when careful inspection of the vagina and cervix are performed. Small and moderate-sized hematomas may be spontaneously absorbed and managed expectantly. If the hematoma is small and visible, the edges can be demarcated with a pen, and it can be observed frequently to determine whether it is still growing. If the hematoma is large or possibly continuing to grow (which indicates active bleeding within the hematoma space), a complete blood count can be ordered as soon as the hematoma is identified and an intravenous line started. Vital signs will need to be monitored frequently to observe for signs of shock, and pain

medication prescribed as needed. A physician should be consulted for evaluation and care. Management might include monitoring with hematocrit levels, vaginal packing to produce a counterpressure, or an incision to evacuate blood and blood clots and ensure closure of the cavity. The woman with a diagnosis of a hematoma may also need other surgical interventions, such as interventional radiology, blood replacement, or antibiotics.[5,26]

Postpartum Thrombophlebitis, Deep Vein Thrombosis, and Pulmonary Embolism

During pregnancy and the postpartum period, women have an increased risk (5 to 7 times higher) for venous thrombosis and embolism compared to nonpregnant women.[27–29] The incidence of venous thromboembolism from immediately after birth until 6 weeks postpartum ranges from 0.14 to 3.24 per 1000 births, with the highest risk occurring in the immediate postpartum period.[29]

Postpartum thrombophlebitis is defined as inflammation of a vein with formation of a thrombosis (blood clot) and can occur in both superficial and deep veins. Thrombosis is more common in women with varicosities or who perhaps are genetically susceptible to vein-wall relaxation and venous stasis.

Nearly half of all pregnancy-related thrombosis occurs during the puerperium.[30] Virchow's triad describes the three factors that influence thrombosis formation during pregnancy: (1) stasis, (2) hypercoagulable state, and (3) vascular trauma. Pregnancy fosters venous stasis by virtue of venous-wall relaxation resulting from the effects of progesterone and pressure on the veins by the uterus. Pregnancy is also a hypercoagulable state. Trauma may occur from venous-wall inflammation and endothelial damage secondary to distension, with the hypercoagulable state then predisposing the woman to the creation of a thrombus.[29] Prolonged venous compression during positioning for labor or birth may contribute to the problem as well. Cesarean section is also considered a risk factor for thrombosis. Deep vein thrombosis (DVT) is more common in the left lower extremity (accounting for 70% to 80% cases), presumably due to compression of the left iliac vein from the gravid uterus and the crossing of the right iliac artery.[31–33]

The greatest risk associated with thrombophlebitis is pulmonary embolism. This is true for women who develop deep venous thrombosis, but unlikely in women who have a superficial thrombophlebitis. Tachypnea, dyspnea, and sharp chest pain of sudden onset are the most common symptoms of pulmonary embolism. *Sudden onset of these symptoms mandates urgent physician evaluation.* Many other less specific symptoms may be present, including altered lung or heart sounds and apprehension as the woman's blood oxygen level decreases. Under no circumstances should the leg be massaged. Risk factors for postpartum thrombophlebitis are presented in **Box 35-2**.

Signs and Symptoms of Superficial Thrombophlebitis and Deep Vein Thrombosis

The signs and symptoms of superficial thrombophlebitis and deep vein thrombosis are presented in **Table 35-2**. DVT presents as unilateral edema and increase in leg circumference. Tenderness and a feeling of warmth may be noted over the affected veins. Superficial thrombophlebitis is more localized in appearance, but it may be difficult to distinguish between the two conditions on physical examination.

Management of Superficial Thrombophlebitis and Deep Vein Thrombosis

The management of superficial thrombophlebitis and deep vein thrombosis differ significantly. Superficial thrombophlebitis does not require anticoagulant therapy, whereas DVT is a risk for pulmonary embolism and does require anticoagulation therapy. A woman presenting with clinical signs consistent with superficial thrombophlebitis should also be regarded as a potential candidate for development of DVT.

The differential diagnosis includes superficial thrombophlebitis versus deep vein thrombosis, muscle strain or trauma, ruptured cyst, vasculitis, and lymphedema. Laboratory work-up includes high-sensitivity d-dimer studies, which measure fibrin degradation. Venous ultrasound is the primary diagnostic test (with or without color Doppler imaging).[34] Diagnostic ultrasound is indicated for DVT as well as for superficial thrombophlebitis to rule out underlying DVT.

BOX 35-2 Risk Factors for Venous Thrombosis

Maternal History Risks
- Obesity
- Smoking
- Age > 35 years
- History of thrombosis
- Inherited thrombophilias
- Antiphospholipid antibody syndrome
- Sickle cell disease
- Heart disease
- Diabetes
- Other medical conditions

Pregnancy-Related Risks
- Hypercoaguable state
- Venous stasis
- Multiple pregnancy
- Preeclampsia

Labor- and Birth-Related Risks
- Operative vaginal birth
- Cesarean section
- Infection
- Vascular trauma
- Immobilization
- Postpartum hemorrhage

Eliciting of Homan's sign (pain on dorsiflexion of the foot) was once thought to be a diagnostic sign of deep vein thrombosis. A positive Homan's sign may, in fact, indicate DVT, but it could also indicate a strained calf muscle. A positive Homan's sign is present in fewer than one-third of women who have a confirmed DVT. Conversely, a negative Homan's sign

---

Table 35-2	Signs and Symptoms of Superficial Thrombophlebitis and Deep Vein Thrombosis
Superficial Thrombophlebitis	**Deep Vein Thrombosis**
Leg pain	Possible slight temperature elevation
Localized heat	Mild tachycardia
Tenderness	Abrupt onset, with severe leg pain worsening with motion or when standing
Palpation of a knot or cord	Generalized edema of the ankle, leg, and thigh
Inflammation at the site	Pain with calf pressure
	Tenderness along the entire course of the involved vessel(s) with palpable cord

does not rule out deep vein thrombosis. Furthermore, eliciting Homan's sign could disturb a thrombosis; thus this test is no longer recommended for evaluation of leg pain in the postpartum period.

Treatment of superficial thrombophlebitis includes leg rest, elevation of the affected extremity, supportive stockings, and analgesia (nonsteroidal anti-inflammatory drugs) as needed. Deep vein thrombosis treatment is similar, albeit with the addition of anticoagulants and bed rest. Ambulation resumes gradually once acute symptoms have resolved. Supportive stockings are indicated for deep vein thrombosis when ambulation resumes. Anticoagulation therapy is usually continued for at least 6 months or longer if needed. Warfarin (Coumadin) is considered safe during lactation.

Postpartum Thyroiditis and Thyroid Storm

Postpartum thyroiditis (inflammation of the thyroid gland) is an unusual condition characterized by both hyperthyroid and hypothyroid phases. Pregnancy results in a physiologic immunosuppression, and when this immunosuppression is removed in a woman who has an underlying autoimmune thyroiditis, thyroiditis can become manifest. Postpartum thyroiditis may be difficult to recognize, as its symptoms are similar to those commonly encountered in the postpartum period.

Postpartum thyroiditis may occur anytime during the first year following birth (the first 1 to 4 months is most common), and its incidence varies from 5% to 10%. Women at increased risk for postpartum thyroiditis include those with gestational diabetes, autoimmune disorders such as type 1 diabetes, previous thyroid dysfunction, and those with a history of thyroid disorders.[35]

The clinical course of this disorder is characterized by excessive thyroid hormone release, followed by release of insufficient amounts of thyroid hormone. Consequently, "hyper" thyroiditis occurs first, followed by "hypo" thyroiditis. The hyperthyroid phase typically occurs around 3 months postpartum and resolves spontaneously within 2 to 3 months.

Signs and Symptoms of Postpartum Thyroiditis

Signs and symptoms of postpartum thyroiditis resemble the common symptoms familiar to women during the postpartum period. In addition, there is usually no recognizable pain or swelling of the thyroid. Common symptoms of postpartum thyroiditis depend on the phase (hyper or hypo) of the illness. **Table 35-3** compares and contrasts common signs and symptoms of both hyperthyroiditis and hypothyroiditis.

Because thyroiditis does not become manifest until later in the postpartum period, its symptoms may go unnoticed in either phase of the disorder and misdiagnosis may occur. In the hyperthyroid phase, low levels of thyroid-stimulating hormone (TSH), the presence of thyroid peroxidase antibodies, and a lack of TSH receptor antibodies suggest the diagnosis of postpartum thyroiditis. In the hypothyroid phase, an elevated TSH level and a positive test for anti-thyroid peroxidase antibodies are pathognomonic for this disorder. Postpartum depression and anxiety have similar symptoms, however, so they should be included in the differential diagnosis. Women experiencing thyroiditis can have an episode of mild dysphoria that could be mistaken for psychosis.

Management of Postpartum Thyroiditis

Treatment depends on the phase and degree of symptoms. Beta blockers are the treatment of choice for hyperthyroiditis if the symptoms are bothersome, whereas thyroid supplementation with levothyroxine (Synthroid) is prescribed for hypothyroid symptoms.[36] Physician management is indicated. There is no consensus on criteria for treatment, dose of medication, or duration of treatment.

Thyroid Storm

Thyroid storm or clinical thyrotoxicosis is a rare but life-threatening acute exacerbation of hyperthyroidism. It occurs earlier than thyroiditis (usually during the first month postpartum) and is distinguished by an abrupt onset of symptoms. This disorder, which

Table 35-3	Signs and Symptoms of Postpartum Thyroiditis	
Hyperthyroidosis (1–4 Months Postpartum)	**Hypothyroiditis (4–8 Months Postpartum)**
Fatigue	Fatigue
Palpitations	Impaired concentration
Anxiety	Depression
Insomnia	Dry skin
Irritability and nervousness	Constipation
Weight loss	Weight gain
Goiter	Goiter

results from overproduction of thyroid hormone, is characterized by the sudden onset of a hypermetabolic state. Signs and symptoms include nausea and vomiting, diarrhea, fever(> 41°C), tachycardia, and tremor. Potential outcomes include dehydration, seizures, coma, and death if thyroid storm goes untreated. Increased T_4 levels can lead to cardiomyopathy and heart failure.[37]

The diagnosis of thyroid storm is made clinically, and treatment is initiated prior to obtaining the results of confirmatory laboratory studies. Women in thyroid storm usually present to an emergency room acutely ill and may initially be assumed to have preeclampsia. The presence of neuropsychiatric symptoms and hyperpyrexia distinguish thyroid storm from postpartum preeclampsia or eclampsia. Women in thyroid storm will be hospitalized for intensive care management.

Postpartum Preeclampsia/Eclampsia

Preeclampsia most often resolves within 24 to 48 hours postpartum. While postpartum onset of preeclampsia usually begins within the same time period, onset of symptoms may be different than the onset of symptoms prenatally. Late postpartum preeclampsia/eclampsia begins after 48 hours postpartum and prior to 4 weeks postpartum.[38]

Risk Factors for Postpartum Preeclampsia/Eclampsia

Women with gestational hypertension are at increased risk for developing postpartum preeclampsia/eclampsia. In addition, pulmonary edema is an increased risk owing to the normal extravascular-to-intravascular fluid shift, an effect that is particularly enhanced if intravenous fluids were administered during labor and birth. If renal function is already compromised from severe preeclampsia, pulmonary edema risk increases as well. Along with increasing the chance of pulmonary edema, postpartum preeclampsia increases the risk for eclampsia, stroke, and thromboembolism.[39,40]

It is important to note that postpartum preeclampsia/eclampsia may still develop despite intrapartum treatment with magnesium sulfate.

Clinical Presentation of Postpartum Preeclampsia/Eclampsia

Postpartum preeclampsia or hypertension often presents more subtly than onset of the corresponding condition during the prenatal period. Women may exhibit headaches, nausea, vomiting, epigastric pain, or visual changes. Hypertension and proteinuria are not always present in postpartum preeclampsia, however, and should not be considered the defining symptoms. Neurologic indicators (e.g., visual disturbance, headache), nausea, and vomiting appear more frequently during postpartum-onset preeclampsia compared to the prenatal-onset or intrapartum-onset condition.

Management of Postpartum Preeclampsia/Eclampsia

Physician referral is indicated for hospitalization and 24-hour intravenous administration of magnesium sulfate, as well as additional antihypertensive initiation. Midwives can provide education about signs and symptoms of postpartum preeclampsia, as early recognition is key to prevention of eclampsia or worsening of the woman's condition.

Cultural Influences on Complications of the Puerperium

The postpartum period is a time steeped in rich traditions and cultural influences that differ within any given community. Recognition of these cultural influences should guide all treatment plans. Diverse cultures recognize different time frames for postpartum, which can provide additional or reduced time for recovery. Decision making may include other family members or one particular family member. For this reason, when possible, all educational discussions and management plans should include the family healthcare decision maker. Understanding variations in beliefs and traditions will increase trust between the healthcare provider, the woman, and family members.[41]

Conclusion

Most women experience a normal postpartum recovery period that is free from complications. Comprehensive postpartum education is essential for early recognition of problems by women and family members. Postpartum education (about both normal changes and complications) begins during prenatal care and continues into the postpartum period. Family members should be included whenever possible.

Midwives who are astute in assessing the normal physiology of the puerperium will readily recognize pathologic processes to initiate early treatment and prevent worsening illness. Despite the fact that most postpartum complications require physician management, midwives will initiate the diagnostic work-up and recognize occasions when it is appropriate to consult, collaborate, or refer. While physicians medically manage some complications, the midwife will continue to manage other aspects of the woman's postpartum course and adjustments.

• • • References

1. The Joint Commission. Preventing maternal death. January 26, 2010; issue 44. Available at: http://www .jointcommission.org/sentinel_event_alert_issue_44_ preventing_maternal_death/. Accessed September 24, 2012.

2. King JC. Maternal mortality in the United States: why is it important and what are we doing about it? *Semin Perinatol*. 2012;36:14-18.

3. Hankins GDV, Clark SL, Pacheco LD, et al. Maternal mortality, near misses, and severe morbidity: lowering rates through designated levels of maternity care. *Obstet Gynecol*. 2012;120:929-934.

4. Berg CJ, Callaghan WM, Syverson C, Henderson Z. Pregnancy-related mortality in the United States, 1998 to 2005. *Obstet Gynecol*. 2010;116:1302-1309.

5. Cunningham FG, Leveno KJ, Bloom SL, et al. *Williams Obstetrics*. 23rd ed. New York: McGraw-Hill; 2010.

6. World Health Organization, UNICEF, UNFPA, World Bank. *Trends in Maternal Mortality: 1990 to 2010 WHO, UNICEF, UNFPA and the World Bank Estimates*. Geneva: World Health Organization; 2012.

7. Xu J, Kochanek K, Murphy S, Tejada-Vera B. *Deaths: Final Data for 2007*. National Vital Statistics Reports No. 58:19, Hyattsville, MD: National Center for Health Statistics; 2010.

8. Tucker MJ, Berg CJ, Callaghan WM, Hsia J. The black–white disparity in pregnancy-related mortality from 5 conditions: differences in prevalence and case-fatality rates. *Am J Pub Health*. 2007;97:247-251.

9. Belfort MA, Clark SL, Saade GR, et al. Hospital readmission after delivery: evidence for an increased incidence of nonurogenital infection in the immediate postpartum period. *Am J Obstet Gynecol*. 2010;202(1):35.e1-35.e7.

10. Maharaj D. Puerperal pyrexia: a review. Part II. *Obstet Gynecol Surv*. 2007;62:400.

11. Baxter JK, Berghella V, Mackeen AD, et al. Timing of prophylactic antibiotics for preventing postpartum infectious morbidity in women undergoing cesarean delivery. *Cochrane Database System Rev*. 2011;12:CD009516. doi: 10.1002/14651858. CD009516.

12. Ahnfeldt-Mollerup P, Petersen LK, Kragstrup J, et al. Postpartum infections: occurrence, health care contacts and association with breastfeeding. *Acta Obstet Gynecol Scand*. 2012;91(12):1440-1444.

13. Sweet RL, Gibbs RS. *Infectious Diseases of the Female Genital Tract*. 5th ed. Baltimore, MD: Lippincott Williams & Wilkins; 2009.

14. American College of Obstetricians and Gynecologists. Antimicrobial prophylaxis for cesarean delivery: timing of administration. Committee Opinion No. 465. *Obstet Gynecol*. 2010;116:791-792.

15. Smaill FM, Gyte GM. Antibiotic prophylaxis versus no prophylaxis for preventing infection after cesarean section. *Cochrane Database System Rev*. 2010;1:CD007482.pub2. doi: 10.1002/14651858.

16. Duggal N, Mercado C, Daniels K, Bujor A, Caughey AB, El-Sayed Y. Antibiotic prophylaxis for prevention of postpartum perineal wound complications: a randomized controlled trial. *Obstet Gynecol*. 2008; 111(6):1268-1273.

17. Tharpe N. Postpregnancy genital tract and wound infections. *J Midwifery Women's Health*. 2008;53(3): 236-246.

18. Weydent JA. Subinvolution of the placental site as an anatomic cause of postpartum uterine bleeding. *Arch Path Lab Med*. 2006;130:1538-1552.

19. Petrovitch I, Jeffrey RB, Heerema-McKenney A. Subinvolution of the placental site. *J Ultrasound Med*. 2009;28(8):1115-1119.

20. Shen O, Rabinowitz R, Eisenberg VH, Samueloff A. Transabdominal sonography before uterine exploration as a predictor of retained placental fragments. *J Ultrasound Med*. 2003;22(6):561-564.

21. Alexander J, Thomas PW, Sanghera J. Treatments for secondary postpartum haemorrhage. Cochrane Pregnancy and Childbirth Group. 2008. doi: 10.1002 /14651858.CD002867.

22. American College of Obstetricians and Gynecologists. *Postpartum Hemorrhage*. Practice Bulletin 76. *Obstet Gynecol*. 2006;108:1039-1047.

23. Mannucci PM. Treatment of von Willebrand's disease. *N Engl J Med*. 2004;351:683.

24. Pacheco LD, Costantine MM, Saade GR, et al. von Willebrand disease and pregnancy: a practical approach for the diagnosis and treatment. *Am J Obstet Gynecol*. 2010;203(3):194-200.

25. Katz V. Postpartum care. In: *Obstetrics: Normal and Problem Pregnancies*. Gabbe SG, Niebyl JR, Simpson JL, et al., eds. 6th ed. Philadelphia, PA: Churchill Livingstone; 2012: 517-532.

26. You WB, Zahn CM. Postpartum hemorrhage: abnormally adherent placenta, uterine inversion, and puerperal hematomas. *Clin Obstet Gynecol*. 2006;49(1):184-197.

27. Heit JA, Kobbervig CE, James AH, Petterson TM, Bailey KR, MElton LJ 3rd. Trends in the incidence of

venous thromboembolism during pregnancy or post-partum: a 30-year population-based study. *Ann Intern Med.* 2005;143:697-706.

28. Jackson E, Curtis KM, Gaffield ME. Risk of venous thromboembolism during the postpartum period: a systematic review. *Obstet Gynecol.* 2011;117:691-703.

29. Davis SM, Branch DW. Thromboprophylaxis in pregnancy: who and how? *Obstet Gynecol Clin North Am.* 2010;37:333-343.

30. Jacobsen AF, Skjeldestad FE, Sandset PM. Incidence and risk patterns of venous thromboembolism in pregnancy and puerperium: a register-based case-control study. *Am J Obstet Gynecol.* 2008;198:233.

31. Ray JG, Chan WS. Deep vein thrombosis during pregnancy and the puerperium: a meta-analysis of the period of risk and the leg of presentation. *Obstet Gynecol Surv.* 1999;54:256-271.

32. Bourjeily G, Paidas M, Khalil H, Rosene-Montella K, Rodger M. Pulmonary embolism in pregnancy. *Lancet.* 2010;375(9713):500-512.

33. Marik PE. Thromboembolism in pregnancy. *Clin Chest Med.* 2010;31:731-740.

34. Pettker C, Lockwood C. Thromboembolic disorders. In: *Obstetrics: Normal and Problem Pregnancies.* Gabbe SG, Niebyl JR, Simpson JL, et al., eds. 6th

ed. Philadelphia, PA: Churchill Livingstone; 2012: 980-993.

35. Kennedy RL, Malabu UH, Jarrod G, Nigam P, Kannan K, Rane A. Thyroid function and pregnancy: before, during and beyond. *J Obstet Gynaecol.* 2010;30(8): 774-783.

36. Stagnaro-Green A. Postpartum thyroiditis. *J Clin Endocrin Met.* 2002;87(9):4042-4047.

37. Neville MW. Thyroid disorders. In: King TL, Brucker MC, eds. *Pharmacology for Women's Health.* Sudbury, MA: Jones and Bartlett; 2011:539-559.

38. Sibai BM, Stella CL. Diagnosis and management of atypical preeclampsia–eclampsia. *Am J Obstet Gynecol.* 2009;200:481.e1-481.e7.

39. Hirshfeld-Cytron J, Lam C, Karumanchi SA, Lindheimer M. Late postpartum eclampsia: examples and review. *Obstet Gynecol Surv.* 2006;61(7): 471-480.

40. Sibai BM. Hypertension. In: *Obstetrics: Normal and Problem Pregnancies.* Gabbe SG, Niebyl JR, Simpson JL, et al., eds. 6th ed. Philadelphia, PA: Churchill Livingstone; 2012:779-824.

41. Purnell LD. The Purnell Model for cultural competence. In: *Transcultural Health Care: A Culturally Competent Approach.* 4th ed. Philadelphia, PA: F. A. Davis; 2012:19-55.

CHAPTER

36

Breastfeeding and the Mother–Newborn Dyad

ERIN M. WRIGHT

Breastfeeding: A Call to Action

In 2011, the U.S. Department of Health and Human Services issued a publication entitled *The Surgeon General's Call to Action to Support Breastfeeding*, urging clinicians, employers, researchers, government leaders, and communities to help women to meet the *Healthy People 2020* goals for breastfeeding, as well as their personal breastfeeding goals.[1] Included in this publication is a stepwise blueprint of specific actions to be taken to facilitate this goal. These include actions directed toward systemwide improvements for women and their infants, employers, communities, healthcare systems, research and surveillance entities, and the public health infrastructure (**Box 36-1**). The rationale behind this support is based on the plethora of health benefits for both mother and child that are associated with breastfeeding.

Federal support for breastfeeding echoes multiple position statements and recommendations from maternal and child health professional organizations, including the American Academy of Pediatrics (AAP),[2] the Association of Women's Health, Obstetrical, and Neonatal Nurses (AWHONN),[3] and the American College of Nurse-Midwives (ACNM).[4] Each of these organizations considers breastfeeding the "optimal infant nutrition."

Benefits of Breastfeeding

Infant Benefits

The significant health advantages when the nutritive norm is human milk consumption have been repeatedly demonstrated. Children who are breastfed experience dose-related reductions in otitis media (recurrent and nonrecurrent), asthma, type 1 and type 2 diabetes, obesity, upper and lower respiratory tract infections, atopic dermatitis, inflammatory bowel

---

BOX 36-1 The Surgeon General's Call to Action to Support Breastfeeding

Actions for Health Care

1. Ensure that maternity practices around the United States are fully supportive of breastfeeding
2. Develop systems to guarantee continuity of skilled support for lactation between hospitals and healthcare settings in the community
3. Provide education and training in breastfeeding for all health professionals who care for women and children
4. Include basic support for breastfeeding as a standard of care for midwives, obstetricians, family physicians, nurse practitioners, and pediatricians
5. Ensure access to services provided by international board-certified lactation consultants
6. Identify and address obstacles to greater availability of safe banked donor milk for fragile infants

Source: U.S. Department of Health and Human Services. *The Surgeon General's Call to Action to Support Breastfeeding.* Washington, DC: U.S. Department of Health and Human Services, Office of the Surgeon General; 2011.

disease, celiac disease, gastroenteritis, childhood leukemias, lymphomas, and sudden infant death syndrome (SIDS).[5,6] Preterm infants experience even greater benefits from consuming their mother's milk, including a significant reduction in the incidence of necrotizing enterocolitis (a leading cause of infant morbidity and mortality), neonatal sepsis, metabolic syndrome in adolescence, and hospital readmission. Preterm infants who are breastfed also have improved neurodevelopmental outcomes.[5-7] Not only are there benefits to breastfeeding, but such benefits tend to be magnified the longer a woman breastfeeds. Conversely, not breastfeeding has been associated with various health risks.[5] The list of benefits from breastfeeding continues to grow as additional research is conducted.

Maternal Benefits

Women who breastfeed their infants experience faster uterine involution and, subsequently, a reduction in postpartum bleeding. As women continue to breastfeed, they experience longer periods of lactational amenorrhea, providing the potential for extended child spacing. While it is commonly known that women who breastfeed experience a greater caloric expenditure, research regarding a faster return to pre-pregnancy weight has been inconclusive owing to a multitude of confounding variables, such as maternal diet choices and maternal BMI prior to and at the birth of the infant.[6,8] Nevertheless, research has demonstrated that women who breastfeed have reduced rates of a number of conditions, including breast and ovarian cancer, rheumatoid arthritis, diabetes mellitus, hypertension, hyperlipidemia, and cardiovascular disease.[6,9-12]

In addition to the physical maternal benefits obtained through breastfeeding, this practice confers psychological benefits. Women who breastfeed have lower rates and decreased duration of postpartum depression, and breastfeeding is associated with significantly lower rates of child abuse and neglect.[6,13,14]

Definitions

Breastfeeding initiation is a term that refers to the first episode of breastfeeding after the birth of an infant. It may take place in any setting but ideally should begin within the first hour of birth, as this is when infants are most alert.

Breastfeeding exclusivity indicates that no source of nutrition is being given to the infant other than breast milk. If the infant is receiving any formula, water, or foods in addition to breast milk, it is referred to as *partial breastfeeding*.

Breastfeeding Prevalence

The *Healthy People* goals are a set of objectives set forth for a 10-year period with the intention of improving the U.S. public health. One of the topic areas in *Healthy People 2020* is maternal, infant, and child health. "To increase the proportion of breast-fed infants" has always been an objective of *Healthy People*.[15] To assess whether this objective is being met, one of the important metrics is the number of women initiating breastfeeding. Because most women in the United States give birth in a hospital, attention has been devoted to the percentage of women who breastfeed in a hospital; researchers found that this rate rose from 74.6% in 2008 to 76.9% in 2009—the largest increase in the past decade.[15] However, despite continued increases in the 6-month and 1-year breastfeeding continuation rates in the United States, the continuation rates remain well below the *Healthy People 2020* goals. **Table 36-1** provides the most recent data from the Centers for Disease Control and Prevention's (CDC) breastfeeding report card, which assesses U.S. progress toward increasing rates of breastfeeding.[15,16]

In addition to collecting total prevalence rates, the CDC stratifies breastfeeding data by racial and ethnic groups. The latest data, related to births reported in

Table 36-1	Breastfeeding Prevalence in the United States	
	***Healthy People 2020* Goal**	**Breastfeeding Report Card 2012**
Initiation rate	81.9%	76.9%
At 6 months	60.6%	47.2%
At 1 year	34.1%	25.5%
Exclusively through 3 months	46.2%	36.0%
Exclusively through 6 months	25.5%	16.3%

Source: Centers for Disease Control and Prevention. *Breastfeeding Report Card—United States, 2012.* Atlanta, GA: U.S. Department of Health and Human Services, Centers for Disease Control and Prevention; 2012. Available at: http://www.cdc.gov/breastfeeding/data/reportcard.htm.

2007,[17] demonstrate that African American women continue to have the lowest rates for breastfeeding initiation (59.7%), while Asian Americans currently account for the greatest proportion of breastfed infants immediately following birth (83%). White women initiate breastfeeding at a rate of 77.7%, and Latina women's initiation rates are even higher, at 80.6%. **Figure 36-1** summarizes these findings.

Economics of Breastfeeding

In addition to saving dollars associated with purchasing milk alternatives for an infant, breastfeeding eliminates waste from bottles and preparations. However, family savings are simply some of the positive economics when societal health is considered. In a 2010 study, Bartick et al. examined the current costs of healthcare expenditures for a variety of conditions, including necrotizing enterocolitis, otitis media, asthma, respiratory tract illnesses resulting in hospitalizations, gastroenteritis, type 1 diabetes, childhood lymphoma, and obesity. Based on this analysis, the researchers estimated the potential cost reduction: if 80% to 90% of families fed their babies human milk exclusively for 6 months, the United States could save 13 billion dollars per year and prevent 911 deaths annually.[18]

Promotion, Protection, and Support

Promotion

According to a report from the Agency for Healthcare Research and Quality (AHRQ), efforts designed to improve breastfeeding outcomes should include three features: promotion, protection, and support.[5]

Promotion

Breastfeeding promotion efforts focus on the physical, immunologic, and psychologic advantages of breastfeeding for each mother–baby dyad. Promotion can be accomplished through provider-driven perinatal education about breastfeeding and effective communication of the maternal and infant benefits from breastfeeding.

Protection

Breastfeeding protection pertains to the legal rights of women and children. In the United States, there

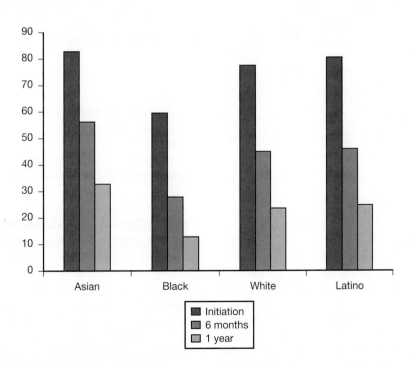

Figure 36-1 Breastfeeding initiation and continuation rates by demographic.
Source: Centers for Disease Control and Prevention. Breastfeeding among U.S. children born 2004–2008, CDC National Immunization Survey. 2009. Available at: http://www.cdc.gov/breastfeeding/data/nis_data. Accessed August 2, 2012.

has been considerable, and increasing, legislative support for breastfeeding at federal, state, and local levels. Federal laws emphasize the rights of the woman and infant to breastfeed freely on any public property and designate that breastfeeding is not considered a lewd or indecent act. The 2010 Patient Protection and Affordable Care Act states that one component of the required health plan guidelines is provision of comprehensive lactation support and counseling by a trained provider during pregnancy and/or in the postpartum period.[19] This includes coverage of the costs of renting breastfeeding equipment. Other state laws address a woman's right to breastfeed in the workplace, adequate maternity leave policies from employers, and appropriate childcare options. Government agencies have designed priority goals and activities to increase breastfeeding initiation and duration.

Responsible marketing practices from infant formula manufacturers are also required to support breastfeeding. As a part of the International Code of Marketing of Breast-milk Substitutes, adopted by the World Health Assembly, governments joined together to regulate the marketing practices related to infant breast milk substitutes as well as devices used to aid in artificial feeding, such as bottles and artificial nipples.[20] To date, the United States is the only member state not to have signed on to the International Code of Marketing of Breast-milk Substitutes.

One example of marketing practices is the common distribution of hospital "gift bags" given to women as they leave the hospital after giving birth. The bags, sponsored by formula companies, include formula and artificial feeding supplies. Women who receive commercial hospital discharge packs are significantly less likely to be exclusively breastfeeding at the 10-week mark when compared to women who do not receive these hospital discharge packs.[21]

Support

Baby-Friendly Hospital Initiative

Support of breastfeeding is accomplished through evidence-based hospital policies such as those outlined in the Baby-Friendly Hospital Initiative. This initiative is based on the World Health Organization's (WHO) Ten Steps to Successful Breastfeeding as outlined in **Box 36-2**.[22]

The Baby-Friendly Hospital Initiative is successful. In a study that surveyed the exposure of women (*n* = 1082) to five of the Ten Steps—namely, breastfeeding initiation within 1 hour of birth, encouraging breastfeeding on demand, no supplementation, rooming-in, and no artificial nipples or pacifiers—the

---

> ### BOX 36-2 Ten Steps to Successful Breastfeeding
>
> Each facility providing maternity and newborn care services should:
>
> 1. Have a written policy that is routinely communicated to staff
> 2. Train all healthcare staff in skills necessary to implement this policy
> 3. Inform all pregnant women about the benefits and management of breastfeeding
> 4. Help all mothers initiate breastfeeding within 1 hour of birth
> 5. Show mothers how to breastfeed and how to maintain lactation even if they should be separated from their infants
> 6. Give newborn infants no food or drink other than breast milk unless medically indicated
> 7. Practice rooming-in to allow mothers and infants to remain together 24 hours a day
> 8. Encourage breastfeeding on demand
> 9. Give no artificial teats or pacifiers to breastfeeding infants
> 10. Foster the establishment of breastfeeding support groups, and refer mothers to them on discharge from the hospital or clinic.
>
> *Source:* World Health Organization, UNICEF. *Protecting, Promoting and Supporting Breastfeeding: The Special Role of Maternity Services.* Geneva, Switzerland: WHO; 1989. http://whqlibdoc.who.int/publications/9241561300.pdf. Reprinted by permission of World Health Organization Press.

---

researchers found that only 7% of women surveyed experienced all five steps. Women who experienced none of the steps were approximately 8 times more likely to discontinue breastfeeding before 6 weeks postpartum. The more steps that women experienced, the greater the likelihood of continuation of breastfeeding after 6 weeks postpartum. The strongest risk factors for early breastfeeding termination were late breastfeeding initiation and supplementation of the newborn, with or without maternal knowledge.[23]

Implementation of WHO's Ten Steps has been shown to positively affect both rates of initiation and rates of exclusivity.[24] Infants who are breastfed for 6 months exclusively experience less morbidity from gastrointestinal infection than do infants who become partially breastfed at 3 to 4 months of age.[25]

In 2011, the CDC issued a press release offering funds to increase the number of Baby-Friendly hospitals in the United States, with the ultimate goal being to support breastfeeding and improve maternity practices. Barriers to implementing the Baby-Friendly Hospital Initiative include the influences of formula company marketing, lack of training of healthcare staff, inadequate leadership of the practice change process, and lack of endorsement by establishment and local government.[25]

Peer Support

La Leche League is a community peer support group that provides mother-to-mother support for those who are breastfeeding their infants. Seven women founded this organization in the 1950s with the idea of providing peer support, information, and education for women within the communities they served. Today, La Leche League is an international organization and has helped to improve the rates of breastfeeding worldwide, thereby improving global health.[26]

Anatomy and Physiology of Lactation

Prior to 2005, midwives tended to share information with women about breastfeeding based on knowledge derived from a 140-year-old model of breast anatomy. The Cooper model of anatomy was first published in 1860 and relied primarily on postmortem analysis of the breast. In the twenty-first century, ultrasound-guided anatomy studies of the human breast of a living woman have demonstrated vast differences between the actual breast and the previous operational model of breast anatomy. **Figure 36-2** compares the old and new breast anatomy models.

Anatomy of the Lactating Breast

Today's model describes the breast tissue as including two major divisions: the parenchyma and the stroma. The parenchyma includes the milk ducts. Rather than being a symmetrical tree-like system of ducts as previously believed, the ductal system is random and intertwined, with ducts often intersecting as they reach the nipple–areolar complex. There are far fewer ducts than previously assumed—approximately 9 to 10 per breast, rather than the 22 ducts the Cooper model describes. The ducts open onto the surface of the nipple and the lobular alveolar structure.

Contrary to the Cooper model, there is no evidence of a lactiferous sinus, and this structure is no longer referred to or accepted as a part of breast anatomy. It is likely that this misconception was born out of the methodology used for Cooper's study of the breast, which involved injecting colored wax into the milk ducts in anatomic studies of cadaver breasts.

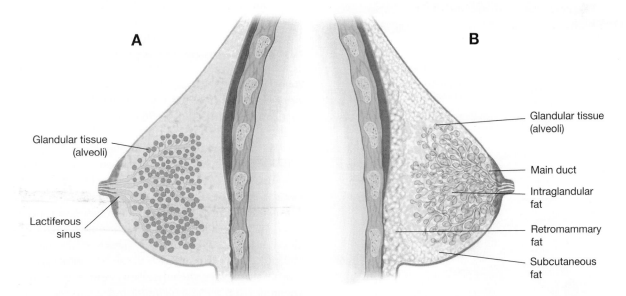

Figure 36-2 Drawing of the gross anatomy of the lactating breast based on ultrasound observations made of the milk duct system and distribution of different tissues within the breast. (A) Traditional schematic with presence of lactiferous sinuses near the nipple and glandular tissue deeper in the breast. (B) Ductal anatomy based on the findings of Ramsey et al. Milk ducts are small and branch a short distance from the base of the nipple. The glandular tissue is distributed superficially beneath the nipple and extending back toward the chest wall.

Source: © Medela 2008. Used with permission.

This wax subsequently collected at the base of the ducts closest to the nipple, where it distended the duct both by weight and positive pressure of the wax injection. From this larger and distended area, the concept of the lactiferous sinus was theorized.

The stroma includes the connective tissue, fat (adipose) tissue, blood vessels, lymphatics, and Cooper's ligaments. The glandular tissue where the milk is formed is interspersed throughout the breast, with more than 65% of the glandular tissue being located in a 30-mm radius from the base of the nipple.

The functional unit of milk making is the alveolus. The alveolar epithelial cells produce milk and excrete it into the lumen of the alveolar sac. The alveoli are surrounded by myoepithelial cells, which contract under the influence of oxytocin. The contraction then causes the milk to be ejected into the ductules and ducts that connect to the nipple pores (**Figure 36-3**).[27]

The skin of the breast includes the nipple and the areola, the area that surrounds the nipple. The nipple is composed of elastic tissue that contains smooth muscle fibers and is innervated by both sensory and autonomic nerve endings. The composition of the nipple enables it to become smaller and firmer in response to cold, touch, and sexual stimulation under the influence of oxytocin. Surrounding the nipple, the areola is a circular area, also elastic and usually more darkly pigmented than the general skin of the breast. The size of the areola varies from woman to woman.

Montgomery's tubercles have the appearance of small pimples on the areola that appear during pregnancy and lactation. They secrete a substance that is both lubricating and antimicrobial.

During pregnancy, the weight of the breast increases by approximately 200 g to an average of 400–600 grams, whereas the lactating breast weighs an average of 600–800 grams. In the first trimester of pregnancy, the woman's breasts respond to the changing levels of circulating hormones with rapid ductular–lobular–alveolar growth. This can happen even before abdominal girth begins to increase and is part of the first phase of lactogenesis.

Lactogenesis

Milk production, referred to as lactogenesis, occurs in four separate stages (**Table 36-2**).

Lactogenesis I

During the third month of pregnancy, a secretory material known as colostrum begins to appear under the influence of prolactin, and in the last trimester the alveoli become filled with colostrum. By weeks 16 to 18 of pregnancy, the breast is fully prepared for lactation, the physiologic completion of the reproductive cycle. Lactogenesis I takes place during the last half of pregnancy, when lobules increase in number and size, and alveoli epithelial cells become secretory cells.

Lactogenesis II

The sudden drop in progesterone levels that occur once the placenta is delivered is the trigger for the second stage of lactogenesis. Lactogenesis II is referred to as onset of copious milk secretion. Lactogenesis II is noted clinically as a sudden fullness or "engorgement" of the breasts approximately 30 to 72 hours postpartum, although if a woman has had a cesarean birth it may take as long as 96 hours and occasionally longer for milk secretion to be clinically apparent.

Lactogenesis II involves both milk synthesis and milk ejection. Two different hormones work in tandem to coordinate the functions. Suckling stimulates the secretion of prolactin by the anterior pituitary. Plasma concentrations of prolactin increase rapidly once suckling starts. Prolactin initiates milk production by the alveolar cells. Suckling also causes the posterior pituitary to release oxytocin, which causes the myoepithelial cells to contract, ejecting the milk from the alveoli and lobules into the ducts. Oxytocin has many complex roles , many of which are not yet fully elucidated. This hormone promotes mother–infant bonding by having a calming effect on mother and infant, lowers maternal blood pressure, decreases cortical levels, and decreases anxiety and aggressive behaviors.[28]

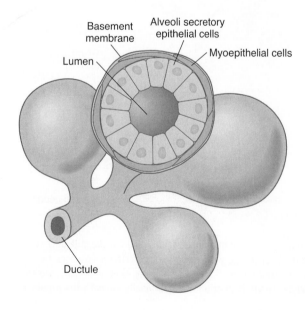

Figure labels: Lumen, Basement membrane, Alveoli secretory epithelial cells, Myoepithelial cells, Ductule

Figure 36-3 Anatomy of the alveoli of the breast.

Table 36-2	Stages of Lactogenesis	
Stage	Description	When This Stage Occurs
Lactogenesis I	Cytologic and enzymatic differentiation of alveolar cells; uptake of the substrates for milk begins, small fat droplets and some proteins are produced that become colostrum	Starts at approximately 16 weeks' gestation and ends approximately 2 days after birth
Lactogenesis II	Colostrum ends and mature milk begins to form	Takes place from approximately 30 to 72 hours postpartum; may take up to 96 hours after cesarean birth
Lactogenesis III	Formation of large amounts of breast milk	End of lactogenesis II until weaning
Lactogenesis IV	Involution of mammary gland and apoptosis of alveolar cells	Begins when the woman chooses to wean; ends after approximately 40 days, with variation based on the abruptness of the weaning process

Several factors are implicated in delayed onset of lactogenesis II including maternal intravenous fluid loads in labor, type 1 diabetes, gestational diabetes, polycystic ovary syndrome, cesarean birth, retained placental fragments, ovarian theca lutein cysts, hypothyroidism, certain types of breast surgery, and severe maternal anemia.[29,30]

Obesity is also associated with delayed lactogenesis.[31] Women who are obese have a lowered prolactin response to suckling. In addition they are at higher risk for several interventions that delay lactogenesis such as prolonged labor and cesarean birth. The larger nipples may be difficult for the newborn to grasp. Without nipple stimulation, prolactin levels drop to those of nonpregnant, nonlactating women within 2 weeks postpartum. Thus women who are obese can need intensive support in the early postpartum period.[31]

In addition, several fetal conditions can result in delayed lactogenesis II, including ineffective or weak suck, palate abnormalities, tongue-tie, and congenital heart defects.[31] Proper evaluation through laboratory studies and physical examination may yield some information about the cause of the delayed lactogenesis. Proper management of the underlying causes, as well as supportive care for the mother–baby dyad, can help to ensure a healthy nursing relationship.

Lactogenesis III

Lactogenesis III, which is also referred to as galactopoiesis, refers to the establishment of mature milk and a switch to autocrine or local control of lactation. Nipple stimulation occurs through infant suckling and provides the impetus for continued prolactin release. Milk removal stimulates milk synthesis; alternatively, if milk is not removed, secretion slows and ceases over a period of days. The rate of milk synthesis and the amount of milk produced may vary from one breast to the other, according to the frequency of suckling and the amount of milk removed.

During suckling, oxytocin is released as the nipple is stimulated and stretched as well as through sensory pathways when the mother sees, feels, touches, or hears stimuli that remind her of the infant and breastfeeding. If the infant does not suckle, the levels of oxytocin return to baseline.

Lactogenesis IV

The mammary gland involutes, or regresses, during and after weaning but never fully returns to its prepregnancy state. During involution, the alveolar cells undergo apoptosis, any remaining secretion is absorbed, and adipose tissue increases within the breast. Complete involution occurs approximately 40 days after cessation of breastfeeding, although variations may occur depending on whether the weaning process is abrupt or gradual.

Prenatal Assessment

Items to be addressed the prenatal evaluation for breastfeeding are listed in **Box 36-3**. The initial opportunity to assess and prepare a woman for breastfeeding is during a woman's initial visit for pregnancy care. This visit includes a history, physical examination, and assessment of psychosocial factors that may present challenges to breastfeeding or require additional resources for support. Such factors may include

---

BOX 36-3 Prenatal Assessment for Breastfeeding

I. History
   a. Past medical history
      i. History of breast surgery: augmentation or reduction
      ii. Breast cancer: mastectomy or lumpectomy
      iii. Breast pain
      iv. Galactorrhea
   b. Psychosocial history
      i. History of abuse
      ii. Prior unsuccessful breastfeeding
      iii. Family or support persons attitudes toward breastfeeding
      iv. Cultural beliefs about breastfeeding
II. Physical examination
   a. Inspection
      i. Breast symmetry and shape
      ii. Nipple type
   b. Palpation
      i. Four-quadrant breast examination
      ii. Presence or absence of breast tissue in axilla
      iii. Nipple discharge

---

current health conditions, as well as partner, family, and community attitudes toward breastfeeding.

Any history of sexual trauma or abuse should be discussed with regard to the plan for breastfeeding once a therapeutic relationship has been established because it may trigger underlying stressors that could affect the breastfeeding relationship. As many as 1 in 3 women have been sexually assaulted in their lifetime, and this type of trauma affects the function of at least 20% of adult survivors.[32] As part of the discussion of breastfeeding, the healthcare provider can emphasize the functional role of the breast rather than the sexualization of the breast, as often seen in American culture.[32] Women and their families may benefit from community support services and/or mental health services in addition to the support provided at prenatal visits, to prepare for a healthy breastfeeding relationship.

A bilateral examination of each of the four quadrants of the breast—upper outer, upper inner, lower outer, and lower inner—is essential. Clear or milky nipple discharge noted for the first time during later pregnancy is generally benign and signals normal changes consistent with preparation for lactation. Breast symmetry, noting size and shape, should be documented during the physical examination. Asymmetry may be a marker of one breast lacking in functional tissue.

Wide variations exist in nipple type. Some types of nipples are more likely to facilitate successful breastfeeding than others.[33] **Figure 36-4** illustrates several types of nipples.

Prenatal Counseling Regarding Breastfeeding

A direct question such as "Do you plan to breastfed or bottle-feed?" should be avoided. This closed-ended question implies equality of the methods and often results in a monosyllabic answer that makes further discussion difficult. Instead, the midwife should begin the discussion of infant feeding plans with an open-ended question such as "What have people told you about breastfeeding?" or "What do you think breastfeeding will be like for you?" Pregnancy is the optimal time to deal with misconceptions and to explore information gaps. Listen carefully for indications of self-doubt or misinformation—for example, comments such as "No one in my family makes enough milk," "My breasts are too big [or too small]," or "I tried before and the baby never latched on"—and provide support to the pregnant woman by clarifying and teaching.

If a woman has experienced difficulty initiating or continuing breastfeeding with a prior infant, it may be wise to refer her to a lactation consultant during the prenatal period for a consultation. Even if the reason for the difficulty in breastfeeding does not appear to have been physical in nature, but rather an issue of support, referral may provide the psychological support she needs to breastfeed successfully following her current pregnancy. If a woman has had positive previous breastfeeding experiences, these should be discussed as well. How did breastfeeding work out before? What was positive about the experience? What would she do differently this time? This discussion is especially important if the woman stopped breastfeeding before she intended to wean her child.

Ask the pregnant woman what she is doing to prepare for breastfeeding. Preparation of the nipple tissue is unnecessary and should be discouraged. Such activities would include nipple stimulation such as "rolling" or scrubbing with washcloths or the improper use of nipple shields or pumps. These measures are not helpful for protractility of the nipple for breastfeeding, and they may cause tissue trauma that serves as a subsequent route of infection.

Type of Nipple	Before Stimulation	After Stimulation
The majority of mothers have what is referred to as a **common nipple**. It protrudes slightly when at rest and becomes erect and more graspable when stimulated. A baby has no trouble finding and grasping this nipple to pull in a large amount of breast tissue and stretch it to the roof of his or her mouth.	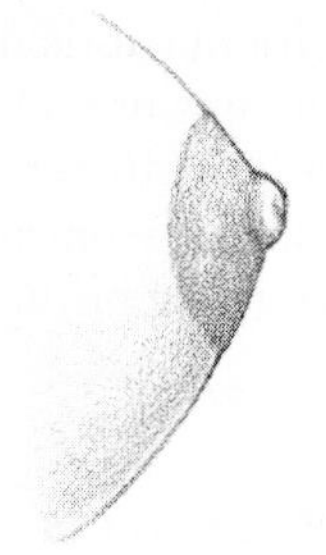	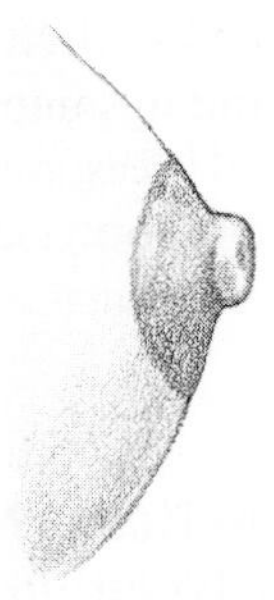
The **flat nipple** has a very short shank that makes it less easy for the baby to find and grasp. In response to stimulation, slight movement inward or outward may be present, but not enough to aid the baby in finding and initially grasping the breast on center.	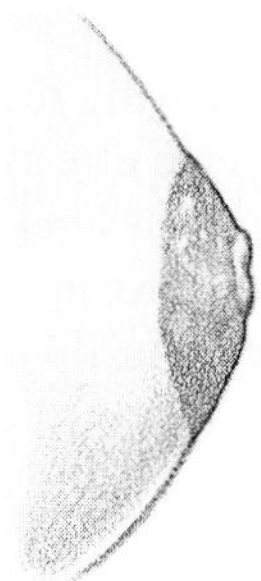	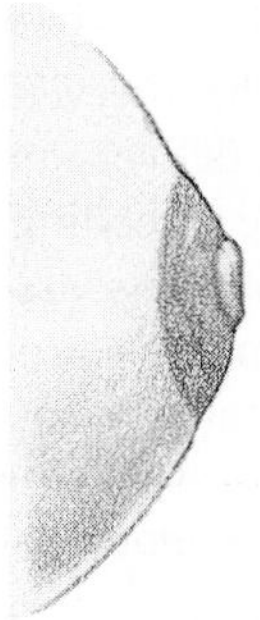
An **inverted-appearing nipple** may appear inverted but becomes erect and easily graspable after stimulation.	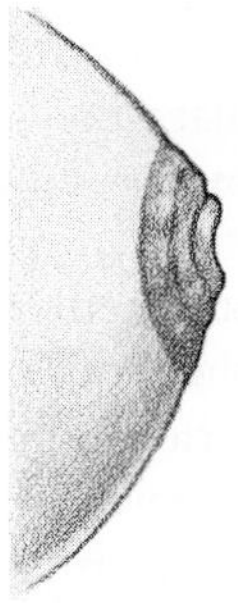	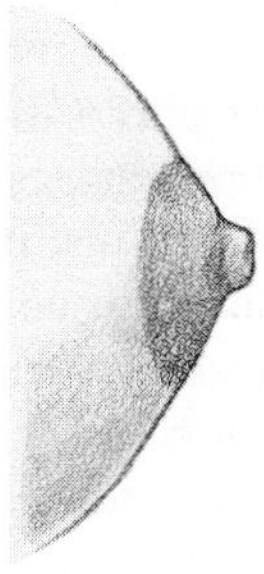
The **retracted nipple** is the most common type of inverted nipple. On stimulation it retracts, making attachment difficult.	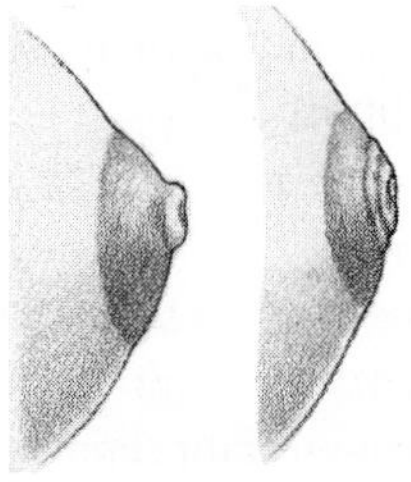	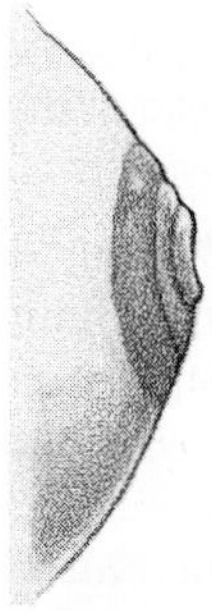
The truly **inverted nipple** is retracted both at rest and when stimulated. Such a nipple is very uncommon and more difficult for the baby to grasp.	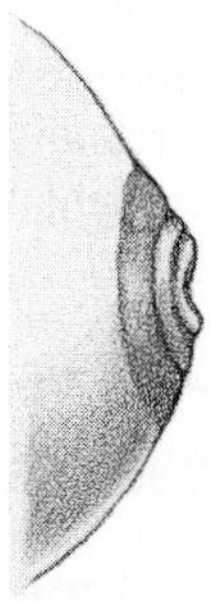	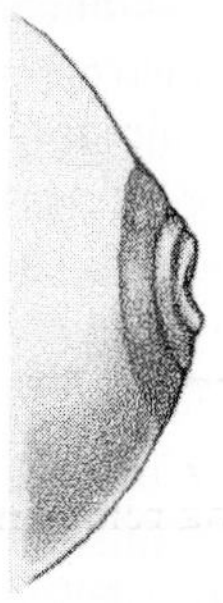

Figure 36-4 Five basic types of nipples.

Source: International Lactation Consultant Association; Mannel R, Martens PJ, Walker M, eds. *Core Curriculum for Lactation Consultant Practice.* 3rd ed. Burlington, MA: Jones & Bartlett Learning; 2013.

If the woman has limited financial resources, she will benefit from a referral to the local Women, Infants, and Children (WIC) program for nutritional support, and in some states, from programs providing optional breast pumps and supplies. Anticipatory guidance and strategizing may be of value for women who have to return to work soon after giving birth.

Birth Practices That Have Adverse Effects on Breastfeeding

Many of the interventions routinely used during the labor and delivery process can have adverse effects on the breastfeeding relationship. Often, these effects are not discussed either during the informed decision-making process for birth or prior to their implementation.

Epidural Analgesia

The relationship between epidural analgesia and breastfeeding initiation and continuation is controversial. Observational studies have found that women with epidural analgesia are less likely to successfully breastfeed,[34,35] but the studies are confounded by many factors that could have an independent effect on breastfeeding such as oxytocin use, longer duration of labor, maternal–newborn separation, and varying doses and varying drugs used in the epidural. Although it is not possible to state conclusively that epidural analgesia adversely affects breastfeeding, women who have epidural analgesia may have many reasons to need extra lactation support.[34,35]

Operative Vaginal Delivery

Delivery of the infant with the assistance of vacuum or forceps often necessitates immediate evaluation of the newborn, resulting in maternal–infant separation. In addition, operative vaginal birth increases the risk of impaired suckling reflex, newborn intracranial hemorrhage, and headache.[36] Women who have undergone an instrumented vaginal delivery have often had difficult labors, leaving them exhausted and fatigued—conditions that also can have a detrimental impact on breastfeeding initiation.

Suctioning

Routine bulb or DeLee suctioning of the newborn should be minimized unless clearly indicated, as it can cause physical injury to the nares, inadvertently cause infant electrolyte imbalances if gastric contents are suctioned, and result in injury to the oropharynx, including perforation of the soft palate. Such injury can affect the newborn's desire for latch for several days as a result of discomfort or pain.[37] A difficulty with latch may, in turn, affect milk production and prevent appropriate levels of oxytocin secretion for let-down. Ultimately this may have an effect on overall milk supply.

Cesarean Birth

Delivery of an infant by cesarean section can adversely affect breastfeeding for several reasons.[38] Newborns delivered via cesarean section are routinely suctioned to get rid of fluid in the upper respiratory passages that is normally excreted during the vaginal birth process. In addition, these newborns have a higher risk of developing transient tachypnea, which can result in prolonged separation of mother and infant. Women who have an indicated cesarean section are more likely to have had a prolonged labor, longer exposure to epidural analgesia, and are more likely to develop chorioamnionitis. Cesarean sections are associated with more blood loss, which can delay lactogenesis II. A key problem is that women undergoing cesarean section may not be offered skin-to-skin care in the critical first hour after birth.[39] Finally, women who experience cesarean section have incisional pain, which can make positioning for breastfeeding challenging.

Birth Practices That Facilitate Breastfeeding

Breastfeeding Initiation in the First Hour After Birth

Breastfeeding should be initiated within the first hour after birth, when neonates are most alert. Shortly after the first 2 hours of life, infants go into a state of prolonged sleep. When at all possible, breastfeeding should be initiated during this time.

Skin-to-Skin Contact

Skin-to-skin contact (also called kangaroo care) between the woman and her newborn has been proven to result in better and faster regulation of temperature, heart rate, and breathing than use of radiant warmers and is a common policy implemented in out-of-hospital births.[39,40] It is performed by placing the infant with bare skin directly upon the mother's bare skin, then covering the remaining exposed areas of the infant with a towel or blanket and a cap for the infant's head. Significant elevations of oxytocin have been found to occur in the first hour if the newborn is placed in skin-to-skin contact with the mother and skin-to-skin care is associated with improved rates of breastfeeding initiation. Skin-to-skin contact should occur immediately after birth and for the first few hours after birth. If the woman has had a cesarean birth, skin-to-skin care can be offered with the assistance of a person to help support the newborn (**Figure 36-5**). This practice has also been found to provide beneficial effects for preterm infants.[39,40]

Continuous Labor Support

In addition to being an invaluable tool to facilitate normal physiologic birth, women who have continuous labor support experience higher rates of breastfeeding.[41] Many hospitals have implemented in-hospital labor support programs. Schools of nursing and midwifery have also begun to develop community-based doula programs, which have met with high demand.

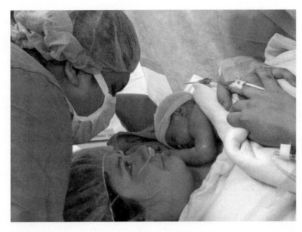

Figure 36-5 Skin-to-skin in the operating room after cesarean section.
Source: Reprinted with permission from Hung KJ, Berg O. Early skin-to-skin after cesarean to improve breastfeeding. *Matern Child Nurs.* 2011;36(5):318.

Breastfeeding: Getting Started

Assessment of the maternal–infant feeding dyad includes evaluation of five aspects: (1) prefeeding behaviors in the infant, (2) latch-on and infant suckle, (3) transfer of milk, (4) maternal comfort, and (5) signs of infant satiety.[42] Several assessment tools are available for clinicians.[43] Although none of the available tools has demonstrated superiority over others, they do help the clinician conduct a systematic assessment. Each of the tools relies on some aspect of the key assessments discussed in this section.

Prefeeding Behaviors

Neonates are extraordinarily adept at communicating when they need to breastfeed (**Table 36-3**). Newborns use their senses of touch, sight, smell, and hearing to ascertain the location of the breast, and they send cues that they are hungry through the reflexes of rooting, sucking, and wiggling their arms and legs—all early signs of breastfeeding desire. If these cues go unheeded, the infant will become increasingly frustrated and move on to different and more intense cues such as fussing and restlessness. Active crying is one of the last cues of hunger and a problematic signal of desperation. When an infant is actively crying, he or she becomes disorganized and is not easily calmed and coaxed to latch on the nipple.

There are six states of consciousness, which are defined based on the categorical variables of infant body activity, eye movements, facial movements, breathing patterns, and response to stimuli. Infants are more likely to breastfeed well when in the active alert state of consciousness. Sleep states are restorative states. While an infant may often become drowsy and fall asleep while nursing, it can be difficult to rouse an infant from a deep restorative sleep state specifically for the purposes of breastfeeding.[44]

Parents may at first be overwhelmed by the idea of reading infant readiness-to-feed cues, but with encouragement and support they can quickly adapt and immediately spot a hungry newborn when they see one. The clearer the cues are for parents, the more confidence is built in the maternal mind, and the stronger the breastfeeding dyad becomes.

Latch-on and Infant Suck

One of the most essential components of breastfeeding success is a good infant latch onto the breast. Good latch is essential for adequate milk transfer as well as the prevention of maternal nipple pain. It is most effectively facilitated with proper positioning of the infant. Physical comfort of the woman is paramount when initiating breastfeeding and implies more than a comfortable physical posture. The breastfeeding woman should have all things she may find she needs within easy reach, such as reading materials, glasses, water, or telephone. She also may find it helpful to have the aid of breastfeeding devices such as a specially designed pillow to rest the infant on during breastfeeding (although other pillows may work equally as well). The goal of optimal positioning is to bring the infant close to the breast

Table 36-3	Infant Feeding Cues and Prefeeding Behaviors	
Feeding Cue	**Timing of Cue**	**Description**
Increasing alertness	Early	Especially rapid eye movement (REM) under closed eyelids
Rooting	Early	Turning the head, especially with searching movements of the mouth
Flexing	Early	Legs and arms
Flexed arm or closed fist	Early	May bring hand toward mouth
Sucking	Early, mic	Fist or finger
Mouthing	Early	Motions made with the lips and tongue
Fussing or restlessness	Mid	
Full cry	Late	Turns red, high-pitched scream

Sources: Adapted from Cadwell K. Latching on and suckling of the healthy term neonate: breastfeeding assessment. *J Midwifery Women's Health.* 2007;52(6):638-642; Riordan J, Wambach K. *Breastfeeding and Human Lactation.* 4th ed. Sudbury, MA: Jones and Bartlett; 2010.

and prevent maternal slouching, and subsequent maternal back or nipple pain. Once a comfortable position that can be maintained is found, the process of breastfeeding can begin. The infant and mother should lay belly to belly to facilitate both comfort of the infant and effective swallowing.

Alignment is a critical component of a proper latch. The most effective alignment occurs when the infant's nose is aligned with mother's nipple. An effective technique to elicit the wide-open gape most effective in latching on is to tickle the infant's mouth with the mother's nipple. Through the senses of touch, smell, and sight, the infant begins to understand the cues for breastfeeding. Once the infant's mouth is in a wide-open gape, as demonstrated in **Figure 36-6**, the mother draws her infant to the breast. The jaw should be at a 130–150° angle with both lips flared outward.[44] There is controversy about determining whether the latch should be centered on the areola or asymmetrical, and no consensus on this issue has been reached.[42]

The infant's mouth should be completely full of breast tissue, but it may not be possible to have the entire areola in the infant's mouth given the large variety of areolar anatomy. The infant uses lips, tongue, oral cavity, jaw, facial muscles, and buccal fat pads to generate both negative and positive pressure, drawing the milk forward. The mother's hormonal response to nipple stretching and stimulation increases oxytocin circulation, which causes the myoepithelial cells to eject milk into the milk ducts; through negative and positive pressure, this milk is transferred into infant's mouth.

Important actions to avoid in latch-on include bringing the breast to the infant, moving the breast from its resting position, forcing the infant's mouth open, flexing or extending the infant's neck, and allowing the infant's arms to flail. Positions that can be used for breastfeeding are described in **Table 36-4**.

Transfer of Milk

Breastfeeding has a visible and audible rhythm. The infant suckles in a burst of short, rapid, piston-like motions of the jaw at the beginning of the feeding, followed by a slower, deeper, rocking motion as the jaw indents the breast, drawing out milk. The ratio of sucks to swallows is high in the initial piston-like phase, but then falls to 1:1 or 2:1 as the milk flows rapidly in the slower rocking phase. One can denote the presence of milk transfer from the following signs: a puff of air from the nose, a "ca" sound from the throat, deeper jaw excursion preceding each swallow, and the top of areola moving inward toward the infant's mouth.[45]

Signs of Infant Satiety: Breastfeeding Frequency

New mothers often struggle to know how often to breastfeed. While establishing a milk supply, infants should be fed on demand, as galactopoiesis operates on a positive feedback mechanism: The more an infant nurses, the more the body will make the supply needed to meet that demand. Until approximately the first month of life, infants should be nursed approximately 8 to 12 times each day. During the first days of life, it is not uncommon for an infant to cluster feed—that is, to sleep for several hours, then wake up and nurse every 30 to 60 minutes for a period of time. Feeding frequency becomes more predictable once the milk supply is established and the infant

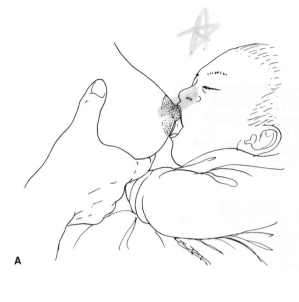

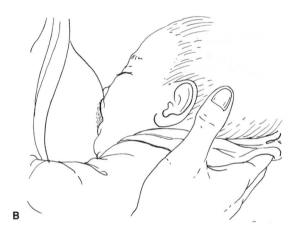

Figure 36-6 Latch-on. (A) Mouth gaped open. (B) Grasping breast.

Source: Riordan J, Wambach K. *Breastfeeding and Human Lactation.* 4th ed. Sudbury, MA: Jones and Bartlett; 2010.

ages. By the end of the second month of life, infants nurse 7 to 9 times each day. Some women report that breastfed babies eat more frequently than their bottle-fed counterparts, which may be explained by the easy digestibility of breast milk, which, therefore, requires more frequent feeding sessions.

Common Breastfeeding Problems

Pain is one of the most common reasons given for why women discontinue breastfeeding.[46] Consequently, prompt evaluation, treatment, and support are essential whenever a woman reports pain associated with breastfeeding.

Engorgement

Breast engorgement is a swelling of the breast tissue due to congestion of breast milk. Engorgement occurs most commonly during the initiation of breastfeeding and during times of weaning. An engorged breast is edematous and often painful. Engorged breasts due to milk stasis should be carefully monitored and steps taken to avoid progression to mastitis, which is an inflammation—either infective or noninfective—of the breast tissue.

The best remedy for engorgement is prevention, which entails frequent nursing of the infant to keep the breast empty. Some lactation consultants recommend emptying one breast in its entirety first before offering the opposite breast, then offering the other breast first at the next nursing session to ensure proper and complete drainage.

If prevention is not possible and the breast becomes severely engorged, it will cause the nipple to flatten and make latch difficult. This edema can also cause inhibition of milk duct dilation, preventing appropriate milk flow. In such a case, it will be necessary to relieve some of the edema preventing proper milk flow, which may be achieved by applying ice packs prior to nursing, using anti-inflammatory medication, and using massage to mobilize lymph drainage through hand expression of the milk just until the nipple is soft. Overstimulation of the breast may prolong engorgement. Heat is not appropriate for relieving engorgement or for encouraging milk flow. Once milk is flowing, the best method of milk removal and relief of the edema is to nurse the infant directly. If for some reason the infant cannot successfully nurse, then a manual or electric pump may be employed.[47]

Plugged Ducts

Plugged ducts are a fairly common occurrence in the early weeks of breastfeeding and are usually attributed to restriction of milk flow due to internal or external pressure (e.g., engorgement, tight bras and clothing). Women should be encouraged to feed their infants frequently, preferentially offering the affected breast first, when the infant is hungriest, to attempt to drain the plugged areas. Many clinicians suggest changing the orientation of the infant's position so that the infant's chin points to the plugged segment of the breast. This approach is thought to focus the massaging action of the tongue on the plugged area.

When assessing the lactating breast that has a plugged duct, a close assessment of a woman's breast for signs of bra indentations, bruises, and other trauma is indicated. Watching the woman and infant

Table 36-4	Common Body Positions for Breastfeeding		
Position	**Description**	**Advantages**	**Graphic**
Cradle or Madonna position	The infant is side-lying, facing the mother, with the side of the head and body resting on the mother's forearm of the arm next to the breast to be used.	This is the most commonly used nursing position and tends to feel most natural for the mother. However, it offers the least amount of control over the infant's head.	
Cross-cradle posture	The infant is side-lying, facing the mother, with the side resting on the mother's forearm of the arm on the opposite side of the breast being used.	This posture is considered especially useful for the mother of a newborn or preterm infant. It offers greater control over the infant's head	
Football or clutch	A sitting position in which the infant lies on her or his back, curled between the side of the mother's chest and her arm. The infant's upper body is supported by the mother's forearm. The mother's hand supports the infant's neck and shoulders. The infant's hips are flexed up along the chair back or other surface that the mother is leaning against.	This position is helpful for women post cesarean section and those who have large pendulous breasts or are nursing multiple infants.	
Semi-reclining	The mother leans back and the infant lies against her body, in chest-to-chest contact, usually prone.	This is the most comfortable position for women recovering from a cesarean section, those who have large pendulous breasts, and those who choose to co-sleep with their infants.	
Side-lying	The mother lies on her side. The infant is side-lying, chest to chest with the mother. The mother's arm closest to the mattress supports the infant's back.	This position is helpful for women who have had a cesarean section or have large or pendulous breasts.	
Australian	The mother is "down-under," lying on her back, with the infant supported on her chest.	This posture allows the infant to be in maximal control of the feeding and is especially valuable when the milk flow is faster than the infant can handle.	

Source: Adapted from International Lactation Consultant Association; Mannel R, Martens PJ, Walker M, eds. *Core Curriculum for Lactation Consultant Practice*. 3rd ed. Burlington, MA: Jones & Bartlett; 2013.

closely throughout a feeding may demonstrate mal-positioning or breast compression. Most problems are multifactorial. Rarely, plugs that do not respond to treatment may be unrelated to breastfeeding; if they do not resolve within 24 to 48 hours, the woman should be referred for further evaluation, including ultrasound imaging. Breast cancer has been detected in the lactating breast. Milk retention cysts, known as galactoceles, are thought to be unusual products of plugged ducts and may be visualized by ultrasound. Upon aspiration, these cysts are found to contain milk. They will typically refill with milk after aspiration. Galactoceles are not a contraindication to breastfeeding.

Nipple Pain

While initial nipple pain during the first week of breastfeeding is normal, nipple pain in women who have established lactation is not normal. Nipple pain can variously be reported as stinging, itching, burning, or even dull and stabbing pain. The usual cause of nipple pain is an improper latch. Additional differential diagnoses include atopic dermatitis, eczema, damage from irritation from nipple shields or other breastfeeding devices, yeast or bacterial infections, Raynaud's syndrome, or, very rarely, Paget's disease.

Nipples infected with *C. albicans* usually appear very shiny red and may have flaking of the skin around the nipple or cracks in the areola.[48] Because women with severe nipple infections can have a concurrent bacterial infection in nipple fissures, treatment is three-pronged:

1. A topical azole cream is used to treat a *C. albicans* infection of the nipple and areola. Nystatin (Mycostatin) has been the first-line treatment for many years, but approximately 40% of *C. albicans* infections are now resistant to nystatin.[48] Therefore miconazole (Monistat-Derm) or clotrimazole (Lotrimin) are better choices.

2. A topical antibiotic such as mupirocin (Bactroban) is added to cover *Staphylococcus aureus*.

3. A low- or mid-corticosteroid cream can be added to treat inflammation and facilitate healing.

The mother–infant dyad should be treated together, so a prescription for nystatin is also given for treating infant thrush.

Ductal Candida

While one traditionally thinks of *Candida* infections as related to nipple pain, such an infection can also proliferate and infiltrate the milk ducts, resulting in severe, primarily bilateral breast pain in addition to the usual nipple pain. Women report itching, burning, and sometimes a shooting pain through the nipple upon let-down described as "shards of glass."

Ductal *Candida* is more challenging to treat than the same infection on the nipple or areola. Although not approved by the Food and Drug Administration (FDA) for this use, oral fluconazole (Diflucan) may be prescribed. A regimen consisting of a loading dose of 200–400 mg followed by 100–200 mg daily for 10 to 14 days has been effective.[48] One must have a high suspicion for ductal *Candida* based on the clinical features of the infection—which include shiny, flaky skin of the areola, stabbing or non-stabbing pain of the breast, and sore nipples—prior to prescribing fluconazole, given that there are limited studies on the safety and efficacy of this medication.[48]

Breastfeeding Complications

Inadequate Milk Supply

Perceived lack of milk supply is the most common reason for discontinuation of breastfeeding.[49] In the absence of significant infant weight loss suggesting failure to thrive, this is often not an appropriate assessment.

One method to determine whether the milk supply and transfer is appropriate is to assess the infant's elimination patterns. Within the first 2 days of life, a newborn should have at least one thick, tarry bowel movement each day, as infants eliminate their meconium. During days 3–4, the infant should have one to three black to green to yellow stools, which become progressively looser and increase in volume. By days 4–7, infants should have one to four bowel movements each day of a yellow, seedy consistency that appear loose or runny. The frequency of bowel movements increases to three to six or more times each day for babies of 1 to 6 weeks of age. By 6 months of life, infants may have three to five or more bowel movements each day. At this point it is not uncommon for bowel elimination not to occur every day. If an infant is still passing meconium on day 5 or is not urinating or stooling at all regardless of day of life, the neonatal provider should be alerted.

Urination patterns also increase as the mother's milk supply is established. The first 2 days of life should yield at least 2 wet diapers. By day 6, newborns should produce 6 to 8 wet diapers or more in a 24-hour period. The newer and highly absorbent disposable diapers can make it difficult to determine the amount of urine the newborn has eliminated. One way of helping this is to place a tissue in the bottom of the infant's diaper to assess moisture content. One may also consider using cloth diapers or weighing the diapers before and after use.

Perceived milk insufficiency is a common concern for women whose infants are hospitalized in the neonatal intensive care unit. These mother–infant dyads, given the severity of prematurity and ability of the infant to suckle, may have problems establishing lactogenesis. This problem can be addressed with the help of an electric breast pump and perhaps, if appropriate, a supplemental nursing system and consultation with a lactation consultant. "Hands-on pumping," which entails manual stimulation of the breasts while using an electric pump, has been shown to increase milk supply more than use of the electric pump without manual stimulation.

Women who have undergone breast surgery often have concerns regarding milk production and capacity. While it is generally accepted that augmentation surgery poses no issues with breastfeeding, reduction mammoplasty has been considered a surgical procedure that can impair breastfeeding. Healthcare workers have often counseled that it is possible to breastfeed depending on the type of surgical technique used with reduction mammoplasty. The belief has been that if the nipple and milk ducts were on a pedicle and were not severed during the surgery, then milk production and delivery will be preserved. However, should the ducts have been severed, the prediction has been that no or limited breastfeeding will be possible. According to a 2010 systematic review that examined the effects of reduction mammoplasty from 1950 to 2008, this is not the case.[50] Thibodeaux et al. found that there was no difference in milk production or capacity regardless of surgical technique.[50] Furthermore, the authors cited healthcare workers' advice and counseling related to the breast surgery as a barrier to effective breastfeeding.[50] They concluded that women should be counseled that it is possible and advisable to breastfeed for the first 6 months of life.[50]

Additionally, women who have adopted infants may wish to engage in a breastfeeding experience. Unfortunately, these women do not have the benefit of any of the stages of lactogenesis on which they can rely the same way as if their body had carried the pregnancy. Efforts toward lactation are more likely to be effective if they have breastfed before.

Failed or Delayed Lactogenesis

Some women do experience delayed or failed lactogenesis despite early interventions. Diagnosing failed or delayed lactogenesis is done by assessing a number of criteria, including fewer than the appropriate number of stools or wet diapers per day of life, more than 7% infant weight loss or continued weight loss after day 3 postpartum, no audible swallowing form the infant, minimal or absent breast changes by day 5 postpartum, or an irritable or lethargic infant.[50]

Women who are at risk for delayed or failed lactogenesis include women who have an underlying endocrine condition, such as diabetes, thyroid disease, or a pituitary problem, as well as those who may have retained placental fragments, theca-lutein cysts, or polycystic ovary syndrome (PCOS).[51] There is some evidence that women with very little breast tissue may have difficulty supporting the infant's nutritional needs and increasing evidence that women who are obese may experience delayed lactogenesis. One sign of insufficient glandular tissue is a lack of breast growth during pregnancy.

Treatment for true failed lactogenesis is not available. Treatments for delayed lactogenesis may have more effectiveness. Above all, infant nutrition should be provided as the mother continues to promote breastfeeding practices, keep milk-pumping logs, and perform infant test weights prior to and after each feeding.[51]

Galactagogues

At this time, the American Academy of Breastfeeding Medicine does not recommend any specific pharmacologic or herbal remedies due to these preparations' untoward side effects or lack of evidence regarding their effectiveness. Commonly used galactagogues are listed in **Table 36-5**. Domperidone (Motilium), a dopamine agonist, is a medication that has been used in the past with the goal of increasing milk supply, particularly with pump-dependent mothers. While evidence exists that it may be an extremely effective agent for increasing milk production,[52] the FDA has recommended that domperidone not be used, as it has shown to result in QT-segment elevation on EKG, which in rare cases may be fatal.

Metoclopramide (Reglan) is another pharmacologic agent frequently used to increase milk supply, although its reliability in doing so is based on studies of poorer strength. This medication increases prolactin levels, which in turn increases milk production. There is controversy regarding whether the dose should be tapered at the time of cessation. Rare and more severe side effects of metoclopramide include central nervous system (CNS) effects, such as tardive dyskinesia, which prompted the FDA to use issue a "black box" warning to be placed on the drug's

Table 36-5	Commonly Used Galactagogues		
Medication Generic (Brand)	**Drug Classification**	**Dose**	**Comments**
Metoclopramide (Reglan)	Central dopamine antagonist	10 mg orally three times a day for 10 days or 10 mg orally once on day 1, 10 mg twice on day 2, 10 mg three times on days 3–10, 10 mg twice on day 11, 10 mg once on day 12 or 15 mg three times per day orally days 1–7, 10 mg three times on day 8, 5 mg three times on day 9	On regimen 1, after a mean interval 3.4 days, 8 of 12 women with complete lactation failure and 20 of 20 mothers with partial failure responded with increased milk production. Those with complete failure maintained improved lactation throughout an 8-week follow-up period. However, supplementation was required. Thirty-five percent of mothers with partial failure eliminated supplemental feedings completely within 11 days of therapy. Women may have fewer side effects with regimen 2.
Fenugreek	Greek hayseed	2–3 capsules orally three times per day until adequate milk production occurs or 1 cup of tea 3 times a day until adequate milk production occurs	The capsules are usually considered to be more effective than the tea. Fenugreek is commonly used as a culinary spice by Eastern Indian women.
Oxytocin	Endogenous nonapeptide hormone	1 spray of 40 U/mL in each nostril (3 units) prior to breast milk expression for 7 days	Use of the nasal spray resulted in a 3- to 5-fold increase in milk production in primiparas and a 2-fold increase in multiparas. Chronic use of the nasal spray has led to dependence. Limit use to 7 days.
Domperidone (Motilium)	Peripheral dopamine antagonist	Ranges from 10 mg to 30 mg orally tid for 7 days. Usually 10–20 mg is given.	Domperidone is contraindicated for use as a galactagogue in the United States secondary to the possibility that this drug can induce cardiac arrhythmias.

Source: Adapted from Betzold CM. Galactagogues. *J Midwifery Women's Health.* 2004;49:151-154. Reprinted with permission of Wiley.

label, advising against prolonged use or high doses of the drug.

Fenugreek is an herbal remedy that is often used to boost milk production. This herb comes in formulations such as teas and herbal capsules. Studies have suggested there is a placebo effect with its use, rather than an actual increase in milk production. Usual doses are 3 capsules 3 times a day.[53]

More commonly accepted and effective methods for increasing milk supply include, first and foremost, improved breastfeeding practice. Included in these interventions are evaluation of the mother–baby pair for proper latch, increased skin-to-skin contact,

alleviation of any nipple pain that may be present, encouraging the woman to perform breast self-massage to promote release of oxytocin, cessation of unnecessary supplementation, use of an electric breast pump between feedings to mimic autocrine response, and evaluation of preexisting medical conditions, such as abnormal thyroid-stimulating hormone (TSH) levels, diabetes, use of medications that may inhibit milk production, smoking, or excessive alcohol use.[54]

Women have exclusively breastfed twins, triplets, and quadruplets. The demand of multiple infants suckling appears to drive the milk supply, just as it does with singletons. Early, frequent breastfeeding (or expressing milk if the infants are premature) will optimize the woman's long-term ability to produce milk. Midwives may refer women to a lactation consultant or La Leche League for assistance with positioning and caring for multiple infants.

Mastitis

Mastitis refers to an inflammation in which one or more segments of the breast appear to be hot, red, and inflamed. The clinical presentation of mastitis ranges in severity. Some women present with only focal painful inflammation, whereas others present with systemic symptoms that include elevated temperatures and a feeling of malaise. Rarely mastitis will present as septicemia. In addition, the role of pathogenic bacteria in mastitis is unclear. Mastitis is frequently classified as infective or noninfective, but it is not clear if this distinction is real. Some authors suggest mastitis is actually a spectrum of pathology that starts with milk stasis and subsequent inflammation, which may then progress to infection depending on the pathogenic potential of colonized bacteria and host response.[55,56] **Table 36-6** presents signs and symptoms associated with common breast conditions in lactating women.

Noninfective mastitis is purported to result from plugged ducts, milk stasis, and reabsorption of milk from the duct into the interstitial spaces in the breast tissue where the inflammatory response occurs. Milk contains many pro-inflammatory substances, including cytokines, as well as proteins not seen elsewhere in the body. In addition, the inflammatory response stimulated by milk stasis can cause systemic symptoms, which add to the difficulty in discerning noninfectious versus infectious mastitis.[56] Infective mastitis is often associated with nipple fissure or other trauma creating an entryway to the breast, but it can occur without a preexisting history of skin abrasion. The infective agents most commonly implicated in this type of mastitis include *Staphylococcus aureus* and coagulase-negative *Staphylococcus* (CoNS), although *Candida albicans*, *Escherichia coli*, *Enterobacteriaceae*, and *Mycobacterium tuberculosis* have also been cultured from infected breasts. Bilateral mastitis rarely occurs, but when it does, it is likely to be associated with *Streptococcus* infection. Methicillin-resistant *Staphylococcus aureus* (MRSA) mastitis has been noted in communities with a high prevalence of these bacteria.[57]

The incidence of mastitis in lactating women is reported to range from 9.5% to 30% within the first 3 months postpartum. This range probably reflects differing definitions and populations.[58,59] Regardless of the exact incidence, mastitis is a common postpartum condition that is associated with significant morbidity for those affected.

Diagnosis of Mastitis

The diagnosis of mastitis is made clinically on the basis of a localized, unilateral area of erythema with associated fever ($\geq$ 38.5°C [101°F]) and feelings of malaise, flu-like symptoms, and fatigue.

Breast milk cultures are rarely helpful in making the diagnosis of mastitis, for several reasons. Breast milk has antibacterial components, milk expression can dilute colony counts, and women without symptoms of mastitis frequently have breast milk colonized with the bacteria commonly found on skin. The one exception occurs when a woman has recurrent mastitis despite adequate treatment. In this situation, MRSA should be considered, and culturing the breast milk is indicated to determine the etiologic agent and plan appropriate antibiotic treatment.

Because it is difficult to distinguish between infective and noninfective mastitis, treatment of mastitis in the United States starts with empirical treatment using dicloxacillin (Dycill) in doses of 500 mg four times daily for 10 to 14 days. Shorter courses have been shown to result in higher risk of reinfection[60] (**Table 36-7**). Women should be encouraged to complete a full course of antibiotic treatment, as mastitis has been noted to reoccur following incomplete treatment.

Ensuring adequate drainage of the affected breast is crucial for the resolution of this condition and is accomplished through continued breastfeeding. Women should be assisted to improve and/or maintain appropriate latch and attachment. A sudden change in feeding frequency, such as a delay or a skipped feeding, with subsequent milk stasis is enough to trigger mastitis in some women.[56]

Breast Abscess

An abscess is a localized collection of pus in the breast, formed by disintegrated cells and surrounded by an inflamed area (**Figure 36-7**). Unresolved mastitis can result in the formation of one or several abscesses within the breast as diagnosed via ultrasound. Most abscesses require surgical lancing and may be drained to the exterior. Exudate from the abscess should be cultured to determine appropriate antibiotic treatment. Breastfeeding on the opposite breast is desirable throughout treatment, although feeding from the affected breast is possible in many cases. The safety of breastfeeding on the affected breast is likely to depend on the location of the drain(s) and the causative agent. Milk expression via hand or pump

Table 36-6	Signs and Symptoms Associated with Common Breast Conditions in Lactating Women						
Condition	**Definition**	**Description**	**Systemic Symptoms**	**Fever**	**Pain**	**Unilateral vs. Bilateral**	**Other**
Breast fullness	The breast is full of milk but without obstruction of venous or lymphatic drainage and the milk flows readily with suckling or pumping.	Firm, heavy, no erythema	No	No	No	Usually bilateral	Occurs between postpartum days 3–5 when the "milk comes in"
Engorgement	The breast is "engorged" with milk and there is obstruction of venous and lymphatic drainage.	Hard, enlarged, shiny, bilateral erythema	May have "milk fever"	< 38.5°C	Yes	Usually bilateral	Often confused with breast fullness
Blocked ducts[a]	The breast has an area of localized milk stasis.	Single lumpy area that with erythema	Unlikely	Unlikely and if present < 38.5°C	Tender or localized pain	Usually unilateral	May occur with a painful white bleb on the nipple[b]
Galactocele	A milk-retention cyst that is thought to result from a plugged duct.	Smooth, rounded swelling	No	No	No	Usually unilateral	Compression of the cyst may cause milky fluid to exude from the nipple
Noninfectious mastitis[c]	Secondary to ineffective and/or obstructed drainage of milk from the breast.	Erythematous	Yes in 50–66% of women	Mild: < 37.5 °C Acute: > 37.5°C and < 38.5°C Hyperacute: > 38°C	Yes, localized	Usually unilateral	See note[d]
Infectious mastitis	Results from untreated milk stasis and/ or colonization with pathogenic bacteria.	Hard, usually wedged shaped. May or may not be erythematous	No in 33–50% of women	Mild: < 37.5 °C Acute: > 37.4°C and < 38.5°C Hyperacute: > 38°C	Usually	Usually unilateral but may be bilateral	See note[d]
Breast abscess	A localized area of infection that has formed a barrier of granulation tissue.	Swollen lump, possibly fluctuant, with erythema	May or may not be present		Severe	Often unilateral but may be bilateral	

[a]It may be referred to as "focal breast engorgement," "caked breast," or "plugged duct."

[b]The bleb may be opened up with a sterile needle to relieve discomfort.

[c]Also termed obstructive mastitis.

[d]The clinician cannot reliably differentiate non-infectious mastitis clinically from infectious mastitis. Treat with antibiotics if mother is toxic/acutely ill, there are severe or bilateral symptoms, there are nipple fissures, or symptom resolution doesn't occur within 12–24 hours of improved milk removal.

Source: Betzold CM. An update on the recognition and management of lactational breast inflammation. *J Midwifery Women's Health.* 2007;52:595-605. Reprinted with permission of Wiley.

Table 36-7 Treatment Options for Various Causes of Breast Inflammation

Disease	Antibiotics	Antifungal*	Other Therapy
Blocked duct/ nipple blebs	Mupirocin 2% ointment (not cream) if blocked pore (bleb) is opened.	Only if recurrent or persistent; then culture the nipple/areola, bleb if present, and milk. First-line: fluconazole (Diflucan) 200–400 mg STAT followed by 100–200 mg daily for 2–3 weeks or until blocked duct has resolved for 1 week. Consider undiagnosed maternal IgA deficiency.	If no improvement within 24–48 hours, then order therapeutic ultrasound of 2 W/cm², continuous, for 5 minutes once a day to the affected region. It may be repeated once the next day. Lecithin 1 tablespoon per day or 1200 mg 3–4 times per day can be used to prevent or treat recurrences. If problem is recurrent, have the mother limit her intake of saturated fats and increase her rest. Lecithin can also be rubbed into a bleb to soften it.
Noninfectious mastitis	If symptoms do not resolve within 12–24 hours, then treat for infectious mastitis as described next.	No.	Hot compresses, massage of affected area, frequent milk removal on affected side.
Infectious mastitis	First-line choices: Dicloxacillin (Dynapen) 500 mg qid for 10–14 days or Cephalexin (Keflex) 500 mg qid for 10–14 days If penicillin allergic, use clindamycin 300 mg qid or erythromycin 250 mg or 500 mg qid for 10–14 days.	If indicated based on cultures or the development of burning breast pain.	Same as previous entry. Cultures of milk and nipple are indicated for maternal acute illness, failure to respond to treatment, high suspicion of MRSA, and bilateral mastitis. The infant may need to be treated concurrently, particularly if group A or B Streptococcus suspected.
Recurrent mastitis	Culture and treat as appropriate for 14–30 days.	Culture and treat as appropriate for 14–30 days.	Low-dose erythromycin or clindamycin may be given on a daily or weekly basis. Consider cultures and treatment with nasal mupirocin (Bactroban) if S. aureus carrier state is suspected.
Ductal infections	Culture and treat as appropriate for at least 14 days. May be prudent to treat until symptoms resolved for at least 1 week. Can empirically start treatment with Clindamycin 300 mg qid or sulfamethoxazole-trimethoprim (Bactrim) double strength bid.	Treat with antifungals if any signs of yeast on infant. First-line: fluconazole (Diflucan) 200–400 mg STAT followed by 100–200 mg daily for 2–3 weeks or until symptoms have resolved for 1 week. Ketoconazole (Nizoral) may also be used.	Sterilize any object that comes in contact with the maternal breast, breast milk, or infant mouth (e.g., pumping parts, bottles, pacifiers, toys). Consider other family members as carriers if yeast infection is recurrent.

(continues)

Table 36-7	Treatment Options for Various Causes of Breast Inflammation *(continued)*		
Disease	**Antibiotics**	**Antifungal**[*]	**Other Therapy**
Nipple infections	Mupirocin 2% ointment (not cream): 15 g. If no improvement, culture and treat based on sensitivity results or treat empirically for yeast or consider other etiologies. Polymyxin B sulfate (Bacitracin): Apply mupirocin or polymyxin after each nursing or pumping.	Nystatin (Nilstat): • Neonate: 100,000 units/mL. Place 1 mL in cup, then swab inside of infant's mouth qid. 2 mL qid for older infants. Have infant drink what is left. • Maternal: May treat topically with nystatin (Nilstat) suspension or with cream. Apply cream or suspension after each nursing. Allow suspension to air dry or, if using cream, rub in small amount. Gentian violet 1% in 10% alcohol can be applied to the infant's mouth with a Q-tip before feeding so that the mother's nipple will be coated during the feeding. It should be used daily for 4 days, although treatment length may be extended to 7 days if there is improvement but no resolution. Clotrimazole cream (preferably Gyne-Lotrimin): Apply after each feeding/pumping and rub in well.	The topical treatment known as Dr. Newman's Famous "All-Purpose Nipple Ointment" (APNO) will treat bacterial and yeast infections. APNO is compounded and contains the following ingredients: • Mupirocin 2% ointment (not cream): 15 g • Betamethasone 0.1% ointment (not cream): 15 g Add miconazole powder to formulate a final concentration of 2% miconazole. If unavailable, substitute clotrimazole powder added to a final concentration of 2%/ Sparingly apply APNO after each feeding and use until nipple soreness has dissipated.
Abscess (puerperal)	Outpatient: dicloxacillin (Dynapen) 500 mg po qid for 10–14 days or clindamycin (Cleocin) 300 mg po qid Inpatient: nafcillin or oxacillin 2.0 g every 4 hours IV or cefazolin 1.0 g every 6 hours IV or vancomycin 1.0 g every 12 hours IV	If indicated based on cultures or if burning breast pain develops.	Incision and drainage, or use ultrasound-guided needle for aspiration. Send aspirate or discharge for culture. Infants may continue nursing on the affected side unless the area of incision involves the areola. May want to treat infant concurrently if the mother has S. aureus or streptococcal disease.

[*] If *Candida* is suspected or diagnosed, both mother and infant must be treated concurrently even if one is asymptomatic.

Source: From Betzold CM. An update on the recognition and management of lactational breast inflammation. *J Midwifery Women's Health.* 2007;52:595-605. Reprinted with permission of Wiley.

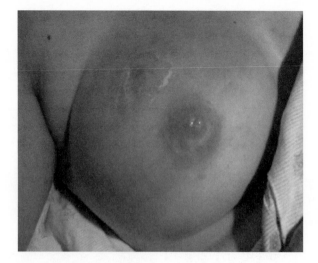

Figure 36-7 Breast abscess.

Source: Betzold CM. An update on the recognition and management of lactational breast inflammation. *J Midwifery Women's Health.* 2007;52:595-605. Reprinted with permission of Wiley.

should continue when feeding is suspended on the affected breast. Breastfeeding on the affected breast may resume after the treatment course is completed.

Breastfeeding Discontinuation

Weaning is a process of change that begins with the introduction of the first supplemental food to the infant. Weaning—whether from the breast or from the bottle—can be a stressful process for families. A gradual process of weaning is best. Weaning continues as the woman gradually replaces an increasing number of daily feedings with acceptable substitutes. Breastfeeding women will need to monitor their breasts for possible over-fullness, plugged ducts, and inflamed areas during the weaning process, as engorgement and mastitis occur most commonly during times of reduction of breastfeeding.

Contraindications for Breastfeeding

While uncommon, some situations and conditions make the choice to breastfeed inadvisable. Contraindication to breastfeeding are listed in **Table 36-8**.[61]

Infant Conditions

There are a few rare disorders wherein breastfeeding is contraindicated for the infant. Infants with galactosemia are unable to metabolize the milk sugar known as galactose. Infants with phenylketonuria

Table 36-8	Contraindications for Breastfeeding
Neonatal Contraindications	**Maternal Contraindications**
Infant diagnosed with galactosemia	Active tuberculosis
	HIV positive
	Infected with human T-cell lymphotrophic virus 1 or 2 infection
	Active use of and/or dependence on an illicit drug
	Taking prescribed chemotherapy agents for cancer (e.g., anti-metabolites that interfere with DNA replication and cell division)
	Undergoing radiation therapy (for temporary cessation)
	Taking antiretroviral medications

Source: Adapted from Centers for Disease Control and Prevention. When should a mother avoid breastfeeding? October 9, 2009. Available from: www.cdc.gov/breastfeeding/disease/index.htm. Accessed February 21, 2013.

(PKU) require special diets, but some may be partially breastfed in addition to receiving a phenylalanine-free formula.[61]

Maternal Conditions

Maternal medications may affect breastfeeding by decreasing the volume of milk, affecting the infant's behavior, or exposing the infant to undesirable concentrations of the medication. Even so, very few medications taken by breastfeeding women require complete weaning.

Breastfeeding may also need to be withheld temporarily if a lesion on the breast is suspected to be herpes simplex virus (HSV). A culture should be obtained in this situation. If the lesion is remote from the nipple–areolar complex and does not come into contact with the breast pump components, the milk may be pumped and given to the infant with a cup or bottle. In contrast, if the lesion is near the areolar complex or in any way comes in contact with the pump components, the infant should be fed formula or banked milk (from a donor milk bank) during diagnosis and treatment. The woman will need to pump for comfort and to maintain her milk supply. The pumped milk and the pump kit should be discarded once the infection has resolved.[62]

Women who are HIV positive can transmit the virus to their infant via breast milk. Current recommendations regarding HIV and breastfeeding vary from country to country and are based on perceived risks and benefits. In the United States, women who are HIV positive are advised not to breastfeed.

Formulations of Breast Milk Substitutes

Breast milk alone—that is, exclusive breastfeeding—is recommended for infants for the first 6 months of life, continuing with the addition of complementary foods for the first year and beyond.[2–4] In the event that breastfeeding is not possible or the woman chooses not to breastfeed, formula should be recommended for the first year with the addition of solid foods after about 6 months. Formula-fed infants should receive a breast milk substitute throughout the first year, then switch to whole milk until they reach 2 years of age, as the fats in whole milk are required for nerve development.

Formulas based on cow's milk are considered standard and should be the choice for formula-fed infants except those with a known allergy to cow's milk. There has been no benefit shown that justifies the use of a cow's milk substitute without iron supplementation.[63]

Soy-based formulas are reserved for infants with a proven allergy to cow's milk or if the family is adverse to the use of animal products. However, many infants who are allergic to bovine proteins will also be allergic to soy. Special formulas should be recommended only when the infant's condition is such that a standard formula cannot be tolerated—for example, if the infant has been diagnosed with phenylketonuria.

Hydrolysate formulas have had cow's milk proteins modified in varying manners depending on the manufacturer. Two types of hydrolyzed formula are available: infant formula with partially hydrolyzed protein and infant formula with extensively hydrolyzed protein. Partially hydrolyzed protein formulas are intended for feeding the normal term infant. However, because the cow's milk protein is not extensively hydrolyzed, such products are contraindicated for the infant with a cow's milk protein allergy. Extensively hydrolyzed protein formulas do not contain lactose as the carbohydrate. These products are intended for the infant with a cow's milk allergy.[63]

Docosahexaenoic acid (DHA) and arachidonic acid (ARA) formulas have added ingredients that purport to make them more like breast milk. The goal when adding these amino acids is to increase the infant's visual acuity and cognition. However, clinical trials have failed to show any efficacy in terms of improved mental and motor development. There is little evidence to support adding DHA/ARA for the improvement of visual development.[64,65]

Donor milk banks provide screened and pasteurized human milk. A processing fee is charged, and the distributing milk bank may prioritize recipients according to medical need. Informal sharing of milk (without a milk bank) should be discouraged due to the lack of screening for infectious diseases. Even if one assumes the health history of a well-meaning friend or family member is benign, it can take time for latent infections to become detectable through currently available testing.

Formula Feeding Methods

Formula should be prepared according to the manufacturer's instructions. Caretakers for the infant will need to recognize the difference between ready-to-feed, concentrated, and powdered formulations and dilute them (or not) appropriately. The water supply should also be considered; if well water is used, it should be checked for the presence of organisms and heavy metals, especially lead.

Formula should be stored according to the manufacturer's directions. Generally speaking, ready-to-feed liquid formula, once opened, may be covered and stored in a refrigerator for no longer than 48 hours. Unopened bottles of the prepared formula should not be left unrefrigerated for longer than 2 hours. Once the feeding has commenced, the formula in the bottle should be used within 1 hour or discarded. Powdered formula should be stored in a cool, dry environment, rather than the refrigerator. Once opened, it may be stored with the cap in place for as long as 4 weeks if precautions are taken to avoid microbiological contamination. Once formula is prepared, it should not be left out of the refrigerator. All bottles prepared should be used within 24 hours.

Cup feeding and bottle feeding have been found to take approximately the same amount of time. Infants fed formula when there are inadequate resources available to clean the equipment are advised to cup feed with an open, easily cleaned cup.

Research does not support the use of one type of bottle nipple over another or indicate that the shape of the bottle influences infant behavior. Feeding implements should be cleaned carefully, especially the tip of the nipple. Bisphenol A (BPA)–free bottles should be used. In July 2012, the FDA banned the production of bottles and toddler sippy cups containing BPA due to concerns regarding this compound's effects on the brain, behavior, and prostate glands of infants. Any borrowed or passed-down items from friends should be verified as BPA free prior to use.

Parents and other caretakers should hold the infant closely while feeding the child from a cup or bottle, maintaining eye-to-eye contact. It has also been suggested that the infant be switched from side to side, as happens when the infant is fed at the breast. Babies should never be fed "propped" bottles or given a bottle in the crib to hold because doing so carries a risk of choking and potential aspiration. Stroking, talking, and interaction are important components of feeding that all babies should receive. When teeth have erupted, formula or juice should be carefully wiped away before the baby sleeps to prevent the development of "bottle mouth" caries.

• • • References

1. U.S. Department of Health and Human Services. *The Surgeon General's Call to Action to Support Breastfeeding*. Washington, DC: U.S. Department of Health and Human Services, Office of the Surgeon General; 2011.

2. American Academy of Pediatrics Work Group on Breastfeeding. Breastfeeding and the use of human milk. *Pediatrics*. 2005;115:496.

3. Association of Women's Health, Obstetric, and Neonatal Nurses. *Breastfeeding: Clinical Position Statement*. Washington, DC: AWHONN; 2007.

4. American College of Nurse Midwives. *Position Statement: Breastfeeding*. Washington, DC: ACNM; 2011.

5. Ip S, Chung M, Raman G, Trikalinos TA, Lau J. A summary of the Agency for Healthcare Research and Quality's evidence report on breastfeeding in developed countries. *Breastfeed Med* 2009;4(suppl 1):S17-S30.

6. American Academy of Pediatrics. Breastfeeding and the use of human milk. *Pediatrics*. 2012;129:600-603.

7. Isaacs EB, Fischl BR, Quinn BT, et al. Impact of breast milk on intelligence quotient, brain size, and white matter development. *Pediatr Res*. 2010;67:357-362.

8. Ip S, Chung M, Raman G, et al. Breastfeeding and maternal and infant health outcomes in developed countries. *Evid Rep Technol Assess (Full Rep)*. 2007; 153:1-186.

9. Schwarz EB, Ray RM, Stuebe AM, et al. Duration of lactation and risk factors for maternal cardiovascular disease. *Obstet Gynecol*. 2009;113:974-982.

10. Karlson EW, Mandl LA, Hankinson SE, Grodstein F. Do breast-feeding and other reproductive factors influence future risk of rheumatoid arthritis? Results from the Nurses' Health Study. *Arthritis Rheum*. 2004;503:3458-3467.

11. Schwarz EB, Brown JS, Creasman JM, et al. Lactation and maternal risk of type 2 diabetes: a population-based study. *Am J Med*. 2010;123:863.e1, 863.e6.

12. Collaborative Group on Hormonal Factors in Breast Cancer. Breast cancer and breastfeeding: collaborative reanalysis of individual data from 47 epidemiological studies in 30 countries, including 50302 women with breast cancer and 96973 women without the disease. *Lancet*. 2002;360:187-195.

13. Watkins S, Meltzer-Brody S, Zolnoun D, Stuebe A. Early breastfeeding experiences and postpartum depression. *Obstet Gynecol*. 2011;118:214-221.

14. Strathearn L, Mamun AA, Najman JM, O'Callaghan MJ. Does breastfeeding protect against substantiated child abuse and neglect? A 15-year cohort study. *Pediatrics*. 2009;123:483-493.

15. U.S. Department of Health and Human Services, Office of Disease Prevention and Health Promotion. Healthy people 2020. Washington, DC. Available at: http://www.usbreastfeeding.org/Legislation Policy/FederalPoliciesInitiatives/HealthyPeople 2020BreastfeedingObjectives/tabid/120/Default.aspx. Accessed August 2, 2012.

16. Centers for Disease Control and Prevention. *Breastfeeding Report Card—United States, 2012*. Atlanta, GA: U.S. Department of Health and Human Services, Centers for Disease Control and Prevention; 2012. Available at: http:// www.cdc.gov/breastfeeding /data/reportcard.htm.

17. Centers for Disease Control and Prevention. Breastfeeding among U.S. children born 2004-2008, CDC National Immunization Survey. 2009. Available at: http://www.cdc.gov/breastfeeding/data/nis_data. Accessed August 2, 2012.

18. Bartick M, Reinhold A. The burden of suboptimal breastfeeding in the United States: a pediatric cost analysis. *Pediatrics*. 2010;125:e1048-e1056.

19. Patient Protection and Affordable Care Act. 42 USC §18001 (2010).

20. World Health Organization, UNICEF. *Protecting, Promoting and Supporting Breastfeeding: The Special Role of Maternity Services*. Geneva, Switzerland: WHO; 1989.

21. Rosenberg KD, Eastham CA, Kasehagen LJ, Sandoval AP. Marketing infant formula through hospitals: the impact of commercial hospital discharge packs on breastfeeding. *Am J Public Health*. 2008;98:290-295.

22. Kyenkya-Isabirye M. UNICEF launches the Baby-Friendly Hospital Initiative. *Am J Matern Child Nurs*. 1992;17:177-179.

23. DiGirolamo AM, Grummer-Strawn LM, Fein S. Maternity care practices: implications for breastfeeding. *Birth*. 2001;28:94-100.

24. Semenic S, Childerhose JE, Lauziere J, Groleau D. Barriers, facilitators, and recommendations related

to implementing the Baby-Friendly Initiative (BFI): an integrative review. *J Hum Lact.* 2012;28:317-334.

25. Renfrew MJ, McCormick FM, Wade A, Quinn B, Dowswell T. Support for healthy breastfeeding mothers with healthy term babies. *Cochrane Database Syst Rev.* 2012;5:CD001141.

26. Eglash A. La Leche League International (LLLI) is foundational to all aspects of breastfeeding. *Breastfeed Med.* 2009;4:51.

27. Ramsay DT, Kent JC, Hartmann RA, Hartmann PE. Anatomy of the lactating human breast redefined with ultrasound imaging. *J Anat.* 2005;206:525-534.

28. Galbally M, Lewis AJ, Ijzendoorn M, Permezel M. The role of oxytocin in mother–infant relations: a systematic review of human studies. *Harv Rev Psychiatry.* 2011;19(1):1-14.

29. Jevitt C, Hernandez L, Goer M. Lactation complicated by obesity. *J Midwifery Womens Health* 2007; 52(6):606-613.

30. Betzold CM, Hoover KL, Snyder CL. Delayed lactogenesis II: a comparison of four cases. *J Midwifery Women's Health.* 2004;49:132-137.

31. Hurst NM. Recognizing and treating delayed or failed lactogenesis II. *J Midwifery Women's Health.* 2007;52:588-594.

32. Kendall-Tackett K. Breastfeeding and the sexual abuse survivor. *J Hum Lact.* 1998;14:125, 130; quiz 131-133.

33. Lauwers J, Swisher A. *Counseling the Nursing Mother: A Lactation Consultant's Guide.* 4th ed. Sudbury, MA: Jones and Bartlett; 2005.

34. Jonas K, Johansson LM, Nissen E, Ejdeback M, Ransjo-Arvidson AB, Uvnas-Moberg K. Effects of intrapartum oxytocin administration and epidural analgesia on the concentration of plasma oxytocin and prolactin, in response to suckling during the second day postpartum. *Breastfeed Med.* 2009;4:71-82.

35. Szabo AL. Intrapartum neuraxial analgesia and breastfeeding outcomes: limitations of current knowledge. *Anesth Analg.* 2013;116:399-405.

36. Doumouchtis SK, Arulkumaran S. Head trauma after instrumental births. *Clin Perinatol.* 2008;35(1):69-83, viii.

37. Widström AM, Ransjö-Arvidson AB, Christensson K, Matthiesen AS, Winberg J, Uvnäs-Moberg K. Gastric suction in healthy newborn infants: effects on circulation and developing feeding behavior. *Acta Paediatr Scand.* 1987;76(4):566-572.

38. Dewey KG, Nommsen-Rivers LA, Heinig MJ, Cohen RJ. Risk factors for suboptimal breastfeeding behavior, delayed onset of lactation, and excess neonatal weight loss. *Pediatrics* 2003;112(3 Pt 1):607-619.

39. Hung KJ, Berg O. Early skin-to-skin after cesarean to improve breastfeeding. *Matern Child Nurs.* 2011;36(5):318.

40. Charpak N, Ruiz-Pelaez JG, Figueroa de CZ, Charpak Y. A randomized, controlled trial of kangaroo mother care: results of follow-up at 1 year of corrected age. *Pediatrics.* 2001;108:1072-1079.

41. Renfrew MJ, McCormick FM, Wade A, Quinn B, Dowswell T. Support for healthy breastfeeding mothers with healthy term babies. *Cochrane Database Syst Rev.* 2012;5:CD001141. doi: 10.1002/14651858. CD001141.pub4.

42. Cadwell K. Latching on and suckling of the healthy term neonate: breastfeeding assessment. *J Midwifery Women's Health.* 2007;52(6):638-642.

43. International Lactation Consultant Association; Mannel R, Martens PJ, Walker M, eds. *Core Curriculum for Lactation Consultant Practice.* 3rd ed. Burlington, MA: Jones & Bartlett; 2013.

44. Hill PD. Assessment of breastfeeding and infant growth. *J Midwifery Women's Health.* 2007;52(6):571-578.

45. Riordan J, Wambach K. *Breastfeeding and Human Lactation.* 4th ed. Sudbury, MA: Jones and Bartlett; 2010.

46. Morrill JF, Heinig MJ, Pappagianis D, Dewey KG. Risk factors for mammary candidosis among lactating women. *J Obstet Gynecol Neonatal Nurs.* 2005;34:37-45

47. Academy of Breastfeeding Medicine Protocol Committee, Berens P. ABM clinical protocol #20: Engorgement. *Breastfeed Med.* 2009;4:111-113.

48. Wiener S. Diagnosis and management of *Candida* of the nipple and breast. *J Midwifery Women's Health.* 2006;51:125-128.

49. Gatti L. Maternal perceptions of insufficient milk supply in breastfeeding. *J Nurs Scholarsh.* 2008;40: 355-363.

50. Thibaudeau S, Sinno H, Williams B. The effects of breast reduction on successful breastfeeding: a systematic review. *J Plast Reconstr Aesthet Surg.* 2010; 63(10):1688-1693.

51. Hurst NM. Recognizing and treating delayed or failed lactogenesis II. *J Midwifery Women's Health.* 2007;52(6):588-594.

52. Osadchy A, Moretti ME, Koren G. Effect of domperidone on insufficient lactation in puerperal women: a systematic review and meta-analysis of randomized controlled trials. *Obstet Gynecol Int.* 2012;2012: 642893.

53. Betzold CM. Galactagogues. *J Midwifery Women's Health.* 2004;49:151-154.

54. Academy of Breastfeeding Medicine Protocol Committee. ABM clinical protocol #9: use of galactogogues in initiating or augmenting the rate of maternal milk secretion (first revision, January 2011). *Breastfeed Med.* 2011;6:41-49.

55. Miche C. The challenge of mastitis. *Arch Dis Child.* 2003;88:818-821.

56. Betzold CM. An update on the recognition and management of lactational breast inflammation. *J Midwifery Women's Health.* 2007;52:595-605.

57. Berens P, Swaim L, Peterson B. Incidence of methicillin-resistant *Staphylococcus aureus* in postpartum breast abscesses. *Breastfeed Med.* 2010;5(3):113-115.

58. Department of Child and Adolescent Health and Development. *Mastitis: Causes and Management.* Geneva, Switzerland: World Health Organization; 2000. Available at: http://whqlibdoc.who.int/hq/2000/WHO_FCH_CAH_00.13.pdf.

59. Foxman B, D'Arcy H, Gillespie B, Bobo JK, Schwartz K. Lactation mastitis: occurrence and medical management among 946 breastfeeding women in the United States. *Am J Epidemiol.* 2002;155(2):103-114.

60. ABM clinical protocol #4: mastitis. Revision, May 2008. *Breastfeed Med.* 2008;3(3):177-180.

61. Centers for Disease Control and Prevention. When should a mother avoid breastfeeding? October 9, 2009. Available from: www.cdc.gov/breastfeeding/disease/index.htm. Accessed February 21, 2013.

62. U.S. Department of Health and Human Services, Office on Women's Health. *Genital Herpes.* Washington, DC; 2009. Available at: http://www.womenshealth.gov/faq/genital-herpes.cfm.

63. American Academy of Pediatrics Committee on Nutrition. *Pediatric Nutrition Handbook.* Elk Grove, IL: American Academy of Pediatrics; 2009.

64. Wright K, Coverston C, Tiedeman M, Abegglen JA. Formula supplemented with docosahexaenoic acid (DHA) and arachidonic acid (ARA): a critical review of the research. *J Spec Pediatr Nurs.* 2006;11:100, 112; discussion 112-113.

65. Simmer K. Long-chain polyunsaturated fatty acid supplementation in infants born at term. *Cochrane Database Syst Rev.* 2001;4:CD000376.

VII

Newborn

Welcoming the Newborn

The moment a newborn enters the world, a lusty cry connotes an instant and unconditional welcome to the family. That initial, spontaneous wail reassures the newborn's mother, midwife, and family that this infant is off to a safe and healthy journey through extrauterine transition and adaptation. Everyone present at the birth can now take a deep breath and feel at ease as congratulations are extended all around.

As the newborn and mother bond, the midwife performs an initial head-to-toe examination in front of the family—a quick way to confirm that the infant's appearance and behavior are normal. Any concerns that arise during this process call for an in-depth evaluation of any variations that are present, including immediate intervention when necessary.

Midwives caring for women and newborns during the first 28 days of life must maintain currency in the basic knowledge necessary for systematic evaluation and management of neonates, including a solid grounding in the physiology of the transition from intrauterine to extrauterine life. This requires the reliable, validated, evidence-based techniques and standards for evaluation contained in this text.

The midwife is privileged to serve women and families at some of the most vulnerable times in their lives. To serve competently, compassionately, and with respect, the midwife seeks to strengthen the family by providing them with advocacy, support, resources, and understanding that enable them to make informed choices. Benefiting from the midwife's commitment in the form of educational and emotional nourishment, the family can move forward freely and securely in their adaptive process as they grow and flourish.

Lily Hsia

CHAPTER

37

Anatomy and Physiology of the Newborn

MARY KATHLEEN MCHUGH

TEKOA L. KING

The first few moments and hours of extrauterine life are among the most dynamic of the entire life cycle. At birth, the newborn moves from complete dependence to physiologic independence. This complex process of change is known as the transitional period—a period that starts prenatally with fetal breathing activity and lung fluid shifts, and then continues. Some organs, such as the lungs, make rapid changes that are fully accomplished within days of birth. Other organ systems, such as the hepatic system, take longer to convert to extrauterine function. Overall, the transition to extrauterine life is an ongoing process and part of a continuum that starts with conception and extends through infancy.

Extrauterine transition can be profoundly influenced by prenatal factors as well as intrapartum events. At each birth, the midwife considers prenatal or intrapartum factors that could cause compromise in the first extrauterine hours of newborn life. Events during conception and the prenatal period that might cause compromise include fetal growth restriction, congenital malformations, genetic disorders, prenatal infections (especially viral), chronic poor nutrition, prematurity or postmaturity, maternal chronic disease (cardiac, renal, hepatic, diabetes), the residual effect of environmental or workplace teratogens, substance use by the mother, and any condition causing blood loss. Labor and birth events that might influence extrauterine transition include prolonged labor, maternal fever, hypoxic uterine conditions, birth trauma, infection, passage of meconium, fetal blood loss, use of medications during labor, and difficult birth or operative birth. Accurate risk prediction is essential for selection of the appropriate site and personnel for the birth.

Immediate Extrauterine Transition

The newborn's most dramatic and most rapid extrauterine transitions occur in four areas: the respiratory system, the circulatory system, the ability to thermoregulate, and the ability to maintain euglycemia. These four areas of transition are interdependent—failure of one can lead to impairment of others, and all must occur successfully for neonatal transition to happen smoothly. Whenever a neonate struggles with one area of transition, prompt support is needed to avoid a cascade of problems.

Respiratory Changes

The respiratory system is quickly challenged in the change from an intrauterine to extrauterine environment, as the newborn must begin respiration immediately upon arrival in the atmosphere. Prior to birth, the fetus receives oxygen from the maternal circulation via the placenta and umbilical artery.

During gestation, numerous developments provide the infrastructure for the onset of respiration. A fetus develops the musculature needed to breathe and has demonstrated breathing movements throughout the second and third trimesters. Fetal breathing activity may have circadian properties and change in response to maternal meals and caffeine intake.[1] The alveoli develop throughout gestation, as does the fetal ability to produce surfactant, the phospholipid that becomes available by 34 weeks' gestation and reduces surface tension at the alveolar–air interface. As pregnancy approaches its end, the interstitial space between the alveoli markedly thins, which allows for maximum contact between the capillaries and the alveoli for air exchange.

Prior to labor, the lungs are full of fluid, which is produced in alveolar cells secondary to stimulation by chloride ion secretion The term fetus experiences a decrease in lung fluid in the days before labor mediated by the expression of genes, which in turn leads to increased activity of epithelial sodium channels (ENaC) that transport fluid away from the alveoli. Activation of ENaC is correlated with gestational age, so preterm and near-term infants are born with lower activation in their ENaC, which accentuates the possibility of respiratory distress.[2,3]

During normal labor, fetal plasma levels of catecholamines and glucocorticoids increase. These stress hormones cause reabsorption of lung fluid during labor.[3-5] On a mechanical level, animal models have demonstrated that the constricted fetal posture during labor causes increased transpulmonary pressure and a significant release of lung fluid from the airways during the first stage of labor, long before the final thoracic squeeze of second-stage labor.[5] Neonates who experience a cesarean section birth, especially in the absence of labor, do not receive the benefit of the diminution of lung fluid and have an increased risk for transient tachypnea of the newborn (TTN) or respiratory distress syndrome (RDS).

In spite of decades of investigation, the phenomena that stimulate the neonate to take the first breath are only partially understood (**Figure 37-1**). Some biochemical events have been implicated in the processes. For example, the relative hypoxia of the end of labor and physical stimuli to which the neonate is subjected, such as cold, gravity, pain, light, and noise, cause excitation of the respiratory center. The release of the thoracic pressure at birth may help stimulate a breath. The squeezing of the thorax that occurs in the last minutes of second-stage labor when the fetus is in the birth canal helps extrude some upper airway fluid, although this effect is small. With the neonate's first breath, fluid filling the mouth and trachea is partially released, and air begins to fill the tracheal column.

The first active breaths set in motion a seamless chain of events that (1) assists with the conversion from fetal to adult circulation, (2) empties the lungs of liquid, (3) establishes neonatal lung volume and the characteristics of pulmonary function in the newly born infant, and (4) decreases pulmonary artery pressure.

When the head is born, mucus drains from the nares and mouth. Many newborns gasp and even cry at this time. The first few breaths require some

pressure because room air is flowing into a fluid-filled space. However, the use of a bulb syringe or other device to suction the mouth or nares of a vigorous newborn is unnecessary. Conversely, newborns who are exhausted and compromised by the birth process may need assistance in clearing the fluid and mucus from the upper airway. Use of a suctioning device such as a bulb syringe or wall suction should be limited to situations in which the newborn's respiratory efforts are diminished. In addition, suctioning of the oropharynx and nasopharynx on the perineum does not prevent meconium aspiration.[6,7]

With the first few breaths, room air starts to fill the large airways of the neonate's trachea and bronchi. Fetal lung fluid remaining in the alveoli is pushed to the lung periphery, where it is absorbed. Although it has been widely believed that the first few breaths involve a higher opening pressure to force air into the lungs, there is little current evidence to confirm this relationship.[8]

All of the alveoli expand with air over time. Maximum function of the alveoli occurs in the presence of adequate surfactant and adequate blood flow through the pulmonary microcirculation. After 34 weeks of gestation, sufficient quantities of surfactant helps to stabilize the walls of the alveoli so that they do not collapse onto themselves at the end of a breath. This effect reduces the pressure needed to expand the alveoli during subsequent breaths, thereby decreasing the workload of breathing. It is also important to remember that adequate oxygenation is a critical factor in *maintenance* of adequate air exchange. In the presence of hypoxia, the pulmonary vasculature vasoconstricts and oxygen in the alveoli cannot be transported into blood vessels for oxygenation of other areas of the body.

If the first breaths are of adequate volume and pressure, they establish the functional residual capacity (FRC) of the neonate—that is, the gas volume left in the lungs at the end of each expiration. Maintenance of the FRC is critical for survival. Crying has been found to have a functional purpose.[9] In a crying neonate, expiration is slowed by resistance from the narrowed glottis, which helps maintain end-expiratory pressure within the lungs. The muscles of the diaphragm also slow the rate of lung deflation. Control of expiration ensures a slower lung deflation that minimizes the chance of alveolar collapse and loss of the FRC.[10]

Continuation of breathing occurs secondary to central brain stem activity and specialized cells within the carotid body. In the term newborn, the chemoreceptors in the carotid body initiate increases in ventilatory effort in response to acidosis and hypercapnia, and decreases in ventilatory effort in response to hypocapnia. Respirations fluctuate; they are not stable and rhythmic for any extended period of time in the neonate. Breathing in a newborn may sound noisy and wet during this period of transition. Additionally, there may be short periods of apnea or sighing in the term newborn.[11] Lack of persistent rhythm and occasional periodic breathing (irregular rhythm with short periods of apnea) is common in a near-term newborn.

There are, however, certain normal and abnormal responses to look for in the newborn. A respiratory rate consistently higher than 60 breaths per minute, with or without flaring, grunting, or retractions, is clearly abnormal at 2 hours of life. Significant episodes of periodic breathing signal the need for medical intervention before major apnea occurs.[1] Other normal and abnormal responses are summarized in **Table 37-1**.

When a newborn does need resuscitation and respiratory support, room air rather than oxygen should be used initially. The switch to 100% oxygen should only be made if room air is not sufficient. Although historically 100% oxygen has been used for respiratory resuscitation, it is now known that 100% oxygen can create free oxygen radicals that exacerbate reperfusion injury and decreases cerebral perfusion. Therefore, room air is now preferred.

Circulatory Changes

The blood flow from the placenta stops with the clamping of the umbilical cord. This action eliminates the maternal supply of oxygen and causes a subsequent series of reactions. These reactions are complemented by those occurring in the lungs in response to the first breath.

Fetal circulation is characterized by three shunts: the foramen ovale, ductus arteriosus, and ductus venosus (**Figure 37-1**). Because the lungs are a closed, fluid-filled organ, they need minimal blood flow and the fetal circulation has high pulmonary vascular resistance. Oxygenated blood bypasses the lungs by flowing through the opening between the right and left atria called the foramen ovale and then into the descending aorta. In the second shunt, blood in the right ventricle does not flow into the high-pressure pulmonary vasculature, but rather flows through the ductus arteriosus into the descending aorta. Placental prostaglandin, prostacyclin, and low oxygen tension keep the ductus arteriosus open.[12] The third fetal shunt, the ductus venosus, connects the umbilical vein to the inferior vena cava, which allows a portion of fetal blood to bypass the circulation through the liver.

At birth, the oxygen tension rises, and placental prostaglandins and prostacyclin no longer enter the system via the umbilical vein. This causes constriction of the ductus arteriosus. Blood from the right ventricle is then able to enter the pulmonary circulation, and the oxygenated blood now routinely passing by the ductus arteriosus also causes it to constrict. Within 48 hours, the ductus arteriosus functionally closes.

Clamping the umbilical cord shuts down the low-pressure system that characterizes the fetal–placental unit, so that the newborn circulatory system becomes a freestanding, closed system. The immediate effect of the cord clamping is a rise in the systemic vascular resistance (SVR). Most importantly, this rise occurs at the same time the newborn takes the initial breaths. The oxygen in those breaths causes the pulmonary vasculature to relax and open. The pulmonary vasculature resistance (PVR) decreases just as the SVR increases, and this shift in pressure, in combination with closure of the ductus arteriosus, encourages blood flow into the pulmonary system. A transitional period ensues during which kinked pulmonary vessels straighten and decrease resistance to blood flow. Over time, the development of elongated and thinner cell walls also increases vessel flexibility.[13]

The combination of increased SVR and lower PVR also changes the pressure of blood flow within the heart. As blood flow increases in the left side of the heart, the foramen ovale closes. The results of the change in SVR and PVR and the closure of the three fetal shunts complete the radical changes in the anatomy and physiology of the heart. Deoxygenated blood enters the neonatal heart, becomes fully

Table 37-1	Normal and Abnormal Respiratory Characteristics in the Newborn	
Characteristic	**Normal**	**Abnormal**
Respiratory rate	40–60 bpm	< 30 bpm or > 60 bpm
Diaphragm	Diaphragmatic and abdominal breathing	Grunting
Nasal	Obligate nasal breather	Flaring

bpm = breaths per minute.

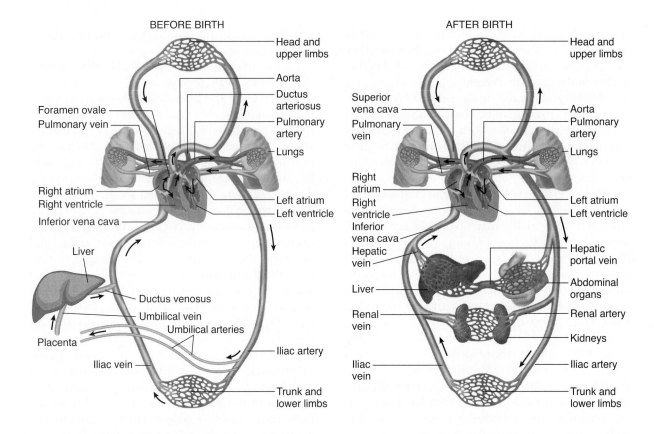

Figure 37-1 Fetal and neonatal circulation.

oxygenated in the lungs, and is distributed to all other body tissues.

Clinical evidence of these tremendous changes in circulation is manifested as increasingly pink color, normal heart rate, and strong pulses. Although these changes are not anatomically complete for weeks, the functional closure of the foramen ovale and the ductus arteriosus occurs soon after birth. The change from fetal to newborn circulation is intimately related to adequate respiratory function and oxygenation. The term newborn stressed by hypoxia, hypoglycemia, cold, or infection may not make the transition smoothly and can develop persistent pulmonary hypertension.[13]

Thermoregulation

The newborn can become rapidly stressed by changes in environmental temperature. The fetal temperature is typically 0.6°C higher than the maternal temperature. Factors that contribute to heat loss in the newborn include the large surface area of a newborn (the ratio of surface area to body weight ratio in a neonate is two times higher than that of an adult), limited

subcutaneous fat insulation, and the inability to generate heat via shivering.

Prevention of Hypothermia

Newborns can lose heat through four mechanisms: (1) convection, (2) conduction, (3) radiation, and (4) evaporation. Skin-to-skin contact between the neonate and mother is recommended as the initial method for maintaining neonatal body temperature for healthy term infants.[14] Skin-to-skin contact minimizes heat loss via conduction and results in better short-term temperature stability than bundling or placing the neonate under a warmer. Skin-to-skin contact should be the first line of treatment for hypothermia, especially in low-resource environments.[15,16] Box 37-1 lists other methods used to prevent hypothermia.

Coping with Cold Stress

The neonate can create heat in three ways: shivering, voluntary muscle activity, and nonshivering thermogenesis. Shivering in term neonates is seen only in the most severe cold stress. Muscle activity can generate heat but is of limited benefit in increasing

<table>
<tr><td>

BOX 37-1 Interventions to Prevent Newborn Hypothermia

- Prewarm the newborn resuscitation area.
- Set the birth room temperature at 23.9°C (75°F).
- Prewarm any blankets, hats, or clothing prior to the birth.
- Gently dry the newborn after birth and then immediately replace wet blankets with dry ones.
- Do not evaluate the newborn on wet sheets or towels.
- Postpone the newborn's bath until newborn temperature has been stable for 2 hours.
- Place the newborn care areas away from windows, outside walls, and doorways.
- Keep the newborn's head covered and body well wrapped for 48 hours.

</td></tr>
</table>

temperature, even in term infants with sufficient muscle strength.

Nonshivering thermogenesis refers to utilization of brown fat for heat production. Brown adipose tissue contains more lipids, mitochondria, and capillaries than does white adipose tissue. The primary purpose of brown adipose tissue is to generate heat; such tissue is a nonrenewable resource of the newborn. Brown adipose tissue is located in and around the upper spine, the clavicles and sternum, the kidneys, and major blood vessels. The amount of brown adipose tissue depends on gestational age and is relatively sparse in growth-retarded newborns and preterm infants.

Creation of heat through utilization of brown adipose stores starts at birth with a surge of catecholamines and withdrawal of the placental suppressors prostaglandin and adenosine. The cold stimulus of leaving the mother's warm body triggers activity in the newborn hypothalamus that leads to oxidation of stored lipids in brown fat and subsequent production of heat.[17] Through the mediation of glucose and glycogen, the brown fat cells convert multiple small intracellular fat vacuoles into heat energy. The heat produced warms the blood before it circulates to peripheral areas of the neonate's body and ensures a stable temperature for other biochemical reactions.[18] In a newborn experiencing hypoglycemia or thyroid dysfunction, however, the use of brown fat stores does not proceed efficiently.

The sequelae of heat loss in the neonate can cascade quickly into effects that include hypoglycemia, hypoxia, acidosis, and respiratory distress (**Figure 37-2**). These effects are consequences of the increased metabolic demands that result from the newborn's attempts to create a neutral thermal zone.

The World Health Organization defines hypothermia as a core temperature less than 36.5°C (97.7°F). Clinical symptoms of hypothermia may be subtle and include a low core temperature and cold skin, pale skin, pallor, hypotonia, lethargy or irritability, poor feeding or vomiting tachypnea, and an increased heart rate.[15] Any newborn who is hypothermic should be evaluated for hypoglycemia because of the high caloric demands associated with nonshivering thermogenesis.[19] The rewarming process will take a number of hours. Attempts to rapidly rewarm a newborn may lead to apnea. Head coverings should be removed during the rewarming process in an incubator or radiant warmer. Because the head is a large surface area, temporarily uncovering it during the rewarming maximizes heat gain from the warming source.

The newborn's temperature can be assessed at various sites with different types of thermometers. Although historically rectal temperatures were commonly performed in newborns, this technique had some disadvantages: These temperatures can remain high after the core temperature drops, they can be affected by the presence of stool, and rectal perforation is possible. Thus rectal temperatures are no longer recommended. Axillary temperatures are normally in the range of 36.5–37.5°C (97.7–99.0°F) but may be falsely elevated in a cold-stressed infant secondary to metabolism of brown fat. Abdominal skin temperature is normally in the range of 36–36.5°C (96.8–97.7°F). Infrared tympanic thermometers (2 seconds in the ear) can be used to measure temperature but are likely the least reliable method for a newborn.

Noncontinuous temperature assessment is accurate only if the thermometer remains in place for an adequate time. If temperature is assessed with an abdominal skin sensor, the sensor must be in good contact with the skin and covered with a reflective shield. Skin temperatures should be slightly lower than core temperatures.

Glucose Regulation

Prior to birth, the fetus is exposed to nearly constant blood glucose levels that are approximately 60% to 70% of maternal levels. In preparation for extrauterine life, the healthy fetus stores glucose as glycogen, especially in the liver. Most glycogen storage occurs

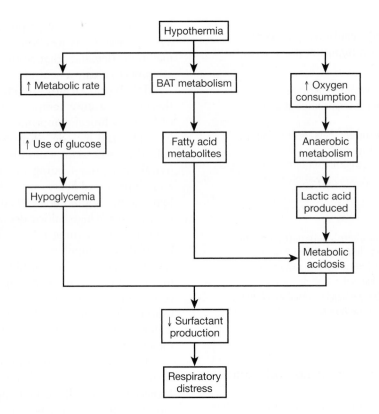

Figure 37-2 Hypothermia in the newborn.

in the third trimester. Although any infant can develop symptomatic or asymptomatic hypoglycemia, newborns with fetal growth restriction, post-term infants, preterm infants, and those who have experienced some form of distress prior to birth are at particular risk.[20] In all of these neonates, less glycogen may have been stored. The large for gestational age (LGA) neonate is also at risk for hypoglycemia, whether or not the mother has diabetes, with the newborn's risk increasing as birth weight increases.[21]

The moment the cord is clamped, the newborn must find a way to maintain a serum glucose level that is essential for neonatal brain function. Blood levels of glucose initially fall to a nadir at approximately 1 to 2 hours after birth. The physiologic low occurs at approximately 1 to 1.5 hours after birth, with levels subsequently stabilizing at 3 to 4 hours. In a meta-analysis of term newborns, Alkakaly et al. recommended that low thresholds for plasma glucose levels in full-term newborns be 28 mg/dL at 1 to 2 hours, 40 mg/dL at 3 to 23 hours, 41 mg/dL at 24 to 47 hours, and 48 mg/dL at 48 to 72 hours.[22] Their analysis included newborns fed via both bottle and breast. These researchers also noted that further study is needed on exclusively breastfed newborns.

The healthy newborn maintains blood glucose levels in one of three ways: (1) through utilization of breast milk or a substitute; (2) utilization of the glycogen stores; or (3) creation of glucose via glycogenolysis and gluconeogenesis. The healthy newborn generates glucose in the amount of 4–8 mg/kg/min.

The healthy newborn should be encouraged to feed as soon as possible after birth. Many newborns are active feeders during the first period of reactivity. This is an ideal time to imprint the infant with a breastfeeding experience. Newborns who are exhausted and stressed from long labor may show minimal interest in feeding. Even if the newborn feeds successfully, the amount of calories taken in will be minimal and may not be adequate for the glucose needs of a stressed newborn.

Newborns who cannot ingest adequate food will create glucose from glycogen. However, glycogenolysis can occur only if the infant has adequate stores of glycogen. Although it is possible for the newborn to create glucose from fats or proteins, the process of gluconeogenesis is inefficient and creates many metabolic by-products.

There is no indication for routine blood glucose testing of term newborns after an uncomplicated birth.[23,24] At the same time, all newborns should be monitored for signs of hypoglycemia. Symptoms of hypoglycemia can be vague and nonspecific and can include jitteriness, cyanosis, apnea, weak cry, lethargy, limpness, and refusal to feed. Hypoglycemia may be asymptomatic at first. Long-term sequelae of persistent hypoglycemia include damage to the occipital area of the brain manifesting as seizures, mental retardation, and attention-deficit disorder.[25] Damage is accentuated if hypoglycemia is accompanied by neonatal asphyxia.

Evaluation of hypoglycemia is done via capillary blood sample. It is no longer recommended to warm the heel prior to sampling, as research has not revealed any benefit from heel warming with regard to blood flow, collection time, or newborn comfort.[26,27] When performing this blood test, care should be taken to avoid puncturing the sensitive structures on the back of the heel (**Figure 37-3**).[26] Use of an automated blood collection device may cause less trauma and lead to more successful sample collection results than use of manual lancets and squeezing the heel, which creates hemolysis.[28] To prevent infection, the infant's heel should be cleansed with antiseptic, followed by sterile water, and allowed to air dry. Alcohol should be avoided, as it is drying and can leave residue. Newborn discomfort may be diminished by swaddling, being held in the arms of the neonate's mother or other family member, and non-nutritive sucking.[29]

Any glucose level below the recommended threshold for normal requires intervention. Initially feeding the infant is the first step. A repeat test is performed in 30 minutes and if the borderline level persists, a venous sample should be checked. Low values should be evaluated immediately with a venous sample drawn from a scalp vein or the antecubital fossa. If the low value is confirmed, pediatric consultation is needed and treatment is indicated.

Venous samples can be analyzed using either whole blood or plasma (serum). Samples should be chilled during transport to the laboratory. Most laboratories report the plasma result, which will be close to 15% higher than a sample run on whole blood. Thus it is important to know the testing method and reference ranges used by a particular lab to accurately interpret results.

Normal values for a term newborn's blood components are listed in **Table 37-2**. At birth, newborns have higher values for hemoglobin and hematocrit compared to adult values. Neonatal blood contains both fetal hemoglobin (HbF), which contains 2 alpha subunits and 2 gamma subunits, and adult hemoglobin (HbA), which contains 2 alpha subunits and 2 beta subunits. HbF has a higher affinity for oxygen than does HbA, is more stable in an acidic environment, and has a shorter lifespan. After birth, HbA gradually replaces HbF. Because HbF breaks down faster than erythropoiesis, however, newborns experience a physiologic anemia approximately 6 to 8 weeks after birth. The hemoglobin level decreases slowly over the first 7 to 9 weeks after birth, reaching an average of 12.0 g/dL in a 2-month-old infant.

The initial hemoglobin/hematocrit values in a newborn can be influenced by the timing of clamping of the cord and the newborn's position immediately after birth. Delay in clamping the umbilical cord (more than 30 seconds after birth) allows a passive placental transfusion, which increases the neonate's blood volume by 80 mL.[30] Delaying cord clamping has several benefits: (1) a bolus of oxygenated blood during the first breaths, (2) volume expansion that promotes pulmonary capillary perfusion, (3) a more rapid achievement of adequate oxygenation leading to closure of fetal structures such as the ductus arteriosus, and (4) decreased risk of iron-deficiency anemia at 4 to 6 months of life.[31–33] Delaying cord clamping has been shown to be safe and is recommended to increase neonatal iron storage at birth despite being associated with a slightly increased risk for hyperbilirubinemia.[32,33,35]

To support the physiologic transfusion that occurs over the first 1 to 3 minutes of life, the newborn is placed on the mother's abdomen with the cord intact. This position promotes modest amounts

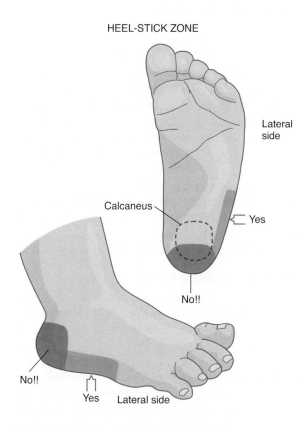

HEEL-STICK ZONE

Lateral side

Calcaneus

Yes

No!!

No!!

Yes   Lateral side

Figure 37-3 Anatomic landmarks for heel sticks.

Table 37-2	Cord Blood Values of a Full-Term Newborn
Component	**Optimal Range**
Hemoglobin concentration	14.0–20.0 g/dL
Red blood cell (RBC) count	4,200,000–5,800,000/mm³
Hematocrit	43–63%
Mean cell diameter	8.0–8.3 μm
Mean corpuscular volume (MCV)	100–120 μm³
Mean corpuscular hemoglobin (MCH)	32–40 pg
Mean corpuscular hemoglobin concentration (MCHC)	30–34%
Reticulocyte count	3–7%
Nucleated red blood cell count	200–600/mm³
White blood cell count	10,000–30,000/mm³
Granulocytes	40–80%
Lymphocytes	20–40%
Monocytes	3–10%
Platelet count	150,000–350,000/mm³
Serum iron concentration	125–225 mcg/dL
Total iron-binding capacity	150–350 mcg/dL

Source: This table was published in Fanaroff A, Martin R. *Neonatal and Perinatal Medicine: Diseases of the Fetus and Infant.* 7th ed. St. Louis, MO: Mosby, p. 1661, Copyright Mosby 2002. Reprinted with permission of Elsevier.

of blood flow to the newborn without the potential danger of a forced and large bolus of blood. By 3 minutes, most of the blood flow from the cord to the neonate is accomplished.

The custom of immediate cord clamping is related to modern obstetrical practices and is not a universal practice globally. Proponents of early clamping cite concerns about the potential of side effects from placental transfusion, including respiratory distress, polycythemia, and hyperviscosity syndrome. Lowering the neonate markedly below the introitus and actively stripping the cord toward the newborn can cause an excessively large transfusion and subsequent adverse effects. Although it is possible for blood flow to reverse from infant to placenta, this situation is unusual because the umbilical arteries (carrying blood from the fetus back to the placenta) spasm quickly in the ambient temperature of the

birthing room. If reverse flow occurs, the newborn could become profoundly hypovolemic. Therefore, the midwife should make every effort to minimize extremes of position of the infant in relation to the vaginal introitus.

Red Blood Cells and Hyperbilirubinemia

The newborn's red blood cells (RBCs) have a short lifespan of 80 days on average (the adult RBC lifespan averages 120 days). This rapid cell turnover creates more by-products of cell breakdown, including bilirubin, which must be metabolized. Newborns also have a reduction in activity of the protein known as uridine diphosphate glucuronosyltransferase (UGT), which helps to conjugate bilirubin and prepare it for excretion. These two factors are most instrumental in development of the physiologic jaundice seen in many newborns.

Total serum bilirubin peaks at the approximately 3 days of postnatal life. Ninety-six percent of term newborns will have a total serum bilirubin of less than 17 mg/dL at 96 hours of age, so levels higher than this are considered pathological.[35] Significant jaundice before day 3 may be pathological, and any visible jaundice in the first 24 hours of life is of significant concern. There is a correspondingly high reticulocyte count in newborns, reflecting the high rate of formation of new red blood cells.

White Blood Cells

The average white blood cell (WBC) levels in a newborn range from 10,000 to 26,000/mm³. There can be a further elevation in the WBC count in a normal newborn during the first 24 hours of life, with this level then gradually decreasing over the next 3 to 5 days. Because of these physiologic shifts, it is more useful to focus on neutrophils as a marker for infection. Limits for normal neutrophil shifts in term newborns have recently been changed to reflect a normal peak of 28,500/mm³ at 8 hours of age and 13,000/mm³ at 72 hours.[36] Labor, meconium aspiration, prolonged periods of crying, and maternal fever can cause a shift upward in the neutrophil count.

Platelets and Clotting Factors

Platelet counts in newborns are within the same range as adult values. Levels lower than 150,000/mm³ should prompt further medical evaluation. However, platelet aggregation can vary in term newborns. In the first month of life, there is an overall deficiency of many of the clotting factors that are dependent on vitamin K. Because of this general deficiency, it is customary to give newborns supplementary vitamin K after birth. Intramuscular vitamin K is the common route, as studies have not fully explored the therapeutic effect of oral administration.[37] Prothrombin time, thrombin time, and partial thromboplastin time are slightly prolonged.

The Newborn Immune System

The neonatal immune system is immature in a number of ways. This functional immaturity makes the neonate vulnerable to many infections and allergic responses. The neonate has limited adaptive immunity, using B and T lymphocytes as protective mechanisms secondary to the lack of antigenic stimulation in fetal life. However, innate immunity remains the main defense for the neonate.[38]

Innate Immunity

Innate immunity consists of cellular and noncellular first responders to infection and bodily structures that prevent or minimize infection. Innate immunity is the first line of defense to an infection. Some examples of innate immunity include (1) the barrier protection offered by the skin and mucous membranes; (2) the sieve-like action of the respiratory passages; (3) the colonization of skin and intestine by protective microbes; (4) the chemical protection offered by the acidic environment of the stomach; and (5) the physical barrier made by cells that line the intestinal tract.

Skin and mucous membranes are colonized as the fetus passes through the vaginal canal. The vernix caseosum contains antimicrobial proteins and peptides (APPs) and forms a "microbial shield" on the newborn body.[39,40] The presence of vernix also moistens the skin and increases its acidity, which inhibits growth of pathogenic bacteria.[41] The inflammatory skin reaction of normal newborns called erythema toxicum contains the antimicrobial peptide LL-37, indicating that this skin condition may be a manifestation of bacterial colonization.[38,40,42] Intestinal colonization occurs as the infant begins to ingest normal bacterial flora through the diet as well as through exposure to the flora in natural environment.

Breastfeeding in the first month of life is a powerful stimulant of the innate immune response, as it influences the concentrations of innate immune cell and cytokine responses via expression of immune molecules including toll-like receptors (TLRs). Other environmental triggers that stimulate the innate immune response include vaginal birth and exposure to pets and siblings. Innate immunity is also provided at the cellular level. Three cell types—polymorphonuclear neutrophils (PMNs), monocytes, and macrophages—act via phagocytosis to engulf and kill foreign antigens.

The PMNs will eventually become the primary phagocytes in the defense of the host. However, in the neonate, the PMN is compromised both in ability to mobilize and move in the right direction and in ability to adhere to inflammatory sites.[40,43] These deficiencies do not reflect inadequate numbers of the PMN cells but rather inadequate chemotaxis and opsonization. Chemotaxis refers to the organized movement of a phagocytic cell—that is, its actual travel around the body. Opsonization is the alteration, or "marking," of the cell surface of a foreign microbe or antigen; it promotes the destruction of foreign cells. The immaturity of chemotaxis and opsonization in the newborn decreases the effectiveness of the phagocytic response and leads to one of the main weaknesses of the neonatal immune system: the inability to localize infection. Thus the risk for systemic infection is higher in newborns than in adults.

The innate immune system also includes numerous noncellular proteins, such as complement molecules, acute-phase reactants, cytokines, chemokines, coagulation proteins, and vasoactive substances.[42] The process of phagocytosis is enhanced if the foreign cells are prepared by complement components. Natural killer (NK) cells contribute to innate immunity, but their function is compromised in the neonate, as they have limited cytolytic ability.[44]

In the newborn, signs of infection can be subtle, such as changes in activity, tone, color, or feeding. In addition, lack of fever does not exclude the possibility of infection. Thus observation for symptoms of systemic infection is one of the most important aspects of monitoring the newborn.

Adaptive Immunity

Adaptive immunity is acquired as a response to specific pathogens. It is divided into two components: cellular and antibody mediated (humoral). The cellular adaptive immune response is modulated through T-cell and B-cell lymphocytes. T cells have two main roles: killing infected cells and aiding other cells by stimulation of cytokines. These cells are found in high levels in the newborn, but are slow to respond and require increased stimulus to generate their activity compared to later in life.[43] The T cells that develop immunological memory, CD8 and CD4 cells, are present in low levels in the neonate and increase slowly throughout childhood. Until the newborn has been exposed to some antigens, these T cells do not offer significant protection. Thus it is not until 4 to 6 weeks after birth that the infant will experience minimal protection by these cells.[45]

The activation of the antibody-mediated B cells is dependent on T-cell activity. Thus, as a consequence of diminished T-cell functionality in the newborn, B-cell responses are also deficient, having a delayed onset and shorter duration. Bacteria may also trigger B-cell development. Recent evidence indicates that B cells are also activated by early intestinal colonization by maternal intestinal bacteria.[46]

Passive Immunity

The neonate is born with passive immunity to viruses and bacteria via transplacental passage of immunoglobulin G (IgG) from the mother, which continues to protect the infant for approximately 6 months.[43] The newborn is dependent on this passive immunity because significant amounts of IgG are not produced by the infant until 6 months of age.

Other immunoglobulins, such as IgM and IgA, are much larger than IgG and do not cross the placenta. Identification of IgM or IgA in cord blood is an indication that the fetus has actively responded to an infection while in utero.

Gradually, the young infant will begin to produce adequate circulating antibodies of the IgG class. This process takes time, and the full antibody response to a foreign antigen is not possible until well into early childhood. The full antibody response corresponds with the diminution of the IgG acquired prenatally.

In summary, because of a variety of deficiencies in both natural and acquired immunities, the neonate is vulnerable to infection. Neonatal response to infection is sluggish and inadequate, leading to a predisposition to systemic rather than localized infections. Vaginal birth and breastfeeding both help establish healthy microbial colonization, an effect that persists throughout infancy.

The Newborn Gastrointestinal Tract

The gastrointestinal system in a term newborn exhibits varying levels of maturity. Prior to birth, the term fetus exhibits sucking and swallowing motions. Mature gag and cough reflexes are intact at birth. Meconium, although sterile, contains debris from the amniotic fluid, which confirms that the fetus ingests amniotic fluid and that the fluid passes through the gastrointestinal passage.

The ability of the term newborn to ingest and digest exogenous food sources is limited secondary to varying amounts of digestive enzymes and hormones in all portions of the gastrointestinal tract. Newborns are less able to digest proteins and fats than adults. Carbohydrate absorption is relatively efficient but still less than the adult ability. The newborn is particularly efficient in absorbing monosaccharides such as glucose, as long as the amount of glucose is not too large.

The cardiac sphincter—the juncture of the lower esophagus and the stomach—is incomplete, which contributes to frequent regurgitation of stomach contents in newborns and young infants. The capacity of the stomach itself is limited, holding less than 30 cc for a term newborn.

The newborn's intestines are also relatively immature. Prior to birth, this organ is semi-dormant. Normal extrauterine transition includes a striking increase in blood flow and a decrease in vascular resistance that results in increased blood flow to the neonate's rapidly growing intestines.[47] The underlying musculature is thinner and less efficient in the newborn than in the adult, leading to unpredictable peristaltic waves. The folds and villi of the intestinal wall are not fully developed. The epithelial cells lining the newborn's small intestine do not have the rapid cell turnover that promotes most effective absorption. This immaturity of the intestinal epithelium affects the ability of the intestine to be protected from harmful substances, and the decreased vascular resistance increases the risk of damage subsequent to hypoxia should hypoxia occur.[47]

At birth, the rapid colonization of the sterile fetal intestine with commensal bacteria performs valuable functions and prevents some pathogenic bacteria from dominating. Following a vaginal birth, the first colonization is with maternal vaginal bacteria. Following a cesarean section birth, the first colonization is with bacteria from the operating room environment. Although the intestinal epithelium is exposed to trillions of bacteria, the intestinal epithelium makes an effective barrier against bacteria in a process known as mucosal host–microbial homeostasis.[48] This physiological process is the start of the development of an intestinal microbiota that recognizes healthy bacteria and repels harmful ones.

In humans, the entire gastrointestinal tract serves as part of the natural immune system, a system of defense for the host. During early infancy, the newborn faces the substantial task of "gut closure," the process by which the epithelial surfaces of the intestine become impermeable to antigens. Prior to gut closure, the infant is vulnerable to bacterial/viral infection as well as to allergenic stimulation through intestinal absorption of large molecules.

Among the defenses present in the GI tract are the chemical barriers of increased acidity, the digestive enzymes that break down large molecules, and the secretory IgA that lines the small intestine. Secretory IgA dampens inappropriate immune activation and binds with harmful antigens.[48,49] In the breastfed newborn, maternal secretory IgA restricts immune activation and bacterial attachments.[49] Unlike other types of immunoglobulin, secretory IgA is not absorbed but rather works at the local level in the intestine.[50]

The beginning of oral feedings stimulates the intestinal lining to mature via promotion of rapid cell turnover and production of microvillus enzymes such as amylase, trypsin, and pancreatic lipase. All enteral feedings, even in very small amounts, lead to helpful surges in gastrointestinal trophic factors—mainly hormones that lead to a full maturation in functioning.[51] The colon in the newborn conserves water less efficiently than that in the adult, which predisposes the newborn to complications from water loss. This makes a diarrheal illness potentially serious in a young infant.

The Renal System

The term newborn has some structural and functional immaturity in the renal system, most of which resolves spontaneously during the first month of life. Thus this issue is only a problem for sick or stressed newborns. If the newborn needs intravenous fluids or medications, the limitations of the still developing renal system increase the risk of iatrogenic fluid overload.

The newborn kidney has decreased renal blood flow and glomerular filtration rate. Tubular function is immature, which can lead to large sodium losses and other electrolyte imbalances. The newborn is unable to concentrate urine very well, which is reflected in a low specific gravity (as low as 1.004) and urine osmolality. All of these renal limitations are accentuated in the preterm infant.

The newborn excretes a small quantity of urine in the first 48 hours of life, often as little as 30 to 60 mL. This urine should not include any protein or blood. Large amounts of cellular debris may indicate injury or irritation within the renal system.

Conclusion

Newborn physiology comprises a fascinating, dynamic, and rapidly changing system that both protects the newborn during adjustment to life and exhibits significant vulnerabilities to certain stressors such as cold and infection. Basic knowledge of newborn physiology can help midwives care for newborns and teach parents how to care for their infants as well.

● ● ● ● **References**

1. Darnall RA. The role of CO_2 and central chemoreception in the control of breathing in the fetus and the neonate. *Resp Physiol Neurobiol.* 2010;173(3): 201-212.

2. Helve O, Pitkanen O, Janer C, Andersson S. Pulmonary fluid balance in the human newborn infant. *Neonatology.* 2009;95(4):347-352.

3. Katz C, Bentur L, Elias N. Clinical implication of lung fluid balance in the perinatal period. *J Perinatol.* 2011;31(4):230-235.

4. Jain L, Eaton DC. Physiology of fetal lung fluid clearance and the effect of labor. *Semin Perinatol.* 2006;1(30):34-43.

5. Te Pas AB, Davis PG, Hooper SB, Morley CJ. From liquid to air: breathing after birth. *J Pediatr.* 2008;5(152):607-611.

6. Aguilar AM, Vain NE. The suctioning in the delivery room debate. *Early Hum Develop.* 2011;87(suppl 1): S13-S15.

7. Roggensack A, Jefferies A, Farine D, et al. Management of meconium at birth. *J Obstet Gynaecol Can.* 2009; 31(4):355-357.

8. Stenson BJ, Boyle DW, Szyld EG. Initial ventilation strategies during newborn resuscitation. *Clin Perinatol.* 2006;33(1):65-82.

9. Te Pas AB, Wong C, Kamlin CF, Dawson JA, Morley CJ, Davis PG. Breathing patterns in preterm and term infants immediately after birth. *Pediatr Res.* 2009;3(65):352-356.

10. Hutten GJ, van Eykern LA, Latzin P, Kyburz M, van Aalderen WM, Frey U. Relative impact of respiratory muscle activity on tidal flow and end expiratory volume in healthy neonates. *Pediatr Pulmonol.* 2008;43(9):882-891.

11. Gauda EB, Martin RJ. Control of breathing. In: *Avery's Diseases of the Newborn.* 9th ed. Philadelphia: W. B. Saunders; 2012:584-597.

12. Schneider DJ, Moore JW. Patent ductus arteriosus. *Circulation.* 2006;114(17):1873-1882.

13. Dakshinamurti S. Pathophysiologic mechanisms of persistent pulmonary hypertension of the newborn. *Pediatr Pulmonol.* 2005;6(39):492-503.

14. Mercer J, Erickson-Owens D, Graves B, Haley M. Evidence-based practices for the fetal to newborn transition. *J Midwifery Women's Health.* 2007;52(3):262.

15. Lunze K, Hamer DH. Thermal protection of the newborn in resource-limited environments. *J Perinatol.* 2012;32(5):317-324.

16. World Health Organization. *Reproductive Health: Managing Newborn Problems: A Guide for Doctors, Nurses, and Midwives.* Geneva, Switzerland: WHO; 2003.

17. Ravussin E, Galgani JE. The implication of brown adipose tissue for humans. *Annu Rev Nutr.* 2012; 31(1):33-47.

18. Tews D, Wabitsch. Renaissance of brown adipose tissue. *Hormone Res Pediatr.* 2011;75:231-239.

19. Soll RF. Heat loss prevention in neonates. *J Perinatol.* 2008;28(suppl 1):S57-S59.

20. DePuy A, Coassolo K, Som D, Smulian J. Neonatal hypoglycemia in term, nondiabetic pregnancies. *Am J Obstet Gynecol.* 2009;5(200):45-51.

21. Weissmann-Brenner A, Simchen MJ, Zilberberg E, et al. Maternal and neonatal outcomes of large for gestational age pregnancies. *Acta Obstet Gynecol Scand.* 2012;91(7):844-849.

22. Alkalay A, Sarnat H, Flores-Sarnat L, Elashoff J, Farber S, Simmons C. Population meta-analysis of low plasma glucose thresholds in full-term normal newborns. *Am J Perinatol.* 2006;2(23):115-119.

23. Milcic TL. Neonatal glucose homeostasis. *Neonatal Netw.* 2008;3(27):203-207.

24. Taylor JA, Wright JA, Woodrum D. Routine newborn care. In: Gleason CA, Devaskar SU, eds. *Avery's Diseases of the Newborn.* Philadelphia, PA: Elsevier; 2012:300-315.

25. Straussman S, Levitsky LL. Neonatal hypoglycemia. *Curr Opin Endocrinol Diab Obesity.* 2010;17(1): 20-24.

26. Folk L. Guide to capillary heelstick blood sampling in infants. *Adv Neonatal Care.* 2007;7(4):171-178.

27. Janes M, Pinelli J, Landry S, Downey S, Paes B. Comparison of capillary blood sampling using an automated incision device with and without warming the heel. *J Perinatol.* 2002;22(2):154-158.

28. Phillips C, Clifton-Koeppel R, Sills J, et al. Capillary blood draws in the NICU: The use of the Innovac quick-draw whole blood collection system versus traditional capillary blood draws. *Neonatal Netw J Neonatal Nurs.* 2011;30(3):175-178.

29. Morrow C, Hidinger A, Wilkinson-Faulk D. Reducing neonatal pain during routine heel lance procedures. *Am J Matern Child Nurs.* 2010;35(6):346-354.

30. Davis PG, Dawson JA. New concepts in neonatal resuscitation. *Curr Opin Pediatr.* 2012;24:147-153.

31. McDonald SJ, Middleton P, Dowswell T, Morris PS. Effect of timing of umbilical cord clamping of term infants on maternal and neonatal outcomes. *Cochrane Database Syst Rev.* 2013;7:CD004074. doi: 10.1002/14651858.CD004074.pub3.

32. Mercer JS, Skovgaard RL. Neonatal transitional physiology: a new paradigm. *J Perinatal Neonatal Nurs.* 2002;15(4):56-75.

33. Chaparro CM. Timing of umbilical cord clamping: effect on iron endowment of the newborn and later iron status. *Nutr Rev.* 2011;69:S30-S36.

34. Cernadas J, Carroli G, Pellegrini L, et al. The effect of timing of cord clamping on neonatal venous hematocrit values and clinical outcome at term: a randomized, controlled trial. *Pediatrics.* 2006;4(117):779-786.

35. Lauer B, Spector ND. Hyperbilirubinemia in the newborn. *Pediatr Rev.* 2011;32:341-349.

36. Schmutz N, Henry E, Jopling J, Christensen RD. Expected ranges for blood neutrophil concentrations of neonates: the Manroe and Mouzinho charts revisited. *J Perinatol.* 2008;28(4):275-281.

37. Puckett RM, Offringa M. Prophylactic vitamin K for vitamin K deficiency bleeding in neonates. *Cochrane Database Syst Rev.* 2000;4:CD002776. doi: 10.1002/14651858.CD002776.

38. Yoshio H, Lagercrantz H, Gudmundsson GH, Agerberth B. First line of defence in early human life. *Semin Perinatol.* 2004;28:304-311.

39. Tollin M, Bergsson G, Kai-Larsen Y, et al. Vernix caseosa as a multi-component defence system based on polypeptides, lipids and their interactions. *Cell Molecul Life Sci.* 2005;62(19):2390-2399.

40. Levy O. Innate immunity of the newborn: basic mechanisms and clinical correlates. *Nat Rev Immunol.* 2007;7(5):379-390.

41. Visscher MO, Narendran V, Pickens W, et al. Vernix caseosa in neonatal adaptation. *J Perinatol.* 2005; 25(7):440-446.

42. Wynn JL, Levy O. Role of innate host defenses in susceptibility to early-onset neonatal sepsis. *Clin Perinatol.* 2010;37(2):307-337.

43. Ygberg S, Nilsson A. The developing immune system: from foetus to toddler. *Acta Paediatr.* 2012; 101(2):120-127.

44. Guilmot A, Hermann E, Braud VM, Carlier Y, Truyens C. Natural killer cell responses to infections in early life. *J Innate Immun.* 2011;3(3):280-288.

45. Blackburn S. Cytokines in the perinatal and neonatal periods: selected aspects. *J Perinatal Neonatal Nurs.* 2008;22(3):187-190.

46. Lundell AC, Björnsson V, Ljung A, et al. Infant B cell memory differentiation and early gut bacterial colonization. *J Immunol.* 2012;188(9):4315-4322.

47. Reber KM, Nankervis CA, Nowicki PT. Newborn intestinal circulation: physiology and pathophysiology. *Clin Perinatol.* 2002;29(1):23-39.

48. Stockinger S, Hornef MW, Chassin C. Establishment of intestinal homeostasis during the neonatal period. *Cell Molecul Life Sci.* 2011;68(22):3699-3712.

49. Renz H, Brandtzaeg P, Hornef M. The impact of perinatal immune development on mucosal homeostasis and chronic inflammation. *Nat Rev Immunol.* 2012;12(1):9-23.

50. Harris NL, Spoerri I, Schopfer JF, et al. Mechanisms of neonatal mucosal antibody protection. *J Immunol.* 2006;177(9):6256-6262.

51. Neu J. Gastrointestinal maturation and implications for infant feeding. *Early Hum Develop.* 2007;83:767-775.

C H A P T E R

38

Examination of the Newborn

MARY KATHLEEN MCHUGH

JANET L. LEWIS

CYNTHIA JENSEN

Introduction

Immediately after birth, the newborn is assessed to determine if there is a need for resuscitation. The components and resuscitation techniques that all midwives need are reviewed in **Appendix 38B**. This chapter reviews the basic newborn examination. An extensive guide to the content and findings of the newborn physical examination is provided in Appendix 38A.

Components of the Newborn Examination

The complete newborn examination is composed of three parts: (1) a newborn history, (2) the gestational age assessment, and (3) the physical examination. From these results, the midwife will ascertain a newborn's level of wellness and identify potential or existing problems. A plan of care appropriate for that newborn and family can then be developed.

Appreciation for the role of the newborn history and the gestational age assessment has grown in recent years. With new knowledge of genetic inheritance, fetal development, and the effect of maternal conditions on fetal well-being, it is now recognized that birth is merely a continuation of a life already influenced by many variables. An accurate history of these variables becomes a critical piece of the full assessment of the newborn.

The development of gestational age assessment in the 1960s revolutionized neonatal care. Prior, gestational age was determined by maternal recollection and newborn birth weight. The clinical implications were enormous: A small newborn might be treated as preterm even though the neonate could be suffering from fetal growth restriction at an advanced gestational age. Conversely, a preterm infant of a woman with diabetes might be classed as being at term solely based on birth weight. With the ability to determine gestational age accurately came the ability to predict newborn health risks more precisely.

Approach to the Newborn Examination

The goal in examination of the newborn is to maximize the amount of information gathered while minimizing distress to the newborn and parents. Parents usually show appropriate concern about any handling or examinations that cause their child to cry. It is best to examine the newborn approximately 1 hour after a feeding, when the infant is most likely to be content. The general order of the examination also should be modified based on infant status at the time of the examination. For example, if the infant is asleep or in a quiet alert phase, collection of assessments that benefit from this status (e.g., heart rate and respiratory rate) should be obtained first. Once these data are collected, more potentially upsetting examination techniques can follow.

Prior to starting a physical examination and gestational age assessment, the maternal records during pregnancy, labor and birth records, and neonatal records should be reviewed. The examination should be performed in an environment that provides proper lighting, cleanliness, and warmth. All equipment needed for the examination should be organized before beginning, including gestational age and physical examination forms (or access to an electronic health record), measuring tape and length growth chart, stethoscope, and ophthalmoscope. Familiarity with the correct use of equipment and the guidelines for accurate measurement is essential. As a case in point, a study published in 2009 reported that of 200 children admitted to a large, urban hospital, only 24% had their linear measurement plotted correctly.[1] Prior to making any physical contact with the newborn, the midwife should perform a 3-minute scrub of hands and forearms with a bactericidal soap. Nonsterile gloves also frequently are used by midwives to perform the examination, especially in hospital settings.

Before beginning the examination, the midwife will explain the goal and purpose of the examination and identify estimated length of time to perform to the mother and/or family members. During the examination, feedback can be offered to the parents about the strengths and attributes of their newborn as well as any significant findings. As part of this exchange, the midwife can provide the parents with information and further assess their readiness for infant care.

Newborn History

The history of a newborn is gathered through chart review and interviews with the mother and possibly other members of the newborn's family. As the information is gathered, the midwife develops a mental list of areas of potential concern, including environmental, genetic, social, maternal medical, perinatal, and neonatal factors.

Environmental and Genetic Factors

Environmental factors that influence the newborn can include occupational exposure of the mother or father to hazardous materials such as X rays, other radiation, solvents, infectious agents, fumes, and gases. In the home, environmental factors that can cause fetal or neonatal damage or illness include unsafe drinking water, ingestion of raw or undercooked meats, exposure to paints or solvents, infections transmitted by house pets or gardening activities, poorly ventilated heaters, living near a hazardous waste site, and exposure to toxins brought to the home from a family member's workplace.

Inquiring about the well-being of other children in the home and their ages is important to assess for exposure to illnesss that could affect the fetus prenatally such as varicella, cytomegalovirus (CMV), parvovirus, or other viral illness.

The genetic history should include information about any family members, alive or deceased, with physical or mental disorders or inherited diseases. Any family members with unexplained multiple pregnancy losses also should be noted. Current health status of the newborn's parents, siblings, and second-degree relatives (aunts, uncles) should be included.

Social Factors

The social history includes information about the mother's place of residence, extent of prenatal care, and socioeconomic status. Other important information includes who else lives in the home and the designated caregiver identified for this newborn. At a discreet time, the midwife should ask the mother to clarify who is the biological father of the newborn. If the mother is in a lesbian relationship, the midwife should inquire whether the biological father is known to her or her partner and what role (if any) he will take in the child's life. It is important to learn whether the mother's relationship with her current partner is stable, because this aspect of her life could affect her ability to safely care for her infant. Identification of the decision maker in the household (e.g., mother, father, partner, grandmother, foster parent) is important so he or she may be included in discussions if needed.

If the mother has other children, there should be an attempt to determine whether or not they live with her and, if not, the reason for their absence. Inquiring about the health and well-being of the children, paying particular attention to any accident pattern that may indicate abuse or neglect, also is important. A key question used in the past to indicate the status of care received by other children in the home was the immunization status of those children. As more families choose among various immunization schedules, the decision making regarding this topic should be further explored (e.g., is the family making an informed decision regarding the immunization of their children, or is a lack of immunization due to neglect or other problem such as lack of access to healthcare services).

It is important to screen for substance abuse by the mother and other members of the newborn's household. Maternal exposure to even passive cigarette smoke may affect fetal development and growth,[2] while newborns and small children exposed to passive smoke are at risk for respiratory illness, including sudden infant death syndrome (SIDS).[3] Newborns living in an environment where there is regular substance abuse may also be vulnerable to neglect. The possibility for exposure to violence, direct or secondary, is also increased in such a setting. Some information about substance abuse screening may be found in the prenatal record.

Maternal Medical and Perinatal Factors

Basic data about the newborn's mother includes maternal age, last normal menstrual period, and expected date of birth. The number of prenatal visits is noted, along with any prenatal problems listed in the prenatal record. All lab work and prenatal testing, including ultrasound reports, should be reviewed.

A wide variety of maternal medical, prenatal, and intrapartum conditions can adversely affect the newborn's health and well-being. **Table 38-1** lists maternal medical conditions and indicates their possible fetal and newborn implications.

Neonatal Factors

Valuable data from the immediate neonatal period include the Apgar scores at 1 and 5 minutes and duration of any resuscitation efforts performed immediately after the birth. Information that indicates an increased risk for perinatal asphyxia is important, as is evidence suggesting an increased risk for hypothermia/hyperthermia and hypoglycemia.

Often the notes of the nurse or birth assistant regarding vital signs and the newborn's behavior in the time since birth provide insight into the newborn's health. Behaviors indicative of a healthy newborn transition include sucking, the ability to feed, alertness, voiding, and passage of meconium; behaviors of concern include jitteriness, lethargy, poor or absent sucking, and unusual cry.[4]

The results of lab tests performed in the birth room should be noted in the newborn history. Typically these tests include peripheral glucose samples, hematocrit, and blood gases. The site from which blood samples were obtained should be noted, as this site will be assessed during the physical examination.

Recording the Newborn History

Most institutions have forms, if not electronic health record systems, for newborn records. These forms may not allow the collection of the social or environmental information that is part of a thorough assessment. A blank progress note or section of the chart for narrative notes to record these pertinent areas of the history can be used.

Gestational Age Assessment

The Art of Observation

Observation is particularly powerful and useful in newborn assessment. Judicious use of observation minimizes handling of the newborn and subsequent newborn agitation. If the newborn is sick, less turning and handling will allow the infant to conserve oxygen and glucose.

Key components of both the gestational age assessment and the physical examination can be achieved by observation alone (**Box 38-1**).

Scales for Gestational Age Assessment

Standardized forms of gestational assessment achieved a wide level of use after the publication of research by Dubowitz in 1970, which described a detailed examination, named after the major researcher.[5] The Dubowitz examination combined assessment of both physical and neurologic characteristics.

In 1979, Ballard published a simplified method for assessing gestational age based on physical examination and neuromuscular assessment.[6] The Ballard Scale, based on the work of Dubowitz and others, involves less handling of sick newborns and relies less on a quiet, rested newborn for accurate results. This scale was revised in 1991 in an attempt to more accurately assess extremely premature newborns and provide more accuracy for term newborns.[7] It is now known as the New Ballard Scale, and has become the universal scale used to assess the gestational age of the newborn.

The New Ballard Scale (**Figure 38-1**) is accurate within a range of 2 weeks and can determine the gestational age of newborns as early as 20 weeks. This test is standardized and best performed by a trained examiner. Older studies have found that prior knowledge of the obstetric assessment of gestational age does not bias the examiner performing the New Ballard Scale.[8] Other studies have validated the New Ballard Scale as a reliable clinical tool until day 7 in the life of the moderately preterm infant, with neurologic signs being more reliable than strictly physical ones.[9] The New Ballard Scale does have some limitations, most notably, it may overestimate gestational age compared with ultrasound or last menstrual period among infants with lower weight or gestational age, and among those newborns whose mothers received prenatal corticosteroid therapy.[10]

The proper procedure for both the neuromuscular evaluation and assessment of physical maturity is included in Appendix 38A. Accurate assessment using the New Ballard Scale requires practice, and new examiners should have their examinations validated by a preceptor for several gestational age assessments with infants of different gestational ages.

The New Ballard Scale takes approximately 2 or 3 minutes to perform and its results should be recorded directly on the standardized form. It is best to record findings as the assessment is made, rather than

Table 38-1	Medical and Perinatal Factors and Neonatal Impact
Factor	**Possible Implications for the Newborn**
Maternal Medical Factors	
Cardiac disease	Chronic intrauterine hypoxia
Diabetes	Large for gestational age; trauma; hyperbilirubinemia
Kidney disease	Prematurity; fetal growth restriction
Hypertension	Fetal growth restriction; prematurity; abruptio placentae
Sexually transmitted infections	Perinatal transmission
Substance abuse	Neonatal withdrawal syndrome
Rh or other isoimmunization	Anemia; jaundice; hydrops fetalis
History of prior pregnancy losses	Genetic syndromes
Prenatal Factors	
No prenatal care	Maternal substance abuse; lack of social supports
Size–dates discrepancy	Fetal growth restriction; large newborn; birth trauma
Gestational diabetes	Macrosomia; birth trauma
Polyhydramnios	Neonatal kidney problems, tracheoesophageal fistula; other congenital anomalies
Oligohydramnios	Fetal growth restriction; amniotic band defects; dehydration syndromes, neonatal kidney/bladder abnormalities
Infection	Perinatal transmission
Perinatal Factors	
Preterm/post-term labor	RDS; metabolic acidemia at birth (BE > 12)
Prolonged labor	Neonatal trauma
Drug use in labor	Neonatal respiratory distress
Fetal intolerance of labor	Metabolic acidemia at birth (BE > 12)
Elevated maternal temperature	Perinatal transmission of infection
Abnormal presentation or position of fetus	Neonatal trauma
Meconium-stained fluid	Meconium aspiration pneumonia
Prolonged rupture of membranes	Perinatal transmission of infection
Excess bleeding in labor (e.g., abruption, uterine rupture)	Newborn hypovolemia; hypoxia
Prolapsed cord	Metabolic acidemia at birth (BE > 12)
Maternal hypotension	Metabolic acidemia at birth (BE > 12)
Fetal acidosis	Metabolic acidemia at birth (BE > 12)
Assisted vaginal delivery	Cephalohematoma; subgaleal hemorrhage
Cesarean section	Increased risk for transient respiratory problems in the newborn period
Shoulder dystocia	Erb's palsy

BE = base excess; RDS = respiratory distress syndrome.

BOX 38-1 Information Gathered by Observation

Gestational Age Assessment

- Skin attributes
- Genital maturation (female)
- Posture
- Lanugo

Physical Assessment

- Central and peripheral body color
- Muscle tone; resting posture
- Characteristics of cry
- Characteristics of respirations
- Body proportions and formation of visible body parts
- Abdominal contours
- Presence of hair, fingernails, toenails
- Symmetry of eyes; movements of mouth, arms, legs
- Presence of normal external genitalia
- Straight, intact spine

---

relying on memory. After scores for each category of physical and neuromuscular maturity have been assigned, they are summed and the aggregate score is plotted to obtain gestational age.

Application of Gestational Age Assessment

When the physical maturity score and the neuromuscular maturity score on the New Ballard Scale form are added, the sum yields a gestational age determination. The newborn will then be classified into one of the following categories:[11]

1. *Preterm*: gestational age of less than 37 weeks
2. *Term*: gestational age of 37 to 42 weeks
3. *Post-term*: gestational age of more than 42 weeks

Small, Appropriate, and Large for Gestational Age

It is possible to estimate newborn health risks solely based on gestational age. A more sophisticated relationship exists between gestational age and birth weight.[12] Within each of the three categories of gestational age, there will be some newborns who are larger and some who are smaller. The extremes of accelerated and diminished growth are associated with certain newborn problems and predispositions.

At any gestational age, birth weights vary with altitude, race, country of origin, and socioeconomic class.[13,14] Thus there is no international standard for normal birth weights for specific gestational ages.

The older charts that graph weight in relation to gestational age have limited utility because they determine gestational age based on the menstrual history alone. More recent research has studied birth weight in comparison to a gestational age assigned by Ballard scores and ultrasound.[15] Assessing birth weight in relation to gestational age will characterize the newborn as being in one of three categories:

1. Small for gestational age (SGA)
2. Appropriate for gestational age (AGA)
3. Large for gestational age (LGA)

Combining the gestational age categories with the weight/gestational age categories classifies the newborn as being term, preterm, or posterm and either small, average, or large for gestational ages. There are therefore nine possible assessments.

After accurately categorizing the newborn into one of these nine categories, a plan can be developed to assess and manage potential problems that are associated with each of these categories. This approach initially was based on publications from Lubchenco in the 1960s regarding newborn management.[11,12]

Midwives frequently care for late preterm newborns, the most common category of preterm infants. Late preterm infants are at higher risk for multiple respiratory conditions, problems with feeding, thermoregulation issues, and jaundice.[16] A study involving more than 300,000 neonates found that late preterm, SGA infants were 44 times more likely than term, AGA infants to die in their first month of life and 22 times more likely to die in their first year.[17] These differences in mortality rate ratios persisted for SGA infants, even when controlling for congenital conditions.

Physical Examination of the Newborn

Basic Approach to the Examination

The physical examination of the newborn is designed to screen for physical variations, malformations, and the overall health of the newborn. There are many differences between the components of an adult physical examination and that of a newborn.

During examination of the newborn, the four basic techniques of physical examination are used—inspection, palpation, auscultation, and percussion—in addition to observation. The complete examination will involve three types of evaluation:

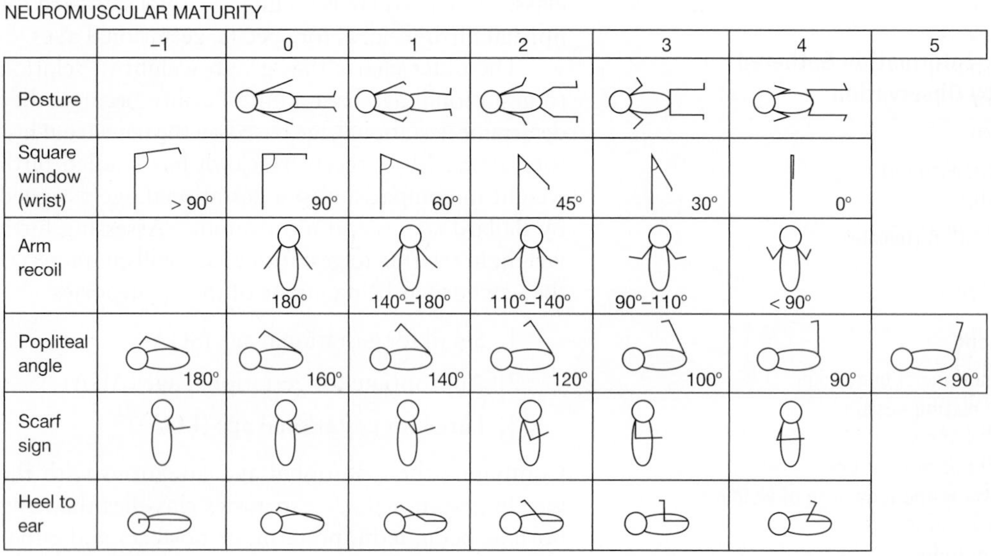

NEUROMUSCULAR MATURITY

	−1	0	1	2	3	4	5
Posture							
Square window (wrist)	> 90°	90°	60°	45°	30°	0°	
Arm recoil		180°	140°–180°	110°–140°	90°–110°	< 90°	
Popliteal angle	180°	160°	140°	120°	100°	90°	< 90°
Scarf sign							
Heel to ear							

PHYSICAL MATURITY

Skin	Sticky, friable, transparent	Gelatinous, red, translucent	Smooth, pink, visible veins	Superficial peeling and/or rash, few veins	Cracking, pale areas, rare veins	Parchment, deep cracking, no vessels	Leathery, cracked, wrinkled
Lanugo	None	Sparse	Abundant	Thinning	Bald areas	Mostly bald	
Plantar surface	Heel-toe 40–50 mm: −1 < 40 mm: −2	> 50 mm, no crease	Faint red marks	Anterior tranverse crease only	Creases anterior two-thirds	Creases over entire sole	
Breast	Imperceptible	Barely perceptible	Flat areola, no bud	Stippled areola, 1–2 mm bud	Raised areola, 3–4 mm bud	Full areola, 5–10 mm bud	
Eye/Ear	Lids fused loosely: −1 tightly: −2	Lids open; pinna flat, stays folded	Slightly curved pinna, soft, slow recoil	Well-curved pinna, soft but ready recoil	Pinna formed and firm, instant recoil	Thick cartilage, ear stiff	
Genitals (male)	Scrotum flat, smooth	Scrotum empty, faint rugae	Testes in upper canal, rare rugae	Testes descending, few rugae	Testes down, good rugae	Testes pendulous, deep rugae	
Genitals (female)	Clitoris prominent, labia flat	Clitoris prominent, labia minora small	Clitoris prominent, labia minora enlarged	Labia majora and minora equally prominent	Labia majora large, labia minora small	Labia majora cover clitoris and labia minora	

MATURITY RATING

Score	Weeks
−10	20
−5	22
0	24
5	26
10	28
15	30
20	32
25	34
30	36
35	38
40	40
45	42
50	44

Figure 38-1 The New Ballard Scale (NBS).

Source: Ballard J, Khoury J, Wedig K, Wang L, Eilers-Walsman BL, Lipp R. New Ballard Scale, expanded to include extremely premature infants. *J Pediatr.* 1991;119:417. Reproduced by permission.

(1) anthropomorphic measurements, (2) evaluation of organ systems, and (3) neurologic evaluation.

When documenting findings it is important to note during the physical examination, name any variations present, and avoid use of the nondescript phrase "within normal." There are also many minor newborn physical and behavioral variations that fall within the normal range and therefore it is important to know all the relevant terms and descriptions for newborn characteristics.

Most textbooks and physical examination records assume an examination that proceeds from head to toe. This approach is not absolute. For example, if the newborn is quiet or sleeping, many examiners start the hands-on examination with auscultation of heart and bowel sounds and palpation of the femoral pulses. In an awake, alert newborn, the examiner may check the red reflex first.[18] A crying newborn presents the opportunity for inspection of the mouth and throat. Excessive handling can overstimulate the newborn. Many times the newborn can be calmed during an examination by being given a non-latex gloved finger or pacifier to suck on if the mother gives permission.

Anthropomorphic Measurements

Anthropomorphic measurements include the infant's length, and chest and head circumferences. The newborn body has a unique appearance. Normally, the head circumference is larger than the chest circumference, the abdomen is protuberant, and the tone is flexed (**Figure 38-2**). Measurements should be performed using a standardized technique. The newborn length is most accurately assessed if the head of the newborn is flush against a firm surface. A mark often is made on the table paper to designate the top of the neonate's head. The newborn's legs are then extended and a mark made on the table paper where the heels rest when the legs are completely extended. After the newborn is moved, the distance between the mark from the top of the head and the mark placed at the heel is measured and documented in centimeters.

The newborn head circumference is measured around the head at the level of the occiput, parietal bosses, and just above the eyebrows. This measurement may decrease in the first week of life as caput succedaneum, cephalohematoma, or soft facial tissue swelling from birth recedes.[19] Chest circumference is measured under the arms and across the nipple line. The newborn's weight should be assessed on a scale with a drape between the newborn and the metal or plastic. This covering prevents conductive heat loss

and minimizes infection from cross-contamination. The scale should be calibrated to account for the weight of the drape. **Table 38-2** lists mean birth weights, lengths, and head circumferences of term newborns (37–42 weeks) born in North America.[20]

Assessment for Birth Defects

Variations in physical appearance may be due to inconsequential human variation or familial traits. However, approximately 3% to 4% of live births involve some congenital defect—most minor, but some serious. Many genetic, chromosomal, multifactorial disorders are initially suspected or even diagnosed based on the newborn's physical appearance.

Many parents believe that normal prenatal tests provide assurance that their fetus is normal. Unfortunately, all prenatal tests have limitations, and it is important to explain to new parents that most prenatal tests are screening tools meant to identify an increased risk for specific common disorders rather than being either diagnostic or able to detect all possible birth defects. Although no caregiver wishes to be the bearer of bad news to parents, the newborn examiner must inform parents about any potential problems and refer them to a specialist for more extensive evaluation.

Most minor malformations (**Box 38-2**), when found in isolation, are simple physical variants. However, the presence of three or more minor malformations is suggestive of a major underlying

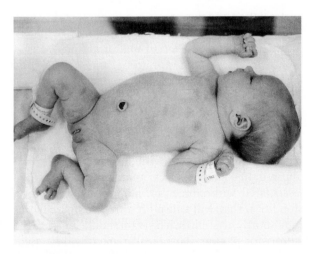

Figure 38-2 Normal newborn body proportions.

> ### BOX 38-2 Common Minor Malformations Noted on a Newborn Examination
>
> - Large fontanel
> - Epicanthal folds
> - Hair whorls
> - Widow's peak
> - Low posterior hair line
> - Preauricular tags and pits
> - Minor ear anomalies: protruding, rotated, low-set
> - Darwinian tubercle
> - Digital anomalies: clinodactyly (curved finger); camptodactyly (bent finger); syndactyly (webbed finger)
> - Transverse palmar crease
> - Shawl scrotum
> - Redundant umbilicus
> - Widespread nipples
> - Supernumerary nipples

Table 38-2	Mean (and Standard Deviation) for Birth Weight, Length, and Head Circumference by Sex, Gestational Age at Birth, and Ethnicity					
	European Descent		**Chinese Descent**		**South Asian Descent**	
Gestational Age	**Weight (g) Mean (SD)**	**Length (cm) Mean (SD)**	**Weight (g) Mean (SD)**	**Length (cm) Mean (SD)**	**Weight (g) Mean (SD)**	**Length (cm) Mean (SD)**
Boys						
37	3336.4 (434.3)	49.4 (2.0)	3119.0 (361.9)	48.3 (1.6)	3060.0 (346.1)	48.7 (3.9)
38	3359.4 (416.3)	49.4 (1.7)	3209.5 (356.5)	48.4 (2.0)	3201.8 (397.8)	50.2 (2.2)
39	3586.0 (460.3)	50.5 (1.9)	3359.0 (390.4)	49.4 (2.0)	3361.2 (383.5)	50.2 (1.7)
40	3687.6 (410.5)	50.8 (1.7)	3500.4 (343.5)	50.1 (1.6)	3452.5 (399.1)	50.4 (2.5)
41	3877.1 (384.4)	51.4 (2.2)	3724.1 (522.3)	50.9 (2.9)	3674.7 (363.1)	51.4 (1.5)
Girls						
37	3050.7 (414.1)	47.4 (2.5)	3048.4 (402.9)	47.6 (1.7)	2956.8 (436.3)	48.2 (2.2)
38	3993.5 (423.3)	48.6 (1.8)	3190.2 (377.1)	48.2 (1.6)	3118.4 (371.4)	48.8 (1.8)
39	3455.8 (434.0)	49.4 (1.7)	3271.0 (424.1)	48.7 (1.7)	3311.7 (458.5)	49.5 (1.9)
40	3639.5 (458.2)	50.2 (1.8)	3373.3 (362.3)	49.2 (2.2)	3376.1 (389.4)	50.0 (2.6)
41	3696.8 (448.0)	50.5 (1.6)	3451.0 (344.5)	49.4 (2.7)	3411.4 (401.6)	50.6 (1.6)

Source: Adapted from Janssen PA, Thiessen P, Klein MC, et al. Standards for the measurement of birth weight, length and head circumference at term in neonates of European, Chinese and South Asian ancestry. *Open Med.* 2007;1(2), Table 2. Available at: http://www.openmedicine.ca/article/view/47/45. Reprinted by permission.

malformation, and requires further evaluation.[21] For example, epicanthal folds may be normal by themselves, especially for infants of certain Asiatic descent. In combination with a transverse palmar crease and low-set ears, however, genetic evaluation for a possible trisomy is warranted.

With the routine use of prenatal ultrasound, many physical malformations of the fetus may already have been detected during the prenatal period. However, the accuracy of ultrasonography can be compromised by numerous factors (e.g., technician experience level, fetal position during sonogram), which may lead to many subtle malformations going undetected until the infant's birth. **Table 38-3** lists visual clues that may be noted during physical

examination and the serious conditions that they may indicate. Early evaluation and intervention can help prevent serious sequelae of malformations such as infection, intestinal perforation, spinal cord injury, or intellectual disability.

Newborns with ambiguous genitalia present a challenge. These newborns present with external genital characteristics of both males and females. If the examiner has doubts about the genitalia, an immediate consultation with a neonatal team is indicated. In some instances, ambiguous genitalia are associated with congenital adrenal hyperplasia, a condition that will cause life-threatening dehydration shortly after birth. The team should measure the clitoris or phallus. This measurement will be used,

Table 38-3	Visual Clues That Suggest Birth Defects and Genetic Conditions
Diagnosis	**Possible Visual Clues**
Mendelian Inheritance	
Autosomal Dominant (Mendelian Inheritance)	
Neurofibromatosis I	Café-au-lait spots
Tuberous sclerosis	Ash leaf spot
Myotonic dystrophy	Myopathic facies
Multiple epiphyseal dysplasia	Bumps at end of long bones
Waardenburg syndrome	White forelock
Peutz-Jehger syndrome	Brown lip macules
Van der Woude syndrome	Lip pits
Holt-Oram syndrome	Thumb anomaly
Autosomal Recessive (Mendelian Inheritance)	
Tay-Sachs disease	Cherry red spot
Galactosemia	Cataracts and neonatal jaundice
Cystic fibrosis	Meconium ileus, rectal prolapse
Congenital adrenal hyperplasia	Ambiguous genitalia
Mucopolysaccharidoses	Corneal clouding, joint contracture
Meckel-Gruber syndrome	Polydactyly, encephalocele
Rhizomelia chondrodysplasia	Short proximal limbs, cataracts
X-Linked Recessive (Mendelian Inheritance)	
Fragile X syndrome	Large testes
Duchenne muscular dystrophy	Large calf muscle
Menke kinky hair syndrome	Steel-wool like hair
Usher syndrome	Retinitis pigmentosa
Lesch-Nyhan syndrome	Gravel urine
X-Linked Dominant (Mendelian Inheritance)	
Incontinentia pigmenti	Pigmented skin swirls
Rett syndrome	Hand wringing
Vitamin D–resistant rickets	Bowed legs
Mitochondrial (Non-Mendelian Inheritance)	
Kearns-Sayre syndrome	Muscle weakness, ophthalmoplegia
Leber's hereditary optic neuropathy	Muscle weakness, ophthalmoplegia
MELAS syndrome (mitochondrial encephalopathy, lactic acidosis, and stroke-like seizures)	Muscle weakness, ophthalmoplegia
MERRF syndrome (myoclonic epilepsy with ragged red fibers)	Muscle weakness, ophthalmoplegia
Uniparental Disomy (Non-Mendelian Inheritance)	
Prader-Willi syndrome	Obesity, small hands and feet

Table 38-3	Visual Clues That Suggest Birth Defects and Genetic Conditions *(continued)*
Diagnosis	**Possible Visual Clues**
Gonadal Mosaicism (Non-Mendelian Inheritance)	
Osteogenesis imperfecta	Blue sclera
Teratogen(s)	
Alcohol	Microcephaly, short palpebral fissures
Dilantin	Nail hypoplasia
Hyperpyrexia	Neural tube defects
Tegretol	Neural tube defects
Coumadin	Flat nasal bridge
Accutane	Facial and limb anomalies
Multifactorial	
Clubfoot	Same as diagnosis
Cleft lip/palate	Same as diagnosis
Neural tube defects	Same as diagnosis
Dislocated hip	Same as diagnosis
Congenital heart	Same as diagnosis
Hypospadias	Same as diagnosis
Chromosomal	
Trisomy 21	Hypotonia, single palmar crease, prominent tongue
Trisomy 18	Finger and joint contracture, webbed neck
Trisomy 13	Polydactyly, cleft palate, scalp defects
Turner syndrome (45 XO)	Short stature, webbed neck
Klinefelter syndrome (47XXY)	Small testes, gynecomastia
Cri-du-chat syndrome (chromosome 5p deletion syndrome)	Natal mewing
Sporadic Multiple Pattern Syndrome	
Cornelia de Lange syndrome	Synophrys, phocomelia
Rubinstein-Taby syndrome	Large thumbs and great toes
Williams syndrome	Elfin facies
Sturge-Weber syndrome	Nevus flammeus
VACTERL association (VATER syndrome)	Tracheo-esophageal fistula, imperforate anus, limb defects
Congenital Defects: Minor and Major Malformations	
Deafness and renal disease	Preauricular tags and sinus tracts
Nasal sinus tract to septum and to brain in some cases	Nasal dermoids
Cleft lip and palate	Lip pits
Submucous cleft	Bifid uvula
Hypothyroidism	Enlarged tongue
Renal disease	Two-vessel cord
Spinal cord lesions	Lumbar hair tuft

Source: Adapted from Wardinsky T. Visual clues to diagnosis of birth defects and genetic disease. *J Pediatr Health Care.* 1994;8(2):63.

along with other physical characteristics of the genitalia, to describe the virulization as in categorized in Praderstaging.[22] Families should be informed of the examiner's concern and be encouraged not to assign a sex to the newborn.

Complete assessment of an infant with physical variations should be performed by a team that includes specialists such as a neonatologist, a geneticist, an endocrinologist, and the nurse who is caring for the child. Some common abnormalities may be confirmed with rapid testing within 48 hours, but unfortunately it may take weeks before a comprehensive genetic karyotype is complete. Extensive additional testing may be necessary to evaluate the type and extent of the malformation. When a physical variation of concern is detected, the midwife's role is to support the anxious family. It is very helpful to the family if a known and trusted clinician stays in touch with them during the period of testing and uncertainty.

The Neurologic Examination

The procedure of assessing reflexes, cranial nerves, and special senses is integrated into the overall physic examination outlined in Appendix 38A. The neurologic examination is an indicator of the integrity of the nervous system. Both diminished (hypo) and accentuated (hyper) responses are cause for concern. Diminished response can result from a congenital absence of a nerve, damage to sensory or motor pathways, or infection. Diminished or accentuated response to stimulation can also reflect a central neurologic deficit.

During the neurologic examination, assessments are made of the newborn's senses, including sight, hearing, and smell. Poor or absent response to oral, auditory, or olfactory stimulation may indicate nerve damage.

An absent or diminished response to an elicited reflex may be an indication of a variety of conditions.[23,24] Sometimes the reflex is partial or diminished because of newborn depression secondary to medications or infection. In other cases, the response may not be optimal because the sensory pathway conducting the stimulation has been damaged, reflecting a spinal or central nervous system lesion. Sometimes a reflex cannot be elicited because of temporary motor nerve damage that prevents the muscles in the affected area from responding to stimulation, as with a weak palmar grasp after a breech delivery or facial nerve paralysis after a forceps delivery (**Figure 38-3**). Sometimes damage is permanent, as in some brachial plexus injuries and some spinal cord defects. The following reflexes are elicited as part of

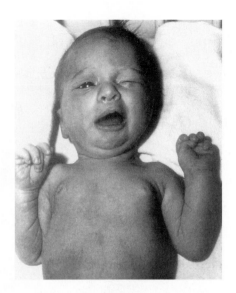

Figure 38-3 Facial nerve paralysis.

the physical examination and are described in detail in Appendix 38A:

1. *Eyes*: pupillary reflex, red reflex, doll's eye reflex, blink reflex
2. *Upper extremities*: palmar grasp reflex
3. *Lower extremities*: patellar reflex, plantar reflex, Babinski reflex (**Figures 38-4 and 38-5**)
4. *Torso*: anal wink, tonic neck reflex

Absent, markedly diminished, or accentuated reflexes and asymmetrical reflexes should be noted on the physical examination form and consultation with a pediatric provider about further testing and follow-up initiated.

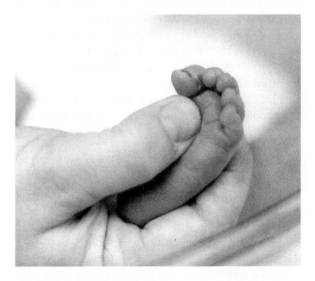

Figure 38-4 Plantar reflex.

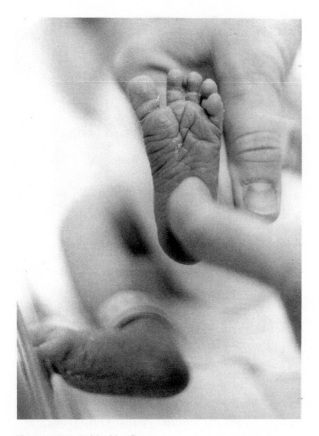

Figure 38-5 Babinski reflex.

One of the most commonly used evaluations of the neurologic status of the newborn is the Moro reflex, also known as the embracing reflex. As is true for the other primitive reflexes, the Moro reflex is mediated by the brain stem and becomes apparent at approximately 25 to 26 weeks' gestational age.[24] Once thought to reflect an infant's effort to cling to or "embrace" its caregiver, it is now more commonly seen as an involuntary motor response meant to protect the infant from sudden changes in body displacements.[24–26] In normal infants, the response is symmetrical and disappears by 3 to 4 months. The Moro reflex consists predominantly of abduction and extension of the arms with hands open, and the thumb and index finger semiflexed to form a "C". Leg movements may occur, but they are not as uniform as the arm movements. With return of the arms toward the body, the infant either relaxes or cries. In comparison, a "startle pattern" (or reaction) is primarily a flexion rather than an extension response to sudden stimulation, and becomes more pronounced and regular as the infant matures, rather than diminishing.[23,25]

Acceptable ways to elicit a Moro reflex that avoid eliciting a "startle pattern" include the following:

1. While the child is in a semi-sitting position, allow the infant to fall backward onto the examiner's open hand from an angle of 30 degrees.
2. While holding the infant in a horizontal position with both hands, quickly lower the infant approximately 10 to 20 cm, and come to sudden halt.[23]

As one of the primary primitive reflexes, any deviations found in the Moro reflex necessitates a pediatric consultation at a minimum and possibly a full neurologic work-up, especially if deviations in other reflex tests are also found. Sample deviations of the Moro reflex and their possible etiologies include:

1. Absence of the reflex may indicate intracranial lesions.
2. Asymmetrical response may indicate birth injury involving the brachial plexus, clavicle, or humerus.
3. Abnormal persistence of embrace gesture may indicate hypertonicity.
4. Persistence of entire Moro reflex after 4 months may indicate delay in neurologic maturation.

Becoming Confident at Newborn Physical Examination

Many intricacies and nuances are involved in conducting and assessing a complete newborn examination. Recognition of normal as well as possible deviations is an essential skill for any clinician involved in the care of infants. While many academic sources are available for reference and review,[27,28] they cannot substitute for multiple clinical experiences involving the observation and examination of many newborns.

● ● ● **References**

1. Lipman TH, Euler D, Markowitz GR, Ratcliffe SJ. Evaluation of linear measurement and growth plotting in an in-patient pediatric setting. *J Pediatr Nurs.* 2009;24(4):323-329.
2. Suarez L, Ramadhani T, Felkner M, et al. Maternal smoking, passive tobacco smoke, and neural tube defects. *Birth Defects Res.* 2011;91(1):29-33.
3. Adams SM, Good MW, deFranco GM. Sudden infant death syndrome. *Am Fam Physician.* 2009;79(10): 870-874.

4. Tappero EP, Honeyfield ME. *Physical Assessment of the Newborn: A Comprehensive Approach to the Art of Physical Examination.* 4th ed. Santa Rosa, CA: NICU Ink Book Publishers; 2011.

5. Dubowitz L, Dubowitz V, Goldberg C. Clinical assessment of gestational age in the newborn infant. *Pediatrics.* 1970;77:1.

6. Ballard J, Novak K, Driver M. A simplified score for assessment of fetal maturation of newly born infants. *J Pediatr.* 1979;95(5):771.

7. Ballard J, Khoury J, Wedig K, Wang L, Eilers-Walsman BL, Lipp R. New Ballard Scale, expanded to include extremely premature infants. *J Pediatr.* 1991;119:417.

8. Smith LN, Dayal VH, Monga M. Prior knowledge of obstetrical gestational age and possible bias of Ballard score. *Obstet Gynecol.* 1999;93(5):712-714.

9. Sasidharan K, Dutta S, Narang A. Validity of New Ballard Score until 7th day of postnatal life in moderately preterm neonates. *Arch Dis Child Fetal Neonatal Ed.* 2009;94:39-44.

10. Marín Gabriel MA, Martín Moreiras J, Lliteras Fleixas G, et al. Assessment of the New Ballard Score to estimate gestational age. *Anales de Pediatria.* 2006;64(2):140-145.

11. Battaglia F, Lubchenco L. A practical classification of newborn infants by weight and gestational age. *J Pediatr.* 1967;71:159.

12. Lubchenco L, Hansman C, Boyd E. Intrauterine growth in length and head circumference as estimated from live births at gestational ages from 26 to 42 weeks. *Pediatrics.* 1966;37:403.

13. Davidson S, Sokolover N, Erlich A, Litwin A, Linder N, Sirota L. New and improved Israeli reference of birth weight, birth length, and head circumference by gestational age: a hospital-based study. *Israeli Med Assoc J.* 2008;10:13-134.

14. Niermeyer S, Andrade Mollinedo P, Huicho L. Child health and living at high altitude. *Arch Dis Child.* 2009;94(10):806-811.

15. Dombrowski MP, Wolfe HM, Brans YW, Saleh AA, Sokol RJ. Neonatal morphometry: relation to obstetric, pediatric, and menstrual estimates of gestational age. *Arch Pediatr Adolesc Med.* 1992;146(7):852-856.

16. Ramachandrappa A, Jain L. Health issues of the late preterm infant. *Pediatr Clin North Am.* 2009;56(3):565-577.

17. Pulver LS, Guest-Warnick G, Stoddard GJ, Byington CL, Young PC Weight for gestational age affects the mortality of late preterm infants. *Pediatrics.* 2009;123:1072-1077.

18. American Academy of Pediatrics, Section on Ophthalmology. Red reflex examination in neonates, infants, and children. *Pediatrics.* 2008;122(6):1401-1404.

19. Gleason C, Devaskar S. *Avery's Diseases of the Newborn.* 9th ed. Philadelphia, PA: Elsevier Saunders; 2012.

20. Janssen PA, Thiessen P, Klein MC, Whitfield MF, Macnab YC, Cullis-Kuhl SC. Standards for the measurement of birth weight, length and head circumference at term in neonates of European, Chinese and South Asian ancestry. *Open Med.* 2007;1(2). Available at: http://www.openmedicine.ca/article/view/47/45.

21. Wardinsky T. Visual clues to the diagnosis of birth defects and genetic disease. *J Pediatr Health Care.* 1994;8(2):63.

22. Murphy C, Allen L, Jamieson MA. Ambiguous genitalia in the newborn: an overview and teaching tool. *J Pediatr Adolesc Gynecol.* 2011;24(5):236-250.

23. Futagi Y, Toribe Y, Suzuki Y. The grasp reflex and Moro reflex in infants: hierarchy of primitive reflex responses. *Int J Pediatr.* 2012;2012:191562.

24. Zafeiriou D. Primitive reflexes and postural reactions in neurodevelopmental examination. *Pediatr Neurol.* 2004;31:1-8.

25. Goldstein K, Landis C, Hunt W, et al. Moro reflex and startle pattern. *Arch Neur Psych.* 1938;40(2):322-327.

26. Sohn M, Ahn Y, Lee S. Assessment of primitive reflexes in high-risk newborns. *J Clin Med Res.* 2011;3(6):285-290.

27. Jones K. *Smith's Recognizable Patterns of Human Malformation.* 6th ed. Philadelphia, PA: Elsevier Saunders; 2006.

28. Zitelli BJ, McIntire SC, Nowalk AJ. *Zitelli and Davis' Atlas of Pediatric Physical Diagnosis.* 6th ed. Philadelphia, PA: Elsevier Saunders; 2012.

38A

Physical Examination of the Newborn

MOE: Method of Evaluation (I: Inspection; A: Auscultation; Pa: Palpation; Pe: Percussion)

NBS: New Ballard Scale

Findings	Significance	MOE	Notes
Color			Indicative of overall status of infant, especially cardiopulmonary system
In light-skinned infants: Body and mucous membranes should be pink	No cardiopulmonary compromise	I	
In dark-skinned infants: Mucous membranes should be pink			
Acrocyanosis of hands and feet during first 24 hours of life	Sluggish peripheral circulation caused by transition to the cool extrauterine life	I	*Definition:* Acrocyanosis—a blue or purple mottled discoloration of the extremities, especially the fingers, toes, or nose
Reddish hue	Adjustment in oxygen levels in extrauterine environment	I	Especially noted immediately after birth
Ecchymosis over presenting part	Pressure over presenting part, causing bruising and trapping of blood in external tissue layers	I	*Definition:* Ecchymosis—the escape of blood into the tissues from ruptured blood vessels marked by a livid black-and-blue or purple spot or area
			Technique: To differentiate between cyanosis and ecchymosis, apply pressure to darkened area; cyanotic area will blanche, ecchymotic area will remain dark
Mongolian spots over buttocks, with possible extension to sacral region	Hyperpigmentation	I	*Normal variation*, especially if found in dark-skinned infants
Jaundice after first 48 hours of age, receding by days 4–5	Physiologic jaundice	I	*Definition*: Physiologic jaundice—transition of blood supply to liver, increased RBC count with decreased lifespan of cells, decreased plasma protein level, and decreased glucuronyl transferase that aids in bilirubin conjugation
			Prematurity: Peak in jaundice may occur later

(continues)

Findings	Significance	MOE	Notes
General Appearance			Indicative of nutritional status, infant maturity, and general well-being
Well-formed and rounded, with presence of subcutaneous tissue	Good nutritional status; generally healthy	I	
No obvious anomalies			
Vernix	Increases with gestational age	I	*Definition:* Vernix—a pasty covering chiefly of dead cells and sebaceous secretions that protects the skin of the fetus
Lanugo	Decreases with gestational age	I	*Definition:* Lanugo—a dense cottony or downy growth of hair; specifically, the soft downy hair that covers the fetus of some mammals
			Technique (NBS): Check lanugo on the back with a direct light to get a clear view
Posture			
Newborn position: • Fists clenched • Arms adducted, flexed • Hips abducted • Knees flexed • Flexion moves upward to arms • Spinal column straight		I	*Technique (NBS):* With the infant supine and quiet, score as indicated on Figure 38-1 *Prematurity:* "Frog position" of legs
Movement: • Spontaneous, symmetrical, may be slightly tremulous • Flexion and extension should be equal bilaterally	Full-term newborn activity	I	*Definition:* Tremulous—jerky motions, unequal movement. *Prematurity:* No movement or asymmetrical, irregular, tremulous
Muscle Strength and Tone			
Strength and tone: Strong	May be full term	I	*Prematurity:* Strength and tone weak, hypotonia, or flaccid
Palmar grasp: Strong	Good overall strength; may be full term	I	*Prematurity:* Palmar grasp weak
Alertness and Cry			
Mood: • Ranges from quiet to alert • Consolable when upset	Normal newborn activity	I	*Prematurity:* Not easily aroused, not very alert
Cry: Strong	No increased intracranial pressure	I	
Moro (embracing) reflex: • Symmetrical • Disappears by 2 to 4 months		I/Pa	*Definition:* Consists predominantly of abduction and extension of the arms with hands open and the thumb and index finger semiflexed to form a "C". Leg movements may occur, but they are not as uniform as the arm movements. With return of the arms toward the body, the infant either relaxes or cries.

Findings	Significance	MOE	Notes
Moro (embracing) reflex: *(continued)*			*Technique:* Acceptable ways to elicit a Moro reflex include the following: 1. While the child is in a semi-sitting position, allow the infant to fall backward onto the examiner's open hand from an angle of 30 degrees 2. While holding the infant in a horizontal position with both hands, quickly lower the infant approximately 10–20 cm and come to sudden halt

Cardiopulmonary System

Findings	Significance	MOE	Notes
Respiratory effort: • Easy, unlabored rhythm • May be irregular, but periods of apnea < 15 seconds • Abdominal breathing	No respiratory distress or difficulty	I	
Respiratory rate: 40–60 breaths per minute	Normal rate	I	*Variation on normal:* Tachypnea in cesarean section or in full-term infants may be transient from retention of lung fluid *Prematurity:* Apnea > 15 seconds and accompanied by duskiness, cyanosis, or respiratory rate > 60 breaths per minute
Thorax: Symmetrical excursion	Normal respiratory pattern	I	*Definition:* Excursion—one complete movement of expansion and contraction of the lungs and their membranes (as in breathing)
Anteroposterior diameter: Normal	Normal respiratory pattern	I	
Breath sounds: • Clear • Equal bilaterally, anteriorly, and posteriorly • Occasional rales in first 24 hours	Clear lung fields	A	*Variation on normal:* Occasional rales may be present the first few hours after birth because of residual fetal lung fluid; no color changes or cyanosis should accompany this finding
Heart rate: • 100–160 bpm • Regular rate and rhythm • Without murmurs or only initial slight murmur	Normal cardiac rhythm without significant abnormalities	A	*Variation on normal:* Initial, slight murmur, usually heard at left sternal border or above apical pulse; may persist until the ductus arteriosus closes *Prematurity:* Bradycardia < 100 beats per minute or tachycardia > 160 beats per minute; murmur
Cranium/abdomen: No bruit Apical pulse: At fourth or fifth intercostal space, mid-clavicular line, left anterior chest	No arteriovenous malformation Normal position of cardiac pulse; no shifting; without cardiomegaly	Pa	*Definition:* Bruit—any of several generally abnormal sounds heard on auscultation *Variation on normal:* Point of maximum impulse at the fourth intercostal space just right of the mid-clavicular line may be shifted to the right during the first few hours of life

(continues)

Findings	Significance	MOE	Notes
Thrill: None present after first few hours of life	No increased cardiac activity	Pa	*Definition*: Thrill—an abnormal fine tremor or vibration in the respiratory or circulatory systems felt on palpation

Blood pressure:
• Average systolic rate
  ◆ 28–32 weeks: 52
  ◆ 32–36 weeks: 56
  ◆ Full term: 63
• Equal in all 4 extremities
	Normal cardiac output; good circulation; possibly no cardiac defect	Pa	

Tympany: Not increased over lung fields	Normal lung field borders	Pe	*Definition:* Tympany—a resonant sound heard in percussion
Skin			
Moist Warm to touch No peeling, wrinkles, edematous or shiny/taut skin	Normal, well hydrated	I	*Technique (NBS):* With the infant supine and quiet, score as indicated on Figure 38-1 *Variation on normal* (unless other abnormal findings are also present): Nevus flammeus; meconium staining; petechiae; skin tags *Prematurity*: Gelatinous with visible veins (transparent skin and visible veins disappear with increasing gestational age) *Postmaturity*: Dry, peeling, cracked
Vernix: Present	Increases with gestational age	I	*Definition:* See above *Prematurity:* No vernix
Lanugo: Scant	Full term Decreases with gestational age	I	*Definition:* See above *Prematurity:* Abundant lanugo
Milia	Common in newborns	I	*Definition:* Milia—a small, pearly, firm, non-inflammatory elevation of the skin due to retention of keratin in an oil gland duct blocked by a thin layer of epithelium
Erythema toxicum	Newborn rash over body, usually on days 1–3	I	
Mottling	May be normal reaction to immaturity of organ systems, if infant is of normal temperature, without color changes or bradycardia	I	
Temperature: • Warm • Axillary temperature 35.5–37.0°C	Normal range	P	*Prematurity:* Temperature may be cool (< 35.5°C) or warm (> 37°C)
Head			
Normocephalic in proportion to body (head circumference for average full-term newborn is 32–38 cm)	Normal	I	

Findings	Significance	MOE	Notes
Head *(continued)*			
Molding: Cranial distortion lasting < 5–7 days	Excessive pressure on cranium during vaginal delivery	I	
Overriding sutures	Excessive pressure on cranium during vaginal delivery	I	
Caput succedaneum	Edematous region of scalp extending over suture lines, resulting from pressure on the presenting part during vaginal delivery	I	
Head lag: ≥ 10 degrees in full-term infant Able to support head	Head lag: Decreases with maturity	I	*Technique*: Pull newborn up, supporting the arms, from supine to sitting position; grade degree of head lag by position of head in relationship to trunk *Prematurity*: Head lag > 10 degrees; little or no support of head
Hair distribution: Over top of head, with single strands identifiable	Full term	I	*Prematurity*: Fine, fuzzy, may be over entire head
Without masses or soft areas over skull bones	Normal	Pa	*Variation on normal*: Masses or soft areas such as craniotabes over parietal bones may be normal if no abnormality is present *Definition*: Craniotabes—thinning and softening of the infantile skull in spots
Bruit: None	Normal	A	*Definition*: See above
Fontanelles			
Anterior fontanelle: • Open until 12–18 months • Diamond shaped • Approximately 5 × 4 cm • Found along the coronal and sagittal sutures	Normal	I/A	
Posterior fontanelle: • Triangle shaped • Approximately 1 × 1 cm • Found along sagittal and lambdoidal suture lines	Normal May be closed at birth	I/A	
Facies			
Eyes: • On line with ears • Normal distance between eyes (approximately 2.5 cm) • Unworried expression	Normal	I	
Nose: Midline	Normal	I	

(continues)

Findings	Significance	MOE	Notes
Oral Cavity			
Mouth: • Midline on face, symmetrical without drooping or slanting unilaterally with crying or other movement of mouth • Shape and size in proportion with face	Normal	I	
Mucous membranes: Moist, pink	Well hydrated and oxygenated	I	
Chin: Shape and size in proportion with face	Normal	I	
Lips: Completely formed, pink, moist	Normal	I	
Palate: No arching; intact	Normal	I/Pa	
Tongue: • Size in proportion with mouth • Midline	Normal No neurologic dysfunction	I	
Uvula: Midline rises with crying	Normal function of glossopharyngeal and vagus nerves	I	
Gag reflex: Present	Normal neurologic function of glossopharyngeal and vagus nerves	I	*Physiology:* Reflexes generally develop from head to toe during gestation
Sucking reflex: Present and strong	Normal maturity and intact hypoglossal nerve	I	*Technique:* Offer non-latex gloved finger or nipple to test *Prematurity:* May be absent
Rooting reflex: Present	Normal maturity and intact trigeminal nerve	I	*Technique:* When cheek is stroked, infant turns toward stroking *Prematurity:* May be absent
Salivation: Without excess	Normal	I	
Nose			
Position: Midline	Normal	I	
Nares: Bilaterally present	Intact	I	
Nares: Patent	Normal	I	*Technique:* Occlude neonate's nostrils one at a time while holding mouth closed; infant should be able to breathe through one side at a time; passing a catheter into newborn's nares, one at a time, also demonstrates patency
Nares: Grimace or cry in response to strong odors passed under nose	Normal; intact olfactory nerve	I	
Nares: Breathing detected bilaterally	Patent	A	*Technique:* With a stethoscope, auscultate for breathing one side at a time

Findings	Significance	MOE	Notes
Eyes			*Technique (NBS):* With the infant supine and quiet, score as indicated on Figure 38-1
Sclera: Clear	Normal	I	
Conjunctiva: Clear	Normal	I	
Iris: Colored evenly, bilaterally	Normal	I	*Variation on normal*: Brushfield's spots (these gold flecks may be normal if not found with other anomalies)
Pupils: Equal bilaterally and reactive to light	Normal; intact oculomotor nerve	I	*Technique:* Examination is done in a darkened room with penlight or flashlight; if done with a newborn in an incubator or in the nursery, shield the infant's eyes as much as possible
Cornea: Clear	Normal; intact	I	*Prematurity:* Hazy
Retina: Transparent	Normal; intact	I	
Lacrimal duct: Patent	Normal	I	*Definition:* Lacrimal duct—any of several small ducts that carry tears from the lacrimal gland to the fornix of the conjunctiva
Blink reflex: Reactive	Intact optic nerve	I	*Technique:* Responds to bright light
Red reflex: Present	Lens intact	I	*Technique:* Hold a direct ophthalmoscope close to the examiner's eye with the ophthalmoscope lens power set at 0. In a darkened room, the ophthalmoscope light should then be projected onto both eyes of the child simultaneously from approximately 18 inches away. To be considered normal, a red reflex should emanate from both eyes and be symmetric in character.
			Variation on normal: Transient opacity from mucus in the tear film that is mobile and completely disappears with blinking
Eyelids: Without edema, ptosis, or epicanthal folds	Normal; intact oculomotor nerve	I	*Definition:* Ptosis—a drooping of the upper eyelid
			Definition: Epicanthic fold—a prolongation of a fold of the skin of the upper eyelid over the inner angle or both angles of the eye
Doll's-eye response: Present	Normal: Intact trochlear, abducens, and oculomotor nerves	I	*Technique:* With the infant in supine position, turn the head from one side to the other: eyes move to the side opposite the side to which the head is turned
Eye position: Without slant	Normal	I	
Ears			*Technique (NBS):* With the infant supine and quiet, score as indicated on Figure 38-1
Position: In straight line with eyes; vertical angle that is greater than straight vertical line; without slant	Normal	I	
Skin tags: Absent	Normal	I	
Cartilage formation: Well-curved pinna, sturdy, stiff cartilage, instant recoil	Normal	I/Pa	*Technique:* Palpate the entire pinna of the ear for the presence of cartilage
			Prematurity: Cartilage flattened or folded with slow recoil

(continues)

Findings	Significance	MOE	Notes
Ears *(continued)*			
Hearing: Neonate startles or cries in reaction	Normal; intact auditory nerve	I	*Technique:* Use a loud noise or snapping fingers to elicit response
Otoscopic examination: • Umbo (cone) of light present, pearl-gray tympanic membrane may have vernix • Membrane is movable without bulging	Normal; intact ear without infection	I	*Technique:* This exam is often omitted because it is difficult to perform and may be potentially harmful if the examiner is not skilled; ear should be pulled down and back for examination
Neck			
Shape: Symmetrical	Normal	I	*Variation on normal:* Asymmetrical shape may be due to fetal position in utero
Head: • Turns from side to side equally, full range of joint motion • Shape symmetrical	Normal	I	
Length: Short, without excessive skin	Normal	I	
Tonic neck reflex: Asymmetrical and present but decreases	Normal	I	*Technique:* Place the infant in supine position; turn the head to one side with the body restrained; extremities on the side to which the head is turned are extended, but extremities on the other side are flexed: newborn's attempt to right the head when turned to the side tests the accessory nerve *Prematurity:* May be asymmetrical and strongly present
Thyroid: Midline	Normal	P	
Lymph nodes: Not palpable	Normal	P	
Masses: None	Normal	P	
Carotid: Pulse rate strong and regular	Normal cardiac and circulatory function	P	*Technique:* Do not massage the carotid artery or neck, as this action can result in reflex bradycardia
Clavicles: • Even and without "lumps" along bones • Symmetrical	No fractures	P	
Abdomen and Thorax			
Chest circumference: 30–36 cm	Average for full-term neonate	I	*Prematurity:* Chest circumference < 30 cm
Diaphragm: Equal excursion	Normal	I	
Ribs: Symmetrical	Normal	I	
Breast: Nipple spacing on line without extra nipples	Normal	I	*Variation on normal:* Extra nipple
Areola: Raised and without discharge	Full term	I	*Variations on normal:* Flat areola, discharge, or hypertrophy may be due to maternal hormonal influence *Prematurity:* Flat areola and/or discharge

Findings	Significance	MOE	Notes
Abdomen and Thorax (continued)			
Abdomen: Rounded, contoured, symmetrical	Normal	I	_Technique:_ To document distension accurately, measure the abdominal girth every 4 hours to detect changes _Prematurity:_ Abdominal edema or distension may be present
Umbilical cord: • 3 vessels (2 arteries, 1 vein) • Bluish white color	Normal	I	_Variation on normal_: 2 vessels (1 artery, 1 vein)
Abdominal musculature: Strong	Normal	I	
Peristaltic waves: Not visible	Normal bowel activity	I	
Bowel sounds: Present	Normal	A	
Abdomen: No bruit	Normal	A	
Renal: No bruit	Normal	A	
Xiphoid process: Present	Normal; intact	Pa	
Ribs: Without masses or crepitus	Intact, without defects or "air leaks"	Pa	_Definition:_ Crepitus—grating or crackling sound or sensation (like that produced by the fractured ends of a bone moving against each other)
Breast tissue: 1 cm	Normal: Full term	Pa	_Technique (NBS):_ Palpate to accurately assess breast tissue _Prematurity:_ Breast tissue may be < 1 cm and as little as 5 mm
Abdomen: • Soft • Nontender • Without masses	Normal	Pa	_Prematurity_: Separation of abdomino-rectus muscles (diastasis recti) is common
Kidneys: • 4–5 cm in length • Right kidney lower than left • Found in abdomen and posteriorly in lumbar or flank area	Normal	Pa	_Technique:_ Palpate with the newborn's legs flexed in a fetal position to relax the infant
Liver: • Sharp edge just above right costal margin • Firm	Normal	Pa	
Spleen: 1 cm below left costal margin	Normal	Pa	
Bladder: Not distended	Normal kidney and urinary tract system	Pa	_Technique:_ Be sure to evaluate immediately post void or may be falsely evaluated as distension

(continues)

Findings	Significance	MOE	Notes
Abdomen and Thorax *(continued)*			
Groin: • Femoral pulse rate strong and regular bilaterally • No hernias or masses	Normal	Pa	
Gastric bubble: • Just below left costal margin and toward midline • Tympanic	Normal	Pe	
Abdomen: Tympanic except dull over liver, spleen, and bladder	Normal liver, spleen, bladder, no masses (indicated by dullness)	Pe	*Technique:* Be sure to examine post-void
Genitourinary Tract, Female			
Labia majora: Present and extend beyond labia minora	Full term	I	*Technique (NBS):* With the infant supine and quiet, score as indicated on Figure 38-1 *Prematurity:* Labia majora smaller than labia minora
Labia minora: Present and well formed	Full term	I	*Technique (NBS):* With the infant supine and quiet, score as indicated on Figure 38-1 *Prematurity:* Labia minora larger than labia majora
Clitoris: Present, may be enlarged	Full term	I	*Technique (NBS):* With the infant supine and quiet, score as indicated on Figure 38-1 *Prematurity:* May also be enlarged
Urethral meatus: Present in front of vaginal orifice	Normal	I	
Vagina: Patent with or without white discharge	Normal	I	*Variation on normal:* Slight bleeding related to maternal (?) hormonal influence
Genitalia: Distinguishable as female or male	Normal	I	
Perineum: Smooth	Normal	I	
Anus: Midline, patent	Normal	I	*Technique:* Test by gently attempting to insert small non-latex gloved finger
Anal wink: Present	Normal sphincter	I	*Technique:* Light stroking of anal area produces constriction of sphincter
Genitourinary Tract, Male			
Penis: • Straight • Proportionate to body • Length: 2.8–4.3 cm	Normal	I	
Urinary meatus: • Midline • At tip of glans	Normal	I	*Technique:* If male neonate is uncircumcised, gently retract the foreskin. If circumcised, also check for edema or bleeding.

Findings	Significance	MOE	Notes
Genitourinary Tract, Male *(continued)*			
Urinary stream: Straight from penis	Normal urinary pattern	I	First void should occur within 24 hours after birth
Testes and scrotum: Full, numerous rugae	Full term	I	*Technique (NBS):* With the infant supine and quiet, score as indicated on Figure 38-1 *Prematurity:* Testes and scrotum may be flaccid, smooth, or with few rugae
Pigmentation: Dark	Normal	I	
Perineum: Smooth	Normal	I	
Anus: • Midline • Patent	Normal	I	*Technique:* Test by inserting small non-latex gloved finger
Anal wink: Present	Normal sphincter	I	*Technique:* Light stroking of anal area produces constriction of sphincter
Testes: Descended on at least one side	Full term	Pa	*Variation on normal:* Undescended testes *Prematurity:* Testes not palpable, though they may be found high in the inguinal canal
Upper Extremities			
Length: • In proportion to each other • Lower extremities and body symmetrical	Normal	I	
Full range of joint motion, including: • Abduction • Adduction • Internal and external rotation • Flexion • Extension as applicable to joint	Normal	I	*Physiology:* Full flexion of upper extremities comes with maturity *Prematurity:* • Limited range of joint motion • Limited range of flexion
Shoulder: Full range of motion and flexion	Normal	I	
Clavicles: Full range of motion and flexion	Normal	I	
Elbow: Full range of motion and flexion	Normal	I	*Variation on normal:* Limited range of motion or flexion of the elbow may be related to fetal position in utero
Wrist: Square window test	Normal	I	*Technique (NBS):* Test for square window by flexing the infant's wrist on the forearm, then measure the angle according to gestational examination chart (i.e., 0-degree angle for term neonate); exert pressure sufficient to get as much flexion as possible *Variation on normal:* Limited range of motion or flexion of the wrist may be due to fetal position in utero *Prematurity:* • Limited range of motion or flexion of the wrist • Square window angle > 0 degrees

(continues)

Findings	Significance	MOE	Notes
Upper Extremities (continued)			
Hand—grasp reflex: Present, strong, equal bilaterally	Normal; maturity	I	*Variation on normal*: Weak, absent, or unequal grasp reflex may be due to fetal position in utero *Prematurity*: Hand—grasp reflex may be weak or absent, or unequal bilaterally
Scarf sign: Elbow short of midline	Maturity	I	*Technique (NBS):* With the infant supine, take the infant's hand and draw it across the neck and as far across the opposite shoulder as possible. Assist the elbow by lifting it across the body. Observe the position of the elbow to the chest. Grade the position according to the gestational chart. *Prematurity:* Scarf sign—elbow beyond midline
Arm recoil	Maturity	I	*Technique (NBS):* With the infant supine, fully flex the forearm for 5 seconds, then fully extend by pulling the hands, and release; recoil time is graded *Prematurity:* Arm recoil—slow
Palm: No simian creases	Normal	I	*Definition:* Simian crease—a deep crease extending across the palm that results from the fusion of the two normally occurring horizontal palmar creases and is found especially in individuals with Down syndrome
Fingers: • 10 digits and without webbing • Equal spacing	Normal	I	
Carpals and metacarpals: • Present • Equal bilaterally	No fractures; bone formation normal	I	
Nails: Extend beyond nailbeds	Normal; full term	I	
Nailbeds: • Pink • Brisk capillary refill (< 3 seconds) • Equal bilaterally	Normal peripheral perfusion, normal oxygenation	Pa	
Clavicles: • Symmetrical • Without fractures or pain	Normal	Pa	
Humerus, radius, and ulna: • Present • Symmetrical • Without fractures	Normal bone formation	Pa	
Pulses: • Brachial and radial strong and equal bilaterally • Brachial and radial strong and equal in comparison with femoral pulses	Good peripheral perfusion, without obvious cardiac defects	Pa	

Findings	Significance	MOE	Notes
Lower Extremities			
Legs: • Length in proportion to body • Equal bilaterally • Limbs straight	Normal extremity length	I	
Toes: • 10 digits • Without webbing • Equal spacing	Normal	I	
Feet: Straight	Normal	I	*Variations on normal*: • Valgus (turned outward) or varus (turned inward) position of the foot may be related to fetal position in utero and usually resolves • Pedal edema may be due to pressure exerted by fetal position in utero
Ankle dorsiflexion: 0-degree angle	Maturity	I	*Technique*: Foot is flexed back on ankle, then angle between foot and ankle is measured *Prematurity*: Ankle dorsiflexion angle > 0 degrees, may be up to 90 degrees in very premature neonates
Popliteal angle: < 90 degrees	Maturity	I	*Technique (NBS):* With the infant supine and the pelvis flat on the examining surface, the leg is flexed on the thigh and the thigh fully flexed using one hand; with the other hand, the leg is then extended *Prematurity*: Popliteal angle: > 90 degrees and < 180 degrees in very immature infant
Heel-to-ear maneuver	Maturity		*Technique (NBS):* With the infant supine, hold the infant's foot with one hand and move it as near to the head as possible without forcing it; keep the pelvis flat on the examining surface. The heel will not reach the ear but only near the shoulder area in a full-term infant. *Prematurity*: The heel reaches the ear, or just short of the ear
Nails: Extend to end of nailbed	Normal; maturity	I	*Prematurity*: Nails do not extend to end of nailbed
Nailbeds: • Pink • Brisk capillary refill (< 3 seconds)	Good peripheral perfusion	I/Pa	
Plantar creases: Cover the sole of foot	Maturity	I	*Technique (NBS):* With the infant supine and quiet, score as indicated on Figure 38-1 *Prematurity*: Plantar creases are few or cover only the anterior third of the sole of the foot
Buttocks: Creases symmetrical	Normal hips	I	

(continues)

Findings	Significance	MOE	Notes
Lower Extremities _(continued)_			
Fibula, tibia, trochanter, and femur: • Present • Equal bilaterally	No fractures; bone formation normal	Pa	
Tarsals and metatarsals: • Present • Equal bilaterally	No fractures; bone formation normal	Pa	
Full range of joint motion (includes abduction, adduction, internal and external rotation, flexion, and extension as applicable to respective joints of legs, knees, ankles, feet, and toes)	Normal; maturity	Pa	_Prematurity_: Limited range of joint motion; flexion of legs, knees, ankles, feet, and toes is limited
Hips: Without clicks and full range of joint motion	Normal range of joint motion and no clicks	Pa	_Technique_: Ortolani's maneuver—flex the newborn's hips and knees, then abduct and adduct the hip to detect a slipping of the hip out of the acetabulum or an uneven motion unilaterally _Technique_: Barlow's maneuver—flex the newborn's hips and knees, then place a finger on the femur and trochanter, put the hip through full range of joint motion, and listen for an audible click
Knee jerk or patellar reflex: • Present • Symmetrical	Normal; mature	Pa	_Prematurity_: Knee jerk or patellar reflex absent, weak, or asymmetrical
Flexor plantar reflex: • Present • Symmetrical	Normal; mature	Pa	_Technique_: Stroking the lateral part of the sole of the foot with a fairly sharp object produces plantar flexion of the big toe; often there is also flexion and adduction of the other toes _Prematurity_: Plantar reflex absent, weak, or asymmetrical
Extensor plantar (Babinski) reflex: • Present • Symmetrical	Normal; mature	Pa	_Technique_: When the sole of the foot is firmly stroked, the big toe extends (bends back toward the top of the foot) and the other toes fan out; this is a normal reflex up to about 2 years of age
Back			
Spinal column: Straight	Normal alignment	I	_Variation on normal_: A curved spinal column should gradually resolve if it results from fetal positioning while in utero
No visible deviations or defects	Intact	I	_Definition_: Pilonidal cysts—containing hair nested in a cyst; used to describe congenitally anomalous cysts in the sacrococcygeal area that often become infected and emit discharge through a channel near the anus
Vertebrae: Present, without enlargement or pain	Normal spinal column	Pa	
Anus: See genitourinary tract		Pa	
Buttocks: See lower extremities		Pa	

Sources: Data from American Academy of Pediatrics, Section on Ophthalmology, American Association for Pediatric Ophthalmology and Strabismus, et al. Red reflex examination in neonates, infants, and children. _Pediatrics._ 2008; 122:1401; Kenner C, Lott JW, Flandermeyer AA. _Comprehensive Neonatal Nursing; A Physiological Perspective._ 2nd ed. Philadelphia, PA: W. B. Saunders; 1998: Table 17-2, pp. 237–249; Tappero EP, Honeyfield ME. _Physical Assessment of the Newborn: A Comprehensive Approach to the Art of Physical Examination._ 4th ed. Santa Rosa, CA: NICUInk Book Publishers; 2009.

38B

Newborn Resuscitation

CYNTHIA JENSEN

Resuscitation of the Newborn

Approximately 10% of newborns need some form of resuscitation at birth and 1% will require extensive intervention to transition to extrauterine life.[1] Any midwife attending births has a moral and ethical obligation to provide a birth environment in which resuscitation of the newborn can be effectively accomplished. To achieve that goal, the midwife needs standardized training in resuscitation techniques, available and functional resuscitation equipment, adequate support personnel, and a clear-cut system for escalation and transfer of care.

The midwife making resuscitation decisions follows the same critical management process used in every area of midwifery care: data collection, problem identification, formulation of a plan, action, and evaluation/reevaluation. Failure to follow the management framework can lead to resuscitation that is needlessly vigorous—or worse, woefully inadequate.

Standardized Education

Midwives, as well as any personnel attending births, should complete a neonatal resuscitation course. Two available evidence-based programs exist to train providers to care for newborns needing resuscitation. Helping Babies Breathe (HBB) is an initiative from the American Academy of Pediatrics (AAP) and the World Health Organization (WHO) to teach evidence-based resuscitation techniques for resource-limited settings. Information on Helping Babies Breathe can be found at www.helpingbabiesbreathe.org.

The American Heart Association and the AAP jointly developed the Neonatal Resuscitation

Program (NRP). NRP is the international standard for newborn resuscitation. Midwives, especially those attending births, can find information regarding accessing the course on the AAP website (www.aap.org/nrp) or find a course provided by a regional trainer in the community.

After completion of required study, students take an online exam and participate in "hands-on" facilitated simulation scenarios. Renewal is required every 2 years. Passing a multiple choice exam and satisfactory performance in a "megacode" does not guarantee competency or retention of course content and skills.[2] High-risk, low-frequency events such as resuscitation of a compromised newborn require rapid intervention and coordinated care. For this reason, in 2011, the format of NRP changed to allow participants to demonstrate not only the cognitive knowledge gained by study of the textbook but also active application of the technical and behavioral skills needed for the resuscitation of a depressed newborn.[3] Regular participation in simulated resuscitations or mock codes may increase content retention through repetition and exposure to uncommon events.

Simulated learning environments offer opportunities for interdisciplinary teams to practice effective communication techniques. The need to emphasize team communication as part of the training for newborn resuscitation is highlighted in the Joint Commission's *Sentinel Event Alert 30* titled "Preventing Infant Death and Injury During Delivery."[4] The report's root-cause analysis noted communication breakdown as a factor in 72% of cases that culminated in neonatal death or permanent disability. The Joint Commission's report emphasized the importance of communication over technical skills alone and their analysis even prompted it to recommend institutions regularly conduct training exercises to improve communication among team members in addition to practicing high-risk, low-frequency skills that might arise during newborn resuscitation or an obstetric emergency.[5,6]

Ten key behavioral skills known as Crew Resource Management (CRM) have been integrated into the NRP curriculum. These were adapted from the aerospace industry with the goal of improving team performance and safety for compromised neonates during resuscitation.[1,7] These principles and possible applications for midwives are listed in **Table 38B-1** and reflect the fact that the birth of a compromised newborn always is a possibility.

Table 38B-1	Behavioral Principles Adapted to Neonatal Resuscitation
Principle	**Application to Practice**
1. Know the environment	Know location of equipment and how to use it Know process to call for help if needed Know the standards and guidelines for care in the setting
2. Anticipate and plan	Use a checklist to ensure equipment is available, ready and functioning Be certain support personnel are immediately available to assist with care for the newborn Have a clear process for escalation and transfer of care
3. Assume the leadership role	Take control of the situation The midwife may need to initiate and guide the resuscitation until pediatric expert help arrives
4. Communicate effectively	Speak calmly and clearly Elucidate exactly what you need by making eye contact with assistants while assigning tasks Foster collaboration; anyone involved with the care of the newborn should speak up if there are any concerns with the resuscitation
5. Delegate workload optimally	At least one person should be devoted solely to the care of the newborn in distress Avoid attempting to do everything alone Avoid trying to do multiple tasks at once Delegate tasks such as: • Airway management • "Runner" to gather supplies • Chest compressions • Recorder
6. Allocate attention wisely	Focus care on the newborn; another person should be assigned to care for the mother and family Maintain overall awareness of the newborn's status and response to interventions Avoid fixating on tasks
7. Use all available information	Gather pertinent information about factors that may have contributed to the compromised newborn Be prepared to share this information clearly and succinctly with others who assume care of the newborn
8. Use all available resources	The person with the most expertise in neonatal care should assume care of the newborn Know who can be called for help and what they can do
9. Call for help when needed	Help should be summoned without delay as soon as there is suspicion that a newborn needs resuscitation
10. Maintain professional behavior	Maintain a calm environment Maintain personal composure Keep communication professional; avoid nervous laughter or use of foul language

Preparation for Neonatal Resuscitation

Neonatal Resuscitation Supplies and Equipment

The equipment necessary for basic resuscitation of the newborn should be available in all sites. Certain medications and equipment for advanced life support may only be available at a hospital site where trained neonatal and pediatric providers will make use of them. In a hospital setting, nursing staff are usually responsible for checking and maintaining equipment and supplies. In a birth center or home birth practice this responsibility may remain with the midwife or a nurse. It is imperative that all providers in all settings familiarize themselves with the location of resuscitation equipment, and know how to use it. Equipment should be checked at frequent intervals to be certain that all components are present and functioning, particularly before each delivery. A checklist is a useful tool to ascertain that all necessary equipment is available.

Equipment for birth in a home, a free-standing birth center, or a resource-limited setting will differ from the hospital. At a *minimum*, the equipment listed in **Box 38B-1** and illustrated in **Figure 38B-1** should be available. Discussion of additional equipment, especially for use in hospitals, can be found in the NRP course.

BOX 38B-1 Basic Equipment Necessary for Resuscitation of the Newborn at an Out-of-Hospital Site

- Gloves and personal protective equipment
- Firm, padded surface for resuscitation
- Towel and blankets for drying and covering/wrapping newborn
- Newborn hat
- Bulb syringe
- Cord clamps or cord ties
- Sterile scissors for cutting cord
- Stethoscope
- Self-inflating bag with pressure release valve, oxygen reservoir, and tubing
- Infant masks in term and preterm sizes
- Access to oxygen source if needed
- A cognitive instrument such as a card or poster with the NRP or HBB algorithm outlining critical steps

---

Immediate Assessment of the Newborn and Initial Steps

This appendix serves as a general guideline of initial steps that can be undertaken in any environment. However, it is not a substitute for formal neonatal resuscitation training (NRP, HBB) that is the standard of care, and it is the responsibility of every midwife to practice according to that standard. In addition, midwives should avail themselves of the information in the NRP textbook regarding resuscitation of the preterm infant, care for the infant with congenital anomalies, and the use of advanced resuscitation techniques.

1. Goals for resuscitation
   a. Establishment of effective respiratory effort
   b. Cardio respiratory stabilization
   c. Minimize heat loss and maintain normothermia

2. Immediately dry the newborn on the mother's abdomen, remove wet linen, and assess:
   a. General appearance
   b. Respiratory effort: Is the infant breathing or crying?
   c. Check the newborn heart rate by palpating at the base of the umbilical cord and abdomen or by auscultation. Communicate heart rate to other team members so everyone is clear on the status of the newborn.
   d. Does the newborn have appropriate tone?
   e. Note for an infant born in a setting where personnel are available to intubate: An infant born through meconium-stained fluid who is nonvigorous with poor tone, apnea, and heart rate < 100 bpm should not be dried or stimulated prior to tracheal suction.

3. If the heart rate is less than 100 bpm and the newborn is not making respiratory effort, briefly attempt to stimulate by rubbing the back or flicking the soles of the feet. If the neonate does not respond, is apneic, or is gasping, prepare to administer positive pressure ventilation (PPV) via self-inflating bag, flow-inflating bag, or T-piece resuscitator. These actions may necessitate moving the newborn to a flat surface with easy access for the resuscitation activities.
   a. Designate someone to call for help as soon as additional assistance is needed, but do not delay initiation of PPV
   b. Place infant supine

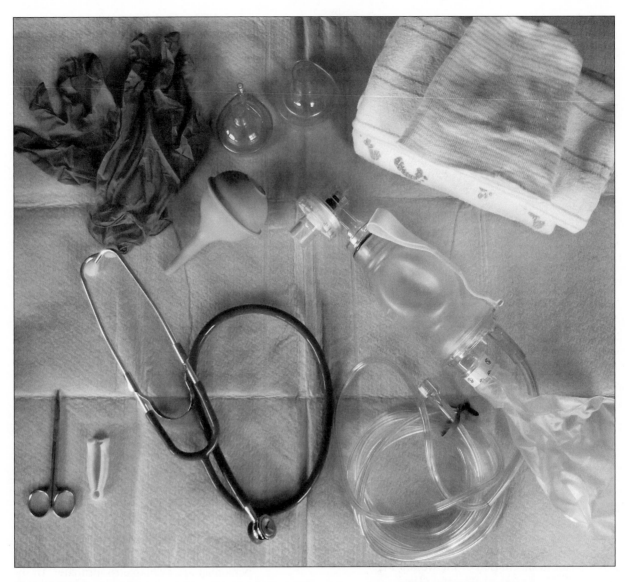

Figure 38B-1 Basic equipment necessary for resuscitation of the newborn at an out-of-hospital site.

c. Open airway with head in "sniffing" position as illustrated in **Figure 38B-2**.

d. Clear airway if necessary with towel, bulb syringe, or suction catheter. Suction mouth first, then nose as illustrated in **Figure 38B-3**. Deep suctioning is contraindicated and may induce a vagal response.

e. Place appropriate-sized mask over newborn's mouth and nose and ensure seal as illustrated in **Figure 38B-4**. It should be noted that mask ventilation is one of the most difficult skills to master and the most critical. If a seal cannot be obtained, assistance should be requested immediately. It may be necessary for one person to hold a seal initially while the other administers breaths.

f. Administer 40–60 breaths per minute while watching for gentle chest rise. Bilateral breath sounds should be heard throughout the lung fields on auscultation.

g. Initial distending breaths may require pressure up to 30 cm H_2O.

h. Maintain positive end-expiratory pressure (PEEP) of at least 5 cm H_2O when using a flow-inflating bag or T-piece resuscitator to prevent alveolar collapse on expiration. PEEP cannot be delivered via self-inflating bag.

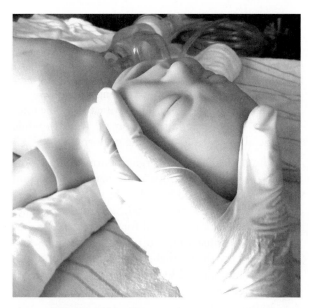

Figure 38B-2 Head in sniffing position with open mouth using shoulder roll.

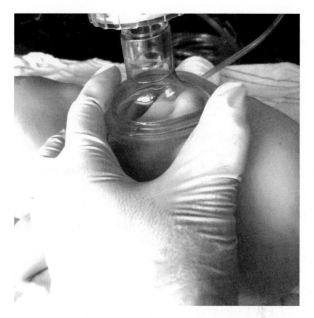

Figure 38B-4 Mask positioning.

i. Continue to ventilate for 30 seconds. Increasing heart rate, chest rise, and improvement in overall condition are indicators that PPV is effective.

j. If chest is not rising, take the following steps, sometimes referred to by the acronym "Mr. Sopa":[1]

  i. **Mask:** Make sure mask is positioned correctly and there is no leak

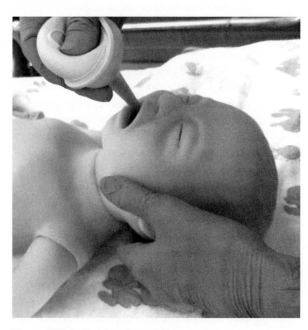

Figure 38B-3 Clearing the oropharynx.

  ii. **Reposition:** Maintain newborn's head in neutral position, avoiding flexion or hyperextension

  iii. **Suction:** Mouth, then nose

  iv. **Open:** Mouth

  v. **Pressure:** Increase pressure of administrated breaths, but do not exceed 40 cm H_2O

  vi. **Airway:** Consider alternative airway (intubation, oral airway, laryngeal mask airway)

k. Guidelines for use of supplemental oxygen have changed recently and the most recent version of NRP has recommendations based on current evidence. Pre-ductal oxygen saturation readings are used to guide decision making for administration of oxygen, and this is applicable to the hospital setting. In many cases room air resuscitation (21% oxygen) is adequate, but supplemental oxygen should be administered in the case of a severely compromised neonate. The NRP handbook includes additional information.

l. Gastric insufflation is a consequence of PPV and abdominal distension may impede lung inflation. If the newborn receives PPV for an extended period of time, air can be released from the infant's stomach via a 20- to 30-mL syringe attached to a 6–8 French orogastric tube (OG). If the newborn already is bradycardic, passage of an OG tube may exacerbate this phenomenon by inducing a vagal response; therefore, it may be advisable to wait until the initial steps are completed and the heart rate has stabilized before placing the OG.

4. If heart rate is < 60 bpm after 30 seconds of *effective* PPV, chest compressions should be initiated. Chest compressions require two people, one to compress and one to ventilate.

    a. Use ratio of 3:1 compressions to breaths. There should be 90 compressions to 30 breaths/minute, or 120 events per minute.

    b. The two-thumb technique is preferred and it is illustrated in **Figure 38B-5**

    c. Place thumbs one on top of the other on the lower third of the sternum above the xiphoid process

    d. Thumbs should remain in contact with chest at all times

    e. Compression depth should be one third the anterior–posterior diameter of the chest

    f. Compressions and breaths via bag mask need to be coordinated so breaths are administered during chest recoil. The compressor should audibly count "One and two and three and breathe"

    g. If room air is used for initial resuscitation, increase to 100% once chest compressions begin if it has not already been done. A self-inflating bag requires a reservoir to deliver 100% oxygen.

    h. Reevaluate heart rate and respiratory effort every 30 seconds

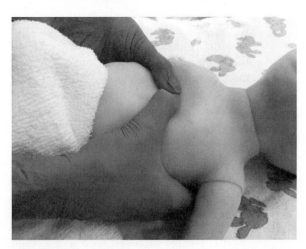

Figure 38B-5 Two-thumb technique for chest compressions.

i. Stop compressions when the heart rate is > 60 bpm

j. Continue to provide PPV if the infant is not making adequate respiratory effort

5. Maintain normothermia during and following resuscitation. This action is critical, and the midwife can be facilitating neonatal warmth while the above actions are being performed.

The World Health Organization defines normothermia as a temperature between 36.5 and 37.5°C (97.7 and 99.5°F).[8] In this range, metabolic demands are minimal. Skin-to-skin contact with the mother is ideal for the well infant, but a compromised newborn will need to be separated from the mother during resuscitation. Both hypothermia and hyperthermia increase energy demands and may complicate resuscitation and stabilization.[9]

Methods to promote normothermia include:

a. Prewarming the room to at least 25°C (77°F)[8]

b. Placement on a prewarmed surface to prevent conductive heat loss

c. Immediate drying to prevent evaporative heat loss

d. Removal of wet linens

e. Use of warmed linens to dry and cover newborn. In the hospital setting, a commercial blanket warmer may be used. In the home environment, a clothes dryer or hot water bottle may be used to heat blankets, but the temperature must be checked prior using on the newborn. A microwave should never be used to heat any item that will be used on a newborn because of uneven heating and case reports of extensive burns from this method. Bottles and gloves filled with hot water and placed in direct contact with the newborn's skin have also been implicated in severe burns.[9]

f. Covering the infant's head

g. Protection from drafts to prevent convective heat loss

h. Keep neonate away from windows to prevent radiant heat loss or gain

i. In the hospital setting, use of radiant warmer in servo mode when temperature probe placed on infant

j. For the preterm infant, additional measures may include use of a thermal mattress and covering the body entirely except for face with food-grade polyethylene wrap

6. Postresuscitation: A newborn who has required extensive resuscitation will need transfer to a higher level of care for observation and monitoring. The S.T.A.B.L.E. Program is an excellent course for anyone who cares for newborns and addresses the most critical needs during post resuscitation care. Information can be found at www.stableprogram.org.

   Documentation of the resuscitation efforts should be meticulous. Debriefing of all staff assists in identifying actions that were positive as well as changes to be made in similar situations in the future.

Endotracheal Intubation: To Perform or Not

Major resuscitation is a low-frequency event; however, the need for intubation is even less commonly employed. Midwives in tertiary care practices rarely may find themselves without a colleague skilled in this technique. Thus, they may not include this in their repertoire. Other midwives, especially in small hospitals, birth centers, or home birth practices remote from pediatric experts may find this an essential skill. The NRP program includes education about the procedure. It is critical that if the midwife learns this skill, the professional must regularly practice. It is better to continue ventilation by skillful use of bag and mask than inept intubation resulting in long periods of neonatal apnea.

Neonatal intubation is performed to establish airway access and to facilitate ventilation with an endotracheal tube (ET tube) with a bag, continuous positive end-expiratory pressure, or mechanical ventilation. Medications can be administered by the ET tube. For a newborn, only oral endotracheal intubation should be performed, not nasotracheal. If the newborn has thick meconium, intubation allows aspiration of the particulates under visualization before ventilation. When a newborn has a known congenital diaphragmatic hernia, intubation may be preferable to bag and mask ventilation.

Materials needed for the procedure minimally include:

1. Laryngoscope with appropriate straight blade size based on birth weight

   a. Miller 0 if preterm or less than 3500 grams

   b. Miller 1 if term infant 3500 grams or greater

2. Endotracheal tube of the appropriate size based on birth weight

   a. Weight of 2001–3500 grams usually requires 3.5 French tube size

   b. Weight greater than 3500 grams usually requires 4.0 French tube size

3. A stylet or endotracheal tube guide to provide rigidity of the tube in order to facilitate insertion. Should be at least 0.5 cm shorter than the tube to prevent inadvertent injury

4. Tape to stabilize the tube after insertion

5. Suction catheters to aspirate through the tube with suction

6. Bag and mask or other ventilator device

7. Oxygen

8. Stethoscope

General Guidelines

Note that the following guidelines provide an *overview* of this procedure. Any midwife who anticipates performing intubation should complete the NRP program and continually practice/update skills. The usual steps include:

1. Securely hold the laryngoscope in the left hand, position the device, and stabilize it with the right hand

2. Visualize the anatomic structures

3. Slide the ET tube with the right hand into the trachea

4. Note: Discontinue and initiate bag and mask ventilation if intubation is unsuccessful after 20 seconds and ventilate for 2 minutes. Repeat attempt only once more.

5. When ET tube is inserted, advance it to 1.0 to 1.5 below the vocal cords

6. Verify positioning with the stethoscope by listening to airflow

7. Secure the tube with tape after rotating it so lettering faces middle of lower lip and blue line is on the left. Note the number along the side of the ET tube

8. Use skin prep as appropriate

9. Verify positioning through X ray

● ● ● **References**

1. Kattwinkel J, ed. *Textbook of Neonatal Resuscitation.* 6th ed. Elk Grove Village, Illinois: American Academy of Pediatrics; 2011.

2. Halamek LP. The simulated delivery-room environment as the future modality for acquiring and maintaining skills in fetal and neonatal resuscitation. *Semin Fetal Neonatal Med.* 2008;13(6):448-453.

3. Zaichkin J, Weiner GM. Neonatal Resuscitation Program (NRP) 2011: new science, new strategies. *Neonatal Netw.* 2011 Jan-Feb 1;30(1):5-13.

4. The Joint Commission. Sentinel event alert: preventing infant death and injury during delivery. 2004 July 21;30. Available at: http://www.jointcommission.org/assets/1/18/SEA_30.PDF. Accessed August 21, 2013.

5. Yaeger KA, Arafeh JM. Making the move: from traditional neonatal education to simulation-based training. *J Perinat Neonatal Nurs.* 2008 Apr-Jun; 22(2):154-158.

6. Miller KK, Riley W, Davis S, Hansen HE. In situ simulation: a method of experiential learning to promote safety and team behavior. *J Perinat Neonatal Nurs.* 2008 Apr-Jun;22(2):105-113.

7. Halamek LP, Kaegi DM, Gaba DM, et al. Time for a new paradigm in pediatric medical education: teaching neonatal resuscitation in a simulated delivery room environment. *Pediatrics.* 2000 Oct;106(4):E45.

8. World Health Organization. *Thermal Control of the Newborn: A Practical Guide.* Geneva, Switzerland: Maternal and Safe Motherhood Programme, Division of Family Health; 1993.

9. Karlsen KA. *The S.T.A.B.L.E. Program: Post-resuscitation/Pre-transport Stabilization Care of Sick Infants.* 6th ed. Salt Lake City, UT: S.T.A.B.L.E., Inc; 2013.

CHAPTER

39

Neonatal Care

MARY C. BRUCKER

MARY KATHLEEN MCHUGH

Introduction

The role of the midwife in caring for the neonate during the first month of life varies markedly. In some locales, the midwife has little formal role once the newborn leaves the birthing room. In other practices, the midwife will continue care of the woman and newborn throughout the first several weeks of life. Newborns undergo profound physiologic transformations after birth, so midwives must be prepared to manage their care effectively.

The *Core Competencies for Basic Nurse-Midwifery Practice*, revised in late 2012, states that certified nurse-midwives and certified midwives "independently manages the care of the newborn immediately after birth and continue to provide care to well newborns up to 28 days of life."[1] Regardless of the formal scope of practice in specific settings, parents often call their midwife with questions related to the care and well-being of their newborn. Thus knowledge of normal newborn behavior(s) and signs of newborn disorders is an important component of midwifery practice for all midwives who care for families during the maternity cycle.

The First Golden Hour

The initial examination of the newborn is performed by the midwife, who places the neonate on the mother's abdomen immediately after birth. Although this is a very short period of time and it is not usually considered a formal physical examination, many important assessments are made. While the newborn nestles on the mother's skin and her arms encompass her baby, most likely the parents view the infant through the lens of the family connections, even to the point of noting how much the newborn looks like a previous child or other family member. The midwife, however, is identifying various neonatal parameters of health such as tone, color, and heartbeat (palpated through touching the umbilical cord) and identifying any congenital abnormalities. In addition, the midwife observes the basic physiologic responses of the newborn and corresponding parental behaviors, all while maintaining vigilance regarding maternal well-being. This initial complex set of observations and assessments takes place in the first minute of life before a formal Apgar score is awarded. Resuscitation is initiated if required, before the 1-minute Apgar score is given.

To be effective in verifying the normality of the newborn and intervening when abnormal findings are suspected, the midwife must be willing to accept the inevitable fact that not all newborns will be healthy at birth. Occasionally a newborn exhibits signs and symptoms that may indicate a deviation from health, either minor or major. The role of the midwife includes recognition of abnormal signs and symptoms, provision of adequate supportive care, and parent education.

The second assessment is assignment of the Apgar score, preferably by someone other than the person conducting the birth in order to decrease bias. Discussion of the Apgar score is found in more detail in *The Second Stage of Labor and Birth* chapter. Depending on the site, umbilical artery blood gases may be drawn and blood obtained for cord blood banking at this time.

During the first hour after birth, a newborn must successfully navigate the physiologic transition from an intrauterine environment to an extrauterine one. This process is described in the *Anatomy and Physiology of the Newborn* chapter. The concept of the Golden Hour originated in the care of trauma victims, for whom the first 60 minutes of care tended to predict death or survival. Today this term also has been applied to the important hours and actions immediately after birth.[2]

The First Hours: Initial Newborn Assessments and Care

In past decades, umbilical cords were immediately clamped and cut, after which a newborn was whisked away from the mother and sent to a central nursery. More recently, the newborn might remain in the room but still be separated from the mother by being placed into a warmer where professionals could perform the "necessary" immediate care measures, including injections, ointments, and, in some sites, routine supplemental oxygen. Various well-conducted studies have called into question this need for immediate care and separation from the mother.[3] Oxygen, in particular, is potentially hazardous to the newborn. Today, the American Heart Association, American Academy of Pediatrics, and Neonatal Resuscitation Program recommend resuscitation with room air (21% oxygen) for the term neonate instead of 100% oxygen, as no advantage from the latter has been demonstrated and possible risks of delayed alveolar septation and development of bronchopulmonary dysplasia have been suggested with the use of oxygen.[4–6]

Skin-to-Skin Contact

In lieu of separating mother and child, placing the newborn on the mother's abdomen provides several advantages. The infant is dried while on the mother, and her warmth decreases neonatal chilling. Early skin-to-skin contact (SSC), also known as kangaroo care, promotes longer breastfeeding and has been found to result in less crying among newborns when compared to infants who are separated from their mothers immediately after birth.[7] Other potential advantages of SSC are purported to be related to the establishment of a trusting relationship between mother and child at a sensitive period, although long-term studies about this hypothesis have not proven that SSC improves maternal–infant bonding over time.

Cord-Clamping

Within the next 2 to 5 minutes after initial SCC is initiated, the umbilical cord is clamped and cut. Often the midwife performs this task, but the woman's significant other or partner also may cut the cord. Waiting for these few minutes before clamping and cutting the cord is known as delayed cord-clamping. This practice decreases the incidence of iron deficiency during the first 6 months of life. Delayed cord-clamping has not been found to increase the incidence of postpartum hemorrhage, although there is some evidence of a potential increase in the risk of neonatal jaundice.[8] The advantage of delayed cord-clamping in preventing anemia appears to be apparent even among preterm infants.[9]

Instead of immediately placing the newborn on the mother's skin, some clinicians hold the infant below the level of the woman's perineum to facilitate a "placental transfusion" of more blood. However, there are reasons not to perform this maneuver, including no current evidence recommending this activity, it delays SCC, and most women are anxious to see and touch their offspring.[10]

Neonatal Hypothermia

Newborns have a predilection for developing hypothermia, as they have a large surface area per unit of body weight. As discussed in the *Anatomy and Physiology of the Newborn* chapter, brown fat is the major site for production of heat and serves as the circulatory route for heat production, or nonshivering thermogenesis. Hypothermia is associated with depression of the central nervous system, hypoglycemia, metabolic acidosis, tachypnea, respiratory distress, and decreased peripheral perfusion. The best treatment for hypothermia is prevention, and SSC is the best source of heat for the newborn. Many practices provide hats for the newborn after initial drying because the head has a large surface area from which heat can be lost. Temperatures usually are obtained by the axilla route and should be higher than 36.5°C (approximately 98°F). Not only has SSC been associated with a decreased risk of hypothermia, but it has also been found to be at least equal to incubators for rewarming infants who already have experienced chilling.[11]

Neonatal Hypoglycemia

Hypoglycemia may appear in the infant at any time, but is especially likely to occur during the first few days of life. Early and frequent feeding during the first week of life is an important preventive measure. After a nonmedicated birth, when the newborn is in skin-to-skin contact with the mother, a phenomenon known as the "breast crawl" has been observed in which the newborn can be observed actively moving, seeking the breast and, when finding it, suckling.[12] Breastfeeding decreases the risk of hypoglycemia and provides long-term advantages, as discussed in the *Breastfeeding and the Mother–Newborn Dyad* chapter.

Newborns born to women who have diabetes, preterm infants, and newborns who are small for gestational age are at increased risk for hypoglycemia. Common symptoms of hypoglycemia include jitteriness, irritability, lethargy, or poor feeding. Blood glucose levels obtained by heel stick can be of value in diagnosing hypoglycemia. Any glucose value of 45 to 50 mg/dL or lower should be immediately verified via a venous sample, and notification of the pediatric provider should follow promptly. The exact degree of hypoglycemia that requires formula feeding or intravenous glucose depends on other clinical factors such as feeding ability, weight, and risk factors for hypoglycemia. Although hypoglycemia can be easily treated, in extreme circumstances prolonged hypoglycemia is associated with neurodevelopmental delays.

Initial Newborn Treatments

Two prophylactic treatments are recommended for newborns within the first 4 hours of life: ophthalmic treatment for prevention of ophthalmic neonatorum and administration of vitamin K to prevent hemorrhagic disease of the newborn.

Ophthalmic Treatments

Eye prophylaxis is pharmacologic treatment originally intended to prevent blindness associated with undiagnosed maternal *Neisseria gonorrhoeae* infection. Neonatal conjunctivitis (also known as ophthalmia neonatorum) is more commonly caused by the *Chlamydia trachomatis* organism in the United States today.

Neonatal conjunctivitis secondary to *C. trachomatis* usually becomes symptomatic 5 to 14 days after birth and the risk that the infant will acquire conjunctivitis is 20% to 60% if the mother is infected when she gives birth. Conjunctivitis secondary to *N. gonorrhoeae* becomes symptomatic 1 to 5 days after birth and the risk that the infant will acquire conjunctivitis is 30% to 40%.

In years past, silver nitrate or tetracyclines were employed as treatments. Today, an erythromycin ophthalmic ointment is used for neonatal ocular prophylaxis throughout the United States. Infants may develop a chemical conjunctivitis after eye prophylaxis, but that condition resolves spontaneously within 24 to 48 hours. Some legal jurisdictions mandate that the eye prophylaxis be performed within the first hour of life, but in those situations many professionals wait until the end of the hour to apply this treatment in order to promote better *en face* interactions between parents and newborns. In developing countries, small studies of the use of povidone-iodine eventually may provide an alternative treatment.[13]

Prophylactic Administration of Vitamin K

Newborns do not have a major store of vitamin K. In addition, the levels of vitamin K are low in breast milk, and the neonate's gut flora, which usually includes bacteria that produce vitamin K, tends to be immature. A deficiency of this vitamin can result in the condition termed hemorrhagic disease of the newborn (HDN) or vitamin K–deficiency bleeding (VKDB). HDN commonly is categorized as either early (within 24 hours of life), classic (days 1–7), or late (2–12 weeks). Early HDN is rare and requires immediate pediatric consultation when the infant is bleeding, especially from injection sites or the umbilicus. Early HDN is most commonly found among infants whose mothers have taken pharmacologic agents such as anticonvulsant drugs. Classic HDN is most commonly found among infants who have not received prophylactic vitamin K injection during the first day of life, with the most common bleeding sites being gastrointestinal, cutaneous, or penile (subsequent to a circumcision). Late HDN is most common among newborns who are being exclusively breastfed and have not received prophylaxis; it is potentially the most serious type of vitamin K deficiency, as many infants affected with this variation develop intracranial bleeding.

A single injection of vitamin K, 1.0 mg given intramuscularly, has been found to prevent classic HDN.[14] For exclusively breastfed infants, the intramuscular injection also is protective, although some evidence exists that an oral administration of 1 mg vitamin K may be effective as well.[15] Controversy exists regarding the best route of administration for prophylaxis of infants at risk of late HDN. Intramuscular injection appears effective, but a single oral dose may be subtherapeutic.[16]

Vitamin K soon may not be the only recommended prophylactic treatment for a neonate. Some sources have suggested that newborns might benefit from several days of augmentation with vitamin D in an attempt to decrease deficiency of the vitamin and potential rickets.[17]

The First Hours: The Newborn with an Unexpected Immediate Health Condition

Various methods of assessment of the fetus are commonly used during a woman's pregnancy and birth today in the United States. When a newborn is anticipated to have a major health risk, such as preterm birth, a known genetic anomaly, or an overt congenital anomaly, plans regarding place of birth, route of delivery, and presence of a pediatric/neonatal team are often made in advance.

No single method of prenatal evaluation of the fetus assessment is perfect, however, and in spite of multiple prenatal assessments, a neonate may be born with an unexpected health problem. Major conditions include unsuspected congenital anomalies and birth injuries, although some "birth injuries" may occur prior to labor. When the unexpected occurs, the midwife should be able to accurately assess the situation and expedite appropriate pediatric transfer.

Congenital Defects

Some anomalies, such as cleft lip and extra digits, can cause emotional turmoil for parents. Parents often may be reassured that these conditions can be surgically corrected without long-term sequelae. Other types of congenital defects can result in rapid deterioration in the newborn and may lead to significant morbidity and mortality if not properly managed. Of these, abdominal wall defects and spinal cord defects pose particular challenges.

Abdominal wall defects are subdivided into gastroschisis and omphalocele, both of which have unclear etiologies.[18,19] Gastroschisis is a condition in which the eviscerated abdominal organs are not covered by a sac. In an omphalocele, the abdominal organs are external but are covered by a sac. In both cases, there is a high likelihood of infection, hypothermia, and dehydration because of the large surface area that is exposed.

Management of the newborn with an abdominal wall defect includes an immediate call for pediatric assistance and transport to a tertiary pediatric hospital or unit. The newborn is placed in a radiant warmer in as sterile an environment as possible. Sterile, warmed saline is applied to the eviscerated abdominal contents via sterile gauze pads. The infant's torso is then wrapped in sterile gauze to keep the saline in place. The infant is not fed via breast or a bottle; instead, a feeding tube is inserted and any stomach contents are aspirated. This neonate has an acute need for intravenous fluids.

The two most common neural tube defects are meningocele and meningomyelocele.[20] Meningocele is a bony defect of the spinal cord. With meningomyelocele, the vertebra is defective and the spinal cord and spinal roots are externally located in a sac. Meningomyeloceles are commonly found in the lower spine, lumbar, and sacral areas. The principles

for immediate management of spinal cord defects are similar to those described for abdominal wall defects: application of a sterile, warm saline dressing with a dry sterile overwrap, thermoregulation, and fluid maintenance. In addition, the infant is positioned prone and fecal contamination is scrupulously avoided.

Diaphragmatic hernias are surgical emergencies in the newborn because herniation of abdominal contents into the chest cavity may have caused pulmonary hypoplasia. These hernias are usually unilateral on the left. The degree of respiratory distress is directly related to the amount of lung tissue that has been compromised. In some newborns, the herniation is so severe that there has been stunted, if any, lung growth on the affected side. Signs of diaphragmatic hernia include decreased left-sided breath sounds, heart sounds on the right side, and severe respiratory distress at birth secondary to persistent pulmonary hypertension. Depending on the degree of the defect, the abdominal contents may be in the chest cavity, which causes a concave (scaphoid) abdominal contour. An endotracheal tube should be placed because use of bag and mask ventilation will worsen the situation. A feeding tube, preferably attached to low suction, should be passed and taped in place to vent the infant's stomach of air. Skilled pediatric care should be sought immediately.

Birth Injuries

Birth injuries may occur during a long, protracted labor or a difficult birth. For example, they can be associated with situations in which the fetus is large or the fetal presentation/position is abnormal. Palsies and plexus conditions generally are categorized as birth injuries and traditionally have been assumed to be associated with an event such as shoulder dystocia. Nevertheless, injury may sometimes occur in utero, such that parents and professionals are surprised when the child is born with a palsy or injury after an uneventful labor and birth.[21]

Facial Palsy and Brachial Plexus Injuries

Injuries to the face include bruising from forceps or facial palsy caused by either forceps or pressure from the maternal sacrum. The signs of facial palsy—a temporary condition—include asymmetry of the face. Consultation may be needed, and use of an eye patch and lubricating eye drops are common treatments.

Injuries to the brachial plexus may occur prenatally or during a birth when traction is applied to the neck. Such injuries can occur during breech births or births involving shoulder dystocia. The newborn with a brachial plexus injury may be in pain. The manifestations of the injury will depend on the nerve root that was injured and the degree of the injury. Nerve roots involved can include the cervical roots C5 and C6 (Erb-Duchenne paralysis), roots C8 and T1 (Klumpke's paralysis), or both. The physical signs of Erb-Duchenne paralysis include a generalized loss of movement in the affected arm with an adduction of the lower part of the arm. This leads to the characteristic "waiter's tip" sign, involving an internal rotation of the lower portion of the arm with the finger and wrist flexed. The grasp reflex is intact, but the Moro reflex is weak on the affected side. In Klumpke's paralysis, the grasp reflex is absent and the infant's hand is kept in a claw-like posture.

Management includes referral for splinting of the affected arm close to the body and consultation with the pediatric team. Parents should be encouraged to minimize handling the affected extremity for the first week because of the pain involved. Parents can be reassured that in the vast majority of cases, paralysis disappears in 3 to 6 months, with initial improvement becoming evident within a few weeks. Physical therapy is helpful after the first swelling subsides.

Injuries to nerve roots higher in the brachial plexus (C3–C5) can lead to signs of significant respiratory compromise because of paralysis of the phrenic nerve and diaphragmatic compromise. Newborns with this type of nerve injury take very shallow breaths with limited respiratory excursion and need aggressive respiratory support after birth.

Bone Fractures

Pressure and manipulation during the birth process may cause fractures of bones, although occasionally intrauterine fractures may occur.[22] The bones most frequently affected include the clavicles and the extremities. Signs of bone fracture include swelling, skin discoloration, lack of movement, abnormal positioning, and pain with movement. Crepitus occasionally can be elicited on palpation. The Moro reflex will be asymmetric. Management includes obtaining a pediatric consultation and splinting. If a clavicle or arm fracture is suspected, parents can be assured that newborn bones usually heal well and quickly.

Cephalhematomas and Skull Fractures

Injuries to the head include cephalohematomas, subgaleal hematoma, intracranial hemorrhage, scalp abrasions, retinal hemorrhage, and skull fractures. Cephalohematomas occur in approximately 16% of newborns who are delivered by vacuum extraction and they occur less often following a spontaneous vaginal birth. More severe cranial hemorrhages are more often associated with forceps deliveries. A cephalohematoma is a collection of blood under the periosteum of one of the cranial bones, usually the parietal bone. Unlike caput succedaneum or general edema, the blood does not cross the suture lines of the newborn skull, because the bleeding is under the periosteum (**Figure 39-1**). Some cephalohematomas occur with linear skull fractures, most of which heal well. A subgaleal hemorrhage is an accumulation

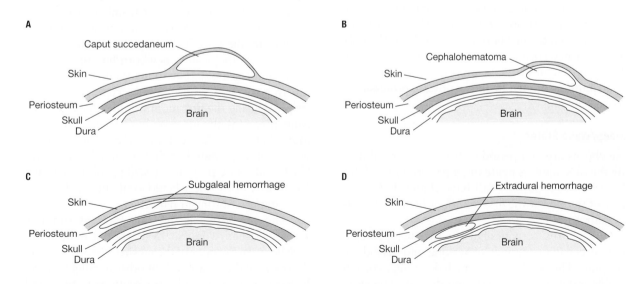

Figure 39-1 Cephalohematoma versus caput succedaneum.

Source: Sawyer SS. *Pediatric Physical Examination & Health Assessment.* Sudbury, MA: Jones & Bartlett; 2012.

of blood below the scalp but above the periosteum. A subgaleal hemorrhage is rare but life-threatening because this space is large and the newborn can lose a great deal of blood very quickly. Signs are a diffuse swelling in the head that shifts independent of movement. The newborn will display symptoms of shock and hypovolemia. Pediatric support is needed urgently if symptoms of a subgaleal hemorrhage are present. Symptoms of intracranial hemorrhage generally appear a few hours after birth and include irritability, apnea, poor feeding, or lethargy, and possibly a bulging fontanelle. A clear sign of a skull fracture is a depressed area of fetal skull, particularly over the parietal bones. An area of skull depression increases the possibility that fragments of skull bone have penetrated through the dura, the covering of the brain. Management includes careful positioning of the newborn on the side opposite the affected area and consultation with the pediatric team, who will order imaging tests.

The First Golden Days: Normal Newborn Behavior

Parents of newborns are particularly interested in the behavior and sensory capabilities of their children. Parents with exaggerated views of newborn abilities may become more easily frustrated. Parental advice from professionals, websites, social media, and even family frequently assumes that all newborns act similarly, but each neonate is an individual and all information, especially about behavior, should be viewed in that light. The midwife can help parents develop realistic expectations about normal newborn behavior during the newborn period. If this is the only aspect of newborn care the midwife is involved in, it may be one of the most important and significant contributions offered by the healthcare professional to the new family.

Sleep/Wake States

Newborns are in a period of behavioral instability. By the time parents figure out a pattern of newborn behavior, that pattern will have changed. A good rule of thumb for the first month of life is "There is no pattern."

Newborns' activities fall into two major categories of behavior: periods of waking and periods of sleeping. The waking states include crying, considerable motor activity, alert, and drowsy. The sleep states include active (light) sleep and deep sleep.

Table 39-1 summarizes these states, along with their implications for care.[23]

During the first month of life, the percentage of time spent in each of these states changes. Healthy newborns spend as much as 60% of their time sleeping. However, much of this sleeping takes the form of short naps. As the first month of life progresses, infants shift away from active (light) sleep and toward more extended periods of deep sleep. Similarly, there is a shift in the waking states toward an increase in alertness.

Newborn Reflexes

The newborn has two categories of reflexes: proprioceptive and exteroceptive. The exteroceptive reflexes are best evoked when the infant is quiet and alert, as they are stimulated by light touch. They include the rooting, grasping, plantar, and superficial abdominal reflexes. The proprioceptive reflexes include gross motor reflexes such as the Moro reflex, which can be checked at any time. Complete absence of any of these reflexes is a cause for alarm. An incomplete elicitation of a reflex may occur in some circumstances, however—for example, owing to neurologic depression secondary to medication. The loss of a previously strong reflex in the first month of life is a cause for alarm and should be reported to a pediatric provider.

Sensory Capabilities

Sensory capabilities are strongly related to gestational age. Dramatic increases in the sensory stimulation that occur just after birth can lead to neonatal exhaustion, evidenced as fussiness or aversion. Crying infants and fatigued mothers are frequently associated.[24]

At term, the healthy newborn has an ability to fix on and track objects visually. Many studies have shown a strong newborn preference for patterns of stripes. During the first month of life, newborns become preferentially interested in patterns with contours that resemble the human face. The ability to see in color is limited at first, so newborns prefer black-and-white patterns or strong colors like red. Newborns in the alert behavioral state will spend some minutes staring at patterns.

The newborn has the ability to discriminate among distinctive odors.[25] A newborn can discriminate between the odor of the mother's breast pad and the odors of the breast pads of other nursing women. Newborns react strongly to variations in taste and show a strong preference for sweet liquids. They suck

Table 39-1 Infant States

State	Appearance	Eye/Facial Movements	Breathing	Response to Stimuli	Implications
Sleep States					
Quiet sleep (deep sleep)	Essentially still with occasional startle	Occasional regular sucking, otherwise still	Smooth and regular	Tolerates stimuli well; only responds to intense stimuli	Avoid trying to feed at this time; will lead to frustration
Active sleep (light sleep/REM sleep)	Some body movements	REM fluttering of eyes with occasional smiling or crying sounds	Irregular	More responsive to hunger and handling than in quiet sleep; if stimulated, may return to active sleep to progress to quiet sleep or arousal	Highest proportion of newborn sleep Usually occurs before arousal Although may provide evidence of hunger, will not eat well in this state
Awake States					
Drowsy	Activity varies	Eyes may open and close or be slit-like in appearance Although often no facial movement, may have some smiling or sounds	Irregular	Will respond to stimuli, although response may be delayed	To promote awakening, provide some stimulation such as visual, auditory, or sucking stimulus
Quiet alert	Minimal movements	Eyes widen Face appears bright and attentive	Regular	Very responsive	Often occurs immediately after nonmedicated birth and can be positive for parent–child interactions As baby ages, spends more time in this state Good state in which to feed baby
Active alert	Smooth movements but variable activity	Eyes are open, but appearance is more dull Although often no facial movement, may have some smiling or sounds	Irregular	Will respond to stimuli, although response may be delayed	More sensitive to stimuli (e.g., hunger, handling) May move into crying state If fatigued, may move into drowsy or sleep state
Crying	Increased body movements, often with darkening skin tones	Eyes may be open or closed Grimaces	More irregular than other states	Very responsive, especially to negative stimuli	Sometimes crying infants can self-console May need swaddling, cuddling, or other measures to resolve crying

Source: Adapted from Blackburn S, Bakewell-Sachs S. *Understanding the Behavior of Term Infants.* White Plains, NY: March of Dimes Birth Defects Foundation. Available at: http://www.marchofdimes.com/nursing/modnemedia/othermedia/states.pdf. Accessed March 25, 2013.

longer and with an increase in heart rate when presented with a sweet liquid in a bottle.

Newborns have acute hearing and are able to localize sound in the environment. They can discriminate finely among sounds and show a preference both for real voices as opposed to synthesized voices. By the end of 1 month, neonates prefer sound with a pattern similar to speech.

Prior to birth, the fetus experienced touch in the shifting of the amniotic fluid. At birth, the newborn is dry for the first time and is subject to many and varied forms of touch. The ability of the newborn to respond to touch is well demonstrated with the elicitation of the various exteroceptive reflexes such as rooting, grasping, abdominal reflexes, and spinal curving.

Regulation of Behavior

Each infant has a unique ability to react to stimulation presented by the environment and personal bodily functions. Infants vary in their ability to cope with these stimuli. The newborn learns best in the alert state. At times, parental intervention in the form of rousing the infant or decreasing environmental stimuli may be essential if the newborn is to achieve the alert state.

Infants also disengage from interaction with adults when they are unable to tolerate more stimulation. They may convey their inability to engage by a variety of neurobehavioral cues. In contrast to the quiet alert phase, newborns may demonstrate extremes such as either crying or sleepiness, or either staring or averting gaze. **Table 39-2** summarizes common neurobehavioral cues.[26]

On occasion, a midwife may recommend to parents that the Brazelton Neonatal Behavioral Assessment Scale (NBAS) be performed.[27] This test generates a picture of the infant's communication via responses to stimuli and neurologic reflexes. The results are used to help parents interpret their newborn's behaviors. The test is standardized and can only be reliably administered by a trained examiner. The NBAS begins with the newborn in a sleeping state. Repeated stimulations are offered, and the examiner observes how the newborn adjusts to the stimuli. The behavioral components of the NBAS assess the infant's ability to perform the six tasks listed in **Box 39-1**.[27]

Several other assessment instruments exist regarding infant behaviors and development. For example, the Denver Developmental Screening Test (Denver Scale) assesses children from birth to age 6.[28]

Similar to the NBAS, this test observes the actions of the child and can assist in identifying conditions suggestive of cerebral palsy. The Broussard Neonatal Perception Inventory explores how mothers perceive their infants and assesses the attachment of the mother to child.[29] A number of other assessment tests exist, although most—if not all—cannot be used as diagnostic instruments.

Psychological Tasks of Early Infancy

During the first months after birth, a profound psychodynamic develops between the infant and the principal caregiver (usually the mother). The infant is performing the psychological task of differentiation: identifying herself or himself as a separate being in relation to other beings. Infancy and childhood for humans, unlike the corresponding periods for other species, are lengthy and dependent periods of life. Young infants must be able to prompt their caregivers

Table 39-2	Infant Neurobehavioral Cues
Stability/ Engagement Cues	**Distress/ Disengagement Cues**
Raises head, turns head	Facial changes (gaze aversion, grimace, hyperalert face, open mouth, slack jaw, tongue thrusting, frowning)
Searches for source of sound	
Facial gaze (eye-to-eye contact with alert eyes)	Startle, jerky movements
Sucking, mouthing	Sneezing
Smiling vocalization	Eyes staring, glassy eyed, aversion of stare, eyelids partially closed
Feeding posture	
Flexion of arms and legs	Change in color (mottled, dusky, cyanosis)
Stable heart rate	
Stable respiratory rate	Change in respirations/ pulse (e.g., tachypnea, bradycardia)
Smooth movements	
Finger folding or grasping	Grunting, crying, arching, sighing, hiccoughs
Smooth state transitions	Jitteriness, flaccidity, tremors
	GI changes (stooling, vomiting, regurgitation)
	Fingers splay, interlacing
	Limb extension, hyperextension, flaccidity

Source: Adapted from Hotelling BA. Newborn capabilities: parent teaching is a necessity. *J Perinat Educ.* 2004;13(4):43-49.

to feed, clothe, and shelter them. They trigger these protective reactions in adult humans by their sweet, physical appearance, their cuddliness, their social smiles, and their cries. A growing body of research implicates the maternal hormone oxytocin in the initiation and maintenance of human attachment behaviors. The brain is a target organ for oxytocin activity, as it is known to contain oxytocin receptors.

The midwife can assist the new parents in understanding the importance of forming this secure attachment. Some women need validation of their desire to spend time with their infant. The midwife can explain to both parents the critical importance of parental response to infant cues. This advice can help shape the parents' response to crying and the infant's attempts to communicate through smiling and eye contact. Mothering capability and desire to build this attachment can be undermined by failures at soothing or feeding. Women who *perceive* themselves as successful develop a feeling of confidence and competence. Therefore it is very important to take the time to talk with the woman about her perception of herself as a caregiver, and help to reframe expectations that may be unrealistic. Although most of the literature discusses maternal–infant attachment, it is also important to be cognizant of other possible "secure bases" for infants, including fathers and grandparents. If the infant is to learn the basic human emotion of trust, it is imperative that attempts to communicate receive an appropriate response.

Some women did not experience quality mothering when they were children. As a consequence, they may not have any memory or imprint of a secure attachment. The task of mothering may seem overwhelming to these women, and they are at high risk for frustration during the early months of motherhood. Whenever possible, attempt to refer these women to a counselor or parenting group during the weeks immediately after birth.

The First Golden Days of Life: Care of the Healthy Neonate

Breastfeeding

The *Breastfeeding and the Mother–Newborn Dyad* chapter provides an overview of the evidence in favor of the importance of establishing early breastfeeding. The mother–newborn dyad should be supported, especially during the early days when lactation is initiated.

Newborn Bathing

As with some of the other previously accepted "routines," bathing has been scrutinized since evidence-based care has become popular. Several studies have found that water alone is as effective as mild soaps in cleansing infants.[30,31] Antimicrobial soaps tend to be harsh and should be avoided.[32] However, there is a need for more rigorous dermatologic studies of the effect bathing methods have on neonatal skin integrity and hydration.[33]

Cord Treatments

In years past, treatment of the umbilical cord stump was initiated immediately or shortly after birth. Various antiseptic solutions were used, including rubbing alcohol, iodine, goldenseal, and echinacea. Today, the prevailing advice is to simply keep the area dry. A Cochrane systematic review found that newborns with cords treated with antiseptic solutions were no more or less likely to develop omphalitis when compared to neonates who received no treatment or placebo.[34] Conversely, some evidence suggests that treatment with an antiseptic solution may prolong adherence of the cord. The Cochrane review was primarily based on studies in developed countries where births occurred in clean conditions. Few studies have explored treatments in low-resource countries where newborns frequently die from such conditions as neonatal tetanus. In those areas, additional research is needed, especially regarding the potential advantages of antiseptic solutions used to treat the umbilical cord stump.[35]

Hospital Rooming-in

The healthy infant born at home or in a birth center has the advantage of constant maternal–newborn contact. This connection has not always been the case in hospitals. It was not until the 1940s that newborns were allowed to stay in a mother's room—that is, to room-in. By the middle of the twentieth century, rooming-in and the family-centered maternity care movement had begun.[36] This approach later served as the organized theme for a well-known maternity nursing textbook authored by a prominent midwife and nurse that contains basic tenets of the midwifery philosophy of care that are pertinent even today.[37]

Care of the newborn in hospital settings, including the full examination, can be conducted with the family in the room and may be conducted with the infant resting on a parent's lap. Including the family also provides invaluable opportunities to educate the family and answer questions as well as provide anticipatory guidance.

Newborn Screening

Increase in Number of Screening Tests

More than a half-century ago, it was discovered that a newborn could be accurately tested for phenylketonuria (PKU), an autosomal recessive metabolic disorder.[38] When PKU is untreated, children develop a range of debilitating neurologic conditions, including mental retardation, microcephaly, and seizures. Early diagnosis, however, allows dietary interventions to be initiated that can result in a normal life for the child. Newborn screening for PKU ushered in a new era in neonatal care, and its adoption was rapidly followed by identification of a number of potential disorders for which screening could be performed.

PKU and other conditions require whole blood that is obtained from the newborn and allowed to dry on absorbent filter paper. In some sites, the midwife collects the blood and places it onto the correct absorbent material. Proper technique and timing are important considerations. The test should be performed after the newborn has had a few feedings, as PKU will not be evident to the laboratory until some protein has been digested and metabolized. More than 50 core and minor conditions can be included in the basic newborn screening test, including hypothyroidism, cystic fibrosis, congenital adrenal hyperplasia, and various inborn errors of metabolism.[39]

Newborn screening programs are state specific; that is, not all states include the same list of conditions in the newborn screening test. In the past, lists could be obtained of the different state requirements for the test and those conditions that are included

in the test. Today, changes are occurring rapidly and clinicians have to make a concerted effort to understand current state laws. For example, a particular state may mandate testing for one condition that another state may not include in its newborn screening program. Parental education may be included in the state newborn screening programs; however, in some states it may not be reimbursed. Some states mandate testing of only newborns who are born in hospitals and do not address neonates born in out-of-hospital settings. Midwives who practice in out-of-hospital settings may either invest in the appropriate equipment for newborn screening or refer new parents to facilities wherein they can obtain the necessary screening.

There is a general consensus that no test should be included in a state newborn screening program unless treatments—albeit not necessarily cures—exist.[40] Factors such as financial and family costs of false-positive results have been discussed as important considerations regarding whether to include a particular test in a state program. Privacy of the newborn's genetic material also has been noted as a concern, especially after it was found that the state of Texas retained blood spots for research testing without informed consent—a realization that ultimately led to changes in the laws of that state.[41,42]

Point-of-Care Testing

Newborn screening has expanded to include hearing and pulse oximetry. As opposed to dried-blood testing that is performed in a central laboratory, hearing and pulse oximetry are performed and interpreted outside of a laboratory and at, or close, to the site of direct care. This type of screening, which is also known as point-of-care testing, presents myriad legal problems regarding oversight, standards, follow-up, and programmatic evaluation. In 2012, the Secretary's Advisory Committee on Heritable Disorders in Newborns and Children held a conference and recommended to the Secretary of the U.S. Department of Health and Human Services that quality control problems with point-of-care testing be addressed for safety and consistency reasons.[43]

Hearing

Approximately half of children with hearing loss have no identifiable risk factors; thus risk-based screening has been problematic. Universal hearing screening has been found to be useful, however, and newborns with hearing conditions identified in this manner have benefited from early intervention and ultimately fewer communication disorders.[44] In the United

States, universal hearing screening is advocated for all infants younger than the age of 1 month.[45]

Hearing programs often follow a two-step process, beginning with otoacoustic emissions (OAE) testing in the first few days of life. If a newborn fails the OAE test, an auditory brain stem response (ABR) should be conducted. In some sites, both tests are regularly performed. False-positive results occur occasionally, so confirmatory testing by pediatric providers is necessary. Midwives who conduct out-of-hospital births may find the equipment needed for such testing and its maintenance to be costly, and instead refer parents to sites such as hospitals that will administer the testing.

Pulse Oximetry

Although a number of studies in the early twenty-first century found that pulse oximetry is a good screening method to identify undiagnosed critical congenital heart defects (CCHDs) among otherwise healthy newborns, the initial research had few participants and a low prevalence of CCHDs.[46] However, by 2013, a systematic review of almost 250,000 infants found that the screening is highly specific, moderately sensitive, and likely to be cost-effective.[46–48]

Pulse oximetry targets several major and secondary CCHDs, including hypoplastic left heart syndrome, pulmonary atresia with intact septum, tetralogy of Fallot, coarctation of the aorta, and transposition of the great vessels. Oxygenation should be higher than 95%, and less than a 3% difference should be apparent when the pulse oximetry results for the foot and results for the hand are compared. As with hearing testing, midwives who conduct out-of-hospital births may need to find alternative sites that will conduct pulse oximetry testing.

The Circumcision Decision

In the United States, circumcising male newborns became prevalent in the 1950s. A complex web of religious, cultural, and family traditions surrounds each family in making this decision. Certain religious traditions (e.g., Jewish, Muslim) have practiced male circumcision for centuries. The type of practitioner who performs a circumcision varies. In many sites the obstetrician is the clinician who is responsible for this procedure, while in other areas it is a pediatric provider or a family physician. If the reason for the procedure is religious, a cleric such as a rabbi or a midwife who also is a Mohel may perform the circumcision. Circumcision is not a core competency in midwifery education but midwives can learn and offer this procedure as an advanced procedure following the recommended steps outlined in the *ACNM Standards for the Practice of Midwifery*.

The circumcision procedure involves the surgical removal of adhesions and retraction of the foreskin covering the glans of the penis (prepuce). This procedure usually occurs in the hospital or within the first 2 weeks of life as a religious ceremony. Complications from circumcision are unusual but can be serious, with the most common being infection and bleeding. Although the foreskin of male newborns is rarely able to be retracted, within the first few years the foreskin can be spontaneously retracted for the vast majority of male children who are not circumcised.

The contemporary rationale for circumcision is a source of controversy. Arguments exist both for and against male circumcision, although true benefits and hazards are relatively rarely cited.[49] Proponents of circumcision note that circumcised males experience lower incidence of medical problems including cancer of the penis, urinary tract infection (UTI), and sexually transmitted disease or infection (STI). Cancer of the penis is an unusual malignancy, especially in the cooler climates of the Northern Hemisphere. UTIs are similarly uncommon in infants. A number of studies have found a positive correlation between men who were uncircumcised and increased incidence of STIs, including HIV, although other contributing factors such as socioeconomic class and sexual practices have clouded the association, especially in developed countries. Routinely circumcising newborns does prevent the small percentage of men with phimosis (inability to retract the foreskin) from developing problems with edema and inflammation of the glans, and male circumcision does not interfere with reproductive functioning of the penis.[50] When circumcision is chosen by a mother or family, anesthesia is indicated for the newborn.

Opponents of circumcision maintain that modern sanitary conditions in the United States diminish the need for this procedure and argue that the procedure is a painful violation of a nonconsenting infant to remove a functional body part. For some, this topic inspires passionate debate, in which they may even liken male circumcision to female circumcision/genital mutilation. Parents who choose not to circumcise their sons should be taught the normal anatomy of the penis and its development. As the child matures, he should be taught to retract the foreskin gently while bathing to clear any collection of smegma. Parents should be counseled not to retract a foreskin forcefully, as the resultant irritation and edema may cause further adhesions.

Just as conflicting opinions have arisen in the general population regarding circumcision, so the

American Academy of Pediatrics (AAP) has issued statements on this practice that have varied over the years. Based on research studies from 2005 to 2010, the most recent AAP statement notes that the health benefits of circumcision outweigh the risks and justify access to the process for families who choose it.[51] A critical component of this statement is the informed desire of families. Information about circumcision should be included in prenatal care so women and their families have adequate time to make this decision. Some practices develop their own culturally sensitive documents to help individuals with this decision-making process. A nonprofit consumer-based group that uses evidence-based information to develop interactive instruments that aid individuals in making a variety of decisions is the Healthwise website; that website has an interactive program for parents considering whether to circumcise their sons.[52]

Hepatitis B Vaccine

For several decades, the Centers for Disease Control and Prevention (CDC) has recommended that all newborns be immunized against hepatitis B.[53] Although there is some controversy about the need for the hepatitis B vaccine (HBV) for this age group, seroprotection has been confirmed.[54] The current recommendation is that all infants receive the first dose of HBV within 12 hours of birth. **Table 39-3** summarizes the CDC recommendation based on whether the mother has a negative, positive, or unknown hepatitis B surface antigen (HBsAg) test.[53] According to the CDC, licensed vaccines contain 10 to 40 mcg of HBsAg protein per milliliter and either do not contain thimerosal or contain a trace amount of no more than 1.0 mcg mercury per milliliter. Only a single-antigen HBV is used for the birth dose.

The HBV administered at birth is the first of a series of vaccines that are completed during infancy, with the last dose being given at age of 6 months. The series is composed of either three or four injections, based on the type of HBV employed. In some parts of the world, a combination vaccine including vaccination against hepatitis B, diphtheria, tetanus, pertussis, and influenza is administered during the first year of life.[55]

Maternal Conditions That Influence Newborn Care

The schedule for hepatitis B immunization of a newborn/infant varies based on maternal status. With mothers who are HBsAg positive, the infant receives both HBV and hepatitis B immune globulin (HBIG) within the first 12 hours of birth. These injections should be administered in separate sites. Although the majority of states have laws requiring obstetric providers to screen women for hepatitis B, occasionally a woman presents for care and her HBsAg status is unknown. Neonates born to these women should receive HBV within the first 12 hours of life, and maternal blood should be tested as soon as possible. If the maternal HBsAg test is positive, HBIG should be immediately administered to the newborn within the first week of life.

Some parents decline HBV for their infants. This decision reflects maternal autonomy, although there is evidence of the advantages of primary prevention of disease through immunization, as discussed in the *Health Promotion and Health Maintenance* chapter. However, for women who are HBsAg positive, there are distinct risks to the infant regarding development of chronic hepatitis B and potentially fatal hepatic carcinoma or cirrhosis. Thus the ethical concerns in such situations are more complex, and in some situations, legal authorities have advocated to protect the child.[56]

Women with HIV

Although no longer an automatic death sentence, infection with HIV remains a major perinatal threat. This condition is described in detail in the *Reproductive Tract and Sexually Transmitted Infections* chapter. In the late 1990s, a major breakthrough occurred when a study found that treatment of newborns born to HIV-positive mothers with zidovudine (AZT, Retrovir) reduced their risk of developing the infection.[57] In 2013, it was reported that a newborn with evidence of HIV shortly after birth was treated with a short course of multiple antivirals and later was found to be free of any infection.[58] Today, there is no controversy about whether to treat children born to women with HIV, but the drug, dosing, and follow-up have yet to be codified. In any case, a newborn whose mother has HIV is best treated by a pediatric provider with expertise in this area.

In the United States, it is recommended that HIV-positive women not breastfeed their infants because the virus is transmitted through breast milk. However, in areas where safe breast milk substitutes are lacking, the risks of HIV must be weighed against the risks of newborn diarrhea and nutritional deficits associated with bottle feeding; thus the recommendation to breastfeed or not is a more complex decision in such locations.[59]

Table 39-3	Hepatitis B Vaccine Schedules for Newborn Infants, by Maternal Hepatitis B Surface Antigen (HBsAg) Status				
	Single-Antigen Vaccine			**Single-Antigen + Combination Vaccine**	
Maternal HBsAg Status	**Dose**	**Age**		**Dose**	**Age**
Negative	1[a,e]	Birth (12 hours or before)		1[a,e]	Birth (12 hours or before)
	2	1–2 months		2	2 months
	3	6 months		3	4 months
				4[c]	6 months (Pediarix) or 12–15 months (Comvax)
Positive	1[a]	Birth (12 hours or before)		1[a]	Birth (12 hours or before)
	HBIG[b]	Birth (12 hours or before)		HBIG[b]	Birth (12 hours or before)
	2	1–2 months		2	2 months
	3	6 months		3	4 months
				4[c]	6 months (Pediarix) or 12–15 months (Comvax)
Unknown[d]	1[a]	Birth (12 hours or before)		1[a]	Birth (12 hours or before)
	2	1–2 months		2	2 months
	3			3	4 months
				4	6 months (Pediarix) or 12–15 months (Comvax)

[a] Recombivax HB or Engerix-B should be used for the birth dose. Comvax and Pediarix cannot be administered at birth or before age 6 weeks.

[b] Hepatitis B immune globulin (0.5 mL) is administered intramuscularly in a separate site from the vaccine.

[c] The final dose in the vaccine series should not be administered before age 24 weeks (164 days).

[d] Mothers should have blood drawn and tested for HBsAg as soon as possible after admission for delivery; if the mother is found to be HBsAg positive, the infant should receive HBIG as soon as possible but no later than 7 days of age.

[e] On a case-by-case basis and only in rare circumstances, the first dose may be delayed until after hospital discharge for an infant who weighs 2000 g or more and whose mother is HBsAg negative. When such a decision is made, an order to withhold the birth dose and a copy of the original laboratory report indicating that the mother was HBsAg negative during this pregnancy should be placed in the infant's medical record.

Source: Mast EE, Margolis HS, Fiore AE, et al. Advisory Committee on Immunization Practices. A comprehensive immunization strategy to eliminate transmission of hepatitis B virus infection in the United States: recommendations of the Advisory Committee on Immunization Practices (ACIP). Part 1: immunization of infants, children, and adolescents. *MMWR Recomm Rep.* 2005;54(RR-16):1-31.

Vaginal Colonization with Group B *Streptococcus*

Group B *Streptococcus* (GBS) infection is a leading cause of neonatal sepsis in the United States.[60] Approximately 1 in 100 to 200 newborns born to women who are are colonized with GBS will develop newborn sepsis if the woman is not treated in labor. Because newborn sepsis has a significant risk of morbidity and mortality, efforts to prevent GBS-related newborn disease have been a standard part of maternity care in the United States since 1996.

The term infant whose mother received thorough intrapartum GBS prophylaxis, defined as 4 hours or more of penicillin, ampicillin (Principen), or cefazolin (Ancef) during labor in the hours immediately before the birth, should be observed for 24 to 48 hours but these newborns do not require special diagnostic testing unless they have signs or symptoms of illness.[61] Conversely, all infants who have signs of sepsis and all infants whose mothers have developed chorioamnionitis should have a full or limited evaluation and antimicrobial therapy. **Figure 39-2** provides an algorithm for treatment of neonates whose mothers are colonized with GBS under different clinical circumstances. The CDC publishes and updates recommended guidelines for GBS prophylaxis. The CDC guidelines are recommended by all obstetric professional associations.

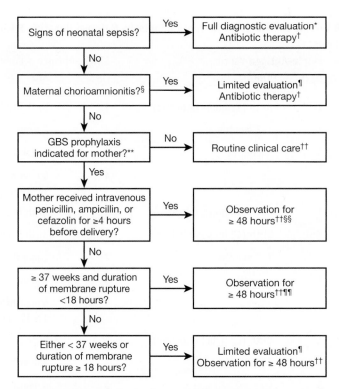

* Full diagnostic evaluation includes a blood culture, a complete blood count
  (CBC) including white blood cell differential and platelet counts, chest
  radiograph (if respiratory abnormalities are present), and lumbar puncture (if
  patient is stable enough to tolerate procedure and sepsis is suspected).
† Antibiotic therapy should be directed toward the most common causes of
  neonatal sepsis, including intravenous ampicillin for GBS and coverage for
  other organisms (including *Escherichia coli* and other gram-negative
  pathogens) and should take into account local antibiotic resistance patterns.
§ Consultation with obstetric providers is important to determine the level of
  clinical suspicion for chorioamnionitis. Chorioamnionitis is diagnosed
  clinically and some of the signs are nonspecific.
¶ Limited evaluation includes blood culture (at birth) and CBC with differential
  and platelets (at birth and/or at 6–12 hours of life).
** See table 3 for indications for intrapartum GBS prophylaxis.
†† If signs of sepsis develop, a full diagnostic evaluation should be conducted
  and antibiotic therapy initiated.
§§ If ≥ 37 weeks' gestation, observation may occur at home after 24 hours if
  other discharge criteria have been met, access to medical care is readily
  available, and a person who is able to comply fully with instructions for home
  observation will be present. If any of these conditions is not met, the infant
  should be observed in the hospital for at least 48 hours and until discharge
  criteria are achieved.
¶¶ Some experts recommend a CBC with differential and platelets at age 6–12
  hours.

Figure 39-2 Algorithm for secondary prevention of early-onset group B streptoccocal disease among newborns.

Source: Verani JR, McGee L, Schrag SJ; Division of Bacterial Diseases, National Center for Immunization and Respiratory Diseases, Centers for Disease Control and Prevention. Prevention of perinatal group B streptococcal disease: revised guidelines from CDC, 2010. *MMWR Recomm Rep.* 2010;59(RR-10):1-36.

Women with Diabetes

Infants of women who have diabetes are at risk for low or high birth weight, congenital anomalies, birth injuries, polycythemia, and hypoglycemia.[62] The hypoglycemia may result from hyperinsulinemia characterized by accelerated use of exogenous glucose and diminished endogenous glucose production, but is temporary for the newborn. Hypoglycemia is less common if the woman had good diabetic control during pregnancy and stable blood glucose levels. Newborns who are born to women who have diabetes may be either macrosomic or growth restricted, depending on the type and severity of the woman's diabetes.

Because of the risk of hypoglycemia, early feeding is important for these newborns. These neonates should have a blood glucose level obtained during the first 2 hours of life. Some controversy exists about interpretation of newborn blood glucose levels, but in general a prefeeding blood glucose level equal to or greater than 47 mg/dL (2.6 mmol/L) is normal; 40 to 46 mg/dL (2.2 to 2.5 mmol/L) is mild hypoglycemia; 30 to 39 mg/dL (1.7 to 2.1 mmol/L) is moderate hypoglycemia; and severe hypoglycemia occurs when the glucose level is less than 30 mg/dL (1.7 mmol/L).[63] Any heel stick value of 50 mg/dL or lower should immediately be verified by drawing a central venous sample. A consultation with a member of the pediatric team is needed if any abnormal blood glucose levels are reported because intravenous fluids may be indicated.

Examination of the Newborn

Although the midwife will initiate a brief immediate assessment of the newborn at the time of birth, a full examination is necessary to identify subtle abnormalities. Usually this exam is deferred for the healthy newborn who is spending some immediate time as a new member of a family. However, the examination should be conducted within the first few hours, even if the newborn appears grossly normal. In all cases, it should be complete before either neonatal discharge from a hospital or birth center or before the midwife leaves the home after a birth. Most minor anomalies are of little consequence, but other variations may indicate serious underlying disease. The *Examination of the Newborn* chapter provides details about conduct of the examination and common findings.

Maternal Drug Use and Neonatal Abstinence Syndrome

The term *drug exposure*, when used in reference to a newborn, covers a wide variety of substances and situations, ranging from the most casual exposure to daily and repeated in utero exposures. Many attempts have been made to quantify the effects of substance exposure on the fetus and newborn. Most of these studies have yielded equivocal results or results that were contradicted by other studies.

Major limitations of studies are that many women who use illicit drugs may be polydrug users. In addition, drugs of abuse often vary in terms of their additives and purity. Women who abuse drugs also may suffer from malnutrition, poverty, and chronic stress. Some women who use illicit drugs

lack prenatal care and folate supplementation. Thus, in addition to potential teratogenic effects, the mother's lifestyle can have negative effects on fetal well-being. Newborns who have had significant exposure to a teratogenic or fetotoxic agent during pregnancy frequently will be small for gestational age and may have dysmorphic physical characteristics. Neonatal withdrawal symptoms include a wide spectrum of physiologic and neurobehavioral symptoms. Any infant suspected of being at risk for neonatal abstinence syndrome should be observed carefully for the first 72 hours of life. Some infants may require hospitalization for as long as a week after birth.

Nicotine

Historically, smoking has been termed a fetotoxic agent because of its relationship to low birth weight. Data now suggest that the delay in normal development may begin during the embryonic period.[64] This phenomenon results from the effects of both carbon monoxide (leading to relative fetal hypoxia) and nicotine (leading to placental vasoconstriction). The effect on the fetus appears to be dose related and will cease if the woman stops smoking during pregnancy. Infants who are born to women who smoke should be evaluated for gestational size and, if they are small for gestational age, treated accordingly.

Alcohol

Newborns born to women who abuse alcohol can suffer serious and permanent damage.[65] Because ethanol readily crosses the placenta, the amount of fetal exposure can be high. Damage is characterized as a continuum, and two terms are used to describe the damage: fetal alcohol syndrome (FAS) and fetal alcohol spectrum disorders (FASD). FASD encompasses FAS but also includes individuals with milder effects of alcohol.

Newborns exhibiting signs of FAS may have both physical and cognitive damage. Physical damage includes dysmorphic features that are congruent with a midline defect, which occurs early in fetal life. The manifestations of FASD are more subtle and will become obvious when the child is older and has trouble with school or socialization.

The dysmorphic features of the newborn with FAS are primarily facial and include a narrow forehead, flat midface, low nasal bridge, short nose, thin upper lip with indistinct philtrum (indentation between top lip and nose), epicanthal folds, and micrognathia. Other signs include palmar creases and low birth weight. Affected newborns may exhibit behavioral signs including irritability, poor feeding, tremors, and hypersensitivity to stimuli. **Figure 39-3** provides an illustration of some of the dysmorphic features associated with FAS.[66]

The signs of FAS may or may not be obvious during the newborn period. Damage varies with timing and dose of exposure. If physical or behavioral signs that are possibly indicative of FAS or FASD are noted, consultation with a pediatric team is necessary. These newborns need careful monitoring because of their risk for failure to thrive. Their behavioral characteristics may make it a challenge for parents to care for them, rendering them vulnerable to abuse by caregivers.

Opiates and Other Illicit Drugs

Neonatal abstinence syndrome long has been associated with use of opiates such as heroin and cocaine. More recently, neonatal withdrawal symptoms have been found among the children of women using various psychotropic drugs.[67,68] Maternal use of cocaine has been suspected as a cause of many fetal problems, most of them related to the intense vasoconstrictive properties of cocaine, which can cause placental and cord accidents. The known effects of cocaine exposure include behavioral problems that are secondary to central nervous system irritability. Cocaine-exposed newborns may be irritable, tremulous, and hard to comfort. They may favor a rigid, hyperextended posture. The manifestations of cocaine exposure are related to the amount, duration, and timing of fetal exposure. Third-trimester use is more likely to result in residual behavioral effects.

In the case of opiates and potentially other drugs of abuse, the fetus becomes tolerant and can show evidence of severe withdrawal symptoms in utero if the mother stops using the drug during pregnancy. At birth, most newborns of women who are addicted to illicit drugs will exhibit some withdrawal symptoms.[69] These start in the first few days after birth and can persist for many weeks. If a woman used drugs by the intravenous route, her newborn will also be at risk of infection with the hepatitis and HIV viruses.

The symptoms of neonatal abstinence syndrome involve many neonatal systems, including central nervous system irritability, tremors, excess hunger and salivation, sweating, yawning, sneezing, fist sucking, and temperature regulation problems. Some infants progress to seizures and profuse vomiting and diarrhea. These newborns need to be managed by the pediatric team during an inpatient stay. Management considerations include providing a quiet, nonstimulating environment, a possible increased need for calories and fluids, and potential need for pharmacotherapy to control symptoms. Traditionally methadone (Dolophine) has been the drug used to support withdrawal; however, buprenorphine (Buprenex) now is gaining popularity for this indication.[70]

Meconium is a particularly attractive medium for drug testing because of the ease of specimen collection from the diaper and the ability to obtain accurate drug sampling of opiates and other prescriptive drugs that often are abused.[71] In some states and localities, a positive toxicology screen must be reported to child welfare officials.

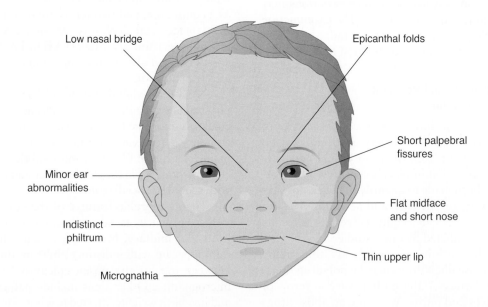

Figure 39-3 Facial characteristics of an infant affected by intrauterine alcohol.

Source: Warren KR, Hewitt BG, Thomas JD. *Fetal alcohol spectrum disorders: research challenges and opportunities.* National Institutes of Health, National Institute on Alcohol Abuse and Alcoholism. Available at: http://pubs.niaaa.nih.gov/publications/arh341/4-14.htm. Accessed March 29, 2013.

Newborns experiencing withdrawal need an environment that is not too stimulating. The mother should be taught the swaddling and calming techniques. Healthcare providers have a particular obligation to help this mother identify resources that she can rely upon if she has difficulty coping with the newborn's behaviors.

The First Golden Month: Primary Care of the Newborn

The Midwife's Role in Neonatal Well-Child Care

The role of the midwife during the newborn's first month of life varies markedly. In some locales, the midwife has little formal role once the newborn leaves a birthing room. In other practices, the midwife will continue care of the mother and newborn throughout the first 4 to 6 weeks after birth. These midwives may work in a collegial relationship with pediatric providers, with the well-child care gradually shifting to pediatric or family healthcare providers.

Regardless of any formal expectation regarding the role of the midwife, the reality is that many parents will call the midwife with questions related to the care and well-being of their newborn. The midwife, conscious of the special connection between mother and child, promotes family well-being by her involvement in care and evidence-based advice.

Well-Child Surveillance: Physical Care of the Newborn

Parents have many concerns regarding the physical care of their newborn. Overall, they should be reassured that there is more than one right way to approach many physical aspects of their child's care. Many midwives help mothers learn about their infants by working with the mother–newborn dyad during a home visit (**Figure 39-4**). Various common conditions about which parents may have concerns are summarized in **Table 39-4**.

For example, an infant does not need a full bath daily. Newborns need to have their heads and diaper areas sponged whenever appropriate using a mild, nondeodorized soap, with the area then being completely dried. A full bath can be given occasionally when the parent has the time to make it a relaxing event for the newborn. Parents should be urged never to leave a newborn unattended in the bath. The soap, towels, shampoo, and clean clothes should all be organized before starting the bath. Slip-proof bath mats are inexpensive and helpful.

Parents frequently have strong feelings about which type of diaper to use—paper disposable or cloth—and the best type to use is controversial. Disposable diapers present environmental problems related to paper/plastic waste. Conversely, commercial diaper services often use large amounts of bleach and the delivery trucks create pollution. A few parents will choose to wash their child's diapers themselves. If so, they should presoak dirty diapers using bleach and detergent and wash them twice in very hot water without packing the washer too full, to ensure that bacteria are destroyed.

Parents often are encouraged by family members to dress infants in excessive layers of clothing. A general rule of thumb is to clothe the infant with as many layers as other persons in the room are wearing, plus one layer. Because infants cannot sweat effectively, symptoms of overheating are mainly a red skin color, irritability, and body warmth. Eventually the overheated infant will appear lethargic. Infants also cool rapidly through inspired cold air. When taken outside on windy cold days, newborns should have a nonrestrictive covering near their faces.

From the earliest moments at home with a newborn, parents should evaluate the environment for safety risks. In the first months of life, these risks are primarily related to falling or becoming impinged in small places such as between the bars on the sides of cribs. Parents should also consider removing soft pillows, mobiles, and toys that may lead to suffocation from the site in which the newborn sleeps.

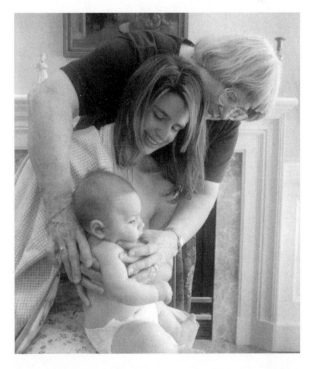

Figure 39-4 Midwife illustrating care of a child with a mother.
Source: Courtesy of Helen Varney Burst

Table 39-4	Common Neonatal Conditions and Parental Concerns in the First Month of Life	
Conditions/Questions	**Comments**	**Treatments/Advice**
Skin conditions	Diaper simple dermatitis	Flat, reddened areas	Gentle cleaning with water
		Minimal skinfold involvement	Frequent diaper changes
		Neonate may demonstrate distress during cleaning/diaper changes	Use of protectants (e.g., zinc oxide)
	Diaper dermatitis secondary to fungus	Usually due to *Candida albicans*	Topical antifungals (e.g., miconazole)
		Confluent erythematous lesions	Topical steroids (e.g., hydrocortisone)
		Often lesions remote from main area (satellite lesions)	
		Painful to neonate, even when not touched	
	Diaper dermatitis with secondary infection	Usually due to *Staphylococcus* or *Streptococcus* microorganisms	Treatment based on type of microorganism involved
		Peeling skin	
		Vesicles	
		Exudates	
	Cradle cap	Seborrheic exudates	Gently comb hair/scalp with oil (e.g., vegetable, olive)
			Remove exudate with shampoo
			Regular shampooing usually resolves issue
	Erythema toxicum neonatorum and milia	Various eruptions, small vesicles or generalized rash	These dermatologic conditions are common in the first week of life and will spontaneously resolve. No treatment is necessary and the condition does not appear to be painful to the newborn. Parents can be reassured that this is a normal transient finding in newborns.
Oral conditions	Thrush	Adherent white plaques on tongue, gums, and/or palate	Oral antifungals
			Also rule out mastitis if the mother is breastfeeding
	Nasal discharge	Discharge may be apparent	Counsel parents to avoid bulb syringes; they can cause trauma and edema
		Occasional periods of irregular breathing	Saline drops
		Crusting around nares may or may not be present	Differentiate between nasal congestion and apnea (apnea is associated with low heart rate, pauses of 20 seconds or more)

(continues)

Table 39-4 Common Neonatal Conditions and Parental Concerns in the First Month of Life *(continued)*

Conditions/Questions	Comments	Treatments/Advice
Behavior	"Fussiness"	Crying "Colicky" behavior Difficult to console Reasons unknown and likely to be unique to individual parent–newborn dyad	Multiple suggestions to console a baby—although no research that one method is better than another: • Swaddling • Talk with baby *en face* • Cuddle, reposition, walk, or move with baby • Attempt to feed or give pacifier • Reduce environment sensory stimulation • *Never shake a baby!*
Sleep	Timing of sleep	Usually sleep 16–18 hours in first few days Variation more profound as baby grows, ranging from as few as 8 hours or as much as almost 20 hours by 4 weeks Newborns are less governed by circadian rhythms than adults Sleep is associated with feeding; more likely to sleep during day	Reassure parents that newborns do not necessarily have days and nights confused Most likely will take 12 weeks at least to start sleeping more during nighttime and may take 3–5 months based on melatonin and cortisol production
	Safe sleep	Newborns who sleep on their backs are less likely to experience sudden infant death syndrome (SIDS) Originally part of the national campaign "Back to Sleep"; now termed "Safe Sleep"	Newborns should be placed on their backs for sleep Should have "tummy time" or interactions when on abdomen only when the newborn is awake
Feeding*	Adequate feeding	Newborn should feed multiple times daily (e.g., approximately every 2–4 hours) May lose 5–7% of birth weight in first few days of life	Surrogates for adequate intake include: • Weight gain at end of first week or beginning of the second week (usually 150–200 g per week) • Stools and urine in diapers at least 1–3 times during each of the first few days of life • Once lactation established, 3–4 stools and 5–6 wet diapers every day If difficult to ascertain if diaper is wet, place a soft tissue inside the absorbent diaper If no bowel movement or urine within 24–48 hours, consult pediatric provider
Car safety	Car seats	Newborns should travel in rear-facing car seats	Never leave a baby alone in a car Because multiple car seats/multiple models of cars exist, have the car seat installed by or verified by a car seat technician (may be found at the local fire station) Do not use a previously used seat or one not made by a manufacturer

*More details can be found in the *Breastfeeding and the Mother–Newborn Dyad* chapter.

Many families use pacifiers to help calm newborns. If parents choose to use a pacifier, the pacifier should be cleaned regularly and checked for signs of dirt or mold. Most pacifiers today have a design that promotes proper development of the muscles of the mouth. Pacifiers should never be placed around the baby's neck because of the risk of strangulation. Some newborns do not accept a pacifier, so parents devise other methods to help the newborn become calm (walking the baby, distracting the baby, encouraging thumb sucking).

When an infant sucks on a bottle for a prolonged period of time, the residual sugars from the milk or juice may contribute to childhood dental caries, also known as "baby bottle mouth." The accumulation of milk in the back of the oropharynx may lead to ear infections as well. Therefore, prolonged bottle feeding, especially by propping a bottle, should never be used to calm an infant.

Parents also need to recognize situations in which immediate pediatric care is needed for the newborn. **Table 39-5** lists some situations in which a pediatric provider should be contacted promptly.

Well-Child Care Visits

When a midwife is the provider for a newborn during the first 28 days of life, the neonate may be seen in an ambulatory setting, often at the same time the woman is seen for a postpartum examination. The purpose of this visit is fourfold: (1) to monitor normal growth and development, (2) to identify symptoms of disease, (3) to offer screening measures, and (4) to educate and support the parents. When a parent brings a newborn in for a well-child visit, every effort should be made to keep the infant from exposure to others, especially anyone who is ill. Whenever possible, the parents should be escorted into an exam room as soon as they arrive with their child. **Box 39-2** summarizes the components of a newborn visit.

The visit starts with a brief interview of the parent(s) or primary caregiver. Particular attention should be paid to unresolved problems related to the birth or the immediate care of the newborn following birth. The midwife should assess the well-being of the parents and look for signs of depression or inability to cope with the demands of the newborn. Inquiries should be made about help in the home,

Table 39-5	Neonatal Signs and Symptoms Requiring Prompt Parental Reporting/Pediatric Referral[a]
Grade	**Suggestions for Practice**
Temperature instability	Axillary temperature higher than 37.4°C or 99.3°F or less than 36.5°C or 97.5°F
Abnormal respirations	Tachypnea (more than 60 breaths/min) for more than 60 seconds
	Pauses more than 20 seconds
	Regular retractions, wheezing, grunting
Infection of umbilicus	Odor, drainage, or bleeding from umbilical stump
Infection of eyes	Purulent discharge from eyes
Jaundice	Icteric changes of eyes, chest, or extremities
Gastrointestinal	Projectile vomiting
	Bile-stained vomit
	No stools/no urination since birth
	Marked color changes during eating
	Taut, swollen abdomen
	More than six stools per 24 hours/bloody or very watery stools
General signs of illness	Cough
	Diarrhea
	Poor muscle tone
	Sleepiness/refusal to feed/inability to rouse
	Poor suck
	Neurologic signs such as bulging fontanelle, irritability, abnormal reflexes

[a]This list is not comprehensive. Midwives who provide well-baby care should have a list of conditions that require pediatric referral as part of the practice guidelines developed jointly with pediatric providers.

sibling reactions, and reaction of other relatives to the newborn. Particular emphasis should be paid to the infant's feeding patterns, levels of alertness, bowel and bladder patterns, and crying patterns.

A complete physical exam is performed, as described in the appendix of the *Examination of the Newborn* chapter. During the physical examination, the midwife has an opportunity to observe the parent–newborn relationship. If there is an opportunity to observe a feeding, this can be particularly valuable. The greatest part of the initial well-child visit should be spent soliciting parental concerns and offering guidance and anticipatory advice. Any midwife providing well-child care should have a clear relationship established for pediatric consultation or referral of any infant presenting with signs or symptoms of illness.

Early Recognition of Clinically Significant Newborn Conditions

Several other newborn conditions may adversely affect newborn health. In addition to jaundice and other specific conditions, one of the great challenges facing providers who care for newborns is the non-specificity of signs and symptoms of some serious conditions. Because of the nonspecific nature of some of these signs and symptoms, a careful history and physical examination to gather the maximum amount of data to report to pediatric caregivers is needed. The midwife practicing far from a pediatric inpatient facility should become familiar with techniques for starting a peripheral intravenous line in the neonate. If the neonate's condition deteriorates, it will be more difficult to find a vein.

Jaundice

As many as 50% of newborns develop clinically evident jaundice.[72] Management of jaundice depends on whether the jaundice is determined to be within the norm for physiologic jaundice or is hyperbilirubinemia that is indicative of a pathophysiologic process. **Table 39-6** provides a list to help distinguish physiologic jaundice from hyperbilirubinemia.

Newborn physiologic jaundice is the result of bilirubin deposits in the dermis. As described in the *Anatomy and Physiology of the Newborn* chapter, bilirubin levels rise during the first few days after birth. This occurs secondary to three aspects of newborn physiology: (1) The newborn has more red blood cells than does an adult and these red blood cells have a shorter lifespan. As fetal red blood cells break down so fetal hemoglobin can be replaced with adult hemoglobin, bilirubin is produced as a byproduct of heme catabolism. (2) Bilirubin must be converted from an unconjugated (indirect) non-water-soluble form to a conjugated (direct) form that is water-soluble in order to be excreted via the kidney and stool. The hepatic metabolism pathway that conjugates bilirubin is immature in the newborn and is not effective for a few weeks. (3) Conjugated bilirubin must be broken down further by intestinal bacteria in order to be excreted. Because the newborn has an essentially sterile gastrointestinal tract, conjugated bilirubin is reabsorbed and recirculated via the enterohepatic system more than it would be in an adult. Thus, physiologic jaundice is the result of increased production of bilirubin at a time when elimination is delayed.

All newborns exhibit rising total bilirubin levels for the first few days after birth and it is not uncommon to have some bilirubin deposited in the skin that is evident as newborn jaundice. The mean peak of total bilirubin plasma levels occur between 48 and 92 hours after birth and the average values are between 7 mg/dL and 9 mg/dL.

Table 39-6	Newborn Jaundice
Type of Jaundice	**Signs and Symptoms**
Physiologic jaundice	Jaundice appears day 2–4 after birth
	Total bilirubin rises slowly and peaks at day 3 or 4 of life
	Total bilirubin peaks < 13 mg/d L
Hyperbilirubinemia	Jaundice visible during first 24 hours after birth
	Total bilirubin rise quickly, up to > 5mg/dL/24 hours
	Total bilirubin > 13 mg/dL
	Visible jaundice persists after one week of life
	Newborn may have risk factors such as cephalohematoma or ABO or Rh incompatibility, polycythemia
Breast milk failure jaundice	Jaundice appears in first week after birth
	Total bilirubin levels may rise to > 13 mg/dL
	Exclusively breastfed: feeds poorly, weight loss and signs of dehydration, infrequent urine output
	Delayed passage of meconium
Breast milk jaundice	Jaundice appears after first week of life and persists for up to 12 weeks
	Mildly elevated bilirubin levels that do not rise
	Feeds well, normal weight gain, normal urine output

Physiologic jaundice usually becomes apparent between days 2 to 4, when newborns are usually at home. Some hospitals screen all newborns with serum total bilirubin levels at 1 day of age, and those infants with a level less than 5 mg/dL are not re-screened unless the clinical picture changes. Infant care practices that enhance clearance of bilirubin, such as early and frequent feedings to promote the passage of meconium, should be advocated. Delayed passage of meconium promotes reabsorption of bilirubin as part of the enterohepatic circulation. All parents should be educated about newborn jaundice and taught to assess the newborn in a well-lighted room or near a sunny window by blanching the skin to reveal the underlying color.

Hyperbilirubinemia in newborns who are equal to or more than 35 weeks gestation at birth is defined as a total bilirubin level that is higher than the 95% on the hour-specific Bhutani nomogram. This nomogram is used in a standardized bilirubin calculator that accounts for gestational age at birth, risk factors, number of hours since birth, and bilirubin values. The bilirubin calculator is available on the Internet or as a medical app for smartphones or personal computers. The calculator determines the risk for hyperbilirubinemia and presents recommended management based on the degree of risk.

A total bilirubin level that is higher than 25 to 30 mg/dL is associated with a risk for bilirubin-induced neurologic dysfunction (BIND). This disorder occurs when bilirubin crosses the blood–brain barrier and binds to brain tissue. Unconjugated bilirubin is highly neurotoxic and the term *acute bilirubin encephalopathy* (ABE) refers to cerebral symptoms such as irritability, high-pitched cry, hyper or hypotonia, seizures, and possibly death if left untreated. The term *kernicterus* is used to describe the chronic and permanent sequelae of ABE in infants who sustain permanent cerebral damage as the result of hyperbilirubinemia. The incidence of kernicterus in full-term newborns is exceedingly rare even when in those who develop ABE.

Newborns at increased risk for hyperbilirubinemia include those who have a hemolytic process such as an ABO blood-type incompatibility, or accelerated red blood cells break down from a large cephalohematoma. Other risk factors include inherited red blood cell membrane defects, enzyme defects such as glucose-6-phosphate dehydrogenase (G6PD) deficiency, newborn sepsis, and newborns born to women with diabetes.

In addition to physiologic jaundice and hyperbilirubinemia, there are two additional forms of newborn jaundice related to breastfeeding. Infants diagnosed with *breast milk jaundice* have mild hyperbilirubinemia that persists beyond the first week of life and slowly declines between 3 and 12 weeks of life. These infants need to be monitored but rarely need treatment and continued breastfeeding should be encouraged. Although the etiology is not clearly known, it appears some women have a substance in their breast milk that stimulates reabsorption of bilirubin from the neonate's intestine. Conversely *breastfeeding failure jaundice* is secondary to exclusive breastfeeding but inadequate intake. In this case, the infant loses weight and has slower bilirubin elimination and higher levels of reabsorption via enterohepatic circulation. Breastfeeding failure jaundice is not the result of breast milk per se; rather, it is the result of too little fluid and dehydration. This form of newborn jaundice appears in the first week of life and may need specific treatment for the jaundice in addition to interventions designed to establish lactation.

Bilirubin can be measured via a central venous sample, a point-of-care transcutaneous meter, or estimated via physical examination. Jaundice appears first in the face and has a cephalo-caudal progression. Although bilirubin levels can be visually estimated based on the level of jaundice in the newborn, visual estimation is not sufficiently predictive to be relied upon for management decisions.

The treatment for newborn jaundice is phototherapy and in severe cases exchange transfusion. The light from the phototherapy converts bilirubin to a water-soluble form that can be excreted. Phototherapy is effective and can be performed at home. The American Academy of Pediatrics (AAP) has issued guidelines for newborn jaundice that, although not all evidence-based, are generally followed throughout the United States, especially regarding indications for phototherapy.[73] The following symptoms may indicate that the jaundice is not physiologic and the newborn needs a more extensive medical evaluation: vomiting, lethargy, poor feeding, weight loss, hepatosplenomegaly, apnea, temperature instability, tachypnea, dark urine or urine positive for bilirubin, light-colored stools, and jaundice that persists for more than 3 weeks.

Home phototherapy is not as effective as the technology available in the hospital, and one recommendation is to initiate therapy at home when a newborn has a serum total bilirubin level 2 to 3 mg/dL lower than when phototherapy is initiated in a hospital.[74] Home therapy is less expensive than hospitalization and allows mothers and neonates to stay together, especially for breastfeeding. Occasionally a woman is unable to manage the process at home.

Outside the United States, a cholesterol-lowering agent, clofibrate, has been used in conjunction with phototherapy to reduce unconjugated bilirubin more rapidly, but additional studies are needed to assess its effectiveness.[75]

Respiratory Conditions

Respiratory signs are the most common abnormal finding in newborns. The most common pulmonary causes of neonatal respiratory distress in term infants are pneumothorax, aspiration of meconium, neonatal pneumonia, and transient tachypnea of the newborn (**Table 39-7**). Signs of respiratory distress include tachypnea (> 60/min), nasal flaring, retractions of intercostal muscles or sternum if severe, or grunting. Cyanosis, rales, or rhonchi are possible. Central cyanosis (of the trunk, lips, tongue, and oral mucous membranes) is a sign of serious compromise of the neonate's hemoglobin oxygen saturation and requires supplemental oxygen.

If the newborn is having respiratory distress, continued monitoring of heart rate and respiratory rate is necessary while awaiting pediatric consultation or transport. If possible, blood pressure should be checked. Oxygen levels can be assessed by continuous pulse oximetry attached to one of the neonate's fingers or toes. This method computes arterial oxygen saturation (SaO_2), with an acceptable level being between 92% and 95%.

Newborn Infection

The newborn may have a congenital infection or may become infected with a virus or bacterium during labor, birth, or the immediate postpartum period. The viruses most likely to cause congenital infection are toxoplasmosis, parvovirus, varicella, syphilis, rubella, CMV, and herpes. Infants with such infections are often small for gestational age. They may present with signs that include early jaundice, hepatosplenomegaly, petechiae, and palpable lymph nodes. Some viruses cause cataracts, limb or cardiac defects, microcephaly, rash, or vesicles.[76] Thrombocytopenia may be evident on a complete blood count (CBC). The visible effects of infection will vary according to the timing of fetal exposure and the severity of the infection.

Management may include isolation of the newborn from other newborns and from pregnant healthcare workers until the virus is identified. Usually the mother and infant can be isolated together. Cord blood should be saved for further testing. Historically, TORCH testing has been a routine component of the assessment of infants who are small for gestational

Table 39-7	Common Neonatal Respiratory Conditions
Associated Conditions	**Comments**
Transient tachypnea of newborn (TTN) due to longer period of time transitioning from fluid-filled to air-filled lungs	TTN lasts 48–72 hours with spontaneous resolution, although the newborn may need assistance with feedings and extra oxygen. Generally these infants are monitored in the hospital until TTN resolves.
Meconium aspiration that can result in pneumonitis, hypoxia, respiratory failure and persistent pulmonary hypertension	Requires support from a respirator and occasionally extracorporeal membrane oxygenation (ECMO)
Neonatal pneumonia caused by bacteria, viruses, or other microorganisms	Anti-inflammatory agents and supportive therapy
Pneumothorax (unilateral or bilateral), often after mechanical ventilation and overdistension	A large pneumothorax is a pediatric emergency
Congenital anomalies causing airway obstruction or pulmonary obstruction	May require surgical intervention
Sepsis	Evaluate other signs of sepsis such as temperature variations

age. TORCH is an acronym for "toxoplasmosis, other, rubella, CMV, and herpes"; the "other" category includes tests for syphilis, varicella, and parvovirus as indicated.[77] Although the presence of IgM antibodies in the cord blood will help to confirm a suspected viral infection, it is rare that IgM antibodies are present to aid diagnosis. Often the diagnosis of congenital infection does not become clear until the infant is older. Treatment in the newborn period is symptomatic.

Infections caused by *Staphylococcus aureus* and *Staphylococcus epidermidis* are usually acquired after birth in hospital settings. Signs of neonatal sepsis include respiratory distress, vomiting, lethargy, apnea, and irritability. Common causes of bacterial infections acquired in labor are group B beta-hemolytic *Streptococcus* and *Escherichia coli*.

Cardiac Conditions

Cardiac problems in newborns result from a variety of causes and mimic a number of other problems, especially respiratory disease and sepsis. Pulse oximetry is advocated for all infants, as described earlier.

Some newborns will quickly demonstrate signs of an underlying congenital defect. These are usually structural in nature and may affect the heart valves, the walls between the atrium and the ventricles, or the heart muscle itself. The primary signs of heart disease include central cyanosis, murmurs, and other cardiac sounds.[78] Depending on the defect, pulses may be bounding or diminished. Pulses can vary in intensity

from the upper to lower extremities. Similarly, based on the defect, a loud murmur may be present at birth or may not be heard until 1 to 2 weeks after birth. The cyanosis of heart disease may be present over the entire body, which differentiates this condition from the peripheral cyanosis often found among normal newborns. For infants with a ventral septal defect, oxygenated blood crosses over the opening in the septum and recirculates through the lungs. In this case, cyanosis often is not present and a murmur may not be heard until 2 or more weeks of age as the compensatory measure of increased pulmonary vascular resistance diminishes and more blood flows from left to right. This is characteristic of a large defect and may be associated with a subtle onset of congestive heart failure evidenced by tachypnea, feeding problems, and failure to thrive. A parent may describe troubling symptoms during a postpartum visit or during calls about breastfeeding. In smaller ventricular septal defects, the systolic murmur is heard soon after birth but will not lead to congestive heart failure.

Some newborns will not make the transition from intrauterine to extrauterine circulation. In these neonates, the pulmonary resistance remains so high that blood flow through the newborn lungs is decreased. This relatively rare phenomenon results in persistent pulmonary hypertension (formerly called persistent fetal circulation). Signs include tachypnea, nasal flaring, and intercostal retractions. Because of the high level of resistance from the lungs, the ductus arteriosus and the foramen ovale may stay open to provide right-to-left shunting. In this case, peripheral pulses will be bounding, the precordium will be active, and a murmur will be heard.[79]

Midwifery management of newborns with acute signs of heart disease includes immediate consultation with the pediatric team and supportive care for the resulting respiratory distress. The newborn's heart rate and respiratory rate are constantly monitored. If heart disease is suspected, the blood arterial oxygen saturation of an upper extremity can be compared to that of a lower extremity. In persistent pulmonary hypertension, the saturation is lower in the descending aorta. Warm, humidified oxygen is provided via hood at high concentrations. When there is a cardiac problem, however, even high concentrations of oxygen may not yield normal results. If the newborn is tachypneic, oral feedings are withheld. The metabolic demands of respiratory distress will predispose the newborn to hypoglycemia.

Signs of Neurologic Disease

The most common sign of neurologic compromise in the newborn period is seizure activity. There are many causes of neonatal seizures, ranging from hypoglycemia to neonatal encephalopathy. Treatment is based on the etiology of the seizure. Prognosis is also related to the etiology more than the seizure activity itself unless the seizures are prolonged or frequent.[80] In rare cases, a congenital abnormality in the brain may be present.[81] In the older newborn, seizures can be an indicator of an inborn error of metabolism.

Newborns may evidence various types of seizure activity. The most common is the subtle seizure. Signs of subtle seizures include sucking motions, chewing, bicycling of limbs, drooling, apnea, deviation of the eyes, and eyelid fluttering. These seizures are evidenced as short, repetitive bursts of activity. Such repetitive behavioral patterns can be observed during a newborn examination. Because there is an association between hypoglycemia and seizure activity, it is recommended to perform a point-of-care glucose screening when seizure is suspected. Because of the risk of apnea, the newborn with possible seizure activity usually is carefully monitored by professionals with expertise in the area. Current treatment for a newborn with seizures secondary to hypoxia-ischemic encephalopathy includes therapeutic hypothermia or brain cooling.[82]

Other types of seizures (multifocal, focal) are less common in newborns. The signs of these seizures include movement of one limb with progression to other limbs or movement of both limbs on one side of the body.

Nonvisible Congenital Defects

Tracheoesophageal fistula and esophageal atresia are not visible on physical examination and may not present immediately at birth. However, signs such as excess salivation, respiratory distress, swallowing problems, and abdominal distension will be present. If esophageal fistula is suspected, a sterile feeding tube can be introduced into the newborn's esophagus but will not be able to be passed more than 10 to 12 centimeters.[83] The newborn should be positioned in a prone position with the head elevated and oral feedings withheld. Aspiration of the esophageal contents by feeding tube attached to a syringe helps to minimize the chance of aspiration into the lungs. Tracheoesophageal fistula and esophageal atresia often occur together.

A variety of congenital defects can lead to intestinal obstruction in the newborn. Among these are malrotation and midgut volvulus, meconium plugs, meconium ileus, Hirschsprung's disease (megacolon), and imperforate anus. The major diagnostic signs of all these anomalies are bile-stained emesis and failure to pass stool. Significant abdominal distension will be present with meconium ileus, meconium plug, and Hirschsprung's disease. Studies exploring genetic predisposition for some of these conditions are ongoing.[84] Newborns with these signs should be evaluated immediately by a pediatric caregiver. No oral feedings should be given if bile-stained emesis is observed. If neglected, any of these defects can lead to intestinal perforation.

Conclusion

The first extrauterine touch a newborn feels usually are the hands of the healthcare provider who attended the birth. Although midwives are not commonly viewed as primary pediatric providers, in many cases midwives provide the first assessment of the newborn during this initial newborn period. Thus midwives have an important role during the first Golden Hour. Even in areas where pediatric care quickly is assumed by other professionals, the relationship between a midwife and a woman and her family often means that as questions arise about the infant, the midwife may be the first person to be called. Through their acceptance of this responsibility, midwives have an integral role in caring for the health of society's future generations.

● ● ● **References**

1. American College of Nurse-Midwives. Core competencies for basic midwifery practice. 2012. Available at: http ://www.midwife.org/ACNM/files/ACNMLibraryData /UPLOADFILENAME/000000000050/Core%20 Comptencies%20Dec%202012.pdf. Accessed April 4, 2013.

2. Doyle KJ, Bradshaw WT. Sixty golden minutes. *Neonatal Netw.* 2012;31(5):289-294.

3. Mercer JS, Erickson-Owens DA, Graves B, Haley MM. Evidence-based practices for the fetal to newborn transition. *J Midwifery Women's Health.* 2007;52(3): 262-272.

4. Harach T. Room air resuscitation and targeted oxygenation for infants at birth in the delivery room. *J Obstet Gynecol Neonatal Nurs.* 2013;42:227-232.

5. Tan A, Schulze AA, O'Donnell CPF, Davis PG. Air versus oxygen for resuscitation of infants at birth. *Cochrane Database Syst Rev.* 2005;2:CD002273. doi: 10.1002/14651858.CD002273.pub3.

6. Jobe AH, Kallapur SG. Long term consequences of oxygen therapy in the neonatal period. *Semin Fetal Neonatal Med.* 2010;15(4):230-235.

7. Moore ER, Anderson GC, Bergman N, Dowswell T. Early skin-to-skin contact for mothers and their healthy newborn infants. *Cochrane Database Syst Rev.* 2012;5:CD003519. doi: 10.1002/14651858. CD003519.pub3.

8. McDonald SJ, Middleton P. Effect of timing of umbilical cord clamping of term infants on maternal and neonatal outcomes. *Cochrane Database Syst Rev.* 2008;2:CD004074. doi: 10.1002/14651858. CD004074.pub2.

9. Rabe H, Diaz-Rossello JL, Duley L, Dowswell T. Effect of timing of umbilical cord clamping and other strategies to influence placental transfusion at preterm birth on maternal and infant outcomes. *Cochrane Database Syst Rev.* 2012;8:CD003248. doi: 10.1002/14651858. CD003248.pub3.

10. Palethorpe RJ, Farrar D, Duley L. Alternative positions for the baby at birth before clamping the umbilical cord. *Cochrane Database Syst Rev.* 2010;10:CD007555. doi: 10.1002/14651858.CD007555.pub2.

11. Christensson K, Bhat GJ, Amadi BC, Eriksson B, Höjer B. Randomised study of skin-to-skin versus incubator care for rewarming low-risk hypothermic neonates. *Lancet.* 1998;352(9134):1115.

12. Widström AM, Lilja G, Aaltomaa-Michalias P, Dahllöf A, Lintula M, Nissen E. Newborn behaviour to locate the breast when skin-to-skin: a possible method for enabling early self-regulation. *Acta Paediatr.* 2011;100(1):79-85.

13. Hammerschlag MR. Chlamydial and gonococcal infections in infants and children. *Clin Infect Dis.* 2011; 53(suppl 3):S99-S102.

14. Puckett RM, Offringa M. Prophylactic vitamin K for vitamin K deficiency bleeding in neonates. *Cochrane Database Syst Rev.* 2000;4:CD002776. doi: 10. 1002/14651858.CD002776.

15. Van Winckel M, De Bruyne R, Van De Velde S, Van Biervliet S. Vitamin K: an update for the paediatrician. *Eur J Pediatr.* 2009;168(2):127-134.

16. Ipema HJ. Use of oral vitamin K for prevention of late vitamin K deficiency bleeding in neonates when injectable vitamin K is not available. *Ann Pharmacother.* 2012;46(6):879-883.

17. Lauer B, Spector N. Vitamins. *Pediatr Rev.* 2012; 33(8):339-351.

18. Feldkamp ML, Carey JC, Sadler TW. Development of gastroschisis: review of hypotheses, a novel hypothesis, and implications for research. *Am J Med Genet A.* 2007;143(7):639-652.

19. Sadler TW. The embryologic origin of ventral body wall defect. *Semin Pediatr Surg.* 2010;19(3):209-214.

20. Adzick NS, Walsh DS. Myelomeningocele: prenatal diagnosis, pathophysiology and management. *Semin Pediatr Surg.* 2003;12(3):168-174.

21. Gilbert WM, Nesbitt TS, Danielsen B. Associated factors in 1611 cases of brachial plexus injury. *Obstet Gynecol.* 1999;93(4):536-540.

22. Morgan JA, Marcus PS. Prenatal diagnosis and management of intrauterine fracture. *Obstet Gynecol Surv.* 2010;65(4):249-259.

23. Blackburn S, Bakewell-Sachs S. *Understanding the behavior of term infants.* White Plains, NY: March of Dimes Birth Defects Foundation. Available at: http ://www.marchofdimes.com/nursing/modnemedia /othermedia/states.pdf. Accessed March 25, 2013.

24. Kurth E, Kennedy HP, Spichiger E, Hösli I, Stutz EZ. Crying babies, tired mothers: what do we know? A systematic review. *Midwifery.* 2011;27(2):187-194.

25. Winberg J. Mother and newborn baby: mutual regulation of physiology and behavior: a selective review. *Dev Psychobiol.* 2005;47(3):217-229.

26. Hotelling BA. Newborn capabilities: parent teaching is a necessity. *J Perinat Educ.* 2004;13(4):43-49.

27. Brazelton TB, Nugent JK. *Neonatal Behavioral Assessment Scale.* 4th ed. London: Mac Keith Press; 2011.

28. Nelson HD, Nygren P, Walker M, Panoscha R. *Screening for Speech and Language Delay in Preschool Children.* U.S. Preventive Services Task Force Evidence Syntheses (formerly Systematic Evidence Reviews). Rockville, MD: Agency for Healthcare Research and Quality; February 2006.

29. Povedrano MCA, Noto IS, Pinhiero MDS, Guinsburg R. Mothers' perceptions and expectations regarding their newborn infants: the use of Broussard's neonatal perception inventory. *Rev Paul Pediatr.* 2011; 29(2):239-244.

30. Lavender T, Bedwell C, O'Brien E, Cork MJ, Turner M, Hart A. Infant skin-cleansing product versus water: a pilot randomized, assessor-blinded controlled trial. *BMC Pediatr.* 2011;13(11):35.

31. Lavender T, Bedwell C, Roberts SA, et al. Randomized, controlled trial evaluating a baby wash product on skin barrier function in healthy, term neonates. *J Obstet Gynecol Neonatal Nurs.* 2013;42(2):203-214.

32. Ness MJ, Davis DMR, Care WA. Neonatal skin care: a concise review. *Int J Dermatol.* 2013;52:14-22.

33. Blume-Peytavi U, Hauser M, Stamatas GN, Pathirana D, Garcia Bartels N. Skin care practices for newborns and infants: review of the clinical evidence for best practices. *Pediatr Dermatol.* 2012;29(1):1-14.

34. Zupan J, Garner P, Omari AAA. Topical umbilical cord care at birth. *Cochrane Database Syst Rev.* 2004;3:CD001057. doi: 10.1002/14651858.CD001057.pub2.

35. Soofi S, Cousens S, Imdad A, Bhutto N, Ali N, Bhutta ZA. Topical application of chlorhexidine to neonatal umbilical cords for prevention of omphalitis and neonatal mortality in a rural district of Pakistan: a community-based, cluster-randomised trial. *Lancet.* 2012;17;379(9820):1029-1036.

36. Young, D. Family centered maternity care. *Int J Childbirth Educ.* 1987;5-7.

37. Weidenbach, E. *Family-Centered Maternity Care.* New York: G. P. Putnam; 1959.

38. DeLuca J, Zanni KL, Bonhomme N, Kemper AR. Implications of newborn screening for nurses. *J Nurs Scholar.* 2013;45(1):25-33.

39. American College of Medical Genetics Newborn Screening Expert Group. Newborn screening: toward a uniform screening panel and system: executive summary. *Pediatrics.* 2006;117(5 Pt 2):S296-S307.

40. President's Council on Bioethics. *The Changing Moral Focus of Newborn Screening: An Ethical Analysis by the President's Council on Bioethics.* Washington, DC: December 2008. Available at: http://bioethics.georgetown.edu/pcbe/reports/newborn_screening. Accessed March 24, 2013.

41. Andermann A, Blancquaert I, Beauchamp S, Costea I. Guiding policy decisions for genetic screening: developing a systematic and transparent approach. *Public Health Genomics.* 2011;14(1):9-16.

42. Lewis MH, Goldenberg A, Anderson R, Rothwell E, Botkin J. State laws regarding the retention and use of residual newborn screening blood samples. *Pediatrics.* 2011;127(4):703-712.

43. Kemper AR, Kus CA, Ostrander RJ, et al., on behalf of the United States Secretary of Health and Human Services Advisory Committee on Heritable Disorders in Newborns and Children. Implementing point-of-care newborn screening. 2012. Available at: http://www.hrsa.gov/advisorycommittees/mchbadvisory/heritabledisorders/recommendations/correspondence/implementpocnewbornscreen.pdf. Accessed March 24, 2013.

44. Wolff R, Hommerich J, Riemsma R, Antes G, Lange S, Kleijnen J. Hearing screening in newborns: systematic review of accuracy, effectiveness, and effects of interventions after screening. *Arch Dis Child.* 2010;95(2):130-135.

45. Melnyk BM, Grossman DC, Chou R, et al. USPSTF perspective on evidence-based preventive recommendations for children. *Pediatrics.* 2012;130(2):e399-e407.

46. Ewer AK. Review of pulse oximetry screening for critical congenital heart defects in newborn infants. *Curr Opin Cardiol.* 2013;28(2):92-96.

47. Ewer AK, Middleton LF, Furnston AT, et al. Pulse oximetry screening for congenital heart defects in newborn infants. *Lancet.* 2011;378:785-794.

48. Thangaratinam S, Brown K, Zamora J, Khan KS, Ewer AK. Pulse oximetry screening for critical congenital heart defects in asymptomatic newborn babies: a systematic review and meta-analysis. *Lancet.* 2012;379(9835):2459-2464.

49. Robinson JD, Ortega G, Carrol JA, et al. Circumcision in the United States: where are we? *JAMA.* 2012;104(9-10):455-458.

50. American Academy of Pediatrics Task Force on Circumcision. Male circumcision. *Pediatrics.* 2012;130(3):e756-e785.

51. American Academy of Pediatrics Task Force on Circumcision. Circumcision policy statement. *Pediatrics.* 2012;130(3):585-586.

52. Healthwise. Circumcision: should I keep my son's penis natural? Available at: https://www.healthwise.net/cochranedecisionaid/Content/StdDocument.aspx?DOCHWID=aa41834. Accessed March 28, 2013.

53. Mast EE, Margolis HS, Fiore AE, et al. Advisory Committee on Immunization Practices. A comprehensive immunization strategy to eliminate transmission of hepatitis B virus infection in the United States: recommendations of the Advisory Committee on Immunization Practices (ACIP). Part 1: immunization of infants, children, and adolescents. *MMWR Recomm Rep.* 2005;54(RR-16):1-31.

54. Schillie SF, Murphy TV. Seroprotection after recombinant hepatitis B vaccination among newborn infants: a review. *Vaccine.* 2013;31(21):2506-2516.

55. Bar-On ES, Goldberg E, Hellmann S, Leibovici L. Combined DTP-HBV-HIB vaccine versus separately administered DTP-HBV and HIB vaccines for primary prevention of diphtheria, tetanus, pertussis, hepatitis B and *Haemophilus influenzae* B (HIB).

Cochrane Database Syst Rev. 2012;4:CD005530. doi: 10.1002/14651858.CD005530.pub3.

56. Isaacs D, Kilham HA, Alexander S, Wood N, Buckmaster A, Royle J. Ethical issues in preventing mother-to-child transmission of hepatitis B by immunisation. *Vaccine.* 2011;29(37):6159-6162.

57. Sperling RS, Shapiro DE, Coombs RW, et al. Maternal viral load, zidovudine treatment, and the risk of transmission of human immunodeficiency virus type 1 from mother to infant. Pediatric AIDS Clinical Trials Group Protocol 076 Study Group. *N Engl J Med.* 1996; 335(22):1621-1629.

58. Cohen J. HIV/AIDS: Early treatment may have cured infant of HIV infection. *Science.* 2013;339(6124):1134.

59. World Health Organization. *HIV Transmission Through Breast-Feeding: A Review of Available Evidence.* Geneva, Switzerland: World Health Organization; 2008.

60. Verani JR, Schrag SJ. Group B streptococcal disease in infants: progress in prevention and continued challenges. *Clin Perinatol.* 2010;37(2):375-392.

61. Verani JR, McGee L, Schrag SJ; Division of Bacterial Diseases, National Center for Immunization and Respiratory Diseases, Centers for Disease Control and Prevention. Prevention of perinatal group B streptococcal disease: revised guidelines from CDC, 2010. *MMWR Recomm Rep.* 2010;59(RR-10):1-36.

62. Hay WW Jr. Care of the infant of the diabetic mother. *Curr Diab Rep.* 2012;12(1):4-15.

63. Maayan-Metzger A, Lubin D, Kuint J. Hypoglycemia rates in the first days of life among term infants born to diabetic mothers. *Neonatology.* 2009;96(2):80-85.

64. Fréour T, Dessolle L, Lammers J, Lattes S, Barrière P. Comparison of embryo morphokinetics after in vitro fertilization–intracytoplasmic sperm injection in smoking and nonsmoking women. *Fertil Steril.* February 25, 2013. pii: S0015-0282(13)00192-1.

65. Pruett D, Waterman EH, Caughey AB. Fetal alcohol exposure: consequences, diagnosis, and treatment. *Obstet Gynecol Surv.* 2013;68(1):62-69.

66. Warren KR, Hewitt BG, Thomas JD. Fetal alcohol spectrum disorders: research challenges and opportunities. National Institutes of Health, National Institute on Alcohol Abuse and Alcoholism. Available at: http://pubs.niaaa.nih.gov/publications/arh341/4-14.htm. Accessed March 29, 2013.

67. Jansson LM, Velez M. Neonatal abstinence syndrome. *Curr Opin Pediatr.* 2012;24(2):252-258.

68. Källén B, Reis M. Neonatal complications after maternal concomitant use of SSRI and other central nervous system active drugs during the second or third trimester of pregnancy. *J Clin Psychopharmacol.* 2012;32(5):608-614.

69. Shainker SA, Saia K, Lee-Parritz A. Opioid addiction in pregnancy. *Obstet Gynecol Surv.* 2012;67(12): 817-825.

70. Jones HE, Finnegan LP, Kaltenbach K. Methadone and buprenorphine for the management of opioid dependence in pregnancy. *Drugs.* 2013;5(7):529-533.

71. Launiainen T, Nupponen I, Halmesmäki E, Ojanperä I. Meconium drug testing reveals maternal misuse of medicinal opioids among addicted mothers. *Drug Test Anal.* 2013;5(7):529-533.

72. Woodgate P, Jardine LA. Neonatal jaundice. *Clin Evid (Online).* September 15. 2011. pii: 0319.

73. American Academy of Pediatrics Subcommittee on Hyperbilirubinemia. Management of hyperbilirubinemia in the newborn infant 35 or more weeks of gestation. *Pediatrics.* 2004;114:297-316.

74. Maisels MJ, McDonagh AF. Phototherapy for neonatal jaundice. *N Engl J Med.* 2008;358:920-928.

75. Gholitabar M, McGuire H, Rennie J, Manning D, Lai R. Clofibrate in combination with phototherapy for unconjugated neonatal hyperbilirubinaemia. *Cochrane Database Syst Rev.* 2012;12:CD009017. doi: 10.1002/14651858.CD009017.pub2.

76. de Jong EP, Vossen AC, Walther FJ, Lopriore E. How to use neonatal TORCH testing. *Arch Dis Child Educ Pract Ed.* 2013;98(3):93-98.

77. Stegmann BJ, Carey JC. TORCH infections: toxoplasmosis, other (syphilis, varicella-zoster, parvovirus B19), rubella, cytomegalovirus (CMV), and herpes infections. *Curr Women's Health Rep.* 2002;2(4):253-258.

78. Gandhi A, Sreekantam S. Evaluation of suspected congenital heart disease. *Paediatr Child Health.* 2011; 21(1);7-12.

79. D'cunha C, Sankaran K. Persistent fetal circulation. *Paediatr Child Health.* 2001;6(10):744-750.

80. Tekgul H, Gauvreau K, Soul J, et al. The current etiologic profile and neurodevelopmental outcome of seizures in term newborn infants. *Pediatrics.* 2006; 117:1270.

81. Khajeh L, Cherian PJ, Swarte RM, Smit LS, Lequin MH. The puzzle of apparent life-threatening events in a healthy newborn. *J Child Neurol.* March 25, 2013. [Epub ahead of print.]

82. Jacobs SE, Berg M, Hunt R, Tarnow-Mordi WO, Inder TE, Davis PG. Cooling for newborns with hypoxic ischaemic encephalopathy. *Cochrane Database Syst Rev.* 2013;1:CD003311. doi: 10.1002/14651858. CD003311.pub3.

83. Pinheiro PF, Simões e Silva AC, Pereira RM. Current knowledge on esophageal atresia. *World J Gastroenterol.* 2012;28;18(28):3662-3672.

84. Bergeron KF, Silversides DW, Pilon N. The developmental genetics of Hirschsprung's disease. *Clin Genet.* 2013;3(1):15-22.

Index

Note: Page numbers followed by *b*, *f*, or *t* indicate material in boxes, figures, or tables, respectively.